MERRITT'S NEUROLOGY

TENTH EDITION

MERRITT'S NEUROLOGY

TENTH EDITION

Edited by

LEWIS P. ROWLAND, M.D.

Professor of Neurology
Columbia University College of Physicians and Surgeons
Neurological Institute of New York-Presbyterian Hospital
Columbia-Presbyterian Medical Center
New York, New York

LIPPINCOTT WILLIAMS & WILKINS
A **Wolters Kluwer** Company

Philadelphia · Baltimore · New York · London
Buenos Aires · Hong Kong · Sydney · Tokyo

Acquisitions Editor: Charles W. Mitchell
Developmental Editor: Joyce A. Murphy
Production Editor: Robin E. Cook
Manufacturing Manager: Tim Reynolds
Cover Designer: Christine Jenny
Compositor: Maryland Composition
Printer: Courier Westford

© 2000 by LIPPINCOTT WILLIAMS & WILKINS
530 Walnut Street
Philadelphia, PA 19106 USA
www.LWW.com

All rights reserved. This book is protected by copyright. No part of this book may be reproduced in any form or by any means, including photocopying, or utilized by any information storage and retrieval system without written permission from the copyright owner, except for brief quotations embodied in critical articles and reviews. Materials appearing in this book prepared by individuals as part of their official duties as U.S. government employees are not covered by the above-mentioned copyright.

Printed in the USA

Library of Congress Cataloging-in-Publication Data

Merritt's neurology—10th ed./editor, Lewis P. Rowland.
   p.; cm.
  Includes bibliographical references and index.
  ISBN 0-683-30474-7
   1. Nervous system—Diseases. 2. Neurology. I. Title: Neurology. II. Merritt, H.
Houston (Hiram Houston), 1902–1979. Textbook of neurology. III. Rowland, Lewis P.
  [DNLM: 1. Nervous System Diseases. WL 140 M572 2000]
  RC346.M4 2000
  616.8—dc21
                      99-046827

Care has been taken to confirm the accuracy of the information presented and to describe generally accepted practices. However, the authors, editors, and publisher are not responsible for errors or omissions or for any consequences from application of the information in this book and make no warranty, expressed or implied, with respect to the currency, completeness, or accuracy of the contents of the publication. Application of this information in a particular situation remains the professional responsibility of the practitioner.

The authors, editors, and publisher have exerted every effort to ensure that drug selection and dosage set forth in this text are in accordance with current recommendations and practice at the time of publication. However, in view of ongoing research, changes in government regulations, and the constant flow of information relating to drug therapy and drug reactions, the reader is urged to check the package insert for each drug for any change in indications and dosage and for added warnings and precautions. This is particularly important when the recommended agent is a new or infrequently employed drug.

Some drugs and medical devices presented in this publication have Food and Drug Administration (FDA) clearance for limited use in restricted research settings. It is the responsibility of the health care provider to ascertain the FDA status of each drug or device planned for use in their clinical practice.

10 9 8 7 6 5 4 3 2 1

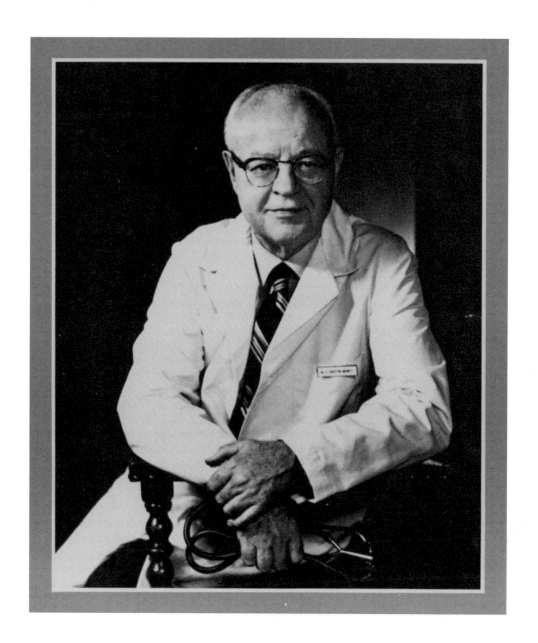

Dedicated to
H. Houston Merritt
(1902–1979)

CONTENTS

CONTRIBUTORING AUTHORS

Gary M. Abrams, M.D.
Associate Professor
Department of Neurology
University of California
505 Parnassus Avenue
San Francisco, California 94143, and
Chief, Department of Neurology/Rehabilitation
University of California, San Francisco/Mt. Zion Medical
  Center
1600 Divisadero Street
San Francisco, California 94115

Alan M. Aron, M.D.
Professor of Pediatrics and Clinical Neurology
Departments of Neurology and Pediatrics
Mount Sinai-New York University Medical Center, and
Director, Attending Neurologist, and Attending Pediatrician
Department of Pediatric Neurology
Mount Sinai Hospital
One Gustave Levy Place
New York, New York 10029

Casilda M. Balmaceda, M.D.
Assistant Professor of Neurology
Columbia University College of Physicians and Surgeons
Assistant Attending Neurologist
New York-Presbyterian Hospital
Neurological Institute
Columbia-Presbyterian Medical Center
710 West 168th Street
New York, New York 10032

Carl W. Bazil, M.D., Ph.D.
Assistant Professor of Neurology
Columbia University College of Physicians and Surgeons
Assistant Attending Neurologist
New York-Presbyterian Hospital
Neurological Institute
Columbia-Presbyterian Medical Center
710 West 168th Street
New York, New York 10032

Myles M. Behrens, M.D.
Professor of Clinical Ophthalmology
Columbia University College of Physicians and Surgeons
Attending Ophthalmologist
New York-Presbyterian Hospital
Eye Institute Room 114
635 165th Street, Box 71
New York, New York 10032

Gary L. Bernardini, M.D., Ph.D.
Associate Professor of Neurology
Albany Medical College
Director
Neurological Intensive Care Unit
Albany Medical Center
47 New Scotland Avenue
Albany, New York 12208

Susan B. Bressman, M.D.
Chair
Department of Neurology
Beth Israel Hospital
Phillips Ambulatory Care Center
10 Union Square East, Suite 2Q
New York, New York 10032

Carolyn Barley Britton, M.D.
Associate Professor of Clinical Neurology
Columbia University College of Physicians and Surgeons
Associate Attending Neurologist
New York-Presbyterian Hospital
Neurological Institute
Columbia-Presbyterian Medical Center
710 West 168th Street
New York, New York 10032

Jeffrey N. Bruce, M.D.
Associate Professor of Neurological Surgery
Associate Attending Neurological Surgeon
Neurological Institute
Columbia-Presbyterian Medical Center
710 West 168th Street
New York, New York 10032

John C. M. Brust, M.D.
Professor of Clinical Neurology
Department of Neurology
Columbia University College of Physicians and Surgeons
Attending Neurologist
New York-Presbyterian Hospital
710 West 168th Street
New York, New York 10032, and
Director, Department of Neurology
Harlem Hospital Center
506 Lenox Avenue
New York, New York 10037

Robert E. Burke, M.D.
Professor of Neurology
Attending Neurologist
Columbia University College of Physicians and Surgeons
Black Building
650 West 168th Street, 3rd Floor
New York, New York 10032

Abba L. Cargan, M.D.
Assistant Professor of Neurology
Columbia University College of Physicians and Surgeons
Assistant Attending Neurologist
New York-Presbyterian Hospital
Neurological Institute
Columbia-Presbyterian Medical Center
710 West 168th Street
New York, New York 10032

Stephen Chan, M.D.
Assistant Professor of Radiology
Assistant Attending Neurologist (Neuroradiology)
Columbia University College of Physicians and Surgeons
Milstein Hospital Building
177 Fort Washington Avenue
New York, New York 10032

Claudia A. Chiriboga, M.D.
Assistant Professor of Neurology
Columbia University College of Physicians and Surgeons
Assistant Attending Neurologist
New York-Presbyterian Hospital
Neurological Institute
Columbia-Presbyterian Medical Center
710 West 168th Street
New York, New York 10032

Massimo Corbo
Assistant Professor of Neurology
Department of Neurology
San Raffaele Hospital
Scientific Institute of Milan
20132 Milan, Italy

Darryl C. De Vivo, M.D.
Sidney Carter Professor of Neurology
Professor of Pediatrics
Columbia University College of Physicians and Surgeons
Attending Neurologist and Pediatrician
Chief, Division of Pediatric Neurology
Neurological Institute
Columbia-Presbyterian Medical Center
710 West 168th Street
New York, New York 10032

Robert DeLaPaz, M.D.
Professor of Radiology
Columbia University College of Physicians and Surgeons
Attending Radiologist
Director, Division of Neuroradiology
New York-Presbyterian Hospital
Milstein Hospital Building
Columbia-Presbyterian Medical Center
177 Fort Washington Avenue
New York, New York 10032

Stefano Di Donato, M.D.
Department of Pediatric Neurology
Istituto Nazionale Neurologico C. Besta
Via Celoria, 11
Milano, 20133
Italy

Salvatore DiMauro, M.D.
Lucy G. Moses Professor
Department of Neurology
Columbia University College of Physicians and Surgeons
630 West 168th Street
New York, New York 10032

Mitchell S.V. Elkind, M.D.
Assistant Professor of Neurology
Columbia University College of Physicians and Surgeons
Assistant Attending Neurologist
New York-Presbyterian Hospital
Neurological Institute
Columbia-Presbyterian Medical Center
710 West 168th Street
New York, New York 10032

Ronald G. Emerson, M.D.
Professor of Clinical Neurology and Clinical Pediatrics
Columbia University College of Physicians and Surgeons
Attending Neurologist
New York-Presbyterian Hospital
Columbia-Presbyterian Medical Center
Neurological Institute
710 West 168th Street
New York, New York 10032

Stanley Fahn, M.D.
H. Houston Merritt Professor of Neurology
Columbia University College of Physicians and Surgeons
Attending Neurologist
Chief, Division of Movement Disorder
New York-Presbyterian Hospital
Neurological Institute
710 West 168th Street
New York, New York 10032

Neil A. Feldstein, M.D.
Assistant Professor of Neurological Surgery
Assistant Attending Neurosurgeon
Neurological Institute
Columbia-Presbyterian Medical Center
710 West 168th Street
New York, New York 10032

Michael R. Fetell, M.D.
Professor of Clinical Neurology and Neurosurgery
Attending Neurologist
Neurological Institute
Columbia-Presbyterian Medical Center
710 West 168th Street
New York, New York 10032

Robert L. Fine, M.D.
Herbert Irving Associate Professor of Medicine
Director, Medical Oncology Division
Columbia University College of Physicians and Surgeons
Associate Attending Physician in Medicine
New York-Presbyterian Hospital
650 West 168th Street
New York, New York 10032

Matthew E. Fink, M.D.
Department of Neurology
Albert Einstein College of Medicine
President, Chief Executive Officer, and Attending Neurologist
Beth Israel Medical Center
First Avenue at 16th Street
New York, New York 10003

Robert A. Fishman, M.D.
Professor Emeritus
Department of Neurology
University of California, San Francisco, and
Attending Neurologist
Department of Neurology
University of California, San Francisco Hospitals
505 Parnassus Avenue
San Francisco, California 94143

Pamela U. Freda
Associate Professor of Clinical Medicine
Department of Medicine
Columbia University College of Physicians and Surgeons
630 West 168th Street
New York, New York 10032, and
Assistant Attending Physician
Department of Medicine
New York-Presbyterian Hospital
622 West 168th Street
New York, New York 10032

June M. Fry, M.D., Ph.D.
Professor
Department of Neurology
MCP Hahnemann University
3200 Henry Avenue
Philadelphia, Pennsylvania 19129, and
Director of Sleep Medicine
Department of Neurology
Medical College of Pennsylvania Hospital
3300 Henry Avenue
Philadelphia, Pennsylvania 19129

James H. Garvin, Jr., M.D., Ph.D.
Professor of Clinical Pediatrics
Columbia University College of Physicians and Surgeons
Attending Pediatrician
New York-Presbyterian Hospital
630 West 168th Street
New York, New York 10032

Sid Gilman, M.D.
William J. Herdman Professor and Chair
Department of Neurology
University of Michigan, and
Chief, Neurology Service
University of Michigan Hospitals
1500 East Medical Center Drive
Ann Arbor, Michigan 48109-0316

Arnold P. Gold, M.D.
Professor of Clinical Neurology and Professor of Clinical Pediatrics
Columbia University College of Physicians and Surgeons
Attending Neurologist and Pediatrician
New York-Presbyterian Hospital
Neurological Institute
Columbia-Presbyterian Medical Center
710 West 168th Street
New York, New York 10032

Paul E. Greene, M.D.
Assistant Professor of Neurology
Columbia University College of Physicians and Surgeons
Assistant Attending Neurologist
New York-Presbyterian Hospital
Neurological Institute
Columbia-Presbyterian Medical Center
710 West 168th Street
New York, New York 10032

Melvin Greer, M.D.
Professor and Chairman
Department of Neurology
University of Florida College of Medicine
Box 100236
Gainesville, Florida 32610

Alexander Halim, Ph.D.
Department of Neurology
Columbia University College of Physicians and Surgeons
Neurological Institute
Columbia-Presbyterian Medical Center
710 West 168th Street
New York, New York 10032

James H. Halsey, M.D.
Professor of Clinical Neurology
Department of Neurology
Columbia University College of Physicians and Surgeons
710 West 168th Street
New York, New York 10032

Arthur P. Hays, M.D.
Associate Professor of Clinical Neuropathology
Department of Pathology
Columbia University College of Physicians and Surgeons
630 West 168th Street
New York, New York 10032, and
Associate Attending in Pathology
Department of Pathology
New York Presbyterian Hospital
622 West 168th Street
New York, New York 10032

Eric J. Heyer, M.D.
Associate Professor of Clinical Anesthesiology and Clinical
 Neurology
Associate Attending Anesthesiologist
Columbia University College of Physicians and Surgeons
630 West 168th Street
New York, New York 10032

Michio Hirano, M.D.
Herbert Irving Assistant Professor of Neurology
Assistant Attending Neurologist
Department of Neurology
Columbia University College of Physicians and Surgeons
630 West 168th Street
New York, New York 10032

Stephen R. Isaacson
Associate Professor
Department of Radiation Oncology
Columbia University College of Physicians and Surgeons
622 West 168th Street
New York, New York 10032

William G. Johnson, M.D.
Professor of Neurology
University of Medicine and Dentistry of New Jersey
Robert Wood Johnson Medical School
675 Hoes Lane
Piscataway, New Jersey 08854-5635

Burk Jubelt, M.D.
Professor and Chairman
Department of Neurology
Professor
Department of Microbiology/Immunology
SUNY Upstate Medical University
Chief
Department of Neurology
University Hospital
750 East Adams Street
Syracuse, New York 13210

Ram Kairam, M.D.
Assistant Professor of Clinical Pediatrics and Clinical
 Neurology
Columbia University College of Physicians and Surgeons
Lincoln Hospital
234 E. 149th Street
Bronx, New York 10451

M. Richard Koenigsberger, M.D.
Professor of Clinical Neurosciences
University of Medicine and Dentistry of New Jersey
185 S. Orange Avenue
Newark, New Jersey 07103

Dale J. Lange, M.D.
Associate Professor of Clinical Neurology
Associate Attending Neurologist
Neurological Institute
Columbia-Presbyterian Medical Center
710 West 168th Street
New York, New York 10032

Norman Latov, M.D., Ph.D.
Professor of Neurology
Attending Neurologist
Director, Peripheral Neuropathy Division
Neurological Institute
Columbia-Presbyterian Medical Center
710 West 168th St.
New York, New York 10032

Robert B. Layzer, M.D.
Professor of Neurology Emeritus
University of California, San Francisco
Box 0114
San Francisco, California 94143

Laura Lennihan, M.D.
Associate Professor of Clinical Neurology
Associate Attending Neurologist
New York-Presbyterian Hospital
710 West 168th Street
New York, New York 10032, and
Chief, Department of Neurology
Helen Hayes Hospital
Route 9W
West Haverstraw, New York 10993

Elan D. Louis, M.D.
Assistant Professor of Neurology
Columbia University College of Physicians and Surgeons
Assistant Attending Neurologist
New York-Presbyterian Hospital
Neurological Institute
Columbia-Presbyterian Medical Center
710 West 168th Street
New York, New York 10032

Robert E. Lovelace, M.D.
Professor of Neurology
Attending Neurologist
Neurological Institute
Columbia-Presbyterian Medical Center
710 West 168th Street
New York, New York 10032

Timothy Lynch, M.R.C.P.I., M.R.C.P. (London)
Consultant Neurologist
The Mater Misericordiae Hospital
Eccles Street
Dublin 7, Ireland

Mia MacCollin, M.D.
Assistant Professor
Department of Neurology
Harvard Medical School
Boston, Massachusetts 02115, and
Assistant Professor
Department of Neurology
Massachusetts General Hospital
Neuroscience Center, MGH East
Building 149, 13th Street
Charlestown, Massachusetts 02129

Elliott L. Mancall, M.D.
Professor and Interim Chairman
Department of Neurology
Jefferson Medical College
Thomas Jefferson University Hospital
1025 Walnut Street, Suite 310
Philadelphia, Pennsylvania 19107

Joseph T. Marotta, M.D., F.R.C.P. (C)
Professor Emeritus of Neurology
Department of Neurological Sciences
University of Western Ontario
London Health Sciences Centre
London, Ontario N6A 5C1
Canada

Randolph S. Marshall
Assistant Professor
Neurological Institute
Columbia-Presbyterian Medical Center
710 West 168th Street
New York, New York 10032

Thornton B.A. Mason, II, M.D.
Assistant Professor of Neurology and Pediatrics
Assistant Attending Neurologist and Pediatrician
Neurological Institute
Columbia-Presbyterian Medical Center
710 West 168th Street
New York, New York 10032

Stephan A. Mayer, M.D.
Assistant Professor of Neurology (in Neurological Surgery)
Assistant Attending Neurologist
Director, Columbia-Presbyterian Neuro-Intensive Care Unit
Neurological Institute
Columbia-Presbyterian Medical Center
710 West 168th Street
New York, New York 10032

Richard Mayeux, M.D.
Gertrude H. Sergievsky Professor of Neurology, Psychiatry, and
*   Public Health*
Attending Neurologist
New York-Presbyterian Hospital
Columbia University College of Physicians and Surgeons
Sergievsky Center
622 West 168th Street
New York, New York 10032

Paul C. McCormick, M.D.
Associate Professor of Clinical Neurological Surgery
Associate Attending Neurosurgeon
Neurological Institute
Columbia-Presbyterian Medical Center
710 West 168th Street
New York, New York 10032

John H. Menkes, M.D.
Professor Emeritus
Departments of Neurology and Pediatrics
University of California, Los Angeles
Director of Pediatric Neurology
Cedars Sinai Medical Center
Los Angeles, California 90212

James R. Miller, M.D.
Associate Professor of Clinical Neurology
Associate Attending Neurologist
Director, Multiple Sclerosis Care Center
Neurological Institute
Columbia-Presbyterian Medical Center
710 West 168th Street
New York, New York 10032

J. P. Mohr, M.D.
Sciarra Professor of Clinical Neurology
Attending Neurologist
Director, Columbia-Presbyterian Stroke Unit
Neurological Institute
Columbia-Presbyterian Medical Center
710 West 168th Street
New York, New York 10032

Martha J. Morrell, M.D.
Professor of Clinical Neurology
Attending Neurologist and Director
Comprehensive Epilepsy Center
New York-Presbyterian Hospital
Neurological Institute
Columbia-Presbyterian Medical Center
710 West 168th Street
New York, New York 10032

Douglas R. Nordli, Jr., M.D.
Director of Pediatric Epilepsy
Associate Professor of Neurology
Children's Memorial Hospital
Northwestern University
2300 Children's Plaza, Room 51
Chicago, Illinois 60614

Alison M. Pack, M.D.
Fellow in Neurology
Neurological Institute
Columbia-Presbyterian Medical Center
710 West 168th St.
New York, New York 10032

Kyriakos P. Papadopoulos, M.D.
Assistant Professor of Medicine
Division of Medical Oncology/Hematology
Columbia University College of Physicians and Surgeons, and
Assistant Attending Physician
New York-Presbyterian Hospital
177 Fort Washington Avenue
New York, New York 10032

Timothy A. Pedley, M.D.
Henry and Lucy Moses Professor of Neurology
Chairman of Neurology
Columbia University College of Physicians and Surgeons, and
Director, Neurological Service
New York-Presbyterian Hospital
Neurological Institute
Columbia-Presbyterian Medical Center
710 West 168th Street
New York, New York 10032

Audrey S. Penn, M.D.
Deputy Director
National Institute of Neurological Disorders and Stroke
National Institutes of Health
31 Center Drive, MSC 2540, Room 8A52
Bethesda, Maryland 20892–2540

John Pile-Spellman
Professor of Radiology
Vice Chair of Research
Director of Interventional Neuroradiology
Columbia University College of Physicians and Surgeons
Milstein Hospital Building
177 Fort Washington Avenue
New York, New York 10032

Leon D. Prockop, M.D.
Professor
Department of Neurology
College of Medicine, University of South Florida
12901 Bruce B. Downs Boulevard, Box 55
Tampa, Florida 33629

Serge Przedborski, M.D., Ph.D.
Associate Professor of Neurology and Pathology
Associate Attending Neurologist
Columbia University College of Physicians and Surgeons
630 West 168th Street
New York, New York 10032

Isabelle Rapin, M.D.
Professor of Neurology and Pediatrics (Neurology)
Albert Einstein College of Medicine
Room 807 Kennedy Center
1410 Pelham Parkway South
Bronx, New York 10461

Neil H. Raskin, M.D.
Professor
Department of Neurology
University of California, San Francisco, and
Attending Physician
Department of Neurology
Moffitt/Long Hospital
505 Parnassus Ave.
San Francisco, California 94143

Roger N. Rosenberg, M.D.
Zale Distinguished Chair and Professor
Department of Neurology
University of Texas Southwestern Medical Center
5323 Harry Hines Boulevard
Dallas, Texas 75235-9036, and
Attending Neurologist
Department of Neurology
Zale-Lipsky University Hospital and Parkland Hospital
5300 Harry Hines Boulevard
Dallas, Texas 75235

Lewis P. Rowland, M.D.
Professor of Neurology
Attending Neurologist
Neurological Institute
Columbia-Presbyterian Medical Center
710 West 168th Street
New York, New York 10032-2603

Ralph L. Sacco, M.S., M.D.
Associate Professor of Neurology and Public Health
  (Epidemiology)
Assistant Attending Neurologist
Neurological Institute
Columbia-Presbyterian Medical Center
710 West 168th Street
New York, New York 10032-2603

Eric A. Schon, Ph.D.
Professor of Genetics and Development (in Neurology)
Department of Neurology
Columbia University College of Physicians and Surgeons
630 West 168th Street
New York, New York 10032

Glenn M. Seliger, M.D.
Assistant Professor of Neurology
Assistant Attending Neurologist
New York-Presbyterian Hospital
710 West 168th Street
New York, New York 10032, and
Director of Head Injury Services
Helen Hayes Hospital
Route 9W
West Haverstraw, New York 10993

Michael B. Sisti, M.D.
Assistant Professor of Clinical Neurological Surgery
Assistant Attending Neurosurgeon
Neurological Institute
Columbia-Presbyterian Medical Center
710 West 168th Street
New York, New York 10032

Scott A. Small, M.D.
Assistant Professor of Neurology
Columbia University College of Physicians and Surgeons
Assistant Attending Neurologist
New York-Presbyterian Hospital
Neurological Institute
Columbia-Presbyterian Medical Center
710 West 168th Street
New York, New York 10032

Robert A. Solomon
Byron Stookey Professor and Chairman
Department of Neurological Surgery
Columbia University College of Physicians and Surgeons
Director of Neurosurgery
New York-Presbyterian Hospital
Neurological Institute
Columbia-Presbyterian Medical Center
710 West 168th Street
New York, New York 10032

Christian Stapf, M.D.
Visiting Research Scientist in Neurology
Columbia University College of Physicians and Surgeons
Fellow, Stroke Center
New York-Presbyterian Hospital
710 West 168th Street
New York, New York 10032, and
Clinical Fellow
Stroke Unit/Department of Neurology
Universitaetsklinikum Benjamin Franklin
Hindenburgdamm 30
D-12203 Berlin, Germany

Leonidas Stefanis, M.D.
Assistant Professor of Neurology
Assistant Attending Neurologist
Neurological Institute
Columbia-Presbyterian Medical Center
710 West 168th Street
New York, New York 10032

Bennett M. Stein, M.D., F.A.C.S.
Chairman and Professor Emeritus
Department of Neurosurgery
Columbia University College of Physicians and Surgeons, and
Director Emeritus
Department of Neurosurgery
Neurological Institute
Columbia-Presbyterian Medical Center
710 West 168th Street
New York, New York 10032

Yaakov Stern, Ph.D.
Professor of Neurology and Psychiatry
Columbia University College of Physicians and Surgeons
Professional Neuropsychologist
New York-Presbyterian Hospital
630 West 168th Street
New York, New York 10032

Eveline C. Traeger, M.D.
Assistant Professor
Departments of Pediatrics and Neurology
Robert Wood Johnson School of Medicine
University of Medicine and Dentistry of New Jersey, and
Attending Physician
Robert Wood Johnson University Hospital
New Brunswick, New Jersey 08903

Rosario R. Trifiletti, M.D.
Assistant Professor of Neurology, Neuroscience, and Pediatrics
Weill Medical College of Cornell University
Assistant Attending Neurologist and Pediatrician
Cornell-New York Center
New York-Presbyterian Hospital
525 East 68th Street, Box 91
New York, New York 10021

Werner Trojaborg, M.D.
Special Lecturer in Neurology
Columbia University College of Physicians and Surgeons
Attending Neurologist
New York-Presbyterian Hospital
Neurological Institute
Columbia-Presbyterian Medical Center
710 West 168th Street
New York, New York 10032

Graziella Uziel, M.D.
Assistant
Department of Pediatric Neurology
Istituto Nazionale Neurologico C. Besta
Via Celoria, 11
Milano, 20133
Italy

Thaddeus S. Walczak, M.D.
Associate Professor of Neurology
University of Minnesota, Twin Cities Campus
5775 Wayzata Boulevard
Minneapolis, Minnesota 55416

Ching H. Wang, M.D., Ph.D.
Assistant Professor
Department of Neurology and Biochemistry
University of Missouri, and
Attending Neurologist
Department of Neurology and Child Health
University Hospitals and Clinics
M741, MSB
One Hospital Drive
Columbia, Missouri 65212

Jack J. Wazen, M.D.
Associate Professor
Department of Otolaryngology-Head and Neck Surgery
Columbia-Presbyterian Medical Center
Atchley Pavilion (AP 5512)
161 Fort Washington Avenue
New York, New York 10032

Louis H. Weimer, M.D.
Assistant Professor
Department of Neurology
Columbia University College of Physicians and Surgeons, and
Assistant Attending Neurologist
New York-Presbyterian Hospital
710 West 168th Street
New York, New York 10032

Leon A. Weisberg, M.D.
Director
Department of Neurology
Vice-Chairman
Department of Psychiatry and Neurology
Tulane Medical School
1430 Tulane Avenue, SL 28
New Orleans, Louisiana 70112

Bradford P. Worrall, M.D.
Clinical Instructor
Department of Neurology and Health Evaluation Sciences
University of Virginia
Health System #394
Charlottesville, Virginia 22908

Frank M. Yatsu, M.D.
Professor and Chairman Emeritus
Department of Neurology
University of Texas
6431 Fannin Street
Houston, Texas 77030

Dewey K. Ziegler, M.D.
Professor Emeritus
Department of Neurology
University of Kansas Medical School
3901 Rainbow Boulevard
Kansas City, Kansas 66103

Earl A. Zimmerman, M.D.
Professor and Chairman
Department of Neurology
Oregon Health Sciences University, and
Chief, Neurology Service
Oregon Health Sciences University Hospital
3181 S.W. Sam Jackson Park Road
Portland, Oregon 97201-3098

PREFACE

H. Houston Merritt first published this *Textbook of Neurology* in 1955. He was the sole author. The book became popular, and he revised it himself through the fourth edition. As the mass of information increased, he finally accepted contributions from colleagues for the fifth edition. Even then, he wrote most of the book himself, and he continued to do so for the sixth edition despite serious physical disability. He died in 1979, just as the sixth edition was released for distribution.

The seventh edition, published in 1984, was prepared by seventy of Merritt's students. Thirty of them headed neurology departments and others had become distinguished clinicians, teachers, and investigators. That edition was a landmark in the history of neurology. It documented the human legacy of a singular and great leader whose career set models for clinical investigation (when it was just beginning), clinical practice, teaching, editing books and journals, administering schools and departments, and commitment to national professional and voluntary organizations.

We now provide the tenth edition. The list of authors has changed progressively, as a dynamic book must do. Yet the ties to Merritt persist. Many of his personal students are still here and their students, Merritt's intellectual grandchildren, are appearing in increasing numbers.

Merritt's Neurology is intended for medical students, house officers, practicing neurologists, non-neurologist clinicians, nurses, and other healthcare workers. We hope it will be generally useful in providing the essential facts about common and rare diseases or conditions that are likely to be encountered.

We have tried to maintain Merritt's literary attributes: direct, clear, and succinct writing; emphasis on facts rather than unsupported opinion (now called "evidence-based medicine"); and ample use of illustrations and tables.

The book now faces competition from other books, including electronic textbooks, but its success is based on several attributes. A book, unlike a computer, can be taken and used almost anywhere. A one-volume textbook is handier, more mobile, and less expensive than the multivolume sets that now dot the scene. Briefer paperbacks provide less information and fewer references.

This edition includes comprehensive revisions demanded by the progress of research in epilepsy, Parkinson disease and other movement disorders, stroke, dementia, critical care, multiple sclerosis, ataxias, neurology of pregnancy, prion diseases, mitochondrial diseases, autonomic diseases, neuro-oncology, neurotoxicology, peripheral neuropathies, muscular dystrophies, cerebral complications of cardiac surgery, transplantation and imaging. New chapters have been added on prion diseases, CSF hypotension, superficial siderosis, glucose transporter deficiency, and end-of-life issues.

In almost every chapter, the impact of molecular genetics has left its mark in much updating. The progress of medical science has produced monographs on each of these subjects; a challenge to our authors has been the need to transmit the essential information without unduly enlarging the textbook.

We have retained the general organization of previous editions, including arbitrary decisions about the placement of some subjects. Does the discussion of seizures or multiple sclerosis in pregnancy belong in chapters on pregnancy, epilepsy or multiple sclerosis? Is the Lambert-Eaton syndrome best described in a chapter on neuromuscular disorders or one on paraneoplastic syndromes? We have opted for redundancy on these issues. It makes the book a bit longer than it might be otherwise, but the reader does not have to keep flipping pages to find the information.

The impact of molecular genetics has left other marks. Do we continue to organize the book by clinical syndromes and diseases or do we group by the nature of the mutation? "Channelopathies" or "neuromuscular disease" for Lambert-Eaton disease? "Channelopathy for familial hemiplegic migraine" or a form of headache? "Nondystrophic myotonia" or periodic paralysis for the hyperkalemic type? Triplet repeat or ataxia or spinobulbar muscular atrophy? We have opted for the clinical classification while recognizing that we are on the verge of understanding the pathogenesis of these increasingly scrutable diseases.

Another uncertainty involves eponyms: use apostrophe or not? There is no consensus in medical publishing because not everyone recognizes there is a problem. Neurology journals and the influential *New England Journal of Medicine* have not changed, but journals devoted to genetics or radiology have dropped the apostrophe and even the AMA journals are coming around. The Council of Biology Editors has taken a strong stand against the use of the possessive form.

It is not only the possessive inference that is objectionable. The legendary humorist A. J. Liebling once wrote: "I had Bright's disease and he had mine." In other usage, the nominal adjective is not the possessive; no one objects to Madison Avenue, Harvard University, Nobel Prize, or Kennedy Center. And there are other challenges, including the grating sibilance of "Duchenne's dystrophy" and the inconsistency of people who use that term, sometimes with the apostrophe and sometimes without. In the neuromuscular community, "Duchenne dystrophy" is surely preferred. And consider our hapless heroes whose names end in an "s": Graves, Kufs, Gowers, Menkes and others become incorrectly singular when the apostrophe is inserted (creating the nonexistent "Kuf's disease"). If the possessive is added at the end, something sounds wrong in "Graves's disease."

We have therefore followed the general rules of Victor McKusick in dealing with eponyms, giving general preference to the nonpossessive form without being totally rigid about it. Often, an inserted "the" can smoothly precede the eponym, especially in hyphenated compounds such as "the Guillain-Barré syndrome." Nevertheless, as McKusick states: "some nonpossessive terms, because of long usage in the possessive, roll off the tongue awkwardly—e.g., the Huntington disease, the Wilson disease, the Hodgkin disease, etc." I myself have a hard time saying "Bell palsy." But Huntington disease, Alzheimer disease, Parkinson disease, and Hodgkin disease are heard with increasing frequency, even without a preceding "the". Once the nonpossessive form is used in conversation, it is more likely to sound natural.

In another tribute to the tremendous impact of Victor McKusick, we have retained the practice of giving his catalog numbers for genetic diseases. Readers can then find the history of the syndrome and current research data in the catalog, which is now online. In this day of gender-neutral writing, it is awkward to use the acronym MIM for *Mendelian Inheritance in Man.* It seems too late to change that historic title, but "Human Mendelian Inheritance" would be euphonic.

On the other hand, the stiff-man syndrome remains a problem. Papers entitled "stiff-man syndrome in a woman" or "in a boy" ought to be fixed and "stiff-person syndrome" is just plain awkward. My personal attempts to use the eponym, "Moersch-Woltman syndrome" have had zero success, partly because the names do not trip lightly off the lip, and reversing the order is no better.

We thank all the authors for their devoted and skillful work. In the editor's office, Sheila Crescenzo has once again kept her head when I was losing mine, and she remained patient when I misplaced pages. She has been remarkably skillful in tracking correspondence and keeping multiple revisions of the same chapter in order. Terrance Gabriel was again a valuable resource in updating references throughout the book. At Lippincott Williams & Wilkins, Joyce Murphy supervised editing and production. Robin Cook was an excellent production editor. Charles Mitchell has had overall responsibility for the publisher. Their combined efforts have resulted in the handsome volume.

We formally dedicate the book to H. Houston Merritt. I personally dedicate it also to all the spouses and children of all the contributors, especially to Esther E. Rowland; our children, Andrew, Steven, and Joy; and our grandchildren, Mikaela, David Liam, Cameron Henry, and Mariel Rowland. All of them, Rowlands and others, have suffered neglect because of the contributors' clinical research and writing that provide the substance and content of this book.

REFERENCES

American Medical Association. *Manual of style. A guide for authors and editors,* 9th ed. Chicago: American Medical Association, 1998:469–472.

McKusick VA. *Mendelian inheritance in man. A catalog of human genes and genetic disorders.* 12th ed. Baltimore, Johns Hopkins University Press, 1998.

McKusick VA. On the naming of clinical disorders, with particular reference to eponyms. *Medicine* 1998;77:1–2.

ABBREVIATIONS

AchR   Acetyl choline receptor
AIDS   Acquired immunodeficiency syndrome
ALS   Amyotrophic lateral sclerosis
BAER   Brainstem auditory evoked response
BMD   Becker muscular dystrophy
C3   A specific component of complement
CIDP   Chronic inflammatory demyelinating Polyneuropathy
CJD   Creutzfeldt-Jakob disease
CK   Creatine kinase
CMT   Charcol-Marie-Tooth disease
CMV   Cytomegalovirus
CNS   Central nervous system
CPS   Complex partial seizures
CSF   Cerebrospinal fluid
CT   Computed tomography
DMD   Duchenne muscular dystrophy
DNA   Deoxyribonucleic acid
ECG   Electrocardiogram
EEK   Electroencephalography
EMG   Electromyography
ESR   Erythrocyte sedimentation rate
FSH   Facioscapulohumeral muscular Dystrophy
GBS   Guillain-Barré syndrome
GM1   A specific neural ganglioside
GSS   Gerstmann-Sträussler-Scheinker Disease

HD   Huntington disease
HIV   Human immunodeficiency virus
IVIG   Intravenous immunoglobulin therapy
KSS   Kearns-Sayre-syndrome
LHON   Leber hereditary optic neuropathy
MAG   Myelin-associated glycoprotein
MELAS   Mitochondrial encephalopathy with lactic acidosis and stroke
MERRF   Myoclonus epilepsy with ragged red fibers
MRA   Magnetic resonance angiography
MRI   Magnetic resonance imaging
MS   Multiple sclerosis
mtDNA   Mitochondrial DNA
MyD   Myotomic muscular dystrophy
NARP   Neuropathy, ataxia, retinitis pigmentosa
NPH   Normal pressure hydrocephalus
PET   Positron emission tomography
PML   Progressive multifocal leukoencephalopahy
POEMS   Syndrome of polyneuropathy, organomegaly, endocrinopathy, monoclonal paraproteinemia, and skin changes
RNA   Ribonucleic acid
SPECT   Single-photon emission computed tomography
SSER   Somatosensory evoked response
TIA   Transient ischemic attack
VER   Visual evoked response

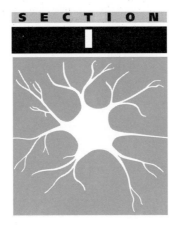

SYMPTOMS OF NEUROLOGIC DISORDERS

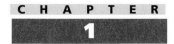

DELIRIUM AND DEMENTIA

SCOTT A. SMALL
RICHARD MAYEUX

Delirium and dementia are two of the most common disorders of elderly patients, although both conditions may occur at any age. *Delirium* is the acute confusional state that may accompany infections, fever, metabolic disorders, and other medical or neurologic diseases. *Dementia,* in contrast, is usually chronic and progressive, and is usually caused by degenerative diseases of the brain, multiple strokes, or chronic infection. The most significant difference, however, is that delirium manifests itself by a fluctuating mental state, whereas patients suffering from dementia are usually alert and aware until late in the course of the disease.

DELIRIUM

The features of delirium were originally described by Hippocrates. Delirium refers to a global mental dysfunction marked by a disturbance of consciousness, especially reduced awareness of the environment and inability to maintain attention. Associated features include disruption of the sleep–wake cycle, drowsiness, restlessness, incoherence, irritability, emotional lability, perceptual misinterpretations (illusions), and hallucinations. Symptoms appear within hours or days and fluctuate, often worsening at night. Other characteristics that lead to the classification of a mental state as delirium include impairment of memory and intellectual function, the presence of a medical or neurologic condition to which the mental impairment is secondary, the disappearance of mental impairment if the primary medical or neurologic disorder is reversed, and the effect of the primary disorder on the brain, which is diffuse rather than focal.

Delirium is involved in a wide range of clinical states. Almost any severe acute medical or surgical condition, under the right circumstances, can cause delirium. Common causes can be divided into primary cerebral disease and systemic illness. Primary brain disorders include head injury, stroke, raised intracranial pressure, infection, and epilepsy. Systemic illnesses may be infectious, cardiovascular, endocrine, or toxic-metabolic.

Delirium tremens occurs only in people addicted to alcohol. It develops 24 to 48 hours after withdrawal from alcohol. Onset is marked by confusion, agitation, and hyperactivity. Memory is affected, and hallucinations are prominent. Autonomic hyperactivity results in tachycardia and high fever. If untreated, delirium tremens can be fatal.

The following drugs can cause delirium:

Atropine and related compounds
Barbiturates
Bromides
Chlordiazepoxide (Librium)
Chloral hydrate
Cimetidine and related compounds
Clonidine
Cocaine
Diazepam
Digitalis
Dopamine agonists
Ethanol
Flurazepam
Glutethimide
Haloperidol and other neuroleptics
Lithium
Mephenytoin (Mesantoin)
Meprobamate
Methyldopa
Opioids
Phencyclidine hydrochloride (PCP)
Phenytoin sodium (Dilantin)
Prednisone
Propranolol
Tricyclic antidepressants

In elderly patients, anticholinergic and hypnotic agents are particularly common causes of drug-induced delirium.

Delirium is a medical emergency because the disease or drug intoxication may be fatal if untreated, especially in the elderly. The appearance of delirium may double the risk of death within hours or weeks. Successful treatment of delirium eliminates much of this excess mortality. The two best predictors of fatal outcome are advanced age and the presence of multiple physical diseases.

The diagnostic evaluation is dictated by evidence in the patient's history and physical examination. First-line investigations include electrolytes, complete blood cell count, erythrocyte sedimentation rate (ESR), liver and thyroid function tests, toxicology screen, syphilis serology, blood cultures, urine culture, chest x-ray, and electrocardiogram (ECG). If the cause cannot be determined from these tests, additional investigations to consider include neuroimaging, cerebrospinal fluid (CSF) analysis, electroencephalogram (EEG), human immunodeficiency virus (HIV) antibody titer, cardiac enzymes, blood gases, and autoantibody screen.

The fluctuating state of awareness in delirium is accompanied by characteristic EEG changes. The varying level of attention parallels slowing of the background EEG rhythms. Triphasic waves may also be present. Appropriate treatment of the underlying disease improves both the patient's mental state and the EEG.

The management of delirium includes general supportive and symptomatic measures, as well as treatment of the specific underlying conditions.

DEMENTIA

Dementia is characterized by progressive intellectual deterioration that is sufficiently severe to interfere with social or occupational functions. Memory, orientation, abstraction, ability to learn, visuospatial perception, language function, constructional praxis, and higher executive functions, such as planning, organizing, and sequencing, are all impaired in dementia. In contrast to patients with delirium, those with dementia are alert and aware until late in the disease. Delirium is most often associated with intercurrent systemic diseases or drug intoxication, but dementia is usually due to a primary degenerative or structural disease of the brain. Alzheimer disease (AD) (see Section XIII: Dementias) accounts for more than 50% of cases of dementia in both clinical and autopsy series. In a community-based disease registry in New York City limited to people older than 65 years, the relative frequency of AD was similar to that in other clinical and autopsy series (Table 1.1). Parkinsonism (see Chapter 114) is sometimes associated with dementia, and diffuse Lewy body disease (see Chapter 106) is incorporated into this group. Huntington disease (see Chapter 108) is much less common but is still an important cause in the presenium. Less common degenerative diseases include Pick disease and frontotemporal dementia (see Chapter 106), progressive supranuclear palsy (see Chapter 115), and the hereditary ataxias (see Chapter 107).

Cerebrovascular dementia may be defined as a clinical syndrome of acquired intellectual impairment resulting from brain injury due to either ischemic or hemorrhagic cerebrovascular disease. Of cases of dementia, 15% to 20% are attributed to vascular disease. An essential requirement for the concept of cerebrovascular dementia is that cerebrovascular disease causes the cognitive loss. Features that support causality include a temporal relationship between stroke and dementia; abrupt or, less commonly, stepwise deterioration in mental function; fluctuating course; or radiologic evidence of damage to regions important for higher cerebral function, such as angular gyrus, inferomedial temporal lobe, medial frontal lobe, thalamus, caudate, anterior internal capsule, and the border-zone infarction territory between the superior frontal and parietal convexities.

Intracranial mass lesions, including brain tumors and subdural hematomas, cause dementia without focal neurologic signs in as many as 5% of patients with dementia. With computed tomography (CT), these patients are rapidly identified and treated. Future series of dementia cases will probably include fewer patients with dementia caused by intracranial mass lesions.

The frequency of chronic communicating hydrocephalus (*normal pressure hydrocephalus*) as a cause of dementia in adults

TABLE 1.1. DISEASES THAT CAUSE DEMENTIA

	Number of subjects	Clinical series[a]	Autopsy series[b]	Washington Heights community series[c]
Depressed; psychotic; no dementia		42	—	522
Patients with dementia		474	1000	514
Degenerative				
Alzheimer disease	267	56.3%	50.3%	54.6%
Vascular; multiinfarct	40	8.4	22.3	7.0
Mixed (Alzheimer with vascular/multiinfarct)	23	4.9	13.4	17.1
Other degenerative				
Huntington disease	26	5.5	—	0
Parkinson disease	7	1.5	1.0	5.6
Progressive supranuclear palsy	6	1.2	—	0.2
Amyotrophic lateral sclerosis with dementia	3	0.6	—	0
Progressive hemiatrophy	2	0.4	—	0
Pick disease	1	0.2	2.1	0
Olivopontocerebellar atrophy	—	—	0.5	0
Epilepsy	1	0.2	—	0
Metabolic; toxic; nutritional; alcoholism; Wernicke-Korsakoff	17	3.6	1.1	8.8
Drug toxicity	8	1.7	—	0
Metabolic (thyroid; B12; hepatic; hypercalcemia)	8	1.7	—	0
Infectious				
Creutzfeldt-Jakob disease	3	0.6	0.9	0
Acquired immunodeficiency syndrome	24	5.1	—	0
Other infections or inflammatory neurosyphilis; multiple sclerosis; encephalitis	2	0.4	1.3	0
Vasculitis	3	0.6	—	0
Hydrocephalus	8	3.8	1.1	0
Intracranial tumors	12	2.5	4.5	0
Posttraumatic; subdural	3	0.6	1.5	0
Cause undetermined	—	—	—	6.7

PA, pernicious anemia.
[a]Combined series. Data from Wells, 1977; Katzman R, personal series.
[b]Data from Jellinger, 1976.
[c]Data from Mayeux R, personal New York City community series, the Washington Heights-Inwood Community Aging Project, 1993.

varies from 1% to 5% in different series. Diagnosis is usually straightforward when the hydrocephalus follows intracranial hemorrhage, head injury, or meningitis, but in idiopathic cases it is often difficult to differentiate communicating hydrocephalus from ventricular enlargement due to brain atrophy.

At the turn of the 20th century, the most common cause of dementia was neurosyphilis. Today, however, general paresis and other forms of neurosyphilis are rare. HIV-associated dementia is now among the most common infectious causes of dementia, as well as among the most common causes of dementia in young adults. Creutzfeldt-Jakob disease (CJD) is another cause of transmissible dementia. Nonviral infections rarely cause chronic rather than acute encephalopathy. Fungal meningitis occasionally manifests itself as dementia.

Nutritional, toxic, and metabolic causes of dementia are particularly important because they may be reversible. Korsakoff psychosis, usually found in alcoholics and attributed to thiamine deficiency, remains an important problem in the United States. In contrast, the dementia of pellagra, a disorder produced by niacin and tryptophan deficiencies, has been almost entirely eliminated in the United States. Vitamin B_{12} deficiency occasionally causes dementia without anemia or spinal cord disease. Among the metabolic disorders that may cause dementia, hypothyroidism is the most important. Inherited metabolic disorders that can lead to dementia in adults include Wilson disease, the adult form of ceroid lipofuscinosis (Kufs disease), cerebrotendinous xanthomatosis, adrenoleukodystrophy, and mitochondrial disorders. Finally, prolonged administration of drugs or heavy metal exposure may cause chronic intoxication (due to inability to metabolize the drug or to idiosyncratic reactions) that may be mistaken for dementia.

Differential Diagnosis

The first symptoms of progressive dementia may be occasional forgetfulness, misplacing objects, or difficulties in finding objects. The distinction between cognitive decline in old age and early dementia may be difficult. To improve the identification of cognitive changes associated with aging, varying sets of criteria have resulted in multiple terms, including age-associated memory impairment, age-related cognitive change, and mild cognitive impairment. It is likely that demonstrable changes in cognition are not an inevitable result of aging and that early dementing illnesses are one contributing cause.

Another difficult diagnostic problem is the differentiation of dementia and secondary depression from depression and a secondary memory problem that will improve with treatment of the depression. This problem is dramatized by the misdiagnosis rate of 25% to 30% in dementia series; the errors resulted chiefly from failure to recognize that older depressed people may show cognitive changes in the mental status examination. Furthermore, depression may be an early manifestation of AD. In depression, the memory problem usually follows the mood change. The onset of memory loss may be more abrupt than it usually is in dementia, and is often mild, tending to plateau. Neuropsychologic test results may be atypical for dementia.

The differential diagnosis of dementia requires an accurate history and neurologic and physical examinations. In AD, the onset of symptoms is typically insidious and the course is slowly progressive but relentless in an otherwise healthy person; in contrast, the history of a patient with vascular dementia may include an abrupt onset of memory loss, history of an obvious stroke, or the presence of hypertension or cardiac disease. A history of alcoholism raises suspicion of Korsakoff psychosis.

Examination of a patient with AD is usually normal, except for the presence of extrapyramidal signs such as rigidity, bradykinesia, and change in posture, and primitive reflexes, such as the snout reflex. Conversely, a vascular syndrome may include hemiparesis or other focal neurologic signs. Huntington disease is readily recognized by chorea and dysarthria. Patients with Parkinson disease (PD) show the characteristic extrapyramidal signs. Dementia in PD usually occurs with advanced age and includes depression and severe motor manifestations. Progressive supranuclear palsy is recognized by the limitation of vertical eye movements and extrapyramidal signs. Myoclonus occurs most often in CJD but may be seen in advanced AD and other dementias. Unsteadiness of gait is a hallmark of communicating hydrocephalus, but it may be even more severe in CJD, hereditary ataxias, or Korsakoff psychosis.

Diagnostic tests to differentiate AD from other dementias are still in their infancy. Amyloid-beta protein and tau protein can be measured in CSF, and hypersensitivity to pupillary dilation in response to tropicamide, a potent cholinergic antagonist, may help identify AD. However, none of these tests has shown improved accuracy over the clinical criteria of the National Institute of Neurological and Communicative Disorders and Stroke and the Alzheimer's Disease and Related Disorders Association (NINCDS-ADRDA). Several genes have been associated with forms of familial dementia, and a single gene has been associated with sporadic AD; nonetheless, it is difficult to use any particular gene as a diagnostic test, unless the patient is a member of one of the few identified families with that mutation. The apolipoprotein E genotype alone is insufficient to make the diagnosis, but the haplotype may improve diagnostic specificity in conjunction with NINCDS-ADRDA clinical criteria. The NINCDS-ADRDA clinical criteria make the diagnosis of AD reasonably accurate and reliable.

Neuropsychologic testing is the best way to establish the presence of dementia. Age, education, socioeconomic background, and premorbid abilities must be considered in the interpretation of the test scores. CT and magnetic resonance imaging are important for establishing the cause of dementia. Atrophy, strokes, brain tumor, subdural hematoma, and hydrocephalus are readily diagnosed by neuroimaging. Changes in white matter intensity must be interpreted with caution. Intensity changes may be due to small-vessel ischemic disease, normal aging, or dilated Virchow-Robin spaces from generalized atrophy in AD. Functional brain imaging with single-photon emission computed tomography may also be helpful. Bilateral temporoparietal hypometabolism is suggestive of AD or idiopathic PD with dementia. Bilateral frontal hypometabolism suggests Pick disease, progressive supranuclear palsy, or depression. Multiple hypometabolic zones throughout the brain suggest vascular dementia or HIV-associated dementia. In addition, the EEG is useful in identifying CJD, which is characterized by periodic discharges.

Blood tests are essential to identify dementia with endocrine disease and liver or kidney failure. Hypothyroidism is a reversible cause of dementia. Vitamin B_{12} deficiency may be present without anemia, as determined by serum vitamin B_{12} levels. Neurosyphilis is a rare but a reversible cause, so serologic testing for syphilis is mandatory. Blood levels of drugs may detect intoxication. The ESR and screens for connective tissue disease (e.g., antinuclear antibodies and rheumatoid factor) are performed if the clinical picture suggests evidence of vasculitis or arthritis. In any young adult with dementia, an HIV titer should be considered, and if an associated movement disorder is present, a test for ceruloplasmin should be performed.

Details of the differential diagnosis of diseases that cause dementia are provided in subsequent chapters. An exhaustive evaluation of patients with dementia is warranted. Although effective treatment for the primary degenerative diseases is limited, many other disorders that cause dementia are amenable to treatment that may arrest, if not reverse, the cognitive decline.

Mental Status Examination

The mental status evaluation is an essential part of every neurologic examination. It includes evaluation of awareness and consciousness, behavior, emotional state, content and stream of thought, and sensory and intellectual capabilities. Intellectual impairment is obvious in such florid conditions as delirium tremens or advanced dementia, but cognitive loss may not be evident in early delirium or dementia, unless the physician specifically tests mental status.

Traditionally, mental status examinations test *information* (e.g., where were you born? what is your mother's name? who is the president? when did World War II occur?), *orientation* (e.g., what place is this? what is the date? what time of day is it?), *concentration* (by use of serial reversals, e.g., spelling "world" backwards, naming the months of the year backwards beginning with December), *calculation* (e.g., doing simple arithmetic, making change, counting backwards by threes or sevens), and *reasoning, judgment,* and *memory* (e.g., identifying three objects and asking the patient to recall their names or telling a short story and asking the patient to try to recall it after a few minutes). The most important and sensitive items are probably orientation to time, serial reversals, and a memory phrase. The mini–mental status examination (MMSE) was introduced as a standard measure of cognitive function for both research and clinical purposes. This short examination can be administered at the bedside and completed in 10 minutes. Scores are assigned for each function (Table 1.2); the maximum score is 30 points. A score less than 24 is considered consistent with dementia. The MMSE, like all other brief mental status examinations, is not precise. Some investigators use a score of 26 as the cutoff to include milder forms of dementia and improve specificity. The MMSE tends to underdiagnose dementia in well-educated people and overdiagnose it in those with little schooling. Therefore, the MMSE should be used only as a first step. It does not replace the history or a more detailed examination of neuropsychologic function (see Chapter 19).

In addition to testing mental status, it is necessary to test higher intellectual functions, including disorders of language (dysphasias); constructional apraxia; right–left disorientation; inability to carry out complex commands, especially those requiring crossing the midline (e.g., touching the left ear with the right thumb); inability to carry out imagined acts (ideomotor apraxia; e.g., "pretend that you have a book of matches and show

---

TABLE 1.2. MINI–MENTAL STATUS EXAMINATION

Cognitive domain	Specific questions	Scoring
Orientation	1. What is the (year) (day) (month) (date) (season)?	1. 1 point for each correct response (maximum 5 points)
	2. What is the (name of this place) (address) (floor) (city) (state)?	2. 1 point for each correct response (maximum 5 points)
Registration	Name three objects (Take 1 second to say each; then ask the patient to name all three after you have said them; then repeat them until all three are learned)	3 points if all three objects are repeated on first trial; deduct 1 point for each repetition required
Attention/calculation	Serial sevens, or spelling "word" backwards	1 point for each correct response (maximum 5 points)
Recall	Ask for the three objects repeated for registration	1 point for each correct response (maximum 3 points)
Language	1. Ask patient to name a pencil and a watch	1. 1 point for each correct response (maximum 2 points)
	2. Ask patient to repeat the following: "no ifs, ands, or buts"	2. 1 point for correct response
	3. Ask patient to "take a paper in your right hand, fold it in half, and put it on the floor"	3. 1 point for each correct response (maximum 3 points)
	4. Ask patient to read and obey the following: "close your eyes"	4. 1 point for correct response
		5. 1 point for correct response
Visuospatial	5. Ask patient to write a sentence Copy a design	1 point for correct response

Modified from Folstein et al., 1975.

me how you would light a match"); unilateral neglect; or inattention on double stimulation. These abnormalities are often associated with more focal brain lesions but may also be impaired in delirium or dementia. Examination of aphasia, apraxia, and agnosia is described in detail in Chapter 2.

SUGGESTED READINGS

Arai H, Terajima M, Miura M, et al. Tau in cerebrospinal fluid: a potential diagnostic marker in Alzheimer's disease. *Ann Neurol* 1995;38:649–652.

Cummings JL, Benson DB. *Dementia: a clinical approach,* 2nd ed. Boston: Butterworth–Heinemann, 1992.

Devanand DP, Sano M, Tang MX, et al. Depressed mood and the incidence of Alzheimer's Disease in the elderly living in the community. *Arch Gen Psychiatry* 1996;53:175–182.

Diagnostic and statistical manual of mental disorders: DSM-IV. Washington, DC: American Psychiatric Association, 1994.

Folstein MF, Folstein S, McHugh P. "Mini-mental state:" a practical method for grading the cognitive state of patients for the clinician. *J Psychiatr Res* 1975;12:189–198.

Hachinski VC, Iliff LE, Ziljka E, et al. Cerebral blood flow in dementia. *Arch Neurol* 1975;32:632–637.

Jellinger K. Neuropathological aspects of dementia resulting from abnormal blood and cerebrospinal fluid dynamics. *Acta Neurol Belg* 1976;76:83–102.

Kahn RL, Goldfarb AI, Pollack M, et al. Brief objective measures for the determination of mental status in the aged. *Am J Psychiatry* 1960;117:326–328.

Katzman R, Brown T, Fuld P, et al. Validation of a short orientation-memory-concentration test of cognitive impairment. *Am J Psychiatry* 1983;140:734–739.

Lipowski ZJ. Delirium (acute confusional state). *JAMA* 1987;258:1789–1792.

Mayeux R, Foster NL, Rosser M, et al. The clinical evaluation of patients with dementia. In: Whitehouse PJ, ed. *Dementia.* Philadelphia: FA Davis Co, 1993:92–117.

Mayeux R, Saunders AM, Shea S, et al. Utility of the apolipoprotein E genotype in the diagnosis of Alzheimer's disease: the Alzheimer's Disease Centers Consortium on Apolipoprotein E and Alzheimer's Disease. *N Engl J Med* 1998;338:506–511. Erratum: *N Engl J Med* 1998;30:1325.

McHugh PR, Folstein MF. Psychopathology of dementia: implications for neuropathology. In: Katzman R, ed. *Congenital and acquired disorders.* New York: Raven Press, 1979:17–30.

McKhann G, Drachman D, Folstein M, Katzman R, Price D, Stadlan EM. Clinical diagnosis of Alzheimer's disease: report of the NINCDS-ADRDA Work Group under the auspices of Department of Health and Human Services Task Force on Alzheimer's Disease. *Neurology* 1984;34:939–944.

Neary D, Snowden JS, Gustafson L, et al. Frontotemporal lobar degeneration: a consensus on clinical diagnostic criteria. *Neurology* 1998;51:1546–1554.

Pirttila T, Kim KS, Mehta PD, et al. Soluble amyloid beta-protein in the cerebrospinal fluid from patients with Alzheimer's disease, vascular disease and controls. *J Neurol Sci* 1994;127:90–95.

Roman CG, Tatemichi TK, Erkinjuntti T, et al. Vascular dementia: diagnostic criteria for research studies. Report of NINDS-AIREN International Work Group. *Neurology* 1993;43:250–260.

Romano J, Engel GL. Delirium. I. Electro-encephalographic data. *Arch Neurol* 1944;51:356–377.

Scinto LF, Daffner KR, Dressler D, et al. A potential noninvasive neurobiological test for Alzheimer's disease. *Science* 1994;266:1051–1054.

Senility reconsidered: treatment possibilities for mental impairment in the elderly. Task force sponsored by the National Institute on Aging. *JAMA* 1980;244:259–263.

Small SA, Stern Y, Tang M, Mayeux R. Selective decline in memory function among healthy elderly. *Neurology* 1999;52:1392–1396.

Small SA, Perera GM, DeLaPaz R, Mayeux R, Stern Y. Differential regional dysfunction of the hippocampal formation among elderly with memory decline and Alzheimer's disease. *Ann Neurol* 1999;45:466–472.

Tatemichi TK, Sacktor N, Mayeux R. Dementia associated with cerebrovascular disease, other degenerative diseases, and metabolic disorders. In: Terry RD, Katzman R, Bick KL, eds. *Alzheimer disease.* New York: Raven Press, 1994:123–166.

Taylor D, Lewis S. Delirium. *J Neurol Neurosurg Psychiatry* 1993;56:742–751.

Van Heertum RL, Miller SH, Mosesson RE. SPECT brain imaging in neurologic disease. *Radiol Clin North Am* 1993;31:881–907.

Wells CE, ed. *Dementia,* 2nd ed. New York: Raven Press, 1977.

Wolfson LW, Katzman R. Neurological consultation at age 80. In: Katzman R, Terry RD, eds. *Neurology of aging.* Philadelphia: FA Davis Co, 1983:221–224.

Merritt's Neurology, 10th ed., edited by L.P. Rowland. Lippincott Williams & Wilkins, Philadelphia © 2000.

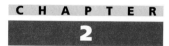

CHAPTER 2

APHASIA, APRAXIA, AND AGNOSIA

J. P. MOHR

APHASIA

Left-hemisphere dominance for speech and language applies to more than 95% of all populations studied. Right-hemisphere dominance in a right-handed person is rare enough to prompt case reports in the literature. Most left-handed persons show some disturbance in speech and language from either left- or right-hemisphere lesions, making predictions for hemisphere dominance for left-handed persons difficult to predict on an individual basis. The most predictable site for disturbances in speech and language are the regions in and bordering on the sylvian fissure of the hemisphere controlling the hand preferred for skilled movements. The farther from this zone that the lesion occurs, the less the lesion disturbs speech and language. The disturbances in speech and language resulting from a lesion form a group of disorders known as the *aphasias.*

The popular classifications of aphasia are based on classic views that the front half of the brain performs motor or executive functions and the back half sensory or receptive functions, with the two regions connected by pathways in the white matter. Classically, frontal lesions have been inferred to cause *motor aphasia,* those affecting the posterior regions cause *sensory aphasia,* and those interrupting the pathways between the frontal and posterior regions cause *conduction aphasia.* This formulation posits an anatomic functional loop with an afferent portion from the eyes and ears connecting to the visual and auditory system, an intrahemispheral portion through the white matter connecting the temporal with the frontal lobes (the arcuate fasciculus), and an efferent portion from the frontal lobes to the mouth and hand permitting, in its simplest function, words heard to be repeated aloud and words seen to be copied manually. Apart from the crude replication of sounds heard and shapes seen, of which any person even ignorant of the language conveyed by the sounds or forms is capable, meaning is thought to be conveyed to these shapes and sounds by access of the perisylvian region to the rest of the brain through intrahemispheral and transcallosal pathways. Interruption of these linkage pathways is postulated to produce *transcortical sensory aphasia,* in which words heard are repeated aloud or copied without comprehension, or *transcortical motor aphasia,* in which words can be repeated and copied but no spontaneous communication by conversation or writing occurs. Other "disconnections" have also been proposed for pathways to or from the periphery, which presumably would be in the subcortical white matter. Disconnections of incoming pathways bearing visual lexical information yield *pure alexia;* those of pathways conveying auditory material cause *pure word deafness.* The combination of these two disconnections causes *subcortical sensory aphasia.* Disconnections of efferent pathways from the motor speech zones produce *pure word mutism* or *subcortical motor aphasia.*

Although these generalizations are widely held to account for the major principles of cerebral organization, uncritical acceptance of the expected effects of certain lesion locations or prediction of lesion locations by the clinical features, as based on the classical formulas, often proves misleading for clinicians seeking the site and cause of a clinical disorder of speech and language. To avoid this problem, the material that follows emphasizes the clinical features that aid in local lesion diagnosis, with less emphasis on the classical concepts.

Motor Aphasias

An acute focal lesion (the most frequent and best known being an infarct) involving any portion of the insula or the individual gyrus forming the upper banks of the opercular cortex (from the anteroinferior frontal region to the anterior parietal) acutely disrupts the acquired skills involving the oropharyngeal, laryngeal, and respiratory systems that mediate speech, causing *mutism.* Writing may be preserved, although it is usually confined to a few simple words. Comprehension of words heard or seen is generally intact because these functions are largely subserved by posterior regions. The speech that emerges within minutes or days of the onset of motor aphasia consists mostly of crude vowels (*dysphonia*) and poorly articulated consonants (*dysarthria*). Disturbed coordination (*dyspraxia*) of speaking and breathing alters the rhythm of speech (*dysprosody*). This faulty intonation, stress, and phrasing of words and sentences is known collectively as *speech dyspraxia.* The language conveyed through this speech is usually only slightly disturbed, but the grammatic forms used in speaking or writing are sometimes simplified.

The more anterior that the lesion is along the operculum, the more speech dyspraxia predominates, especially with involvement of the inferior frontal region (Broca area) located adjacent to the sensorimotor cortex. When the sensorimotor cortex itself is affected, dysarthria and dysphonia are more prominent than dysprosody and dyspraxia. The errors in pronunciation may make it impossible to understand the language conveyed by the patient's speech, but they are not, strictly speaking, a language disorder.

When an acute lesion occurs more posteriorly along the sylvian operculum, the precise sensorimotor control over the positioning of the oropharynx may be impaired, causing unusual mispronunciations as well as mild dysphasia. The disturbed pronunciation is not simple dysarthria. Instead, the faulty oropharyngeal positionings yield sounds that differ from those intended (e.g., "dip" is said instead of "top"). The errors, analogous to the typing errors of a novice unfamiliar with the typewriter keyboard, are called *literal paraphasias.* The listener may mistake the utterances as language errors (*paraphasias*) or may be impressed with some of the genuine paraphasias and give the condition the name *conduction aphasia* (see the following). The patient's comprehension is intact despite the disordered pronunciation.

Stroke is the most common cause of acute lesions. The arrangement of the individual branches of the upper division of the sylvian artery favors the wide variety of focal embolic obstructions that produce this remarkable array of syndromes. The more specific that the speech abnormality is, the more limited is the focal infarction. Because the sensorimotor cortex is part of the same arterial supply of the upper division of the middle cerebral artery, the larger infarcts and other disorders such as *basal ganglia hemorrhages, abscesses, large tumors,* and *acute encephalitis* usually cause accompanying contralateral hemiparesis and hemisensory syndromes, making the diagnosis of perisylvian disease fairly easy. One disorder, known as *primary progressive aphasia,* appears to be an unusual form of atrophy, causing mainly a relentless decline in speech and language function without the accompanying motor, sensory, visual, or other clinical evidence of a large lesion affecting the main pathways serving these functions.

For speech and language, the smaller and more superficial that the injury is, the briefer and less severe is the disruption. Rapid improvement occurs even when the lesion involves sites classically considered to cause permanent speech and language disturbances, such as the foot of the third frontal gyrus (Broca area). The larger the acute lesion, the more evident is dysphasia and the longer is the delay before speech improves. In larger sylvian lesions, dysphasia is evident in disordered grammar, especially when tests involve single letters, spelling, and subtleties of syntax. Problems with syntax occur not only in speaking and writing but also in attempts to comprehend the meaning of words heard or seen. For example, the word "ear" is responded to more reliably than is "'are," "cat" more than "act," and "eye" more than "I." The language content of spontaneously uttered sentences is condensed, missing many of the filler words, causing *telegraphic speech,* or *agrammatism.* Agrammatism is an important sign of a major lesion of the operculum and insula. When the causative lesion involves many gyri, as with large infarcts, hemorrhages, and neoplasms or abscesses large enough to produce unilateral weakness, the reduction of both speech and comprehension is profound and is called *total aphasia.* Within weeks or months in cases of infarction and hemorrhage, comprehension improves, especially for nongrammatic forms, and speaking and writing seem to be affected more than listening and reading. This last syndrome, in which dysphasia is most evident in speaking and writing, is known as motor aphasia; the eponym *Broca aphasia* is often used. This syndrome emerges from an initial total aphasia as a late residual. It is not the usual acute syndrome of a circumscribed infarction, even when the lesion is confined to the pars opercularis of the inferior frontal gyrus (Broca area).

Sensory Aphasias

A different set of acute symptoms follows acute focal lesions of the posterior half of the temporal lobe and the posterior parietal and lateral occipital regions. Infarction is also the usual cause of the discrete syndromes, while hemorrhage, epilepsy, and acute encephalitis may account for sudden major syndromes. Even large lesions in these areas are usually far enough removed from the sensorimotor cortex so that hemiparesis and speech disturbances (e.g., dysprosody, dysarthria, or mutism) are only occasionally part of the clinical picture.

In patients with large posterior lesions, the effects are almost the reverse of the insular-opercular syndromes: Syntax is better preserved than semantics; speech is filled with small grammatic words, but the predicative words (i.e., words that contain the essence of the message) are omitted or distorted. Patients vocalize easily, engage in simple conversational exchanges, and even appear to be making an effort to communicate; however, little meaning is conveyed in the partial phrases, disjointed clauses, and incomplete sentences. In the most severe form, speech is incomprehensible gibberish. Errors take the form of words that fail to occur (*omissions*), are mispronounced as similar-sounding words (*literal paraphasias*), or are replaced by others that have a similar meaning (*verbal paraphasias*). A similar disturbance affects understanding words heard or seen. These language disturbances may require prolonged conversation to be revealed in mild cases. Because this disturbance in language contrasts with motor aphasia, it is often labeled as sensory aphasia, or *Wernicke aphasia,* but neither syndrome is purely motor or sensory.

The posterior portions of the brain are more compact than the anterior portions. As a result, large infarctions or mass lesions from hemorrhage, abscess, encephalitis, or brain tumors in the posterior brain tend to cause similar clinical disorders with few variations in syndrome type. Contralateral hemianopia usually implies a deep lesion. When hemianopia persists for longer than about 1 week, the aphasia is likely to persist.

Highly focal lesions are uncommon and, when present, usually mean focal infarction. Those limited to the posterior temporal lobe usually produce only a part of the larger syndrome of sensory aphasia. Speech and language are only slightly disturbed, reading for comprehension may pass for normal, but auditory comprehension of language is grossly defective. This syndrome was classically known as *pure word deafness.* Patients with this disorder also usually reveal verbal paraphasias in spontaneous speech and disturbed silent reading comprehension. This syn-

drome might be better named the *auditory form of sensory aphasia.* It has a good prognosis, and useful clinical improvement occurs within weeks; some patients are almost normal.

A similarly restricted dysphasia may affect reading and writing, more so than auditory comprehension, because of a more posteriorly placed focal lesion that damages the posterior parietal and lateral occipital regions. Reading comprehension and writing morphology are strikingly abnormal. This syndrome has traditionally been known as *alexia with agraphia,* but spoken language and auditory comprehension are also disturbed (although less than reading and writing). A better label might be the *visual form of sensory aphasia.* It also has a good prognosis.

The more limited auditory and visual forms of Wernicke aphasia are rarely produced by mass lesions from any cause and tend to blend in larger lesions. Whether the major syndrome of sensory aphasia is a unified disturbance or a synergistic result of several separate disorders has not been determined.

Amnestic Aphasia

Anomia or its more limited form *dysnomia* is the term applied to errors in tests of naming. Analysis requires special consideration because the mere occurrence of naming errors is of less diagnostic importance than is the type of error made. In all major aphasic syndromes, errors in language production cause defective naming (dysnomia), taking the form of paraphasias of the literal (e.g., "flikt" for "flight") or verbal (e.g., "jump" for "flight") type. For this reason, it is not usually of diagnostic value to focus a clinical examination on dysnomias alone, as they have little value as signs of focal brain disease.

A pattern known as *amnestic dysnomia* has a greater localizing value. Patients act as though the name has been forgotten and may give functional descriptions instead. Invoking lame excuses, testimonials of prowess, claims of irrelevance, or impatience, patients seem unaware that the amnestic dysnomia is a sign of disease. The disturbance is common enough in normal individuals, but in those with disease it is prominent enough to interfere with conversation. Amnestic aphasia, when fully developed, is usually the result of disease of the deep temporal lobe gray and white matter. A frequent cause is Alzheimer disease, in which atrophy of the deep temporal lobe occurs early, and forgetfulness for names may be erroneously attributed to old age by the family. Identical symptoms may occur in the early stages of evolution of mass lesions from neoplasms or abscess but are rarely a sign of infarction in the deep temporal lobe. Other disturbances in language, such as those involving grammar, reading aloud, spelling, or writing, are usually absent, unless the responsible lesion encroaches on the adjacent temporal parietal or sylvian regions. When due to a mass lesion, the disturbance often evolves into the full syndrome of Wernicke aphasia.

Thalamic Lesions and Aphasia

An acute deep lesion on the side of the dominant hemisphere may cause dysphasia if it involves the posterior thalamic nuclei that have reciprocal connections with the language zones. Large mass lesions or slowly evolving thalamic tumors distort the whole hemisphere, making it difficult to recognize the components of the clinical picture. Small lesions are most often hematomas and are the usual cause of the sudden syndrome. As in delirium, consciousness fluctuates widely in this syndrome. As it fluctuates, language behavior varies from normal to spectacular usage. The syndrome may be mistaken for delirium due to metabolic causes (e.g., alcohol withdrawal). It is also important in the theory of language because the paraphasic errors are not due to a lesion that affects the cerebral surface, as was claimed traditionally. Prompt computed tomography usually demonstrates the thalamic lesion.

APRAXIA

The term *apraxia* (properly known as *dyspraxia* because the disorder is rarely complete) refers to disturbances in the execution of learned movements other than those disturbances caused by any coexisting weakness. These disorders are broadly considered to be the body-movement equivalents of the dysphasias and, like them, have classically been categorized into motor, sensory, and conduction forms.

Limb-kinetic or Innervatory Dyspraxia

This motor form of dyspraxia occurs as part of the syndrome of paresis caused by a cerebral lesion. Attempts to use the involved limbs reveal a disturbance in movement beyond that accounted for simply by weakness. Because attempted movements are disorganized, patients appear clumsy or unfamiliar with the movements called for in tasks such as writing or using utensils. Although difficult to demonstrate and easily overlooked in the presence of the more obvious weakness, innervatory dyspraxia is a useful sign to elicit because it indicates that the lesion causing the hemiparesis involves the cerebrum, presumably including the premotor region and other association systems. Dyspraxias of this type are thought to be caused by a lesion involving the cerebral surface or the immediately adjacent white matter; apraxia is not seen in lesions that involve the internal capsule or lower parts of the neuraxis.

Ideational Dyspraxia

Ideational dyspraxia is a different type of disorder altogether. Movements of affected body parts appear to suffer from the absence of a basic plan, although many spontaneous actions are easily carried out. This disorder is believed to be analogous to sensory aphasia (which features a breakdown of language organization despite continued utterance of individual words). The term is apparently derived from the simplistic notion that the lesion disrupts the brain region containing the motor plans for the chain of individual movements involved in complex behaviors such as feeding, dressing, or bathing. To the observer, patients appear uncertain about what to do next and may be misdiagnosed as confused. The lesion causing ideational dyspraxia is usually in the posterior half of the dominant hemisphere. The coexisting sensory aphasia often directs diagnostic attention away from the dyspraxia, which, like innervatory dyspraxia, is only rarely prominent enough to result in separate clinical recognition.

Ideomotor Dyspraxia

This form of dyspraxia is frequently encountered. The term derives from the notion that a lesion disrupts the connections between the region of the brain containing ideas and the region involved in the execution of movements. The disturbance is analogous to conduction aphasia: Motor behavior is intact when executed spontaneously, but faulty when attempted in response to verbal command. For movements to be executed by the nondominant hemisphere in response to dictated commands processed by the dominant hemisphere, the lesion could involve the presumed white-matter pathways through the dominant hemisphere to its motor cortex, the motor cortex itself, or the white matter connecting to the motor cortex of the nondominant hemisphere through the corpus callosum. Because so many presumed pathways are involved, ideomotor dyspraxia is common. The syndrome is most frequently encountered in the limbs served by the nondominant hemisphere when the lesion involves the convexity of the dominant hemisphere. Concomitant right hemiparesis and dysphasias, usually of the motor type, often occupy the physician's attention so that the ideomotor dyspraxia of the nondominant limbs passes without notice. Dysphasia may make it impossible to determine whether ideomotor dyspraxia is present, but, when mild, dyspraxia can be demonstrated by showing that patients cannot make movements on command, although they can mimic the behavior demonstrated by the examiner and execute it spontaneously at other times. The disturbances are most apparent for movements that involve the appendages (e.g., fingers, hands) or oropharynx. Axial and trunk movements are often spared.

AGNOSIA

When patients with a brain lesion respond to common environmental stimuli as if they had never encountered them previously, even though the primary neural pathways of sensation function normally, this disorder is called an *agnosia*. Because the disturbance seen in response to a few stimuli is assumed to apply to others with similar properties, agnosias embrace specific classes of stimuli (e.g., agnosia for colors) or more global disturbances for a form of sensation (e.g., visual or auditory agnosia).

Such sweeping generalizations are usually unjustified in practice because careful examination often shows that the abnormality can be explained in some other way, including genuine unfamiliarity with the stimuli, faulty discrimination due to poor lighting, poor instructions from the examiner, or an overlooked end-organ failure (e.g., peripheral neuropathy, otosclerosis, cataracts). Faulty performance may also result from a dysphasia or dyspraxia. Errors arising from a dysphasia are easily understood; a dyspraxia may be more difficult to recognize. Sometimes, it is not clear whether dyspraxia produces agnosia, or vice versa. Posterior parietal lesions arising from cardiac arrest, neoplasm, or infections may impair cerebral control of the precise eye movements involved in the practiced exploration of a picture or other complex visual stimuli; the resulting chaotic but conjugate eye movements prevent the victim from naming or interacting properly with the stimuli. This abnormality seems to be a form of cerebral blindness (which patients may deny) and is an essential element of *Balint syndrome* (biparietal lesions causing disordered ocular tracking, bilateral hemineglect, and difficulties deciphering complex thematic pictures). Similar disturbances in skilled manual manipulation of objects may be documented in anterior parietal lesions that interfere with the ability to name or use an object properly.

When all these variables have been taken into account, a small group of patients may remain for whom the term *agnosia* may apply. Some neurologists deny that such a state exists, the errors presumably resulting from a combination of dementia and impaired primary sensory processing; others postulate anatomic disconnections due to lesions that lie between intact language areas and intact cerebral regions responsible for processing sensory input.

Two claimed clinical subtypes of visual agnosia embrace these differing theories of agnosia: *Apperceptive agnosia* refers to abnormality in the discrimination process, and *associative agnosia* implies an inability to link the fully discriminated stimulus to prior experience in naming or matching the stimulus to others. Clinically, patients with apperceptive visual agnosia are said to fail tests of copying a stimulus or cross-matching a stimulus with others having the same properties (i.e., different views of a car), whereas patients with the associative form can copy and cross-match; neither type can name the stimulus as such. Disturbances of the ability to respond to stimuli have been described for colors (*color agnosia*) and for faces (*prosopagnosia*). Although the definition of agnosia requires that a patient treat the stimuli as unfamiliar, the errors often pass almost unnoticed (i.e., dark colors are misnamed for other dark colors; names of famous people are mismatched with their pictures). In the auditory system, a similar disturbance may occur with a normal audiogram in discrimination of sounds (cortical deafness or *auditory agnosia*), including words (*pure word deafness* or *auditory agnosia for speech*). A patient's inability to recognize familiar objects by touch while still being able to recognize them by sight is referred to as *tactile agnosia*.

In practical clinical terms, the clinical diagnosis of agnosia warrants consideration when patients respond to familiar stimuli in an unusually unskillful manner, treat them as unfamiliar, or misname them for other stimuli having similar hue, shape, or weight, but do not show other signs of dysphasia or dyspraxia in other tests. The special testing is time-consuming but may yield a diagnosis of a disorder arising from lesions of the corpus callosum, the deep white matter, or the cerebrum adjacent to the main sensory areas. The usual cause is atrophy or metastatic or primary tumor. When the disorder develops further, the more obvious defects occur in formal confrontation visual field testing, and the "agnosia" is even more difficult to demonstrate.

SUGGESTED READINGS

Albert ML. Treatment of aphasia. *Arch Neurol* 1998;55:1417–1419.

Alexander MP, Baker E, Naeser MA, et al. Neuropsychological and neuroanatomical dimensions of ideomotor apraxia. *Brain* 1992;115:87–107.

Balint R. Seelenlähmung des "Schauens," optische Ataxia und räumliche Störung der Aufmerksamkeit. *Monatsschr Psychiatr Neurol* 1909;25:51–81.

Binder JR, Mohr JP. The topography of callosal reading pathways: a case-control analysis. *Brain* 1992;115:1807–1826.

Carlesimo GA, Casadio P, Sabbadini M, Caltagirone C. Associative visual agnosia resulting from a disconnection between intact visual memory and semantic systems. *Cortex* 1998;34:563–576.

Damasio AR. Aphasia. *N Engl J Med* 1992;326:531–539.

Geschwind N. Disconnection syndromes in animals and man. *Brain* 1965;88:585–644.

Graff-Radford NR, Damasio H, Yamada T, et al. Nonhemorrhagic thalamic infarction: clinical, neuropsychological and electrophysiological findings in four anatomical groups defined by computerized tomography. *Brain* 1985;108:485–516.

Heilman KM, Valenstein E. *Clinical neuropsychology.* New York: Oxford University Press, 1979.

Karbe H, Thiel A, Weber-Luxenburger G, Herholz K, Kessler J, Heiss WD. Brain plasticity in poststroke aphasia: what is the contribution of the right hemisphere? *Brain Lang* 1998;64:215–230.

Kertesz A, Hudson L, Mackenzie IR, Munoz DG. The pathology and nosology of primary progressive aphasia. *Neurology* 1994;44:2065–2072.

Mohr JP, Pessin MS, Finkelstein S, et al. Broca aphasia: pathologic and clinical aspects. *Neurology* 1978;28:311–324.

Naezer MA, Hayward RW. Lesion localization in aphasia with cranial computed tomography and Boston Diagnostic Aphasia Examination. *Neurology* 1978;28:545–551.

Tranel D. Neurology of language. *Curr Opin Neurol Neurosurg* 1992;5:77–82.

Victor M, Angevine JB, Mancall EL, et al. Memory loss with lesions of the hippocampal formation. *Arch Neurol* 1961;5:244–263.

Merritt's Neurology, 10th ed., edited by L.P. Rowland. Lippincott Williams & Wilkins, Philadelphia © 2000.

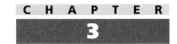

SYNCOPE AND SEIZURE

TIMOTHY A. PEDLEY
DEWEY K. ZIEGLER

Unexplained loss of consciousness is a common clinical problem. Seizure and syncope usually figure high on the list of diagnostic possibilities. The distinction is critical. This chapter considers clinical features that help discriminate among various causes of loss of consciousness and other episodic alterations in behavior and responsiveness.

SYNCOPE

Syncope refers to the transient alteration of consciousness accompanied by loss of muscular tone that results from an acute, reversible global reduction in cerebral blood flow. It is one of the most common causes of fading or complete loss of consciousness and accounts for about 3% of visits to emergency rooms. The prevalence of syncope has been as high as 47% in surveys of college students or young military flying personnel, and is equally high or higher in the elderly. In all forms of syncope, symptoms result from a sudden and critical decrease in cerebral perfusion. The causes of syncope are diverse (Table 3.1), and there is no uniformly satisfactory classification. Clinical features distinguish different types of syncope (Table 3.2).

Although syncope is generally a benign condition, nearly one-third of persons who experience syncope sustain injuries, including fractures of the hip or limbs. Additional morbidity may relate to the underlying cause of syncope.

Cardiovascular causes are most often encountered, although the exact mechanisms vary and include hypotension, arrhythmias, or direct cardiac inhibition (Table 3.3). Direct cardiac inhibition is responsible for the common *vasovagal* forms of syncope; bradycardia and hypotension are abnormal responses arising from activation of myocardial mechanoreceptors. Syncope can also occur when vasomotor tone is altered.

In reporting syncope, many patients say that they "passed out" or "had a spell." Careful history taking, with attention to the meaning patients attach to words, is the cornerstone of differentiating syncope from other conditions. Important differential points for syncope include precipitating stimuli or situations, the nature of the fall, the character and evolution of prodromal symptoms, and the absence of any true postictal phase.

The following description is typical of most syncopal events. In the premonitory phase, the person feels light-headed and often apprehensive with a strong but ill-defined sensation of malaise. Peripheral vasoconstriction imparts a pale or ashen appearance, and the pulse is rapid. Profuse sweating is often accompanied by nausea and an urge to urinate or defecate. At this point, some individuals hyperventilate, which results in hypocapnia and further reduction in cerebral blood flow. Vision blurs and characteristically fades or "grays out" before consciousness is lost, but no alterations or distortions suggest an epileptic aura; there are no visual or olfactory hallucinations, or metamorphopsia. Response times slow, and the patient may feel detached or floating just before losing consciousness. Attacks usually occur when the person is standing or sitting and may be aborted if one can lie down or at least lower the head below the level of the heart.

If the attack proceeds, the patient loses tone in the muscles of the legs and trunk as consciousness is lost, but the fall is more of a swoon or limp collapse. While unconscious, the patient continues to be pale and sweaty; the limbs are flaccid. The period of unconsciousness is brief, lasting only seconds or a few minutes. If the hypoxia associated with syncope is severe, brief tonic posturing of the trunk or a few clonic jerks of the arms and legs (*convulsive syncope*) may be seen as the episode ends. Although these involuntary movements may superficially suggest a seizure, the absence of a typical tonic-clonic sequence, the prompt recovery, and other features of the attack lead to the correct diagnosis.

Pulse and blood pressure rapidly return to normal, and symptoms resolve promptly and completely if the patient is allowed to remain recumbent. Some patients feel weak and are briefly confused on recovery; incontinence is rare.

Neurocardiogenic (Vasovagal) Syncope

This type of syncope most often occurs in adolescents and young adults and is especially common in individuals with some emotional lability. There is usually some provoking stimulus, such as

---

TABLE 3.1. CAUSES OF SYNCOPE

I. *Neurocardiogenic syncope* (direct cardiac inhibition)
   1. Vasovagal syncope
   2. Carotid sinus syndrome
   3. Micturition syncope
   4. Cough and other Valsalva-induced syncopes
   5. Emotional states

II. *Vasomotor syncope* (inability to maintain peripheral vascular tone)
   1. Medications
   2. Postural changes
   3. Autonomic and peripheral neuropathies
   4. Peripheral vascular disease
   5. Neurodegenerative disease with orthostatic hypotension
   6. Blood loss

III. *Cardiac syncope*
   1. Tachyarrhythmias
   2. Asystole and heart block
   3. Outflow obstruction
   4. Failing myocardium

TABLE 3.2. DIFFERENTIAL DIAGNOSIS OF TYPES OF SYNCOPE

Type	Autonomic dysfunction before and during	Onset of symptoms	Relation to posture	Movement during episode	ECG during episode	Age of patient	Recovery of consciousness	Urinary incontinence during episode
Neurocardio-genic (vasovagal)	Usually, marked (pallor, sweating) preceding loss of consciousness	May be rapid or with premonitory sensation of "faintness"	Usually occurs with patient sitting or standing	Usually none; occasionally a few myoclonic jerks, tonic extension	Bradycardia, occasional arrhythmia	Usually adoles-cents, young adults	Rapid	Rare
Vasomotor	Frequent except with multiple system atrophy (e.g., Shy-Drager syndrome)	May be rapid or with premonitory sensation of "faintness"	Invariably erect posture	Usually none; occasionally a few myoclonic jerks, tonic extension	Tachycardia common	All ages	Rapid	Rare
Cardiac	Variable, not as severe as in neurocardio-genic or vasovagal syncope	May or may not be rapid	Inconstant	Usually none; occasionally a few myoclonic jerks, tonic extension	Arrhythmia frequent; tachycardia, asystole, or heart block	All ages, older most common	Rapid	Rare
Psychogenic	None	Slow or rapid	None	Wide variety of involuntary movements or none	Normal	Usually young	Slow or rapid	Rare

TABLE 3.3. CAUSES OF SYNCOPE

Cause	Patients (n)
Neurocardiogenic syncope	28
Vasovagal syncope	9
Carotid sinus syncope	1
Reflex syncope (cough, micturition)	15
Vagal reaction with trigeminal neuralgia	1
Bradycardia (unspecified)	2
Vasomotor syncope	23
Orthostatic hypotension	14
Drug-induced	6
Subclavian steal	2
Dissecting aortic aneurysm	1
Cardiac syncope	49
Ventricular tachycardia	20
Sick-sinus syndrome	10
Supraventricular tachycardia	3
Complete heart block	3
Mobitz II atrioventricular block	2
Pacemaker malfunction	1
Aortic stenosis	5
Failing myocardium	5
Other	7
Seizure disorder	3
Psychogenic	1
Transient ischemic attacks	3
Unknown	97
Total	204

Modified from Kapoor, et al., 1983.

severe pain, apprehension of pain, or sudden emotional shock. A variety of background states, such as fasting, hot overcrowded rooms, prolonged standing, and fatigue, may add to the likelihood of vasovagal syncope.

Carotid sinus syncope arises when the carotid sinus displays unusual sensitivity to normal pressure stimuli. In elderly patients, this sensitivity is probably related to atherosclerosis of the carotid sinus region. Because the carotid sinus is abnormally sensitive even to slight pressure, syncope can be caused by a tight collar or inadvertent pressure on the side of the neck. The result is direct cardiac inhibition with bradycardia and occasionally even cardiac arrest. If carotid sinus syndrome is suspected, light massage of the neck area can be performed one side at a time as a diagnostic maneuver. This procedure should be done only by an experienced clinician with electrocardiograph (ECG) monitoring and, preferably, electroencephalograph (EEG) recording, as well.

Syncope can occur after emptying a distended urinary bladder (*micturition syncope*). This syndrome is confined to men and may be the result of both vagal stimuli and orthostatic hypotension. It occurs especially after ingestion of excess fluid and alcohol.

Syncope after prolonged coughing (*tussive syncope*) is usually seen in stocky individuals with chronic lung disease. In children with asthma, tussive syncope may mimic epilepsy. Increased intrathoracic pressure may decrease cardiac output, and vagal stimuli presumably play a role. Syncope with weight lifting probably results from similar mechanisms.

Vasomotor Syncope

A mild orthostatic fall in blood pressure often occurs in normal individuals without causing symptoms. However, syncope results when vascular reflexes that maintain cerebral blood flow with upright posture are impaired. In the United States, prescribed drugs may be the most common cause, but susceptibility varies markedly from one individual to the another. The frail and elderly are particularly vulnerable to this effect. Use of phenothiazines to control agitation in elderly patients often results in hypotension, syncope, a fall, and hip fracture. Other agents frequently implicated in orthostatic hypotension include antihypertensive drugs, diuretics, arterial vasodilators, levodopa, calcium channel blockers, tricyclic antidepressants, beta-blockers, and lithium. Orthostatic hypotension may also follow prolonged standing or an illness that leads to prolonged bed rest. Conditions that cause debilitation or lower blood pressure, such as malnutrition, anemia, blood loss, or adrenal insufficiency, also predispose to orthostatic hypotension.

Finally, several diseases of the central nervous system (CNS) or peripheral nervous system lead to failure of the vasomotor reflexes that are normally activated by standing, and may cause orthostatic hypotension. These conditions include peripheral neuropathy, especially diabetic peripheral neuropathy; diseases that affect the lateral columns of the spinal cord, such as syringomyelia; and multiple system atrophy, including the Shy-Drager syndrome.

Cardiac Syncope

Cardiac arrhythmias occur at all ages, but they are particularly frequent in the elderly. Attacks can be produced by many types of cardiac disease, and both tachyarrhythmias and bradyarrhythmias can produce syncope. The most commonly diagnosed arrhythmias are atrioventricular and sinoatrial block, and paroxysmal supra- and infraventricular tachyarrhythmias. When cardiac arrhythmia is suspected, a chest x-ray and routine ECG should first be obtained. Frequently, however, the resting ECG is normal, and thus longer periods of recording are then necessary. Minor and clinically insignificant disturbances in heart rhythm are common under such circumstances, and firm diagnosis requires concurrence of typical syncopal symptoms with a recorded arrhythmia. For a select group of patients, exercise testing and intracardiac electrophysiologic recordings may be necessary for diagnosis. Invasive electrophysiologic testing is also usually necessary when the conduction disturbance must be localized precisely. Other cardiac conditions that can cause syncope include a failing myocardium from cardiomyopathy or multiple infarctions, aortic and mitral stenosis, myxoma, congenital heart diseases, and pulmonary stenosis or emboli. Clues to a cardiac origin for syncope include attacks with little relation to posture, position, or specific triggers, as well as frequent "presyncopal" symptoms. Patients are often aware of a chest sensation that is difficult to describe. Syncope after exertion is typical of outflow obstruction. Finally, although cardiac syncope is usually of rapid onset, some tachyarrhythmias produce prolonged premonitory symptoms. Diagnosis of a cardiac cause of syncope is especially important because the 5-year mortality rate can exceed 50% in this group of patients.

Treatment

Treatment must be based on accurate diagnosis of the underlying cause of syncope. Isolated syncopal episodes require no treatment other than reassurance. Refractory vasovagal syncope, confirmed by tilt-table testing, responds best to beta-blockers, which suppress overactive cardiac mechanoreceptors. Disopyramide phosphate (Norpace), an antiarrhythmic drug, may be an alternative for some patients. Anticholinergic drugs may be effective but are poorly tolerated, especially by the elderly. In patients with orthostatic hypotension and autonomic insufficiency, initial measures should expand the intravascular volume by increasing fluid and salt intake. Fludrocortisone acetate (Florinef Acetate) is a mineralocorticoid that can be a useful adjunct in volume expansion. It must be used with caution in patients at risk for congestive heart failure. Compression stockings or other support garments may be required in more severe cases.

Differential Diagnosis

Episodic vertigo is a sudden violent sensation of movement, either of the self or the environment. The patient may interpret this as loss of consciousness. The diagnostic problem is complicated by prominent autonomic symptoms, such as sweating, nausea, and, occasionally, light-headedness, that frequently accompany vertiginous episodes. The critical element is the intensity of the vertigo.

Occasionally, transient loss of tone in the legs (e.g., in atonic seizures or with "drop attacks") may be mistaken for syncope.

Transient ischemic attacks (TIAs) due to severe atherosclerotic disease of the vertebrobasilar system are a rare cause of loss of consciousness. Episodic ischemia of the reticular formation of the brainstem is the presumptive cause. Vertebrobasilar TIAs causing loss of consciousness usually occur in patients who at other times have additional manifestations of brainstem, cerebellar, or occipital lobe dysfunction (i.e., cranial nerve palsies, Babinski sign, ataxia, hemianopia, or cortical blindness).

Hypoglycemia may cause feelings of faintness or dizziness, but only rarely with rapid loss of consciousness and rapid recovery. Characteristic of hypoglycemia are states of impaired consciousness of varying degrees and altered behavior of insidious onset. Symptoms last from minutes to hours, and if the hypoglycemia is prolonged or severe, generalized tonic-clonic seizures usually occur. Diagnosis depends on documenting profound hypoglycemia with the symptoms and reversing them by intravenous injection of glucose. Borderline or mild degrees of hypoglycemia do not cause CNS dysfunction.

SEIZURES AND EPILEPSY

Many nonepileptic events may be mistaken for seizures, depending on patient age, the nature of the symptoms, and the circumstances of the attacks (Table 3.4). Syncope has been reviewed in the foregoing section, but additional points may be

TABLE 3.4. DIFFERENTIAL DIAGNOSIS OF SEIZURES

Neonates and infants
    Jitteriness and benign myoclonus
    Apnea
    Shuddering attacks
    Gastroesophageal reflux

Young children
    Breathholding spells
    Infantile syncope
    Parasomnias
    Benign paroxysmal vertigo
    Tics and habits spasms
    Rage attacks

Adolescents and adults
    Movement disorders
        Myoclonus
        Paroxysmal choreoathetosis
    Migraine
        Confusional
        Vertebrobasilar
    Syncope and cardiac arrhythmias
    Hyperventilation syndrome
    Panic attacks
    Narcolepsy and sleep apnea
        Automatic behavior syndrome
        Partial cataplexy
    Transient global amnesia
    Transient ischemic attacks
    Acute confusional states
    Psychogenic seizures

pertinent. Epileptic seizures, unlike syncope, are never consistently related to head or body posture. In complex partial seizures, impaired or lost consciousness is usually accompanied by automatisms or other involuntary movements. Falls are unusual, unless the seizure becomes generalized. Urinary incontinence and postictal confusion or lethargy are common with seizures; both are rare with syncope. Likewise, warning feelings described as faintness or light-headedness are uncommon in seizures, and preictal diaphoresis is rare in contrast to the sequence of events in syncope. Atonic seizures, which may be confused with syncope, most often occur in children and young adults and tend to be much more energetic, even propulsive, than the fall experienced with syncope.

A few generalizations about other disorders that can be confused with epilepsy are warranted.

Panic Attacks

Panic attacks and anxiety attacks with hyperventilation are often unrecognized by neurologists. In both conditions, symptoms may superficially mimic partial seizures with affective or special sensory symptoms. In panic attacks, patients typically describe a suffocating sensation or "lack of oxygen," racing heart beat or palpitations, trembling or shaking, feelings of depersonalization or detachment, gastrointestinal discomfort, and fear, especially of dying or "going crazy." Hyperventilation episodes can be similar, and the overbreathing may not be obvious unless specifically considered.

The most common complaints are dizziness, a sense of floating or levitation, feelings of anxiety, epigastric or substernal discomfort, muscle twitching or spasms (tetany), flushing or chills, and sometimes "feeling like my mind goes blank." If sufficiently prolonged and intense, hyperventilation may result in syncope.

Psychogenic Seizures

In epilepsy-monitoring units, psychogenic seizures account for about 30% of admissions. Definite diagnosis of psychogenic seizures on the basis of historical data alone is usually not possible. However, the diagnosis may be suggested by atypical attacks with consistent precipitating factors that include a strong emotional or psychologic overlay, a history of child abuse or incest, and a personal or family history of psychiatric disease. Repeatedly normal interictal EEGs in the presence of frequent and medically refractory seizures also raise the possibility of psychogenic seizures.

Violent flailing or thrashing of arms and legs, especially when movements are asynchronous or arrhythmic, and pelvic thrusting are widely considered to be signs of hysteric seizures, but similar phenomena may be observed in complex partial seizures of frontal lobe origin. Preserved consciousness with sustained motor activity of the arms and legs is rare in epilepsy. Even experienced observers cannot distinguish epileptic from psychogenic seizures more than 50% to 80% of the time. Thus, for many patients, a secure diagnosis of psychogenic seizure can be made only by inpatient monitoring with simultaneous video-EEG recording. Careful analysis of the patient's behavior during a typical attack and correlation of the behavior with time-locked EEG activity permit classification of most episodes (Table 3.5).

The situation, however, may be more complicated because psychogenic seizures and epileptic seizures frequently coexist in the same patient. Therefore, recording nonepileptic attacks in a patient with uncontrolled seizures does not, by itself, prove that all the patient's seizures are psychogenic. Before reaching a final conclusion in these circumstances, one must verify with the patient and family that the recorded events are typical of the habitual and disabling seizures experienced at home.

Serum prolactin measurements may help classify a seizure as psychogenic or epileptic if the clinical behavior includes bilateral convulsive movements that last more than 30 seconds, if the prolactin measurements are obtained within 15 minutes of the event and compared with interictal baseline levels drawn on a different day at the same time, and if values are established for what constitutes a significant elevation.

Sleep Disorders

Some sleep disorders mimic seizures. In children, diagnostic difficulty is most often encountered with the *parasomnias:* sleep talking (somniloquy), somnambulism, night terrors, and enuresis. Confusion with complex partial seizures arises because all these conditions are paroxysmal, may include automatic behavioral mannerisms, and tend to be recurrent. In addition, the patient is usually unresponsive during the attacks and amnesic for them afterward. Parasomnias occur during the period of deepest slow-wave sleep, especially just before or during the transition

TABLE 3.5. DISTINGUISHING FEATURES OF EPILEPTIC AND PSYCHOGENIC SEIZURES

	Epileptic seizures		
	Generalized tonic-clonic seizures	Complex partial seizures	Psychogenic seizures
Comparison of questionable seizure with known seizure types	Relatively little variation in events	Wide range of events, but most common are well described	Extremely wide range of events with bizarre and unusual behavior
EEG during seizure	Abnormal and changed from preictal	Almost always abnormal and changed from preictal	Usually normal and unchanged from preictal
EEG immediately after seizure	Almost always abnormal and changed from preictal	Frequently abnormal and changed from preictal	Usually normal and unchanged from preictal
Relation of attacks to medication regimen	Prominent, especially in severely affected patients	Usually related	Usually unrelated
Onset	Usually paroxysmal, but may be preceded by seizure of different type	Usually paroxysmal, but may be preceded by aura of only few seconds	Often gradual, prolonged nonspecific warning period may occur
Primary or secondary gain	Rare; a few patients use seizures for secondary gain	Unusual, but a few patients use seizures for secondary gain	Common
Postictal confusion lethargy, sleepiness	Prominent	Almost always present and often prominent, but may be mild	Often conspicuously absent; patient may be normal immediately after attack
Gross tonic-clonic motor phenomena	Always	Rare; seen only in secondarily generalized attacks	None, but resemblance is related to sophistication of mimicry
Tongue biting	Frequent	Rare	Rare
Urinary incontinence	Frequent	Unusual, but not rare	Rare
Abnormal neurologic signs during sleep	May be present	May be present	None
Nocturnal occurrence	Common	May occur	Rare
Injuries sustained	Common	Common	Rare, but occasionally occur
Stereotypy of attacks	Relatively little variation	Attacks may or may not be varied, but usually have some consistent patterns	Attacks may or may not be varied; occasionally patterns may be widely divergent

Modified from Desai, et al., 1982.

into the first rapid eye movement period. They tend to occur in the early part of the night. Seizures are less predictable, although they tend to occur shortly after going to sleep or in the early morning hours. Finally, the pace of observed movements in parasomnias is usually slow and trancelike; motor activity lacks the complex automatisms, stereotyped postures, and clonic movements typical of epileptic seizures.

In adults, the *automatic behavior syndrome* may result in periods of altered mental function, awareness of "lost time" having elapsed, detached behavior that seems out of touch with the environment, and amnesia. This syndrome is usually associated with excessive daytime sleepiness and is caused by repeated episodes of microsleep that impair performance and vigilance. Attacks due to the automatic behavior syndrome lack an aura, a change in affect, oroalimentary automatisms, and a postictal period. In addition, stimulation usually stops the episode, unlike an epileptic seizure.

Migraine

Some migraine events may be mistaken for seizures, especially when the headache is mild or inconspicuous. *Basilar artery migraine* may include episodic confusion and disorientation, lethargy, mood changes, vertigo, ataxia, bilateral visual disturbances, and alterations in, or even loss of, consciousness. In children, migraine can occur as a confusional state that resembles absence status or as paroxysms of cyclic vomiting with signs of vasomotor instability (flushing, pallor, mydriasis) and photophobia.

Transient Ischemic Attack

TIAs are not usually confused with seizures. Diagnosis is occasionally difficult when a TIA is apparent only by dysphasia or disturbed sensation over part or all of one side of the body, or when muscle weakness results in a fall. In general, focal sensory symptoms associated with epilepsy show sequential spread from one body area to another, whereas ischemic paresthesias lack this segmental spread, instead developing simultaneously over affected areas. Absence of clonic motor activity and confusion favor focal ischemia more than epilepsy. Furthermore, the "negative" nature of the predominant symptoms generally argue against epilepsy.

SUGGESTED READINGS

Day SC, Cook EF, Funkenstein H, Goldman L. Evaluation and outcome of emergency room patients with transient loss of consciousness. *Am J Med* 1982;73:15–23.

Delanty N, Vaughan CJ, French JA. Medical causes of seizures. *Lancet* 1998;352:383–390.

Desai BT, Porter RJ, Penry JK. A study of 42 attacks in six patients with intensive monitoring. *Arch Neurol* 1982;39:202–209.

Devinsky O. Nonepileptic psychogenic seizures: quagmires of pathophysiology, diagnosis and treatment. *Epilepsia* 1998;39:458–462.

Fogoros RN. Cardiac arrhythmias: syncope and stroke. *Neurol Clin* 1993;11:375–390.

Hannon DW, Knilams TK. Syncope in children and adolescents. *Curr Probl Pediatr* 1993;23:358–384.

Kapoor WN. Evaluation and outcome of patients with syncope. *Medicine* 1990;69:160–175.

Kapoor WN. Evaluation and management of the patient with syncope. *JAMA* 1992;268:2553–2560.

Kapoor WN, Karpf M, Wieand S, et al. A prospective evaluation and follow-up of patients with syncope. *N Engl J Med* 1983;309:197–203.

Kaufmann H. Neurally mediated syncope and syncope due to autonomic failure: differences and similarities. *J Clin Neurophysiol* 1997;14:183–196.

Lempert T. Recognizing syncope: pitfalls and surprises. *J R Soc Med* 1996;89:372–375.

Lempert T, Bauer M, Schmidt D. Syncope: a videometric analysis of 56 episodes of transient cerebral hypoxia. *Ann Neurol* 1994;36:233–237.

Pedley TA. Differential diagnosis of episodic symptoms. *Epilepsia* 1983;24[Suppl 1]:S31–S44.

Pritchard PB, Wannamaker BB, Sagel J, Daniel CM. Serum prolactin and cortisol levels in evaluation of pseudoepileptic seizures. *Ann Neurol* 1985;18:87–89.

Saygi S, Katz A, Marks DA, Spencer S. Frontal lobe partial seizures and psychogenic seizure: comparison of clinical and ictal characteristics. *Neurology* 1992;43:1274–1277.

Sneddon JF, Camm AJ. Vasovagal syncope: classification, investigation and treatment. *Br J Hosp Med* 1993;49:329–334.

Sra JS, Mohammad RJ, Boaz A, et al. Comparison of cardiac pacing with drug therapy in the treatment of neurocardiogenic (vasovagal) syncope with bradycardia or asystole. *N Engl J Med* 1993;328:1085–1090.

Sra JS, Jazayeri MR, Dhala A, et al. Neurocardiogenic syncope: diagnosis, mechanisms, and treatment. *Cardiol Clin* 1993;11:183–191.

Sturzenegger MH, Meienberg O. Basilar artery migraine: a follow-up study in 82 cases. *Headache* 1985;25:408–415.

Merritt's Neurology, 10th ed., edited by L.P. Rowland. Lippincott Williams & Wilkins, Philadelphia © 2000.

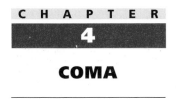

CHAPTER 4

COMA

JOHN C.M. BRUST

Consciousness, the awareness of self and environment, requires both arousal and mental content; the anatomic substrate includes both reticular activating system and cerebral cortex. Coma is a state of unconsciousness that differs from syncope in being sustained and from sleep in being less easily reversed. Cerebral oxygen uptake (cerebral metabolic rate of oxygen [$CMRO_2$]) is normal in sleep or actually increases during the rapid eye movement stage, but $CMRO_2$ is abnormally reduced in coma.

Coma is clinically defined by the neurologic examination, especially responses to external stimuli. Terms such as *lethargy, obtundation, stupor,* and coma usually depend on the patient's response to normal verbal stimuli, shouting, shaking, or pain. These terms are not rigidly defined, and it is useful to record both the response and the stimulus that elicited it. Occasionally, the true level of consciousness may be difficult or impossible to determine (e.g., when there is catatonia, severe depression, curarization, or akinesia plus aphasia).

Confusional state and *delirium* are terms that refer to a state of inattentiveness, altered mental content, and, sometimes, hyperactivity rather than to a decreased level of arousal; these conditions may presage or alternate with obtundation, stupor, or coma.

EXAMINATION AND MAJOR DIAGNOSTIC PROCEDURES

In the assessment of a comatose patient, it is first necessary to detect and treat any immediately life-threatening condition: Hemorrhage is stopped; the airway is protected, with intubation when necessary (including the prevention of aspiration in a patient who is vomiting); circulation is supported; and an electrocardiogram is obtained to detect dangerous arrhythmia. If the diagnosis is unknown, blood is drawn for glucose determination, after which 50% dextrose is given intravenously with parenteral thiamine. (Administering glucose alone to a thiamine-deficient patient may precipitate Wernicke-Korsakoff syndrome.) When opiate overdose is a possibility, naloxone hydrochloride (Narcan) is given. If trauma is suspected, damage to internal organs and fracture of the neck should be taken into consideration until radiographs determine otherwise.

The next step is to ascertain the site and cause of the lesion. The history is obtained from whoever accompanies the patient, including ambulance drivers and police. Examination should include the following: skin, nails, and mucous membranes (for pallor, cherry redness, cyanosis, jaundice, sweating, uremic frost, myxedema, hypo- or hyperpigmentation, petechiae, dehydration, decubiti, or signs of trauma); the breath (for acetone, alcohol, or fetor hepaticus); and the fundi (for papilledema, hypertensive or diabetic retinopathy, retinal ischemia, Roth spots, granulomas, or subhyaloid hemorrhages). Fever may imply infection or heat stroke; hypothermia may occur with cold exposure (especially in alcoholics), hypothyroidism, hypoglycemia, sepsis, or, infrequently, a primary brain lesion. Asymmetry of pulses may suggest dissecting aneurysm. Urinary or fecal incontinence may signify an unwitnessed seizure, especially in patients who awaken spontaneously. The scalp should be inspected and palpated for signs of trauma (e.g., Battle sign), and the ears and nose are examined for blood or cerebrospinal fluid (CSF). Resistance to passive neck flexion but not to turning or tilting suggests meningitis, subarachnoid hemorrhage, or foramen magnum herniation, but may be absent early in the course of the disorder and in patients who are deeply comatose. Resistance in all directions suggests bone or joint disease, including fracture.

In their classic monograph, Plum and Posner (1980) divided the causes of coma into supra- and infratentorial structural lesions and diffuse or metabolic diseases. By concentrating on motor responses to stimuli, respiratory patterns, pupils, and eye movements, the clinician can usually identify the category of coma.

The patient is observed to assess respiration, limb position, and spontaneous movements. Myoclonus or seizures may be subtle (e.g., twitching of one or two fingers or the corner of the mouth). More florid movements, such as facial grimacing, jaw gyrations, tongue protrusion, or complex repetitive limb movements, may defy ready interpretation. Asymmetric movements or postures may signify either focal seizures or hemiparesis.

Asymmetry of muscle tone suggests a structural lesion, but it is not always clear which side is abnormal. *Gegenhalten,* or *paratonia,* is resistance to passive movement that, in contrast to parkinsonian rigidity, increases with the velocity of the movement and, unlike clasp-knife spasticity, continues through the full range of the movement; it is attributed to diffuse forebrain dysfunction and is often accompanied by a grasp reflex.

Motor responses to stimuli may be appropriate, inappropriate, or absent. Even when patients are not fully awake, they may be roused to follow simple commands. Some patients who respond only to noxious stimuli (e.g., pressure on the sternum or supraorbital bone, pinching the neck or limbs, or squeezing muscle, tendon, or nailbeds) may make voluntary avoidance responses. The terms "decorticate" and "decerebrate" posturing are physiologic misnomers but refer to hypertonic flexion or extension in response to noxious stimuli. In *decorticate rigidity,* the arms are flexed, adducted, and internally rotated, and the legs are extended; in *decerebrate rigidity,* the arms and legs are all extended. These postures are most often associated with cerebral hemisphere disease, including metabolic encephalopathy, but may follow upper brainstem lesions or transtentorial herniation.

Flexor postures generally imply a more rostral lesion and have a better prognosis than extensor posturing, but the pattern of response may vary with different stimuli, or there may be flexion of one arm and extension of the other. When these postures seem to occur spontaneously, there may be an unrecognized stimulus (e.g., airway obstruction or bladder distention). With continuing rostrocaudal deterioration, there may be extension of the arms and flexion of the legs until, with lower brainstem destruction, there is flaccid unresponsiveness. However, lack of motor response to any stimulus should always raise the possibility of limb paralysis caused by cervical trauma, Guillain-Barré neuropathy, or the locked-in state.

Respiration

In Cheyne-Stokes respiration (CSR), periods of hyperventilation and apnea alternate in a crescendo-decrescendo fashion. The hyperpneic phase is usually longer than the apneic, so that arterial gases tend to show respiratory alkalosis; during periods of apnea, there may be decreased responsiveness, miosis, and reduced muscle tone. CSR occurs with bilateral cerebral disease, including impending transtentorial herniation, upper brainstem lesions, and metabolic encephalopathy. It usually signifies that the patient is not in imminent danger. Conversely, "short-cycle CSR" (*cluster breathing*) with less smooth waxing and waning is often an ominous sign of a posterior fossa lesion or dangerously elevated intracranial pressure.

Sustained hyperventilation is usually due to metabolic acidosis, pulmonary congestion, hepatic encephalopathy, or stimulation by analgesic drugs (Fig. 4.1). Rarely, it is the result of a lesion in the rostral brainstem. *Apneustic breathing,* consisting of inspiratory pauses, is seen with pontine lesions, especially infarction; it occurs infrequently with metabolic coma or transtentorial herniation.

Respiration having an variably irregular rate and amplitude (*ataxic* or *Biot breathing*) indicates medullary damage and can progress to apnea, which also occurs abruptly in acute posterior fossa lesions. Loss of automatic respiration with preserved voluntary breathing (*Ondine curse*) occurs with medullary lesions; as the patient becomes less alert, apnea can be fatal. Other ominous respiratory signs are end-expiratory pushing (e.g., coughing) and "fish-mouthing" (i.e., lower-jaw depression with inspiration). Stertorous breathing (i.e., inspiratory noise) is a sign of airway obstruction.

Pupils

Pupillary abnormalities in coma may reflect an imbalance between input from the parasympathetic and sympathetic nervous systems or lesions of both. Although many people have slight pupillary inequality, anisocoria should be considered pathologic in a comatose patient. Retinal or optic nerve damage does not cause anisocoria, even though there is an afferent pupillary defect. Parasympathetic lesions (e.g., oculomotor nerve compression in uncal herniation or after rupture of an internal carotid artery aneurysm) cause pupillary enlargement and ultimately full dilatation with loss of reactivity to light. Sympathetic lesions, either intraparenchymal (e.g., hypothalamic injury or lateral medullary

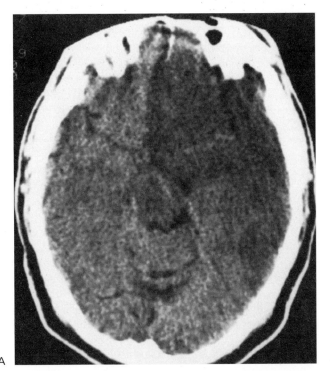 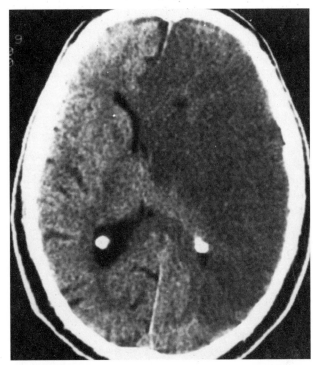

A   B

FIG. 4.1. Cerebral herniation secondary to hemispheral infarction. Noncontrast axial CT demonstrates an extensive area of decreased density within the left frontal, temporal, and parietal lobes with relative sparing of the left thalamus and left occipital lobe. A dense left middle cerebral artery is seen, consistent with thrombosis. **A:** Obliteration of the suprasellar cistern by the medial left temporal lobe indicates uncal herniation. **B:** Left-to-right shift of the left frontal lobe, left caudate nucleus, and left internal capsule denote severe subfalcine herniation. (Courtesy of Dr. S. Chan, Columbia University College of Physicians and Surgeons, New York, N.Y.)

infarction) or extraparenchymal (e.g., invasion of the superior cervical ganglion by lung cancer), cause Horner syndrome with miosis. With involvement of both systems (e.g., midbrain destruction), one or both pupils are in midposition and are unreactive. Pinpoint but reactive pupils following pontine hemorrhage are probably the result of damage to descending intraaxial sympathetic pathways, as well as to a region of the reticular formation that normally inhibits the Edinger-Westphal nucleus.

With few exceptions, metabolic disease does not cause unequal or unreactive pupils. Fixed, dilated pupils after diffuse anoxia-ischemia carry a bad prognosis. Anticholinergic drugs, including glutethimide, amitriptyline, and antiparkinsonian agents, abolish pupillary reactivity. Hypothermia and severe barbiturate intoxication can cause not only fixed pupils but a reversible picture that mimics brain death. Bilateral or unilateral pupillary dilatation and unreactivity can accompany (or briefly follow) a seizure. In opiate overdose, miosis may be so severe that a very bright light and a magnifying glass are necessary to detect reactivity. Some pupillary abnormalities are local in origin (e.g., trauma or synechiae).

Eyelids and Eye Movements

Closed eyelids in a comatose patient mean that the lower pons is intact, and blinking means that reticular activity is taking place; however, blinking can occur with or without purposeful limb movements. Eyes that are conjugately deviated away from hemiparetic limbs indicate a destructive cerebral lesion on the side toward which the eyes are directed. Eyes turned toward paretic limbs may mean a pontine lesion, an adversive seizure, or the wrong-way gaze paresis of thalamic hemorrhage. Eyes that are dysconjugate while at rest may mean paresis of individual muscles, internuclear ophthalmoplegia, or preexisting tropia or phoria.

When the brainstem is intact, the eyes may rove irregularly from side to side with a slow, smooth velocity; jerky movements suggest saccades and relative wakefulness. Repetitive smooth excursions of the eyes first to one side and then to the other, with 2- to 3-second pauses in each direction (*periodic alternating* or *ping-pong gaze*), may follow bilateral cerebral infarction or cerebellar hemorrhage with an intact brainstem.

If cervical injury has been ruled out, oculocephalic testing (the *doll's-eye maneuver*) is performed by passively turning the head from side to side; with an intact reflex arc (vestibular–brainstem–eye muscles), the eyes move conjugately in the opposite direction. A more vigorous stimulus is produced by irrigating each ear with 30 to 100 mL of ice water. A normal awake person with head elevated 30 degrees has nystagmus with the fast component in the direction opposite the ear stimulated, but a comatose patient with an intact reflex arc has deviation of the eyes toward the stimulus, usually for several minutes. Simultaneous bilateral irrigation causes vertical deviation, upward after warm water and downward after cold water.

Oculocephalic or caloric testing may reveal intact eye movements, gaze palsy, individual muscle paresis, internuclear ophthalmoplegia, or no response. Cerebral gaze paresis can often be overcome by these maneuvers, but brainstem gaze palsies are usually fixed. Complete ophthalmoplegia may follow either extensive brainstem damage or metabolic coma, but except for barbiturate or phenytoin sodium (Dilantin) poisoning, eye movements are preserved early in metabolic encephalopathy. Unexplained dysconjugate eyes indicate a brainstem or cranial nerve lesion (including abducens palsy due to increased intracranial pressure).

Downward deviation of the eyes occurs with lesions in the thalamus or midbrain pretectum and may be accompanied by pupils that do not react to light (*Parinaud syndrome*). Downward eye deviation also occurs in metabolic coma, especially in barbiturate poisoning, and after a seizure. Skew deviation, or vertical divergence, follows lesions of the cerebellum or brainstem, especially the pontine tegmentum.

Retraction and convergence nystagmus may be seen with midbrain lesions, but spontaneous nystagmus is rare in coma. *Ocular bobbing* (conjugate brisk downward movements from the primary position) usually follows destructive lesions of the pontine tegmentum (when lateral eye movements are lost) but may occur with cerebellar hemorrhage, metabolic encephalopathy, or transtentorial herniation. Unilateral bobbing (nystagmoid jerking) signifies pontine disease.

Tests

Computed tomography (CT) or magnetic resonance imaging (MRI) is promptly performed whenever coma is unexplained. Unless meningitis is suspected and the patient is clinically deteriorating, imaging should precede lumbar puncture. If imaging is not readily available, a spinal tap is cautiously performed with a no. 20 or no. 22 needle. If imaging reveals frank transtentorial or foramen magnum herniation, the comparative risks of performing a lumbar puncture or of treating for meningitis without CSF confirmation must be weighed individually for each patient.

Other emergency laboratory studies include blood levels of glucose, sodium, calcium, and blood urea nitrogen (or creatinine); determination of arterial pH and partial pressures of oxygen and carbon dioxide; and blood or urine toxicology testing (including blood levels of sedative drugs and ethanol). Blood and CSF should be cultured, and liver function studies and other blood electrolyte levels determined. Coagulation studies and other metabolic tests are based on index of suspicion.

The electroencephalogram (EEG) can distinguish coma from psychic unresponsiveness or locked-in state, although alphalike activity in coma after brainstem infarction or cardiopulmonary arrest may make the distinction difficult. In metabolic coma, the EEG is always abnormal, and early in the course, it may be a more sensitive indicator of abnormality than the clinical state of the patient. The EEG may also reveal asymmetries or evidence of clinically unsuspected seizure activity. Infrequently, patients without clinical seizures demonstrate repetitive electrographic seizures or continuous spike-and-wave activity; conversely, patients with subtle motor manifestations of seizures sometimes display only diffuse electrographic slowing. Distinguishing true status epilepticus from myoclonus (common after anoxic-ischemic brain damage) is often difficult, both clinically and electrographically; and if any doubt exists, anticonvulsant therapy should be instituted.

COMA FROM SUPRATENTORIAL STRUCTURAL LESIONS

Coma can result from bilateral cerebral damage or from sudden large unilateral lesions that functionally disrupt the contralateral hemisphere (*diaschisis*). CT studies indicate that with acute hemisphere masses, early depression of consciousness correlates more with lateral brain displacement than with transtentorial herniation. Eventually, however, downward brain displacement and rostrocaudal brainstem dysfunction ensue. Transtentorial herniation is divided into lateral (uncal) or central types. In *uncal herniation* (as in subdural hematoma), there is early compression of the oculomotor nerve by the inferomedial temporal lobe with ipsilateral pupillary enlargement. Alertness may not be altered until the pupil is dilated, at which point there may be an acceleration of signs with unilaterally and then bilaterally fixed pupils and oculomotor palsy, CSR followed by hyperventilation or ataxic breathing, flexor and then extensor posturing, and progressive unresponsiveness. Aqueductal obstruction and posterior cerebral artery compression may further raise supratentorial pressure. If the process is not halted, there is progression to deep coma, apnea, bilaterally unreactive pupils, ophthalmoplegia, and eventually circulatory collapse and death.

In *central transtentorial herniation* (as in thalamic hemorrhage), consciousness is rapidly impaired, pupils are of normal or small diameter and react to light, and eye movements are normal. CSR, gegenhalten, and flexor or extensor postures are also seen. As the disorder progresses, the pupils become fixed in midposition, and this is followed by the same sequence of unresponsiveness, ophthalmoplegia, and respiratory and postural abnormalities as seen in uncal herniation. During the downward course of transtentorial herniation, there may be hemiparesis ipsilateral to the cerebral lesion, attributed to compression of the contralateral midbrain peduncle against the tentorial edge (*Kernohan notch*). The contralateral oculomotor nerve is occasionally compressed before the ipsilateral oculomotor nerve.

The major lesions causing transtentorial herniation are traumatic (epidural, subdural, or intraparenchymal hemorrhage), vascular (ischemic or hemorrhagic), infectious (abscess or granuloma, including lesions associated with acquired immunodeficiency syndrome), and neoplastic (primary or metastatic). CT or MRI locates and often defines the lesion.

COMA FROM INFRATENTORIAL STRUCTURAL LESIONS

Infratentorial structural lesions may compress or directly destroy the brainstem. Such lesions may also cause brain herniation, either transtentorially upward (with midbrain compression) or downward through the foramen magnum, with distortion of the medulla by the cerebellar tonsils. Abrupt tonsillar herniation causes apnea and circulatory collapse; coma is then secondary, for the medullary reticular formation has little direct role in arousal. In coma, *primary infratentorial lesions* are suggested by bilateral weakness or sensory loss, crossed cranial nerve and long tract signs, miosis, loss of lateral gaze with preserved vertical eye movements, dysconjugate gaze, ophthalmoplegia, short-cycle CSR, and apneustic or ataxic breathing. The clinical picture of pontine hemorrhage (i.e., sudden coma, pinpoint but reactive pupils, and no eye movement) is characteristic, but if the sequence of signs in a comatose patient is unknown, it may not be possible without imaging to tell whether the process began supratentorially or infratentorially. Infrequent brainstem causes of coma include multiple sclerosis and central pontine myelinolysis.

COMA FROM METABOLIC OR DIFFUSE BRAIN DISEASE

In metabolic, diffuse, or multifocal encephalopathy, mental and respiratory abnormalities occur early; there is often tremor, asterixis, or multifocal myoclonus. Gegenhalten, frontal release signs (snout, suck, or grasp), and flexor or extensor posturing may occur. Except in anticholinergic intoxication, the pupils remain reactive. The eyes may be deviated downward, but sustained lateral deviation or dysconjugate eyes argue against a metabolic disturbance. Metabolic disease, however, can cause both focal seizures and lateralizing neurologic signs, often shifting but sometimes persisting (as in hypoglycemia and hyperglycemia).

Arterial gas determinations are especially useful in metabolic coma. Of the diseases listed in Table 4.1, psychogenic hyperventilation is more likely to cause delirium than stupor, but may coexist with hysterical coma. Mental change associated with metabolic alkalosis is usually mild.

Metabolic and diffuse brain diseases causing coma are numerous but not unmanageably so. Most entities listed in Table 4.2 are described in other chapters.

HYSTERIA AND CATATONIA

Hysterical (conversion) unresponsiveness is rare and probably overdiagnosed. Indistinguishable clinically from malingering, it is usually associated with closed eyes, eupnea or tachypnea, and normal pupils. The eyelids may resist passive opening and, when released, close abruptly or jerkily rather than with smooth descent; lightly stroking the eyelashes causes lid fluttering. The eyes do not slowly rove but move with saccadic jerks, and ice-water caloric testing causes nystagmus rather than sustained deviation. The limbs usually offer no resistance to passive movement yet demonstrate normal tone. Unless organic disease or drug effect is also present, the EEG pattern is one of normal wakefulness.

In catatonia (which may occur with schizophrenia, depression, toxic psychosis, or other brain diseases), there may be akinetic mutism, grimacing, rigidity, posturing, catalepsy, or excitement. Respirations are normal or rapid, pupils are large but reactive, and eye movements are normal. The EEG is usually normal.

TABLE 4.1. CAUSES OF ABNORMAL VENTILATION IN UNRESPONSIVE PATIENTS

Hyperventilation
  Metabolic acidosis
    Anion gap
      Diabetic ketoacidosis[a]
      Diabetic hypersomolar coma[a]
      Lactic acidosis
      Uremia[a]
      Alcoholic ketoacidosis
      Acidic poisons (ethylene glycol, methyl alcohol, paraldehyde)[a]
    No anion gap
      Diarrhea
      Pancreatic drainage
      Carbonic anhydrase inhibitiors
      NH$_4$Cl ingestion
      Renal tubular acidosis
      Ureteroenterostomy
  Respiratory alkalosis
    Hepatic failure[a]
    Sepsis[a]
    Pneumonia
    Anxiety (hyperventilation syndrome)
  Mixed acid–base disorders (metabolic acidosis and respiratory alkalosis)
    Salicylism
    Sepsis[a]
    Hepatic failure[a]

Hypoventilation
  Respiratory acidosis
    Acute (uncompensated)
      Sedative drugs[a]
      Brainstem injury
      Neuromuscular disorders
      Chest injury
      Acute pulmonary disease
    Chronic pulmonary disease
  Metabolic alkalosis
    Vomiting or gastric drainage
    Diuretic therapy
    Adrenal steroid excess (Cushing syndrome)
    Primary aldosteronism
    Bartter syndrome

[a]Common causes of stupor or coma. From Plum and Posner, 1980, with permission.

TABLE 4.2. DIFFUSE BRAIN DISEASES OR METABOLIC DISORDERS THAT CAUSE COMA

Deprivation of oxygen, substrate, or metabolic cofactor
 Hypoxia
 Diffuse ischemia (cardiac disease, decreased peripheral circulatory resistance, increased cerebrovascular resistance, widespread small vessel occlusion)
 Hypoglycemia
 Thiamine deficiency (Wernicke-Korsakoff syndrome)

Disease of organs other than brain
 Liver (hepatic coma)
 Kidney (uremia)
 Lung (carbon dioxide narcosis)
 Pancreas (diabetes, hypoglycemia, exocrine pancreatic encephalopathy)
 Pituitary (apoplexy, sedative hypersensitivity)
 Thyroid (myxedema, thyrotoxicosis)
 Parathyroid (hypo- and hyperparathyroidism)
 Adrenal (Addison or Cushing disease, pheochromocytoma)
 Other systemic disease (cancer, porphyria, sepsis)

Exogenous poisons
 Sedatives and narcotics
 Psychotropic drugs
 Acid poisons (e.g., methyl alcohol, ethylene glycol)
 Others (e.g., anticonvulsants, heavy metals, cyanide)

Abnormalities of ionic or acid–base environment of central nervous system
 Water and sodium (hypo- and hypernatremia)
 Acidosis
 Alkalosis
 Magnesium (hyper- and hypomagnesemia)
 Calcium (hyper- and hypocalcemia)
 Phosphorus (hypophosphatemia)

Disordered temperature regulation
 Hypothermia
 Heat stroke

Central nervous system inflammation or infiltration
 Leptomeningitis
 Encephalitis
 Acute toxic encephalopathy (e.g., Reye syndrome)
 Parainfectious encephalomyelitis
 Cerebral vasculitis
 Subarachnoid hemorrhage
 Carcinomatous meningitis

Primary neuronal or glial disorders
 Creutzfeldt-Jakob disease
 Marchiafava-Bignami disease
 Adrenoleukodystrophy
 Gliomatosis cerebri
 Progressive multifocal leukoencephalopathy

Seizure and postictal states

Modified from Plum and Posner, 1980.

TABLE 4.3. CRITERIA FOR DETERMINATION OF VEGETATIVE STATE

1. No evidence of awareness of self or surroundings. Reflex or spontaneous eye opening may occur.
2. No communication between examiner and patient, auditory or written, that is meaningful and consistent. Target stimuli not usually followed visually, but sometimes visual tracking present. No emotional response to verbal stimuli.
3. No comprehensible speech or mouthing of words.
4. Smiling, frowning, or crying inconsistently related to any apparent stimulus.
5. Sleep–wake cycles present.
6. Brainstem and spinal reflexes variable, e.g., preservation of sucking, rooting, chewing, swallowing, pupillary reactivity to light, oculocephalic responses, and grasp or tendon reflexes.
7. No voluntary movements or behavior, no matter how rudimentary; no motor activity suggesting learned behavior; no mimicry. Withdrawal or posturing can occur with noxious stimuli.
8. Usually intact blood pressure control and cardiorespiratory function. Incontinence of bladder and bowel.

ments, including blinking. (Even with facial paralysis, inhibition of the levator palpebrae can produce partial eye closure.) Communication is possible with blinking or eye movements to indicate "yes," "no," or letters.

VEGETATIVE STATE

The terms *akinetic mutism* and *coma vigil* have been used to describe a variety of states, including coma with preserved eye movements following midbrain lesions, psychomotor bradykinesia with frontal lobe disease, and isolated diencephalic and brainstem function after massive cerebral damage. For this last condition, the term *vegetative state* is preferred to refer to patients with sleep–wake cycles, intact cardiorespiratory function, and primitive responses to stimuli, but without evidence of inner or outer awareness (Table 4.3). Patients who survive coma usually show varying degrees of recovery within 2 to 4 weeks; those who enter the vegetative state may recover further, even fully. *Persistent vegetative state* is defined as a vegetative state present for at least 1 month. Although further improvement is then unlikely, anecdotal reports exist of recovery after many months. The technologic feasibility of indefinitely prolonging life without consciousness has generated considerable ethical debate.

BRAIN DEATH

Unlike vegetative state, in which the brainstem is intact, the term *brain death* means that neither the cerebrum nor the brainstem is functioning. The only spontaneous activity is cardiovascular, apnea persists in the presence of hypercarbia sufficient for respiratory drive, and the only reflexes present are those mediated by the spinal cord (Table 4.4). In adults, brain death rarely lasts

LOCKED-IN SYNDROME

Infarction or central pontine myelinolysis may destroy the basis pontis, producing total paralysis of the lower cranial nerve and limb muscles with preserved alertness and respiration. At first glance, the patient appears unresponsive, but examination reveals voluntary vertical and sometimes horizontal eye move-

TABLE 4.4. CRITERIA FOR DETERMINATION OF BRAIN DEATH

1. Coma, unresponsive to stimuli above foramen magnum.

2. Apnea off ventilator (with oxygenation) for a duration sufficient to produce hypercarbic respiratory drive (usually 10–20 minutes to achieve PCO_2 of 50–60 mm Hg).

3. Absence of cephalic reflexes, including pupillary, oculocephalic, oculovestibular (caloric), corneal, gag, sucking, swallowing, and extensor posturing. Purely spinal reflexes may be present, including tendon reflexes, plantar responses, and limb flexion to noxious stimuli.

4. Body temperature above 34°C.

5. Systemic circulation may be intact.

6. Diagnosis known to be structural disease or irreversible metabolic disturbance; absence of drug intoxication, including ethanol, sedatives, potentially anesthetizing agents, or paralyzing drugs.

7. In adults with known structural cause and without involvement of drugs or ethanol, at least 6 hours of absent brain function; for others, including those with anoxic-ischemic brain damage, at least 24 hours' observation plus negative drug screen.

8. Diagnosis of brain death inappropriate in infants younger than 7 days. Observation of at least 48 hours for infants aged 7 days to 2 months, at least 24 hours for those aged 2 months to 1 year, and at least 12 hours for those aged 1–5 years (24 hours if anoxic-ischemic brain damage). For older children, adult criteria apply.

9. Optional confirmatory studies include:
   EEG isolectric for 30 minutes at maximal gain
   Absent brainstem evoked responses
   Absent cerebral circulation demonstrated by radiographic, radioisotope, or magnetic resonance angiography.

more than a few days and is always followed by circulatory collapse. In the United States, brain death is equated with legal death. When criteria are met, artificial ventilation and blood pressure support are appropriately discontinued, whether or not organ harvesting is intended.

SUGGESTED READINGS

American Neurological Association Committee on Ethical Affairs. Persistent vegetative state. *Ann Neurol* 1993;33:386–390.

Childs NL, Mercer WN. Late improvement in consciousness after post-traumatic vegetative state. *N Engl J Med* 1996;334:24–25.

Feldmann E, Gandy SE, Becker R, et al. MRI demonstrates descending transtentorial herniation. *Neurology* 1988;38:697–701.

Fisher CM. Some neuro-ophthalmological observations. *J Neurol Neurosurg Psychiatry* 1967;30:383–392.

Fisher CM. The neurological examination of the comatose patient. *Acta Neurol Scand* 1969;45[Suppl 36]:1–56.

Grindal AB, Suter C, Martinez AJ. Alpha-pattern coma: 24 cases with 9 survivors. *Ann Neurol* 1977;1:371–377.

Guidelines for the determination of brain death in children. *Ann Neurol* 1987;21:616–617.

Guidelines for the determination of death: report of the medical consultants on the diagnosis of death to the President's Commission for the Study of Ethical Problems in Medicine and Biomedical and Behavioral Research. *Neurology* 1982;32:395–399.

Levy DE, Caronna JJ, Knill-Jones R, et al. Predicting outcome from hypoxic-ischemic coma. *JAMA* 1985;253:1420–1426.

Levy DE, Dates D, Coronna JJ, et al. Prognosis in nontraumatic coma. *Ann Intern Med* 1981;94:293–301.

Lowenstein DH, Aminoff MJ. Clinical and EEG features of status epilepticus in comatose patients. *Neurology* 1992;42:100–104.

Malouf R, Brust JCM. Hypoglycemia: causes, neurological manifestations, and outcome. *Ann Neurol* 1985;17:421–430.

Marks SJ, Zisfein J. Apneic oxygenation in apnea tests for brain death: a controlled trial. *Arch Neurol* 1990;47:1066–1068.

Multi-society Task Force on PVS. Medical aspects of the persistent vegetative state. *N Engl J Med* 1994;330:1499–1508, 1572–1579.

Payne K, Taylor RM, Stocking C, et al. Physicians' attitudes about the care of patients in the persistent vegetative state: a national survey. *Ann Intern Med* 1996;125:104–110.

Plum F, Posner JB. *The diagnosis of stupor and coma,* 3rd ed. Philadelphia: FA Davis Co, 1980.

Ropper AH. Lateral displacement of the brain and level of consciousness in patients with an acute hemispheral mass. *N Engl J Med* 1986;314:953–958.

Merritt's Neurology, 10th ed., edited by L.P. Rowland. Lippincott Williams & Wilkins, Philadelphia © 2000.

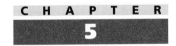

CHAPTER 5

DIAGNOSIS OF PAIN AND PARESTHESIAS

LEWIS P. ROWLAND

All pain sensations are carried by nerves and therefore concern neurology; however, not all pain is relevant to neurologic diagnosis. The pain of any traumatic lesion is a separate concern. Except for attacks of herpes zoster or diabetic radiculopathy, pain in the thorax or abdomen almost always implies a visceral disorder rather than one of the spinal cord or nerve roots. Headache and other head pains, in contrast, are a major neurologic concern (see Chapters 8 and 139). This chapter considers pain in the neck, low back, and limbs.

Pain syndromes often include another sensory aberration, *paresthesia,* a spontaneous and abnormal sensation. The problem may arise from an abnormality anywhere along the sensory pathway from the peripheral nerves to the sensory cortex. A paresthesia is often described as a *pins-and-needles sensation* and is recognizable by anyone who has ever had an injection of local anesthetic for dental repairs. Central nervous system disorders may cause particular kinds of paresthesias: focal sensory seizures with cortical lesions, spontaneous pain in the thalamic syndrome, or bursts of paresthesias down the back or into the arms on flexing the neck (*Lhermitte symptoms*) in patients with multiple sclerosis or other disorders of the cervical spinal cord. Level lesions of the spinal cord may cause either a band sensation or a girdle sensation, a vague sense of awareness of altered sensation encircling the abdomen, or there may be a *sensory level* (i.e., altered sensation below the level of the spinal cord lesion). Nerve root lesions or isolated peripheral nerve lesions may also cause paresthesias, but the most intense and annoying paresthesia encountered is due to multiple symmetric peripheral neuropathy (polyneuropathy). *Dysesthesia* is the term for the disagreeably abnormal sensations evoked when an area of abnormal sensation is touched; sometimes even the pressure of bedclothes cannot be tolerated by a patient with dysesthesia.

Beginning students are often confused by reports of paresthesias when the review of systems is recorded, or when they find abnormalities in the sensory examination that do not conform to normal anatomic patterns. Two general rules may help:

1. If paresthesias do not persist, they are likely to imply a neurologic lesion. (Pressure on a nerve commonly causes transient paresthesias in normal people who cross their legs, sit too long on a toilet seat, drape an arm over the back of a chair, or lean on one elbow while holding a newspaper in that hand. Many people have fleeting paresthesias of unknown cause and no significance.)
2. If paresthesias persist and the examiner fails to find a corresponding abnormality to explain it, the patient should be reexamined. Persistent paresthesias reliably imply an abnormality of sensory pathways.

NECK PAIN

Most chronic neck pain is caused by bony abnormalities (cervical osteoarthritis or other forms of arthritis) or by local trauma. If pain remains local (i.e., not radiating into the arms), it is rarely of neurologic significance unless there are abnormal neurologic signs. It may be possible to demonstrate overactive tendon reflexes, clonus, or Babinski signs in a patient who has no symptoms other than neck pain. These signs could be evidence of compression of the cervical spinal cord and might be an indication for cervical magnetic resonance imaging (MRI) or myelography to determine whether the offending lesion is some form of arthritis, tumor, or a congenital malformation of the cervical spine; however, neck pain is rarely encountered as the only symptom of a compressive lesion.

Neck pain of neurologic significance is more commonly accompanied by other symptoms and signs, depending on the location of the lesion: *Radicular* distribution of pain is denoted by radiation down the medial (ulnar) or lateral (radial) aspect of the arm, sometimes down to the corresponding fingers. Cutaneous sensation is altered within the area innervated by the compromised root, or below the level of spinal end compression. The motor disorder may be evident by weakness and wasting of hand muscles innervated by the affected root, and the gait may be abnormal if there are corticospinal signs of cervical spinal cord compression. When autonomic fibers in the spinal cord are compromised, abnormal urinary frequency, urgency, or incontinence may occur, there may be bowel symptoms, and men may note sexual dysfunction. Reflex changes may be noted by the loss of tendon reflexes in the arms and overactive reflexes in the legs. Cervical pain of neurologic significance may be affected by movement of the head and neck, and it may be exaggerated by natural Valsalva maneuvers in coughing, sneezing, or straining during bowel movements.

Cervical spondylosis is a more common cause of neck pain than is spinal cord tumor, but it is probably not possible to make the diagnostic distinction without MRI or myelography because the pain may be similar in the two conditions. In young patients (i.e., younger than 40 years), tumors, spinal arteriovenous malformations, and congenital anomalies of the cervicooccipital region are more common causes of neck pain than cervical spondylosis.

LOW BACK PAIN

The most common cause of low back pain is herniated nucleus pulposus, but it is difficult to determine the exact frequency because acute attacks usually clear spontaneously and chronic low back pain is colored by psychologic factors. The pain of an acute herniation of a lumbar disc is characteristically abrupt in onset and brought on by heavy lifting, twisting, or Valsalva maneuvers (sneezing, coughing, or straining during bowel movements). The patient may not be able to stand erect because paraspinal muscles contract so vigorously, yet the pain may be relieved as soon as the patient lies down, only to return again on any attempt to stand. The pain may be restricted to the low back or may radiate into one or both buttocks or down the posterior aspect of the leg to the thigh, knee, or foot. The distribution of pain sometimes gives a precise delineation of the nerve root involved, but this is probably true in only a minority of cases. The pain of an acute lumbar disc herniation is so stereotyped that the diagnosis can be made even if there are no reflex, motor, or sensory changes.

Chronic low back pain is a different matter. If neurologic abnormalities are present on examination, MRI or myelography is often indicated to determine whether the problem is caused by tumor, lumbar spondylosis with or without spinal stenosis, or arachnoiditis. If there are no neurologic abnormalities or if the patient has already had a laminectomy, chronic low back pain may pose a diagnostic and therapeutic dilemma. This major public health problem accounts for many of the patients who enroll in pain clinics.

ARM PAIN

Pain in the arms takes on a different significance when there is no neck pain. Local pain arises from musculoskeletal diseases (e.g., bursitis or arthritis), which are now common because of widespread participation in sports by people who are not properly prepared.

Chronic pain may arise from invasion of the brachial plexus by tumors that extend directly from lung or breast tissue or that metastasize from more remote areas. The brachial plexus may also be affected by a transient illness (e.g., *brachial plexus neuri-*

tis) that includes pain in the arm that is often poorly localized. The combination of pain, weakness, and wasting has given rise to the name *neuralgic amyotrophy*. (Amyotrophy is taken from Greek words meaning loss of nourishment to muscles; in practice, it implies the wasting of muscle that follows denervation.)

Thoracic outlet syndromes are another cause of arm pain that originates in the brachial plexus. The pain of a true thoracic outlet syndrome is usually brought on by particular positions of the arm and is a cause of diagnostic vexation because there may be no abnormality on examination (see Chapter 69). In a true thoracic outlet syndrome, the neurologic problems are often caused by compressed and distended blood vessels that in turn secondarily compress nerves or lead to ischemia of nerves.

Single nerves may be involved in *entrapment neuropathies* that cause pain in the hands. Carpal tunnel syndrome of the median nerve is the best known entrapment neuropathy. The ulnar nerve is most commonly affected at the elbow but may be subject to compression at the wrist. The paresthesias of entrapment neuropathies are restricted to the distribution of the affected nerve and differ from the paresthesias of areas innervated by nerve roots, although the distinction may be difficult to make if only a portion of the area supplied by a particular nerve root is affected.

Causalgia (see Chapter 70) is the name given to a constant burning pain accompanied by trophic changes that include red glossy skin, sweating in the affected area, and abnormalities of hair and nails. The trophic changes are attributed to an autonomic disorder. Causalgia was described in the 19th century in a monograph by Mitchell, Morehouse, and Keen when they reviewed gunshot wounds and other nerve injuries of American Civil War veterans. The basic mechanisms of causalgia are still poorly understood. The traumatic lesions of peripheral nerves are usually incomplete, and several nerves are often involved simultaneously. Causalgia usually follows high-velocity missile wound (bullets or shrapnel). It is less commonly caused by traction injury and is only rarely seen in inflammatory neuropathy or other types of peripheral nerve disease. The arms are more often involved than the legs, and the lesions are usually above the elbow or below the knee. Symptoms usually begin within the first few days following injury. Causalgic pain most often involves the hand. The shiny red skin, accompanied by fixed joints, is followed by osteoporosis. Both physical and emotional factors seem to play a role. Causalgia may be relieved by sympathectomy early in the course of treatment and may be due to *ephaptic transmission* through connections between efferent autonomic fibers at the site of partial nerve injury. This concept of "artificial synapses" after nerve injury has been widely accepted; however, there has been no convincing anatomic or physiologic corroboration.

Reflex sympathetic dystrophy refers to local tissue swelling and bony changes that accompany causalgia. Similar changes may be encountered after minor trauma or arthritis of the wrist. In the shoulder–hand syndrome, inflammatory arthritis of the shoulder joint may be followed by painful swelling of the hand, with local vascular changes, disuse, and atrophy of muscle and bone. Sympathectomy has been recommended.

A major problem in the management of causalgic syndromes is the lack of properly controlled comparison of placebo with sympathetic blockade, as well as the difficulty in evaluating psychogenic factors and the confusion caused by incomplete syndromes (with or without preceding trauma, with or without attendant vascular abnormalities, and with or without response to sympathetic block).

LEG PAIN AND PARESTHESIAS

Leg pain due to occlusive vascular disease, especially with diabetes, varies markedly in different series but seems to be related to the duration of the diabetes and shows increasing incidence with age. Pain may be a major symptom of diabetic peripheral neuropathy of the multiple symmetric type. Diabetic mononeuritis multiplex, attributed to infarcts of the lumbosacral plexus or a peripheral nerve, is a cause of more restricted pain, usually of abrupt onset. Diabetic mononeuropathy may be disabling and alarming at the onset, but both pain and motor findings improve in a few months to 1 or 2 years. Nutritional neuropathy is an important cause of limb pain, especially in the legs, in some parts of the world. This condition was striking in prisoner-of-war camps in World War II and has also been noted in patients on hemodialysis. Sudden fluid shifts may cause peripheral nerve disease symptoms for a time after dialysis.

Barring intraspinal disease, the most common neurologic cause of leg pain and paresthesias is probably multiple symmetric peripheral neuropathy. The paresthesias usually take on a glove-and-stocking distribution, presumably because the nerve fibers most remote from the perikaryon are most vulnerable. The feet are usually affected, sometimes alone or sometimes with the hands; the hands are rarely affected alone. Mixed sensorimotor neuropathies show motor abnormalities with weakness and wasting, as well as loss of tendon reflexes. Some neuropathies are purely sensory. Pain is characteristic of severe diabetic neuropathy, alcoholic neuropathy, amyloid neuropathy, and some carcinomatous neuropathies, but it is uncommon in inherited neuropathies or the Guillain-Barré syndrome. The pain of peripheral neuropathy, for unknown reasons, is likely to be more severe at night.

Entrapment neuropathy rarely affects the legs; however, diabetic mononeuropathy, especially femoral neuropathy, may cause pain of restricted distribution and abrupt onset, with later improvement of the condition that may take months.

Another major cause of leg pain is invasion of the lumbosacral plexus by tumor, but this is rarely an isolated event and other signs of the tumor are usually evident. The problem of distinguishing between spinal and vascular claudication is discussed in Chapter 67.

Limb pain and paresthesias are important in neurologic diagnosis not only because they persist for prolonged periods. They also become the object of symptomatic therapy by analgesics, tricyclic antidepressant drugs, and monoamine oxidase inhibitors (which may affect abnormal sensations by actions other than antidepressant effects), transcutaneous nerve stimulation, dorsal column stimulation, cordotomy, acupuncture, and other procedures. The long list of remedies attests to the limitations of each. Psychologic factors cannot be ignored in chronic pain problems.

SUGGESTED READINGS

Bowsher D. Neurogenic pain syndromes and their management. *Br Med Bull* 1991;19:644–646.

Chapman CR, Foley KM. *Current and emerging issues in cancer pain: research and practice.* New York: Raven Press, 1993.

Deyo RA, Rainville J, Kent DL. What can the history and physical examination tell us about low back pain? *JAMA* 1992;268:760–765.

Dotson RM. Causalgia—reflex sympathetic dystrophy—sympathetically maintained pain: myth and reality. *Muscle Nerve* 1993;16:1049–1055.

Fields HL, ed. *Pain syndromes in neurology.* London: Butterworth, 1990.

Fields HL. *Pain mechanisms and management.* New York: McGraw-Hill, 1999.

Frank A. Low back pain. *BMJ* 1993;306:901–909.

Frymoyer JW. Back pain and sciatica. *N Engl J Med* 1988;318:291–300.

Hanks GW, Justins DM. Cancer pain: management. *Lancet* 1992;339:1031–1036.

Haerer AF. *DeJong's the neurologic examination,* 3rd ed. Philadelphia: JB Lippincott Co, 1992.

Illis LS. Central pain: much can be offered from a methodical approach. *BMJ* 1993;300:1284–1286.

Livingston WK; Fields HL, ed. *Pain and suffering.* Seattle, WA: IASP Press, 1998.

Mitchell SW, Morehouse GR, Keen WW. *Gunshot wounds and other injuries of nerves.* Philadelphia: JB Lippincott, 1864.

Payne R, Patt RB, Hill S, eds. *Assessment and treatment of cancer pain.* Seattle, WA: IASP Press, 1998.

Pither CE. Treatment of persistent pain. *BMJ* 1989;299:1239–1240.

Schwartzman RJ, Maleki J. Postinjury neuropathic pain syndromes. *Med Clin North Am* 1999;83:597–626.

Wall PD, Melzack R, eds. *Textbook of pain,* 3rd ed. Edinburgh: Churchill Livingstone, 1994.

Woolf CJ, Mannion RJ. Neuropathic pain: aetiology, symptoms, mechanisms, and management. *Lancet* 1999;353:1959–1964.

Merritt's Neurology, 10th ed., edited by L.P. Rowland. Lippincott Williams & Wilkins, Philadelphia © 2000.

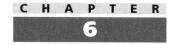

CHAPTER 6

DIZZINESS AND HEARING LOSS

JACK J. WAZEN

The peripheral auditory system is composed of the outer ear, the middle ear, the inner ear (cochlea and vestibular system), and the eighth cranial nerve. Lesions of these structures cause three major symptoms: hearing loss, vertigo, and tinnitus. Vertigo usually implies a lesion of the inner ear or the vestibular portion of the eighth nerve. Tinnitus and hearing loss may arise from lesions anywhere in the peripheral or central auditory pathways.

TINNITUS

Tinnitus is an auditory sensation that arises within the head and is perceived in one or both ears, or inside the head. The sound may be continuous, intermittent, or pulsatile. Tinnitus should be divided into *objective tinnitus,* heard by the examiner as well as the patient, or *subjective tinnitus,* heard only by the patient. Objective tinnitus is uncommon, but it is associated with several serious conditions that mandate early diagnosis.

Objective Tinnitus

This condition results from intravascular turbulence, increased blood flow, or movement in the eustachian tube, soft palate, or temporomandibular joint. Bruits due to vascular turbulence may arise from aortic stenosis, carotid stenosis, arteriovenous malformations of the head and neck, vascular tumors (e.g., glomus jugulare), or aneurysms of the abdomen, chest, head, or neck. A continuous hum may result from asymmetric enlargement of the sigmoid sinus and the jugular vein. Pulsatile objective tinnitus may result from high blood pressure, hyperthyroidism, or in-

creased intracranial pressure. As part of the diagnostic evaluation of objective tinnitus, the stethoscope should be used for auscultation of the ear, head, and neck in all patients who note noises in the head or ear. Anyone with pulsatile tinnitus should also have blood pressure and funduscopic evaluation.

Subjective Tinnitus

Unless of brief duration, subjective tinnitus results from damage or abnormality somewhere in the auditory system. The abnormality can be in the external ear, middle ear, inner ear, eighth cranial nerve, or central auditory connections. Tinnitus may be an early warning signal, such as pain arising from a lesion in or near a sensory peripheral nerve. For example, tinnitus after exposure to loud noise is due to cochlear injury, usually resulting in a temporary shift of the threshold in hearing sensitivity. Repeated exposure to noise may result in permanent cochlear damage and permanent hearing loss. Unilateral tinnitus is an early symptom of acoustic neuroma, often years before there is overt loss of hearing or unsteadiness of gait. Persistent tinnitus therefore requires otologic evaluation, including hearing tests. The basic hearing tests for evaluation of patients with tinnitus comprise pure tone and speech audiometry, as well as middle ear impedance measures, including tympanometry and measurement of the threshold and decay of the stapedial reflex. Auditory evoked potentials are often necessary, even in the absence of a significant difference in the hearing thresholds. Auditory evoked potentials, however, do not replace conventional audiometry and must be interpreted in light of the audiogram. These tests help localized the site of the lesion.

HEARING LOSS

Hearing loss can be divided into two anatomic types on the basis of the site of the lesion: conductive and sensorineural. Conductive hearing loss is due to middle ear disease. Sensorineural hearing loss is most often due to a lesion in the cochlea or the cochlear nerve. It rarely results from central auditory dysfunctions.

Conductive Hearing Loss

This type of hearing loss results from conditions in the external or middle ear that interfere with movement of the oval or round window. Patients with conductive hearing loss speak with a soft voice or with normal loudness because to them their own voices sound louder than background sounds in the environment. External ear or middle ear abnormalities are usually evident on physical examination, except when there is ossicular fixation (e.g., with otosclerosis), ossicular discontinuity from trauma, or erosion from chronic otitis media with or without cholesteatoma. In tuning-fork tests, best carried out with a 256- or 512-Hz tuning fork, sound conveyed by bone conduction is as loud as or louder than air conduction (negative Rinne test). In contrast, sound conveyed by air conduction is perceived as louder than bone conduction sound in patients with normal hearing or with sensorineural hearing loss. In conductive hearing loss, a tuning fork placed at midline of the forehead is heard louder in the ear on the side of the hearing loss (Weber test lateralizes to the abnormal side).

The diagnosis of conductive hearing loss can be confirmed by testing middle ear impedance, which measures the resistance of the middle ear to the passage of sound and can differentiate ossicular discontinuity from stiffness or mass effects that interfere with movement of the oval window. The severity of hearing loss and the conductive component should be assessed by audiometry, which determines sound conduction by air and bone. Conductive hearing loss most commonly affects children and is usually due to otitis media with effusion. Conductive hearing loss should be treated vigorously in children because persistent hearing loss, even if slight, may interfere with speech and cognitive development. Chronic forms of conductive hearing loss can usually be restored to functional levels of hearing by reconstructive microsurgery. Hearing aids are also effective in rehabilitating patients with conductive hearing loss.

Sensorineural Hearing Loss

This condition is due to defects in the cochlea, cochlear nerve, or the brainstem and cortical connections. Patients with sensorineural hearing loss tend to speak with a loud voice. Findings on physical examination are normal. Tuning-fork tests show that air conduction exceeds bone conduction (positive Rinne test); in the Weber test, the tuning fork seems louder in the better ear.

Patients with sensorineural hearing loss require a battery of audiometric tests to determine the site of the abnormality. Patients with cochlear damage may show low-frequency hearing loss, a flat audiometric configuration, or, more commonly, high-frequency hearing loss. The main causes are excessive exposure to noise, ototoxic drugs, age-related cochlear degeneration, congenital cochlear defects, and viral or bacterial infections. Speech discrimination remains relatively preserved, compared to the extent of pure-tone hearing loss. The stapedial reflex threshold, as determined by impedance measurements, is present at reduced sensation levels; that pattern implies *recruitment,* an abnormal increase in the subjective sensation of loudness as the amplitude of the test sounds increases above the threshold. Brainstem audi-

tory evoked responses show a delay in the first brainstem wave, but a normal or shortened interpeak latency.

Patients with damage to the cochlear nerve, such as the neural form of presbycusis or compression of the nerve by an acoustic neuroma, usually show high-frequency hearing loss, as do patients with cochlear lesions. In nerve lesions, however, speech discrimination tends to be more severely affected than pure-tone hearing loss. The stapedial reflex either is absent or shows abnormal adaptation or decay. The test is carried out as part of impedance audiometry and is useful in determining the site of the lesion. Stapedial reflex threshold and decay, along with tympanometry, must be considered part of the diagnostic workup for all patients with asymmetric sensorineural hearing loss. Brainstem auditory evoked response testing in neural forms of hearing loss shows no waves at all, poorly formed waves, or normal or increased interpeak latency, either absolute or in comparison with the opposite ear.

Central lesions, such as recurrent small strokes or multiple sclerosis, often cause no detectable pure-tone hearing loss because the central auditory pathways are bilateral. Some patients, however, do note hearing loss. For them, hearing should be evaluated by brainstem auditory evoked response testing, which may show bilateral conduction delay despite normal pure-tone hearing. Central auditory testing may show abnormalities.

Most patients with sensorineural hearing loss can be helped by amplification; hearing aids are becoming smaller and more effective. The narrow range between speech and noise is being ameliorated by improved microcircuitry. The latest in hearing aid technology, including digital and programmable devices, allows individuals to change the hearing aid parameters under different acoustical conditions for better hearing, particularly in noisy backgrounds. Patients with profound bilateral sensorineural hearing loss not responding to hearing aids may be candidates for a cochlear implant.

DIZZINESS

Complaints of dizziness must be separated into three different categories: vertigo, disequilibrium, and dizziness. *Vertigo* is a hallucination of movement involving the patient or the environment. Vertigo often implies a spinning sensation but may also be experienced as a feeling of swaying back and forth or falling. All such characteristics are most often related to a peripheral vestibular lesion. Vertigo of peripheral origin is usually episodic, with normal periods between spells. It is accompanied by horizontal or rotatory-horizontal nystagmus with nausea and vomiting. *Disequilibrium* or *ataxia* is a feeling of unsteadiness on walking. Patients may feel normal when they are stationary, but they notice difficulty in walking. Often, they have no symptoms of vertigo or dizziness. Disequilibrium suggests a central lesion. Patients with severe bilateral peripheral vestibular dysfunction may also note unsteady gait and oscillopsia, the symptom of nystagmus in which objects seem to be jumping from side to side or up and down while the patient is walking. *Dizziness* without spinning or disequilibrium is difficult for patients to describe. They mention light-headedness, sensations of swimming and floating, or giddiness. These symptoms have no localizing value and may be due to circulatory, metabolic, endocrine, degenerative, or psychologic factors. Peripheral vestibular and central lesions must be ruled out.

The sense of equilibrium and position in space is an integrated function of multiple peripheral sensory inputs into the brain, including the visual, vestibular, and proprioceptive systems. The vestibular system plays a dual role, responding to gravity and linear acceleration through the utricle and saccule, and to angular acceleration through the semicircular canals. If insufficient or conflicting information is presented to the central nervous system, different degrees of dizziness result. Spinning vertigo, associated with nystagmus, nausea, and vomiting and aggravated by head and body movement, suggests a peripheral vestibular lesion, especially if it is episodic and recurrent. Other symptoms suggesting a peripheral origin of these symptoms are accompanying hearing loss or tinnitus.

COMMON CAUSES OF DIZZINESS AND HEARING LOSS

Benign Positional Paroxysmal Vertigo

This condition is characterized by recurrent momentary episodes of vertigo that are brought on by changing head position, mainly with extension of the neck, by rolling over in bed from side to side, by rising from bed, or by bending down. The vertigo starts after a latency of a few seconds after the stimulating position is assumed. Vertigo builds to a peak before it subsides, usually lasting less than 1 minute. It is associated with rotatory nystagmus, beating toward the floor if the patient is lying down with the head turned toward the offending ear. As the patient sits up or turns to a neutral position, a few beats of nystagmus are experienced, with the rapid phase toward the opposite side. These symptoms can be reproduced in the office by positional testing. The patient is asked to lie down quickly from a sitting position, with the head extended and turned all the way to one side. Benign paroxysmal vertigo is fatigable. Repeating the positional test abolishes the response.

Known causes of the syndrome include head trauma, labyrinthitis, and aging. Histologic sections of temporal bones from affected patients have shown otoconia in the posterior semicircular canal ampulla. These calcium carbonate crystals are normally found in the utricle and the saccule; they are thought to have been dislodged into the posterior canal and consequently to stimulate the vertigo, thus the term *cupulolithiasis*.

The natural history of benign positional vertigo is spontaneous resolution. Most patients are free of symptoms within a few weeks or months. Symptoms can be abolished by a variety of positioning exercises, the most successful and frequently performed being the Epley maneuver. Labyrinthine suppressants, such as meclizine hydrochloride (Antivert) and diazepam, may reduce the intensity of the vertigo. Avoiding the offending position is highly effective in avoiding the symptoms. If disabling positional vertigo persists for more than 1 year despite multiple maneuvers and conservative medical management, section of the posterior ampullary nerve (singular neurectomy) through a middle ear approach often abolishes the vertigo while preserving hearing. Another highly successful procedure is obliteration of the posterior semicircular canal through a transmastoid approach. Hearing and the remainder of the vestibular function are preserved through either procedure.

The syndrome must be differentiated from other positional vertigo conditions (Table 6.1). Otologic evaluation with audiologic and vestibular testing may be necessary for final diagnosis.

Vestibular Neuronitis

In this condition, vertigo occurs suddenly and severely with vomiting and nystagmus; it may last several days. There are no cochlear symptoms, and audiologic tests are normal. Caloric tests show a reduced response on the affected side. The patient may feel unsteady for several weeks after an attack. Recurring attacks usually seem less severe than the first and may continue for several months. The syndrome results from a sudden loss of function of one vestibular system; it is analogous to sudden loss of hearing. Vestibular neuronitis may follow an overt viral illness. In most cases, however, the cause is unknown. A brief course of vestibular suppressants followed by encouragement of physical activity may shorten the duration of disability by enhancing vestibular compensation.

Meniere Syndrome

This illness is characterized by recurrent attacks of tinnitus, hearing loss, and vertigo accompanied by a sense of pressure in the ear, distortion of sounds, and sensitivity to noise. All the symptoms may not occur at the same time in the same spell. Hearing loss or vertigo may even be absent for several years. Symptoms occur in clusters with variable periods of remission that may last for several years. Major attacks of vertigo with nausea and vomiting last from a few minutes to many hours and may force ces-

TABLE 6.1. DIFFERENTIATION BETWEEN PERIPHERAL AND CENTRAL PAROXYSMAL POSITIONAL NYSTAGMUS

	Appearance	Latency	Duration (sec)	Fatigability	Mechanism	Localization
Peripheral	Torsional upbeat disconjugate	Usual	<30	Usual	Change in cupula specific gravity	Labyrinth
Central	Conjugate, pure horizontal or vertical	Unusual	>30	Unusual	Damage to central otolithocular pathways	Brainstem or cerebellum

From Baloh and Honrubia, 1990, with permission.

sation of all usual activities. Minor spells are characterized by unsteadiness, giddiness, or light-headedness. Hearing loss begins as a low-frequency cochlear type of hearing loss that improves between attacks. In severe cases, hearing loss becomes slowly progressive and persistent, with a flat configuration on the audiogram. Symptoms are usually unilateral but become bilateral in 20% to 30% of patients with long-term follow-up. The pathogenesis is unknown.

A typical histopathologic feature of Meniere syndrome, *endolymphatic hydrops,* consists of an increase in the endolymphatic fluid pressure and volume with ballooning of the cochlear duct, utricle, and saccule. As in other conditions characterized by increased extracellular fluid volume, symptoms are aggravated by salt-loading and may be helped by reducing dietary intake of salt or by giving diuretics. In the few patients who are incapacitated by major spells of vertigo, ablative surgery is used through either a labyrinthectomy, when there is no useful hearing, or a vestibular nerve section that spares the cochlear nerve in patients with serviceable hearing. Endolymphatic sac decompression and shunt are another commonly performed procedure when hearing preservation is desired. However, the long-term success rates in vertigo control are better with vestibular neurectomy.

Meniere syndrome must be separated from congenital or tertiary syphilis, which also causes endolymphatic hydrops, vertigo, and hearing loss. In syphilis, hearing loss is progressive and usually bilateral. Cogan syndrome also resembles Meniere syndrome with endolymphatic hydrops, hearing loss, and vertigo. In Cogan syndrome, in addition, ocular inflammation occurs without evidence of syphilis. Cogan syndrome is thought to be an autoimmune condition, which may also be true of Meniere syndrome.

Perilymphatic Fistula

Hearing loss with or without vertigo may follow sudden changes of pressure in the middle ear or cerebrospinal fluid that may be due to weight lifting, barotrauma from scuba diving or flying, or even forceful coughing or nose blowing. Perilymphatic fistula may arise spontaneously, especially in children with congenital defects of the inner ear. Stapedectomy also increases the risk for perilymphatic fistula. Surgery to patch the fistula may be necessary in selected patients to stop progression of the symptoms.

Cerebellopontine Angle Tumors

The most common tumor involving the cerebellopontine angle is the acoustic neuroma (schwannoma). By the time loss of corneal reflex, cerebellar signs, gross nystagmus, and facial weakness are seen, the tumor is large. Because the earliest symptoms are tinnitus, hearing loss, and dizziness, this tumor must always be considered in the evaluation of a patient with any of these symptoms. Early diagnosis is particularly important because improvement in microsurgical techniques has made possible complete removal of the tumor without damaging the facial nerve, and even preservation of useful hearing if the tumor is small. "Dizziness" is rarely true vertigo and does not occur in recurrent attacks; rather, there is a persistent sense of unsteadiness or light-

headedness. All patients with tinnitus, hearing loss, or dizziness must have audiometric testing, including impedance testing with stapedial reflex evaluation. If the initial evaluation suggests a neural site of hearing loss, then electronystagmography with a caloric test and a brainstem auditory evoked response test should be carried out. Magnetic resonance imaging with gadolinium enhancement is the definitive test in the diagnosis of acoustic neuroma.

Drug Toxicity

Salicylates, aminoglycoside antibiotics, furosemide (Lasix), anticonvulsants, and alcohol can cause dizziness in the form of vertigo, disequilibrium, and light-headedness. Tinnitus and hearing loss may also occur. These symptoms are bilateral and are often accompanied by ataxic gait, as they variously affect the vestibular and cochlear apparatuses. Sedatives (e.g., diazepam, phenobarbital), antihistamines, mood elevators, and antidepressants can also cause light-headedness and disequilibrium. Recent intake of possibly toxic drugs should be reviewed with any patient complaining of "dizziness." Cessation of use of a drug usually causes clearing of the symptoms in a few days, although vestibular and cochlear damage due to aminoglycosides and other ototoxic drugs can result in permanent ataxia or hearing loss.

Craniocerebral Injuries

Loss of hearing, tinnitus, and vertigo (often postural) can be sequelae of head injury. Hearing loss may be due to a fracture in the middle ear ossicles or the cochlea. Vertigo may be due to concussion or hemorrhage into the labyrinth or a perilymphatic fistula. Postural vertigo may be a nonspecific reaction to concussion and part of the postconcussion syndrome, or may be secondary to posttraumatic cupulolithiasis and benign paroxysmal vertigo.

Cardiac Arrhythmia

Cardiac arrhythmias sufficient to lower cardiac output can cause dizziness. The patient may not notice palpitations. If a cardiac arrhythmia is suspected, 24- to 48-hour continuous electrocardiograph monitoring (Holter monitor) may help establish the relationship of arrhythmias to episodes of dizziness.

End-organ Degeneration

With the increase in life expectancy, many patients now reach ages at which degenerative losses cause disequilibrium. Past a certain age (which is different for each patient), there is an almost linear decline in the numbers of hair cells in the cochlea and of nerve fibers in the vestibular nerve; deterioration of other sensory systems (i.e., visual, proprioceptive, exteroceptive, and auditory) and of the ability to integrate information from those sensory systems causes disequilibrium in older patients. Older patients also lose cerebral adaptive functions and cannot compensate for the loss of sensory function.

Psychophysiologic Causes of Vertigo: Hyperventilation

Acute anxiety attacks or panic attacks can cause vertigo. It is not always easy to differentiate psychophysiologic cause and effect because vertigo can sometimes trigger acute anxiety or panic attacks. The history usually includes a period of external stress, fear of blacking out, fear of dying, shortness of breath, palpitations, tingling or weakness in the hands, mouth, or legs, and frequent or daily occurrence. Whirling vertigo is uncommon. These spells are often induced by hyperventilation. Asking the patient to hyperventilate for 2 minutes will evoke the typical symptoms. Patients with anxiety, depression, and panic attacks may respond to specific therapy and the appropriate psychopharmacologic agents.

Other Causes of Dizziness

Dizziness may be a secondary effect of a variety of disorders, including the following:

Migraine (vertebrobasilar type)
Multiple sclerosis
Neurosyphilis
Cervical spondylosis
Sensory deprivation (e.g., polyneuropathy, visual impairment)
Vertebrobasilar insufficiency (e.g., transient ischemic attack, infarction)
Cerebellar hemorrhage
Anemia
Orthostatic hypotension
Intralabyrinthine hemorrhage (e.g., leukemia, trauma)
Carotid sinus syncope
Diabetes mellitus
Hypoglycemia

TAKING THE HISTORY

The first step in taking the patient's history is to determine whether the patient is suffering from vertigo, disequilibrium, light-headedness, motor incoordination, seizure, syncope, or a combination of these. It is necessary to determine the time of onset, temporal pattern, associated symptoms, and factors that seem to precipitate, aggravate, or relieve symptoms. If there are episodes, the sequence of events needs to be known, including activities at onset, possible aura, quality, severity, sequence of symptoms, and the patient's response during the attack. Does the patient have to sit or lie down? Is consciousness lost? Can someone communicate with the patient during an attack? What other symptoms occur? After an attack, how does the patient feel? Can the patient remember the events that occurred during an attack? Can the patient function normally following an attack? These considerations suggest specific questions that must be asked in taking the history. The following list contains examples of the kinds of specific questions that should be put to the patient:

1. Is the dizziness precipitated by head movement? (Benign positional vertigo is characteristically precipitated by head movement, but orthostatic hypotension causes dizziness on rising from sitting or lying. Neck movements may precipitate dizziness in cervical osteoarthritis or muscle spasm. Head turning may precipitate dizziness with carotid sinus syncope if the patient is wearing a tight collar.)
2. If there is vertigo, is it rotational? Does the patient have a veering gait or an unsteady stance with nausea, perspiration, and tachycardia? In which direction does the vertigo occur?
3. Are cochlear and vestibular symptoms associated? (This pattern would suggest a peripheral lesion affecting both portions of the inner ear or eighth cranial nerve.)
4. Has there been recent head trauma?
5. Are there other neurologic symptoms, such as visual changes, paralysis, sensory alterations, altered consciousness, or headaches? (These symptoms might suggest a more generalized neurologic disorder in which dizziness and hearing loss are only a part.)
6. Is there numbness in the hands and feet, visual impairment, or a history of diabetes or anemia? (Sensory loss in the elderly or chronically debilitated patient can lead to environmental disorientation that is interpreted as dizziness.)
7. Are there cardiac symptoms (e.g., tachycardia, palpitation, or angina) that suggest a cardiac disorder?
8. Are there psychiatric symptoms (e.g., thought disorders, delusions, hallucinations, bizarre behavior, or depression) that suggest dizziness of a psychic nature? Do symptoms of anxiety suggest possible hyperventilation?
9. Transient ischemic attacks may cause recurrent dizziness. Inquiry should include questions about other recurrent symptoms of vertebrobasilar ischemia, as well as risk factors (e.g., hypertension and cardiovascular disease).
10. Is there a familial history of dizziness or hearing loss?

CONCLUSION

Diagnosing dizziness, disequilibrium, or vertigo can be a challenging task. The differential diagnosis is spread across medical specialties and may require multiple consultations. If symptoms are persistent, neurologic and neurootologic evaluations are indicated. An accurate clinical history, appropriate examinations, and tests of audiologic and vestibular systems are needed for accurate diagnosis and effective treatment.

SUGGESTED READINGS

Baloh RW, Honrubia V. *Clinical neurophysiology of the vestibular system,* 2nd ed. Contemporary Neurology Series. Philadelphia: FA Davis Co, 1990.

Barber HO. Current ideas on vestibular diagnosis. *Otolaryngol Clin North Am* 1978;11:283–300.

Coles RRA, Hallan RS. Tinnitus and its management. *Br Med Bull* 1987;43:983–998.

Dobie RA, Berlin CI. Influence of otitis media on hearing and development. *Ann Otol Rhinol Laryngol* 1979;88:48–56.

Drachman DA, Hart CW. A new approach to the dizzy patient. *Neurology* 1972;22:323–334.

Gacek RR. Transection of the posterior ampullary nerve for the relief of benign paroxysmal positional vertigo. *Ann Otol Rhinol Laryngol* 1974;83:596–605.

Grundfast KM, Bluestone CD. Sudden or fluctuating hearing loss and vertigo in children due to perilymph fistula. *Ann Otol Rhinol Laryngol* 1978;87:761–779.

Lambert PR. Evaluation of the dizzy patient. *Compr Ther* 1997;23:719–723.

Schuknecht HF. Cupulolithiasis. *Arch Otolaryngol* 1969;90:113–126.

Schuknecht HF. *Pathology of the ear*, 2nd ed. Philadelphia: Lea & Febiger, 1994.

Shulman A. Neuroprotective drug therapy: a medical and pharmacological treatment for tinnitus control. *Int Tinnitus J* 1997;3:77–93.

Merritt's Neurology, 10th ed., edited by L.P. Rowland. Lippincott Williams & Wilkins, Philadelphia © 2000.

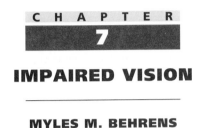

CHAPTER 7

IMPAIRED VISION

MYLES M. BEHRENS

Impaired vision may be due to a lesion within the eyes, in the retrobulbar visual pathway (including the optic nerve and optic chiasm), or in the retrochiasmal pathway. The retrochiasmal pathway includes the optic tract, geniculate body (where synapse occurs), the visual radiation through the parietal and temporal lobes, and the occipital cortex. The pattern of visual loss may identify the site of the lesion. The course and accompanying symptoms and signs may clarify its nature.

OCULAR LESIONS

Impaired vision of ocular origin may be caused by refractive error, opacity of the ocular media (which may be seen by external inspection or ophthalmoscopy), or a retinal abnormality (e.g., retinal detachment, inflammation, hemorrhage, vascular occlusion). There may be associated local symptoms or signs, such as pain or soft tissue swelling.

OPTIC NERVE LESIONS

A visual defect may originate in the optic nerve, particularly if the symptoms affect only one eye. The hallmarks of optic nerve dysfunction include blurred vision (indicated by decreased visual acuity), dimming or darkening of vision (usually with decreased color perception), and decreased pupillary reaction to light. This pupillary sign is not seen if the problem is media opacity, minor retinal edema, or nonorganic visual loss. It may be present to a mild degree in simple amblyopia.

The *relative afferent pupillary defect* results from an optic nerve lesion in one eye; the sign is best shown by the swinging-flashlight test. A bright flashlight is swung from one eye to the other just below the visual axis while the subject stares at a distant object in a dark room. Constriction of the pupils should be the same when either eye is illuminated. However, if an eye

with optic nerve dysfunction is illuminated, the pupils constrict less quickly in response to the light, less completely, and less persistently than when the normal fellow eye is illuminated. If the expected constriction does not occur or if the pupils actually dilate after an initial constriction on stimulation of one eye, the test is positive. Both pupils are equal in size at all times in purely afferent defects because there is hemidecussation of all afferent light input to the midbrain with equal efferent stimulation through both third cranial nerves. Therefore, if one pupil is fixed to light because of an efferent defect, the other one can be observed throughout the performance of this test.

The patient may be aware of, or the examiner may find, a *scotoma* (blind spot) in the visual field. This is often central or centrocecal (because the lesion affects the papillomacular bundle that contains the central fibers of the optic nerves), or altitudinal (because arcuate or nerve-fiber-bundle abnormalities respect the nasal horizontal line, corresponding to the separation of upper and lower nerve-fiber bundles by the horizontal raphe in the temporal portion of the retina). These abnormalities are often evident on confrontation tests of the visual fields.

In a central scotoma of retinal origin (e.g., due to macular edema affecting photoreceptors), the patient may report that lines seem to be distorted *(metamorphopsia)* or objects may seem small *(micropsia)*. Recovery of visual acuity may be delayed (e.g., in comparison to a normal fellow eye) after photostress, such as a flashlight stimulus for 10 seconds.

Bilateral optic nerve abnormalities, in particular those with centrocecal scotomas (Fig. 7.1A), suggest a hereditary, toxic, nutritional, or demyelinating disorder; unilateral optic nerve disease is usually ischemic, inflammatory, or compressive. The course and associated symptoms and signs help differentiate these possibilities.

Optic nerve infarction (anterior ischemic optic neuropathy) usually affects patients older than 50 years. The visual defect is usually primarily altitudinal, occasionally centrocecal, sudden in onset, and stable (occasionally progressive during the initial weeks). There is pallid swelling of the optic disc with adjacent superficial hemorrhages. The swelling resolves in 4 to 6 weeks, leaving optic atrophy and arteriolar narrowing on the disc (Fig. 7.2). The cause may be arteritis (giant cell or temporal arteritis, often with associated symptoms and signs) but is usually idiopathic, painless, and only rarely associated with carotid occlusive disease. In the idiopathic nonarteritic variety, the discs are characteristically crowded, with small,

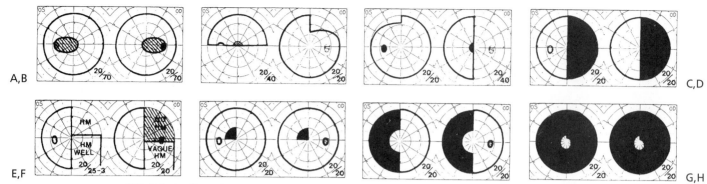

FIG. 7.1. A: Bilateral centrocecal scotoma. **B:** Inferior altitudinal defect with central scotoma O.S. (left eye) and upper temporal hemianopic (junctional) defect O.D. (right eye). **C:** Bitemporal hemianopia. **D:** Total right homonymous hemianopia. **E:** Incongruous right homonymous hemianopia. **F:** Congruous left homonymous hemianopic scotoma. **G:** Left homonymous hemianopia with macular sparing. **H:** Bilateral congruous homonymous hemianopia.

if any, physiologic cup, thus suggesting structural susceptibility. The fellow eye is often similarly affected after months or years.

Optic neuritis usually affects young adults. It typically begins with a central or centrocecal scotoma and subacute progression of the defect that is followed by a gradual resolution; there may be residual optic atrophy. Initially, the disc may be normal (retrobulbar neuritis) or swollen (papillitis). Local tenderness or pain on movement of the eye is usually present and suggests such an intraorbital inflammatory disorder. The *Pulfrich phenomenon* is a stereo illusion that may be caused by delayed conduction in one optic nerve, making it difficult to localize moving objects. This is not specific and may occur with retinal abnormality or media defect. The *Uhthoff symptom* is an exacerbation of a symptom after exercise or exposure to heat; it is not specific but occurs most often in demyelinating disorders. If in a case suggesting op-

tic neuritis there is evidence of preexisting optic atrophy in either eye or optic neuropathy in the fellow eye (e.g., if the degree of relative afferent pupillary defect is less than anticipated, suggesting subclinical involvement of the other eye), demyelinating disease is also suggested.

In *compressive optic neuropathy,* there is usually steady progression of visual defect, although it may be stepwise or even remitting. The disc may remain relatively normal in appearance for months before primary optic atrophy is indicated funduscopically by decrease in color of the disc, visible fine vessels on the disc, and peripapillary nerve fibers (best seen with a bright ophthalmoscope with red-free light). This form of optic atrophy must be distinguished from other specific types (e.g., glaucoma, in which the nerve head has an excavated or cupped appearance; postpapilledema [secondary] atrophy with narrowing and sheathing of vessels and often indistinct mar-

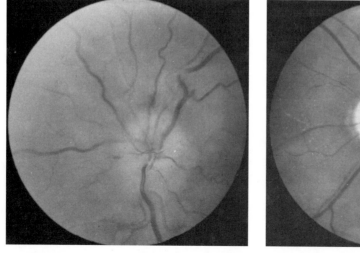
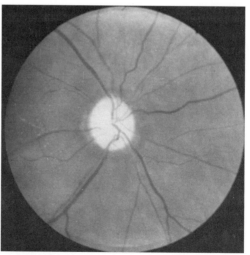

FIG. 7.2. A: Pallid swelling of the disc with superficial hemorrhages in a patient with acute anterior ischemic optic neuropathy. **B:** Optic atrophy with arteriolar narrowing after anterior ischemic optic neuropathy.

gins; retinal pigmentary degeneration with narrowed vessels, which may also be seen after central retinal artery occlusion or optic nerve infarction; and congenital defects, such as coloboma or hypoplasia of the disc, with a small nerve head and a peripapillary halo that corresponds to the expected normal size of the disc).

LESIONS OF THE OPTIC CHIASM

In a patient with optic neuropathy, recognition of an upper temporal hemianopic visual-field defect (which may be asymptomatic) in the other eye is evidence of a chiasmal lesion that affects the anteriorly crossing lower fibers (see Fig. 7.1B). In contrast to optic nerve lesions, the majority of chiasmal lesions are compressive. The typical visual-field defect is bitemporal hemianopia (see Fig. 7.1C). Because the macular fibers permeate the chiasm, any compressive lesion of the chiasm with a visual-field defect is accompanied by temporal hemianopic dimming of red objects of any size in a pattern that respects the vertical line and permits secure confrontation testing.

RETROCHIASMAL LESIONS

Homonymous hemianopia results from a retrochiasmal lesion. There may be varying awareness of the defect. It may be mistakenly attributed to the eye on the side of the defect, or the patient may be aware only of bumping into things on that side or of trouble reading (slowness and difficulty seeing the next word with right homonymous hemianopia, or difficulty finding the next line with left hemianopia). The patient may ignore that side of the visual acuity test chart that corresponds to the hemianopia, but can see 20/20 unless there is another defect (see Fig. 7.1D).

With subtotal lesions, the congruity of the visual-field defect in the two eyes helps in localization. Optic tract and geniculate lesions tend to have grossly incongruous visual-field defects (see Fig. 7.1E). The farther posterior that the lesion is, the more congruous is the defect because the fibers from corresponding retinal loci in the two eyes converge on the same occipital locus.

With optic tract lesions anterior to the geniculate synapse, *optic atrophy* may develop. The eye with a temporal field defect develops a bow-tie pattern of atrophy, which may also occur with chiasmal lesions. The nasal portion of the disc is pale due to loss of the nasal fibers; the usual mild temporal pallor is more evident due to loss of the nasal half of the papillomacular bundle. An imaginary vertical line through the macula corresponds to the vertical line that separates the nasal and temporal halves of the visual field. There is a relatively pink appearance above and below where fibers from the temporal retina reach the disc.

With optic tract lesions, afferent pupillary input is impaired. When the lesion is grossly incongruous, a relative afferent pupillary defect may occur on the side with the greater deficit. It is found in the eye with temporal hemianopia when homonymous hemianopia is total, because the temporal half-field is more extensive than the nasal half-field. The *Wernicke hemianopic pupillary phenomenon* may be difficult to elicit: Pupillary constriction is more vigorous when the unaffected portion of the retina is stimulated. When an optic tract lesion is close to and encroaches on the chiasm, visual acuity in the ipsilateral eye diminishes. There may be a relative afferent pupillary defect on that side, as well.

Retrogeniculate lesions are not accompanied by clinical impairment of pupillary reactivity or optic atrophy. The homonymous hemianopic visual-field defect tends to be superior when the temporal lobe radiations are affected, and the defect is denser below if the lesion is parietal. Occipital lesions result in precisely congruous defects, often scotomas with preserved peripheral vision (see Fig. 7.1F). If the scotoma is large enough, the area of preserved peripheral vision may be present only in the eye with the loss of temporal field (a preserved temporal crescent). This corresponds to the most anterior portion of the occipital cortex. The central portion of the visual field is represented in the posterior striate cortex, a marginal perfusion zone of both posterior and middle cerebral arteries. When the posterior cerebral artery is occluded, collateral supply from the middle cerebral artery may allow gross *macular sparing* (see Fig. 7.1G), preserving central vision. Homonymous hemianopia of occipital origin is often total. Isolated homonymous hemianopia is due to an infarct in 90% of patients. *Cerebral blindness* (bilateral homonymous hemianopia [see Fig. 7.1H]) may require distinction from hysterical blindness; opticokinetic nystagmus (OKN) can be elicited in psychogenic disorders, but not after bilateral occipital lesions when they are complete.

Irritative visual phenomena include formed visual hallucinations (usually of temporal lobe origin) and unformed hallucinations (usually of occipital origin), including the *scintillating homonymous scotoma* of migraine. *Amaurosis fugax* of one eye is occasionally due to vasospasm in migraine but is usually due to ophthalmic-carotid hypoperfusion or embolization, or cardiogenic emboli. Formed or unformed hallucinations may be release phenomena when there is visual loss due to a lesion anywhere along the visual pathway. *Phosphenes* (light flashes) may occur in several kinds of optic nerve lesions, including demyelinating optic neuritis, or they may occur with movement of the eye. Vitreoretinal traction is a frequent and nonsinister cause of light flashes, especially with advancing age, although a retinal tear premonitory to retinal detachment may occur and must be ruled out.

IMPAIRMENT OF OCULAR MOTILITY

Impairment of ocular motility is often a clue to diagnosis in many neurologic disorders. It may reflect a supra-, inter-, or infranuclear (fascicular or peripheral nerve) neurogenic lesion, neuromuscular transmission defect, myopathy, or mechanical restriction in the orbit. *Diplopia* (double vision) indicates malalignment of the visual axes if it is relieved by occlusion of either eye. Diplopia of monocular origin is psychogenic or due to a disturbance of the refractive media in the eye (e.g., astigmatism or opacity of the cornea or lens). Malalignment of the visual axes may occur in psychogenic convergence spasm (suggested by associated miosis due to the near response), in decompensation of strabismus (including convergence insufficiency, usually of no pathologic import), and, less frequently, in divergence insufficiency (possibly due to bilateral sixth cranial nerve paresis, occasionally caused by increased intracranial pressure). The diplopia and malalignment of the visual axes in these cases are usually commitant, that is, equal in all directions of gaze. If strabismus begins in early childhood, there may be habitual suppression of the image of one eye, with impaired development of vision in that eye (*amblyopia*) rather than diplopia.

Incommitance, or inequality in the alignment of the visual axes in the direction of gaze, suggests limitation of action of one or more muscles. The deviation is generally greater if the paretic eye is fixing. The patient may use one eye or adopt a head-turn or tilt to avoid diplopia (e.g., turning to the right when the right lateral rectus is limited, or tilting to the left if the right superior oblique is affected, to avoid the need for the intortional effect of that muscle). The patient may not be aware of either the diplopia or these adaptations.

To determine which muscle is impaired, the examiner obtains information from the history and examination (including use of a red glass). It is important to know whether the diplopia is vertical or horizontal, whether it is crossed (if the visual axes are divergent) or uncrossed (if convergent), whether greater near (if adducting muscles are involved) or at a distance (if abducting muscles are involved), and the direction of gaze in which the diplopia is maximal.

If the pattern of motility limitation conforms to muscles innervated by a single nerve, the lesion probably affects that nerve. With a third cranial nerve palsy, there is ptosis, limitation of action of the medial, inferior, and superior rectus muscles and of the inferior oblique muscle; that is, all the extraocular muscles are affected except the lateral rectus (sixth cranial nerve) and superior oblique (fourth cranial nerve). *Internal ophthalmoplegia* (i.e., pupillary enlargement with defective constriction and defective accommodation) may be evident. When the ptotic lid is lifted, the eye is abducted (unless the sixth cranial nerve is also affected), and on attempted downward gaze the globe can be seen to intort (by the observation of nasal episcleral vessels) if the fourth cranial nerve is intact. If more than one of these nerves is affected, the lesion is probably in the cavernous sinus, superior orbital fissure, or orbital apex. There may also be fifth cranial nerve (ophthalmic division) and oculosympathetic defect (*Horner syndrome*). The latter is indicated by relative miosis, mild ptosis, and incomplete and delayed dilation of the pupil. Such involvement is usually due to tumor, aneurysm, or inflammation, whereas isolated involvement of one of the ocular motor nerves may be ischemic.

Mechanical limitation of ocular motility may occur with orbital lesions, such as thyroid ophthalmopathy, orbital fracture, or tumor. It is indicated by limitation on forced duction, such as an attempt to rotate the globe with forceps (traction test), or by elevation of intraocular pressure on the attempted movement with relatively intact velocity *saccades* (i.e., rapid eye movements). Other symptoms or signs of orbital lesions include proptosis (or enophthalmos in the case of fracture) beyond acceptable normal asymmetry of 2 mm, resistance to retropulsion, vascular congestion, tenderness, and eyelid abnormality other than ptosis (e.g., retraction, lid-lag, swelling).

Myasthenia gravis (see Chapter 120) is suggested when affected muscles do not conform to the distribution of a single

nerve (although they may) and when symptoms vary, including diurnal fluctuation and fatigability. A demonstrable increase in paresis or a slowing of saccades may occur after sustained gaze or repetitive movement. Ptosis may similarly increase after sustained upward gaze (or lessen after rest in sustained eye closure) or a momentary lid twitch may be seen on return of gaze from downward to straight ahead. There is no clinical abnormality of the pupils in myasthenia gravis.

Analysis of saccadic function is of particular value in the analysis of supra- and internuclear ocular motility defects. The supranuclear control mechanisms of ocular movements include the *saccadic system* of rapid conjugate eye movement of contralateral frontal lobe origin to achieve foveal fixation on a target (a combination of *pulse,* burst discharge in agonist with total inhibition of antagonist, and *step,* increased level of agonist and decreased level of antagonist discharge to maintain the new eccentric position); the *pursuit system* of slow conjugate movement of ipsilateral occipital lobe origin to maintain foveal fixation on a slowly moving target; the *vestibular system* of slow conjugate movement to maintain stability of the retinal image if the head moves in relation to the environment; and the *vergence system* of dysconjugate slow movement to maintain alignment of the visual axes for binocular single vision. *OKN* is the normal response to a sequence of objects moving slowly across the field of vision and can be considered a combination of pursuit and refixation saccades (to allow continuous pursuit, because vision is suppressed during the saccadic phase).

The polysynaptic saccadic pathway crosses at the level of the fourth cranial nerve nucleus to enter the *pontine paramedian reticular formation* (PPRF), where ipsilateral saccades and other horizontal movements are generated by stimulation of neurons in the sixth cranial nerve nucleus and also interneurons therein that travel up the opposite *medial longitudinal fasciculus* (MLF) to stimulate the contralateral subnucleus for the medial rectus in the third cranial nerve nucleus to assure normal conjugate gaze. Pathways for vertical movement seem to require bilateral stimuli. The immediate supranuclear apparatus for generating vertical gaze is in the midbrain, the rostral interstitial nucleus of the MLF.

General dysfunction of saccades (with limitation, slowing, or hypometria) is seen in several disorders, including Huntington disease (see Chapter 108), hereditary cerebellar degeneration (see Chapter 107), progressive supranuclear palsy (see Chapter 115), and Wilson disease (see Chapter 89). *Congenital ocular motor apraxia* is a benign abnormality of horizontal saccades that resolves with maturity. Infants with this abnormality are unable to perform horizontal saccades and substitute characteristic head thrusts past the object of regard, achieving fixation by the contraversive vestibular doll's-head movement and then maintaining it while slowly rotating the head back. Focal dysfunction of saccades is manifested by lateral gaze paresis after contralateral frontal or ipsilateral pontine lesions; vestibular stimuli may overcome frontal gaze palsies but do not affect pontine lesions.

Internuclear ophthalmoplegia is the result of a lesion in the MLF that interrupts adduction in conjugate gaze (but convergence may be intact). Abduction nystagmus is seen in the contralateral eye. When the defect is partial, adducting saccades are slow, with resultant dissociation of nystagmus again more marked in the abducting eye, as when OKN is elicited. When the lesion is unilateral, an ischemic lesion is likely; a bilateral syndrome suggests multiple sclerosis. Vertical gaze-evoked nystagmus and *skew deviation* (one eye higher than the other) may be seen. The latter is a supranuclear vertical divergence of the eyes, seen with brainstem or cerebellar lesions.

A unilateral pontine lesion that involves both the MLF and PPRF causes the combination of ipsilateral gaze palsy and internuclear ophthalmoplegia on contralateral gaze, a pattern called the *1 1/2 syndrome*. The only remaining horizontal movement is abduction of the contralateral eye. The eyes are straight or exodeviated (if there is gaze preference away from the side of the gaze palsy). Superimposed esodeviation with related diplopia may occur if there is sixth cranial nerve (fascicular) involvement, as well.

Vertical gaze disorders are seen with midbrain lesions (the *sylvian aqueduct syndrome*). Characteristic dyssynergia on attempted upward saccades is best demonstrated by downward moving OKN stimuli: Failure of inhibition leads to cofiring of oculomotor neurons with convergence-retraction nystagmus and related fleetingly blurred vision or diplopia. This may also occur, to a lesser extent, with horizontal saccades, causing excessive adductor discharge and "pseudo sixth cranial nerve paresis." There is usually pupillary sluggishness in response to light (often with light-near dissociation) due to interruption of the periaqueductal afferent light input to the third cranial nerve nuclei. Concomitant abnormalities may include lid retraction (*Collier sign*), defective or excess accommodation or convergence, and skew deviation or monocular elevator palsy.

Oscillopsia is a sensation of illusory movement of the environment that is unidirectional or oscillatory; it is seen with acquired nystagmus of various types. *Nystagmus* is an involuntary rhythmic oscillation of the eyes, generally conjugate and of equal amplitude but occasionally dysconjugate (as in the sylvian aqueduct syndrome) or dissociated in amplitude (as in internuclear ophthalmoplegia). The oscillations may be pendular or jerk in type; the latter is more common in acquired pathologic nystagmus. In jerk nystagmus, the slow phase is operative and the fast phase is a recovery movement. The amplitude usually increases on gaze in the direction of the fast phase.

Horizontal and upward gaze-evoked nystagmus may be due to sedative or anticonvulsant drugs. Otherwise, *vertical nystagmus* indicates posterior fossa disease. Extreme end-gaze physiologic nystagmus, which may be of greater amplitude in the abducting eye, must be distinguished. It occurs only horizontally. *Jerk nystagmus* in the primary position, or rotatory nystagmus, usually indicates a vestibular disorder that may be either central or peripheral. In a destructive peripheral lesion, the fast phase is away from the lesion; the same pattern is seen with a cold stimulus when the horizontal canals are oriented vertically (i.e., with the head elevated 30 degrees in the supine position). *Downbeating nystagmus* in the primary position, often more marked on lateral gaze to either side, frequently indicates a lesion at the cervicomedullary junction. *Ocular bobbing* is usually associated with total horizontal pontine gaze palsy; it is not rhythmic, is coarser than nystagmus, may vary in amplitude, and is occasionally asymmetric; the initial movement is downward with a slower return. *Upbeating nystagmus* in the primary position may indicate a lesion of the cerebellar vermis or medulla but most commonly the pons. *Seesaw nystagmus* is vertically dysconjugate with a rotatory element, so that there is intortion of the elevating eye and simultaneous extortion of the falling eye. This pattern is often seen with parachiasmal lesions and is probably a form of alternating skew deviation due to involvement of vertical and tortional oculomotor control regions around the third ventricle. *Periodic alternating nystagmus* implies a nonsinister lesion of the lower brainstem; in effect, it is a gaze-evoked nystagmus to either side of a null point that cycles back and forth horizontally. In the primary position, there is nystagmus of periodically alternating direction. *Rebound nystagmus,* which may be confused with periodic alternating nystagmus, is a horizontal jerk nystagmus that is transiently present in the primary position after sustained gaze to the opposite side; it implies dysfunction of the cerebellar system.

Other ocular oscillations that follow cerebellar system lesions include *ocular dysmetria* (overshoot or terminal oscillation of saccades), *ocular flutter* (bursts of similar horizontal oscillation, actually back-to-back saccades without usual latency), *opsoclonus* (chaotic multidirectional conjugate saccades), and *fixation instability* (square-wave jerks), in which small saccades interrupt fixation, with movement of the eye away from the primary position and then its return after appropriate latency for a saccade. *Ocular myoclonus* is a rhythmic ocular oscillation that often is vertical and associated with synchronous palatal myoclonus.

When oscillopsia is monocular, there may be dissociated pathologic nystagmus of posterior fossa origin, including the jellylike, primarily vertical, pendular nystagmus akin to myoclonus that is occasionally seen in multiple sclerosis. There may be benign myokymia of the superior oblique muscle, in which the patient is often aware of both a sensation of ocular movement and oscillopsia. Monocular nystagmus may also result from monocular visual loss in early childhood or from the insignificant and transient acquired entity of *spasmus nutans,* which is of uncertain etiology. It begins after 4 months of age and disappears within a few years. The nystagmus of spasmus nutans is asymmetric and rapid and may be accompanied by head nodding. It may be similar to congenital nystagmus. The latter begins at birth, persists, and is usually horizontal, either gaze-evoked or pendular, often with jerks to the sides, and there may be a null with head turn adopted for maximal visual acuity. It originates in a motor disorder, although it may be mimicked by the nystagmus of early binocular visual deprivation.

SUGGESTED READINGS

Behrens MM. *Neuro-ophthalmic motility disorders.* American Academy of Ophthalmology and Otolaryngology CETV videotape, 1975;1(5).

Burde RM, Savino PJ, Trobe JD. *Clinical decisions in neuro-ophthalmology,* 2nd ed. St. Louis, MO: CV Mosby, 1992.

Glaser JS. *Neuro-ophthalmology,* 2nd ed. Philadelphia: JB Lippincott Co, 1990.

Leigh RJ, Zee DS. *The neurology of eye movements,* 2nd ed. Philadelphia: FA Davis Co, 1991.

Miller NR, Newman NJ. The essentials. *Walsh and Hoyt's clinical neuro-ophthalmology,* 5th ed. Baltimore: Lippincott Williams & Wilkins, 1998.

Miller NR, Newman NJ, eds. *Walsh and Hoyt's clinical neuro-ophthalmology,* 5th ed, vols 1–5. Baltimore: Lippincott Williams & Wilkins, 1998.

Merritt's Neurology, 10th ed., edited by L.P. Rowland. Lippincott Williams & Wilkins, Philadelphia © 2000.

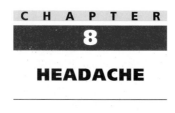

HEADACHE

NEIL H. RASKIN

Nearly everyone is subject to headache from time to time; moreover, 40% of persons experience severe headaches annually. The mechanism generating headaches may be activated by worry and anxiety, but emotional stress is not necessary for the symptom to appear. Genetic factors may augment this system, so that some people are susceptible to more frequent or more severe head pain. The term *migraine* is increasingly being used to refer to a mechanism of this kind, in contradistinction to prior usage of the term as an aggregation of certain symptoms. Thus, stress-related or *tension* headaches, perhaps the most common syndrome reported by patients, is an example of the expression of this mechanism when it is provoked by an adequate stimulus; it may also be activated in some people by the drinking of red wine, by exposure to glare or pungent odors, or premenstrually.

Headache is usually a benign symptom and only occasionally is a manifestation of a serious illness, such as brain tumor or giant cell arteritis. The first issue to resolve in the care of a patient with headache is to make the distinction between benign and more ominous causes. If the data supporting a benign process are strong enough, as reviewed in this chapter, neuroimaging can be deferred. If a benign diagnosis cannot be made, magnetic resonance imaging is a better choice than computed tomography (CT) for visualizing the posterior fossa; posterior fossa tumors are far more likely than forebrain tumors to cause headache as the only symptom. Moreover, the Arnold-Chiari malformation, an important structural cause of headache, cannot be visualized with CT.

GENERAL PRINCIPLES

The quality, location, duration, and time course of the headache and the conditions that produce, exacerbate, or relieve it should be elicited.

Most headaches are dull, deeply located, and aching in quality. Superimposed on such nondescript pain may be other elements that have greater diagnostic value; for example, jabbing, brief, sharp pain, often occurring multifocally (*ice-picklike* pain), is the signature of a benign disorder. A throbbing quality and tight muscles about the head, neck, and shoulder girdle are common nonspecific accompaniments of headache that suggest that intra- and extracranial arteries and skeletal muscles of the head and neck are activated by a generic mechanism that generates head pain. Tight, pressing "hat-band" headaches were once believed to indicate anxiety or depression, but studies have not supported this view.

Pain *intensity* seldom has diagnostic value, nor does response to placebo medication provide any useful information. Administration of placebo simply identifies placebo responders, a group that includes about 30% of the population. No evidence reveals that placebo responders have lower pain levels than nonresponders or that they do not really have pain. Patients entering emergency departments with the most severe headache of their lives usually have migraine. Meningitis, subarachnoid hemorrhage, and cluster headache also produce intense cranial pain. Contrary to common belief, the headache produced by a brain tumor is not usually severe.

Data regarding headache *location* is occasionally informative. If the source is an extracranial structure, as in giant cell arteritis, correspondence with the site of pain is fairly precise. Inflammation of an extracranial artery causes scalp pain and extensive tenderness localized to the site of the vessel. Posterior fossa lesions cause pain that is usually occipitonuchal, and supratentorial lesions most often induce frontotemporal pain. *Multifocality* alone is a strong indicator of benignity.

Time-intensity considerations are particularly useful. A ruptured aneurysm results in head pain that peaks in an instant, *thunderclap*-like manner; much less often, unruptured aneurysms may similarly signal their presence. *Cluster headache* attacks peak over 3 to 5 minutes, remain at maximal intensity for about 45 minutes, and then taper off. Migraine attacks build up over hours, are maintained for several hours to days, and are characteristically relieved by sleep. Sleep disruption is characteristic of headaches produced by brain tumors.

The relationship of a headache to certain biologic events or to physical environmental changes is essential information for triage of patients. The following exacerbating phenomena have high probability value in asserting that a headache syndrome is benign: provocation by red wine, sustained exertion, pungent odors, hunger, lack of sleep, weather change, or menses. The association of diarrhea with attacks is pathognomonic of a benign disorder (migraine). Cessation or amelioration of headache during pregnancy, especially in the second and third trimesters, is similarly pathognomonic. Patients with continuous benign headache often observe a pain-free interlude of several minutes on waking before the head pain begins once again. This phenomenon, wherein the cessation of sleep seems to unleash the headache mechanism, also occurs with other centrally mediated pain syndromes, such as thalamic pain, but does not occur among patients with somatic disease as the cause of pain.

A history of amenorrhea or galactorrhea leads to the possibility that the polycystic ovary syndrome or a prolactin-secreting pituitary adenoma is the source of headache (Table 8.1). Headache arising *de novo* in a patient with a known malignancy suggests either cerebral metastasis or carcinomatous meningitis. When the accentuation of pain is striking with eye movement, a systemic infection, particularly meningitis, should be considered. Head pain appearing abruptly after bending, lifting, or coughing can be a clue to a posterior fossa mass or the Arnold-Chiari malformation. Orthostatic headache arises after lumbar puncture and also occurs with subdural hematoma and benign intracranial hypertension. The eye itself is seldom the cause of acute orbital pain if the sclerae are white and noninjected; red eyes are a sign of ophthalmic disease. Similarly, acute sinusitis

TABLE 8.1. STUDIES PERFORMED TO INVESTIGATE CHRONIC HEADACHE

Erythrocyte sedimentation rate
Antinuclear antibody titer
Thyroid microsomal antibody titer
Cardiolipin antibody titer
Serum prolactin level
Lumbar puncture (pressure, malignant cells)
Neuroimaging
Muscle biopsy (mitochondrial disorders, arteritis)
Temporal artery biopsy

nearly always declares itself through a dark green, purulent nasal exudate.

The analysis of facial pain requires a different approach. Trigeminal and glossopharyngeal neuralgias are common causes of facial pain, especially the trigeminal syndrome. *Neuralgias* are painful disorders characterized by paroxysmal, fleeting, often electric shocklike episodes; these conditions are caused by demyelinative lesions of nerves (the trigeminal or glossopharyngeal nerves in cranial neuralgia) that activate a pain-generating mechanism in the brainstem. *Trigger* maneuvers characteristically provoke paroxysms of pain. However, the most common cause of facial pain by far is dental; provocation by hot, cold, or sweet foods is typical. Application of a cold stimulus repeatedly induces dental pain, whereas in neuralgic disorders a refractory period usually occurs after the initial response so that pain cannot be induced repeatedly. The presence of refractory periods nearly always can be elicited in the history, thereby saving the patient from a painful experience.

Mealtimes offer the physician an opportunity to gain needed insight into the mechanism of a patient's facial pain. Does chewing, swallowing, or the taste of a food elicit pain? Chewing points to trigeminal neuralgia, temporomandibular joint dysfunction, or giant cell arteritis (*jaw claudication*), whereas the combination of swallowing *and* taste provocation points to glossopharyngeal neuralgia. Pain on swallowing is common among patients with *carotidynia* (facial migraine), because the inflamed, tender carotid artery abuts the esophagus during deglutition.

As in other painful conditions, many patients with facial pain do not describe stereotypic syndromes. These patients have sometimes had their syndromes categorized as "atypical facial pain," as though this were a well-defined clinical entity. Only scant evidence shows that nondescript facial pain is caused by emotional distress, as is sometimes alleged. Vague, poorly localized, continuous facial pain is *characteristic* of the condition that may result from nasopharyngeal carcinoma and other somatic diseases; a burning painful element often supervenes as deafferentation occurs and evidence of cranial neuropathy appears. Occasionally, the cause of a pain problem cannot be promptly resolved, thus necessitating periodic follow-up examinations until further clues appear (and they usually do). *Facial pain of unknown cause* is a more reasonable tentative diagnosis than "atypical facial pain."

PAIN-SENSITIVE STRUCTURES OF THE HEAD

The most common type of pain results from activation of peripheral nociceptors in the presence of a normally functioning nervous system, as in the pain resulting from scalded skin or appendicitis. Another type of pain results from injury to or activation of the peripheral or central nervous system. Headache, formerly believed to originate peripherally, may originate from either mechanism. Headache may arise from dysfunction or displacement of, or encroachment on, pain-sensitive cranial structures. The following are sensitive to mechanical stimulation: the scalp and aponeurosis, middle meningeal artery, dural sinuses, falx cerebri, and the proximal segments of the large pial arteries. The ventricular ependyma, choroid plexus, pial veins, and much of the brain parenchyma are insensitive to pain. On the other hand, electrical stimulation near midbrain dorsal raphe cells may result in migrainelike headaches. Thus, most of the brain is insensitive to electrode probing, but a particular midbrain site is nevertheless a putative locus for headache generation.

Sensory stimuli from the head are conveyed to the brain by the trigeminal nerves from structures above the tentorium in the anterior and middle fossae of the skull. The first three cervical nerves carry stimuli from the posterior fossa and infradural structures. The ninth and tenth cranial nerves supply part of the posterior fossa and refer pain to the ear and throat.

Headache can occur as the result of the following:

1. Distention, traction, or dilation of intracranial or extracranial arteries,
2. Traction or displacement of large intracranial veins or their dural envelope,
3. Compression, traction, or inflammation of cranial and spinal nerves,
4. Spasm, inflammation, and trauma to cranial and cervical muscles,
5. Meningeal irritation and raised intracranial pressure,
6. Perturbation of intracerebral serotonergic projections.

By and large, intracranial masses cause headache when they deform, displace, or exert traction on vessels, dural structures, or cranial nerves at the base of the brain; these changes often happen long before intracranial pressure rises. Such mechanical displacement mechanisms do not explain headaches resulting from cerebral ischemia, benign intracranial hypertension after reduction of the pressure, or febrile illnesses and systemic lupus erythematosus. Impaired central inhibition as a result of perturbation of intracerebral serotonergic projections has been posited as a possible mechanism for these phenomena.

APPROACH TO THE PATIENT WITH HEADACHE

Entirely different diagnostic possibilities are raised by the patient who has the first severe headache ever and the one who has had recurrent headaches for many years. The probability of finding a potentially serious cause is considerably greater in patients with their first severe headache than in those with chronic recurrent headaches. Acute causes include meningitis, subarachnoid hemorrhage, epidural or subdural hematoma, glaucoma, and purulent sinusitis. In general, acute, severe headache with stiff neck and fever means meningitis, and without fever means subarachnoid hemorrhage; when the physician is confronted with such a patient, lumbar puncture is mandatory. Acute, persistent headache and fever are often manifestations of an acute systemic viral infection; if the neck is supple, lumbar puncture may be deferred. A first attack of migraine is always a possibility, but fever is a rare associated feature. Nearly all illnesses have been an occasional cause of headache; however, some illnesses are *characteristically* associated with headache. These include infectious mononucleosis, systemic lupus erythematosus, chronic pulmonary failure with hypercapnia (early morning headaches), Hashimoto thyroiditis, corticosteroid withdrawal, oral contraceptives, ovulation-promoting agents, inflammatory bowel disease, many illnesses associated with human immunodeficiency virus infection, and acute blood pressure elevation that occurs in pheochromocytoma and malignant hypertension. Pheochromocytoma and malignant hypertension are the exceptions to the generalization that hypertension *per se* is an uncommon cause of headache; a diastolic pressure of at least 120 mm Hg is requisite for hypertension to cause headache.

Adolescents with chronic daily frontal or holocephalic headache pose a special problem. Extensive diagnostic tests, including psychiatric assessment, are most often unrevealing. Fortunately, the headaches tend to stop after a few years, so that structured analgesic support can enable these teenagers to move through secondary school and enter college. By the time they reach their late teens, the cycle has usually ended.

The relationship of head pain to depression is not straightforward. Many patients in chronic daily pain cycles become depressed (a reasonable sequence of events); moreover, there is a greater-than-chance coincidence of migraine with both bipolar (manic-depressive) and unipolar depressive disorders. Studies of large populations of depressed patients do not reveal headache prevalence rates that are different from those in the general population. The physician should be cautious about assigning depression as the cause of recurring headache; drugs with antidepressant action are also effective in migraine.

Finally, note must be made of recurring headaches that may be pain-driven. As an example, *temporomandibular joint (TMJ) dysfunction* generally produces preauricular pain that is associated with chewing food. The pain may radiate to the head but is not easily confused with headache *per se.* Conversely, headache-prone patients may observe that headaches are more frequent and severe in the presence of a painful TMJ problem. Similarly, headache disorders may be activated by the pain attending otologic or endodontic surgical procedures. Treatment of such headaches is largely ineffectual until the cause of the primary pain is treated. Thus, pain about the head as a result of somatic disease or trauma may reawaken an otherwise quiescent migrainous mechanism.

SUGGESTED READINGS

Day JW, Raskin NH. Thunderclap headache: symptom of unruptured cerebral aneurysm. *Lancet* 1986;2:1247–1248.

Lance JW, Goadsby PJ. *Mechanism and management of headache,* 6th ed. London: Butterworth, 1998.

Raskin NH. On the origin of head pain. *Headache* 1988;28:254–257.

Raskin NH. *Headache,* 2nd ed. New York: Churchill Livingstone, 1988.

Rasmussen BK, Olesen J. Symptomatic and nonsymptomatic headaches in a general population. *Neurology* 1992;42:1225–1231.

Merritt's Neurology, 10th ed., edited by L.P. Rowland. Lippincott Williams & Wilkins, Philadelphia © 2000.

C H A P T E R
9

INVOLUNTARY MOVEMENTS

STANLEY FAHN

Although convulsions, fasciculations, and myokymia are involuntary movements, these disorders have special characteristics and are not classified with the types of abnormal involuntary movements described in this chapter. The disorders commonly called abnormal involuntary movements, or *dyskinesias,* are usually evident when a patient is at rest, are frequently increased by action, and disappear during sleep. There are exceptions to these generalizations. For example, palatal myoclonus may persist during sleep, and mild torsion dystonia may be present only during active voluntary movements (action dystonia), but not when the patient is at rest. The known dyskinesias are distinguished mainly by visual inspection of the patient. Electromyography can occasionally be helpful by determining the rate, rhythmicity, and synchrony of involuntary movements. Sometimes, patients have a dyskinesia that bridges the definitions of more than one disorder; this leads to compound terms such as choreoathetosis, which describes features of both chorea and athetosis.

Most abnormal involuntary movements are continual or easily evoked, but some are intermittent or paroxysmal, such as tics, the *paroxysmal dyskinesias,* and *episodic ataxias.* Gross movements of joints are highly visible, unlike the restricted muscle twitching of fasciculation or myokymia.

Tremors are rhythmic oscillatory movements. They result from alternating contractions of opposing muscle groups (e.g., parkinsonian tremor at rest) or from simultaneous contractions of agonist and antagonist muscles (e.g., essential tremor). A useful way to clinically differentiate tremor to aid in diagnosis is to determine whether the tremor is present under the following conditions: when the affected body part is at rest, as in parkinsonian disorders of the extrapyramidal system; when posture is maintained (e.g., with arms outstretched in front of the body), as in essential tremor (see Chapter 113); when action is undertaken (e.g., writing or pouring water from a cup), as in essential tremor, which increases with action; or when intention is present (e.g., finger-to-nose maneuver), as in cerebellar disease (see Chapter 107).

The term *myoclonus* (see Chapter 110) refers to shocklike movements due to contractions or inhibitions (negative myoclonus). *Chorea* delineates brief, irregular contractions that, although rapid, are not as lightninglike as myoclonic jerks. In classic choreic disorders, such as Huntington disease (see Chapter 108) and Sydenham chorea (see Chapter 109), the jerks affect individual muscles as random events that seem to flow from one muscle to another. They are not repetitive or rhythmic. *Ballism* is a form of chorea in which the choreic jerks are of large amplitude, producing flinging movements of the affected limbs. Chorea is presumably related to disorders of the caudate nucleus but sometimes involves other structures. Ballism is related to lesions of the subthalamic nucleus.

Dystonia (see Chapter 112) is a syndrome of sustained muscle contraction that frequently causes twisting and repetitive movements or abnormal postures. Dystonia is represented by (1) sustained contractions of both agonist and antagonist muscles, (2) an increase of these involuntary contractions when voluntary movement in other body parts is attempted ("overflow"), (3) rhythmic interruptions (*dystonic tremor*) of these involuntary, sustained contractions when the patient attempts to oppose them, (4) inappropriate or opposing contractions during specific voluntary motor actions (*action dystonia*), and (5) torsion spasms that may be as rapid as chorea but differ because the movements are continual and of a twisting nature in contrast to the random and seemingly flowing movements of chorea. Torsion spasms may be misdiagnosed as chorea; the other characteristics frequently lead to the misdiagnosis of a conversion reaction.

Tics are patterned sequences of coordinated movements that appear suddenly and intermittently. The movements are occasionally simple and resemble a myoclonic jerk, but they are usually complex, ranging from head shaking, eye blinking, sniffing, and shoulder shrugging to complex facial distortions, arm waving, touching parts of the body, jumping movements, or making obscene gestures (*copropraxia*). Most often, tics are rapid and brief, but occasionally they can be sustained motor contractions (i.e., dystonic). In addition to motor tics, vocalizations may be a manifestation of tics. These range from sounds, such as barking, throat-clearing, or squealing, to verbalization, including the utterance of obscenities (*coprolalia*) and the repetitions of one's own sounds (*palilalia*) or the sounds of others (*echolalia*). Motor and vocal tics are the essential features of Tourette syndrome (see Chapter 111).

One feature of tics is the compelling need felt by the patient to make the motor or phonic tic, with the result that the tic movement brings relief from unpleasant sensations that develop in the involved body part. Tics can be voluntarily controlled for brief intervals, but such a conscious effort is usually followed by more intense and frequent contractions. The milder the disorder is, the more control the patient can exert. Tics can sometimes be suppressed in public. The spectrum of severity and persistence of tics is wide. Sometimes, tics are temporary, and sometimes they are permanent.

Many persons develop personalized mannerisms. These physiologic tics may persist after repeated performances of motor habits and have therefore been called *habit spasms.* As a result, unfortunately, all tics have been considered by some physicians as habit spasms of psychic origin. Today, however, the trend is to consider pathologic tics a neurologic disorder.

Stereotypic movements (*stereotypies*) can resemble tics, but these are usually encountered in persons with mental retardation, autism, or schizophrenia. However, bursts of stereotypic shaking movements, especially of the arms, can be encountered in otherwise normal children. Stereotypic movements are also encountered in the syndrome of drug-induced tardive dyskinesia (see Chapter 116) and refer to repetitive movements that most often affect the mouth; in *orobuccolingual dyskinesia,* there are constant chewing movements of the jaw, writhing and protrusion movements of the tongue, and puckering movements of the mouth. Other parts of the body may also be involved.

Athetosis is a continuous, slow, writhing movement of the limbs (distal and proximal), trunk, head, face, or tongue. When these movements are brief, they merge with chorea (*choreoathetosis*). When the movements are sustained at the peak of the contractions, they merge with dystonia, and the term *athetotic dystonia* can be applied.

Akathitic movements are those of restlessness. They commonly accompany the subjective symptom of *akathisia,* an inner feeling of motor restlessness or the need to move. Today, akathisia is most commonly seen as a side effect of antipsychotic drug therapy, either as acute akathisia or tardive akathisia, which often accompanies tardive dyskinesia. Akathitic movements (e.g., crossing and uncrossing the legs, caressing the scalp or face, pacing the floor, and squirming in a chair) can also be a reaction to stress, anxiety, boredom, or impatience; it can then be termed *physiologic* akathisia. Pathologic akathisia, in addition to that induced by antipsychotic drugs, can be seen in the encephalopathies of confusional states, in some dementias and in Parkinson disease. Picking at the bedclothes is a common manifestation of akathitic movements in bedridden patients.

Two other neurologic conditions in which there are subjective feelings of the need to move are *tics* and the *restless legs syndrome.* The latter is characterized by formication in the legs, particularly in the evening when the patient is relaxing and sitting or lying down and attempting to fall asleep. These sensations of ants crawling under the skin disappear when the patient walks around. This disorder is not understood but may respond to opioids, levodopa, and dopamine agonists.

Continued muscle stiffness due to continuous muscle firing can be the result of neuromyotonia, encephalomyelitis with rigidity and myoclonus (spinal interneuronitis), the stiff limb syndrome, and the stiff person syndrome (see Chapter 129). The last tends to involve axial and proximal limb muscles.

Paroxysmal movement disorders are syndromes in which the abnormal involuntary movements appear for brief periods out of a background of normal movement patterns. They can be divided into four distinct groups: (1) the *paroxysmal dyskinesias,* (2) *paroxysmal hypnogenic dyskinesias,* (3) *episodic ataxias,* and (4) *hy-*

perekplexias. The molecular genetics of the episodic ataxias implicate abnormalities of membrane ionic channels as underlying mechanisms for the paroxysmal movement disorders.

Three types of paroxysmal dyskinesias are recognized (Table 9.1). All three consist of bouts of any combination of dystonic postures, chorea, athetosis, and ballism. They can be unilateral, always on one side or on either side, or bilateral. Unilateral episodes can be followed by a bilateral one. The attacks can be severe enough to cause a patient to fall down. Speech is often affected, with inability to speak due to dystonia, but there is never any alteration of consciousness. Very often, patients report variable sensations at the beginning of the paroxysms. *Paroxysmal kinesigenic dyskinesia* is the easiest to recognize. Attacks are very brief, usually lasting seconds, and always less than 5 minutes. They are induced by sudden movements, startle, or hyperventilation, and can occur many times a day; they respond to anticonvulsants. The primary forms of paroxysmal dyskinesias are inherited in an autosomal-dominant pattern, but secondary causes are common, particularly multiple sclerosis. Attacks of *paroxysmal nonkinesigenic dyskinesia* last minutes to hours, sometimes longer than a day. Usually, they range from 5 minutes to 4 hours. They are primed by consuming alcohol, coffee, or tea, as well as by psychologic stress, excitement, and fatigue. There are usually no more than three attacks per day, and often attacks may be months apart. No consistent response to therapeutic interventions is yet available. This form can sometimes be the major presentation of a psychogenic movement disorder. *Paroxysmal exertional dyskinesia* is triggered by prolonged exercise; attacks last from 5 to 30 minutes.

Paroxysmal hypnogenic dyskinesias are divided into short- and long-duration attacks. Short-duration attacks are often the result of supplementary sensorimotor seizures that occur during sleep. Three types of episodic ataxias have been distinguished (Table 9.2). *Hyperekplexia* (excessive startle syndrome) consists of dramatic complex motor responses to a sudden tactile or verbal stimulus. Echolalia and echopraxia are sometimes seen. The syndrome was originally described with local names, such as jumping Frenchmen of Maine, Myriachit, and Latah. Hyperekplexia can be hereditary (glycine receptor on chromosome 5q) or sporadic. When it is severe, the patient's movements must be curtailed because a sudden attack can lead to injury from falling.

Although most of the involuntary movements described are the result of central nervous system disorders, particularly in the basal ganglia, some dyskinesias arise from the brainstem, spinal cord, or peripheral nervous system. Dyskinesias attributed to peripheral disorders are hemifacial spasm (see Chapter 68), painful legs–moving toes, jumpy stumps, belly-dancer's dyskinesia, and the sustained muscle contractions seen in reflex sympathetic dystrophy (see Chapter 70). Psychogenic movement disorders seem to be increasingly more common. Usually, they appear with a mixture of different types of movements, particularly shaking, paroxysmal disorders, fixed postures, or bizarre gaits. Careful evaluation for inconsistency, incongruity, false weakness or sensory changes, sudden onset, deliberate slowness, and the appearance of marked fatigue and exhaustion from the "involuntary" movements helps suggest the diagnosis, which is best established by relief of the signs and symptoms using psychotherapy, suggestion, and physiotherapy.

TABLE 9.1. CLINICAL FEATURES OF PAROXYSMAL KINESIGENIC (PKD), NONKINESIGENIC (PNKD), AND EXERTIONAL DYSKINESIA (PED)

Feature	PKD	PNKD	PED
Male:female	4:1	1.4:1	10:12 (n=22)
Inheritance	Autosomal dominant	Autosomal dominant	Autosomal dominant
Genetic mapping	?	Mount-Reback syndrome (2q33-35) with diplopia and spasticity chromosome 1p	?
Age at onset (yr)	<1–40	<1–30	2–30
Range	12	12	11.5
Median	12	12	12
Mean			
Attack	<5 min	2 m in to 4h	5 min to 2 hr
Duration	100/d to 1/mo	3/d to 2/yr	1/d to 2/mo
Frequency			
Trigger	Sudden movement, startle, hyperventilation	Nil	Prolonged exercise
Movement pattern	Any combination of dystonic postures, chorea, athetosis, and ballism; unilateral or bilateral		
Precipitant	Stress	Ethanol, stress, caffeine, fatigue	Stress
Treatment	Anticonvulsants	Clonazepam, benzodiazepines, acetazolamide, antimuscarinics	Acetazolamide, antimuscarinics, benzodiazepines

TABLE 9.2. CLINICAL AND GENETIC FEATURES OF EPISODIC ATAXIAS

Type	Age at Onset (yr)	Clinical	Acetazolamide Response	Precipitant	Frequency/ Duration	Interictal	Gene
Myokymia, neuromyotonia (EA-1)	2–15	Aura of weightlessness or weakness, then ataxia, dysarthria, tremor, facial twitching	In some kindreds, anticonvulsants may help	Startle, movement, exercise, excitement, fatigue	Up to 15/d; usually ≤1/d; seconds to minutes, usually 2–10 min	Myokymia, shortened Achilles tendon; PKD	12p13, K$^+$ channel, different point mutations in KCNA1
Vestibular (EA-2)	0–40, usually 5–15	Ataxia, vertigo, nystagmus, dysarthria, headache, ptosis, ocular palsy, vermis atrophy	Very effective	Stress, alcohol, fatigue, exercise, caffeine	Daily to every 2 mo; usually hours; 5 min to weeks	Nystagmus, mild ataxia; less common: dysarthria and progressive cerebellar	19p13, Ca$^+$ channel, CACNL1A4 familial hemiplegic migraine?
Ocular	20–50	Ataxia, diplopia, vertigo, nausea	No response	Sudden change in head position	Daily to yearly; minutes to hours	Symptoms gradually become constant	Unknown

SUGGESTED READINGS

Baloh RW, Yue Q, Furman JM, Nelson SF. Familial episodic ataxia: clinical heterogeneity in four families linked to chromosome 19p. *Ann Neurol* 1997;41:8–16.

Bhatia KP, Bhatt MH, Marsden CD. The causalgia-dystonia syndrome. *Brain* 1993;116:843–851.

Brown P. Physiology of startle phenomena. In: Fahn S, Hallett M, Luders HO, Marsden CD, eds. *Negative motor phenomena.* Advances in Neurology, vol 67. Philadelphia: Lippincott–Raven Publishers, 1995:273–287.

Dressler D, Thompson PD, Gledhill RF, Marsden CD. The syndrome of painful legs and moving toes: a review. *Mov Disord* 1994;9:13–21.

Fahn S. Motor and vocal tics. In: Kurlan R, ed. *Handbook of Tourette's syndrome and related tic and behavioral disorders.* New York: Marcel Dekker, 1993:3–16.

Fahn S. Paroxysmal dyskinesias. In: Marsden CD, Fahn S, eds: *Movement disorders*, 3rd ed. Oxford: Butterworth-Heinemann, 1994;310–345.

Fahn S. Psychogenic movement disorders. In: Marsden CD, Fahn S, eds. *Movement disorders*, 3rd ed. London: Butterworth, 1994:358–372.

Iliceto G, Thompson PD, Day BL, et al. Diaphragmatic flutter, the moving umbilicus syndrome, and belly dancers' dyskinesia. *Mov Disord* 1990;5:15–22.

Kulisevsky J, Marti-Fabregas J, Grau JM. Spasms of amputation stumps. *J Neurol Neurosurg Psychiatry* 1992;55:626–627.

Marsden CD, Fahn S, eds. *Movement disorders.* London: Butterworth, 1982.

Marsden CD, Fahn S, eds. *Movement disorders*, 2nd ed. London: Butterworth, 1987.

Marsden CD, Fahn S, eds. *Movement disorders*, 3rd ed. London: Butterworth, 1994.

Tan A, Salgado M, Fahn S. The characterization and outcome of stereotypic movements in nonautistic children. *Mov Disord* 1997;12:47–52.

Walters AS, Wagner ML, Hening WA, et al. Successful treatment of the idiopathic restless legs syndrome in a randomized double-blind trial of oxycodone versus placebo. *Sleep* 1993;16:327–332.

Merritt's Neurology, 10th ed., edited by L.P. Rowland. Lippincott Williams & Wilkins, Philadelphia © 2000.

LEWIS P. ROWLAND

C H A P T E R 10

SYNDROMES CAUSED BY WEAK MUSCLES

Weakness implies that a muscle cannot exert normal force. Neurologists use the words *paralysis* or *plegia* to imply total loss of contractility; anything less than total loss is *paresis.* In practice, however, someone may mention a *partial hemiplegia,* which conveys the idea even if it is internally inconsistent. *Hemiplegia* implies weakness of an arm and leg on the same side. *Crossed hemiplegia* is a confusing term, generally implying unilateral cranial nerve signs and hemiplegia on the other side, a pattern seen with brainstem lesions above the decussation of the corticospinal tracts. *Monoplegia* is weakness of one limb; *paraplegia* means weakness of both legs.

This chapter describes syndromes that result from pathologically weak muscles, so that a student new to neurology can find the sections of the book that describe specific diseases. There is more than one approach to this problem, because no single approach is completely satisfactory. Elaborate algorithms have been devised, but the flowchart may be too complicated to be useful unless it is run by a computer.

It may be simpler to determine first whether there is pathologic weakness, then to find evidence of specific syndromes that depend on recognition of the following characteristics: distribution of weakness, associated neurologic abnormalities, tempo of disease, genetics, and patient age.

RECOGNITION OF WEAKNESS OR PSEUDOWEAKNESS

Patients with weak muscles do not often use the word "weakness" to describe their symptoms. Rather, they complain that they cannot climb stairs, rise from chairs, or run or that they note footdrop (and may actually use that term). They may have difficulty turning keys or doorknobs. If proximal arm muscles are affected, lifting packages, combing hair, or working overhead may be difficult. Weakness of cranial muscles causes ptosis of the eyelids, diplopia, dysarthria, dysphagia, or the cosmetic distortion of facial paralysis. These specific symptoms will be analyzed later.

Some people use the word "weakness" when there is no neurologic abnormality. For instance, aging athletes may find that they can no longer match the achievements of youth, but that is not pathologic weakness. Weakness in a professional athlete causes the same symptoms that are recognized by other people when the disorder interferes with the conventional activities of daily life. Losing a championship race, running a mile in more than 4 minutes, or jogging only 5 miles instead of a customary 10 miles are not symptoms of diseased muscles.

Others who lack the specific symptoms of weakness may describe *"chronic fatigue."* They cannot do housework; they have to lie down to rest after the briefest exertion. If they plan an activity in the evening, they may spend the entire day resting in advance. Employment may be in jeopardy. Myalgia is a common component of this syndrome, and there is usually evidence of depression.

The chronic fatigue syndrome affects millions of people and is a major public health problem. Vast research investments have been made to evaluate possible viral, immune, endocrine, autonomic, metabolic, and other factors, None, however, seems as consistent as depression and psychosocial causes. It is not, as some put it, a "diagnosis of exclusion." Instead, the characteristic history is recognizable, and on examination there is no limb weakness or reflex alteration.

Fading athletes and depressed, tired people with aching limbs have different emotional problems, but both groups lack the specific symptoms of muscle weakness, and they share two other characteristics: No abnormality appears on neurologic examination, and no true weakness is evident on manual muscle examination. That is, there is no weakness unless the examiner uses brute force. A vigorous young adult examiner may outwrestle a frail octogenarian, but that does not imply pathologic weakness in the loser. Students and residents must use reasonable force in tests of strength against resistance.

Fatigue and similar symptoms may sometimes be manifestations of systemic illness due to anemia, hypoventilation, congestive heart failure with hypoxemia and hypercapnia, cancer, or systemic infection. There is usually other evidence of the underlying disease, however, and that syndrome is almost never mistaken for a neurologic disorder.

Other patients have *pseudoweakness.* For instance, some patients attribute a gait disorder to weak legs, but it is immediately apparent on examination or even before formal examination that they have parkinsonism. Or a patient with peripheral neuropathy may have difficulty with fine movements of the fingers, not because of weakness but because of severe sensory loss. Or a patient may have difficulty raising one or both arms because of bursitis, not limb weakness. Or a patient with arthritis may be reluctant to move a painful joint. These circumstances are explained by findings on examination.

Examination may also resolve another problem in the evaluation of symptoms that might be due to weakness. Sometimes, when limb weakness is mild, it is difficult for the examiner to know how much resistance to apply to determine whether the apparent weakness is "real." Then, the presence or absence of wasting, fasciculation, or altered tendon reflexes may give the crucial clues. Symptomatic weakness is usually accompanied by some abnormality on examination. Even in myasthenia gravis, symptoms may fluctuate in intensity, but there are always objective signs of abnormality on examination if the patient is currently having symptoms. There is a maxim: A normal neurologic examination is incompatible with the diagnosis of symptomatic myasthenia gravis.

Finally, examination may uncover patients with pseudoweakness that may be due to deceit, deliberate or otherwise. Hysteric patients and Munchausen deceivers or other malingerers who feign weakness all lack specific symptoms. Or they may betray inconsistencies in the history because they can participate in some activities but not in others that involve the same muscles. On examination, their dress, cosmetic facial makeup, and behavior may be histrionic. In walking, they may stagger dramatically, but they do not fall or injure themselves by bumping into furniture. In manual muscle tests, they abruptly give way, or they shudder in tremor rather than apply constant pressure. Misdirection of effort is one way to describe that behavior. Some simply refuse to participate in the test. The extent of disorder may be surprising, however. I and others have seen psychogenic impairment of breathing that led to use of a mechanical ventilator.

PATTERNS OF WEAKNESS

In analyzing syndromes of weakness, the examiner uses several sources of information for the differential diagnosis. The pattern of weakness and associated neurologic signs delimit some of the anatomic possibilities to answer the question of *where* the lesion is located. Patient age and the tempo of evolution aid in deciding *what* the lesion is.

The differential diagnosis of weakness encompasses much of clinical neurology, so the reader will be referred to other sections for some of the review. For instance, the first task in the analysis of a weak limb is to determine whether the condition is due to a lesion of the upper or lower motor neuron, a distinction that is made on the basis of clinical findings. Overactive tendon reflexes with clonus, Hoffmann signs, and Babinski signs denote an upper motor neuron disorder. Lower motor neuron signs include muscle weakness, wasting, and fasciculation, with loss of tendon reflexes. These distinctions may seem crude, but they have been passed as reliable from generation to generation of neurologists.

If the clinical signs imply a lower motor neuron disorder, the condition could be due to problems anywhere in the motor unit (motor neuron or axon, neuromuscular junction, or muscle). This determination is guided by principles stated in Chapter 124. Diseases of the motor unit are also covered in that chapter, so the following information will be concerned primarily (but not entirely) with central lesions.

Hemiparesis

If there is weakness of the arm and leg on the same side and upper motor neuron signs imply a central lesion, the lesion could be in the cervical spinal cord or in the brain. Pain in the neck or in the distribution of a cervical dermatome might be clues to the site of the lesion. Unilateral facial weakness may be ipsilateral to the hemiparesis, placing the lesion in the brain and above the nucleus of the seventh cranial nerve; or a change in mentation or speech may indicate that the lesion is cerebral, not cervical. Sometimes, however, there are no definite clinical clues to the site of the lesion, and the examiner must rely on magnetic resonance imaging (MRI), computed tomography (CT), electroencephalography, cerebrospinal fluid (CSF) findings, or myelography to determine the site and nature of the lesion together.

The course of hemiparesis gives clues to the nature of the disorder. The most common cause in adults is cerebral infarction or hemorrhage. Abrupt onset, prior transient attacks, and progression to maximal severity within 24 hours in a person with hypertension or advanced age are indications that a stroke has occurred. If no cerebral symptoms are present, there could conceivably be transverse myelitis of the cervical spinal cord, but that condition would be somewhat slower in evolution (days rather than hours) and more likely to involve all four limbs. Similarly, multiple sclerosis is more likely to be manifest by bilateral corticospinal signs than by a pure hemiplegia.

If hemiparesis of cerebral origin progresses for days or weeks, it is reasonable to suspect a cerebral mass lesion, whether the patient is an adult or a child. If the patient has had focal seizures, that possibility is the more likely. In addition to brain tumors, other possibilities include arteriovenous malformation, brain abscess, or other infections. Infectious or neoplastic complications of acquired immunodeficiency syndrome are constant considerations these days. Metabolic brain disease usually causes bilateral signs with mental obtundation and would be an unusual cause of hemiparesis, even in a child.

Hemiparesis of subacute evolution could arise in the cervical spinal cord if there were, for instance, a neurofibroma of a cervical root. That condition would be signified by local pain in most cases, and because there is so little room in the cervical spinal canal, bilateral corticospinal signs would probably be present.

In general, hemiparesis usually signifies a cerebral lesion rather than one in the neck, and the cause is likely to be denoted by the clinical course and by CT or MRI.

Paraparesis

Paresis means weakness, and *paraparesis* is used to describe weakness of both legs. The term has also been extended, however, to include gait disorders caused by lesions of the upper motor neuron, even when there is no weakness on manual muscle examination. The disorder is then attributed to *spasticity* or the clumsiness induced by malfunction of the corticospinal tracts. In adults, the most common cause of that syndrome, *spastic paraparesis of middle life,* is multiple sclerosis. The differential diagnosis includes tumors in the region of the foramen magnum, Chiari malformation, cervical spondylosis, arteriovenous malformation, and primary lateral sclerosis (all described in other sections of this book). The diagnosis cannot be made on clinical grounds alone and requires information from CSF examination (protein, cells, gamma globulin, oligoclonal bands), evoked potentials, CT, MRI, and myelography.

When there are cerebellar or other signs in addition to bilateral corticospinal signs, the disorder may be multiple sclerosis or an inherited disease, such as olivopontocerebellar degeneration. The combination of lower motor neuron signs in the arms and upper motor neuron signs in the legs is characteristic of amyotrophic lateral sclerosis; the same syndrome has been attributed without proof to cervical spondylosis. That pattern may also be seen in syringomyelia, but it is exceptional to find syringomyelia without typical patterns of sensory loss.

Other clues to the nature of spastic paraparesis include cervical or radicular pain in neurofibromas or other extraaxial mass lesions in the cervical spinal canal. Or there may be concomitant cerebellar signs or other indication of multiple sclerosis.

It is said that brain tumors in the parasagittal area may cause isolated spastic paraparesis by compressing the leg areas of the motor cortex in both hemispheres. This possibility seems more theoretical than real, however, because no well documented cases have been reported.

Chronic paraparesis may also be due to lower motor neuron disorders. Instead of upper motor neuron signs, there is flaccid paraparesis, with loss of tendon reflexes in the legs. This differential diagnosis includes motor neuron diseases, peripheral neuropathy, and myopathy as described in Chapter 124.

Paraparesis of acute onset (days rather than hours or weeks) presents a different problem in diagnosis. If there is back pain and tendon reflexes are preserved or if there are frank upper motor neuron signs, a compressive lesion may be present. As the population ages, metastatic tumors become an increasingly more common cause. In children or young adults, the syndrome may be less ominous, even with pain, because the disorder is often due to acute transverse myelitis. This may be seen in children or adults, and in addition to the motor signs, a sensory level usually designates the site of the lesion. Spinal MRI or myelography is needed to make this differentiation. In the elderly population, a rare cause of acute paraplegia is infarction of the spinal cord. That syndrome is also sometimes seen after surgical procedures that require clamping of the aorta.

If the tendon reflexes are lost and there is no transverse sensory level in a patient with an acute paraparesis, the most common cause is Guillain-Barré syndrome, at any age from infancy to the senium. Sensory loss may facilitate that diagnosis, but sometimes little or no sensory impairment occurs. Then, the diagnosis depends on examination of the CSF and electromyography (EMG). The Guillain-Barré syndrome, however, may also originate from diverse causes. In developing countries, acute paralytic poliomyelitis is still an important cause of acute paraplegia. Rarely, an acute motor myelitis may be due to some other virus. In China, for instance, there have been summertime outbreaks of an acute motor axonopathy that differs from both Guillain-Barré syndrome and poliomyelitis, in particular, but, like the other syndromes, causes paraparesis.

The "reverse" of paraplegia would be weakness of the arms with good function in the legs, or *bibrachial paresis*. Lower motor neuron syndromes of this nature are seen in some cases of amyotrophic lateral sclerosis (with or without upper motor neuron signs in the legs). The arms hang limply at the side while the patient walks with normal movements of the legs. Similar patterns may be seen in some patients with myopathy of unusual distribution. It is difficult to understand how a cerebral lesion could cause weakness of the arms without equally severe weakness of the legs, but this "man-in-the-barrel syndrome" is seen in comatose patients who survive a bout of severe hypotension. The

site of the lesion is not known, but it could be bilateral and prerolandic.

Monomelic Paresis

If one leg or one arm is weak, the presence of pain in the low back or the neck may point to a compressive lesion. Whether acute or chronic, herniated nucleus pulposus is high on the list of possibilities if radicular pain is present. Acute brachial plexus neuritis (neuralgic amyotrophy) is another cause of weakness in one limb with pain; a corresponding syndrome of the lumbosacral plexus is much less common. Peripheral nerve entrapment syndromes may also cause monomelic weakness and pain, but the pain is local, not radicular. Mononeuritis multiplex may also cause local pain, paresthesia, and paresis.

In painless syndromes of isolated limb weakness in adults, motor neuron disease is an important consideration if there is no sensory loss. Sometimes, in evaluating a limb with weak, wasted, and fasciculating muscle, the examiner is surprised because tendon reflexes are preserved or even overactive, instead of being lost. This apparent paradox implies lesions of both upper and lower motor neurons, almost pathognomonic of amyotrophic lateral sclerosis. The signs may be asymmetric in early stages of the disease.

Although rare, it is theoretically possible for strokes or other cerebral lesions to cause monomelic weakness with upper motor neuron signs. Weakness due to a cerebral lesion may be more profound in the arm, but abnormal signs are almost always present in the leg, too; that is, the syndrome is really a hemiparesis.

Neck Weakness

Difficulty holding up the head is seen in some patients with diseases of the motor unit, probably never in patients with upper motor neuron disorders. Usually, patients with neck weakness also have symptoms of disorder of the lower cranial nerves (dysarthria and dysphagia) and often also of adjacent cervical segments, as manifest by difficulty raising the arms. Amyotrophic lateral sclerosis and myasthenia gravis are probably the two most common causes.

Rarely, there is isolated weakness of neck muscles, with difficulty holding the head up, but no oropharyngeal or arm symptoms. This *floppy head syndrome* or *dropped head syndrome* is a disabling disorder that is usually due to one of three conditions: motor neuron disease, myasthenia gravis, or polymyositis. I have seen one such patient with a Chiari malformation. Some cases, however, are idiopathic.

New terms have been introduced to explain this syndrome: the bent spine syndrome and isolated myopathy of the cervical extensor muscles, which may be variations of the same condition. EMG shows a myopathic pattern in affected paraspinal muscles, and MRI may show replacement of muscle by fat in cervical, thoracic, or both areas.

Weakness of Cranial Muscles

The syndromes due to weakness of cranial muscles are reviewed in Chapters 7 and 68. The major problems in differential diagnosis involve the site of local lesions that affect individual nerves of ocular movement, facial paralysis, or the vocal cords. Pseudobulbar palsy due to upper motor neuron lesions must be distinguished from bulbar palsy due to lower motor neuron disease and then almost always a form of amyotrophic lateral sclerosis. This distinction depends on associated signs of upper or lower motor neuron lesions. Myasthenia gravis can affect the eyes, face, or oropharynx (but only exceptionally the vocal cords); in fact, the diagnosis of myasthenia gravis is doubtful if there are no cranial symptoms. Brainstem syndromes in the aging population may be due to stroke, meningeal carcinomatosis, or brainstem encephalitis.

SUGGESTED READINGS

Adams RW. The distribution of muscle weakness in upper motor neuron lesions affecting the lower limb. *Brain* 1990;113:1459–1476.

Asher R. Munchausen's syndrome. *Lancet* 1954;1:339–341.

Ashizawa T, Rolak LA, Hines M. Spastic pure motor monoparesis. *Ann Neurol* 1986;20:638–641.

Blackwood SK, MacHale SM, Power MJ, Goodwin GM, Lawrie SM. Effects of exercise on cognitive and motor function in chronic fatigue syndrome and depression. *J Neurol Neurosurg Psychiatry* 1998;65:541–546.

Bourbanis D. Weakness in patients with hemiparesis. *Am J Occup Ther* 1989;43:313–319.

Goshorn RK. Chronic fatigue syndrome: a review for clinicians. *Semin Neurol* 1998;18:237–242.

Hopkins A, Clarke C. Pretended paralysis requiring artificial ventilation. *BMJ* 1987;294:961–962.

Kennedy HG. Fatigue and fatigability. *Lancet* 1987;1:1145.

Knopman DS, Rubens AB. The value of CT findings for the localization of cerebral functions: the relationship between CT and hemiparesis. *Arch Neurol* 1986;43:328–332.

Lange DJ, Fetell MR, Lovelace RE, Rowland LP. The floppy-head syndrome. *Ann Neurol* 1986;20:133 [abstract].

Layzer RB. Asthenia and the chronic fatigue syndrome. *Muscle Nerve* 1998;21:1609–1611.

Marsden CD. Hysteria—a neurologist's view. *Psychol Med* 1986;16:277–288.

Maurice-Williams RS, Marsh H. Simulated paraplegia: an occasional problem for the neurosurgeon. *J Neurol Neurosurg Psychiatry* 1985;48:826–831.

Myer BV. Motor responses evoked by magnetic brain stimulation in psychogenic limb weakness: diagnostic value and limitations. *J Neurol* 1992;239:251–255.

Oerlemans WG, de Visser M. Dropped head syndrome and bent spine syndrome: two separate clinical entities or different manifestations of axial myopathy? *J Neurol Neurosurg Psychiatry* 1998;65:258–259.

Rutherford OM. Long-lasting unilateral muscle wasting and weakness following injury and immobilization. *Scand J Rehabil Med* 1990;22:33–37.

Sage JI, Van Uitert RL. Man-in-the-barrel syndrome. *Neurology* 1986;36:1102–1103.

Serratrice G, Pouget J, Pellissier JF. Bent spine syndrome. *J Neurol Neurosurg Psychiatry* 1996;65:51–54.

Seyal M, Pedley TA. Sensory evoked potentials in adult-onset progressive spastic paraparesis. *N Y State J Med* 1984;84:68–71.

Thijs RD, Notermans NC, Wokke JH, van der Graaf Y, van Gijn J. Distribution of muscle weakness of central and peripheral origin. *J Neurol Neurosurg Psychiatry* 1998;65:794–796.

Merritt's Neurology, 10th ed., edited by L.P. Rowland. Lippincott Williams & Wilkins, Philadelphia © 2000.

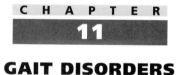

CHAPTER 11

GAIT DISORDERS

SID GILMAN

Observation of the stance and gait of patients with neurologic symptoms can provide important diagnostic information and may immediately suggest particular disorders of motor or sensory function, or even specific diseases. Some types of gait are so characteristic of certain diseases that the diagnosis may be obvious at the initial encounter with a patient. An example of this is the typical posture and gait of patients with Parkinson disease.

In normal bipedal locomotion, one leg and then the other alternately supports the erect moving body. Each leg undergoes brief periods of acceleration and deceleration as body weight shifts from one foot to the other. When the moving body passes over the supporting leg, the other leg swings forward in preparation for its next support phase. One foot or the other constantly contacts the ground, and when support of the body is transferred from the trailing leg to the leading leg, both feet are on the ground momentarily.

Normal bipedal locomotion requires two processes: continuous ground reaction forces that support the body's center of gravity, and periodic movement of each foot from one position of support to the next in the direction of progression. As a consequence of these basic requirements, certain displacements of the body segments regularly occur in walking. To start walking, a person raises one foot and accelerates the leg forward; this is the *swing phase* of walking. Muscle action in the supporting leg causes the center of gravity of the body to move forward, creating a horizontal reaction force at the foot. The greater this reaction force is, the greater is the acceleration of the body, because the amount of force equals the body mass multiplied by the amount of acceleration. The swing phase ends when the leg that has swung forward makes contact with the ground, which is when the *stance phase* of walking begins. During the stance phase, the body weight shifts to the opposite leg and another swing phase can begin. The major groups of muscles of the leg are active at the beginning and the end of the stance and swing phases. As the body passes over the weight-bearing leg, it tends to be displaced toward the weight-bearing side, causing a slight side-to-side movement. In addition, the body rises and falls with each step. The body rises to a maximum level during the swing phase and descends to a minimum level during the stance phase. As the body accelerates upward during the swing phase, the vertical floor reaction increases to a value that exceeds the body weight. The vertical floor reaction falls to a minimum during downward acceleration, reducing the total vertical reaction to a value less than the body weight.

EXAMINING STANCE AND GAIT

When examining patients' stance and gait, the physician should observe them from the front, back, and sides. Patients should rise quickly from a chair, walk normally at a slow pace and then at a fast pace, and then turn around. They should walk successively on their toes, on their heels, and then in tandem (i.e., placing the heel of one foot immediately in front of the toes of the opposite foot and attempting to progress forward in a straight line). They should stand with their feet together and the head erect, first with open eyes and then with closed eyes, to determine whether they can maintain their balance.

When a person walks normally, the body should be held erect with the head straight and the arms hanging loosely at the sides, each moving rhythmically forward with the opposite leg. The shoulders and hips should be approximately level. The arms should swing equally. The steps should be straight and about equal in length. The head should not be tilted, and there should be no appreciable scoliosis or lordosis. With each step, the hip and knee should flex smoothly, and the ankle should dorsiflex with a barely perceptible elevation of the hips as the foot clears the ground. The heel should strike the ground first, and the weight of the body should be transferred successively onto the sole of the foot and then onto the toes. The head and then the body should rotate slightly with each step, without lurching or falling.

Although there are gross similarities in the way that normal people walk, each person walks in a distinctive fashion. The distinctions between people reflect both their individual physical characteristics and their personality traits. Among the variables that compose the physical characteristics are speed, stride length, positions of the feet (e.g., with the toes pointing outward or pointing inward), characteristics of the walking surface, and the type of footwear worn. Perhaps, more important are the goals to be accomplished in walking, as well as the person's aspirations, motivations, and attitudes. For some situations, speed is the most important factor. In other situations, safe arrival or the minimal expenditure of energy may be more important. Some people learn to walk gracefully or in the least obtrusive manner possible and consequently may expend extra energy. Others learn to walk ungracefully but as effectively as possible for the amount of energy expended. The manner of walking may provide clues to personality traits (e.g., aggressiveness, timidity, self-confidence, aloofness).

GAIT IN HEMIPARESIS

Hemiparesis from an upper motor neuron lesion results in a characteristic posture and gait owing to the combined effects of spasticity and weakness of the affected limbs. Patients with hemiparesis usually stand and walk with the affected arm flexed and the leg extended. In walking, they have difficulty flexing the hip and knee and dorsiflexing the ankle; the paretic leg swings outward at the hip to avoid scraping the foot on the floor. The leg maintains a stiff posture in extension and rotates in a semicircle, first away from and then toward the trunk, with a circumduction movement. Despite the circumduction, the foot may scrape the floor so that the toe and outer side of the sole of the shoe become worn first. The upper body often rocks slightly to the opposite side during the circumduction movement. The arm on the hemiparetic side usually moves little during walking, remaining adducted at the shoulder, flexed at the elbow, and partially flexed at the wrist and fingers. In a person without a previous motor disorder, loss of the swinging motion of an arm may be the first sign of a progressive upper motor neuron lesion that will result in a hemiparesis.

GAIT IN PARAPARESIS

Paraparesis usually results from lesions of the thoracic portion of the spinal cord. The gait of these patients results from the combined effects of spasticity and weakness of the legs and consists of slow, stiff movements at the knees and hips with evidence of considerable effort. The legs are usually maintained extended or slightly flexed at the hips and knees and are often adducted at the hips. In some patients, particularly those with severe spasticity, each leg may cross in front of the other during the swing phase of walking, causing a *scissors gait*. The steps are short, and patients may move the trunk from side to side in attempts to compensate for the slow, stiff movements of the legs. The legs circumduct at the hips, and the feet scrape the floor, so that the soles of the shoes become worn at the toes.

GAIT IN PARKINSONISM

The gait in Parkinson disease reflects a combination of akinesia (difficulty in initiating movement), dystonia (relatively fixed abnormal postures), rigidity, and tremor. These patients stand in a posture of general flexion, with the spine bent forward, the head bent downward, the arms moderately flexed at the elbows, and the legs slightly flexed. They stand immobile and rigid, with a paucity of automatic movements of the limbs and a masklike fixed facial expression with infrequent blinking. Although the arms are held immobile, often a rest tremor involves the fingers and wrists at 4 to 5 cycles per second. When these patients walk, the trunk bends even farther forward; the arms remain immobile at the sides of the body or become further flexed and carried somewhat ahead of the body. The arms do not swing. As patients walk forward, the legs remain bent at the knees, hips, and ankles. The steps are short so that the feet barely clear the ground and the soles of the feet shuffle and scrape the floor. The gait, with characteristically small steps, is termed *marche à petits pas.* Forward locomotion may lead to successively more rapid steps, and the patient may fall unless assisted; this increasingly rapid walking is called *festination.* If patients are pushed forward or backward, they cannot compensate with flexion or extension movements of the trunk. The result is a series of propulsive or retropulsive steps. Parkinsonian patients can sometimes walk with surprising rapidity for brief intervals. These patients often have difficulty when they start to walk after standing still or sitting in a chair. They may take several very small steps that cover little distance before taking longer strides. The walking movements may stop involuntarily, and the patient may freeze on attempts to pass through a doorway or into an elevator.

GAIT IN CEREBELLAR DISEASE

Patients with disease of the cerebellum stand with their legs farther apart than normal and may develop *titubation,* a coarse fore-and-aft tremor of the trunk. Often, they cannot stand with their legs so close that the feet are touching; they sway or fall in attempts to do so, whether their eyes are open or closed. They walk cautiously, taking steps of varying length, some shorter and others longer than usual. They may lurch from one side to another. Because of this unsteady or *ataxic gait,* which they usually attribute to poor balance, they fear walking without support and tend to hold onto objects in the room, such as a bed or a chair, moving cautiously between these objects. When gait ataxia is mild, it can be enhanced by asking the patient to attempt tandem walking in a straight line, successively placing the heel of one foot directly in front of the toes of the opposite foot. Patients commonly lose their balance during this task and must quickly place one foot to the side to avoid falling.

When disease is restricted to the vermal portions of the cerebellum, disorders of stance and gait may appear without other signs of cerebellar dysfunction, such as limb ataxia or nystagmus. This pattern is seen in alcoholic cerebellar degeneration. Diseases of the cerebellar hemispheres, unilateral or bilateral, may also affect gait. With a unilateral cerebellar-hemisphere lesion, ipsilateral disorders of posture and movement accompany the gait disorder. Patients usually stand with the shoulder on the side of the lesion lower than the other; there is accompanying scoliosis. The limbs on the side of the cerebellar lesion show decreased resistance to passive manipulation (*hypotonia*). When these patients attempt to touch their nose and then the examiner's finger (the finger-nose-finger test), they miss their target and experience a side-to-side tremor generated from the shoulder. When they attempt to touch the knee of one leg with the heel of the other leg and then move the heel smoothly down along the shin (the heel-knee-shin test), a side-to-side tremor of the moving leg develops, generated from the hip. On walking, patients with cerebellar disease show ataxia of the leg ipsilateral to the cerebellar lesion; consequently they stagger and progressively deviate to the affected side. This can be demonstrated by asking them to walk around a chair. As they rotate toward the affected side, they tend to fall into the chair; rotating toward the

normal side, they move away from the chair in a spiral. Patients with bilateral cerebellar-hemisphere disease show a disturbance of gait similar to that seen in disease of the vermis, but signs of cerebellar dysfunction also appear in coordinated limb movements. Thus, these patients show abnormal finger-nose-finger and heel-knee-shin tests bilaterally.

GAIT IN SENSORY ATAXIA

Another characteristic gait disorder results from loss of proprioceptive sensation in the legs due to lesions of the afferent fibers in peripheral nerves, dorsal roots, dorsal columns of the spinal cord, or medial lemnisci. Patients with such lesions are unaware of the position of the limbs and consequently have difficulty standing or walking. They usually stand with their legs spread widely apart. If asked to stand with their feet together and eyes open, they remain stable, but when they close their eyes, they sway and often fall (*Romberg sign*). They walk with their legs spread widely apart, watching the ground carefully. In stepping, they lift the legs higher than normal at the hips and fling them abruptly forward and outward. The steps vary in length and may cause a characteristic slapping sound as the foot contacts the floor. They usually hold the body somewhat flexed, often using a cane for support. If vision is impaired and these patients attempt to walk in the dark, the gait disturbance worsens.

PSYCHOGENIC GAIT DISORDERS

Psychogenic disorders of gait often appear in association with many other neurologic complaints, including "dizziness," loss of balance, and weakness of both legs or the arm and leg on one side of the body. The gait is usually bizarre, easily recognized, and unlike any disorder of gait evoked by organic disease. In some patients, however, hysteric gait disorders may be difficult to identify. The key to the diagnosis is the demonstration that objective organic signs of disease are missing. In hysteric hemiplegia, patients drag the affected leg along the ground behind the body and do not circumduct the leg, scraping the sole of the foot on the floor, as in hemiplegia due to an organic lesion. At times, the hemiplegic leg may be pushed ahead of the patient and used mainly for support. The arm on the affected side does not develop the flexed posture commonly seen with hemiplegia from organic causes, and the hyperactive tendon reflexes and Babinski sign on the hemiplegic side are missing.

Hysteric paraplegic patients usually walk with one or two crutches or lie helplessly in bed with the legs maintained in rigid postures or at times completely limp. The term *astasia-abasia* refers to patients who cannot stand or walk but who can carry out natural movements of the limbs while lying in bed. At times, patients with hysteric gait disorders walk only with seemingly great difficulty, but they show normal power and coordination when lying in bed. On walking, patients cling to the bed or objects in the room. If asked to walk without support, they may lurch dramatically while managing feats of extraordinary balance to avoid falling. They may fall, but only when a nearby physician or family member can catch them or when soft objects are available to cushion the fall. The gait disturbance is often dramatic, with the patient lurching wildly in many directions and finally falling, but only when other people are watching the performance. They often demonstrate remarkable agility in their rapid postural adjustments when they attempt to walk.

GAIT IN CEREBRAL PALSY

The term *cerebral palsy* includes several different motor abnormalities that usually result from perinatal injury. The severity of the gait disturbance varies, depending on the nature of the lesion. Mild limited lesions may result in exaggerated tendon reflexes and extensor plantar responses with a slight degree of talipes equinovarus but no clear gait disorder. More severe and extensive lesions often result in bilateral hemiparesis; patients stand with the legs adducted and internally rotated at the hips, extended or slightly flexed at the knees, with plantar flexion at the ankles. The arms are held adducted at the shoulders and flexed at the elbows and wrists. Patients walk slowly and stiffly with plantar flexion of the feet, causing them to walk on the toes. Bilateral adduction of the hips causes the knees to rub together or to cross, causing a scissors gait.

The gait in patients with cerebral palsy can be altered by movement disorders. Athetosis is common and consists of slow, serpentine movements of the arms and legs between the extreme postures of flexion with supination and extension with pronation. On walking, patients with athetotic cerebral palsy show involuntary limb movements that are accompanied by rotatory movements of the neck and constant grimacing. The limbs usually show the bilateral hemiparetic posture described previously; however, superimposed on this posture may be partially fixed asymmetric limb postures with, for example, flexion with supination of one arm and extension with pronation of the other. Asymmetric limb postures commonly occur in association with rotated postures of the head, generally with extension of the arm on the side to which the chin rotates and flexion of the opposite arm.

GAIT IN CHOREA

Chorea literally means the dance and refers to the gait disorder seen most often in children with Sydenham chorea or adults with Huntington disease. Both conditions are characterized by continuous and rapid movements of the face, trunk, and limbs. Flexion, extension, and rotatory movements of the neck occur with grimacing movements of the face, twisting movements of the trunk and limbs, and rapid piano-playing movements of the digits. Walking generally accentuates these movements. In addition, sudden forward or sideward thrusting movements of the pelvis and rapid twisting movements of the trunk and limbs result in a gait resembling a series of dancing steps. With walking, patients speed up and slow down at unpredictable times, evoking a lurching gait.

GAIT IN DYSTONIA MUSCULORUM DEFORMANS

The first symptom of this disorder often consists of an abnormal gait resulting from inversion of one foot at the ankle. Patients walk initially on the lateral side of the foot; as the disease progresses, this problem worsens, and other postural abnormalities develop, including elevation of one shoulder and hip and twisted postures of the trunk. Intermittent spasms of the trunk and limbs then interfere with walking. Eventually, there is torticollis, tortipelvis, lordosis, or scoliosis. Finally, patients may become unable to walk.

GAIT IN MUSCULAR DYSTROPHY

In muscular dystrophy, weakness of the muscles of the trunk and the proximal parts of the legs produces a characteristic stance and gait. In attempting to rise from the seated position, patients flex the trunk at the hips, put their hands on their knees, and push the trunk upward by working their hands up the thighs. This sequence of movements is termed *Gowers sign*. Patients stand with exaggerated lumbar lordosis and a protuberant abdomen because of weakness of the abdominal and paravertebral muscles. They walk with the legs spread widely apart, showing a characteristic waddling motion of the pelvis that results from weakness of the gluteal muscles. The shoulders often slope forward, and winging of the scapulae may be seen as the patients walk.

SENILE GAIT DISORDERS

Many disorders of gait have been observed in elderly persons, including some people who have overt neurologic disease.

Cautious Gait

This gait is often seen in normal elderly people. It is characterized by a slightly widened base, shortened stride, slowness of walking, and turning in a block. There is no hesitancy in the initiation of gait and no shuffling or freezing. The rhythm of walking and foot clearance are normal. There is mild disequilibrium in response to a push and difficulty in balancing on one foot.

Subcortical Disequilibrium

This gait disorder is seen with progressive supranuclear palsy and multiinfarct dementia. Patients have marked difficulty maintaining the upright posture and show absent or poor postural adjustments in response to perturbations. Some patients hyperextend the trunk and neck and fall backward or forward, thus impairing locomotion. These patients commonly show ocular palsies, dysarthria, and the parkinsonian signs of rigidity, akinesia, and tremor.

Frontal Disequilibrium

Many patients with frontal disequilibrium cannot rise, stand, or walk; some cannot even sit without support. Standing and walking are difficult or impossible. When they try to rise from a chair, they lean backward rather than forward, and they cannot bring their legs under their center of gravity. When they attempt to step, their feet frequently cross and move in a direction that is inappropriate to their center of gravity. Clinical examination usually reveals dementia, signs of frontal release (suck, snout, and grasp reflexes), motor perseveration, urinary incontinence, pseudobulbar palsy, exaggerated muscle stretch reflexes, and extensor plantar responses.

Isolated Gait Ignition Failure

Patients with this disorder have difficulty starting to walk and continuing walking, even though they have no impairment of equilibrium, cognition, limb praxis, or extrapyramidal function. Once they start to walk, the steps are short and their feet barely clear the ground, thereby creating a shuffling appearance. With continued stepping, however, the stride lengthens, foot clearance is normal, and the arms swing normally. If their attention is diverted, their feet may freeze momentarily and shuffling may recur. Postural responses and stance base are normal, and falls are rare. The terms *magnetic gait* or *apraxia of gait* pertain to both isolated gait ignition failure and frontal gait disorder.

Frontal Gait Disorder

This disturbance is often seen with multiinfarct dementia or normal pressure hydrocephalus. Characteristically, these patients stand on a wide base (though sometimes a narrow base) and take short steps with shuffling, hesitate in starting to walk and in turning, and show moderate disequilibrium. Associated findings include cognitive impairment, pseudobulbar palsy with dysarthria, signs of frontal release (e.g., suck, snout, and grasping reflexes), paratonia, signs of corticospinal tract disease, and urinary dysfunction. In patients who have this gait disorder in association with normal pressure hydrocephalus, ventricular shunting may restore a normal gait.

GAIT IN LOWER MOTOR NEURON DISORDERS

Diseases of the motor neurons or peripheral nerves characteristically cause distal weakness, and footdrop is a common manifestation. In motor neuron disease and in the hereditary neuropathies (e.g., Charcot-Marie-Tooth disease), the disorder is likely to be bilateral. If the patient has a compressive lesion of one peroneal nerve, the process may be unilateral. In either case, patients cannot dorsiflex the foot in walking, as is normal each time the swinging leg begins to move. As a result, the toes are scuffed along the ground. To avoid this awkwardness, patients raise the knee higher than usual, resulting in a "steppage" gait. If the proximal muscles of the legs are affected (in addition to or instead of distal muscles), the gait also has a waddling appearance.

SUGGESTED READINGS

Alexander NB. Differential diagnosis of gait disorders in older adults. *Clin Geriatr Med* 1996;12:689–703.

Alexander NB. Gait disorders in older adults. *J Am Geriatr Soc* 1996;44:434–451.

Dietz V. Neurophysiology of gait disorders: present and future applications. *Electroencephalogr Clin Neurophysiol* 1997;103:333–355.

Gilman S. Cerebellar disorders. In: Rosenberg R, Pleasure DE, eds. *Comprehensive neurology*, 2nd ed. New York: John Wiley & Sons, 1998:415–433.

Keane JR. Hysterical gait disorders: 60 cases. *Neurology* 1989;39:586–589.

Morris M, Iansek R, Matyas T, Summers J. Abnormalities in the stride length-cadence relation in parkinsonian gait. *Mov Disord* 1998;13:61–69.

Nutt JG, Marsden CD, Thompson PD. Human walking and higher-level gait disorders, particularly in the elderly. *Neurology* 1993;43:268–279.

Rubino FA. Gait disorders in the elderly: distinguishing between normal and dysfunctional gaits. *Postgrad Med* 1993;93:185–190.

Tyrrell PJ. Apraxia of gait or higher level gait disorders: review and description of two cases of progressive gait disturbance due to frontal lobe degeneration. *J R Soc Med* 1994;87:454–456.

Merritt's Neurology, 10th ed., edited by L.P. Rowland. Lippincott Williams & Wilkins, Philadelphia © 2000.

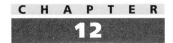

SIGNS AND SYMPTOMS IN NEUROLOGIC DIAGNOSIS

LEWIS P. ROWLAND

An anonymous sage once said that 90% of the neurologic diagnosis depends on the patient's medical history and that the remainder comes from the neurologic examination and laboratory tests. Sometimes, of course, findings in blood tests, magnetic resonance imaging (MRI), or computed tomography (CT) are pathognomonic, but students have to learn which tests are appropriate and when to order them. It is therefore necessary to know which diagnostic possibilities are reasonable considerations for a particular patient. In the consideration of these different diagnostic possibilities, specific symptoms are not the only ingredient in the analysis of a patient's history, as this chapter briefly reviews.

It is commonly taught that neurologic diagnosis depends on answers to two questions that are considered separately and in sequence:

1. *Where is the lesion?* Is it in the cerebrum, basal ganglia, brainstem, cerebellum, spinal cord, peripheral nerves, neuromuscular junction, or muscle?
2. *What is the nature of the disease?*

If the site of the lesion can be determined, the number of diagnostic possibilities is reduced to a manageable number. An experienced clinician, however, is likely to deal with both questions simultaneously; site and disease are identified at the same time. Sometimes, the process is reversed. To take an obvious example, if a patient suddenly becomes speechless or awakens with a hemiplegia, the diagnosis of stroke is presumed. The location is then deduced from findings on examination, and both site and process are ascertained by CT or MRI. If there are no surprises in the imaging study (e.g., demonstration of a tumor or vascular malformation), further laboratory tests might be considered to determine the cause of an ischemic infarct.

The specific nature of different symptoms and findings on examination are reviewed in preceding chapters and in teaching manuals on the neurologic examination. Other considerations that influence diagnosis are briefly described here.

PATIENT AGE

The symptoms and signs of a stroke may be virtually identical in a 10-year-old, a 25-year-old, and a 70-year-old; however, the diagnostic implications are vastly different for each patient. Some brain tumors are more common in children, and others are more common in adults. Progressive paraparesis is more likely to be due to spinal cord tumor in a child, whereas in an adult it is more likely to be due to multiple sclerosis. Focal seizures are less likely to be fixed in pattern and are less likely to indicate a specific structural brain lesion in a child than in an adult. Myopathic weakness of the legs in childhood is more likely to be caused by muscular dystrophy than polymyositis; the reverse is true in patients older than 25 years. Muscular dystrophy rarely begins after age 35. Multiple sclerosis rarely starts after age 55. Hysteria is not a likely diagnosis when neurologic symptoms start after age 50. (These ages are arbitrary, but the point is that age is a consideration in some diagnoses.)

SEX

Only a few diseases are sex-specific. X-linked diseases (e.g., Duchenne muscular dystrophy) occur only in boys or, rarely, in girls with chromosome disorders. Among young adults, autoimmune diseases are more likely to affect women, especially systemic lupus erythematosus and myasthenia gravis, although young men are also affected in some cases. Women are exposed to the neurologic complications of pregnancy and may be at increased risk of stroke because of oral contraceptives. Men are more often exposed to head injury.

ETHNICITY

Stating the race of the patient in every case history is an anachronism of modern medical education. In neurology, race is important only when sickle cell disease is considered. Malignant hypertension and sarcoidosis may be more prevalent in blacks, but whites are also susceptible. Other ethnic groups, however, are more susceptible to particular diseases: Tay-Sachs disease, familial dysautonomia, and Gaucher disease in Ashkenazi Jews; thyrotoxic periodic paralysis in Japanese and perhaps in other Asians; nasopharyngeal carcinoma in Chinese; Marchiafava-Bignami disease in Italian wine drinkers (a myth?); and hemophilia in descendants of the Romanovs. Ethnicity is rarely important in diagnosis.

SOCIOECONOMIC CONSIDERATIONS

In general, social deprivation leads to increased mortality, and the reasons are not always clear. Ghetto dwellers, whatever their race, are prone to the ravages of alcoholism, drug addiction, and trauma. Impoverishment is also accompanied by malnutrition, infections, and the consequences of medical neglect. Within the ghetto and in other social strata, the acquired immunodeficiency syndrome epidemic has generated concern about the risk factors of male homosexuals, intravenous drug users, prostitutes, and recipients of blood transfusions. For most other neurologic disorders, however, race, ethnicity, sex, sexual orientation, and socioeconomic status do not affect the incidence.

TEMPO OF DISEASE

Seizures, strokes, and syncope are all abrupt in onset but differ in manifestations and duration. Syncope is the briefest. There are usually sensations that warn of the impending loss of consciousness. After fainting, the patient begins to recover consciousness in a minute or so. A seizure may or may not be preceded by warning symptoms. It can be brief or protracted and is manifested by alteration of consciousness or by repetitive movements, stereotyped behavior, or abnormal sensations. A stroke due to cerebral ischemia or hemorrhage "strikes out of the blue" and is manifest by hemiparesis or other focal brain signs. The neurologic disorder that follows brain infarction may be permanent, or the patient may recover partially or completely in days or weeks. If the signs last less than 24 hours, the episode is called a transient ischemic attack (TIA). Sometimes, it is difficult to differentiate a TIA from the postictal hemiparesis of a focal motor seizure, especially if the seizure was not witnessed. Another syndrome of abrupt onset is subarachnoid hemorrhage, in which the patient often complains of "the worst headache of my life;" this is sometimes followed by loss of consciousness.

Symptoms of less than apoplectic onset may progress for hours (intoxication, infection, or subdural hematoma), days (Guillain-Barré syndrome), or longer (most tumors of the brain or spinal cord). The acute symptoms of increased intracranial pressure or brain herniation are sometimes superimposed on the slower progression of a brain tumor. Progressive symptoms of brain tumor may be punctuated by seizures. Heritable or degenerative diseases tend to progress slowly, becoming most severe only after years of increasing disability (e.g., Parkinson disease or Alzheimer disease).

Remissions and exacerbations are characteristic of myasthenia gravis, multiple sclerosis, and some forms of peripheral neuropathy. Bouts of myasthenia tend to last for weeks at a time; episodes in multiple sclerosis may last only days in the first attacks and then tend to increase in duration and to leave more permanent neurologic disability. These diseases sometimes become progressively worse without remissions.

The symptoms of myasthenia gravis vary in a way that differs from any other disease. The severity of myasthenic symptoms may vary from minute to minute. More often, however, there are differences in the course of a day (usually worse in the evening than in the morning, but sometimes vice versa) or from day to day.

Some disorders characteristically occur in bouts that usually last minutes or hours, rarely longer. Periodic paralysis, migraine headache, cluster headaches, and narcolepsy are examples of such disorders.

To recognize the significance of these differences in tempo, it is necessary to have some notion of the different disorders.

DURATION OF SYMPTOMS

It may be of diagnostic importance to know how long the patient has had symptoms before consulting a physician. Long-standing headache is more apt to be a tension or vascular headache, but headache of recent onset is likely to imply intracranial structural disease and should never be underestimated. Similarly, seizures or drastic personality change of recent onset implies the need for CT, MRI, and other studies to evaluate possible brain tumor or encephalopathy. If no such lesion is found or if seizures are uncontrolled for a long time, perhaps video-electroencephalographic monitoring should be carried out to determine the best drug therapy or surgical approach.

MEDICAL HISTORY

It is always important to know whether any systemic disease is in the patient's background. Common disorders, such as hypertensive vascular disease or diabetes mellitus, may be discovered for the first time when the patient is examined because of neurologic symptoms. Because they are common, these two disorders may be merely coincidental, but depending on the neurologic syndrome, either diabetes or hypertension may actually be involved in the pathogenesis of the neural signs. If the patient is known to have a carcinoma, metastatic disease is assumed to be the basis of neurologic symptoms until proved otherwise. If the patient is taking medication for any reason, the possibility of intoxication must be considered. Cutaneous signs may point to neurologic complications of von Recklinghausen disease or other phakomatoses or may suggest lupus erythematosus or some other systemic disease.

IDENTIFYING THE SITE OF DISORDER

Aspects of the history may suggest the nature of the disorder; specific symptoms and signs suggest the site of the disorder. *Cerebral disease* is implied by seizures or by focal signs that can be attributed to a particular area of the brain; hemiplegia, aphasia, or hemianopia are examples. Generalized manifestations of cerebral disease are seizures, delirium, and dementia. *Brainstem disease* is suggested by cranial nerve palsies, cerebellar signs of ataxia of gait or limbs, tremor, or dysarthria. Dysarthria may be due to incoordination in disorders of the cerebellum itself or its brainstem connections. Cranial nerve palsies or the neuromuscular disorder of myasthenia gravis may also impair speech. Ocular signs have special localizing value. Involuntary movements suggest *basal ganglia disease.*

Spinal cord disease is suggested by spastic gait disorder and bilateral corticospinal signs with or without bladder symptoms. If there is neck or back pain, a compressive lesion should be suspected; if there is no pain, multiple sclerosis is likely. The level of a spinal compressive lesion is more likely to be indicated by cutaneous sensory loss than by motor signs. The lesion that causes spastic paraparesis may be anywhere above the lumbar segments.

Peripheral nerve disease usually causes both motor and sensory symptoms (e.g., weakness and loss of sensation). The weakness is likely to be more severe distally, and the sensory loss may affect only position or vibration sense. A more specific indication of peripheral neuropathy is loss of cutaneous sensation in a glove-and-stocking distribution.

Neuromuscular disorders and *diseases of muscle* cause limb or cranial muscle weakness without sensory symptoms. If limb weakness and loss of tendon jerks are the only signs (with no sensory loss), electromyography and muscle biopsy are needed to determine whether the disorder is one of motor neurons, peripheral nerve, or muscle.

The diseases that cause these symptoms and signs are described later in this volume.

SUGGESTED READINGS

Angel M. Privilege and health—what is the connection? *N Engl J Med* 1993;329:126–127.

Fried R. *The hyperventilation syndrome: research and clinical treatment.* Baltimore: Johns Hopkins University Press, 1987.

Haerer AF. *Dejong's the neurologic examination,* 5th ed. Philadelphia: JB Lippincott Co, 1992.

Mayo Clinic and Foundation. *Clinical examinations in neurology,* 5th ed. Philadelphia: WB Saunders, 1981.

Navarro N. Race or class versus race and class: mortality differences in the United States. *Lancet* 1990;336:1238–1240.

Wiebers DO, ed. *Mayo Clinic examinations in neurology,* 7th ed. St. Louis, MO: Mosby-Year Book, 1998.

Merritt's Neurology, 10th ed., edited by L.P. Rowland. Lippincott Williams & Wilkins, Philadelphia © 2000.

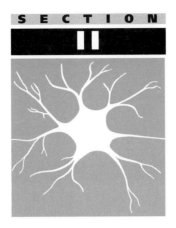

HOW TO SELECT DIAGNOSTIC TESTS

COMPUTED TOMOGRAPHY AND MAGNETIC RESONANCE IMAGING

ROBERT DELAPAZ
STEPHEN CHAN

Computed tomography (CT) and magnetic resonance imaging (MRI) are the core imaging methods in neurodiagnosis. CT is quicker and less expensive, but MRI is now the "gold standard" for detecting and delineating intracranial and spinal lesions. Given the advances in MR technology, including magnetic resonance angiography (MRA), MR spectroscopy (MRS), and functional MRI, the usefulness of MRI will continue to grow. CT technology has also advanced. For instance, spiral or helical CT now permits scanning an entire body part, such as the neck, in less than 1 minute; it also makes CT suitable for angiographic and dynamic studies. In the past, the major advantage of CT was the speed of imaging, which reduced patient discomfort and motion artifact. New ultrafast MR methods such as echo-planar imaging (EPI) are now bringing MRI into the same arena.

COMPUTED TOMOGRAPHY

CT is based on image reconstruction from sets of quantitative x-ray measurements through the head from multiple angles. A fan beam of x-rays emitted from a single source passes through the head to an array of detectors. The x-ray source rotates around the patient's head, and the x-ray attenuation through the section plane is measured in compartments called pixels. The computer reconstructs the image from about 800,000 measurements and assigns a number to each pixel according to its x-ray attenuation (which is proportional to tissue electron density). These values are displayed along a gray scale from black for low density (low attenuation) to white for high density. Iodinated water-soluble contrast agents, which have high x-ray density, can be given intravenously to enhance differences in tissue density, show vascular structures, or detect areas of blood–brain barrier breakdown. CT differentiates between white and gray matter, shows the main divisions of the basal ganglia and thalamus and, after infusion of a contrast agent, depicts the major arteries and veins. CT is especially useful for identifying acute hemorrhage, which appears as much higher density than normal brain or cerebrospinal fluid (CSF).

A scanner gantry houses the x-ray source and detectors; it can be tilted to perform scans at a range of angles from axial to coronal, depending on head position, but not in the sagittal plane. Scan time can be shortened to less than 1 second to minimize motion artifact if the patient is restless. The major limitation of CT is in the posterior fossa, where linear artifacts appear because bone selectively attenuates the x-ray beam; the resulting "beam hardening" creates dense or lucent streaks that project across the brainstem and may obscure underlying lesions.

MAGNETIC RESONANCE IMAGING

A magnetic field causes alignment of atomic nuclei, such as hydrogen protons, into one of two (or more) magnetic states. In proton-based MRI, radiowaves (the radiofrequency pulse) are applied at a frequency that resonates with the hydrogen nucleus in tissue water, resulting in a shift of a small percentage of protons into higher energy states. Following the radiofrequency pulse, relaxation of these protons back to their original energy state is accompanied by the emission of radiowave signals that are characteristic of the particular tissue. Two tissue-specific relaxation-time constants are important. T1 is the longer time constant, generally from 500 to 2,000 milliseconds in the brain, and is a measure of the rate of proton reorientation back along the Z-axis of the magnetic field. T2 is the shorter time constant, usually 40 to 100 milliseconds in the brain, and is a measure of the interaction of protons during the relaxation process. The differences in tissue T1 and T2 relaxation times enable MRI to distinguish between fat, muscle, bone marrow, and gray or white matter of the brain. Most lesions in the brain prolong these relaxation times by increasing the volume or changing the magnetic properties of tissue water.

MR images are displayed as maps of tissue signal intensity values. Spatial localization is achieved by application of a magnetic field gradient across the magnet bore, creating slight variations in radiofrequency across the object being imaged. The specific location of the radiowave emissions can be determined by measurement of the exact radiofrequency. In addition, MR images can be modified for T1 or T2 relaxation characteristics or proton-density characteristics. Factors that influence the results include (1) the imaging technique or pulse sequence (e.g., spin echo, gradient echo, or inversion recovery), (2) the repetition time (the interval between repeated pulse sequences), and (3) the echo time (the interval between radiofrequency excitation and measurement of the radiowave emission or signal). T1-weighted images are most useful for depicting anatomy and show CSF and most lesions as low signal, except for areas of fat, subacute hemorrhage, or gadolinium (Gd) enhancement, which appear as high signal. T2-weighted images are more sensitive for lesion detection and show CSF and most lesions as high signal, except areas of acute hemorrhage or chronic hemosiderin deposits, which appear as low signal. Proton-density images show mixed contrast characteristics, reflecting both T1 and T2 weighting. All three types of images show rapidly flowing blood, dense calcification, cortical bone, and air as signal voids because of flow effects or absence of protons.

The most useful basic MRI technique is the *spin-echo* (SE) pulse sequence, which repeats the sequence of 90- and 180-degree pulses and measures the signal after each 180-degree pulse. The 90-degree pulse creates the radiowave perturbation of the tissue, and the following 180-degree pulse rephases the signal to produce an "echo," which is the signal used for image reconstruction. A double SE method allows both proton-density and

T2-weighted images to be obtained at the same time. *Fast spin-echo* (FSE) methods have reduced 8- to 10-minute acquisition times to 2 to 3 minutes for high-resolution images through the entire brain. The addition of an *inversion* 180-degree pulse before the 90-degree pulse, timed to suppress CSF signal, results in the fluid-attenuated inversion recovery (FLAIR) pulse sequence. FLAIR images are T2-weighted with low-signal CSF and are more sensitive in detecting lesions than SE or FSE pulse sequences. Gradient-echo (GRE) images are created by angles of less than 90 degrees without the 180-degree pulse; gradient switching generates the signal echoes. GRE imaging allows fast acquisition and is useful for detecting subtle magnetic field variations around hemorrhage; it is used primarily for specialized applications, such as MRA.

USES OF COMPUTED TOMOGRAPHY

For reasons of cost, speed, and availability, CT is still widely used for screening in the acute evaluation of stroke, head injury, or acute infections. It is especially useful for patients who are neurologically or medically unstable, uncooperative, or claustrophobic, as well as for patients with pacemakers or other metallic implants. If a mechanical ventilator is being used, CT is used for imaging because most respirators will not function in the high magnetic field of the MR scanner. Although some MR methods are sensitive to acute hemorrhage, its appearance is variable, and in daily clinical practice CT remains superior to MRI for detecting acute extravascular collections of blood, especially subarachnoid hemorrhage (Fig. 13.1). CT is also superior for evaluating cortical bone of the skull and spine, although MRI is superior in studying the bone marrow.

Contrast-enhanced CT (CECT) is used to detect lesions that involve breakdown of the blood–brain barrier, such as brain or spinal tumors, infections, and other inflammatory conditions. CECT is often used to rule out cerebral metastases. However, it is less sensitive than Gd-enhanced MRI (Gd-MRI), which is also better for detection of other intracranial tumors and infections.

Intravenous CT contrast agents are based on iodine, and the older and cheaper agents are classified as high-osmolar contrast media (HOCM). Newer, nonionic agents, classified as low-osmolar contrast media (LOCM), are more expensive but less allergenic, and they cause less morbidity than do HOCM. LOCM are especially useful in patients at high risk for adverse reaction, such as those with severe heart disease, renal insufficiency, asthma, severe debilitation, or previous allergic reaction to iodinated contrast (HOCM).

Spiral or *helical* scanning increases scanning speed to less than 1 second per section and provides large-volume acquisitions that can be used for *three-dimensional* (3D) presentation of anatomic information. Single and multislice spiral scanning is now fast enough to allow acquisition of the entire neck or head during intravenous infusion of a bolus of contrast agent for reconstruction of CT angiography (CTA). Maximum intensity projection (MIP) reformations, often with 3D surface shading, display vascular features such as stenosis or aneurysm. Advantages of CTA over catheter angiography include more widely available technology, less specialized skill requirements, and less invasive intravenous administration of contrast material. However, the use of CTA has been growing slowly because of competition from existing MRA. In contrast to MRA, the iodinated contrast used is potentially more toxic because of allergic reactions and direct cardiac volume stress, as well as renal toxicity. Another limitation of CTA is the time-consuming processing required to edit out bone and cal-

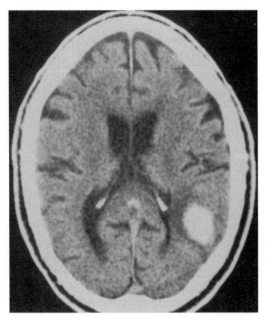
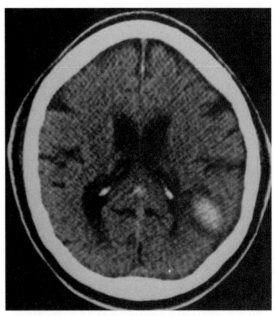

A   B

FIGURE 13.1. Acute intracerebral hemorrhage with resorption over 6 weeks. **A:** Noncontrast axial CT in acute phase shows left parietal hyperdensity with mild mass effect and mild sulcal and ventricular effacement. **B:** Follow-up noncontrast axial CT 1 week later. Note the decrease in density of hemorrhage. Surrounding lucency is due to edema with persistent mass effect.

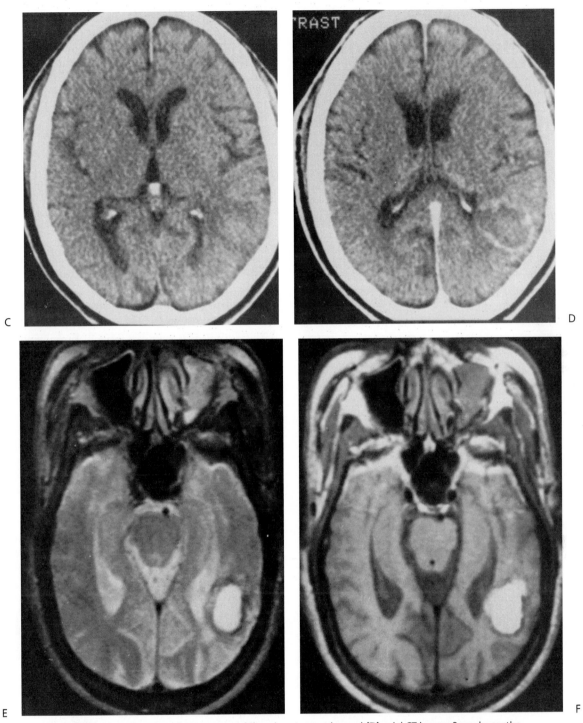

C

D

E

F

FIGURE 13.1. *(Continued)* Noncontrast **(C)** and contrast-enhanced **(D)** axial CT images 3 weeks posthemorrhage show further decrease in density of hemorrhage, which appears isodense in this phase with less surrounding lucency and mass effect. **D:** Peripheral ring enhancement postcontrast. T2-weighted **(E)** and T1-weighted **(F)** axial MR scans 6 weeks posthemorrhage demonstrate near-complete resolution of mass effect. In this subacute phase, hemorrhage typically appears hyperintense on both T2 and T1 pulse sequences, surrounded by a hypointense hemosiderin ring. (Courtesy of Dr. J.A. Bello and Dr. S.K. Hilal.)

cium and to generate 3D surface renderings. Rapid CT is also used to generate brain perfusion studies during a bolus contrast injection. This method suffers from limited volume coverage and the risks of iodinated contrast injection, in contrast to MRI tissue perfusion methods.

USES OF MAGNETIC RESONANCE IMAGING

MRI is the neuroimaging method of choice for most intracranial and intraspinal abnormalities. The technical advantages of MRI are threefold: (1) Greater soft tissue contrast provides better definition of anatomic structures and greater sensitivity to pathologic lesions; (2) multiplanar capability displays dimensional information and relationships that are not readily available on CT; and (3) MRI can better demonstrate physiologic processes such as blood flow, CSF motion, and special properties of tissue such as water diffusion or biochemical makeup (using MRS). Other advantages include better visualization of the posterior fossa, lack of ionizing radiation, and better visualization of intraspinal contents.

There are some disadvantages of MRI. The most practical problem is the need for cooperation from the patient because most individual MRI sequences require several minutes and a complete study lasts 20 to 60 minutes. However, EPI and single-shot FSE methods can acquire low-resolution images in as little as 75 milliseconds and whole brain studies in 30 to 40 seconds. These can be used to salvage an adequate study for identifying or excluding major lesions in uncooperative patients. In addition, about 5% of all persons are claustrophobic inside the conventional MR unit. Oral or intravenous sedation can be used to ensure cooperation, but closer patient monitoring is then required. Development of low-magnetic-field, "open" MRI systems has improved patient acceptance, but these systems sacrifice image quality because of the lower signal-to-noise ratio. High-field (1.5 T), short-bore MR systems reduce patient perception of a closed tube while maintaining full MR capabilities.

MRI is absolutely contraindicated in patients with some metallic implants, especially cardiac pacemakers, cochlear implants, older-generation aneurysm clips, metallic foreign bodies in the eye, and implanted neurostimulators. Newer aneurysm clips have been designed to be nonferromagnetic and non-torqueable at high-magnetic-field strengths, but the U.S. Food and Drug Administration still urges caution in performing MRI in all patients with aneurysm clips. Individual clips may develop unpredictable magnetic properties during manufacture, and careful observation of initial images for magnetic artifacts should be used as an additional precaution. Published lists of MR-compatible clips and metallic objects provide advice about specific clip types and any unusual metallic implants.

Some authorities consider pregnancy (especially in the first trimester) a relative contraindication to MRI, primarily because safety data are incomplete. To date, no harmful effect of MRI has been demonstrated in pregnant women or fetuses, and late-pregnancy fetal MRI has been used clinically. An additional unknown risk to the fetus is the effect of intravenous MR contrast agents such as Gd- and iron-based agents. The urgency, need, and benefits of the MRI study for the patient should be considered in relation to potential unknown risks to the fetus in early pregnancy.

Indications for Gadolinium-enhanced MRI

Most intravenous contrast agents for MRI are chelates of gadolinium, a rare-earth heavy metal. The most commonly used agent is gadopentetate dimeglumine (Gd-DTPA), which is water-soluble and crosses the damaged blood–brain barrier in a manner similar to that of iodinated CT contrast media. The local accumulation of Gd-DTPA shortens both T1 and T2 relaxation times, an effect best seen on T1-weighted images. Lesions that accumulate extravascular Gd-DTPA appear as areas of high signal intensity on T1-weighted images. Comparison with pre-contrast images is needed to exclude preexisting high signal, such as hemorrhage, fat, and, occasionally, calcification. Specialized MR methods can improve detection of Gd-DTPA enhancement. For instance, magnetization transfer improves contrast enhancement, and fat suppression helps in the evaluation of the skull base and orbital regions. Unlike iodinated contrast material, Gd-DTPA administration is associated with few adverse reactions.

Gd-MRI has been most useful in increasing sensitivity to neoplastic and inflammatory lesions. This high sensitivity can show brain tumors that are often difficult to detect on CT, such as small brain metastases, schwannomas (especially within the internal auditory canal), optic nerve or hypothalamic gliomas, and meningeal carcinomatosis. In addition, the multiplanar capability of Gd-MRI delineates the extent of neoplastic lesions so well that the images can be used directly to plan neurosurgery and radiation therapy (Fig. 13.2).

Gd-MRI is superior to CECT in detecting cerebral metastases, but even Gd-MRI at standard dosages can miss metastatic lesions. Newer nonionic Gd-based contrast agents allow up to three times as much contrast agent to be used. In some cases, triple-dose Gd-MRI detects metastases not seen with the standard method. Similar high detection rates can be achieved with standard-dose Gd-DTPA when it is combined with magnetization-transfer MRI. Maximizing lesion sensitivity is especially significant in patients with solitary metastases, for whom surgical resection is a therapeutic option, in contrast to multiple lesions, for which radiation or chemotherapy may be better options.

MRI is the imaging method of choice for detecting the demyelinating plaques of multiple sclerosis in both the brain and spinal cord. Multiple sclerosis plaques are characteristically seen on T2-weighted images as multifocal hyperintense lesions within the periventricular white matter and corpus callosum. They appear ovoid and oriented along medullary veins, perpendicular to the long axis of the lateral ventricles (*Dawson fingers*). Gd-MRI can identify active inflammation by contrast enhancement of acute demyelinating plaques and distinguish them from nonenhancing chronic lesions. Serial Gd-MRI studies allow the progress of the disease to be monitored. Magnetization-transfer imaging, without Gd contrast injection, has also been used to identify abnormal white matter regions that appear normal on T2-weighted images.

Gd-MRI is vastly superior to CECT in the detection of meningitis, encephalitis (especially herpes simplex encephalitis and acute disseminated encephalomyelitis), and myelitis. Epidural abscess or empyema may also be better delineated on Gd-MRI. In acquired immunodeficiency syndrome, many kinds of

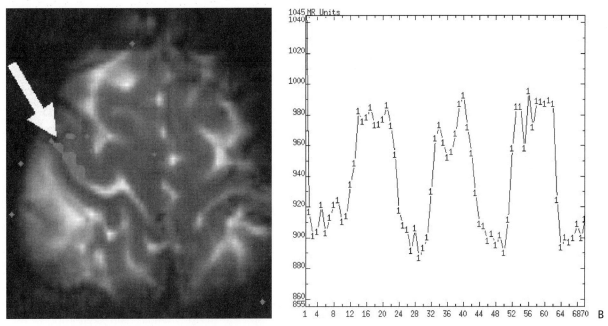

FIGURE 13.2. Functional MRI for surgical planning. **A:** Axial T2*-weighted EPI image acquired during a left-hand grasping task shows activation of the precentral gyrus *(arrow)* immediately anterior to a region of high-signal cortical dysplasia scheduled for surgical resection. **B:** Time–intensity curves show three phases of increased signal, each during a 30-second period of repeated hand grasping separated by 30-second periods of rest. The rise in signal is produced by the BOLD effect, as local increases in blood flow in areas of cortical activation produce increased levels of oxyhemoglobin (decreased levels of de-oxyhemoglobin) in capillaries and venules. (Y-axis represents signal intensity; X-axis shows sequential image numbers, each separated by 3 seconds. EPI GRE pulse sequence with TR 3000 ms, TE 90 ms, flip 90 degrees.)

lesions show increased signal intensity within the cerebral white matter on noncontrast T2-weighted images. These lesions can be further characterized by Gd-MRI. For example, if a single large or dominant enhancing mass is seen on Gd-MRI, the favored diagnosis is cerebral lymphoma. If multiple, small enhancing nodules are found, the possible diagnoses include cerebral toxoplasmosis, granulomas, or fungal infection. When no enhancement is present, the white matter lesions may be the result of human immunodeficiency virus encephalitis (if symmetric) or progressive multifocal leukoencephalopathy (if asymmetric). Thus, the presence or absence of contrast enhancement, the character of contrast enhancement, and the pattern of signal abnormality are all important features in the differential diagnosis.

Gd-MRI is also useful in evaluation of the spine. Herniated discs and degenerative spondylosis can be well evaluated on noncontrast MRI in the unoperated patient, but Gd-MRI is needed in patients with a "failed back syndrome" to separate nonenhancing recurrent disc herniation from enhancing postsurgical scarring or fibrosis. Identification and delineation of spinal tumors and infections are also improved with Gd-MRI. However, Gd enhancement of vertebral bone marrow metastases may make them isointense with normal fatty marrow. Screening precontrast T1-weighted images of the spine should always be obtained. MRI is much more sensitive to bone marrow metastases than conventional radionuclide bone scans. The emergency evaluation of spinal cord compression is also best done with pre- and postcontrast Gd-MRI because multilevel disease can be directly visualized and definitive characterization of lesions can be

done immediately (i.e., intra- versus extramedullary, dural and spinal involvement). For these reasons, the indications for conventional and CT-myelography are decreasing. Outside the spine, fat-suppressed MRI of spinal nerve roots and peripheral nerves, known as MR *neurography,* identifies compressive or traumatic nerve injuries.

Appropriate Utilization of Gadolinium-Enhanced MRI

Some experts have proposed universal administration of Gd for MRI. The use of Gd, however, adds to the direct costs of MRI and increases imaging time, as well as patient discomfort from the intravenous injection. Others recommend that Gd-MRI should be restricted to specific clinical situations in which efficacy has been demonstrated (except when a significant abnormality on routine noncontrast MRI requires further characterization).

In some clinical situations, Gd-MRI is not very useful because relatively few contrast-enhancing lesions are typically found. These clinical situations include complex partial seizures, headache, dementia, head trauma, psychosis, low back or neck pain (in unoperated patients), and congenital craniospinal anomalies. MRI evaluation in many of these conditions would be improved by special MR pulse sequences directed to the structures of greatest interest. For example, patients with temporal lobe epilepsy or Alzheimer disease benefit most by high-resolution imaging of the temporal lobes for evidence of hippocampal atrophy or sclerosis (Fig. 13.3). Patients who have experienced remote head trauma or child abuse might be best served by a T2-weighted GRE pulse sequence, which is more sensitive than the SE pulse sequence in detecting lesions associated with hemosiderin deposition, such as axonal shear injuries or subarachnoid hemosiderosis from repeated subarachnoid hemorrhages.

Magnetic Resonance Angiography

On standard SE images, the major arteries and veins of the neck and brain are usually seen as areas of signal void because of relatively fast blood flow. A GRE pulse sequence can show flowing blood as areas of increased signal intensity known as *flow-related enhancement* (not to be confused with Gd contrast enhancement). In these images, the soft tissues appear relatively dark. After a series of contiguous thin sections is obtained with either two-dimensional or 3D GRE techniques, a map of the blood vessels is reconstructed as a set of MIP angiograms that can be viewed in any orientation and displayed with 3D surface shading. These MRA images, like a conventional angiogram, can show the vascular anatomy but also have the advantage of multiple viewing angles that provide oblique and other nonstandard angiographic views. An advantage of MRA over CTA is that it is completely noninvasive, requiring no contrast injection. MRA does not require specialized catheter skills and avoids the 0.5% to 3% risk of neurologic complications associated with arterial catheter angiography.

In the evaluation of the carotid arteries in the neck or the arteries of the circle of Willis, the most commonly used MRA technique is the *time-of-flight* (TOF) method. TOF is sensitive to T1 relaxation effects and may produce false-positive or obscuring high-signal artifacts from orbital fat, hemorrhage, or areas of Gd enhancement. Another important MRA technique, the *phase-contrast* (PC) technique, depends on the phase (rather than magnitude) of the MR signal. PC technique shows the direction and velocity of blood flow, may be adjusted to low or high flow sensitivity, and is useful for evaluating altered hemodynamics, such as flow reversal after major vessel occlusion or stenosis.

MRA occasionally overestimates cervical carotid stenosis because of local turbulent flow, but it compares favorably with conventional angiography in detecting carotid stenosis. Conventional angiography is still the "gold standard" for cerebrovascular imaging, but extracranial carotid evaluation is now done primarily with ultrasound and MRA.

Indications for MRA include stroke, transient ischemic attack (TIA), possible venous sinus thrombosis, arteriovenous malformation (AVM), and vascular tumors (for delineation of vascular supply and displacements). It is thought that MRA reliably detects aneurysms as small as 3 mm. Conventional angiography, however, is still the most sensitive examination for evaluation of intracranial aneurysms or AVMs because of its higher spatial resolution and ability to observe the rapid sequence of vascular filling, especially the early venous filling seem with AVMs.

Functional MRI

The term *functional* is used here in a broad sense to encompass several MRI methods that are used to image physiologic processes such as tissue blood flow, water diffusion, and biochemical makeup (with MRS), as well as cerebral activation with sensory, motor, and cognitive tasks. Tissue blood flow is most commonly imaged with MRI using a *first-pass* or *bolus-tracking* method that records the signal changes occurring when rapidly repeated images are acquired during the first passage of an intravascular bolus of paramagnetic contrast material through the

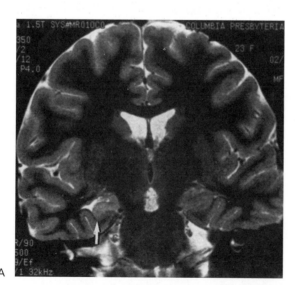 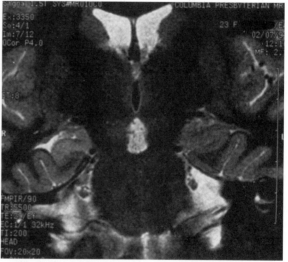

FIGURE 13.3. High-resolution image of the temporal lobes. **A:** High-resolution (512 × 512 matrix) coronal MR scan through the temporal lobes obtained with the use of short-tau inversion recovery (STIR) pulse sequence shows increased signal intensity within the right hippocampus *(arrow)*. The normal left hippocampus is well visualized, with clear definition of internal architecture. **B:** Magnification view allows close inspection of the hippocampi with no significant distortion because a high-resolution image was obtained. Patient has presumed right mesial temporal sclerosis associated with a clinical and electroencephalogram-defined syndrome of right temporal lobe epilepsy.

brain, usually Gd-DTPA. Using T2*- or T2-weighted EPI or fast GRE techniques, MR images are acquired every 1 to 3 seconds over the whole brain, and the signal decreases that occur in each tissue with passage of the contrast bolus are plotted against time. The area under this time–intensity curve is proportional to cerebral blood volume (CBV), and other manipulations of the data can give cerebral blood flow (CBF), mean transit time (MTT), and other measures of tissue perfusion. This method has been used most extensively with primary brain tumors, where CBV seems to correlate well with histologic tumor grade and demonstrates responses to treatment of the tumor. The obvious application to cerebral ischemic disease has become more widespread, and measures of perfusion delay, such as MTT and time to peak, are sensitive indicators of small reductions in cerebral perfusion. A second method of MR perfusion imaging is called *spin tagging* or *TOF* imaging and, like TOF MRA, depends on T1 relaxation and flow enhancement phenomena, without the use of injected contrast agents. This method is less widely used than bolus tracking but gives more quantitative CBF measurements.

A second important functional MRI technique is *diffusion-weighted imaging* (DWI). This is most commonly performed using an EPI SE pulse sequence with gradients added before and after the 180-degree pulse. On DW images, areas of high diffusion show up as low signal, and those with low diffusion appear as high signal. Quantitative *apparent diffusion coefficient* (ADC) maps can be generated to display diffusion with the opposite polarity: high ADC as high signal and low ADC as low signal. Severe cerebral ischemia causes a rapid decrease in intracellular diffusion, and high signal appears on DWI within minutes of cell injury. After the initial reduction in diffusion, there is a gradual rise through normal to prolonged diffusion rates during the 1 to 2 weeks after infarction, as cells disintegrate and freely diffusible water dominates the encephalomalacic tissue. A minor pitfall of DWI is called "T2 shine-through," where high signal on T2-weighted images may produce high signal on DWI, falsely indicating reduced diffusion. This error can be avoided by the use of calculated ADC maps. DWI is an essential part of acute stroke imaging, and because it takes less than 1 minute to acquire a whole-brain study, it is widely used. DWI can be combined with perfusion imaging to identify the so-called *penumbra zone* of potentially salvageable tissue within the area of reduced perfusion but outside the unrecoverable infarct, represented by DWI high signal.

MRS can be performed with clinical high-field MR scanners. Proton spectroscopy is most widely used and produces semi-quantitative spectra of common tissue metabolites, including *N*-acetylaspartate (NAA; a marker of healthy neurons and axons), creatine (the molecular storage depot for high-energy phosphates), choline (a component of cell membranes and myelin), and lactate (elevated with normal tissue energetic stress and in many pathologic tissues). Proton spectra can be obtained from as little as 0.5 cc of tissue at 1.5 T and MRS images can be generated to show metabolite distributions, albeit at lower spatial resolution than anatomic MR images. The most widely accepted clinical use of proton MRS is the identification of brain neoplasms that tend to show a characteristic but not completely specific pattern of elevated choline, reduced NAA, and elevated lactate. MRS is also used to characterize multiple sclerosis plaques,

degenerative diseases such as Alzheimer disease or amyotrophic lateral sclerosis, and metabolic disorders such as MELAS.

Using MRI to map cerebral activation is specifically called *functional MRI* (fMRI). The technique most widely used is the *blood-oxygen-level-dependent* (BOLD) method, which is based on local increases in CBF and the consequent shift from deoxyhemoglobin to oxyhemoglobin in areas of cerebral activation. With T2*- or T2-weighted EPI or fast GRE images and rapidly repeated acquisitions (every 1 to 3 seconds), MR images show small increases in signal in areas of cerebral activation. BOLD fMRI has been used in research on motor, sensory, and cognitive activation. Growing clinical applications of fMRI include mapping of motor, sensory, and language function prior to surgery, radiation therapy, or embolization procedures; monitoring recovery of function after brain injury or stroke; and mapping specific cognitive changes in degenerative brain diseases.

PARADIGM: DIAGNOSTIC WORKUP FOR STROKE

In the first evaluation of patients with stroke, either CT or MRI can be used. In many centers, CT is the primary choice because of availability, immediate access, less need for patient cooperation, and lower cost. In addition, hemorrhage, calcification, and skull fracture are easy to recognize on CT. CT is less sensitive than MRI, however, in showing nonhemorrhagic infarction in the first 24 hours after the ictus. In addition, infarcts within the brainstem and cerebellum are usually better demonstrated by MRI.

MRI is the modality of choice for acute ischemic stroke because of the high sensitivity and specificity of DWI. As noted above, DWI can specifically identify cerebral infarction within minutes of onset, and, when combined with quantitative ADC maps, can specify the age of a lesion to within a few days. FLAIR imaging also shows high signal in acute infarcts and is sensitive to lesions within the first 6 to 12 hours. A comparison of T2-weighted and proton-density MRI to CT found that within the first 24 hours 82% of lesions were seen on MRI, whereas only 58% were seen on CT. The earliest changes are seen on proton-density-weighted images, with hyperintensity present within the affected cortical gray matter. During the first 5 days after stroke onset, Gd enhancement may be seen within the small arteries of the ischemic vascular territory, with gyral cortical enhancement present 5 days to several months after onset. The focal reversible lesions of TIAs are also more frequently seen on MRI than on CT.

MRA and duplex ultrasonography of the carotid arteries are then used to evaluate possible underlying carotid stenosis. If necessary, invasive angiography can corroborate the presence of carotid stenosis and may depict ulcerations that are not well seen on MRA or duplex ultrasonography.

MRA of the brain is also useful in determining patency of the vessels of the circle of Willis. Acute occlusions of the major vessels of the circle of Willis or of the superior portions of the internal carotid arteries and basilar artery can be detected, but occlusion of small distal branches is not as well demonstrated (Fig. 13.4). Arterial and venous flow can be separated to identify ve-

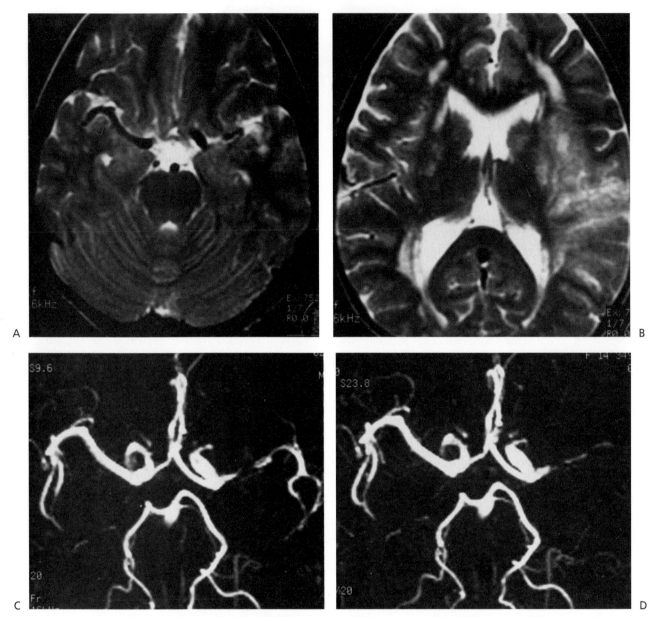

FIGURE 13.4. A,B: T2-weighted axial MR scans demonstrate increased signal intensity within the opercular areas of the left frontal and temporal lobes, consistent with acute ischemia or infarction. Note the decreased visualization of left middle cerebral artery flow void as compared to right. **C:** Collapsed (base) view of an MR angiogram of the circle of Willis shows marked stenosis of the M1 (first) segment of the left middle cerebral artery (MCA). **D:** Follow-up collapsed (base) view of an MR angiogram of the circle of Willis demonstrates virtually complete occlusion of the left MCA. Progression occurred despite aggressive medical therapy, including anticoagulation.

nous occlusion. MRA can also be used serially for evaluation of therapy, such as intraarterial thrombolysis, but conventional angiography may still be useful in early diagnostic evaluation and is necessary for intraarterial thrombolytic therapy.

SUGGESTED READINGS

Adamson AJ, Rand SD, Prost RW, Kim TA, Schultz C, Haughton VM. Focal brain lesions: effect of single-voxel proton MR spectroscopic findings on treatment decisions. *Radiology* 1998;209:73–78.

Akeson P, Larsson EM, Kristoffersen DT, Jonsson E, Holtas S. Brain metastases—comparison of gadodiamide injection-enhanced MR imaging at standard and high dose, contrast-enhanced CT and non-contrast-enhanced MR imaging. *Acta Radiol* 1995;36:300–306.

Anderson CM, Saloner D, Lee RE, et al. Assessment of carotid artery stenosis by MR angiography: comparison with x-ray angiography and color-coded Doppler ultrasound. *AJNR* 1992;13:989–1008.

Atlas SW, Mark AS, Grossman RI, Gomori JM. Intracranial hemorrhage: gradient-echo MR imaging at 1.5 T. *Radiology* 1988;168:803–807.

Atlas SW, Sheppard L, Goldberg HI, Hurst RW, Listerud J, Flamm E. Intracranial aneurysms: detection and characterization with MR angiography with use of an advanced postprocessing technique in a blinded-reader study. *Radiology* 1997;203:807–814.

Baird AE, Warach S. Magnetic resonance imaging of acute stroke. *J Cereb Blood Flow Metab* 1998;18:583–609.

Brant-Zawadzki M, Heiserman JE. The roles of MR angiography, CT angiography, and sonography in vascular imaging of the head and neck. *AJNR* 1997;18:1820–1825.

Bryan RN, Levy LM, Whitlow WD, et al. Diagnosis of acute cerebral infarction: comparison of CT and MR imaging. *AJNR* 1991;12:611–620.

Carmody RF, Yang PJ, Seeley GW, Seeger JF, Unger EC, Johnson JE. Spinal cord compression due to metastatic disease: diagnosis with MR imaging versus myelography. *Radiology* 1989;173:225–229.

Castillo M, Kwock L, Scatliff J, Mukherji SK. Proton MR spectroscopy in neoplastic and non-neoplastic brain disorders. *Magn Reson Imaging Clin N Am* 1998;6:1–20.

Davis PC, Hudgins PA, Peterman SB, Hoffman JC. Diagnosis of cerebral metastases: double-dose delayed CT vs. contrast-enhanced MR imaging. *AJNR* 1991;12:293–300.

De Coene B, Hajnal JV, Gatehouse P, et al. MR of the brain using fluid-attenuated inversion recovery (FLAIR) pulse sequences. *AJNR* 1992;13:1555–1564.

DeLaPaz RL. Echo planar imaging. *Radiographics* 1994;14:1045–1058.

Edelman RR, Warach S. Magnetic resonance imaging. *N Engl J Med* 1993;328:708–716.

Gonzalez RG, Schaefer PW, Buonanno FS, et al. Diffusion-weighted MR imaging: diagnostic accuracy in patients imaged within 6 hours of stroke symptom onset. *Radiology* 1999;210:155–162.

Grossman RI, Gomori JM, Ramer KN, Lexa FJ, Schnall MD. Magnetization transfer: theory and clinical applications in neuroradiology. *Radiographics* 1994;14:279–290.

Heinz R, Wiener D, Friedman H, Tien R. Detection of cerebrospinal fluid metastasis: CT myelography or MR? *AJNR* 1995;16:1147–1151.

Heldmann U, Myschetzky PS, Thomsen HS. Frequency of unexpected multifocal metastasis in patients with acute spinal cord compression: evaluation by low-field MR imaging in cancer patients. *Acta Radiol* 1997;38:372–375.

Jack CR, Petersen RC, O'Brien PC, Tangalos EG. MR-based hippocampal volumetry in the diagnosis of Alzheimer's disease. *Neurology* 1992;42:183–188.

Jack CR, Sharbrough FW, Twomey CK, et al. Temporal lobe seizures: lateralization with MR volume measurements of the hippocampal formation. *Radiology* 1990;175:423–429.

Jensen MC, Brant-Zawadski M. MR imaging of the brain in patients with

AIDS: value of routine use of IV gadopentetate dimeglumine. *AJR* 1993;160:153–157.

Katayama H, Yamaguchi K, Kozuka T, et al. Adverse reactions to ionic and nonionic contrast media: a report from the Japanese committee on the safety of contrast media. *Radiology* 1990;175:621–628.

Mathews VP, Caldemeyer KS, Ulmer JL, Nguyen H, Yuh WT. Effects of contrast dose, delayed imaging, and magnetization transfer saturation on gadolinium-enhanced MR imaging of brain lesions. *J Magn Reson Imaging* 1997;7:14–22.

Miller DH, Grossman RI, Reingold SC, McFarland HF. The role of magnetic resonance techniques in understanding and managing multiple sclerosis. *Brain* 1998;121:3–24.

Murphy KJ, Brunberg JA, Cohan RH. Adverse reactions to gadolinium contrast media: a review of 36 cases. *AJR* 1996;167:847–849.

Mushlin AI, Detsky AS, Phelps CE, et al. The accuracy of magnetic resonance imaging in patients with suspected multiple sclerosis. *JAMA* 1993;269:3146–3151.

Ogawa S, Menon RS, Kim SG, Ugurbil K. On the characteristics of functional magnetic resonance imaging of the brain. *Annu Rev Biophys Biomol Struct* 1998;27:447–474.

Ross B, Michaelis T. Clinical applications of magnetic resonance spectroscopy. *Magn Reson Q* 1994;10:191–247.

Ross JS, Masaryk TJ, Schrader M, et al. MR imaging of the postoperative lumbar spine: assessment with gadopentetate dimeglumine. *AJNR* 1990;11:771–776.

Schwartz RB, Tice HM, Hooten SM, Hsu L, Stieg PE. Evaluation of cerebral aneurysms with helical CT: correlation with conventional angiography and MR angiography. *Radiology* 1994;192:717–722.

Shellock FG. *Pocket guide to MR procedures and metallic objects.* New York: Raven Press, 1995.

Shellock FG, Kanal E. *Magnetic resonance bioeffects, safety and patient management.* New York: Raven Press, 1994.

Sorenson AG, Copen WA, Ostergard L, et al. Hyperacute stroke: simultaneous measurement of relative cerebral blood volume, relative cerebral blood flow, and mean tissue transit time. *Radiology* 1999;210:519–527.

Sze G, Zimmerman RD. The magnetic resonance imaging of infectious and inflammatory diseases. *Radiol Clin North Am* 1988;26:839–885.

Merritt's Neurology, 10th ed., edited by L.P. Rowland. Lippincott Williams & Wilkins, Philadelphia © 2000.

CHAPTER 14

ELECTROENCEPHALOGRAPHY AND EVOKED POTENTIALS

RONALD G. EMERSON
THADDEUS S. WALCZAK
TIMOTHY A. PEDLEY

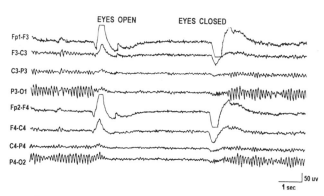

FIGURE 14.1. Normal EEG in an awake 28-year-old man.

Electroencephalography (EEG) and evoked potentials (EPs) are measures of brain electric activity. EEG reflects spontaneous brain activity, whereas EPs reflect activity of the central nervous system in response to specific stimuli. In contrast to anatomic imaging techniques, such as computed tomography and magnetic resonance imaging, which provide information about brain structure, EEG and EP studies provide information about brain function. Functional and structural investigations are often complementary. Electrophysiologic studies are particularly important when neurologic disorders are unaccompanied by detectable alteration in brain structure. This chapter provides an overview of the current capabilities and limitations of these techniques in clinical practice.

ELECTROENCEPHALOGRAPHY

Normal Adult EEG

EEG activity is characterized by the frequency and voltage of the signals. A major feature of the EEG during wakefulness is the alpha rhythm, an 8- to 12-cycles-per-second (cps) parietooccipital rhythm (Fig. 14.1). The alpha rhythm is best seen when the patient is awake and relaxed with eyes closed. It attenuates when the eyes are opened, or the subject is alerted. Beta activity, between 13 and 25 cps, is usually maximal in the frontal and central regions. High-voltage beta activity suggests the effect of sedative-hypnotic medication. A small amount of slower frequencies may be diffusely distributed.

Sleep is divided into five stages on the basis of the combinations of EEG patterns, eye movements, and axial electromyography (EMG). Stage 1 is a transitional period between wakefulness and sleep. The alpha rhythm disappears during stage 1 and is replaced by low-voltage, slower activity. Vertex waves, high-voltage, "sharp" transients, are recorded maximally at the vertex. Stage 2 sleep is characterized by sleep spindles (symmetric 12- to 14-cps sinusoidal waves). The EEG in stages 3 and 4 is composed of high-voltage, widely distributed, slow-wave activity. Rapid eye movement (REM) sleep is characterized by low-voltage, mixed-frequency activity, similar to that in early stage 1, together with REM and generalized atonia. REM occurs about 90 minutes after sleep onset in adults and is not usually seen in routine studies. The presence of REM in a daytime EEG suggests sleep deprivation, withdrawal

from REM-suppressant drugs, alcohol withdrawal, or narcolepsy (Chapter 145).

Common EEG Abnormalities

Diffuse slowing of background rhythms is the most common EEG abnormality (Fig. 14.2). This finding is nonspecific and is present in patients with diffuse encephalopathies of diverse causes, including toxic, metabolic, anoxic, and degenerative. Multiple structural abnormalities can also cause diffuse slowing.

Focal slowing suggests localized parenchymal dysfunction (Fig. 14.3). Focal neuroradiologic abnormalities are found in 70% of patients with significant focal slowing and must always be suspected in this situation. Focal slowing may also be seen in patients with focal seizure disorders, even when no lesions are found. Focal voltage attenuation usually indicates localized lesions of gray matter but may also be seen with focal subdural, epidural, or even subgaleal fluid collections (Fig. 14.3).

Triphasic waves typically consist of generalized synchronous waves occurring in brief runs (Fig. 14.4). Approximately one-half the patients with triphasic waves have hepatic encephalopathy, and the remainder have other toxic-metabolic encephalopathies.

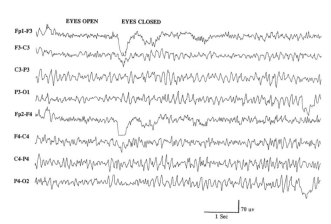

FIGURE 14.2. Diffuse slowing in a 67-year-old patient with dementia. Six- to seven-cps activity predominates over the parietooccipital regions. Although reactive to eye closure, the frequency of this rhythm is abnormally slow.

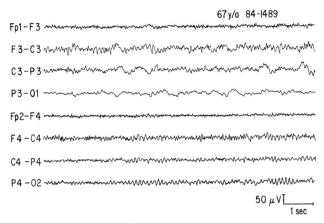

FIGURE 14.3. Focal slow activity with attenuation of the alpha rhythm over the left hemisphere in a 67-year-old patient with an acute left hemispheral infarction.

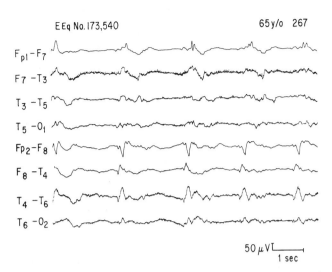

FIGURE 14.5. Right hemispheral PLEDs in a 65-year-old patient with herpes simplex encephalitis. (From Pedley TA, Emerson RG. Clinical neurophysiology. In: Bradley WG, Daroff RB, Fenichel GM, Marsden CD, eds. *Neurology in clinical practice*, 2nd ed. Boston: Butterworth-Heinemann, 1996:460; with permission.)

Epileptiform discharges (EDs) are the interictal hallmark of epilepsy. They are strongly associated with seizure disorders and are uncommon in normal adults. The type of ED may also suggest a specific epileptic syndrome (see the following).

Periodic lateralizing epileptiform discharges (PLEDs) suggest the presence of an acute destructive cerebral lesion. Focal EDs recur at 1 to 2 cps in the setting of a focally slow or attenuated background (Fig. 14.5). In a study of nearly 600 patients with PLEDs, the finding was related to an acute cerebral infarction in 35%, to other mass lesions in 26%, and to cerebral infection, anoxia, or other causes in the the remainder. Clinically, PLEDs are associated with seizures, obtundation, and focal neurologic signs.

Generalized periodic sharp waves typically recur at 0.5 to 1 cps on an attenuated background. This pattern is most commonly seen following cerebral anoxia. It is also recorded in about 90% of patients with Creutzfeldt-Jakob disease.

CLINICAL UTILITY OF ELECTROENCEPHALOGRAPHY

Epilepsy

The EEG is the most useful laboratory test to help establish the diagnosis of epilepsy and assist in the accurate classification of specific epileptic syndromes. Characteristic interictal EDs strongly support the diagnosis of epilepsy, but absence of EDs does not rule out this diagnosis. EDs are recorded in 30% to 50% of epileptic patients on the first routine EEG and in 60% to 90% by the third routine EEG. Further EEGs do not appreciably increase the yield. Thus, 10% to 40% of patients with epilepsy do not demonstrate interictal discharges, even on several EEGs. Sleep, sleep deprivation, hyperventilation, and photic stimulation increase the likelihood of recording EDs in some patients.

Conversely, interictal EDs are infrequent in healthy normal subjects or patients without epilepsy. EDs occur in only 1.5% to 3.5% of healthy normal children. Siblings of children with benign focal epilepsy or petit mal absence without seizures may also have interictal EDs recorded incidentally. EDs occur in 2.7% of adult patients with various illnesses, including neurologic diseases, but with no history of seizures. The presence of EDs with the appropriate clinical findings strongly supports the diagnosis of epilepsy but does not establish it unequivocally.

The type of interictal ED, together with the patient's clinical features, often allows diagnosis of a specific epileptic syndrome. Confident diagnosis of an epileptic syndrome leads to proper treatment and provides information regarding prognosis. Table 14.1 summarizes specific characteristics of epileptiform abnormalities in some common epileptic syndromes. Clinical features of the syndromes are summarized in Chapter 140. A useful example is the distinction between generalized 3-cps spike and wave and temporal spike and

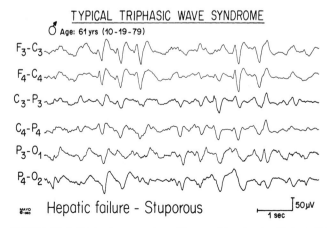

FIGURE 14.4. Triphasic waves in a 61-year-old patient with hepatic failure. (Courtesy of Bruce J. Fisch.)

TABLE 14.1. EPILEPTIFORM ABNORMALITIES IN THE COMMON EPILEPSY SYNDROMES

West syndrome (hypsarrhythmia)	No organized background rhythm Random high-voltage slow activity Multifocal epileptiform discharges Abrupt attenuation (infantile spasm)
Lennox Gastaut syndrome	Slow generalized spike and wave (<2 cps) Significantly slowed background rhythm
Childhood absence epilepsy	Generalized spike and wave (>3 cps) Usually precipitated by hyperventilation Normal background rhythm
Benign rolandic epilepsy	Focal centrotemporal epileptiform discharge Normal background rhythm
Juvenile myoclonic epilepsy	Generalized polyspike wave (often >3 cps) May be precipitated by photic stimulation Normal background rhythm
Localization-related epilepsy (e.g., temporal lobe seizures)	Focal epileptiform discharges Occasional focal slowing Occasional mild slowing of background

wave. Three-cps spike and wave is seen in childhood absence epilepsy, an epileptic syndrome with early age of onset, absence and tonic-clonic seizures, and relatively good prognosis (Fig. 14.6). Either ethosuximide (Zarontin) or valproic acid (Depakene) is the medication of choice. In contrast, temporal-lobe spikes are seen in complex partial seizures or complex partial seizures with secondary generalization (Fig. 14.7). Prognosis is poorer, and phenytoin sodium (Dilantin), carbamazepine (Tegretol), or barbiturates are the medications of choice.

Dementia and Diffuse Encephalopathies

The EEG provides useful clues in obtunded patients. Triphasic waves suggest a toxic-metabolic cause. High-voltage beta activity suggests the presence of sedative-hypnotic medications. Generalized voltage attenuation is seen in Huntington disease. Generalized periodic sharp waves are seen in about 90% of patients with Creutzfeldt-Jakob disease within 12 weeks of clinical onset. EEG is critical when spike-wave stupor is the cause of obtundation. EEG may be normal early in the course of Alzheimer disease, when cognitive changes are minor and the diagnosis is still uncertain. As moderate to severe symptoms appear, diffuse slowing is seen (see Fig. 14.2). Almost all patients with biopsy-proven Alzheimer disease have unequivocal EEG abnormalities within 3 years of the onset of symptoms. Focal slowing is uncommon and, if present, suggests multiinfarct dementia or another multifocal cause.

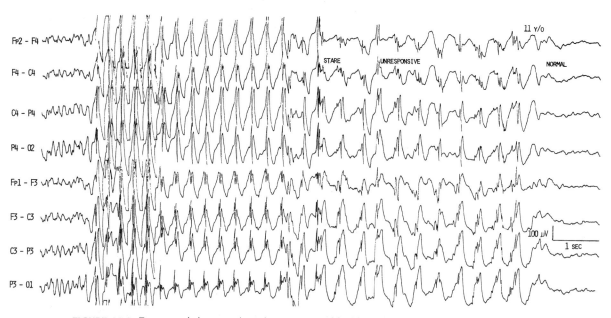

FIGURE 14.6. Ten-second absence seizure in an 11-year-old with staring spells. Three- to four-cps generalized spike wave is seen at the beginning of the seizure. The rate gradually slows toward the end of the seizure. Then patient was asked to follow a simple command 6 seconds after seizure onset and was unable to do so.

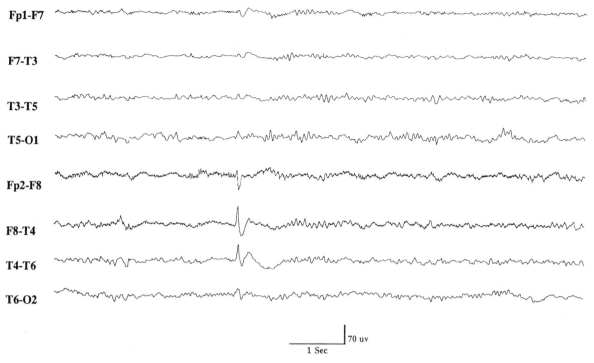

FIGURE 14.7. Right anterior temporal epileptiform discharge in a 32-year-old patient with complex partial seizures emerging from the right temporal lobe.

Focal Brain Lesions

As neuroimaging has become widely available, EEG has come to play a less important role in the diagnosis of structural lesions. EEG is necessary, however, to assess the epileptogenic potential of mass lesions. Focal EEG abnormalities accompany one-half of hemispheral transient ischemic attacks. Normal EEG in a patient with a neurologic deficit strongly suggests a lacunar infarction. EEG slowing in hemispheral infarcts gradually improves with time, whereas focal slowing in neoplasms remains the same or worsens. This difference can be useful when neuroradiologic findings do not distinguish between semiacute infarction and neoplasm.

Cerebral Infections

Focal changes are noted in more than 80% of patients with herpes encephalitis, and PLEDs are seen in more than 70% (see Fig. 14.5). PLEDs typically appear 2 to 15 days after onset of illness, but the interval may be as long as 1 month. Serial EEG is therefore useful if early studies are nonfocal. Early focal findings strongly suggest this diagnosis if the clinical picture is compatible, and may indicate the appropriate site for biopsy. Virtually diagnostic EEG changes are seen in subacute sclerosing panencephalitis: stereotyped bursts of high-voltage delta waves at regular intervals of 4 to 10 seconds. Early in the disease, slow-wave bursts may be infrequent or confined to sleep, so serial EEG may be useful. EEG findings in patients infected with human immunodeficiency virus are nonspecific. Diffuse slowing may precede clinical neurologic manifestations. The slowing becomes more persistent in patients with dementia related to acquired immunodeficiency syndrome. Focal slowing suggests the presence of a superimposed cerebral lesion, such as lymphoma or toxoplasmosis.

EVOKED POTENTIALS

Principles of Evoked Potential Recording

Visual, auditory, and somatosensory stimuli cause small electric signals to be produced by neural structures along the corresponding sensory pathways. These EPs are generally of much lower voltage than ongoing spontaneous cortical electric activity. They are usually not apparent in ordinary EEG recordings and are detected with the use of averaging techniques. Changes in EPs produced by disease states generally consist of delayed responses, reflecting conduction delays in responsible pathways, or attenuation or loss of component waveforms, resulting from conduction block or dysfunction of the responsible generator.

Clinically, EP tests are best viewed as an extension of the neurologic examination. Abnormalities identify dysfunction in specific sensory pathways and suggest the location of a responsible lesion. They are most useful when they identify abnormalities that are clinically inapparent or confirm abnormalities that correspond to vague or equivocal signs or symptoms.

Visual Evoked Potentials

The preferred stimulus for visual evoked potential (VEP) testing is a checkerboard pattern of black and white squares. *Pattern re-*

versal (i.e., change of the white squares to black and the black squares to white) produces an occipital positive signal, the P100, approximately 100 milliseconds after the stimulus. Because fibers arising from the nasal portion of each retina decussate at the optic chiasm (Fig. 14.8), an abnormality in the P100 response to stimulation of one eye necessarily implies dysfunction anterior to the optic chiasm on that side. Conversely, delayed P100 responses following stimulation of both eyes separately may result from bilateral abnormalities either anterior or posterior to the chiasm or at the chiasm. Unilateral hemispheral lesions do not alter the latency of the P100 component because of the contribution of a normal response from the intact hemisphere.

Acute optic neuritis is accompanied by loss or severe attenuation of the VEP. Although the VEP returns, the latency of the P100 response almost always remains abnormally delayed, even if vision returns to normal (Fig. 14.9). Pattern-reversal VEPs (PRVEPs) are abnormal in nearly all patients with a definite history of optic neuritis. More important, PRVEPs are abnormal in about 70% of patients with definite multiple sclerosis who have no history of optic neuritis.

Despite the sensitivity of PRVEPs to demyelinating lesions of the optic nerve, the VEP changes produced by plaques are often not distinguishable from those produced by many other diseases that affect the visual system; these include ocular disease (major refractive error, media opacities, glaucoma, retinopathies), compressive lesions of the optic nerve (extrinsic tumors, optic nerve tumors), noncompressive optic nerve lesions (ischemic optic neuritis, nutritional and toxic

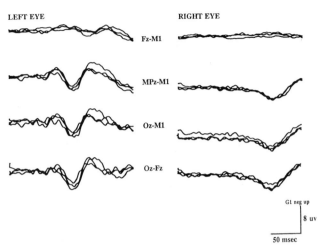

FIGURE 14.9. Pattern shift VEP in a patient with right optic neuritis. The response to left eye stimulation is normal. Right eye stimulation produces a marked delay of the P100 response. The relative preservation of waveform morphology despite pronounced latency prolongation is typical of demyelinating optic neuropathies. Unless otherwise specified, electrode positions are standard locations of the International 10–20 System. *MPz* corresponds to an electrode positioned midway between *Oz* and *Pz. M1* is an electrode on the left mastoid process.

amblyopias), and diseases affecting the nervous system diffusely (adrenoleukodystrophy, Pelizaeus-Merzbacher disease, spinocerebellar degenerations, Parkinson disease). VEPs can help distinguish blindness from hysteria and malingering. If a patient reports visual loss, a normal VEP strongly favors a psychogenic disorder.

Brainstem Auditory Evoked Potentials

Brainstem auditory evoked potentials (BAEPs) are generated by the auditory nerve and the brainstem in response to a "click" stimulus. The normal BAEP includes a series of signals that occurs within 7 milliseconds after the stimulus, comprising three components important to clinical interpretation (Fig. 14.10): wave I arising from the peripheral portion of the auditory nerve; wave III generated in the tegmentum of the caudal pons, most likely the superior olive or the trapezoid body; and wave V generated in the region of the inferior colliculus. Although brainstem auditory pathways decussate at multiple levels, unilateral abnormalities of waves III and V are most often associated with ipsilateral brainstem disease.

BAEPs in Neurologic Disorders

The clinical utility of BAEPs derives from (1) the close relationship of BAEP waveform abnormalities and structural pathology of their generators and (2) the resistance of BAEPs to alteration by systemic metabolic abnormalities or medications. BAEPs are often abnormal when structural brainstem lesions exist (Fig. 14.11). They are virtually always abnormal in patients with brainstem gliomas. Conversely, brainstem lesions that spare the auditory pathways, such as

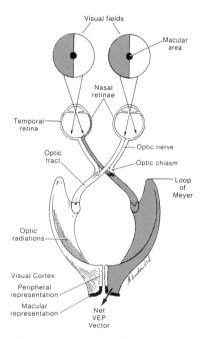

FIGURE 14.8. Primary visual pathways illustrating decussation of nasal retinal fibers at the optic chiasm and projections to the visual cortex. (From Epstein CM. Visual evoked potentials. In: Daly DD, Pedley TA, eds. *Current practice of clinical electroencephalography,* 2nd ed. New York: Raven Press, 1997:565; with permission.)

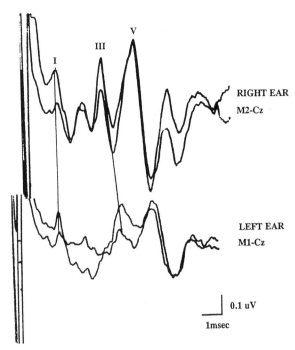

FIGURE 14.10. BAEP study in a patient with a left intracanalicular acoustic neuroma. The BAEP to right ear stimulation is normal. The I to III interpeak latency is prolonged following left ear stimulation, reflecting delayed conduction between the distal eighth nerve and the lower pons.

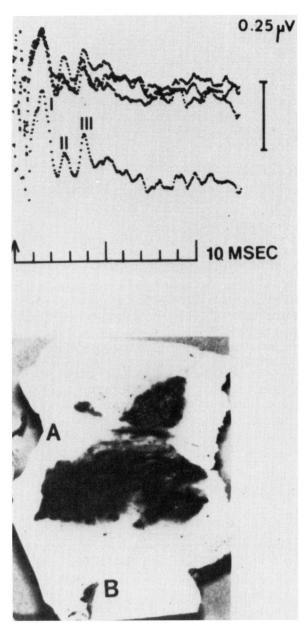

FIGURE 14.11. Abnormal BAEP recorded in a patient with a brainstem hemorrhage sparing the lower one-third of the pons. Waves IV and V are lost, but waves I, II, and III are preserved. (From Chiappa KH. Evoked potentials in clinical medicine. In: Baker AB, Baker LH, eds. *Clinical neurology.* New York: Harper & Row, 1990:22; with permission.)

ventral pontine infarcts producing the locked-in syndrome or lateral medullary infarcts, do not produce abnormal BAEPs. Barbiturate levels high enough to produce an isoelectric EEG leave BAEPs unchanged, as do hepatic and renal failure. BAEPs are therefore useful for demonstrating brainstem integrity in toxic and metabolic perturbations that severely alter the EEG.

BAEPs are sensitive for detection of tumors of the eighth cranial nerve; abnormalities are demonstrated in more than 90% of patients with acoustic neuroma. BAEP abnormalities seen with acoustic neuromas and other cerebellopontine angle tumors range from prolongation of the I to III interpeak interval, thereby indicating a conduction delay between the distal eighth cranial nerve and lower pons (see Fig. 14.10), to preservation of wave I with loss of subsequent components, to loss of all BAEP waveforms. The sensitivity of the BAEP to acoustic nerve lesions can be extended by decreasing the stimulus intensity over a prescribed range and evaluating the effects on the BAEP waveforms (*latency-intensity function*). Some patients with small intracanalicular tumors have normal standard BAEPs, and abnormality is revealed only by latency-intensity function testing.

BAEPs help establish the diagnosis of multiple sclerosis when they detect clinically unsuspected or equivocal brainstem lesions. BAEPs are abnormal in about 33% of patients with multiple sclerosis, including 20% of those who have no other signs or symptoms of brainstem lesions. The BAEP findings in multiple sclerosis consist of the absence or decreased amplitude of BAEP components, or an increase in the III to V interpeak latency.

BAEPs may be useful in demonstrating brainstem involvement in generalized diseases of myelin, such as metachromatic leukodystrophy, adrenoleukodystrophy, and Pelizaeus-Merzbacher disease. BAEP abnormalities may also be demonstrable in asymptomatic heterozygotes for adrenoleukodystrophy.

BAEPs are also used to evaluate hearing in infants and others who cannot cooperate for standard audiologic tests. The latency-intensity test permits determination of the wave V threshold, as well as the relationship of wave V latency to stimulus intensity, and often allows characterization of hearing loss as sensorineural or conductive.

Somatosensory Evoked Potentials

Somatosensory evoked potentials (SSEPs) are generally elicited by electric stimulation of the median and posterior tibial nerves, and reflect sequential activation of structures along the afferent sensory pathways, principally the dorsal columnlemniscal system. The components of median nerve SSEP testing important to clinical interpretation include the Erb point potential, recorded as the afferent volley tranverses the brachial plexus; the N13, representing post-synaptic activity in the central gray matter of the cervical cord; the P14, arising in the lower brainstem, most likely in the caudal medial lemniscus; the N18, attributed to post-synaptic potentials generated in the rostral brainstem; and the N20, corresponding to activation of the primary cortical somatosensory receiving area (Fig. 14.12). The posterior tibial SSEP is analogous to the median SSEP and includes components generated in the gray matter of the lumbar spinal cord, brainstem, and primary somatosensory cortex.

SSEPs are altered by diverse conditions that affect the somatosensory pathways, including focal lesions (strokes, tumors, cervical spondylosis, syringomyelia) or diffuse diseases (hereditary system degenerations, subacute combined degeneration, and vitamin E deficiency). Of patients with multiple sclerosis, 50% to 60% have SSEP abnormalities, even in the absence of clinical signs or symptoms. SSEP abnormalities are also produced by other diseases affecting myelin (adrenoleukodystrophy, adrenomyeloneuropathy, metachromatic leukodystrophy, Pelizaeus-Merzbacher disease). In adrenoleukodystrophy and adrenomyeloneuropathy, SSEP abnormalities may be present in asymptomatic heterozygotes. Abnormally large-amplitude SSEPs, reflecting enhanced cortical excitability, are seen in progressive myoclonus epilepsy, in some patients with photosensitive epilepsy, and in late-infantile ceroid lipofuscinosis.

SSEPs are commonly used to monitor the integrity of the spinal cord during neurosurgical, orthopedic, and vascular procedures that generate risk of injury; SSEPs can detect adverse changes before they become irreversible. Although SSEPs primarily reflect the function of the dorsal columns, they are generally sensitive to spinal cord damage produced by compression, mechanical distraction, or ischemia.

Motor Evoked Potentials

It is possible to assess the descending motor pathways by motor evoked potential (MEP) testing. MEP studies entail stimulation of the motor cortex and recording the compound muscle action potential of appropriate target muscles. The cortex is stimulated either by direct passage of a brief high-voltage electric pulse through the scalp or by use of a time-varying magnetic field to induce an electric current within the brain. Although the clinical utility of this technique is not defined, MEPs evaluate the integrity of the descending motor pathways, complementing data about sensory pathways provided by SSEPs. MEPs also provide information about diseases of the motor system.

DIGITAL EEG TECHNOLOGY AND COMPUTERIZED EEG

Traditional EEG machines record EEG signals as waveforms on paper with pens driven by analog amplifiers. These devices are gradually being replaced by computerized systems that convert EEG data to a digital format, store the transformations on digital media, and display them on computer screens. These systems facilitate interpretation by allowing the physician to manipulate EEG data at the time of interpretation and to supplement standard methods of EEG analysis with display and signal-processing techniques that emphasize particular findings to optimal advantage.

Digital EEG technology has not fundamentally altered the manner in which EEG is interpreted. Rather, it allows standard interpretative strategies to be used more effectively. In conventional paper-based EEG, a technologist sets all recording param-

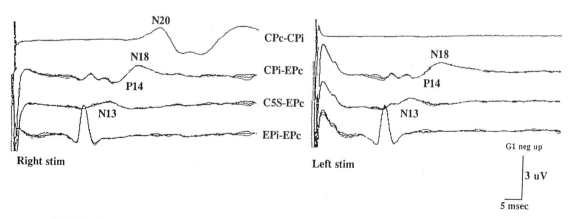

FIGURE 14.12. Median SEPs in a patient with a right putamen hemorrhage. Following right median nerve stimulation, the SEP is normal. Following left median nerve stimulation, the N20 cortical response is absent, while more caudally generated potentials are preserved.

eters, including amplification, filter settings, and montages, at the time EEG is performed. In contrast, digital EEG systems permit these settings to be altered off-line when the EEG is interpreted. The EEG technician can select the best settings for viewing a particular waveform or pattern of interest, or examine it at different instrument settings.

Digital technology has also made it possible to implement computerized pattern-recognition techniques to identify clinically significant electric activities during continuous recordings. For example, automated spike- and seizure-detection algorithms are routinely used in epilepsy monitoring units during video-EEG recording. Currently available software results in a high rate of false-positive detections, and careful manual review of computer-detected events is mandatory. Similar techniques may be useful in intensive care units.

Digital systems also permit use of signal-processing and computer-graphic techniques to reveal features of the EEG that may not be apparent from visual inspection of "raw" waveforms. For example, computer averaging improves the signal-to-noise ratio of interictal spikes, revealing details of the electric-field distributions and timing relationships that cannot be discerned from the routine EEG (Fig. 14.13). The fast Fourier transform (FFT) can quantify frequencies in EEG background activity, and computer-graphic techniques display these data in an appealing and easily understood manner (Fig. 14.14). Dipole source localization has been applied to both interictal spikes and ictal discharges in patients with epilepsy. While these and other forms of processed EEG are at present best used to supplement conventional visual analysis, many computerized techniques are based on specific critical assumptions that, if misapplied,

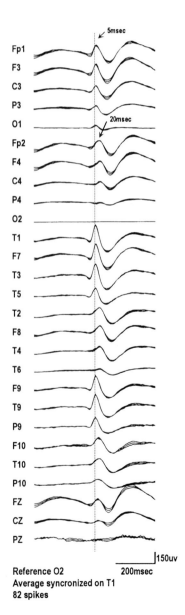

FIGURE 14.13. Averaged left temporal spike in a patient with complex partial seizures associated with mesial temporal sclerosis. Note the time-locked signal over the right frontal–temporal regions occurring after a 20 millisecond delay. This most likely reflects propagation of the spike discharge from the left temporal lobe along neural pathways to the right side. Such time delays cannot be appreciated in routine EEG recordings.

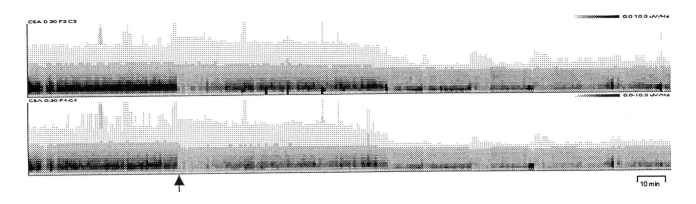

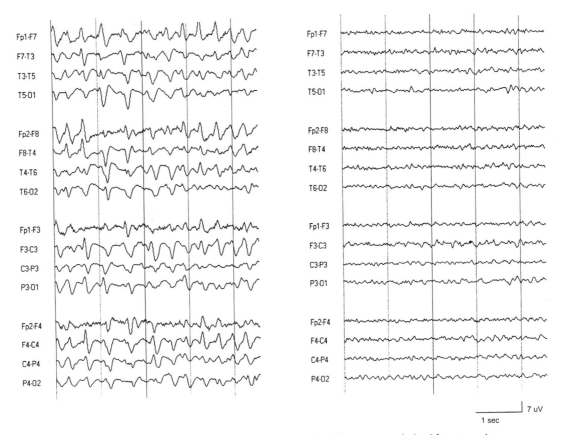

FIGURE 14.14. Compressed spectral array (CSA) depicting the voltage spectra derived from two channels of EEG in a patient in nonconvulsive status epilepticus. The abscissa of each chart represents time as indicated, and the ordinate represents frequency from 0 to 30 Hz. Voltage is encoded with use of a gray scale, as illustrated. There is an abrupt change in the CSA, corresponding to a decrease in the voltage of low-frequency ictal activity when diazepam is administered intravenously *(arrow)*. The accompanying EEG samples correspond to representative epochs before (**left**) and after (**right**) treatment.

may lead to erroneous conclusions. Therefore, at present, findings from computer-processed EEG should be used clinically with caution and generally only when standard visual analysis is supportive and consistent.

SUGGESTED READINGS

Ajmone-Marsan C. Electroencephalographic studies in seizure disorders: additional considerations. *J Clin Neurophysiol* 1984;1:143–157.

American Encephalography Society. Guidelines in EEG and evoked potentials. *J Clin Neurophysiol* 1994;11:1–143.

Chiappa KH. *Evoked potentials in clinical medicine,* 3rd ed. Philadelphia: Lippicott–Raven Publishers, 1997.

Cracco JB, Amassian VE, Cracco RQ, et al. Brain stimulation revisited. *J Clin Neurophysiol* 1990;7:3–15.

Ebersole JS. New applications of EEG/MEG in epilepsy evaluation. *Epilepsy Res* 1996;11[Suppl]:227–237.

Eeg-Olofsson O, Petersen I, Sellden U. The development of the electroencephalogram in normal children from the age of one through fifteen years. *Neuropaediatrie* 1971;4:375–404.

Eisen AA, Shtybel W. Clinical experience with transcranial magnetic stimulation. AAEM minimonograph no.35. *Muscle Nerve* 1990;13:995–1011.

Emerson RG, Adams DC, Nagle, KJ. Monitoring of spinal cord function intraoperatively using motor and somatosensory evoked potentials. In: Chiappa KH, ed. *Evoked potentials in clinical medicine*, 3rd ed. New York: Lippincott–Raven Publishers, 1997:647–660.

Fisch BJ, Klass DW. The diagnostic specificity of triphasic wave patterns. *Electroencephalogr Clin Neurophysiol* 1988;70:1–8.

Fisch BJ, Pedley TA. The role of quantitative topographic mapping or "neurometrics" in the diagnosis of psychiatric and neurological disorders: the cons. *Electroencephalogr Clin Neurophysiol* 1989;73:5–9.

Kellaway P. An orderly approach to visual analysis: characteristics of the normal EEG of adults and children. In: Daly DD, Pedley TA, eds. *Current practice of clinical electroencephalography*, 3rd ed. New York: Raven Press, 1990:139–199.

Lai CW, Gragasin ME. Electroencephalography in herpes simplex encephalitis. *J Clin Neurophysiol* 1988;5:87–103.

Lee EK, Seyal M. Generators of short latency human somatosensory evoked potentials recorded over the spine and scalp. *J Clin Neurophysiol* 1998;15:227–234.

Lerman P. Benign partial epilepsy with centro-temporal spikes. In: Roger J,

Bureau M, Dravet C, et al., eds. *Epilepsy syndromes in infancy, childhood, and adolescence,* 2nd ed. London: John Libbey & Co, 1992:189–200.

Levy SR, Chiappa KH, Burke CJ, Young RR. Early evolution and incidence of electroencephalographic abnormalities in Creutzfeldt-Jakob disease. *J Clin Neurophysiol* 1986;3:1–21.

Novotny EJ Jr. The role of clinical neurophysiology in the management of epilepsy. *J Clin Neurophysiol* 1998;15:96–108.

Nuwer MR. The development of EEG brain mapping. *J Clin Neurophysiol* 1990;7:459–471.

Pohlmann-Eden B, Hoch DB, Chiappa, KH. Periodic lateralized epileptiform discharges: a critical review. *J Clin Neurophysiol* 1996;13:519–530.

Reeves AL, Westmoreland BF, Klass DW. Clinical accompaniments of the burst-suppression EEG pattern. *J Clin Neurophysiol* 1997;14:150–153.

Salinsky M, Kanter R, Dasheiff RM. Effectiveness of multiple EEGs in supporting the diagnosis of epilepsy: an operational curve. *Epilepsia* 1987;28:331–334.

Zifkin BG, Cracco RQ. An orderly approach to the abnormal EEG. In: Daly DD, Pedley TA, eds. *Current practice of clinical electroencephalography*, 3rd ed. New York: Raven Press, 1990:253–267.

Merritt's Neurology, 10th ed., edited by L.P. Rowland. Lippincott Williams & Wilkins, Philadelphia © 2000.

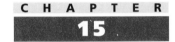

ELECTROMYOGRAPHY AND NERVE CONDUCTION STUDIES IN NEUROMUSCULAR DISEASE

DALE J. LANGE
WERNER TROJABORG

Needle electromyography (EMG) and nerve conduction studies are extensions of the neurologic examination. The primary role for electrophysiologic studies is to separate neurogenic from myogenic disorders. For example, the characteristic EMG findings of stiff-man syndrome (Moersch-Woltman syndrome) and Issac syndrome are the basis for these diagnoses. Repetitive stimulation abnormalities define the Lambert-Eaton syndrome. Characteristic abnormalities in nerve conduction define some entrapment neuropathies or multifocal motor neuropathy with conduction block. EMG and nerve conduction findings may provide important information to confirm a diagnosis, such as myasthenia gravis, Guillain-Barré syndrome, or polymyositis. Even normal EMG and nerve conduction findings may provide essential information for diagnosis. For example, normal sensory studies in an anesthetic limb after trauma suggest nerve root avulsion. Normal repetitive stimulation studies in the presence of severe weakness is strong evidence against myasthenia gravis.

However, EMG and nerve conduction studies are subject to many technical errors that can affect interpretation. For example, low limb temperature can lead to a false diagnosis of neuropathy or may fail to reveal excessive decrement during repetitive nerve stimulation in patients with myasthenia gravis. These and other technical considerations and normal variants, discussed in monographs listed in the references, are essential for performing and interpreting these tests.

Nerve conduction studies are performed on motor and sensory nerves, usually in the distal portions of limbs (hand and feet). Conduction, however, can also be measured to biceps, deltoid, quadriceps, and muscles of the trunk (diaphragm and rectus abdominis). High-voltage electrical and magnetic stimulators activate spinal roots and descending pathways from the brain and spinal cord.

Similar techniques are used for motor and sensory nerve conduction studies (Fig. 15.1). An electrical stimulus is applied to the skin directly over a nerve. One electrical response is recorded from the innervated muscle (motor) or a more proximal portion of the nerve (sensory). The stimulus intensity is increased until the response no longer grows in amplitude (supramaximal response). The interval between the onset of the stimulus and the onset of the evoked response is the latency. Because nerve fibers vary in diameter and speed of conduction, a supramaximal stimulus ensures that all nerve fibers are activated, facilitating comparison of latencies in different people or in serial studies of the same person. The calculated conduction velocity corresponds to the fastest conducting fibers. Conduction studies may therefore fail to show an abnormality in a disease that affects only small-diameter nerve fibers if surface recording methods are used. "Near nerve" recording, however, can assess these slower components of the sensory response from smaller diameter myelinated fibers. Direct recording from the smallest myelinated and unmyelinated fibers is called "microneurography."

The distal motor latency is the time between the onset of the stimulus and the onset of the muscle response. Stimulation at a more proximal point produces an evoked response with a longer

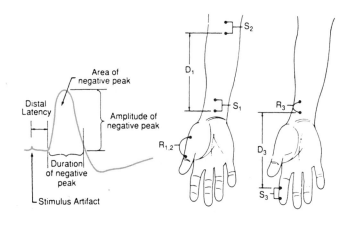

Exam- ination	Segment	Waveform
Motor	S1–R1	ML1
Motor	S2–R2	ML2
Sensory	S3–R3	SL

FIGURE 15.1. Technique for motor and sensory conduction studies of the median nerve. **A:** Components of the evoked compound muscle action potential. **B:** Electrode placement for motor nerve stimulation (S1, S2) and recording (R1, R2). **C:** Electrode placement for sensory nerve stimulation (S3) and recording (R3). S1, motor stimulation at wrist; S2, motor stimulation at elbow; S3, sensory stimulation at finger; R1, motor response after stimulation at S1; R2, motor response after stimulation at S2; R3, sensory nerve evoked response after stimulating finger; ML, motor latency or the time between onset of stimulation and onset of motor response; SL, sensory latency or the time between onset of stimulus to onset of sensory response.

latency (proximal latency). Both distal and proximal motor latencies include the time needed to cross the neuromuscular junction. Therefore, when the distal latency is subtracted from the proximal latency, the effect of neuromuscular transmission is eliminated, and the resulting time represents the speed of conduction of the nerve in that specific segment. The distance between the two points of nerve stimulation is measured to calculate segmental conduction velocity (distance/latency difference = velocity). In contrast, sensory nerve conduction in peripheral nerve does not involve synaptic transmission, so velocity measurements are calculated directly from the distance and latency (Fig. 15.1).

Conduction velocity is determined by the size of the largest diameter (and therefore fastest conducting) axon and the presence of normal myelin, the component of peripheral nerves that provides the structural basis for saltatory conduction. In de-

myelinating diseases, the segmental velocity slows to approximately half of the normal mean. In axonal disease, if the large-diameter fibers are preferentially lost, velocity can also slow but not to less than 50% of the normal mean.

The evoked response has a biphasic (motor) or triphasic (sensory) waveform. The size of the evoked response depends on the number of fibers activated under the electrode, the surface area of the electrode, and the synchrony of firing. If the firing of motor nerve fibers is well synchronized, the muscle response is also synchronized, and the duration of the muscle evoked response is short. If nerve conduction is pathologically slow, nerve fibers that conduct at different speeds may be affected differently, resulting in poorly synchronized arrival of nerve impulses to the muscles, and duration of the waveform increases and the amplitude decreases because of phase cancellation between individual action potentials. In chronic partial denervation, individual axons are not all affected to the same extent, and reinnervation augments the dispersion of conduction velocities. Therefore, in chronic neuropathy or motor neuron disease, proximal stimulation may evoke a response of lower amplitude than distal stimulation even though the same number of fibers is activated.

The excessive loss (>50%) of amplitude between two points of stimulation is a suspicious sign of conduction block, which is pathognomonic of a demyelinating neuropathy (Fig. 15.2). In chronic partial denervation, however, the lower evoked response amplitude may only be due to phase cancellation and temporal dispersion. To differentiate the effects of temporal dispersion from conduction block in chronic partial denervation, the area under the negative phase is measured. Computerized models of conduction in the rat sciatic nerve suggest that a loss of more than 50% of the area of the response indicates that both temporal dispersion and conduction block are present.

If both distal and proximal stimulation result in a response of low amplitude, the pattern implies a diffuse (proximal and distal) process and a generalized loss of axons, as in an axonal neuropathy. Axonal neuropathies usually show normal distal motor latency, normal or borderline normal segmental velocity, no conduction block, or dispersion. Demyelinating neuropathies show prolonged distal latency, slow segmental velocity, normal or reduced evoked response amplitude, conduction block, and increased temporal dispersion.

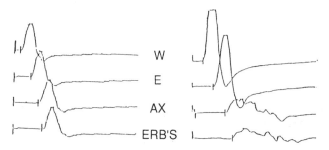

FIGURE 15.2. Motor conduction block. **A:** Normal. Evoked compound muscle action potential amplitude shows little change at all points of stimulation. (Calibration, 1 cm = 10 mV.) **B:** Conduction block with amplitude reduction and temporal dispersion in the nerve segment between axilla and elbow. (Calibration, 1 cm = 5 mV.) W, wrist; E, elbow; Ax, axilla; Erb's, Erb's point.

F response and H reflexes evaluate conduction in the proximal portions of nerve fibers. The F response, so named because it was first observed in small foot muscles, is a measure of conduction along the entire length of nerve from the distal point of stimulation to the anterior horn cells and back to the distal recording electrode. This technique uses the same recording setup as standard motor nerve conduction studies except that the stimulator is rotated 180 degrees (cathode proximal). Normal values depend on limb length but are usually less than 32 ms in the arms and 60 ms in the legs. The waveform is characteristically present at supramaximal stimulation and varies in latency, shape, and presence. Although F responses are often prolonged in neurogenic conditions, they are of most value when distal conduction is normal; that is, if the F response latency is prolonged and velocity in distal segments is normal, slowing occurs in proximal segments. This pattern is seen in proximal polyradiculopathies, such as the Guillain-Barré syndrome. In chronic demyelinating neuropathies, the proximal segments may also be involved, and the F response latency may be longer than expected from the velocity calculated in distal portions.

The H reflex is considered to be the electrical counterpart of the Achilles reflex, although the pathways are not identical. The H reflex is sometimes seen in the absence of the Achilles reflex and vice versa. In contrast to the F response, which uses only the efferent motor nerve pathway, the H reflex is thought to be a monosynaptic reflex with an afferent and efferent limb. It is recorded from multiple muscles in infants, but as the nervous system matures, the H reflex is found only in the tibial nerve or soleus system (absent in 10% of normal subjects) or in the median nerve or flexor carpi radialis system. The H reflex occurs during submaximal stimulation, does not vary in shape, and disappears with supramaximal stimulation. It is one of the few measures of afferent nerve conduction in proximal portions of sensory nerves and identifies dorsal root pathology when the H reflex is prolonged in conjunction with normal F response latency in the same nerve. Additionally, the H reflex may "reappear" in muscle or nerve systems other than the tibial or soleus system as part of upper motor neuron diseases, such as multiple sclerosis or primary lateral sclerosis.

ELECTROMYOGRAPHY

The electrical activity of muscle may be recorded with surface electrodes, but spontaneous electrical activity (fibrillations and positive sharp waves) and individual voluntary motor units cannot be seen with surface electrodes. EMG is therefore performed with a needle electrode (either monopolar or concentric) placed directly in the muscle for extracellular recording of action potentials generated by the muscle fibers spontaneously or during voluntary movement. Needle recording can also be used to measure evoked potentials after motor nerve stimulation when the surface recorded potential is too low for reliable measurements. Needle recording of evoked potentials, however, is less reliable because the waveform is affected by movement of the activated muscle.

Diagnostic information includes the type and amount of spontaneous activity, evaluation of motor unit form with minimal volitional activity, and the density of motor units during maximal activation. After denervation, muscle fibers discharge spontaneously. These extracellular potentials recorded at rest are called positive sharp waves and fibrillation potentials. Although characteristic of denervating conditions (peripheral neuropathy, traumatic neuropathy, plexopathy, radiculopathy, and motor neuron disease), spontaneous potentials are also seen in some myogenic disorders (polymyositis and even in dystrophinopathies) but rarely in disorders of neuromuscular transmission (myasthenia gravis, Lambert-Eaton syndrome, and botulism). Fibrillation potentials are biphasic or triphasic and of short duration and are generated by discharges of single muscle fibers. Positive sharp waves are thought to have the same implications as fibrillation potentials but are differently shaped because the traveling wave terminates at the point of needle recording, so there is no upward negative phase.

Fasciculations are spontaneous discharges of an entire motor unit that comprise all the muscle fibers innervated by a single axon. The amplitude and duration of the fasciculation potential are therefore greater than the fibrillation. Fibrillations are never seen clinically, but fasciculations can usually be seen with the naked eye. Fasciculations are of neurogenic origin and are most often associated with proximal diseases, such as anterior horn cell disease or radiculopathy. They are occasionally found, however, in generalized peripheral neuropathy and even in normal individuals (benign fasciculations).

Other types of spontaneous activity include myotonia (high-frequency muscle fiber discharge of waxing and waning amplitude), complex repetitive discharges (which are spontaneous discharges of constant shape and frequency with abrupt onset and abrupt cessation), and myokymia and neuromyotonia (bursts of muscle activity that often, but not always, are associated with cramps and visible twitching). Clinically, these electrical phenomena occur in Isaac syndrome and myokymia. EMG is useful in the difficult clinical differentiation of facial myokymia and facial hemispasm.

Motor unit configuration changes depending on the particular disease. In neurogenic disease, the motor unit territory increases and the motor unit potentials increase in duration and amplitude. Standard monopolar and concentric needles record only from a portion of the motor unit, but the change in amplitude and duration is diagnostic. In myogenic disease, motor unit potentials decrease in amplitude and duration. Quantitative motor unit potential analysis provides more reliable correlation with muscle and nerve disease than muscle biopsy. Normal extracellularly recorded motor unit potentials are triphasic in shape; polyphasic motor units occur in both neurogenic and myogenic disease and are normally found in small numbers in all muscles. They are therefore nonspecific findings.

The recruitment pattern refers to the electrical activity generated by all activated motor units within the recording area of a maximally contracting muscle. Normally, the recruitment pattern on maximal effort is dense with no breaks in the baseline. The amplitude of the envelope (excluding single high-amplitude spikes) is normally 2 to 4 mV using a concentric needle with standard recording area (0.07 mm^2). In neurogenic disease, the density of the recruitment is reduced and the firing frequency of the remaining units increases. Sometimes only one unit can be recruited by maximal effort, and this unit may fire faster than 40 Hz (discrete recruitment). In myogenic disease, the number of motor units is unchanged by the disease, but the amplitude and duration of the motor units are reduced. Therefore, recruitment density is normal, but the envelope amplitude is reduced, leading to the pathognomonic finding of myopathy: full recruitment in a weak wasted muscle.

NEUROMUSCULAR TRANSMISSION DISORDERS

Weakness occurs only if muscle fibers fail to contract or generate less than normal tension. Muscle fibers may fail to contract because of impaired nerve conduction, neuromuscular transmission, or muscle conduction. If muscle fibers are not activated because neuromuscular transmission fails, the abnormality is called blocking. If a sufficient number of muscle fibers is blocked, the amplitude of the evoked response is reduced. For example, in myasthenia gravis, repetitive electrical stimulation at 2 to 3 Hz causes progressive loss of the compound muscle action potential amplitude until the fourth or fifth response because of increasing numbers of neuromuscular junctions with blocking (Fig. 15.3). After the fifth potential, the compound muscle action potential usually shows no further decline or may slightly increase. Decrement also improves immediately after 10 to 15 seconds of intense exercise (postactivation facilitation; Fig. 15.3). If the muscle is exercised manually for 1 minute, the decrement becomes more pronounced at 3 to 4 minutes (postactivation exhaustion; Fig. 15.3).

In Lambert-Eaton syndrome and botulism, release of acetylcholine is impaired at rest, but during exercise or rapid rates of stimulation, acetylcholine release is facilitated. This is reflected

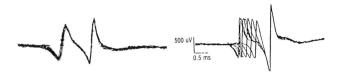

FIGURE 15.4. Single-fiber EMG recordings showing normal **(A)** and increased **(B)** jitter.

by a positive edrophonium test and electrophysiologic decrement at low rates of stimulation and increment at fast rates.

Single-fiber EMG is a technique that identifies dysfunction of the muscle fibers before any blocking or overt weakness occurs (Fig. 15.4). When weakness appears, blocking is usually demonstrable. A normal single-fiber EMG study in a weak muscle rules out a disorder of neuromuscular transmission.

SUGGESTED READINGS

Albers JW, Allen AA, Balstron JA, et al. Limb myokymia. *Muscle Nerve* 1981;4:494–504.

Aminoff MJ, ed. *Electrodiagnosis in clinical neurology*, 4th ed. New York: Churchill Livingstone, 1999.

Anderson K. Surface recording of orthodromic sensory nerve potentials in median and ulnar nerves in normal subjects. *Muscle Nerve* 1985;8:402–408.

Bolton CF, Sawa GM, Carker K. The effects of temperature on human compound action potentials. *Neurol Neurosurg Psychiatry* 1981;44:407–413.

Bornstein S, Desmedt JE. Local cooling in myasthenia. *Arch Neurol* 1975;32:152–157.

Buchthal F, Rosenfalck A. Evoked action potentials and conduction velocity in human sensory nerves. *Brain Res* 1966;3:1–122.

Buchthal F, Rosenfalck P. Spontaneous electrical activity of human muscle. *Electroencephalogr Clin Neurophysiol* 1966;20:321–326.

Dumitru D, King JC, Stegeman DF. Normal needle electromyographic insertional activity morphology: a clinical and simulation study. *Muscle Nerve* 1998;21:910–920.

Franssen H, Wieneke GH, Wokke JHJ. The influence of temperature on conduction block. *Muscle Nerve* 1999;22:166–173.

Gassell MM. Sources of error in motor nerve conduction velocity determinations. *Neurology* 1964;14:825–835.

Gilliatt RW, LeQuesne PM, Logue V, Sumner AJ. Wasting of the hand associated with a cervical rib or band. *Neurol Neurosurg Psychiatry* 1970;32:615–624.

Kelly JJ. The electrodiagnostic findings in peripheral neuropathy associated with monoclonal gammopathy. *Muscle Nerve* 1983;6:504–509.

Kimura J. *Electrodiagnosis in disease of nerve and muscle: principles and practice*, 2nd ed. Philadelphia: FA Davis, 1988.

King D, Ashby P. Conduction velocity in the proximal segments of a motor nerve in the Guillain Barré syndrome. *J Neurol Neurosurg Psychiatry* 1976;39:538–544.

Krarup C, Stewart JD, Sumner AJ, et al. A syndrome of asymmetric limb weakness with motor conduction block. *Neurology* 1990;40:118–127.

Lewis RA, Sumner AJ. The electrodiagnostic distinctions between chronic familial and acquired demyelinative neuropathies. *Neurology* 1982;32:592–596.

McLeod JG. Electrophysiological studies in Guillain Barré syndrome. *Ann Neurol* 1981;9[Suppl]:20–27.

Nardin RA, Raynor EM, Rutkove SB. Fibrillations in lumbosacral paraspinal muscles of normal subjects. *Muscle Nerve* 1998;21:1347–1349.

Parry GJ, Clarke S. Multifocal acquired demyelinating neuropathy masquerading as motor neuron disease. *Muscle Nerve* 1988;11:103–107.

Preston DC, Shapiro BE. *Electromyography and neuromuscular disorders*. Boston: Butterworth-Heinemann, 1998.

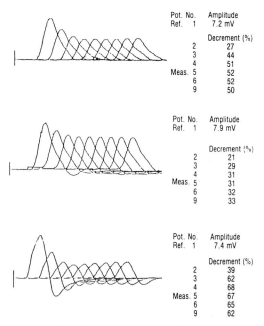

Pot. No.	Amplitude
Ref. 1	7.2 mV
	Decrement (%)
2	27
3	44
4	51
Meas. 5	52
6	52
9	50

Pot. No.	Amplitude
Ref. 1	7.9 mV
	Decrement (%)
2	21
3	29
4	31
Meas. 5	31
6	32
9	33

Pot. No.	Amplitude
Ref. 1	7.4 mV
	Decrement (%)
2	39
3	62
4	68
Meas. 5	67
6	65
9	62

FIGURE 15.3. Muscle action potentials evoked by repetitive stimulation at 3 Hz in myasthenia gravis. **A:** Showing decrement at rest. **B:** Postactivation facilitation. **C:** Postexercise exhaustion. (Calibration, 1 cm = 5 mV.)

Roleveld K, Sandberg A, Stålberg EV, Stegeman DF. Motor unit size estimation of enlarged motor units with surface electromyography. *Muscle Nerve* 1998;21:878–886.

Rowland LP. Cramps, spasm, and muscle stiffness. *Rev Neurol (Paris)* 1985;141:261–273.

Sacco G, Buchthal F, Rosenfalck P. Motor unit potentials at different ages. *Arch Neurol* 1966;6:44–51.

Sanders DB, Howard JF. Single fiber electromyography in myasthenia gravis. *Muscle Nerve* 1986;9:809–819.

Stalberg E, Andreassen S, Falck B, et al. Quantitative analysis of individual motor unit potentials: A proposition for standardized terminology and criteria for measurement. *J Clin Neurophysiol* 1986;3:313–348.

Stalberg E. Macro EMG: a new recording technique. *J Neurol Neurosurg Psychiatry* 1980;43:475–482.

Trojaborg W. Prolonged conduction block with axonal degeneration: an electrophysiological study. *J Neurol Neurosurg Psychiatry* 1977;40:50–57.

Trojaborg W, Buchthal F. Malignant and benign fasciculations. *Acta Neurol Scand* 1965;41[Suppl 13]:251–255.

Walsh JC, Yiannikas C, McLeod JG. Abnormalities of proximal conduction in acute idiopathic polyneuritis: comparison of short latency evoked potentials and F waves. *J Neurol Neurosurg Psychiatry* 1984;47:197–200.

Warren J. Electromyographic changes of brachial plexus avulsion. *J Neurosurg* 1969;31:137–140.

Wiederholt W. Stimulus intensity and site of excitation in human median nerve sensory fibers. *J Neurol Neurosurg Psychiatry* 1970;40:982–986.

Zalewska E, Rowinska-Marcinska K, Hausmanowa-Petrusewicz I. Shape irregularity of motor unit potentials in some neuromuscular disorders. *Muscle Nerve* 1998;21:1181–1187.

Merritt's Neurology, 10th ed., edited by L.P. Rowland. Lippincott Williams & Wilkins, Philadelphia © 2000.

CHAPTER 16

NEUROVASCULAR IMAGING

J. P. MOHR
ROBERT DELAPAZ

Brain imaging plays a central role in the diagnosis, classification, and prognosis of stroke. As technology advances, so do the applications. Conventional radiology plays little role now, and current techniques include computed tomography (CT) and magnetic resonance imaging (MRI) with or without contrast enhancement, MR diffusion and perfusion imaging, CT or MR angiography (MRA), ultrasonic Doppler insonation of blood flowing in the extra- or intracranial arteries and veins, MR spectroscopy (MRS), and single photon emission computed tomography (SPECT) by agents that assess blood flow or specific chemical reactions or receptors of the brain.

COMPUTED TOMOGRAPHY

Acute hematomas have a characteristic high-density (high-attenuation) appearance (bright) on CT in the first week; CT reliably differentiates the low-attenuation lesion (dark) typical of bland infarction from the high-attenuation of hematoma or grossly hemorrhagic infarction (Figs. 16.1 and 16.2). The volume of an acute parenchymal hematoma can be estimated accurately by CT. As the high signal of fresh blood is lost in days or weeks (hemoglobin breakdown) at the site, the CT appearance evolves from initial hyperdensity through an isodense (subacute) phase to hypodensity in the chronic state (see Fig. 13.1). In the subacute phase, contrast administration may result in ring enhancement around the hemorrhage (Fig. 16.3), a pattern different from the gyral enhancement typical of infarction (Fig. 16.1). This ring or rim enhancement may appear

similar to tumor or abscess, a pitfall that is especially misleading with isodense or hypodense late hematomas. In the chronic state, a hematoma is usually reduced to a slitlike cavity after phagocytic clearing of hemorrhagic and tissue debris. Many hematomas disappear without creating a cavity, leaving isodense tissue. Subarachnoid hemorrhage is even more transient and may not be visible unless it is particularly dense; lumbar puncture can make the diagnosis of subarachnoid bleeding in those with normal CTs.

With nonhemorrhagic infarction, CT may appear normal for several days. When there is collateral supply to the region, CT is usually positive within 24 hours, showing hypodensity due to edema. Ischemic infarcts with little collateral flow or edema may remain isodense or may not enhance for days or weeks, later appearing only as focal atrophy. Although CT may overestimate the size of deep lesions, it better approximates the volume of discrete surface infarcts, especially after several months when the acute effects of edema and necrotic tissue reabsorption have subsided (Fig. 16.4). Contrast-enhanced infarction is usually seen within 1 week and may persist for 2 weeks to 2 months. A characteristic gyriform enhancement pattern is often seen when cortical gray matter is involved.

Standard CT techniques do not distinguish partial ischemia from actual infarction. In the early stages, the physician may be frustrated by the difficulty determining how much tissue is viable and how much damage is permanent. Spiral CT provides serial scans during the first pass of an intravenous contrast bolus and can give relative measures of ischemia from derived blood volume and perfusion delay maps. Stable xenon-enhanced CT may also be useful.

Spiral CT can also scan the entire neck or head with a bolus intravenous infusion of contrast agent for a "CT angiogram." Maximum intensity projection reformations, often with three-dimensional surface shading, display vascular features such as stenosis or aneurysm. Advantages of CT angiogram over catheter angiography include more widely available technology, less specialized skill requirements, and relatively noninvasive intravenous administration of contrast material. However, use of CT angiogram has been growing slowly because of competition from MRA. In contrast to MRA, the iodinated contrast agent is po-

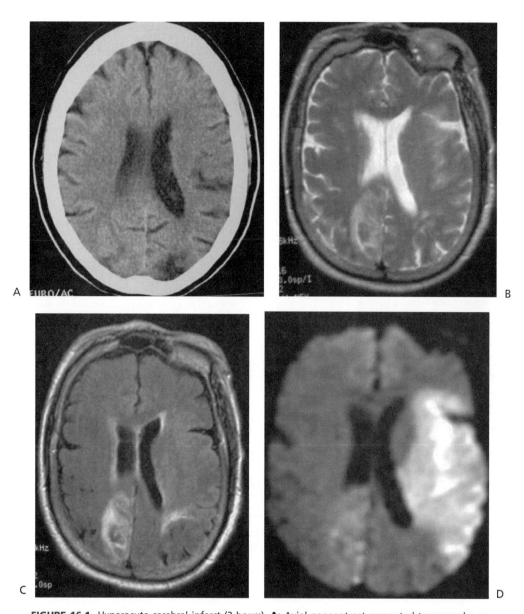

FIGURE 16.1. Hyperacute cerebral infarct (3 hours). **A:** Axial noncontrast computed tomography appears normal except for the low density in the left medial parietal cortex representing a chronic infarct. **B:** Axial T2-weighted fast spin echo magnetic resonance (MR) image shows slight elevation of signal in the left insular cortex, high curvilinear signal at the deep margin of the chronic left parietal infarct, and high signal with central low signal in a subacute hemorrhagic infarct in the medial right parietal lobe. **C:** Axial fluid attenuated inversion recovery MR image shows slightly increased signal in the left periventricular region and high signal at the margin of the chronic infarct and mixed signal in the subacute infarct. **D:** Axial diffusion-weighted image (b = 1,000) shows a large region of high signal, representing low water proton diffusion rates, in the large middle cerebral artery infarct produced by carotid dissection 3 hours before the study. (Courtesy of Dr. R. L. DeLaPaz.)

FIGURE 16.2. Acute cerebral infarct (24 hours). **A:** Axial diffusion-weighted image (DWI, b = 1,000) shows a patchy region of high signal, representing low water proton diffusion rates, in an acute deep left basal ganglia and corona radiata infarct. **B:** The exponential apparent diffusion coefficient (ADC) map represents the ratio of signal on the DWI to the T2-weighted (b = 0) image. This map corrects for high signal on the DWI produced by high signal on the T2-weighted image, the T2 "shine through" effect. This acute infarct produces high signal on both the DWI and exponential ADC maps, confirming reduced tissue water diffusion. **C:** This map of relative perfusion delay, time to peak, was produced by rapid scanning with T2*-weighted images during an intravenous gadolinium contrast bolus injection.

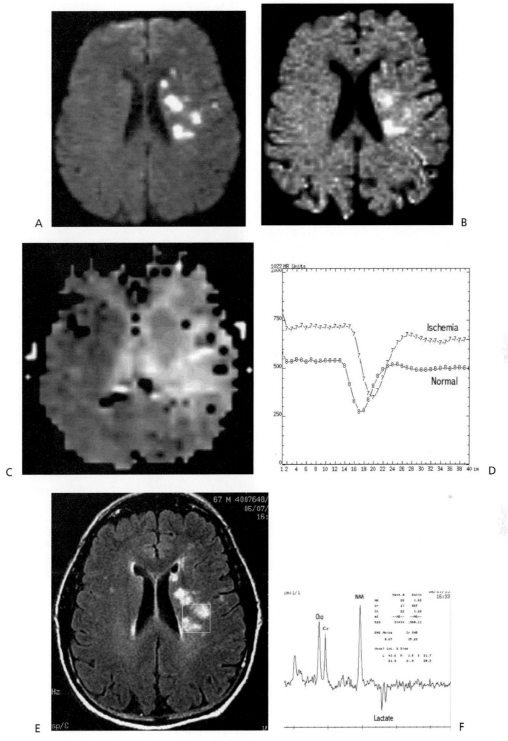

The high signal area in the region of the left-sided infarct represents a large zone of relatively delayed arrival of the peak signal change produced by the gadolinium bolus as it passes through the tissue capillary bed. **D:** The time-intensity curves show the transient drop in signal on T2*-weighted images as the gadolinium bolus passes through and indicate a substantial delay in the left-sided ischemic zone (9-second peak arrival delay; x-axis is image number with TR = 3 seconds and y-axis is signal intensity). **E:** Axial fluid attenuated inversion recovery magnetic resonance (MR) image shows patchy increased signal in the infarct. The square outline represents the voxel used for proton MR spectroscopy. **F:** Proton MR spectrum (TR 2,000, TE 144) shows a slight elevation of choline (Cho), a slight decrease in *N*-acetylaspartate (NAA), and a marked elevation of lactate (peak inversion is due to J-coupling of lactate doublet). Peak areas represent relative concentrations of tissue metabolites. (Courtesy of Dr. R. L. DeLaPaz.)

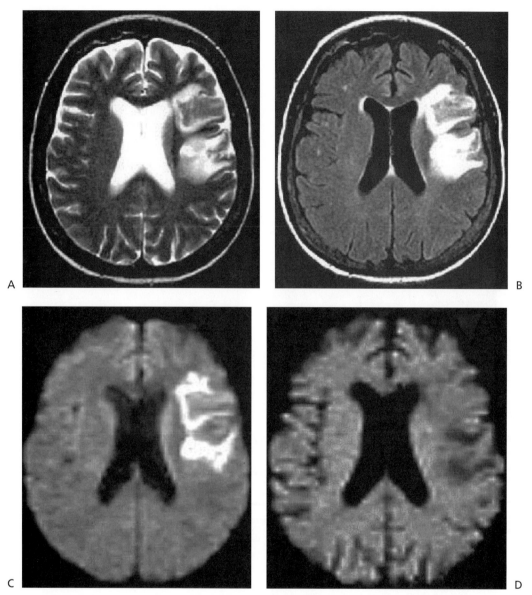

FIGURE 16.3. Chronic cerebral infarct with T2 "shine through." **A:** Axial T2-weighted fast spin echo (FSE) magnetic resonance (MR) image shows high signal in a chronic left middle cerebral artery (MCA) territory infarct. **B:** Axial fluid attenuated inversion recovery (FLAIR) MR image also shows high signal in the chronic left MCA territory infarct. **C:** Axial diffusion-weighted image (DWI, b = 1,000) shows a region of high signal corresponding to the MCA infarct and the high signal seen on the FSE and FLAIR images. **D:** The exponential apparent diffusion coefficient (ADC) map represents the ratio of signal on the DWI to the T2-weighted (b = 0) image. This map corrects for high signal on the DWI produced by high signal on the T2-weighted image, the T2 "shine through" effect. The exponential ADC map shows low signal in the lesion, indicating high water diffusion rates, as would be expected in a chronic infarct. Acute infarcts produce high signal on both the DWI and exponential ADC maps, indicating reduced tissue water diffusion (see Fig. 16.2). (Courtesy of Dr. R. L. DeLaPaz.)

tentially more toxic because of allergic reactions, direct cardiac volume stress, or renal toxicity. Another limitation of CT angiogram is the time-consuming postprocessing required to edit out bone and calcium and to generate three-dimensional surface rendering.

Within the brain, CT may differentiate abnormal from normal soft tissues, particularly after intravenous administration of iodinated contrast agents; abnormal enhancement implies a breakdown of the blood–brain barrier. MRI is more sensitive than CT in demonstrating parenchymal abnormalities and can also be augmented by a contrast agent, gadolinium.

MAGNETIC RESONANCE IMAGING

MRI is rapidly overtaking CT in imaging of both hemorrhagic and ischemic stroke. The physics of MRI are discussed in Chapter 13. Selection of the pulse sequence and plane of imag-

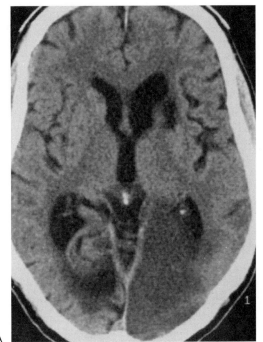

A

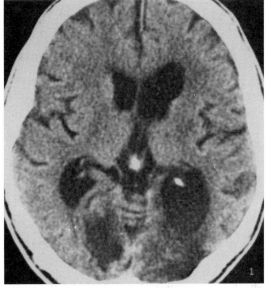

B

FIGURE 16.4. Cerebral infarction, acute and chronic phases. **A:** Axial noncontrast computed tomography reveals focal regions of discrete lucency in left basal ganglia and right occipital regions without mass effect, suggesting nonacute infarcts. A "fainter" less well-defined left occipital lucency is also noted, with effacement of cortical sulci and the atrium of the ventricle, suggesting more recent infarction. **B:** Follow-up noncontrast scan 2 months later demonstrates interval demarcation of the left occipital infarct with evidence of focal atrophy, "negative mass effect" on the atrium, which appears larger. Similar change is noted in left frontal horn. (Courtesy of Drs. J. A. Bello and S. K. Hilal.)

ing is necessary to achieve the maximum utility of the technique. To diagnose and date hemorrhage, T1- and T2-weighted images are necessary (Figs. 13.1 and 16.5). The appearance of parenchymal hemorrhage on MRI is much more complicated than on CT and varies as the hemorrhage evolves. Hyperacute hemorrhage, within the first 12 to 24 hours, usually appears as isointense to slightly hypointense on T1-weighted images and isointense to hypointense on T2-weighted images (also hypointense on fluid attenuated inversion recovery [FLAIR] and gradient echo [GRE] images). This pattern arises because a clot is first composed of intact red blood cells with fully oxygenated hemoglobin, giving it the same signal characteristics as brain tissue. Rapid deoxygenation generates deoxyhemoglobin, which is paramagnetic and produces low signal on T2-weighted images (shortens T2 relaxation) with little effect on T1-weighted images. After this hyperacute period, the hemoglobin within the red cells evolves into methemoglobin, which has a stronger paramagnetic effect and produces high signal on T1-weighted images (shortens T1 relaxation) with persistent low signal on T2-weighted images. After several days, the red cells break down in the subacute hematoma, resulting in a more uniform distribution of methemoglobin and dominance of the shortened T1 relaxation time, producing high signal on T1-weighted and T2-weighted images. This appearance remains stable for weeks to months until the hemorrhagic debris is cleared by phagocytes, leaving only hemosiderin at the site of the hemorrhage. The chronic hemorrhagic site

is isointense on T1-weighted images and hypointense to isointense on T2-weighted images. GRE images are especially sensitive to hemosiderin deposits and often show sites of chronic hemorrhage as low signal when both T1-weighted and T2-weighted images are isointense. GRE images are particularly useful as a screen for occult prior hemorrhage associated with suspected vascular malformations, amyloid angiopathy, trauma, or anticoagulation.

The appearance of subarachnoid and other extraaxial hemorrhage follows similar stages of signal change but may evolve more rapidly or slowly, depending on location and cerebrospinal fluid dilution effects. The diagnosis of acute subarachnoid hemorrhage is still made most reliably with CT; recent experience with FLAIR indicates a high sensitivity to subarachnoid hemorrhage. FLAIR may identify subarachnoid hemorrhage as abnormal high signal in sulci that appear normal on CT. However, this high signal is less specific than high density on CT and may also represent cells or elevated protein content in cerebrospinal fluid caused by infection or meningeal neoplasm. GRE images are not sensitive or specific for acute subarachnoid hemorrhage but may show signs of repeated prior subarachnoid hemorrhage as low signal along the pial surface caused by deposition of hemosiderin ("hemosiderosis").

MRI is unquestionably more sensitive and more specific than CT for the diagnosis of acute brain ischemia and infarction. The multiplanar capability, lack of artifact from bone, and the greater sensitivity to tissue changes provide MRI a par-

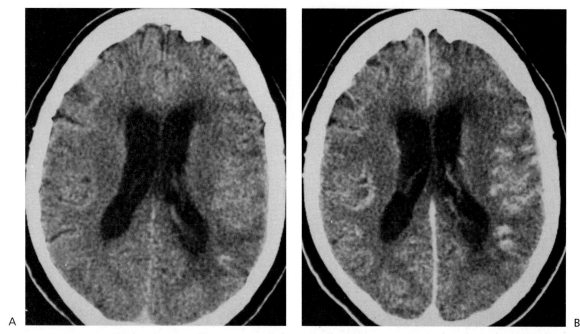

A   B

FIGURE 16.5. Hemorrhagic infarction. **A:** Axial precontrast computed tomography shows focal left parietal gyral density consistent with hemorrhagic infarction. Note edema and sulcal effacement in left frontoparietal cortical region. **B:** Postcontrast enhancement in area of recent hemorrhagic infarction. (Courtesy of Drs. J. A. Bello and S. K. Hilal.)

ticular advantage over CT for imaging infarcts in the brainstem (Fig. 16.6). Diffusion weighted imaging (DWI), described in more detail in Chapter 13, has revolutionized acute infarct detection. Severe cerebral ischemia and infarction cause a rapid decrease in intracellular diffusion that consistently produces high signal on DWI within minutes of cell injury. T2-weighted and FLAIR images show high signal in acute infarction only after a delay of 6 to 12 hours. DWI is also more specific for acute infarction. High signal lesions on FLAIR or T2-weighted images may represent acute, subacute, or chronic infarction, whereas the DWI shows high signal only in acute lesions. After the initial reduction in diffusion, there is a gradual rise through normal to prolonged diffusion rates during the 1 to 2 weeks after infarction, as cells disintegrate and freely diffusable water dominates the encephalomalacic tissue. A minor pitfall of DWI in subacute infarcts is the phenomenon called "T2 shine through," where high signal on T2-weighted images may produce high signal on DWI, falsely indicating reduced diffusion. This pitfall can be avoided by the use of calculated apparent diffusion coefficient maps. DWI has become an essential part of acute stroke imaging and, because it takes less than a minute to acquire a whole brain study, is being used for screening a variety of clinical presentations for possible ischemic injury.

MRI methods for assessing cerebral perfusion, described in more detail in Chapter 13, have also transformed the evaluation of acute cerebral ischemia. Tissue blood flow is most commonly imaged with MRI using a "first pass" or "bolus tracking" method that records the signal changes that occur when rapidly repeated images are acquired during the first passage of an intravascular bolus of paramagnetic contrast

material through the brain, usually gadolinium-diethylenetriamine pentaacetic acid. This rapid imaging can be done during routine contrast administration, adding minimal time to the routine examination. This method provides maps of relative cerebral blood volume, cerebral blood flow, and bolus mean transit time or time to peak. Measures of perfusion delay such as mean transit time and time to peak are proving to be sensitive indicators of subtle reductions in cerebral perfusion. A second method of MR perfusion imaging is called "spin tagging" or "time of flight" imaging and, like time-of-flight MRA, depends on T1 relaxation and flow enhancement phenomena without the use of injected contrast agents. This method is less widely used than bolus tracking but is capable of giving more quantitative cerebral blood flow measurements but with more limited coverage of the brain. These methods can be used to identify relatively underperfused brain regions distal to arterial stenoses or occlusions. They can also give an indication of the potentially salvageable "penumbra" of ischemic, but not yet infarcted, brain around an infarction, as indicated by high signal on DWI.

MRS (also described in Chapter 13), using either proton (^{1}H) or phosphorus (^{31}P), has limited application in the evaluation of acute ischemia. Although changes characteristic of injured or dead tissue can be seen, such as reduced *N*-acetylaspartate and elevated lactate on proton MRS and reduced energy metabolites on phosphorus MRS, the long duration (3 to 20 minutes) and low resolution (2 to 8 cm voxel size) of these methods limit practical application in the acute stroke patient. Proton MRS may be helpful with enhancing subacute infarction in deep white matter where routine imaging may suggest primary brain tumor. Al-

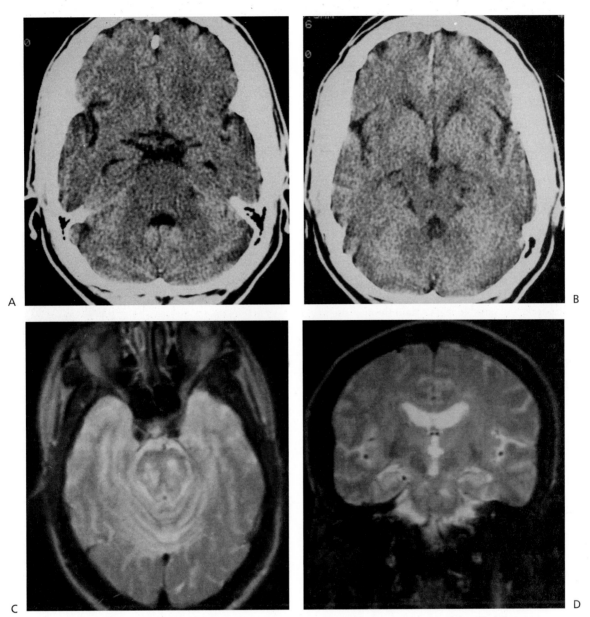

FIGURE 16.6. Brainstem infarction. Noncontrast axial computed tomographies reveal possible infarcts in left brachium pontis **(A)** and right midbrain **(B)**. Axial **(C)** and coronal **(D)** T2-weighted magnetic resonance scans of the same patient clearly show these and additional small infarcts not seen on CT. (Courtesy of Drs. J. A. Bello and S. K. Hilal.)

though both infarct and tumor may show reduced *N*-acetylaspartate and elevated lactate, a markedly elevated choline peak is strong evidence for tumor and against infarction. Adding DWI may also be helpful because diffusion rates are usually normal to prolonged in tumor (iso to low signal on DWI) in contrast to low diffusion rates in acute to subacute infarction (high signal on DWI).

MAGNETIC RESONANCE ANGIOGRAPHY

MRA, also described in Chapter 13, is rapidly becoming the method of choice for screening the extracranial and intracranial vasculature. MRA, with Doppler ultrasound, is commonly used for the initial evaluation of carotid bifurcation stenosis. Depending on the institution and surgeon, these may be the only preoperative imaging studies done. Although MRA generally depicts a similar degree of stenosis to that on the Doppler ultrasound, there are artifacts on MRA that can be misleading. High flow rates can produce signal loss within the lumen, exaggerating the degree of stenosis, and turbulent flow can mimic complex plaque anatomy or ulceration. When the MRA and Doppler disagree substantially, catheter angiography is indicated for a definitive diagnosis.

MRA is also used for screening the intracranial circulation. Large vessels of the circle of Willis can be imaged effectively and rapidly, but current resolution precludes detailed observation of vessels more distal than the second-order branches of the middle cerebral artery. Conventional angiography remains the gold standard for evaluation of subtle segmental stenoses produced by arteritis, especially in small distal branches. Although MRA images are not as sharp as those of conventional angiography, all vessels are visualized simultaneously and can be viewed from any angle; most important, MRA is completely safe, noninvasive, and can be added to the routine MRI examination. The use of MRA as a screening technique for intracranial aneurysms is also increasing. Although MRA can detect aneurysms as small as 3 mm under optimal conditions, a practical lower limit in clinical usage is probably 5 mm diameter. A pitfall with time-of-flight MRA is the high signal produced by subacute parenchymal or subarachnoid hemorrhage that can mimic an aneurysm or AVM. Phase contrast MRA may be a better choice in patients with known hemorrhage. Conventional angiography is the definitive examination for evaluation of intracranial aneurysms and arteriovenous malformations. Other indications for screening MRA include stroke, transient ischemic attack, and possible venous sinus thrombosis.

CATHETER ANGIOGRAPHY

Analysis of cerebrovascular disease has become increasingly precise with new technologies. As a result, many changes have occurred in practice, especially in the use of cerebral catheter angiography, once the mainstay of vascular imaging. Before the availability of CT and MRI, angiography was used routinely to outline intra- and extraaxial hematomas, evaluate vasospasm after ruptured aneurysms, and estimate degree of extracranial arterial stenosis. With the advent of CT, MRI, and Doppler studies, the diagnostic role of angiography is now more restricted. In many centers, angiography is used only to study intracranial vascular disease that is not visualized by MRI, MRA, or Doppler techniques. Catheter angiography involves the intraarterial injection of water-soluble iodinated contrast agents; transient opacification of the arterial lumen is filmed by conventional radiographic or digital subtraction techniques. Angiography is unsurpassed in the detailed anatomic depiction of stenosis, occlusion, recanalization, ulceration, or dissection of large and small intra- and extracranial arteries (Fig. 16.7).

Because catheter angiography is expensive, requires specialized catheter skills, and carries a 0.5% to 3% risk of embolic stroke, it is often undertaken only once in the course of hemorrhage or infarct evaluation. For a diagnosis of embolism, angiography should be carried out within hours of the ictus because the embolic particle may fragment early, changing the appearance of the affected vessel from occlusion to stenosis or a normal lumen, depending on the delay time. When atheromatous stenosis of large arteries is suspected, preangiographic studies of central retinal artery pressure or Doppler ultrasound (see the following) help to tailor the angiographic study and enable the angiographer to concentrate on the major territories thought to be affected. Catheter angiography is the primary method for preoperative evaluation of intracranial aneurysms and arteriovenous malformations, especially if interventional catheter therapies are being considered.

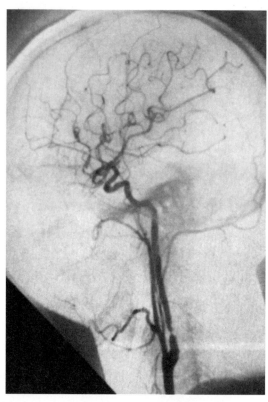

FIGURE 16.7. Proximal internal carotid stenosis. Lateral arteriogram of the common carotid shows an ulcerated plaque of the proximal internal carotid with hemodynamically significant stenosis. Anterior circulation failed to fill and cross-filled from the contralateral side. (Courtesy of Drs. J. A. Bello and S. K. Hilal.)

Catheter angiography techniques have become more sophisticated and now include interventional methods for the treatment of neurovascular disease. Thrombolytic agents can be delivered directly to intravascular clots, including higher order intracranial vessel branches using superselective microcatheter techniques and to major dural sinuses using retrograde venous approaches. Arterial stenosis can be treated with angioplasty, which involves catheter placement of an intravascular balloon at the stenotic site and then inflating the balloon to expand the vessel. Angioplasty is used mostly for atherosclerotic disease in the extracranial vessels, sometimes followed by placement of a wire mesh stent to help keep the lumen patent. Angioplasty is also used to expand a stenosis caused by vasospasm with subarachnoid hemorrhage. Occlusion of abnormal vessels and aneurysms can also be performed using intravascular techniques. Arteriovenous malformations and fistulas can be treated by occlusion of the feeding arteries with coils (flexible metal spiral coils that induce local thrombosis), and the AVM nidus can be occluded with bucrylate, a rapidly setting polymer glue. Aneurysms can be treated by catheter placement of coils and occasionally balloons within them when surgical treatment is not feasible because of aneurysm anatomy, location, or the patient's medical status. Emergency arterial occlusions are also performed for uncontrollable epistaxis and postoperative hemorrhage in the neck, paranasal sinus, and skull base regions.

DOPPLER MEASUREMENTS

The simplest Doppler devices pass a high-frequency continuous wave sound signal over the tissues in the neck, receive the reflected signal, and process them through a small speaker. Technicians using a *continuous wave Doppler* listen for the pitch of the sound and make a rough judgment of the degree of the Doppler shift to infer whether the blood moving through the artery beneath the probe is normal, decreased, or increased and, if increased, whether blood flow is smooth or turbulent. Little experience is required to separate the high-frequency arterial signal from the low-frequency venous sound or to recognize the extremely high frequencies of severe stenosis. More effort is required to quantitate the signal for comparison with a test at a later date. Because the Doppler shift equation depends on the cosine of the beam versus the flowing blood within the artery, casual angulation of the probe can have major effects on signal production.

To assist in proper probe angulation, *duplex Doppler* devices have two crystals, one atop the other, in a single probe head; one crystal handles the Doppler shift for spectral analysis and the other, the B-mode image of the vessel walls. Improvement in crystal designs have reduced the size of the probe, but it is still so bulky that it is difficult to image and insonate the carotid artery high up under the mandible. The Doppler shift crystal has an adjustable range gate to permit analysis of flow signals from specific depths in the tissues, eliminating conflicting signals where arteries and veins overlie one another. Some even have two range gates, providing an adjustable "volume" or "window" to insonate the moving blood column in an artery at volumes as small as 0.6 mm, the size of the tightest stenosis. The capacity to interrogate the flow pattern from wall to wall across the lumen has made this technique useful for detecting, measuring, and monitoring degrees of stenosis (Fig. 16.8). Because duplex Doppler is sensitive to cross-sectional area and not to wall anatomy, if it is used before angiography, it can alert

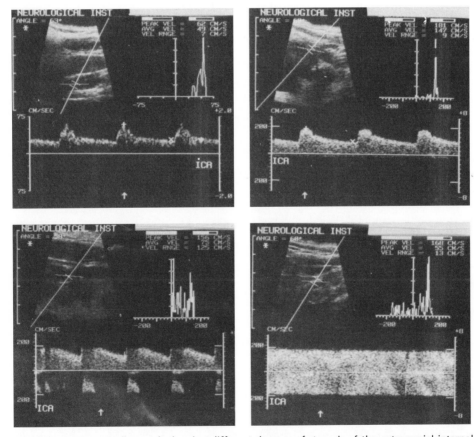

FIGURE 16.8. Four studies, each showing different degrees of stenosis of the extracranial internal carotid. The studies, obtained with the Diasonics DRF 400 instrument, image the carotid by B-mode ultrasound (upper left-hand corner of each of the four pictures) by passing the ultrasound beam through the tissues (*angled line*) and sampling the flow velocity at a point within the lumen of the vessel (*horizontal bracketed line*). From this sample, the device displays the waveforms representing the velocity profile calculated from the Doppler shift (waveforms shown with velocity in cm/s in each picture). The mean velocities are then calculated from a sample taken near the peak of each waveform (small *arrow* under each waveform line) and the spectrum of velocities (i.e., degree of turbulence) is displayed as "peak vel" (i.e., velocity), "mean vel," and "vel range" (shown in graphic form in the upper right-hand corner of each picture). Examples of varying degrees of stenosis are shown: normal flow, left upper corner; moderate (60% to 80%) stenosis with moderate turbulence, right upper corner; severe (80% to 90%) stenosis with marked turbulence, left lower corner; extremely severe (90% to 99%) stenosis with extreme turbulence, right lower corner.

the angiographer to seek stenotic lesions that might be missed on a survey angiogram. Unfortunately, B-mode vessel imaging is insensitive to most minor ulcerations, which are better seen by conventional angiography. Although duplex Doppler methods were developed to insonate the carotid, they can assess the extracranial vertebral artery through the intervertebral foramina.

Using a probe with great tissue penetration properties, it is possible to insonate the major vessels of the circle of Willis, the vertebrals, and the basilar. Current transcranial Doppler devices are range gated, and the latest models give a color-coded display of the major intracranial arteries (Fig. 16.9). The signals accurately document the direction and velocity of the arterial flow insonated by the narrow probe beam. Spectrum analysis of the signal allows estimation of the degree of stenosis as does extracranial duplex Doppler. Hemodynamically important extracranial stenosis may damp the waveform in the ipsilateral arteries above, allowing the effect of the extracranial disease to be measured and followed serially. A challenge test of contralateral compression can be done to determine whether the effects of unilateral extracranial stenosis are compensated or lack anatomic collaterals. Care must be taken to determine which artery is being insonated; the middle cerebral and posterior cerebral are often misinsonated. The technique is user sensitive, requiring patience to detect the signal and then find the best angle for insonation at a given depth. Minor anatomic variations can cause misleading changes in signal strength. Because the procedure is safe, fast, and uses a probe and microprocessor of tabletop size, the device can be taken to the bedside even in an intensive care unit and used to diagnose developing vasospasm, collateral flow above occlusions, recanalization of an embolized artery, and the presence of important basilar or cerebral artery stenosis. When combined with MRI, it is possible to make a noninvasive diagnosis of stenosis of the basilar artery on the stem of the middle cerebral artery.

REGIONAL CEREBRAL BLOOD FLOW

This oldest and least expensive of the techniques uses ^{133}Xe, inhaled or injected, to generate precise measurements of cortical blood flow. This is one method that can be used at the bedside, in the operating room, or in the intensive care unit, but its spatial resolution is inferior to that of positron emission tomography (PET) or SPECT and it provides no information about subcortical perfusion. It is commonly used with hypercapnia or hypotension to test autoregulatory capacity of resistance vessels. For instance, focal failure of vasodilatory response, if distributed in the territory of a major vessel, has been taken as evidence of maximal dilatation and therefore reduced perfusion pressure. This finding is correlated with elevated cerebral blood volume by SPECT and oxygen extraction fraction by PET and may indicate hemodynamic insufficiency.

STABLE-XENON COMPUTED TOMOGRAPHY

CT can measure changes in tissue density over a period of minutes when nonradioactive xenon gas (essentially a freely diffusible high-attenuation contrast agent) is inhaled and circulates through the capillary bed. This method measures flow in both deep and surface structures at high resolution and provides automatic registration to the anatomic information in the baseline CT. It is limited by problems of signal-to-noise ratio and also by the physiologic and anesthetic effects of the high xenon concentrations (approximately 30%).

SINGLE PHOTON EMISSION COMPUTED TOMOGRAPHY

Like PET, SPECT consists of tomographic imaging of injected radioisotopes. However, these isotopes emit single photons

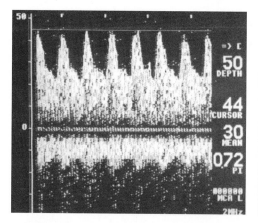 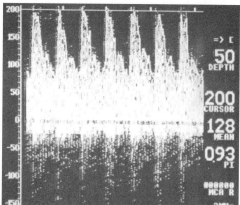

FIGURE 16.9. Two examples of transcranial Doppler insonations of the middle cerebral artery, obtained at a depth of 50 mm from the side of the head overlying the temporal bone, using the Carolina Medical Electronics TC-64B device. The velocity profile of the Doppler shift is insonated at this depth from the blood in the middle cerebral artery flowing toward the probe (upper *arrow* directed to the right in each picture). The left picture shows a normal peak (cursor 44 [cm/s], **left**) and mean (30) and pulsatility index (0.72 PI, i.e., the difference between the peak systolic velocity and the end diastolic velocity divided by the mean velocity). **Right:** The peak (200 cursor) and mean (128 mean) velocities and the pulsatility index (0.93) are higher, consistent with local stenosis at this point in the course of the middle cerebral artery.

rather than positrons, a difference that gives SPECT a more favorable cost-to-benefit ratio and makes it more widely available and clinically useful. However, SPECT is limited in application and is used widely only for imaging cerebral perfusion. Cerebral blood volume imaging is also available, and combined flow and volume scans are possible. Metabolic and receptor agents are being developed. SPECT imaging of infarction and ischemia appears to offer high sensitivity and early detection, but specificity is not yet established. In contrast to PET, SPECT can be used hours after an injection of the tracer; cerebral blood flow can be assessed under unique circumstances (e.g., during an epileptic seizure). Another promising use may be determination of cerebrovascular reserve through dilatory challenge (CO_2 or acetazolamide) or combined flow and volume imaging (Fig. 16.10). These techniques may identify the areas where blood flow is reduced because of perfusion pressure, and therefore possibly of causal relevance, as opposed to the areas where flow is reduced because of diminished metabolic demand (e.g., due to infarction) and therefore of less therapeutic significance. Similar to cardiac methods, these techniques may indicate regions of tissue viability.

POSITRON EMISSION TOMOGRAPHY

PET generates axial images using physical and mathematical principles similar to those used in CT, but the source of radiation is internal to the imaged organ, originating in injected or inhaled radioisotopes. The radioisotopes are short lived and require an adjacent cyclotron. The expense and technical complexity limit the availability of PET. On the other hand, the biochemical flexibility and sensitivity of PET are unparalleled. PET is superior to any other technique in imaging specific receptors or protein synthesis and turnover.

DISCUSSION

All these laboratory methods can be summarized with respect to their information content under four headings: vascular anatomy, tissue damage, hemodynamics, and biochemistry (Table 16.1). Although most techniques provide information in many domains, Table 16.1 indicates only the predominant ap-

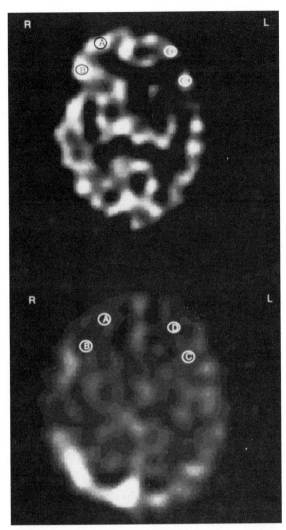

FIGURE 16.10. Single photon emission computed tomography (SPECT) study of a 64-year-old woman after 2 weeks of progressive saltatory aphasia and right hemiparesis. The syndrome was attributed to a distal field infarct in the left hemisphere, and the left internal carotid artery was occluded. SPECT simultaneously imaged cerebral blood flow (CBF) with ^{123}I-IMP and cerebral blood volume (CBV) with ^{99m}Tc-labeled red blood cells. **Top:** CBF; **bottom:** CBV. Four areas of interest (**A–D**) were selected on the CBF image and samples on the CBV image. In the frontal cortex, blood flow was reduced and volume was increased on the left. The CBV/CBF ratio was 0.76 for **A** and **D** and 0.66 for **B** and **C**, thus implying a lower perfusion pressure on the left. (As is conventional for computed tomography and magnetic resonance imaging figures, the left side of brain is on the right of the figure.)

TABLE 16.1. PREDOMINANT APPLICATIONS OF NEUROVASCULAR IMAGING TECHNIQUES

	Tissue Damage	Vascular Anatomy	Hemodynamics	Biochemistry
CT	✓			
MR imaging	✓		✓	
MR angiography		✓		
MR spectroscopy				✓
Positron emission tomography			✓	✓
^{133}Xe regional cerebral blood flow			✓	
Stable xenon CT			✓	
Single proton CT emission			✓	
Angiography		✓		
Doppler		✓	✓	

MC, magnetic resonance; CT, computed tomography.

plications. All cerebrovascular laboratory techniques can be assigned to one or more of the four main categories, but overlap is common and the boundaries are sometimes diffuse. For instance, tissue damage visualized by CT or MRI can be either hemorrhagic or ischemic infarction. Although the information may be useful in suggesting the more likely cause, vascular anatomy and local hemodynamics are usually more informative. For example, carotid occlusion or local absence of vascular reserve are two distinctly different causes of ischemic infarction and may lead to distinctly different treatment options. Finally, the assessment of local metabolism and biochemistry, best performed by PET and MRS, is not known to be clinically useful, but it is an area of active research.

SUGGESTED READINGS

Beauchamp NJ Jr, Ulug AM, Passe TJ, van Zijl PC. MR diffusion imaging in stroke: review and controversies. *Radiographics* 1998;18:1269–1283; discussion 1283–1285.

Brant-Zawadzki M, Heiserman JE. The roles of MR angiography, CT angiography, and sonography in vascular imaging of the head and neck. *AJNR Am J Neuroradiol* 1997;10:1820–1825.

Bryan RN, Levy LM, Whitlow WD, et al. Diagnosis of acute cerebral infarction: comparison of CT and MR imaging. *AJNR Am J Neuroradiol* 1991;12:611–620.

Go JL, Zee CS. Unique CT imaging advantages. Hemorrhage and calcification. *Neuroimaging Clin N Am* 1998;8:541–558.

Gomori JM, Grossman RI. Mechanisms responsible for the MR appearance and evolution of intracranial hemorrhage. *Radiographics* 1988;8:427–440.

Gonzalez RG, Schaefer PW, Buonanno FS, et al. Diffusion-weighted MR imaging: diagnostic accuracy in patients imaged within 6 hours of stroke symptom onset. *Radiology* 1999;210:155–162.

Hacein-Bey L, Kirsch CF, DeLaPaz R, et al. Early diagnosis and endovascular interventions for ischemic stroke. *New Horizons* 1997;5:316–331.

Hagen T, Bartylla K, Piepgras U. Correlation of regional cerebral blood flow measured by stable xenon CT and perfusion MRI. *J Comput Assist Tomogr* 1999;23:257–264.

Hunter GJ, Hamberg LM, Ponzo JA, et al. Assessment of cerebral perfusion and arterial anatomy in hyperacute stroke with three-dimensional functional CT: early clinical results. *AJNR Am J Neuroradiol* 1998;19:29–37.

Irino T, Tandea M, Minami T. Angiographic manifestations in postrecanalized cerebral infarction. *Neurology* 1977;27:471.

Kaps M, Damian MS, Teschendorf U, Dorndorf W. Transcranial Doppler ultrasound findings in middle cerebral artery occlusion. *Stroke* 1990;21:532–537.

Koenig M, Klotz E, Luka B, Venderink DJ, Spittler JF, Heuser L. Perfusion CT of the brain: diagnostic approach for early detection of ischemic stroke. *Radiology* 1998;209:85–93.

Kushner MJ, Zanette EM, Bastianello S, et al. Transcranial Doppler in acute hemispheric brain infarction. *Neurology* 1990;41:109–113.

Lennihan L, Petty GW, Mohr JP, et al. Transcranial Doppler detection of anterior cerebral artery vasospasm. *Stroke* 1989;20:151.

Mattle HP, Kent KC, Edelman RR, et al. Evaluation of the extracranial carotid arteries: correlation of magnetic resonance angiography, duplex ultrasonography, and conventional angiography. *J Vasc Surg* 1991;13:838.

Mohr JP, Biller J, Hilal SK, et al. MR vs CT imaging in acute stroke. Presented at the 17th International Conference on Stroke and the Cerebral Circulation, Phoenix, 1992.

Nussel F, Wegmuller H, Huber P. Comparison of magnetic resonance angiography, magnetic resonance imaging and conventional angiography in cerebral arteriovenous malformation. *Neuroradiology* 1991;33:56–61.

Pessin MS, Hinton RC, Davis KR, et al. Mechanisms of acute carotid stroke: a clinicoangiographic study. *Ann Neurol* 1979;6:245.

Ricci PE Jr. Proton MR spectroscopy in ischemic stroke and other vascular disorders. *Neuroimaging Clin N Am* 1998;8:881–900.

Schwartz RB, Tice HM, Hooten SM, Hsu L, Stieg PE. Evaluation of cerebral aneurysms with helical CT: correlation with conventional angiography and MR angiography. *Radiology* 1994;192:717–722.

Singer MB, Atlas SW, Drayer BP. Subarachnoid space disease: diagnosis with fluid-attenuated inversion-recovery MR imaging and comparison with gadolinium-enhanced spin-echo MR imaging—blinded reader study. *Radiology* 1998;208:417–422.

Sorensen AG, Copen WA, Ostergaard L, et al. Hyperacute stroke: simultaneous measurement of relative cerebral blood volume, relative cerebral blood flow, and mean tissue transit time. *Radiology* 1999;210:519–527.

Steinke W, Hennerici M, Rautenberg W, Mohr JP. Symptomatic and asymptomatic high-grade carotid stenosis in Doppler color flow imaging. *Neurology* 1992;42:131–138.

Tatemichi TK, Chamorro A, Petty GW, et al. Hemodynamic role of ophthalmic artery collateral in internal carotid artery occlusion. *Neurology* 1990;40:461–464.

Zyed A, Hayman LA, Bryan RN. MR imaging of intracerebral blood: diversity in the temporal pattern at 0.5 and 1.0 T. *AJNR Am J Neuroradiol* 1991;12:469–474.

Merritt's Neurology, 10th ed., edited by L.P. Rowland. Lippincott Williams & Wilkins, Philadelphia © 2000.

LUMBAR PUNCTURE AND CEREBROSPINAL FLUID EXAMINATION

ROBERT A. FISHMAN

INDICATIONS

Lumbar puncture (LP) should be performed only after clinical evaluation of the patient and consideration of the potential value and hazards of the procedure. Cerebrospinal fluid (CSF) findings are important in the differential diagnosis of the gamut of central nervous system (CNS) infections, meningitis, and encephalitis and subarachnoid hemorrhage, confusional states, acute stroke, status epilepticus, meningeal malignancies, demyelinating diseases, and CNS vasculitis. CSF examination usually is necessary in patients with suspected intracranial bleeding to establish the diagnosis, although computed tomography (CT), when available, may be more valuable. For example, primary intracerebral hemorrhage or posttraumatic hemorrhage is often readily observed with CT, thus making LP an unnecessary hazard. In primary subarachnoid hemorrhage, however, LP may establish the diagnosis when CT is falsely negative. LP can ascertain whether the CSF is free of blood before anticoagulant therapy for stroke is begun. (Extensive subarachnoid or epidural bleeding is a rare complication of heparin anticoagulation that starts several hours after a traumatic bloody tap. Therefore, heparin therapy should not commence for at least 1 hour after a bloody tap.) LP has limited therapeutic usefulness (e.g., intrathecal therapy in meningeal malignancies and fungal meningitis).

CONTRAINDICATIONS

LP is contraindicated in the presence of infection in skin overlying the spine. A serious complication of LP is the possibility of aggravating a preexisting, often unrecognized brain herniation syndrome (e.g., uncal, cerebellar, or cingulate herniation) associated with intracranial hypertension. This hazard is the basis for considering papilledema to be a relative contraindication to LP. The availability of CT has simplified the management of patients with papilledema. If CT reveals no evidence of a mass lesion or edema, then LP is usually needed in the presence of papilledema to establish the diagnosis of pseudotumor cerebri and to exclude meningeal inflammation or malignancy.

HAZARDS OF BLEEDING DISORDERS

Thrombocytopenia and other bleeding diatheses predispose patients to needle-induced subarachnoid, subdural, and epidural hemorrhage. LP should be undertaken only for urgent clinical indications when the platelet count is depressed to about 50,000/mm^3 or below. Platelet transfusion just before the puncture is recommended if the count is below 20,000 mm^3 or dropping rapidly. The administration of protamine to patients on heparin and of vitamin K or fresh frozen plasma to those receiving warfarin is recommended before LP to minimize the hazard of the procedure.

COMPLICATIONS

Complications of LP include worsening of brain herniation or spinal cord compression, headache, subarachnoid bleeding, diplopia, backache, and radicular symptoms. Post-LP headache is the most common complication, occurring in about 25% of patients and usually lasting 2 to 8 days. It results from low CSF pressures caused by persistent fluid leakage through the dural hole. Characteristically, the head pain is present in the upright position, promptly relieved by the supine position, and aggravated by cough or strain. Aching of the neck and low back, nausea, vomiting, and tinnitus are common complaints. Post-LP headache is avoided when a small styletted needle is used and if multiple puncture holes are not made. The management of the problem depends on strict bedrest in the horizontal position, adequate hydration, and simple analgesics. If conservative measures fail, the use of a "blood patch" is indicated. The technique uses the epidural injection of autologous blood close to site of the dural puncture to form a fibrinous tamponade that apparently seals the dural hole.

CEREBROSPINAL FLUID PRESSURE

The CSF pressure should be measured routinely. The pressure level within the right atrium is the reference level with the patient in the lateral decubitus position. The normal lumbar CSF pressure ranges between 50 and 200 mm (and as high as 250 mm in extremely obese subjects). With the use of the clinical manometer, the arterially derived pulsatile pressures are obscured, but respiratory pressure waves reflecting changes in central venous pressures are visible. Low pressures occur after a previous LP, with dehydration, spinal subarachnoid block, or CSF fistulas. Intracranial hypotension may be a technical artifact when the needle is not inserted in the subarachnoid space. Increased pressures occur in patients with brain edema, intracranial mass lesions, infections, acute stroke, cerebral venous occlusions, congestive heart failure, pulmonary insufficiency, and hepatic failure. Benign intracranial hypertension (pseudotumor cerebri) and spontaneous intracranial hypotension are discussed elsewhere.

CEREBROSPINAL FLUID CELLS

Normal CSF contains no more than 5 lymphocytes or mononuclear cells/mm^3. A higher white cell count is pathognomonic of disease in the CNS or meninges. A stained smear of the sediment must be prepared for an accurate differential cell count. Various centrifugal and sedimentation techniques have been used. A pleocytosis occurs with the gamut of inflammatory disorders. The changes characteristic of the various meningitides are listed in Table 17.1. The heterogeneous forms of neuro-AIDS are associated with a wide range of cellular responses. Other disorders associated with a pleocytosis include brain infarction, subarachnoid bleeding, cerebral vasculitis, acute demyelination, and brain tumors. Eosinophilia most often accompanies parasitic infections, such as cysticercosis, and may reflect blood eosinophilia. Cytologic studies for malignant cells are rewarding with some CNS neoplasms.

Bloody CSF due to needle trauma contains increased numbers of white cells contributed by the blood. A useful approximation of a true white cell count can be obtained by the following correction for the presence of the added blood: If the patient has a normal hemogram, subtract from the total white cell count (cells/mm^3) 1 white cell for each 1,000 red blood cells present. Thus, if bloody fluid contains 10,000 red cells/mm^3 and 100 white cells/mm^3, 10 white cells would be accounted for by the added blood and the corrected leukocyte

TABLE 17.1. CEREBROSPINAL FLUID FINDINGS IN MENINGITIS

Meningitis	Pressure (mm H$_2$O)	Leukocytes (mm^3)	Protein (mg/dL)	Glucose (mg/dL)
Acute bacterial	Usually elevated	Several hundred to more than 60,000; usually few thousand; occasionally less than 100 (especially meningococcal or early in disease); polymorphonuclear leukocytes predominate	Usually 100–500, occasionally more than 1,000	5–40 in most cases (in absence of hyperglycemia)
Tuberculous	Usually elevated; may be low with dynamic block in advanced stages	Usually 25–100; rarely more than 500; lymphocytes predominate except in early stages when polymorphonuclear leukocytes may account for 80% of cells	Nearly always elevated, usually 100–200; may be much higher if dynamic block	Usually reduced; less than 45 in 75% of cases
Cryptococcal	Usually elevated	0–800; average 50; lymphocytes predominate	Usually 20–500; average 100	Reduced in most cases; average 30 (in absence of hyperglycemia)
Viral	Normal to moderately elevated	5 to few hundred but may be more than 1,000, particularly with lymphocytic choriomeningitis; lymphocytes predominate but may be more than 80% polymorphonuclear leukocytes in first few days	Frequently normal or slightly elevated; less than 100; may show greater elevation in severe cases	Normal (reduced in 25% of cases of mumps and herpes simplex)
Syphilitic (acute)	Usually elevated	Average 500; usually lymphocytes; rarely polymorphonuclear leukocytes	Average 100	Normal (rarely reduced)
Cysticercosis	Often increased; low with dynamic block	Increased mononuclear and polymorphonuclear leukocytes with 2–7% eosinophilia in about 50% of cases	Usually 50–200	Reduced in 20% of cases
Sarcoid	Normal to considerably elevated	0 to less than 100 mononuclear cells	Slight to moderate elevation	Reduced in 50% of cases
Tumor	Normal or elevated	0 to several hundred mononuclear leukocytes plus malignant cells	Elevated, often to high levels	Normal or greatly reduced (low in 75% of carcinomatous meningitis cases)

Cerebrospinal fluid (CSF) immunoglobulins are commonly increased in all described conditions (including carcinomatous meningitis) and in multiple sclerosis. CSF immunoglobulins are assessed by the IgG index:

$$\frac{\text{IgG(CSF)} \times \text{albumin(serum)}}{\text{IgG(serum)} \times \text{albumin (CSF)}}$$

The normal index is less than about 0.65. The presence of multiple oligoclonal bands (with gel electrophoresis) is also a measure of abnormally increased CSF immunoglobulins.

count would be 90/mm³. If the patient's hemogram reveals significant anemia or leukocytosis, the following formula may be used to determine more accurately the number of white cells (W) in the spinal fluid before the blood was added:

$$W = \frac{\text{blood WBC} \times \text{CSF RBC}}{\text{blood RBC}} \times 100.$$

The presence of blood in the subarachnoid space produces a secondary inflammatory response, which leads to a disproportionate increase in the number of white cells. After an acute subarachnoid hemorrhage, this elevation in the white cell count is most marked about 48 hours after onset, when meningeal signs are most striking.

To correct CSF protein values for the presence of added blood resulting from needle trauma, subtract 1 mg for every 1,000 red blood cells. Thus, if the red cell count is 10,000/mm³ and the total protein is 110 mg/dL, the corrected protein level would be about 100 mg/dL. The corrections are reliable only if the cell count and total protein are both made on the same tube of fluid.

BLOOD IN THE CEREBROSPINAL FLUID: DIFFERENTIAL DIAGNOSIS AND THE THREE-TUBE TEST

To differentiate between a traumatic spinal puncture and pre-existing subarachnoid hemorrhage, the fluid should be collected in at least three separate tubes (the "three-tube test"). In traumatic punctures, the fluid generally clears between the first and the third collections. This change is detectable by the naked eye and should be confirmed by cell count. In subarachnoid bleeding, the blood is generally evenly admixed in the three tubes. A sample of the bloody fluid should be centrifuged and the supernatant fluid compared with tap water to exclude the presence of pigment. The supernatant fluid is crystal clear if the red count is less than about 100,000 cells/mm³. With bloody contamination of greater magnitude, plasma proteins may be sufficient to cause minimal xanthochromia, an effect that requires enough serum to raise the CSF protein concentration to about 150 mg/dL.

After an acute subarachnoid hemorrhage, the supernatant fluid usually remains clear for 2 to 4 hours or even longer after the onset of subarachnoid bleeding. The clear supernatant may mislead the physician to conclude erroneously that the observed blood is the result of needle trauma in patients who have had an LP within 4 hours of aneurysmal rupture. After an especially traumatic puncture, some blood and xanthochromia may be present for as long as 2 to 5 days. In pathologic states associated with a CSF protein content exceeding 150 mg/dL and in the absence of bleeding, faint xanthochromia may be detected. When the protein is elevated to much higher levels, as in spinal block, polyneuritis, or meningitis, the xanthochromia may be considerable. A xanthochromic fluid with a normal protein level or a minor elevation to less than 150 mg/dL usually indicates a previous subarachnoid or intracerebral hemorrhage. Xanthochromia may be caused by severe jaundice, carotenemia, or rifampin therapy.

Pigments

The two major pigments derived from red cells that may be observed in CSF are oxyhemoglobin and bilirubin. Methemoglobin is seen only spectrophotometrically. Oxyhemoglobin, released with lysis of red cells, may be detected in the supernatant fluid within 2 hours after subarachnoid hemorrhage. It reaches a maximum in about the first 36 hours and gradually disappears over the next 7 to 10 days. Bilirubin is produced in vivo by leptomeningeal cells after red cell hemolysis. Bilirubin is first detected about 10 hours after the onset of subarachnoid bleeding. It reaches a maximum at 48 hours and may persist for 2 to 4 weeks after extensive bleeding. The severity of the meningeal signs associated with subarachnoid bleeding correlates with the inflammatory response (i.e., the severity of the leukocytic pleocytosis).

Total Protein

The normal total protein level of CSF ranges between 15 and 50 mg/dL. Although an elevated protein level lacks specificity, it is an index of neurologic disease reflecting a pathologic increase in endothelial cell permeability. Greatly increased protein levels, 500 mg/dL and above, are seen in meningitis, bloody fluids, or spinal cord tumor with spinal block. Polyneuritis (Guillain-Barré syndrome), diabetic radiculoneuropathy, and myxedema also may increase the level to 100 to 300 mg/dL. Low protein levels, below 15 mg/dL, occur most often with CSF leaks caused by a previous LP or traumatic dural fistula and uncommonly in pseudotumor cerebri.

Immunoglobulins

Although many proteins may be measured in CSF, only an increase in immunoglobulins is of diagnostic importance. Such increases are indicative of an inflammatory response in the CNS and occur with immunologic disorders and bacterial, viral, spirochetal, and fungal diseases. Immunoglobulin assays are most useful in the diagnosis of multiple sclerosis, other demyelinating diseases, and CNS vasculitis. The CSF level is corrected for the entry of immunoglobulins from the serum by calculating the IgG index (Table 17.1). More than one oligoclonal band in CSF with gel electrophoresis (and absent in serum) is also abnormal, occurring in 90% of multiple sclerosis cases and in the gamut of inflammatory diseases.

Glucose

The CSF glucose concentration depends on the blood level. The normal range of CSF is between 45 and 80 mg/dL in patients with a blood glucose between 70 and 120 mg/dL (i.e., 60% to 80% of the normal blood level). CSF values between 40 and 45 mg/dL are usually abnormal, and values below 40 mg/dL are invariably so. Hyperglycemia during the 4 hours before LP results in a parallel increase in CSF glucose. The CSF glucose approaches a maximum, and the CSF-to-blood ratio may be as low as 0.35 in the presence of a greatly elevated blood glucose level and in the absence of any neurologic disease. An increase in CSF glucose is of no diagnostic significance apart from reflecting hyperglycemia within the 4 hours before LP.

The CSF glucose level is abnormally low (hypoglycorrhachia) in several diseases of the nervous system apart from hypoglycemia. It is characteristic of acute purulent meningitis and is a usual finding in tuberculous and fungal meningitis. It is usually normal in viral meningitis, although reduced in about 25% of mumps cases and in some cases of herpes simplex and zoster meningoencephalitis. The CSF glucose is also reduced in other inflammatory meningitides, including cysticercosis, amebic meningitis (*Naegleria*), acute syphilitic meningitis, sarcoidosis, granulomatous arteritis, and other vasculitides. The glucose level is also reduced in the chemical meningitis that follows intrathecal injections and in subarachnoid hemorrhage, usually 4 to 8 days after the onset of bleeding. The major factor responsible for the depressed glucose levels is increased anaerobic glycolysis in adjacent neural tissues and to a lesser degree by a polymorphonuclear leukocytosis. Thus, the decrease in CSF glucose level is characteristically accompanied by an inverse increase in CSF lactate level. A low CSF glucose with a decreased lactate level indicates impairment of the glucose transporter responsible for the transfer of glucose across the blood–brain barrier.

MICROBIOLOGIC AND SEROLOGIC REACTIONS

The use of appropriate stains and cultures is essential in cases of suspected infection. Tests for specific bacterial and fungal antigens and countercurrent immunoelectrophoresis are useful in establishing a specific cause. DNA amplification techniques using polymerase chain reaction have improved diagnostic sensitivity. Serologic tests on CSF for syphilis include the reagin antibody tests and specific treponemal antibody tests. The former are particularly useful in evaluating CSF because positive results occur even in the presence of a negative blood serology. There is no logical basis for applying specific treponemal antibody tests to CSF because these antibodies are derived from the plasma, where they are present in greater concentration.

SUGGESTED READING

Fishman RA. *Cerebrospinal fluid in diseases of the nervous system*, 2nd ed. Philadelphia: W.B. Saunders, 1992.

Merritt's Neurology, 10th ed., edited by L.P. Rowland. Lippincott Williams & Wilkins, Philadelphia © 2000.

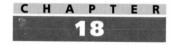

CHAPTER 18

MUSCLE AND NERVE BIOPSY

ARTHUR P. HAYS

Biopsy of skeletal muscle or peripheral nerve is performed in patients with neuromuscular disorders, chiefly those with myopathy or peripheral neuropathy. At the least, the findings may indicate whether a syndrome of limb weakness is neurogenic or myopathic. This determination is made in conjunction with the findings on electromyography and nerve conduction studies; the interpretations based on biopsy and physiologic study are usually congruent with each other and also with clinical indicators from the history and examination. At best, the biopsy of muscle and nerve may give a specific tissue diagnosis. Sometimes, however, the findings are not diagnostic because the defining lesion has been missed in the biopsy, which is only a tiny sample of a voluminous tissue, and the lesions may be present in one area but not in another. Also, the pathologic changes may be too mild to distinguish from normal or too advanced to draw conclusions ("end-stage" muscle, for instance).

The yield of a specific diagnosis is low, but the percentage has increased through the application of technologic innovations. In myopathies, histochemical and immunohistochemical stains applied to frozen tissue sections and

biochemical analysis of enzymes, structural proteins, or DNA have transformed the prospects of tissue-based diagnosis. Precise diagnoses in peripheral nerve disorders often require immunohistochemical stains to localize human antigens, resin histology (semithin plastic sections), electron microscopy, and teased preparations of myelinated nerve fibers.

The performance and analysis of a muscle and nerve biopsy are time-consuming and expensive. Therefore, the decision for biopsy is made only after a thorough evaluation that includes neurologic examination, family history, laboratory tests, cerebrospinal fluid examination, and electrodiagnostic studies. This workup obviates the need for biopsy in typical cases of myasthenia gravis, myotonic dystrophy, dermatomyositis, amyotrophic lateral sclerosis, Guillain-Barré syndrome, diabetic neuropathy, or any defined toxic neuropathy. Additionally, a rapidly expanding number of diseases can be diagnosed by DNA analysis of blood leukocytes without recourse to tissue analysis (e.g., McArdle disease, Duchenne or Becker muscular dystrophy, mitochondrial disorders, and Charcot-Marie-Tooth disease type IA, as described in Chapters 84, 96, 102, and 125).

If a biopsy is deemed necessary, the neurologist should formulate a preliminary diagnosis and inform the pathologist to direct evaluation of the specimen most efficiently. The surgical procedure should be performed by an experienced neurologist or surgeon, identifying the tissue correctly and avoiding mechanically induced artifacts or insufficient quantity for examination. If special methods are not available locally, the service usually can be provided by a regional research center.

SKELETAL MUSCLE BIOPSY

Muscle biopsy is performed in patients with limb weakness, infantile hypotonia, exercise intolerance, myoglobinuria, or cramps. Evaluation should include serum creatine kinase assay, family history, and electromyography. A biopsy is also indicated in the final assessment of patients with a presumptive diagnosis of a muscular dystrophy, polymyositis, inclusion body myositis, congenital myopathy, or spinal muscular atrophy; glycolytic or oxidative enzyme defect; or myopathies associated with alcohol, electrolyte disturbance, drug toxicity, carcinoma, endocrine overactivity or underactivity, or long-term treatment with steroids. It is also justified in polymyalgia rheumatica and eosinophilic fasciitis and to show the extent of denervation associated with peripheral neuropathy in conjunction with sural nerve biopsy.

Muscles preferred for biopsy are the vastus lateralis, biceps, or deltoid in disorders of proximal limb weakness and the gastrocnemius, tibialis anterior, or peroneus brevis when symptoms are pronounced distally. The muscle should be affected clinically and electrophysiologically. However, to avoid obtaining an end-stage picture, the muscle should not be severely wasted and paralyzed.

Routine histology of muscle can demonstrate groups of atrophic myofibers in a neurogenic disorder or myopathic features that include necrotic fibers, regenerating fibers, excessive sarcoplasmic glycogen, or centrally located myonuclei. Lymphocytic infiltration of connective tissue is seen in dermatomyositis, polymyositis, and inclusion body myositis. The diagnosis of vasculitis or amyloidosis is occasionally established by finding changes in the muscle biopsy, even if neuropathy is evident clinically and physiologically.

Histochemical techniques applied to cryosections of muscle permit the recognition of fiber-type grouping; target fibers; fiber-type predominance; selective fiber atrophy; central cores; nemaline rods; excessive sarcoplasmic glycogen, lipid, or mitochondria (ragged red fibers) as a result of a disorder of metabolism; deficiency of phosphorylase, phosphofructokinase, adenylate deaminase, or cytochrome *c* oxidase activity; and other structurally specific abnormalities that are not visible by conventional light microscopy of paraffin-embedded tissue. An example is provided by the finding of rimmed vacuoles and the intracellular amyloid inclusions of inclusion body myositis.

Biochemical assays of muscle can detect a quantitative reduction of enzymes of intermediary metabolism, including enzymes of the glycolytic pathway, acid maltase, adenylate deaminase, and enzymes of mitochondria (carnitine palmitoyl transferase, enzymes of the citric acid cycle, and electron transport chain).

Immunohistochemical stains can detect the absence of dystrophin in Duchenne muscular dystrophy and a mosaic pattern of dystrophin in girls or women who carry the mutation. Discontinuities of sarcolemmal dystrophin are found in Becker dystrophy. These dystrophinopathies must be confirmed by DNA analysis of blood leukocytes or by electrophoresis of a muscle homogenate (Western blot) to show quantitative or qualitative abnormalities of the protein. Dystrophin analysis is indicated in any syndrome of limb weakness of unknown cause, including possible limb-girdle dystrophy, polymyositis, inclusion body myositis, myoglobinuria, or spinal muscular atrophy. Genetic lack of sarcoglycans, merosin, emerin, or other proteins can be demonstrated by immunohistochemistry in the appropriate muscular dystrophies and confirmed by DNA analysis. Also, evaluation of mitochondrial DNA of muscle or blood can detect deletions in Kearns-Sayre syndrome and point mutations in other mitochondrial encephalomyopathies.

PERIPHERAL NERVE BIOPSY

Nerve biopsy is indicated in patients with peripheral neuropathy when additional information about the nature and severity of the disorder is needed. The biopsy is most likely helpful in mononeuritis multiplex or in patients with palpably enlarged nerves; biopsy is often uninformative in distal symmetric axonal neuropathies. In children, the pathologic features in nerve can be diagnostic in three diseases (metachromatic leukodystrophy, adrenoleukodystrophy, and Krabbe disease), but the biopsy can usually be avoided by making a diagnosis with tests of a blood sample. Several central nervous system disorders are also expressed pathologically in nerve: neuronal ceroid lipofuscinosis, Lafora disease, infantile neuroaxonal dystrophy, and lysosomal storage diseases. The best source of tissue, however, is not a nerve but rather skin and conjunctiva, which may show distinctive features in terminal nerve fibers and skin appendages.

The human sural nerve is the most widely studied nerve in health and disease, and it is most frequently recommended for biopsy. If mononeuritis multiplex spares the sural nerve, other cutaneous nerves can be selected (e.g., a branch of the superficial peroneal nerve at the head of the fibula or the radial sensory nerve at the wrist). Motor nerve fibers can be examined specifically in a nerve that supplies a superfluous or accessory muscle, such as the gracilis muscle in the medial thigh. Neurologists often choose simultaneous biopsy of both sural nerve and gastrocnemius muscle in patients with neuropathy because vasculitis, amyloidosis, sarcoid, lymphoma, and other systemic disorders are focal and lesions may be encountered in either tissue. The muscle also can demonstrate the degree of denervation.

Diagnosis can often be established by microscopic examination of paraffin-embedded tissue in nine conditions: vasculitis, amyloidosis, leprosy, sensory perineuritis, cholesterol emboli, infiltration of nerve by leukemic or lymphoma cells, malignant angioendotheliomatosis (intravascular lymphoma), giant axonal neuropathy, or adult polyglucosan body disease. Amyloid deposits in plasma cell dyscrasia can be identified by antibodies to immunoglobulin light chains. Amyloid deposits in the familial neuropathy resulting from transthyretin mutations can be distinguished by antibodies to the mutant protein. Small cell lymphoma and chronic lymphocytic leukemia can be separated from inflammatory reactions by application of lymphocyte markers.

Most neuropathies do not have distinctive pathologic findings and usually require examination of semithin sections of epoxy-resin–embedded tissue. Teased nerve fibers and electron microscopy are necessary to identify the focal thickening of myelin sheaths (*tomacula*) of hereditary neuropathy with liability to pressure palsy, and they can detect subtle degrees of demyelination, remyelination, or axonal degeneration and regeneration.

These features occur in normal nerves with increasing age, and evaluation may require formal quantitative study (morphometry). Electron microscopy also demonstrates accumulation of neurofilaments, widened myelin lamellae, and various intracellular inclusions in neuropathies, and it is needed to assess unmyelinated nerve fibers.

Axonal neuropathy is recognized by marked depletion of fibers and interstitial fibrosis, with or without myelin debris or regeneration of axons. It is most likely caused by a toxic or metabolic disorder, such as alcoholism or diabetes. Other axonopathies include vasculitis, amyloidosis, paraneoplastic syndromes, and infection (including the distal symmetric neuropathy of AIDS). Segmental demyelination and remyelination, recognized by thinly myelinated fibers and onion bulbs, are most often the result of an immunologically mediated or hereditary neuropathy. If demyelination is not pronounced in semithin plastic sections, it may be proved by electron microscopy or analysis of teased myelinated nerve fibers. Sural nerve biopsy is recommended in all patients with a clinical diagnosis of chronic inflammatory demyelinating polyneuropathy to confirm the suspected demyelination before commencing therapy with intravenous gamma globulin, plasmapheresis, or steroids. The pathologic findings do not distinguish chronic inflammatory demyelinating polyneuropathy from Charcot-Marie-Tooth disease type I, but an acquired myelinopathy is favored by finding prominent variability of abnormalities among nerve fascicles, inflammatory infiltrates, and endoneurial edema. The neuropathies associated with IgM paraproteinemia and antibody to myelin-associated glycoprotein resemble chronic inflammatory demyelinating polyneuropathy clinically and pathologically; deposits of the C3 component of complement may be seen along the periphery of myelin sheaths, usually with IgM located at the same site. Other demyelinative neuropathies include diphtheria, hereditary disorders other than Charcot-Marie-Tooth disease

type I, Guillain-Barré syndrome, and acute or chronic inflammatory neuropathies in the early phase of human immunodeficiency virus infection. The inflammatory neuropathies are multifocal, and the sural nerve may be normal or show only axonal degeneration.

Complications of sural nerve biopsy include annoying causalgia in about 5% of patients. Many patients experience twinges of pain when bending forward for several days caused by stretching of the nerve. All patients should anticipate permanent loss of discriminative sensation in the lateral border of the foot extending to the fifth toe, heel, and lateral malleolus. In weeks or months, however, the sensory symptoms subside completely or to a tolerable level.

SUGGESTED READINGS

Asbury AK, Johnson PC. *Pathology of peripheral nerve.* Philadelphia: W.B. Saunders, 1978.

Dubowitz V. *Muscle biopsy. A practical approach.* London: Churchill Livingstone, 1984.

Dubowitz V. *Muscle disorders in childhood,* 2nd ed. Philadelphia: W.B. Saunders, 1995.

Dyck PJ, Thomas PK, Griffin JW, et al. *Peripheral neuropathy,* 3rd ed. Philadelphia: W.B. Saunders, 1993.

Engel AG, Franzini-Armstrong C. *Myology,* 2nd ed. New York: McGraw-Hill, 1994.

Graham DI, Lanatos PI. *Greenfield's neuropathology,* 6th ed. New York: Oxford University Press, 1997.

Midroni G, Bilbao JM. *Biopsy diagnosis of peripheral neuropathy.* Boston: Butterworth-Heinemann, 1995.

Schaumburg HH, Berger AR, Thomas PK. *Disorders of peripheral nerves,* 2nd ed. Philadelphia: FA Davis, 1992.

Merritt's Neurology, 10th ed., edited by L.P. Rowland. Lippincott Williams & Wilkins, Philadelphia © 2000.

C H A P T E R

19

NEUROPSYCHOLOGIC EVALUATION

YAAKOV STERN

Neuropsychologic testing is a valuable adjunct to neurologic evaluation, especially for the diagnosis of dementia and to evaluate or quantify cognition and behavior in other brain diseases. The tests are therefore important in research as well.

STRATEGY OF NEUROPSYCHOLOGIC TESTING

Conditions that affect the brain often cause cognitive, motor, or behavioral impairment that can be detected by appropriately de-

signed tests. Defective performance on a test may suggest specific pathology. Alternately, patients with known brain changes may be assessed to determine how the damaged brain areas affect specific cognitive functions. Before relating test performance to brain dysfunction, however, other factors that can affect test performance must be considered.

Typically, performance is compared with values derived from populations similar to the patient in age, education, socioeconomic background, and other variables. Scores significantly below mean expected values imply impaired performance. Performance sometimes can be evaluated by assumptions about what can be expected from the average person (e.g., repeating simple sentences or simple learning and remembering).

Comparable data may not exist for the patient being tested. This problem is common in older populations or for those with language and cultural differences. This situation may be addressed by collecting "local norms" that are more descriptive of the served clinical population or by evaluating the cognitive areas that remain intact. In this way, the patient guides the clinician in terms of the level of performance that should be expected in possibly affected domains.

Other factors that also influence test performance must be considered, including depression or other psychiatric disorders, medication, and the patient's motivation.

Patterns of performance, such as strengths in some cognitive domains and weaknesses in others, have been associated with specific conditions based on empirical observation and knowledge of the brain pathology associated with those conditions. Observation of these patterns can aid in diagnosis.

TEST SELECTION

Neuropsychologic tests in an assessment battery come from many sources. Some were developed for academic purposes (e.g., intelligence tests), and others from experimental psychology. The typical clinical battery consists of a series of standard tests that have been proved useful and are selected for the referral issue. A trade-off exists between the breadth of application and ease of interpretation available from standard batteries and the ability to pinpoint specific or subtle disorders offered by more experimental tasks that are useful in research but have not been standardized.

Most tests are intended to measure performance in specific cognitive or motor domains, such as memory, spatial ability, language function, or motor agility. These domains can be subdivided (e.g., memory can be considered verbal or nonverbal; immediate, short-term, long-term, or remote; semantic or episodic; public or autobiographic; or implicit or explicit). No matter how focused a test is, however, multiple cognitive processes are likely to be invoked. An ostensibly simple task, such as the Wechsler Adult Intelligence Scale Digit Symbol—Coding subtest (using a table of nine digit–symbol pairs to fill in the proper symbols for a series of numbers), taps learning and memory, visuospatial abilities, motor abilities, attention, and speeded performance. In addition, tests can be failed for more than one reason: Patients may draw poorly because they cannot appreciate spatial relationships or because they plan the construction process poorly. Relying solely on test scores can lead to spurious conclusions.

TESTS USED IN A NEUROPSYCHOLOGICAL EVALUATION

Intellectual Ability

Typically, the Wechsler Adult Intelligence Scale-III (WAIS-III) or the Wechsler Intelligence Scale for Children-III is used to assess the present level of intellectual function. These tests yield a global intelligence quotient (IQ) score and verbal and performance IQ scores that are standardized, so that 100 is the mean expected value at any age with a standard deviation of 15. The WAIS-III also groups some of the subtests, based on "more refined domains of cognitive functioning," into four index scales: Verbal Comprehension, Perceptual Organization, Working Memory, and Processing Speed. The index scales have the same psychometric properties as the traditional IQ scores.

The WAIS-III consists of seven verbal and seven performance subtests. Scaled scores range from 1 to 19, with a mean of 10 and a standard deviation of 3; the average range for subtest scaled scores is from 7 to 13 (Table 19.1).

The overall IQ score supplies information about the level of general intelligence, but the neuropsychologist is usually more interested in the "scatter" of subtest scores, which indicate strengths and weaknesses. The subtests are better considered as separate tests, each tapping specific areas of cognitive function. There are also other tests of general intelligence, including some that are nonverbal.

TABLE 19.1. SUBTESTS OF THE WECHSLER ADULT INTELLIGENCE SCALE-III

Verbal subtests	
Vocabulary	Defining 33 words. Typically represents "premorbid" level of ability.
Similarities	Deriving relevant superordinate category or similarity for 19 word pairs. Assesses abstract reasoning.
Arithmetic	20 verbal arithmetic problems.
Digit span	Standardized assessment of digits forward and backward. Primarily assesses attention and working memory.
Information	28 general information items. Assesses "old stores" of information.
Comprehension	18 items assessing appreciation of social norms and standards and proverb interpretation.
Letter-number sequencing[a]	New. Listening to a combination of numbers and letters and recalling the numbers first in ascending order and then the letters in alphabetical order. Assesses working memory.
Performance subtests	
Picture completion	Determining the missing feature in 25 pictures.
Digit symbol–coding	Using a table of nine digit-symbol pairs to fill in the proper symbols for a series of numbers. Taps new learning, visuospatial abilities, and speeded performance.
Block design	Arranging blocks with red, white, and half-red and half-white sides to form 14 designs. A complex visuospatial task.
Matrix reasoning	New. Identifying the picture that completes a pattern, using pattern completion, classification, analogy, or serial reasoning. A nonverbal intelligence test.
Picture arrangement	Arranging sets of comic-strip pictures so that they tell a coherent story.
Symbol search[a]	New. Visually scanning a target group of items (composed of two symbols) and a search group (composed of five symbols) and indicating whether either of the target symbols match any of the symbols in the search group.
Object assembly	Assembling five jigsaw puzzles.

[a]Contributes to index scores but not to intelligence quotient scores.

Memory

The subclassifications of memory have evolved from clinical observation and experimentation; most are important to the assessment (Table 19.2). Preservation of remote memories despite inability to store and recall new information is the hallmark of specific amnestic disorders. Other subclassifications are used to evaluate different clinical syndromes.

Construction

Construction, typically assessed by drawing or assembly tasks, requires both accurate spatial perception and an organized motor response. The Block Design and Object Assembly subtests of the WAIS-R are examples of assembly tasks. In the Rosen Drawing Test, the patient is asked to copy 15 drawings that range in difficulty from simple shapes to complex three-dimensional figures. In addition to the scores these tests yield, the clinician attends to the patient's construction performance to determine factors that may underlie poor performance (e.g., a disorganized impulsive strategy may be more related to anterior brain lesions, whereas difficulty aligning angles may arise in parietal lobe injury).

TABLE 19.2. TYPICAL SUBCLASSIFICATIONS OF MEMORY ADDRESSED BY NEUROPSYCHOLOGIC TESTS

Verbal and nonverbal	Memory for material that is or is not verbally encoded.
Immediate, short-term, long-term, and remote	Length of time between exposure to material and recall. The length of time has implications for how the memory may be stored and retrieved.
Semantic and episodic	Memory for encodeable knowledge, such as vocabulary or facts about the world, as opposed to memory for events.
Public and autobiographic	Memory for public commonly known events versus events that occurred in one's own life.
Implicit and explicit	Memory tested on tasks that do not require conscious explicit recollection of recent exposures (such as motor skills, procedural skills, classical conditioning, or priming) versus tasks that demand explicit recall of prior information (such as recall or recognition tasks).
Working	Similar to what in the past has been called short-term memory, working memory provides a buffer for briefly holding on to information, such as a telephone number or the name of a newly met person. It is also important for tasks that require mental manipulation of information, such as multistep arithmetic problems. For many theorists, working memory also has a more important role as the work space where recalled information is actually used, manipulated, and related to other information, allowing complex cognitive processes such as comprehension learning and reasoning to take place.

Language

"Mapping" of different aphasic disorders to specific brain structures was one of the early accomplishments of behavioral neurology. In neuropsychologic assessment, this model is often followed. Comprehension, fluency, repetition, and naming are assessed in spoken or written language.

Perceptual

Neuropsychologists may provide a standardized version of the neurologists' perceptual tasks: double simultaneous stimulation in touch, hearing, or sight; stereognosis; graphesthesia; spatial perception; or auditory discrimination.

Executive

The ability to plan, sequence, and monitor behavior has been called "executive function." These functions, linked to the prefrontal cortex, rely on and organize other intact cognitive functions that are required components for performance. Formal tests of executive function may be divided into set switching and set maintenance. For set switching, the Wisconsin Card Sort uses symbols that can be sorted by color, number, or shape. Based only on feedback about whether each card was or was not correctly placed, the subject must infer an initial sort rule. At intervals, the sort rule is changed without the subject's knowledge; subjects must switch based only on their own observation that the current rule is no longer effective.

The Stroop Color-Word Test assesses set maintenance. The subject is given a series of color names printed in contrasting ink colors (e.g., the word "blue" printed in red ink) and is asked to name the color of the ink. The response set must be maintained while the subject suppresses the alternate (and more standard) inclination to read words without regard to the color of the print.

Motor

Tests of motor strength, such as grip strength, and of motor speed and agility, such as tapping speed and peg placement, establish laterality and focality of impairment. In some diseases, such as the dementia of AIDS, reduced motor agility is part of the diagnosis. Higher order motor tasks, such as double alternating movements or triple sequences, are used to assess motor sequencing or programming as opposed to pure strength or speed.

Attention

The ability to sustain attention is often tested by cancellation tasks in which the patient must detect and mark targets embedded in distractors or by reaction time tasks. Speed and accuracy are the outcome measures.

Mood

Mood may affect test performance. At minimum, the neuropsychologist notes the psychiatric history and probes for current psychiatric symptoms. Standardized mood rating scales are also available.

Clinical Observation

Along with the formal scores, testing affords an extensive period to observe the patient under controlled conditions. These clinical observations are valuable for diagnosis. Formal test scores capture only certain aspects of performance. The patient's problem-solving approach or the nature of the errors made can be telling. Also important in timed tasks is whether the patient can complete them with additional time or is actually incapable of solving them. Another important dimension is the ability to learn and follow directions for the many tests.

More subtle aspects of behavior include responses or coping abilities when confronted with difficult tasks, ability to remain socially appropriate as the session progresses, and the subjects' appreciation of their own capacities.

REFERRAL ISSUES

Neuropsychologic testing is useful for the diagnosis of some conditions and is a tool for evaluating or quantifying the effects of disease on cognition and behavior. The tests can assess the beneficial or adverse effects of drug therapy, radiation, or surgery. Serial evaluations give quantitative results that may change with time. In temporal lobectomy for intractable epilepsy, tests are required in presurgical evaluation to minimize the possibility of adverse effects. Specific referral issues are summarized in the following paragraphs.

Dementia

Testing can detect early dementing changes and discriminate them from "normal" performance; obtain information contributing to differential diagnosis either between dementia and nondementing illness, such as depression versus dementia, or between alternate forms of dementia (e.g., Alzheimer disease, dementia with Lewy bodies, or vascular dementia); or confirm or quantify disease progression and measure efficacy of clinical interventions.

Other Brain Disease

The effects of stroke, cancer, head trauma, or other conditions on cognitive function can be investigated. This typical reason for testing may be prompted by the patient's complaints. The evaluation helps to clarify the cause or extent of the condition.

Epilepsy

Testing is needed for presurgical evaluation, because lateralization of memory and language, as well as focality of cognitive impairments, is an important concern. Pre- and postoperative evaluations after other types of neurosurgery are also common.

Toxic Exposure

Testing can evaluate consequences of toxic or potentially toxic exposures, either on an individual basis or for particular exposed groups (e.g., factory workers). Exposures can include metals, solvents, pesticides, alcohol and drugs, or any other compounds that may affect the brain.

Medication

The potential effect of medications on the central nervous system can be evaluated in therapeutic trials or clinical practice. For example, in trials of agents to treat Alzheimer disease, neuropsychologic tests are typically primary measures of drug efficacy. In clinical practice, adverse or therapeutic effects of newly introduced medications can be evaluated.

Psychiatric Disorders

Testing can help in the differential diagnosis of psychiatric and neurologic disorders, especially affective disorders and schizophrenia.

Learning Disability

Testing will evaluate learning disabilities and the residua of these disabilities in later life. Behavioral disorders, attention deficit disorder, autism, dyslexia, and learning problems are common referral issues.

EXPECTATIONS FROM A NEUROPSYCHOLOGIC EVALUATION

The minimum that a neuropsychologic evaluation yields is an extensive investigation of the abilities of the patient. In these cases, although the studies do not lead to a definite diagnosis, they help to determine the patient's capacities, track the future, and advise the patient and family.

Sometimes the evaluation suggests that additional diagnostic tests would be useful. For example, if a patient's pattern of performance deviates substantially from that typically expected at the current stage of dementia, a vascular contribution may be considered. Similarly, evaluation can suggest the value of psychiatric consultation or more intensive electroencephalographic recording.

Many times the neuropsychologist can offer a tentative diagnosis or discuss the possible diagnoses compatible with the test findings. Neuropsychologic evaluation cannot yield a diagnosis without appropriate clinical and historical information. In the context of a multidisciplinary testing, however, it may provide evidence to confirm or refute a specific diagnosis. Testing might best be considered an additional source of information to be used by the clinician for diagnosis in conjunction with the neurologic examination and laboratory tests.

HOW TO REFER

The more information the examiner has at the start, the more directly the issues can be addressed. For example, if magnetic resonance imaging has revealed a particular lesion, tests can be tailored specifically. The examination is not an exploration of ability to detect a lesion, but a contribution to understanding the implications of the lesion. Similarly, the more explicit the referral question, the more likely the evaluation can yield useful information. A useful referral describes the differential diagnosis being entertained. Alternately, the neurologist or the family may simply want to document the current condition or explore some specific aspect of performance, such as language.

SUGGESTED READINGS

Berg E. A simple objective test for measuring flexibility in thinking. *J Gen Psychol* 1948;39:15–22.

Ron MA, Toone BK, Garralda ME, Lishman WA. Diagnostic accuracy in presenile dementia. *Br J Psychiatry* 1979;134:161–168.
Rosen WG. *The Rosen drawing test.* New York: Veterans Administration Medical Center, 1981.
Stroop JR. Studies of interference in serial verbal reactions. *J Exp Psychol* 1935;18:643–662.
Wechsler D. *Wechsler intelligence scale for children*, 3rd ed. San Antonio, TX: The Psychological Corp., 1991.
Wechsler D. *Wechsler adult intelligence scale*, 3rd ed. San Antonio, TX: The Psychological Corp., 1997.

Merritt's Neurology, 10th ed., edited by L.P. Rowland. Lippincott Williams & Wilkins, Philadelphia © 2000.

C H A P T E R
20

DNA DIAGNOSIS

LEWIS P. ROWLAND

We are still in the midst of the whirlwind created by molecular genetics. A little more than a decade ago, the diagnosis of an inherited disease depended primarily on clinical recognition. For some diseases, biochemical tests were available that identified the disease by the excretion or storage of an abnormal metabolite or, best of all, by finding decreased activity of the responsible enzyme.

That was the era of biochemical genetics, and one of the clinical lessons we learned was the recognition of genetic heterogeneity. The same enzyme abnormality might be associated with totally different clinical manifestations. For instance, the original clinical concept of muscle phosphorylase deficiency was a syndrome of muscle cramps and myoglobinuria induced by exertion, usually starting in adolescence. Later, however, we recognized totally different disorders as manifestations of phosphorylase deficiency. Infantile and late-onset forms have symptoms of limb weakness but no myoglobinuria.

Biochemical analysis in these diseases, as described in the chapters on metabolic diseases, is still important. Even in those conditions (mostly autosomal recessive), however, evidence from DNA analysis now reveals that different point mutations can result in the same biochemical abnormality. Already, 16 mutations in the muscle phosphorylase gene are known. Moreover, DNA analysis of circulating white blood cells may obviate the need for muscle biopsy.

Also, we can now diagnose autosomal dominant diseases by DNA analysis. For some conditions, we are in the peculiar position of trying to decide whether the disease should be named according to the change in DNA or, as in the past, by the clinical features. The problem arises because of two kinds of genetic heterogeneity. One is called *allelic heterogeneity*, which results from mutations in the same gene locus on one or both chromosomes. As a result, more than one clinical syndrome can be caused by mutations in the same gene. Conversely, the second type is *locus heterogeneity*, that is, the same clinical syndrome may be caused by mutations in different genes on different chromosomes.

DNA analysis is used in either of two ways to diagnose an individual who is at risk. In one way, *haplotype analysis, gene tracking, or linkage analysis* is applied when linked markers indicate the region of the disease gene but the gene itself has not been identified. Under these circumstances, we depend on DNA "markers" that are "polymorphic," that is, there are two alleles for the particular marker, and many individuals are heterozygous so that the marker is "informative." Using a set of markers, investigators define different types, one pattern labeled A, another B, and so on, depending on the number of markers. In this way, maternal and paternal genes can be identified, and one pattern tracks consistently with the disease (phenotype). In this way, an asymptomatic individual or a carrier of the gene can be identified. The method was used fruitfully for the study of families with Huntington disease or Duchenne dystrophy, among others. Chromosome maps of neurologic diseases indicate which diseases are amenable to this approach.

Haplotype analysis, however, has several drawbacks as a diagnostic test. Most important, it cannot be used for an individual, only for families. Moreover, the family must include people who are both affected by the disease and also alive. The more, the better. For such late-onset or rapidly fatal diseases as Parkinson disease, amyotrophic lateral sclerosis, or Alzheimer disease, however, many affected individuals in a family are no longer alive; sometimes, no affected family member is alive, only those at risk. If DNA is available from only one affected person, the investigation should include samples from at least three generations. Moreover, the test is labor intensive and expensive. Therefore, banking of DNA from affected people in families with heritable diseases is important.

The second kind of DNA analysis is more precise and can be used for individuals who may have a particular disease. This analysis can be done when the gene has been cloned and sequenced so that point mutations can be identified. Other mutations of diagnostic value include deletions, insertions, amplifications, and trinucleotide repeats. The number of diseases so identified has increased vastly in the past decade and seems to be augmented daily. In the ninth edition of this book, we provided a list of 41 individual diseases. Now several hundred individual diseases are amenable to DNA diagnosis, and it would take a booklet to tabulate them one by one. Instead, they can be grouped into 22 broad clinical categories (Table 20.1). More information is given in the specific chapters about these diseases.

TABLE 20.1. DNA DIAGNOSIS IN NEUROLOGIC DISEASE

Ataxias (SCA, FA)
Dementia: Alzheimer disease, Pick disease; FTD tauopathy)
Dystonia musculorum deformans
Epilepsy
Episodic ataxia
Hemiplegic migraine
Huntington disease
Inclusion body myositis
Mental retardation, developmental disorders: Down syndrome, fragile X, Williams syndrome
Mitochondrial encephalomyopathies: KSS, PEO, MELAS, MERRF, NARP, LHON
Motor neuron diseases: FALS, SMA, XSBMA
Muscular dystrophies (DMD, BMD, DM, EDMD, FSHMD, LGMD, congenital, distal forms)
Myasthenia gravis, congenital
Myotonia congenita; nondystrophic myotonias
Myotonic muscular dystrophies: DM, PROMM
Parkinson disease
Periodic paralysis (HoPP, HyPP, Andersen syndrome)
Peripheral neuorpathies (CMT, DSS, FAP, HNPP, HSMN)
Prion diseases (CJD, GSS)
Spastic paraplegia
Stroke syndromes (CADASIL, DCH)
Tumor syndromes (NF1, NF2, xeroderma pigmentosum)

BMD, Becker muscular dystrophy; CADASIL, cerebral autosomal dominant arteriopathy with subcortical infarcts and leucoencephalopathy; CJD, Creutzfeldt-Jakob disease; CMT, Charcot-Marie-Tooth; DCH, Dutch cerebral hemorhage; DM, myotonic muscular dystrophy (dystrophia myotonica); DMD, Duchenne muscular dystrophy; DSS, Dejerine-Sottas syndrome; EDMD, Emery-Dreifuss muscular dystrophy; FA, Friedreich ataxia; FAD, familial Alzheimer disease; FALS, familial amyotrophic lateral sclerosis; FAP, familial amyloidotic polyneuropathy; FSHMD, facioscapulohumeral muscular dystrophy; FTD, frontotemporal dementia (familial tauopathy, Wilhelmsen-Lynch disease); GSS, Gerstmann-Straussler-Scheinker disease; HNPP, hereditary neuropathy with liability to pressure palsies; HoPP, hypokalemic periodic paralysis; HSMN, hereditary sensorimotor neuropathies; HyPP, hyperkalemic periodic paralysis; KSS, Kearns-Sayre syndrome; LGMD, limb-girdle muscular dystrophy; LHON, Leber hereditary optic atrophy; MELAS, mitochondrial encephalomyopathy and stroke; MERRF, myoclonus epilepsy and ragged red fibers; NARP, neuropathy, ataxia, retinitis pigmentosa; NF1, neurofibromatosis type 1 (Von Recklinghausen disease); NF2, neurofibromatosis type 2, familial acoustic neuroma; PEO, progressive external ophthalmoplegia; PROMM, proximal myotonic myopathy (Ricker syndrome); SCA, spinocerebellar atrophy; SMA, spinal muscular atrophy (Werdnig-Hofmmann, Kugelberg-Welander syndromes); XSBMA, X-linked spinobulbar muscular atrophy (Kennedy syndrome).
From Harding AE. The DNA laboratory and neurological practice. J Neurol Neurosurg Psychiatry 1993; 56:229–233.

Cloning a gene has more than diagnostic value; for many of these diseases, candidate gene products were suggested because they were mapped close to the position of the disease gene, were then linked to the gene, and are presumed to account for the manifestations of the disease. These characteristics are described in the chapters on specific diseases.

As a result of both locus heterogeneity and allelic heterogeneity, several different types of syndromes have been identified. Relying on the molecular differences, there are seven different forms of spinocerebellar atrophy, SCA 1 through SCA 7. It is difficult for clinicians to communicate about numerical names like these, but no alternative is in sight unless clinical manifestations emerge to provide old-fashioned names for diseases (i.e., in plain words).

Another problem of nomenclature arises from the diverse clinical syndromes caused by similar mutations, such as expansion of trinucleotide repeats or mutations in ion channel genes. Although the molecular changes are similar, there is little clinical similarity, for instance, between hemiplegic migraine and periodic paralysis (except that they are intermittent).

At present, there are still major impediments to widespread applicability of DNA analysis for diagnosis. First, reimbursement for the test is not established in many parts of the United States or elsewhere. Second, as a result, a systematic development of diagnostic laboratories has not yet emerged, not even commercially. Consequently, testing is often left to research laboratories, which is an inefficient use of resources; finding the appropriate laboratory may be a problem for the clinician and the patients. In time, this should be corrected.

SUGGESTED READINGS

Conneally PM. *Molecular basis of neurology.* Boston: Blackwell Scientific Publications, 1993.

DiMauro S, Schon EA. Mitochondrial DNA and diseases of the nervous system. *The Neuroscientist* 1998;4:53–63.

Emery AEH, ed. *Neuromuscular disorders: clinical and molecular genetics.* New York: John Wiley & Sons, 1998.

Harding AE. The DNA laboratory and neurological practice. *J Neurol Neurosurg Psychiatry* 1993;56:229–233.

Martin JB. Molecular basis of the neurodegenerative disorders. *N Engl J Med* 1999;340:1970–1980.

Martin JB, ed. *Molecular neurology.* New York: Scientific American, 1998.

McKusick VA. *Mendelian inheritance in man,* 12th ed. Baltimore: Johns Hopkins University Press, 1997.

Online Mendelian Inheritance in Man, updated quarterly (http://www3.ncbi.nlm.nih.gov/Omin).

Rosenberg RN, Prusiner SB, DiMauro S, et al. *The molecular and genetic basis of neurological disease,* 2nd ed. Boston: Butterworth-Heinemann, 1997.

Rowland LP. The first decade of molecular genetics in neurology; changing clinical thought and practice. *Ann Neurol* 1992;32:207–214.

Rowland LP. Molecular basis of genetic heterogeneity: role of the clinical neurologist. *J Child Neurol* 1998;13:122–132.

Merritt's Neurology, 10th ed., edited by L.P. Rowland. Lippincott Williams & Wilkins, Philadelphia © 2000.

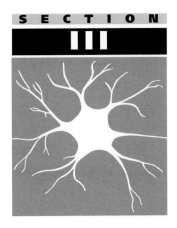

SECTION III

INFECTIONS OF THE NERVOUS SYSTEM

21

BACTERIAL INFECTIONS

JAMES R. MILLER
BURK JUBELT

The parenchyma, coverings, and blood vessels of the nervous system may be invaded by virtually any pathogenic microorganism. It is customary, for convenience of description, to divide the syndromes produced according to the major site of involvement. This division is arbitrary because the inflammatory process frequently involves more than one of these structures.

Involvement of the meninges by pathogenic microorganisms is known as *leptomeningitis*, because the infection and inflammatory response are generally confined to the subarachnoid space and the arachnoid and pia. Cases are divided into acute and subacute meningitis, according to the rapidity with which the inflammatory process develops. This rate of development, in part, is related to the nature of the infecting organism.

ACUTE PURULENT MENINGITIS

Bacteria may gain access to the ventriculosubarachnoid space by way of the blood in the course of septicemia or as a metastasis from infection of the heart, lung, or other viscera. The meninges may also be invaded by direct extension from a septic focus in the skull, spine, or parenchyma of the nervous system (e.g., sinusitis, otitis, osteomyelitis, and brain abscess). Organisms may gain entrance to the subarachnoid space through compound fractures of the skull and fractures through the nasal sinuses or mastoid or after neurosurgical procedures. Introduction by lumbar puncture is rare. The pathologic background, symptoms, and clinical course of patients with acute purulent meningitis are similar regardless of the causative organisms. The diagnosis and therapy depend on the isolation and identification of the organisms and the determination of the source of the infection.

Acute purulent meningitis may be the result of infection with almost any pathogenic bacteria. Isolated examples of infection by the uncommon forms are recorded in the literature, In the United States, *Streptococcus pneumoniae* now accounts for about one-half of cases when the infecting organism is identified and *Neisseria meningitidis* about one-fourth (Table 21.1). In recent years, there has been an increase in the incidence of cases in which no organism can be isolated. These patients now comprise the third major category of purulent meningitis. This may be due to the administration of therapy before admission to the hospital and the performance of lumbar puncture. In the neonatal period, *Escherichia coli* and group B streptococci are the most common causative agents. Approximately 60% of the postneonatal bacterial meningitis of children used to be due to *Hemophilus influenzae*. The impact of *H. influenzae* B vaccine has been dramatic. In the past decade there has been a 100-fold decrease in incidence. In 1997 there were less that 300 cases reported. Overall fatality rate from bacterial meningitis is now 10% or less. Many deaths occur during the first 48 hours of hospitalization.

For convenience, special features of the common forms of acute purulent meningitis are described separately. Neonatal infections are reviewed in Chapter 74.

Meningococcal Meningitis

Meningococcal meningitis was described by Vieusseux in 1805, and the causative organism was identified by Weichselbaum in 1887. It occurs in sporadic form and at irregular intervals in epidemics. Epidemics are especially likely to occur during large shifts in population, as in time of war.

Pathogenesis

Meningococci *(N. meningitidis)* may occasionally gain access to the meninges directly from the nasopharynx through the cribriform plate. The bacteria, however, usually are recovered from blood or cutaneous lesions before the meningitis, thus indicating that spread to the nervous system is hematogenous in most instances. The ventricular fluid may be teeming with organisms before the meninges become inflamed.

Recent studies have defined more clearly the role of bacterial elements in the initiation of meningitis with meningococcus and other bacteria. The bacterial capsule appears most important in the attachment and penetration to gain access to the body. Elements in the bacterial cell wall appear critical in penetration into the cerebrospinal fluid (CSF) space through vascular endothelium and the induction of the inflammatory response.

Pathology

In acute fulminating cases, death may occur before there are any significant pathologic changes in the nervous system. In the usual case, when death does not occur for several days after the onset of the disease, an intense inflammatory reaction occurs in the meninges. The inflammatory reaction is especially severe in the subarachnoid spaces over the convexity of the brain and around the cisterns at the base of the brain. It may extend a short distance along the perivascular spaces into the substance of the brain and spinal cord but rarely breaks into the parenchyma. Meningococci, both intra- and extracellular, are found in the meninges and CSF. With progress of the infection, the pia-arachnoid becomes thickened, and adhesions may form. Adhesions at the base may interfere with the flow of CSF from the fourth ventricle and may produce hydrocephalus. Inflammatory reaction and fibrosis of the meninges along the roots of the cranial nerves are thought to be the cause of the cranial nerve palsies that are seen occasionally. Damage to the auditory nerve often occurs suddenly, and the auditory defect is usually permanent. Such damage may result from extension of the infection to the inner ear or thrombosis of the nutrient artery. Facial paralysis frequently occurs after the meningeal reaction has subsided. Signs and symptoms of parenchymatous damage (e.g., hemiplegia, aphasia, and cerebellar signs) are infrequent and are probably due to infarcts as the result of thrombosis of inflamed arteries or veins.

TABLE 21.1. CAUSES OF 248 CASES OF BACTERIAL MENINGITIS IN 1995 AND OVERALL FATALITY RATE ACCORDING TO ORGANISM

Organism	No. of Cases Reported	Percentage of Total[a]	Incidence[b]	Case Fatality Rate (%)[c]
Hemophilus influenzae	18	7	0.2	6
Streptococcus pneumoniae	117	47	1.1	21
Neisseria meningitidis	62	26	0.6	3
Group B streptococcus	31	12	0.3	7
Listeria monocytogenes	20	8	0.2	15

[a]Because of rounding, the percentages do not total 100.
[b]The incidence is the number of cases per 100,000 population.
[c]Outcome data were missing for 11 cases of meningitis (4%). The fatality rates are based on cases with known outcome.
From Schuchat A, Robinson K, Werger J, et al., 1997.

With effective treatment, and in some cases without treatment, the inflammatory reaction in the meninges subsides, and no evidence of the infection may be found at autopsy in patients who die months or years later.

In the past, the inflammation in meningitis had been attributed mainly to the toxic effects of the bacteria. In all types of meningitis, the contribution to the inflammatory process of various cytokines released by phagocytic and immunoactive cells, particularly interleukin 1 and tumor necrosis factor, has been recognized. These studies have formed the basis for the use of anti-inflammatory corticosteroids in the treatment of meningitis. Several studies in both *H. influenzae* and *S. pneumonia* meningitis have suggested an improved outcome with the use of corticosteroids, particularly if the steroids are given shortly before the initiation of antibiotics. Treatment usually continues for 2 to 4 days. The use of corticosteroids in meningitis is still not considered the standard of practice, but many infectious disease specialists advocate it, particularly when clinical signs are severe.

Incidence

Meningococcus is the causative organism in about 25% of all cases of bacterial meningitis in the United States. Serogroup B is now the most commonly reported causative type (50%). Although both the sporadic and the epidemic forms of the disease may attack individuals of all ages, children and young adults are predominantly affected. The normal habitat of the meningococcus is the nasopharynx, and the disease is spread by carriers or by individuals with the disease. A polysaccharide vaccine for groups A, C, Y, and W-B5 meningococci has reduced the incidence of meningococcal infection among military recruits.

Symptoms

The onset of meningococcal meningitis, similar to that of other forms of meningitis, is accompanied by chills and fever, headache, nausea and vomiting, pain in the back, stiffness of the neck, and prostration. The occurrence of herpes labialis, conjunctivitis, and a petechial or hemorrhagic skin rash is common with meningococcal infections. At the onset, the patient is irritable. In children, there is frequently a characteristic sharp shrill cry (meningeal cry). With progress of the disease, the sensorium becomes clouded and stupor or coma may develop. Occasionally, the onset may be fulminant and accompanied by deep coma. Convulsive seizures are often an early symptom, especially in children, but focal neurologic signs are uncommon. Acute fulminating cases with severe circulatory collapse are relatively rare.

Signs

The patient appears acutely ill and may be confused, stuporous, or semicomatose. The temperature is elevated at 101° to 103°F, but it may occasionally be normal at the onset. The pulse is usually rapid and the respiratory rate is increased. Blood pressure is normal except in acute fulminating cases when there may be profound hypotension. A petechial rash may be found in the skin, mucous membranes, or conjunctiva but never in the nail beds. It usually fades in 3 or 4 days. There is rigidity of the neck with positive Kernig and Brudzinski signs. These signs may be absent in newborn, elderly, or comatose patients. Increased intracranial pressure causes bulging of an unclosed anterior fontanelle and periodic respiration. The reflexes are often decreased but occasionally may be increased. Cranial nerve palsies and focal neurologic signs are uncommon and usually do not develop until several days after the onset of the infection. The optic disks are normal, but papilledema may develop if the meningitis persists for more than a week.

Laboratory Data

The blood white cell count is increased, usually in the range of 10,000 to 30,000/mm^3, but occasionally may be normal or higher than 40,000/mm^3. The urine may contain albumin, casts, and red blood cells. Meningococci can be cultured from the nasopharynx in most cases, from the blood in more than 50% of the cases in the early stages, and from the skin lesions when these are present.

The CSF is under increased pressure, usually between 200 and 500 mm H$_2$O. The CSF is cloudy (purulent) because it contains a large number of cells, predominantly polymorphonuclear leukocytes. The cell count in the fluid is usually between 2,000 and 10,000/mm^3. Occasionally, it may be less than 100 and infrequently more than 20,000/mm^3. The protein content is increased. The sugar content is decreased, usually to levels below 20 mg/dL. Gram-negative diplococci can be seen intra- and extracellularly in stained smears of the fluid, and meningococci can be cultured in more than 90% of untreated patients. Particle agglutination may rapidly identify bacterial antigens in the CSF. It cannot be relied on for definite diagnosis, however, because of relatively low specificity and sensitivity. For meningococcus, the capsular polysaccharide is the antigen detected. In unusual instances, the CSF may demonstrate minimal or no increase in cell count and no bacteria on the Gram stain, but *N. meningitidis* may be isolated. Clear CSF in a patient with suspected bacterial meningitis must be cultured carefully.

Complications and Sequelae

The complications and sequelae include those commonly associated with an inflammatory process in the meninges and its blood vessels (i.e., convulsions, cranial nerve palsies, focal cerebral lesions, damage to the spinal cord or nerve roots, hydrocephalus) and those that are due to involvement of other portions of the body by meningococci (e.g., panophthalmitis and other types of ocular infection, arthritis, purpura, pericarditis, endocarditis, myocarditis, pleurisy, orchitis, epididymitis, albuminuria or hematuria, adrenal hemorrhage). Disseminated intravascular coagulation may complicate the meningitis. Complications may also arise from intercurrent infection of the upper respiratory tract, middle ear, and lungs. Any of these complications may leave permanent residua, but the most common sequelae are due to injury of the nervous system. These include deafness, ocular palsies, blindness, changes in mentality, convulsions, and hydrocephalus. With the available methods of treatment, complications and sequelae of the meningeal infection are rare, and the complications due to the involvement of other parts of the body by the meningococci or other intercurrent infections are more readily controlled.

Diagnosis

Meningococcal meningitis can be diagnosed with certainty only by the isolation of the organism from the CSF. The diagnosis can be made, however, with relative certainty before the organisms are isolated in a patient with headache, vomiting, chills and fever, neck stiffness, and a petechial cutaneous rash, especially if there is an epidemic of meningococcal meningitis or if there has been exposure to a known case of meningococcal meningitis.

To establish the diagnosis of meningococcal meningitis, cultures should be made of the skin lesions, nasopharyngeal secretions, blood, and CSF. The diagnosis can be established in many cases by examination of smears of the sediment of the CSF after application of the Gram stain.

Prognosis

The mortality rate of untreated meningococcal meningitis varied widely in different epidemics but was usually between 50% and 90%. With present-day therapy, however, the overall mortality rate is about 10%, and the incidence of complications and sequelae is low.

Features of the disease that influence the mortality rate are the age of the patient, bacteremia, rapidity of treatment, complica-

tions, and general condition of the individual. The lowest fatality rates are seen in patients between the ages of 5 and 10. The highest mortality rates occur in infants, in elderly debilitated individuals, and in those with extensive hemorrhages into the adrenal gland.

Treatment

Antibiotic therapy for bacterial meningitis usually commences before the nature of the organism is assured. Therefore, the initial regimen should be appropriate for most likely organisms, the determination of which depends to some extent on the patient's age and the locale. Third-generation cephalosporins, usually ceftriaxone or cefotaxime, have become the first choice of treatment for bacterial meningitis. Their spectrum is broad, and they have become particularly useful since the occurrence of *H. influenzae* and *S. pneumoniae* strains that are resistant to penicillin or ampicillin and amoxicillin. They also require less frequent administration than the penicillins. In circumstances when *S. pneumoniae* resistance to cephalosporins is an issue, vancomycin should be added. If the Gram stain or epidemic setting clearly suggests that meningococcus is the infectious agent, penicillin or ampicillin may be used. Chloramphenicol remains an acceptable choice if allergy to the penicillins and cephalosporins is a problem. Unless a dramatic response to therapy occurs, the CSF should be examined 24 to 48 hours after the initiation of treatment to assess the effectiveness of the medication. Posttreatment examination of the CSF is not a meaningful criterion of recovery, and the CSF does not need to be reexamined if the patient is clinically well.

Dehydration is common, and fluid balance should be monitored carefully to avoid hypovolemic shock. Hyponatremia frequently occurs and may be caused either by overzealous free water replacement or inappropriate antidiuretic hormone secretion. Heparization should be considered if disseminated intravascular coagulation occurs.

Anticonvulsants should be used to control recurrent seizures. Cerebral edema may require the use of osmotic diuretics or the administration of corticosteroids, but only if early or impending cerebral herniation is evident.

Persons who have had intimate contact with patients with meningococcal meningitis may be given rifampin as a prophylactic measure.

Hemophilus influenzae Meningitis

Infections of the meninges by *H. influenzae* were reported as early as 1899. In the United States and other countries where *H. influenzae* B vaccination is widespread, the incidence of meningitis is now negligible. It remains an important disease elsewhere, however. Where it is still prevalent, *H. influenzae* meningitis is predominantly a disease of infancy and early childhood; more than 50% of the cases occur within the first 2 years of life and 90% before the age of 5. In the United States, *H. influenzae* meningitis is now more common in adults. Serotype B is the most common.

In adults, *H. influenzae* meningitis is more commonly secondary to acute sinusitis, otitis media, or fracture of the skull. It is associated with CSF rhinorrhea, immunologic deficiency, diabetes mellitus, and alcoholism. Currently, cases tend to occur in the autumn and spring, with fewest occurring in the summer months.

The pathology of *H. influenzae* meningitis does not differ from that of other forms of acute purulent meningitis. In patients with a protracted course, localized pockets of infection in the meninges or cortex, internal hydrocephalus, degeneration of cranial nerves, and focal loss of cerebral substance secondary to thrombosis of vessels may be found.

The symptoms and physical signs of *H. influenzae* meningitis are similar to those of other forms of acute bacterial meningitis. The disease usually lasts 10 to 20 days. It may occasionally be fulminating, and frequently it is protracted and extends over several weeks or months.

The CSF changes are similar to those described for the other acute meningitides. The organisms can be cultured from the CSF. Blood cultures are often positive early in the illness.

The mortality rate in untreated cases of *H. influenzae* meningitis in infants is greater than 90%. The prognosis is not so grave in adults, in whom spontaneous recovery is more frequent. Adequate treatment has reduced the mortality rate to about 10%, but sequelae are not uncommon. These include paralysis of extraocular muscles, deafness, blindness, hemiplegia, recurrent convulsions, and mental deficiency. Recent studies have indicated that treatment with anti-inflammatory corticosteroids reduces the frequency of the sequelae, particularly if started just before the initiation of antibiotic treatment.

The diagnosis of *H. influenzae* meningitis is based on the isolation of the organisms from the CSF and blood. *H. influenzae* capsular antigens may be detected in the CSF by particle agglutination, which may rapidly provide information, but is less sensitive and specific than is culture identification.

Because of resistance to ampicillin, third-generation cephalosporins are commonly used in initial therapy of meningitis and are an effective treatment.

Subdural effusion, which may occur in infants with any form of meningitis, is most commonly seen in connection with *H. influenzae* meningitis. Persistent vomiting, bulging fontanelles, convulsion, focal neurologic signs, and persistent fever should lead to consideration of this complication. Prompt relief of the symptoms usually follows evacuation of the effusion by tapping the subdural space through the fontanelles. Persistent or secondary fever without worsening of meningeal signs may be due to an extracranial focus of infection, such as a contaminated urinary or venous catheter, or to drug administration.

Pneumococcal Meningitis

Pneumococcus (*S. pneumoniae*) is about equal in frequency to meningococcus as a cause of meningitis, except that it is more frequent in the elderly population. Meningeal infection is usually a complication of otitis media, mastoiditis, sinusitis, fractures of the skull, upper respiratory infections, and infections of the lung. Alcoholism, asplenism, and sickle cell disease predispose patients to developing pneumococcal meningitis. The infection may occur at any age, but more than 50% of the patients are younger than 1 or older than 50 years of age.

The clinical symptoms, physical signs, and laboratory findings in pneumococcal meningitis are the same as those in other forms of acute purulent meningitis. The diagnosis is usually made without difficulty because the CSF contains many of the organisms. When gram-positive diplococci are seen in smears of the CSF or its sediment, a positive quellung reaction serves to identify both the pneumococcus and its type. Particle agglutination of CSF and serum may be helpful in demonstrating pneumococcal antigen.

Before the introduction of sulfonamides, the mortality rate in pneumococcal meningitis was almost 100%. It is now approximately 20% to 30%. The prognosis for recovery is best in cases that follow fractures of the skull and those with no known source of infection. The mortality rate is especially high when the meningitis follows pneumonia, empyema, or lung abscess or when a persisting bacteremia indicates the presence of an endocarditis. The triad of pneumococcal meningitis, pneumonia, and endocarditis (Austrian syndrome) has a particularly high fatality rate.

The prevalence of penicillin resistant *S. pneumoniae* in the United States has made a third-generation cephalosporin the initial treatment for *S. pneumoniae* until sensitivities are established. Because some strains may also be relatively resistant to the cephalosporins, vancomycin is often used initially as well. The treatment should be continued for 12 to 15 days. Chloramphenicol is an alternative drug for adults who are sensitive to the penicillins and cephalosporins. Any primary focus of infection should be eradicated by surgery if necessary. Persistent CSF fistulas after fractures of the skull must be closed by craniotomy and suturing of the dura. Otherwise, the meningitis will almost certainly recur.

Staphylococcal Meningitis

Staphylococci (*S. aureus* and *S. epidermidis)* are a relatively infrequent cause of meningitis. Meningitis may develop as a result of spread from furuncles on the face or from staphylococcal infections elsewhere in the body. It is sometimes a complication of cavernous sinus thrombosis, epidural or subdural abscess, and neurosurgical procedures involving shunting to relieve hydrocephalus. Endocarditis may be found in association with staphylococcal meningitis. Intravenous treatment with a penicillinase-resistant penicillin (oxacillin) is the preferred treatment. Therapy must be continued for 2 to 4 weeks. In nosocomial infections or other situations in which resistance to oxacillin is likely, treatment with vancomycin is appropriate. Complications, such as ventriculitis, arachnoiditis, and hydrocephalus, may occur. The original focus of infection should be eradicated. Laminectomy should be performed immediately when a spinal epidural abscess is present, and cranial subdural abscess should be drained through craniotomy openings.

Streptococcal Meningitis

Infection with streptococcus accounts for 1% to 2% of all cases of meningitis. Streptococcal meningitis is usually caused by group A organisms. The symptoms are not distinguished from other forms of meningitis. Members of other groups may occasionally be isolated from CSF. It is always secondary to some septic focus, most commonly in the mastoid or nasal sinuses. Treatment is the same as outlined for the treatment of pneumococcal meningitis together with surgical eradication of the primary focus.

Meningitis Caused by Other Bacteria

Meningitis in the newborn infant is most often caused by coliform gram-negative bacilli, especially *E. coli* and group B hemolytic streptococci. It often accompanies septicemia and may show none of the typical signs of meningitis in children and adults. Instead, the infant shows irritability, lethargy, anorexia, and bulging fontanelles. Meningitis caused by gram-negative enteric bacteria also occurs frequently in immunosuppressed or chronically ill hospitalized adult patients and in persons with penetrating head injuries, neurosurgical procedures, congenital defects, or diabetes mellitus. In these circumstances, meningitis may be difficult to recognize because of altered consciousness related to the underlying illness.

A third-generation cephalosporin and an aminoglycoside are currently used for treatment of gram-negative meningitides. If *Pseudomonas aeruginosa* is present or suspected, ceftazidime is preferred. If initial response is poor, intraventricular administration of the aminoglycoside can be considered. Care also must be taken to ensure that the organism is sensitive to the agents chosen; if not, some other antibiotic should be selected. Gram-negative bacillary meningitis has a high mortality (40% to 70%) and a high morbidity.

Meningitis caused by *Listeria monocytogenes* may occur in adults with chronic diseases (e.g., renal disease with dialysis or transplantation, cancer, connective tissue disorders, chronic alcoholism) and in infants. It may occur, however, without any predisposing factor, and the incidence of such appears to be increasing. Occasionally, *L. monocytogenes* meningitis occurs with prominent brainstem findings (rhomboencephalitis). A laboratory report of "diphtheroids" seen on Gram stain or isolated in culture should suggest the possible presence of *L. monocytogenes*. *Listeria* septicemia occurs in about 65% of patients, and the organism may be isolated from blood cultures even when not recoverable from the CSF. The treatment of choice for *L. monocytogenes* meningitis is ampicillin. If *Listeria* is considered a reasonable possibility, ampicillin should be added to initial therapy, because the bacterium is resistant to cephalosporins. High-dose aqueous penicillin and gentamicin is preferred treatment. Trimethoprim/sulfasoxazole is an acceptable alternative. The illness has a mortality rate of 30% to 60%, with the highest fatality rate among elderly patients with malignancies.

Acute Purulent Meningitis of Unknown Cause

Patients may have clinical symptoms indicative of an acute purulent meningitis but with atypical CSF findings. These patients have usually manifested nonspecific symptoms and have often been treated for several days with some form of antimicrobial therapy in dosages sufficient to modify the CSF abnormalities but not sufficient to eradicate the infection. Their symptoms are of longer duration, and the patients have less marked alterations of mental status and die later in their hospitalization than do patients with proven bacterial meningitis. In these cases, the CSF pleocytosis is usually only moderate (500 to 1,000 cells/mm^3 with predominance of polymorphonuclear leukocytes), and the sugar content is normal or only slightly decreased. Organisms are not seen on stained smears and are cultured with difficulty. Repeated lumbar puncture may be helpful in arriving at the correct diagnosis. Antibiotics should be selected on the basis of epidemiologic or clinical factors. The age of the patient and the setting in which the infection occurred are the primary considerations. In patients with partially treated meningitis and in those with meningitis of unknown etiology, third-generation cephalosporins and vancomycin are now considered the antibiotics of choice for initial therapy. Ampicillin should be added in neonates or if *L. monocytogenes* is considered. Therapy should be modified if an organism different from that originally suspected is isolated or if the clinical response is less than optimal. The mortality and frequency of neurologic complications of these patients are similar to those of patients in whom the responsible bacteria have been identified.

Recurrent Bacterial Meningitis

Repeated episodes of bacterial meningitis signal a host defect, either in local anatomy or in antibacterial and immunologic defenses. They usually follow trauma; several years may pass between the trauma and the first bout of meningitis. *S. pneumoniae* is the usual pathogen. Bacteria may enter the subarachnoid space through the cribriform plate, a basilar skull fracture, erosive bony changes in the mastoid, congenital dermal defects along the craniospinal axis, penetrating head injuries, or neurosurgical procedures. CSF rhinorrhea or otorrhea is often present but may be transient. It may be detected by testing for a significant concentration of glucose in nasal or aural secretions. Treatment of recurrent meningitis is similar to that for first bouts. Cryptic CSF leaks can be demonstrated by polytomography of the frontal and mastoid regions by monitoring the course of radioiodine-labeled albumin instilled intrathecally or by computed tomography (CT) after intrathecal injection of metrizamide. Patients with recurrent pneumococcal meningitis should be vaccinated with pneumococcal vaccine. Long-term prophylactic treatment with penicillin should be considered. Surgical closure of CSF fistulas is indicated to prevent further episodes of meningitis.

SUBACUTE MENINGITIS

Subacute meningitis is usually due to infection with tubercle bacilli or mycotic organisms. The clinical syndrome differs from that of acute purulent meningitis in that the onset of symptoms is usually less acute, the degree of inflammatory reaction less severe, and the course more prolonged.

Tuberculous Meningitis

Tuberculous meningitis differs from that caused by most other common bacteria in that the course is more prolonged, the mortality rate is higher, the CSF changes are acutely less severe, and treatment is less effective in preventing sequelae.

Pathogenesis

Tuberculous meningitis is always secondary to tuberculosis elsewhere in the body (Figs. 21.1 and 21.2). The primary focus of infection is usually in the lungs but may be in the lymph glands, bones, nasal sinuses, gastrointestinal tract, or any organ in the body. The onset of meningeal symptoms may coincide with signs of acute miliary dissemination, or there may be clinical evidence of activity in the primary focus; however, meningitis is often the only manifestation of the disease.

Tubercular meningitis usually occurs after the rupture of a meningeal or parenchymal tubercle into the ventricular or subarachnoid space. Tubercles in the nervous system of any appreciable size are rare in the United States, but dissemination may be from minute or microscopic granulomas near the meningeal surfaces. When meningitis is a manifestation of miliary dissemi-

nation, it suggests that the meningitis is due to lodgement of bacteria directly in the choroid plexus or meningeal vessels.

Pathology

The meninges over the surface of the brain and the spinal cord are cloudy and thickened, but the process is usually most intense at the base of the brain. A thick collar of fibrosis may form around the optic nerves, cerebral peduncles, and basilar surface of the pons and midbrain. The ventricles are moderately dilated and the ependymal lining is covered with exudate or appears roughened (granular ependymitis). Minute tubercles may be visible in the meninges, choroid plexus, and cerebral parenchyma.

On microscopic examination, the exudate in the thickened meninges is composed chiefly of mononuclear cells, lymphocytes, plasma cells, macrophages, and fibroblasts with an occasional giant cell. The inflammatory process may extend for a short distance into the cerebral substance where microscopic granulomas may also be found. Proliferative changes are fre-

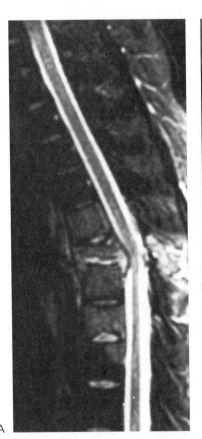
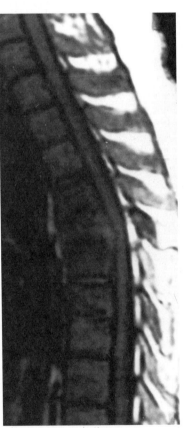
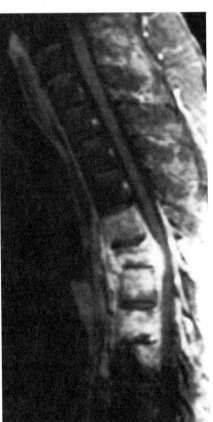

A   B and C

FIG. 21.1. Potts disease (spinal tuberculosis). **A:** T2-weighted sagittal magnetic resonance (MR) scan of the thoracic spine shows abnormally increased signal intensity within four to five consecutive vertebral bodies of the lower thoracic spine. Also evident is a compression fracture of one of the thoracic vertebral bodies with apparent impingement upon the lower thoracic spinal cord. **B and C:** T1-weighted sagittal MR scans of thoracic spine before and after gadolinium enhancement show marked enhancement of affected thoracic vertebral bodies with mild epidural extension, especially at the level of the compression fracture. (Courtesy of Dr. S. Chan.)

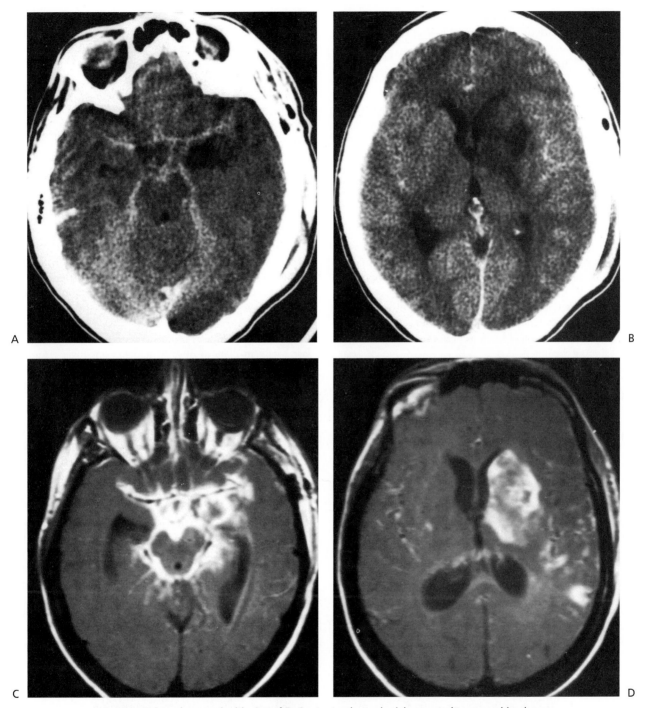

FIG. 21.2. Tuberculous meningitis. **A and B:** Contrast-enhanced axial computed tomographies demonstrate large nonenhancing hypodense lesion in the left temporal lobe **(A)** and left basal ganglia **(B)** most consistent with infarcts. Significant cisternal enhancement is seen consistent with meningitis. **C and D:** T1-weighted axial magnetic resonance scans after gadolinium enhancement show florid contrast enhancement within basal cisterns most consistent with exudative meningitis of tuberculosis. Enhancement of the left temporal lobe and left basal ganglia lesions suggests persistent inflammation within these infarcts. (Courtesy of Dr. S. Chan.)

quently seen in the inflamed vessels of the meninges, producing a panarteritis. These arteritic changes may lead to thrombosis of the vessel and cerebral infarcts.

Incidence

Until the 1980s, the incidence of tuberculosis and tubercular meningitis had been declining steadily in the United States because of hygienic improvements and later the development of antibiotic therapy. The incidence, however, is now slowly increasing, in part a result of the propensity of human immunodeficiency virus (HIV)-infected individuals to develop tuberculosis and in part because of the increased immigration from Asian, Latin American, and African countries, which have a high incidence of the disease. Although tuberculous meningitis may occur at any age, it is most common in childhood and early adult life. In areas with a high incidence of tuberculosis, tuberculous meningitis is seen most commonly in infants and young children. In areas of low incidence, such as the United States, tuberculous meningitis is more common in adults. Until recently, adult cases occurred mainly over the age of 40. With the increased incidence of tuberculosis, however, younger adults are again developing the illness.

Symptoms

The onset is usually subacute, with headache, vomiting, fever, bursts of irritability, and nocturnal wakefulness as the most prominent symptoms. Anorexia, loss of weight, and abdominal pain may be present. The prodromal stage lasts for 2 weeks to 3 months in most cases. In young children, a history of close contact with a person known to have tuberculosis is a diagnostic help. Stiffness of the neck and vomiting become evident within a few days. Convulsive seizures are not uncommon in children during the first days of the disease. The headache becomes progressively more severe; there is bulging of the fontanelles in infants. The pain often causes the infant to emit a peculiarly shrill cry (meningeal cry). With progress of the disease, patients become stuporous or comatose. Blindness and signs of damage to other cranial nerves may appear, or there may be convulsive seizures or focal neurologic signs.

Physical Findings

The physical findings in the early stages are those associated with meningeal infection (i.e., fever, irritability, stiffness of the neck, and Kernig and Brudzinski signs). Tendon reflexes may be exaggerated or depressed. Signs of increased intracranial pressure and focal brain damage are rarely present at the onset. The initial irritability is gradually replaced by apathy, confusion, lethargy, and stupor. Papilledema, cranial nerve palsies, and focal neurologic signs are common in the late stages of the disease. There may be external ophthalmoplegia, usually incomplete, unilateral, and involving chiefly the oculomotor nerve. Ophthalmoscopy may demonstrate choroid tubercles. Clinical evidence of tuberculosis elsewhere in the body is usually present. Convulsions, coma, and hemiplegia occur as the disease advances. The temperature, which is only moderately elevated (100° to 102°F) in the early stages, rises to high levels before death. The respiratory and pulse rates are increased. In the terminal stages, respirations become irregular and of the Cheyne-Stokes type.

Diagnosis

The diagnosis of tuberculous meningitis can be established by recovery of the organisms from the CSF. The CSF findings are, however, quite characteristic, and a presumptive diagnosis can be made when the typical abnormalities are present. These include increased pressure; slightly cloudy or ground-glass appearance of the CSF with formation of a clot on standing; moderate pleocytosis of 25 to 500 cells/mm^3, with lymphocytes as the predominating cell type; increased protein content; decreased sugar content with values in the range of 20 to 40 mg/dL; a negative serologic test for syphilis or cryptococcal antigen; and absence of growth when the CSF is inoculated on routine culture media. Although none of these abnormalities is diagnostic, their occurrence in combination is usually pathognomonic and is sufficient evidence to warrant intensive therapy until the diagnosis can be confirmed by stained smears of the sediment or pellicle or by culture of the CSF. Smears of the CSF sediment demonstrate acid-fast bacilli in 20% to 30% of patients on single examination; with repeated examinations, the yield of positive smears is increased to 75%. The yield is probably lower in HIV-infected patients, because the illness tends to be more indolent.

Diagnosis is ultimately based on the recovery of the mycobacterium from culture, which may require several weeks. However, detection of mycobacterial DNA in the CSF by polymerase chain reaction (PCR) is highly sensitive and specific and faster. It is not, however, foolproof. Histologic analysis of the CSF sediment is also still useful for detecting the organism and provides the most rapid result.

Other diagnostic aids include a thorough search for a primary focus, including radiographs of the chest and tuberculin skin tests. Patients with tuberculous meningitis may have hyponatremia due to inappropriate secretion of antidiuretic hormone. CT or magnetic resonance imaging (MRI) of the brain in tuberculous meningitis may disclose enhancing exudates in the subarachnoid cisterns, hydrocephalus, areas of infarction, and associated tuberculomas.

Tuberculous meningitis must be differentiated from other forms of acute and subacute meningitis, viral infections, and meningeal reactions to septic foci in the skull or spine.

Acute purulent meningitis is characterized by a high cell count and the presence of the causative organisms in the CSF. Preliminary antibiotic therapy of purulent meningitis may cause the CSF findings to mimic those of tuberculous meningitis.

The CSF in syphilitic meningitis may show changes similar to those of tuberculous meningitis. The normal or relatively normal sugar content and the positive serologic reactions make the diagnosis of syphilitic meningitis relatively easy.

The clinical picture and CSF findings in cryptococcus meningitis may be identical with those of tuberculous meningitis. The differential diagnosis can be made by finding the budding yeast organisms in the counting chamber or in stained smears, by detecting cryptococcal antigen in CSF by the latex agglutination test, and by obtaining a culture of the fungus. Much less frequently, other mycotic infections may involve the meninges.

Meningeal involvement in the course of viral infections, such as mumps, lymphocytic choriomeningitis, or other forms of viral encephalitis, may give a clinical picture similar to that of tuberculous meningitis. In these cases, the CSF sugar content is usually normal or only minimally depressed.

Diffuse involvement of the meninges by metastatic tumors (carcinoma or sarcoma) or by gliogenous tumors may produce meningeal signs. The CSF may contain numerous lymphocytes and polymorphonuclear leukocytes and a reduced sugar content. The triad of mental clarity, lack of fever, and hyporeflexia suggests neoplastic meningitis. A protracted course or the finding of neoplastic cells in the CSF excludes the diagnosis of tuberculous meningitis.

Central nervous system (CNS) sarcoidosis may also cause meningitis with CSF changes similar to those of tuberculous meningitis. Failure to detect microbes by smear or culture and a protracted course are clues to the diagnosis of sarcoidosis. Leptomeningeal biopsy may be needed to establish the diagnosis, but most patients show systemic signs of sarcoidosis in lymph nodes, liver, lung, or muscle (see Chapter 26).

Prognosis and Course

The natural course of the disease is death in 6 to 8 weeks. With early diagnosis and appropriate treatment, the recovery rate approaches 90%. Delay in diagnosis is associated with rapid progression of neurologic deficits and a poorer prognosis. Prognosis is worst at the extremes of life, particularly in the elderly person. The presence of cranial nerve abnormalities on admission, confusion, lethargy, and elevated CSF protein concentration are associated with a poor prognosis. The presence of active tuberculosis in other organs or of miliary tuberculosis does not significantly affect the prognosis if antitubercular therapy is given. Relapses occasionally occur after months or even years in apparently cured patients.

Sequelae

Minor or major sequelae occur in about 25% of the patients who recover. These vary from minimal degree of facial weakness to severe intellectual and physical disorganization. Physical defects include deafness, convulsive seizures, blindness, hemiplegia, paraplegia, and quadriplegia. Intracranial calcifications may appear 2 to 3 years after the onset of the disease.

Treatment

Treatment should be started immediately without waiting for bacteriologic confirmation of the diagnosis in a patient with the characteristic clinical symptoms and CSF findings. It is generally agreed that the prognosis for recovery and freedom from sequelae are directly related to the promptness of the initiation of therapy. Concomitant with the resurgence of tuberculosis in the United States has been the emergence of multidrug-resistant organisms. Treatment is now commonly started with four drugs, usually isoniazid, rifampin, pyrazinamide, and ethambutol; streptomycin is an alternative if one of the preferred antibiotics cannot be used. Other second-line drugs may be substituted if

absolutely necessary. The regimen later can be modified and the number of agents reduced if the sensitivities of the isolated bacterium allow. Treatment is usually for 18 to 24 months. Corticosteroids may prove beneficial in the early phases of the disease when there is evidence of subarachnoid block or impending cerebral herniation. Peripheral neuropathy secondary to isoniazid treatment can be prevented by giving pyridoxine. Intrathecal therapy is not indicated.

In association with the HIV epidemic has been an increased incidence of infection with nontubercular mycobacteria, particularly of the avium-intracellulare group. Although these organisms are occasionally isolated from the CSF, the meningeal reaction related to their presence is a mild and indolent process. Treatment of the infections is difficult.

SUBDURAL AND EPIDURAL INFECTIONS

Cerebral Subdural Empyema

A collection of pus between the inner surface of the dura and the outer surface of the arachnoid of the brain is known as *subdural empyema.*

Etiology

Subdural empyema may result from the direct extension of injection from the middle ear, the nasal sinuses, or the meninges. It may develop as a complication of compound fractures of the skull or in the course of septicemia. An acute attack of sinusitis just before the development of subdural empyema is common. The mechanism of the formation of subdural empyema after compound fractures of the skull is easily understood, but the factors that lead to subdural infection rather than leptomeningitis or cerebral abscess in patients with infections of the nasal sinuses or mastoids are less clear. Chronic infection of the mastoid or paranasal sinuses with thrombophlebitis of the venous sinuses or osteomyelitis and necrosis of the cranial vault commonly precedes the development of the subdural infection.

The infection is most often due to streptococcus. Other bacteria frequently recovered from subdural pus are staphylococci and gram-negative enteric organisms.

Pathology

The pathologic findings depend on the mode of entry of the infection into the subdural space. In traumatic cases, there may be osteomyelitis of the overlying skull, with or without accompanying foreign bodies. When the abscess is secondary to infection of the nasal sinuses or middle ear, thrombophlebitis of the venous sinuses or osteomyelitis of the frontal or temporal bone is a common finding. Dorsolateral and interhemispheric collections of pus are common; collections beneath the cerebral hemispheres are uncommon. After paranasal infections, subdural pus forms at the frontal poles and extends posteriorly over the convexity of the frontal lobe. After ear infection, the subdural pus passes posteriorly and medially over the falx to the tentorium and occipital poles. The brain beneath the pus is molded in a manner similar to that seen in cases of subdural hematoma. Thrombosis or thrombophlebitis of the superficial cortical veins, especially in the frontal region, is common and produces a hemorrhagic softening of the gray and white matter drained by the thrombosed vessels. The subarachnoid spaces beneath the subdural empyema are filled with a purulent exudate, but there is no generalized leptomeningitis in the initial stage.

Incidence

Subdural empyema is a relatively rare form of intracranial infection, occurring less than half as frequently as brain abscess. It may develop at any age but is most common in children and young adults. Males are more frequently affected than females.

Symptoms and Signs

Symptoms include those associated with the focus or origin of the infection and those due to the intracranial extension. Local pain and tenderness are present in the region of the infected nasal sinus or ear. Orbital swelling is usually present when the injection is secondary to frontal sinus disease. Chills, fever, and severe headache are common initial symptoms of the intracranial involvement. Neck stiffness and Kernig sign are present. With progress of the infection, the patient lapses into a confused, somnolent, or comatose state. Thrombophlebitis of the cortical veins is manifested by jacksonian or generalized convulsions and by the appearance of focal neurologic signs (e.g., hemiplegia, aphasia, paralysis of conjugate deviation of the eyes, cortical sensory loss). In the late stages, the intracranial pressure is increased and papilledema may occur. The entire clinical picture may evolve in as little as a few hours or as long as 10 days.

Laboratory Data

A marked peripheral leukocytosis is usually present. Radiographs of the skull may show evidence of infection of the mastoid or nasal sinuses or of osteomyelitis of the skull. The CSF is under increased pressure. It is usually clear and colorless, and there is a moderate pleocytosis, varying from 25 to 500 cells/mm^3 with 10% to 80% polymorphonuclear leukocytes. In some patients, the CSF cellular response may be composed chiefly of lymphocytes or mononuclear cells. CSF pleocytosis may be absent. The protein content is increased, with values commonly in the range of 75 to 150 mg/dL. The sugar content is normal, and the CSF is sterile unless the subdural infection is secondary to a purulent leptomeningitis. Spinal puncture should be done with caution because instances of transtentorial herniation within 8 hours after lumbar puncture have been described in this condition. Lumbar puncture should be avoided if the diagnosis can be established in other ways.

CT of the head characteristically demonstrates a crescent-shaped area of hypodensity at the periphery of the brain and mass displacement of the cerebral ventricles and midline structures. There usually is contrast enhancement between the empyema and cerebral cortex. CT may fail to define the pus collection in some patients with typical clinical presentations, however. MRI appears to be more sensitive. Arteriography is no longer required.

Diagnosis

The diagnosis of subdural empyema should be considered whenever meningeal symptoms or focal neurologic signs develop in patients presenting evidence of a suppurative process in nasal sinuses, mastoid process, or other cranial structures.

Subdural empyema must be differentiated from other intracranial complications of infections in the ear or nasal sinus. These include extradural abscess, sinus thrombosis, and brain abscess. The presence of focal neurologic signs and neck stiffness is against the diagnosis of epidural abscess.

The differential diagnosis between subdural empyema and septic thrombosis of the superior longitudinal sinus is difficult because focal neurologic signs and convulsive seizures are common to both conditions. In fact, thrombosis of the sinus or its tributaries is a frequent complication of subdural empyema. Factors in favor of the diagnosis of sinus thrombosis are a septic temperature and the absence of signs of meningeal irritation. Subdural empyema can also be confused with viral encephalitis or various types of meningitis. The diagnosis may be obscured by early antibiotic therapy. Brain abscess can be distinguished by the relatively insidious onset and the protracted course.

Clinical Course

The mortality rate is high (25% to 40%) because of failure to make an early diagnosis. If the disorder is untreated, death commonly follows the onset of focal neurologic signs within 6 days. Uncontrollable cerebral edema contributes to a lethal outcome. The causes of death are dural venous sinus thrombosis, fulminant meningitis, and multiple intracerebral abscesses. With prompt evacuation of the pus and chemotherapy, recovery is possible even after focal neurologic signs have appeared. Gradual improvement of the focal neurologic signs may occur after recovery from the infection. Seizures, hemiparesis, and other focal deficits may be long-term sequelae, however.

Treatment

The treatment of subdural empyema is prompt surgical evacuation of the pus through trephine operation, carefully avoiding passage through the infected nasal sinuses. Systemic antibiotic therapy should commence before surgery and should be tailored to any suspected organism. If *S. aureus* is suspected, penicillin G and metronidazole with vancomycin are suitable as a broad-spectrum treatment before culture reports. Sometimes a third-generation cephalosporin also is added. Treatment is usually 3 to 4 weeks. Instillation of antibiotics into the subdural space during surgery is of uncertain efficacy but commonly is done. Treatment of cerebral edema is also a necessity.

Intracranial Epidural Abscess

Abscesses confined to the epidural space are frequent and are almost always associated with overlying infection in the cranial bones. Penetration from chronic sinusitis or mastoiditis is most common, but infection after head trauma or neurosurgery may also cause this problem. Occasionally, no source is apparent. Frequently, intracranial epidural abscess is associated with deeper penetration of the infection and subdural empyema, meningitis, or intraparenchymal abscess. Severe headache, fever, malaise, and findings referable to the initial site of infection are the features of isolated intracranial epidural abscess. Focal neurologic findings are rarely present. Diagnosis is made most conveniently by CT or MRI, which usually demonstrate a characteristic extradural defect (Fig. 21.3). MRI appears to be more sensitive when the lesion is small. If no abnormality is detected, repeat scanning should be performed when headache persists after antibiotic treatment of an infected sinus or other focus. Evaluation of CSF is not of great help. The protein may be modestly ele-

vated and a mild pleocytosis may be present, but organisms are not seen on Gram stain and cultures are routinely negative. Lumbar puncture is certainly discouraged until after scanning has established that significant mass effect is not present. As with most abscesses, surgical drainage is usually necessary to ensure cure. If, however, the scan and lack of neurologic findings suggest that the infection is confined to the epidural space, trephination may suffice and a craniotomy can be avoided. Appropriate antibiotic treatment is the same as that for subdural empyema, because the sources of infection are similar. It is not clear whether irrigation of the epidural space with antibiotic is useful.

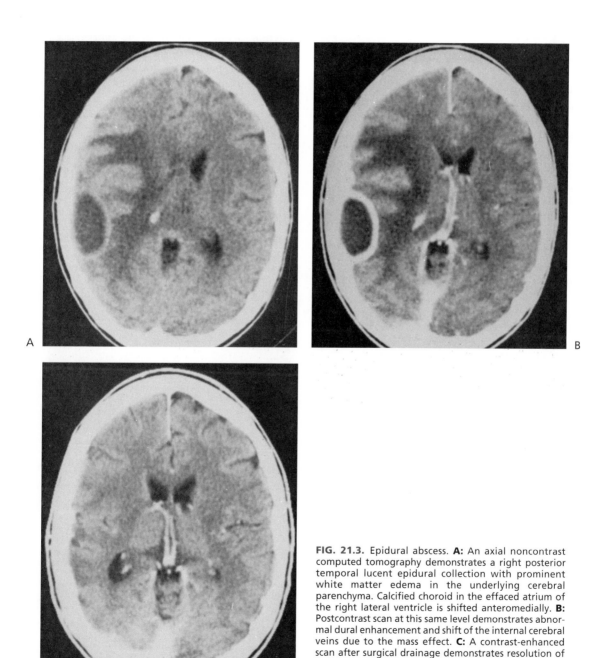

FIG. 21.3. Epidural abscess. **A:** An axial noncontrast computed tomography demonstrates a right posterior temporal lucent epidural collection with prominent white matter edema in the underlying cerebral parenchyma. Calcified choroid in the effaced atrium of the right lateral ventricle is shifted anteromedially. **B:** Postcontrast scan at this same level demonstrates abnormal dural enhancement and shift of the internal cerebral veins due to the mass effect. **C:** A contrast-enhanced scan after surgical drainage demonstrates resolution of the abscess, edema, mass effect, and shift. (Courtesy of Drs. J. A. Bello and S. K. Hilal.)

Spinal Epidural Abscess

Spinal epidural abscess is a collection of purulent material located outside the dura mater within the spinal canal. Infections of the spinal epidural space are accompanied by fever, headache, pain in the back, weakness of the lower extremities, and, finally, complete paraplegia.

Etiology

Infections may reach the fatty tissue in the spinal epidural space by one of three routes: direct extension from inflammatory processes in adjacent tissues, such as decubitus ulcers, carbuncles, or perinephric abscesses; metastasis through the blood from infections elsewhere in the body; and perforating wounds, spinal surgery, or lumbar puncture. The first route of infection accounts for most cases. The primary site of infection is often a furuncle on the skin, but septic foci in the tonsils, teeth, lungs, uterus, or other organ may metastasize to the epidural fat. Chronic debilitating diseases, diabetes mellitus, immunosuppressive therapy, and heroin abuse are contributing factors.

S. aureus accounts for 50% to 60% of epidural abscesses. Other bacteria responsible include *E. coli*, other gram-negative organisms, and hemolytic and anaerobic streptococci.

Pathology

No region of the spine is immune to infection, but the midthoracic vertebrae are most frequently affected. The character of the osteomyelitis in the vertebra is similar to that encountered in other bones of the body. The laminae are most commonly involved, but any part of the vertebra, including the body, may be the seat of the infection. The infection in the epidural space may be acute or chronic.

In acute cases, which are by far the most common, a purulent necrosis of the epidural fat extends over several segments of the entire length of the cord. The pus is usually posterior to the spinal cord but may be on the anterior surface. When the infecting organism is of low virulence, the infection may localize and assume a granulomatous nature.

The lesions in the spinal cord depend on the extent to which the infection has progressed before treatment is begun. Necrosis in the periphery of the cord may result from pressure of the abscess, or myelomalacia of one or several segments may occur when the veins or arteries are thrombosed. There is ascending degeneration above and descending degeneration below the level of the necrotic lesion. The substance of the spinal cord occasionally may be infected by extension through the meninges, with the formation of a spinal cord abscess.

Incidence

Spinal epidural abscesses account for approximately 1 of every 20,000 admissions to hospitals in the United States. They can occur at all ages; 60% affect adults between 20 and 50 years of age.

Symptoms and Signs

The symptoms of acute spinal epidural abscess develop suddenly, several days or weeks after an infection of the skin or other parts of the body. The preceding infection occasionally may be so slight that it is overlooked. Severe back pain is usually the presenting symptom. Malaise, fever, neck stiffness, and headache may be present or follow in a few days. Usually within hours, but sometimes not for several weeks, initial symptoms are followed by radicular pain. If the abscess is untreated, muscular weakness and paralysis of the legs may develop suddenly.

Fever and malaise are usually present in the early phase; lethargy or irritability develops as the disease progresses. There is neck stiffness and a Kernig sign. Local percussion tenderness over the spine is an important diagnostic sign. Tendon reflexes may be increased or decreased, and the plantar responses may be extensor. With thrombosis of the spinal vessels, a flaccid paraplegia occurs with complete loss of sensation below the level of the lesion and paralysis of the bladder or rectum. Immediately after the onset of paraplegia, tendon reflexes are absent in the paralyzed extremities. There is often erythema and swelling in the area of back pain.

In chronic cases in which the infection is localized and there is granuloma formation, the neurologic signs are similar to those seen with other types of extradural tumors. Fever is rare; weakness and paralysis may not develop for weeks or months.

Laboratory Data

In acute cases, leukocytosis is present in the blood. The erythrocyte sedimentation rate is usually elevated. Radiographs of the spine are usually normal but may show osteomyelitis or a contiguous abscess (Fig. 21.4).

Myelography is almost invariably abnormal. Complete extradural block is found in 80% of patients; the others demonstrate partial block. It is critically important to consider the pos-

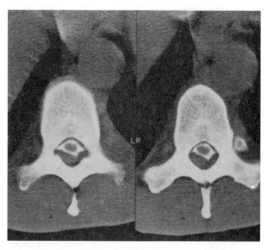

FIG. 21.4. Epidural abscess. Axial computed tomography myelography demonstrates abnormal epidural soft-tissue density posterior to and deforming the thecal sac, with anterior displacement of the cord at this lower thoracic level. (Courtesy of Dr. S. K. Hilal.)

sibility of epidural abscess in any case of acute or subacute myelopathy, because lumbar puncture may penetrate the pus and carry infection into the subarachnoid space. When complete block or a lower thoracic-lumbar abscess is suspected, myelography should be performed by cervical puncture. The needle should be advanced slowly and suction applied with a syringe as the epidural space is approached. If the abscess has extended to the level of the puncture, pus may be withdrawn for culture and the procedure terminated.

Epidural abscesses can be demonstrated by spinal CT, with or without use of intravenous contrast material. MRI, especially with gadolinium enhancement, is even more sensitive (Fig. 21.5). When lesions are clearly defined by either of these techniques, myelography is not necessary.

CSF pressure is normal or increased and there is complete or almost complete subarachnoid block. The CSF is xanthochromic or cloudy in appearance. There is usually a slight or moderate pleocytosis in the CSF, varying from a few to several hundred cells per cubic millimeter. Rarely, no cells may be present. The protein content is increased with values commonly between 100 and 1,500 mg/dL. The CSF sugar content is normal, and CSF cultures are sterile unless meningitis has developed.

Diagnosis

A presumptive diagnosis can be made when subarachnoid block is found in a patient with back and leg pain of acute onset with back tenderness and signs of meningeal irritation. This is true when there is a history of recent pyogenic infection. The diagnosis should be made before signs of transection of the cord develop.

Acute spinal epidural abscess must be differentiated from acute or subacute meningitis, acute poliomyelitis, infectious polyneuritis, acute transverse myelitis, multiple sclerosis, and epidural hematoma. The clinical, CSF, and myelography findings are sufficient to differentiate these conditions. Chronic epidural abscess may be confused with chronic adhesive arachnoiditis or tumors in the epidural space.

The diagnosis of granulomatous infection is rarely made before operation. The signs are those of chronic cord compression. Operation is indicated by the presence of these signs and evidence of spinal subarachnoid block.

Course and Prognosis

If treatment is delayed in acute spinal epidural abscess, complete or incomplete transection syndrome almost invariably develops. Flaccid paraplegia, sphincter paralysis, and sensory loss below the level of the lesion persist throughout the life of the individual.

The mortality rate is approximately 30% in the acute cases and 10% in the chronic cases. Death may occur in acute cases as a direct result of the infection or secondary to complications. Total recovery may occur in patients who do not have total paralysis or who have weakness lasting less than 36 hours. Of patients paralyzed for 48 hours or more, 50% progress to permanent paralysis and death.

Treatment

The treatment of spinal epidural abscess is prompt surgical drainage by laminectomy. Antibiotics should be administered before and after the operation. Aerobic and anaerobic cultures should be obtained at operation. The area of suppuration should be irrigated with an antibiotic solution. Delay in draining the abscess may result in permanent paralysis. Little improvement can be expected in acute cases with signs of transection if the operation is performed after they occur because these signs are caused by softening of the spinal cord secondary to thrombosis of the spinal vessels. In chronic cases where compression of the cord plays a role in the production of the signs, considerable improvement in the neurologic symptoms and signs may be expected after the operation.

When there is back pain with minimal or no neurologic abnormality, surgery may not be needed, but epidural aspiration for culture is used to guide antibiotic therapy, followed by MRI monitoring of the course. This is potentially perilous because progression of neurologic dysfunction can be rapid and irreversible. Close observation and immediate surgical drainage are necessary if neurologic deterioration occurs.

Infective Endocarditis

The etiologic causes of infective endocarditis have changed remarkably in the antibiotic era. Rheumatic heart disease now accounts for fewer than 25% of cases, whereas it once accounted for nearly 75%. Endocarditis secondary to prosthetic valves or other intravascular devices, intravenous drug addiction, and degenerative cardiac disease related to aging has become more prominent. Congenital heart abnormalities remain an important cause, especially in children. Unfortunately, morbidity and mortality rates have not been affected much by these etiologic changes and the use of antibiotics, thus probably reflecting more severe infections associated with these newer causes. In the past, the terms acute or subacute were used to describe infective endocarditis. These subdivisions, however, are artificial; the underlying cause of the endocarditis and the specific organism involved are more useful considerations when determining prognosis and treatment.

Neurologic complications of infective endocarditis are important because of their frequency and severity. They may be the first manifestation of the underlying intracardiac infection. Cerebral infarcts, either bland or less often hemorrhagic, are most common. Infarcts of cranial or peripheral nerves and of the spinal cord rarely occur. Intracranial hemorrhage caused by mycotic aneurysms, brain abscess, and meningitis also are frequent. These complications presumably result from emboli of infective material from the heart. Inflammatory arteritis also has been implicated as a cause, particularly of intracranial hemorrhage when no mycotic aneurysm is apparent. An encephalopathy sometimes with prominent psychiatric features can occur and may be related to microemboli with or without microabscess formation, vasculitis, toxic effects of medications, or metabolic derangements associated with the illness occurring either individually or concurrently. Seizures may occur in association with any of the cerebral complications.

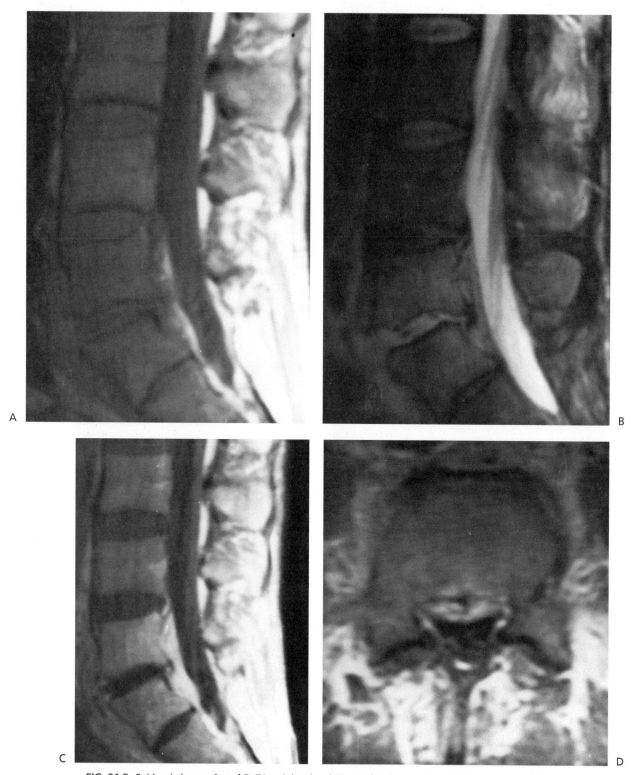

FIG. 21.5. Epidural abscess. **A and B:** T1-weighted and T2-weighted saggital magnetic resonance (MR) scans demonstrate a vague area of mixed signal intensity within the anterior epidural space extending from the top of the L5 vertebral level down to the S1 level, suggestive of an underlying epidural process. Also noted is mild increased signal intensity within the L5 and S1 vertebral bodies on the T2-weighted images suggestive of adjacent vertebral inflammation or degeneration. (Degenerative disc disease is present at the L4-L5 disc space.) **C and D:** T1-weighted saggital and axial MR scans demonstrate significant contrast enhancement within the anterior epidural space between L5 and S1 levels, consistent with epidural infection. Axial view shows compression upon spinal sac anteriorly. Patient had known *Staphylococcus aureus* sepsis; epidural abscess receded with intravenous antibiotics. (Courtesy of Dr. S. Chan.)

Infective endocarditis always should be considered in sudden neurologic vascular events, particularly when known predisposing factors exist, such as cardiac disease, drug addiction, fever, or infection elsewhere in the body. The frequency of neurologic events is between 20% and 40% in most reported series of endocarditis. They appear to occur more frequently in the elderly patient. As might be anticipated, neurologic complications are more frequent in endocarditis that affects the left side of the heart. Right-sided lesions usually cause meningitis, intracerebral abscesses, or encephalopathy rather than embolic-related events, although these still rarely occur. The type of organism is also important in determining the frequency of neurologic events. *S. aureus* and *S. pneumoniae* in particular are associated with a high risk of nervous system complications.

Diagnostic evaluation of neurologic events depends in part on whether the presence of infective endocarditis already has been established. Imaging studies are important to define the nature of lesions that have focal neurologic findings. Differentiation of infarcts from hemorrhages or abscesses may be accomplished by either CT or MRI. On occasion, both techniques may be necessary to define clearly the nature of the lesion. Analysis of the CSF is mandatory in cases of meningitis regardless of whether the diagnosis of infective endocarditis already has been made. Such analysis also is useful in encephalopathic conditions to evaluate for low-grade meningitic infection. Lumbar puncture also should be considered strongly in stroke associated with fever even if endocarditis is not yet documented. It is probably not useful in known infective endocarditis with focal CNS presentations and a clearly defined lesion with imaging studies. Demonstration of suspected mycotic aneurysms can be made by arteriography. The usefulness of magnetic resonance angiography has not been established yet. Some practitioners have advocated arteriography in all cases of infective endocarditis. No controlled studies have been done to determine the indications for arteriography, and indications for surgical treatment of detected aneurysms also are uncertain.

Treatment of infective endocarditis with nervous system complications is primarily treatment of the cardiac lesion. Prolonged antibiotic treatment is required, and surgical replacement of infected valves may be appropriate. In most instances, treatment of nervous system events is nonspecific and supportive. Brain abscesses that do not resolve rapidly with systemic antibiotics should be drained. As noted, indications for surgical management of mycotic aneurysms is uncertain and must be decided on an individual basis. The aneurysms usually do not have a neck and cannot be conveniently clipped. Sacrifice of the distal vessel usually is necessary, and further cerebral damage is possible.

Leprosy

Leprosy (Hansen disease) is a chronic disease due to infection by *Mycobacterium leprae*, which has a predilection for the skin and the peripheral nerves. The bacillus has this predilection for mucous membranes and skin, including superficial nerves, because these are the cooler areas of the body where the temperature is ideal for multiplication. Two major clinical types are recognized: lepromatous and tuberculoid. The type that predominates ap-

pears to depend on the nature of the immunologic response to the organism.

Etiology

M. leprae is an acid-fast rod-shaped organism morphologically similar to the tubercle bacillus. The organism can be demonstrated in the cutaneous lesion and is sometimes present in the blood of lepromatous patients. The disease is transmitted by direct contact, which must be intimate and prolonged because the contagiousness is low. The portal of entry is probably through abrasions in the skin or mucous membranes of the upper respiratory tract. The incubation period is long, averaging 3 to 4 years in children and longer in adults. Transmission from patients with tuberculoid leprosy is rare.

Pathology

The affected nerve trunks are diffusely thickened or are studded with nodular swellings. There is an overgrowth of connective tissue with degeneration of the axon and myelin sheath. Bacilli are present in the perineurium and endoneural septa. They also have been found in dorsal root ganglia, spinal cord, and brain, but they do not produce any significant lesions within the CNS. Degenerative changes in the posterior funiculi of the cord, which are found in some cases, can be attributed to the peripheral neuritis.

Incidence

Leprosy is most common in tropical and subtropical climates, and it is estimated that 10 to 20 million people are infected. The disease is prevalent in South and Central America, China, India, and Africa. It is uncommon in Europe or North America. In the United States, the disease is mostly confined to Louisiana, Texas, Florida, Southern California, Hawaii, and New York. The number of new cases in the United States has increased in recent years because of immigration from endemic areas.

Children are especially susceptible to the disease, but it may occur in adults. In childhood, the disease is evenly distributed between the two sexes, but among adults, men are more frequently affected than women.

Symptoms and Signs

In most cases, a mixture of cutaneous and peripheral nerve lesions occurs. Neurologic involvement is more frequent and occurs early in the tuberculoid form. The earliest manifestation of neural leprosy is an erythematous macule, the lepride. This lesion grows by peripheral extension to form an annular macule. The macule has an atrophic depigmented center that is partially or completely anesthetic. These lesions may attain an enormous size and cover the major portion of one extremity or the torso. Infection of the nerve may result in the formation of nodules or fusiform swelling along its course. Although any of the peripheral nerves may be affected, the disease has a predilection for the ulnar, great auricular, posterior tibial, common peroneal, and the Vth and VIIth cranial nerves. These nerves are involved at locations where their course is superficial. Repeated attacks of neuralgic pains often precede the onset of weakness or sensory loss.

Cranial Nerves

Involvement of the Vth cranial nerve is evident by the appearance of patches of anesthesia on the face. Involvement of the entire sensory distribution of the nerve or its motor division is rare. Keratitis, ulceration, and blindness may ensue as results of injury to the anesthetic cornea. Complete paralysis of the facial nerve is rare, but weakness of a portion of one or several muscles is common. The muscles of the upper half of the face are most severely affected. Partial paralysis of the orbicularis and other facial muscles may result in lagophthalmos, ectropion, and facial asymmetry. Involvement of the oculomotor or other cranial nerves is rare.

Motor System

Weakness and atrophy develop in the muscles innervated by the affected nerves. There is wasting of the small muscles of the hands and feet, with later extension to the forearm and leg, but the proximal muscles usually are spared. Clawing of the hands or feet is common, but wrist drop and foot drop are late manifestations. Fasciculations may occur and contractures may develop.

Sensory System

Cutaneous sensation is impaired or lost in the distribution of the affected nerves in a somewhat irregular or patchy fashion. Various types of dissociated sensory impairment are seen. The sensory impairment may be of a nerve or root distribution but more commonly it is of a glove-and-stocking type. Deep sensation, pressure pain, the appreciation of vibration, and position sense usually are spared or are affected less severely than is superficial cutaneous sensation.

Reflexes

Tendon reflexes are usually preserved until late advanced stages of nerve damage when they are reduced or lost. The abdominal skin reflexes and plantar responses are normal.

Other Signs

Vasomotor and trophic disturbances are usually present. Anhidrosis and cyanosis of the hands and feet are common. Trophic ulcers develop on the knuckles and on the plantar surface of the feet. There may be various arthropathies and resorption of the bones of the fingers, starting in the terminal phalanges and progressing upward. The skin shrinks as digits become shorter, and finally the nail may be attached to a small stump.

Laboratory Data

There are no diagnostic changes in the blood, although mild anemia and an increased erythrocyte sedimentation rate may be seen. As many as 33% of lepromatous patients have false-positive serologic tests for syphilis. The only CSF abnormality is a slight increase in the protein content.

Diagnosis

The diagnosis of leprosy is made without difficulty from the characteristic skin and neuritis lesions. The clinical picture occasionally may have a superficial similarity to that of syringomyelia, hypertrophic interstitial neuritis, or von Recklinghausen disease. The correct diagnosis usually is not difficult if the possibility of leprosy is kept in mind and scrapings from cutaneous lesions and nerve biopsy specimens are examined for acid-fast bacilli.

Course and Prognosis

The prognosis in the neural form (primarily tuberculoid) of the disease is less grave than that in the cutaneous form (primarily lepromatous), in which death within 10 to 20 years is the rule. Neural leprosy is not necessarily fatal. The progress of the neuritis is slow, and the disease may come to a spontaneous arrest or may be controlled by therapy. Incapacitation may result from the paralyses and disfigurement.

Treatment

Dapsone (4,4-diamino-diphenylsulphone), a folate antagonist, is the primary drug for treatment, supplemented by a single dose of rifampin once a month for the tuberculoid form. Treatment continues for at least 6 months. For the lepromatous form, dapsone and rifampin are supplemented with clofazimine, and treatment continues for at least 2 years.

RICKETTSIAL INFECTIONS

Rickettsiae are obligate intracellular parasites about the size of bacteria. They are visible in microscopic preparations as pleomorphic coccobacilli. Each rickettsiae pathogenic for humans is capable of multiplying in arthropods and in animals and humans. They have a gram-negative–like cell wall and an internal structure similar to that of bacteria (i.e., with a prokaryotic DNA arrangement and ribosomes). Diseases due to rickettsiae are divided into five groups on the basis of their biologic properties and epidemiologic features: typhus, spotted fever, scrub typhus, Q fever, and trench fever. Invasion of the nervous system is common only in infections with organisms of the first three groups. Infection with Rocky Mountain spotted fever is the most important rickettsial infection currently in the United States. A sixth group of rickettsiae in the genus *Ehrlichia* have come to be recognized as significant pathogens in humans in the past 10 years. Ehrlichial infections have also been associated with CNS symptoms, but the frequency of nervous system infection is still not certain.

Rocky Mountain Spotted Fever

Rocky Mountain spotted fever is an acute endemic febrile disease produced by infection with the *Rickettsia rickettsii*. It is transmitted to humans by various ticks, the most common of which are the *Dermacentor andersoni* (wood tick) in the Rocky Mountain and Pacific Coast states and the *Dermacentor variabilis* (dog tick) in the East and South. Rabbits, squirrels, and other small rodents serve as hosts for the ticks and are responsible for maintaining the infection in nature. Diseases of the Rocky Mountain spotted fever group are present throughout the world.

Pathology

The pathologic changes are most severe in the skin, but the heart, lungs, and CNS also are involved. The brain is edematous, and minute petechial hemorrhages are present. The characteristic microscopic lesions are small round nodules composed of elongated microglia, lymphocytes, and endothelial cells. These are scattered diffusely through the nervous system in close relation to small vessels. Vessels in the center of the lesions show severe degeneration. The endothelial cells are swollen, and the lumen may be occluded. Minute areas of focal necrosis are common as the result of thrombosis of small arterioles. Some degree of perivascular infiltration without the presence of nodules may be seen in both the meninges and the brain parenchyma.

Incidence

The disease has been reported from almost all states and from Canada, Mexico, and South America. Approximately 1,000 cases are reported annually in the United States, mostly from rural areas. Most cases are seen during the period of maximal tick activity—the late spring and early summer months.

Symptoms and Signs

A history of tick bite is elicited in 80% of affected patients. The incubation period varies from 3 to 12 days. The onset is usually abrupt, with severe headache, fever, chills, myalgias, arthralgias, restlessness, prostration, and, at times, delirium and coma. A rose-red maculopapular rash appears between the second and sixth day (usually on the fourth febrile day) on the wrists, ankles, palms, soles, and forearms. The rash rapidly spreads to the legs, arms, and chest. The rash becomes petechial and fails to fade on pressure by about the fourth day.

Neurologic symptoms occur early and are frequently a prominent feature. Headache, restlessness, insomnia, and back stiffness are common. Delirium of coma alternating with restlessness is present during the height of the fever. Tremors, athetoid movements, convulsions, opisthotonos, and muscular rigidity may occur. Retinal venous engorgement, retinal edema, papilledema, retinal exudates, and choroiditis may occur. Deafness, visual disturbances, slurred speech, and mental confusion may be present and may persist for a few weeks following recovery.

Laboratory Data

The white cell count is either normal or mildly elevated. Proteinuria, hematuria, and oliguria commonly occur. CSF pressure and glucose are usually normal. The CSF is clear, but a slight lymphocytic pleocytosis and protein elevation may occur. Eosinophilic meningitis has been reported.

Diagnosis

The diagnosis is made on the basis of the development of the characteristic rash and other symptoms of the disease after exposure to ticks. Clinical distinction from typhus fever may be impossible. The onset of the rash in distal parts of the limbs favors a diagnosis of Rocky Mountain spotted fever. In rare instances, however, neurologic signs may occur before the rash appears. A rise in antibody titer during the second week of illness can be detected by specific complement fixation, immunofluorescence and microagglutination tests, or by the Weil-Felix reaction with *Proteus* OX-19 and OX-2.

Course and Prognosis

In patients who recover, the fever falls at about the end of the third week, although mild cases may become afebrile before the end of the second week. Convalescence may be slow, and residuals of damage to the nervous system may persist for several months.

In untreated cases, the overall case fatality is about 20%. Prognosis depends on the severity of the infection, host factors (e.g., age, the presence of other illness), and the promptness with which antimicrobial treatment is started.

Treatment

Control measures include personal care and vaccination. Tick-infested areas should be avoided. If exposure is necessary, high boots, leggings, or socks should be worn outside the trouser legs. Body and clothing should be inspected after exposure, and attached ticks should be removed with tweezers. The hands should be carefully washed after handling the ticks. Workers whose occupations require constant exposure to tick-infested regions should be vaccinated yearly, just before the advent of the tick season.

The treatment of Rocky Mountain spotted fever is the prompt administration of tetracycline or doxycycline. In children, chloramphenicol is preferred to avoid tooth discoloration. Any patient seriously considered to have Rocky Mountain spotted fever should be treated promptly while diagnostic tests proceed.

The other rickettsial infections that may affect the nervous system directly either are rare or do not occur in the United States. Except for some variation in their incubation times, the pathology and clinical picture are similar to those of Rocky Mountain spotted fever and need not be described again. All such infections respond to tetracyclines or chloramphenicol.

Typhus Fever

Three types of infection with rickettsiae of the typhus group are recognized: primary louse-borne epidemic typhus; its recrudescent form, Brill-Zinsser disease; and flea-borne endemic murine typhus.

Incidence

Since its recognition in the 16th century, typhus has been known as one of the great epidemic diseases of the world. It is especially prevalent in war times or whenever there is a massing of people in camps, prisons, or ships.

Epidemic typhus (caused by *R. prowazekii*) is spread among humans by the human body louse (*Pediculus humanus corporis*). Outbreaks of epidemic typhus last occurred in the United States in the 19th century. The freedom of the population from lice explains the absence of epidemics in the United States. Sporadic cases in the United States have been associated with flying squirrel contact. The location of the disease is now limited to the Balkans and Middle East, North Africa, Asia, Mexico, and the Andes. In the epidemic form, all age groups are affected.

Rickettsiae may remain viable for as long as 20 years in the tissues of recovered patients without manifest symptoms. Brill-Zinsser disease is a recrudescence of epidemic typhus that occurs years after the initial attack and may cause a new epidemic.

Murine typhus (*R. typhi*) is worldwide in distribution and is distributed to humans by fleas. The disease is most prevalent in southeastern and Gulf Coast states and among individuals whose occupations bring them into rat-infested areas. The disease is most common in the late summer and fall months.

Diagnosis

A presumptive diagnosis of typhus fever can be made on the basis of the characteristic skin rash and signs of involvement of the nervous system. The diagnosis is established by the Weil-Felix reaction, which becomes positive in the fifth to eighth day of the disease. The titer rises in the first few weeks of the convalescence and then falls. Antibodies to specific rickettsiae can be demonstrated by complement fixation, microagglutination, or immunofluorescence reactions.

Course and Prognosis

The course of typhus fever usually extends over 2 to 3 weeks. Death from epidemic typhus usually occurs between the 9th and 18th day of illness. In patients who recover, the temperature begins to fall after 14 to 18 days and reaches normal levels in 2 to 4 days. Complications include bronchitis and bronchopneumonia, myocardial degeneration, gangrene of the skin or limbs, and thrombosis of large abdominal, pulmonary, or cerebral vessels.

The prognosis of epidemic typhus depends on the patient's age and immunization status. The disease is usually mild in children younger than 10. After the third decade, mortality increases steadily with each decade. Death is usually due to the development of pneumonia, circulatory collapse, and renal failure. The mortality rate for murine typhus in the United States is low (less than 1%). There are no neurologic residua in patients who recover.

Scrub Typhus

Scrub typhus is an infectious disease caused by *R. tsutsugamushi* (*R. orientalis*), which is transmitted to humans by the bite of larval trombiculid mites (chiggers). It resembles the other rickettsial diseases and is characterized by sudden onset of fever, cutaneous eruption, and the presence of an ulcerative lesion (eschar) at the site of attachment of the chigger.

Epidemiology

The disease is limited to eastern and southeastern Asia, India, and northern Australia and adjacent islands.

Symptoms and Signs

The disease begins abruptly, after an incubation period of 10 to 12 days, with fever, chills, and headache. The headache increases in intensity and may become severe. Conjunctival congestion, moderate generalized lymphadenopathy, deafness, apathy, and anorexia are common symptoms. Delirium, coma, restlessness, and muscular twitchings are present in severe cases. A primary lesion (the eschar) is seen in nearly all cases and represents the former site of attachment of the infected mite. There may be multiple eschars. The cutaneous rash appears between the fifth and eighth day of the disease. The eruption is macular or maculopapular and nonhemorrhagic. The trunk is involved first with later extension to the limbs.

Diagnosis

The diagnosis is made on the basis of the development of typical symptoms, the presence of the characteristic eschar, and a rising titer to *Proteus* OXK in the Weil-Felix test during the second week of illness. Immunofluorescence testing with specific antigens may be diagnostic.

Course and Prognosis

In fatal cases, death usually occurs in the second or third week as a result of pneumonia, cardiac failure, or cerebral involvement. In the preantibiotic era, mortality could reach 60%, depending on geographic locale and virulence of the strain. Deaths are rare with appropriate antibiotic treatment.

In patients who recover, the temperature begins to fall at the end of the second or third week. Permanent residua are not common, but the period of convalescence may extend over several months.

Human Ehrlichiosis

The nature and extent of infections in humans with rickettsia of the genus *Ehrlichia* is still not fully determined. These organisms appear to infect leukocytes. Two forms of human infection have been identified. One species, *E. chaffeensis*, is associated with human monocytic ehrlichiosis (HME) and the organism can be preferentially found in these cells. The agent of human granulocytic ehrlichiosis (HGE) has not yet been assigned a species. Serologically it cross-reacts with *E. equus*, but it is not clear if it is the same species. Both human infections are detectable in the appropriate cells as coccobacillary forms. It has become possible to cultivate the organisms, and PCR reactions are also coming into use to detect infection. Most studies still rely on antibody detection. *E. chaffeensis* appears to be transmitted by *Amblyomma americanum* (lone star tick) and possibly by *D. variabilis*, whereas the human granulocytic ehrlichiosis agent is transmitted by *Ixodid* ticks and probably *Dermacentor andersonii*.

Epidemiology

The epidemiologic range for both agents appears to be extending. Whether this is an actual phenomenon or due to an heightened awareness of the infection is still unclear. HME is more common in the South and Southeast, whereas HGE was first found in the Midwest. Now cases have been reported from New England and New York State, in keeping with the distribution of *Ixodes scapularis*. Coinfection of HGE with *Borrelia burgdorferi* and HME with Rocky Mountain spotted fever has already been reported.

Symptoms and Signs

Infection of both agents usually presents as a febrile systemic process often associated with myalgias and headaches. Changes in mental status and ataxia have also been noted and are correlated with more serious illness. Rashes have been reported in about 20% of cases. This makes it difficult to distinguish the illness from Rocky Mountain spotted fever, whose distribution overlaps with *E. chaffeensis*. CSF pleocytosis and elevated proteins have been reported and appear to correlate with altered mental status.

Diagnosis

Because of the nonspecific nature of the symptoms and signs, a high index of suspicion is required. A history of exposure to ticks may be helpful, but epidemiologic studies have shown serologic evidence of infection usually is not correlated with known tick bites. As might be anticipated, lymphopenia is often a feature of *E. chaffeensis* infection, whereas granulocytopenia is usually noted with the HGE agent. Elevated hepatic enzymes are usually present. The rickettsiae can often be found in infected leukocytes. Confirmation of the diagnosis is by antibody titers or immunofluorescent detection of the intracellular organisms. PCR detection of the organisms' DNA, when it is more widely available, will be an important technique because of sensitivity and rapidity. Culturing of the agents is now also possible but is not as sensitive as PCR.

Course and Prognosis

A complete understanding of the course of both HME and HGE has yet to be determined. Initially, a high proportion of reported cases was fatal in both HME and HGE. However, serologic studies indicate asymptomatic or minor infections are common. Clinically, it has also been found that some cases may be self-limited, even without treatment. Treatment with tetracycline or doxycycline results in rapid improvement. Therefore, prognosis appears to be good, if the diagnosis is promptly made and treatment started. Whether chloramphenicol will be an acceptable alternative antibiotic has yet to be established.

OTHER BACTERIAL INFECTIONS

Brucellosis

Brucellosis (undulant fever) is a disease with protean manifestation due to infection with short, slender, rod-shaped, gram-negative microorganisms of the genus *Brucella*. The infection is transmitted to humans from animals, usually cattle or swine. The illness is prone to occur in slaughterhouse workers, livestock producers, veterinarians, and persons who ingest unpasteurized milk or milk products. An acute febrile illness is characteristic of the early stages of the disease. The common symptoms include chilly sensations, sweats, fever, weakness, and generalized malaise; 70% of patients experience body aches and nearly 50% complain of headache. Physical signs of lymphadenopathy, splenomegaly, hepatomegaly, and tenderness of the spine, however, are infrequent, occurring in less than 25% of cases. The early constitutional symptoms are followed by the subacute and chronic stages in about 15% to 20% of patients with localized infection of the bones, joints, lungs, kidneys, liver, lymph nodes, and other organs.

Involvement of the nervous system is not common. Cases have been reported with meningitis and sometimes with accompanying cranial nerve paresis, meningoencephalitis, meningomyelitis, optic neuritis, and peripheral neuritis. Brain abscesses also have been reported.

The CSF in reported cases is under increased pressure, with a pleocytosis varying from a few to several hundred cells. The protein content is moderately to greatly increased, and the sugar content is decreased. The CSF has increased gamma globulin levels and often contains *Brucella*-agglutinating antibodies.

In the few patients with CNS involvement who came to autopsy, there was a subacute meningitis with perivascular infiltrations, thickening of the vessels in the brain and spinal cord, and degenerative changes in the white and gray matter. Organisms have been cultured from the CSF of a few patients.

The diagnosis is made from a history of previous symptoms of the disease, culture of the organisms from the blood or CSF, and serologic testing. Treatment is with doxycycline or other tetracycline plus an aminoglycoside. Trimethoprim/sulfoxazole is an alternative to the tetracycline.

Behçet Syndrome

An inflammatory disorder of unknown cause, characterized by the occurrence of relapsing uveitis and recurrent genital and oral ulcers, was described by Behçet in 1937. The disease may involve the nervous system, skin, joints, peripheral blood vessels, and other organs. Evidence of CNS involvement is present in 25% to 30% of patients. Neurologic symptoms antedate the more diagnostic criteria of aphthous stomatitis, genital ulcerations, and uveitis in only 5% of cases. Pathologic confirmation of cerebral involvement has been obtained in a few cases. The disease appears to have a predilection for young adult men.

Etiology and Pathology

The cause of Behçet syndrome is unknown. No infectious agent has been isolated consistently, although there have been several reports of a virus having been recovered from patients with the disease. Circulating immune complexes of the IgA and IgG variety may be detected in patients' serums. The disease is associated with HLA-B5 tissue type in Japan and the Mediterranean nations.

In patients studied at necropsy, there was a mild inflammatory reaction in the meninges and in the perivascular spaces of the cerebrum, basal ganglia, brainstem, and cerebellum and degenerative changes in the ganglion cells. Inflammatory changes were also found in the iris, choroid, retina, and optic nerve.

Incidence

The disease is common in northern Japan, Turkey, and Israel; the incidence in Japan is 1 in 10,000. The syndrome is seen less commonly in the United States. An annual incidence of 1 in 300,000 was determined for Olmstead County, Minnesota. The age at onset is in the third and fourth decades of life; men are more frequently affected than women. The exact incidence of neurologic symptoms is not known, but it approximates 10% of affected individuals.

Symptoms and Signs

The ocular signs include keratoconjunctivitis, iritis, hypopyon, uveitis, and hemorrhage into the vitreous. Ocular symptoms occur in 90% of patients and may progress to total blindness in one or both eyes. The cutaneous lesions are in the nature of painful recurrent and indolent ulcers, which are most commonly found on the genitalia or the buccal mucosa. Virtually all patients have recurrent oral aphthous ulcers. Arthritis occurs in about 50% of patients. Furunculosis, erythema nodosum, thrombophlebitis, and nonspecific skin sensitivity are also common. Patients with Behçet syndrome often develop a pustule surrounded by erythema at the site of a needle puncture; when present, the finding is considered virtually pathognomonic.

Any portion of the nervous system may be affected. Cranial nerve palsies are common. Other symptoms and signs include papilledema, convulsions, mental confusion, coma, aphasia, hemiparesis, quadriparesis, pseudobulbar palsy, and evidence of involvement of the basal ganglia, cerebellum, or spinal cord.

Laboratory Data

A low-grade fever is common during the acute exacerbations of the disease. Fever may be accompanied by an elevation of the sedimentation rate, anemia, and a slight leukocytosis in the blood. A polyclonal increase in serum gamma globulin may be present. Coagulation profile may disclose elevated levels of fibrinogen and factor VIII.

The CSF pressure may be slightly increased. There is a pleocytosis of a mild or moderate degree and a moderate increase in the protein content. CSF sugar, when reported, has been normal. The serologic tests for syphilis are negative in the blood and CSF. Elevation of the CSF gamma globulin content has been reported. CSF cultures have been negative. Mild diffuse abnormalities may be found on the electroencephalogram. CT may demonstrate lesions of decreased density that may be contrast enhancing.

Diagnosis

The diagnosis is based on the occurrence of signs of a meningoencephalitis in combination with the characteristic cutaneous and ocular lesions. The disease may simulate multiple sclerosis with multifocal involvement of the nervous system, including the brainstem, cerebellum, and corticospinal tract. Syphilis is excluded by the negative serologic tests. Sarcoidosis is excluded by the absence of other signs of this disease: lack of characteristic histologic changes in biopsied lymph node, liver, or other tissues and the presence of serum angiotensin-converting enzyme.

Course

The course of the disease is characterized by a series of remissions and exacerbations extending over several years. During the period of remission, all symptoms may improve greatly. Unilateral amblyopia or complete blindness may result from the ocular lesions. Residuals of the neurologic lesions are not uncommon.

Neurologic and posterior uveal tract lesions indicate a poor prognosis. Death has occurred from the disease, chiefly when the CNS became involved. Permanent remission of symptoms has not been reported.

Treatment

Various antibiotics, chemotherapy, and corticosteroids have been used in the treatment, but there is no evidence that any of these forms of therapy have any effect on the course of the disease. When the neurologic components of the disease are life threatening, immunosuppressive therapy may be considered. Therapy is difficult to assess because of the variable natural course.

Vogt-Koyanagi-Harada Syndrome

A relatively rare disease characterized by uveitis, retinal hemorrhages and detachment, depigmentation of the skin and hair, and signs of involvement of the nervous system was reported by Vogt, Koyanagi, and Harada in the 1920s. The dermatologic signs include poliosis and canities (patchy whitening of eyelashes, eyebrows, and scalp hair), alopecia (patchy loss of hair), and vitiligo (patchy depigmentation of skin).

The nervous system is affected in practically all cases. The neurologic symptoms are caused by an inflammatory adhesive arachnoiditis. The most common patient complaint is headache, sometimes accompanied by dizziness, fatigue, and somnolence. Neurosensory deafness, hemiplegia, ocular palsies, psychotic manifestations, and meningeal signs may occur. The CSF is under increased pressure. There is a moderate degree of lymphocytic pleocytosis. The CSF protein content is normal or slightly elevated; an elevated gamma globulin has been reported. The CSF glucose level is normal. The period of activity of the process lasts for 6 to 12 months and is followed by a recrudescence of the ophthalmic and neurologic signs.

The cause of the disease is unknown. It has been suggested that it is caused by a viral infection, but proof for this is lacking. The eye lesions are similar to those of sympathetic ophthalmia.

There is no specific therapy, but some reports suggest that administration of corticosteroids may be of value.

Mollaret Meningitis

Patients with recurrent episodes of benign aseptic meningitis were first described by Mollaret in 1944. The disease is characterized by repeated, short-lived, spontaneous, remitting attacks of headache and by nuchal rigidity. Between attacks, the patient enjoys good health. The meningitis episodes usually last 2 or 3 days. Most are characterized by a mild meningitis without associated neurologic abnormalities. Transient neurologic disturbances (coma, seizures, syncope, diplopia, dysarthria, disequilibrium, facial paralysis, anisocoria, and extensor plantar responses) have been reported. The patient's body temperature is moderately elevated with a maximum of 104°F (40°C). Neck stiffness and the signs of meningeal irritation are present. The first attack may appear at any age between childhood and late adult years. Both sexes are equally affected. The episodes usually last for 3 to 5 years.

During the attacks, there is a CSF pleocytosis and a slight elevation of the protein content. The CSF sugar content is normal. The cell counts range from 200 to several thousand/mm³; most cells are mononuclear. Large fragile endothelial cells are found in the CSF in the early phases of the disease; their presence is variable and is not considered essential for the diagnosis.

Proposed etiologic agents in individual cases have included herpes simplex type I, epidermoid cyst, and histoplasmosis, but none has been found with consistency. In recent years, detection of herpes simplex type II genome by PCR has been regularly, but not uniformly, reported in recurrent aseptic meningitis to which the name Mollaret meningitis is often applied. It is uncertain whether this constitutes a dilution of the eponym. It is therefore still not possible to determine whether Mollaret meningitis is a syndrome of multiple etiologies or a disease that excludes known causes.

The differential diagnosis of the condition includes recurrent bacterial meningitis, recurrent viral meningitis, sarcoidosis, hydatid cyst, fungal meningitis, intracranial tumors, Behçet syndrome, and the Vogt-Koyanagi-Harada syndrome. The latter two conditions may be differentiated by eye and skin lesions and associated findings.

Patients with Mollaret meningitis always recover rapidly and spontaneously without specific therapy. There is no effective therapy for shortening the attack or preventing fresh attacks.

Aseptic Meningeal Reaction

Aseptic meningeal reaction (sympathetic meningitis, meningitis serosa) is a term used to describe those cases with evidence of a meningeal reaction in the CSF in the absence of any infecting organism. Four general classes of cases fall into this category: those in which the meningeal reaction is due to a septic or necrotic focus within the skull or spinal canal (parameningeal infection), those in which the meningeal reaction is due to the introduction of foreign substances (e.g., air, dyes, drugs, blood) into the subarachnoid space, those in association with connective tissue disorders, and those associated with systemically administered medications (e.g., trimethoprim/sulfoxazole or nonsteroidal anti-inflammatory agents).

The symptoms that are present in the patients in the first group are associated with the infection or morbid process in the skull or spinal cavity. Only occasionally are there any symptoms and signs of meningeal irritation.

In the second group of patients, where the meningeal reaction is due to the introduction of foreign substances into the subarachnoid space, fever, headache, and stiffness of the neck may occur. The appearance of these symptoms leads to the suspicion that an actual infection of the meninges has been produced by the inadvertent introduction of pathogenic organisms. The normal sugar content of the CSF and the absence of organisms on culture establish the nature of the meningeal reaction.

An aseptic meningeal reaction may complicate the course of systemic lupus erythematosus and periarteritis nodosa. In certain instances, the meningeal reaction in patients with systemic lupus erythematosus may be induced by nonsteroidal anti-inflammatory drugs or azathioprine. An aseptic meningeal reaction may also occur in the Sjögren syndrome.

The findings in the CSF that are characteristic of an aseptic meningeal reaction are an increase in pressure, a varying degree of pleocytosis (10 to 4,000 cell/mm³), a slight or moderate increase in the protein content, a normal sugar content, and the absence of organisms on culture. (Exceptionally, and without explanation, the aseptic meningeal reaction of systemic lupus erythematosus may be accompanied by low CSF sugar values.) With a severe degree of meningeal reaction, the CSF may be purulent in appearance and may contain several thousand cells per cubic milliliter with a predominance of polymorphonuclear leukocytes. With a lesser degree of meningeal reaction, the CSF may be normal in appearance or only slightly cloudy and may contain a moderate number of cells (10 to several hundred/mm³), with lymphocytes being the predominating cell type in the CSF with less than 100 cells/mm³.

The pathogenesis of the changes in the CSF is not clearly understood. The septic foci in the head that are more commonly associated with an aseptic meningeal reaction are septic thrombosis of the intracranial venous sinuses; osteomyelitis of the spine or skull; extradural, subdural, or intracerebral abscesses; or septic cerebral emboli. Nonseptic foci of necrosis are accompanied only rarely by an aseptic meningeal reaction. Occasionally, patients with an intracerebral tumor or cerebral hemorrhage that is near to the ventricular walls may show the similar changes in the CSF.

The diagnosis of an aseptic meningeal reaction in patients with a septic or necrotic focus in the skull or spinal cord is important in that it directs attention to the presence of this focus and the necessity for appropriate surgical and medical therapy before the meninges are actually invaded by the infectious process or before other cerebral or spinal complications develop.

Meningism

Coincidental with the onset of any acute infectious diseases in childhood or young adult life there may be headache, stiffness of the neck, Kernig sign, and, rarely, delirium, convulsions, or coma. The appearance of these symptoms may lead to the tentative diagnosis of an acute meningitis or encephalitis.

Meningism refers to the syndrome of headache and signs of meningeal irritation in patients with an acute febrile illness, usually of a viral nature, in whom the CSF is commonly under increased pressure but normal in other respects. The condition may prove diagnostically confusing.

There is no completely satisfactory explanation for the syndrome. Acute hypotonicity of the patient's serum, inappropriate secretion of antidiuretic hormone, and an increased formation of CSF have been considered as possible causes. The characteristic findings on lumbar puncture are a slight or moderate increase in pressure, a clear colorless CSF that contains no cells, and a moderate reduction in the protein content of the CSF.

The condition is brief in duration. Spinal puncture, which is usually performed as a diagnostic measure in these cases, is the only therapy necessary for the relief of the symptoms. The reduction of pressure by the removal of CSF results in the disappearance of symptoms. Rarely is more than one puncture necessary.

Mycoplasma pneumoniae Infection

Mycoplasmas, originally called pleuropneumonia-like organisms, lack a cell wall. Individual mycoplasmas are bounded by a unit membrane that encloses the cytoplasm, DNA, RNA, and other cellular components. They are the smallest of free-living organisms and are resistant to penicillin and other cell wall-active antimicrobials.

Of mycoplasmas that infect humans, *M. pneumoniae* is the only species that has been clearly shown to be a significant cause of disease. It is a major cause of acute respiratory disease, including pneumonia. A variety of neurologic conditions have been described in association with *M. pneumoniae* infection: meningitis, encephalitis, postinfectious leukoencephalitis, acute cerebellar ataxia, transverse myelitis, ascending polyneuritis, radiculopathy, cranial neuropathy, and acute psychosis. The most common neurologic condition appears to be meningitis or meningoencephalitis with alterations in mental status. The neurologic features associated with *M. pneumoniae* infection, however, are so diverse that the correct diagnosis cannot be made on clinical grounds alone. The CSF usually contains polymorphonuclear leukocytes and mononuclear cells in varying proportions. The CSF has a normal or mildly elevated protein content and a normal glucose level. Bacterial, viral, and mycoplasma cultures of the CSF are usually sterile. However, detection of mycoplasma in tissue or CSF has been accomplished. Retrospective diagnosis can be made by cold isohemagglutinins for human type O erythrocytes. These can be detected in about 50% of patients during the second week of illness; they are the first antibodies to disappear. Specific antibodies can also be demonstrated.

Tetracycline and erythromycin are the drugs of choice for *M. pneumoniae* infections of a severe nature. It is not known if the postinfectious neurologic complications benefit from antimicrobial treatment.

Legionella pneumophila Infection

L. pneumophila is a poorly staining gram-negative bacterium that either does not grow or grows very slowly on most artificial media. The organism was first isolated from fatal cases of pneumonia among persons attending an American Legion Convention in Philadelphia in 1976. The bacterium is acquired by inhalation of contaminated aerosols or dust from air-conditioning systems, water, or soil.

Symptoms and Signs

Pneumonia is the most typical systemic manifestation of infection. Upper respiratory infection, a severe influenza-like syndrome (Pontiac fever), and gastrointestinal disease may also occur.

Several neurologic conditions have been described in association with *L. pneumophila* infection (Legionnaires' disease, legionellosis): acute encephalomyelitis, pronounced cerebellar deficit, chorea, and peripheral neuropathy. Confusion, delirium, and hallucinations are common symptoms. The pathophysiology of these syndromes is unclear because bacteria rarely have been demonstrated in the CNS. Myoglobinuria and elevated serum creatine kinase levels also have been reported.

Laboratory Data

L. pneumophila is rarely recovered from pleural fluid, sputum, or blood; it frequently can be isolated from respiratory secretions by transtracheal aspiration or bronchoalveolar lavage and lung biopsy tissue. A retrospective diagnosis can be made by a significant rise in specific serum antibodies detected by immunofluorescence.

Treatment

The treatment of choice is administration of erythromycin. Relapses are uncommon if treatment is continued for 14 days. When relapses occur, they usually respond to a second course of the antibiotic.

The true incidence of neurologic involvement in Legionnaires' disease is still unknown. The neurologic deficit is known to be reversible, but little exact information about recovery is available.

SUGGESTED READINGS

Acute Bacterial Meningitis

Bach MC, Davis KM. *Listeria rhombencephalitis* mimicking tuberculous meningitis. *Rev Infect Dis* 1987;9:130–133.

Benson CA, Harris AA. Acute neurologic infections. *Med Clin North Am* 1986;70:987–1011.

Dunne DW, Quagliarello V. Group B streptococcal meningitis in adults. *Medicine (Baltimore)* 1993;72:1–10.

Gilbert D, Moellering RJ, Sande M. eds. *The Sanford guide to antimicrobial therapy*, 28th ed. Vienna: Antimcrobial Therapy Inc., 1998.

Kennedy WA, Hoyt MJ, McCracken GHJ. The role of corticosteroid therapy in children with pneumococcal meningitis. *Am J Dis Child* 1991;145:1374–1378.

Luby JP. Infections of the central nervous system. *Am J Med Sci* 1992;304:379–391.

Mancebo J, Domingo P, Blanch L, et al. Post-neurosurgical and spontaneous gram-negative bacillary meningitis in adults. *Scand J Infect Dis* 1986;18:533–538.

Mylonakis E, Hohmann EL, Calderwood SB. Central nervous system infection with *Listeria monocytogenes*. 33 years' experience at a general hospital and review of 776 episodes from the literature. *Medicine (Baltimore)* 1998;77:313–336.

Odio CM, Faingezicht I, Paris M, et al. The beneficial effects of early dexamethasone administration in infants and children with bacterial meningitis. *N Engl J Med* 1991;324:1525–1531.

Pomeroy SL, Holmes SJ, Dodge PR, Feigin RD. Seizures and other neurologic sequelae of bacterial meningitis in children. *N Engl J Med* 1990;323:1651–1657.

Pruitt AA. Infections of the nervous system. *Neurol Clin* 1998;16:419–447.

Qayyum Q, Scerpella E, Moreno J, Fischl M. Report of 24 cases of Listeria monocytogenes infection at the University of Miami Medical Center. *Rev Invest Clin* 1997;49:265–270.

Quagliarello V, Scheld W. Treatment of bacterial meningitis. *N Engl J Med* 1997;336:708–716.

Roos K. Pearls and pitfalls in the diagnosis and management of central nervous system infectious diseases. *Semin Neurol* 1998;18:185–196.

Roos KL, Tunkel AR, Scheld WM. Acute bacterial meningitis in children and adults. In: Scheld WM, Whitley RJ, Durack DT, eds. *Infections of the central nervous system.* Philadelphia: Lippincott-Raven, 1997:335–401.

Schaad UB, Lips U, Gnehm HE, Blumberg A, Heinzer I, Wedgwood J. Dexamethasone therapy for bacterial meningitis in children. Swiss Meningitis Study Group. *Lancet* 1993;342:457–461.

Schuchat A, Robinson K, Wenger J, et al. Bacterial meningitis in the United States in 1995. *N Engl J Med* 1997;337:970–976.

Tunkel AR, Scheld WM. Pathogenesis and pathophysiology of bacterial meningitis. *Clin Microbiol Rev* 1993;6:118–136.

Subacute Meningitis

Tuberculous Meningitis

Afghani B, Lieberman JM, Duke MB, Stutman HR. Comparison of quantitative polymerase chain reaction, acid fast bacilli smear, and culture results in patients receiving therapy for pulmonary tuberculosis. *Diagn Microbiol Infect Dis* 1997;29:73–79.

Hosoglu S, Ayaz C, Geyik MF, Kokoglu OF, Ceviz A. Tuberculous meningitis in adults: an eleven-year review. *Int J Tuberc Lung Dis* 1998;2:553–557.

Kent SJ, Crowe SM, Yung A, Lucas CR, Mijch AM. Tuberculous meningitis: a 30-year review. *Clin Infect Dis* 1993;17:987–994.

Kocen RS, Parsons M. Neurological complications of tuberculosis: some unusual manifestations. *Q J Med* 1970;39:17–30.

Shankar P, Manjunath N, Mohan KK, et al. Rapid diagnosis of tuberculous meningitis by polymerase chain reaction. *Lancet* 1991;337(8732):5–7.

Sheller JR, Des Prez RM. CNS tuberculosis. *Neurol Clin* 1986;4:143–158.

Traub M, Colchester ACF, Kingsley DPE, Swash M. Tuberculosis of the central nervous system. *Q J Med* 1984;53:83–100.

Verdon R, Chevret S, Laissy JP, Wolff M. Tuberculous meningitis in adults: review of 48 cases [see comments]. *Clin Infect Dis* 1996;22:982–988.

Zuger A, Lowy FD. Tuberculosis. In: Scheld WM, Whitley RJ, Durack DT, eds. *Infections of the central nervous system.* Philadelphia: Lippincott-Raven, 1997:417–443.

Subdural and Epidural Infections

Cerebral Subdural Empyema

Baum PA, Dillon WP. Utility of magnetic resonance imaging in the detection of subdural empyema. *Ann Otol Rhinol Laryngol* 1992;101:876–878.

Helfgott DC, Weingarten K, Hartman BJ. Sudural empyema. In: Scheld WM, Whitley RJ, Durack DT, eds. *Infections of the central nervous system.* Philadelphia: Lippincott-Raven, 1997:495–505.

Kaufman DM, Litman N, Miller MH. Sinusitis: induced subdural empyema. *Neurology* 1983;33:123–132.

Kaufman DM, Miller MH, Steigbigel NH. Subdural empyema: analysis of 17 recent cases and review of the literature. *Medicine (Baltimore)* 1975;54:485–498.

Sadhu VK, Handel SF, Pinto RS, Glass TF. Neuroradiologic diagnosis of subdural empyema and CT limitations. *AJNR Am J Neuroradiol* 1980;1:39–44.

Intracranial Epidural Abscess

Gellin BG, Weingarten K, Gamache FWJ, Hartman BJ. Epidural abscess. In: Scheld WM, Whitley RJ, Durack DT, eds. *Infections of the central nervous system.* Philadelphia: Lippincott-Raven, 1997:507–522.

Helfgott DC, Weingarten K, Hartman BJ. Sudural empyema. In: Scheld WM, Whitley RJ, Durack DT, eds. *Infections of the central nervous system,* 2nd ed. Philadelphia: Lippincott-Raven, 1997:495–505.

Silverberg AL, DiNubile MJ. Subdural empyema and cranial epidural abscess. *Med Clin North Am* 1985;62:361–374.

Weingarten K, Zimmerman RD, Becker RD, et al. Subdural and epidural empyemas: MR imaging. *AJR Am J Roentgenol* 1989;152:615–621.

Spinal Epidural Abscess

Danner RL, Hartman BJ. Update of spinal epidural abscess: 35 cases and review of the literature. *Rev Infect Dis* 1987;9:265–274.

Darouiche RO, Hamill RJ, Greenberg SB, et al. Bacterial spinal epidural abscess. Review of 43 cases and literature survey. *Medicine (Baltimore)* 1992;71:369–385.

Enberg RN, Kaplan RJ. Spinal epidural abscess in children. Early diagnosis and immediate surgical drainage is essential to forestall paralysis. *Clin Pediatr* 1974;13:247–253.

Nussbaum ES, Rigamonti D, Standiford H, et al. Spinal epidural abscess: a report of 40 cases and review. *Surg Neurol* 1992;38:225–231.

Ravicovitch MA, Spallone A. Spinal epidural abscesses. Surgical and parasurgical management. *Eur Neurol* 1982;21:347–357.

Verner EF, Musher DM. Spinal epidural abscess. *Med Clin North Am* 1985;69:375–384.

Infective Endocarditis

Bertorini TE, Gelfand M. Neurological complications of bacterial endocarditis. *Compr Ther* 1990;16:47–55.

Brust J, Dickinson P, Hughes J, Holtzmann R. The diagnosis and treatment of cerebral mycotic aneurysms. *Ann Neurol* 1990;27:238–246.

Francioli P. Complications of infective endocarditis. In: Scheld WM, Whitley RJ, Durack DT, eds. *Infections of the central nervous system.* Philadelphia: Lippincott-Raven, 1997:523–553.

Garvey GJ, Neu HC. Infective endocarditis—an evolving disease. A review of endocarditis at the Columbia-Presbyterian Medical Center 1968–1973. *Medicine (Baltimore)* 1978;57:105–127.

Heimberger TS, Duma RJ. Infections of prosthetic heart valves and cardiac pacemakers. *Infect Dis Clin North Am* 1989;3:221–245.

Lerner P. Neurologic complications of infective endocarditis. *Med Clin North Am* 1985;69:385–398.

Pelletier LL, Petersdorf RG. Infective endocarditis: a review of 125 cases from the University of Washington hospitals, 1963–72. *Medicine (Baltimore)* 1977;56:287–313.

Salgado AV, Furlan AJ, Keys TF, et al. Neurologic complications of endocarditis. A 12-year experience. *Neurology* 1989;39:173–178.

Leprosy

Brandsma W. Basic nerve function assessment in leprosy patients. *Lepr Rev* 1981;52:111–119.

Browne SG. Leprosy—clinical aspects of nerve involvement. In: Hornabrook RW, ed. *Topics on tropical neurology.* Philadelphia: FA Davis, 1975:1–6.

Canizares O. Diagnosis and treatment of leprosy in the United States. *Med Clin North Am* 1965;49:801–816.

Charosky CB, Gatti JC, Cardama JE. Neuropathies in Hansen's disease. *Int J Lepr Other Mycobact Dis* 1983;51:576–586.

Dastur DK. Leprosy (an infectious and immunological disorder of the nervous system). In: Vinken PJ, Bruyn GW, Klawans HL, eds. *Handbook of clinical neurology.* Vol. 33. New York: Elsevier-North Holland, 1978: 421–468.

Pedley JC, Harman DJ, Waudby H, McDougall AC. Leprosy in peripheral nerves: histopathological findings in 119 untreated patients in Nepal. *J Neurol Neurosurg Psychiatry* 1980;43:198–204.

Reichart PA, Srisuwan S, Metah D. Lesions of the facial and trigeminal nerve in leprosy; an evaluation of 43 cases. *Int J Oral Surg* 1982;11: 14–20.

Turk JL, Curtis J, De-Blaquiere G. Immunopathology of nerve involvement in leprosy [editorial]. *Lepr Rev* 1993;64:1–6.

Rickettsial Infections

Fan MY, Walker DH, Yu SR, Liu QH. Epidemiology and ecology of rickettsial diseases in the People's Republic of China. *Rev Infect Dis* 1987;9:823–840.

Kikuchi M, Tagawa Y, Iwamoto H, Hoshino H, Yuki N. Bickerstaff's brainstem encephalitis associated with IgG anti-GQ1b antibody subsequent to *Mycoplasma pneumoniae* infection: favorable response to immunoadsorption therapy. *J Child Neurol* 1997;12:403–405.

Kim JH, Durack DT. Rickettsiae. In: Scheld WM, Whitley RJ, Durack DT, eds. *Infections of the central nervous system.* Philadelphia: Lippincott-Raven, 1997:403–416.

Marrie TJ, Raoult D. Rickettsial infections of the central nervous system. *Semin Neurol* 1992;12:213–224.

Shaked Y. Rickettsial infection of the central nervous system: the role of prompt antimicrobial therapy. *Q J Med* 1991;79:301–306.

Spach DH, Liles WC, Campbell GL, et al. Tick-borne diseases in the United States. *N Engl J Med* 1993;329:936–947.

Rocky Mountain Spotted Fever

Bell WE, Lascari AD. Rocky Mountain spotted fever. Neurological symptoms in the acute phase. *Neurology* 1970;20:841–847.

Case records of the Massachusetts General Hospital. Weekly clinicopathological exercises. Case 32-1997. A 43-year-old woman with rapidly changing pulmonary infiltrates and markedly increased intracranial pressure. *N Engl J Med* 1997;337:1149–1156.

Helmick CG, Bernard KW, D'Angelo LJ. Rocky Mountain spotted fever: clinical, laboratory, and epidemiological features of 262 cases. *J Infect Dis* 1984;150:480–488.

Latham RH, Schaffner W. Rocky Mountain spotted (and spotless) fever. *Compr Ther* 1992;18:18–21.

Massey EW, Thames T, Coffey CE, Gallis HA. Neurologic complications of Rocky Mountain spotted fever. *South Med J* 1985;78:1288–1290, 1303.

Thorner AR, Walker DH, Petri WA Jr. Rocky mountain spotted fever. *Clin Infect Dis* 1998;27:1353–1359.

Weber DJ, Walker DH. Rocky Mountain spotted fever. *Infect Dis Clin North Am* 1991;5:19–35.

Woodward TE. Rocky Mountain spotted fever: a present-day perspective [comment]. *Medicine (Baltimore)* 1992;71:255–259.

Typhus Fever

Herman E. Neurological syndromes in typhus fever. *J Nerv Ment Dis* 1949;109:25–36.

Scrub Typhus

Ripley MS. Neuropsychiatric observations on tsutsugamushi (scrub typhus). *Arch Neurol Psychiatry* 1946;56:42–54.

Ehrlichiosis

Aguero-Rosenfeld ME, Horowitz HW, Wormser GP, et al. Human granulocytic ehrlichiosis: a case series from a medical center in New York State [see comments]. *Ann Intern Med* 1996;125:904–908.

Dumler JS, Bakken JS. Human ehrlichioses: newly recognized infections transmitted by ticks. *Annu Rev Med* 1998;49:201–213.

Horowitz HW, Aguero-Rosenfeld ME, McKenna DF, et al. Clinical and laboratory spectrum of culture-proven human granulocytic ehrlichiosis: comparison with culture-negative cases. *Clin Infect Dis* 1998;27: 1314–1317.

Nadelman RB, Horowitz HW, Hsieh TC, et al. Simultaneous human granulocytic ehrlichiosis and Lyme borreliosis. *N Engl J Med* 1997;337: 27–30.

Ratnasamy N, Everett ED, Roland WE, McDonald G, Caldwell CW. Central nervous system manifestations of human ehrlichiosis. *Clin Infect Dis* 1996;23:314–319.

Sexton DJ, Corey GR, Carpenter C, et al. Dual infection with Ehrlichia chaffeensis and a spotted fever group rickettsia: a case report. *Emerg Infect Dis* 1998;4:311–316.

Walker DH, Dumler JS. Human monocytic and granulocytic ehrlichioses. Discovery and diagnosis of emerging tick-borne infections and the critical role of the pathologist. *Arch Pathol Lab Med* 1997;121:785–791.

Other Bacterial Infections

Brucellosis

Bahemuka M, Babiker MA, Wright SG, et al. The pattern of infection of the nervous system in Riyadh: a review of 121 cases. *Q J Med* 1988;68:517–524.

Cisneros JM, Viciana P, Colmenero J, et al. Multicenter prospective study of treatment of Brucella melitensis brucellosis with doxycycline for 6 weeks plus streptomycin for 2 weeks. *Antimicrob Agents Chemother* 1990;34:881–883.

McLean DR, Russell N, Khan MY. Neurobrucellosis: clinical and therapeutic features. *Clin Infect Dis* 1992;15:582–590.

Mousa AR, Koshy TS, Araj GF, et al. *Brucella* meningitis: presentation, diagnosis and treatment—a prospective study of ten cases. *Q J Med* 1986;60:873–885.

Shakir RA, Al-Din AS, Araj GF, et al. Clinical categories of neurobrucellosis. A report on 19 cases. *Brain* 1987;110:213–223.

Young EJ. Human brucellosis. *Rev Infect Dis* 1983;5:821–842.

Behçet Syndrome

Alema G. Behçet's disease. In: Vinken PJ, Bruyn GW, Klawans HL, eds. *Handbook of clinical neurology.* Vol. 34. New York: Elsevier-North Holland, 1978:475–512.

Al-Kawi MZ, Bohlega S, Banna M. MRI findings in neuro-Behçet's disease. *Neurology* 1991;41:405–408.

Banna M, el-Ramahl K. Neurologic involvement in Behçet disease: imaging findings in 16 patients. *AJNR Am J Neuroradiol* 1991;12:791–796.

Behçet H. Uber rezidivierende Aphthose durch ein Virusverursachte Geschwur am Mund, am Auge und an den Genitalien. *Dermatol Monatsschr* 1937;105:1152–1157.

Markus HS, Bunker CB, Kouris K, et al. rCBF abnormalities detected, and sequentially followed, by SPECT in neuro-Behçet's syndrome with normal CT and MRI imaging. *J Neurol* 1992;239:363–366.

Namer IJ, Karabudak R, Zileli T, et al. Peripheral nervous system involvement in Behçet's disease. Case report and review of the literature. *Eur Neurol* 1987;26:235–240.

Serdaroglu P, Yazici H, Ozdemir C, et al. Neurologic involvement in Behçet's syndrome. A prospective study. *Arch Neurol* 1989;46:265–269.

Wechsler B, Vidailhet M, Piette JC, et al. Cerebral venous thrombosis in Behçet's disease: clinical study and long-term follow-up of 25 cases. *Neurology* 1992;42:614–618.

Yazici H, Barnes CG. Practical treatment recommendations for pharmacotherapy of Behçet's syndrome. *Drugs* 1991;425:796–804.

Vogt-Koyanagi-Harada Syndrome

Hormigo A, Bravo-Marques JM, Souza-Ramalho P, et al. Uveomeningoencephalitis in a human immunodeficiency virus type 2–seropositive patient. *Ann Neurol* 1988;23:308–310.

Ikeda M, Tsukagoshi H. Vogt-Koyanagi-Harada disease presenting with meningoencephalitis. Report of a case with magnetic resonance imaging. *Eur Neurol* 1992;32:83–85.

Pattison EM. Uveomeningoencephalitic syndrome (Vogt-Koyanagi-Harada). *Arch Neurol* 1965;12:197–205.

Riehl J-L, Andrews JM. Uveomeningoencephalitic syndrome. *Neurology* 1966;16:603–609.

Rubsamen PE, Gass JD. Vogt-Koyanagi-Harada syndrome. Clinical course, therapy, and long-term visual outcome. *Arch Ophthalmol* 1991;109:682–687.

Mollaret Meningitis

Achard JM, Lallement PY, Veyssier P. Recurrent aseptic meningitis secondary to intracranial epidermoid cyst and Mollaret's meningitis: two distinct entities or a single disease? A case report and a nosologic discussion. *Am J Med* 1990;89:807–810.

Crossley GH, Dismukes WE. Central nervous system epidermoid cyst: a probable etiology of Mollaret's meningitis. *Am J Med* 1990;89:805–806.

Jensenius M, Myrvang B, Storvold G, Bucher A, Hellum KB, Bruu AL. Herpes simplex virus type 2 DNA detected in cerebrospinal fluid of 9 patients with Mollaret's meningitis. *Acta Neurol Scand* 1998;98:209–212.

Kwong YL, Woo E, Fong PC, et al. Mollaret's meningitis revisited. Report of a case with a review of the literature. *Clin Neurol Neurosurg* 1988;90:163–167.

Mollaret P. La méningite endothélio-leucocytaire multirecurrente bénigne. Syndrome nouveau ou maladie nouvelle? *Rev Neurol (Paris)* 1944;76:57–76.

Sexton DJ, Corey GR, Carpenter C, et al. Dual infection with *Ehrlichia chaffeensis* and a spotted fever group rickettsia: a case report. *Emerg Infect Dis* 1998;4:311–316.

Aseptic Meningeal Reaction

Alexander EL, Alexander GE. Aseptic meningoencephalitis in primary Sjögren's syndrome. *Neurology* 1983;33:593–598.

Canoso JJ, Cohen AS. Aseptic meningitis in systemic lupus erythematosus. *Arthritis Rheum* 1975;18:369–374.

Meningism

Fishman RA. *Cerebrospinal fluid in diseases of the nervous system*, 2nd ed. Philadelphia: W.B. Saunders, 1992.

Mycoplasma pneumoniae Infection

Abramovitz P, Schvartzman P, Harel D, et al. Direct invasion of the central nervous system by *Mycoplasma pneumoniae*: a report of two cases. *J Infect Dis* 1987;155:482–487.

Behan PO, Feldman RG, Segerra JM, Draper IT. Neurological aspects of mycoplasmal infection. *Acta Neurol Scand* 1986;74:314–322.

Francis DA, Brown A, Miller DH, et al. MRI appearances of the CNS manifestations of *Mycoplasma pneumoniae*: a report of two cases. *J Neurol* 1988;235:441–443.

Ieven M, Demey H, Ursi D, Van Goethem G, Cras P, Goossens H. Fatal encephalitis caused by *Mycoplasma pneumoniae* diagnosed by the polymerase chain reaction. *Clin Infect Dis* 1998;27:1552–1553.

Kikuchi M, Tagawa Y, Iwamoto H, Hoshino H, Yuki N. Bickerstaff's brain-stem encephalitis associated with IgG anti-GQ1b antibody subsequent to *Mycoplasma pneumoniae* infection: favorable response to immunoadsorption therapy. *J Child Neurol* 1997;12:403–405.

Pellegrini M, O'Brien TJ, Hoy J, Sedal L. *Mycoplasma pneumoniae* infection associated with an acute brainstem syndrome. *Acta Neurol Scand* 1996;93:203–206.

Pönka A. Central nervous system manifestations associated with serologically verified Mycoplasma pneumoniae infection. *Scand J Infect Dis* 1980;12:175–184.

Legionella pneumophila Infection

Andersen BB, Sogaard I. Legionnaires' disease and brain abscess. *Neurology* 1987;37:333–334.

Heath PD, Booth L, Leigh PN, Turner AM. Legionella brain stem encephalopathy and peripheral neuropathy without preceding pneumonia [letter]. *J Neurol Neurosurg Psychiatry* 1986;49:216–218.

Johnson DH, Cunha BA. Atypical pneumonias. Clinical and extrapulmonary features of *Chlamydia, Mycoplasma*, and *Legionella* infections. *Postgrad Med* 1993;93:69–72.

Johnson JD, Raff MJ, Van Arsdall JA. Neurologic manifestations of Legionnaires disease. *Medicine (Baltimore)* 1984;63:303–310.

Pendelbury WW, Perl DP, Winn WC Jr, McQuillen JB. Neuropathologic evaluation of 40 confirmed cases of "Legionella" pneumonia. *Neurology* 1983;33:1340–1344.

Weir AI, Bone I, Kennedy DH. Neurological involvement in legionellosis. *J Neurol Neurosurg Psychiatry* 1982;45:604–608.

Merritt's Neurology, 10th ed., edited by L.P. Rowland. Lippincott Williams & Wilkins, Philadelphia © 2000.

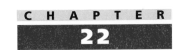

CHAPTER 22

FOCAL INFECTIONS

GARY L. BERNARDINI

MALIGNANT EXTERNAL OTITIS AND OSTEOMYELITIS OF THE BASE OF THE SKULL

Malignant external otitis is an infection that begins in the external auditory canal, penetrates the epithelium, and spreads to the surrounding soft tissue to cause cellulitis and abscess. If untreated, the infection extends to the temporomandibular joint, mastoid, or more commonly soft tissues below the temporal bone. The facial nerve may be affected as the first symptom in up to 30% of patients. Other common symptoms are severe otalgia, purulent otorrhea, hearing loss, and painful swelling of surrounding tissues. Rarely, dysphagia may result from lesions of cranial nerves IX through XII, and the findings may be mistaken for laryngeal carcinoma. Fever and weight loss are uncommon. Mastoid tenderness is evident on examination. The syndrome is most frequently observed in elderly diabetic patients and is also seen in people infected with human immunodeficiency virus.

Laboratory evaluation shows a mildly elevated or normal white blood cell count. The erythrocyte sedimentation rate is almost always elevated (>50 mm/h). Computed tomography (CT) is most useful in evaluating evidence of bony erosion, but films may be normal early in the illness. Magnetic resonance imaging (MRI), with and without gadolinium, is the study of choice. Isotope bone scans are sensitive but not specific. Newer techniques using technetium (^{99m}Tc) methylene diphosphonate and gallium-67 single photon emission CT may be more sensitive and accurate in early detection of malignant external otitis and monitoring response to therapy.

In most cases, *Pseudomonas aeruginosa* is the causative organism. In human immunodeficiency virus-positive individuals or in AIDS, either *P. aeruginosa* or the fungus *Aspergillus fumigatus* may be isolated. In the preantibiotic era, mortality rates were greater than 50% and surgical debridement was the treatment of choice. Standard treatment with intravenous antibiotics consisted of an antipseudomonal penicillin for 4 to 8 weeks combined with an aminoglycoside for at least 2 weeks or, if tolerated, 4 to 6 weeks. Current successful treatment is based on single-drug therapy with either the antipseudomonal third-generation cephalosporin ceftazidime or the fluoroquinolone ciprofloxacin in patients with limited external otitis (i.e., without bony erosion or cranial neuropathy). Double-antibiotic therapy is considered with more extensive lesions. Drug-resistant strains have been found for both ceftazidime and ciprofloxacin. Despite these new treatments, the mortality rate is still 10% to 20% and may be as high as 50% if cranial nerves are involved. If untreated or inadequately treated, malignant external otitis can result in osteomyelitis of the base of the skull, abscess formation, meningitis, and death.

Osteomyelitis of the base of the skull is a rare complication of malignant external otitis, chronic mastoiditis, or paranasal sinus infection. As with malignant otitis, the patients are usually elderly, diabetic, or immunocompromised. Symptoms include headache, otalgia, hearing loss, and otorrhea, but patients are frequently without fever. Osteomyelitis may occur in conjunction with otitis but usually appears weeks or months after starting antibiotics. As the process spreads, cranial nerves may be affected, especially the VII and VIII nerves. Extension of skull base osteomyelitis to the jugular foramen or hypoglossal canal can affect cranial nerves IX through XII, leading to dysphagia. In advanced cases, spread to the petrous pyramid may affect III, IV, V, and VI cranial nerves to cause ocular palsies or trigeminal neuralgia.

Laboratory abnormalities include a normal or slightly elevated white blood cell count and a high erythrocyte sedimentation rate. Thin-cut CT sections through the skull base and temporal bones play an important role in the diagnosis of osteomyelitis and assessing the extent of disease. Carcinoma of the ear canal may cause similar clinical and radiographic findings, and bone biopsy may be needed if there is no response to appropriate antibiotic therapy. MRI is useful in delineating soft tissue involvement. Technetium bone scanning is a sensitive indicator of osteomyelitis but is not helpful in determining resolution of disease. Gallium-67 scans can be useful in tracking resolution of disease over time. Neither bone nor gallium scans are useful in determining the exact extent of the infection. *P. aeruginosa* is the typical causative organism, but *Staphylococcus aureus* or other organisms such as *Staphylococcus epidermidis, Proteus, Salmonella, Mycobacterium, Aspergillus,* and *Candida* have been implicated rarely.

Therapy for osteomyelitis consists of intravenous administration of antibiotics, usually an antipseudomonal penicillin or cephalosporin in combination with an aminoglycoside to provide synergy and to prevent the emergence of drug-resistant bacteria. Ciprofloxacin has been effective when used alone or with other antibiotics. Ceftazidime has bactericidal activity against *Pseudomonas* and may be used as monotherapy. Because the disease is usually extensive, conservative management of skull base osteomyelitis is still an extended course of two-drug therapy. Monthly gallium scans may help to determine the response and duration of antibiotic therapy. In refractory cases, hyperbaric oxygen has been used as adjuvant therapy. Antibiotics should be continued for at least 1 week after the gallium scan becomes normal. Follow-up gallium scans may be performed 1 week after completion of antibiotic therapy to detect early recurrence and at 3 months for late recurrence. Mortality rates of 40% have been reported, but with prolonged antibiotic therapy, complete cure can be achieved.

BRAIN ABSCESS AND SUBDURAL EMPYEMA

Brain Abscess

Incapsulated or free pus in the substance of the brain after an acute focal purulent infection is known as brain abscess. Abscesses vary in size from a microscopic collection of inflammatory cells to an area of purulent necrosis involving the major part of one hemisphere. Abscess of the brain has been known for over 200 years, and surgical treatment started with Macewen in 1880.

Advances in the diagnosis and treatment of brain abscesses have been achieved with the use of CT, stereotactic brain biopsy and aspiration, and new antimicrobials.

Etiology

Brain abscesses are classified on the basis of the likely entry point of the infection. For example, brain abscesses arise most commonly as direct extension from cranial infections (mastoid, teeth, paranasal sinuses, or osteomyelitis of the skull), from infections after fracture of the skull or neurosurgical procedures, or as metastases from infection elsewhere in the body. Brain abscess is only rarely a complication of bacterial meningitis, except in infants. Infections in the middle ear or mastoid may spread to the cerebellum or temporal lobe through involvement of the bone and meninges or by seeding of bacteria through valveless emissary veins that drain these regions, with or without extradural or subdural infection or thrombosis of the lateral sinus. An abscess in one hemisphere can follow infection in the contralateral mastoid, presumably by hematogenous spread of the organism. Infection in the frontal, ethmoid, or rarely the maxillary sinuses spreads to the frontal lobes through erosion of the skull. Subdural or extradural infection or thrombosis of the venous sinuses also may be present. Approximately 20% to 30% of brain abscesses may have no obvious source identified.

Metastatic seeding from a remote site may cause brain abscess (e.g., arising in the lungs, by bronchiectasis or lung abscess) or less frequently in bacterial endocarditis. Other sources include the tonsils and upper respiratory tract, from which the infection can reach the brain along the carotid sheath, or after urinary tract or intraabdominal infections. After metastatic spread, the cerebral lesions are commonly multiple and are found in the distribution of the middle cerebral artery. Congenital heart disease and pulmonary arteriovenous fistulas (as in hereditary hemorrhagic telangiectasia) predispose to brain abscess. In these two disorders, infected venous blood bypasses the pulmonary filtration system and gains access to the cerebral arterial system.

The occurrence of abscesses of the brain after penetrating brain injury is low, although entry of bacteria into the brain is common after such injuries with the introduction of infected missiles or tissues into the brain through compound fractures of the skull. In children, penetration of a lead pencil tip through the thin squamous portion of the temporal bone have resulted in abscess around the foreign material in the frontal lobe.

The infecting organism may be any of the common pyogenic bacteria depending on the site of entry; the most common are *S. aureus*, streptococci (anaerobic, aerobic, or microaerophilic species), *Enterobacteriaceae*, *Pseudomonas*, and anaerobes such as *Bacteroides*. In infants, gram-negative organisms are most frequent offenders. After penetrating head injury, abscess formation is usually due to *S. aureus*, streptococci, *Enterobacteriaceae*, or *Clostridium* species; *S. epidermidis* infection follows neurosurgical procedures. In the immunocompromised host, *Toxoplasma*, fungi, *Nocardia*, and *Enterobacteriaceae* are frequently found. Pneumococci, meningococci, and *Hemophilus influenzae* are major causes of bacterial meningitis but are rarely recovered from a brain abscess. Brain abscess is an infrequent complication of parasitic infection such as *Entamoeba histolytica*. Cultures may be sterile in patients who have received antimicrobial therapy before biopsy, but any material obtained should be sent to the laboratory. A positive Gram stain may guide therapy even when the culture is negative.

Pathology

The pathologic changes in brain abscess are similar regardless of the origin: direct extention to the brain from epidural or subdu-

ral infection, retrograde thrombosis of veins, or arterial metastasis (Fig. 22.1). Four stages of maturation are recognized. Within the first 3 days, suppurative inflammation of brain tissue is characterized by early cerebritis and either a patchy or nonenhancing hypodensity on CT or MRI. The progression from late cerebritis (with an area of central necrosis, edema, and ring enhancement on CT and MRI) to early capsule formation and final maturation of the capsule takes about 2 weeks. When host defenses control the spread of the infection, macroglia and fibroblasts proliferate in an attempt to surround the infected and necrotic tissue, and granulation tissue and fibrous encapsulation develops. The capsule is thicker on the cortical surface than on the ventricular side. If the capsule ruptures, purulent material is released into the ventricular system with a high mortality rate. Edema of adjacent cerebrum or the entire hemisphere is common (Fig. 22.2).

Incidence

Brain abscesses were common in the first half of the 20th century, but the introduction of effective therapy for purulent infection of the mastoid process and nasal sinuses has greatly reduced the incidence of all intracranial complications of these infections, including brain abscess. Brain abscesses constitute less than 2% of all intracranial surgery. Brain abscess may occur at any age but is still encountered in the first to third decades of life as a result of the high incidence of mastoid and nasal sinus disease in those years. Up to 25% of all cases affect children less than 15 years old, with a cluster in the 4- to 7-year-old age group, usually the result of cyanotic congenital heart disease or an otic source.

Symptoms and Signs

The symptoms of brain abscess are those of any expanding lesion in the brain, and headache is the most common symptom. The

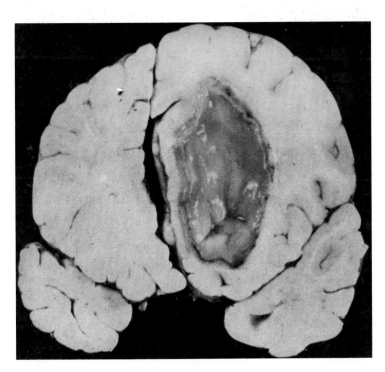

FIG. 22.1. Brain abscess. Fresh abscess in frontal lobe secondary to pulmonary infection. (Courtesy of Dr. Abner Wolf.)

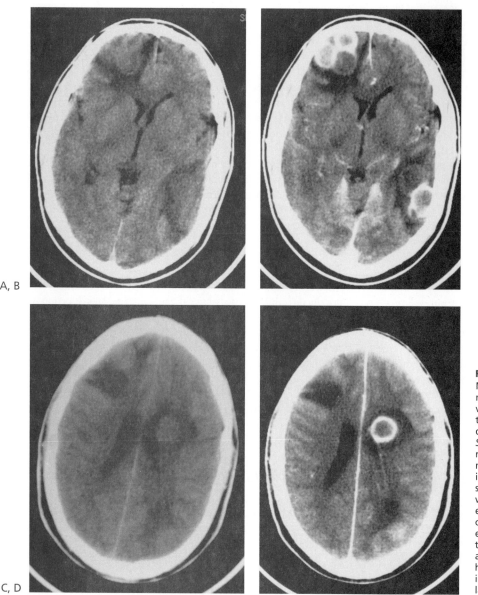

A, B

C, D

FIG. 22.2. Multiple brain abscesses. **A and B:** Multiple brain abscesses seen on computed tomography (CT) both before and after intravenous contrast. Symptoms started 2 weeks after dental cleaning with severe headache and drowsiness; isolates from an abscess revealed *Streptococcus viridans* sp. Note characteristic ring enhancement **(B)** and marked edema with midline shift **(A and B)** around three abscesses in the right frontal lobe; a daughter abscess shows less ring enhancement and is directed inward. In addition, there is a left temporoparietal ring-enhancing lesion, with possible adjacent early cerebritis lesion, with surrounding edema. **C and D:** A periventricular abscess in the same patient seen on a higher cut CT with and without contrast; note ependymal enhancement after the administration of contrast, indicating extension of the abscess into the left lateral ventricle. (Courtesy of Dr. L. Fontana.)

pain is a dull ache that is not localized. Fever is present in less than 50% of patients; many are afebrile. Edema of surrounding brain tissue can rapidly increase intracranial pressure so that worsening headache, nausea, and vomiting are early symptoms. Sudden worsening of preexisting headache with new onset of nuchal rigidity often heralds rupture of brain abscess into the ventricular space. Abrupt onset of a severe headache is less common with abscess and is more often associated with acute bacterial meningitis or subarachnoid hemorrhage. Seizures, focal or generalized, are common with abscess.

Focal signs, including altered mental status and hemiparesis, are seen in approximately 50% of patients depending on abscess location. Hemiparesis may be seen with lesions of the cerebral hemispheres. Apathy and mental confusion have been linked with abscesses in the frontal lobe. Hemianopia and aphasia, particularly anomia, are found when the temporal or parietooccipi-

tal lobes are involved. Ataxia, intention tremor, nystagmus, and other classic symptoms may be seen with cerebellar abscess. Frequently, however, the signs of an abscess in the cerebrum or cerebellum are limited to those of increased intracranial pressure (nausea, vomiting, and headache). Abscesses in the brainstem are rare. The classic findings of a brainstem syndrome are often lacking because the abscess tends to expand longitudinally along fiber tracts rather than transversely. Papilledema is present in only about 25% of all patients. Signs of injury to the III or VI cranial nerve are sometimes the result of increased intracranial pressure.

Subdural or, rarely, epidural infections in the frontal regions may give the same signs and symptoms as those of an abscess in the frontal lobe. Fever and focal seizures favor the diagnosis of subdural rather than intraparenchymal abscess.

Thrombosis of the lateral sinus often follows middle ear or mastoid infection and may be accompanied by seizures and signs of increased intracranial pressure, making the clinical differentiation between this condition and abscess of the temporal lobe or cerebrum difficult. With lateral sinus thrombosis, papilledema may be due to interference with the drainage of blood from the brain. Focal neurologic signs favor the diagnosis of abscess.

Diagnostic Tests

Brain abscess can be suspected clinically when seizures, focal neurologic signs, or increased intracranial pressure develop in a patient with congenital heart disease or with a known acute or chronic infection in the middle ear, mastoid, nasal sinuses, heart, or lungs. The diagnosis is supported by CT or MRI (Figs. 22.2 and 22.3).

Elevated white blood cell count or erythrocyte sedimentation rate is not reliably present. Blood cultures are positive in only 10% of patients but should always be obtained with suspected brain abscess, even in the absence of fever. Lumbar puncture is contraindicated in patients suspected of having a brain abscess because of the clear risk of transtentorial herniation. Older data on the results of cerebrospinal fluid (CSF) examination revealed elevated opening pressures and an aseptic meningeal reaction. In the series of Merritt and Fremont-Smith, opening pressure was over 200 mm H_2O in 70%. The CSF is usually clear but may be cloudy or turbid. The cell count varies from normal to 1,000 or more cells/mm^3. In early unencapsulated abscesses near the ventricular or subarachnoid spaces, the cell count is high, with a high percentage of polymorphonuclear leukocytes. The cell

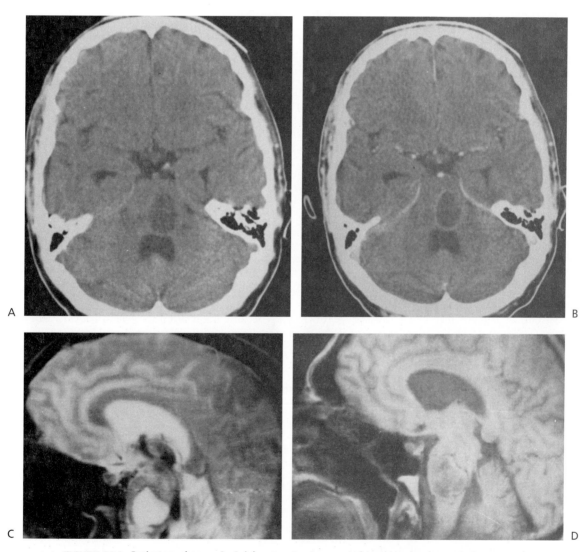

FIGURE 22.3. Brainstem abscess. **A:** Axial noncontrast computed tomography demonstrates a round low-density left pontine lesion with mass effect on the fourth ventricle. **B:** Ring enhancement of the lesion after contrast is typical of an abscess. Sagittal T2-weighted **(C)** and sagittal T1-weighted **(D)** magnetic resonance images (MRIs) demonstrate the lesion to be cystic isointense to cerebrospinal fluid signal (compare with signal within the lateral ventricle). Note definition of the abscess rim in **D**. The sagittal MRIs are useful in planning a surgical approach through the fourth ventricle. (Courtesy of Drs. J. A. Bello and S. K. Hilal.)

count is normal or only slightly increased when the abscess is firmly encapsulated. The cell count in 34 patients at various stages of the disease varied between 4 and 800 cells with an average of 135 cells/mm^3. The protein content is between 45 and 200 mg/dL. The CSF sugar content is normal.

Extension of the abscess to the meninges or ventricles is accompanied by an increase in the CSF cell count and other findings of acute meningitis or ventriculitis. Rupture of an abscess into the ventricles is signaled by a sudden rise of intracranial pressure and the presence of free pus in the CSF with a cell count of 20,000 to 50,000/mm^3. A decrease in sugar content below 40 mg/dL indicates that the meninges have been invaded by bacteria. Only rarely are CSF cultures positive.

MRI and CT are the studies of choice, both for diagnosis and treatment of brain abscess. Plain radiographs of the skull may show separation of sutures in infants or children and an increase in the convolution markings. CT permits accurate localization of cerebritis or abscess and serial assessment of the size of the lesion, its demarcation, the extent of surrounding edema, and total mass effect. MRI with gadolinium is more sensitive and specific than contrast CT in diagnosing early cerebritis. With a mature encapsulated abscess, both contrast CT and MRI with gadolinium reveal the ring-enhancing mass with surrounding vasogenic edema. The differential diagnosis, based on the appearance of the lesion, includes glioblastoma, metastatic tumor, infarct, arteriovenous malformation, resolving hematoma, and granuloma. Features supporting the diagnosis of brain abscess include gas within the center of a ring-enhancing lesion, a thinner rim (<5 mm) than with brain tumors, and ependymal enhancement associated with ventriculitis or ventricular rupture (Fig. 22.2D). Thallium-201 brain single photon emission CT may be useful in differentiating intracerebral lymphoma from toxoplasma encephalitis in patients with AIDS.

Either CT or MRI may be useful in distinguishing abscess from mycotic aneurysms or herpes encephalitis, which may cause similar symptoms and signs. Mycotic aneurysm may arise from bacterial endocarditis with aseptic meningitis. CT or MRI may exclude abscess, but angiography may be necessary to identify the aneurysm before rupture. Herpes simplex encephalitis is manifest by headache, fever, and an acute temporal lobe or frontal lobe syndrome. On CT or MRI, the temporal lobe is swollen, with irregular lucency and patchy contrast enhancement.

Treatment

Before CT, the treatment of brain abscess was surgical, including incision and drainage through a burr hole or open craniotomy with marsupialization, packing the cavity, and complete extirpation. The introduction of CT revolutionized the management of brain abscess. CT made it possible to diagnose and localize cerebritis or abscess, dictate choice of treatment, and monitor patient response. The current recommended treatment for most brain abscesses is CT-guided stereotactic or free-hand needle aspiration with therapeutic drainage and obtaining diagnostic specimens for culture and special studies, along with appropriate antimicrobial therapy. Based on Gram stain results and presumptive source of the abscess, empiric antimicrobial therapy

may be started. Early surgery is recommend, especially in cases with abscesses close to the ventricles into which the lesion may rupture. Nonoperative treatment may be appropriate for some patients who are clinically stable but poor surgical candidates or in those with surgically inaccessible lesions.

Open craniotomy is now performed infrequently and is reserved for patients with multiloculated abscesses that require complete excision or those with more resistant pathogens such as fungi or *Norcardia*.

Choosing the appropriate antimicrobial therapy depends on the ability of the drug to penetrate the abscess cavity and its activity against the suspected pathogen. Chloramphenicol was the standard therapy for brain abscesses at one time, but it lacks bactericidal activity and side effects are serious; it is used infrequently today. Brain abscesses that arise from intracranial extension of sinus infection, with usual isolates of microaerophilic streptococci and anaerobic organisms, can be treated with intravenous high-dose penicillin G (10 to 20 million units per day) and metronidazole. In some cases, cefotaxime or other cephalosporins is given in combination with metronidazole. Additional antibiotic coverage may be needed for some organisms (e.g., *Actinomyces* species) when the abscess is secondary to dental procedures or dental abscess. Special consideration of antimicrobial coverage for *Enterobacteriaceae* and *P. aeruginosa* should be made when an otogenic source of brain abscess is suspected. Vancomycin can be given initially in cases of brain abscess from neurosurgical procedures, likely due to *S. epidermidis*, while awaiting final culture results. It is generally recommended that parenteral antibiotics should be given for a total of 6 to 8 weeks, followed by an additional 2- to 3-month course of oral antibiotic therapy.

Clinical and CT or MRI responses are monitored to assess the effectiveness of medical therapy or the need for repeated surgery. Follow-up CT may show a small area of residual enhancement even after adequate antimicrobial therapy. Occasionally, a previous ring-enhancing lesion on CT disappears with medical management, suggesting that the reversible lesions are forms of suppurative cerebritis.

Seizures occur in up to 50% of patients with brain abscess early in the course. Anticonvulsants such as diphenylhydantoin or carbamazepine can be administered for prophylaxis or to prevent the recurrence of seizures. Generally, these agents are given for at least 3 months after surgery for abscess.

The use of corticosteroids is controversial. In patients with life-threatening cerebral edema or impending herniation, a short course of high-dose corticosteroids may be appropriate. Further deterioration with severe brain edema may require intubation with hyperventilation and the administration of intravenous mannitol to control elevated intracranial pressures. Prolonged use of corticosteroids is not recommended because the steroids may interfere with granulation tissue formation and reduce the concentration of antibiotics within the infected tissue.

Prognosis

The outcome of untreated brain abscess is, with rare exceptions, death. Mortality in pre-CT series varied from 35% to 55%. In the era of advanced neuroimaging with CT or MRI, the mortality rate of brain abscesses is 0 to 30%. Overall morbidity and mortality of brain abscess is related to the rapidity of onset of symptoms, the primary source of infection, the presence of single or multiple abscesses, and the patients neurologic status at the time of diagnosis. If the level of consciousness is depressed, patients tend to do poorly.

Immunocompromised individuals have worse outcomes and higher mortality rates. The highest death rate is found when the primary infection is in the lungs. Intraventricular rupture of a brain abscess is associated with high mortality rates exceeding 80%.

Sequelae of brain abscess include recurrence of the abscess or the development of new abscesses if the primary focus persists. Residual neurologic sequelae with hemiparesis, seizures, or intellectual or behavioral impairment is seen in 30% to 56% of patients.

Subdural Empyema

Subdural empyema is a collection of pus in the subdural space. Symptoms are similar to those of brain abscess. Subdural infection in adults usually arises from contiguous spread of infection; paranasal sinusitis is the most common source. Otitic infection, head trauma, and cranial surgery are other causes. Polymicrobial infection is common with pathogens similar to those of brain abscess, including *S. aureus* and both aerobic and anaerobic streptococci species. The infection spreads to the subdural space through retrograde thrombophlebitis via the venous sinuses or as direct extension through bone and dura. Once the infection develops, it may spread over the convexities and along the falx, although loculation is common. Associated complications include septic cortical vein thrombosis, brain or epidural abscess, and meningitis. The syndrome comprises an initial focal headache, fever, and, in 80% to 90% of patients, focal neurologic signs. The combination of fever, a rapid progressive neurologic deterioration, and focal seizures is particularly suggestive of this disorder. Symptoms of subdural empyema usually begin 1 to 2 weeks after a sinus infection.

Lumbar puncture is risky because of the mass effect. CT reveals a crescent-shaped area of hypodensity over a hemisphere, along the dura or adjoining the falx, with enhancement of the margins around the empyema after administration of contrast. MRI is preferred to CT for the delineation of the presence and extent of the subdural empyema and identifying concurrent intracranial infections.

Treatment of subdural empyema emphasizes rapid institution of antibiotics and early surgery. Intravenous antibiotics are given depending on the organism identified or, if unknown, with the same antibiotics used in brain abscess. Anticonvulsants are frequently required. There is controversy about the neurosurgical technique for drainage of subdural empyema. CT accurately localizes the pus collection, and some advocate drainage through selective burr holes. Others prefer craniotomy for more complete removal of the infection, especially when the empyema is loculated. Limited craniotomy is also used for placement of a tube into the subdural space and local infusion of appropriate antibiotics. Use of either burr hole or craniotomy for drainage of subdural empyema is individualized. The recommended duration of antibiotic therapy is 3 to 4 weeks after surgical drainage.

SUGGESTED READINGS

Osteomyelitis and Malignant External Otitis

Chandler JR. Malignant external otitis and osteomyelitis of the base of the skull. *Am J Otol* 1989;10:108–110.

Damiani JM, Damiani KK, Kinney SE. Malignant external otitis with multiple cranial nerve involvement. *Am J Otol* 1979;1:115–120.

Dinapoli RP, Thomas JE. Neurologic aspects of malignant external otitis: report of three cases. *Mayo Clin Proc* 1971;46:339–344.

Grandis JR, Curtin HD, Yu VL. Necrotizing (malignant) external otitis: prospective comparison of CT and MRI in diagnosis and follow-up. *Radiology* 1995;196:499–504.

Hern JD, Almeyda J, Thomas DM, et al. Malignant otitis externa in HIV and AIDS. *J Laryngol Otol* 1996;110:770–775.

Meyers BR, Mendelson MH, Parisier SC, Hirschman SZ. Malignant external otitis. Comparison of monotherapy vs combination therapy. *Arch Otolaryngol Head Neck Surg* 1987;113:974–978.

Murray ME, Britton J. Osteomyelitis of the skull base: the role of high resolution CT in diagnosis. *Clin Radiol* 1994;49:408–411.

Paramsothy M, Khanijow V, Ong TO. Use of gallium-67 in the assessment of response to antibiotic therapy in malignant otitis externa—a case report. *Singapore Med J* 1997;38:347–349.

Reiter D, Bilaniuk LT, Zimmerman RA. Diagnostic imaging in malignant otitis externa. *Arch Otolaryngol Head Neck Surg* 1982;90:606–609.

Slattery WH, Brackmann DE. Skull base osteomyelitis. Malignant external otitis. *Otolaryngol Clin North Am* 1996;29:795–806.

Tierney MR, Baker AS. Infections of the head and neck in diabetes mellitus. *Infect Dis Clin North Am* 1995;9:195–216.

Brain Abscess and Subdural Empyema

Alderson D, Strong AJ, Ingham HR, Selkon JB. Fifteen-year review of the mortality of brain abscess. *Neurosurgery* 1981;8:1–6.

Clark DB. Brain abscess and congenital heart disease. *Clin Neurosurg* 1966;14:274–287.

Courville CB, Nielsen JM. Fatal complications of otitis media: with particular reference to intracranial lesions in a series of 10,000 autopsies. *Arch Otolaryngol* 1934;19:451–501.

Curless RG. Neonatal intracranial abscess: two cases caused by Citrobacter and a literature review. *Ann Neurol* 1980;8:269–272.

de Falco R, Scarano E, Cigliano A, et al. Surgical treatment of subdural empyema: a critical review. *J Neurosurg Sci* 1996;40:53–58.

Dill ST, Cobbs CG, McDonald CK. Subdural empyema: analysis of 32 cases and review. *Clin Infect Dis* 1995;20:372–386.

Harvey FH, Carlow TJ. Brainstem abscess and the syndrome of acute tegmental encephalitis. *Ann Neurol* 1980;7:371–376.

Heilpern KL, Lorber B. Focal intracranial infections. *Infect Dis Clin North Am* 1996;10:879–898.

Kagawa M, Takeshita M, Yato S, Kitamura K. Brain abscess in congenital cyanotic heart disease. *J Neurosurg* 1983;58:913–917.

Loeser E Jr, Scheinberg L. Brain abscesses: a review of ninety-nine cases. *Neurology* 1957;7:601–609.

Macewen W. *Pyogenic infective diseases of the brain and spinal cord: meningitis, abscess of brain, infective sinus thrombosis.* Glasgow: James Maclehose & Son, 1893.

Mathisen GE, Johnson JP. Brain abscess. *Clin Infect Dis* 1997;25:763–779.

Merritt HH, Fremont-Smith F. *The cerebrospinal fluid.* Philadelphia: W.B. Saunders, 1938.

Pfister HW, Feiden W, Einhaupl KM. Spectrum of complications during bacterial meningitis in adults. Results of a prospective clinical study. *Arch Neurol* 1993;50:575–581.

Rosenblum ML, Hoff JT, Norman D, et al. Decreased mortality from brain abscesses since the advent of computerized tomography. *J Neurosurg* 1978;49:658–668.

Seydoux C, Francioli P. Bacterial brain abscesses: factors influencing mortality and sequelae. *Clin Infect Dis* 1992;15:394–401.

Shaw MDM, Russell JA. Cerebellar abscess: a review of 47 cases. *J Neurol Neurosurg Psychiatry* 1975;38:429–435.

Smith HP, Hendricks EB. Subdural empyema and epidural abscess in children. *J Neurosurg* 1983;58:392–397.

Weingarten K, Zimmerman RD, Becker RD, Heier LA, Haimes AB, Deck MD. Subdural and epidural empyemas: MR imaging. *AJR Am J Roentgenol* 1989;152:615–621.

Weisberg LA. Nonsurgical management of focal intracranial infection. *Neurology* 1981;31:575–580.

Wispelwey B, Dacey RG Jr, Scheld WM: Brain abscess. In: Scheld WM,

Whitley RJ, Durack DT, eds. *Infections of the central nervous system*. New York: Raven Press, 1991.

Zimmerman RA. Imaging of intracranial infections. In: Scheld WM, Whitley RJ, Durack DT, eds. *Infections of the central nervous system*. New York: Raven Press, 1991.

Merritt's Neurology, 10th ed., edited by L.P. Rowland. Lippincott Williams & Wilkins, Philadelphia © 2000.

C H A P T E R 23

VIRAL INFECTIONS

BURK JUBELT
JAMES R. MILLER

Although rabies has been known since ancient times and acute anterior poliomyelitis was recognized as a clinical entity in 1840, our knowledge of the role of viruses in the production of neurologic disease is of recent origin. In 1804, Zinke showed that rabies could be produced in a normal dog by inoculation of saliva from a rabid animal, but the filterable nature of rabies virus was not demonstrated until 1903. In 1908, Landsteiner and Popper produced a flaccid paralysis in monkeys by the injection of an emulsion of spinal cord from a fatal case of poliomyelitis. In the 1930s, filterable viruses were recovered from patients with epidemic encephalitis (arboviruses) and aseptic meningitis (lymphocytic choriomeningitis virus). With the use of electron microscopic, tissue culture, and immunologic techniques, many additional viruses that infect the nervous system have been recovered and characterized.

Although the list of viruses that cause human disease in epidemic or sporadic forms is extensive, most viral infections of the central nervous system (CNS) are uncommon complications of systemic illnesses caused by common human pathogens. After viral multiplication in extraneural tissues, dissemination to the CNS occurs by the hematogenous route or by spread along nerve fibers.

Viruses are *classified* according to their nucleic acid type, size, sensitivity to lipid solvents (enveloped versus nonenveloped), morphology, and mode of development in cells. The principal division is made according to whether the virus contains ribonucleic acid (RNA) or deoxyribonucleic acid (DNA). RNA viruses usually replicate within the cytoplasm of infected cells, whereas DNA viruses replicate in the nucleus. Members of almost every major animal virus group have been implicated in the production of neurologic illness in animals or humans (Table 23.1). The nature of the lesions produced varies with the virus and the conditions of infection. They may include neoplastic transformation, system degeneration, or congenital defects, such as cerebellar agenesis and aqueductal stenosis, as well as the inflammatory and destructive changes often considered

TABLE 23.1. VIRAL INFECTION OF THE NERVOUS SYSTEM

Virus type	Representative viruses responsible for neurologic disease
RNA viruses	
Piconavirus family	
Enterovirus genus	Poliovirus
	Coxsackievirus
	Echovirus
Hepatovirus genus	Enteroviruses 70 and 71
	Hepatitis A virus
Togavirus family	
Alphavirus genus (arbovirus)	Equine encephalitis (eastern, western, Venezuela)
Flavivirus family and genus (arbovirus)	St. Louis encephalitis
	Japanese encephalitis
	Tick-borne encephalitis
Bunyavirus family (arbovirus)	California encephalitis
Reovirus family	Colorado tick fever (coltivirus)
Togavirus family	
Rubivirus genus	Rubella virus
Orthomyxovirus family	Influenza A and B viruses
Paramyxovirus family	Measles and subacute sclerosing panencephalitis
	Mumps
Arenavirus family and genus	Lymphocytic choriomeningitis
Rhabdovirus family	Rabies
Retrovirus family	Human immunodeficiency virus, acquired immunodeficiency syndrome (AIDS)
DNA viruses	
Herpesvirus family	Herpes simplex virus
	Varicella-zoster (virus)
	Cytomegalovirus
	Epstein-Barr virus, infectious mononucleosis
	Human herpesvirus 6
Papovavirus family	Progressive multifocal leukencephalopathy
Poxvirus family	Vaccinia virus
Adenovirus family	Adenovirus

typical of viral infection. In addition, the concept that a viral infection causes only an acute illness that quickly follows infection of the host has been altered by the demonstration that in slow viral infections illness may not appear until many years after exposure to the agent.

ACUTE VIRAL INFECTIONS

CNS Viral Syndromes

Acute viral infections of the nervous system can manifest clinically in three forms: viral (aseptic) meningitis, encephalitis, or myelitis, which is infrequent (Table 23.2). Viral *meningitis* is usually a self-limited illness characterized by signs of meningeal irritation, such as headache, photophobia, and neck stiffness. *Encephalitis* entails involvement of parenchymal brain tissue, as indicated by convulsive seizures, alterations in the state of consciousness, and focal neurologic abnormalities. When both meningeal and encephalitic findings are present, the term *meningoencephalitis* may be used. Viral infections may also localize to the parenchyma of the spinal cord, resulting in *myelitis*. Myelitis may occur from infection of spinal motor neurons (paralytic disease or poliomyelitis), sensory neurons, autonomic neurons (bladder paralysis), or demyelination of white matter (transverse myelitis). When both encephalitis and myelitis occur, the term *encephalomyelitis* is used. The cerebrospinal fluid (CSF) findings in these three acute viral syndromes are usually similar, consisting of an increase in pressure, pleocytosis of varying degree, a moderate protein content elevation, and a normal sugar content.

Common biologic properties of members of a specific virus group may dictate how they attack the CNS and the type of disease that they produce. For example, individual picornaviruses, such as poliovirus and echovirus, can cause similar clinical syndromes. Members of specific virus groups also show different predilections for cell types or regions of the nervous system. Thus, members of the myxovirus group attack ependymal cells, and herpes simplex virus (HSV) shows preference for frontal and temporal lobes.

The tendency for a disease to appear in an epidemic or sporadic form may also be related to the biologic properties of the virus. Most epidemic forms of meningitis, encephalitis, or myelitis are due to infection with enteroviruses or togaviruses. The enteroviruses (picornaviruses) are relatively acid- and heat-resistant, thus resulting in fecal-hand-oral transmission during the hotter months of the year. Many togaviruses require a multiplication phase in mosquitoes or ticks before they can infect people; human epidemics occur when climatic and other conditions favor a large population of infected insect vectors. Neurologic diseases due to members of other virus groups usually occur sporadically or as isolated instances that complicate viral infections of other organs or systems.

Diagnosis

Knowledge of whether an illness is occurring in an epidemic setting and of the seasonal occurrence of the different forms of acute viral infections may indicate the methods to be used in detecting the infective agent. Infection with the picornaviruses or arboviruses tends to occur in the summer and early fall; other viruses, such as mumps, occur in late winter or spring.

The diagnosis can be made by a combination of virus isolation (inoculation of blood, nasopharyngeal washings, feces, CSF, or tissue suspensions into susceptible animals or tissue culture systems), serologic tests, and amplification of viral nucleic acids. Infectious virus particles in human fluids and tissues are usually few in number, and many viruses are easily disrupted and inactivated even at room temperature. Tissues and fluids to be used for virus isolation studies should therefore be frozen unless they can be immediately transferred to the laboratory in appropriate transport media.

The ability to recover virus from the CSF varies according to the nature of the agent. Some viruses, such as mumps virus, can frequently be isolated from the CSF, whereas other viruses, such as poliovirus and HSV type 1, are rarely recovered.

Serologic tests are applicable to all known acute viral diseases of the nervous system. Serum should be frozen and kept at a low temperature until the tests are done. The diagnosis of an acute viral infection and the establishment of the type of virus rest on the development of antibodies to the infection, traditionally a fourfold antibody rise. It is therefore necessary to show that antibodies are not present or are present only in low titer in the early stage of the illness and that they are present in high titer at a proper interval after the onset of symptoms. Several to many days are usually required for the development of antibodies; serum removed in the first few days of the illness can therefore serve as the control (acute-phase serum). Serum withdrawn in the convalescent stage, 3 to 5 weeks after the onset of the illness, may be used to determine whether antibodies have developed (convalescent-phase serum). When there is no change in titer, positive tests merely indicate that the individual has at some time in the past had an infection with this type of virus and that it probably is not the cause of the present illness.

If brain tissue from a patient is available in fatal cases or by brain biopsy, further studies can define the responsible virus. Brain sections can be analyzed by immunostaining techniques (immunofluorescence, immunoperoxidase) to determine whether specific viral antigens are present. Electron microscopy may indicate the presence of virus particles or components of

TABLE 23.2. RELATIVE FREQUENCY OF MENINGITIS AND ENCEPHALITIS OF KNOWN VIRAL ETIOLOGY (NUMBER OF PATIENTS)

	Aseptic meningitis	Encephalitis	Paralytic disease	Total
Mumps	28	11	1	40
Lymphocytic choriomeningitis	7	0	0	7
Herpes simplex virus	2	7	0	9
Poliovirus	18	5	66	89
Coxsackievirus A	18	1	0	19
Coxsackievirus B	71	4	0	75
Echovirus	55	3	1	59
Arbovirus	3	5	0	8

From Buescher, et al. Central nervous system infections of viral etiology: the changing pattern. *Res Publ Assoc Res Nerv Ment Dis* 1968; 44:147–163; with permission.

specific morphology. Suspensions of brain and spinal cord can be injected into susceptible animals and tissue culture cell lines. In special instances, tissue cultures can be initiated from brain tissue itself. Such brain cell cultures can then be examined for the presence of viral antigens or infective virus. If an agent is recovered, final identification can be made by neutralization with known specific antiserum.

Any material used for viral isolation can also be used for amplification of viral nucleic acid by the polymerase chain reaction (PCR). Identification is then made by the use of complimentary probes (hybridization).

Treatment

Antiviral chemotherapeutic agents are now available for several viruses: acyclovir (Zovirax) for HSV; acyclovir, famciclovir (Famvir), and foscarnet sodium (Foscavir) for varicella-zoster virus (VZV); ganciclovir sodium (Cytovene) and foscarnet for cytomegalovirus (CMV), and reverse transcriptase and protease inhibitors for human immunodeficiency virus (HIV).

Immunization procedures with either live attenuated vaccines or inactivated virus are readily available for rabies, poliomyelitis, hepatitis A and B, mumps, influenza, rubella, measles, chickenpox (varicella), and vaccinia. Immunization against the arboviruses is used mainly to protect laboratory workers and military personnel.

Although additional antiviral chemotherapeutic agents will likely become available in the future, vector control and mass immunization now seem to be the most practical means of effective control.

Enterovirus (Picornavirus) Infections

Picornaviruses are small, nonenveloped RNA viruses that multiply in the cytoplasm of cells. They are the smallest RNA viruses, hence the name "pico (small) RNA virus." Human picornaviruses can be divided into three subgroups: enteroviruses, found primarily in the gastrointestinal tract; rhinoviruses, found in the nasopharynx; and hepatitis A viruses (hepatoviruses). The enteroviruses comprise the *polioviruses, coxsackieviruses,* and *echoviruses,* all of which are capable of producing inflammation in the CNS. Recently, identified enteroviruses have been named as *unclassified enteroviruses 68 to 71.* CNS disease has occurred with enteroviruses 70 and 71 and with hepatitis A virus.

The enteroviruses are resistant to the acid and bile of intestinal contents and may survive for long periods in sewage or water. They grow only in primate cells and are highly cytocidal. Virus particles may form crystalline arrays in the cytoplasm of cells, which are recognized as acidophilic inclusions in histologic preparations.

Poliomyelitis

Acute anterior poliomyelitis (infantile paralysis, Heine-Medin disease) is an acute generalized disease caused by poliovirus infection. It is characterized by destruction of the motor cells in the spinal cord, brain, and brainstem and by the appearance of a flaccid paralysis of the muscles innervated by the affected neurons.

Although the disease has probably occurred for many centuries, the first clear description was given by Jacob Heine in 1840, and the foundation of our knowledge of the epidemiology of the disease was laid by Medin in 1890. The studies of Landsteiner, Popper, Flexner, Lewis, and others in the first decade of the 20th century proved that the disease was caused by a virus.

Invasion of the nervous system occurs as a relatively late and infrequent manifestation. Orally ingested virus multiplies in the pharynx and ileum and probably in lymphoid tissue of the tonsils and Peyer patches. The virus then spreads to cervical and mesenteric lymph nodes and can be detected in the blood shortly thereafter. Viremia is accompanied by no symptoms or by a brief minor illness (fever, chills). It is still not definitely known how the virus gains access to the nervous system in paralytic cases. The most likely possibility is via direct spread from the blood at defective areas of the blood–brain barrier. Less likely is neural spread from the intestine or from neuromuscular junctions.

The virus has a predilection for the large motor cells, causing chromatolysis with acidophilic inclusions and necrosis of the cells. Degeneration of the neurons is accompanied by an inflammatory reaction in the adjacent meninges and the perivascular spaces and by secondary proliferation of the microglia. Recovery may occur in partially damaged cells, but the severely damaged cells are phagocytized and removed. The degenerative changes are most intense in the ventral horn cells and the motor cells in the medulla; however, neurons in the posterior horn, the posterior root ganglion, and elsewhere in the CNS are occasionally involved. Rarely, inflammation is also present in the white matter. Although the pathologic changes are most intense in the spinal cord, medulla, and motor areas of the cerebral cortex, any portion of the nervous system may be affected, including the midbrain, pons, cerebellum, basal ganglia, and nonmotor cerebral cortex.

Epidemiology

Acute anterior poliomyelitis is worldwide in distribution but is more prevalent in temperate climates. It may occur in sporadic, endemic, or epidemic form at any time of the year, but it is most common in late summer and early fall. Acute anterior poliomyelitis was formerly the most common form of viral infection of the nervous system. Before 1956, between 25,000 and 50,000 cases occurred annually in the United States.

Since the advent of effective vaccines, the incidence of the disease has dramatically decreased in the United States, as well as in other developed countries. In fact, in these countries, paralytic poliomyelitis is becoming a clinical rarity, except for isolated cases and small epidemics in areas where the population has not been vaccinated. In the United States, fewer than 10 cases of paralytic poliomyelitis occur each year, with most being vaccine-associated. A similar decrease has been reported in other countries in which vaccination has been practiced on a large scale. Paralytic poliomyelitis, however, is still a significant health problem in developing areas of the world. Worldwide in 1991, 12,992 cases of paralytic poliomyelitis were reported to the World Health Organization (WHO), but underreporting is significant. WHO studies have demonstrated that the actual number of cases is about 10 times the number reported.

Three antigenically distinct types of poliovirus have been defined. All three types can cause paralytic poliomyelitis or viral meningitis, but type I appears to be most often associated with paralytic disease.

The disease may occur at any age. It is rare before age 6 months. In the late 19th and early 20th centuries, poliomyelitis changed from an endemic to an epidemic disease. In the early epidemics, 90% of paralytic cases occurred in persons younger than 5 years. As epidemics recurred, there was a shift of paralytic cases to older individuals, so that the majority of cases occurred in children older than 5 years and in teenagers. Paralysis was also seen more frequently in young adults.

Prophylaxis

Oral vaccination with live attenuated virus (oral poliovirus vaccine [OPV], Sabin) is effective in the prevention of paralytic infections. Antibody response depends on multiplication of attenuated virus in the gastrointestinal tract. Significant antibody levels develop more rapidly and persist longer than those that follow intramuscular immunization with formalized polioviruses (inactivated poliovirus vaccine [IPV], Salk). OPV is also capable of spreading and thus immunizing contacts of vaccinated individuals, but it can also cause vaccine-associated poliomyelitis. Because of this, the recommendations for vaccination in the United States have been changed to a sequential vaccination schedule with two doses of IPV followed by two doses of OPV.

Symptoms

The symptoms at the onset of poliomyelitis are similar to those of any acute infection (fever, chills, nausea, prostration). In about 25% of the patients, these initial symptoms subside in 36 to 48 hours, and patients are apparently well for 2 to 3 days until there is a secondary rise in temperature (dromedary type) accompanied by symptoms of meningeal irritation. In most patients, this second phase of the illness directly follows the first without any intervening period of freedom from symptoms. The headache increases in severity and muscle soreness appears, most commonly in the neck and back. Drowsiness or stupor occasionally develops, but patients are irritable and apprehensive, when aroused. Convulsions are occasionally seen at this stage in infants.

Paralysis, when it occurs, usually develops between the second and fifth day after the onset of signs of involvement of the nervous system, but it may be the initial symptom or, in rare instances, may be delayed for as long as 2 to 3 weeks. After the onset of paralysis, there may be extension of the motor loss for 3 to 5 days. Further progress of signs and symptoms rarely occurs after this time. The fever lasts for 4 to 7 days and subsides gradually. The temperature may return to normal before the paralysis develops or while the paralysis is advancing. Limb muscles are usually involved, but in severe cases respiratory and cardiac muscles may be affected. Acute cerebellar ataxia, isolated facial nerve palsies, and transverse myelitis have been observed in poliovirus-infected individuals.

Laboratory Data

Leukocytosis is present in the blood. CSF pressure may be increased. A CSF pleocytosis develops in the period before the onset of the paralysis. Initially, polymorphonuclear (PMN) leuko-

cytes predominate, but a shift to lymphocytes occurs within several days. The CSF protein content is slightly elevated, except in patients with a severe degree of paralysis, when it may be elevated to 100 to 300 mg/dL and may persist for several weeks.

Diagnosis

Acute anterior poliomyelitis can be diagnosed without difficulty in most patients by the acute development of an asymmetric flaccid paralysis accompanied by the characteristic changes in the CSF. A presumptive diagnosis can be made in the preparalytic stage and in nonparalytic cases during an epidemic. The diagnosis can be suspected in patients who have not been vaccinated or have defects in their immune response. The diagnosis of poliovirus infection can be established by recovery of the virus from stool (usually lasts 2 to 3 weeks), throat washings (during the first week), or, rarely, from CSF or blood. Recovery of virus from the throat or feces requires the additional demonstration of a fourfold rise in the patient's antibody titer before a specific viral diagnosis can be made. With recent-generation magnetic resonance imaging (MRI) scanners, imaging studies may show localization of inflammation to the spinal cord anterior horns.

Prognosis

Fewer than 10% of patients die from the acute disease. Death is usually due to respiratory failure or pulmonary complications. The mortality rate is highest in the bulbar form of the disease, where it is often greater than 50%. The prognosis is poor when the paralysis is extensive or when there is a slow progress of paralysis with exacerbations and involvement of new muscles over a period of days. The prognosis with regard to return of function depends on age (infants and children have more recovery) and the extent of paralysis, as muscle groups only partially paralyzed are more likely to recover.

New symptoms develop in about 50% of patients 30 to 40 years after the acute poliomyelitis. These new symptoms have been collectively called the *postpolio syndrome.* In some of these patients, a slowly progressive weakness with atrophy and fasciculations develops, called *postpolio progressive muscular atrophy* (see Chapter 118).

Treatment

Treatment is essentially supportive. Attention should be given to respiration, swallowing, and bladder and bowel functions.

Treatment of patients with paralysis of respiratory muscles or bulbar involvement requires great care. They should be watched carefully for signs of respiratory embarrassment, and as soon as these become apparent, mechanical respiratory assistance should immediately be given. The development of anxiety in a previously calm patient is a serious warning of either cerebral anoxia or hypercarbia and may precede labored breathing or cyanosis.

Treatment in the convalescent stage and thereafter consists of physiotherapy, muscle reeducation, application of appropriate corrective appliances, and orthopedic surgery.

Coxsackievirus Infections

In 1948, Dalldorf and Sickles inoculated specimens obtained from patients with suspected poliomyelitis into the brains of newborn mice and discovered the coxsackieviruses. Two sub-groups, A and B, can be distinguished by their effects on suck-ling mice. In mice, group A viruses cause myositis leading to flac-cid paralysis and death. Group B viruses cause encephalitis, myocarditis, pancreatitis, and necrosis of brown fat; animals ex-perience tremors, spasms, and paralysis before death. Twenty-three group A and six group B serotypes are currently recognized.

When involving the human nervous system, both group A and group B coxsackieviruses usually cause aseptic meningitis. When enteroviral meningitis occurs in infants, residual cogni-tive, language, and developmental abnormalities may occur. Oc-casionally, coxsackievirus infection causes encephalitis, and rarely paralytic disease or acute cerebellar ataxia are seen. Classic extraneural manifestations caused by group A coxsackieviruses are herpangina, hand-foot-and-mouth disease, and other rashes. Group B coxsackieviruses usually cause pericarditis, myocarditis, and epidemic myalgia (pleurodynia, Bornholm disease). They can also cause disseminated infection with severe encephalitis in newborns and may cause congenital anomalies if infection oc-curs in early pregnancy.

The symptoms and signs of meningeal involvement are simi-lar to those that follow infection with other viruses that cause aseptic meningitis. The onset may be acute or subacute with fever, headache, malaise, nausea, and abdominal pain. Stiffness of the neck and vomiting usually begin 24 to 48 hours after the initial symptoms. There is a mild or moderate fever. Muscular paralysis, sensory disturbances, and reflex changes are rare. Paral-ysis, when present, is mild and transient. Meningeal symptoms occasionally occur in combination with myalgia, pleurodynia, or herpangina.

The CSF pressure is normal or slightly increased. There is a mild or moderate pleocytosis in the CSF, ranging from 25 to 250/mm³ with 10% to 50% PMN cells. The protein content is normal or slightly increased, and the sugar content is normal.

Diagnosis of coxsackievirus infection can be established only by recovering the virus from the feces, throat washings, or CSF and by demonstrating an increase in viral antibodies in the serum. Viral genetic amplification (PCR technique) has also been used for diagnosis. Meningitis due to a coxsackievirus can-not be distinguished from aseptic meningitis due to other viral agents, except by laboratory studies. It is differentiated from meningitis due to pyogenic bacteria and yeast by the relatively low cell count and the normal sugar content in the CSF. Differ-entiation must also be made from other diseases associated with lymphocytic pleocytosis in the CSF; these include tuberculous, fungal, or syphilitic meningitis; leptospirosis; Lyme disease; *Lis-teria monocytogenes, Mycoplasma,* or *Rickettsia* infections; toxo-plasmosis; meningitis caused by other viruses; or parameningeal infections. Compared with these entities, coxsackievirus infec-tions are more benign, and the CSF sugar content is normal.

Echovirus Infections

This group of enteroviruses was originally isolated in cell culture from the feces of apparently normal persons. They were consid-ered "orphans" because they apparently did not cause disease. The designation "echo" is an acronym derived from the first let-ters of the term *enteric cytopathogenic human orphans.* Thirty-two

serotypes are now recognized. Many strains cause hemagglutina-tion of human type O erythrocytes.

The echoviruses cause gastroenteritis, macular exanthems, and upper respiratory infections. Echovirus-9 infections may cause a petechial rash that may be confused with meningococ-cemia. When the nervous system is infected, the syndrome of aseptic meningitis usually results.

The clinical picture of infection with the echoviruses is simi-lar to that of other enterovirus infections. Children are more fre-quently affected than adults. The main features are fever, coryza, sore throat, vomiting, and diarrhea. A rubelliform rash is often present. Headache, neck stiffness, lethargy, and irritability indi-cate involvement of the nervous system. The disease usually runs a benign course that subsides in 1 or 2 weeks, but complications similar to those seen with coxsackievirus infections can occur.

Cerebellar ataxia has been reported in children as the result of echovirus infection. The onset of ataxia is acute; the course is be-nign with remission of symptoms within a few weeks. Pupil-sparing oculomotor nerve paralysis and other cranial nerve palsies have rarely been observed. Echoviruses can cause a persis-tent CNS infection in children with agammaglobulinemia; this is an echovirus-induced meningoencephalitis often associated with a dermatomyositis-like syndrome. It can be treated with im-mune globulin.

The CSF pleocytosis may vary from several hundred to a thousand or more cells per cubic millimeter, but it is usually less than 500/mm³. Early in the infection, there may be as many as 90% PMN leukocytes; within 48 hours, however, the response becomes completely mononuclear. The CSF protein content is normal or slightly elevated; the sugar content remains normal.

The echoviruses are commonly recovered from feces, throat swabs, and CSF. Virus typing is carried out by antibody testing. Viral genomic amplification has also been used for diagnosis. The differential diagnosis of echovirus meningitis is similar to that of coxsackievirus infections.

Infections with Enteroviruses 70 and 71 and Hepatitis A Virus

Newly recognized enteroviruses are now named as unclassified enteroviruses. Several of these new enteroviruses have caused CNS infections. Enterovirus 70 has caused epidemics of acute hemorrhagic conjunctivitis (AHC), which initially occurred in Africa and Asia. Neurologic abnormality occurs in about 1 in 10,000 or 1 in 15,000 cases of AHC, primarily in adults. Out-breaks of AHC have recently occurred in Latin America and the southeastern United States, but without any neurologic disease. The most common neurologic picture is a poliolike syndrome of flaccid, asymmetric, and proximal paralysis of the legs accompa-nied by severe radicular pain. Paralysis is permanent in more than 50% of patients. Isolated cranial nerve palsies (primary fa-cial nerve), pyramidal tract signs, bladder paralysis, vertigo, and sensory loss have been reported. Because neurologic involvement usually occurs about 2 weeks after the onset of AHC, it may be difficult to isolate the virus at the time when neurologic signs are seen. Thus, diagnosis often depends on serologic studies. The neurologic disorder has rarely been seen without the preceding conjunctivitis.

Enterovirus 71 has been recognized as causing outbreaks of hand-foot-and-mouth disease. Upper respiratory infections and gastroenteritis also occur. Neurologic involvement may occur in up to 25% of patients, with children and teenagers primarily affected. Neurologic manifestations include aseptic meningitis, cerebellar ataxia, and various forms of poliomyelitis (flaccid monoparesis, bulbar polio). Most of these cases have occurred in Europe and Asia. Two cases of transient paralysis were seen in an outbreak in New York. Diagnosis can be made by virus isolation from throat, feces, or vesicles and by antibody studies.

Hepatitis A virus has apparently caused primarily encephalitis as a distinct entity, although hepatic encephalopathy is obviously more common. It has also been associated with transverse myelitis.

Arbovirus Infections

The arboviruses (*ar*thropod-*bo*rne) are small, spherical, ether-sensitive (enveloped) viruses that contain RNA. More than 400 serologically distinct arboviruses are currently recognized. Although the term *arbovirus* is no longer an official taxonomic term, it is still useful to designate viruses transmitted by vectors. Arboviruses include the alphaviruses (formerly group A arboviruses), flaviviruses (formerly group B arboviruses), bunyaviruses, and some reoviruses (Table 23.1). The alphaviruses are one genus in the togavirus family; the other genus comprises the rubiviruses (rubella viruses). The equine encephalitides are caused by alphaviruses. The flavivirus family is composed of more than 60 viruses, including the viruses that cause yellow fever and St. Louis and Japanese encephalitides. The bunyaviruses include the California encephalitis group. The reovirus family includes the virus causing Colorado tick fever. St. Louis and California encephalitides are the most common arboviral encephalitides in the United States.

Arboviruses multiply in a blood-sucking arthropod vector. In their natural environment, they alternate between the invertebrate vector and a mammal. Mosquitoes and ticks are the most common vectors. Birds seem to be the principal natural hosts, but wild snakes and some rodents are probably a secondary reservoir. People and horses are usually incidental hosts, and human or horse infection in most arbovirus infections terminates the chain of infection (dead-end hosts). Approximately 80 arboviruses are known to cause human disease. The spectrum of disease produced is broad, ranging from hemorrhagic fevers (yellow fever) to arthralgia, rashes, and encephalitis.

Arboviruses are difficult to isolate in the laboratory. The virus may be recovered from blood during the early phases (2 to 4 days) of the illness. In nonfatal cases, the diagnosis usually depends on the demonstration of a fourfold rise in antibodies during the course of the illness. The virus may be isolated from the tissues at necropsy by the intracerebral inoculation of infant mice and susceptible tissue culture cells.

Arbovirus infection of the nervous system may result in viral meningitis but more frequently in moderate or severe encephalitis. Diseases due to arboviruses typically occur in late summer and early fall.

Equine Encephalitis

Three distinct types of equine encephalitis occur in the United States: eastern equine encephalitis (EEE), western equine encephalitis (WEE), and Venezuelan equine encephalitis (VEE). They are due to three serologically distinct alphaviruses. Infection with these viruses was thought to be limited to horses until 1932, when Meyer reported an unusual type of encephalitis in three men who were working in close contact with affected animals. The first cases in which EEE virus was recovered from human brain tissue were reported in Massachusetts in 1938 by Fothergill and coworkers. Many arboviruses take their name from the location in which they were first isolated; they are not confined, however, by specific geographic boundaries. EEE is usually localized to the Atlantic and Gulf coasts and the Great Lakes areas. Infrequently, cases of EEE have been reported in regions west of the Mississippi River, as well as in Central and South America and the Philippines. WEE virus infection is now known to occur in all parts of the United States, although most frequently in the western two-thirds of the country. VEE occurs in Central and South America and the southern half of the United States, but is a rare cause of encephalitis.

Pathology

In EEE, the brain is markedly congested, and there are widespread degenerative changes in nerve cells. The meninges and perivascular spaces of the brain are intensely infiltrated with PMN leukocytes and round cells. Focal vasculitic lesions, often with thrombus formation, may occur. Destruction of myelin is prominent only near the necrotic foci. Lesions are found in both the white and gray matter and are most intensive in the cerebrum and brainstem, but they may also be present in the cerebellum and spinal cord.

In contrast to EEE, the pathology of WEE is less intense, characterized by less inflammation, which is primarily mononuclear, and a paucity of nerve cell changes.

Incidence

Equine encephalitis is a rare human infection, tending to occur as isolated cases or in small epidemics. Epizootics in horses may precede the human cases by several weeks. Equine encephalitis mainly affects infants, children, and adults older than 50 years. Inapparent infection is common in all age groups.

Symptoms

Infection with the EEE virus begins with a short prodrome (approximately 5 days) of fever, headache, malaise, and nausea and vomiting. This is followed by the rapid onset of neurologic manifestations: confusion, drowsiness, stupor, or coma with convulsive seizures and neck stiffness. Cranial nerve palsies, hemiplegia, and other focal neurologic signs are common.

The symptoms of WEE and VEE are less severe. Onset is acute, with general malaise and headache occasionally followed by convulsions and nausea and vomiting. There is moderate fever and neck stiffness. The headaches increase in severity, and there is drowsiness, lethargy, or coma. Paresis and cranial nerve palsies may occur.

Laboratory Data

Leukocytosis may occur in the blood, especially in EEE; white blood cell counts as high as 35,000/mm³ have been reported. CSF changes are greatest in EEE, in which the pressure is always moderately or greatly increased. The CSF is cloudy or purulent, containing 500 to 3,000 cells/mm³. Initially, a predominance of PMN leukocytes usually occurs. The protein content is increased, but the sugar content is normal. With abatement of the acute stage, the cell count drops, and lymphocytes become the predominating cell type, although PMN cells persist as a significant fraction.

The CSF changes in the WEE and VEE are less severe. The pressure is usually normal, and the cellular increase is moderate, with counts varying from normal to 500/mm³, with mononuclear cells as the predominating cell type.

Diagnosis

Isolation of equine encephalitis viruses from blood and CSF is infrequent but should be attempted. Most arboviral infections are diagnosed serologically, with immunoglobulin M (IgM) assays available for rapid diagnosis. MRI may reveal focal lesions in the basal ganglia, thalami, and brainstem in about 50% of patients with EEE (Fig. 23.1). Computed tomography (CT) is less sensitive. A similar distribution of lesions on MRI has been seen in several other arboviral encephalitides (Japanese encephalitis, Central European tick-borne encephalitis).

Equine encephalitis must be differentiated from other acute infections of the CNS. These include postinfectious encephalomyelitis (exanthems, occurrence usually in the late fall and winter, abnormal MRI), advanced bacterial and tuberculous meningitis with parenchymal involvement (low CSF sugar content, positive cultures), brain abscess (abnormal imaging), parasitic encephalitis (detected by serology), and other viral infections. Differentiation from other viral encephalitides, except that caused by HSV, can be made only by isolation of the virus or by serologic tests.

Course and Prognosis

The average mortality rate in EEE is about 50%. The duration of the disease varies from less than 1 day in fulminating cases to more than 4 weeks in less severe cases. In patients who recover, sequelae such as mental deficiency, cranial nerve palsies, hemiplegia, aphasia, and convulsions are common. Children younger than 10 years are more likely to survive the acute infection, but they also have the greatest chance of being left with severe neurologic disability.

The fatality rate in WEE is about 10%. Sequelae among young infants are frequent and severe but are uncommon in adults. The mortality rate in VEE is less than 0.5%; nearly all deaths have occurred in young children.

Treatment

Treatment in the acute stage of equine encephalitis is entirely supportive. Vaccines against the causative viruses have been produced, but their use should be confined to laboratory workers and others who are subject to unusual exposure to the viruses. Vaccination in a large-scale community program is not indicated because of the low incidence of the disease. EEE and WEE have been prevented by controlling the vector by the use of large-scale

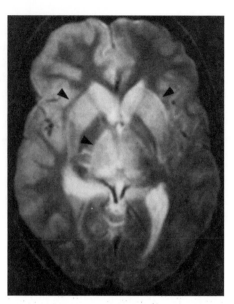

FIG. 23.1. Eastern equine encephalitis. Proton-density MR image 3 days after the onset of neurologic symptoms revealed large bilateral asymmetric lesions of the caudate, putamen, and thalamus *(arrowheads).* Less frequently, lesions can also be seen in the cortex, primarily in the medial temporal cortex and insula (not shown). (From Deresiewicz et al., 1997; with permission. Copyright © 1997 Massachusetts Medical Society. All rights reserved.)

insecticide spraying. However, the key to prevention is avoiding contact with mosquitoes: avoiding endemic areas, wearing appropriate clothing, and using mosquito repellents.

St. Louis Encephalitis

The first outbreak of acute encephalitis in which a virus was definitely established as the causative agent was an epidemic that occurred in St. Louis in 1933. This type of encephalitis probably existed in this area before 1933, as cases of encephalitis had occurred in St. Louis during the previous 14 years. Since 1933, repeated outbreaks have occurred in the United States with increasing frequency and widening geographic distribution.

The virus responsible for St. Louis encephalitis (SLE) is a mosquito-transmitted flavivirus. Epidemics follow two epidemiologic patterns: rural and urban. Rural epidemics tend to occur in the western United States. The rural cycle involves birds as the intermediate host, similar to WEE. Urban epidemics occur primarily in the midwestern United States, the Mississippi River Valley, and the eastern United States. Urban outbreaks can be abrupt and extensive because humans are the intermediate hosts. SLE primarily affects the elderly population. As with other arboviruses, disease in humans usually appears in midsummer to early fall.

Pathology

Grossly, there is a mild degree of vascular congestion and occasional petechial hemorrhages. Microscopic changes include a mild infiltration of the meninges and blood vessels of the brain with mononuclear cells; mononuclear, microglial, and glial cell accumulation in the parenchyma of both the gray and white matter; and degenerative changes in neurons. The nuclear masses of the thalamus and midbrain are more affected than the cortex.

Symptoms and Signs

Infection with the SLE virus usually results in inapparent infection. About 75% of patients with clinical manifestations have encephalitis; the others have aseptic meningitis or nonspecific illness. SLE is a disease of older adults. Encephalitic signs develop in almost all patients older than 40 years with symptoms. The onset of neurologic symptoms may be abrupt or may be preceded by a prodromal illness of 3 or 4 days' duration characterized by headache, myalgia, fever, sore throat, and nausea and vomiting. The headache increases in severity, and neck stiffness develops. Other common signs include pathologic reflexes, intention tremors, ataxia, and cranial nerve abnormalities. In more severe cases, there may be delirium, coma or stupor, focal neurologic signs, and, rarely, seizures, a poor prognostic sign.

Laboratory Data

A mild to moderate leukocytosis occurs in the blood. The CSF is usually abnormal, with a mild pleocytosis in most patients that averages approximately 100 cells/mm^3. Cell counts as high as 500/mm^3 or higher have been reported. Lymphocytes are the predominating cell type, although predominance of PMN cells may be found early in the disease. The sugar content is normal. Hyponatremia due to inappropriate secretion of antidiuretic hormone occurs in 25% to 33% of patients.

Diagnosis

The SLE virus is rarely isolated from the blood or CSF, and diagnosis depends on serologic testing. An IgM assay is available for rapid diagnosis. The differential diagnosis is similar to that of the equine encephalitides.

Course and Prognosis

The disease runs an acute course in most patients and usually results in death or recovery within 2 to 3 weeks. Mortality has varied from 2% to 20%. The most common sequelae of SLE are headaches, insomnia, easy fatigability, irritability, and memory loss, and these usually clear in several years. About 25% of survivors have permanent neurologic sequelae of cranial nerve palsies, hemiplegia, gait disorders, and aphasia.

Treatment

There is no specific treatment or a vaccine for SLE. Supportive care is essential. Vector control and avoidance of contact is preventive.

Japanese Encephalitis

Japanese encephalitis (JE) was first identified as a distinct disease after a large epidemic in 1924, although a form of the encephalitis had been recognized as early as 1871. The causative agent is a mosquito-transmitted flavivirus. Occurrence can be endemic (tropical areas) or epidemic (temperate zones). JE remains a major medical problem throughout Asia, with as many as 10,000 cases annually. The pathologic changes seen with JE are much more intense than those of SLE. In addition to infiltration of lymphocytes, monocytes, and microglial cells, severe neuronal necrosis occurs with neuronophagia in the entire cerebral cortex, basal ganglia, cerebellum, and spinal cord.

The clinical picture and laboratory findings in JE are similar to those of SLE. The disease is most common in children, and the mortality rate in some epidemics has been as high as 50%. This figure is undoubtedly too high because most mild cases are not admitted to hospitals. Severe neurologic residual effects and mental defects are common, especially in the young.

The diagnosis may be established by isolation of the virus from the blood, CSF, or cerebral tissue and by appropriate antibody tests. Neuroimaging studies have revealed findings similar to those reported for EEE (i.e., lesions of the thalami, basal ganglia, and brainstem).

There is no specific treatment. Vector control and vaccination are preventive. An inactivated-virus vaccine is routinely used in Japan, China, and Korea and is available for residents of the United States traveling to endemic or epidemic areas of Asia.

California (La Crosse) Encephalitis

Human neurologic disease associated with California encephalitis virus was first recognized in the early 1960s. Subsequently, La Crosse virus, also a member of the California virus serogroup, has been shown to cause most of these infections. Infection most frequently occurs in the upper midwestern United States, but it is found throughout the eastern half of the continental United States. These viruses are now known to be among the more important causes of encephalitis in the United States; fortunately, the encephalitis is usually mild. The California virus serogroup is now classified among the bunyaviruses, a group of enveloped viruses with segmented, helical, circular ribonucleoproteins.

The virus is transmitted by woodland mosquitoes. Its cycle involves small woodland animals, but not birds. Consequently, rural endemic rather than epidemic disease usually occurs. The disease occurs in the late summer and early fall, and nearly all patients are children. Infants younger than 1 year and adults are rarely affected. Headache, nausea and vomiting, changes in sensorium, meningeal irritation, and upper motor neuron signs have commonly been reported. Unlike in most other viral infections, the peripheral blood count is often quite elevated (20,000 to 30,000 cells/mm^3). The CSF contains an increased number of lymphocytes and shows the other findings typical of viral meningitis or encephalitis. The diagnosis can be established by serologic studies.

The case fatality is low (less than 1%). Recovery usually occurs within 7 to 10 days. Emotional liability, learning difficulties, and recurrent seizures have been reported as sequelae.

Other Arbovirus Encephalitides

Colorado tick fever (CTF) is caused by a coltivirus (reovirus family) transmitted by wood ticks with small animals as intermediate hosts. CTF is confined to the geographic area of the tick in the Rocky Mountains. Infection often involves hikers, foresters, or vacationers in the spring and summer. Three to six days after a tick bite, an abrupt febrile illness develops with headache, myalgia, retroorbital pain, and photophobia. About 50% of patients have a biphasic fever pattern. Peripheral leukopenia and thrombocytopenia are common. Aseptic meningitis occurs in about 20% of patients. This is a benign disease; encephalitis and permanent sequelae are almost never seen. Diagnosis can readily be made by virus isolation from the blood or by serology.

Tick-borne encephalitis (TBE) viruses are closely related flaviviruses transmitted by wood ticks. Disease is seen primarily in the northern latitude woodlands of Siberia and Europe. The Siberian strains cause a severe encephalitis (Russian spring–summer encephalitis virus). The European and Scandinavian strains (Central European encephalitis) tend to cause a milder encephalitis that can present as a biphasic illness with recrudescence several weeks after the initial influenza-like illness. A case of TBE has been seen in Ohio after foreign tick exposure. Powassan virus, a member of the TBE complex, has been isolated from a few patients with severe encephalitis in the United States and Canada. A related virus, louping ill, causes a sporadic, mild encephalitis in the British Isles.

Other arboviruses that have occasionally caused epidemics of encephalitis include West Nile fever and Rift Valley fever in Africa and Murray Valley encephalitis in Australia.

Rubella

Rubella virus is not an arbovirus; it is now classified as a togavirus. It is an enveloped RNA virus that causes rubella (German measles), an exanthematous disease that can produce marked neurologic damage in the unborn child of a mother infected during pregnancy (congenital rubella syndrome [CRS]). Gregg, an Australian ophthalmologist, was the first to correlate the occurrence of congenital cataracts among newborn babies with maternal rubella infection during the first trimester of pregnancy. CRS is now known to produce a variety of defects, including deafness, mental retardation, and cardiac abnormalities. The frequency of congenital defects is highest in the first trimester of pregnancy and falls as gestation advances.

Rubella virus induces a chronic persistent infection in the fetus. For a long time after birth, infants may shed virus from the nasopharynx, eye, or CSF. Virus production continues despite the development of neutralizing and hemagglutinating antibodies by the infected child.

The lesions in the nervous system are those of a chronic leptomeningitis with infiltration of mononuclear cells, lymphocytes, and plasma cells. Small areas of necrosis and glial cell proliferation are seen in the basal ganglia, midbrain, pons, and spinal cord. Microscopic vasculitis and perivascular calcification may also occur.

The infant with rubella encephalitis is usually lethargic, hypotonic, or inactive at birth or within the first few days or weeks after birth. Within the next several months, restlessness, head retraction, opisthotonic posturing, and rigidity may develop. Seizures and a meningitis-like illness may occur. The anterior fontanelle is usually large; microcephaly occurs infrequently. The child may have other associated defects, such as deafness, cardiovascular anomalies, congestive heart failure, cataracts, thrombocytopenia, and areas of hyperpigmentation about the navel, forehead, and cheeks. Improvement of varying degrees may be noted after the first 6 to 12 months of life.

The CSF contains an increased number of cells (lymphocytes), as well as a moderately increased protein content. Rubella virus can be recovered from the CSF of approximately 25% of patients and may persist in the CSF for more than 1 year after birth.

Specific diagnosis can be made by recovery of the virus from throat swab, urine, CSF, leukocytes, bone marrow, or conjunctivae, or by serologic tests. A rubella-specific IgM serologic test can be used for diagnosis in the newborn.

Rubella virus also has caused postinfectious encephalomyelitis with acquired rubella and, rarely, a chronic or slow viral infection termed *progressive rubella panencephalitis* (see below).

The primary method of treatment is prevention of fetal infection. Live rubella virus vaccine should be given to all children between 1 year of age and puberty. Adolescent girls and nonpregnant women should be given vaccine if they are shown to be susceptible to rubella virus by serologic testing. Prevention has been highly effective. Between 1980 and 1996, fewer than 10 cases per year of CRS were reported.

Myxovirus Infections

Mumps Meningitis and Encephalomyelitis

Mumps is a disease caused by a paramyxovirus that has predilection for the salivary glands, mature gonads, pancreas, breast, and the nervous system. It is spread via respiratory droplets. There is only one serotype. Like other paramyxoviruses, mumps is an enveloped virus that develops from the cell surface by a budding process.

Clinical evidence of involvement of the nervous system occurs in the form of a mild meningitis or encephalitis in a small percentage of patients. Other neurologic complications of mumps include encephalomyelitis, myelitis, and peripheral neuritis. During mumps meningitis, virus replicates in choroidal and ependymal cells. It is not clear, however, if the encephalitis results from direct action of the virus or from immune-mediated demyelination (postinfectious encephalomyelitis).

Pathology

The pathology of mumps meningitis and encephalitis has not been clearly elucidated because of the low mortality rate. The pathologic changes are limited to infiltration of the meninges and cerebral blood vessels with lymphocytes and mononuclear cells. The morbid changes in patients with encephalomyelitis include perivenous demyelination with infiltration by lymphocytes and phagocytic microglia. Although pathologic changes are more prominent in white matter, focal areas of neuronal destruction can be seen.

Epidemiology

The incidence of neurologic complications of mumps varies greatly in different epidemics, ranging from a low of less than 1% to a high of about 70%. About two-thirds of patients with mumps parotitis have CSF pleocytosis, but only 50% of those with pleocytosis have CNS symptoms. Conversely, only about 50% of patients with CNS manifestations have parotitis.

Although the two sexes are equally susceptible to mumps, neurologic complications are three times more frequent in males. Children are commonly affected, but epidemics may occur in young adults living under community conditions, such as army camps. Most cases of mumps encephalitis in the United States appear to occur in the late winter and early spring.

Symptoms

In most patients, the symptoms of involvement of the nervous system are those of meningitis (i.e., headache, drowsiness, neck stiffness). These symptoms commonly appear 2 to 10 days after the onset of the parotitis; they occasionally precede the onset of swelling of the salivary glands. These symptoms are benign and disappear within a few days. When encephalitis occurs, it is usually mild.

Complications

Deafness is the most common sequel of mumps. Hearing loss, which is unilateral in more than 65% of patients, may develop gradually, or it may have an abrupt onset accompanied by vertigo and tinnitus. The deafness that follows mumps seems to be due to damage to the membranous labyrinth. Orchitis, oophoritis, pancreatitis, and thyroiditis may also occur. Severe myelitis, polyneuritis, encephalitis, optic neuritis, and other cranial nerve palsies may develop 7 to 15 days after the onset of parotitis, presumably from immune-mediated postinfectious encephalomyelitis.

A few cases of hydrocephalus have been reported in children who have had mumps virus infections. The hydrocephalus seems to be due to aqueductal stenosis induced by mumps virus, replication in aqueductal ependymal cells, and subsequent gliosis.

Laboratory Data

In mumps meningitis, the blood usually shows a relative lymphocytosis and a slight leukopenia. The CSF is under slightly increased pressure. The cell count is increased, usually in the range of 25 to 500 cells/mm^3, but occasionally the counts may be as high as 3,000/mm^3. Lymphocytes usually constitute 90% to 96% of the total, even in CSF with a high cell count, but PMN leukocytes occasionally predominate in the early stages. The degree of pleocytosis is not related to the severity of symptoms, and it may persist for 30 to 60 days. Inclusions of viral nucleocapsid-like material have been recognized by electron microscopic observation of CSF cells from patients with mumps meningitis. The protein content is normal or moderately increased, and mumps-specific oligoclonal immunoglobulin G (IgG) may be present. The sugar content is usually normal but may show a moderate reduction in 5% to 10% of patients. Mumps virus can be recovered from the CSF in a significant number of cases.

Diagnosis

Mumps meningitis is diagnosed on the basis of meningeal symptoms and CSF pleocytosis in a patient with mumps. In patients in whom neurologic symptoms develop during an epidemic of mumps and there is no evidence of involvement of the salivary glands, the diagnosis cannot be made with certainty unless the virus can be recovered from the CSF or there is a significant increase in antibodies in the serum. The presence of IgM antibody in the CSF is diagnostic. Virus can usually be recovered from the saliva, throat, urine, and CSF.

Mumps meningitis must be differentiated from other forms of meningitis, especially tuberculous and fungal, if the CSF glu-

cose is low. A normal sugar content and the absence of organisms in the CSF are important in excluding acute purulent, tuberculous, or fungal meningitis.

Treatment

Since licensure of the live attenuated mumps vaccine in 1967, the incidence of mumps has decreased to less than 5% of the pre-vaccine level. CNS complications (primarily meningitis) from the vaccine, if they occur at all, are rare.

Subacute Measles Encephalitis

Measles virus causes a wide spectrum of neurologic disease ranging from subclinical involvement and acute measles encephalitis (see "Postinfections Encephalomyelitis," below) within days after the onset of a measles exanthem to chronic subacute sclerosing panencephalitis (see below). Toxic encephalopathy and acute infantile hemiplegia rarely occur with measles infections, but these seem to be complications of severe febrile illnesses of childhood and are not specific syndromes caused by measles.

Subacute measles encephalitis (measles inclusion body encephalitis, immunosuppressive measles encephalitis) occurs as an opportunistic infection in immunosuppressed or immunodeficient patients. Most cases have occurred in children, but a few have occurred in adults. Several cases have been reported in patients with no obvious immune defects. A history of measles exposure 1 to 6 months before the onset of neurologic disease can usually be obtained. The disease is characterized by generalized and focal seizures, including epilepsia partialis continua, occasional focal deficits, and a progressive deterioration of mental function leading to coma and death in several weeks to 4 or 5 months. Routine CSF tests are normal. Diagnosis may be difficult because there may not be a history of a rash or even obvious exposure. At the time of presentation, measles antibody may not be present in the serum or CSF. Brain biopsy may be required. Pathology reveals numerous inclusions in neurons and glia with microglial activation, but minimal perivascular inflammation. The role of postexposure immunoglobulin prophylaxis is unclear. In several patients, intravenous ribavirin treatment has resulted in improvement.

Rhabdovirus Infection

Rabies

Rabies (hydrophobia, lyssa, rage) is an acute viral disease of the CNS that is transmitted to humans by the bite of an infected (rabid) animal. It is characterized by a variable incubation period, restlessness, hyperesthesia, convulsions, laryngeal spasms, widespread paralysis, and almost invariably death.

Etiology

Rabies virus is an enveloped bullet-shaped virus that contains single-stranded RNA. Because of its characteristic morphology, rabies has been classified among the *rhabdo* (rod-shaped) viruses. The virus appears capable of infecting every warm-blooded animal. Rabies virus is present in the saliva of infected animals and is transmitted to humans by bites or abrasions of the skin. The bite of a rabid dog or exposure to bats is the usual circumstance, but the disease may be transmitted by cats, wolves, foxes, raccoons, skunks, and other domestic or wild animals. After inoculation, the virus replicates in muscle cells and then travels to the CNS by way of both sensory and motor nerves by axonal transport. After CNS invasion, dissemination of virus is rapid, with early selective involvement of limbic system neurons.

Several cases of airborne transmission of rabies have occurred in spelunkers of bat-infested caves and in laboratory workers. Unusual human-to-human transmission has occurred in two patients who were recipients of corneal transplants.

The incubation period usually varies between 1 and 3 months, with the extremes of 10 days and more than 1 year. In general, the incubation period is directly related to the severity of the bite or bites and their location. The period is shortest when the wound is on the face and longest when on the leg.

Pathology

The pathology of rabies is that of a generalized encephalitis and myelitis. There is perivascular infiltration of the entire CNS with lymphocytes and, to a lesser extent, PMN leukocytes and plasma cells. The perivascular infiltration is usually mild and may be focal or diffuse. Diffuse degenerative changes occur in the neurons. Pathognomonic of the disease is the presence of cytoplasmic eosinophilic inclusions, with central basophilic granules that are found in neurons (Negri bodies) (Fig. 23.2). These are usually found in pyramidal cells of the hippocampus and cerebellar Purkinje cells, but they may be seen in neurons of the cortex and other regions of the CNS, as well as in the spinal ganglia. These inclusions contain rabies virus antigen, as demonstrated by immunofluorescence. Rabies virus nucleocapsids have been found in electron microscopic studies of the inclusions. These inclusion bodies are occasionally absent. There is proliferation of microglia with the formation of rod cells, which may be collected into small nodules (Babès nodules). In cases with a long incubation period, the degenerative changes in neurons may be quite severe with little or no inflammatory reaction.

Incidence

The incidence of rabies is inversely proportional to the control of rabid animals. Wildlife rabies has become an increasingly serious problem in the United States during the 1990s. However, the disease in wildlife is almost nonexistent in Great Britain, where strict animal regulations are enforced. Human rabies is a clinical rarity in the United States and most of the countries of central Europe, but it is still common in southeastern Europe and Asia. There have been 36 cases of human rabies in the United States from 1980 through 1997. About 50% of the cases were imported.

The incidence of the disease in individuals who have been bitten by rabid dogs is low (15%), but it is high (40%) when the bite is inflicted by a rabid wolf. The incidence is highest when the wounds are severe and near the head. It is low when the bite is inflicted through clothing, which cleans some or most of the infecting saliva from the teeth.

Symptoms

Onset is denoted by pain or numbness in the region of the bite in about 50% of patients. Other initial symptoms include fever, apathy, drowsiness, headache, and anorexia. This period of

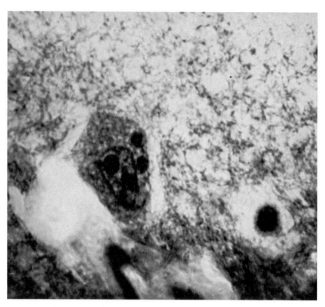

FIG. 23.2. Rabies. Inclusion bodies (Negri bodies) in cytoplasm of a ganglion cell of cerebral cortex.

lethargy passes rapidly into a state of excitability in which all external stimuli are apt to cause localized twitchings or generalized convulsions. There may be delirium with hallucinations and bizarre behavior (thrashing, biting, severe anxiety). A profuse flow of saliva occurs; spasmodic contractions of the pharynx and larynx are precipitated by any attempt to consume liquid or solid food. As a result, the patient violently refuses to accept any liquids, hence, the name hydrophobia. The body temperature is usually elevated and may reach 105° to 107°F (40.6° to 41.7°C) in the terminal stages. The stage of hyperirritability gradually passes into a state of generalized paralysis and coma. Death results from paralysis of respiration.

The disease occasionally begins with paralysis (paralytic form or dumb rabies) without convulsive phenomena or laryngeal spasm. The paralysis is a flaccid type and may start in one limb and spread rapidly to involve the others. The paralysis is more often symmetric than asymmetric. Symptoms and signs of a transverse myelitis may develop.

Laboratory Data

Leukocytosis occurs in the blood, and albumin may be present in the urine. The CSF is under normal pressure, and a lymphocytic pleocytosis is present, varying from five to several hundred cells per cubic millimeter in only about 50% of patients. The protein content is usually increased.

Diagnosis

Rabies is often diagnosed from the appearance of the characteristic symptoms after the bite of a rabid animal. The diagnosis can occasionally be made by fluorescent antibody staining of corneal smears or skin biopsies from the back of the neck, although both false-negative and false-positive results occur. Serum and CSF should also be tested for rabies antibodies. However, negative results for these tests do not rule out the possibility of rabies. The presence of rabies antibodies in the CSF is diagnostic. Virus isolation from the saliva, throat, tears, and CSF should also be attempted, although this is rarely successful. With the recent introduction of PCR techniques, virus detection in these specimens appears to be more successful. The only sure way of making the diagnosis while the patient is alive is by brain biopsy. The differential diagnosis includes all forms of encephalitis and, for the paralytic form of rabies, those viruses causing lower motor neuron paralysis.

Course and Prognosis

The disease is almost always fatal and usually runs its course in 2 to 10 days. Death within 24 hours of the onset of symptoms has been reported. Several cases with recovery have been reported.

Treatment

There is no specific antiviral therapy. Treatment during the encephalitic phase is supportive and, as noted, rarely successful. Specific treatment is entirely prophylactic and includes both passive antibody and vaccine. Passive immunization is by use of human rabies immune globulin. Immune globulin is infiltrated into the wound and given intramuscularly. A full course of active immunization with rabies vaccine should be given.

Arenavirus Infections

Lymphocytic Choriomeningitis

Lymphocytic choriomeningitis (LCM) is a relatively benign viral infection of the meninges and CNS. The clinical features of the disease were described by Wallgren in 1925 (under the term *aseptic meningitis*). The disease is of historic importance because it was the first in which a virus was proved to be the cause of a benign meningitis with a predominance of lymphocytes in the CSF. The role of the virus in human disease was established by Rivers and Scott in 1935, when they isolated it from the CSF of two patients with the clinical syndrome described by Wallgren.

LCM virus is an enveloped RNA virus. It causes less than 0.5% of cases of viral meningitis. Neurologic disease develops in only about 15% of those infected. Mice are the major reservoir of the virus and are implicated as the intermediate host. Both pet and laboratory hamsters have also been a source of infection. Ingestion of food contaminated by animal excreta and wound exposure to contaminated dirt are thought to be the modes of transmission. Human-to-human transmission does not occur. The disease is most common in the winter, when mice move indoors.

Onset of the infection is characterized by fever, headache, malaise, myalgia, and symptoms of upper respiratory infection or pneumonia. In a few patients, meningeal symptoms develop within 1 week after the onset. Occasionally, there is a remission in the prodromal symptoms, and the patient is apparently in good health when meningeal symptoms develop. Severe headache, nausea, and vomiting mark the beginning of neurologic involvement, most often aseptic meningitis. The temperature is moderately elevated (99° to 104°F [37.2° to 40.0°C]). The usual signs of meningitis (stiff neck, Kernig and Brudzinski signs) are present. The parenchyma is occasionally involved (encephalitic or meningoencephalitic forms), but good restoration of function usually occurs. Fewer than 12 deaths have been reported.

In the early influenza-like stages, leukopenia and thrombocytopenia may be seen. Later, the leukocyte count may be elevated with a predominance of PMN leukocytes. The CSF findings are similar to those of other viral causes of meningitis.

A definitive viral diagnosis may be made by recovery of the virus from blood or CSF, but in most patients the diagnosis is made by serology. The differential diagnosis is similar to that of enterovirus infection, the most common cause of viral meningitis.

The duration of the meningeal symptoms varies from 1 to 4 weeks with an average of 3 weeks. The mortality rate is low, and complete recovery is the rule, except in the rare patients with encephalitis in whom residuals of focal lesions in the brain or spinal cord may be present. There is no specific treatment.

Other Arenavirus Infections

Junin (Argentinian hemorrhagic fever) and Machupo (Bolivian hemorrhagic fever) viruses and Lassa fever virus of Africa cause severe hemorrhagic fevers. Although hemorrhage and shock are the usual causes of death from these severe systemic infections, neurologic involvement is not unusual.

Adenovirus Infections

Adenoviruses are nonenveloped (ether-resistant), icosahedral DNA containing viruses of which there are more than 30 serotypes. These viruses were not discovered until 1953 when they were isolated from tissue culture of surgically removed tonsils and adenoids, thus the name. Adenoviruses can be spread by both respiratory and gastrointestinal routes and cause a variety of clinical syndromes. Respiratory infection is most often seen, manifested by coryza, pharyngitis, and, at times, pneumonia. Pharyngoconjunctival fever, epidemic keratoconjunctivitis, pertussis-like syndrome, and hemorrhagic cystitis are other manifestations. Most infections occur in children; about 50% of these infections are asymptomatic. Epidemics of respiratory diseases have occurred among military personnel. Opportunistic infections have occurred in both adults and children.

Neurologic involvement has occurred mostly in children as an encephalitis or meningoencephalitis and is quite rare. Only a few pathologic studies have been performed, and the encephalitis appears to be of the primary type with virus invasion of the brain. Histologic changes include perivascular cuffing and mononuclear cell parenchyma infiltrates, but in some patients, little or no inflammation is seen. Virus has been isolated from the brain and CSF in several patients. The encephalitis is usually of moderate to severe intensity with meningism, lethargy, confusion, coma, and convulsions. Ataxia has also been reported. Death occurs in up to 30% of patients. CSF pleocytosis often, but not always, occurs and can be PMN or mononuclear. The protein content may be normal or elevated. Diagnosis can be made by serology or by isolation of virus from the CSF, throat, respiratory secretions, and feces. There is no specific treatment.

Herpesvirus Infections

The herpesvirus group is composed of DNA-containing viruses that have a lipid envelope and multiply in the cell nucleus. Members of this group share the common feature of establishing latent infections. Herpesviruses may remain quiescent for long periods of time, being demonstrable only sporadically or not at all until a stimulus triggers reactivated infection. Within cells, accumulations of virus particles can often be recognized in the nucleus in the form of acidophilic inclusion bodies. There are at present eight recognized members of the human herpesvirus family: herpes simplex virus (HSV) types 1 and 2, varicella-zoster virus (VZV), Epstein-Barr virus (EBV), cytomegalovirus (CMV), human herpesvirus 6 (HHV-6), HHV-7, and HHV-8, also known as Kaposi sarcoma herpesvirus. All of these viruses are capable of causing neurologic disease, but only a few cases have been reported in association with HHV-7 and HHV-8.

Herpes Simplex Encephalitis

Encephalitis caused by HSV is the single most important cause of fatal sporadic encephalitis in the United States. Early diagnosis is crucial because there is effective antiviral treatment.

Etiology

Two antigenic types of HSV are distinguished by serologic testing. Type 1 strains (HSV-1) are responsible for almost all cases of HSV encephalitis in adults and cause oral herpes. Type 2 strains (HSV-2) cause genital disease. In the neonatal period, HSV-2 encephalitis occurs as part of a disseminated infection or as localized disease acquired during delivery. In adults, HSV-2 is spread by venereal transmission and causes aseptic meningitis.

Pathogenesis

HSV-1 is transmitted by respiratory or salivary contact. Primary infection usually occurs in childhood or adolescence. It is usually subclinical or may present as stomatitis, pharyngitis, or respiratory disease. About 50% of the population has antibody to HSV-1 by age 15 years, whereas 50% to 90% of adults have antibody, depending on socioeconomic status. HSV-1 encephalitis can occur at any age, but more than 50% of cases occur in patients older than 20 years. This finding suggests that encephalitis most often occurs from endogenous reactivation of virus rather than from primary infection. Neurologic involvement is a rare complication of reactivation. During the primary infection, virus becomes latent in the trigeminal ganglia. Years later, nonspecific stimuli cause reactivation, which is usually manifested as herpes labialis (cold sores). Presumably, virus can reach the brain through branches of the trigeminal nerve to the basal meninges, resulting in localization of the encephalitis to the temporal and orbital frontal lobes. Alternatively, serologic studies suggest that about 25% of cases of HSV-1 encephalitis occur as part of a primary infection. Experimental studies indicate that this could occur by spread of virus across the olfactory bulbs to the orbital frontal lobes and subsequently the temporal lobes. The encephalitis is sporadic without seasonal variations. HSV-1 encephalitis rarely occurs as an opportunistic infection in immunocompromised hosts.

Except when infantile infection occurs at delivery, HSV-2 is spread by sexual contact. Thus, primary infection usually occurs during the late teenage or early adult years. As noted previously,

TABLE 23.3. MANIFESTATIONS OF HERPES SIMPLEX ENCEPHALITIS AT PRESENTATION

	NIAID Collaborative Study[a]	Swedish Study[b]
Symptoms		
Altered consciousness	97% (109/112)	100% (53/53)
Fever	90% (101/112)	100% (53/53)
Headache	81% (89/110)	74% (39/53)
Seizures	67% (73/109)	—
Vomiting	46% (51/111)	38% (20/53)
Hemiparesis	33% (33/100)	—
Memory loss	24% (14/59)	—
Signs		
Fever	92% (101/110)	—
Personality alteration (confusion, disorientation)	85% (69/81)	57% (30/53)
Dysphasia	76% (58/76)	36% (19/53)
Autonomic dysfunction	60% (54/88)	—
Ataxia	40% (22/55)	—
Hemiparesis	38% (41/107)	40% (21/33)
Seizures	38% (43/112)	62% (33/53)
Focal	(28/43)	—
Generalized	(10/43)	—
Both	(5/43)	—
Cranial nerves deficits	32% (34/105)	—
Papilledema	14% (16/111)	—

[a]Data from Whitley, et al. Herpes simplex encephalitis: vidarabine versus acyclovir therapy. *N Engl J Med* 1986;314:144–149.
[b]Data from Skoldenberg, et al. Acyclovir vs. vidarobine in herpes simplex encephalitis: randomised multicentre study in consecutive Swedish patients. *Lancet* 1984;2:707–711.

HSV-2 causes aseptic meningitis in adults, which probably occurs as part of the primary infection. As with HSV-1, opportunistic infections may also occur in immunocompromised patients.

Pathology

In fatal cases, intense meningitis and widespread destructive changes occur in the brain parenchyma. Necrotic, inflammatory, or hemorrhagic lesions may be found. These lesions are maximal, most often in the frontal and temporal lobes. There is often an unusual degree of cerebral edema accompanying the necrotic lesions. Eosinophilic intranuclear inclusion bodies (Cowdry type A inclusions) are present in neurons. These inclusions containing herpesvirus particles are recognized on electron microscopic examination.

Symptoms and Signs

The most common early manifestations are fever, headache, and altered consciousness and personality (see Table 23.3). Onset is most often abrupt and may be ushered in by major motor or focal seizures. The encephalitis may evolve more slowly, however, with aphasia or mental changes preceding more severe neurologic signs. Most patients have a temperature between 101° and 104°F (38.4° and 40.0°C) at the time of admission. Nuchal rigidity or other signs of meningeal irritation are often found. Mental deficits include confusion and personality changes varying from withdrawal to agitation with hallucinations. A progres-

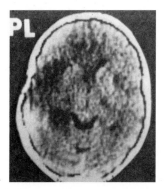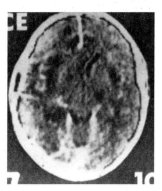

A, B

FIG. 23.3. Herpes simplex encephalitis. **A:** Axial CT on day 10 shows a low-density lesion in the right temporal amd basal frontal lobes. **B:** Corresponding contrast-enhanced CT shows gyral enhancement in the sylvian fissure and insular regions, which is greater on the right. An abnormal CT is not usually seen until day 6 or 7 after the onset of manifestations. Eventually, a majority of scans show gyral enhancement in the sylvian fissure area. These findings should raise the suspicion of an underlying infectious lesion such as herpes, early infarction from emboli or vasculitis, or metastatic tumors. (From Davis JM, et al. Computed tomography of herpes simplex encephalitis with clinicopathological correlation. *Radiology* 1978;129:409–417; with permission.)

Laboratory Data

There is a moderate leukocytosis in the blood. The CSF pressure may be moderately or greatly increased. Pleocytosis in the CSF varies from less than 10 to 1,000 cells/mm^3; lymphocytes usually predominate, but occasionally PMN leukocytes may predominate early in the infection, followed by a shift to lymphocytes. Red blood cells are frequently seen, but their presence or absence is not diagnostic. The CSF sugar content is usually normal but may be low. Virus is rarely recovered from the CSF. In 5% to 10% of patients, the initial CSF examination is normal.

The electroencephalogram (EEG) and MRI are the most likely diagnostic studies to be abnormal at onset and during the first week of infection. The EEG is usually abnormal (about 80% in biopsy-proven cases) with diffuse slowing or focal changes over temporal areas; periodic complexes against a slow-wave background may be seen. CT may demonstrate low-density abnormality, mass effect, or linear contrast enhancement in more than 90% of patients, but it is often entirely normal during the first week of disease (Fig. 23.3). Thus, CT cannot be relied on for early diagnosis. MRI often reveals focality during the first week of disease when the CT scan is normal (Fig. 23.4).

Diagnosis

Because HSV encephalitis has a high mortality rate and the outcome of therapy is affected by the patient's level of consciousness and neurologic deficits, diagnostic measures leading to a presumptive diagnosis should be initiated as soon as possible. Presumptive diagnosis for treatment can be made based on clinical, CT, CSF, EEG, and MRI findings. Definitive diagnosis can be established only by recovery of virus from the CSF (rare) or brain, demonstration of viral DNA in the CSF or brain by PCR amplification, or the finding of viral antigen in the brain. Be-

sive course ensues within hours to several days, with an increasing impairment of consciousness and the development of focal neurologic signs. Rarely, the course may be subacute or chronic, lasting several months. Focal signs, such as hemiplegia, hemisensory loss, focal seizures, and ataxia, are considered distinguishing features of herpes encephalitis but are seen in less than 50% of affected patients on initial examination. Herpetic skin lesions are seen in only a few patients but are also seen with other diseases. A history of cold sores is not helpful because the incidence is similar to that of the general population.

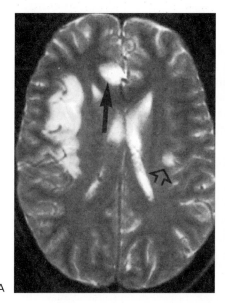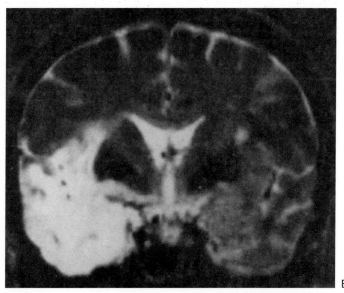

A

B

FIG. 23.4. Herpes simplex encephalitis. **A:** T2-weighted axial MRI reveals high signal intensity in the right insular cortex, medial right frontal cortex *(solid arrow)*, and left insular cortex *(open arrow)*. (From Runge VM. *Magnetic resaonance imaging of the brain.* Philadelphia: JB Lippincott Co, 1994:190; with permission.) **B:** T2-weighted coronal MRI shows increased signal in the left temporal lobe and early involvement of the right side. (From Schroth et al., l987; with permission.) An abnormal MR image is usually seen by day 1 or 2 after the onset of manifestations. Coronal images are the most useful for detecting the herpes simplex lesions.

cause patients may show a rise in antibody titer with recurrent HSV cutaneous lesions or with inapparent infection, a fourfold rise in the serum antibody titer to herpesvirus may occur in patients with encephalitis from other causes. The appearance of herpes antibodies in the CSF is a useful retrospective diagnostic test, but these antibodies occur too late in the disease to aid in therapy.

The differential diagnosis of HSV-1 encephalitis includes other viral and postinfectious encephalitides; bacterial, fungal, and parasitic infections; and tumors. Brain abscess is often the most difficult diagnosis to exclude. Before the advent of MRI, about 25% of biopsy-negative patients had another treatable disease.

Prognosis and Treatment

Without treatment, the disease is fatal in about 70% to 80% of patients, and patients who survive the acute disease are usually left with severe neurologic residuals. Measures to decrease life-threatening brain edema, including the administration of corticosteroids, are indicated. Vidarabine (Vira-A), a DNA polymerase inhibitor, has been demonstrated to decrease mortality to 44% at 6 months compared to 70% for patients receiving placebo. Subsequently, acyclovir was demonstrated to be more efficacious than vidarabine in two controlled trials. In the National Institute of Allergy and Infectious Disease study, acyclovir reduced mortality to 28% compared to 55% for vidarabine at 18 months. It selectively inhibits virus-specific polymerase, has less toxicity than vidarabine, and is now the drug of choice. Outcome depends on patient age, level of consciousness, and the rapidity with which treatment is instituted. After presumptive diagnosis, acyclovir treatment should be instituted even if MRI cannot be performed until the next day. If deterioration in the clinical course occurs over the next 48 to 72 hours, brain biopsy is indicated. Because relapses have occurred after a 10-day treatment regimen, a 14-day course is now recommended.

Herpes Zoster

Herpes zoster (shingles) is a viral disease that produces inflammatory lesions in the posterior root ganglia and is characterized clinically by pain and a skin eruption in the distribution of the affected ganglia. Involvement of motor roots or the CNS occurs in a small percentage of patients.

Etiology

The virus of herpes zoster is identical to VZV, the causative agent of chickenpox (varicella). VZV is a large, enveloped, DNA-containing virus that has the same structure as that of other herpesviruses. Children can catch chickenpox from exposure to adults with shingles, but adults are subject to herpes zoster only if they have had chickenpox earlier in life. The CNS complications (acute cerebellar ataxia, encephalitis, myelitis, meningitis) of varicella are thought to occur by a postinfectious autoimmune mechanism (see "Acute Disseminated Encephalomyelitis" below), although direct viral invasion may occur less frequently. Epidemiologic considerations led Hope-Simpson to speculate that zoster infection is a reactivation of latent VZV originally acquired in a childhood attack of chickenpox. Herpes zoster fre-

quently occurs in connection with systemic infections, immunosuppressive therapy, and localized lesions of the spine or nerve roots (e.g., acute meningitides, tuberculosis, Hodgkin disease, metastatic carcinoma, trauma to the spine).

Pathology

Although symptoms are usually confined to the distribution of one or two sensory roots, the pathologic changes are usually more widespread. The affected ganglia of the spinal or cranial nerve roots are swollen and inflamed. The inflammatory reaction is chiefly of a lymphocytic nature, but a few PMN leukocytes or plasma cells may also be present. The inflammatory process commonly extends to the meninges and into the root entry zone (posterior poliomyelitis). Not infrequently, some inflammatory reaction occurs in the ventral horn and in the perivascular space of the white matter of the spinal cord. The pathologic changes in the ganglia of the cranial nerves and in the brainstem are similar to those in the spinal root and spinal cord.

Incidence

Herpes zoster is a relatively common disease with an incidence that varies from 1 to 5 cases per 1,000 people each year. Rates are higher in patients with malignancies and in those receiving immunosuppressive therapy. Symptoms of involvement of the nervous system, with the exception of pain, are rare, only occurring in about 10% of patients. Zoster is more common in middle or later life.

Symptoms and Signs

The initial symptom is usually a neuralgic pain or dysesthesia in the distribution of the affected root. The pain is followed in 3 to 4 days by reddening of the skin and the appearance of clusters of vesicles in part of the area supplied by the affected roots. These vesicles, which contain clear fluid, may be discrete or may coalesce. Within 10 days to 2 weeks, the vesicles are covered with a scab, which after desquamation leaves a pigmented scar. These scars are usually replaced by normally colored skin in the ensuing months. Permanent scarring may occur if there is ulceration or secondary infection of the vesicles. Coincidental to the eruption is adenopathy that is usually painless.

Herpes zoster is primarily an infection of the spinal ganglia, but the cranial ganglia are affected in about 20% of patients. The thoracic, lumbar, cervical, and sacral segments are involved in descending order of frequency. Involvement is almost always unilateral.

Among the less common symptoms are impairment of cutaneous sensation and muscle weakness in the distribution of the affected root, malaise, fever, headache, neck stiffness, and confusion. The latter symptoms indicate involvement of the meninges. Involvement of the cervical or lumbar segments may be accompanied by weakness and, occasionally, subsequent atrophy of isolated muscle groups in the arm or leg (zoster paresis). The rare involvement of sacral segments may result in bladder paralysis with urinary retention or incontinence. Oculomotor palsies may also occur.

Ophthalmic Zoster. Involvement of the trigeminal ganglion occurs in about 20% of patients. Any division of the ganglion may be involved, but the first division (ophthalmic) is by far the most commonly affected. The seriousness of the involvement of this ganglion is due to the changes that develop in the eyes secondary to panophthalmitis or scarring of the cornea. There may be a temporary or permanent paresis of the muscles supplied by the oculomotor nerves as a complication of ophthalmic zoster.

Geniculate Herpes. Otic zoster with involvement of the geniculate ganglion (Ramsay Hunt syndrome), although rare, assumes prominence because of paralysis of the facial muscles. The rash is usually confined to the tympanic membrane and the external auditory canal. It may spread to involve the outer surface of the lobe of the ear, and when it is combined with cervical involvement, vesicles are found on portions of the neck. Loss of taste over the anterior two-thirds of the tongue occurs in more than 50% of patients. Partial or complete recovery is the rule. Involvement of the ganglia of Corti and Scarpa is accompanied by tinnitus, vertigo, nausea, and loss of hearing.

Complications
Although the CSF shows a lymphocytic pleocytosis, meningeal symptoms are uncommon. Signs of involvement of the tracts of the spinal cord in the form of a Brown-Séquard syndrome or a transverse or ascending *myelitis* have occurred. Mental confusion, ataxia, and focal cerebral symptoms have been attributed to involvement of the brain by VZV (herpes zoster *encephalitis*). *Polyneuritis* of the so-called infectious or Guillain-Barré type has been reported as a sequela of herpes zoster. Involvement of the anterior roots may result in zoster paresis. A more recently recognized complication of ophthalmic zoster is acute contralateral hemiplegia and at times other ipsilateral hemispheral deficits, such as aphasia, that occur several weeks to several months later (herpes zoster ophthalmicus with delayed contralateral hemiparesis). An *arteritis,* apparently with viral invasion, develops in the carotid and other vessels ipsilateral to the zoster ophthalmicus, resulting in hemispheral infarction.

Postherpetic neuralgia is most common in elderly debilitated patients and chiefly affects the ophthalmic or intercostal nerves. The pains are persistent, sharp, and shooting in nature. The skin is sensitive to touch. These pains may persist for months or years and are often refractory to all forms of treatment.

Laboratory Data
The abnormalities in the laboratory findings are confined to the CSF. Even in uncomplicated herpes zoster, there is an inconstant lymphocytic pleocytosis, which may be found before the onset of the rash. The CSF may be normal in patients with symptoms of involvement of only one thoracic segment, but it is usually abnormal when the cranial ganglia are involved or when paralysis or other neurologic signs is present. The cell count varies from 10 to several hundred per cubic millimeter, with lymphocytes as the predominating cell type. The protein content is normal or moderately increased; the sugar content is normal.

Diagnosis
Herpes zoster is diagnosed without difficulty when the characteristic rash is present. In the preeruptive stage, the pain may lead to the erroneous diagnosis of disease of the abdominal or thoracic viscera. The possibility of herpes zoster should be considered in all patients with root pains of sudden onset that have existed for less than 4 days. Difficulties in diagnosis may also be encountered when the vesicles are widespread or when they are scant or entirely absent (zoster sine herpete). It is possible that herpes zoster may cause intercostal neuralgia or facial palsy without any cutaneous eruption, but a careful search usually reveals a few vesicles.

If necessary, VZV may be cultured from vesicular fluid, detected by electron microscopic examination of vesicular fluid, and identified by immunohistochemical staining of cells from vesicular scrapings. PCR amplification techniques should become available for detecting viral DNA in vesicular fluid and CSF.

Treatment
There is still no effective means of preventing herpes zoster. Treatment of uncomplicated zoster includes only the use of analgesics and nonspecific topical medications for the rash. Use of topical antiviral agents is of questionable benefit. Although antibiotics have no effect on the virus, they may be indicated to control secondary infection. Systemic acyclovir (oral or intravenous) has been the agent of choice for the treatment of acute herpes zoster. Several new antiviral agents (valacyclovir [Valtrex], famciclovir) have also been shown to decrease pain, virus shedding, and healing time of acute herpes zoster. In addition, famciclovir significantly reduced the duration of postherpetic neuralgia. All of these agents decrease viral dissemination and its complications. For this reason, they are indicated for systemic complications, especially in immunosuppressed patients, and for zoster encephalomyelitis and arteritis. Because the arteritis may be due to an allergic response, it has been treated with a combination of corticosteroids and an antiviral agent. Zoster immune globulin is useful in prophylaxis of varicella in immunosuppressed children, but it is not helpful for zoster.

Postherpetic neuralgia is difficult to treat. It is refractory to the usual analgesics. Sectioning the affected posterior roots is usually not successful in relieving pain. The efficacy of corticosteroids is minimal (decreases in duration of acute neuritis and time to healing, but not in the incidence or duration of postherpetic neuralgia). Their use would seem risky because of immunosuppression and possible virus dissemination. Amitriptyline, other tricyclic antidepressants, and anticonvulsants (carbamazepine [Tegretol], phenytoin sodium [Dilantin], gabapentin [Neurontin]) are the mainstays of therapy.

Cytomegalovirus Infection

Cytomegalic inclusion body disease is an infection that occurs *in utero* by transplacental transmission. The responsible agent is CMV, a member of the herpesvirus family. CMV infection results in the appearance of large, swollen cells that often contain large eosinophilic intranuclear and cytoplasmic inclusions.

Intrauterine infection of the nervous system may result in stillbirth or prematurity. The cerebrum is affected by a granulomatous encephalitis with extensive subependymal calcification. Hydrocephalus, hydranencephaly, microcephaly, cerebellar hypoplasia, or other types of developmental defects of the brain may be found. Convulsive seizures, focal neurologic signs, and mental retardation are common in infants who survive (Table 23.4). Jaundice with hepatosplenomegaly, purpuric lesions, and hemolytic anemia may be present. Periventricular calcification is often seen in radiographs of the skull. Affected infants often succumb in the neonatal period, but prolonged periods of survival are possible. Subclinical or silent congenital infections may result in deafness and developmental abnormalities. There may also be progressive nervous system damage and, presumably, a persistent infection for months after birth.

CMV infections may also occur in adults (see Table 23.4), producing a mononucleosis-like syndrome, but involvement of the nervous system is uncommon in this acute adult form of the disease. CNS infection in immunodeficient patients, including those with acquired immunodeficiency syndrome (AIDS), is probably more frequent, however. CNS involvement in immunocompromised patients is often asymptomatic, although fa-

TABLE 23.4. CYTOMEGALOVIRUS NEUROLOGIC INFECTIONS

Diseases and features	Host and frequency
Cytomegalic inclusion body disease	Neonates, congenital disease; rare

Encephalitis
  Microcephaly
  Seizures
  Mental retardation
  Periventricular calcifications
  Disseminated disease	

Encephalitis/ventriculitis
  Subacute course
  Progressive mental status changes
  Disseminated disease in immunocompromised-compromised patients
  MRI: periventricular hyperintensities, meningeal enhancement
	Immunocompromised patients (described primarily in AIDS patients); uncommon
	Immunocompetent patients; rare

Polyradiculitis/polyradiculomyelitis
  Pain and paresthesia in legs and perineum
  Sacral hypesthesia
  Urinary retention
  Subacute ascending hypotonic paraparesis
  Eventually ascends to cause myelitis
  CSF: pleocytosis (PMNs > lymphocytes), low glucose, high protein level,
  CMV positive by culture or PCR
  Usually disseminated disease
  MRI: lumbosacral leptomeningeal enhancement
	Immunocompromised patients (described only in AIDS patients); common

Multifocal neuropathy
  Markedly asymmetric
  Numbness, painful paresthesia for months, followed by sensorimotor neuropathy
  Usually disseminated disease
  CMV positive in CSF by culture or PCR
	Immunocompromised patients (described only in AIDS); uncommon

From Jubelt B. Ropka S. Infectious diseases of the nervous system. In: Rosenberg RN, ed., *Atlas of Clinical Neurology*. Philadelphia: Current Medicine, 1998:12.1–12.71; with permission.

tal encephalitis may occur. The encephalitis has a subacute or chronic course and is clinically indistinguishable from HIV encephalitis (HIV dementia). MRI demonstrates either diffuse or focal white matter abnormalities in about 25% of patients. CMV infection has also been implicated as a cause of both a subacute polyradiculomyelopathy and a multifocal neuropathy that have been seen only in AIDS patients. The polyradiculomyelopathy has a subacute onset of leg weakness and numbness leading to a flaccid paraplegia.

For cytomegalic inclusion body disease, CMV can be recovered from urine, saliva, or liver biopsy specimens. Complement-fixation and neutralization tests are available. A presumptive diagnosis can be made by finding typical cytomegalic cells in stained preparations of urinary sediment or saliva.

In adult infections, virus may be cultured from extraneural sites. Antibody testing is usually not helpful in immunodeficient patients. CMV cannot be cultured from the CSF; PCR amplification is the best microbiologic test. In polyradiculomyelopathy, PMN cells are often seen in the CSF, and there may be meningeal enhancement on MRI.

Both ganciclovir and foscarnet have been reported to be beneficial for some postnatally acquired infections. Recent case reports have noted successful treatment with cidofovir.

Epstein-Barr Virus Infection

Infectious mononucleosis (glandular fever) is a systemic disease of viral origin with involvement of the lymph nodes, spleen, liver, skin, and, occasionally, the CNS. It occurs sporadically and in small epidemics. It is most common in children and young adults. The usual symptoms and signs are headache, malaise, sore throat, fever, enlargement of the lymph nodes in the cervical region, occasionally enlargement of the spleen, and changes in the blood. Unusual manifestations include a cutaneous rash, jaundice, and symptoms of involvement of the nervous system.

Although neurologic complications rank first as a cause of death, there have been few autopsy studies of the brain in fatal cases of infectious mononucleosis. Acute cortical inflammation similar to that seen in other viral infections has been observed. Atypical cells, probably lymphocytes, have been found in the inflammatory exudate.

The exact incidence of involvement of the nervous system is unknown, but it is probably less than 1%. A lymphocytic pleocytosis in the CSF may be found in the absence of any neurologic symptoms or signs. Severe headache and neck stiffness may be the initial or only symptoms of cerebral involvement (aseptic meningitis). Signs of encephalitis (delirium, convulsions, coma, and focal deficits) are rare manifestations. Optic neuritis, paralysis of the facial and other cranial nerves, acute autonomic neuropathy, infectious polyneuritis (Guillain-Barré syndrome), and transverse myelitis have been reported in a few patients. Acute cerebellar ataxia has also been associated with infectious mononucleosis.

CNS manifestations may appear early in the course of the disease in the absence of any other findings, but usually occur 1 to 3 weeks after onset. The prognosis for EBV encephalitis is excellent with few fatalities and minimal residua.

In the laboratory examination, the important findings are leukocytosis in the blood with an increase in lymphocytes and the appearance of abnormal mononuclear cells (atypical lymphocytes). Liver function tests are often abnormal, and heterophil antibody is present in 90% of patients. With involvement of the meninges, the CSF shows a lymphocytic pleocytosis (10 to 600 cells/mm^3) with or without a slight increase in protein content. The sugar content is normal, and CSF serologic tests for syphilis are negative. False-positive tests for syphilis are occasionally obtained on the serum.

The diagnosis is established by the appearance of neurologic symptoms in patients with other manifestations of the disease. The differential diagnosis includes other viral diseases that cause a lymphocytic meningeal reaction. The diagnosis can be made by a study of the blood, the heterophil antibody reaction, and measurement of specific antibodies to EBV antigens. At times, EBV can be isolated from the oropharynx. MRI abnormalities have been reported, with both gray and white matter lesions, in about 25% of patients.

There is no specific therapy. Treatment with steroids may be indicated in certain patients with severe pharyngotonsillitis or other complications.

Human Herpesvirus-6 Infection

HHV-6 was first isolated from AIDS patients in 1986. Two years later it was shown to be the etiologic agent for roseola infantum (exanthema subitum, sixth disease). HHV-6 has also been found to cause opportunistic CNS disease in immunocompromised individuals.

Roseola is an acute, self-limited disease of infants and children. It is caused by an HHV-6 primary infection. It begins with abrupt onset of high fever, lasting 3 to 4 days. Febrile convulsions commonly occur with a high fever. As the temperature rapidly falls, a transient maculopapular rash appears on the neck and trunk. The rash fades in 1 to 3 days. Other physical findings are minimal but include mild injection of the pharynx and tympanic membranes and postoccipital and postauricular lymphadenopathy.

The most common CNS complication of roseola is febrile seizures, which occur in up to one-third of patients. Several studies suggest that recurrent seizures may develop in a small percentage of these patients. Meningoencephalitis has also occurred as a complication of roseola. Manifestations include persistent fever, a depressed level of consciousness, and seizures. The prognosis is variable. There is usually a mild mononuclear pleocytosis in the CSF. Less frequently, encephalopathy (no CSF pleocytosis) and demyelination have been reported.

Recurrent HHV-6 infections have been associated with a range of illnesses (pneumonia, bone marrow suppression, possibly lymphoma and encephalitis) in immunocompromised patients. The encephalitis occurring in these patients is usually more severe than that seen during roseola, and is more likely to result in death.

Diagnosis

During roseola, initially the peripheral white blood cell count may be slightly elevated, but with disease progression, leukopenia is invariably present. This finding, along with the characteristic presentation and course, makes a presumptive diagnosis of roseola. Diagnosis is confirmed by isolation of virus (throat, saliva, blood) and seroconversion. Since HHV-6 appears to be latent in the brain, it is not clear what role CSF PCR amplification and CSF antibody assays will have in diagnosis. The diagnosis of reactivated infection is also confirmed by virus isolation and, at times, with a concomitant fourfold rise in IgG titer.

Treatment

For roseola, antipyretics are important for controlling the fever, which should decrease the incidence of febrile seizures. Anticonvulsants may be needed for recurrent seizures. Systemic antiviral agents should be used for CNS or systemic disease occurrence with roseola or with reactivation. *In vitro,* HHV-6 resembles CMV in its antiviral susceptibilities. It is resistant to acyclovir but susceptible to ganciclovir and foscarnet. No clinical trials have been undertaken.

Acute Disseminated Encephalomyelitis

Acute disseminated encephalomyelitis (ADE) may occur in the course of various infections, particularly the acute exanthematous diseases of childhood, and following vaccinations; thus, ADE is also known by the terms *post-* or *parainfectious encepholomyelitis* (PIE) and *postvaccinal encephalomyelitis.* The clinical symptoms and the pathologic changes are similar in all of these cases, regardless of the nature of the precipitating infection or vaccination.

Etiology and Pathogenesis

The list of diseases that may be accompanied or followed by signs and symptoms of an encephalomyelitis is probably not yet complete, but it includes measles, rubella, varicella, smallpox, mumps, influenza, parainfluenza, infectious mononucleosis, typhoid, mycoplasmal infections, and upper respiratory and other obscure febrile diseases, as well as vaccination against measles, mumps, rubella, influenza, and rabies. Reactions in the nervous system may also follow inoculations with typhoid vaccine and with sera, particularly that against tetanus. In these latter conditions, the clinical picture is more likely to be that of a mononeuritis or generalized polyneuritis.

The pathogenesis of ADE is not known. Because virus is not usually isolated from the nervous system of patients, an allergic or autoimmune reaction appears to be most likely. Presumably, the virus triggers an immune-mediated reaction against CNS myelin, causing a disease similar to experimental allergic encephalomyelitis. This could possibly involve an extraneural interaction of a virus with the immune system without viral invasion of the nervous system.

Pathology

Little or no change occurs in the external appearance of the brain or spinal cord. On sectioning, many small yellowish-red lesions are present in the white matter of the cerebrum, cerebellum, brainstem, and spinal cord. The characteristic feature of these lesions is a loss of myelin, with relative sparing of the axis cylinders. Brain lesions are oval or round and usually surround a distended vein. Lesions are usually found in large numbers in almost all parts of the CNS, but in some cases they may be concentrated in the white matter of the cerebrum, while in others the cerebellum, brainstem, or spinal cord may be most severely affected. On microscopic examination, there is perivenular lymphocytic and mononuclear cell infiltration and demyelination. On myelin-stained specimens, there is destruction of myelin sheaths within the lesions, with a fairly sharp margin between the affected and normal areas. Axis cylinders are affected secondarily to a much lesser extent than the myelin sheaths. Phagocytic microglial cells may also be found within lesions and in perivascular spaces of adjacent vessels. Although lesions are concentrated in the white matter, a few patches may be found in the gray matter. Occasionally, nerve cells in these areas may be destroyed or may show various degenerative changes. ADE and PIE are monophasic diseases, as lesions have a similar age of onset. *Acute hemorrhagic leukoencephalitis* appears to be a fulminant form of ADE or PIE. Pathologic lesions are similar to those of ADE with the addition of microscopic hemorrhages and perivascular PMN cell infiltrates.

Epidemiology

Previously, smallpox vaccination (vaccinia virus) was one of the more frequent causes of PIE or postvaccinal encephalomyelitis. The exact frequency has not been accurately established because of the wide range reported, varying from more than 1 case per 100 to less than 1 case per 100,000 vaccinees. Because smallpox has apparently been eradicated as a natural disease, vaccination is no longer recommended. Thus, vaccinia virus is no longer a common cause of PIE. The smallpox virus (variola virus) also probably caused this syndrome in the past.

The incidence of encephalomyelitis following vaccination against rabies with the old nerve-tissue-prepared vaccines ranged as high as 1 in 600 persons, with a mortality rate of 10% to 25%. With the duck-embryo vaccine, this complication has decreased to approximately 1 in 33,000 recipients. This complication has rarely been reported with the new human diploid cell vaccine (several cases); there have also been a few cases of Guillain-Barré syndrome.

Damage to the nervous system with the acute exanthems occurs most commonly following measles, for which the incidence is approximately 1 in 1,000 persons. In countries using measles vaccination, however, measles is no longer a common cause of PIE. The incidence following measles vaccine is only about 1 in 1 million recipients. PIE followed rubella or mumps much less frequently than it did natural measles, but even this occurrence has decreased with vaccination. VZV infections are now probably the more common cause of PIE, although the exact incidence is not known. Nonspecific upper respiratory infections are probably the most common overall cause.

Symptoms and Signs

The symptoms and signs of ADE or PIE are related to the portion of the nervous system that is most severely damaged. Because any portion of the nervous system may be affected, it is not surprising that variable clinical syndromes may occur. In some cases, there are signs and symptoms of generalized involvement (ADE), but one or more portions of the neuraxis may suffer the brunt of the damage, resulting in various clear-cut clinical syndromes: meningeal, encephalitic, brainstem, cerebellar, spinal cord, or neuritic.

Symptoms of involvement of the meninges (headaches, neck stiffness) are common early in the course of all types. In some cases, no further symptoms are present. In others, these initial symptoms and signs may be followed by evidence of damage to the cerebrum. In this *encephalitic form,* there may be convulsions, stupor, coma, hemiplegia, aphasia, or other signs of focal cerebral involvement. Cranial nerve palsies, especially *optic neuritis,* or signs and symptoms of cerebellar dysfunction predominate in a few cases. *Acute cerebellar ataxia* constitutes about 50% of cases of PIE following varicella, whereas cerebral and spinal involvement are more common with measles and vaccinia.

Overall, spinal cord involvement is more common than involvement of either the brainstem or cerebellum. This may be disseminated in the cord or, more commonly, may take the form of an *acute transverse myelitis* or *acute transverse myelopathy* (ATM), a syndrome of multiple causes. It may be acute, developing over hours to several days, or subacute, developing over 1 to 2 weeks. The most common picture is a transverse myelitis interrupting both motor and sensory tracts at one level, usually thoracic. It usually begins with localized back or radicular pain followed by abrupt onset of bilateral paresthesia in the legs, an ascending sensory level, and a paraparesis that often progresses to paraplegia. Urinary bladder and bowel involvement occurs early and is prominent. In general, patients with rapid progression and flaccidity below the level of the lesion have the worst prognosis. The syndrome may also take the form of an ascending myelitis, a diffuse or patchy myelitis, or a partial myelitis (Brown-Séquard syndrome, anterior spinal artery distribution lesion, posterior column myelopathy). Only about 25% to 33% of cases of ATM are caused by viral infections or vaccinations via a demyelinating process. Less frequently, a complete transverse myelitis may result from direct virus invasion of the cord (e.g., poliovirus or herpesviruses). Other less frequent causes of ATM include systemic lupus erythematosus, other vasculitides, other causes of spinal cord infarction, multiple sclerosis, and trauma. Idiopathic ATM is most frequent. Obviously, it is important to exclude cord compression by epidural abscess or tumor, intrinsic cord bacterial or fungal infections, tumors, and treatable vascular diseases.

Other parainfectious syndromes may also be seen. Acute toxic encephalopathy and Reye syndrome are seen more frequently after varicella, influenza, and rubella. Peripheral nerve involvement with an acute ascending paralysis of the Guillain-Barré type is more frequent with rabies vaccine, especially with the older preparations, and after influenza and upper respiratory infections. Brachial neuritis is the usual neurologic complication of antitetanus vaccine.

Laboratory Studies

The CSF pressure may be slightly elevated. There is a mild to moderate increase in white cells (15 to 250 cells/mm^3), with lymphocytes as the predominating cell type. The protein content is normal or slightly elevated (35 to 150 mg/dL); the sugar content is within normal limits. The CSF myelin basic protein level is usually increased. The EEG is abnormal in most patients, usually with slow frequency of 4 to 6 Hz and high voltage. The abnormalities are usually generalized and symmetric, but focal or unilateral changes may be found. The abnormalities persist for several weeks after apparent clinical recovery. Persisting abnormalities correlate well with permanent neurologic damage or convulsive disorders. After several days, CT may show diffuse or scattered low-density lesions in the white matter, some of which may enhance with contrast. MRI usually reveals an increased signal intensity on T2-weighted images (Fig. 23.5).

Diagnosis

Because there is no specific diagnostic test, the diagnosis of PIE or postvaccinal encephalomyelitis should be considered when neurologic signs develop 4 to 21 days following onset of acute exanthems or an upper respiratory tract infection, or after vaccination. The differential diagnosis includes practically all the acute infectious diseases of the nervous system, particularly acute or subacute encephalitis, and acute diffuse multiple sclerosis.

Prognosis and Course

The mortality rate is high (10% to 30%) in patients with severe involvement of the cerebrum in measles or rubella, or after rabies vaccination with the old brain-derived vaccine. It is low in patients with acute cerebellar ataxia or involvement only of the peripheral nerves. Death may occur as a result of cerebral damage in the acute stage or following intercurrent infections, bed sores, or urinary sepsis in late stages. In patients who survive, the neurologic signs usually improve considerably, with about 90% having complete recovery. The exception is measles, in which sequelae may occur in 20% to 50% of patients. Sequelae include seizures, mental syndromes, and hemiparesis. Delayed postencephalitic sequelae, such as parkinsonism, do not occur; as a rule, there are no new symptoms after recovery from an acute attack.

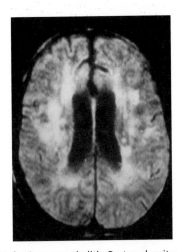

FIG. 23.5. Postinfectious encephalitis. Proton-density MR image shows a lesion that began 2 weeks after a nonspecific upper respiratory tract infection. There is prominent diffuse cerebral white matter disease. (From Jubelt B, Ropka S. Infectious diseases of the nervous system. In: Rosenberg RN, ed., *Atlas of clinical neurology.* Philadelphia: Current Medicine, 1998:12.1–12.71; with permission.)

Treatment

Several reports suggest that the administration of adrenocorticotropic hormone or intravenous corticosteroids reduces the severity of the neurologic defects.

CHRONIC VIRAL INFECTIONS

Chronic or slow viral infections that result in chronic neurologic disease are caused by both conventional viruses and the unconventional transmissible spongiform encephalopathy agents. However, the transmissible spongiform encephalopathy agents, or prions, as presently understood, are not true viruses (see Chapter 33). Conventional agents cause chronic inflammatory or demyelinating disease; in humans, these include subacute sclerosing panencephalitis (SSPE), progressive rubella panencephalitis (PRP), progressive multifocal leukoencephalopathy (PML), human T-cell lymphotropic virus (HTLV)-associated myelopathy (HAM)/tropical spastic paraparesis (TSP), and AIDS. In SSPE, a chronic inflammatory disease is caused by a defect in the production of measles virus, which results in a cell-associated infection. With PRP, both inflammation and demyelination may be seen. The pathogenic mechanisms have not yet been defined, but the virus does not appear to be defective. PML is a noninflammatory demyelinating disease that occurs in immunocompromised hosts; it is caused by an opportunistic papovavirus infection. HAM/TSP is an inflammatory demyelinating disease caused by HTLV, a retrovirus. AIDS is reviewed in Chapter 24. Other conventional viruses (enteroviruses, HSV, VZV, CMV, measles virus, adenovirus) can cause chronic opportunistic infections in immunocompromised patients.

Subacute Sclerosing Panencephalitis

SSPE (Dawson disease or subacute inclusion body encephalitis) is a disease caused by a defective measles virus. It is characterized by progressive dementia, incoordination, ataxia, myoclonic jerks, and other focal neurologic signs. First described by Dawson in 1933 and 1934 as "subacute inclusion encephalitis," it was thought to be of viral origin because of the presence of type A intranuclear inclusions. Numerous cases have since been reported, but recovery of a viral agent was not possible until the advent of specialized techniques of viral isolation by cocultivation of brain cells with extraneural cells capable of replicating fully infectious virus. The cases reported by Pette and Doring in 1939 as "nodular panencephalitis" and by Van Bogaert in 1945 as "subacute sclerosing leukoencephalitis" appear to involve the same disease. The name of this disease reflects a combination of the three terms.

Pathology

In severe long-standing cases, the brain may feel unduly hard. A perivascular infiltration occurs in the cortex and white matter with plasma and other mononuclear cells. Patchy areas of demyelination and gliosis occur in the white matter and deeper layers of the cortex. The neurons of the cortex, basal ganglia, pons, and inferior olives show degenerative changes. Intranuclear and intracytoplasmic eosinophilic inclusion bodies are found in neurons and glial cells. When examined with the electron microscope, these inclusions are seen to be composed of hollow tubules similar to the nucleocapsids of paramyxoviruses. Staining of inclusions by the fluorescent antibody method shows that they are positive for measles virus.

Incidence

Children younger than 12 years are predominantly affected, although a few cases in adults in their 20s have been reported. Boys are more often affected than girls, and more cases have occurred in rural than in urban settings. The incidence of SSPE has decreased markedly in the United States since the introduction of the live attenuated measles vaccine. After natural measles infection, the incidence of SSPE is 5 to 10 cases per 1 million clinical measles infections. After vaccine, the rate is less than 1 case per 1 million vaccine recipients.

Symptoms

SSPE has a gradual onset without fever. Forgetfulness, inability to keep up with schoolwork, and restlessness are common early symptoms. These are followed in the course of weeks or months by incoordination, ataxia, myoclonic jerks of the trunk and limbs (often noise-induced), apraxia, and loss of speech; seizures and dystonic posturing may occur. Vision and hearing are preserved until the terminal stage, in which there is a rigid quadriplegia simulating complete decortication.

Laboratory Data and Diagnosis

Elevated levels of measles antibody can be found in serum and CSF. The CSF is under normal pressure, and the cell count is normal or, rarely, only slightly increased. The protein content is normal, but a striking increase in the CSF immunoglobulin content is found, even in an otherwise normal fluid. Oligoclonal IgG bands, representing measles virus-specific antibodies, can be demonstrated by agarose electrophoresis of CSF. The EEG often shows a widespread abnormality of the cortical activity with a "burst suppression" pattern of high-amplitude slow-wave (or spike and slow-wave) complexes occurring at a rate of every 4 to 20 seconds synchronous with or independent of the myoclonic jerks. CT may show cortical atrophy and focal or multifocal low-density lesions of the white matter.

Pathogenesis

A defect in measles virus production seems to occur because the viral M (membrane) protein cannot be found in the brain tissue of affected patients. The M protein is necessary for alignment of nucleocapsids under viral proteins in the cell membrane so that budding of virus can take place. Thus, in SSPE there is no budding and no release of extracellular virus. There is accumulation of measles virus nucleocapsids within cells (cell-associated infection), and virus spread occurs by cell fusion. Brain cells may be

incapable of synthesizing the M protein, or selective antibody pressure might cause a restricted cell-associated infection, because more than 50% of patients with SSPE have had an acute measles infection before reaching 2 years of age, when maternal antibody may still have been present.

Course, Prognosis, and Treatment

The course of the disease is prolonged, usually lasting several years. Both rapidly progressive disease, leading to death in several months, and protracted disease, lasting more than 10 years, have occurred. Spontaneous long-term improvement or stabilization occurs in about 10% of patients. There is no definite specific therapy. Intrathecal interferon alfa with or without isoprinosine (inosine pranobex, Imunovir) may induce remissions. No controlled studies have been performed.

Progressive Rubella Panencephalitis

Rubella virus, like measles virus, has been recognized to cause slowly progressive rubella panencephalitis. This is a rare disease of children and young adults. Fewer than a dozen cases have been reported. Most cases have occurred in patients with the congenital rubella syndrome, but several cases have appeared following postnatally acquired rubella. None has been ascribed to rubella vaccine. There does not appear to be a defect in rubella virus production, as occurs in SSPE. Unlike measles virus, rubella virus does not have an M protein. Because of the recognition that immune complexes are in the serum and CSF, it is thought that immune complex deposition in vascular endothelium results in vasculitis.

The pathologic condition is characterized by inflammation and demyelination. The inflammation consists of lymphocytic and plasma cell infiltration of the meninges and perivascular spaces of the gray and white matter. Extensive demyelination with atrophy and gliosis of the white matter is usually seen, together with vasculitis involving arterioles with fibrinoid degeneration and mineral deposition. Arterioles may be thrombosed, and there are adjacent microinfarcts. IgG deposits have been demonstrated in vessels.

PRP usually occurs in the second decade of life, beginning with dementia similar to that of SSPE. Cerebellar ataxia, however, is more prominent. Gait ataxia is initially seen, but the arms subsequently become involved. Later, pyramidal tract involvement is seen. Optic atrophy and retinopathy similar to those seen in congenital rubella occur. Seizures and myoclonus are not prominent. Symptoms and signs suggestive of infection (headache, fever, nuchal rigidity) are not seen.

Routine blood tests are normal. The EEG reveals diffuse slowing; periodicity is rare. CT may demonstrate ventricular enlargement, which is most prominent in the fourth ventricle and cisterna magna because of cerebellar atrophy. The CSF is under normal pressure. There is usually a lymphocytic pleocytosis with up to 40 cells/mm^3, but the fluid is occasionally acellular. The protein is increased in the range of 60 to 150 mg/dL, with the IgG fraction being up to 50% of this. Most of the IgG is composed of oligoclonal bands directed against rubella virus. Conventional serologic techniques demonstrate elevated serum and

CSF antibody titers against rubella virus. Recovery of the virus is difficult and requires cocultivation.

The diagnosis can easily be made in a patient with the congenital rubella syndrome. In postnatally acquired cases, SSPE is the other major diagnostic consideration. Other dementing illnesses of childhood should be considered; however, the combined data of the clinical picture (especially when ataxia ensues), the CSF findings, and serology should be diagnostic. The course is protracted over 8 to 10 years. There is no specific treatment.

Retrovirus Infections

HIV Infection

See Chapter 24.

HTLV-associated Myelopathy/Tropical Spastic Paraparesis

Etiology

HTLV is a retrovirus that causes adult T-cell leukemia and a chronic progressive myelopathy, hereditary and acquired spastic paraplegia (see Chapter 117). This chronic HTLV-associated myelopathy (HAM) has been referred to as tropical spastic paraparesis (TSP) in tropical areas, hence the abbreviation HAM/TSP. Of the two serotypes of HTLV, most cases of HAM/TSP are caused by HTLV-I.

Pathology and Pathogenesis

Patients have a mild chronic meningoencephalomyelitis with mononuclear infiltrates of the meninges and perivascular cuffing primarily in the spinal cord. In addition, there are proliferation of smaller parenchymal vessels, thickening of the meninges, and a reactive astrocytic gliosis. A second prominent feature is demyelination in the pyramidal tracts and posterior columns.

Like HIV, HTLV apparently enters the CNS via infected peripheral blood mononuclear cells, thereby causing secondary infection of glial cells. Presumably, demyelination is caused by cytotoxic T cells rather than by direct infection with HTLV.

Epidemiology

TSP occurs in tropical islands (including the Caribbean), as well as in tropical areas of the United States, Central and South America, India, and Africa. The prevalence is quite variable, ranging from 12 to 128 cases per 100,000 population. HAM is found on the southwestern and northern islands of Japan; the prevalence is not known. The temporal behavior of HAM/TSP reflects an endemic myelopathy. Most cases occur after age 30 years, but childhood cases have been reported. There is a female preponderance.

More cases of HAM/TSP are being recognized throughout the United States, in both immigrants and native residents. As in HIV infection, exposure is related to intravenous drug use, sexual transmission, and blood transfusions.

Symptoms and Signs

Onset is usually gradual, with weakness of one leg followed in several months by weakness of the other leg. Other complaints include numbness and dysesthesia, bladder dysfunction, and impotence. Infrequently, more abrupt onset may occur. Examination reveals spastic paraparesis with overactive tendon reflexes (legs more than arms) and Babinski signs. Posterior column dysfunction is common, and hypesthesia is often noted diffusely below the midthoracic level. Less frequently, a distinct sensory level or peripheral neuropathy (25%) is found. Cerebral involvement caused by white matter disease and made evident by encephalopathy and seizures has been described in several patients. Neurogenic muscular atrophy and polymyositis occur rarely.

Laboratory Studies

CSF examination may be entirely normal, but a mild lymphocytic pleocytosis may be seen. About 50% of patients have an elevated CSF protein content in the 50- to 90-mg/dL range. Increased CSF IgG levels and oligoclonal bands are found in most patients. Antibodies to HTLV are increased in both serum and CSF. The ratio of helper to suppressor T cells is increased. MRI may show white matter lesions in the brain, even in asymptomatic patients.

Diagnosis

Diagnosis depends on the appropriate clinical and CSF manifestations and a positive antibody response in the serum and CSF. The differential diagnosis includes other causes of spastic paraparesis, including multiple sclerosis (see Chapters 117 and 133).

Course, Prognosis, and Treatment

Most patients progress slowly over months to a few years and may stabilize. Responses to corticosteroids and danazol (Danocrine) have been reported in uncontrolled studies. In a recent double-blind, controlled trial, two-thirds of patients reported benefit from interferon alfa.

Progressive Multifocal Leukoencephalopathy

PML is a rare subacute demyelinating disease caused by an opportunistic papovavirus. The disease occurs in patients with defective cell-mediated immunity. Cases have primarily occurred in patients with reticuloendothelial diseases, such as Hodgkin disease, other lymphomas, and leukemia before the AIDS epidemic. Cases have also occurred in patients with carcinoma or sarcoidosis and in those immunosuppressed therapeutically. In most of these disorders, PML is a rare complication; it occurs in 2 to 5% of AIDS patients. A few cases have occurred in the apparent absence of an underlying disease.

Pathology

The condition is characterized by the presence of multiple, partly confluent areas of demyelination in various parts of the nervous system, accompanied at times by a mild degree of perivascular infiltration. These multifocal areas of demyelination are most prominent in the subcortical white matter, whereas involvement of cerebellar, brainstem, or spinal cord white matter is less common. As the disease progresses, the demyelinated areas coalesce to form large lesions. Hyperplasia of astrocytes into bizarre giant forms that may resemble neoplastic cells is found. There is loss of oligodendroglia with relative sparing of axons in the lesions. Eosinophilic intranuclear inclusions are seen in oligodendroglial cells at the periphery of the lesions. Electron microscopic studies have shown that these inclusions are composed of papovavirus particles (Fig. 23.6). It is presumed that the demyelination is due to destruction of oligodendroglia by the virus. Most cases have been caused by the JC strain and possibly several by the SV-40 strain. Isolation of these agents requires special techniques of cocultivating brain cultures from patients with permissive cell lines; human fetal brain tissue could also be used to induce virus replication.

Symptoms and Signs

The clinical manifestations are diverse and are related to the location and number of lesions. Onset is subacute to chronic with focal or multifocal signs (hemiplegia, sensory abnormalities, field cuts, and other focal signs of lesions in the cerebral hemispheres). Cranial nerve palsies, ataxia, and spinal cord involvement are less common. As the number of lesions increases, dementia ensues.

Laboratory Data and Diagnosis

A definite diagnosis of PML can be made only by pathologic investigation (brain biopsy). Eventually, PCR amplification of JC virus RNA in the CSF should obviate brain biopsy. Virus isolation techniques are difficult and time-consuming. More rapid identification can be made by immunofluorescence or by immune electron microscopy. The CSF is usually normal. The EEG often demonstrates nonspecific diffuse or focal slowing. CT reveals nonenhancing multiple lucencies in the white matter. MRI may demonstrate additional white matter abnormalities (Fig. 23.7). Serology is not helpful because most people have been exposed to the JC strain in the first two decades of their lives. A presumptive diagnosis can be made on the basis of the clinical presentation and the appropriate CT findings in an immune-compromised patient.

Pathogenesis

Apparently, the virus is latent in the kidney and in B lymphocytes and enters the CNS in activated B lymphocytes. Once virus enters the brain, glial cells (astrocytes and oligodendroglia) support virus replication because viral transcription factors are selectively expressed in these cells.

Course, Prognosis, and Treatment

The course usually lasts months, and 80% of patients die within 9 months. Rarely, the course may last several years, with the longest verified course recorded at 6 years. In most patients with AIDS, the inflammatory response has been prominent and the course longer than that noted with other underlying disease. If possible, treatment should include an attempt to improve immune function. There is no definite treatment. Spontaneous improvement has been reported.

Encephalitis Lethargica

Encephalitis lethargica (sleeping sickness, von Economo disease) is a disease of unknown cause that occurred in epidemic form from 1917 to 1928. Clinically, the disease was characterized by signs and symptoms of diffuse involvement of the brain and the development of various sequelae in a large percentage of recovered patients. Although the disease spread rapidly over the entire world, the epidemic form is apparently extinct. It may now occur as very rare isolated cases. Encephalitis lethargica affected patients of all ages and both sexes equally, including people of all races and occupations.

The etiology of encephalitis lethargica is unknown. It is presumed that the disease was caused by a virus, but proof is lacking. Because of the concurrence of encephalitis lethargica and the pandemic of influenza beginning in 1918, there has been speculation about a common etiology; this has not been resolved but is probably unlikely.

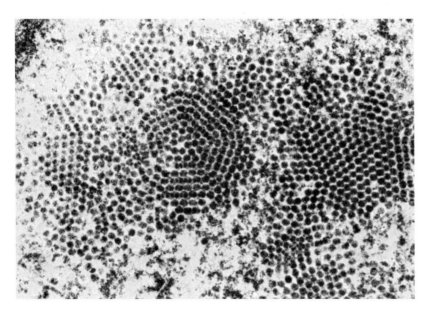

FIG. 23.6. Progressive multifocal leukoencephalopathy. Papovavirus-like particles are present in a glial nucleus (×65,000). (Courtesy of Dr. G.M. Zu Rhein.)

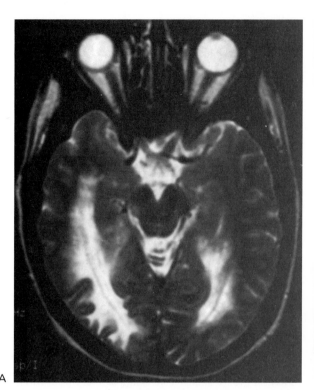
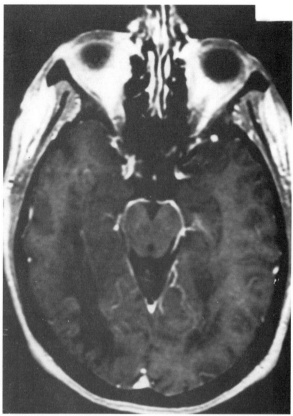

FIG. 23.7. Progressive multifocal leukoencephalopathy. **A:** T2-weighted spin-echo axial MR image shows increased signal intensity of the temporooccipital white matter, which is greater on the right than the left. Relative cortical sparing is seen. **B:** T1-weighted gradient-echo axial MR image after gadolinium administration shows decreased signal intensity in the same areas with no evidence of abnormal enhancement. Note the normal enhancement of both internal carotid arteries and posterior cerebral arteries on the gradient-echo enhanced images. (Courtesy of Dr. S. Chan, Columbia University College of Physicians and Surgeons, New York, N.Y.)

The pathologic lesions in the subacute stages were similar to those of other encephalitides, with inflammation in the meninges, around blood vessels, and in the parenchyma (both gray and white matter) of the brain and spinal cord. Acute degenerative changes of neurons also occurred.

The symptoms and signs were usually of acute or subacute onset. Fever was usually present at the outset and was usually mild. In fatal cases, a rise to 107°F (41.7°C) or higher often occurred in the terminal stages. Headache and lethargy were common early symptoms. Disorders of eye movements were present in about 75% of patients. An acute organic psychosis was not uncommon. The most frequent motor symptoms were all categories of basal ganglia diseases.

Pertinent laboratory studies showed a lymphocytic pleocytosis in the CSF and an abnormal CSF protein content in about 50% of patients.

The diagnosis of encephalitis lethargica may be justified in any patient with signs and symptoms of encephalitis with special features of disturbed sleep rhythm and diplopia in the acute stage, and the development of signs of injury of the basal ganglia at that time or in subsequent years. The duration of the acute stage was about 4 weeks and merged gradually into the so-called postencephalitic phase of the disease. The mortality rate was

about 25% and was highest among infants and elderly persons.

The frequency of sequelae is unknown. In some instances, symptoms were merely a continuation of those present in the acute stage. In others, the symptoms developed after an interval of several months or many years, during which the patient was apparently well. The parkinsonian syndrome that develops after encephalitis lethargica can often be distinguished from idiopathic parkinsonism because of an early age of onset and unusual features, such as grimaces, torticollis, torsion spasms, myoclonus, oculogyric crises, facial and respiratory tics, and bizarre postures and gaits. Behavior disorders and emotional instability without evidence of intellectual impairment were common sequelae in children.

SUGGESTED READINGS

General

Bale JF Jr. Viral encephalitis. *Med Clin North Am* 1993;77:25–42.
Bell WE, McCormick WF. *Neurologic infections in children,* 2nd ed. Philadelphia: WB Saunders, 1981.
Evans AS, Kaslow RA, eds. *Viral infections of humans,* 4th ed. New York: Plenum Publishing, 1997.
Fields BN, Knipe PM, Howley PM, eds. *Virology,* 3rd ed. Philadelphia: Lippincott–Raven Publishers, 1996.

Hanshaw JB, Dudgeon JA. *Viral diseases of the fetus and newborn,* 2nd ed. Philadelphia: WB Saunders, 1985.

Jeffery KJM, Read SJ, Pete TEA, Mayon-White RT, Bangham CRM. Diagnosis of viral infections of the central nervous system: clinical interpretation of PCR results. *Lancet* 1997;349:313–317.

Johnson RT. *Viral infections of the nervous system,* 2nd ed. New York: Lippincott–Raven Publishers, 1998.

Koskiniemi M, Korppi M, Mustonen K, et al. Epidemiology of encephalitis in children: a prospective multicentre study. *Eur J Pediatr* 1997;156:541–545.

Koskiniemi M, Rautonen J, Lehtokoski-Lehtiniemi E, Vaheri A. Epidemiology of encephalitis in children: a 20-year survey. *Ann Neurol* 1991;29:429–497.

Lennette EH, Lennette DA, Lennette ET, eds. *Diagnostic procedures for viral, rickettsial and chlamydial infections,* 7th ed. Washington, DC: American Public Health Association, 1995.

Lennette EH, Magoffin RL, Knouf EG. Viral central nervous system disease: an etiologic study conducted at the Los Angeles County General Hospital. *JAMA* 1962;179:687–695.

Lepow ML, Coyne N, Thompson LB, et al. A clinical, epidemiologic and laboratory investigation of aseptic meningitis during the four-year period 1955–1958. II. The clinical disease and its sequelae. *N Engl J Med* 1962;266:1188–1193.

McKendall RR, Stroop WC, eds. *Handbook of neurovirology.* New York: Marcel Dekker, 1994.

Meyer HM Jr, Johnson RT, Crawford IP, et al. Central nervous system syndromes of "viral" etiology: a study of 713 cases. *Am J Med* 1960;29:334–347.

Nathanson N, ed. *Viral pathogenesis.* Philadelphia: Lippincott–Raven Publishers, 1997.

Nicolosi A, Hauser WA, Beghi E, Kurland LT. Epidemiology of central nervous system infections in Olmsted County, Minnesota, 1950–1981. *J Infect Dis* 1986;154:399–408.

Scheld WM, Whitley RJ, Durack DT, eds. *Infections of the central nervous system,* 2nd ed. Philadelphia: Lippincott–Raven Publishers, 1997.

Tyler KL, Martin JB, eds. *Infectious diseases of the central nervous system.* Philadelphia: FA Davis Co, 1993.

Vinken PJ, Bruyn GW, Klawans HL, McKendall RR, eds. *Viral disease. Handbook of clinical neurology, vol 56.* New York: Elsevier Science, 1989.

Enterovirus (Picornavirus) Infections

Baker RC, Kummer AW, Schultz JR, Ho M, Gonzalez del Rey J. Neurodevelopmental outcome of infants with viral meningitis in the first three months of life. *Clin Pediatr (Phila)* 1996;35:295–301.

Berlin LE, Rorabaugh ML, Heldrich F, et al. Aseptic meningitis in infants less than 2 years of age: diagnosis and etiology. *J Infect Dis* 1993;168:888–892.

Jubelt B, Lipton HL. Enterovirus infection. In: Vinken PJ, Bruyn GW, Klawans HL, McKendall RR, eds. *Viral disease. Handbook of clinical neurology, vol 56.* New York: Elsevier Science, 1989:307–347.

Sawyer MH, Holland D, Aintablian N. Diagnosis of enteroviral central nervous system infection by polymerase chain reaction during a large community outbreak. *Pediatr Infect Dis J* 1994;13:177–182.

Poliomyelitis

Centers for Disease Control and Prevention. Poliomyelitis prevention in the United States: introduction of a sequential vaccination schedule of inactivated poliovirus vaccine followed by oral poliovirus vaccine. Recommendations of the Advisory Committee on Immunization Practices. *MMWR* 1997;46(RR-3):1–25.

Centers for Disease Control and Prevention. Paralytic poliomyelitis—United States, 1980–1994. *MMWR* 1997;46:79–83.

Davis LE, Bodian D, Price D, et al. Chronic progressive poliomyelitis secondary to vaccination of an immunodeficient child. *N Engl J Med* 1977;297:241–245.

Jubelt B, Drucker JS. Poliomyelitis and the postpolio syndrome. In: Younger DS, ed. *The motor disorders textbook.* Philadelphia: Lippincott–Raven Publishers, 1998:381–395.

Kornreich L, Dagan O, Grunebaum M. MRI in acute poliomyelitis. *Neuroradiology* 1996;38:371–372.

Patriarca PA, Sutter RW, Oostvogel PM. Outbreaks of paralytic poliomyelitis, 1976–1995. *J Infect Dis* 1997;175[Suppl 1]:S165–S172.

Price RW, Plum F. Poliomyelitis. In: Vinken PJ, Bruyn GW, Klawans HL, eds. *Infections of the nervous system. Handbook of clinical neurology, vol 34.* New York: Elsevier/North-Holland, 1978:93–132.

Wyatt HV. Poliomyelitis in hypogammaglobulinemics. *J Infect Dis* 1972;128:802–806.

Coxsackievirus Infections

Farmer K, MacArthur BA, Clay MM. A follow-up study of 15 cases of neonatal meningoencephalitis due to coxsackie virus B5. *J Pediatr* 1975;87:568–571.

Gauntt CJ, Gudvangen RJ, Brans YW, Marlin AE. Coxsackievirus group B antibodies in the ventricular fluid of infants with severe anatomic defects of the central nervous system. *Pediatrics* 1985;76:64–68.

Kaplan MH, Klein SW, McPhee J, Harper RG. Group B coxsackievirus infections in infants younger than three months of age: a serious illness. *Rev Infect Dis* 1983;5:1019–1032.

Medlin JF, Dagan R, Berlin LE, et al. Focal encephalitis with enterovirus infections. *Pediatrics* 1991;88:841–845.

Echovirus Infections

Ashwell MJS, Smith DW, Phillips PA, Rouse IL. Viral meningitis due to echovirus types 6 and 9: epidemiological data from Western Australia. *Epidemiol Infect* 1996;117:507–512.

McKinney RE, Katz SL, Wilfert CM. Chronic enteroviral meningoencephalitis in agammaglobulinemic patients. *Rev Infect Dis* 1987;9:334–356.

Modlin JF. Perinatal echovirus infection: insights from a literature review of 61 cases of serious infection and 16 outbreaks in nurseries. *Rev Infect Dis* 1986;8:918–926.

Rice SK, Heinl RE, Thornton LL, Opal SM. Clinical characteristics, management strategies, and cost implications of a statewide outbreak of enterovirus meningitis. *Clin Infect Dis* 1995;20:931–937.

Enteroviruses 70 and 71 Infections

Alexander JP, Baden L, Pallansch MA, Anderson LJ. Enterovirus 71 infections and neurologic disease—United States, 1977–1991. *J Infect Dis* 1994;169:905–908.

Gilbert GL, Dickson KE, Waters MJ, et al. Outbreak of enterovirus 71 infections in Victoria, Australia, with a high incidence of neurologic involvement. *Pediatr Infect Dis J* 1988;7:484–488.

Hayward JC, Gillespie SM, Kaplan KM, et al. Outbreak of poliomyelitis-like paralysis associated with enterovirus 71. *Pediatr Infect Dis J* 1989;8:611–616.

Vejjajiva A. Acute hemorrhagic conjunctivitis with nervous system complications. In: Vinken PJ, Bruyn GW, Klawans HL, McKendall RR, eds. *Viral disease. Handbook of clinical neurology, vol 56.* New York: Elsevier Science, 1989:349–354.

Arbovirus Infections

Aguilar MJ, Calanchini PR, Finley KH. Perinatal arbovirus encephalitis and its sequelae. *Res Publ Assoc Nerv Ment Dis* 1968;44:216–235.

Centers for Disease Control and Prevention. Arboviral infections of the central nervous system—United States, 1996–1997. *MMWR* 1998; 47:517–522.

Lowry PW. Arbovirus encephalitis in the United States and Asia. *J Lab Clin Med* 1997;129:405–411.

Tsai TF. Arboviral infections in the United States. *Infect Dis Clin North Am* 1991;5:73–102.

Equine Encephalitides

Deresiewicz RL, Thaler SJ, Hsu L, Zamani AA. Clinical and neuroradiographic manifestations of eastern equine encephalitis. *N Engl J Med* 1997;336:1867–1874.

Earnest MP, Goolishian HA, Calverley JR, et al. Neurologic, intellectual, and psychologic sequelae following western encephalitis. *Neurology* 1971;21:969–974.

Ehrenkranz NJ, Ventura AK. Venezuelan equine encephalitis virus infection in man. *Annu Rev Med* 1974;25:9–14.

Przelomski MM, O'Rourke E, Grady GF, et al. Eastern equine encephalitis in Massachusetts: a report of 16 cases: 1970–1984. *Neurology* 1988;38:736–739.

Rozdilsky B, Robertson HE, Charney J. Western encephalitis: report of eight fatal cases, Saskatchewan epidemic, 1965. *Can Med Assoc J* 1968;98:79–86.

St. Louis Encephalitis

Brinker KR, Paulson G, Monath TP, et al. St. Louis encephalitis in Ohio, September 1975: clinical and EEG studies in 16 cases. *Arch Intern Med* 1979;139:561–566.

Marfin AA, Bleed DM, Lofgren JP, et al. Epidemiologic aspects of a St. Louis encephalitis epidemic in Jefferson County, Arkansas, 1991. *Am J Trop Med Hyg* 1993;49:30–37.

Monath TP, Tsai TF. St. Louis encephalitis: lessons from the last decade. *Am J Trop Med Hyg* 1987;37[Suppl]:S40–S59.

Reyes MG, Gardner JJ, Poland JD, Monath TP. St. Louis encephalitis: quantitative histologic and immunofluorescent studies. *Arch Neurol* 1981;38:329–334.

Japanese Encephalitis

Centers for Disease Control and Prevention. Inactivated Japanese encephalitis virus vaccine. Recommendations of the Advisory Committee on Immunization Practices. *MMWR* 1993;42(RR-1):1–15.

Johnson RT, Intralawan P, Puapanwatton S. Japanese encephalitis: identification of inflammatory cells in cerebrospinal fluid. *Ann Neurol* 1986;20:601–695.

Kumar S, Misra UK, Kalita J, et al. MRI in Japanesse encephalitis. *Neuroradiology* 1997;39:180–184.

Monath TP. Japanese encephalitis—a plague of the Orient. *N Engl J Med* 1988;319:641–643.

Richter RW, Shimpjyo S. Neurologic sequelae of Japanese B encephalitis. *Neurology* 1961;11:553–559.

California (La Crosse) Encephalitis

Balfour HH, Siem RA, Bauer H, Quie PG. California arbovirus (La Crosse) infections. *Pediatrics* 1973;52:680–691.

Centers for Disease Control. La Crosse encephalitis in West Virginia. *MMWR* 1988;37:79–82.

Chun RWM, Thompson WH, Grabow JD, Mathews CG. California arbovirus encephalitis in children. *Neurology* 1968;18:369–375.

Clark GG, Pretula HL, Langkop CW, Martin RJ, Calisher CH. Occurrence of La Crosse (California serogroup) encephalitis viral infections in Illinois. *Am J Trop Med Hyg* 1983;32:838–843.

Demikhov VG, Chaitsev VG, Butenko AM, et al. California serogroup virus infections in the Ryazan region of the USSR. *Am J Trop Med Hyg* 1991;45:371–376.

McJunkin JE, Khan RR, Rsai TF. California-La Crosse encephalitis. *Infect Dis Clin North Am* 1998;12:83–93.

Other Arbovirus Encephalitides

Bennett NM. Murray Valley encephalitis, 1974: clinical features. *Med J Aust* 1976;2:446–450.

Cruse RP, Rothner AD, Erenberg G, Calisher CH. Central European tick-borne encephalitis: an Ohio case with a history of foreign travel. *Am J Dis Child* 1979;133:1070–1071.

Embil JA, Camfield P, Artsob H, Chase DP. Powassan virus encephalitis resembling herpes simplex encephalitis. *Arch Intern Med* 1983;143:341–343.

Gadoth N, Weitzman S, Lehmann EE. Acute anterior myelitis complicating West Nile fever. *Arch Neurol* 1979;36:172–173.

Goodpasture HC, Poland JD, Francy DB, et al. Colorado tick fever: clinical, epidemiologic, and laboratory aspects of 228 cases in Colorado in 1973–1974. *Ann Intern Med* 1978;88:303–310.

Meegen JM, Niklasson B, Bengtsson E. Spread of Rift Valley fever virus from continental Africa. *Lancet* 1979;2:1184–1185.

Smorodintsev AA. Tick-borne spring–summer encephalitis. *Prog Med Virol* 1958;1:210–247.

Rubella

Centers for Disease Control and Prevention. Rubella and congenital rubella syndrome–United States, 1994–1997. *MMWR* 1997;46:350–354.

Desmond MM, Wilson GS, Melnick JL, et al. Congenital rubella encephalitis. *J Pediatr* 1967;71:311–331.

Ishikawa A, Murayama T, Sakuma N, et al. Computed cranial tomography in congenital rubella syndrome. *Arch Neurol* 1982;39:420–421.

Miller E, Cradock-Watson JE, Pollock TM. Consequence of confirmed maternal rubella at successive stages of pregnancy. *Lancet* 1982;2:781–784.

Waxham NR, Wolinsky JS. Rubella virus and its effects on the central nervous system. *Neurol Clin* 1984;2:367–385.

Mumps Meningitis and Encephalomyelitis

Black S, Shinefield H, Ray P, et al. Risk of hospitalization because of aseptic meningitis after measles-mumps-rubella vaccination in one- to two-year-old children: an analysis of the Vaccine Safety Datalink (VSD) Project. *Pediatr Infect Dis J* 1997;16:500–503.

Colville A, Pugh S. Mumps meningitis and measles, mumps, and rubella vaccine [Letter]. *Lancet* 1992;340:786. Errata: *Lancet* 1992;340:986; *Lancet* 1992;340:1420.

Johnstone JA, Ross CAC, Dunn M. Meningitis and encephalitis associated with mumps infection: a 10-year study. *Arch Dis Child* 1972;47:647–651.

Jubelt B. Enterovirus and mumps virus infections of the nervous system. *Neurol Clin* 1984;2:187–213.

Koskiniemi M, Donner M, Pettay O. Clinical appearance and outcome in mumps encephalitis in children. *Acta Paediatr Scand* 1983;72:603–609.

Levitt LP, Rich RA, Kinde SW, et al. Central nervous system mumps: a review of 64 cases. *Neurology* 1970;20:829–834.

Thompson JA. Mumps: a cause of acquired aqueductal stenosis. *J Pediatr* 1979;94:923–924.

Subacute Measles Encephalitis

Hughes I, Jenney MEM, Newton RW, et al. Measles encephalitis during immunosuppressive treatment for acute lymphoblastic leukaemia. *Arch Dis Child* 1993;68:775–778.

Kim TM, Brown HR, Lee SH, et al. Delayed acute measles inclusion body encephalitis in a 9-year-old girl: ultrastructural, immunohistochemical, and *in situ* hybridization studies. *Mod Pathol* 1992;5:348–352.

Mustafa MM, Weitman SD, Winick NJ, et al. Subacute measles encephalitis in the young immunocompromised host: report of two cases diagnosed by polymerase chain reaction and treated with ribavirin, and review of the literature. *Clin Infect Dis* 1993;16:654–660.

Rabies

Alvarez L, Fajardo R, Lopez E, et al. Partial recovery from rabies in a nine-year-old boy. *Pediatr Infect Dis J* 1994;13:1154–1155.

Baer GM, Shaddock JH, Houff SA, et al. Human rabies transmitted by corneal transplant. *Arch Neurol* 1982;39:103–107.

Bernard KW, Smith PW, Kader FJ, Moran MJ. Neuroparalytic illness and human diploid cell rabies vaccine. *JAMA* 1982;248:3136–3138.

Centers for Disease Control and Prevention. Human rabies–Texas and New Jersey, 1997. *MMWR* 1998;47:1–5.

Chopra JS, Banerjee AK, Murthy JMK, Pal SR. Paralytic rabies: a clinico-pathological study. *Brain* 1980;103:789–802.

Dupont JR, Earle KM. Human rabies encephalitis: a study of forty-nine fatal cases with a review of the literature. *Neurology* 1965;15:1023–1034.

Fishbein DB, Robinson LE. Rabies. *N Engl J Med* 1993;329:1632–1638.

Hemachudha T. Rabies. In: Vinken PJ, Bruyn GW, Klawans HL, McKendall RR, eds. *Viral disease. Handbook of clinical neurology, vol 56.* New York: Elsevier Science, 1989:383–404.

Lymphocytic Choriomeningitis

Biggar RJ, Woodall JP, Walter PD, Haughie GE. Lymphocytic choriomeningitis outbreak associated with pet hamsters: fifty-seven cases from New York State. *JAMA* 1975;232:494–500.

Chesney PJ, Katcher ML, Nelson DB, Horowitz SD. CSF eosinophilia and chronic lymphocytic choriomeningitis virus meningitis. *J Pediatr* 1979;94:750–752.

Lehmann-Grube F. Diseases of the nervous system caused by lymphocytic choriomeningitis virus and other arenaviruses. In: Vinken PJ, Bruyn GW, Klawans HL, McKendall RR, eds. *Viral disease. Handbook of clinical neurology, vol 56.* New York: Elsevier Science, 1989:355–381.

Rousseau MC, Saron MF, Brouqui P, Bourgeade A. Lymphocytic choriomeningitis virus in southern France: four case reports and a review of the literature. *Eur J Epidemiol* 1997;13:817–823.

Thacker WL, Lewis VF. Prevalence of lymphocytic choriomeningitis virus antibodies in patients with acute central nervous system disease. *J Infect* 1982;5:309–310.

Adenovirus Infections

Anders KH, Park CS, Cornford ME, Vinters HV. Adenovirus encephalitis and widespread ependymitis in a child with AIDS. *Pediatr Neurosurg* 1990–1991;16:316–320.

Davis D, Henslee J, Markesbery WR. Fatal adenovirus meningoencephalitis in a bone marrow transplant patient. *Ann Neurol* 1988;23:385–389.

Kelsey SD. Adenovirus meningoencephalitis. *Pediatrics* 1978;61:291–293.

Kim KS, Gohd RS. Acute encephalopathy in twins due to adenovirus type 7 infection. *Arch Neurol* 1983;40:58–59.

Roos R. Adenovirus. In: Vinken PJ, Bruyn GW, Klawans HL, McKendall RR, eds. *Viral disease. Handbook of clinical neurology, vol 56.* New York: Elsevier Science, 1989:281–293.

Herpes Simplex Encephalitis

Britton CB, Mesa-Tejada R, Fenoglio CM, et al. A new complication of AIDS: thoracic myelitis caused by herpes simplex virus. *Neurology* 1985;35:1071–1074.

Cinque P, Cleator GM, Weber T, Monteyne P, Sindic CJ, van Loon AM. The role of laboratory investigation in the diagnosis and management of patients with suspected herpes simplex encephalitis: a consensus report. The EU Concerted Action on Virus Meningitis and Encephalitis. *J Neurol Neurosurg Psychiatry* 1996;61:339–345.

Dennett C, Cleator GM, Klapper PE. HSV-1 and HSV-2 in herpes simplex encephalitis: a study of sixty-four cases in the United Kingdom. *J Med Virol* 1997;53:1–3.

Dix RD, Waitzman DM, Follansbee S, et al. Herpes simplex virus type 2 encephalitis in two homosexual men with persistent lymphadenopathy. *Ann Neurol* 1985;17:203–206.

Koskiniemi M, Vaheri A, Taskinen E. Cerebrospinal fluid alterations in herpes simplex encephalitis. *Rev Infect Dis* 1984;6:608–618.

Lakeman FD, Whitley RJ. Diagnosis of herpes simplex encephalitis: application of polymerase chain reaction to cerebrospinal fluid from brain-biopsied patients and correlation with disease. National Institute of Allergy and Infectious Disease Collaborative Antiviral Study Group. *J Infect Dis* 1995;171:857–863.

McGrath N, Anderson NE, Croxson MC, Powell KF. Herpes simplex encephalitis treated with acyclovir: diagnosis and long-term outcome. *J Neurol Neurosurg Psychiatry* 1997;63:321–326.

McKendall RR. Herpes simplex. In: Vinken PJ, Bruyn GW, Klawans HL, McKendall RR, eds. *Viral disease. Handbook of clinical neurology, vol 56.* New York: Elsevier Science, 1989:207–227.

Sage, JI, Weinstein MP, Miller DC. Chronic encephalitis possibly due to herpes simplex virus: two cases. *Neurology* 1985;35:1470–1472.

Schlageter N, Jubelt B, Vick NA. Herpes simplex encephalitis without CSF leukocytosis. *Arch Neurol* 1984;41:1007–1008.

Schroth G, Gawehn J, Thron A, et al. Early diagnosis of herpes simplex encephalitis by MRI. *Neurology* 1987;37:179–183.

Whitley RJ, Cobbs CG, Alford CA Jr, et al. Diseases that mimic herpes simplex encephalitis: diagnosis, presentation, and outcome. *JAMA* 1989;262:234–239.

Herpes Zoster

Balfour HH Jr, Bean B, Laskin DL, et al. Acyclovir halts progression of herpes zoster in immunocompromised patients. *N Engl J Med* 1983;308:1448–1453.

Berrettini S, Bianchi MC, Segnini G, Sellari-Franceschini S, Bruschini P, Montanaro D. Herpes zoster oticus: correlations between clinical and MRI findings. *Eur Neurol* 1998;39:26–31.

deSilva SM, Mark AS, Gilden DH, et al. Zoster myelitis: improvement with antiviral therapy in two cases. *Neurology* 1996;47:929–931.

Eidelberg D, Sotrel A, Horoupian S, et al. Thrombotic cerebral vasculopathy associated with herpes zoster. *Ann Neurol* 1986;19:7–14.

Gilden DH. Varicella-zoster virus infections. In: Vinken PJ, Bruyn GW, Klawans HL, McKendall RR, eds. *Viral disease. Handbook of clinical neurology, vol 56.* New York: Elsevier Science, 1989:229–247.

Gilden DH, Wright RR, Schneck SA, et al. Zoster sine herpete: a clinical variant. *Ann Neurol* 1994;35:530–533.

Hope-Simpson RE. The nature of herpes zoster: a long-term study and a new hypothesis. *Proc R Soc Med* 1965;58:9–20.

Jackson JL, Gibbons R, Meyer G, Inouye L. The effect of treating herpes zoster with oral acyclovir in preventing postherpetic neuralgis. *Arch Intern Med* 1997;157:909–912.

Jemsek J, Greenberg SB, Tabor L, et al. Herpes zoster-associated encephalitis: clinicopathologic report of 12 cases and review of the literature. *Medicine* 1983;62:81–97.

Mulder RR, Lumish RM, Corsello GR. Myelopathy after herpes zoster. *Arch Neurol* 1983;40:445–446.

Ryder JW, Croen K, Kleinschmidt-DeMasters BK, et al. Progressive encephalitis three months after resolution of cutaneous zoster in a patient with AIDS. *Ann Neurol* 1986;19:182–188.

Thomas JE, Howard FM Jr. Segmental zoster paresis: a disease profile. *Neurology* 1972;22:459–466.

Whitley RJ, Weiss H, Gnann JW Jr, et al. Acyclovir with and without prednisone for the treatment of herpes zoster: a randomized, placebo-controlled trail. The National Institute of Allergy and Infectious Diseases Collaborative Antiviral Study Group. *Ann Intern Med* 1996;125:376–383.

Cytomegalovirus Infection

Arribas JR, Storch GA, Clifford DB, Tselis AC. Cytomeglavirus encephalitis. *Ann Intern Med* 1996;125:577–587.

Bale JF Jr, Jordon C. Cytomegalovirus infections. In: Vinken PJ, Bruyn GW, Klawans HL, McKendall RR, eds. *Viral disease. Handbook of clinical neurology, vol 56.* New York: Elsevier Science, 1989:263–279.

Cohen BA. Prognosis and response to therapy of cytomegalovirus encephalitis and meningomyelitis in AIDS. *Neurology* 1996;46:444–450.

Cohen BA, McArthur JC, Grohman S, et al. Neurologic prognosis of cytomegalovirus polyradiculomyelopathy in AIDS. *Neurology* 1993;43:493–499.

Holland NR, Power C, Mathews VP, et al. Cytomegalovirus encephalitis in acquired immunodeficiency syndrome (AIDS). *Neurology* 1994;44:507–514.

Miller RF, Lucas SB, HallCraggs MA, et al. Comparison of magnetic resonance imaging with neuropathological findings in the diagnosis of HIV- and CMV-associated CNS disease in AIDS. *J Neurol Neurosurg Psychiatry* 1997;62:346–351.

Perlman JM, Argyle C. Lethal cytomegalovirus infection in preterm infants: clinical, radiological, and neuropathological findings. *Ann Neurol* 1992;31:64–68.

Pierelli F, Tilia G, Damiani A, et al. Brainstem CMV encephalitis in AIDS: clinical case and MRI features. *Neurology* 1997;48:529–530.

Talpos D, Tien RD, Hesselink JR. Magnetic resonance imaging of AIDS-related polyradiculopathy. *Neurology* 1991;41:1995–1997.

Wildemann B, Haas J, Lynen N, et al. Diagnosis of cytomegalovirus encephalitis in patients with AIDS by quantitation of cytomegalovirus genomes in cells of cerebrospinal fluids. *Neurology* 1998;50:693–697.

Epstein-Barr Virus Infection

Bray PF, Culp KW, McFarlin DE, et al. Demyelinating disease after neurologically complicated primary Epstein-Barr virus infection. *Neurology* 1992;42:278–282.

Domachowske JB, Cunningham CK, Cummings DL, Crosley CJ, Hannan WP, Weiner LB. Acute manifestations and neurologic sequelae of Epstein-Barr virus encephalitis in children. *Pediatr Infect Dis J* 1996;15:871–875.

Erzurum S, Kalavsky SM, Watanakanakorn C. Acute cerebellar ataxia and hearing loss as initial symptoms of infectious mononucleosis. *Arch Neurol* 1983;40:760–762.

Gottlieb-Stematsky T, Arlazoroff A. Epstein-Barr virus infection. In: Vinken PJ, Bruyn GW, Klawans HL, McKendall RR, eds. *Viral disease. Handbook of clinical neurology, vol 56*. New York: Elsevier Science, 1989:249–261.

Grose C, Henle W, Henle G, Feorino PM. Primary Epstein-Barr virus infections in acute neurologic disease. *N Engl J Med* 1975;292:392–395.

Russell J, Fisher M, Zivin JA, et al. Status epilepticus and Epstein-Barr virus encephalopathy. *Arch Neurol* 1985;42:789–792.

Silverstein A, Steinberg G, Nathanson M. Nervous system involvement in infectious mononucleosis: the heralding and/or major manifestation. *Arch Neurol* 1972;26:353–358.

Tselis A, Duman R, Storch GA, et al. Epstein-Barr virus encephalomyelitis diagnosed by polymerase chain reactions: detection of the genome in the CSF. *Neurology* 1997;48:1351–1355.

Human Herpesvirus-6 Infection

Carrigan DR, Harrington D, Knox KK. Subacute leukoencephalitis caused by CNS infection with human herpesvirus-6 manifesting as acute multiple sclerosis. *Neurology* 1996;47:145–148.

Kamei A, Ichinohe S, Onoma R, Hiraga S, Fujiwara T. Acute disseminated demyelination due to primary human herpesvirus-6 infection *Eur J Pediatr* 1997;56:709–712.

Knox KK, Carrigan DR. Active human herpesvirus (HHV-6) infection of the central nervous system in patients with AIDS. *J Acquir Immune Defic Syndr Hum Retrovirol* 1995;9:69–73.

McCullers JA, Lakeman FD, Whitley RJ. Human herpesvirus 6 is associated with focal encephalitis. *Clin Infect Dis* 1995;21:571–576.

Mookerjee BP, Vogelsang G. Human herpesvirus-6 encephalitis after bone marrow transplantation: successful treatment with ganciclovir. *Bone Marrow Transplant* 1997;20:905–906.

Sing N, Carrigan DR. Human herpesvirus-6 in transplantation: an emerging pathogen. *Ann Intern Med* 1996;124:1065–1071.

Suga S, Yoshikawa T, Asano Y, et al., Clinical and virological analyses of 21 infants with exanthem subitum (roseola infantum) and central nervous system complications. *Ann Neurol* 1993;33:597–603.

Acute Disseminated Encephalomyelitis

Alvord ED Jr. Disseminated encephalitis: its variations in form and their relationships to other diseases of the nervous system. In: Vinken PJ, Bruyn GW, Klawans HL, Koetsier JC, eds. *Demyelinating diseases. Handbook of clinical neurology, vol 47*. New York: Elsevier Science, 1985:467–502.

Arnason BGW. Neuroimmunology. *N Engl J Med* 1987;316:406–408.

Case records of the Massachusetts General Hospital. Case 37-1995. *N Engl J Med* 1995;333:1485–1493.

Decaux G, Szyper M, Ectors M, Cornil A, Franken L. Central nervous system complications of *Mycoplasma pneumoniae. J Neurol Neurosurg Psychiatry* 1980;43:883–887.

Fenichel GM. Neurological complications of immunization. *Ann Neurol* 1982;12:119–128.

Hirtz DG, Nelson KB, Ellenberg JH. Seizures following childhood immunizations. *J Pediatr* 1983;102:14–18.

Jeffrey DR, Mandler RN, Davis LE. Transverse myelitis: retrospective analysis of 33 cases, with differentiation of cases associated with multiple sclerosis and parainfectious events. *Arch Neurol* 1993;50:532–535.

Johnson RT, Griffin DE, Hirsch RL, et al. Measles encephalitis: clinical and immunological studies. *N Engl J Med* 1984;310:137–141.

Kepes JJ. Large focal tumor-like demyelinating lesions of the brain: intermediate entity between multiple sclerosis and acute disseminated encephalomyelitis? A study of 31 patients. *Ann Neurol* 1993;33:18–27.

Kesselring J, Miller DH, Robb SA, et al. Acute disseminated encephalomyelitis: MRI findings and the distinction from multiple sclerosis. *Brain* 1990;113:291–302.

Miller HG, Stanton JB, Gibbons JL. Parainfectious encephalomyelitis and related syndromes. *Q J Med* 1956;25:427–505.

Pellegrini M, O'Brien TJ, Hoy J, Sedal L. *Mycoplasma pneumoniae* infection associated with an acute brainstem syndrome. *Acta Neurol Scand* 1996;93:203–206.

Peters ACB, Versteeg J, Lindeman J, Bots GTAM. Varicella and acute cerebellar ataxia. *Arch Neurol* 1978;35:769–771.

Straub J, Chofflon M, Delavalle J. Early high-dose intravenous methylprenisolone in acute disseminated encephalitis: a successful recovery. *Neurology* 1997;49:1145–1147.

Ziegler DK. Acute disseminated encephalitis: some therapeutic and diagnostic considerations. *Arch Neurol* 1966;14:476–488.

Subacute Sclerosing Panencephalitis

Anlar B, Yalaz K, Oktem F, Kose G. Long-term follow-up of patients with subacute sclerosing panencephalitis treated with intraventricular alpha-interferon. *Neurology* 1997;48:526–528.

Begeer JH, Haaxma R, Snoek JW, et al. Signs of focal posterior cerebral abnormality in early subacute sclerosing panencephalitis. *Ann Neurol* 1986;19:200–202.

Case Records of the Massachusetts General Hospital. Case 25-1986. *N Engl J Med* 1986;314:1689–1700.

Freeman JM. The clinical spectrum and early diagnosis of Dawson's encephalitis. *J Pediatr* 1969;75:590–603.

Risk WS, Haddad FS. The variable natural history of subacute sclerosing panencephalitis: a study of 118 cases from the Middle East. *Arch Neurol* 1979;36:610–614.

Singer C, Lang AE, Suchowersky O. Adult-onset subacute sclerosing panencephalitis: case reports and review of the literature. *Mov Disord* 1997;12:342–353.

SSPE in the developing world [Editorial]. *Lancet* 1990;336:600.

Swoveland PT, Johnson KP. Subacute sclerosing panencephalitis and other paramyxovirus infections. In: Vinken PJ, Bruyn GW, Klawans HL, McKendall RR, eds. *Viral disease. Handbook of clinical neurology, vol 56*. New York: Elsevier Science, 1989:417–437.

Progressive Rubella Panencephalitis

Guizzaro A, Volpe E, Lus G, et al. Progressive rubella panencephalitis: follow-up EEG study of a case. *Acta Neurol (Napoli)* 1992;14:485–492.

Townsend JJ, Stroop WG, Baringer JR, et al. Neuropathology of progressive rubella panencephalitis after childhood rubella. *Neurology* 1982;32:185–190.

Weil ML, Itabashi HH, Cremer NE, et al. Chronic progressive panencephalitis due to rubella virus simulating subacute sclerosing panencephalitis. *N Engl J Med* 1975;292:994–998.

Wolinsky JS. Progressive rubella panencephalitis. In: Vinken PJ, Bruyn

GW, Klawans HL, McKendall RR, eds. *Viral disease. Handbook of clinical neurology, vol 56.* New York: Elsevier Science, 1989:405–446.

HTLV-associated Myelopathy/Tropical Spastic Paraparesis

Bartholomew C, Cleghorn F, Jack N, et al. Human T-cell lymphotropic virus type I-associated facial nerve palsy in Trinidad and Tobago. *Ann Neurol* 1997;41:806–809.

Dooneief G, Marlink R, Bell K, et al. Neurologic consequences of HTLV-II infection in injection-drug users. *Neurology* 1996;46:1556–1560.

Dover AG, Pringle E, Guberman A. Human T-cell lymphotropic virus type 1 myositis, peripheral neuropathy, and cerebral white matter lesions in the absence of spastic paraparesis. *Arch Neurol* 1997;54:896–900.

Harrison LH, Vaz B, Taveira DM, et al. Myelopathy among Brazilians coinfected with human T-cell lymphotropic virus type I and HIV. *Neurology* 1997;48:13–18.

Izumo S, Goto MD, Itoyama MD, et al. Interferon-alpha is effective in HTLV-I-associated myelopathy: a multicenter, randomized, double-blind, controlled trial. *Neurology* 1996;46:1016–1021.

Janssen RS, Kaplan JE, Khabbaz RF, et al. HTLV-I-associated myelopathy/tropical spastic paraparesis in the United States. *Neurology* 1991;41:1355–1357.

Lehky TJ, Flerlage N, Katz D, et al. Human T-cell lymphotropic virus type II-associated myelopathy: clinical and immunologic profiles. *Ann Neurol* 1996;40:714–723.

McKendall RR, Oas J, Lairmore MD. HTLV-I-associated myelopathy endemic in Texas-born residents and isolation of virus from CSF cells. *Neurology* 1991;41:831–836.

Murphy EL, Fridey J, Smith JW, et al. HTLV-associated myelopathy in a cohort of HTLV-I- and HTLV-II-infected blood donors. *Neurology* 1997;48:315–320.

Roman GC, Vernant JC, Osamc M, eds. *HTLV-I and the nervous system.* New York: Alan R. Liss, 1989.

Shermata WA, Berger JR, Harrington WJ Jr, et al. Human T lymphotropic virus type I-associated myelopathy: a report of 10 patients born in the United States. *Arch Neurol* 1992;49:1113–1118.

Progressive Multifocal Leukoencephalopathy

Brooks BR, Walker DL. Progressive multifocal leukoencephalopathy. *Neurol Clin* 1984;2:299–313.

Chang L, Ernst T, Torratore C, et al. Metabolite abnormalities in progressive multifocal leukoencephalopathy by proton magnetic resonance spectroscopy. *Neurology* 1997;48:836–845.

Gillespie SM, Chang Y, Lemp G, et al. Progressive multifocal leukoencephalopathy in persons infected with human immunodeficiency virus, San Francisco, 1981–1989. *Ann Neurol* 1991;30:597–604.

Hair LS, Nuovo G, Powers JM, et al. Progressive multifocal leukoencephalopathy in patients with human immunodeficiency virus. *Hum Pathol* 1992;23:663–667.

Hall CD, Dafni U, Simpson D, et al. Failure of cytarabine in progressive multifocal leukoencephalopathy associated with human immunodeficiency virus infection. AIDS Clinical Trials Group 243 Team. *N Engl J Med* 1998;338:1345–1351.

Holman RC, Janssen RS, Buehler JW, et al. Epidemiology of progressive multifocal leukoencephalopathy in the United States: analysis of mortality and AIDS surveillance data. *Neurology* 1991;41:1733–1736.

Matsushima T, Nakamura K, Oka T, et al. Unusual MRI and pathologic findings of progressive multifocal leukoencephalopathy complicating adult Wiskott-Aldrich syndrome. *Neurology* 1997;48:279–282.

McGuire D, Barhite S, Hollander H, Miles M. JC virus DNA in cerebrospinal fluid of HIV-infected patients: predictive value for progressive multifocal leukoencephalopathy. *Ann Neurol* 1995;37:395–399.

Richardson EP Jr. Progressive multifocal leukoencephalopathy 30 years later. *N Engl J Med* 1988;318:315–317.

Whiteman ML, Post MJ, Berger JR, et al. Progressive multifocal leukoencephalopathy in 47 HIV-seropositive patients: neuroimaging with clinical and pathologic correlation. *Radiology* 1993;187:233–240.

Zunt JR, Tu RR, Anderson DM, et al. Progressive multifocal leukoencephalopathy presenting as human immunodeficiency virus type 1 (HIV)-associated dementia. *Neurology* 1997;49:263–265.

Encephalitis Lethargica

Blunt SB, Lane RJ, Turjanski N, Perkin GD. Clinical features and management of two cases of encephalitis lethargica. *Mov Disord* 1997;12:354–359.

Calne DB, Lees AJ. Late progression of postencephalitic Parkinson's syndrome. *Can J Neurol Sci* 1988;15:135–138.

Howard RS, Lees AJ. Encephalitis lethargica: a report of four recent cases. *Brain* 1987;110:19–33.

Pearce JM. Baron Constantin von Economo and encephalitis lethargica. *J Neurol Neurosurg Psychiatry* 1996;60:167.

Reavenholt RT, Foege WH. 1918 influenza, encephalitis lethargica, parkinsonism. *Lancet* 1982;2:860–864.

Wenning GK, Jellinger K, Litvan I. Supranuclear gaze palsy and eyelid apraxia in postencephalitic parkinsonism. *J Neural Transm* 1997;104:845–865.

Yahr MD. Encephalitis lethargica (von Economo's disease, epidemic encephalitis). In: Vinken PJ. Bruyn GW. Klawans HL, eds. *Infections of the nervous system. Handbook of Clinical Neurology, vol 34.* New York: Elsevier/North-Holland, 1978:451–457.

Merritt's Neurology, 10th ed., edited by L.P. Rowland. Lippincott Williams & Wilkins, Philadelphia © 2000.

24

ACQUIRED IMMUNODEFICIENCY SYNDROME

CAROLYN BARLEY BRITTON

HISTORY

Acquired immunodeficiency syndrome (AIDS) was first recognized clinically in 1981. In 1982, the Centers for Disease Control (CDC) proposed epidemiologic surveillance criteria for the diagnosis of AIDS as the occurrence of unusual opportunistic infections (OIs) or malignancies indicative of a defect in cell-mediated immunity without a known cause.

In 1983, human immunodeficiency virus type 1 (HIV-1), the retrovirus that causes AIDS, was isolated from human peripheral blood lymphocytes. An explosive pace of research followed. The virus was sequenced and its structure elucidated by x-ray crystallography. There were rapid advances in understanding of the viral life cycle, mechanisms of human infection and pathogenesis, and development of successful drug therapies. The cellular immune defect of AIDS was attributed to HIV infection of CD4 (T4 helper) lymphocytes. Soon after infection, HIV replicates vigorously in peripheral blood lymphocytes and lymphoid tissues throughout the body, including gut-associated lymphoid, brain microglial, and macrophage cells. Disseminated viral infection causes systemic and neurologic disorders, such as the wasting syndrome and dementia that are now recognized as AIDS-defining illnesses, even in the absence of OIs or neoplasia.

Serologic studies showed that there can be a latency of several years between HIV infection and AIDS, the latter indicative of advanced immunosuppression. Direct viral nucleic acid detection (viral load) and viral replication assays showed that there is no virologic latency after initial infection. Despite ongoing viral replication, most infected people are asymptomatic or experience transient self-limited illnesses. Some have chronic lymphadenopathy or the AIDS-related complex of adenopathy, weight loss, fever, and diarrhea.

CLASSIFICATION OF HIV DISEASE

The CDC proposed staging criteria for HIV infection in 1986, which were modified in 1987 to include the neurologic syndromes of AIDS dementia and myelopathy among 23 AIDS-defining illnesses (Table 24.1). Future revisions were anticipated, based on improved understanding of HIV biology. The 1993 revisions added three laboratory categories stratified by CD4 cell counts and three clinical categories (Table 24.2). AIDS-defining illnesses were expanded to include positive HIV serology and pulmonary tuberculosis, recurrent bacterial pneumonia, invasive cervical carcinoma, or a CD4 lymphocyte count less than 200/mm³. The revisions defined the end stage of HIV

TABLE 24.1. RELCLASSIFICATION OF HIV INFECTION

Group I	Acute infection (transient symptoms with seroconversion)
Group II	Asymptomatic infection (seropositive only)
Group III	Persistent generalized lymphadenopathy
Group IV	Other disease
Subgroup A	Chronic constitutional disease
Subgroup B	Neurologic disease
Subgroup C	Specified secondary infections
Category C–1	Diseases listed in the CDC definition for AIDS
Category C–2	Other specified secondary infections
Subgroup D	Specified secondary cancers (includes cancers fulfilling CDC definition of AIDS)
Subgroup E	Other conditions

From Centers for Disease Control. *MMWR* 1986;35:334–339.

infection and clarified the relationship of specific clinical syndromes that are not diagnostic of AIDS, especially neurologic disease, to advanced immunosuppression.

The classification system guides medical management of HIV-infected persons. The Walter-Reed classification system has not gained wide acceptance.

HIV replication (*viral load*) is the determining factor in progression to clinical endpoints such as AIDS or death. Viral load assays have supplanted staging criteria for decisions about antiretroviral therapy. Staging is still useful for prognosis and decisions about OI prophylaxis.

TABLE 24.2. CDC CLASSIFICATION OF HIV INFECTION

Laboratory categories	
1	CD4 lymphocyte count >500 cells/mm³
2	CD4 lymphocyte count from 200–499 cells/mm³
3	CD4 lymphocyte count <200 cells/mm³
Clinical categories	
A	Asymptomatic infection, persistent generalized lymphadenopathy, and acute primary HIV infection
B	Symptomatic conditions not included in the CDC's 1987 surveillance case definition of AIDS that are judged by a physician to be HIV-related or where medical management is complicated by HIV infection (e.g., sepsis, bacterial endocarditis, pulmonary tuberculosis, cervical dysplasia or carcinoma, vulvovaginal candidiasis)
C	Any of the 23 conditions listed in the CDC's 1987 case definition for AIDS

Modified from US Congress. CDC's case definition of AIDS: implications of the proposed revisions background paper. Washington, DC: US Government Printing Office, 1992. OTA-BP-H-89.

EPIDEMIOLOGY

General Picture

HIV infection is a worldwide pandemic affecting virtually all population groups, with especially rapid spread in developing countries, where 90% of new cases occur. Transmission occurs through homosexual or heterosexual contact, exposure to contaminated blood or blood products, or perinatally. Worldwide, heterosexual activity is the most common mode of transmission. In the United States, homosexual activity is slightly more frequent than injection-drug use (IDU) as the most common exposure but seroconversion is more common in IDU. In western Europe, IDU accounts for 40% of cases and homosexual activity for 35%.

Retrospective analysis of banked blood showed that HIV was present in the United States in the 1970s. By September 1997, the cumulative total of AIDS cases reported to the CDC was 626,334; cases in New York, Florida, New Jersey, California, and Puerto Rico accounted for 64% of the total. Eighty percent of cases were in the Northeast (44%) and the South (36%); 85% of cases had a defined transmission risk. Of 91,837 cumulative cases reported by 1997 without a known transmission category, 41,391 (31,190 men, 10,201 women) were assigned to one of the recognized categories. Homosexual activity was the most common unrecognized risk for 57% of men and heterosexual activity for 67% of women. Recipients of blood products or clotting factor for hemophilia or other coagulation or blood disorders accounted for less than 1% of adult AIDS cases in 1997. Routine testing of blood products has largely eliminated this source of infection in the United States.

Occupational exposure with documented transmission and seroconversion has occurred in 52 health care workers: 45 had percutaneous exposure, five had mucocutaneous exposure, and two had both mucocutaneous and percutaneous exposure. Most exposures were to blood or bloody fluid. Possible occupational transmission has occurred in 114 additional health care workers who were exposed to HIV-contaminated blood, body fluids, or laboratory solutions, but HIV seroconversion after a specific occupational exposure was not documented. Prospective studies of known exposures estimate the average risk for HIV transmission after a percutaneous exposure to HIV-infected blood as approximately 0.3% and after mucous membrane exposure 0.09%. There were no documented cases of seroconversion after isolated skin exposure.

The first 100,000 AIDS cases were reported in 8 years; more than 500,000 cases were reported in the second 8-year period. Changes in the case definition were responsible for a transient increase in AIDS cases. The AIDS case definition may become less relevant as more states require integrated HIV/AIDS case reporting. Dual reporting allows accurate assessment of the scope and demographics of the epidemic, appropriate funding initiatives, and identification of persons for counseling about treatment. There are also increased efforts to identify contacts. The fastest growing populations with AIDS in the United States are women, African-American and Hispanic minorities, and injection-drug users (Table 24.3). A rise in seroconversion among some young homosexual male populations implies a need for continued vigilance in targeted education. In 1994, AIDS be-

TABLE 24.3. EPIDEMIOLOGY OF AIDS: THE FIRST AND SECOND 100,000 CASES

	First 100,000 Cases (%)	Second 100,000 Cases (%)
Homosexual/bisexual men	61	55
Intravenous drug users, men and women	20	24
Heterosexual transmission	5	7
Women	9	12
Children	1.6	1.7
African-American adults	27	31
Hispanic adults	15	17

Modified from Centers for Disease Control. *MMWR* 1991; 4:164.

came the leading cause of death among men and African-American women. The disproportionate representation of African-American and Hispanic men is related to drug use. Minority women are also directly or indirectly affected by drug use, but unprotected heterosexual activity has become the predominant transmission risk.

HIV infection has been reported in virtually every country. In developing countries, rapid spread is related to inadequate public health and health care infrastructures. The World Health Organization estimated that 30,000,000 people worldwide are currently infected. There were 2.3 million deaths from AIDS by 1997, 50% higher than in 1996. Globally, there are an estimated 16,000 new cases of HIV infection daily. Although unprotected heterosexual activity is the predominant transmission risk, there are substantial risks in health care settings due to contaminated blood or needles.

AIDS in Children

By September 1997, 7,310 children younger than 13 with HIV infection were reported to the CDC, slightly more than 1% of all AIDS cases, most infected perinatally. Perinatal infection disproportionately affects African-Americans and Hispanics, a measure of their disproportionate number among seropositive women. Since 1992, perinatal transmission in the United States has declined 43% due to successful implementation of CDC guidelines for maternal zidovudine (Retrovir) treatment. Worldwide, perinatal transmission unfortunately continues because treatment is not available. Children account for more than 1,000,000 of worldwide AIDS cases, with 350,000 annual infections. Millions of uninfected children will be orphaned by the loss of both parents to AIDS.

ETIOLOGY

Virologic, serologic, and epidemiologic data support the conclusion that AIDS is caused by HIV infection. HIV is an enveloped ribonucleic acid (RNA) virus. It contains an RNA-dependent, DNA polymerase (reverse transcriptase) that produces a provirus capable of integrating into host-cell DNA. In the target cell, the virus exists in both free and integrated states. It is a lentivirus. The best-known of this family is visna virus, which, like HIV, demonstrates cellular tropism, establishes persistent infection, and after long clinical latency establishes a slowly progressive demyelinating disease in ovines.

Human HIV infection is considered a cross-species (zoonotic) infection arising from monkeys infected with simian immunodeficiency virus (SIV) through multiple independent transmissions. Of the two recognized viral species, HIV-1 is found worldwide and is more prevalent, whereas HIV-2 is found in western Africa and in Europe among African immigrants and their sexual partners. Sporadic cases of HIV-2 infection occur in the United States. HIV-2 less frequently causes immunodeficiency and AIDS than HIV-1. There are phylogenetic groups of HIV-1 (M, N, and O), and each comprises several viral strains. Group M (the main group) is responsible for the global epidemic. Group O (the outlier) is found in Cameroon, Gabon, and Equatorial Guinea. Group N (non-M/non-O) was isolated from two individuals in Cameroon.

SIV was first isolated from macaque monkeys in captivity and later found in African green monkeys. The sooty mangabey is the primate host suspected of transmitting HIV-2. This subspecies is infected with a strain of SIV that is genomically and phylogenetically related to HIV-2. Its natural habitat is the epicenter of the HIV-2 epidemic, and large numbers of wild animals are infected. The chimpanzee seems to be the primate host for HIV-1. The recognition of HIV infection as a zoonosis raises concern for animal-to-human transmission of other potentially pathogenic retroviruses.

Although scientific data overwhelmingly support the view that HIV is the cause of AIDS, other theories have been proposed, including toxic drug exposure or an as yet unidentified agent. In 1992, 35 cases of HIV-negative CD4 cell lymphopenia or AIDS were reported in the United States and six other countries. Some patients had risk factors associated with HIV; others had no reported risk factors. Alternative theories of infection lack substantial scientific support.

PATHOGENESIS

Infection of CD4 lymphocytes by HIV, mediated by viral attachment to the cell-surface CD4 receptor, leads to cell death. In humans, the CD4 receptor is expressed on several cell types, including neurons and glia in the brain, yet there is no evidence of viral replication in cells other than lymphocytes, macrophages, monocytes, and their derivatives. A coreceptor necessary for viral entry into cells was identified in 1996 as a chemokine receptor. In acute and early HIV infection, a macrophage-tropic viral strain predominates and uses the chemokine receptor CCR5 (R5 virus). In chronic infection, T-cell tropic strains predominate and use the receptor CXCR4 (X4 virus). Other chemokine receptors are sometimes used. Genetic variation in the chemokine receptor may affect susceptibility to HIV infection. Relative resistance to infection is observed in persons who are homozygous for a 32-base-pair deletion in CCR5.

Primary HIV infection may be asymptomatic or, as in 50% to 70% of patients, result in an acute, self-limited mononucleosis-like illness with fever, headaches, myalgia, malaise, lethargy, sore throat, lymphadenopathy, and maculopapular rash. Painful ulceration of the buccal mucosa may impede swallowing (odynophagia).

Acute infection is characterized by viremia, a high viral replication rate, ease of viral isolation from peripheral blood lymphocytes, and a high serum level of a viral core antigen, p24. Initial viral load in acute infection may be as high as 10^6 RNA molecules per milliliter. Cytotoxic lymphocytes and soluble factors from CD8 lymphocytes are effective in reducing viral load to a set point that differs for each individual. Despite the effective early immune response, there is almost simultaneous immune dysfunction. Neutralizing antibodies of the immunoglobulin (Ig) M and, later, IgG type appear in 2 to 6 weeks, resulting in clearance of viremia and a decrease in serum p24 levels. Rarely, antibodies do not appear for several months and exceptionally not at all.

Adverse immunologic effects occur early and are more severe in symptomatic persons. An early absolute lymphopenia affects both CD4 helper and CD8 suppressor cells, with lymphocyte hyporesponsiveness to mitogens and antigens, and with thrombocytopenia. Lymphocytosis usually follows, especially of CD8 lymphocytes, with inversion of the CD4/CD8 ratio. Atypical lymphocytes are sometimes seen. Early changes in the CD4/CD8 ratio are usually transient, with reversion to more normal values but with persistent functional abnormalities. Cutaneous anergy is a direct result of the viral effects on CD4 cells.

After acute infection and seroconversion, clinical latency may last several years before the onset of symptoms of secondary infection, malignancy, or neurologic disease appears. There is no biologic latency, however; HIV infection is a chronic, persistent infection of variable viral replication rate.

The viral load set point after acute infection correlates with the rate of progression to symptomatic infection or AIDS. Several proprietary assays provide quantitative measurement of plasma HIV RNA. The branched (b)DNA assay detects as few as 20 to 50 copies/mL. Recognition of acute infection is important because early antiretroviral treatment may prevent extensive seeding of lymphoid tissues or may eliminate infection. Without treatment, viral replication is robust. It is estimated that 10^9 virions enter plasma daily in untreated people. Productively infected peripheral blood lymphocytes turn over rapidly with a half-life of 1.6 days. Most of the total viral load is in tissues, not plasma. In lymphoid tissue, virus is contained in two compartments: CD4+ lymphocytes or macrophages, and follicular dendritic cells within germinal centers, where virus is passively adherent. The total lymphoid viral burden is three times that of plasma, the majority in follicular dendritic cells. The total-body viral load is 10^{11} HIV-RNA copies. Approximately 10% of latently infected cells contain replication-competent provirus. Cellular destruction of lymphoid tissue is mediated by direct HIV cytopathic effects, autoimmunity, and other mechanisms. Eventually, the lymphoid system is overwhelmed by the viral burden, which increases with advancing disease, culminating in AIDS.

Other factors that may augment HIV replication and the onset of symptoms are biologic variability of HIV and the appearance of increasingly virulent strains; host immunogenetics; interaction with concomitant infection by cytomegalovirus (CMV), herpes simplex virus (HSV), hepatitis B (HBV) and C viruses, human herpesvirus 6, or human T-cell lymphotropic virus type 1, which upregulates expression of HIV; and upregulation of infection and cell-killing ability by cytokines. Cytokines are released by immune cells in response to infection and may upregulate or downregulate viral replication.

Other immunologic abnormalities in AIDS are caused by effects of HIV on immune cells other than the CD4 lymphocyte, such as B cells or macrophage. These include hypergammaglobulinemia; impaired antibody responses to new antigens, including encapsulated bacteria; and increased levels of immune complexes. Antibodies to platelets may cause thrombocytopenia. Loss of cellular immune function and impairment of B-cell and macrophage function increase susceptibility to some bacterial infections, opportunistic organisms, and rare neoplasms.

Highly active antiretroviral treatment (HAART) and specific prophylaxis have reduced the incidence of AIDS-related OIs and neoplasms in the United States. In untreated HIV infection, *Pneumocystis carinii* is the most common opportunistic pathogen. Other pathogens causing OIs are often multiple: fungal (candidiasis, cryptococcosis, aspergillosis, histoplasmosis, coccidioidomycosis, and others), viral (CMV, disseminated HSV, varicella-zoster virus [VZV]), or parasitic (toxoplasmosis, cryptosporidiosis, strongyloidiasis, isosporiasis, and *Acanthamoeba* infection). Mycobacteria (tuberculosis and atypical forms), *Salmonella, Treponema pallidum,* and *Staphylococcus aureus* are common causes of pulmonary and systemic bacterial infections. Many of these infections involve the central nervous system (CNS), secondarily in most cases, but sometimes as the primary infection. The papovavirus that causes progressive multifocal leukoencephalopathy (PML) infects brain primarily. Common pathogens in developing countries, such as *Trypanosoma,* are sometimes seen in recent immigrants to the United States.

Kaposi sarcoma, Hodgkin lymphoma, and non-Hodgkin lymphoma are the most commonly encountered neoplasms.

CNS PATHOGENESIS

HIV enters the CNS at the time of primary infection and may result in no apparent disease, acute self-limited syndromes, or chronic disorders. These are caused by HIV itself, secondary OIs, or neoplasia, metabolic abnormalities, medical treatment, or nutritional disorders. Neurologic disorders are found in up to 70% of patients with AIDS in clinical series and in more than 80% of autopsy series. In 10% to 20% of patients, the neurologic disorder is the first manifestation of AIDS. Uncommonly, a neurologic disorder is the sole evidence of chronic HIV infection and the cause of death. Early, effective antiretroviral treatment has decreased the incidence of secondary OI of the nervous system and may decrease the incidence of primary HIV-related syndromes.

Evidence of early CNS invasion includes isolation of virus from cerebrospinal fluid (CSF) or neural tissues (brain, spinal cord, peripheral nerve) and intrathecal production of antibodies to HIV. How HIV enters the CNS is not known. Possible mechanisms include intracellular transport across the blood–brain barrier within infected macrophages, free virus seeding the leptomeninges, or free virus after replication within the choroid plexus or vascular epithelium. In the brain, viral infection is detected only in microglial cells or macrophages by *in situ* hybridization techniques; it is not found in neurons or glial cells, even though these cells have CD4 and chemokine receptors.

The high frequency of neurologic disorders in HIV infection has led to the designation of HIV as a neurotropic virus. The term *neurotropic* implies selective vulnerability and homing of the virus to neurons. Alternatively, the high frequency of neurologic disorders may be explained by the chronicity of infection that results in continued seeding of the CNS. Specific neurotropism is not needed for continued accrual of neurologic damage. It has been difficult to establish correlation of neurologic syndromes with productive viral replication in the affected tissue. There is an increase, however, in the viral burden or viral load with advancing disease, which parallels dementia and other neurologic syndromes.

The mechanism of neurologic injury is believed to be indirect. Potential mechanisms include immune-mediated indirect injury; restricted persistent cellular infection; cellular injury due to cytokines released by infected monocytes and macrophages; excitotoxic amino acid injury; voltage-mediated increase of intracellular calcium; free radical damage; potentiation of inflammatory damage by chemokines and lipid inflammatory mediators (arachidonic acid and platelet activating factor); direct cellular toxicity of HIV gene products, such as the envelope glycoprotein gp120; and cross-reacting antibody to an HIV glycoprotein binding a cell membrane epitope, resulting in cell receptor blockade. More than one mechanism may be important. Genetic changes in the virus in the host may result in noncytopathic CNS virus with enhanced replicative capacity in monocytes and macrophages, leading to a greater viral burden in the CNS than is apparent in the periphery. Phenotypic and viral load discordance are documented in several studies of plasma and CSF. This compartmentalization of virus may explain the occurrence of neurologic syndromes when peripheral viral replication appears well controlled.

CLINICAL SYNDROMES

HIV-related Syndromes

Neurologic disorders may occur at any stage from first infection and seroconversion to AIDS. Even without other manifestations of HIV infection, some are diagnostic of AIDS (dementia and myelopathy). All levels of the neuraxis may be affected, including multisystem disorders. Neurologic disorders are likely to be transient in early HIV infection; in chronic infection, they are more prevalent and more often chronic or progressive.

The neurologic syndromes in early HIV infection are indistinguishable from disorders that occur with infection by other viruses (Table 24.4). These include aseptic meningitis, reversible encephalopathy, leukoencephalitis, seizures, transverse myelitis, cranial and peripheral neuropathy (Bell palsy, Guillain-Barré syndrome), polymyositis, and myoglobinuria. Brachial neuritis and ganglioneuritis are rarely reported. The course is typically self-limited and often with full neurologic recovery.

TABLE 24.4. PRIMARY HIV-RELATED NEUROLOGIC SYNDROMES: ACUTE INFECTION

Acute aseptic meningitis
Acute encephalopathy
Leukoencephalitis
Seizures, generalized or focal
Transverse myelitis
Cranial and peripheral neuropathy
    Bell palsy
    Acute inflammatory demyelinating polyneuropathy of the Guillain-Barré type
Polymyositis
Myoglobinuria

From Britton CB. In: Rowland LP, ed. *Merritt's textbook of neurology. Update 11.* Philadelphia: Lea & Febiger, 1992; with permission.

CSF abnormalities (pleocytosis up to 200 cells/mm^3 and oligoclonal bands) differentiate HIV syndromes from postinfectious disorders. Tests for HIV antibody may be negative because these syndromes may precede or accompany seroconversion, and the tests must be repeated in several weeks. If acute HIV infection is strongly suspected, p24 antigen and viral load assay should be considered if serology is negative. Early antiretroviral therapy may be offered to quickly lower the high viral load typical of acute infection, thereby lowering the viral load set point. The long-term efficacy of this approach is unknown. No specific treatment is indicated for these self-limited disorders, except that plasmapheresis or immune globulin is used for the Guillain-Barré syndrome and steroids for polymyositis.

TABLE 24.5. PRIMARY HIV-RELATED NEUROLOGIC SYNDROMES: CHRONIC INFECTION

Persistent or recurrent meningeal pleocytosis with or without meningeal symptoms

Organic brain syndromes
    Dementia, static or progressive with or without motor signs
    Mild cognitive impairment, neuropsychologic test criteria only
    Organic psychiatric disorder

Cerebrovascular syndromes

Cerebellar ataxia

Seizure disorder

Multisystem degeneration

Chronic progressive myelopathy

Anterior horn cell disease

Cranial and peripheral neuropathy
    Bell palsy
    Hearing loss
    Chronic inflammatory demyelinating polyneuropathy
    Distal symmetric sensory neuropathy
    Mononeuritis multiplex

Autonomic neuropathy

Myopathy

From Britton CB. In: Rowland LP, ed. *Merritt's textbook of neurology. Update 11.* Philadelphia: Lea & Febiger, 1992; with permission.

In chronic HIV infection, neurologic disorders may accompany systemic HIV disease or secondary disorders (Table 24.5). Chronic or recurrent meningeal pleocytosis may occur, sometimes with meningeal symptoms, but it is often asymptomatic. Chronic pleocytosis does not predict any specific neurologic complication. Ascribing CSF pleocytosis to HIV infection requires exclusion of secondary pathogens or tumor.

Cognitive impairment is a well-recognized complication of chronic HIV infection; it may be mild or severe (Table 24.6). Mild cognitive impairment, detected by neuropsychologic tests, does not significantly impair daily function. Minor motor signs, usually motor slowness, may be present. Severe dementia, HIV-1-associated dementia complex (HADC), or AIDS dementia complex (ADC) is diagnostic of AIDS. Other designations are subacute encephalitis, subacute encephalopathy, or HIV encephalitis. The word *complex* is used to denote the association of dementia with motor and behavioral signs. Myelopathy and peripheral neuropathy coexist in 25% of patients.

HADC or ADC is an insidiously progressive subcortical dementia. Early symptoms include apathy, social withdrawal, diminished libido, slow thinking, poor concentration, and forgetfulness. Psychiatric syndromes are sometimes profound and may be the first manifestation of HIV infection, expressed as psychosis, depression, or mania. Motor signs include slow movements, leg weakness, and gait ataxia. There may be headache, tremor, seizures, parkinsonian features, or frontal release signs. Although the disorder is usually progressive, a static level of disability develops in some patients, and some improve in response to medical treatment for HIV or complicating disorders. Complete reversal is exceptional. When progressive, the disease culminates in akinetic mutism, an immobile, bedridden state with global cognitive impairment and urinary incontinence.

In children, there may be a similar static or progressive encephalopathy. Most affected children meet criteria for AIDS, but progressive encephalopathy may occur before immunologic dysfunction is severe, as in adults. Neurologic findings include intellectual deterioration, microcephaly, loss of developmental milestones, and progressive motor impairment that may culminate in spastic quadriparesis and pseudobulbar palsy. Seizures are usually due to fever. Myoclonus and extrapyramidal rigidity are rare.

The CSF is usually normal or shows mild pleocytosis, protein elevation, and oligoclonal bands. CSF gamma globulin content is increased owing to intrathecal synthesis of antibody to HIV antigens. Virus may be cultured from CSF. Both CSF and plasma viral load correlate with dementia occurrence but may be discordant in some cases, with the load being greater in CSF than

TABLE 24.6. HIV-1-ASSOCIATED COGNITIVE/MOTOR COMPLEX AIDS DEMENTIA COMPLEX

Severe manifestations
    HIV-1-associated dementia complex
    HIV-1-associated myelopathy

Mild manifestations
    HIV-1-associated minor cognitive/motor disorder

From American Academy of Neurology AIDS Task Force, 1991; with permission.

in plasma. Phenotypic discordance is also observed, sometimes causing different patterns of drug resistance. CSF markers of immune activation may correlate with severity of dementia and include HIV p24 antigen, β_2-microglobulin, tumor necrosis factor, and antimyelin basic protein. None of these is predictive of or specific for dementia. Other CSF and serum markers also lack predictive value or specificity but may correlate with severity of dementia; the list includes serum neopterin and tryptophan levels, CSF tryptophan and serotonin metabolites, and CSF quinolinic acid levels.

In adults, computed tomography (CT) or magnetic resonance imaging (MRI) may show cortical atrophy and ventricular dilatation, sometimes with white matter changes. On CT, there is attenuation of white matter; T2-weighted and proton-density MRI shows hyperintense white matter lesions ranging from discrete foci to large confluent periventricular lesions (Fig. 24.1). CT in children shows basal ganglia calcification and cerebral atrophy. MRI white matter changes may not correlate with dementia and may disappear spontaneously or with antiretroviral therapy.

Abnormalities in functional neuroimaging are detected in HIV-infected persons with and without dementia. The abnormalities become worse or change with progressive cognitive impairment. Positron emission tomography using fluorodeoxyglucose shows relative hypermetabolism in the thalamus and basal ganglia in HIV-infected persons. Progressive dementia is accompanied by cortical and subcortical hypometabolism. Single-photon emission computed tomography (SPECT) shows multifocal cortical perfusion deficits in the frontal lobes, which are worse in those with dementia. Cerebral metabolite abnormalities demonstrated by magnetic resonance spectroscopy (MRS) include elevated myoinositol and choline levels in frontal white matter, indicative of glial proliferation in patients with mild cognitive

impairment. Severe dementia is associated with decreased levels of *N*-acetylaspartate, a neuronal marker. Dynamic cerebral blood volume (CBV) studies by functional MRI in HIV-positive persons show increased CBV in deep and cortical gray matter and even greater increases in deep gray matter of those with dementia.

Pathologic abnormalities in brain include microglial nodules, giant cells, focal perivascular demyelination and gliosis, and neuronal loss in the frontal cortex. There is often no correlation between the severity of pathologic changes and the severity of dementia.

The incidence of AIDS dementia is less than the frequency of pathologic abnormalities. The CDC reported a prevalence of 7.3% for the diagnosis of HIV encephalopathy in 1987 through 1991. The Multicenter AIDS Cohort Study Group reported a 4% prevalence of dementia diagnosis with a 7% annual rate and a 15% overall probability of dementia before death. There may be excess mortality in demented patients.

The diagnosis of HADC or ADC requires exclusion of secondary OIs or neoplasms. Other confounding variables include drug use and vitamin B_{12} deficiency. Although some investigators report improvement in dementia and a lower incidence since the introduction of azidothymidine (zidovudine), others find transient or no effect of the drug on progressive dementia. The impact of protease inhibitors and HAART on dementia is not yet known. Clinical trials of selegiline hydrochloride (also known as deprenyl) (Eldepryl), a monoamine oxidase type B inhibitor, and nimodipine (Nimotop) suggest a trend for improvement in cognitive impairment. Antioxidants and agents that block gp120 are ineffective.

Longitudinal cohort studies have shown no neuropsychologic deterioration in asymptomatic individuals. Neuropsychologic

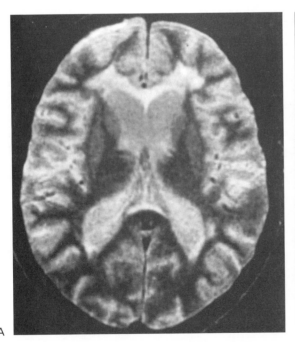
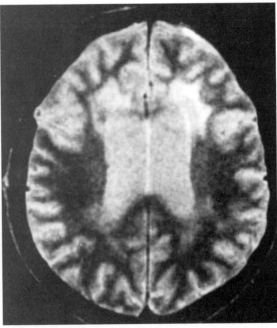

A   B

FIG. 24.1. A,B: T2-weighted MR images from a patient with progressive dementia show ventricular dilatation, cortical atrophy, and periventricular frontal lobe white matter hyperintensity.

test abnormalities do accrue with advancing disease but not necessarily with overt dementia. Those showing a decline in neuropsychologic test performance, however, have an excessive risk of death. The strongest predictors of significant dementia identified in a multiinstitution study of 19,462 HIV-infected persons are a CD4+ T-lymphocyte count of less than 100 cells/μL, anemia, and an AIDS-defining infection or neoplasm (18.6% to 24.9% risk in 2 years).

Stroke syndromes occur in 0.5% to 8% of patients in clinical studies, and infarcts are more frequent at autopsy. Stroke syndromes may follow secondary infections or neoplasms, such as cryptococcosis or other fungal infections, toxoplasmosis, tuberculosis, herpes zoster, CMV infection, syphilis, or Kaposi sarcoma. Other causes include HIV-related vasculitis, cardiogenic emboli, and thrombogenic conditions such as hyperviscosity, disseminated intravascular coagulopathy, and lupus anticoagulant. Cerebral hemorrhage may follow HIV-associated thrombocytopenia or toxoplasmosis.

Evaluation of cerebrovascular syndromes includes imaging; CSF examination; cultures for viruses, bacteria, mycobacteria, and fungi; serum and CSF antibodies for cryptococcosis, syphilis, and toxoplasmosis; plasma and CSF HIV viral load; polymerase chain reaction (PCR) amplification of CSF for suspected pathogens; echocardiography; Doppler ultrasound; coagulation profiles; platelet count; and determination of procoagulants. If vasculitis is suspected, angiography or brain or meningeal biopsy may be useful.

Seizures may occur at any stage of HIV infection and may be focal or generalized. The incidence is uncertain, but in one study of 100 consecutive cases, secondary pathogens were identified in 53% and HIV encephalopathy in 24%; there was no identified cause in 23%. All patients with seizures should be evaluated for other pathogens or tumor.

Leukoencephalopathies in acute or chronic HIV infection include acute fulminating and fatal leukoencephalitis, multifocal vacuolar leukoencephalopathy presenting as rapid dementia, and a relapsing-remitting leukoencephalitis that may simulate multiple sclerosis. The pathogenesis of these syndromes is uncertain.

Chronic progressive myelopathy, an AIDS-defining illness, is characterized by progressive spastic, ataxic paraparesis with bowel and bladder disorders. Although most patients rapidly become wheelchair-bound, others progress indolently for years. Subclinical myelopathy may be detected by electrophysiologic studies in otherwise asymptomatic subjects. Pathologic findings are similar to those of subacute combined degeneration owing to vitamin B_{12} deficiency and include vacuolar change with intramyelin swelling or demyelination that is most severe in the lateral and posterior columns. Microglial nodules and giant cells are sometimes seen, and HIV may be detected by hybridization techniques or cultured. Pathologic abnormalities are more commonly detected than clinical symptoms. The diagnosis of HIV myelopathy requires exclusion of cord compression, secondary infections, and nutritional deficiency. Contrast MRI may show gadolinium-enhanced lesions of myelitis.

No specific treatment is available for myelopathy. Improvement on zidovudine therapy has been reported, but the drug is generally ineffective. The impact of protease inhibitors and HAART is unknown.

Peripheral and *autonomic neuropathy* occur in otherwise asymptomatic HIV-infected persons, especially with advancing disease. Clinical syndromes include mononeuritis multiplex, chronic inflammatory demyelinating polyneuropathy (CIDP), distal symmetric polyneuropathy, and ganglioneuritis.

CIDP is distinguished from Guillain-Barré syndrome by a subacute or progressive course and variable response to steroids or plasmapheresis. Electrodiagnostic studies show demyelination with variable axonal damage. Histopathologic studies reveal epineurial inflammatory cell infiltrates and primary demyelination with variable axonal degeneration. HIV is sometimes cultured from nerve. CSF findings are nondiagnostic, although pleocytosis is sometimes found.

Distal sensorimotor neuropathy is the most common peripheral nerve disorder of AIDS, increasing in frequency with advancing disease. The incidence of neuropathy is also increasing because of longer survival of HIV-infected persons. Symptoms include painful, burning dysesthesia that is often confined to the soles of the feet. Signs include stocking-glove sensory loss, mild muscle wasting and weakness, and loss of ankle jerks. Conduction studies show sensorimotor neuropathy with mixed axonal and demyelinating features. Pathologic findings include axonal degeneration, loss of large myelinated fibers, and variable inflammatory cell infiltration. Vasculitis is sometimes found. CSF may be normal or show mild pleocytosis and elevated protein content. HIV may be cultured from nerve, but the cellular localization of the virus is not known. The neuropathy may be mediated by the binding of gp120 envelope viral glycoprotein to sensory ganglion cells.

The *pain syndrome* may be disabling, sometimes responsive to tricyclic antidepressants, anticonvulsants, and nonsteroidal or narcotic analgesia. Pain control may be difficult. Peptide T was ineffective in clinical trials. Immune globulin is sometimes used in refractory cases, with anecdotal reports of success. Vasculitis may respond to prednisone.

Myopathy is uncommon, characterized by proximal limb weakness, mild creatine kinase elevation, and myopathic features on electromyography (EMG). Pathologic findings include muscle fiber degeneration with or without inflammatory cell infiltrates. An HIV-related cause is suspected after exclusion of other causes. Zidovudine causes a clinically similar myopathy related to effects on mitochondria, with ragged red fibers. Cytochrome oxidase is deficient in zidovudine myopathy but not in HIV myopathy. Some patients respond well to steroid therapy without accelerated progression of HIV disease.

Opportunistic Infections and Neoplasms

Secondary OIs and neoplasia are diagnostic of AIDS (Table 24.7). Their incidence and severity have declined since 1996 because of potent combination antiretroviral regimens that include protease inhibitors. Even before the use of HAART for HIV, prophylactic therapy had lowered the incidence of many infections.

Meningitis may be due to viruses (herpesvirus group: HSV, VZV, CMV, HBV, and Epstein-Barr virus [EBV]), fungi (*Cryptococcus, Histoplasma, Coccidioides, Candida*), bacteria (*Listeria, T. pallidum, Salmonella, S. aureus,* pyogenic bacteria, and atypi-

TABLE 24.7. SECONDARY NEUROLOGIC SYNDROMES IN HIV INFECTION AND AIDS: OPPORTUNISTIC INFECTIONS AND NEOPLASMS

Leptomeninges
Viral	CMV, HSV, VZV, EBV, HBV
Fungal	*Cryptococcus, Histoplasma, Coccidioides, Candida*
Bacterial	*Listeria, Treponema pallidum*, pyogenic bacteria (*Salmonella, Staphylococcus aureus*), atypical or conventional mycobacteria
Neoplasm	Lymphoma

Cerebral syndromes: diffuse encephalopathy or encephalitis
Viral	CMV, HSV, VZV
Bacterial	Atypical mycobacterium
Parasitic	*Acanthamoeba, Toxoplasma*
Neoplasm	Lymphoma

Focal cerebral syndromes
Viral	HSV, VZV, PML
Fungal	Abscess due to *Cryptococcus, Candida, Zygomycetes, Histoplasma, Aspergillus*
Bacterial	Abscess due to pyogenic bacteria,
Parasitic	mycobacteria (tuberculoma), *Listeria, Nocardia Trypanosoma cruzei, Taenia solium, Toxoplasma*
Neoplasm	Primary or metastatic lymphoma, glioma, metastatic Kaposi sarcoma

Cerebrovascular syndromes and seizures
Viral	VZV, HSV, rarely PML
Fungal	*Cryptococcus* or other fungi
Bacterial	*T. pallidum, Mycobacterium* tuberculosis
Parasitic	*Toxoplasma*
Neoplasm	Lymphoma, lymphomatoid granulomatosis, metastatic Kaposi sarcoma
Other	Cerebral hemorrhage, cardiac emboli, vasculitis

Movement disorders
Bacterial	CNS Whipple disease
Parasitic	*Toxoplasma*

Spinal cord syndromes
Viral	VZV, CMV, HSV
Bacterial	Mycobacteria
Parasitic	*Toxoplasma*
Neoplasm	Lymphoma

Cranial and peripheral neuropathy
Viral	CMV (retinitis, polyradiculitis, mononeuritis multiplex)
Fungal	*Candida* (retinitis)
Parasitic	*Toxoplasma* (retinitis)

Myositis
Bacterial	*S. aureus*, mycobacteria
Parasitic	*Toxoplasma*

cal or conventional mycobacteria), and neoplasm (lymphoma). Cryptococcal infection is the most common cause of meningitis in AIDS, reported in 6% to 11% of patients in clinical series. There are no specific distinguishing features, except that meningeal signs may be mild or absent. The diagnosis is made by detecting cryptococcal antigen in serum and CSF or by CSF culture. CSF cell count and chemistries may be normal or nondiagnostic when antigen is present. CT may show normal patterns, atrophy, mass lesion (cryptococcoma), hydrocephalus, or diffuse edema. Lifelong suppressive therapy, necessary to eradicate infection and prevent relapse, may not be necessary if immune reconstitution occurs with antiretroviral therapy (see Chapter 25).

Oral agents (fluconazole [Diflucan] and itraconazole [Sporanox]) have generally replaced amphotericin B in management. Oral prophylaxis in late-stage HIV disease may prevent most fungal infections.

The clinical course of *neurosyphilis* may be altered by concomitant HIV infection. Occasionally, the CSF Venereal Disease Research Laboratory test is nonreactive, and baseline CSF abnormalities render interpretation of CSF data difficult when the diagnosis is suspected. Intravenous penicillin therapy is required for documented neurosyphilis. Relapse is more common in HIV-infected persons, and follow-up is needed after cessation of therapy. Serology is tested monthly for 3 months and at 3-month intervals thereafter. If serologic titers rise, retreatment is indicated. The best treatment for late lues in dually infected patients is controversial. Some argue that intravenous therapy should be used in all dually infected patients, even when the CSF is normal. At our institution, intravenous therapy is reserved for symptomatic patients with positive serum and CSF serology, with monitoring of those who do not meet criteria for neurosyphilis (see Chapter 27).

Tuberculous meningitis, atypical mycobacterial infections of the brain, and *tuberculomas* are risks in HIV-infected persons. Conventional antituberculous therapy is usually effective for conventional mycobacteria. Prophylaxis with clarithromycin (Biaxin) or rifabutin (Mycobutin) is reasonably effective for infections with atypical organisms, which otherwise require multidrug regimens. The incidence of tuberculous disease and drug resistance in AIDS has declined dramatically due to effective treatment strategies that include directly observed therapy. Atypical organisms are less common because of potent HIV therapy.

Viral encephalitis may be due to a virus of the herpesvirus group: CMV most commonly and HSV and VZV infrequently. *Mycobacterium avium-intracellulare* complex infection, toxoplasmosis, and lymphoma may also cause diffuse encephalopathy.

Focal brain syndromes are caused by toxoplasmosis, PML, and abscesses owing to *Nocardia, Listeria, Trypanosoma cruzei, Taenia solium, Candida, Cryptococcus, Histoplasma, Aspergillus, Coccidioides, Mycobacterium tuberculosis*, atypical mycobacteria, and pyogenic bacteria.

Toxoplasmosis, the most common cause of intracranial mass lesion in AIDS, typically causes chronic progressive focal signs and seizures. In some patients, the clinical disorder is a subacute encephalopathy. CT or MRI discloses enhancing lesions with mass effect that typically involve the basal ganglia (Fig. 24.2). Although the radiographic findings are not diagnostic, multiple lesions in the basal ganglia in patients with anti-*Toxoplasma* antibodies are presumptive evidence. CSF is nondiagnostic; PCR amplification may detect *Toxoplasma* DNA. Toxoplasmosis antibodies are found in more than 95% of patients. Seronegative toxoplasmosis is rare. Differential diagnosis is mainly lymphoma or, rarely, pyogenic abscess. Toxoplasmosis is treated in patients at risk for HIV, multiple lesions, and antibodies to the organism. Biopsy is reserved for those who show no clinical or radiographic response after 1 week of therapy.

Before AIDS, *PML* was a rare infection seen in immunosuppressed persons. After PML was recognized as a complication of AIDS in 1982, the death rate increased in the general population from 1.5 to 6.1 per 10 million population. The reported incidence in AIDS is 1.0% to 5.3%. Lytic viral infection of oligo-dendrocytes causes demyelination and progressive focal signs. Localization is hemispheral in 85% to 90% of patients; the posterior fossa is affected in the remainder. Focal or generalized seizures occur in 6% of patients. PML may be the first AIDS-

defining illness and may occur when immunosuppression is not severe. Prognosis is generally poor, with death in 4 to 6 months.

The diagnosis may be suspected in a patient with focal signs, hypodense nonenhancing lesions on CT, and no mass effect. MRI is more sensitive, with high-signal-intensity lesions on T2-

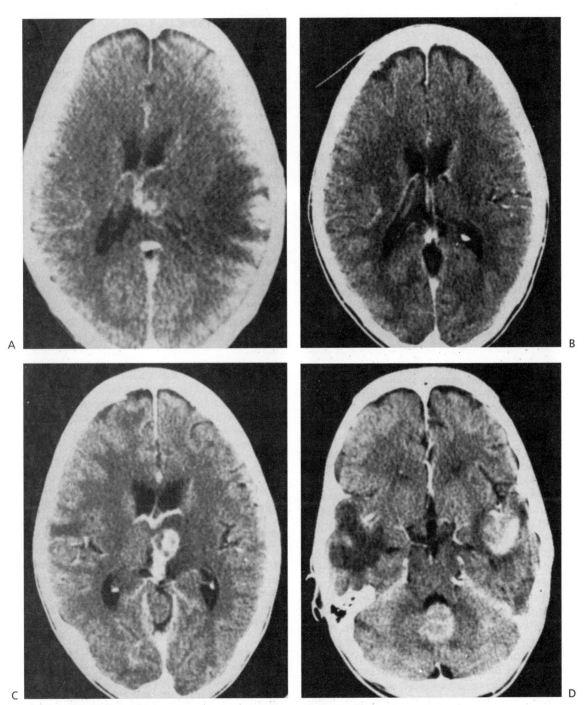

FIG. 24.2. Toxoplasmosis in AIDS. **A:** Contrast-enhanced axial CT shows left thalamic parietal and nodular enhancing lesions with adjacent edema and mass effect, consistent with toxoplasmosis. **B:** A follow-up contrast-enhanced scan 6 weeks later demonstrates resolution of the lesions and mass effect with therapy. Contrast-enhanced axial CT obtained at the same **(C)** and lower **(D)** levels 11 weeks later demonstrates recurrent nodular and ring enhancement in the left thalamus with adjacent edema and mass effect. The edema in the right frontal and temporal regions **(C,D)** is related to another lesion. Additional enhancing lesions are present in the left temporal region and vermis **(D)**. (Courtesy of Drs. J.A. Bello and S.K. Hilal.)

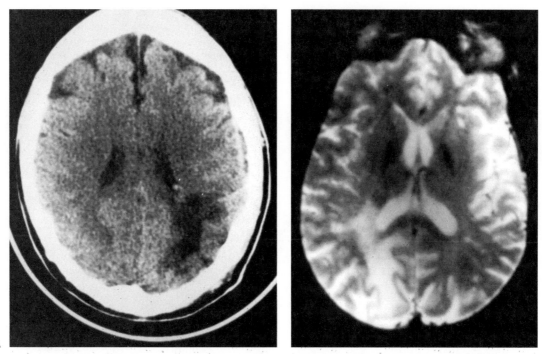

FIG. 24.3. A: CT in a patient with biopsy-proven PML shows a hypointense parietooccipital lesion without mast effect. **B:** T2- weighted MR image from a patient with biopsy-proven PML shows a hyperintense parietooccipital lesion.

weighted studies without mass effect or enhancement (Fig. 24.3). The causative virus may be detected in CSF by PCR, but a negative study does not exclude the diagnosis. Diagnosis requires brain biopsy because imaging abnormalities are similar to those of toxoplasmosis, fungal infection, and lymphoma.

There may be spontaneous stabilization of PML lesions in HIV infection, and there may be a response to zidovudine therapy or potent combination therapy that includes protease inhibitors. Clinical trials failed to show beneficial effect of intravenous or intrathecal cytarabine (Cytosar-U). There are anecdotal reports of efficacy, however. Topetecan, a topoisomerase inhibitor, is currently being studied.

Lymphoma is the most common neoplasm in AIDS, occurring in 0.6% to 3% of patients. Clinical signs are nonspecific and include focal neurologic signs, seizures, cranial neuropathy, and headache. CT may be normal or show hypodense lesions and single or multiple lesions with patchy or nodular enhancement. EBV DNA is found in PCR studies of CSF. Brain biopsy is required for diagnosis. The prognosis is poor; most patients succumb in 6 months. Some, however, respond to radiotherapy, chemotherapy, and management of coexistent OIs. There are reports of complete tumor regression after potent antiretroviral therapy. Other neoplasms reported in AIDS include metastatic Kaposi sarcoma and, rarely, primary glial tumors.

Movement disorders in patients with HIV infection are usually symptomatic of underlying cerebral infection, most commonly toxoplasmosis.

Infection of the spinal cord has been reported with the herpesvirus group, including HSV, CMV, and VZV, as well as with mycobacteria, pyogenic bacteria, and *Toxoplasma*. Spinal cord biopsy is necessary for definitive diagnosis and may be consid-

ered if systemic infection suggests metastatic foci in the spinal cord.

Infectious *retinopathy* may be caused by toxoplasmosis, CMV infection, or candidiasis. Cranial neuropathy may complicate meningitis. Polyradiculopathy or cauda equina syndrome may be due to CMV infection. The diagnosis may be suspected clinically in patients with disseminated CMV and may respond to ganciclovir sodium (Cytovene) and foscarnet sodium (Foscavir). Antiviral therapy may be given to patients with an otherwise typical syndrome, even before CMV infection is confirmed. PCR studies of CSF are helpful if positive, but negative studies do not exclude the diagnosis. Quantitative plasma PCR may identify persons at risk for CMV disease. Without treatment, the syndrome is progressive and fatal. Both the incidence and severity of CMV disease are lessened by HAART for HIV. In some cases, lifelong prophylaxis is no longer necessary. Pyomyositis may be due to infection with *S. aureus*, *Toxoplasma*, or atypical mycobacteria.

Drug-induced Syndromes

The nucleoside analogs used to treat HIV infection cause dose- and duration-related neurologic complications. Chronic zidovudine therapy may cause myopathy with ragged red fibers. Symptoms usually improve following cessation of the drug. The nucleoside antiretrovirals didanosine (ddI; Videx), zalcitabine (ddC; Hivid), stavudine (d4T; Zerit), and lamivudine (3TC; Epivir) can cause dose-related severe, painful sensory neuropathy that often improves after dose reduction or drug withdrawal. Failure to improve may indicate the cooccurrence of HIV-related neuropathy.

Patients with HIV infection experience hypersensitivity to many drugs, including the neuroleptics, which may cause secondary parkinsonism or the neuroleptic malignant syndrome. Nutritional deficiencies may include thiamine, vitamin B_{12}, folic acid, and glutathione, which may lead to encephalopathy, dementia, neuropathy, or spinal cord disorders. Metabolic abnormalities often occur in late disease and are reversible causes of encephalopathy.

DIAGNOSTIC EVALUATION

The diagnostic evaluation of patients with a suspected HIV-related disease includes an enzyme-linked immunosorbent assay for HIV serology. Positive results are confirmed by Western blot test. Depending on local laws, serologic tests may require informed consent and counseling. In patients with otherwise typical viral syndromes, such as aseptic meningitis or transverse myelitis, HIV infection must be suspected, even in the absence of known risk behavior. Absence of antibodies during the acute illness does not negate the diagnosis, because these disorders typically occur with seroconversion. A convalescent titer should be obtained at least 6 weeks later and possibly again at 3 and 6 months to ensure true seronegativity. Rarely, patients may be seronegative for prolonged periods. Repeat testing or studies to detect viral antigen or nucleic acid is based on risk behavior or other clinical information.

Other diagnostic studies include determination of CD lymphocyte subset ratio, plasma viral load, serum protein electrophoresis, quantitative immunoglobulins, and enumerated platelets. An anergy panel can assess functional immune status.

Evaluation for specific neurologic syndromes should be preceded by general physical examination to exclude OIs or tumor. Evaluation may include biopsy of skin, lymph nodes, or bone marrow, as well as chest film. Blood culture for viruses and fungi may be necessary. Accurate neurologic diagnosis requires systematic evaluation, including the possibility of multiple diseases. Electroencephalography may show evidence of a focal lesion when scans are still nondiagnostic. CSF is most helpful in syphilis and fungal or tuberculous infection. In lymphoma meningitis, tumor cells are rarely recognized by cytologic studies. Viruses are infrequently cultured from CSF; HIV may be detected but may be a copassenger and not responsible for the disorder in question. CMV may be cultured in CMV-related polyradiculopathy. PCR amplification of CSF may be helpful for diagnosis of CMV infection, toxoplasmosis, or PML; but negative results do not exclude these infections. CSF abnormalities are common in asymptomatic HIV infection and must be interpreted with caution in the consideration of other possible conditions. CT or MRI is useful in distinguishing focal from diffuse brain lesions. MRS and thallium-SPECT may distinguish tumor from infection.

Brain biopsy may be required for diagnosis. Stereotactic biopsy is a low-risk procedure in experienced hands. For solitary lesions, it is reasonable to treat for toxoplasmosis when serology or PCR is positive; biopsy is reserved for failure to respond to treatment and for PCR- and seronegative cases.

Myelopathy is evaluated by MRI with gadolinium enhancement or by myelography. CSF may be helpful in evaluating peripheral neuropathies, especially CMV polyneuropathy. EMG and nerve conduction studies are useful in evaluating myelopathy, peripheral neuropathy, and myopathy. Nerve or muscle biopsy may be required.

TREATMENT, COURSE, AND PROGNOSIS

Potent combination antiretroviral therapy has transformed AIDS from a fatal disease to a chronic illness. In the United States, AIDS diagnosis and AIDS deaths have declined since 1996. Even before potent drug therapy for HIV, prophylactic therapy of common OIs reduced their incidence. Improved medical care has reduced the need for hospital admissions in this population.

Antiretroviral drugs improve morbidity owing to HIV and extend survival. Fifteen drugs in three classes have been approved for use, and more are in clinical trials or development: nucleoside reverse transcriptase (RT) inhibitor, nonnucleoside RT inhibitor, nucleotide RT inhibitor, and protease inhibitor. Nucleoside RT inhibitors block viral replication by incorporation into the DNA copy of the RNA genome and termination of the DNA synthesis. This class includes zidovudine, didanosine, zalcitabine, stavudine, lamivudine, and abacavir (Ziagen). Nonnucleoside RT inhibitors include nevirapine (Viramune), delavirdine mesylate, and efavirenz (Sustiva). Adefovir dipivoxil is the sole nucleotide analog RT inhibitor. Protease inhibitors include ritonavir (Norvir), saquinavir mesylate (Invirase, Fortovase), indinavir (Crixivan), nelfinavir (Viracept), and amprenavir. Combination drug therapy that includes a protease inhibitor is recommended.

Despite improved therapy, HIV infection is a serious diagnosis and rapidly fatal in developing countries, where there is no access to effective treatment. Moreover, therapy does not eliminate latent provirus and may fail if resistant mutants arise. Efforts continue in attempts to develop an effective vaccine. Candidate vaccines are in clinical trials in areas of high seroprevalence and seroconversion. The complex biology of the virus and the host immunogenetic response to infection pose significant challenges to successful vaccine development.

PRECAUTIONS FOR CLINICAL AND LABORATORY SERVICES

Strict observation of contamination procedures or universal precautions is mandatory. The hospital patient with known or suspected HIV infection is not isolated, unless there is a respiratory infection, such as tuberculosis, or severe neutropenia. Strict precautions should be observed in the handling of all waste, body fluids, and surgical specimens. Gloves are worn to prevent mucous membrane contact with blood, excretions, secretions, and tissues of infected patients. Goggles or glasses should be used if heavy aerosol contamination with blood or other secretions is anticipated, for example, in the operating room. Masks are not needed, unless the patient requires respiratory isolation for other reasons. Needles and other sharp instruments in contact with infected blood should be disposed in proper containers. Health care workers should not recap needles to avoid needle-stick injury.

The risks to health care workers are small but real. At least 52 people have been documented with HIV seroconversion following needle-stick injury or mucocutaneous exposure. The converse risk, to patients from infected workers, is exceedingly small, but HIV-positive workers should not engage in invasive procedures in which cuts may occur.

HIV is readily inactivated by heat in standard sterilization solutions including 70% alcohol. Special sterilization procedures may not be necessary but are often used.

HIV-infected people may survive 10 to 20 years or longer before succumbing. During this time, many complications are likely to ensue. Patients need rigorous evaluation for systemic and neurologic syndromes at all stages of infection because of the risk for multiple, coexistent, or sequential problems.

SUGGESTED READINGS

Albrecht H, Hoffmann C, Degen O, et al. Highly active antiretroviral therapy significantly improves the prognosis of patients with HIV-associated progressive multifocal leukoencephalopathy. *AIDS* 1998;12:1149–1154.

American Academy of Neurology AIDS Task Force. Nomenclature and research case definition for neurologic manifestations of human immunodeficiency virus-type (HIV-1) infection. *Neurology* 1991;41:778–785.

Antinori A, Ammassari A, De Luca A, et al. Diagnosis of AIDS-related focal brain lesions: a decision-making analysis based on clinical and neuroradiologic characteristics combined with polymerase chain reaction assays in CSF. *Neurology* 1997;48:687–694.

Behar R, Wiley C, McCutchan JA. Cytomegalovirus polyradiculoneuropathy in acquired immune deficiency syndrome. *Neurology* 1987;37:557–561.

Bencherif B, Rottenberg DA. Neuroimaging of the AIDS dementia complex. *AIDS* 1998;12:233–244.

Berger JR, Svenningsson A, Raffanti S, et al. Tropical spastic paraparesis-like illness occurring in a patient dually infected with HIV-I and HTLV-II. *Neurology* 1991;41:85–87.

Berger JR, Tornatore C, Major EO, et al. Relapsing and remitting human immunodeficiency virus-associated leukoencephalomyelopathy. *Ann Neurol* 1992;31:34–38.

Bishburg E, Sunderam G, Reichman LB, et al. Central nervous system tuberculosis with the acquired immunodeficiency syndrome and its related complex. *Ann Intern Med* 1986;105:210–213.

Britton CB, Mesa-Tejada R, Fenoglio CM, et al. A new complication of AIDS: thoracic myelitis caused by herpes simplex virus. *Neurology* 1985;35:1071–1074.

Buchacz KA, Wilkinson DA, Krowka JF, et al. Genetic and immunological host factors associated with susceptibility to HIV-1 infection. *AIDS* 1998;12[Suppl A]:S87–S94.

Centers for Disease Control. 1993 revised classification system for HIV infection and expanded surveillance case definition for AIDS among adolescents and adults. *MMWR* 1992;41(RR-17):1–19.

Chalmers AC, Greco CM, Miller RG. Prognosis in AZT myopathy. *Neurology* 1991;41:1181–1184.

Chang L, Ernst T, Leonido-Yee M, et al. Cerebral metabolite abnormalities correlate with clinical severity of HIV-1 cognitive motor complex. *Neurology* 1999;52:100–108.

Cinque P, Vago L, Ceresa D, et al. Cerebrospinal fluid HIV-1 RNA levels: correlation with HIV encephalitis. *AIDS* 1998;12:389–394.

The Dana Consortium on the Therapy of HIV Dementia and Related Cognitive Disorders. A randomized, double-blind, placebo-controlled trial of deprenyl and thioctic acid in human immunodeficiency virus-associated cognitive impairment. *Neurology* 1998;50:645–651.

De la Monte SM, Ho DD, Schooley RT, et al. Subacute encephalomyelitis

of AIDS and its relation to HTLV-III infection. *Neurology* 1987;37:562–569.

Eilbott DJ, Peress N, Burger H, et al. Human immunodeficiency virus type 1 in spinal cords of acquired immunodeficiency syndrome patients with myelopathy: expression and replication in macrophages. *Proc Natl Acad Sci U S A* 1989;86:3337–3341.

Epstein LG, Gendelman HE. Human immunodeficiency virus type 1 infection of the nervous system: pathogenetic mechanisms. *Ann Neurol* 1993;33:429–436.

Epstein LG, Sharer LR, Oleske JM, et al. Neurologic manifestations of human immunodeficiency virus infection in children. *Pediatrics* 1986;78:678–687.

Flexner C. HIV-protease inhibitors. *N Engl J Med* 1998;338:1281–1292.

Freeman R, Roberts MS, Friedman LS, et al. Autonomic function and human immunodeficiency virus infection. *Neurology* 1990;40:575–580.

Gao F, Bailes E, Robertson DL, et al. Origin of HIV-1 in the chimpanzee *Pan troglodytes troglodytes*. *Nature* 1999;397:436–441.

Goldstein JD, Dickson DW, Moser FG, et al. Primary central nervous system lymphoma in acquired immune deficiency syndrome: a clinical and pathologic study with results of treatment with radiation. *Cancer* 1991;67:2755–2765.

Gray F, Chimelli L, Mohr M, et al. Fulminating multiple sclerosis-like leukoencephalopathy revealing human immunodeficiency virus infection. *Neurology* 1991;41:105–109.

Haase AT, Henry K, Zupancic M, et al. Quantitative tissue analysis of HIV-1 infection in lymphoid tissue. *Science* 1996;274:985–989.

Hammer AM, Yeni P. Antiretroviral therapy: where are we? *AIDS* 1998;12[Suppl A]:S181–S188.

Hengge UR, Brockmeyer NH, Esser S, et al. HIV-1 RNA levels in cerebrospinal fluid and plasma correlate with AIDS dementia. *AIDS* 1998;12:818–820.

Ho DD, Rota TR, Schooley RT, et al. Isolation of HTLV-III from cerebrospinal fluid and neural tissues of patients with neurologic syndromes related to the acquired immunodeficiency syndrome. *N Engl J Med* 1985;313:1493–1497.

Hoffman TL, Doms RW. Chemokines and coreceptors in HIV/SIV-host interactions. *AIDS* 1998;12[Suppl A]:S17–S26.

Hollander H, Stringari S. Human immunodeficiency virus-associated meningitis: clinical course and complications. *Am J Med* 1987;83:813–816.

Holtzman DM, Kaku DA, So YT. New onset seizures associated with human immunodeficiency virus infection: causation and clinical features in 100 cases. *Am J Med* 1989;87:173–177.

Husstedt IW, Grotemeyer KH, Busch H, et al. Progression of distal-symmetric polyneuropathy in HIV infection: a prospective study. *AIDS* 1993;7:1069–1073.

Jacobson MA, French M. Altered natural history of AIDS-related opportunistic infections in the era of potent combination antiretroviral therapy. *AIDS* 1998;12[Suppl A]:S157–S163.

Kahn JO, Walker BD. Acute human immunodeficiency virus type 1 infection. *N Engl J Med* 1998;339:33–39.

Kinloch-De Loes S, Hirschel BJ, Hoen B, et al. A controlled trial of zidovudine in primary human immunodeficiency virus infection. *N Engl J Med* 1995;333:408–413.

Lange DJ, Britton CB, Younger DS, et al. The neuromuscular manifestations of human immunodeficiency virus infections. *Ann Neurol* 1988;45:1084–1088.

Luft BJ, Haffner R, Korzun AH, et al. Toxoplasmic encephalitis in patients with the acquired immunodeficiency syndrome. *N Engl J Med* 1993;329:995–1000.

Mahe A, Bruet A, Chabin E, et al. Acute rhabdomyolysis coincident with primary HIV infection [Letter]. *Lancet* 1989;2:1454–1455.

Mayeux R, Stern Y, Tang MX, et al. Mortality risks in gay men with human immunodeficiency virus infection and cognitive impairment. *Neurology* 1993;43:176–182.

McArthur JC, Cohen BA, Farzedegan H, et al. Cerebrospinal fluid abnormalities in homosexual men with and without neuropsychiatric findings. *Ann Neurol* 1988;23[Suppl]:S34–S37.

McArthur JC, Hoover DR, Bacellar H, et al. Dementia in AIDS patients: incidence and risk factors. *Neurology* 1993;38:2245–2252.

McGowan JP, Shah S. Long-term remission of AIDS-related primary central nervous lymphoma associated with highly active antiretroviral therapy [Letter]. *AIDS* 1998;12:952–954.

Mellors JW, Rinaldo CR Jr, Gupta P, et al. Prognosis in HIV-1 infection predicted by the quantity of virus in plasma. *Science* 1996;272:1167–1170.

Michelet C, Arvieux C, Francois C, et al. Opportunistic infections occurring during highly active antiretroviral treatment. *AIDS* 1998;12:1815–1822.

Miller EN, Selnes OA, McArthur JC, et al. Neuropsychological performance in HIV-1-infected homosexual men: the Multicenter AIDS Cohort Study (MACS). *Neurology* 1990;40:197–203.

Miller JR, Barrett RE, Britton CB, et al. Progressive multifocal leukoencephalopathy in a male homosexual with T-cell immune deficiency. *N Engl J Med* 1982;307:1436–1438.

Nath A, Jankovic J, Pettigrew LC. Movement disorders and AIDS. *Neurology* 1987;37:37–41.

Navia BA, Cho ES, Petito CK, Price RW. The AIDS dementia complex. II. Neuropathology. *Ann Neurol* 1986;19:525–535.

Navia BA, Jordan BD, Price RW. The AIDS dementia complex. I. Clinical features. *Ann Neurol* 1986;19:517–524.

Navia BA, Price RW. The acquired immunodeficiency syndrome dementia complex as the presenting or sole manifestation of human immunodeficiency virus infection. *Arch Neurol* 1987;44:65–69.

Petito CK, Cho ES, Lemann W, et al. Neuropathology of acquired immunodeficiency syndrome (AIDS): an autopsy review. *J Neuropathol Exp Neurol* 1986;45:635–646.

Petito CK, Navia BA, Cho ES, et al. Vacuolar myelopathy pathologically resembling subacute combined degeneration in patients with the acquired immunodeficiency syndrome. *N Engl J Med* 1985;312:874–879.

Portegeis P, Enting RH, deGans J, et al. Presentation and course of AIDS dementia complex: 10 years of follow-up in Amsterdam, the Netherlands. *AIDS* 1993;7:669–675.

Price RW, Perry SW, eds. *HIV, AIDS and the brain. Research publication of the Association for Research in Nervous and Mental Disease, vol 72.* New York: Raven Press, 1994.

Qureshi AI, Hanson DL, Jones JL, et al. Estimation of the temporal probability of human immunodeficiency virus (HIV) dementia after risk stratification for HIV-infected persons. *Neurology* 1998;50:392–397.

Redfield RR, Wright DC, Tramont EC. The Walter Reed staging classification for HTLV-III/LAV infection. *N Engl J Med* 1986;314:131–132.

Resnick L, diMarzo-Veronese F, Schupbach J, et al. Intra-blood-brain-barrier synthesis of HTLV-III-specific IgG in patients with neurologic symptoms associated with AIDS or AIDS-related complex. *N Engl J Med* 1985;313:1498–1504.

Seirlean D, Duyckaerts C, Vazeux R, et al. HIV-1-associated cognitive motor complex: absence of neuronal loss in the cerebral neocortex. *Neurology* 1993;43:1492–1499.

Selnes OA, Galai N, McArthur JC, et al. HIV infection and cognition in intravenous drug users: long-term follow-up. *Neurology* 1997;48:223–230.

Simpson DM, Bender AN. Human immunodeficiency virus-associated myopathy: analysis of 11 patients. *Ann Neurol* 1988;24:79–84.

Snider WD, Simpson DM, Nielsen S, et al. Neurological complications of acquired immune deficiency syndrome: analysis of 50 patients. *Ann Neurol* 1983;14:403–418.

So YT, Olney RK. Acute lumbosacral polyradiculopathy in acquired immunodeficiency syndrome: experience in 23 patients. *Ann Neurol* 1994;35:53–58.

Steinman RM, Germain RN. Antigen presentation and related immunological aspects of HIV-1 vaccines. *AIDS* 1998;12[Suppl A]:S97–S112.

Telzak EE, Zweig-Greenberg MS, Harrison J, et al. Syphilis treatment response in HIV-infected individuals. *AIDS* 1991;5:591–595.

Wildemann B, Haas J, Lynen N, et al. Diagnosis of cytomegalovirus encephalitis in patients with AIDS by quantitation of cytomegalovirus genomes in cells of cerebrospinal fluid. *Neurology* 1998;50:693–697.

Wiley CA, Masliah E, Morey M, et al. Neocortical damage during HIV infection. *Ann Neurol* 1991;29:651–657.

Wiley CA, Schrier RD, Nelson JA, et al. Cellular localization of human immunodeficiency virus infection within the brains of acquired immune deficiency syndrome patients. *Proc Natl Acad Sci U S A* 1986;83:7089–7093.

Yankner BA, Sklonik PR, Shoukimas GM, et al. Cerebral granulomatous angiitis associated with isolation of human T-lymphotropic virus type III from the central nervous system. *Ann Neurol* 1986;20:362–364.

Yerba M, Garcia-Merino A, Albarrán F, et al. Cerebellar disease without dementia and infection with the human immunodeficiency virus (HIV). *Ann Intern Med* 1988;108:310–311.

Merritt's Neurology, 10th ed., edited by L.P. Rowland. Lippincott Williams & Wilkins, Philadelphia © 2000.

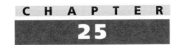

CHAPTER 25

FUNGAL AND YEAST INFECTIONS

LEON D. PROCKOP

Fungal infection, or mycosis, of the central nervous system (CNS) results in one or more of the following tissue reactions: meningitis, meningoencephalitis, abscess or granuloma formation, or arterial thrombosis. Subacute or chronic meningitis and meningoencephalitis are most common, but granulomatous lesions and abscesses typify the response to some fungi; thrombotic occlusions occur with other fungal infections. The lungs, skin, and hair are usually the primary sites of involvement by fungi.

Fungi exist in two forms: molds and yeasts. *Molds* are composed of tubular filaments called hyphae that are sometimes branched. *Yeasts* are unicellular organisms that have a thick cell wall surrounded by a well-defined capsule. Infecting fungi comprise two groups: pathogenic and opportunistic.

The *pathogenic* fungi are those few species that can infect a normal host after inhalation or implantation of the spores. Naturally, chronically ill or other immunologically compromised persons are more susceptible to infection than normal persons. Acquired immunodeficiency syndrome (AIDS) has become a major cause of fungal infection. In nature, fungi grow as saprophytic soil-inhabiting mycelial units that bear spores. During infection, they adapt to higher temperatures and lower oxidation-reduction potentials of tissues. They also overcome host defenses by increased growth rate and by relative insensitivity to host defense mechanisms (e.g., phagocytosis).

The pathogenic fungi cause histoplasmosis, blastomycosis, coccidioidomycosis, and paracoccidioidomycosis. The first three are endemic to some areas of North America, and the last is endemic to areas of Central and South America. Neurologic disorders are rare in patients with systemic North American blastomycosis or histoplasmosis. Coccidioidomycosis is a more common disease, especially in Arizona and California, and meningitis is a dreaded, often fatal complication.

The second group of systemically infecting fungi, the *opportunistic* organisms, is not thought to incite infection in the normal host. Diseases include aspergillosis, candidiasis, cryptococcosis, mucormycosis (phycomycosis), nocardiosis, and even rarer fungal diseases. With some of these fungi, minor changes in host defenses may cause disease (e.g., candidal overgrowth in mucous membranes). With most opportunistic fungi, the CNS is infected only after major changes have occurred in the host, such as extensive use of antimicrobial agents that destroy normal nonpathogenic bacterial flora, administration of immunosuppressive agents or corticosteroids that lower host resistance, and existence of systemic illness, such as Hodgkin disease, leukemia, diabetes mellitus, AIDS, or other diseases that interfere with immune responses of the host. Prolonged therapeutic use of deep venous lines also seems to be a contributing factor.

Except in some regions of Asia, CNS manifestations of aspergillosis are uncommon. CNS nocardiosis is rare. Although clinically apparent meningeal infection with candidae is rare, candidiasis has become an increasingly common postmortem brain finding, although it is not often revealed clinically. In autopsy studies, candidiasis occurs in compromised patients and produces intracerebral microabscesses and noncaseating granulomas without diffuse leptomeningitis. In contrast to most mycoses, in which neurologic disease is secondary to systemic involvement, cryptococcal meningitis may be a primary infection. Although this fungus is considered opportunistic, the factors that predispose to cryptococcal infection in some apparently normal individuals are unknown.

In mucormycosis, primary infection of the nasal sinuses and eye often extends to the brain or cranial nerves in the compromised patient. Rare fungal causes of neurologic disorders include allescheriosis, alternariasis, cephalosporiosis, cladosporiosis, diplorhinotrichosis, drechsleriasis, fonsecaeasis, madurellosis, paecilomycosis, penicilliosis, sporotrichosis, streptomycosis, torulopsosis, trichophytosis, and ustilagomycosis.

Diagnosis of fungal infections is often difficult and depends on the alertness of the physician. The characteristic findings in radiographs of the lungs and other organs, skin tests, antibody tests of serum and CSF, and isolation of organisms from lesions and CSF are important diagnostic aids. Serial monitoring of serum antigen (e.g., *Aspergillus*) shows promise in early diagnosis. Brain computed tomography (CT) and magnetic resonance imaging (MRI) may document mass lesions caused by granulomas or abscess. Likewise, in meningitis, CT or MRI may demonstrate obliteration of subarachnoid spaces or hydrocephalus, findings that are useful in management and prognosis.

Treatment of human fungal infections is at best unsatisfactory. Penicillin and other commonly used antimicrobial agents are useless and may lead to spread of the infection, except in actinomycosis or nocardiosis. Actinomycosis is curable by either tetracycline antibiotics or penicillin, and nocardiosis responds to sulfonamides. Amphotericin B is the most effective therapeutic

preparation for most neurologic fungal disease, although important roles for miconazole, ketoconazole (Nizoral), fluconazole (Diflucan), and itraconazole (Sporanox) are being recognized.

CRYPTOCOCCOSIS

Cryptococcosis is the most common mycotic infection that directly involves the CNS and is a major cause of morbidity and mortality among immunosuppressed patients. The disease may simulate tuberculous meningitis, brain tumor, encephalitis, or psychosis.

Pathogenesis

Cryptococcus neoformans (*Torula histolytica* or *Torulopsis neoformans*) is a fungus found throughout the world. Infections by the small yeastlike spherule have been described under various terms such as torulosis, yeast meningitis, and European blastomycosis. Although the skin and mucous membranes may be the primary sites of infection, the respiratory tract is usually the portal of entry. The organism has been recovered in fruit, milk, soil, wasps' nests, some grasses and plants, human skin and mucous membranes, and the manure of pigeons and other birds. The manure serves as a reservoir from which human infection may occur.

In 30% to 60% of reported cases, cryptococcosis is associated with debilitating diseases, such as AIDS, lymphosarcoma, reticulum-cell sarcoma, leukemia, Hodgkin disease, multiple myeloma, sarcoidosis, tuberculosis, diabetes mellitus, renal disease, and lupus erythematosus. CNS infection may occur independently of, or in association with, systemic disease. By the time the diagnosis of systemic cryptococcosis is firmly established, however, 70% of patients have neurologic abnormalities.

Pathology

The changes in the nervous system include infiltration of the meninges by mononuclear cells and cryptococcal organisms. The organisms may be scattered diffusely throughout the parenchyma of the brain with little or no local inflammatory reaction. Occasionally, an abscess or small granulomas form in the meninges of the brain or spinal cord.

Symptoms and Signs

Symptomatic onset of nervous system involvement is subacute. Meningeal symptoms usually predominate, but occasionally focal neurologic signs or mental symptoms are in the foreground. The usual clinical picture is that of subacute meningitis or encephalitis. The diagnosis of tuberculous meningitis is often entertained until the correct diagnosis is revealed by the peculiar appearance of some of the "cells" in the CSF. The diagnosis of yeast meningitis can be established by culture of the organism on Sabouraud medium.

Large granulomas in the cerebrum, cerebellum, or brainstem cause the same clinical syndromes as do other expanding lesions in these sites. Before the availability of CT and MRI, the diagnosis of a granuloma was rarely made before operation. Nonetheless, definitive diagnosis can be made only when meningeal involvement is also present and organisms are recovered from the CSF.

Laboratory Data

The CSF findings in infections with cryptococci are similar to those of tuberculous meningitis. The CSF is usually under increased pressure. There is a slight or moderate pleocytosis of 10 to 500 cells/mm³. The protein content is increased. The sugar content is decreased, with values commonly between 15 and 35 mg/dL. The diagnosis is made by finding the organisms in the counting-chamber centrifuge sediment of the fluid (Fig. 25.1), by growth on Sabouraud medium, or by the results of animal inoculation. The organisms also may be cultured from the urine, blood, stool, sputum, and bone marrow. They are usually visible on smear or growth in cultures. Diagnosis can be established by the detection of cryptococcal antigen in serum and CSF.

Course

The disease in untreated patients is usually fatal within a few months, but occasionally it persists for several years with recurrent remissions and exacerbations (Fig. 25.2). Occasionally, yeast organisms in the CSF have been noted for 3 years or longer. Spontaneous cure has been reported in a few cases.

Treatment

Treatment with amphotericin B has a definite beneficial effect. Butler and associates reported improvement in 31 of 36 treated patients. Of the 31 patients who showed improvement, 17 remained well, three died of unrelated causes, and 11 had one or more relapses of meningitis. In this era of epidemic AIDS, cryp-

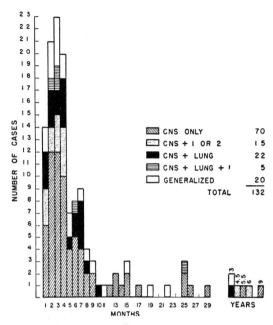

FIG. 25.2. Duration of life (in months) for 132 patients with untreated cryptococcal meningitis, from onset to death. *Stippled areas 1* and *2* indicate cases in which skin or bones were also involved. (Courtesy of Dr. Charles Carton.)

tococcosis is reported even more frequently. Many authorities now consider fluconazole to be the drug of choice for AIDS-associated cryptococcal infection. Fluconazole should be continued for 3 months after the CSF is sterilized. Suppressive therapy with 200 mg orally once daily is employed in relapsing cases. Liver function studies must be monitored if phenytoin sodium (Dilantin) is given concomitantly.

Alternative therapy employs amphotericin B and flucytosine (Ancobon). Combined treatment may be used to prevent failure resulting from emergence of flucytosine resistance. Ampho-

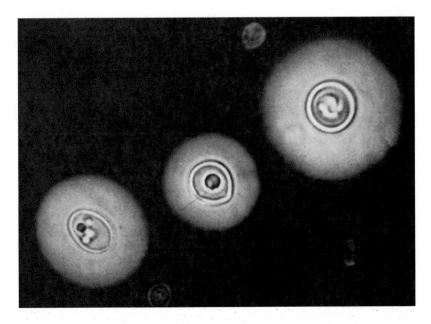

FIG. 25.1. *Cryptococcus neoformans* meningitis. Fresh preparation of sediment from CSF stained with India ink. The capsule is three times the diameter of the cell. (Courtesy of Dr. Margarita Silva.)

tericin B has sometimes been given by cisternal injection or by administration into the lateral ventricle through an Ommaya reservoir. Sterility of the CSF is probably the best endpoint of successful treatment. The course of treatment should be repeated if a relapse occurs.

Side effects of amphotericin B include thrombophlebitis, nausea and vomiting, fever, anemia, hypokalemia, and elevation of the blood urea level. Aspirin and antihistamines, blood transfusions, and temporary reduction in the drug dosage are of value in control of side effects.

MUCORMYCOSIS

Cerebral mucormycosis (phycomycosis) is an acute, rarely curable disease caused by fungi of the class Phycomycetes, especially of the genus *Rhizopus*. A common contaminant of laboratory cultures, it is not ordinarily pathogenic. Cases have been reported in all parts of the United States, in Canada, and in England. The disease probably exists worldwide. It usually occurs as a complication of diabetes mellitus or a blood dyscrasia, particularly leukemia. Use of antibiotics and adrenocortical steroids may also predispose patients to mucormycosis.

The fungi enter the nose and, in susceptible persons, cause sinusitis and orbital cellulitis. Subsequently, they may penetrate arteries to produce thrombosis of the ophthalmic and internal carotid arteries, and may later invade veins and lymphatics. Ocular, cerebral, pulmonary, intestinal, and disseminated forms of the disease exist.

Proptosis, ocular palsies, and hemiplegia are common neurologic signs associated with the involvement of the orbital and internal carotid arteries. The organisms may invade the meninges to cause meningitis or may extend into the brain to produce a mycotic encephalitis.

Diagnosis is made by examination of the sputum, CSF, or exudate of tissue from the nasal sinuses. Culture of *Rhizopus* is corroborative but not diagnostic because it is a common contaminant.

A dramatic improvement in prognosis has been noted in recent years, with 73% survival of patients diagnosed since 1970 compared to 6% survival before 1970. Treatment consists of the administration of amphotericin B and control of predisposing factors (e.g., diabetes). Local drainage and early surgery of the necrotic tissue should be performed to prevent spread of disease.

SUGGESTED READINGS

General

Chandler FW, Watts JC. *Pathologic diagnosis of fungal infections.* Chicago: ASCP Press, 1987.

Chimelli L, Rosemberg S, Hahn MD, et al. Pathology of the central nervous system in patients infected with the human immunodeficiency virus (HIV): a report of 252 autopsy cases from Brazil. *Neuropathol Appl Neurobiol* 1992;18:478–488.

Khanna N. Chandramuki A. Desai A. Ravi V. Cryptococcal infections of the central nervous system: an analysis of predisposing factors, laboratory findings and outcome in patients from South India with special reference to HIV infection. *J Med Microbiol* 1996;45:376–379.

Kurstak E, Marquis G. *Immunology of fungal diseases.* New York: Marcel Dekker, 1989.

Malik R, Malhortra V, Gondal R, et al. Mycopathology of cerebral mycosis. *Acta Neurochir (Wien)* 1985;78:161–163.

Mori T, Ebe T. Analysis of cases of central nervous system fungal infections reported in Japan between January 1979 and June 1989. *Intern Med* 1992;31:174–179.

Ostrow TD, Hudgins PA. Magnetic resonance imaging of intracranial fungal infections. *Top Magn Reson Imaging* 1994;6:22–31.

Rippon JW. Mycosis. In: Vinken PH, Bruyn GW, Klawans HL, eds. *Infections of the nervous system. Handbook of clinical neurology, vol 35.* Amsterdam: Elsevier/North-Holland, 1978.

Treseler CB, Suga AM. Fungal meningitis. *Infect Dis Clin North Am* 1990;4:789–808.

Verweij PE, Dompeling EC, Donnelly JP, Schattenberg AV, Meis JF. Serial monitoring of *Aspergillus* antigen in the early diagnosis of invasive aspergillosis: preliminary investigation with two examples. *Infection* 1997;25:86–89.

Walsh TJ, Hier DB, Caplan LR. Fungal infections of the central nervous system: comparative analysis of risk factors and clinical signs in 57 patients. *Neurology* 1985;35:1654–1657.

Wang F, So Y, Vittinghoff E, et al. Incidence proportion of and risk factors for AIDS patients diagnosed with HIV dementia, central nervous system toxoplasmosis, and cryptococcal meningitis. *J Acquir Immune Defic Syndr Hum Retrovirol* 1995;8:75–82.

Actinomycosis

Dailey AT, LeRoux PD, Grady MS. Resolution of an actinomycotic abscess with nonsurgical treatment. *Neurosurgery* 1993;31:134–136.

Smego RA Jr. Actinomycosis of the central nervous system. *Rev Infect Dis* 1987;9:855–865.

Aspergillosis

Ashdown BC, Tien RD, Felsberg GJ. Aspergillosis of the brain and paranasal sinuses in immunocompromised patients: CT and MR imaging findings. *AJR* 1994;162:155–159.

Camarata PJ, Dunn DL, Farney AC, et al. Continual intracavitary administration of amphotericin B as an adjunct in the treatment of *Aspergillus* brain abscess: case report and review of the literature. *Neurosurgery* 1992;31:575–579.

Cox J, Murtagh FR, Wilfong A, Brenner J. Cerebral aspergillosis: MR imaging and histopathologic correlation. *AJNR* 1992;13:1489–1492.

Darras-Joly C, Veber B, Bedos JP, Gachot B, Regnier B, Wolff M. Nosocomial cerebral aspergillosis: a report of 3 cases. *Scand J Infect Dis* 1996;28:317–319.

Mikolich DJ, Kinsella LJ, Skowron G, Friedman J, Sugar AM. *Aspergillus* meningitis in an immunocompetent adult successfully treated with itraconazole. *Clin Infect Dis* 1996;23:1318–1319.

Minaux Y, Ribaud P, Williams M, et al. MR of cerebral aspergillosis in patients who have had bone marrow transplantation. *AJNR* 1995;16:555–562.

Rhine WD, Arvin AM, Stevenson DK. Neonatal aspergillosis. *Clin Pediatr* 1986;25:400–403.

Walsh TJ, Hier DB, Caplan LR. Aspergillosis of the central nervous system: clinicopathological analysis of 17 patients. *Ann Neurol* 1985;18:574–582.

Blastomycosis

Roos KL, Bryan JP, Maggio WW, et al. Intracranial blastomycoma. *Medicine* 1987;66:224–235.

Taillan B, Ferrari E, Cosnefroy JY, et al. Favourable outcome of blastomycosis of the brain stem with fluconazole and flucytosine treatment. *Ann Med* 1992;24:71–72.

Candida (Moniliasis)

Coker SM, Beltran RS. *Candida* meningitis: clinical and radiographic diagnosis. *Pediatr Neurol* 1988;4:317–319.

Moyer DV, Edwards JE. *Candida* endophthalmitis and central nervous system infection. In: Bodey G, ed. *Candidiasis: pathogenesis, diagnosis and treatment.* New York: Raven Press, 1993.

Parker JC, McCloskey JJ, Lee RS. Human cerebral candidosis: a postmortem evaluation of 19 patients. *Hum Pathol* 1981;12:23–28.

Ruchel R, Zimmerman F, Boning-Stutzer B, Helmchen U. Candidiasis visualized by proteinase-directed immunofluorescence. *Pathol Anat Histopathol* 1991;419:199–202.

Coccidioidomycosis

Lababie EL, Hamilton RH. Survival improvement in coccidioidal meningitis by high-dose intrathecal amphotericin B. *Arch Intern Med* 1986;146:2013–2018.

Tucker RM, Galgiani JN, Denning DW, et al. Treatment of coccidioidal meningitis with fluconazole. *Rev Infect Dis* 1990;3:5380–5389.

Williams PL, Johnson R, Pappagianis D, et al. Vasculitic and encephalitic complications associated with *Coccidioides immitis* infection of the central nervous system in humans: report of 10 cases and review. *Clin Infect Dis* 1992;14:673–682.

Wrobel CJ, Meyer S, Johnson RH, Hesselink JR. MR findings in acute and chronic coccidioidomycosis meningitis. *AJNR* 1992;13:1241–1245.

Histoplasmosis

Bradsher RW. Histoplasmosis and blastomycosis. *Clin Infect Dis* 1996;22[Suppl 2]:S102–S111.

Rivera IV, Curless RG, Indacochea FJ, Scott GB. Chronic progressive CNS histoplasmosis presenting in childhood: response to fluconazole therapy. *Pediatr Neurol* 1992;8:151–153.

Tan V, Wilkins P, Badve S, et al. Histoplasmosis of the central nervous system. *J Neurol Neurosurg Psychiatry* 1992;55:619–622.

Nocardiosis

Barnicoat MJ, Wierzbicki AS, Norman PM. Cerebral nocardiosis in immunosuppressed patients: five cases. *Q J Med* 1989;72:689–698.

Bross JE, Gordon G. Nocardial meningitis: case reports and review. *Rev Infect Dis* 1991;13:160–165.

Paracoccidioidomycosis

De Freitas MR, Nascimento OJ, Chimelli L. Tapia's syndrome caused by *Paracoccidioidis brasiliensis. J Neurol Sci* 1991;103:179–181.

Teive HA, Arruda WO, Ramina R, et al. Paracoccidioidomycosis granuloma simulating posterior fossa tumour. *J R Soc Med* 1991;84:562–563.

Uncommon Fungal Diseases

Fetter BF, Klintworth GK. Uncommon fungal diseases of the nervous system. In: Vinken PH, Bruyn GW, Klawans HL, eds. *Infections of the nervous system. Handbook of clinical neurology, vol 35.* Amsterdam: Elsevier/North-Holland, 1978.

Cryptococcosis

Andreula CF, Burdi N, Carlla A. CNS cryptococcosis in AIDS: spectrum of MR findings. *J Comput Assist Tomogr* 1993;17:438–441.

Bozzette SA, Larsen RA, Chiu J, et al. A placebo-controlled trial of maintenance therapy with fluconazole after treatment of cryptococcal meningitis in the acquired immunodeficiency syndrome. California Collaborative Treatment Group. *N Engl J Med* 1991;324:580–584.

Brown RW, Clarke RJ, Gonzales MF. Cytologic detection of *Cryptococcus neoformans* in cerebrospinal fluid. *Acta Cytol* 1985;29:151–153.

Chan KH, Mann KS, Yue CP. Neurosurgical aspects of cerebral cryptococcosis. *Neurosurgery* 1989;25:44–47.

Chen SC, Miller M, Zhou JZ, Wright LC, Sorrell TC. Phospholipase activity in *Cryptococcus neoformans:* a new virulence factor? *J Infect Dis* 1997;175:414–420.

De Wytt CN, Dickson PL, Holt GW. Cryptococcal meningitis: a review of 32 years' experience. *J Neurol Sci* 1982;53:283–292.

Lees SC, Dickson DW, Casadevall A. Pathology of cryptococcal meningoencephalitis: analysis of 27 patients with pathogenic implications. *Hum Pathol* 1996;27:839–847.

Mathews VP, Alo PL, Glass JD, et al. AIDS-related CNS cryptococcosis: radiologic-pathologic correlation. *AJNR* 1992;13:1477–1486.

Ruiz A, Post MJ, Bundschu CC. Dentate nuclei involvement in AIDS patients with CNS cryptococcosis: imaging findings with pathologic correlation. *J Comput Assist Tomogr* 1997;21:175–182.

Speed B, Dunt D. Clinical and host differences between infections with the two varieties of *Cryptococcus neoformans. Clin Infect Dis* 1995;21:28–34.

Mucormycosis

Abril V, Ortega E, Segarra P, Pedro F, Sabter V, Herrera A. Rhinocerebral mucormycosis in a patient with AIDS: a complication of diabetic ketoacidosis following pentamidine therapy. *Clin Infect Dis* 1996;23:845–946.

Adam RD, Hunter G, DiTomasso J, Comerci G Jr. Mucormycosis: emerging prominence of cutaneous infections. *Clin Infect Dis* 1994;19:67–76.

Anand VK, Alemar G, Griswold JA Jr. Intracranial complications of mucormycosis: an experimental model and clinical review. *Laryngoscope* 1992;102:656–662.

McLean FM, Ginsberg LE, Stanton CA. Perineural spread of rhinocerebral mucormycosis. *AJNR* 1996;17:114–116.

Ochi JW, Harris JP, Feldman JI, Press GA. Rhinocerebral mucormycosis: results of aggressive surgical debridement and amphotericin B. *Laryngoscope* 1988;98:1339–1342.

Terk MR, Underwood DJ, Zee CS, Colletti PM. MR imaging in rhinocerebral and intracranial mucormycosis with CT and pathologic correlation. *Magn Reson Imaging* 1992;10:81–87.

Merritt's Neurology, 10th ed., edited by L.P. Rowland. Lippincott Williams & Wilkins, Philadelphia © 2000.

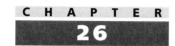

NEUROSARCOIDOSIS

JOHN C.M. BRUST

TABLE 26.1. SYMPTOMS AND SIGNS IN NEUROSARCOIDOSIS

Cranial neuropathy	53% (range, 37%–73%)
CNS parenchymal disease	48% (range, 14%–100%)
Aseptic meningitis	22% (range, 8%–40%)
Peripheral neuropathy	17% (range, 6%–40%)
Myopathy	15% (range, 7%–26%)
Hydrocephalus	7% (range, 0–14%)

Sarcoidosis is a multisystem granulomatous disease of unknown cause. Sarcoid granulomas resemble those of tuberculosis but lack tubercle bacilli, caseation, or characteristic necrosis. Active lesions contain epithelioid and multinucleate giant cells; such lesions may resolve but more often become fibrotic.

Sarcoidosis occurs worldwide, with estimated prevalence ranging from 3 to 50 per 100,000 population. In the United States, it occurs more frequently in blacks. Onset is most often in the fourth or fifth decade, but the disease also affects children and the elderly. An infectious cause remains elusive. Immunologic features include concentration at disease sites of activated CD4 lymphocytes, which secrete cytokines that in turn lead to accumulation of monocytes and macrophages to form granulomas. Lesions can affect any organ, especially lung, lymph nodes, skin, bone, eyes, and salivary glands. The nervous system is clinically involved in about 5% of patients, one-half of whom have central or peripheral nervous system disease at presentation. Although nearly 20% of such patients have only neurologic symptoms or signs, workup reveals evidence of systemic disease in as many as 97%. When nervous system disease complicates systemic sarcoidosis, it usually does so within 2 years of onset.

In the central nervous system (CNS), sarcoid granulomas most often involve the meninges, especially at the base of the brain, with secondary infiltration of cranial nerves and obstruction of CSF flow. Lesions tend to be perivascular and thereby can spread intraparenchymally, thus frequently affecting the hypothalamus and less often other CNS structures, including the spinal cord. Granulomas also occur in peripheral nerves and muscle.

Given the unpredictable dispersal of lesions, sarcoidosis is a clinically protean disease, systemically and neurologically. Nearly 50% of patients with neurosarcoidosis have more than one neurologic complication, with relative frequencies varying among different clinical series (Table 26.1).

Although any cranial nerve can be affected, the most frequently affected is the seventh, sometimes in association with uveitis and parotitis (uveoparotid fever) but usually alone, thus suggesting Bell palsy. Facial weakness can be bilateral and either simultaneous or sequential, and can recur after recovery. Optic nerve involvement causes papillitis or retrobulbar neuritis and eventually optic atrophy. Trigeminal nerve involvement causes either sensory loss or neuralgia, and eighth cranial nerve lesions produce auditory and vestibular symptoms.

Granulomas involve the hypothalamus more often than the pituitary, thereby producing combinations of endo-crinologic and nonendocrinologic symptoms that include diabetes insipidus, decreased libido, galactorrhea, amenorrhea, abnormal sleep patterns, altered appetite, temperature dysregulation, and abnormal behavior. Cerebral granulomas may be scattered diffusely, some too small to be detected on computed tomography (CT) or magnetic resonance imaging (MRI), or they may consist of one or more large masses that mimic a brain neoplasm. Seizures are common in such patients. Symptomatic subdural granulomas have occurred. Rarely, sarcoid vasculitis causes cerebral infarction in a pattern clinically and pathologically indistinguishable from so-called granulomatous angiitis of the nervous system. Autoantibodies to endothelial cells have been identified in patients with neurosarcoid.

Meningeal infiltration can be asymptomatic or produce symptomatic aseptic meningitis. Complications include cauda equina signs, hydrocephalus, and ependymitis with encephalopathy.

Peripheral nerve lesions cause mononeuropathy, mononeuropathy multiplex, and sensory, motor, or sensorimotor polyneuropathy, either chronically progressive or resembling Guillain-Barré neuropathy. A positive muscle biopsy has been reported in as many as 75% of patients with sarcoidosis. However, muscle granulomas are usually asymptomatic, although they sometimes cause palpable nodules or progressive diffuse polymyositis.

In patients known to have sarcoidosis, the appearance of neurologic symptoms usually poses no diagnostic problem, but the possibility of unrelated disease must be kept in mind, especially potential complications of corticosteroid treatment such as infection (tuberculosis, mycosis, toxoplasmosis, or progressive multifocal leukoencephalopathy), mental change, or myopathy. Patients with neurologic symptoms require both systemic and neurologic investigation. CNS granulomas, symptomatic or asymptomatic, are apparent on either T2-weighted MRI or contrast-enhanced CT; they are sometimes calcified. Leptomeningeal CT enhancement is common, and imaging can reveal hydrocephalus and spinal cord, cauda equina, or optic nerve involvement. The CSF may contain as many as a few thousand white cells (usually with lymphocytic preponderance), elevated protein levels, and low sugar content, as well as elevated immunoglobulin (Ig) G and IgG index, oligoclonal bands, and elevated angiotensin-converting enzyme (ACE) (also found in infection and malignancy).

Other studies, tailored to individual patients, include chest radiographs (revealing either asymptomatic hilar adenopathy or, more ominously, fibronodular disease), pulmonary function studies, bronchiolar lavage for lymphocytes, serum calcium (elevated in about 20% of patients with sarcoidosis), urinary calcium (elevated in 50%), serum ACE (elevated in 65%), serum gamma globulin (elevated in 50%), serum sodium, and endocrinologic studies (thyroid function tests, cortisol, gonadotropins, testosterone or estradiol, and prolactin). About two-thirds of patients are anergic to tuberculin purified protein derivative, mumps, and other antigens, and those who are positive are usually only weakly so. Ophthalmologic or otolaryngologic consultation may disclose unsuspected lesions. Systemic or brain gallium scanning can be positive but is nonspecific. Diagnosis ultimately depends on histology; biopsy sites include lymph nodes (including transbronchial), salivary gland, conjunctiva, skin, liver, and, as a last resort, meninges or brain. Kveim testing can be diagnostic, but the antigen, unavailable in many centers and not well standardized, is not approved by the U.S. Food and Drug Administration for general use.

About two-thirds of patients with neurosarcoidosis have a self-limited monophasic illness; the rest have a chronic remitting-relapsing course. With treatment, death from neurologic disease is unusual. Although controlled studies are lacking, corticosteroids appear to reduce symptoms and size of granulomas, and it is unclear whether they affect the natural history. Their use depends on the clinical setting. Short-term therapy can be given to patients with aseptic meningitis or isolated facial palsy; long-term treatment is often necessary for intraparenchymal lesions, hydrocephalus, optic or other cranial nerve involvement, peripheral neuropathy, or symptomatic myopathy. Prednisone, 40 to 80 mg daily, can be given for a few weeks and then slowly tapered either to a lowest possible maintenance dose or, if possible, to discontinuation. Higher initial doses may be necessary in some patients. Adjunctive immunosuppressive treatment for refractory patients includes azathioprine (Imuran), methotrexate, cyclophosphamide, chlorambucil (Leukeran), and cyclosporine (Sandimmune). Radiation therapy has been used with uncertain benefit.

SUGGESTED READINGS

Agbogu BN, Stern BJ, Sewell C, et al. Therapeutic considerations in patients with refractory neurosarcoidosis. *Arch Neurol* 1995;52:875–879.

Brust JCM, Rhee RS, Plank CR, et al. Sarcoidosis galactorrhea, and amenorrhea: two autopsy cases, one with Chiari-Frommel syndrome. *Ann Neurol* 1977;2:130–137.

Case records of the Massachusetts General Hospital. *N Engl J Med* 1998;339:1534–1551.

Challenor Y, Brust JCM, Felton C. Electrodiagnostic studies in sarcoidosis. *J Neurol Neurosurg Psychiatry* 1984;46:1219–1222.

Chapelon C, Ziza JM, Piette JC, et al. Neurosarcoidosis: signs, course and treatment in 35 confirmed cases. *Medicine* 1990;69:261–276.

Colover JJ. Sarcoidosis with involvement of the nervous system. *Brain* 1948;71:451–455.

Cordingley G, Navarro C, Brust JCM, Healton EB. Sarcoidosis presenting as senile dementia. *Neurology* 1981;31:1148–1151.

Delaney P. Neurologic manifestations in sarcoidosis: review of the literature, with a report of 23 cases. *Ann Intern Med* 1977;87:336–345.

Healton EB, Zito G, Chauhan P, Brust JCM. Subdural sarcoid granuloma. *J Neurosurg* 1982;32:776–778.

Krumholz A, Stern BJ, Stern EG. Clinical implications of seizures in neurosarcoidosis. *Arch Neurol* 1991;48:842–844.

Luke RA, Stern BJ, Krumholz A, Johns CJ. Neurosarcoidosis: the long-term clinical course. *Neurology* 1987;37:461–463.

Okasanen V. Neurosarcoidosis: clinical presentations and course in 50 patients. *Acta Neurol Scand* 1986;73:283–290.

Newman LS, Rose CS, Maier LA. Sarcoidosis. *N Engl J Med* 1997;336:1224–1234.

Sauter MK, Panitch HS, Krist DA. Myelopathic neurosarcoidosis: diagnostic value of enhanced MRI. *Neurology* 1991;41:150–151.

Scott TF. Neurosarcoidosis: progress and clinical aspects. *Neurology* 1993;43:8–12.

Sharma OP, Sharma AM. Sarcoidosis of the nervous system: a clinical approach. *Arch Intern Med* 1991;151:1317–1321.

Stern BJ, Krumholz A, Johns C, et al. Sarcoidosis and its neurological manifestations. *Arch Neurol* 1985;42:909–917.

Tsukada N, Yanegisawa N, Mochizuki I. Endothelial cell damage in sarcoidosis and neurosarcoidosis: autoantibodies to endothelial cells. *Eur Neurol* 1995;35:108–112.

Von Brevern M, Lempert T, Bronstein AM, et al. Selective vestibular damage in neurosarcoidosis. *Ann Neurol* 1997;42:117–120.

Zuniga G, Ropper AH, Frank J. Sarcoid peripheral neuropathy. *Neurology* 1991;41:1558–1561.

Merritt's Neurology, 10th ed., edited by L.P. Rowland. Lippincott Williams & Wilkins, Philadelphia © 2000.

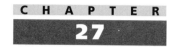

SPIROCHETE INFECTIONS: NEUROSYPHILIS

LEWIS P. ROWLAND
LEONIDAS STEFANIS

DEFINITION

Neurosyphilis comprises several different syndromes that result from infection of the brain, meninges, or spinal cord by *Treponema pallidum* (Table 27.1). It is not known how much damage is caused by direct effects of the organism and how much by other immune mechanisms.

A clinical definition must include the results of diagnostic laboratory tests. Accordingly, neurosyphilis is defined by three findings: a syndrome consistent with neurosyphilis, abnormal blood titer of a treponemal antibody test, and positive nontreponemal antibody test in the cerebrospinal fluid (CSF). All three must be present.

HISTORY

Neurosyphilis, recognized for about 100 years, has played an important role in the evolution of modern neurology. Paretic neurosyphilis was the first "mental disorder" for which specific cerebral pathology was found. Erb described spinal syphilis (tabes dorsalis) in 1892. Quincke introduced lumbar puncture, and CSF examination was used to diagnose infection, even in asymptomatic people. The organism was identified in the brain by Noguchi and Moore in 1913. The first effective treatment came in 1918 when Wagner Jaurregg gave fever therapy for paresis. He was the first neurologist to be given a Nobel Prize. Then came arsenical chemotherapy, the first planned use of a drug that would attack the organism without harming host tissues; this was Ehrlich's concept of "the magic bullet." Safer and more effective therapy came in 1945 with the introduction of penicillin, which has been used since.

Syphilis was also important in the evolution of this textbook. The subject has been allotted many pages because the disease was a major research interest of Houston Merritt and it was still prevalent when he wrote the first edition. His chapters were revised only slightly in subsequent editions, but now neurosyphilis is inextricably linked to acquired immunodeficiency syndrome (AIDS). Classic clinical syndromes are now exceptional, and both diagnosis and therapy have become more complicated; these changes require a recasting of the description.

EPIDEMIOLOGY

Following the introduction of penicillin, the incidence of neurosyphilis declined for two main reasons: (1) Fewer people spread the disease because those affected were being identified and treated, and (2) many neurosyphilitic infections were prevented because penicillin was being used to treat gonorrhea and other infections. For instance, the frequency of neurosyphilis as a cause of first admission to a psychiatric hospital plummeted from 5.9 per 100,000 population in 1942 to 0.1 per 100,000 in 1965. New cases became so rare that many hospitals discarded routine testing to detect syphilis.

During the next few decades, some investigators detected a shift in the clinical patterns, but this finding was debated. The segment of the population with the highest incidence was young homosexual men. Then, in 1981, came AIDS. The incidence of primary and secondary syphilis rose from 13.7 per 100,000 in 1981 to 18.4 per 100,000 in 1989, an increase of 34%. Between 1985 and 1989, the increase was 61%. Since then, there has been further decline in the incidence of syphilis. In 1997, fewer than 8,000 cases of early syphilis were reported in the United States, representing the lowest rates in 38 years and a sixfold decline since 1990.

Neurosyphilis ultimately develops in about 10% of untreated persons with early syphilis. Among those infected with human immunodeficiency virus (HIV), about 15% have serologic evidence of syphilis, and about 1% have neurosyphilis.

Even before the HIV era, there had been a shift in clinical manifestations because of the widespread use of antibiotics. Previously common parenchymal forms became rare, while the incidence of meningeal and vascular syndromes rose (Table 27.2). The diagnosis of neurosyphilis is often delayed because there are other, more common causes of stroke and meningitis. From 1985 to 1992 in San Francisco, parenchymal forms of neurosyphilis accounted for only 5% of 117 cases.

PATHOLOGY

In early neurosyphilis, lymphocytes and other mononuclear cells infiltrate the meninges. The inflammatory reaction also involves the cranial nerves and provokes axonal degeneration. When the inflammation affects small meningeal vessels, occlusion due to endothelial proliferation may lead to ischemic necrosis of brain and spinal cord. This process may cause demyelination, myelomalacia at the periphery of the cord, or transverse myelitis.

The pathology of dementia paralytica develops slowly. After an inflammatory meningeal reaction, lymphocytes and plasma cells infiltrate small cortical vessels and sometimes extend into the cortex itself. The cortical inflammatory response provokes loss of cortical neurons and glial proliferation. Spirochetes can be demonstrated in the cortex in dementia paralytica, but only rarely in other forms of neurosyphilis.

In tabes dorsalis, the mononuclear inflammation of meninges and blood vessels is followed by insidious degeneration of the posterior roots and posterior fiber columns of the spinal cord (Fig. 27.1), as well as the cranial nerves occasionally.

TABLE 27.1. CLASSIFICATION OF NEUROSYPHILIS

Type	Clinical Symptoms	Pathology	CSF WBC	Brain CT or MRI
I. Asymptomatic	No symptoms; CSF abnormal	Various. Chiefly, leptomeningitis; arteritis or encephalitis may be present	<5 >5	Normal Meningeal enhancement
II. Meningeal and vascular Cerebral meningeal Diffuse	Increased intracranial pressure; cranial nerve palsies	Leptomeningitis with hydrocephalus; degeneration of cranial nerves; arteritis	≥5	Meningeal enhancement
Focal	Increased intracranial pressure; focal cerebral symptoms and signs of slow onset	Granuloma formation (gumma)	Any	Mass lesion
Cerebrovascular	Focal cerebral symptoms and signs of sudden onset	Endarteritis with infarcts	Any	Subcortical or cortical infarct
Spinal meningeal and vascular	Paresthesias, weakness, atrophy, and sensory loss in limbs and trunk	Admixture of endarteritis and meningeal infiltration and thickening with degeneration of nerve roots and substance of the cord (myelomalacia)	Any	NA
III. Parenchymatous Tabetic	Pain, paresthesia, crises, ataxia, impairment of pupillary reflexes, loss of tendon reflexes, impaired proprioceptive sensation, and trophic changes	Leptomeningitis and degenerative changes in posterior roots, dorsal funiculi, and brainstem	Any	NA
Paretic	Personality changes, convulsions, and dementia	Meningoencephalitis	Any	Optic atrophy
Optic atrophy[a]	Loss of vision, pallor of optic discs	Leptomeningitis and atrophy of optic nerves	Any	NA

NA, not applicable.
[a] Rarely occurs alone; usually found in tabetic or paretic neurosyphilis.
Data from Merritt et al., 1946; and Katz et al., 1993.

CLINICAL DIAGNOSIS

The three most common forms of neurosyphilis are asymptomatic, meningeal, and vascular. Often, the meninges and cerebral vessels are affected together in meningovascular neurosyphilis. The once prominent parenchymal forms, including general paresis (dementia paralytica) and tabes dorsalis, are rarely seen now. The major clinical syndromes are differentiated from other causes of the same manifestations only by finding blood and CSF changes indicative of syphilis. Of course, the patient with serologic evidence of syphilis and concomitant HIV or other viral meningitis poses a diagnostic dilemma. Therefore, the efficacy of diagnostic tests must be considered.

TABLE 27.2. FREQUENCY OF DIFFERENT FORMS OF SYMPTOMATIC NEUROSYPHILIS*

	Preantibiotic Era (%)			Antibiotic Era (%)		AIDS Era (%)	
						HIV (−)	HIV (+) or AIDS
	1	2	3	4	5	6	7
Tabetic	45	48	45	15	11	5	0
Paretic	17	18	8	12	4	9	4
Taboparetic	4	7	9	23	23	—	—
Vascular	15	19	9	19	61	41	38
Meningeal	8	8	19	23	0	23	46
Optic neuritis	4	—	—	—	—	14	42
Spinal cord	4	—	10	8	—	—	—

1. Merritt et al., 1946 (457 patients).
2. Kierland et al. Symptomatic neurosyphilis. *Ven Dis Inform* 1942;22:350–377 (2,019 patients).
3. Wolters, 1987 (518 patients, 1930–1940).
4. Wolters, 1987 (121 patients, 1970–1984).
5. Burke and Schaberg, 1985 (26 patients).
6. and 7. Katz et al., 1993 (HIV negative, 22 patients; HIV positive and AIDS, 24 patients).

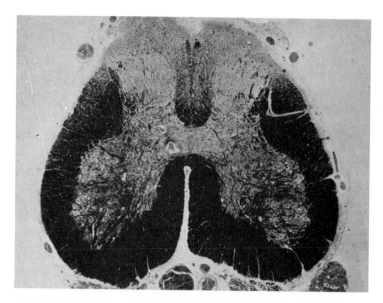

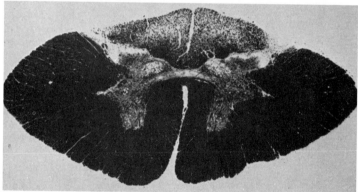

FIG. 27.1. Tabes dorsalis. Degeneration of the posterior column in the sacral and thoracic cord (myelin sheath stain). (From Merritt et al., 1946.)

Serology

Isolation of *T. pallidum* is difficult and impractical for clinical diagnosis, which rests on two categories of antibodies that are used as serologic tests for syphilis (STS). *Nontreponemal* antibodies react with reagin, a complex of cardiolipin, lecithin, and cholesterol. This complex was the basis for the original complement-fixation Wasserman test, for the more sensitive Kolmer test, and then for the Venereal Disease Research Laboratory (VDRL) test and a variation called the rapid plasma reagin (RPR) test, a flocculation test that is macroscopically visible on a glass slide. The RPR test is not suitable for CSF.

The CSF VDRL test is highly specific, but false-positive reactions can result from contamination of CSF by blood, high CSF protein content, or the presence of paraproteinemia or autoimmune disease. Some clinicians believe that the CSF VDRL test may be negative in some cases of neurosyphilis, but if so, the clinical syndrome of neurosyphilis would then be difficult to prove, especially if the manifestations were not typical. Although accurate in diagnosis, the CSF VDRL test is not as reliable in following treatment (because the titer may not change); CSF pleocytosis is a more useful guide.

An even more specific treponemal antibody test is the *fluorescent treponemal antibody* (FTA) test. The antigen preparation is made from the spirochete and can be absorbed (FTA-ABS) to remove sources of nonspecific and false reactions. A positive FTA-ABS test in plasma has high specificity for diagnosis, but not for activity because it may remain positive for years after successful treatment. In addition, the test is so sensitive that it cannot be used on CSF because as little as 0.8 μL blood in 1 mL CSF can give a positive reaction. A diagnosis of syphilis requires a high titer in the blood on VDRL testing, ascertained by a positive FTA-ABS. In some centers, a variation of the FTA is the *microhemagglutination test* for *T. pallidum*.

Problems arise when the specific treponemal tests are applied to CSF. They lack specificity because positive results appear with minor contamination by blood or with diffusion of serum immunoglobulins into CSF. Attempts to increase the reliability have included indices of intrathecal production (intrathecal *T. pallidum* antibody and *T. pallidum* hemagglutination assay); still it is difficult to be confident of the diagnosis of neurosyphilis if other CSF measures are normal. The specific treponemal antibody tests for CSF are more reliable in excluding neurosyphilis than in confirming it.

Another promising technique is the polymerase chain reaction that amplifies treponemal deoxyribonucleic acid in CSF. However, the test is not yet fully developed.

Therefore, the diagnosis of neurosyphilis requires appropriate blood serology and a reactive CSF VDRL test, which is also a measure of disease activity. A reactive FTA-ABS in the blood indicates that the CSF VDRL result is not a false-positive.

CSF Abnormalities

CSF pleocytosis is the best measure of disease activity, and the number of cells is roughly proportionate to the clinical syndrome. In an untreated patient, the white blood cell (WBC) count should be at least 5 cells/mm³ for secure diagnosis. The pleocytosis should respond to penicillin therapy within 12 weeks. The CSF protein content is usually increased, and the sugar content may be low or normal. The CSF content of gamma globulin may be increased and oligoclonal bands may be present, but these findings are nonspecific.

CLINICAL SYNDROMES

In the following discussion of clinical syndromes, we assume positive VDRL or FTA-ABS in serum, positive CSF VDRL, and CSF pleocytosis. These findings constitute the modern diagnostic triad of neurosyphilis, even in HIV-positive patients.

Asymptomatic Neurosyphilis

This diagnosis depends entirely on the serologic findings in blood and CSF. If there are more than 5 WBCs/mm³, the disorder could be called "asymptomatic meningeal syphilis," and there may be meningeal enhancement on MRI.

Meningeal Neurosyphilis

This syndrome is seen within a year of the primary infection. The clinical manifestations are those of any acute viral or aseptic meningitis: malaise, fever, stiff neck, and headache. The CSF cell count may rise to several hundred, CSF pressure may be increased, and CSF glucose may be low but is usually greater than 25 mg/dL. The protein content may exceed 100 mg/dL. The syndrome may subside spontaneously and is recognized by positive blood and CSF STS reactions.

Signs may not appear on examination, or there may be cranial nerve abnormalities, with facial diplegia or hearing loss. Occlusion of CSF pathways may cause obstructive or communicating hydrocephalus, and the course may be punctuated by cerebral infarction (meningovascular lues).

Cerebrovascular Neurosyphilis

Cerebral infarct syndromes of syphilis are similar to those of other, more common causes; the diagnosis rests on typical findings in blood and CSF. Patients are younger than those with atherosclerosis and are more likely to have risk factors for venereal disease. Clinical evidence may imply concomitant meningeal disease (meningovascular disease), with a prodromal syndrome of headache or personality change for weeks before the ictus, and signs may progress for several days. MRI may show meningeal enhancement. Symptoms appear 5 to 30 years after the primary infection.

Meningovascular Syphilis of the Spinal Cord

Conventional symptoms and signs of transverse myelitis (meningomyelitis) usually affect both sensory and motor pathways, as well as bladder control. The syndrome must be differentiated from tabes, a parenchymal infection. Syphilis has not reliably been implicated as a cause of motor neuron disease, and it is doubted that syphilis ever causes "spastic paraplegia of Erb," an anterior spinal artery syndrome.

Gumma

This mass lesion is now rare. This avascular granuloma was attached to the dura and was considered a localized form of meningeal syphilis.

Paretic Neurosyphilis

This form of neurosyphilis has also been called dementia paralytica, general paresis of the insane, or syphilitic meningoencephalitis. Spirochetes cause the chronic meningoencephalitis. The leptomeninges are opalescent to opaque, thickened, and adherent to the cortex; the cortical gyri are atrophic (Fig. 27.2). The sulci are widened and filled with CSF. When the brain is sectioned, the ventricles are enlarged. The walls are covered with sandlike granulations termed *granular ependymitis* (Fig. 27.3).

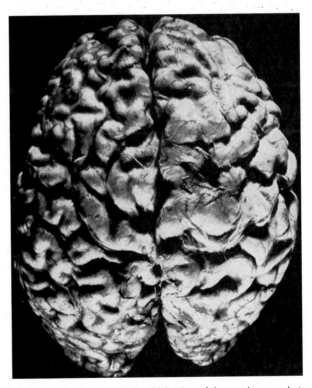

FIG. 27.2. Paretic neurosyphilis. Thickening of the meninges and atrophy of the cerebral convolutions. (From Merritt et al., 1946.)

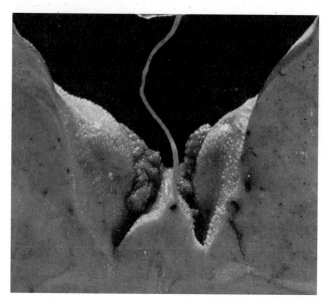

FIG. 27.3. Paretic neurosyphilis. Granular ependymitis of the floor of lateral ventricles. (From Merritt et al., 1946.)

TABLE 27.3. SYMPTOMS AND SIGNS IN TABETIC NEUROSYPHILIS: ANALYSIS OF 150 CASES

Symptoms	%	Signs	%
Lancinating pains	75	Abnormal pupils	94
Ataxia	42	Argyll-Robertson	48
Bladder disturbance	33	Other abnormalities	64
Paresthesia	24	Reflex abnormalities	
Gastric or visceral crises	18	Absent ankle jerks	94
Visual loss	16	Absent knee jerks	81
Rectal incontinence	14	Absent reflexes	11
Deafness	7	Romberg sign	55
Impotence	4	Impaired sensation	
		Impaired vibratory sense	52
		Impaired vision	43
		Impaired touch and pain	13
		Optic atrophy	20
		Ocular palsy	10
		Charcot joints	7

From Merritt et al., 1946.

Behavioral changes may suggest a psychosis, but the most common problem is dementia, with loss of memory, poor judgment, and emotional lability. In the final stages, dementia and quadriparesis are severe (general paresis of the insane). Seizures may occur.

If untreated, paretic neurosyphilis is fatal in 3 to 5 years. Penicillin is an effective treatment, but ultimately clinical results depend on the nature and extent of neuropathology when treatment is started. If inflammatory reaction is the only cause of the cerebral dysfunction, cure is likely. If spirochetal infection has already destroyed enough cerebral neurons, the infection may be arrested, but cerebral functions will not be restored.

Tabes Dorsalis

Tabes dorsalis, also called progressive locomotor ataxia, is manifested by lancinating or lightninglike pains, progressive ataxia, loss of tendon reflexes, loss of proprioception, dysfunction of sphincters, and impaired sexual function in men. The chief signs are loss of tendon reflexes at the knees and ankles, impaired vibratory and position sense in the legs, and abnormal pupils (Table 27.3).

In 94% of patients with tabes dorsalis, the pupils are irregular or unequal, or show impaired responses to light. In 48%, Argyll-Robertson pupils are present, with loss of the light reaction but with preservation of pupillary constriction in accommodation. Other findings include impaired superficial and deep sensation; weakness, wasting, and hypotonia of muscles; optic atrophy with visual loss; other cranial nerve palsies; and trophic changes, including Charcot joints or "mal perforant." Dysfunction of bowel, bladder, or genitals is also frequent.

Tabes dorsalis is seldom fatal. Ataxia or blindness may be incapacitating. Atonic bladder may lead to urinary tract infection and death. Progression may be arrested spontaneously or with treatment, but the lancinating pains and ataxia often continue.

Congenital Neurosyphilis

Congenital syphilis has been recognized since the 16th century. The spirochete is transmitted from the mother to the fetus between the fourth and seventh months of pregnancy. Mothers who have had syphilis for a longer time are less likely to give birth to an infected infant. The incidence of congenital neurosyphilis in North America has continued to decline with the improved detection and treatment of syphilis in adults, and it is now rare. The clinical types are similar to those in adults except that tabes dorsalis is uncommon. Additional features of congenital neurosyphilis are hydrocephalus and the Hutchinson triad (interstitial keratitis, deformed teeth, and hearing loss). The penicillin treatment schedule is similar to that in adults. Although the infection may be arrested, preexisting damage and neurologic signs may persist.

TREATMENT

Early Syphilis

The treatment of neurosyphilis begins with the treatment of early syphilis. The standard treatment has been a single intramuscular injection of 2.4 million U of penicillin G benzathine (Tables 27.4 and 27.5). In early studies, the failure rate was about 4%.

There is no prompt and reliable way to determine the adequacy of treatment. Instead, patients must return for repeat testing at 3, 6, and 12 months, or until serologic tests give negative results. Criteria for treatment failure (in the absence of reinfection) include the following: (1) persistent clinical signs of syphilis, (2) a fourfold rise in VDRL titer, and (3) a positive VDRL after 1 year in patients treated for primary syphilis or 2 years after treatment for secondary syphilis. The Centers for Disease Control and Prevention criterion is failure of the VDRL titer to drop by a factor of 2 within 6 to 12 months.

The occasional failure of this regimen has been documented when symptoms of neurosyphilis appeared after a few patients

TABLE 27.4. RECOMMENDED TREATMENT FOR SYPHILIS

Stage	Treatment
Primary, secondary, and early latent syphilis	Penicillin G benzathine, 2.4 million U i.m.
	For patients allergic to penicillin: doxycycline, 100 mg p.o. b.i.d. for 14 d; or tetracycline, 500 mg p.o. q.i.d. for 14 d
Late latent syphilis or duration unknown	Penicillin G benzathine, 7.2 million U i.m. given as 2.4 million U weekly for 3 wk
	For patients allergic to penicillin: doxycycline, 100 mg p.o. b.i.d. for 28 d; or tetracycline, 500 mg p.o. q.i.d. for 28 d
Tertiary disease other than neurosyphilis	As for late latent
Neurosyphilis	Penicillin G sodium, 12–24 million U daily i.v. (2–4 million U q4h) for 10–14 d; or penicillin G procaine, 2–4 million U/d i.m., plus probenecid, 500 mg p.o. q.i.d. for 10–14 d

Modified from Hook and Marra, 1992.

TABLE 27.5. RECOMMENDATIONS FOR USE OF DIAGNOSTIC TESTS FOR SYPHILIS

Immediate Diagnostic or Therapeutic Action	Further Investigation or Action
Primary syphilis Dark-field or direct fluorescent test	VDRL titer for follow-up
Secondary syphilis VDRL titer	VDRL titer for follow-up
Selected asymptomatic persons[a] VDRL titer	FTA-ABS if VDRL positive
Adequacy of treatment for early or late syphilis VDRL titer 3, 6, 12 mo after treatment	Retreat if high titer does not fall by 12 mo or if titer increases after initial fall
Seropositive persons[b] CSF VDRL, CSF cell count	Treat for neurosyphilis if CSF VDRL positive or pleocytosis
Follow-up after treatment for asymptomatic neurosyphilis CSF cell count 6 wks, 3 mo, and 6 mo after treatment	CSF cell count at 12 mo, 24 mo if normal at 6 mo
Suspected syphilis[c] Treat as for early syphilis	VDRL titer 1, 3, and 6 mo after treatment

[a]Includes all pregnant women, proven contacts of people with infectious syphilis, and people in high-risk groups.
[b] Includes people with neurologic abnormalities, before treatment with nonpenicillin regimens, before retreatment after treatment failure.
[c]Includes women with newly discovered syphilis seropositivity late in pregnancy, infants of mothers with inadequately treated syphilis, proven contacts of those with infectious syphilis.
From Hart, 1986; with permission.

had received the standard dose of penicillin G benzathine. To avoid this problem, a fourth criterion for retreatment is being considered: a fourfold drop in VDRL titer at 3 months and an eightfold drop at 6 months. The general belief is that neurosyphilis can be prevented only if CSF is normal 2 years after treatment of early syphilis.

Neurosyphilis

Penicillin G benzathine does not provide therapeutic levels of the drug in CSF. Therefore, the recommended therapy for established neurosyphilis is intravenous administration of aqueous penicillin G, 12 to 24 million U daily for 10 to 14 days, or intramuscular aqueous penicillin G, 2.4 million U daily, with probenecid (Benemid), 2 g given orally each day. Probenecid enhances serum levels of penicillin by reducing renal excretion.

Penicillin may provoke allergic reactions of rash or anaphylaxis. The Jarisch-Herxheimer fever reaction may occur with any form of antisyphilitic treatment but seems to be less common in neurosyphilis. Effective alternatives for patients who are allergic to penicillin are doxycycline, 300 mg orally, given in divided doses daily for 30 days; or tetracycline, 500 mg four times daily for 14 days.

Gummas have responded to treatment with penicillin alone, penicillin plus steroids, and even steroids alone. If the clinical circumstances make that diagnosis likely, and if the clinical condition of the patient permits, a trial of conservative treatment is warranted. If the diagnosis is doubtful, or if the circumstances dictate more immediate attention, biopsy and excision may be appropriate.

For patients with both AIDS and any form of syphilis, some authorities advocate treatment with a regimen recommended for neurosyphilis.

After a course of therapy, quantitative blood serology is determined at 3-month intervals and usually shows a decline in titer if it had previously been elevated. Clinical neurologic examination should be performed regularly. The CSF is examined at 6 and 12 months. If not normal, CSF is reexamined in 2 years. After 3 years, if the patient has improved and is clinically stable and if the CSF and serologic tests are normal, neurologic and CSF examinations are discontinued.

Retreatment is recommended with high doses of intravenous penicillin G in the following situations: if the clinical neurologic findings progress without the discovery of another cause, especially if CSF pleocytosis persists; if the CSF cell count is not normal at 6 months; if the VDRL test in serum or CSF fails to shows a decline or shows a fourfold increase; or if the first course of treatment was suboptimal.

NEUROSYPHILIS AND AIDS

Neurosyphilis now probably occurs more often in HIV-positive persons than in those not HIV-infected. At least one-third of HIV-infected persons are coinfected with *T. pallidum*. How HIV infection affects neurosyphilis is a matter of debate, but suspicions abound about concomitant HIV infection. For example, some authorities state that immunodeficiency reduces resistance to acquisition of syphilis and that the disease is more aggressive, with more frequent and more rapid progression to neurosyphilis and with increased severity, less response to therapy, and more frequent relapse. In one series, 20% of penicillin-treated patients had rising STS titers or new clinical signs. Some authors state that current treatment recommendations may be inadequate. Ophthalmic syphilis is more frequent. CSF cell counts and protein levels are higher, and the incidence of luetic meningitis has increased.

These views, however, are virtually all subjects of argument. The frequency of neurosyphilis in an HIV-positive population is probably less than 2%. In addition, *T. pallidum* is not more likely to invade the CNS. Postmortem examination showed no pathologic differences in neurosyphilis, regardless of whether or not the subjects were HIV-infected. There is no major difference in the clinical syndromes of neurosyphilis, and claims about more aggressive disease have been difficult to substantiate. Serologic responses to syphilis seem undiminished, and the infections respond to treatment as well. Penicillin therapy may be somewhat less effective in HIV-infected patients, but the clinical significance of this is uncertain. A reactive CSF VDRL test does not impair treatment responses.

The practical question is whether special syphilis treatment schedules are required for HIV-infected patients. A large trial of enhanced treatment of early syphilis included the addition of amoxicillin and probenecid to the conventional regimen; there was no decrease in the rate of treatment failure.

Therefore, there are no data to warrant enhanced treatment regimens for syphilis in HIV-infected people. The questions, however, reinforce the need for careful follow-up after treatment, so that retreatment can be given when needed. For patients who seem unlikely to comply, intravenous penicillin therapy (10 to 20 million U daily for 10 to 14 days) is an option. The declining incidence of syphilis and HIV infection may leave many of the questions unanswered because there may not be enough patients for large clinical trials.

SUGGESTED READINGS

Adie WJ. Argyll-Robertson pupils, true and false. *BMJ* 1931;2:136–138.

Argyll-Robertson D. Four cases of spinal miosis with remarks on the action of light on the pupil. *Edinburgh Med J* 1869;15:487–493.

Berger JR. Neurosyphilis in HIV-I seropositive individuals: a prospective study. *Arch Neurol* 1991;48:700–702.

Berry CD, Hooton TM, Collier AC, Lukehart SA. Neurologic relapse after benzathine penicillin therapy for secondary syphilis in a patient with HIV infection. *N Engl J Med* 1987;316:1587–1589.

Brandon WR, Boulos LM, Morse A. Determining the prevalence of neurosyphilis in a cohort co-infected with HIV. *Int J STD AIDS* 1993;4:99–101.

Burke JM, Schaberg DR. Neurosyphilis in the antibiotic era. *Neurology* 1985;35:1368–1371.

Dans PE, Cafferty L, Otter SE, Johnson RJ. Inappropriate use of the CSF VDRL test to exclude neurosyphilis. *Ann Intern Med* 1986;104:86–89.

Dowell ME, Ross PG, Musher DM, et al. Response of latent syphilis or neurosyphilis to ceftriaxone therapy in persons infected with HIV. *Am J Med* 1992;93:481–488.

Feraru ER, Aronow HA, Lipton RB. Neurosyphilis in AIDS patients: initial CSF-VDRL may be negative. *Neurology* 1990;40:541–543.

Fichter RR, Aral SO, Blount JH, et al. Syphilis in the United States, 1967–1979. *Sex Transm Dis* 1983;10:77–80.

Fleet WS, Watson RT, Ballinger WE. Resolution of a gumma with steroid therapy. *Neurology* 1986;36:1104–1107.

Flood JM, Weinstock HS, Guroy ME, et al. Neurosyphilis during the AIDS epidemic, San Francisco, 1985–1992. *J Infect Dis* 1998;177:931–940.

Gourevich MN, Selwyn PA, Davenny K, et al. Effects of HIV infection on the serologic manifestations and response to treatment of syphilis in intravenous drug users. *Ann Intern Med* 1993;118:350–355.

Guinam ME. Treatment of primary and secondary syphilis: defining failure at 3- and 6-month follow-up. *JAMA* 1987;257:359–360.

Hahn RD, Cutler JC, Curtis AC, et al. Penicillin treatment of asymptomatic central nervous system syphilis. I. Probability of progression to symptomatic neurosyphilis. *Arch Dermatol* 1956;74:355–366.

Harrigan EP, MacLaughlin TJ, Feldman RG. Transverse myelitis due to meningovascular syphilis. *Arch Neurol* 1984;41:337–338.

Hart G. Syphilis tests in diagnostic and therapeutic decision making. *Ann Intern Med* 1986;104:368–376.

Holmes MD, Brant-Zawadzki MM, Simon RP. Clinical features of meningovascular syphilis. *Neurology* 1984;34:553–556.

Hook EW III. Management of syphilis in HIV-infected individuals. *Am J Med* 1992;93:477–479.

Hook EW. Editorial response: diagnosing neurosyphilis. *Clin Infect Dis* 1994;18:295–297.

Hook EW, Marra CM. Acquired syphilis in adults. *N Engl J Med* 1992;326:1060–1069.

Hotson JR. Modern neurosyphilis: a partially treated chronic meningitis. *West J Med* 1981;135:191–200.

Jaffe HW, Kabins SA. Examination of CSF in patients with syphilis. *Rev Infect Dis* 1982;4[Suppl]:S842–S847.

Johns DR, Tierney M, Felsenstein D. Alteration in the natural history of neurosyphilis by concurrent infection with HIV. *N Engl J Med* 1987;316:1569–1572.

Jordan KG, Simon RP, Miller JN, et al. Modern neurosyphilis: immunobiology, pathogenesis, and clinical features. In: *Merritt's textbook of neurology. Update 4, 3–13.* Philadelphia: Lea & Febiger, 1992.

Katz DA, Berger JR, Duncan RC. Neurosyphilis: a comparative study of the effects of infection with human immunodeficiency virus. *Arch Neurol* 1993;50:243–249.

Lanska MJ, Lanska DJ, Schmidley JW. Syphilitic polyradiculopathy in an HIV-positive man. *Neurology* 1988;38:1297–1301.

Lukehart SA, Hook EW III, Baker-Zander SA, et al. Invasion of the CNS by *Treponema pallidum*: implications for diagnosis and treatment. *Ann Intern Med* 1988;113:872–881.

Marra CM, Crithlow CW, Hook EW, et al. Cerebrospinal fluid treponemal antibodies in untreated early syphilis. *Arch Neurol* 1995;52:68–72.

Marra CM, Gary DW, Kuypers J, Jacobson MA. Diagnosis of neurosyphilis in patients infected with HIV type 1. *J Infect Dis* 1996;174:219–221.

Marra CM, Longstreth WT, Maxwell CL, Lukeheart SA. Resolution of serum and cerebrospinal fluid abnormalities after treatment of neurosyphilis. *Sex Transm Dis* 1996;:184–189.

Merritt HH, Adams RD, Solomon HC. *Neurosyphilis.* New York: Oxford University Press, 1946.

Musher DM, Hammill RJ, Baughn RE. Syphilis, the response to penicillin therapy, neurosyphilis, and the human immunodeficiency virus. *Ann Intern Med* 1990;113:872–881.

Noguchi H, Moore JW. A demonstration of *Treponema pallidum* in the brain of general paresis. *J Exp Med* 1913;17:232–238.

Rolfs RT, Joesoef MR, Hendershot EF, et al. A randomized trial of enhanced therapy for early syphilis in patients with and without human immunodeficiency virus infection. *N Engl J Med* 1997;337:307–314.

Rolfs RT, Nakashima AK. Epidemiology of primary and secondary syphilis in the United States, 1981 through 1989. *JAMA* 1990;264:1432–1437.

Roos KL. Neurosyphilis. *Semin Neurol* 1992;112:209–212.

Simon RP. Neurosyphilis. *Neurology* 1994;44:2228–2230.

Tomberlin MG, Holton PD, Owens JL, Larsen RA. Evaluation of neurosyphilis in HIV-infected individuals. *Clin Infect Dis* 1994;18:288–294.

Vartdal F, Vandvik B, Michaelsen T, et al. Neurosyphilis: intrathecal synthesis of oligoclonal antibodies to *Treponema pallidum*. *Ann Neurol* 1982;11:35–40.

Wagner-Jauregg J. Über die Einwirkung der Malaria auf die progressive Paralyse. *Psychiatr Neurol Wochenschr* 1918–1919;20:132–151.

Wolters EC. Neurosyphilis: a changing diagnostic problem? *Eur Neurol* 1987;26:23–28.

Merritt's Neurology, 10th ed., edited by L.P. Rowland. Lippincott Williams & Wilkins, Philadelphia © 2000.

CHAPTER 28

SPIROCHETE INFECTIONS: LEPTOSPIROSIS

JAMES R. MILLER

Leptospirosis is caused by a group of closely related spirochetes belonging to the genus *Leptospira.* The organisms that cause human disease are now thought to belong to a single species, *L. interrogans,* with subtypes such as *canicola, pomona,* and *icterohaemorrhagiae* recognized serologically. More than 170 serovariants are arranged in 18 serogroups.

Previously, specific serovariants were linked with particular clinical syndromes. Different serovariants, however, have been associated with the same or different clinical manifestations. Humans are incidental hosts for these spirochetes, which are enzootic in both wild and domestic animals, including cats, dogs, and cattle. Animals can become clinically sick, and asymptomatic carriers can excrete the spirochete in urine for months or years. Human infection comes from contact with infested animal tissue or urine or from exposure to contaminated groundwater, soil, or vegetation. Leptospira can survive for prolonged periods outside of hosts in appropriate environmental conditions. The spirochete is thought to enter humans through mucocutaneous abrasions; it is not known whether the organism can penetrate intact skin. Infection is not limited to specific human populations, but the incidence is probably higher in those who work with animal tissue, such as slaughterhouse employees, farmers, biologic laboratory workers, and persons preparing foods.

Symptoms usually appear abruptly 1 to 2 weeks after exposure, with chills, fever, myalgia, headache, and meningismus. Gastrointestinal symptoms include nausea, emesis, anorexia, and diarrhea. There may be cough and chest pain. Cardiac manifestations, including bradycardia and hypotension, can be severe. Conjunctival suffusion is typical but not constant. There may be pharyngeal injection, cutaneous hemorrhages, or maculopapular rash. Hepatosplenomegaly and lymphadenopathy may occur. In the acute first stage, there is septicemia, and the organism can be isolated from cerebrospinal fluid (CSF).

A second wave of symptoms may appear after the acute illness has apparently resolved. Original symptoms recur, sometimes with meningeal signs. Rarely, encephalitis, myelitis, optic neuritis, or peripheral neuritis develops. During the second phase of illness, immunoglobulin (Ig) M antibody to the *Leptospira* microorganisms and immune complexes can be found. Because the spirochete can no longer be isolated at this time, it is thought that the clinical disease of this phase is immune-mediated.

Leptospiral infection can be manifest clinically as aseptic meningitis. Although the agent can be recovered early in the syndrome, pleocytosis is not found until the second phase. Usually, cell counts are in the range of 10 to several hundred per cubic millimeter, but they can be higher. Neutrophils might be present early, but mononuclear cells predominate from the outset. Unlike most forms of viral meningitis, CSF protein can exceed 100 mg/dL in leptospirosis. Probably, all pathogenic serovariants (*canicola, icterohaemorrhagiae,* and *pomona*) can cause aseptic meningitis.

Other specific syndromes associated with leptospiral infection are pretibial (Fort Bragg) fever. Culture of the organism is possible if special facilities are available. Dark-field examination of blood, urine, or CSF is unreliable. Serologic studies usually confirm the clinical diagnosis, but the antibody is not detected until the second phase of the illness.

Various antibiotics can effectively treat leptospiral infection. They must be administered early in the illness. High-dose penicillin is most generally used; tetracycline is the alternative for those who are allergic to penicillin. Spontaneous recovery is the rule for younger patients without other illnesses. Mortality is greater than 50% after age 50 years, however, and is usually associated with severe liver disease and jaundice.

SUGGESTED READINGS

Arean VM. The pathologic anatomy and pathogenesis of fatal human leptospirosis (Weil's disease). *Am J Pathol* 1962;40:393–423.

Centers for Disease Control and Prevention. Update: leptospirosis and unexplained acute febrile illness among athletes participating in triathlons—Illinois and Wisconsin, 1998. *JAMA* 1998;280:1474–1475.

Coyle PK, Dattwyler R. Spirochetal infection of the central nervous system. *Infect Dis Clin North Am* 1990;4:731–746.

Edwards GA, Domm BM. Human leptospirosis. *Medicine* 1960;39:117–156.

Farr RW. Leptospirosis. *Clin Infect Dis* 1995;21:1–6.

Feigin RD, Anderson DC. Human leptospirosis. *Crit Rev Clin Lab Sci* 1975;5:413–467.

Gollop JH, Katz AR, Rudoy RC, et al. Rat-bite leptospirosis. *West J Med* 1993;159:76–77.

Jackson LA, Kaufmann AF, Adams WG, et al. Outbreak of leptospirosis associated with swimming. *Pediatr Infect Dis J* 1993;12:48–54.

Sperber SJ, Schleupner CJ. Leptospirosis: a forgotten cause of aseptic meningitis and multisystem febrile illness. *South Med J* 1989;82:1285–1288.

Starr SR, Wheeler DS. Index of suspicion. Case 1. Diagnosis: leptospirosis. *Pediatr Rev* 1998;19:385–387.

Merritt's Neurology, 10th ed., edited by L.P. Rowland. Lippincott Williams & Wilkins, Philadelphia © 2000.

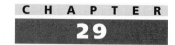

SPIROCHETE INFECTIONS: LYME DISEASE

JAMES R. MILLER

In 1975, a cluster of arthritis cases in children was recognized in Old Lyme, Connecticut. Many patients had had a migratory rash called erythema chronicum migrans (ECM), and some had neurologic or myocardial dysfunction. Affected adults also were seen. The syndrome was subsequently found to be caused by a previously unrecognized spirochete transmitted to humans by ixodid ticks. The spirochete has some characteristics of treponemes, but it is classified among the borreliae (*Borrelia burgdorferi*). In the northeastern United States, the vector, *Ixodes scapularis,* regularly infests deer and mice. Other animals are also hosts for the tick.

EPIDEMIOLOGY

The disease occurs throughout the United States in regions where ixodid ticks are found, although all ixodid populations do not appear to be equal in supporting the presence of the spirochete. The extent of human infection is unknown, but in the Lyme area antibodies are found in 4% of the population. In Europe, a *B. burgdorferi* strain is associated with a similar clinical disorder called *Bannwarth syndrome* or tick-borne *meningopolyneuritis* (Garin-Bujadoux, Bannwarth). Although the manifestations of the disease were described in Europe earlier in the century and were associated with ixodid ticks, the nature of the infection was determined only after the spirochete was identified in North America.

Genetic variation of the spirochete probably accounts for differences between the syndromes described in Europe and in the United States. In the narrow sense, *B. burgdorferi* refers to the American isolate, but broadly it represents a more inclusive term, referring to all the variants that cause similar syndromes. The worldwide distribution of the spirochetes and associated illnesses is still being defined, but symptomatic infection seems to occur throughout the world wherever appropriate ticks reside. *Neuroborreliosis* is sometimes used synonymously with Lyme disease. However, other borreliae that cause relapsing fever may also cause similar neurologic manifestations.

SIGNS AND SYMPTOMS

B. burgdorferi is most frequently transmitted to humans by the nymph stage of the tick, which is active in early summer, but transmission earlier or later can occur from contact with the adult arthropod. The organism can also be isolated from the tick larva, but it is difficult to recover from infected humans.

The course of infection in humans is variable. It has been divided into three stages, but overlaps in symptoms and in timing are common. Usually, a migrating erythematous ring (ECM) develops 3 to 32 days after exposure; the center of the rash is at the site of the tick bite. Smaller secondary rings often appear later, whose centers are less indurated than that of the primary lesion. At this stage, headache, myalgia, stiff neck, and even cranial nerve palsies (almost invariably the seventh nerve) can occur, but cerebrospinal fluid (CSF) is usually normal. The ECM usually resolves in 3 to 4 weeks, although transitory erythematous blotches and rings that do not migrate may occur later.

More prominent neurologic and cardiac manifestations are seen in the second stage, several weeks after the onset of ECM. Heart problems are usually confined to conduction defects, but there may be myopericarditis with left ventricular dysfunction. Meningeal symptoms and signs constitute the major features of the neurologic illness, with headache and stiff neck. Fever is not a regular feature. Radiculitis, multiple or isolated, is common and can cause severe root pain or focal weakness. Cranial nerves, usually the seventh, are frequently involved. Both sides of the face may become paralyzed simultaneously or sequentially. Polyneuritis or mononeuritis multiplex may also occur. Identifying the cause requires a sensitive index of suspicion in areas where the disease is endemic. Neurologic disease may also occur without previous ECM or recognized tick bite.

In original descriptions, *encephalopathic features* were noted, including ataxia, altered consciousness, and myelitis. Later, however, central nervous system (CNS) manifestations were less prominent, with decreased concentration, irritability, emotional lability, and memory and sleep disorders most usually noted. Because the disease is not fatal, the lesions that cause the neurologic syndromes have not been defined. *Immune-mediated processes,* including vasculitis, may be important.

The third stage of Lyme disease is characterized by chronic arthritis in patients with HLA-DR2 antigen. It usually appears several months after the original infection, but it can be present at the time of the subacute neurologic disease. The spirochete has not been isolated from joint fluid, and the arthritis could be an autoimmune disorder, although successful treatment of the arthritis with an antibiotic has been reported.

Although neurologic abnormalities have been mostly associated with the subacute second stage of the disease, a later chronic encephalomyelopathy has been associated with the infection. Often, white matter disease is evident on computed tomography (CT) or magnetic resonance imaging (MRI), usually in association with elevated Lyme disease spirochete antibody titers in blood or CSF. The syndrome is one of progressive long-tract dysfunction that may include optic nerve and sphincters. Cases characterized by only memory loss and cognitive dysfunction have also been reported. Response to antibiotic treatment has been variable. A syndrome of acral dysesthesias has been described in the late stage of Lyme disease. Electrophysiologic evidence reveals a neuropathic process, and the sensory symptoms respond to appropriate antibiotic therapy.

DIAGNOSIS

The combination of meningitis, radiculitis, and neuritis without fever occurs in virtually no other circumstance. If the appropriate history of tick exposure and ECM is obtained, the diagnosis is assured. Partial syndromes and absence of appropriate early findings, however, might require differentiation from a wide variety of illnesses ranging from herniated disc to other causes of acute aseptic or subacute meningitis. Brain MRI and CT scans are normal, and the electroencephalogram is usually normal or nonspecific. CSF pressure is normal. Abnormalities in the CSF formula are usually, but not always, present (Table 29.1). Oligoclonal bands are often present. *B. burgdorferi* has been isolated from the CSF, a rare technical feat that cannot be relied on for routine diagnosis. Demonstration of elevated levels of spirochete-specific immunoglobulin (Ig) M or IgG in the serum or of CSF by enzyme-linked immunosorbent assay or, less reliably, by immunofluorescent antibody test constitutes the basis of diagnosis in clinically appropriate circumstances. Specific confirmation of elevated titers is often sought by Western blot reaction to spirochetal proteins. The procedure is complicated by frequent cross-reactions with other proteins, and strict criteria of interpretation are required for the test to be useful.

The diagnosis of Lyme disease, particularly chronic encephalomyelopathy, is complicated by vagaries of the immune response and the indefinite clinical picture. Rapid treatment of Lyme disease in the early stages, or perhaps even intercurrent use of antibiotics for other purposes, may result in the absence of agent-specific antibody response when the more chronic syndromes become apparent. In addition, antibody carriers in endemic areas may be asymptomatic, making the presence of antibodies inconclusive in questionable cases. Brain single-photon emission CT has been suggested as a method for determining abnormality when other imaging procedures are normal. The specificity of the abnormalities for Lyme disease as opposed to other encephalopathies, however, is not yet determined. The ambiguities in diagnosis of chronic encephalomyelopathies have led to a generous use of prolonged antibiotic treatment in doubtful circumstances, sometimes when other neurologic problems,

such as multiple sclerosis, are clearly the cause. Polymerase chain reaction technology and sensitive immunoassays have been applied to the detection of *B. burgdorferi* deoxyribonucleic acid and antigens in the CSF, but their usefulness is still undetermined.

TREATMENT

Doxycycline, amoxicillin, and clarithromycin (Biaxin) have become the common medications for treatment of Lyme disease during the early stage characterized by ECM. Tetracycline or azithromycin (Zithromax) are also still used. These agents usually prevent the development of subsequent stages. Intravenously administered third-generation cephalosporins, usually ceftriaxone sodium (Rocephin) or cefuroxime axetil (Ceftin), are now generally employed for treatment of neurologic symptoms. Before antibiotic therapy, the second-stage neurologic syndrome lasted for a mean of 30 weeks, although the intensity fluctuated. Intravenous antibiotics usually cause acute symptoms to resolve as the agents are being given. Motor signs last a mean of 7 to 8 weeks, irrespective of the use of antibiotics.

It is now recognized that even with mild CNS involvement, a prolonged period of subtle to moderate memory, emotional, and cognitive problems may follow successful treatment. In the best documented late encephalomyelopathy cases, several months were required after treatment before clinical improvement was noted. The proper length of treatment is uncertain. For most straightforward cases, 2 to 3 weeks seems sufficient. As more chronic and less well documented cases have been treated, the tendency is to treat longer, even up to several months. The efficacy of prolonged treatment has not been established. Antibiotic doses appropriate for ECM therapy are sufficient to treat isolated nerve palsies associated with elevated spirochete antibody levels.

The U.S. Food and Drug Administration has approved the use of a vaccine constituted against the spirochete's outer-surface protein A (OspA). A second vaccine against the same antigen is likely to be approved. Both vaccines require three inoculations for full efficacy and protection, and are about 80% effective after the full series. The length of protection following a single series is not yet known. The vaccines are not yet approved for children younger than 12 years. Recommendations are for those who live in areas where the ticks are endemic and for those who are frequently outdoors in these areas.

TABLE 29.1. CSF ANALYSIS IN LYME DISEASE ENCEPHALOMYELITIS

Test	CSF
Opening pressure[a]	Normal
Total white cells/mm³	166 (15–700)[b]
Lymphocytes (%)	93 (40–100)
Glucose (mg/dL)[c]	49 (33–61)
Proteiun (mg/dL)	79 (8–400)
IgG/albumin ratio (n=20)	0.18 (0.9–0.44)
Oligoclonal bands (n=4)	Present
Myelin basic protein (n=5)	Absent
VDRL (n=20)	Negative

[a] n=38 except where noted
[b] Median (range)
[c] Serum glucose = 95 mg/dL (87–113)
From Pachner and Steere, 1985; with permission.

SUGGESTED READINGS

Ackermann R, Horstrup P, Schmidt R. Tick-borne meningopolyneuritis (Garin-Bujadoux, Bannwarth). *Yale J Biol Med* 1984;57:485–490.

Benke T, Gasse T, Hittmair-Delazer M, Schmutzhard E. Lyme encephalopathy: long-term neuropsychological deficits years after acute neuroborreliosis. *Acta Neurol Scand* 1995;91:353–357.

Bloom BJ, Wyckoff PM, Meissner HC, Steere AC. Neurocognitive abnormalities in children after classic manifestations of Lyme disease. *Pediatr Infect Dis J* 1998;17:189—196.

Cadavid D, Barbour AG. Neuroborreliosis during relapsing fever: review of the clinical manifestations, pathology, and treatment of infections in humans and experimental animals. *Clin Infect Dis* 1998;26:151–164.

Haass A. Lyme neuroborreliosis. *Curr Opin Neurol* 1998;11:253–258.

Halperin JJ. Nervous system Lyme disease. *J Neurol Sci* 1998;153:182–191.

Halperin JJ, Little BW, Coyle PK, Dattwyler RJ. Lyme disease: cause of a treatable peripheral neuropathy. *Neurology* 1987;37:1700–1706.

Halperin JJ, Logigian EL, Finkel MF, Pearl RA. Practice parameters for the diagnosis of patients with nervous system Lyme borreliosis (Lyme disease). Quality Standards Subcommittee of the American Academy of Neurology. *Neurology* 1996;46:619–627.

Halperin JJ, Luft BJ, Anand AK, et al. Lyme neuroborreliosis: central nervous system manifestations. *Neurology* 1989;39:753–759.

Hubalek Z, Halouzka J. Distribution of *Borrelia burgdorferi sensu lato* genomic groups in Europe: a review. *Eur J Epidemiol* 1997;13:951–957.

Nadelman RB, Wormser GP. Lyme borreliosis. *Lancet* 1998;352:557–565.

Nowakowski J, Schwartz I, Nadelman RB, Liveris D, Aguero-Rosenfeld M, Wormser GP. Culture-confirmed infection and reinfection with *Borrelia burgdorferi*. *Ann Intern Med* 1997;127:130–132.

Oksi J, Kalimo H, Marttila RJ, et al. Inflammatory brain changes in Lyme borreliosis: a report on three patients and review of literature. *Brain* 1996;119:2143–2154.

Pachner AR, Steere AC. The triad of neurologic manifestations of Lyme disease: meningitis, cranial neuritis and radiculoneuritis. *Neurology* 1985;35:47–53.

Pacuzzi RM, Younger DS, eds. Lyme disease issue. *Semin Neurol* 1997;17(1).

Reik LJ. Lyme disease. In: Scheld WM, Whitley RJ, Durack DT, eds. *Infections of the central nervous system*, 2nd ed. Philadelphia: Lippincott–Raven Publishers, 1997:685–718.

Schmidt BL. PCR in laboratory diagnosis of human *Borrelia burgdorferi* infections. *Clin Microbiol Rev* 1997;10:185–201.

Sigal LH, Zahradnik JM, Lavin P, et al. A vaccine consisting of recombinant *Borrelia burgdorferi* outer-surface protein A to prevent Lyme disease. Recombinant Outer-Surface Protein A Lyme Disease Vaccine Study Consortium. *N Engl J Med* 1998;339:216–222. Erratum: *N Engl J Med* 1998;339:571.

Steere AC, Grodzicki RL, Kornblatt AN, et al. The spirochetal etiology of Lyme disease. *N Engl J Med* 1983;308:733–740.

Steere AC, Malawista SE, Snydman DR, et al. Lyme arthritis: an epidemic of oligoarticular arthritis in children and adults in three Connecticut communities. *Arthritis Rheum* 1977;20:7–17.

Steere AC, Sikand VK, Meurice F, et al. Vaccination against Lyme disease with recombinant *Borrelia burgdorferi* outer-surface lipoprotein A with adjuvant. Lyme Disease Vaccine Study Group. *N Engl J Med* 1998;339:209–215.

Merritt's Neurology, 10th ed., edited by L.P. Rowland. Lippincott Williams & Wilkins, Philadelphia © 2000.

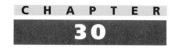

CHAPTER 30

PARASITIC INFECTIONS

BURK JUBELT
JAMES R. MILLER

Disease caused by parasites is uncommon in developed countries. In tropical and less-developed areas, however, parasitic infections exact a heavy toll on society. Poverty and poor living conditions play a significant role in the pathogenesis of these infections, but an appropriate climate for vectors to facilitate transmission is also necessary. The combination of increased international travel to and immigration from endemic areas has increased the likelihood of encountering tropical parasitic infections in the United States. Indigenous parasites are being encountered more frequently because of long-term survival of immunosuppressed patients who have increased susceptibility to infection.

Parasitic infections can be divided into two categories: those caused by worms (helminths) and those caused by protozoa.

HELMINTHIC INFECTION

Helminths are large complex organisms that frequently elicit systemic allergic responses (eosinophilia) and more often cause focal, rather than diffuse, involvement of the nervous system. Helminths are divided into tapeworms (cestodes), flukes (trematodes), and roundworms (nematodes) (Table 30.1).

Cysticercosis

Cysticercosis is the result of encystment of the larvae of *Taenia solium*, the pork tapeworm, in the tissues. The infestation is acquired by ingestion of the ova usually by fecal contamination of food or less often by autoinfection via anal–oral transfer or reverse peristalsis of proglottids into the stomach. The larvae are not acquired by eating infected pork, and cysticercosis regularly occurs in vegetarians in endemic areas. Ingestion of infected pork results in the adult tapeworm infection.

TABLE 30-1. COMMON HELMINTHIC INFECTIONS OF THE NERVOUS SYSTEM

Disease/Parasite	Geographic Location
Cestodes (tapeworms)	
Cysticercosis	Asia, Africa, Central and South
Taenia solium	America, Eastern Europe
Echinococcosis (hydatid cyst disease)	Worldwide
Trematodes (flukes)	
Schistosomiasis	
S. japonicum	Far East
S. mansoni	South America, Carribbean, Africa, and Middle East
S. haimatobium	Africa, Middle East
Paragonimiasis	Asia, Central Africa, Central and South America
Nematodes (roundworms)	
Trichinosis	Worldwide
Eosinophilic meningitis	Southeast Asia, Pacific Islands,
Angiostrongylus contoneasis	Hawaii, Cuba, and Africa
Gnathastoma spinigerum	
Toxocariasis (visceral larva migrans)	Worldwide
Strongyloidiasis	Tropical and Subtropical regions, including United States

Incidence

Central nervous system (CNS) involvement occurs in 50% to 70% of all cases. Virtually all symptomatic patients have CNS involvement. It is the most common parasitic infection of the CNS. Cerebral cysticercosis is common in Mexico, Central and South America, Southeast Asia, China, and India. The disease has again become relatively common in the United States because of immigration from Mexico. The disease may occur in other areas where a reservoir of infected pigs exists. In Mexico, cerebral cysticercosis is found in 2% to 4% of the population in unselected autopsy studies.

Pathology

Typical cysts measure 5 to 10 mm and may be discrete and encapsulated or delicate, thin-walled, and multicystic. The miliary form with hundreds of cysticerci is most common in children. Meningeal cysts cause a chronic cerebrospinal fluid (CSF) pleocytosis. Live encysted larvae in the parenchyma cause little inflammation. Inflammation occurs when the larvae die, usually years after ingestion, and often correlates with the onset of symptoms.

Symptoms and Signs

Clinical manifestations can be divided into four basic types, depending on anatomic site: parenchymal, subarachnoid (or meningitic), intraventricular, and spinal. The most common presenting manifestations are seizures, increased intracranial pressure with headaches and papilledema, and meningitis.

In the parenchymal form, symptoms are related to the site of encystment. Cortical cysts frequently give rise to focal or generalized seizures. Other focal deficits may appear suddenly or may be more chronic. Signs include hemiparesis, sensory loss, hemianopsia, aphasia, or ataxia from cerebellar cysts. Stroke, which occurs secondary to vessel involvement, and dementia are occasionally seen. Rarely, an acute diffuse encephalitis, with confusion to coma, is seen at the time of the initial infection.

The subarachnoid form may be the result of the rupture or death of an arachnoidal cyst or its transformation into the racemose form of the organism, which can enlarge within the basal cisterns and cause obstructive hydrocephalus. Symptoms of meningeal involvement vary from mild headache to a syndrome of chronic meningitis with meningism and communicating hydrocephalus. Spinal involvement may occur and may evolve into arachnoiditis and complete spinal subarachnoid block.

Cysts in the third or fourth ventricle (intraventricular form) obstruct the flow of CSF and can result in obstructive hydrocephalus. The cyst may move within the ventricular cavity and produce a "ball-valve" effect, resulting in intermittent symptoms. Sudden death may occur in these patients, occasionally without prior symptoms. This form frequently occurs in conjunction with the subarachnoid form.

The spinal form is rare. Extramedullary intradural lesions, which are usually cervical, and intramedullary lesions, which are usually thoracic, may be present.

Laboratory Data and Diagnosis

The diagnosis of cysticercosis should be considered in all patients who have ever resided in endemic areas and who have epilepsy, meningitis, or increased intracranial pressure. Computed tomography (CT) and magnetic resonance imaging (MRI) are useful in evaluating such patients. Hydrocephalus may be observed and the exact site of obstruction determined. Intravenous contrast material may demonstrate intraventricular cysts. Parenchymal cysts may calcify, revealing single or multiple punctate calcifications on CT. Viable cysts appear as small lucent areas that may be enhanced either diffusely or in a ring pattern after the infusion of intravenous contrast material (Fig. 30.1). CSF examination may be normal or may reveal a moderate pleocytosis and elevated pressure. In more severe meningitis, the CSF may contain several hundred to several thousand white blood cells (usually mononuclear), elevated protein content, and low glucose, presenting a clinical picture similar to that for fungal or tuberculous meningitis. Eosinophilic meningitis is occasionally seen but is uncommon. The presence of eosinophilia in the blood suggests another parasitic infestation and does not occur in pure neurocysticercosis. CSF or serum antibody (complement fixation, ELISA, Western blot) are usually positive.

Treatment

Ventricular shunting is usually adequate for treatment of hydrocephalic forms of this disorder. Seizures can be controlled with anticonvulsants. Intractable seizures may develop, and surgical removal of cysts may be beneficial. Corticosteroids have been used to relieve the meningitic symptoms, but their value has not

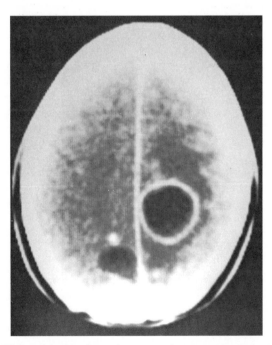

FIG. 30.1. Cerebral cysticercosis: computed tomography. Patient with partial seizures and normal examination. A large lucent lesion with rim enhancement is seen on the left. A nonenhancing lucency with small calcification appears in the right parietal region. Other small lesions are seen bilaterally. (Courtesy of Drs. Verity Grinnell and Mark A. Goldberg.)

been established. Praziquantel, effective in stopping the progression of the parenchymal form of cysticercosis, was the first drug used successfully against the cysts. It is less effective for the chronic meningitic form with arachnoiditis. Albendazole has greater anticysticercal activity and is now the drug of choice. Concomitant use of corticosteroids may be required to prevent severe inflammatory reactions and edema in response to the dying cysticerci.

Echinococcosis (Hydatid Cysts)

Echinococcosis is a tissue infection of humans caused by the larvae of *Echinococcus granulosus*, a tapeworm parasite of the dog family. There is an intermediate phase of development with hydatid cyst formation in other mammals. Sheep and cattle are usually the intermediate hosts, but humans may be infected, especially by ova shed in dog feces. The disease is most common in countries where herd dogs assist with sheep and cattle raising. It is rare in the United States. Several other *Echinococcus* species rarely infect the human CNS.

The cysts are most commonly found in the liver and the lungs. If the embryos pass the pulmonary barrier, cyst formation may occur in any organ. The brain is involved in about 2% of the cases, and neurologic symptoms may develop in patients with cysts in the skull or spine.

Cerebral cysts are usually single. They are most common in the cerebral hemispheres but may develop in the ventricles or cerebellum. The infestation may occur at any age but is most common in children from rural areas.

The signs and symptoms that develop with enlarging cysts in the brain are similar to those of tumor in the affected region. Seizures and increased intracranial pressure may also occur. Involvement of the spine may result in spinal cord compression. The diagnosis of hydatid cyst as the cause of cerebral symptoms is rarely made before operation. CT and MRI should be used to localize the lesions, which are usually single, nonenhancing, and of CSF density. Needle biopsy usually is precluded, because rupture of a cyst results in allergic manifestations, including anaphylaxis. In spinal disease, vertebral collapse is common and is evident on x-rays. Eosinophilia is uncommon except after cyst rupture. Liver enzymes are usually normal. Serologic tests are positive in 60% to 90% of infected individuals.

Treatment is complete surgical removal without puncturing the cyst. Drug treatment with albendazole may decrease the size of cysts and prevent allergic reactions and secondary hydatidosis at the time of surgery.

Schistosomiasis (Bilharziasis)

Involvement of the nervous system by the ova of trematodes is rare. In most reported cases, the lesions were associated with infection with *Schistosoma japonicum*, but isolated cases of *S. haematobium* and *S. mansoni* have also been recorded. *S. japonicum* has a predilection for the cerebral hemispheres; *S. haematobium* and *S. mansoni* more frequently affect the spinal cord. These predilections appear to relate to the location of the adult worms from where ova are released. *S. japonicum* resides in superior mesenteric venules, but the occurrence of ectopic worms

in cerebral venules may explain in part the high incidence of cerebral involvement. *S. mansoni* primarily resides in the inferior mesenteric venules, whereas *S. haematobium* is found in the vesical plexus.

Pathology

The presence of the ova in the nervous system causes an inflammatory exudate containing eosinophils and giant cells (granulomas), necrosis of the parenchyma, and deposition of calcium.

Epidemiology

Schistosomiasis is one of the most important worldwide parasitic diseases, occurring in over 200 million people. *S. japonicum* occurs mainly in Asia and in the Pacific tropics. *S. mansoni* is prevalent in the Caribbean, South America, Africa, and the Middle East. *S. haematobium* occurs in Africa and the Middle East. Symptoms may occur within a few months of exposure or may be delayed for 1 to 2 years. Relapses may occur several or many years after the original infection. The CNS is involved in 3% to 5% of the patients with *S. japonicum* but in fewer patients with other species.

Clinical Manifestations

Schistosomiasis occurs in three phases. The first, or cercarial dermatitis, is an acute reaction to the penetration of the skin by cercariae. The second is a serum sickness reaction, Katayama fever, that occurs 6 to 8 weeks after exposure and manifests as fever, urticaria, abdominal pain, diarrhea, and muscle pain. The third stage is a chronic infection of most internal organs (liver, spleen, bladder, heart, lungs). Cerebral schistosomiasis may be acute during Katayama fever or chronic with the third phase. Acute cases usually present as a diffuse fulminating meningoencephalitis with fever, headache, confusion, lethargy, and coma. Focal or generalized seizures, hemiplegia, and other focal neurologic signs are common. The chronic cerebral form usually simulates the clinical picture of a tumor with localizing signs and increased intracranial pressure with papilledema. Granulomatous masses in the spinal cord almost always present acutely with signs and symptoms of an incomplete transverse lesion, with or without spinal subarachnoid block, depending on the size of the lesion. The conus is the most common site of spinal cord involvement. Granulomatous root involvement may also occur.

Laboratory Data

There is leukocytosis with an increase in eosinophils in the blood, although this may not be the case with the chronic cerebral form. The CSF pressure may be increased with large intracerebral lesions and partial or incomplete subarachnoid block with spinal lesions. A slight or moderate pleocytosis in the CSF (sometimes with eosinophils) and an increased protein content may occur. Cerebral lesions may be seen with CT or MRI. Spinal cord lesions may be demonstrated by myelography, CT, or MRI (Fig. 30.2).

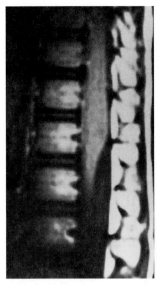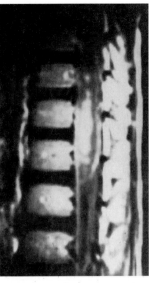

A, B

FIG. 30.2. Spinal cord schistosomiasis: sagittal T1-weighted magnetic resonance images. **A:** Without contrast demonstrates markedly enlarged conus medullaris. **B:** With contrast demonstrates prominent regions of enhancement within the enlarged conus. [From Selwa et al. (1991).]

Diagnosis

The diagnosis is established from the history of gastrointestinal upset, eosinophilia in the blood, and the presence of ova in the stool or urine. Serologic tests and biopsy of the rectal mucosa are also of value in the establishment of the diagnosis.

Treatment

The broad-spectrum drug praziquantel is the drug of choice. It is effective against all three human schistosomes. Oral steroids may decrease swelling. Anticonvulsive drugs should be given to control seizures. Surgical excision of the large granulomatous lesions may be required. Steroids and decompressive laminectomy may be needed when subarachnoid block is present.

Paragonimiasis

Paragonimiasis is the disease caused by the lung flukes *Paragonimus westermani* and *P. mexicanus*. Other *Paragonimus* species may rarely infect humans. These trematodes commonly infect humans in Africa, Southeast Asia, South Pacific areas, India, and Central and South America. Infection occurs by eating uncooked or poorly cooked freshwater crustaceans. Immature flukes exist in the intestines and spread through the body, occasionally reaching the brain and spinal cord. Pulmonary and intestinal symptoms are the most common. Pulmonary involvement includes chronic cough, hemoptysis, and cavitary lesions on chest radiographs, thus simulating tuberculosis.

CNS involvement occurs in 10% to 15% of affected patients. Symptoms and signs of cerebral involvement include fever, headache, meningoencephalitis, focal and generalized seizures, dementia, hemiparesis, visual disturbances, and other focal manifestations. Various syndromes have been recognized: acute meningitis, chronic meningitis, acute purulent meningoencephalitis, infarction, epilepsy, subacute progressive encephalopathy, chronic granulomatous disease (tumorous form), and late inactive forms (chronic brain syndrome). The CSF may be under increased pressure. The pleocytosis is primarily polymorphonuclear in acute forms and lymphocytic in more chronic forms. Eosinophils are occasionally present, and many red blood cells are occasionally seen in the acute cases. The protein content and gamma globulins are usually increased. The glucose content may be decreased. Diagnosis is most often made by detecting ova in the sputum and stool. Peripheral anemia, eosinophilia, leukocytosis, and elevated erythrocyte sedimentation rate and gamma globulins may occur. Serologic and skin tests are available. Positive CSF antibody tests are diagnostic but not very sensitive. CT may also be of assistance in diagnosis, revealing ventricular dilatation and intracranial calcifications, including the characteristic "soap bubble" calcifications. During the early progressive course, mortality may reach 5% to 10%. The later chronic granulomatous state tends to be benign. Therapy includes praziquantel or bithionol for the acute to subacute meningoencephalitis and surgical treatment for the chronic tumorous form.

Trichinosis (Trichinellosis)

Trichinosis is an acute infection caused by the roundworm *Trichinella spiralis*. Infection is acquired by eating larvae (in cysts) in raw or undercooked pork. Bear and walrus meat have also been incriminated. The CNS is involved in 10% to 17% of cases.

Pathology

The pathologic changes in the nervous system include the presence of filiform larvae in the cerebral capillaries and in the parenchyma, perivascular inflammation, petechial hemorrhages, and granulomatous nodules.

Symptoms and Signs

Trichinosis manifests as a systemic infection due to larval migration (larviposition) with fever, headache, muscle pain and tenderness (muscle invasion), periorbital edema, subconjunctival hemorrhages, and myocardial involvement. Gastrointestinal symptoms are less frequent, occurring in about 25% of symptomatic cases. Neurologic involvement occurs in 10% to 25% of symptomatic infections and develops any time within the first few weeks of the infection. There may be a severe diffuse encephalitis with confusion, delirium, coma, seizures, and evidence of focal damage to the cerebrum, brainstem, or cerebellum. Edema of the optic nerve, meningeal signs, spinal cord syndromes, and neuropathies may also occur.

Laboratory Data

The most important laboratory findings are leukocytosis and eosinophilia in the blood. Muscle enzymes may be increased. The CSF is abnormal in about one-third of cases. There may be a slight lymphocyte pleocytosis, but eosinophilia is rare. The protein content and pressure are often elevated. The parasites are found in the CSF of approximately 30% of patients. CTs may reveal single or multiple small hypodensities in the white matter or cortex in about three-fourths of cases, with about half of these lesions enhancing with contrast.

Diagnosis

The diagnosis is usually not difficult when neurologic symptoms appear in a group of individuals who have eaten infected pork and show the other manifestations of the disease (gastrointestinal symptoms, tenderness of the muscles, and edema of the eyelids). Difficulty is encountered in isolated cases when infection results from ingestion of meat other than pork or where the other manifestations of the infection are lacking. Trichinosis should be considered an etiologic factor in all patients with encephalitis of obscure nature. Repeated examination of the blood for eosinophilia and elevated muscle enzymes, biopsy of the muscles, and serologic tests should establish the diagnosis.

Prognosis

Recovery within a few days or weeks is the rule except when there is profound coma or evidence of severe damage to the cerebrum. For those with CNS involvement, mortality is 10% to 20%. Recovery is usually accompanied by complete or almost complete remission of the neurologic signs. Recurrent convulsive seizures have been reported as a late sequel.

Treatment

Thiabendazole is recommended to kill intestinal worms. Mebendazole is used to treat tissue larvae. Corticosteroids are given to reduce inflammation and cerebral edema.

Eosinophilic Meningitis

The human nervous system may be invaded by the nematode rat lungworm, *Angiostrongylus cantonensis*, which uses a molluscan intermediate host and invades the domestic rat and other rodents in the course of its life cycle. Infection in humans (accidental hosts) is usually due to the ingestion of raw snails, shrimp, crabs, and fish, which are the intermediate hosts. Cases have been reported from Hawaii, the Philippines, Pacific Islands, Southeast Asia, Cuba, and Africa.

Involvement of the human nervous system is usually characterized by an acute meningitis (headache 90%, nuchal rigidity 60%, fever 50%), but less frequently there may be encephalitis, encephalomyelitis, radiculomyeloencephalitis, or involvement of cranial nerves (especially VI and VII). Onset occurs 3 to 35 days after the ingestion of the raw intermediate host. Severe dysesthetic pains, probably from posterior root inflammation, occur in about 50% of the patients. The infection is most common in children. Nervous system lesions are due to destruction of tissue by the parasite and to necrosis and aneurysmal dilatation of cerebral vessels, resulting in small or large hemorrhages. A CSF pleocytosis of 100 to 1000 cells/mm^3 with many eosinophils is characteristic. A peripheral blood eosinophilia is almost always seen.

CT is usually normal. Serologic tests are available. Usually, the disease is self-limited. In severe cases, death, which is rare, may be the result of small or large hemorrhagic lesions in the brain. There is no specific therapy.

Not all cases of eosinophilic meningitis are due to *A. cantonensis* infestation; other parasitic infections (cysticerosis, schistosomiasis, paragonimiasis), coccidioidomycosis, foreign bodies, drug allergies, and neoplasms may also cause this syndrome but less frequently. Another nematode of the Far East, *Gnathostoma spinigerum*, usually causes eosinophilic meningitis when it invades the CNS; such invasion occurs much less frequently with *G. spinigerum* than with *A. cantonensis*. It has also caused the clinical syndromes of radiculomyelitis, encephalitis, and subarachnoid and intracranial hemorrhage. When the CNS is involved, the symptoms are more severe and the mortality is higher with *G. spinigerum*, probably because of its larger size, than with *A. cantonensis* infection. Also, with *G. spinigerum*, CT is usually abnormal because parenchymal disease (brain and spinal cord) is more common.

Other Helminths

In toxocariasis, visceral larva migrans is a syndrome of pulmonary symptoms, hepatomegaly, and chronic eosinophilia caused by the larvae of the dog and cat ascarids (roundworms) *Toxocara canis* and *T. cati*. Eggs from the animals' feces may be ingested, especially by children playing with infected dogs or contaminated soil. Although visceral larva migrans is uncommon and nervous system involvement is rare, the disease is always a potential threat due to the ubiquitous infections of domestic animals. Neurologic signs are most often manifest by focal deficits, especially hemiparesis. Encephalopathy and seizures also have occurred. Eosinophils are infrequently seen in the CSF but are common in the periphery. Ocular involvement is more common than CNS disease. Serology is helpful for diagnosis, and hypergammaglobulinemia is common. Larvae may be identified in the sputum or in tissue granulomas from biopsy. Diethylcarbamazine is the drug of choice. Thiabendazole and mebendazole are alternative agents. An association of toxocariasis with pica and lead encephalopathy has been noted. Another ascarid, *Ascaris lumbricoides*, has been reported to cause a similar neurologic syndrome.

Strongyloidiasis is an intestinal infection of humans caused by the nematode *Strongyloides stercoralis*. This infection occurs in tropical and subtropical regions throughout the world but also occurs in most areas of the United States. In the usual infection, the CNS is spared. Disseminated strongyloidiasis (hyperinfection syndrome), however, is not an infrequent complication in the immunosuppressed or immunodeficient host. CNS involvement occurs as part of this disseminated infection. Neurologic signs include meningitis, altered mental states (encephalopathy to coma), seizures, and focal deficits from mass lesions or infarction. CSF abnormalities are nonspecific, and eosinophilia is infrequent. Diagnosis is usually made by finding the larvae in stool, sputum, or duodenal aspirates. Peripheral eosinophilia is not always present. Another clue to the diagnosis is the occurrence in the immunocompromised patient of an unexplained gram-negative bacteremia and meningitis, which is a frequent accompaniment of disseminated strongyloidiasis. Thiabendazole and ivermectin are the drugs of choice.

PROTOZOAN INFECTION

Protozoa are small (microbial size) single-cell organisms that more frequently cause diffuse encephalitic, as opposed to focal, involvement of the nervous system. Protozoa do not elicit allergic reactions or cause eosinophilia.

Toxoplasmosis

Toxoplasmosis is the infection of humans by the protozoan organism *Toxoplasma gondii*. The infection, which has a predilection for the CNS and the eye, may be congenital with encephalitis and chorioretinitis; may cause meningoencephalitis during acquired primary infection in the immunocompetent host; and may cause mass lesions, encephalitis, and chorioretinitis in the immunocompromised host. Toxoplasmosis is especially prevalent in those with acquired immunodeficiency syndrome (AIDS) (see Chapter 24).

Etiology and Pathology

The toxoplasma are minute (about 2×3 μm), oval, pyriform, rounded, or elongated protoplasmic masses with a central nucleus. The important animal host for this organism is the cat. Infection is acquired by ingestion of oocysts from cat feces or contaminated soil. Infection may also occur by eating unwashed vegetables or undercooked meat. The organisms invade the walls of blood vessels in the nervous system and produce an inflammatory reaction. Miliary granulomas are formed. They may become calcified or undergo necrosis. The granulomatous lesions are scattered throughout the CNS and may be found in the meninges and ependyma. Hydrocephalus may develop from occlusion of the aqueduct of Sylvius by the resulting ependymitis. The microorganisms are present in the epithelioid cells of the granulomas, endothelial cells of blood vessels, and nerve cells. Lesions in the retina are common; occasionally, they are also present in the lungs, kidneys, liver, spleen, or skin.

Clinical Manifestations

In the congenital form, the symptoms are usually evident in the first few days of life. Rarely, congenital infections may not manifest for several years. The common manifestations are inanition, microcephaly, seizures, mental retardation, spasticity, opisthotonos, chorioretinitis, microphthalmus, or other congenital defects in development of the eye. Optic atrophy is common, and there may be an internal hydrocephalus. Depending on the extent of systemic disease, the liver and spleen may be enlarged with elevated bilirubin; fever, rash, and pneumonitis may also be present. The presence of calcified nodules in the brain can be demonstrated by CT or radiographs of the skull. Symptoms in the infantile form are similar to those of the congenital form but may not make their appearance until the third or fifth year of life. Cerebral calcifications are not found in postnatally acquired infections.

Acquired toxoplasmosis is most often asymptomatic in the normal host. An infectious mononucleosis-like picture may be seen with lymphadenopathy and fever. Although atypical lymphocytes may be present in the peripheral blood, serologic tests for Epstein-Barr virus are negative. Rarely, meningoencephalitis with headache, confusion, delirium, drowsiness, and coma with seizures can be seen. Signs of meningeal irritation are uncommon.

Severe infection is more likely to occur in immunocompromised patients, and some may be due to reactivation rather than to newly acquired infection. Extraneural manifestations may include pneumonitis, myocarditis, myositis, and choreoretinitis. Neurologic involvement may take one of several forms: subacute to chronic encephalopathic picture with confusion, delirium, obtundation, and coma, occasionally accompanied by seizures; acute meningoencephalitis with headache, nuchal rigidity, and focal or generalized seizures, leading to status epilepticus and coma; and focal signs due to single or multiple mass lesions (toxoplasmic abscess), probably the most common and tends to be chronic. A combination of these three types of neurologic involvement is often seen.

Toxoplasmosis as a complication of neoplastic disease is relatively infrequent. Toxoplasmosis, however, is one of the most frequent CNS opportunistic infection of AIDS patients, accounting for about one-third of all CNS complications.

Laboratory Data

A moderate or severe anemia and a mild leukocytosis or leukopenia may be present. The CSF may be under increased pressure. The protein content is generally increased, and there is an inconstant pleocytosis. Cell counts as high as several thousand per cubic millimeter, mostly lymphocytes, have been recorded. The CSF glucose is normal or mildly reduced. CT may reveal calcifications in congenital infections. Low-density focal lesions may be seen. With contrast, these lesions usually show ring enhancement similar to a brain abscess or, less frequently, diffuse or no enhancement. Often, the lesions are multiple. MRI is more sensitive for demonstrating these lesions (Fig. 30.3).

Diagnosis

The diagnosis of congenital toxoplasmosis is usually considered in the newborn with choreoretinitis, microcephaly, seizures, mental retardation, cerebral calcifications, and evidence of systemic infection. The diagnosis is more difficult to make in older children and adults with either acquired disease or reactivation of a latent infection. Toxoplasma can occasionally be demonstrated in CSF sediment with Wright or Giemsa stain. The organism rarely can be cultivated from CSF sediment by inoculation of laboratory mice. Tissue culture and polymerase chain reaction techniques are still under development but may be available in some locales. Although a definite diagnosis can be made only by isolation of the organism from biopsy of brain or other tissues, a presumptive diagnosis can be made by using readily available serologic tests. Serologic tests include the Sabin-Feldman dye, indirect fluorescent antibody, complement fixation, agglutina-

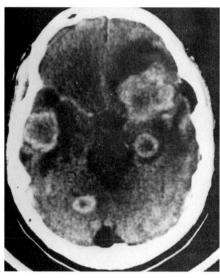

FIG. 30.3. Cerebral toxoplasmosis. Enhanced axial computed tomography demonstrates multiple, bilateral, ring-enhancing hypodense lesions of both temporal, right occipital and left frontal lobes with surrounding edema. (From Farrar WE, Wood MJ, Innes JA, Tubbs H. *Infectious diseases: text and color atlas*, 2nd ed. London: Gower Medical Publishers, 1992:3.30.)

tion, indirect hemagglutination, and ELISA tests. Demonstration of IgM antibodies by ELISA or indirect fluorescent antibody is particularly helpful for diagnosis of a congenital or an acute acquired infection.

In AIDS patients and in most immunocompromised patients, serum IgG antibody is usually positive, although a four-fold rise is infrequent. Serum IgM antibody is not usually detected. The presence of CSF antibodies may be a sensitive indicator of CNS infection.

Course, Prognosis, and Treatment

Prognosis is poor in the congenital form; more than 50% of affected infants die within a few weeks after birth. Mental and neurologic defects are present in the infants who survive. The mortality rate is also high in the infantile form of encephalitis. Most acquired infections in the immunocompetent patient are self-limited and do not require treatment. The severe, acquired, or reactivated infections, which occur more commonly in immunocompromised patients, frequently result in death. These severe infections can at times be treated successfully with pyrimethamine and sulfadiazine. In AIDS patients, if a tissue diagnosis cannot be made but serum IgG titers are positive and the characteristic neuroradiologic abnormalities are present, empiric therapy should be instituted. Indefinite suppression therapy is required for AIDS patients.

Cerebral Malaria

Malaria is the most common human parasitic disease, with 300 million to 500 million infected individuals in the world and about 2 million deaths each year. This disease is endemic in tropical and subtropical areas of Africa, Asia, and Central and South America. The disease can be seen almost anywhere, however, as a result of international travel. Malaria is transmitted by mosquitos.

Involvement of the nervous system occurs in about 2% of affected patients and is most common in infections of the malignant tertian form, almost always caused by *Plasmodium falciparum*.

Pathology and Pathogenesis

The neurologic symptoms are due to congestion or occlusion of capillaries and venules with pigment-laden parasitized erythrocytes and to the presence of multiple petechial hemorrhages. Apparently, parasitized erythrocytes adhere to vascular endothelial cells, thereby obstructing blood flow and causing anoxia. Lymphocytic and mononuclear perivascular inflammation and a microglial cell response may be seen, at times resulting in cerebral edema. Thrombotic occlusion of vessels and large intracranial hemorrhages are rare. It is probable that the pathologic changes in the nervous system are reversible.

Symptoms and Signs

The symptoms and signs are primarily those of an acute diffuse encephalopathy. Spinal cord lesions and a polyneuritis of the Guillain-Barré type have rarely been seen. The neurologic symptoms usually appear in the second or third week of the illness but may be the initial manifestation. The onset of cerebral symptoms has no relationship to the height of the fever. Headache, photophobia, vertigo, convulsions, confusion, delirium, and coma are the most common symptoms. There may be neck stiffness. Focal signs, such as transient hemiparesis, aphasia, hemianopia, and cerebellar ataxia, are uncommon. Myoclonus, chorea, and intention tremors have been observed. Cranial nerve palsies and papilledema are rarely seen, although retinal hemorrhages are common. Psychic manifestations, such as delirium, disorientation, amnesia, or combativeness, are present in a large percentage of the patients. In severe malaria, pulmonary edema, renal failure, and gastrointestinal symptoms occur.

Laboratory Data

Laboratory findings include anemia and the presence in the red blood cells of many parasites. In most cases, the CSF is entirely normal. Elevated pressure, slight xanthochromia, a small or moderate number of lymphocytes, and a moderately increased protein content may be seen. CSF sugar content is normal.

Diagnosis

Cerebral malaria is diagnosed from the appearance of cerebral symptoms and the findings of the organisms of *P. falciparum* by microscopic examination of blood smears. ELISA kits for serologic diagnosis are available. Delirium, convulsions, or coma, probably because of high fever, may occur as symptoms of general infection in patients with *P. vivax* in the absence of cerebral involvement. The symptoms in these cases are transient and respond readily to antimalarial therapy.

Prognosis

The mortality rate is 20% to 40% in cases of cerebral malaria. It is highest (80%) when there is a combination of coma and convulsions. There are few or no residua in the patients who recover.

Treatment

Cerebral malaria is a true medical emergency. In critically ill patients, treatment includes chloroquine, usually given by intramuscular injection, and quinine (or quinidine) given intravenously. In less severe cases, chloroquine alone can be used. If infection occurs in an endemic area of chloroquine-resistant falciparum malaria (now most areas of the world except parts of Central America, Mexico, the Caribbean, and the Middle East), quinine plus pyrimethamine-sulfadoxine (Fansidar), doxycycline, or clindamycin should be used. In Southeast Asia, where multiple drug resistance occurs, various regimens include quinine plus tetracycline, artesunate (or artemether) plus mefloquine, and mefloquine plus doxycycline. Anticonvulsants should be given to control seizures. Transfusions of whole blood or plasma may be required. Other supportive measures include reduction of fever, fluid and glucose replacement, and respiratory support. Sedation may be necessary in excited or delirious patients. The use of dexamethasone is deleterious in the treatment of cerebral malaria. Mannitol should be used for life-threatening cerebral edema. An infrequent possibly corticosteroid-responsive postmalarial encephalopathy has been described.

Trypanosomiasis

Two distinct varieties of infection with trypanosomes are recognized: the African form (sleeping sickness), which is due to infection with *Trypanosoma brucei*, and the South American form (Chagas disease), which is endemic in South America, Central America, and Mexico and is due to infection by *T. cruzi*. Chagas disease occurs as far north as southernmost Texas.

Etiology and Pathology

In the African form of the disease, the organisms retain their trypanosome form and multiply by longitudinal fission. They are transmitted from person to person by the tsetse fly, occasionally by other flies or insects, and by mechanical contact. There are two variants of the species: *T. brucei gambiense* (mid and west Africa) and *T. brucei rhodesiense* (east Africa). The pathologic changes are those of a chronic meningoencephalitis.

The organisms of South American trypanosomiasis, when found in the blood, have an ordinary trypanoform structure. They do not, however, reproduce in the blood but invade tissues and are transformed into typical leishmania parasites. These may later assume the trypanosome form and reenter the blood. The infection is transmitted from an animal host (e.g., rodents, cats, opossum, armadillo) to humans by a blood-sucking reduviid bug known as the "kissing bug."

The pathologic lesion in the nervous system is a meningoencephalitis consisting of miliary granulomas composed of proliferated microglial cells, with lymphocytic-plasmocytic perivascular and meningeal infiltrates. The organisms are present in glial and some nerve cells. The lesions are diffusely scattered throughout the nervous system and are accompanied by a patchy reaction in the meninges and parenchyma.

Symptoms and Signs

African trypanosomiasis (sleeping sickness) passes through two indistinct stages: febrile (hemolymphatic) and lethargic (meningoencephalitic). The incubation period is variable. In some cases, symptoms may have their onset within 2 weeks of the infection. In others, it may be delayed for months or years. The Rhodesian (east African) form usually has an acute to subacute course, whereas the Gambian (west African) disease is usually chronic. The first stage of the disease is characterized by a remitting fever, exanthems, lymphadenitis, splenomegaly, arthralgia, myalgia, and asthenia. During this period, which may last for several months or years, the organisms are present in the blood. The first stage may pass imperceptibly into the second, in which the previous symptoms are exaggerated and involvement of the nervous system is evident in the form of tremors, incoordination, convulsions, paralysis, confusion, headaches, apathy, insomnia or somnolence, and, finally, coma. There is progressive weakness with loss of weight. If the condition is untreated, death usually ensues within a year after the appearance of cerebral symptoms. Death from intercurrent infection is common.

In South American trypanosomiasis, the acute stage generally lasts about 1 month and is characterized by fever; conjunctivitis; palpebral and facial edema; enlargement of the lymph nodes, liver, and spleen; and, rarely, an acute encephalitis. During this stage, trypanosomes are present in the blood, and the leishmaniform bodies are seen in the tissue. The chronic stage is characterized by evidence of involvement of the viscera, particularly the heart and gastrointestinal tract. Neurologic involvement is rare and may be diffuse (mental alterations, seizures, choreoathetosis) or focal (hemiplegia, ataxia, aphasia). The disease is slowly progressive, with occasional acute exacerbations associated with fever. Death usually ensues within a few months or years.

Laboratory Data

Some degree of anemia is common in all forms of trypanosomiasis. The erythrocyte sedimentation rate, liver function tests, serum globulin fraction, and serum IgM may be increased. There is a lymphocytic pleocytosis in the CSF, increased protein content, increased gamma globulin fraction, and increased IgM.

Diagnosis

The diagnosis depends on the development of characteristic symptoms in residents of regions in which forms of the disease are endemic. The diagnosis is established by the demonstration of organisms in the blood or CSF, in material obtained from a biopsied lymph node, or by the inoculation of these substances into susceptible animals. Serologic and CSF antibody tests are also available.

Treatment

Melarsoprol, an organic arsenical, is effective in the treatment of *T. brucei* infections of the nervous system. Suramin or eflornithine are the drugs of choice for the acute stage. No drug treatment is established as safe and effective in chronic Chagas disease, including the CNS component. Nifurtimox or benznidazole are usually effective, however, in the acute stage of infection.

Primary Amebic Meningoencephalitis

It has been known for many years that amebae (*Entamoeba histolytica*) may rarely invade the brain and produce circumscribed abscesses. However, free-living amebae are the species primarily causing meningoencephalitis. *Naegleria fowleri* causes an acute meningoencephalitis, primary amebic meningoencephalitis, whereas *Acanthamoeba* species can cause both acute and granulomatous amebic meningoencephalitis. Another species, *Leptomyxid amebae*, has caused a few cases. Amebic meningoencephalitis is rare but probably has a worldwide distribution. Most cases in the United States are reported from the Southeast.

Naegleria Infections

These infections usually occur in children or young adults who have been swimming in freshwater lakes or ponds. Inhalation of dustborne cysts may also occur in arid regions. Interestingly, the organism apparently invades the nervous system through the olfactory nerves and does not cause a systemic infection. The incubation period is several days to a week. The onset of symptoms of primary amebic meningoencephalitis is abrupt. Mild symptoms of an upper respiratory infection may occur. Fever, headache, and stiff neck are followed within 1 or 2 days by nausea and vomiting, lethargy, disorientation, seizures, increased intracranial pressure, coma, and then death.

The CSF picture is similar to that of an acute bacterial meningitis, with increased pressure, several hundred to thousands of white blood cells per cubic millimeter (primarily neutrophils), as many as several thousand red blood cells, an elevated protein content, decreased glucose, and negative Gram stain. Trophozoites may be recognized in a wet preparation of uncentrifuged CSF or with Wright or Giemsa stains. The organism can be cultured on special media or by mouse inoculation. A serologic test is available at the Centers for Disease Control and Prevention. The disease is rapidly fatal, but recovery with treatment has been reported in some cases. Amphotericin B has been used effectively alone or in combination with several drugs (rifampin, chloramphenicol, ketoconazole).

Acanthamoeba Infections

Acanthamoeba is a ubiquitous organism that can cause a subacute or chronic granulomatous amebic encephalitis as an opportunistic infection in alcoholic and immunocompromised patients. The organism probably causes a systemic infection through the respiratory tract and then seeds the brain by hematogenous spread. The meningoencephalitis may present with chronic fever and headache, followed by the gradual onset of focal neurologic signs (e.g., hemiparesis, aphasia, seizures with focal signature, ataxia) and abnormalities of mentation. Other signs include skin lesions, corneal ulcerations, uveitis, and pneumonitis.

There is CSF pleocytosis that is more often lymphocytic than polymorphonuclear. Protein is usually elevated, and glucose is normal or slightly decreased. Organisms occasionally may be recognized on wet preparations but have never been cultured from CSF. CT and MRI may reveal focal lesions. Biopsy is usually required for diagnosis. Several cases of acute meningoencephalitis, similar to those caused by *Naegleria*, have been reported. The disease is usually fatal. *In vitro*, the organism is usually sensitive to pentamidine, ketoconazole, flucytosine, and less so to amphotericin B.

SUGGESTED READINGS

General

Anonymous. Drugs for parasitic infections. *Med Lett* 1998;40:1–12.

Gutierrez Y. *Diagnostic pathology of parasitic infections with clinical correlations*. Philadelphia: Lea & Febiger, 1990.

Lowichik A, Siegel JD. Parasitic infections of the central nervous system. *J Child Neurol* 1995;10:4–17 (Part I), 77–87 (Part II), 177–190 (Part III).

Scheld WM, Whitle RJ, Durack DT, eds. *Infections of the central nervous system*, 2nd ed. Philadelphia: Lippincott-Raven, 1997.

Strickland GT. *Hunter's tropical medicine*, 8th ed. Philadelphia: W.B. Saunders, 1998.

Warren KS, Mahmound AAF, eds. *Tropical and geographic medicine*, 2nd ed. New York: McGraw-Hill, 1990.

Helminthic Infection

Cysticercosis

Akiguchi I, Fujiwara T, Matsuyama H, et al. Intramedullary spinal cysticercosis. *Neurology* 1979;29:1531–1534.

Barinagarrementeria F, Cantu C. Frequency of cerebral arteritis in subarachnoid cysticercosis: an angiographic study. *Stroke* 1998;29:123–125.

Cantu C, Barinagarrementeria F. Cerebrovascular complications of neurocysticercosis. *Arch Neurol* 1996;53:233–239.

Del Brutto OH. Albendazole therapy for subarachnoid cysticerci: clinical and neuroimaging analysis of inpatients. *J Neurol Neurosurg Psychiatry* 1997;62:659–661.

Del Brutto OH, Santibañez R, Noboa CA, et al. Epilepsy due to cysticercosis: analysis of 203 patients. *Neurology* 1992;42:389–392.

Garcia HH, Gilman RH, Horton J, et al. Albendazole therapy for neurocysticercosis: a prospective double-blind trial comparing 7 versus 14 days of treatment. *Neurology* 1997;48:1421–1427.

Leite CC, Kinkins JR, Escobar BE, et al. MR imaging of intramedullary and intradural-extramedullary spinal cysticercosis. *Am J Roentgenol* 1997;169:1713–1717.

Martinez HR, Rangel-Guerra R, Arredondo-Estrada JH, Marfil A, Onofre J. Medical and surgical treatment in neurocysticercosis: a magnetic resonance study of 161 cases. *J Neurol Sci* 1995;130:25–34.

Mohanty A, Venkatrama SK, Das S, Sas BS, Rao BR, Vasudev MK. Spinal intramedullary cysticercosis. *Neurosurgery* 1997;40:82–87.

Rosenfeld EA, Byrd SE, Shulman ST. Neurocysticercosis among children in Chicago. *Clin Infect Dis* 1996;23:101–113.

Schantz PM, Moore AC, Muñoz JL, et al. Neurocysticercosis in an orthodox Jewish community in New York City. *N Engl J Med* 1992;327:692–695.

Teitelbaum GP, Otto RJ, Lin M, et al. MR imaging of neurocysticercosis. *Am J Roentgenol* 1989;153:857–866.

White AC Jr. Neurocysticercosis: a major cause of neurological disease worldwide. *Clin Infect Dis* 1997;24:101–113.

Echinococcosis

Anderson M, Bickerstaff ER, Hamilton JC. Cerebral hydatid cysts in Britain. *J Neurol Neurosurg Psychiatry* 1975;38:1104–1108.

Copley JB, Fripp PJ, Erasmus AM, Otto DDV. Unusual presentations of cerebral hydatid disease in children. *Br J Neurosurg* 1992;6:203–210.

Hamza R, Touibi S, Jamoussi M, et al. Intracranial and orbital hydatid cysts. *Neuroradiology* 1982;22:211–214.

Pamir MN, Akalon N, Ozgen T, Erbengi A. Spinal hydatid cysts. *Surg Neurol* 1984;21:53–57.

Peter J, Domingo Z, Sinclair-Smith C, de Villiers J. Hydatid infestation of the brain: difficulties with computed tomography diagnosis and surgical treatment. *Pediatr Neurosurg* 1994;20:78–83.

Schistosomiasis

Blunt SB, Boulton J, Wise R. MRI in schistosomiasis of conus medullaris and lumbar spinal cord. *Lancet* 1993;341:557.

Liu LX. Spinal and cerebral schistosomiasis. *Semin Neurol* 1993;13:189–200.

Marcial-Rojas RA, Fiol RE. Neurologic complications of schistosomiasis. *Ann Intern Med* 1963;59:215–230.

Preidler KW, Riepl T, Szolar D, Ranner G. Cerebral schistosomiasis: MR and CT appearance. *Am J Neuroradiol* 1996;17:1598–1600.

Scrimgeour EM, Gajdusek DC. Involvement of the central nervous system in *Schistosoma mansoni* and *S. haematobium* infection. *Brain* 1985;108:1023–1038.

Selwa LM, Brumberg JA, Mandell SH, Garofalo EA. Spinal cord schistosomiasis: a pediatric case mimicking intrinsic cord neoplasm. *Neurology* 1991;41:755–757.

Paragonimiasis

Cha SH, Chang KH, Cho SY, et al. Cerebral paragonimiasis in early active stage: CT and MR features. *AJR Am J Roentgenol* 1994;162:141–145.

Im JG, Chang KH, Reeder MM. Current diagnostic imaging of pulmonary and cerebral paragonimiasis, with pathological correlation. *Semin Roentgenol* 1997;32:301–324.

Kusner DJ, King CH. Cerebral paragonimiasis. *Semin Neurol* 1993;13:201–208.

Toyonaga S, Kurisaka M, Mori K, Suzuki N. Cerebral paragonimiasis—report of five cases. *Neurol Med Chir (Tokyo)* 1992;32:157–162.

Trichinosis

Ellrodt A, Lalfon P, LeBras P, et al. Multifocal central nervous system lesions in three patients with trichinosis. *Arch Neurol* 1987;44:432–434.

Feydy E, Touze E, Miaux Y, et al. MRI in a case of neurotrichinosis. *Neuroradiology* 1996;38:S80–S82.

Fourestie V, Douceron H, Brugieres P, et al. Neurotrichinosis: a cerebrovascular disease associated with myocardial injury and hypereosinophilia. *Brain* 1993;116:603–616.

Mawhorter SD, Kazura JW. Trichinosis of the central nervous system. *Semin Neurol* 1993;13:148–152.

Merritt HH, Rosenbaum M. Involvement of the nervous system in trichinosis. *JAMA* 1936;106:1646–1649.

Eosinophilic Meningitis

Fuller AJ, Munckhof W, Kiers L, et al. Eosinophilic meningitis due to "*Angiostrongylus cantonensis*." *West J Med* 1993;159:78–80.

Koo J, Pien F, Kliks MM. *Angiostrongylus (Parastrongylus)* eosinophilic meningitis. *Rev Infect Dis* 1988;10:1155–1162.

Kuberski T, Wallace GD. Clinical manifestations of eosinophilic meningitis due to *Angiostrongylus cantonensis*. *Neurology* 1979;29:1566–1570.

Punyagupta S, Bunnag T, Juttijudata P. Eosinophilic meningitis in Thailand. Clinical and epidemiological characteristics of 162 patients with myeloencephalitis probably caused by *Gnathostoma spinigerum*. *J Neurol Sci* 1990;96:241–256.

Schmutzhard E, Boongird P, Vejjajiva A. Eosinophilic meningitis and radiculomyelitis in Thailand, caused by CNS invasion of *Gnathostoma spinigerum* and *Angiostrongylus cantonensis*. *J Neurol Neurosurg Psychiatry* 1988;51:80–87.

Weller PF. Eosinophilic meningitis. *Am J Med* 1993;95:250–253.

Toxocariasis (Visceral Larva Migrans)

Duprez TP, Bigaignon G, Delgrange E, et al. MRI of cervical cord lesions and their resolution in toxocara caris myelopathy. *Neuroradiology* 1996;38:792–795.

Gould IM, Newell S, Green SH, George RH. Toxocariasis and eosinophilic meningitis. *Br Med J* 1985;291:1239–1240.

King TD, Moncrief JA, Vingiello R. Hemiparesis and *Ascaris lumbricoides* infection. *J La State Med Soc* 1979;131:5–7.

Zachariah SB, Zachariah B, Varghese B. Neuroimaging studies of cerebral "visceral larva migrans" syndrome. *J Neuroimag* 1994;4:39–40.

Strongyloidiasis

Capello M, Hotez P. Disseminated strongyloidiasis. *Semin Neurol* 1993;13:169–174.

Masdeu JC, Tantulavanich S, Gorelick PP, et al. Brain abscess caused by *Strongyloides stercoralis*. *Arch Neurol* 1982;39:62–63.

Takayanagui OM, Lofrano MM, Araugo MB, Chimelli L. Detection of strongyloides stercoralis in the cerebrospinal fluid of a patient with acquired immunodeficiency syndrome. *Neurology* 1995;45:193–194.

Wachter RM, Burke AM, MacGregor RR. *Strongyloides stercoralis* hyperinfection masquerading as cerebral vasculitis. *Arch Neurol* 1984;41:1213–1216.

Other Helminths

Jeong SC, Bae JC, Hwang SH, Kim HC, Lee BC. Cerebral sparganosis with intracerebral hemorrhage: a case report. *Neurology* 1998;50:503–506.

Kim DG, Paek SH, Chang KH, et al. Cerebral sparganosis: clinical manifestations, treatment, and outcome. *J Neurosurg* 1996;85:1066–1071.

Pau A, Perria C, Turtas S, et al. Long-term follow-up of the surgical treatment of intracranial coenurosis. *Br J Neurosurg* 1990;4:39–43.

Protozoan Infection
Toxoplasmosis

American Academy of Neurology. Evaluation and management of intracranial mass lesions in AIDS. Report of the Quality Standards Subcommittee of the American Academy of Neurology. *Neurology* 1998;50:21–26.

Berlit P, Popescu O, Weng Y, Malessa R. Disseminated cerebral hemorrhages as unusual manifestation of toxoplasmic encephalitis in AIDS. *J Neurol Sci* 1996;141:187–189.

Dina TS. Primary central nervous system lymphoma versus toxoplasmosis in AIDS. *Radiology* 1991;179:823–828.

Gherardi R, Baudriment M, Lionnet F, et al. Skeletal muscle toxoplasmosis in patients with acquired immunodeficiency syndrome: a clinical and pathological study. *Ann Neurol* 1992;32:535–542.

Mitchell CD, Erlich SS, Mastrucci MT, et al. Congenital toxoplasmosis occurring in infants perinatally infected with human immunodeficiency virus 1. *Pediatr Infect Dis J* 1990;9:512–518.

Navia BA, Petito CK, Gold JWM, et al. Cerebral toxoplasmosis complicating the acquired immune deficiency syndrome: clinical and neuropathological findings in 27 patients. *Ann Neurol* 1986;19:224–238.

Porter SB, Sande MA. Toxoplasmosis of the central nervous system in the acquired immunodeficiency syndrome. *N Engl J Med* 1992;327:1643–1648.

Raffi F, Aboulker JP, Michelet C, et al. A prospective study of criteria for the diagnosis of toxoplasmic encephalitis in 186 AIDS patients. *AIDS* 1997;11:177–184.

Strittmatter C, Lang W, Wiestler OD, Kleihues P. The changing pattern of human immunodeficiency virus-associated cerebral toxoplasmosis: a study of 46 postmortem cases. *Acta Neuropathol* 1992;83:475–481.

Townsend JJ, Wolinsky JS, Baringer JR, Johnson PC. Acquired toxoplasmosis: a neglected cause of treatable nervous system disease. *Arch Neurol* 1975;32:335–343.

Vyas R, Ebright JR. Toxoplasmosis of the spinal cord in a patient with AIDS: case report and review. *Clin Infect Dis* 1996;23:1061–1065.

Cerebral Malaria

Bondi FS. The incidence and outcome of neurological abnormalities in childhood cerebral malaria: a long-term follow-up of 62 survivors. *Trans R Soc Trop Med Hyg* 1992;86:17–19.

Crawley J, Smith S, Kirkham F, et al. Seizures and status epilepticus in childhood cerebral malaria. *Q J Med* 1996;89:591–597.

Hoffman SL. Artemether in severe malaria: still too many deaths. *N Engl J Med* 1996;335:124–126.

Mai NTH, Day NPJ, Chueng LV, et al. Post-malaria neurologic syndrome. *Lancet* 1996;348:917–921.

Newton CRJC, Crawley J, Sowumni A, et al. Intracranial hypertension in Africans with cerebral malaria. *Arch Dis Child* 1997;76:219–226.

Newton CRJC, Warrell DA. Neurological manifestations of falciparum malaria. *Ann Neurol* 1998;43:695–702.

Schnorf H, Diserens K, Schnyder H, et al. Corticosteroid-responsive post-malaria encephalopathy characterized by motor aphasia, myoclonus, and postural tremor. *Arch Neurol* 1998;55:417–420.

van Hensbroek MB, Palmer A, Jaffar S, Schneider G, Kwiatkowski D. Residual neurologic sequelae after childhood cerebral malaria. *J Pediatr* 1997;131:125–129.

Wyler DJ. Steroids are out in the treatment of cerebral malaria: what's next? *J Infect Dis* 1988;158:320–324.

Trypanosomiasis

Gluckstein D, Ciferri F, Ruskin J. Chagas' disease: another cause of cerebral mass in the acquired immunodeficiency syndrome. *Am J Med* 1992;92:429–432.

Hunter CA, Jennings FW, Adams JH, et al. Subcurative chemotherapy and fatal post-treatment encephalopathies in African trypanosomiasis. *Lancet* 1992;339:956–958.

Metzek K, Maciel JA Jr. AIDS and Chagas' disease. *Neurology* 1993;43:447–448.

Rocha A, de Meneses AC, da Silva AM, et al. Pathology of patients with Chagas' disease and acquired immunodeficiency syndrome. *Am J Trop Med Hyg* 1994;50:261–268.

Rosemberg S, Chaves CJ, Higuchi ML, et al. Fatal meningoencephalitis caused by reactivation of *Trypanosoma cruzi* infection in a patient with AIDS. *Neurology* 1992;42:640–642.

Villanueva MS. Trypanosomiasis of the central nervous system. *Semin Neurol* 1993;13:209–218.

Primary Amebic Meningoencephalitis

Anonymous. Primary amebic meningoencephalitis—North Carolina, 1991. *MMWR Morb Mortal Wkly Rep* 1992;41:437–440.

Clavel A, Franco L, Letona S, et al. Primary amebic meningoencephalitis in a patient with AIDS: unusual protozoological findings. *Clin Infect Dis* 1996;23:1314–1315.

Darby CP, Conradi SE, Holbrook TW, Chatellier C. Primary amebic meningoencephalitis. *Am J Dis Child* 1979;133:1025–1027.

Gardner HAR, Martinez AJ, Visvesvara GS, Sotrel A. Granulomatous amebic encephalitis in an AIDS patient. *Neurology* 1991;41:1993–1995.

Gordon SM, Steinberg JP, DuPuis MH, et al. Culture isolation of *Acanthamoeba* species and leptomyxid amebas from patients with amebic meningoencephalitis, including two patients with AIDS. *Clin Infect Dis* 1992;15:1024–1030.

Grunnert ML, Cannon GH, Kushner JP. Fulminant amebic meningoencephalitis due to *Acanthamoeba*. *Neurology* 1981;31:174–177.

Martinez AJ, Visvesvara GS. Free-living, amphizoic and opportunistic amebas. *Brain Pathol* 1997;583–598.

Rothrock JF, Buchsbaum HW. Primary amebic meningoencephalitis. *JAMA* 1980;243:2329–2330.

Seidel JS, Harmatz P, Visvesvara GS, et al. Successful treatment of primary amebic meningoencephalitis. *N Engl J Med* 1982;306:346–348.

Merritt's Neurology, 10th ed., edited by L.P. Rowland. Lippincott Williams & Wilkins, Philadelphia © 2000.

BACTERIAL TOXINS

JAMES R. MILLER

The toxins elaborated by several pathogenic bacteria have a special predilection for the nervous system. The exotoxin of the diphtheria bacillus chiefly affects the peripheral nerves, tetanus affects the activity of the neurons in the central nervous system (CNS), and botulism interferes with conduction at the myoneural junction.

DIPHTHERIA

The exotoxin of *Corynebacterium diphtheriae* is a 62,000-Da polypeptide that inhibits protein synthesis in mammalian cells by inactivation of transfer RNA translocase (elongation factor 2). It is composed of two segments: one necessary for binding to the cell and a shorter portion that then is cleaved and enters the cell. The specificity of the exotoxin for heart and peripheral nerve is attributed to receptor binding affinity at the cell surface. The exotoxin is produced by a phage, and strains of the bacterium that do not contain the phage are not pathogenic. The development of neuropathy is proportional to the severity of the primary infection. In pharyngeal infections, palatal and pharyngolaryngoesophageal paralysis is an early and prominent feature. The resistance of the other cranial nerves and brain is unexplained.

The symptoms and course of diphtheritic neuritis are considered in Chapter 105.

TETANUS

Tetanus (lockjaw) causes localized or generalized spasms of muscles due to tetanospasmin, a toxin produced by the bacterium *Clostridium tetani*.

Etiology

C. tetani is commonly shed in the excreta of humans and other animals. Its spores are ubiquitous in the environment. They enter the body through puncture wounds, compound fractures, or wounds from blank cartridges and fireworks. Infection has been reported from contamination of operative wounds, burns, parenteral injections (particularly in heroin addicts), and through the umbilicus of the newborn. The mere deposition of spores of the organism is not sufficient for infection. Necrotic tissue and an associated pyogenic infection are necessary for germination of the bacteria and production of tetanospasmin.

Prevention of tetanus is accomplished by immunization with toxoid (denatured toxin). Children should be routinely immunized and boosters given every 10 years. Immediate booster immunization should be given to patients with penetrating wounds, unless a recent immunization can be documented. Immunity is not conferred by the disease, and patients should receive the toxoid and human tetanus immune globulin (HTIG), but at a different site.

Pathogenesis

Tetanospasmin is made by a single polypeptide chain of 1,315 amino acids by a large bacterial plasmid. The toxin becomes active when nicked by a serine protease into small and large chains held together by a disulfide bridge. The large chain also contains an internal disulfide bridge and appears to be necessary for penetration into the nerve cell. The small chain is responsible for toxin activity. Tetanospasmin prevents synaptic vesicles from fusing with the cell membrane and prevents the release of neurotransmitters. It appears to bind to synaptobrevin, a protein involved in the fusion process. It is active at the neuromuscular junction, autonomic terminals, and most importantly in inhibitory neurons in the CNS. The central effects usually overwhelm the peripheral effects, although autonomic dysfunction may become clinically evident. Access to the CNS is by retrograde transport in alpha motor neurons. Hematogenous spread of the toxin before neuronal transport probably accounts for generalized tetanus.

Pathology

No pathologic changes occur in the central or peripheral nervous system except those caused secondarily by anoxia or other metabolic derangement.

Incidence

The disease is found throughout the world. In the United States, it is most commonly due to infection of puncture wounds of the extremities by nails or splinters.

The incidence in developed countries has been dramatically reduced by immunization with denatured toxin (tetanus toxoid). About 100 to 200 cases probably occur in the United States each year. Worldwide, about 1 million cases occur; 50% are encountered in neonates because of nonsterile birthing technique. In the United States, the infection is most common in narcotic addicts. The narcotic is "cut" by admixing with quinine, which favors the growth of the organisms at the site of the injection.

Symptoms

The incubation period is usually between 5 and 10 days. It may be as short as 3 days or as long as 3 weeks. The severity of the disease usually is greater when the incubation period is short.

The symptoms may be localized or generalized. In the localized form, the spasms are confined to the injured limbs. This form is rare and is most commonly seen in patients who have been partially protected by prophylactic doses of antitetanic serum. When the portal of entrance is in the head (e.g., face, ear, tonsils), symptoms may be localized there (cephalic tetanus), with trismus, facial paralysis, and ophthalmoplegia.

In the generalized form, a prominent symptom is stiffness of the jaw (trismus). This is followed by stiffness of the neck, irritability, and restlessness. As the disease progresses, stiffness of the muscles becomes generalized. Rigidity of the back muscles may become so extreme that the patient assumes the position of opisthotonos. Rigidity of the facial muscles gives a characteristic facial expression, the so-called risus sardonicus. Added to the stiffness of the muscles are paroxysmal tonic spasms, which may occur spontaneously or may be precipitated by an external stimulus. Dysphagia may develop from spasm of the pharyngeal muscles; cyanosis and asphyxia may result from spasm of the glottis or respiratory muscles. Seizures may occur and are probably secondary to anoxia caused by the spasms. Temperature may be normal but more commonly is elevated to 101 to 103°F.

Laboratory Data

No specific changes are found in blood, urine, or cerebrospinal fluid (CSF).

Diagnosis

The diagnosis of tetanus is made by the characteristic signs (i.e., trismus, risus sardonicus, tonic spasms) in a patient with a wound of the skin and deeper tissues. Occasionally, however, a history of an antecedent wound is not obtained. The symptoms of strychnine poisoning differ from those of tetanus in that the muscles are relaxed between spasms and the jaw muscles are rarely involved.

Course and Prognosis

The outlook is grave in all cases of generalized tetanus. The mortality rate is over 50%. Prognosis is best when the incubation period is long. The mortality rate is reduced by the prompt administration of serum and aggressive management of pulmonary and autonomic dysfunction. In fatal cases, death usually occurs in 3 to 10 days. Death is most commonly due to respiratory compromise. In the patients who recover, there is a gradual reduction in the frequency and severity of spasms.

Treatment

The patient should be treated in an intensive care unit. The wound should be surgically cleaned. Antiserum does not neutralize toxins that have been fixed in the nervous system, but it is administered to neutralize toxin that has not yet entered the nervous system. It is customary to administer HTIG in a dose of 3000 to 6000 U intramuscularly as soon as the diagnosis is made, although as little as 500 U may be equally effective. Intrathecal HTIG has been reported to decrease mortality and probably limits transsynaptic spread of the tetanospasmin once it has gained access to the CNS. In the United States, however, HTIG contains potentially neurotoxic preservative.

Penicillin G is the most effective antibiotic for inhibiting further growth of the organisms; dirty wounds should be debrided and cleaned. Tracheostomy should be performed to ensure adequate ventilation. Diazepam is used commonly to control muscle spasms. High doses may be required, and oral dosing is preferred over intravenous administration once initial control has been achieved, because the preservative in the intravenous preparation may be toxic. Diazepam is also useful for immediate control of convulsions, but phenytoin or other suitable long-lasting anticonvulsant should be added if seizures occur. In severe cases, curarization may be necessary with use of a positive pressure respirator. Anticoagulation with heparin then should be considered because the risk of pulmonary embolism is high in curarized patients.

BOTULISM

Botulism is a poisoning by a toxin elaborated by *Clostridium botulinum*, a bacterium widely distributed in soil. Botulinum toxin impairs release of acetylcholine at all peripheral synapses, with resultant weakness of striated and smooth muscles and autonomic dysfunction.

Pathogenesis

Botulinum toxin is a 150-kDa polypeptide with structure and major sequence homologies similar to those of tetanospasmin. It is also activated by nicking of the polypeptide into a larger and smaller chain held together by a disulfide bond. After synthesis, botulinum toxin exists in a macromolecular complex with other bacteria-elaborated proteins. This complex appears necessary for pathogenicity, because the toxin alone is digested in the stomach. After absorption from the gastrointestinal tract, the toxin spreads hematogenously to peripheral presynaptic terminals where it blocks the release of acetylcholine. As with tetanus toxin, botulinum toxin appears to interfere with synaptic vesicle fusion to the presynaptic membrane. Different immune types (see below) bind to different proteins at the fusion site.

Classic botulism is caused by toxin ingested after being produced in inadequately sterilized canned or prepared food. Home-canned or -cured foods are particularly at risk, although commercial products are occasionally implicated. *C. botulinum* growth is inhibited by other common bacteria. Methods of processing that kill those bacteria, but not the resistant *Clostridium* spores, favor germination and growth of the botulinum organism. Infantile botulism, however, is caused by toxin produced by bacteria growing in the intestine.

Six immunologic types of *C. botulinum* have been identified. Human botulism usually results from toxin produced by types A, B, and E. Types A and B botulism follow the eating of tainted food; the same types have been implicated in infantile botulism. Type E is associated with fish and marine mammal products.

The toxin is thermolabile and is easily destroyed by heat. Botulism usually occurs when the preserved food is served uncooked and the rancid taste is obscured by acid dressings.

Symptoms and Signs

The symptoms of poisoning by the toxin appear 6 to 48 hours after the ingestion of contaminated food and may or may not be preceded by nausea, vomiting, or diarrhea. The initial symptom is usually difficulty in convergence of the eyes, soon followed by ptosis and paralysis of the extraocular muscles. The pupils are dilated and may not react to light. The ocular symptoms are followed by weakness of the jaw muscles, dysphagia, and dysarthria. The weakness spreads to involve muscles of the trunk and limbs. Smooth muscle of the intestines and bladder is occasionally affected, with resulting constipation and retention of urine. Mentation is usually preserved, but convulsions and coma may develop terminally. Blood and CSF are normal. In severe cases, symptoms may be those of cardiac or respiratory failure.

Infantile botulism occurs in the first year of life, with a peak incidence at 2 to 4 months of age. About 30% of infantile botulism in the United States appears to follow the ingestion of honey. A period of constipation of about 3 days is followed by the acute onset of hypotonia, weakness, dysphagia, poor sucking, and ptosis. It is estimated that 5% of cases of sudden infant death syndrome are due to botulism, although the true frequency is unknown.

Diagnosis

The diagnosis is not difficult when several members of one household are affected or if samples of the contaminated food can be obtained for testing. Bulbar palsy in acute anterior poliomyelitis can be excluded by the normal CSF. Myasthenia gravis may be simulated, especially if the pupils are not clearly affected in a sporadic case of botulism. In myasthenia gravis, there is a decremental electromyographic response to repetitive stimulation of nerve, but in botulism there is an increasing response that resembles the Lambert-Eaton syndrome.

Course

The course depends on the amount of toxin absorbed from the gut. The symptoms are mild and recovery is complete if only a small amount is absorbed. When large amounts are absorbed, death usually occurs within 4 to 8 days from circulatory failure, respiratory paralysis, or the development of pulmonary complications.

Treatment

Botulism can be prevented by taking proper precautions in the preparation of canned foods and discarding (without sampling) any canned food with a rancid odor or in which gas has formed. The toxin is destroyed by cooking. There are no established means of preventing infant botulism, although honey should not be given in the first year of life.

Patients should be given botulinum antitoxin. In the United States, trivalent (A, B, E) antitoxin is available from the Centers for Disease Control and Prevention. The stomach should be lavaged gently and the lower gastrointestinal tract thoroughly cleansed by enemas and cathartics not containing magnesium. Respiratory assistance may be required. Feedings should be by enteral tube. Some beneficial results on weakness have been reported with the use of guanidine, but the evidence is conflicting. 2,4-Diaminopyridine has also been used.

SUGGESTED READINGS

Arnon SS. Infant botulism. *Annu Rev Med* 1980;31:541–560.

Bleck TP, Brauner J. Tetanus. In: Scheld WM, Whitley RJ, Durack DT, eds. *Infections of the central nervous system*, 2nd ed. Philadelphia: Lippincott-Raven, 1997:629–653.

Cherington M. Clinical spectrum of botulism. *Muscle Nerve* 1998;21:701–710.

Gupta PA, Kapoor R, Goyal S, et al. Intrathecal human immune tetanus immunoglobulin in early tetanus. *Lancet* 1980;2:439–440.

Hughes JM, Hatheway C, Ostroff S. Botulism. In: Scheld WM, Whitley RJ, Durack DT, eds. *Infections of the central nervous system*, 2nd ed. Philadelphia: Lippincott-Raven, 1997:615–628.

Kefer MP. Tetanus. *Am J Emerg Med* 1992;10:445–448.

La Force FM, Young LS, Bennett JV. Tetanus in the United States (1965–1966). Epidemiological and clinical features. *N Engl J Med* 1969;280:569–574.

Lund BM. Foodborne disease due to *Bacillus* and *Clostridium* species. *Lancet* 1990;336:982–986.

Schmidt RD, Schmidt TW. Infant botulism: a case series and review of the literature. *J Emerg Med* 1992;10:713–718.

Shapiro RL, Hatheway C, Swerdlow DL. Botulism in the United States: a clinical and epidemiologic review. *Ann Intern Med* 1998;129:221–228.

Sun KO, Chan YW, Cheung RT, So PC, Yu YL, Li PC. Management of tetanus: a review of 18 cases [see comments]. *J R Soc Med* 1994;87:135–137.

Weber JT, Goodpasture HC, Alexander H, et al. Wound botulism in a patient with a tooth abscess: case report and review. *Clin Infect Dis* 1993;16:635–639.

Merritt's Neurology, 10th ed., edited by L.P. Rowland. Lippincott Williams & Wilkins, Philadelphia © 2000.

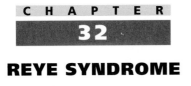

REYE SYNDROME

DARRYL C. DE VIVO

In 1963, Reye et al. reported clinical and pathologic observations in 21 children with encephalopathy and fatty changes in the viscera. Since then, the number of reported cases has increased all over the world with unexplained fluctuations in incidence from decade to decade. The disorder also affects infants and adults, although rarely. White children in suburban or rural environments seem to be more susceptible than urban black children.

Reye syndrome is usually associated with influenza B epidemics or sporadic cases of influenza A and varicella. Characteristically, the encephalopathy develops 4 to 7 days after the onset of the viral illness. It is invariably heralded by recurrent vomiting and often followed by somnolence, confusion, delirium, or coma. These children have frequently been treated with antiemetics, aspirin, or acetaminophen. Epidemiologic studies have shown a statistical association between the ingestion of aspirin-containing compounds and the development of Reye syndrome. These studies, however, do not prove a causal relationship.

Pathologic and metabolic observations suggest a primary injury to mitochondria throughout the body with prominent involvement of the liver and brain. The primary injury may be compounded by many associated insults, including hyperpyrexia, hypoglycemia, hypoxia, hyperammonemia, free fatty acidemia, systemic hypotension, and intracranial hypertension. An appropriate clinical history, characteristic neurologic findings, absence of any other explanation for the encephalopathy, and distinctive laboratory abnormalities are usually sufficient for establishing the diagnosis. Important laboratory abnormalities include elevations of blood ammonia, lactate, and serum transaminases and prolongation of the prothrombin time. Cerebrospinal fluid examination and computed tomography are normal. The electroencephalogram is diffusely abnormal, occasionally displaying paroxysmal epileptiform activity in the more severely ill patients.

Many other conditions can present a similar clinical picture. The differential diagnosis includes bacterial meningitis, viral encephalitis, drug intoxication (e.g., aspirin, valproic acid, and amphetamines), and other metabolic disorders (e.g., inherited defects of fatty acid oxidation, branched-chain amino acid metabolism, and the Krebs-Henseleit urea cycle). Recurrent attacks of a Reye-like syndrome imply an underlying metabolic disorder. The current mainstay of treatment is intensive supportive care. Most patients recover completely within a week after onset.

SUGGESTED READINGS

Arcinue EL, Mitchell RA, Sarnaik AP, et al. The metabolic course of Reye's syndrome: distinction between survivors and nonsurvivors. *Neurology* 1986;36:435–438.

Belay ED, Birsee JS, Holman RC, Khan AS, Shahariari A, Schonberger LB. Reye's syndrome in the United States from 1981 through 1997. *N Engl J Med* 1999;340:1377–1382.

Brown RE, Forman DT: The biochemistry of Reye's syndrome. *CRC Crit Rev Clin Lab Sci* 1982;17:247–297.

Consensus Conference. Diagnosis and treatment of Reye's syndrome. *JAMA* 1981;246:2441–2444.

Corey L, Rubin RJ, Hattwick MAW, et al. A nationwide outbreak of Reye's syndrome. Its epidemiologic relationship of influenza B. *Am J Med* 1976;61:615–625.

Corkey BE, Hale DE, Glennon MC, et al. Relationship between unusual hepatic acyl coenzyme A profiles and the pathogenesis of Reye syndrome. *J Clin Invest* 1988;82:782–788.

DeVivo DC. How common is Reye's syndrome? *N Engl J Med* 1983;309:179–180.

DeVivo DC, Keating JP. Reye's syndrome. *Adv Pediatr* 1976;22:175–229.

Haymond MW, Karl I, Keating JP, DeVivo DC. Metabolic response to hypertonic glucose administration in Reye syndrome. *Ann Neurol* 1978;3: 207–215.

Heubi JE, Daughterty CC, Partin JS, et al. Grade I Reye's syndrome outcome and predictors of progression to deeper coma grades. *N Engl J Med* 1984;311:1539–1542.

Hou JW, Chou SP, Wang TR. Metabolic function and liver histopathology in Reye-like illnesses. *Acta Paediatr* 1996;85:1053–1057.

Hurwitz ES, Barrett MJ, Bregman D, et al. Public health service study on Reye's syndrome and medications: report of the pilot phase. *N Engl J Med* 1985;313:849–857.

Hurwitz ES, Barrett MJ, Bregman D, et al. Public Health Service study of Reye's syndrome and medications. *JAMA* 1987;257:1905–1911.

Huttenlocher PR, Trauner DA. Reye's syndrome in infancy. *Pediatrics* 1978;62:84–90.

Lyon G, Dodge PR, Adams RD. The acute encephalopathies of obscure origin in infants and children. *Brain* 1961;84:680–708.

Monto AS. The disappearance of Reye's syndrome—a public health triumph. *N Engl J Med* 1999;340:1423–1424.

Partin JS, McAdams AJ, Partin JC, et al. Brain ultrastructure in Reye's disease. II. Acute injury and recovery process in three children. *J Neuropathol Exp Neurol* 1978;37:796–819.

Partin JC, Schubert WK, Partin JS. Mitochondrial ultrastructure in Reye's syndrome (encephalopathy and fatty degeneration of the viscera). *N Engl J Med* 1971;285:1339–1343.

Pranzatelli MR, DeVivo DC. The pharmacology of Reye syndrome. *Clin Neuropharmacol* 1987;10:96–125.

Reye BDK, Morgan G, Baral J. Encephalopathy and fatty degeneration of the viscera: a disease entity in childhood. *Lancet* 1963;2:749–752.

Shaywitz SE, Cohen PM, Cohen DJ, et al. Long-term consequences of Reye's syndrome: a sibling-matched, controlled study of neurologic, cognitive, academic, and psychiatric function. *J Pediatr* 1982;100: 41–46.

Stanley CA. New genetic defects in mitochondrial fatty acid oxidation and carnitine deficiency. *Adv Pediatr* 1987;34:59–88.

Stumpf DA. Reye syndrome: an international perspective. *Brain Dev* 1995;17[Suppl]:77–78.

Sullivan-Bolyai JZ, Corey L. Epidemiology of Reye's syndrome. *Epidemiol Rev* 1981;3:1–26.

Trauner DA, Stockard JJ, Sweetman L. EEG correlations with biochemical abnormalities in Reye syndrome. *Arch Neurol* 1977;34:116–118.

Van Coster RN, De Vivo DC, Blake D, et al. Adult Reye's syndrome: a review with new evidence for a generalized defect in intramitochondrial enzyme processing. *Neurology* 1991;41:1815–1821.

You KS. Salicylate and mitochondrial injury in Reye's syndrome. *Science* 1983;221:163–165.

Merritt's Neurology, 10th ed., edited by L.P. Rowland. Lippincott Williams & Wilkins, Philadelphia © 2000.

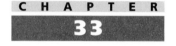

CHAPTER 33

PRION DISEASES

BURK JUBELT

In previous editions of this textbook, the section on viral diseases included a discussion of "unconventional viruses" that cause scrapie, a disease of sheep, and several human diseases: kuru, Creutzfeldt-Jakob disease (CJD), Gerstmann-Straussler syndrome (GSS), and fatal familial insomnia (FFI). All these conditions are rare, but among them, CJD is the most common (Table 33.1). All have characteristic pathologic changes that led to the early designation of *spongiform encephalopathy*. These diseases are now called *prion diseases*. The name has been changed to comply with changing concepts of the agent, which, like a virus, is transmissible. It differs from any known virus, however, because the molecule does not include any detectable nucleic acid. It is resistant to heat, ultraviolet light, and ionizing radiation, which modify nucleic acids. However, the infectivity of the agent is susceptible to treatments that denature proteins (sodium dodecyl sulfate, phenol). The neologism was taken from the two key features of the agent, protein and infectious. Because these agents appear to differ from viruses and because there now is some understanding of the pathogenesis of these diseases, a separate chapter on the prion diseases is appropriate.

The human prion protein is encoded by a gene currently designated *PRNP* on the short arm of chromosome 20. The prion protein (PrP) is found in two isoforms. One is the normal cellular form (PrP^C). The other form differs only in physical characteristics and is found in scrapie (PrP^{Sc}) and other animal prion diseases and in the human prion diseases. PrP^C is an intracellular membrane bound protein. Its normal biological function is unknown. PrP^{Sc} is found not only intracellular but also extracellular in amyloid filaments and amyloid plaques. Delineation of the nature of this new agent gained a Nobel Prize for Stanley Prusiner.

The animal prion diseases include scrapie of sheep, transmissible mink encephalopathy, chronic wasting disease of elk and mule deer, and bovine spongiform encephalopathy (BSE). Scrapie was recognized in ancient times and was considered transmissible or infectious in the 1930s. Scrapie occurs primarily in Europe but has occurred in the United States. In the last decade the prion diseases have become a public health problem because of the epidemic of BSE ("mad cow" disease) in Great Britain. BSE occurred because cattle were fed scrapie-contaminated meat-and-

TABLE 33.1. RELATIVE FREQUENCY OF HUMAN PRION DISEASE: TISSUES REFERRED FOR TRANSMISSION TO PRIMATES

Syndrome	Number of Patients
Creutzfeldt-Jakob disease	278
Sporadic	234
Familial	36
Iatrogenic	8
Kuru	18
Gerstmann-Straussler-Scheinker syndrome	2

Modified from Brown P, Gibbs CJ Jr, Rodgers-Johnson P, et al. Human spongiform encephalopathy: the NIH series of 300 cases of experimentally transmitted disease. *Ann Neurol* 1994;35:513–529.

bone meal. This same mechanism has caused a disease in domestic cats (feline spongiform encephalopathy) and felines in zoos. In addition, atypical CJD ("new variant" CJD) has affected young adults in Great Britain and France infected with the BSE agent.

The human diseases can be sporadic, infectious, or genetic; 80% to 90% of CJD cases are sporadic. Iatrogenic CJD and familial CJD (autosomal dominant) each account for 5% to 10% of CJD cases. GSS and FFI are also genetic and rare (Table 33.1). Sporadic CJD is not spread like an ordinary infection because the agent has low infectivity. Those with prior head and neck trauma and medical personnel may be at higher risk because of increased exposure to the agent. CJD has been transmitted by implanting electrodes or transplanting corneas from affected patients. Iatrogenic disease has also occurred with dura mater grafts and administration of growth hormone extract prepared from pooled human pituitary glands. Gajdusek and colleagues found that all these diseases can be transmitted to chimpanzees or guinea pigs (Brown et al., 1994; see Table 33.1). In that sense the diseases are infectious. Mutations in the *PrP* gene cause the inherited diseases, which are therefore both heritable and transmissible.

There is now debate about nomenclature, whether we should continue to refer to the diseases by the original clinicopathologic designations or whether they should all be lumped as "prion disease" and identified by the specific mutation identified. The latter group points to people in the same family who have different clinical syndromes. They have also identified PrP mutations in atypical syndromes, such as dementia resembling Alzheimer disease, or spastic paraplegia.

The former group, on the other hand, points to a strong tendency for specific mutations to be associated with specific clinical syndromes (Table 33.2) and to differences in transmissibility of the different clinical syndromes. For instance, Brown and colleagues (1994) found that all iatrogenic cases were transmitted to chimpanzees, as were 90% of sporadic CJD but only 68% of the familial cases; 95% of the cases of kuru were transmitted, but only two of four cases of GSS were transmitted. Additional

molecular techniques may be useful for categorizing the prion diseases. Proteinase K digestion of CJD brain homogenates followed by Western blot analysis has demonstrated the presence of protease-resistant prion proteins (PrP^{res}) of different patterns (based on the size and ratio of differently glycosylated isoforms). Thus far, four distinct patterns have been recognized: types 1 and 2 primarily in sporadic CJD; type 3, iatrogenic CJD; type 4, new variant. The prion proteins of the other prion diseases have not as yet been adequately analyzed by this technique.

KURU

This progressive and fatal disorder occurs exclusively among natives (Fore people) of the New Guinea Highlands. It is manifested by incoordination of gait, severe trunk and limb ataxia, abnormal involuntary movements resembling myoclonus or chorea, convergent strabismus, and, later in the disease, dementia. The illness terminates fatally in 4 to 24 months. Cannibalism is considered the principal mode of transmission, affecting children, adolescents, and adult women. Since this practice was eliminated in the 1950s, the disease now is rare and affects only older adults of both sexes. Neuropathologic changes include widespread neuronal loss, neuronal and astrocytic vacuolization, and astrocytic proliferation. Amyloid plaques containing the abnormal prion protein (PrP) were first described in kuru, and called kuru plaques. These pathologic changes are most prominent in the cerebellum, where gross atrophy may be seen. The cerebrum and brainstem are involved to a lesser degree.

The similarity between the clinical and neuropathologic manifestations of kuru and those seen in scrapie-afflicted sheep led Gajdusek and Gibbs to infect higher primates with brain suspensions. Inoculation of chimpanzees was followed by the appearance of a kurulike disease 14 months to several years later. Kuru was the first human-transmissible spongiform encephalopathy (prion disease) to be recognized. Gajdusek was awarded a Nobel Prize for this work.

CREUTZFELDT-JAKOB DISEASE

In 1920 and 1921, Creutzfeldt and Jakob described a progressive disease of the cortex, basal ganglia, and spinal cord that developed in middle-aged and elderly adults. CJD (spastic pseudosclerosis, corticostriatospinal degeneration) was the second human prion disease to be recognized. CJD occurs throughout the world but is relatively rare, with an incidence of about 1 case per 1 million people annually. This incidence is the same throughout the world except for the high incidence among Libyan Jews in Israel and in a few populations elsewhere. The disease affects mainly middle-aged and older individuals, with an average age at onset of about 60 years.

Pathology

The pathologic condition is essentially degenerative with grossly evident cerebral atrophy. Microscopic findings are similar to

TABLE 33.2. MUTATIONS IN THE PRION PROTEIN GENE ASSOCIATED WITH FAMILIAL PRION DISEASES[a]

Codon No.	Normal Amino Acids (s)	Mutant Amino Acid (s)	Familial Prion Disease
51–91	5 octarepeats	Additional 2–9 octarepeats	CJD
178	Asp	Asn	CJD
180	Val	Ile	CJD
200	Glu	Lys	CJD
210	Val	Ile	CJD
232	Met	Arg	CJD
102	Pro	Leu	GSS
105	Pro	Leu	GSS
117	Ala	Val	GSS
145	Tyr	Stop	GSS
198	Phe	Ser	GSS
217	Glu	Arg	GSS
129	Val or Met	Val	178^{Asn} CJD
		Met	178^{Asn} FFI

[a]Other mutations have been described but only in single cases. CJD; Creutzfeldt-Jakob disease; GSS; Gerstmann-Straussler-Scheinker syndrome.

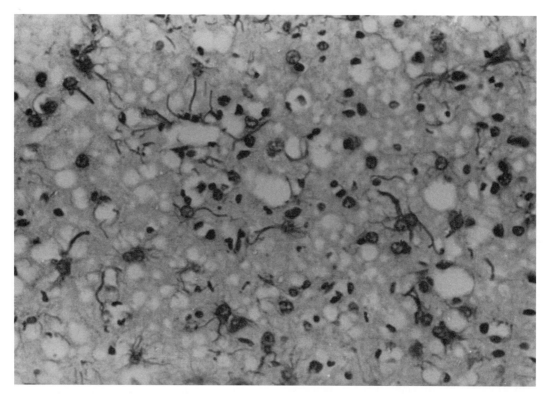

FIG. 33.1. Creutzfeldt-Jakob disease. Section from cortex showing status spongiosis of the neuropil, loss of neurons, and prominent astrocytosis. Phosphotungstic acid hematoxylin stain, ×120. (Courtesy of Dr. Mauro C. Dal Canto.)

other prion diseases with neuronal loss, astrocytosis, and the development of cytoplasmic vacuoles in neurons and astrocytes (status spongiosis, Fig. 33.1). Amyloid plaques that contain the abnormal PrP are found in the areas of infected tissue in most cases. There is no inflammation. The cortex and basal ganglia are most affected, but all parts of the neuraxis may be involved. Early lesions are more severe in the gray matter.

Symptoms and Signs

The clinical features include the gradual onset of dementia in middle or late life, but occasionally in young adults. Vague prodromal symptoms of anxiety, fatigue, dizziness, headache, impaired judgment, and unusual behavior may occur. Once memory loss starts, it progresses rapidly, and other characteristic signs appear, sometimes abruptly. The most frequent signs, aside from dementia, are those of pyramidal tract disease (weakness and stiffness of the limbs with accompanying reflex changes), extrapyramidal signs (tremors, rigidity, dysarthria, and slowness of movements), and myoclonus, which is often stimulus sensitive. Other signs include amyotrophy, cortical blindness, seizures, and those of cerebellar dysfunction (Table 33.3). None of the usual signs of an infection is seen.

Laboratory Data

Routine blood counts and chemistries are normal. Routine cerebrospinal fluid (CSF) tests are usually normal, although the pro-

TABLE 33.3. 232 EXPERIMENTALLY TRANSMITTED CASES OF SPORADIC CREUTZFELDT-JAKOB DISEASE

	Percentage of Patients	
	At Onset	**Later**
Mental deterioration	69	100
Memory loss	48	100
Behavioral change	29	57
Aphasia, agnosia	16	73
Cerebellar signs	33	71
Visual, oculomotor signs	19	42
Headache	11	18
Sensory change	6	11
Involuntary movements	4	91
Myoclonus	1	78
Tremor, other	3	36
Pyramidal signs	2	62
Extrapyramidal signs	0.5	56
Lower motor neuron signs	0.5	12
Seizures	0	19
Pseudobulbar signs	0.5	7
Periodic electroencephalogram	0	60

Modified from Brown P, Gibbs CJ Jr, Rodgers-Johnson P, et al. Human spongiform encephalopathy: the NIH series of 300 cases of experimentally transmitted disease. *Ann Neurol* 1994;35:513–529.

tein content may rarely be elevated. In 1986, Harrington et al. described two abnormal proteins in the CSF of CJD patients on two-dimensional gel electrophoresis. These proteins were also found in acute herpes simplex encephalitis. This assay did not become generally used because of its difficulty. Ten years later, studies from the same laboratory reported the sequence of these two proteins, which matched that of brain proteins known as 14-3-3 neuronal proteins that may play a role in conformational stabilization of other proteins. An immunoassay for the 14-3-3 protein was positive in 96% of CJD CSF samples. The assay was also positive in other diseases with acute massive neuronal dysfunction, especially herpes simplex encephalitis and acute infarction. Still, in the appropriate clinical setting, the immunoassay for the 14-3-3 protein is a highly supportive diagnostic test. The electroencephalogram (EEG) may also be of diagnostic value because periodic complexes of spike or slow wave activity at intervals of 0.5 to 2.0 seconds are characteristic in the middle and late stages of the disease (Fig. 33.2). Computed tomography and magnetic resonance imaging may reveal cerebral atrophy late in the course of the disease. In a few cases, increased signal intensity on T2-weighted magnetic resonance imaging has been seen in the cortex and basal ganglia.

Diagnosis and Differential Diagnosis

A definitive diagnosis of CJD can only be made by neuropathologic, immunologic, or biochemical examination of the brain. In typical cases (dementia, myoclonus, periodic EEG), the diagnosis can be made clinically. However, the diagnosis is difficult to make in atypical cases (no myoclonus, absence of periodic EEG).

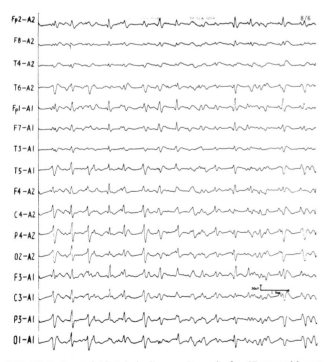

FIG. 33.2. Creutzfeldt-Jakob disease. Record of a 65-year-old man shows spikes of sharp waves at intervals of 0.7 seconds throughout the recording. Such periodicity with 0.5- to 2.0-second intervals occurs in the middle and late stages and may be absent in the early stages of the disease.

In the atypical cases, the diagnosis of Alzheimer disease is often made. Other degenerative diseases, such as Pick disease, corticobasal ganglionic degeneration, familial myoclonic dementia, and multisystem atrophy, and lithium toxicity may also be considered. The CSF test for the 14-3-3 protein may clarify the atypical cases. If not, brain biopsy is needed for evaluation of pathology or demonstration of protease-resistant PrP.

Course and Prognosis

The disease is fatal within 1 year in 90% of patients. Rarely, the course may be prolonged over several years. There is no specific treatment.

Transmissibility and Biohazard Potential

As with kuru, neurologic illness can be produced in primates by the inoculation of brain suspensions prepared from the brains of Creutzfeldt-Jakob patients. The mode of transmission of sporadic CJD is unknown. The agent has been detected in most internal organs (lung, liver, kidney, spleen, and lymph nodes), cornea, and blood but has not been detected in saliva or feces. One isolation from urine may have been a contaminate. These findings suggest a lack of significant spread by respiratory, enteric, or sexual contact. Failure to find an increased incidence in spouses also suggests that these usual modes of transmission of infections are not of major importance. Isolation of Creutzfeldt-Jakob patients does not seem necessary except for body fluids, as in the precautions taken with serum hepatitis. Human-to-human transmission has been reported after corneal transplantation, use of inadequately sterilized stereotactic brain electrodes, parenteral administration of human growth hormone preparations, and the use of human dura mater grafts. Caution must be exercised in operating rooms and pathology laboratories and in the preparation of brain-derived biologicals. Medical personnel should avoid contact of open sores or conjunctiva with these tissues. Caution should be taken to avoid accidental percutaneous exposure to CSF, blood, or tissue. Because the prion agents are highly resistant to ordinary physical or chemical treatment (routine autoclaving or formalin), special autoclaving procedures or special inactivating agents, including sodium hypochlorite (household bleach), are required.

New Variant Creutzfeldt-Jakob Disease

In 1996, 10 cases of "new variant" CJD were reported in Great Britain. These cases were unusual both clinically and pathologically in that they shared many characteristics normally associated with kuru. Symptoms started before age 40; several cases occurred in teenagers. Clinical findings included ataxia and behavioral changes. Myoclonic jerks and the characteristic EEG abnormalities were not seen. The course was slower than conventional CJD, lasting up to 22 months. At least 22 cases have now been reported. The pathologic changes were also unusual with minimal spongiosis but prominent plaque formation in the cerebellum and cerebrum. Transmission experiments of both BSE and new variant CJD brain tissue to animals confirmed the similar strain characteristics. Molecular analysis (proteinase K digestion) of brain homogenates from these new variant CJD cases revealed a Western blot pattern similar to that of BSE rather than that of sporadic CJD.

GERSTMANN-STRÄUSSLER-SCHEINKER DISEASE

GSS disease is the third human disease caused by a prion agent. It has also been referred to as the Gerstmann-Sträussler syndrome. GSS is an autosomal dominant familial disease (Table 33.2). It has a lengthy course with a range of 2 to 10 years. Clinically, it begins with ataxia; dementia eventually supervenes. Brainstem involvement leads to symptoms suggesting olivopontocerebellar degeneration. Less common is the "telencephalic" form with dementia, parkinsonism, and pyramidal tract signs and a variant form with neurofibrillary tangles. Pathologically there is usually spongiform change and prominent amyloid plaque deposition in the cerebellum, cerebrum, and basal ganglia. There is also degeneration of the spinocerebellar and corticospinal tracts. The EEG usually does not show periodicity, only diffuse slowing. As with CJD, there is no treatment.

FATAL FAMILIAL INSOMNIA

FFI is an autosomal dominant disease with a course of 7 to 36 months and an age at onset between 18 to 61 years. Familial thalamic dementia or degeneration appears to be the same disease. The patients have progressive insomnia and dysautonomia (hyperhidrosis, tachycardia, tachypnea, hyperthermia, hypertension) and may develop pyramidal and cerebellar signs, dementia, and myoclonus. However, there may be diverse phenotypic expression of the disease, even in the same family. Some patients do not develop insomnia until later stages. Other patients may present with clinical features of CJD. The EEG usually shows diffuse slowing; periodicity has been described only rarely. These patients have a mutation of the *PrP* gene at codon 178, coupled with a methionine at codon 129 (Table 33.2). Patients who are homozygous for methionine at codon 129 have a much more rapid course than those who are heterozygous. Pathologically, there is prominent neuronal loss and gliosis in the thalamus with little to no spongiform change. Patients with long duration or atypical presentations are more likely to have widespread lesions in cerebral cortex, basal ganglia, brainstem, and cerebellum. Because the clinical manifestations of FFI vary, genotyping is crucial for confirming the diagnosis. There is no specific treatment at this time.

SUGGESTED READINGS

General

Brown P, Gibbs CJ Jr, Rodgers-Johnson P, et al. Human spongiform encephalopathy: the NIH series of 300 cases of experimentally transmitted disease. *Ann Neurol* 1994;35:513–529.

Brown P, Kenney K, Little B, et al. Intracerebral distribution of infectious amyloid protein in spongiform encephalopathy. *Ann Neurol* 1995;38:245–253.

Haywood AM. Transmissible spongiform encephalopathies. *N Engl J Med* 1997;337:1821–1828.

Nitrini R, Rosemberg S, Passos-Bueno MR, et al. Familial spongiform encephalopathy associated with a novel prion protein gene mutation. *Ann Neurol* 1997;42:138–146.

Prusiner SM, Scott MR. Genetics of prions. *Annu Rev Genet* 1997;31:139–175.

Prusiner SM, Scott MR, DeArmond SJ, Cohen FE. Prion protein biology. *Cell* 1998;93:337–348.

Telling GC, Parchi P, DeArmond SJ, et al. Evidence for the conformation of the pathologic isoform of the prion protein enciphering and propagating prion diversity. *Science* 1996;274:2079–2082.

Kuru

Gajdusek DC. Unconventional viruses and the origin and disappearance of kuru. *Science* 1977;197:943–960.

Gajdusek DC, Gibbs CJ Jr, Alpers M. Experimental transmission of a kuru-like syndrome to chimpanzees. Nature 1966;209:794–796.

Hainfellner JA, Liberski PP, Guiroy DC, et al. Pathology and immunocytochemistry of a kuru brain. *Brain Pathol* 1997;7:547–553.

Hornabrook RW. Kuru—a subacute cerebellar degeneration: the natural history and clinical features. *Brain* 1968;91:53–74.

Liberski PP, Gajdusek DC. Kuru: forty years later, a historical note. *Brain Pathol* 1997;7:555–560.

Prusiner SB, Gajdusek DC, Alpers MP. Kuru with incubation periods exceeding two decades. *Ann Neurol* 1982;12:1–9.

Creutzfeldt-Jakob Disease

General

Johnson RT, Gibbs CJ Jr. Creutzfeldt-Jakob disease and related transmissible spongiform encephalopathies. *N Engl J Med* 1998;339:1994–2004.

Clinical and Epidemiologic

Berger JR, David NJ. Creutzfeldt-Jakob disease in a physician: a review of the disorder in health care workers. *Neurology* 1993;43:205–206.

Billette de Villemeur T, Deslys JP, Pradel A, et al. Creutzfeldt-Jakob disease from contaminated growth hormone extracts in France. *Neurology* 1996;47:690–695.

Brown P, Cervenáková L, Goldfarb LG, et al. Iatrogenic Creutzfeldt-Jakob disease: an example of the interplay between ancient genes and modern medicine. *Neurology* 1994;44:291–293.

Brown P, Gibbs CJ Jr, Rodgers-Johnson P, et al. Human spongiform encephalopathy: the NIH series of 300 cases of experimentally transmitted disease. *Ann Neurol* 1994;35:513–529.

Cousens SN, Zeidler M, Esmonde TF, et al. Sporadic Creutzfeldt-Jakob disease in the United Kingdom: analysis of epidemiological surveillance data for 1970–96. *BMJ* 1997;315:389–395.

Will RG, Alperovitch A, Poser S, et al. Descriptive epidemiology of Creutzfeldt-Jakob disease in six European countries, 1993–1995. *Ann Neurol* 1998;43:763–767.

Laboratory Diagnosis

Hsich G, Kenney K, Gibbs CJ, Lee KH, Harrington MG. The 14-3-3 brain protein in cerebrospinal fluid as a marker for transmissible spongiform encephalopathies. *N Engl J Med* 1996;335:924–930.

Kretzschmar HA, Ironside JM, DeArmond SJ, Tateishi J. Diagnostic criteria for sporadic Creutzfeldt-Jakob disease. *Arch Neurol* 1996;53:913–920.

Milton WJ, Atlas SW, Laui E, Mollman JE. Magnetic resonance imaging of Creutzfeldt-Jakob disease. *Ann Neurol* 1991;29:438–440.

Steinhoff BJ, Räcker S, Herrendorf G, et al. Accuracy and reliability of periodic sharp wave complexes in Creutzfeldt-Jakob disease. *Arch Neurol* 1996;53:162–166.

Zerr I, Bodemer M, Gefeller O, et al. Detection of 14-3-3 protein in the cerebrospinal fluid supports the diagnosis of Creutzfeldt-Jakob disease. *Ann Neurol* 1998;43:32–40.

Familial CJD and Genetics

Campbell TA, Palmer MS, Will RG, Gibb WR, Luthert PJ, Collinge J. A prion disease with a novel 96base pair insertional mutation in the prion protein gene. *Neurology* 1996;46:761–766.

Chapman J, Arlazoroff A, Goldfarb LG, et al. Fatal insomnia in a case of familial Creutzfeldt-Jakob disease with the codon 200 (Lys) mutation. *Neurology* 1996;46:758–761.

Cochran EJ, Bennett DA, Cervenakova L, et al. Familial Creutzfeldt-Jakob disease with a five-repeat octapeptide insert mutation. *Neurology* 1996;47:727–733.

Prusiher SM, Scott MR. Genetics of prions. *Annu Rev Genet* 1997;31:139–175.

Molecular Basis, Phenotype, and Pathogenesis

Capellari S, Vital C, Parchi P, et al. Familial prion disease with a novel 144bp insertion in the prion protein gene in a Basque family. *Neurology* 1997;49:133–141.

Parchi P, Castellani R, Capellari S, et al. Molecular basis of phenotypic variability in sporadic Creutzfeldt-Jakob disease. *Ann Neurol* 1996;39:767–778.

Rosenmann H, Halimi M, Kahana I, Biran I, Gabizon R. Differential allelic expression of PrP mRNA in carriers of the E200K mutation. *Neurology* 1997;49:851–856.

New Variant CJD

Bruce ME, Will RG, Ironside JW, et al. Transmissions to mice indicate that 'new variant' CJD is caused by the BSE agent. *Nature* 1997;389:498–501.

Collinge J, Sidle KCL, Meads J, Ironside J, Hill AF. Molecular analysis of prion strain variation and the aetiology of 'new variant' CJD. *Nature* 1996;383:685–690.

Epstein LG, Brown P. Bovine spongiform encephalopathy and a new variant of Creutzfeldt-Jakob disease. *Neurology* 1997;48:569–571.

Hill AF, Desbruslais M, Joiner S, et al. The same prion strain causes vCJD and BSE. *Nature* 1997;389:448–450.

Prusiner SB. Prion diseases and the BSE crisis. *Science* 1997;278:245–251.

Will RG, Ironside JW, Zeidler M, et al. A new variant of Creutzfeldt-Jakob disease in the UK. *Lancet* 1996;347:921–925.

Zeidler M, Stewart GE, Barraclovah CR, et al. New variant Creutzfeldt-Jakob disease: neurological features and diagnostic tests. *Lancet* 1997;350:903–907.

Transmissibility and Tissue Handling

Budka H, Aguzzi A, Brown P, et al. Tissue handling in suspected Creutzfeldt-Jakob disease (CJD) and other human spongiform encephalopathies (prion diseases). *Brain Pathol* 1995;5:319–322.

Brown P. BSE: the final resting place. *Lancet* 1998;351:1146–1147.

Committee on Health Care Issues, American Neurological Association. Precautions in handling tissues, fluids, and other contaminated materials from patients with documented or suspected Creutzfeldt-Jakob disease. *Ann Neurol* 1986;19:75–77.

Manuelidis L. Decontamination of Creutzfeldt-Jakob disease and other transmissible agents. *J Neuro Virol* 1997;3:62–65.

Gerstmann-Sträussler-Scheinker Disease

Barbanti P, Fabbrini G, Salvatore M, et al. Polymorphism at codon 129 or codon 219 of PRNP and clinical heterogeneity in a previously unreported family with Gerstmann-Sträussler-Scheinker disease (PrP-P102L mutation). *Neurology* 1996;47:734–741.

Farlow MR, Yee RD, Dlovhy SR, et al. Gerstmann-Sträussler-Scheinker disease. I. Extending the clinical spectrum. *Neurology* 1989;39:1446–1452.

Masters CL, Gajdusek DC, Gibbs CJ Jr. Creutzfeldt-Jakob disease virus isolations from the Gerstmann-Sträussler syndrome with an analysis of the various forms of amyloid plaque deposition in the virus-induced spongiform encephalopathies. *Brain* 1981;104:559–588.

Mastrianni JA, Curtis MT, Oberholtzer JC, et al. Prion disease (PrP-A117V) presenting with ataxia instead of dementia. *Neurology* 1995;45:2042–2050.

Parchi P, Chen SG, Brown P, et al. Different patterns of truncated prion protein fragments correlate with distance phenotypes in P102L Gerstmann-Straussler-Scheinker disease. *Proc Natl Acad Sci USA* 1998;95:8322–8327.

Fatal Familial Insomnia

Johnson MD, Vnencak-Jones CL, McLean MJ. Fatal familial insomnia: clinical and pathologic heterogeneity in genetic half brothers. *Neurology* 1998;51:1715–1717.

Manetto V, Medori R, Cortelli P, et al. Fatal familial insomnia: clinical and pathologic study of five new cases. *Neurology* 1992;42:312–319.

McLean CA, Storey E, Gardner RJ, Tannenberg AE, Cervenakova L, Brown P. The D178N (cis-129M) "fatal familial insomnia" mutation associated with diverse clinicopathologic phenotypes in an Australian kindred. *Neurology* 1997;49:552–558.

Padovani A, D'Alessandro M, Parchi P, et al. Fatal familial insomnia in a new Italian kindred. *Neurology* 1998;51:1491–1494.

Parchi P, Castellani R, Cortelli P, et al. Regional distribution of protease-resistant prion protein in fatal familial insomnia. *Ann Neurol* 1995;38:21–29.

Rossi G, Macchi G, Porro M, et al. Fatal familial insomnia: genetic, neuropathologic, and biochemical study of a patient from a new Italian kindred. *Neurology* 1998;50:688–692.

Zerr I, Giese A, Windl O, et al. Phenotypic variability in fatal familial insomnia (D178-129M) genotype. *Neurology* 1998;51:1398–1405.

Merritt's Neurology, 10th ed., edited by L.P. Rowland. Lippincott Williams & Wilkins, Philadelphia © 2000.

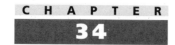

WHIPPLE DISEASE

ELAN D. LOUIS

Whipple disease was originally described as a gastrointestinal disorder with arthralgia. It is caused by a bacilliform bacterium, and infection is evident in many organs, including but not limited to the intestinal tract, heart, lungs, liver, kidneys, and brain. Polymerase chain reaction (PCR) analysis of DNA coding for bacterial ribosomal RNA has led to characterization of the Whipple organism. The organism, *Tropheryma whippelii*, belongs to the Actinomycetaceae family of bacteria. The organism, difficult to culture, has been propagated in cell culture in macrophages that had been deactivated by interleukin-4. Whipple disease has not been reproduced in animals.

The bacillus is rod shaped, 0.2 μm wide by 1.0 to 2.0 μm long, and large enough to be seen under light microscopy. The three-layered cell wall may stain either gram-positive or -negative but more often gram-positive. Bacilli appear both extracellularly and intracellularly in many cell types. The organism produces a cellular rather than a humoral immune response, and this is predominated by macrophage recruitment. Infected macrophages stain strongly with the periodic acid–Schiff (PAS) reaction. Examination by electron microscopy of these macrophages demonstrates that the areas of intense PAS staining are packed with bacilli. These areas usually have a distinctive sickle shape, and the macrophages are often referred to as sickleform particle-containing cells.

EPIDEMIOLOGY

The epidemiology of Whipple disease is not well understood. There seems to be a preponderance of the systemic disorder in males and in whites. Among the nearly 700 patients analyzed by Dobbins (1987), 86.4% were male and 97.8% were white. Individuals who worked with soil or animals accounted for two of every three cases. DNA of the organism was detected in five different sewage treatment plants in Germany, providing the first documented encounter with the organism in the environment and supporting the notion of an environmental source of infection. The route of infection is not known, although an oral route is suspected. There have been reports of clusters of affected individuals within families.

SYSTEMIC DISEASE

Symptoms include weight loss (usually 20 to 30 pounds, occasionally as much as 100 pounds), abdominal pain (often nondescript epigastric pain), diarrhea (often with steatorrhea), and arthritis (often migratory and involving large joints). In 50% of patients, arthritis precedes the intestinal manifestations by 10 to 30 years. Other systemic manifestations include low-grade fever, lymphadenopathy, and increased skin pigmentation.

In systemic disease, blood studies may reveal anemia and hypoalbuminemia. Intestinal absorption studies often reveal steatorrhea and diminished xylose absorption. Diagnosis, however, is usually made by small intestinal biopsy to demonstrate the PAS-staining macrophages. Because PAS-positive macrophages may be found in other diseases and in other tissues of apparently normal individuals, confirmation of the diagnosis is facilitated by detection of the actual bacillus with electron microscopy or by PCR analysis of infected tissue. If intestinal biopsy is PAS-negative, multiple biopsies with electron microscopic examination may be required to establish the diagnoses.

NEUROLOGIC MANIFESTATIONS

In 5% of patients with Whipple disease, the first symptoms are neurologic, but central nervous system (CNS) symptoms may eventually occur in 6% to 43% of cases. Asymptomatic CNS infection occurs as well. In some cases, CNS disease may occur without evidence of infection elsewhere. Neurologic symptoms and signs are protean. Louis et al. (1996) reviewed reports of 84 cases of CNS Whipple disease. The following signs were most prevalent: cognitive changes (including abnormalities of orientation, memory, or reasoning, 71%), supranuclear gaze palsy (more often vertical than horizontal, 51%), altered level of consciousness (including somnolence, lethargy, stupor, or coma, 50%), psychiatric signs (including depression, euphoria, anxiety, psychosis, or personality change, 44%), upper motor neuron signs (37%), and hypothalamic manifestations (including polydipsia, hyperphagia, change in libido, amenorrhea, changes in sleep–wake cycle, insomnia, 31%). Other signs in 20% to 25% of cases included cranial nerve abnormalities, myoclonus, seizures, and ataxia (Table 34.1). The combination of pendular vergence oscillations of the eyes in synchrony with masticatory myorhythmia has been termed "oculomasticatory myorhythmia." When there is myorhythmia of skeletal muscles as well, the term "oculofacial skeletal myorhythmia" has been used. Although

TABLE 34.1. NEUROLOGIC SIGNS IN 84 CASES OF CENTRAL NERVOUS SYSTEM WHIPPLE DISEASE

Signs	Percent
Cognitive change	71
Supranuclear gaze palsy	51
Altered level of consciousness	50
Psychiatric signs	44
Upper motor neuron signs	37
Hypothalamic manifestations	31
Cranial nerve abnormalities	25
Myoclonus	25
Seizures	23
Ataxia	20
Oculomasticatory myorhythmia or oculo-facial-skeletal myorhythmia	20
Sensory deficits	12

these forms of myorhythmia are pathognomonic of CNS Whipple disease, they were noted in only 20% of patients. The classic triad of dementia, supranuclear gaze palsy, and myoclonus was noted in only 15% of cases.

LABORATORY DATA

In CNS Whipple disease, over half of the patients show a focal abnormality on computed tomography or magnetic resonance imaging, ranging from a small focal lesion without mass effect to large numbers of enhancing lesions with mass effect. However, these abnormalities are not specific. A low level cerebrospinal fluid pleocytosis (mean, 91 leukocytes/μL; range, 5 to 900) is found in half the patients with the CNS disorder, and cerebrospinal fluid protein is elevated in half (mean, 75 mg/dL; range, 47 to 158). When CNS Whipple disease is suspected from clinical manifestations, the diagnosis may be confirmed by biopsy of any infected tissue with identification of bacteria or PCR analysis. In Louis et al.'s review (1996), biopsy was a sensitive technique; 70% of intestinal biopsies and 89% of all tissue biopsies (including small bowel, brain, lymph node, vitreous fluid) were positive. Factors that contributed to a negative small-bowel biopsy included absence of chronic diarrhea, lack of endoscopic guidance, specimens not examined by electron microscopy, and biopsy not repeated at least once if initially negative.

TREATMENT

If untreated, CNS disease may have a fulminant course, progressing to death within 1 month. Even when treated, the prognosis is uncertain. Many antibiotics have been used with variable success. The most commonly used agents have been tetracycline, penicillin, and trimethoprim-sulfamethoxazole (TMP-SMX). Many authors recommend oral TMP-SMX, but not all patients respond, and intravenous ceftriaxone or TMP-SMX appears to be more effective. The optimum duration of treatment of acute infection is not known nor is the length of follow-up treatment. Treatment of CNS disease must be prolonged because recurrence has followed months of treatment and apparent disappearance of disease.

SUGGESTED READINGS

Adams M, Rhyner PA, Day J, et al. Whipple's disease confined to the central nervous system. *Ann Neurol* 1987;21:104–108.

Brown AP, Lane JC, Murayama S, Vollmer DG. Whipple's disease presenting with isolated neurological symptoms. Case report. *J Neurosurg* 1990;73:623–627.

Cohen L, Berthet K, Dauga C, Thivart L, Pierrot-Deseilligny C. Polymerase chain reaction of cerebrospinal fluid to diagnose Whipple's disease. *Lancet* 1996;347:329.

Davion T, Rosat P, Sevestre H, et al. MR imaging of CNS replase of Whipple disease. *J Comput Assist Tomogr* 1990;14:815–817.

Dobbins WO III, ed. *Whipple's disease.* Springfield, IL: C Thomas, 1987.

Louis ED, Lynch T, Kaufmann P, Fahn S, Odel J. Diagnostic guidelines in central nervous system Whipple's disease. *Ann Neurol* 1996;40:561–568.

Lynch T, Odel J, Fredericks DN, et al. PCR-based diagnosis of *Tropheryma whippelii* in CNS Whipple's disease. *Ann Neurol* 1997;42:120–124.

Maiwald M, Schuhmacher F, Ditton H-J, von Herbay A. Environmental occurrence of Whipple's disease bacterium (*Tropheryma whippelii*). *Appl Environ Microbiol* 1998;64:760–762.

Relman DA, Schmidt TM, MacDermott RP, Falkow S. Identification of the uncultured bacillus of Whipple's disease. *N Engl J Med* 1992;327:293–301.

Schoedon G, Goldenberger D, Forrer R et al. Deactivation of macrophages with IL-4 is the key to the isolation of *Tropheryma whippelii. J Infect Dis* 1997;176:672–677.

Schwartz MA, Selhort JB, Ochs AL, et al. Oculomasticatory myorhythmia: a unique movement disorder occurring in Whipple's disease. *Ann Neurol* 1986;20:677–683.

Whipple GH. A hitherto undescribed disease characterized anatomically by deposits of fat and fatty acids in the intestinal and mesenteric lymphatic tissues. *Johns Hopkins Hosp Bull* 1907;18:382–391.

Wroe SJ, Pires M, Harding B, et al. Whipple's disease confined to the CNS presenting with multiple intracerebral mass lesions. *J Neurol Neurosurg Psychiatry* 1991;54:989–992.

Merritt's Neurology, 10th ed., edited by L.P. Rowland. Lippincott Williams & Wilkins, Philadelphia © 2000.

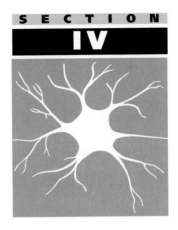

VASCULAR DISEASES

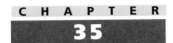

PATHOGENESIS, CLASSIFICATION, AND EPIDEMIOLOGY OF CEREBROVASCULAR DISEASE

RALPH L. SACCO

Stroke continues to be a major public health problem that ranks in the top four causes of death in most countries and is responsible for a large proportion of the burden of neurologic disorders. More often disabling than fatal, stroke is the leading cause of severe neurologic disability and results in enormous costs measured in both health-care dollars and lost productivity. Major strides have been made in understanding the epidemiology, etiology, and pathogenesis of cerebrovascular disease and have led to new approaches to diagnosis and treatment.

DEFINITION AND NOSOLOGY

In the broadest sense, the World Health Organization has defined stroke as "rapidly developing clinical signs of focal (at times global) disturbance of cerebral function, lasting more than 24 hours or leading to death with no apparent cause other than that of vascular origin." By conventional clinical definitions, if the neurologic symptoms continue for more than 24 hours, a person is diagnosed with stroke; otherwise, a focal neurologic deficit lasting less than 24 hours is defined as a transient ischemic attack (TIA). For symptoms that exceed 24 hours and resolve within 3 weeks, another category, reversible ischemic neurologic deficit, has been used to define what is nothing other than a minor stroke. Such terms defined by the duration of neurologic symptoms are being redefined with the more widespread use of sensitive brain imaging that has shown that patients with fleeting symptoms can be found to have an imaged stroke (i.e., cerebral infarction transient symptoms). The most recent definition of stroke for clinical trials has required either symptoms lasting more than 24 hours or imaging of an acute clinically relevant brain lesion in patients with rapidly vanishing symptoms. The duration and severity of the syndrome then can be used to classify patients as those with minor or major stroke. The use of the term "brain attack," which may lack specificity, has been championed by the educational campaigns of national health organizations to help inform the public about the urgency of stroke.

In addition to duration, stroke is classified by the pathology of the underlying focal brain injury into either infarction or hemorrhage. Intracranial hemorrhage can be subdivided into two distinct types based on the site and vascular origin of the blood: subarachnoid, when the bleeding originates in the subarachnoid spaces surrounding the brain, and intracerebral, when the hemorrhage is into the substance or parenchyma of the brain. Ischemic infarction can be classified into various subgroups based on the mechanism of the ischemia and the type and localization of the vascular lesion.

The cardinal feature of stroke is the sudden onset of neurologic symptoms. "Silent stroke" may occur without apparent clinical manifestations, however, because either the patient and family are unaware of minor symptoms or a so-called silent area of brain has been affected. Premonitory stroke symptoms are not always found; fewer than 20% of stroke patients have a prior TIA. Focal premonitory symptoms, when present, usually predate infarction rather than hemorrhage. When they occur, they may be so nonspecific that they are not recognized as signs of an impending stroke.

The neurologic symptoms often reflect the location and size of stroke, but they usually cannot be used to definitively differentiate the type of stroke. When headache, vomiting, seizures, or coma occur, however, hemorrhage is more likely than infarction. Specific neurologic symptoms that may occur in isolation or in various combinations include loss of vision (hemianopia), double vision, weakness or sensory loss on one side of the body, dysarthria, alteration in higher cognitive functions (dysphasia, confusion, spatial disorientation, neglect, dysmemory), difficulty walking, headache, or unilateral deafness. Part of the challenge is to localize precisely the affected anatomic region and the corresponding vascular territory based on the clinical symptoms and signs. This step is reviewed in Chapter 38 in connection with the syndromes of specific cerebral arteries. A prerequisite, however, is a sound understanding of the anatomy of the vascular supply of the brain.

VASCULAR ANATOMY

The brain is perfused by the carotid and vertebral arteries, which begin as extracranial arteries off the aorta or other great vessels and course through the neck and base of the skull to reach the intracranial cavity (Fig. 35.1). The carotid and its branches are referred to as the anterior circulation and the vertebrobasilar as the posterior circulation.

The right common carotid originates from the bifurcation of the innominate, whereas the left originates directly from the aortic arch. The internal carotid arteries stem from the common carotid, usually at the level of the upper border of the thyroid cartilage at the fourth cervical vertebrae, give no branches in the neck and face, and enter the cranium through the carotid canal. The four main segments of the internal carotid are cervical, petrous, cavernous, and supraclinoid. The siphon is the term used to describe the series of turns made by the cavernous and supraclinoid segments. The internal carotid ends by dividing into the middle and anterior cerebral arteries after giving off the ophthalmic, superior hypophyseal, posterior communicating, and anterior choroidal arteries. The carotid system therefore supplies the optic nerves and retina plus the anterior portion of the cerebral hemisphere, which comprises the frontal, parietal, and

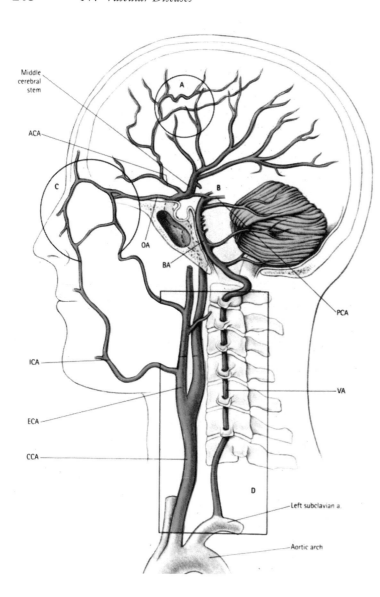

Middle
cerebral
stem

ACA

C

A

B

OA

BA

PCA

ICA

VA

ECA

CCA

D

Left subclavian a.

Aortic arch

FIG. 35.1. Arterial supply to the brain with enlarged detail of the sites of anastomosis in the cerebral circulation. **A:** Over the convexity, subarachnoid interarterial anastomoses link the middle (MCA), anterior (ACA), and posterior cerebral arteries (PCA) through the border zone. **B:** The circle of Willis provides communication between the anterior and posterior cerebral circulation via the anterior and posterior communicating arteries. **C:** Through the orbit, anastomoses occur between the external (ECA) and internal carotid arteries (ICA). **D:** Extracranial anastomoses connect the muscular branches of the cervical arteries to the vertebral arteries (VAs) and the ECAs. OA, ophthalmic artery; BA, basilar artery; CCA, common carotid artery.

anterior temporal lobes. In as many as 15% of adults, the posterior cerebral artery also arises directly from the internal carotid artery so that the entire cerebral hemisphere (including the occipital lobe) is supplied by the internal carotid artery.

The middle cerebral artery is the largest branch of the internal carotid artery and appears almost as a direct continuation. It begins as a single trunk (stem or M1 segment) passing laterally to the sylvian fissure, where it becomes the M2 or insular segment, from which the 12 cerebral surface branches originate. The stem usually ends in either a bifurcation into the upper and lower division or a trifurcation into three major trunks (upper, middle, and lower divisions). The cortical divisions supply almost the entire cortical surface of the brain, including insula, operculum, and frontal, parietal, temporal, and occipital cortices; the frontal pole, the superior and extreme posterior rim of the convex surface, and medial cortical surfaces are not supplied by the middle cerebral artery.

The middle cerebral artery stem gives rise to the medial and lateral lenticulostriates, which supply the extreme capsule, claustrum, putamen, most of the globus pallidus, part of the head and

the entire body of the caudate, and the superior portions of the anterior and posterior limbs of the internal capsule. The upper division usually gives rise to the lateral orbitofrontal, ascending frontal, precentral (prerolandic), central (rolandic), and anterior parietal branches, whereas the lower division usually contains the temporal polar, temporooccipital, anterior, middle, and posterior temporal branches. The posterior parietal and angular branches are more variable.

The anterior cerebral artery begins as a medial branch of the internal carotid artery, forming the proximal or A1 segment to the junction of the anterior communicating artery where it continues as the distal or A2 segment. The largest branch is known as the recurrent artery of Heubner, and several cortical branches supply the medial and orbital surfaces of the frontal lobe.

The vertebral artery usually arises from the subclavian artery, courses through the transverse foramina, pierces the dura, and enters the cranial cavity to join the contralateral vertebral artery. At the distal segment are the origin for the anterior and posterior spinal arteries and posterior inferior cerebellar artery, which supplies the inferior surface of the cerebellum. The lateral medulla is supplied by the multiple perforating branches of the posterior inferior cerebellar artery or direct medullary branches of the vertebral artery.

The basilar artery originates as the merger of the right and left vertebral arteries usually at the level of the pontomedullary junction (Fig. 35.2). Paramedian penetrators, short and long lateral circumferential penetrators, originate from the basilar artery to supply the brainstem. The anterior inferior cerebellar and superior cerebellar arteries perfuse the ventrolateral aspect of the cerebellar cortex, and the internal auditory (labyrinthine) artery arises either directly from the basilar or from the anterior cerebellar artery to supply the cochlea, labyrinth, and part of the facial nerve.

The basilar artery usually terminates into the posterior cerebral arteries. A series of penetrators (posteromedial, thalamoperforates, thalamogeniculate, tuberothalamic) arises from the posterior communicating and posterior cerebral artery to supply the hypothalamus, dorsolateral midbrain, lateral geniculate, and thalamus. The posterior cerebral artery supplies the inferior surface of the temporal lobe and medial and inferior surfaces of the occipital lobe, including the lingual and fusiform gyri.

A rich anastomotic network includes various extracranial intercommunicating systems, intracranial connections through the circle of Willis, and distal intracranial connections through meningeal anastomoses throughout the border zones over the cortical and cerebellar surfaces. These networks protect the brain by providing alternate routes to circumvent obstructions in the main arteries. Obstruction of the extracranial internal carotid may remain asymptomatic if there is adequate perfusion made available through a variety of collateral pathways, such as the external carotid to the ophthalmic to the intracranial internal carotid, the contralateral carotid to the anterior cerebral artery and across the circle of Willis through the anterior communicating artery, the vertebrobasilar to the posterior cerebral artery and anterior through the posterior communicating artery, and distal interconnections between the distal middle cerebral artery with branches of the posterior and anterior cerebral arteries. The small arteries and arterioles (100 μm or less in diameter) that arise from the surface arteries and penetrate the brain parenchyma function as end arteries with few interconnections.

PHYSIOLOGY

The adult brain, which weighs about 1500 g, requires an uninterrupted supply of about 150 g of glucose and 72 L of oxygen every 24 hours. Because the brain does not store these substances, dysfunction results after only a few minutes when either the oxygen or the glucose content is reduced below critical levels. In the resting state, each cardiac contraction delivers about 70 mL of blood into the ascending aorta; 10 to 15 mL are allocated to the brain. Every minute, about 350 mL flows through each internal carotid artery and about 100 to 200 mL through the vertebrobasilar system.

To ensure constant perfusion pressure and blood flow to the brain, the major cerebral arteries have a well-developed muscular

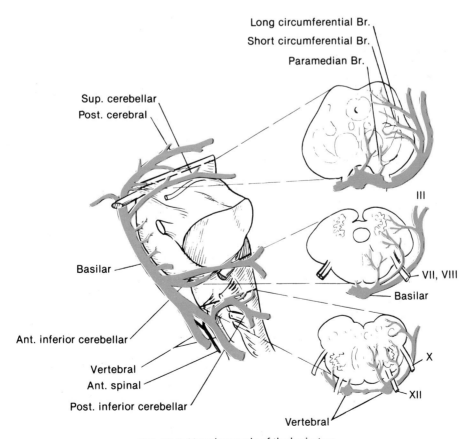

FIG. 35.2. Vascular supply of the brainstem.

coat that allows constriction in response to increased blood pressure and dilation with hypotension. The arterioles are exquisitely sensitive to changes in $Paco_2$ and Pao_2. When the partial pressure of CO_2 increases, the arterioles dilate and cerebral blood flow increases. When CO_2 tension is reduced, the arterioles constrict and blood flow is reduced. Changes in the partial pressure of O_2 have the opposite effect. Focal cerebral activity, such as occurs when moving a limb, is accompanied by accelerated metabolism in the appropriate region, which is accommodated by an increase in the local blood flow. In patients with cerebrovascular disease, this compensatory mechanism may be destroyed.

PATHOGENESIS AND CLASSIFICATION

Brain Infarction

When blood supply is interrupted for 30 seconds, brain metabolism is altered. After 1 minute, neuronal function may cease. After 5 minutes, anoxia initiates a chain of events that may result in cerebral infarction; however, if oxygenated blood flow is restored quickly enough, the damage may be reversible. The following steps occur in the evolution of an infarct: (a) local vasodilatation and (b) stasis of the blood column with segmentation of the red cells are followed by (c) edema and (d) necrosis of brain tissue (Fig. 35.3).

Exciting research into the cellular consequences of ischemia have led to the elucidation of the ischemic cascade. A chain of events at the neuronal level leads to cellular dysfunction and

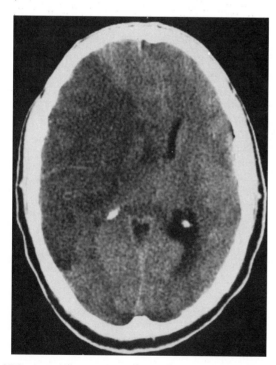

FIG. 35.3. Acute infarct, right middle cerebral artery distribution. Non-contrast axial computed tomography shows right frontal and temporal hypodensity, including cortex and edema producing ventricular effacement and midline shift. Right anterior and posterior cerebral artery territories are spared. Similar appearance could result from occlusion of right internal carotid artery with competent circle of Willis. (Courtesy of Drs. J.A. Bello and S.K. Hilal.)

death starting with the failure of the Na/K pump, the depolarization of the neuronal membrane, the release of excitatory neurotransmitters, and the opening of calcium channels. The influx of calcium is at the root of further neuronal injury with damage to organelles and further destabilization of neuronal metabolism and normal function. Calcium may enter the neuron through various voltage-sensitive and receptor-mediated channels (i.e., the N-methyl-d-aspartate receptor). Excitatory neurotransmitters such as glutamate and glycine can lead to the further influx of calcium through these channels. These events can lead to delayed neuronal death and are the main target of various neuroprotective strategies. The ischemic penumbra has been defined as the region of brain surrounding the core of an infarct in which neuronal function is deranged but potentially salvageable.

Persistently reduced perfusion and the consequences of the ischemic cascade can lead to extension of the core of the infarct to encompass the ischemic penumbra. If the interruption to blood flow is sufficiently prolonged and infarction results, the brain tissue first softens and then liquefies; a cavity finally forms when the debris is removed by the phagocytic microglia. In attempts to fill the defect, astroglia in the surrounding brain proliferate and invade the softened area, and new capillaries are formed.

Although most infarcts are bland, a hemorrhagic infarct occasionally is caused by local hemorrhage into the necrotic tissue, which may be petechial or confluent. Hemorrhagic infarct may occur when the occluding clot or embolus breaks up and migrates, thereby restoring flow through the infarcted area. More widespread use of magnetic resonance imaging (MRI) has shown that petechial hemorrhagic infarction is more frequent than originally suspected and is related to size of the infarct and elevation of blood pressure (Fig. 35.4).

Infarction may be confined to a single vascular territory when the occlusion involves a small penetrant end-artery or distal intracranial branch. If the occlusion is more proximal in the arterial tree, ischemia may be more widespread and may involve more than one vascular territory or border zone ischemia may result with limited infarction in the distal fields of the vascular supply. Intracranial proximal occlusions may result in both penetrant artery ischemia and coexisting surface branch territory infarction.

Multiple mechanisms may lead to brain ischemia. Hemodynamic infarction originates as a result of an impediment to normal perfusion that usually is caused by a severe arterial stenosis or occlusion caused by atherosclerosis and coexisting thrombosis. Embolism occurs when a particle of thrombus originating from a more proximal source (arterial, cardiac, or transcardiac) travels through the vascular system and leads to an arterial occlusion. Small-vessel disease occurs when lipohyalinosis or local atherosclerotic disease leads to an occlusion of a penetrant artery. Less frequent conditions that lead to reductions in cerebral perfusion and result in infarction are arterial dissection, primary or secondary vasculitis (e.g., meningitis caused by tuberculosis or syphilis), hypercoagulable states, vasospasm, systemic hypotension, hyperviscosity (as in polycythemia, dysproteinemia, or thrombocytosis), moyamoya disease, fibromuscular dysplasia, extrinsic compression of the major arteries by tumor, and occlusion of the veins that drain the brain. The four most frequent subtypes of cerebral infarction are atherosclerotic, cardioembolic, small vessel (lacunar), and cryptogenic.

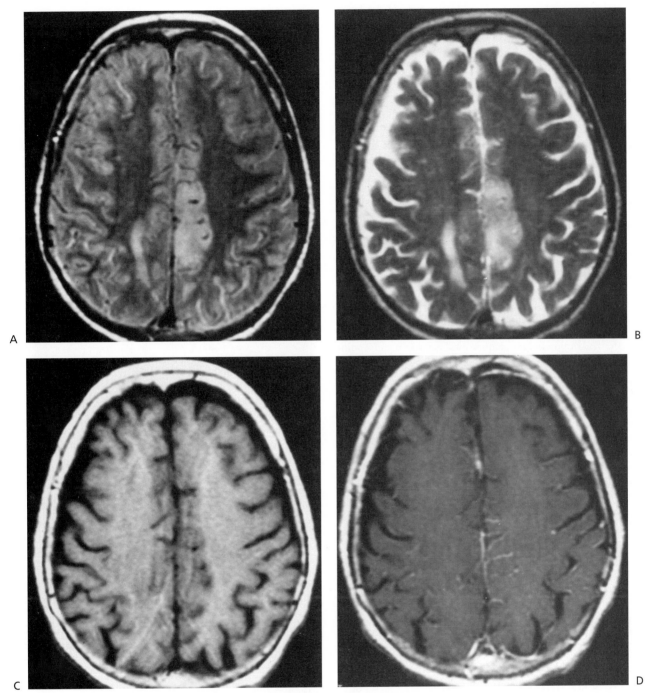

FIG. 35.4. Acute cortical infarction. **A and B:** Proton-density and T2-weighted axial magnetic resonance scans show increased signal intensity within the medial cortex of left frontal and parietal lobes. Note swelling of gray matter and prominence of blood vessels within this lesion. **C and D:** T1-weighted axial magnetic resonance scans before and after gadolinium administration demonstrate several linear foci of contrast enhancement within the area of infarction in the left frontal and parietal lobes, most consistent with enhancing arterial branches. Contrast enhancement of arterial branches is consistent with static blood flow within the infarct and generally is seen only within the first few hours to 5 days after the onset of acute infarction. (Courtesy of Dr. S. Chan.)

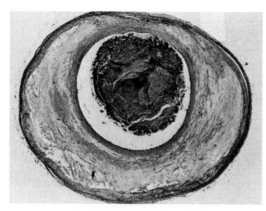

FIG. 35.5. Carotid artery in cross-section. Note atherosclerotic changes and intraluminal thrombus.

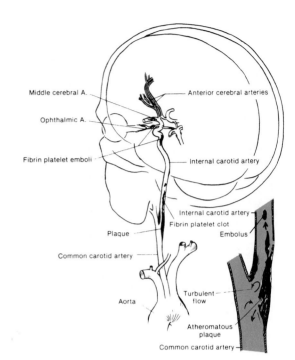

FIG. 35.6. Atheromatous plaques at the carotid bifurcation may be a source of retinal and cerebral emboli.

Atherosclerotic Infarction

Atherosclerotic plaque at a bifurcation or curve in one of the larger vessels leads to progressive stenosis with the final large artery occlusion caused by thrombosis of the narrowed lumen (Fig. 35.5). Arteriosclerotic plaques may develop at any point along the carotid artery and the vertebrobasilar system, but the most common sites are the bifurcation of the common carotid artery into the external and internal carotid arteries, the origins of the middle and anterior cerebral arteries, and the origins of the vertebral from the subclavian arteries (Table 35.1).

Ischemia is attributed to perfusion failure distal to the site of severe stenosis or occlusion of the major vessel. The site of infarction depends on the collateral flow but is usually in the distal fields or border zones. Specifying the degree of stenosis that will lead to perfusion difficulty depends on multiple factors and often is not defined easily. Classification schemes have relied on stenosis greater than 70% to 80% as more predictive of impending hemodynamic compromise.

An atherosclerotic stenosis or occlusion can also lead to a cerebral infarction through an embolic mechanism. In this case, emboli arising from the proximally situated atheromatous lesions occlude otherwise healthy branches located more distal in the arterial tree (Fig. 35.6). Embolic fragments may arise from ex-

tracranial arteries affected by stenosis or ulcer, stenosis of any major cerebral artery stem, the stump of the occluded internal carotid artery, and even from intracranial tail of the anterograde thrombus atop an occluded carotid. The constituents of the offending embolism have earned the labels of "red" (thrombus) and "white" (platelet) clots, but it is nearly impossible to discriminate these based on clinical findings.

Cardiac Embolism

Many strokes caused by embolism originate from a cardiac source of thrombus. A small particle of thrombus breaks off from the source and is carried through the bloodstream until it lodges in an artery too small to allow it to pass, usually a distal intracranial branch. Besides thrombus, other types of particles may embolize, such as neoplasm, fat, air, or other foreign substances. Air embolism usually follows injuries or surgical procedures involving the lungs, the dural sinuses, or jugular veins. It also may be caused by the release of nitrogen bubbles into the general circulation after a rapid reduction in barometric pressure. Fat embolism is rare and almost always arises from a bone fracture. Most emboli are sterile, but some may contain bacteria if emboli arise secondary to subacute or acute bacterial endocarditis. The most common sources of cardiac embolism include valvular heart disease (mitral stenosis, mitral regurgitation, rheumatic heart disease); intracardiac thrombus, particularly along the left ventricular wall (mural thrombus) after anterior myocardial infarction or in the left atrial appendage in patients with atrial fibrillation; ventricular or septal aneurysm; and cardiomyopathies leading to stagnation of blood flow and an increased propensity for the formation of intracardiac thrombus (Table 35.2). A

TABLE 35.1. ANGIOGRAPHIC FINDINGS AMONG 79 PATIENTS WITH ATHEROSCLEROTIC INFARCTION IN THE NINDS STROKE DATA BANK[a]

Angiogram results	n	Percent
ICA occlusion/severe stenosis	49	62.0
MCA occlusion/severe stenosis	8	10.1
ACA stenosis	1	1.3
PCA occlusion	1	1.3
VB (occlusion/severe stenosis)	12	15.2
Other findings	8	10.1

[a]Angiography was performed within a median of 5 days.
ICA, internal carotid artery; MCA, middle cerebral artery; ACA, anterior cerebral artery; PCA, posterior cerebral artery; VB, vertebrobasilar arteries.
Modified from Timsit SG, Sacco RL, Mohr JP, et al. *Stroke* 1992;23: 486–491.

TABLE 35.2. FREQUENCY OF CARDIAC DISEASE AMONG 246 PATIENTS WITH CARDIOEMBOLIC INFARCTION IN THE NINDS STROKE DATA BANK

Abnormalities	n	Percent
History		
Cardiac disease	182	74
Atrial fibrillation	98	40
Abnormal first electrocardiogram	224	91
Echocardiogram done[a]	128	52
Left atrial enlargement	75	58
Left ventricular dilatation	54	42
Akinetic region	34	26
Mitral annulus calcification	20	16
Mitral stenosis (moderate/severe)	13	10
Aortic stenosis (moderate/severe)	11	9
Mural thrombus	8	6

[a]The sum of the various findings on echocardiogram exceeds 100% because many patients had more than 1 abnormality.
Modified from Timsit SG, Sacco RL, Mohr JP, et al. *Stroke* 1992;23:486–491.

"paradoxic" embolus occurs when a thrombus crosses from the venous circulation to the left side of the heart, most often through a patent foramen ovale. Other possible causes of cerebral embolism are atrial myxoma, marantic endocarditis, and severe prolapse of the mitral valve.

Embolism is inferred when the brain image demonstrates an infarction confined to the cerebral surface territory of a single branch, combinations of infarcts involving branches of different divisions of major cerebral arteries, or hemorrhagic infarction. The difficult problem in arriving at a diagnosis of embolism is the identification of the occluding particle and the source. Mural thrombi and platelet aggregates are remarkably evanescent, as has been inferred by findings on angiography. Embolic fragments are found in more than 75% of patients who undergo angiography within 48 hours of onset of the stroke and are then gone when angiogram is repeated later. Embolism is demonstrated in only 11% of clinically similar cases when angiogram is delayed beyond 48 hours from clinical onset of the stroke. Persistence of embolic occlusion is the exception rather than the rule. Embolic obstruction of an arterial lumen is cleared most commonly by recanalization and fibrinolysis. During this process, the lumen may appear "stenotic." The evanescent quality of emboli may explain the wide variation in the frequency with which this subtype is diagnosed in retrospective or prospective studies of stroke. More recently, the improved sensitivities of cerebral and cardiac imaging have led to better detection of sources of thrombus.

Small Vessel Lacunar Infarction

These strokes have distinctive clinical syndromes with a small zone of ischemia confined to the territory of a single vessel. They are understood to reflect arterial disease of the vessels penetrating the brain to supply the internal capsule, basal ganglia, thalamus, corona radiata, and paramedian regions of the brainstem (Fig. 35.7). Disagreements abound about the pathogenesis of lacunar infarcts; some authors favor the use of the term "lacune" to de-

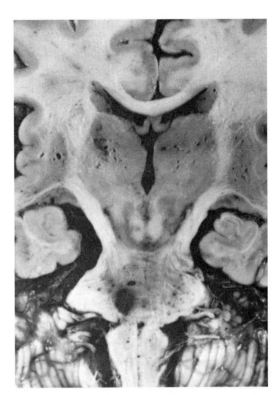

FIG. 35.7. Longitudinal cut through basal ganglia, midbrain, pons, and brainstem shows multiple lacunar infarctions and a small pontine hemorrhage.

scribe size and location without indicating a specific pathology. Only a handful of such infarcts have been studied pathologically by serial section, and only a few studies have documented a tiny focus of microatheroma or lipohyalinosis stenosing one of the deep penetrating arteries. The arterial damage is usually the result of long-standing hypertension or diabetes mellitus. Rare causes include stenosis of the middle cerebral artery stem or microembolization to penetrant arterial territories. Most radiologically defined small deep infarcts do not have significant large-artery atherosclerosis, lack even a potential cardiac source of embolism, and occur in vascular territories less likely to be occluded by emboli.

Many lacunar strokes are diagnosed by clinical characteristics alone. Clinical syndromes include pure motor hemiparesis, pure sensory syndrome, clumsy hand dysarthria, ataxic hemiparesis, and sensorimotor stroke (Table 35.3). When brain imaging is positive, a strategically placed small deep infarct is usually found.

TABLE 35.3. FREQUENCY OF LACUNAR SYNDROMES AMONG 316 LACUNAR INFARCTS IN THE NINDS STROKE DATA BANK

Syndrome	n	Percent
Pure motor hemiparesis	181	57
Sensorimotor	63	20
Ataxic hemiparesis	33	10
Pure sensory	21	7
Dysarthria—clumsy hand	18	6

Because the vascular lesion lies in vessels some 200 to 400 μm in diameter, cerebral angiography understandably is normal. Incidental large vessel disease may be found in some series, but whether it is etiologically related to the site of infarction is often unclear.

Cryptogenic Infarction

Despite efforts to arrive at a diagnosis, the cause of infarction in a discouragingly large number of cases remains undetermined. Some cases may be unexplained because no appropriate laboratory studies are performed, whereas others remain undetermined because of improper timing of the appropriate laboratory studies. The most frequent circumstances, however, are when normal or ambiguous findings are reached despite appropriate laboratory studies performed at the appropriate time. Results from the Stroke Data Bank indicated that large artery atherosclerotic occlusive disease was a less frequent cause of stroke, that small vessel or lacunar and cardioembolic infarction were relatively frequent, and that the cause for most cases of infarction could not be classified into these traditional diagnostic categories. This conclusion forced the creation of a separate diagnostic category for cases whose mechanisms of infarction remained unproven, known as "infarct of undetermined cause" or "cryptogenic infarction."

Cases categorized as cryptogenic infarction have no bruit or TIA ipsilateral to the hemisphere affected by stroke, no obvious history suggestive of cardiac embolism, and usually do not present with a lacunar syndrome. Computed tomography (CT) or magnetic resonance imaging performed within 7 days may be normal, may show an infarct limited to a surface branch territory, or may show a large zone of infarction affecting regions larger than that accounted for by a single penetrant arterial territory. Noninvasive vascular imaging fails to demonstrate an underlying large vessel occlusion or stenosis. No cardiac source of embolism is uncovered by echocardiography, electrocardiography, or Holter monitor. If an angiogram is performed, the study may be normal, may show a distal branch occlusion, or may show occlusion of a major cerebral artery stem or of the top of the basilar. Because these latter occlusions can arise from embolus or thrombosis of an atherosclerotic vessel, their demonstration does not solve the question of mechanism.

Many of these patients present with a hemispheral syndrome, a surface infarction revealed by CT or magnetic resonance imaging, and a corresponding branch occlusion documented by angiography or normal angiogram. This constellation of findings has been considered suggestive of embolism. Ample evidence exists for many occult sources of emboli; the difficulty is in proving their existence and their role in the first or succeeding ischemic strokes. Emerging technologies have led to the suggestion that some cryptogenic infarcts may be explained by hematologic disorders causing hypercoagulable states from protein C, free protein S, lupus anticoagulant, or anticardiolipin antibody abnormalities. Others have implicated paradoxic emboli through a patent foramen ovale and aortic arch atherosclerosis. Rather than reclassifying these cases into embolism as the inferred mechanism, such cases should be labeled as "cryptogenic" until the mechanism, source, and determinants of these unexplained infarcts are clarified.

Intracranial Hemorrhage

Hemorrhage results from rupture of a vessel anywhere within the cranial cavity. Intracranial hemorrhages are classified according to location (extradural, subdural, subarachnoid, intracerebral, intraventricular), according to the nature of the ruptured vessel or vessels (arterial, capillary, venous), or according to cause (primary, secondary). Trauma often is involved in the generation of extradural hematoma from laceration of the middle meningeal artery or vein and subdural hematomas from traumatic rupture of veins that traverse the subdural space.

Intracerebral Hemorrhage

Intracerebral hemorrhage is characterized by bleeding into the substance of the brain, usually from a small penetrating artery. Hypertension has been implicated as the cause of a weakening in the walls of arterioles and the formation of microaneurysms (Charcot-Brouchard). Among elderly nonhypertensive patients with recurrent lobar hemorrhages, amyloid angiopathy has been implicated as an important cause. Other causes include arteriovenous malformations, aneurysms, moyamoya disease, bleeding disorders or anticoagulation, trauma, tumors, cavernous angiomas, and illicit drug abuse. In blood dyscrasias (e.g., acute leukemia, aplastic anemia, polycythemia, thrombocytopenic purpura, scurvy), the hemorrhages may be multiple and of varied size.

The arterial blood ruptures under pressure and destroys or displaces brain tissue. If the hemorrhage is large, the ruptured vessel is often impossible to find at autopsy. The most common sites are the putamen, caudate, pons, cerebellum, thalamus, or deep white matter (Table 35.4). Basal ganglia hemorrhages often extend to involve the internal capsule and sometimes rupture into the lateral ventricle and spread through the ventricular system into the subarachnoid space (Fig. 35.8). Intraventricular ex-

TABLE 35.4. DISTRIBUTION BY LOCATION OF CT-DIAGNOSED PRIMARY INTRACEREBRAL HEMORRHAGE AMONG 203 PATIENTS IN THE NINDS STROKE DATA BANK

Location	Percent
Supratentorial	85
Deep	53
Putamen	25
Thalamus	23
Caudate/other	5
Lobar	32
1 lobe	15
2 lobes	13
3 lobes	4
Intratenlorial	15
Cerebellum	11
Pons	4

CT; Computed tomography. Adapted from Massaro, et al., 1991.

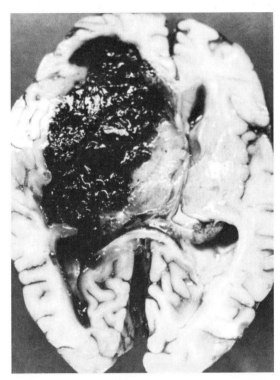

FIG. 35.8. Infarcts of undetermined cause in the Stroke Data Bank. (Reprinted with permission from Sacco RL, et al. Infarction of undetermined cause: the NINCDS Stroke Data Bank. *Ann Neurol* 1989;25:382–390.)

tension increases the likelihood of a fatal outcome. Bleeding into one lobe of the cerebral hemisphere or cerebellum usually remains confined within brain parenchyma. An inferior cerebellar hemorrhage is a neurologic emergency that needs to be diagnosed promptly, because early surgical evacuation of those greater than 3 cm can prevent tonsillar herniation and apnea.

If the patient survives an intracerebral hemorrhage, blood and necrotic brain tissue are removed by phagocytes. The destroyed brain tissue is partially replaced by connective tissue, glia, and newly formed blood vessels, thus leaving a shrunken fluid-filled cavity. Less frequently, the blood clot is treated as a foreign body, calcifies, and is surrounded by a thick glial membrane.

The clinical picture is dictated by the location and size of the hematoma. It is characterized by headache, vomiting, and the evolution of focal motor or sensory signs over minutes to hours. Consciousness is sometimes impaired at the start and often becomes a prominent feature in the first 24 to 48 hours among the moderate and large hematomas. Patients with intracerebral hemorrhage are often younger and more frequently have been men in some series. The diagnosis and localization are established easily with CT, which shows the high density of acute blood.

Subarachnoid Hemorrhage

Subarachnoid hemorrhage occurs when the blood is localized to the surrounding membranes and cerebrospinal fluid. It is most frequently caused by leakage of blood from a cerebral aneurysm. The combination of congenital and acquired factors leads to a degeneration of the arterial wall and the release of blood under arterial pressures into the subarachnoid space and cerebrospinal fluid. Aneurysms are distributed at different sites throughout the base of the brain, particularly at the origin or bifurcations of arteries at the circle of Willis. Other secondary causes that may lead to subarachnoid hemorrhage include arteriovenous malformations, bleeding disorders or anticoagulation, trauma, amyloid angiopathy, or central sinus thrombosis. Signs and symptoms include the abrupt onset of severe headache ("the worst headache of your life"), vomiting, altered consciousness, and sometimes coma; these characteristics often occur in the absence of focal localizing signs.

Subarachnoid hemorrhage afflicts younger patients and women more often than men. Hypertension, oral contraceptive use, and cigarette smoking are some of the known factors associated with this type of stroke. Fatalities are high, ranging from 30% to 70%, and depend on the severity of the initial presentation. Among those who survive, early rebleeding and delayed ischemic neurologic deficits from vasospasm can cause serious morbidity.

Frequency of Stroke Subtypes

Overall, ischemic stroke is three to four times as frequent as hemorrhagic stroke, accounting for 70% to 80% of all strokes. Intracerebral hemorrhage usually accounts for 10% to 30% of the cases, depending on the geographic origin of the patients, with greater relative frequencies reported in Chinese and Japanese series. Frequency of subarachnoid hemorrhage is usually one-third to one-half that of intracerebral hemorrhage. Frequency of infarct subtypes depend on the sample from which cases are drawn (hospital or population based), the geographic region of the study, and the design of investigator-driven diagnostic algorithms. Cardioembolism ranges from 15% to 30% of the cases, atherosclerotic infarction varies from 14% to 40%, and lacunar infarcts account for 15% to 30%. Stroke from other determined causes, such as arteritis or dissection, usually accounts for a small percentage (less than 5%) of the cases. Infarcts of undetermined cause may account for as many as 40% of ischemic infarcts (Fig. 35.9). Clinical features that are observed at stroke onset can help to distinguish cerebral infarction subtypes but are not reliable enough to lead to a definite determination of infarct subtype without confirmatory laboratory data.

STROKE EPIDEMIOLOGY

Incidence, Prevalence, and Mortality

The magnitude of stroke is measured in public health terms by stroke-specific incidence, prevalence, and mortality. Stroke incidence is defined by the number of first cases of stroke over a defined time interval in a defined population, whereas stroke prevalence measures the total number of cases, new and old, at a particular time also in a defined population. Both indices depend on the accurate and complete enumeration of cases and adequate knowledge of the underlying population at risk. Stroke incidence can be viewed as the sum of hospitalized, sudden fatal, and non-hospitalized stroke. Therefore, stroke incidence estimations depend on whether the data are gathered clinically, by CT, or at au-

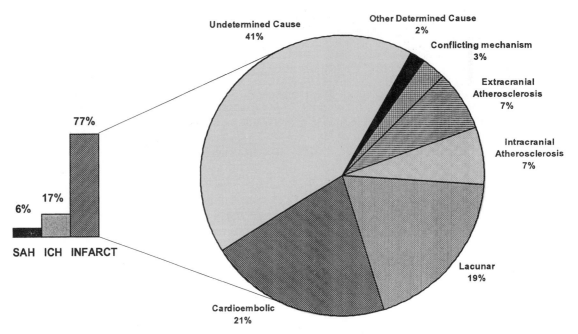

FIG. 35.9. Frequency of stroke and infarct subtypes in the Northern Manhattan Stroke Study, 1993–1997.

topsy and whether the study is hospital or population based. The American Heart Association estimates that in the United States, almost 4 million stroke survivors exist (prevalence) and approximately 600,000 new or recurrent strokes occur per year. Overall, age-adjusted incidence rates range between 100 and 300 per 100,000 population per year and depend on the study methodology, country of origin, and population demographics.

Mortality data are readily available but may underestimate the magnitude of stroke because not all patients with stroke die. Overall, stroke accounts for about 10% of all deaths in most industrialized countries, and most of these deaths are among persons over the age of 65. The average age-adjusted stroke mortality in the United States is 50 to 100 per 100,000 population per year, less than in Japan and China and more than in the Philippines.

Temporal Trends in Mortality

In the United States, stroke mortality has been decreasing since the early 1900s. The rate of decline has been a constant 1% per year until 1969, when it accelerated to nearly 5% per year. The greatest decline has been in the older age groups. The reasons for this mortality trend remain a subject of controversy. Epidemiologic data support various possibilities, including declining stroke incidence, improved survival, reduction in the severity of stroke, changing diagnostic criteria, and better stroke risk factor control. Convincing evidence from National Hospital Discharge Surveys is accumulating in favor of improved survival rather than of declining incidence as the explanation for the drop in stroke mortality. Some investigators have attributed the reduction in stroke mortality to better control of hypertension, whereas others have noted that the decline began before the widespread use of antihypertensive agents and

that indices of hypertension control have not correlated with stroke mortality. More recently, this decline in mortality has ceased, and some have been reporting an increase in mortality.

Determinants of Stroke
Nonmodifiable Risk Factors

Although cerebrovascular disorders may occur at any age, at any time, in either sex, in all families, and in all races, each of these nonmodifiable factors affects the incidence of stroke. The strongest determinant of stroke is age. Stroke incidence rises exponentially with age, with most strokes occurring in persons older than 65. Stroke is less common before age 40, but stroke in young adults is of growing concern because of the impact of early disability. As our population ages, the prevalence and public health impact of stroke will undoubtedly increase.

Stroke incidence is greater among men, those with a family history of stroke, and among certain race-ethnic groups (Fig. 35.10). In a hospital- and community-based cohort study of all cases of first stroke in northern Manhattan, blacks had an overall age-adjusted 1-year stroke incidence rate of 2.4 times that of whites, and Hispanics, predominantly from the Dominican Republic, had an incidence rate 1.6 times that of whites. In Japan, stroke is the leading cause of death in adults, and hemorrhage is more common than atherothrombosis. The predilection of atherosclerosis for the extracranial or intracranial circulation differs by race-ethnic group. Extracranial lesions are more frequent in whites, whereas intracranial lesions are more common in blacks, Hispanics, and Asians. The reasons for these differences have yet to be explained adequately.

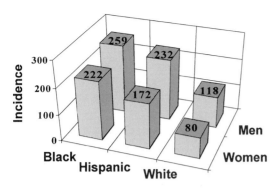

FIG. 35.10. Average age-adjusted incidence rates of stroke (per 100,000 population) among persons aged 20 years in northern Manhattan in white, black, and Hispanic women. (Adapted from Sacco RL, Boden-Abdalla B, Gan R, et al., 1998.)

Modifiable Risk Factors

Nothing is accidental about stroke, as implied by the misnomer "cerebral vascular accident." Instead, stroke is usually the result of predisposing conditions that originated years before the ictus. Epidemiologic investigations, such as prospective cohort and case-control studies, are continuing to identify numerous stroke risk factors. Current modifiable components of the stroke-prone profile include hypertension, cardiac disease (particularly atrial fibrillation), diabetes, hypercholesterolemia, physical inactivity, cigarette use, alcohol abuse, asymptomatic carotid stenosis, and a history of TIAs (Table 35.5).

After age, hypertension is the most powerful stroke risk factor. It is prevalent in the population of the United States in both men and women and is of even greater significance in blacks. The risk of stroke rises proportionately with increasing blood pressure. In Framingham, the relative risk of stroke for a 10-mm Hg increase in systolic blood pressure was 1.9 for men and 1.7 for women after controlling for other known stroke risk factors. Elevated systolic or diastolic blood pressure (or both) increases stroke risk by accelerating the progression of atherosclerosis and predisposing to small vessel disease.

Cardiac disease clearly has been associated with an increased risk of ischemic stroke, particularly atrial fibrillation, valvular heart disease, myocardial infarction, coronary artery disease,

TABLE 35.5. MODIFIABLE RISK FACTORS THAT CAN INCREASE THE PROBABILITY OF STROKE

Risk factors	Modification
Hypertension	Antihypertensives, diet
Heart disease	Antiplatelets
Atrial fibrillation	Anticoagulants, antiarrhythmics
Diabetes melitus	Glucose control
Hypercholesterolemia	Lipid-lowering medication, diet
Physical inactivity	Routine exercise
Smoking	Cessation
Heavy alcohol use	Quantity reduction
Asymptomatic carotid stenosis	Antiplatelets, endarterectomy
Transient ischemic attack	Antiplatelets, endarterectomy, anticoagulants

congestive heart failure, electrocardiographic evidence of left ventricular hypertrophy, and perhaps mitral valve prolapse. Chronic atrial fibrillation affects more than 1 million Americans and becomes more frequent with age. In the Framingham Study, atrial fibrillation was a strong predictor of stroke, with a nearly fivefold increased risk of stroke. In those with coronary heart disease or cardiac failure, atrial fibrillation doubled the stroke risk in men and tripled the risk in women. With coexisting valvular disease, atrial fibrillation had an even greater impact on the relative risk of stroke. Left ventricular dysfunction and left atrial size determined by echocardiography were also predictors of increased thromboembolic risk.

Stroke risk nearly doubles in those with antecedent coronary artery disease and nearly quadruples in subjects with cardiac failure. Even after adjusting for the presence of other risk factors, left ventricular hypertrophy increased the risk of stroke by 2.3 in both men and women, and mitral annular calcification was associated with a relative risk of stroke of 2.1. Improved cardiac imaging has led to the increased detection of such potential stroke risk factors as mitral valve prolapse, patent foramen ovale, aortic arch atherosclerotic disease, atrial septal aneurysms, valvular strands, and spontaneous echo contrast (a smokelike appearance in the left cardiac chambers visualized on transesophageal echocardiography).

Diabetes also has been associated with increased stroke risk, ranging from relative risks of 1.5 to 3.0, depending on the type and severity. The effect was found in both men and women, did not diminish with age, and was independent of hypertension.

Abnormalities of serum lipids (triglyceride, cholesterol, low-density lipoprotein, high-density lipoprotein) are regarded as risk factors, more for coronary artery disease than for cerebrovascular disease. Older meta-analyses of prospective cohort studies among somewhat younger populations have failed to verify an independent relationship between stroke and elevated cholesterol. Part of this is explained by the recognition that not all strokes are due to atherosclerosis. More recent studies have found a protective effect of high-density lipoprotein for stroke, an association between carotid plaque or intima-media thickness and lipoprotein fractions, and a significant reduction in stroke risk among persons treated with the newest class of cholesterol-reducing medicines known as the statins.

Physical inactivity is a definite predictor of cardiac death, and evidence is accumulating regarding the beneficial effects of physical activity for stroke prevention. In the Northern Manhattan Stroke Study, leisure-time physical activity was found to be significantly associated with a reduced risk of stroke among men and women, young and old, and whites, blacks, and Hispanics. Although a dose-response relationship was found, such that heavier activity and longer duration of activity were more beneficial, even light activities in which elderly individuals can engage, such as walking, conferred a significant protective effect.

Cigarette smoking has been established clearly as a biologically plausible independent determinant of stroke. After controlling for other cardiovascular risk factors, cigarette smoking has been associated with relative risks of brain infarction of 1.7. Stroke risk was greatest in heavy smokers and quickly reduced in those who quit. It was an independent determinant of carotid artery plaque thickness. The association of smoking and subarachnoid hemorrhage is particularly striking. A population-based case-control study in Kings County, Washington, demonstrated an odds ratio of 11.1 for heavy smokers (more than one pack per day) and 4.1 for light smokers (no more than one pack per day) compared with nonsmokers. Overall, the stroke risk attributed to cigarette smoking is greatest for subarachnoid hemorrhage; intermediate for cerebral infarction, for which atherosclerotic stroke may be the most related; and lowest for cerebral hemorrhage.

The role of alcohol as a stroke risk factor depends on stroke subtype and dose. Excess drinking has been shown to be a risk factor for both intracerebral and subarachnoid hemorrhage, whereas the relationship between alcohol and cerebral infarction has been more controversial. Results include a definite independent effect in both men and women, an effect only in men, and no effect after controlling for other confounding risk factors, such as cigarette smoking. A J-shaped relationship between alcohol and ischemic stroke has been noted in a few epidemiologic studies. The relative risk of stroke increased with heavy alcohol consumption (five or more drinks per day) and decreased with light to moderate drinking when compared with nondrinkers. In northern Manhattan, drinking up to two drinks per day was significantly protective for ischemic stroke compared with nondrinkers among old and young subjects, both men and women, and in whites, blacks and Hispanics.

Asymptomatic carotid artery disease, which includes nonstenosing plaque or carotid stenosis, has been found to be associated with an increased stroke risk, particularly among those with more than 75% stenosis. The annual stroke risk was 1.3% in those with no more than 75% stenosis and 3.3% in those with more than 75% stenosis, with an ipsilateral stroke risk of 2.5%. The combined TIA and stroke risk was 10.5% per year in those with more than 75% carotid stenosis. Among persons with asymptomatic carotid artery disease, the occurrence of symptoms may depend on the severity and progression of the stenosis, the adequacy of collateral circulation, the character of the atherosclerotic plaque, and the propensity to form thrombus at the site of the stenosis.

TIAs are a strong indicator of subsequent stroke, with annual stroke risks ranging from 1% to 15%. The first year after a TIA seems to have the greatest stroke risk. Amaurosis fugax or transient monocular blindness has a better outcome than hemispheric ischemic attacks. TIAs, however, precede cerebral infarction in fewer than 20% of patients. The stroke risk after TIA probably depends on the presence and severity of underlying atherosclerotic disease, vascular distribution, adequacy of collateral perfusion, and distribution of confounding risk factors. These variables must be considered before comparing different studies or extrapolating results with the individual patient.

Potential Risk Factors

Other potential stroke risk factors identified by some studies need to be confirmed and clarified in further epidemiologic investigations. Migraine, oral contraceptive use, drug abuse, and snoring have been associated with a higher stroke risk. Various laboratory abnormalities, often reflecting an underlying metabolic or hematologic disturbance, have been associated with

stroke and identified as possible stroke precursors. These include hematocrit, polycythemia, sickle cell anemia, white blood count, fibrinogen, hyperuricemia, hyperhomocysteinemia, protein C and free protein S deficiencies, lupus anticoagulant, and anticardiolipin antibodies. Some are clear stroke risk factors, whereas others require further epidemiologic investigations.

Outcome

The immediate period after an ischemic stroke carries the greatest risk of death, with fatality rates ranging from 8% to 20% in the first 30 days. Death is more likely the result of cardiopulmonary complications rather than of brain death from transtentorial herniation. Case fatality rates are worse for hemorrhagic strokes, ranging from 30% to 80% for intracerebral and 20% to 50% for subarachnoid hemorrhage. Characteristics that can be determined at the onset of stroke and used by the clinician to predict early mortality include impaired consciousness, severity of the initial clinical syndrome, hyperglycemia, and age.

Relatively little is known about the predictors of late stroke outcome. Survivors of the initial ictus continue to have a three to five times increased risk of death compared with the age-matched general population. Annual aggregate estimates of death have been 5% for minor stroke and 8% for major stroke. Survival is influenced by age, hypertension, cardiac disease (myocardial infarction, atrial fibrillation, congestive heart failure), and diabetes. Moreover, patients with lacunar infarcts appear to have a better long-term survival than do those with the other infarct subtypes.

Recurrent stroke is frequent and is responsible for major stroke morbidity and mortality. The immediate period after a stroke carries the greatest risk for early recurrence; rates range from 3% to 10% during the first 30 days. Early stroke recurrence is no trivial matter because of significant worsening of neurologic disability, an increased risk of mortality, and clearly a longer hospital stay. Thirty-day recurrence risks varied by infarct subtypes; the greatest rates were found in patients with atherosclerotic infarction and the lowest rates in patients with lacunes. After the early phase, stroke recurrence continues to threaten the quality

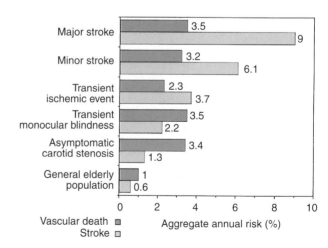

FIG. 35.11. Aggregate estimates of annual vascular events in various subgroups. (Adapted from Wilterdink et al., 1992)

of life after stroke. Long-term stroke recurrence rates range in different studies from 4% to 14% per year, with aggregate annual estimates of 6% for minor stroke and 9% for major stroke (Fig. 35.11).

Universal agreement has not been reached on the predictors of stroke recurrence. Although age is an important predictor of survival after stroke, both young and old are at risk for stroke recurrence. Some studies have found no effect of hypertension and cardiac disease, whereas others have suggested that these factors increased recurrence after stroke. Valvular disease, congestive heart failure, and atrial fibrillation have been found to be determinants of recurrent stroke. In northern Manhattan, hyperglycemia and ethanol abuse, in addition to hypertension, were identified as predictors of stroke recurrence within 5 years. Further studies are required to clarify the predictors of stroke recurrences, which will have increasing public health significance and account for a greater share of the annual cost of stroke-related health care as our population ages and the decline of stroke mortality continues.

SUGGESTED READINGS

Broderick J, Brott T, Kothari R, et al. The Greater Cincinnati/Northern Kentucky Stroke Study: preliminary first-ever and total incidence rates of stroke among blacks. *Stroke* 1998;29:415–421.

Brown RD, Whisnant JP, Sicks RD, et al. Stroke incidence, prevalence, and survival: secular trends in Rochester, Minnesota, through 1989. *Stroke* 1996;27:373–380.

Camargo CA. Moderate alcohol consumption and stroke—the epidemiologic evidence. *Stroke* 1989;20:1611–1626.

Gan R, Sacco RL, Gu Q, Kargman D, Roberts J, Boden-Albala B. Lacunes, lacunar syndromes, and the lacunar hypothesis: the Northern Manhattan Stroke Study experience. *Neurology* 1997;48:1204–1211.

Gorelick PB. Stroke prevention: windows of opportunity and failed expectations—a discussion of modifiable cardiovascular risk factors and a prevention proposal. *Neuroepidemiology* 1997;16:163–173,

Hebert PR, Gaziano JM, Chan KS, Hennekens CH. Cholesterol lowering with statin drugs, risk of stroke, and total mortality. An overview of randomized trials. *JAMA* 1997;278:313–321.

Massaro AR, Sacco RL, Mohr JP, et al. Clinical discriminators between labor and subcortical hemorrhage. *Neurology* 1991;41:1881–1885.

Prospective Studies Collaboration. Cholesterol, diastolic blood pressure, and stroke: 13,000 strokes in 450,000 people in 45 prospective cohorts. *Lancet* 1995;346:1647–1653.

Sacco RL, Benjamin EJ, Broderick JP, et al. Risk Factors Panel—American Heart Association Prevention Conference IV. *Stroke* 1997;28:1507–1517.

Sacco RL, Boden-Albala B, Gan R, et al. Stroke incidence among white, black, and Hispanic residents of an urban community. *Am J Epidemiol* 1998;147:259–268.

Sacco RL, Gan R, Boden-Albala B, et al. Leisure-time physical activity and ischemic stroke risk. The Northern Manhattan Stroke Study. *Stroke* 1998;29:380–387.

Sacco RL, Shi T, Zamanillo MC, Kargman D. Predictors of mortality and recurrence after hospitalized cerebral infarction in an urban community: the Northern Manhattan Stroke Study. *Neurology* 1994;44:626–634.

Sacco RL, Toni D, Mohr JP. Classification of ischemic stroke. In: Barnett HJM, Mohr JP, Stein BM, Yatsu FM, eds. *Stroke—pathophysiology, diagnosis, and management*, 3rd ed. New York: Churchill Livingstone, 1998.

Sacks FM, Pfeffer MA, Moye LA, et al. The effect of pravastatin on coronary events after myocardial infarction in patients with average cholesterol levels. Cholesterol and Recurrent Events Trial Investigators. *N Engl J Med* 1996;335:1001–1009.

Shinton R, Beevers G. Meta-analysis of relation between cigarette smoking and stroke. *Br Med J* 1989;298:789–794.

Wilterdink JL, Easton JD. Vascular event rates in patients with atherosclerotic cerebrovascular disease. *Arch Neurol* 1992;49:857–863.

Wolf PA, D'Agostino RB, Belanger AJ, Kannel WB. Probability of stroke: a risk profile from the Framingham Study. *Stroke* 1991;22:312–318.

Merritt's Neurology, 10th ed., edited by L.P. Rowland. Lippincott Williams & Wilkins, Philadelphia © 2000.

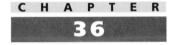

CHAPTER 36

EXAMINATION OF THE PATIENT WITH CEREBROVASCULAR DISEASE

RANDOLPH S. MARSHALL

The goal of the examination of a patient suspected of having a stroke is to gain immediate information about the probable size, location, and etiology of the stroke. Successful treatment depends on starting within a few hours after the onset. Brain imaging has advanced to allow detection of ischemia within minutes to hours after symptoms begin; imaging is necessary to identify hemorrhage before treatment is considered. Nevertheless, the examining physician has the responsibility to identify the symptoms and signs that guide subsequent therapy. For patients who arrive too late, beyond the time window for acute treatment, the neurologic examination is the first step in the diagnostic workup to establish stroke etiology and to start proper treatment aimed at preventing recurrence of stroke.

GENERAL EXAMINATION

Evaluation of the patient with a suspected stroke of large size must first address the level of consciousness and cardiopulmonary status. Irregular or labored breathing and a decreased level of consciousness, particularly if accompanied by gaze deviation, hemiparesis, or unequal pupils, may indicate the need for immediate intubation to treat impending herniation from massive infarction. Reduced alertness is a sign of either extensive hemispheral injury or involvement of the brainstem reticular activating system, which could result from brainstem infarction or from compression on the brainstem by the herniating uncus of the temporal lobe.

The terms "lethargic" and "stuporous" are often used to describe levels of decreasing consciousness, but it is most useful to describe alertness in terms of the minimal stimulus required for a given response (e.g., "opens eyes to voice" or "semipurposeful withdrawal to moderate noxious stimulus"). Subtler impairment of attention and concentration is tested by asking the patient to count backward from 20 to 1 or say the months of the year backward. The level of alertness may fluctuate after injury to the thalamus, often a hemorrhage. Coexisting metabolic derangement such as drug toxicity or hyperglycemia must be ruled out with appropriate laboratory tests. Papilledema is an additional sign of increased intracranial pressure. Cheyne-Stokes respirations with normal level of consciousness may be associated with a smaller territory infarction that involves the insula. Cardiac conduction defects, arrhythmias, subendothelial myocardial infarction, and neurogenic pulmonary edema may occur as a consequence of subarachnoid hemorrhage or large territory infarction, presumably from centrally mediated increase in sympathetic neurotransmitter release. The blood pressure rises acutely in 70% to 80% of stroke patients as a consequence of the infarction or hemorrhage and then returns to baseline spontaneously over the course of a few days. Except for malignant hypertension with encephalopathy or hypertensive cerebral hematoma identified on brain computed tomography, blood pressure is not treated acutely. Nuchal rigidity is often present in subarachnoid hemorrhage. Fever may rarely be caused by brainstem infarction or subarachnoid hemorrhage. A systemic etiology must be sought and treated, however, because fever can exacerbate ischemic brain injury.

Beyond the examination required for emergency management of acute stroke, the general examination should focus on the cardiovascular system to seek a likely stroke etiology. Examination of the neck includes auscultation for carotid bruits, which result from turbulent flow in an artery narrowed by an atherosclerotic plaque. Auscultation of bruits may be misleading if the sound arises from stenosis of the unimportant external carotid artery or if the degree of stenosis in the internal carotid artery is great enough to dampen flow velocity below that which produces an audible bruit. Doppler ultrasound or magnetic resonance angiogram of the neck is needed if carotid stenosis is suspected. Fundoscopy can show retinal arterial narrowing, subhyloid hemorrhages, or cotton wool spots—systemic signs of hypertension or diabetes.

The presence of murmurs or arrhythmia on cardiac examination suggests valvular disease or atrial fibrillation, both independent risk factors and indications for anticoagulation therapy to prevent recurrence of stroke. The presence of fever with a cardiac murmur requires blood culture to rule out bacterial endocarditis. Auscultation of the lungs is important as a means of identifying signs of aspiration pneumonia or pulmonary edema caused by congestive heart failure.

NEUROLOGIC EVALUATION

The neurologic examination can provide valuable clues to the size, location, and etiology of the stroke. A few syndromes are predictive of specific stroke etiologies. For example, Wernicke aphasia, homonymous hemianopia, and the "top-of-the-basilar"

syndrome of cortical blindness, agitation, and amnesia are nearly always caused by embolism from a proximal arterial or cardiac source. The Wallenberg syndrome, due to infarction of the dorsolateral medulla, is typically caused by thrombosis of the vertebral artery. The "lacunar syndromes" (see below) nearly always result from lipohyalinosis and fibrinoid necrosis of small penetrating arterioles arising from the middle cerebral artery stems, the basilar artery, or the first portion of the posterior cerebral arteries. The severity of the clinical syndrome at onset is highly correlated with the ultimate functional outcome. Level of alertness, ocular motility, motor power, and higher cerebral function are the keys to initial assessment. The most common sign of large stroke is the combination of gaze deviation, hemiparesis, and altered mentation. Hyperhydrosis, or excessive sweating, sometimes unilateral, may also occur in brainstem hemorrhage or large hemisphere stroke. In a comatose patient, asymmetry of tendon reflexes supports a diagnosis of unilateral brain injury when motor and sensory testing are not possible. Hypotonia may occur early after stroke, whereas tone often increases only after several days.

Even if fully alert, patients with gaze deviation and hemiparesis who are within the first several hours after stroke onset are at high risk for profound clinical worsening because of an edema-related mass effect that may peak as late as 3 to 5 days after stroke. Gaze palsies often occur with infarction involving the dorsolateral frontal lobes, producing gaze deviation to the opposite side of the hemiparesis. Infarction of the lateral pons, on the other hand, produces hemiparesis on the same side as the direction of forced gaze. Other ocular dysmotility syndromes, including internuclear ophthalmoplegia, vertical gaze palsies, and nystagmus, may also occur with smaller infarcts in the brainstem. Visual fields should be tested by asking the patient to count fingers or identify a moving finger in each of four visual quadrants. Homonymous hemianopia may be the only sign of a large posterior cerebral artery territory infarction. An upper or lower homonymous quadrantanopia is produced by infarction involving the optic radiations hugging the lateral ventricular wall in the temporal or parietal lobe, respectively. A sectoranopia may be produced by injury to the lateral geniculate body of the thalamus due to anterior choroidal artery embolism.

Cortical involvement is suggested when aphasia or hemineglect are present. As a sign of dominant hemisphere injury, aphasia may involve abnormal naming, fluency, comprehension, repetition, reading, or writing. Dysfluency predominates with frontal lobe injury, whereas comprehension deficits predominate with posterior temporal and parietal injury. Severe Wernicke aphasia is characterized by poor auditory and reading comprehension and fluent speech littered with paraphasic errors; the syndrome may be misdiagnosed as delirium in the emergency room. Hemineglect, produced most often by nondominant parietal or frontal lobe injury, can be identified by unilateral extinction of visual or tactile stimuli when bilateral stimuli are presented. Rightward deviation on a line bisection test and failure to identify stimuli on the left side of an array of stimuli are also reliable signs of left hemineglect. Short-term verbal memory may be acutely affected by stroke when one or both anteromedial thalami or medial temporal lobes are involved. Short-term memory is easily tested by asking the patient to recall three objects after a

5-minute delay. Long-term memory impairment may appear as disorientation or dementia in a patient with multiple prior strokes in both hemispheres.

Unilateral weakness is typical of stroke. A complete characterization of the motor loss is important because the distribution and time course of weakness will differ by stroke location and etiology. Proximal and distal upper and lower limbs should be assessed independently on a five-point scale of power. Subtle weakness may be apparent only by the presence of a flattened nasolabial fold or widened palpebral fissure on one side of the face or a unilateral pronator drift when the patient is asked to hold the arms outstretched, palms up. Slowed or clumsy fine movements of one hand or ataxic dysmetria on finger-nose-finger may follow a stroke involving either the contralateral corticospinal tract or the ipsilateral cerebellum or cerebellar connections to the brainstem.

Weakness affecting the face, arm, and leg equally in a fully awake patient implies a small infarct in a deep brain region such as the posterior limb of the internal capsule, where the fibers of the corticospinal tract converge into a small anatomic area. This "pure motor hemiparesis" is one of four classic lacunar syndromes caused by small deep infarcts in the capsule, basal ganglia, thalamus, or pons. Hemicorporeal sensory loss is the syndrome associated with a thalamic lacune. "Clumsy hand dysarthria" or "ataxic hemiparesis" may result from lacunes in the corticospinal tract at any level from the corona radiata to the pons. "Fractionated hemiparesis," for example facio-linguo-brachial paresis with little or no leg weakness, suggests cortical involvement of the perisylvian region due to embolic occlusion of a branch of the middle cerebral artery. An even smaller middle cerebral artery branch occlusion may produce isolated hand weakness, mimicking an ulnar or median neuropathy. Weakness that affects the leg suggests a paramedian infarction due to embolic occlusion of the anterior cerebral artery. Arm and face weakness from anterior cerebral artery infarction may be due to motor neglect as a consequence of injury to the paramedian supplementary motor area and cingulate gyrus. Weakness of the proximal arm and leg sparing facial and lingual function is the most common result of "borderzone" ischemia due to hemodynamic failure from high-grade internal carotid artery stenosis. In patients with severe carotid occlusive disease, an attack of unilateral tremor or limb shaking may rarely be precipitated by standing, a sign that can be mistaken for focal seizure. Weakness due to hemodynamic failure from large vessel atherostenosis may fluctuate before becoming a fixed hemiparesis. Stroke syndromes due to an embolic arterial occlusion are usually maximal at onset. Weakness caused by lacunar disease may sometimes have a stuttering stepwise worsening course over several days.

SUGGESTED READINGS

Barnett HJM, Mohr JP, Stein BM, Yatsu FM, eds. *Stroke: pathophysiology, diagnosis and management*, 3rd ed. New York: Churchill Livingstone, 1998.

Binder JR, Marshall R, Lazar RM, Benjamin JL, Mohr JP. Distinct syndromes of hemineglect. *Arch Neurol* 1992;49:1187–1194.

Chamorro A, Marshall RS, Valls-Solé J, Tolosa E, Mohr JP. Motor behavior in stroke patients with isolated medial frontal ischemic infarction. *Stroke* 1997;28:1755–1760.

Chimowitz MI, Furlan AJ, Sila CA, et al. Etiology of motor or sensory stroke: a prospective study of the predictive value of clinical and radiological features. *Ann Neurol* 1991;30:519–525.

Fisher CM. Lacunar infarcts. A review. *Cerebrovasc Dis* 1991;1:311–320.

Ginsberg MD, Busto R. Combating hyperthermia in acute stroke: a significant clinical concern. *Stroke* 1998;29:529–534.

Mayer SA, LiMandri G, Sherman D, et al. Electrocardiographic markers of abnormal left ventricular wall motion in acute subarachnoid hemorrhage. *J Neurosurg* 1995;83:889–896.

Mohr JP, Foulkes MA, Plois AT, et al. Infarct topography and hemiparesis profiles with cerebral convexity infarction: the Stroke Data Bank. *J Neurol Neurosurg Psychiatry* 1993;56:344–351.

Oxbury JM, Greenhall RCD, Grainger KMR. Predicting the outcome of stroke: acute stage after cerebral infarction. *Br Med J* 1975;3:125–127.

Tatemichi TK, Young WL, Prohovnik I, Gitelman DR, Correll JW, Mohr JP. Perfusion insufficiency in limb-shaking transient ischemic attacks. *Stroke* 1990;21:341–347.

Tijssen CC, van Gisbergen JAM, Schulte BPM. Conjugate eye deviation: side, site, and size of the hemispheric lesion. *Neurology* 1991;41:846–850.

Merritt's Neurology, 10th ed., edited by L.P. Rowland. Lippincott Williams & Wilkins, Philadelphia © 2000.

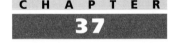

CHAPTER 37

TRANSIENT ISCHEMIC ATTACK

JOHN C.M. BRUST

Transient ischemic attack (TIA) describes neurologic symptoms of ischemic origin that last less than 24 hours. In fact, most attacks last only a few minutes to an hour. TIAs have more than one mechanism. When severe major carotid or vertebrobasilar stenosis is present, transient thrombosis could be operative; such TIAs tend to be brief. Attacks without severe stenosis tend to last longer and often are associated with distal branch occlusion, thereby suggesting embolism from an ulcerated plaque or a more proximal source. Some TIAs, especially vertebrobasilar, may have a hemodynamic basis, including transient hypotension and cardiac arrhythmia, and TIAs responsive to calcium-channel blockers suggest vasospasm. In the *subclavian steal syndrome*, stenosis of the left subclavian artery proximal to the origin of the vertebral artery leads to brainstem, cerebellar, or even cerebral symptoms, often during exertion and accompanied by symptoms of left arm claudication. Other TIAs may be a consequence of primary intraparenchymal vascular disease. They also have been associated with either anemia or polycythemia; such TIAs clear with correction of the underlying disorder.

Symptoms vary with the arterial territory involved. *Transient monocular blindness (amaurosis fugax)* from ischemia in the territory of the central retinal artery, a branch of the ophthalmic artery and ultimately the internal carotid artery, consists of blurring or darkening of vision, peaking within a few seconds, sometimes as if a curtain had descended, and usually clearing within minutes. In some patients, embolic particles (Hollenhorst plaques) are seen in retinal artery branches. Carotid territory TIAs that involve the brain produce varying combinations of limb weakness and sensory loss, aphasia, hemineglect, and homonymous hemianopia. Posterior circulation TIAs cause symptoms referable to the cerebrum (visual field loss or cortical blindness), brainstem (cranial nerve and long tract symptoms, sometimes crossed or bilateral), and cerebellum. Some TIAs consist of pure hemiparesis or pure hemisensory loss, thus suggesting intrinsic disease of small intraparenchymal penetrating vessels. Patients with recurrent TIAs tend to have the same type of attack each time.

The diagnosis of TIA can be difficult when symptoms are ambiguous (e.g., staggering or "drop attacks"; dizziness, light-headedness, or syncope; vertigo; fleeting diplopia; transient amnesia; atypical visual disturbance in one or both eyes such as flashes, distortions, or tunnel vision; a heavy sensation or "tiredness" in one or more limbs; and paresthesias in an area of fixed sensory loss or briefly affecting only one limb). The differential diagnosis of TIAs includes migraine, cardiac arrhythmia, seizures, hypoglycemia, and neurosis.

Although TIAs are defined in terms of their clinical reversibility and are presumed to signify ischemia too brief or incomplete to cause infarction, computed tomography and magnetic resonance imaging frequently demonstrate appropriately located infarcts. Attacks that take longer than 24 hours to clear or that leave mild residua are called reversible ischemic neurologic deficit.

The major significance of TIAs is prognostic. Such patients are at increased risk for both myocardial infarction and major stroke. "Crescendo TIAs"—two or more attacks within 24 hours—represent a medical emergency (see Chapter 44).

SUGGESTED READINGS

Bots ML, van der Wilk EC, Koudstaal PJ, et al. Transient neurological attacks in the general population. Prevalence, risk factors, and clinical relevance. *Stroke* 1997;28:768–773.

Caplan LC. TIAs. *Neurology* 1988;38:791–793.

Dennis M, Bamford J, Sandercock P, Warlow C. Prognosis of transient ischemic attacks in the Oxfordshire Community Stroke Project. *Stroke* 1990;21:848–853.

Evans GW, Howard G, Murros KE, et al. Cerebral infarction verified by cranial computed tomography and prognosis for survival following transient ischemic attack. *Stroke* 1991;22:431–436.

Hanley GJ, Slattery JM, Warlow CP. Transient ischemic attacks: which patients are at high (and low) risk of serious vascular events? *J Neurol Neurosurg Psychiatry* 1992;55:640–652.

Hennerici M, Klemm C, Rautenberg W. The subclavian steal phenomenon: a common vascular disorder with rare neurologic deficits. *Neurology* 1988;38:669–673.

Hornig CR, Lammers C, Buttner T, et al. Long-term prognosis of infratentorial transient ischemic attacks and minor strokes. *Stroke* 1992;23:199–204.

Kappelle LJ, van Latum JC, Koudstaal PJ, van Gijn J. Transient ischemic attacks and small vessel disease. *Lancet* 1991;337:339–341.

Koudstaal PJ, Algra A, Pop GAM, et al. Risk of cardiac events in atypical transient ischemic attack or minor stroke. *Lancet* 1992;340:630–633.

Koudstaal PJ, van Gijn J, Frenken CWGM, et al. TIA, RIND, minor stroke: a continuum, or different subgroups? *J Neurol Neurosurg Psychiatry* 1992;55:95–97.

Shahar A, Sadeh M. Severe anemia associated with transient neurological deficits. *Stroke* 1991;22:1201–1202.

Winterkorn JMS, Kupersmith MJ, Wirtschafter JD, et al. Treatment of vasospastic amaurosis fugax with calcium-channel blockers. *N Engl J Med* 1993;329:396–398.

Merritt's Neurology, 10th ed., edited by L.P. Rowland. Lippincott Williams & Wilkins, Philadelphia © 2000.

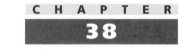

CHAPTER 38

CEREBRAL INFARCTION

JOHN C.M. BRUST

Ischemic syndromes of specific vessels depend not only on the site of the occlusion but on previous brain damage, collateral circulation, and variations in the region supplied by a particular artery, including aberrations in the circle of Willis (e.g., if both anterior cerebral arteries arise from a common trunk, carotid artery occlusion may cause bilateral leg weakness; if one or both posterior cerebral arteries arise from the internal carotid, occlusion of the basilar artery is less likely to cause visual symptoms). Syndromes of specific vessels do not always define the site or the nature of the occlusion (e.g., infarction in the region of the middle cerebral artery is often the result of thrombotic occlusion of the internal carotid artery; occlusion of the middle cerebral artery or its branches is usually embolic). Nonetheless, knowledge of individual artery syndromes helps the clinician to localize a lesion and to determine whether it is vascular (Figs. 38.1 to 38.5 and Table 38.1).

SPECIFIC VESSEL OCCLUSIONS

Middle Cerebral Artery

Infarction in the region of the middle cerebral artery causes contralateral weakness, sensory loss, homonymous hemianopia, and, depending on the hemisphere involved, either language disturbance or impaired spatial perception. If the artery's main trunk

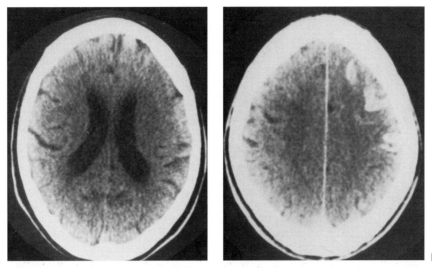

FIG. 38.1. Cerebral infarction, 1 week after stroke. **A:** Before injection of contrast material, computed tomography was normal. **B:** After injection of contrast material, there was gyral enhancement in a pattern conforming to the distribution of the middle cerebral artery. (Courtesy of Drs. S.K. Hilal and S.R. Ganti.)

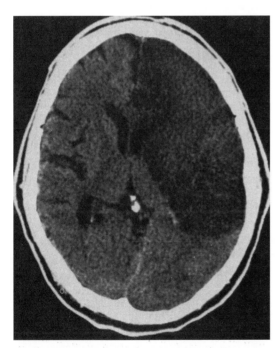

FIG. 38.2. Subacute infarct, anterior and middle cerebral artery distributions. Noncontrast axial computed tomography demonstrates radiolucency in the left basal ganglia and frontal and temporal opercula extending through the cortex. Note sulcal effacement and mild shift due to recent infarction involving the left anterior and middle cerebral artery territories; the left posterior cerebral artery territory is spared. (Courtesy of Drs. J.A. Bello and S.K. Hilal.)

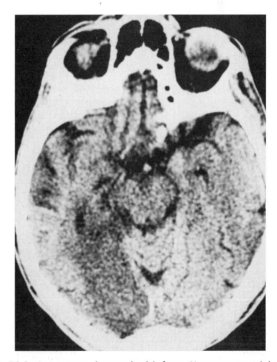

FIG. 38.3. Acute posterior cerebral infarct. Noncontrast axial computed tomography shows right occipital lucency, corresponding to posterior cerebral vascular distribution with mild mass effect (sulcal effacement) due to acute infarction and edema. (Courtesy of Drs. J.A. Bello and S.K. Hilal.)

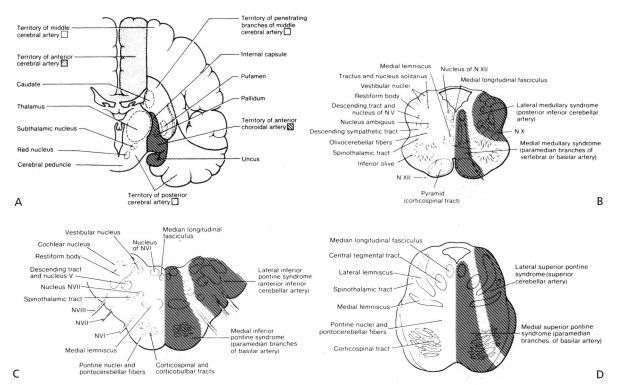

FIG. 38.4. Arterial territories of the cerebrum **(A)**, of the medulla **(B)**, of the lower pons **(C)**, and of the upper pons **(D)**.

is occluded, infarction affects the cerebral convexity and deep structures, including not only the motor and sensory cortices over the cerebral convexity but also the posterior limb of the internal capsule; the face, arm, and leg are equally affected by weakness and sensory loss. If infarction spares the diencephalon after occlusion of the upper division, weakness and sensory loss are greater in the face and arm than in the leg. When infarction is limited to the region of the rolandic branch, such weakness and sensory loss may be the only signs. A small infarct or lacune in the internal capsule (from occlusion of a penetrating lenticulostriate branch of the proximal middle cerebral artery) may cause a syndrome of pure hemiparesis affecting face, arm, and leg but with no other symptoms.

With cerebral lesions, motor and sensory loss tend to be greatest distally, perhaps because the proximal limbs and the trunk are more likely to be represented in both hemispheres. Paraspinal muscles, for example, are rarely weak in unilateral cerebral disease, which also spares muscles of the forehead, pharynx, and jaw. Tongue weakness is variable. If weakness is severe, muscle tone usually decreases initially and then gradually increases in days or weeks to spasticity with hyperactive tendon reflexes. A Babinski sign is usually present from the outset. When weakness is mild or during recovery, there is more clumsiness and incoordination than loss of strength.

There is often paresis of contralateral conjugate gaze after an acute lesion in the so-called frontal gaze center anterior to the prerolandic motor cortex or in its subcortical connections; the gaze palsy usually lasts only 1 or 2 days, even when other signs remain severe. Sensory loss tends to involve discriminative and proprioceptive modalities. Pain and temperature sensation may be impaired but are seldom lost. Joint position sense, however,

TABLE 38.1. SYNDROMES OF CEREBRAL INFARCTION

Artery Occluded	Syndrome
Common carotid	Asymptomatic
Internal carotid	Ipsilateral blindness
	Contralateral hemiparesis and hemianesthesia
	Hemianopia
	Aphasia or denial and hemineglect
Middle cerebral	
Main trunk	Hemiplegia
	Hemianesthesia
	Hemianopia
	Aphasia or denial and hemineglect
Upper division	Hemiparesis and sensory loss (arm and face more affected than leg)
	Broca aphasia or denial and hemineglect
Lower division	Wernicke aphasia or nondominant behavior disorder without hemiparesis
Penetrating artery	Pure motor hemiparesis
Anterior cerebral	Hemiparesis and sensory loss affect leg more than arm
	Impaired responsiveness ("abulia" or "akinetic mutism"), especially if bilateral infarction
	Left-sided ideomotor apraxia or tactile anomia
Posterior cerebral	Cortical, unilateral: isolated hemianopia (or quadrantic field cut); alexia or color anomia
	Cortical, bilateral: cerebral blindness, with or without macular sparing
	Thalamic: pure sensory stroke; may leave anesthesia dolorosa with "spontaneous pain"
	Subthalamic nucleus: hemiballism
	Bilateral inferior temporal lobe: amnesia
	Midbrain: oculomotor palsy and other eye-movement abnormalities

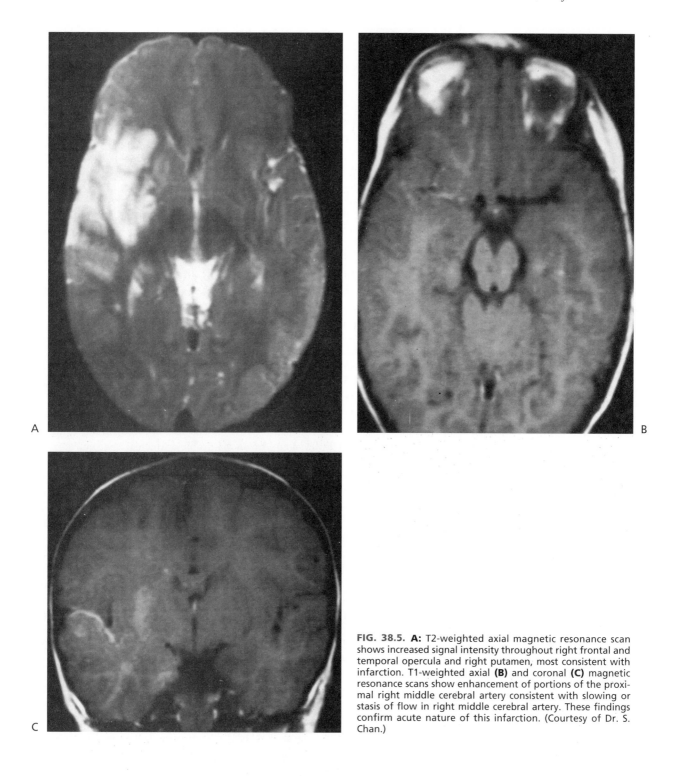

FIG. 38.5. A: T2-weighted axial magnetic resonance scan shows increased signal intensity throughout right frontal and temporal opercula and right putamen, most consistent with infarction. T1-weighted axial **(B)** and coronal **(C)** magnetic resonance scans show enhancement of portions of the proximal right middle cerebral artery consistent with slowing or stasis of flow in right middle cerebral artery. These findings confirm acute nature of this infarction. (Courtesy of Dr. S. Chan.)

may be severely disturbed, causing limb ataxia or pseudoathetosis, and there may be loss of two-point discrimination, astereognosis, or failure to appreciate a touch stimulus if another is delivered simultaneously to the normal side of the body ("extinction"). Homonymous hemianopia is the result of damage to the optic radiations. If the lesion is primarily parietal, the field cut may be an inferior quadrantanopia; with temporal lesions, quadrantanopia is superior.

A lesion of the left opercular (perisylvian) cortex is likely to cause aphasia; when damage is widespread, the aphasia is global,

causing muteness or nonfluent and amelodic speech and severe impairment of speech comprehension, writing, and reading abilities. Restricted damage from branch occlusions can cause an aphasic syndrome. Frontal opercular lesions tend to cause Broca aphasia, with impaired speaking and writing ability but with relative preservation of comprehension. (The relative contributions of cortical and white matter damage to this type of aphasia are controversial.) With posterior periopercular lesions, fluency and prosody are preserved, but paraphasia can reduce speech output to jargon; there may be impairment of speech comprehension and naming, repetition, reading, and writing abilities in different combinations. When aphasia is severe, there is usually some impairment of nonlanguage cognitive functions; when aphasia is global, dementia is obvious. With Broca or global aphasia, hemiparesis is usually severe. When aphasia is the result of a restricted posterior lesion, hemiparesis is mild. Aphasia in left-handed patients, regardless of the hemisphere involved, tends to be milder and resolves more rapidly than in right-handed patients with left hemisphere injury.

Left hemisphere convexity lesions, especially parietal, may cause bilateral ideomotor apraxia, in which the patient cannot perform learned motor acts on command but can describe the act and perform it when the setting is altered (e.g., after the examiner has given the patient an object the use of which the patient could not imitate). Buccolingual apraxia often accompanies Broca aphasia. Ideational apraxia (loss of understanding of the purpose of actions and difficulty manipulating objects) follows bilateral hemisphere damage and associated dementia. Infarction of the angular or supramarginal gyri of the dominant hemisphere can cause Gerstmann syndrome (i.e., agraphia, acalculia, left-right confusion, and finger agnosia).

Right hemisphere convexity infarction, especially parietal, causes disturbances of spatial perception; the patient has difficulty copying simple pictures or diagrams (constructional apraxia or apractognosia), interpreting maps, maintaining physical orientation (topographagnosia), or putting on clothing (dressing apraxia). Difficulty recognizing faces (prosopagnosia) is attributed to bilateral temporooccipital lesions. Hemineglect, a tendency to ignore the contralateral half of one's body or of external space, follows damage to the parietal lobe (or, rarely, the diencephalon), right more often than left. Patients may not recognize the hemiplegia (anosognosia), their arm (asomatognosia), or any external object to the left of their own midline. These phenomena can occur without visual field defects in patients who are otherwise mentally intact. Patients with right hemisphere convexity damage may have difficulty expressing or recognizing nonpropositional aspects of speech ("pragmatics"), such as emotional tone, sarcasm, or jokes. Right hemisphere lesions may also produce an acute confusional state.

Anterior Cerebral Artery

Infarction in the area of the anterior cerebral artery causes weakness, clumsiness, and sensory loss affecting mainly the distal contralateral leg. There may be urinary incontinence. Damage to the "supplementary motor area" may cause a speech disturbance that is considered aphasic by some physicians and a kind of motor inertia by others. There may be motor neglect, an apparent disinclination to use the contralateral limbs despite little or no weakness. Involvement of the anterior corpus callosum may cause tactile anomia or ideomotor apraxia of the left limbs, which is attributed to the disconnection of the left language-dominant hemisphere from the right motor or sensory cortex. If the damage includes the territory supplied by the major diencephalic branch (recurrent artery of Heubner), the anterior limb of the internal capsule is affected and the face or even the arm is also weak. Infarction restricted to structures supplied by the artery of Heubner (caudate nucleus and, variably, head of putamen and

anterior limb of internal capsule) causes unpredictable combinations of dysarthria, abulia, agitation, contralateral neglect, and language disturbance.

Bilateral infarction in the anterior cerebral artery region can cause a severe behavior disturbance, with apathy (abulia), motor inertia, muteness, incontinence, suck and grasp reflexes, and diffuse rigidity (gegenhalten) or total unresponsiveness with open eyes (akinetic mutism). Symptoms and signs are attributed to destruction of the orbitofrontal cortex, deep limbic structures, supplementary motor area, or cingulate gyri.

Posterior Cerebral Artery

Occlusion of the posterior cerebral artery most often causes contralateral homonymous hemianopia by destroying the calcarine cortex. Macular (central) vision tends to be spared because the occipital pole receives a collateral blood supply from the middle cerebral artery. Unilateral lesions are sometimes associated with visual perseveration (palinopsia) or release hallucinations in the blind field.

If the lesion affects the dominant hemisphere and includes the posterior corpus callosum, there may be alexia (without aphasia or agraphia) attributed to disconnection of the right occipital cortex (vision) from the left hemisphere (language). Such patients often have anomia for colors.

When infarction is bilateral, there may be cortical blindness, and sometimes the patient does not recognize or admit the loss of vision (Anton syndrome). Macular sparing, on the other hand, may produce tunnel vision. Other unusual phenomena of bilateral occipital injury are simultanagnosia (inability to synthesize the parts of what is seen into a whole), poor eye–hand coordination, difficulty coordinating gaze, metamorphopsia (distortion of what is seen, associated especially with occipitotemporal lesions), and visual agnosia.

Bilateral (and rarely unilateral) infarction in the posterior cerebral artery's supply to the inferomedial temporal lobe or medial thalamus causes memory disturbance, sometimes so severe and lasting as to resemble Korsakoff syndrome. It is possible that some cases of transient global amnesia represent transient ischemic attacks of this region. Patients with bilateral lesions affecting both the occipital and temporal lobes may present with agitated delirium.

If posterior cerebral artery occlusion is proximal, the lesions may include the thalamus or midbrain, which are supplied by interpeduncular, paramedian, thalamoperforating, and thalamogeniculate branches. Infarction of the ventral posterior nucleus causes severe loss of all sensory modalities on the opposite side or sometimes dissociated sensory loss with relative preservation of touch, proprioception, and discriminative modalities or conversely of pain and temperature sensation. As sensation returns, there may be intractable persistent pain and hyperpathia on the affected side ("thalamic pain," "analgesia dolorosa," or Roussy-Dejerine syndrome). A lesion of the subthalamic nucleus causes contralateral hemiballism.

Several abnormal eye signs may be found when posterior cerebral artery disease affects the midbrain: bilateral (or, less often, unilateral) loss of vertical gaze, convergence spasm, retractatory nystagmus, lid retraction (Collier sign), oculomotor palsy, internuclear ophthalmoplegia, decreased pupillary reactivity, and corectopia (eccentrically positioned pupil). Lethargy or coma follows damage to the reticular activating system. Peduncular hallucinosis, often consisting of formed and vivid hallucinations, can occur with infarcts restricted to either the thalamus or the pars reticulata of the substantia nigra. Posterior cerebral artery occlusion can cause contralateral hemiparesis by damaging the midbrain peduncle; it also causes contralateral ataxia by affecting the superior cerebellar outflow above its decussation.

Anterior Choroidal Artery

Infarction in the area of the anterior choroidal artery produces inconsistent deficits, with varying combinations of contralateral hemiplegia, sensory loss, and homonymous hemianopia that sometimes spares a beaklike zone horizontally (upper and lower homonymous sectoranopia). Responsible structures include the midbrain peduncle or posterior limb of the internal capsule and the lateral geniculate body or early optic radiations. Symptoms are often incomplete and temporary.

Internal Carotid Artery

Internal carotid occlusion may be clinically silent or may cause massive cerebral infarction. Damage occurs most often in the territory of the middle cerebral artery or, depending on collateral circulation, of one of its branches, with syndromes of varying severity. When the anterior communicating artery is not present, infarction may include the territory of the anterior cerebral artery. Internal carotid artery occlusion (or abrupt hypotension in someone with tight stenosis) can also cause infarction in the border zones ("watersheds") between the middle, anterior, and posterior cerebral arteries; syncope at onset, focal seizures, and transcortical aphasia (relatively preserved repetition) are often seen with such lesions. When the posterior cerebral artery arises directly from the internal carotid, there may be symptoms referable to the visual cortex, thalamus, inferior temporal lobe, or upper brainstem. Infrequently, carotid artery disease causes vertebrobasilar transient ischemic attacks.

Emboli dislodged from atherosclerotic plaques in the internal carotid artery reach the retina through the ophthalmic and central retinal arteries to cause partial or complete visual loss. Platelet-fibrin or cholesterol emboli can sometimes be seen ophthalmoscopically in retinal artery branches.

Bilateral border zone infarction after severe hypotension can cause cortical blindness (from parietooccipital damage at the common border zone between the three major arterial territories) or bibrachial palsy (from bilateral rolandic damage at the border zone of the anterior and middle cerebral arteries).

Vertebrobasilar Arteries

Several eponyms have been applied to brainstem syndromes, but except for the lateral medullary syndrome of Wallenberg, most original descriptions concerned patients with neoplasms. Brainstem infarction is more often the result of occlusion of the vertebral or basilar arteries than of their paramedian or lateral branches; classic medial or lateral brainstem syndromes are en-

countered less often than incomplete or mixed clinical pictures (Table 38.1). That an infarct involves posterior fossa structures is suggested by bilateral long tract (motor or sensory) signs; crossed (e.g., left face and right limb) motor or sensory signs; dissociated sensory loss on one half of the body, with pain and temperature sensation more involved than proprioception; cerebellar signs; stupor or coma; dysconjugate eye movements or nystagmus, including internuclear ophthalmoplegia; Horner syndrome; and involvement of cranial nerves not usually affected by single hemispheric infarcts (e.g., unilateral deafness or pharyngeal weakness). Brainstem infarction may cause only unilateral weakness indistinguishable from that seen with lacunes in the internal capsule.

SYNDROMES OF INFARCTION

Lateral Medullary Infarction

This infarction usually follows occlusion of the vertebral or, less often, the posterior inferior cerebellar artery (Fig. 38.6). Manifestations include vertigo, nausea, vomiting, and nystagmus (from involvement of the vestibular nuclei); gait and ipsilateral limb ataxia (cerebellum or inferior cerebellar peduncle); impaired pain and temperature sensation on the ipsilateral face (spinal tract and nucleus of the trigeminal nerve) and the contralateral body (spinothalamic tract); dysphagia, hoarseness, and ipsilateral weakness of the palate and vocal cords and decrease of

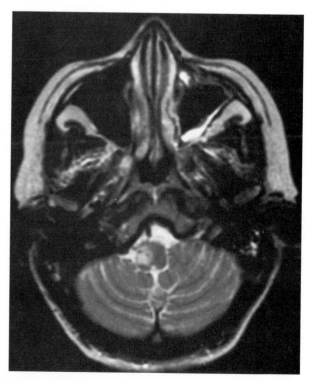

FIG. 38.6. T2-weighted axial magnetic resonance scan demonstrates a single focus of increased signal intensity within the posterior aspect of the right medulla, consistent with an early infarct. This infarct accounted for the patient's acute presentation with the lateral medullary syndrome of Wallenberg, secondary to occlusion of a branch of the right posterior inferior cerebellar artery. (Courtesy of Dr. S. Chan.)

the gag reflex (nucleus ambiguus, or ninth and tenth nerve outflow tracts); and ipsilateral Horner syndrome (descending sympathetic fibers). There may be hiccup and, if the nucleus or tractus solitarius is affected, ipsilateral loss of taste. Some patients have loss of pain and temperature sensation over the contralateral and ipsilateral face (from involvement of the crossed ascending ventral trigeminothalamic tract) and some develop chronic pain, similar to "thalamic pain," in the ipsilateral face or contralateral limbs (Table 38.2).

Infarction of Medial Medulla

An infarction of the medial medulla usually follows an occlusion of a vertebral artery or a branch of the lower basilar artery and involves the pyramidal tract, medial lemniscus, and hypoglossal nucleus or outflow tract. There is ipsilateral tongue weakness (with deviation toward the paretic side) and contralateral hemiparesis and impaired proprioception, but cutaneous sensation is spared.

Lateral Pontine Infarction

This may affect caudal structures when there is occlusion of the anterior inferior cerebellar artery or rostral structures after occlusion of the superior cerebellar artery. The caudal syndrome resembles that of lateral medullary infarction, with vertigo, nystagmus, ataxia, Horner syndrome, and crossed face-and-body pain and temperature loss. There is ipsilateral deafness and tinnitus (from involvement of the cochlear nuclei); if damage includes more medial structures, there is ipsilateral gaze paresis or facial weakness. Rostral lateral pontine infarction causes the same constellation of symptoms except that the seventh and eighth cranial nerves are spared and there is ipsilateral paresis of the jaw muscles.

Medial Pontine Infarction Syndromes

These syndromes occur after occlusion of paramedian branches of the basilar artery and depend on whether the lesion is caudal or rostral. A constant feature is contralateral hemiparesis. When the lesion includes the nucleus of the VIIth nerve, there is ipsilateral facial weakness; when damage is more rostral, facial paresis is contralateral. There also may be dysarthria (corticobulbar projections to the hypoglossal nucleus), ipsilateral gaze palsy (abducens nucleus or paramedian reticular formation), abducens palsy (VIth nerve outflow tract), internuclear ophthalmoplegia (median longitudinal fasciculus), and limb or gait ataxia. Caudal lesions can cause contralateral loss of proprioception. Palatal myoclonus is attributed to involvement of the central tegmental tract and may be accompanied by rhythmic movements of the pharynx, larynx, face, eyes, or respiratory muscles.

Other Posterior Fossa Syndromes

A small infarct in the paramedian basis pontis affecting the pyramidal tract, nuclei of the basis pontis, and crossing pontocerebellar fibers can cause either ataxic hemiparesis, with contralateral weakness and cerebellar ataxia, or dysarthria clumsy-hand syndrome, with dysarthria and contralateral upper limb ataxia. Why the cerebellar signs should be entirely contralateral is unclear.

Symptoms resembling acute labyrinthitis, with vertigo, nausea, vomiting, and nystagmus, may accompany either infarction of the inferior cerebellum or occlusion of the internal auditory artery, which arises from the basilar or anterior inferior cerebellar arteries, with resulting infarction of the inner ear. Large cerebellar infarcts may mimic cerebellar hemorrhage, with headache, dizziness, ataxia, and, if there is brainstem compression, abducens or gaze palsy and progression to coma and death.

TABLE 38.2. SIGNS THAT INDICATE THE LEVEL OF BRAINSTEM VASCULAR SYNDROMES

Syndrome	Artery Affected	Structure Involved	Manifestations
Medial syndromes			
Medulla	Paramedian branches	Emerging fibers of 12th nerve	Ipsilateral hemiparalysis of tongue
Inferior pons	Paramedian branches	Pontine gaze center, near or in nucleus of sixth nerve	Paralysis of gaze to side of lesion
		Emerging fibers of sixth nerve	Ipsilateral abduction paralysis
Superior pons	Paramedian branches	Medial longitudinal fasciculus	Internuclear ophthalmoplegia
Lateral syndromes			
Medulla	Posterior inferior cerebellar	Emerging fibers of 9th and 10th nerves	Dysphagia, hoarseness, ipsilateral paralysis of vocal cord; ipsilateral loss of pharyngeal reflex
		Vestibular nuclei	Vertigo, nystagmus
		Descending tract and nucleus of fifth nerve	Ipsilateral facial analgesia
		Solitary nucleus and tract	Taste loss on ipsilateral half of tongue posteriorly
Inferior pons	Anterior inferior cerebellar	Emerging fibers of seventh nerve	Ipsilateral facial paralysis
		Solitary nucleus and tract	Taste loss on ipsilateral half of tongue anteriorly
		Cochlear nuclei	Deafness, tinnitus
Mid-pons		Motor nucleus of fifth nerve	Ipsilateral jaw weakness
		Emerging sensory fibers of fifth nerve	Ipsilateral facial numbness

Modified from Rowland LP. In: Kandel ER, Schwartz JH, eds. *Principles of neural science*, 3rd ed. New York: Elsevier, 1991.

Drop attacks are caused by fleeting loss of strength or muscle tone without loss of consciousness; bilateral ischemia of the pontine or medullary pyramidal tract is the explanation in some cases. Infarction of the corticobulbar and corticospinal tracts in the basis pontis (sparing the tegmentum) causes the "locked-in syndrome," with paralysis of limbs and lower cranial nerves; communication by preserved eye movements reveals that consciousness is intact.

Midbrain Infarction

This follows occlusion of the posterior cerebral artery, but the classic mesencephalic syndromes (oculomotor palsy with contralateral hemiparesis, the Weber syndrome, or crossed hemiataxia and chorea, the Benedikt syndrome) are infrequently the result of stroke.

Bilateral Upper Brainstem Infarction

Infarction at this site causes coma by destroying the reticular activating system. When the level is pontine, signs mimic those caused by hemorrhage, with reactive miotic pupils and loss of eye movements. When damage is mesencephalic, ophthalmoplegia is accompanied by midposition unreactive pupils. Rostral midbrain lesions cause different kinds of supranuclear vertical gaze palsy—upward, downward, bilateral, or monocular. If there is only partial loss of consciousness, bilateral long tract motor and sensory signs or cerebellar ataxia may be detected.

Pseudobulbar Palsy

This is a syndrome that follows at least two major cerebral infarcts on different sides of the brain (which may occur at different times) or numerous lacunes on both sides. The bilateral hemisphere lesions cause bilateral corticospinal reflex signs (with or without major bilateral hemiparesis), supranuclear dysarthria and dysphagia (with impaired volitional movements but exaggerated reflex movement of the soft palate and pharynx), and emotional incontinence with exaggerated crying (or, less often, laughing) that is attributed to release of limbic functions. Other causes of pseudobulbar palsy are multiple sclerosis and amyotrophic lateral sclerosis.

Vascular Dementia

Cerebral infarction causes dementia by several mechanisms (Table 38.3). Dementia also can follow hemorrhagic stroke, and its frequent occurrence in patients with cerebral amyloid angiopathy suggests possible overlap between that condition and Alzheimer disease. Although some workers have proposed chronic potentially reversible cerebral hypoperfusion as a cause of dementia, most reject such a mechanism.

The diagnosis of vascular dementia is problematic, because the presence, revealed clinically or by imaging studies, of one or more strokes hardly proves causality, and coexisting Alzheimer disease can be excluded only pathologically.

SUGGESTED READINGS

Amarenco P, Hauw J-J. Cerebellar infarction in the territory of the superior cerebellar artery. A clinicopathologic study of 33 cases. *Neurology* 1990;40:1383–1390.

Amarenco P, Rosengart A, DeWitt D, et al. Anterior inferior cerebellar artery territory infarcts. Mechanisms and clinical features. *Arch Neurol* 1993;50:154–161.

Barth A, Bogousslavsky J, Regli F. The clinical and topographic spectrum of cerebellar infarcts: a clinical-magnetic resonance imaging correlation study. *Ann Neurol* 1993;33:451–456.

Bassetti C, Bogousslavsky J, Mattle H, et al. Medial medullary stroke: report of seven patients and review of the literature. *Neurology* 1997;48:882–890.

Bogousslavsky J, Regli F. Anterior cerebral artery territory infarction in the Lausanne Stroke Registry. Clinical and etiologic patterns. *Arch Neurol* 1990;47:144–150.

Bogousslavsky J, Regli F. Capsular genu syndrome. *Neurology* 1990;40:1499–1502.

Brust JCM. Vascular dementia is underdiagnosed. *Arch Neurol* 1988;45:799–801.

Brust JCM, Behrens MM. "Release hallucinations" as the major symptoms of posterior cerebral artery occlusion: a report of 2 cases. *Ann Neurol* 1977;2:432–436.

Brust JCM, Plank C, Burke A, et al. Language disorder in a right-hander after occlusion of the right anterior cerebral artery. *Neurology* 1982;32:492–497.

Brust JCM, Plank CR, Healton EB, Sanchez GF. The pathology of drop attacks: a case report. *Neurology* 1979;29:786–790.

Caplan LR. "Top of the basilar" syndrome. *Neurology* 1980;30:72–79.

Caplan LR, DeWitt LD, Pessin MS, et al. Lateral thalamic infarcts. *Arch Neurol* 1988;45:959–965.

Caplan LR, Schmahmann JD, Kase CS, et al. Caudate infarcts. *Arch Neurol* 1990;47:133–143.

Castaigne P, Lhermitte F, Buge A, et al. Paramedian thalamic and midbrain infarcts: clinical and neuropathological study. *Ann Neurol* 1981;10:127–148.

Damasio AR, Damasio H, Van Hoesen GW. Prosopagnosia: anatomic basis and behavioral mechanisms. *Neurology* 1982;32:331–341.

Devinsky O, Beard D, Volpe BT. Confusional states following posterior cerebral artery infarction. *Arch Neurol* 1988;45:160–163.

Feinberg WM, Rapcsak SZ. "Peduncular hallucinosis" following paramedian thalamic infarction. *Neurology* 1989;39:1535–1536.

TABLE 38.3. PROPOSED MECHANISMS OF VASCULAR DEMENTIA

1. Critically located single infarcts.
   a. Severe aphasia with additional cognitive impairment (middle cerebral artery).
   b. Amnesia with bilateral inferomesial temporal or thalamic damage (posterior cerebral artery).
   c. Abulia, memory impairment, or language disturbance with inferomedial frontal damage (anterior cerebral artery).
   d. Acute confusion or psychosis with nonlanguage dominant parietal lobe damage (middle cerebral artery).
2. Multiinfarct dementia: Multiple large infarcts not necessarily in eloquent locations but usually destroying at least 100 mL of brain volume.
3. Small-vessel disease: Ranging from multiple small deep infarcts (lacunes) to more widespread patchy or diffuse ischemic lesions of the deep cerebral white matter. The latter condition, Binswanger disease, when severe produces abulia, abnormal behavior, pseudobulbar palsy, pyramidal signs, disturbed gait, and urinary incontinence. CT shows periventricular lucencies ("leuko-araiosis") and MRI reveals similarly located signal alterations. Such findings, however, are specific for neither cerebrovascular disease nor dementia.

CT; Computed tomography; MRI, Magnetic resource imaging.

Glass JD, Levey AI, Rothstein JD. The dysarthria-clumsy hand syndrome: a distinct clinical entity related to pontine infarction. *Ann Neurol* 1990;27:487–494.

Ghika JA, Bogousslavsky J, Regli F. Deep perforators from the carotid system. Template of the vascular territories. *Arch Neurol* 1990;47:1097–1100.

Hommel M, Bogousslavsky J. The spectrum of vertical gaze palsy following unilateral brain stem stroke. *Neurology* 1991;41:1229–1234.

Howard R, Trend P, Russell RW. Clinical features of ischemia in cerebral arterial border zones after periods of reduced cerebral blood flow. *Arch Neurol* 1987;44:934–940.

Hupperts RMM, Lodder J, Heuts-van Raak EPM, et al. Infarcts in the anterior choroidal artery territory. Anatomical distribution, clinical syndromes, presumed pathogenesis, and early outcome. *Brain* 1994;117:825–834.

Kataoka S, Hori A, Shirakawa T, et al. Paramedian pontine infarction. Neurological/topographical correlation. *Stroke* 1997;28:809–815.

Kim JS, Lee JH, Lee MC. Pattern of sensory dysfunction in lateral medullary infarction. Clinical-MRI correlation. *Neurology* 1997;49:1557–1563.

Kubik CS, Adams RD. Occlusion of the basilar artery—clinical and pathological study. *Brain* 1946;69:73–121.

McKee AC, Levine DN, Kowall NW, Richardson EP Jr. Peduncular hallucinosis associated with isolated infarction of the substantia nigra pars reticulata. *Ann Neurol* 1990;27:500–504.

Mehler MF. The neuro-ophthalmologic spectrum of the rostral basilar artery syndrome. *Arch Neurol* 1988;45:966–972.

Melo TP, Bogousslavsky J, van Melle G, Regli F. Pure motor stroke: a reappraisal. *Neurology* 1992;42:789–798.

Naeser M, Palumbo CL, Helm-Estabrooks N, et al. Severe nonfluency in aphasia. Role of the medial subcallosal fasciculus and other white matter pathways in recovery of spontaneous speech. *Brain* 1989;112:1–38.

O'Brien MD. Vascular dementia is underdiagnosed. *Arch Neurol* 1988;45:797–798.

Pantoni L, Garcia JH. Pathogenesis of leukoaraiosis. A review. *Stroke* 1997;28:652–659.

Roman GC, Tatemichi TK, Erkinjuntii T, et al. Vascular dementia: diagnostic criteria for research studies. Report of the NINDS-AIREN International Workshop. *Neurology* 1993;43:250–260.

Sacco RL, Bello JA, Traub R, Brust JCM. Selective proprioceptive loss from a thalamic lacunar stroke. *Stroke* 1987;18:1160–1163.

Tatemichi TK. How acute brain failure becomes chronic. A view of the mechanisms of dementia related to stroke. *Neurology* 1990;40:1652–1659.

Tatu L, Moulin T, Bogousslavsky J, et al. Arterial territories of the human brain. Cerebral hemispheres. *Neurology* 1998;50:1699–1708.

Tijssen CC, van Gisbergen JAM, Schulte BPM. Conjugate eye deviation;side, site, and size of the hemispheric lesion. *Neurology* 1991;41:846–850.

van der Zwan A, Hillen B. Review of the variability of the territories of the major cerebral arteries. *Stroke* 1991;22:1078–1084.

Weiller C, Ringelstein EB, Reiche W, et al. The large striatocapsular infarct. A clinical and pathophysiological entity. *Arch Neurol* 1990;47:1085–1091.

Merritt's Neurology, 10th ed., edited by L.P. Rowland. Lippincott Williams & Wilkins, Philadelphia © 2000.

CHAPTER

39

CEREBRAL AND CEREBELLAR HEMORRHAGE

J.P. MOHR
CHRISTIAN STAPF

Most hemorrhages in the brain parenchyma arise in the region of the small arteries that serve the basal ganglia, thalamus, and brainstem and are caused by an arteriopathy of chronic hypertension. This disorder causes either occlusions with lacunar infarction or leakages that are brain hemorrhages. Other well-established risk factors include increasing age, cigarette smoking, alcohol consumption, and low serum cholesterol. Individuals of African, Hispanic, or Asian origin show a higher incidence of brain hemorrhage than do whites. A few hemorrhages arise from *congophilic amyloid angiopathy*, a degenerative disorder affecting the media of the smaller arteries, mainly of the cerebral gray matter in elderly individuals. Brain tumors, sympathomimetic drugs, coagulopathies, and small arteriovenous malformations also cause brain hemorrhages. Although treatment with anticoagulants or fibrinolytic agents encounter a higher risk of hemorrhage with increasing doses, the role of aspirin intake in this context is controversial.

Because most spontaneous hemorrhages arise from tiny vessels, the accumulation of a hematoma takes time and explains the smooth onset of the clinical syndrome over minutes or hours. The progressive course, frequent vomiting, and headache are major points that help to differentiate hemorrhage from infarction. Hemorrhage usually stops spontaneously by 30 minutes but in fatal cases continues until death is caused by brain compression or by disruption of vital structures. The *putamen* is the site most frequently affected. When the expanding hematoma involves the adjacent internal capsule, there is a contralateral hemiparesis, usually with hemianesthesia and hemianopia and, in large hematomas, aphasia or impaired awareness of the disorder. However, small self-limiting hematomas close to the capsular region may occasionally mimic lacunar syndromes featuring pure motor or sensory deficits. When the hemorrhage arises in the *thalamus*, hemianesthesia precedes the hemiparesis. Once contralateral motor, sensory, and visual field signs are established, the main points that distinguish the two sites are conjugate horizontal ocular deviation in putaminal hemorrhage and impaired upward gaze in thalamic hemorrhage.

Pontine hemorrhage usually plunges the patient into coma with quadriparesis and grossly disconjugate ocular motility disorders, although small hemorrhages may mimic syndromes of infarction. Primary spontaneous hemorrhages within the *mesencephalon* or the *medulla* remain objects of debate and are rare curiosities. When they occur, the anatomic involvement is usually secondary to hemorrhage originating in neighboring diencephalic, cerebellar, or pontine regions.

Among the *cerebral lobes*, there is a yet-unexplained predilection for hemorrhages to occur within the posterior two-thirds of the brain. When they affect one or more cerebral lobes, the syndrome is difficult to distinguish clinically from infarction because progressive evolution and vomiting are much less frequent; also, lobar white matter hematomas often result from arteriovenous malformations, amyloid angiopathy, tumors, or other causes that rarely affect the basal ganglia, thalamus, and pons.

Cerebellar hemorrhage warrants separate description because the mode of onset differs from that of cerebral hemorrhage and because it often necessitates surgical evacuation. The syndrome usually begins abruptly with vomiting and severe ataxia (which usually prevents standing and walking); it is occasionally accompanied by dysarthria, adjacent cranial nerve (mostly VIth and VIIth) affection, and paralysis of conjugate lateral gaze to one side, findings that may mislead clinicians into thinking the disease is primarily in the brainstem. However, a cerebellar origin is suggested by the lack of changes in the level of consciousness and lack of focal weakness or sensory loss. Enlargement of the mass does not change the clinical picture until there is enough brainstem compression to precipitate coma, at which point it is too late for surgical evacuation of the hemorrhage to reverse the disorder. This small margin of time between an alert state and an irreversible coma makes it imperative to consider the diagnosis in all patients with this clinical syndrome and a reason to have patients with vomiting of undetermined origin stand and walk when encountered in the emergency room. Computed tomography or magnetic resonance imaging should be carried out promptly, and surgery should be performed within hours on all the larger hemorrhages.

SUGGESTED READINGS

Aring CD, Merritt HH. Differential diagnosis between cerebral hemorrhage and cerebral thrombosis. *Arch Intern Med* 1935;56:435–456.

Broderick JP, Brott TG, Tomsick T, et al. Ultra-early evaluation of intracerebral hemorrhage. *J Neurosurg* 1990;72:195–199.

Broderick J, Brott T, Tomsick T, et al. Intracerebral hemorrhage more than twice as common as subarachnoid hemorrhage. *J Neurosurg* 1993;78:188–191.

Broderick J, Brott T, Tomsick T, Leach A. Lobar hemorrhage in the elderly: the undiminishing importance of hypertension. *Stroke* 1993;24:49–51.

Brott T, Broderick J, Kothari R, et al. Early hemorrhage growth in patients with intracerebral hemorrhage. *Stroke* 1997;28:1–5.

Greenberg SM. Cerebral amyloid angiopathy: prospects for clinical diagnosis and treatment. *Neurology* 1998;51:690–694.

Hier DB, Davis KR, Richardson ER, Mohr JP. Hypertensive putaminal hemorrhage. *Ann Neurol* 1977;1:152–159.

Kase CS. Intracerebral hemorrhage: Non-hypertensive causes. *Stroke* 1986;17:590–595.

Kase CS, Mohr JP, Caplan LR. Intracerebral hemorrhage. In: Barnett HJM, Mohr JP, Stein BM, Yatsu FM, eds. *Stroke. Pathophysiology, diagnosis, and management*, 3rd ed. New York: Churchill Livingstone, 1998:649–700.

Kurata A, Miyasaka Y, Kitahara T, et al. Subcortical cerebral hemorrhage with reference to vascular malformations and hypertension as causes of hemorrhage. *Neurosurgery* 1993;32:505–511.

Levine SR, Brust JCM, Futrell N, et al. Cerebrovascular complications of the use of the "crack" form of alkaloid cocaine. *N Engl J Med* 1990;323:699–704.

Massaro AR, Sacco RL, Mohr JP, et al. Clinical discriminators separate lobar and subcortical hemorrhage: the Stroke Data Bank. *Neurology* 1991;41:1881–1885.

Melo TP, Bogousslavsky J, Regli F, Janzer R. Fatal hemorrhage during anticoagulation of cardioembolic infarction: role of cerebral amyloid angiopathy. *Eur Neurol* 1993;33:9–12.

Okudera T, Uemura K, Nakajima K, et al. Primary pontine hemorrhage: correlations of pathologic features with postmortem microangiographic and vertebral studies. *Mt Sinai J Med* 1978;45:305–321.

Ott KH, Kase CS, Ojemann RG, Mohr JP. Cerebellar hemorrhage: diagnosis and treatment. *Arch Neurol* 1974;31:160–167.

Schutz H, Bodeker R-H, Damian M, et al. Age-related spontaneous intracerebral hematoma in a German community. *Stroke* 1990;21:1412–1418.

NINDS t-PA Stroke Study Group. Intracerebral hemorrhage after intravenous t-PA therapy for ischemic stroke. *Stroke* 1997;28:2109–2118.

WARSS, APASS, PICSS, HAS and GENESIS Study Groups. The feasibility of a collaborative double-blind study using an anticoagulant. *Cerebrovasc Dis* 1997;7:100–112.

Merritt's Neurology, 10th ed., edited by L.P. Rowland. Lippincott Williams & Wilkins, Philadelphia © 2000.

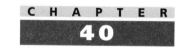

CHAPTER 40

GENETICS OF STROKE

ALEXANDER HALIM
RALPH L. SACCO

Numerous single-gene (Mendelian) disorders associated with ischemic or hemorrhagic stroke have been identified (e.g., sickle cell disease, Marfan syndrome, and Fabry disease). Many of these conditions are discussed elsewhere in this text. Although these disorders represent a direct genetic etiology of stroke, they are rare and do not account for a large proportion of stroke cases.

Genetic factors may also indirectly influence vascular risk factors. Examples include genetic disorders associated with hypercoagulable states that increase the risk of venous thrombosis, metabolic disorders that lead to vasculopathy, and hereditary intracranial aneurysms that cause hemorrhagic stroke.

In 1993, a single gene was identified for the stroke syndrome, cerebral autosomal dominant inherited arteriopathy with subcortical infarcts and leukoencephalopathy (CADASIL). This may be the only stroke condition with a direct genetic etiology. Other types of epidemiologic studies suggest both genetic and environmental factors (Table 40.1).

CADASIL

CADASIL is caused by a Notch3 mutation on chromosome 19. Most CADASIL pedigrees have come from western Europe; sev-

TABLE 40.1. SOME GENETIC ETIOLOGIES OF STROKE

Stroke Subtype	Cytogenetic Map Location	Gene/Protein	MIM
Ischemic stroke			
CADASIL	19p13.2–p13.1	Notch 3 mutation	125310
Activated protein C resistence	1q23	Leiden factor V mutation	227400
Homocystinuria	21q22.3	Cystathionine beta-synthase	236200
Hyperhomocysteinemia	1q36.3	Methylenetetrahydrofolate reductase	236250
Marfan syndrome	15q21.1	Fibrillin 1	134797
Protein C deficiency	2q13–q14	Protein C gene	176860
Protein S deficiency	3p11.1–q11.2	Protein S gene	176880
Sickle cell disease[a]	Multiple	Globin genes	Multiple
ICH			
Carvernous malformations	7q11.2–q21	Cerebral cavernous malformations 1	116860
Hereditary cerebral hemorrhage with amyloidosis			
Dutch type	21q21.3–q22.05	Amyloid precursor protein	104760
Icelandic type	20p11.2	Cystatin C	105150
SAH			134797
Marfan syndrome	15q21.1	Fibrillin 1	601313
Polycystic kidney disease	16p13.3–p13.12	Polycystin 1	173910
	4q21–q23	Polycystin 2	Unknown
	Unknown	Unknown	

[a]Several loci have been identified for sickle cell disease.
MIM, Mendelian inheritence in man number; CADASIL, cerebral autosomal dominant inherited arteriopathy with subcortical infarcts and leukoencephalopathy; ICH, intracerebral hemorrhage; SAH, subarachnoid hemorrhage.

eral pedigrees have been identified in the United States. Linkage to the D19S226 locus on chromosome 19 has been confirmed in over a dozen families, suggesting genetic homogeneity.

CADASIL is characterized by recurrent episodes of subcortical infarcts or transient ischemic attacks and a conspicuous absence of common stroke risk factors such as hypertension. Onset is between ages 30 and 50. The variable clinical manifestations include dementia, pseudobulbar palsy, and migraine. There is no specific treatment, and the mean survival is 20 years from onset.

In symptomatic patients magnetic resonance imaging (MRI) shows deep small infarcts in the subcortical white matter and basal ganglia. The leukoencephalopathy is extensive and can be patchy or diffuse. The U fibers are almost always spared. Skin biopsy can be diagnostic, showing granular, eosinophilic, electron-dense material in the media of the arterial wall. MRI is more sensitive than computed tomography, but the changes may be nonspecific. Skin biopsy is more specific than MRI but may not be more sensitive. Brain biopsy seems most sensitive and specific; granular, eosinophilic, electron-dense, nonamyloid material is found primarily in the walls of penetrating arteries in the white matter and leptomeningeal and basal ganglia arteries.

A phenotypic variant of CADASIL was identified by familial clustering of hemiplegic migraine and labeled CADASILM ("M" for migraine).

INTRACEREBRAL HEMORRHAGE

Intracerebral hemorrhages (ICH) may be caused by amyloid angiopathies. Dutch and Icelandic forms of hereditary cerebral amyloid angiopathy demonstrate the genetic influence in ICH. However, it is unclear how often ICH is hereditary or sporadic.

The Dutch form involves mutations in the amyloid precursor protein gene, and the Icelandic form is caused by a deletion mu-

tation in the cystatin C gene on chromosome 20. Both are rare autosomal dominant diseases characterized by lobar hemorrhages and premature death in young adults without other cause of hemorrhage. The apolipoprotein E $\epsilon2$ and $\epsilon4$ alleles may be directly associated with cerebral amyloid angiopathy, and consequently with an increased risk for and earlier age at first hemorrhage.

Cerebral cavernous malformations often cause hemorrhages. A single abnormal gene causing cerebral cavernous malformation has been localized to chromosome 7q11.2-q21. However, it is difficult to discern whether an individual ICH results from familial or sporadic cavernous malformations.

SUBARACHNOID HEMORRHAGE

Familial aggregation of subarachnoid hemorrhages may be independent of hypertensive vascular disease, suggesting a strong genetic influence. Segregation analysis of intracranial aneurysms indicates the most likely pattern is either autosomal dominant with a rare susceptibility allele or autosomal recessive with a less rare susceptibility allele. The evidence for autosomal inheritance pattern is strong but of insufficient power to detect the true mode of inheritance. Genetic heterogeneity may be important. Cerebral aneurysms have been linked to type III collagen mutations and to several human leukocyte antigens.

ISCHEMIC STROKES

Twin studies suggest a possible genetic etiology of stroke; however, the role of genetics in ischemic strokes is unresolved. Variations in the incidence of ischemic stroke in racial groups support the notion of a genetic component. Alternatively, migration studies among Hawaiian residents of Japanese descent and other epidemiologic studies imply strong environmental risk factors. Relatives of people with ischemic stroke often share the same risk factors, making it difficult to separate genetic factors from shared environment.

Documented risk factors of ischemic stroke are under strong genetic influences. Hypertension, diabetes, heart disease, and obesity all have genetic influences that may or may not interact with environmental factors. Whether a predisposition to cigarette smoking is hereditary is controversial; observed clustering of smoking within families is often attributed to cultural rather than genetic causes. Several polymorphisms modify the effect of cigarette smoking on cancers, and some polymorphisms may influence stroke via an effect on atherogenesis. The observation of multiple cases of ischemic stroke within families could result from a high prevalence of any or all these risk factors in the population, or these may be a familial clustering of hereditary ischemic stroke that is specifically mediated through one or more of these hereditary diseases.

Hypercoagulation states are risk factors for ischemic stroke and are under genetic control. Increased plasma fibrinogen levels, caused by a mutation of the beta-fibrinogen gene, are associated with increased risk of ischemic stroke. Hereditary hypercoagulopathies (protein C deficiency, protein S deficiency, antithrombin III deficiency, and activated protein C resistance due to the Leiden factor V mutation) can cause venous thrombosis, although the association with arterial thrombosis is uncertain.

Ischemic stroke and ischemic heart disease are associated with increased lipoprotein (a) levels that depend on the expression of the apolipoprotein A locus. The role of lipoprotein (a) on a population level and its relation to other stroke risk factors is uncertain.

Homocystinuria and hyperhomocysteinemia increase the risk of ischemic stroke. Both genetic and environmental conditions can cause these disorders. The most common form is homocystinuria, an autosomal recessive disorder caused by a deficiency of the cystathione-beta-synthethase enzyme that catalyzes the conversion of methionine to cysteine. The prevalence of homocystinuria is 1 per 200,000. Other genetic causes of elevated homocysteine levels include reduced plasma concentrations of methyl-tetrahydrofolate and methyl-cobalamine or decreased methylenetetrahydrofolate reductase activity.

SUMMARY

The determination of a genetic etiology for stroke would allow early identification of persons with increased risk of stroke through genetic screening. Except for using skin biopsy to detect CADASIL, genetic screening is not available for most stroke cases. In the case of CADASIL, the absence of effective treatment does not promote disease prevention despite the availability of genetic screening. Stroke prevention would therefore require the early intervention of stroke risk factors that have varying contributions of genetic and environmental influences. Genetic screening of Mendelian disorders may identify asymptomatic or undiagnosed risk factors and potentially prevent stroke.

SUGGESTED READINGS

Alberts MJ, ed. Genetics of cerebrovascular disease. *Futura* 1999.

Alberts MJ. Genetic aspects of cerebrovascular disease. *Stroke* 1991;22:276–280.

Brass LM, Isaacsohn JI, Merikangas KR, Robinette CD. A study of twins and stroke. *Stroke* 1992;23:221–223.

Bromberg JEC, Rinkel GJE, Algra A, et al. Subarachnoid hemorrhage in first and second degree relatives of patients with subarachnoid hemorrhage. *BMJ* 1995;311:228–229.

Chabriat H, Vahedi K, Iba-Zazen MT, et al. The clinical spectrum of CADASIL, cerebral autosomal dominant inherited arteriopathy with subcortical infarcts and leukoencephalopathy. *Lancet* 1995;346:934–939.

Kiely DK, Wolf PA, Cupples LA, et al. Familial aggregation of stroke. The Framingham study. *Stroke* 1993;24:1366–1371.

McKusick VA. *Mendelian inheritance in man. Catalogs of human genes and genetic disorders*, 12th ed. Baltimore: Johns Hopkins University Press, 1998.

Natowicz M, Kelley RI. Mendelian etiologies of stroke. *Ann Neurol* 1987;22:175–182.

Roos RAC, Haan J, Van Broeckhoven C. Hereditary cerebral hemorrhage with amyloidosis B Dutch type: a congophilic angiopathy. *Ann N Y Acad Sci* 1991;640:155–160.

Tournier-Lasserve E, Joutel A, Melki J, et al. Cerebral autosomal dominant inherited arteriopathy with subcortical infarcts and leukoencephalopathy (CADASIL) maps on chromosome 19q12. *Nat Genet* 1993;3:256–259.

Merritt's Neurology, 10th ed., edited by L.P. Rowland. Lippincott Williams & Wilkins, Philadelphia © 2000.

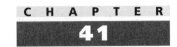

OTHER CEREBROVASCULAR SYNDROMES

FRANK M. YATSU

LACUNAR STROKES

Occlusion of small penetrating arterioles (<500 μm diameter) usually follows sustained hypertension and leads to cystic cerebral degeneration or lacune formation. These small occlusions are frequently located in clinically silent areas, but well-defined lacunar syndromes have been described. These include pure motor hemiplegia, hemisensory stroke, sensorimotor pseudobulbar palsy, ipsilateral ataxia and hemiparesis, and dysarthria–clumsy hand syndrome. Fisher (1982) described over 20 discrete syndromes.

Pure motor hemiplegia usually involves the face, arm, or leg, or their combination, without sensory loss; the lacune disrupts the corticospinal tracts in the internal capsule or pons. As with other lacunar syndromes, diseases other than hypertension may cause identical symptoms; these include emboli and hemorrhage.

Pure hemisensory stroke without motor impairment is characterized clinically by numbness or paresthesias involving typically the face, arm, and leg. The impaired sensation can be explained by a lacune in the sensory nucleus of the thalamus. Pseudobulbar palsy results from multiple bilateral frontal lobe lacunes. Computed tomography may demonstrate lacunar hypodensities. When the lacunar syndrome can be explained adequately by hypertensive disease, no specific therapy other than hypertension control is indicated. The pathologic findings are of "lipohyalinosis," a degenerative process secondary to long-standing hypertension, although occasionally an atheromatous plaque of the feeding vessel can encroach onto the arteriole opening and cause ischemia.

HYPERTENSIVE ENCEPHALOPATHY

In 1928, Oppenheimer and Fishberg introduced the term *hypertensive encephalopathy* to describe encephalopathic symptoms (e.g., headaches, confusion, drowsiness, blurring of vision, occasional seizures, and infrequent focal signs) in association with an accelerated malignant phase of hypertension. The diastolic pressures are usually greater than 140 mm Hg and the fundi usually demonstrate grade IV changes with hemorrhages and disk edema. Children and pregnant or postpartum women show less elevated blood pressures to provoke hypertensive encephalopathy because their starting pressures are usually lower. Because this constellation of clinical findings

may be found with strokes and systemic disorders (e.g., uremia and electrolyte imbalance), the diagnosis of hypertensive encephalopathy is frequently erroneous. The symptoms of hypertensive encephalopathy are reversed when blood pressure is reduced and renal function does not change. The syndrome is attributed to generalized arteriolar constriction with loss of cerebral autoregulation. Because the sustained hypertension may be life threatening, the therapeutic approach has been to treat these patients with hypotensive agents (e.g., sodium nitroprusside, labetalol) as demand therapy, unless stroke or some other conditions clearly explain the encephalopathic symptoms. If the symptoms do not improve, however, establishment of diagnosis is more difficult.

With hypotensive therapy, care must be taken not to reduce the blood pressure excessively because watershed infarcts are possible complications. A 15% to 20% reduction of mean arterial pressure but above the heightened lower end of autoregulation at approximately 125 mm Hg is initially desirable.

FIBROMUSCULAR HYPERPLASIA

Fibromuscular bands of unknown origin form segmental narrowing in large arteries and may cause ischemic symptoms of the brain, including transient ischemic attacks (TIAs) and infarcts, although they most frequently present as asymptomatic carotid bruits. Common involvement of the renal arteries leads to hypertension. Clinical diagnosis of fibromuscular hyperplasia is suggested by the combination of carotid and renal artery bruits in the presence of systemic hypertension. Women are usually affected in middle age. Diagnosis is rarely suspected before the lesions are demonstrated by angiography. Antiplatelet drugs, anticoagulation, and surgical dilatation have all been reported to reduce the frequency of TIAs.

MULTIINFARCT OR VASCULAR DEMENTIA

This syndrome is discussed elsewhere in the book.

CEREBRAL AMYLOID ANGIOPATHY

Cerebral amyloid angiopathy or "congophilic angiopathy" is uncommon; it presents clinically as intracerebral hemorrhages, usually after the fifth decade. Amyloid deposits are found in medium and small cortical and leptomeningeal arteries and are not associated with systemic amyloidosis. Intracerebral hemorrhage, particularly lobar in location, tends to recur within months or years, and multiple hemorrhages may occur simultaneously. Progressive dementia occurs in 30%, and features of Alzheimer disease are seen pathologically in 50%.

No therapy is known for the primary process; indications for hematoma evacuation are similar to those for other causes: location, mass effect, and declining sensorium. A familial Dutch form may be detected by the presence of gamma trace alkaline microprotein in serum.

ANTIPHOSPHOLIPID SYNDROME (LUPUS ANTICOAGULANT AND ANTICARDIOLIPIN ANTIBODY SYNDROME)

Lupus anticoagulants, a double misnomer because thrombosis (arterial and venous) occurs in conditions other than lupus, are immunoglobulins, usually IgG but occasionally IgM and IgA. *In vitro*, they inhibit coagulation by interfering with phospholipid-dependent coagulation tests without inhibiting *in vivo* activity of coagulation factors. Lupus anticoagulants were first described in patients with systemic lupus erythematosis and have been reported with drug-induced lupus, other autoimmune diseases, neoplasm, phenothiazines, and idiopathically. Antiphospholipid syndrome associated with thromboses are both arterial and venous. These conditions may be associated with a false-positive VDRL test and mild thrombocytopenia. When so-called lupus anticoagulants or anticardiolipin antibodies occur without associated diseases, the condition is referred to as "primary antiphospholipid syndrome." Treatment to prevent thrombosis should be directed to the primary underlying condition, but reported therapies to prevent thrombosis include corticosteroids, antiplatelet drugs, and anticoagulation. For anticoagulation, which is perhaps the best therapy, the international normalized ratio (INR) should be kept at at least 3.0 for optimum effects.

HYPERHOMOCYSTEINEMIA

Hyperhomocysteinemia, or the elevation of blood homocysteine, may result from several enzymatic defects either primarily or secondarily from the effects of a number of drugs. For example, impairment of the conversion of homocysteine to cystathionine by cystathionine-β-synthase, which requires vitamin B_6 (pyridoxine) is one example. Other pathways require folate or vitamin B_{12}. Hyperhomocysteinemia is associated with ischemic strokes and myocardial infarction. A prospective study to validate the beneficial effects of these vitamins in preventing strokes and myocardial infarction is in progress.

STROKE IN YOUNG ADULTS

Stroke in young adults is usually defined as those occurring before age 45. The incidence and causes differ from strokes occurring after age 65. Of all strokes, approximately 25% occur before age 65. People younger than 45 account for about 20% of those under age 65, or 5% to 10% of all strokes.

Differential Diagnosis

Strokes in young adults include a wide variety of disorders that are less frequently seen in older adults. The diagnostic approach can be divided into the three major categories: vascular diseases, particularly those other than atherosclerosis related; cardioembolic causes; and blood-element abnormalities, which can be divided into those affecting erythrocytes, proteins, or platelets. Discussion of each disease causing strokes in young adults is be-

yond the scope of this chapter, but the more important entities are discussed (Tables 41.1 and 41.2).

Vascular Diseases

Premature atherosclerosis, migraine, and dissection of the vessel wall are prominent disorders seen in young adults. Premature atherosclerosis is seen with diabetes mellitus or hypertension and other known risks for atherosclerosis, such as smoking and elevated serum lipids; these people show evidence of diffuse vascu-

TABLE 41.1. DIFFERENTIAL DIAGNOSIS OF STROKES IN YOUNG ADULTS

Vascular diseases
  Atherosclerosis
  Arteritides
    Isolated angiitis of the CNS
    Lupus erythematosus
    Polyarteritis nodosa
    Sjögren syndrome
    Behçet disease
    Lymphomatoid granulomatosis
    Drug abuse (heroin, crack, amphetamines)
    Secondary to chronic meningitis
    Sneddon syndrome
    Takayasu arteritis
    Human immunodeficiency virus-associated
  Dissection
  Migraine
  Venous occlusive diseases
  Fibromuscular dysplasia
  Moyamoya syndrome
  Drug-related: oral contraceptives
  Berry or congenital aneurysm
  Arteriovenous malformations/cryptic venous malformations and
    telangiectasias
  Toxemia of pregnancy
  Homocystinuria; Fabry disease
  Hypertensive encephalopathy
  Brain tumors (primary or metastatic)
  Arteriopathies: mitochondrial myopathy-encephalopathy-lactic
    acidosis-strokes (MELAS)

Cardiogenic emboli
  Arrhythmias
  Mitral valve prolapse
  Bacterial endocarditis
  Libman-Sacks (systemic lupus erythematosus)
  Atrial myxoma
  Valvular replacement
  Paradoxic emboli/patent foramen ovale
  Cardiomyopathies (postmyocardial infarction, viral, alcoholic)
  Endocardial fibrosis

Blood element abnormalities
  Erythrocytes
    Sickle cell disease
    Polycythemia vera
  Proteins
    Lupus anticoagulant/antiphospholipid antibodies Protein C and S
    Waldenström macroglobulinemia
  Thrombocytosis
  Coagulation defects: alcohol-induced; antithrombin III inhibitors;
    paroxysmal nocturnal hemoglobinuria; thrombotic
    thrombocytopenic purpura

CNS, Central nervous system.

TABLE 41.2. CAUSES OF BRAIN INFARCTION IN YOUNG ADULTS IN THE LITERATURE

	Cases	%
Atherosclerosis		20
Embolism		20
Nonatherosclerotic arteriopathy		10
Coagulopathy/systemic		10
Peripartum		5
Uncertain causes (including oral contraceptives, migraine, and mitral valve prolapse)		35

Modified from Hart RG, Miller VT. *Stroke* 1983;14:110–114.

lar disease and often have TIAs before the stroke. These attacks are treated just as they are in older subjects, including carotid endarterectomy for symptomatic carotid stenosis and antiatherogenic measures.

Migraine may cause strokes in young adults. Although most have had migraine headaches chronically, the headache may or may not coincide with the stroke. The most common strokelike symptoms associated with migraine or so-called complicated migraine are aphasia, hemiparesis, and vertebrobasilar insufficiency. The goal of the treatment is to prevent the attacks of vasospasm. A young woman who takes oral contraceptives, including low-dose estrogens, seems to be at increased risk for these attacks; if one occurs, oral contraceptive use should be discontinued.

In addition, arteritis and strokes resulting from drug abuse are distinctly more common in young adults. Usually, the arteritides involving cerebral vessels become symptomatic after systemic manifestations of the disease have been present as in polyarteritis nodosa, Sjögren disease, and lupus erythematosus. However, isolated angiitis of the central nervous system or spinal cord is unusual in displaying few peripheral symptoms, signs, or serologic evidence of immune complex disorders; even the cerebral angiogram may be normal. If a young adult experiences multifocal brain disease, with obtundation, severe headaches, and no discernible systemic cause, a brain and leptomeningeal biopsy may be needed to diagnose isolated angiitis of the central nervous system (see Chapter 155).

Drug abuse can lead to strokes from arteritis or occlusive disease. Cerebral hemorrhage can occur with use of amphetamines or cocaine, and intravenous drug use may lead to bacterial endocarditis with bacterial/fibrin emboli or mycotic aneurysms in the brain. For drug-related strokes, both clinical history and drug screening are critical in establishing a diagnosis.

Cardiogenic Emboli

Of the causes of embolic strokes of cardiac origin, mitral valve prolapse is perhaps the most common, except for arrhythmias, although increasing attention is paid to the patent foramen ovale as a cause of cryptogenic strokes. Mitral valve prolapse is found in 10% to 15% of the population and more frequently in women; it is detected by a midsystolic click on auscultation and more specifically by two-dimensional echocardiography. Transesophageal echocardiography may be needed to supplement the transthoracic study by visualizing the posterior mitral leaflets.

Risks of embolization, congestive heart failure, and cardiac arrest are substantially increased in the presence of leaflet redundancy, without which mitral valve prolapse is relatively benign. When redundancy is detected, treatment includes efforts to minimize embolization with antiplatelet drugs or, on occasion, anticoagulation.

With patent foramen ovale, mechanical patency is present in about one-fourth of the population. The pathogenic abnormalities are larger patent foramen ovales with paradoxical emboli with right-to-left shunting of venous emboli. In practice, vigorously shaken saline is injected to observe for the appearance of echogenic bubbles (>25) in the left atrium. Transcranial Doppler studies may detect emboli in the common carotid or middle cerebral arteries. If reembolization occurs despite adequate anticoagulation, surgical closure of the patent foramen ovale may be necessary.

Blood Element Abnormalities

Each constituent of blood may be a source of strokes in young adults, as in other age groups, including the cellular and protein components. The cellular elements include erythrocytes; most notable disorders are sickle cell anemia and polycythemia vera. With the advent of both noninvasive testing of intracranial and extracranial vessels and magnetic resonance imaging, stroke syndromes in sickle cell anemia are found to be complicated by the hyperviscosity state that provokes premature atherosclerosis of larger arteries and causes watershed ischemia and infarcts. Efforts to minimize stroke complications with transfusions and hydroxyurea to increase synthesis of fetal hemoglobin may be helpful.

Abnormalities of protein elements may give rise to stroke syndromes by influencing coagulation or viscosity of platelet aggregation. The role of antiphospholipid antibodies in causing strokes in young adults is reviewed above. As seen in Table 41.1, multiple coagulation defects are associated with ischemic strokes and cortical vein thrombosis, but the most common is resistance to protein C activation. Its primary treatment to avert thrombosis is anticoagulation to keep the INR between 2.0 and 3.0.

SUGGESTED READINGS

Adams RJ, Nichols FT, McKie V, et al. Cerebral infarction in sickle cell anemia. *Neurology* 1988;38:1012–1017.

Alvarez J, Matias Guiu J, Sumalla J, et al. Ischemic stroke in young adults. I. Analysis of the etiological subgroups. *Acta Neurol Scand* 1989;80:28–34.

Bamford JM, Warlow CP. Evolution and testing of the lacunar hypothesis. *Stroke* 1988;19:1074–1082.

Barnett HJM, Boughner DR, Taylor DW, et al. Further evidence relating mitral-valve prolapse to cerebral ischemic events. *N Engl J Med* 1980;302:139–144,

Bogousslavsky J, Pierre P. Ischemic stroke in patients under age 45. *Neurol Clin* 1992;10:113–124.

Brey RL, Hart RG, Sherman DG, et al. Antiphospholipid antibodies and cerebral ischemia in young people. *Neurology* 1990;40:1190–1196.

Carolei A, Marini C, Ferranti E., et al. A prospective study of cerebral ischemia in the young. Analysis of pathogenic determinants. The National Research Council Study Group. *Stroke* 1993;24:362–367.

Collaborative Group for the Study of Stroke in Young Women. Oral contraception and increased risk of cerebral ischemia or thrombosis. *N Engl J Med* 1973;288:871–878.

Coull BM, Levine SR, Brey RL. The role of antiphospholipid antibodies in stroke. *Neurol Clin* 1992;10:125–143.

Di Tullio M, Sacco RL, Gopal A, et al. Patent foramen ovale as a risk factor for cryptogenic stroke. *Ann Intern Med* 1992;117:461–465.

Donaldson JA. *The neurology of pregnancy*. Philadelphia: W.B. Saunders, 1978.

Ellis RJ, Olichney MJ, Thal LJ, et al. Cerebral amyloid angiopathy in the brains of patients with Alzheimer's disease: the CERAD experience, Part XV. *Neurology* 1996;46:1592–1596.

Evers S, Koch HG, Grotemeyer KH, et al. Features, symptoms, and neurophysiological findings in stroke associated with hyperhomocysteinemia. *Arch Neurol* 1997;54:1276–1282.

Feldman E, Levine SR. Cerebrovascular disease with antiphospholipid antibodies: immune mechanisms, significance, and therapeutic options. *Ann Neurol* 1995;37[Suppl 1]:S114–S130.

Ferro D, Quintarelli C, Rasura M, et al. Lupus anticoagulant and the fibrinolytic system in young patients with stroke. *Stroke* 1993;24:368–370.

Fisher CM. Lacunar strokes and infarcts: a review. *Neurology* 1982;321:1–6.

Gan R, Sacco RL, Kargman DE, Roberts JK, Boden-Alabal B, Gu Q. Testing the validity of the lacunar hypothesis: the Northern Manhattan Stroke Study experience. *Neurology* 1997;48:1204–1211.

Gilles C, Brucher JM, Khoubesserian P, et al. Cerebral amyloid angiopathy as a cause of multiple intracerebral hemorrhages. *Neurology* 1984;34:730–773.

Hart RG, Miller VT. Cerebral infarction in young adults: a practical approach. *Stroke* 1983;14:110–114.

Healton EB, Brust JCM, Feinfeld DA, et al. Hypertensive encephalopathy and the neurologic manifestations of malignant hypertension. *Neurology* 1982;32:127–132.

Hinchey JA, Sila CA Cerebrovascular complications of rheumatic disease. *Rheum Dis Clin North Am* 1997;23:293–316.

Hindfelt B, Nilsson O. Long-term prognosis of ischemic stroke in young adults. *Acta Neurol Scand* 1992;86:440–445.

Jura E, Palasik W, Meurer M, et al. Sneddon's syndrome (livedo reticularis and cerebrovascular lesions) with antiphospholipid antibodies and severe dementia in a young man: case report. *Acta Neurol Scand* 1994;89:143–146.

Kaku DA, Lowenstein DH. Emergence of recreational drug abuse as a major risk factor for stroke in young adults. *Ann Intern Med* 1990;113:821–827.

Kityakara C, Guzman NJ. Malignant hypertension and hypertensive emergencies. *J Am Soc Nephrol* 1998;9:133–142.

Larsen BH, Sorensen PS, Marquardsen J. Transient ischemic attacks in young patients: a thromboembolic or migrainous manifestation? A 10 year follow up study of 46 patients. *J Neurol Neurosurg Psychiatry* 1990;53:1029–1033.

Levine S, Welch KMA. Cerebrovascular ischemia and lupus anticoagulant. *Stroke* 1987;18:257–263.

Levine SR, Brey RL, Sawaya KL, et al. Recurrent stroke and thromboocclusive events in the antiphospholipid syndrome. *Ann Neurol* 1995;38:129–134.

Malinow MR. Plasma homocyst(e)ine and arterial occlusive disease: a mini-review. *Clin Chem* 1995;42:173–176.

Manninen HI, Koivisto T, Saari T, et al. Dissecting aneurysms of all four cervicocranial arteries in fibromuscular dysplasia: treatment with self-expanding endovascular stents, coil embolization, and surgical ligation. *Am J Neuroradiol* 1997;18:1216–1220.

Martinez HR, Rangel Guerra RA, Marfil LJ. Ischemic stroke due to deficiency of coagulation inhibitors. Report of 10 young adults. *Stroke* 1993;24:19–25.

Mettinger KL, Ericson K. Fibromuscular dysplasias and the brain. *Stroke* 1982;13:46–58.

Moody CK, Miller BI, McIntryre HB, et al. Neurologic complications of cocaine abuse. *Neurology* 1988;38:1189–1193.

Nencini P, Baruffi MC, Abbate R, et al. Lupus anticoagulant and anticardiolipin antibodies in young adults with cerebral ischemia. *Stroke* 1992;23:189–193.

Nicoll JA, Burnett C, Love S, et al. High frequency of apolipoprotein E epsilon 2 allele in hemorrhage due to cerebral amyloid angiopathy. *Ann Neurol* 1997;41:716–721.

Nishimura RA, McGoon MD, Shub C, et al. Echocardiographically documented mitral-valve prolapse. Long-term follow-up of 237 patients. *N Engl J Med* 1985;313:1305–1309.

Olsen ML, O'Connor S, Arnett FC, et al. Autoantibodies and rheumatic disorders in a neurology inpatient population: a prospective study. *Am J Med* 1991;90:479–488.

Oppenheimer BS, Fishberg AM. Hypertensive encephalopathy. *Arch Intern Med* 1928;41:264–278.

Sandok BA. Fibromuscular dysplasia of the internal carotid artery. *Neurol Clin* 1983;1:17–26.

Vinters HV. Cerebral amyloid angiopathy. Critical review. *Stroke* 1988;19:311–324.

Merritt's Neurology, 10th ed., edited by L.P. Rowland. Lippincott Williams & Wilkins, Philadelphia © 2000.

C H A P T E R

42

DIFFERENTIAL DIAGNOSIS OF STROKE

MITCHELL S.V. ELKIND
J.P. MOHR

The potential for thrombolytic therapy for acute ischemic stroke has made the prompt distinction of cerebral infarction from hemorrhage and other causes of sudden neurologic deficit an important practical matter. Because treatment must be initiated within 3 hours of onset of symptoms, the differential diagnosis must be considered and an accurate diagnosis made very rapidly. Libman et al. (1995) studied 411 patients who received an emergency room diagnosis of stroke. Of those, 81% received a final diagnosis of stroke and a full 19% were determined to have one of several stroke "mimics." These most commonly included seizures, systemic infection, brain tumor, and toxic-metabolic encephalopathy. Less frequent sources of misdiagnosis were positional vertigo, cardiac events, syncope, trauma, subdural hematoma, herpes simplex virus encephalitis, transient global amnesia, dementia, demyelinating disease, C-spine fracture, myasthenia gravis, parkinsonism, hypertensive encephalopathy, and conversion disorder. In multivariate analysis, factors that predicted a "true stroke" were the presence of angina and absence of loss of consciousness.

Within the category of cerebral infarction, a diagnosis of *cerebral embolism* is suggested by a sudden onset and a syndrome of circumscribed focal deficit attributable to cerebral surface infarction, such as in pure aphasia or pure hemianopia. The more complex the neurologic syndrome, the larger the arterial territory involved, the more proximal in the arterial tree that the occlusion occurs, and the more the diagnosis of *thrombosis* must be considered. A diagnosis of embolism is important because the risk of recurrence is high. The source of the embolus may be found in acute or chronic endocarditis, atrial fibrillation, recent myocardial infarction, or patent foramen ovale. The brain is the first site of symptoms in most cases of systemic embolism; clinically recognized embolization at other anatomic sites is rare. When the source of embolization is not obvious on hospital admission, useful procedures include routine blood cultures, electrocardiogram monitoring, and echocardiography. The size of the embolic material sufficient to cause a focal stroke is often too small to allow its exact source to be detected and all too often eludes all efforts at diagnosis. The cause of the embolus cannot be determined in a third or more of cases despite full use of laboratory investigations. Angiography within 24 hours of stroke usually demonstrates a pattern of arterial occlusion that is typical of embolus and permits diagnosis, but angiography is infrequently used. Brain imaging [computed tomography (CT) or magnetic resonance imaging (MRI)] allows the diagnosis of a focal infarction and allows inference of the size of the occluded artery. Modern CT and MRI appear positive for infarction within 24 hours if the artery occluded supplies a brain region sufficiently large to cause a deficit that persists for several days.

A diagnosis of thrombosis is considered first when the stroke has been preceded by transient ischemic attacks (TIAs). When the syndrome is of sudden onset, thrombus is clinically inseparable from embolus. No specific clinical syndrome separates the two mechanisms of infarction.

Hemorrhage has a characteristically smooth onset that is a helpful historical point in differential diagnosis. When the syndrome develops to an advanced stage within minutes or is halted at an early stage with only minor signs, the smooth evolution may not be apparent, and the clinical picture may then be inseparable from that of infarction. The hyperdense signal of blood on CT can immediately separate the clinically inobvious hemorrhage from infarct and should be used whenever treatment with anticoagulants is planned. Exceptional cases have been reported in which the typical hyperdensity characteristic of intracerebral hemorrhage was absent because of severe anemia, but this is unlikely to cause problems clinically. There are no reliable CT findings to distinguish hemorrhagic infarction and frank hematoma. The greater sensitivity to blood signal of MRI enables it to show a higher frequency of hemorrhagic infarction than is seen with CT.

The suddenness of onset and the focal signs give these syndromes the popular term "stroke" and distinguish cerebrovascular disease from other neurologic disorders. Hypertension, cardiac disease, arteriosclerosis, or other evidence of vascular disease are commonly present in cerebrovascular disease as well, unlike in other neurologic causes of focal deficit.

The distinction between TIA and completed stroke has been rendered less important since the advent of MR imaging has allowed detection of small fixed lesions that previously would have been missed. The traditional definition of TIA as a focal deficit lasting up to 24 hours greatly exaggerates the length of time needed for infarction to appear. Recent evidence suggests that 50% of patients with transient deficits lasting less than 24 hours will have evidence of ischemia on diffusion-weighted MR imaging and that 50% of those with diffusion-weighted abnormalities will have evidence of fixed infarction on subsequent T2-weighted images. In the acute state, considerations of differential diagnosis apply equally to TIA and stroke.

Sudden onset also characterizes trauma, epilepsy, and migraine. External signs usually indicate trauma, but when absent, diagnosis depends on a history that is not always easily obtained. It is important to remember that signs of external trauma need not be present for acceleration-deceleration forces to cause focal traumatic injury. The most frequent sites of brain contusions are the frontal and temporal poles, but these lesions neither produce an easily recognized clinical picture nor one often encountered in cases of stroke; however, epidural and subdural hematomas occur in a setting of trauma and may mimic a stroke. Although the trauma itself is sudden, the accumulation of the hematoma takes time: minutes or hours for epidural hemorrhage and as long as weeks for subdural hemorrhages.

Epidural hemorrhage is arterial in origin and usually produces a blood mass large enough to displace the brain and cause coma within hours after the injury. Apart from slower evolution, the clinical picture is otherwise similar to that of putaminal hemorrhage. Radiographs of the skull may reveal a fracture line that passes through the groove of the middle meningeal artery, which is usually a laceration. CT is the most helpful radiologic test; it demonstrates the position of the hematoma in all cases and gives the diagnosis even in comatose patients, when the fine points of clinical examination cannot be used. Surgical evacuation of the hematoma is usually appropriate even in cases with severe deficits because the brain dysfunction is due primarily to compression and the syndrome may be reversible when pressure from the hematoma has been relieved.

Subdural hematoma is typically venous in origin. The bleeding may be recurrent. The precipitating trauma may have been trivial or forgotten, and the blood may have been present long enough (over a week) to become isodense (radiographically inapparent) on CT or MRI. Fluctuating and false localizing signs are frequent. Further, a clot may be found on both sides. These common features often make subdural hematoma difficult to diagnose. Lumbar puncture shows a range of findings from normal to the extremes of xanthochromic cerebrospinal fluid (CSF) under high pressure with increased protein content. MRI has displaced angiography as the best means for showing the displacement of brain away from the skull.

As a sign of acute stroke, *seizures* are rare except in cases of lobar hemorrhage. The immediate postictal deficit mimics that caused by major stroke. Only the obtundation and amnestic state help suggest prior seizure. In a small percentage of cases, seizures develop months or years after a large infarct or hemorrhage. In these, the postictal state often represents a relapse of the original stroke syndrome, which usually resolves toward the chronic preictal state after a few days. Without a proper history, it may be nearly impossible to rule out new stroke. Rarely, seizures occurring in a patient with a prior stroke appear to have caused a long-lasting or permanent worsening or intensification of the prior deficit, without evidence of recurrent infarction. The mechanism by which this unusual event occurs is unknown.

Migraine is increasingly appreciated as a major source of difficulty in the diagnosis of TIA. Migraine may begin in middle age; the aura alone, without headache, is commonly experienced by those who suffer chronic migraine. When symptoms are visual and a diagnosis of transient monocular blindness is considered, the differential diagnosis from migraine is the easiest: Migraine typically produces a visual disorder that marches across the vision of both eyes as an advancing thin scintillating line that takes 5 to 15 minutes to pass out of vision. Subsequent unilateral pounding headache need not occur but makes the diagnosis certain. It is difficult to diagnose migraine as a cause of symptoms of hemisphere dysfunction because the auras of classic migraine only rarely include motor, sensory, language, or behavioral elements. TIA rarely goes from one limb to another like the visual disorder of migraine. A diagnosis of migraine probably should not be seriously considered as an explanation for transient hemisphere attacks unless the patient is young, has repeated attacks, experiences classic visual migraine auras at other times, and has a pounding headache contralateral to the sensory or motor symptoms in the hours after the attack. Recent studies of conditions long-recognized clinically, such as familial hemiplegic migraine and the familial periodic ataxias, have demonstrated mutations in ion channel genes as the cause of some cases of transient strokelike deficits. Familial hemiplegic migraine, for example, is caused by a mutation in a calcium channel gene on chromosome 19. These syndromes are generally recognized by the recurrence of stereotypic episodes throughout life in patients with an appropriate family history. Occasionally, sporadic cases may be seen in which the diagnosis of TIA has been entertained for years.

As indicated above, brain tumor and abscess may mimic TIA or stroke. Both usually evolve in days or weeks, which is longer than stroke, but may present with acute transient symptoms. It is commonly thought but rarely proven that intratumoral hemorrhage or focal seizure is responsible for many of these cases. One helpful historical point is that seizures often occur before focal signs are evident, a sequence that is rare in stroke. CT in tumor or abscess usually demonstrates an enhancing mass even when symptoms are mild. In contrast, CT in ischemic stroke is often negative in the first few days, contrast enhancement may not occur, and there are signs of a mass only when the syndrome is severe. In parenchymatous hemorrhage, the areas around the hematoma do not usually enhance with contrast material, but contrast enhancement is common when hemorrhage has occurred into a tumor. If the CSF is examined, increased pressure and clear or slightly cloudy fluid are encountered equally in tumors, early abscesses, and large infarcts. The CSF usually shows mild or moderate pleocytosis in abscess, but the same findings may be present in large infarcts.

When coma is present, other diagnoses that must be considered include metabolic disturbances of glucose, renal function, electrolytes, alcohol, and drugs. The odor of acetone on the breath and the presence of sugar in the urine favor a diagnosis of diabetes mellitus. Transient mild glycosuria and hyperglycemia often follow cerebral hemorrhage or infarction but do not approach the elevations seen in diabetic coma. In renal failure, high levels of blood urea nitrogen and creatinine often cause coma. Focal signs occasionally occur and then remit when the cause is reversed, often accompanying unrecognized infection or severe disturbances in electrolyte balance. Not uncommonly, however, focal deficits do not reverse themselves immediately, particularly when the metabolic derangement, such as hypoglycemia, has been profound. An alcoholic odor to the breath, normal blood pressure, no evidence of hemiplegia, and a normal CSF are characteristic findings in cases of coma due to acute alcoholism. In barbiturate intoxication, the coma may feature total paralysis of ocular motility and flaccid paralysis of the limbs with preserved pupillary reactions, which is a rare combination in stroke. The CSF pressure may be slightly elevated (200 to 300 mm H_2O) in any form of coma due to hypoventilation and CO_2 retention. Because alcoholics and drug abusers are prone to head injuries, the diagnosis of subdural hematoma should always be considered and excluded with appropriate imaging tests.

SUGGESTED READINGS

Bogousslavsky J, Martin R, Regli F, et al. Persistent worsening of stroke sequelae after delayed seizures. *Arch Neurol* 1992;49:385–388.

Caplan LR. ""Top of the basilar" syndrome. *Neurology* 1980;30:72–79.

Halperin JL, Hart RG. Atrial fibrillation and stroke: new ideas, persisting dilemmas. *Stroke* 1988;19:937–941.

Harrison MJG, Hampton JR. Neurologic presentation of bacterial endocarditis. *Br Med J* 1967;2:148–151.

Hinton RC, Mohr JP, Ackerman RH, et al. Symptomatic middle cerebral artery stem stenosis. *Ann Neurol* 1979;5:152–157.

Homma S, Di Tullio MR, Sacco RL, et al. Characteristics of patent foramen ovale associated with cryptogenic stroke. *Stroke* 1994;25:582–586.

Kasdon DL, Scott RM, Adelman LS, et al. Cerebellar hemorrhage with decreased absorption values on computed tomography: a case report. *Neuroradiology* 1977;13:265–266.

Kooiker JC, MacLean JM, Sumi SM. Cerebral embolism, marantic endocarditis and cancer. *Arch Neurol* 1976;33:260–264.

Libman RB, Wirkowski E, Alvir J, Rao TH. Conditions that mimic stroke in the ED. *Arch Neurol* 1995;52:1119–1122.

Ophoff RA, Terwindt GM, Vergouwe MN. Familial hemiplegic migraine and episodic ataxia type-2 are caused by mutations in the Ca^{2+} channel gene CACNL1A4. *Cell* 1996;87:543–552.

Rogers LR, Cho ES, Kempin S, Posner JB. Cerebral infarction from nonbacterial thrombotic endocarditis. Clinical and pathological study including the effects of anticoagulation. *Am J Med* 1987;83:746–756.

Terwindt GM, Ophoff RA, Haan J, et al. Variable clinical expression of mutations in the P/Q-type calcium channel gene in familial hemiplegic migraine. Dutch Migraine Genetics Research Group. *Neurology* 1998;50:1105–1110.

Wijman CAC, Wolf PA, Kase CS, Kelly-Hayes M, Beiser AS. Migrainous visual accompaniments are not rare in late life. The Framingham Study. *Stroke* 1998;29:1539–1543.

Wolf PA, Dawber TR, Thomas HE, et al. Epidemiologic assessment of chronic atrial fibrillation and risk of stroke: the Framingham Study. *Neurology* 1978;28:973–977.

Merritt's Neurology, 10th ed., edited by L.P. Rowland. Lippincott Williams & Wilkins, Philadelphia © 2000.

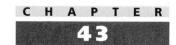

STROKE IN CHILDREN

ARNOLD P. GOLD
ABBA L. CARGAN

Children are not small adults when it comes to the diagnosis of stroke. In contrast to adults, the brain of the fetus or child is rapidly changing in organization and chemical composition. Neurologic functions change with neurologic maturation. The nervous system of a nonverbal relatively spastic newborn is different from that of a school-aged child who has mastered language skills and has purposeful locomotion and prehension.

Strokes in children differ from those in adults in three important ways: predisposing factors, clinical evolution, and anatomic site of pathology.

Cyanotic heart disease is one of the most common childhood conditions that predisposes to cerebral arterial or venous thrombosis. Leukemia commonly leads to cerebral hemorrhage. In contrast, atherosclerosis and hypertension predispose to stroke in adults.

Most stroke-prone children do not die as a direct result of stroke; they often improve much more than an adult with a comparable lesion because of the abundant collateral circulation or because of the differences in response of the immature brain to the lesion. The infant or young child with a new hemiplegia usually recovers to the point of being able to walk. If a child younger than age 4 years has a stroke, speech is invariably recovered and permanent aphasia does not occur. Children, especially before age 2 years, are more prone to behavioral changes, intellectual impairment, and epilepsy.

The anatomic site of the stroke lesion also differs in children. For example, affected children commonly show occlusion of the intracranial portion of the internal carotid artery and its branches, whereas adults more frequently show extracranial occlusions of the internal carotid. Cerebral aneurysms in children usually occur at the peripheral bifurcations of cerebral arteries; in adults, cerebral aneurysms usually occur near the circle of Willis.

INCIDENCE

In a well-defined pediatric population in Rochester, Minnesota, the annual incidence of cerebrovascular disease was 2.52 cases per 100,000 children or about 50% the incidence of primary intracranial neoplasm. This figure did not include conditions associated with birth, infection, or trauma, and there were few African-American children in the study. Cerebrovascular complications occur in 6% to 25% of patients with sickle cell disease; an untreated child with sickle cell disease has a 67% risk of a second stroke. Premature infants weighing less than 1500 g who require intensive care for more

than 24 hours have a 50% incidence of complicating subependymal hemorrhage or intraventricular hemorrhage. Intracranial infections, viral or bacterial, may also precipitate vascular complications. Craniocerebral trauma occurs in 3% of children during the first 7 years of life and cerebrovascular complications are common. Sonography, magnetic resonance imaging (MRI), and computed tomography (CT) (Figs. 43.1 through 43.4) are changing our concepts of the incidence of these disorders in children.

CLINICAL EVALUATION

A variety of studies should be considered in the evaluation of a child with stroke (Table 43.1). Selection of tests is guided by the clinical situation. Coagulopathy should be excluded as the cause of vasoocclusive or hemorrhagic infarctions in the newborn and young infant. Tissue injury occurs much more frequently from hypoxia and ischemia in the asphyxiated newborn. Vasculitis is an uncommon cause of stroke in young children. The possibility of embolic phenomena is increased with cardiac anomaly, particularly in the presence of a midline defect, which acts as a portal for paradoxic emboli. Older infants and children are susceptible to stroke events when there is a coagulopathy, but they also are more susceptible to vasculitides, which may result from immunologic or infectious causes.

ETIOLOGY

A rigid classification of childhood stroke is not possible because a specific cause (e.g., sickle cell disease) may cause hemorrhage in one child and thrombosis in another. Nevertheless, the following

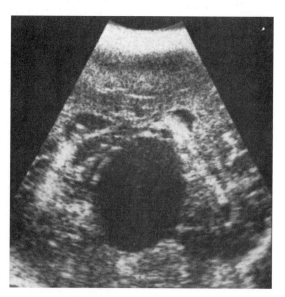

FIG. 43.1. Coronal cranial sonogram of newborn demonstrates aneurysmal dilatation of vein of Galen due to deep midline vascular malformation.

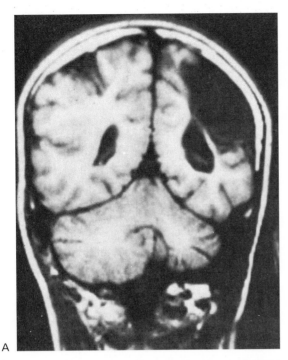
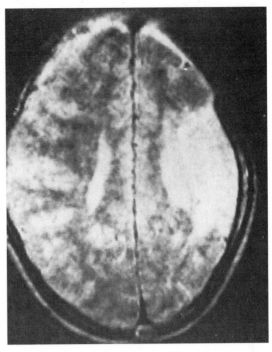

FIG. 43.2. Magnetic resonance images of a child with middle cerebral artery thrombosis and resultant hemiplegia with ischemic infarct. **A:** T1-weighted coronal image. **B:** Axial T2-weighted image of left middle cerebral artery ischemic infarct.

list is a clinically useful classification and includes occlusive vascular disease caused by thrombus or embolus, congenital anomalies (especially aneurysm or vascular malformation), hemorrhage, blood dyscrasias, and disorders that alter the permeability of the vascular wall:

Dural sinus and cerebral venous thrombosis
    Infections—face, ears, paranasal sinuses, meninges
    Dehydration and debilitating states
    Blood dyscrasias—sickle cell, leukemia, thrombotic thrombocytopenia

Neoplasms(neuroblastoma
Sturge-Weber-Dimitri (trigeminal encephaloangiomatosis)
Lead encephalopathy
Vein of Galen malformation
Arterial thrombosis
    Idiopathic
    Dissecting cerebral aneurysm
    Arteriosclerosis—progeria
    Cyanotic heart disease
    Cerebral arteritis
    Collagen disease—lupus erythematosus, periarteritis nodosa, Takayasu, Kawasaki
    Trauma to cervical carotid or cerebral arteries

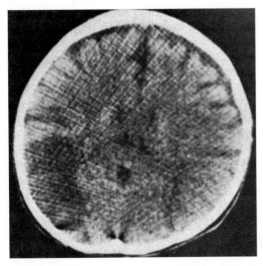

FIG. 43.3. Middle cerebral artery thrombosis of 24-hour duration. Computed tomography reveals inhomogeneous hypodensity with hazy margins in the parietooccipital region (early scanner, right and left reversed).

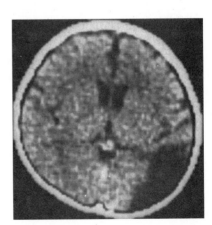

FIG. 43.4. Middle cerebral artery thrombosis, 3-week duration. Computed tomography (same child as in Fig. 43.3 but with different scanner) shows homogeneous lucency with sharp well-defined margins.

TABLE 43.1. CLINICAL EVALUATION OF CHILD WITH STROKE

Laboratory studies
  Serum
    Coagulation profile
    Fibrinogen level
    Protein C
    Protein S
    Antithrombin III
    Anticardiolipin antibody
    Lipid profile
    Antinuclear antibody
    Lupus erythematosus preparation
    Erythrocyte sedimentation rate
    Amino acids
    Blood cultures
    Toxicology screen
    Sickle cell preparation
    Mitochondrial DNA studies
  Urine
    Amino acids
    Organic acids
  Cerebrospinal fluid
    Chemistries (glucose, protein)
    Cell count and differential
    Lactate
    Cultures
Imaging studies
  Radiologic studies
    Computed tomography, head
    MRI, head
    MR, angiogram/MR venogram
    Cerebral angiogram
  Ultrasound studies
    Carotid artery Doppler
    Vertebral artery Doppler
    Transcranial doppler
    Echocardiogram
  Nuclear medicine
    Single-photon emission computed tomography
Electrical studies
  Electroencephalogram
Other studies
  Purified protein derviative (for moyamoya)

MRI, Magnetic resonance imaging.

Inflammatory bowel disease
Delayed radiation
Sickle-cell disease
Extra-arterial disorders—craniometaphyseal dysplasia, mucormycosis, tumors of the base of the skull
Metabolic (diabetes mellitus, hyperlipidemia, homocystinuria)
Oral contraceptives
Drug abuse
Arterial embolism
  Air—complications of cardiac, neck, or thoracic surgery
  Fat complications of long-bone fracture
  Septic complications of endocarditis, pneumonia, lung abscess
  Arrhythmias
  Complications of umbilical vein catheterization
Intracranial hemorrhage
  Neonatal

Premature—subependymal and intraventricular
Full term—subdural
Vascular malformation
Aneurysm
Blood dyscrasias
Trauma
Vitamin-deficiency syndromes
Hepatic disease
Hypertension
Complications of immunosuppressants and anticoagulants
Mitochondrial disease
Mitochondrial myopathy, encephalopathy, lactic acidosis, and strokelike episodes (MELAS)
Migraine

ARTERIAL THROMBOSIS

Cerebral arterial thrombosis in children usually involves the intracranial area of the internal carotid artery, although the cervical portion of the internal carotid artery or a spinal artery may be occluded. Neurologic manifestations vary according to the area involved.

As in adults, systemic diseases, including collagen-vascular diseases and arteritis, may cause cerebral thrombosis in children. Cerebral arteritis usually results from bacterial infections, but other infections may also involve cerebral arteries. Herpes zoster ophthalmica and rarely chickenpox may have complicating vasculitis that causes delayed-onset hemiparesis. Bacterial pharyngitis, cervical adenitis, sinusitis, or pneumonitis may lead to cerebral arteritides. Mucormycosis infection associated with uncontrolled diabetes may extend from the paranasal sinuses to the arteries in the frontal lobe. Both syphilis and tuberculosis may result in cerebral thrombosis in children and adults.

Extrinsic conditions may traumatize or compress the cerebral arteries. Most of these occlusions in children affect the anterior circulation. Vertebrobasilar occlusion may follow cervical dislocations and occlusion of the vertebral artery at the C2 level. Tumors of the base of the skull, craniometaphyseal dysplasia, and retropharyngeal abscesses may compress cerebral arteries.

Sickle cell disease commonly causes thrombosis of large or small arteries; less commonly, it results in dural sinus thrombosis. Approximately 7% to 11% of patients with sickle cell disease have stroke before the age of 20 years. Large cerebral artery thrombosis with telangiectasia (moyamoya) results in acute hemiplegia or alternating hemiplegia (Fig. 43.5). Small arterial thrombosis can produce an altered state of consciousness, convulsions, or visual disturbances. About 65% of untreated children have repeated thromboses with additional impairment of motor and intellectual functions. Radiographic progression in the absence of clinically overt deficits suggests increase in the stroke risk with time and underscores the importance of treatment. Cerebrovascular complications are less common in children with sickle hemoglobin C disease and rarely occur in sickle cell trait. MRI, magnetic resonance angiography, and diffusion-weighted imaging have become invaluable tools in defining stroke events in children, and transcranial Doppler is a useful adjunct for follow-up and screening.

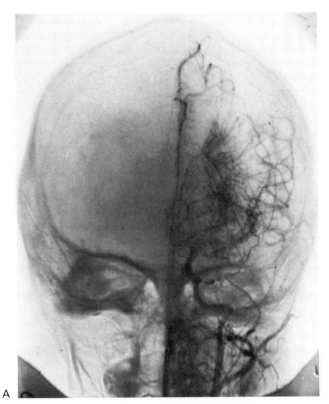

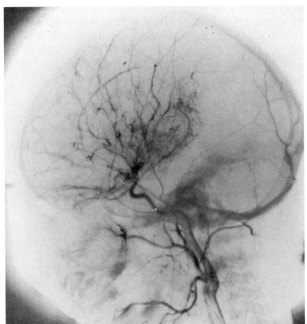

FIG. 43.5. Moyamoya syndrome. Anteroposterior **(A)** and lateral **(B)** views from arterial phase of left common carotid arteriogram demonstrate multiple enlarged and serpentine lenticulostriate arteries, which have a "puff of smoke" appearance. Note occlusions of the proximal segments of the anterior and middle cerebral arteries.

Migraine may be manifested by hemiplegia or visual field defects. MRI changes are nonspecific, but punctate periventricular white matter changes are often attributed to migraine. MELAS should be considered when stroke accompanies migraine in a child.

Inflammatory bowel disease may lead to a hypercoagulable state with or without thrombocytosis. Delayed radiation vasculopathy, juvenile diabetes mellitus, homocystinuria, hyperlipidemias, drug abuse, and oral contraceptives result in acute hemiplegia.

Malignancies, most commonly lymphoreticular tumors, may be complicated by a cerebral infarct. Most often this is a complication of disseminated vascular occlusion or chemotherapy. Stroke may also result from direct metastatic spread or a complicating thrombocytopenia or fungal infection.

Coagulopathies may become evident with a thrombotic event. Protein C and protein S deficiencies increase the risk of stroke in childhood. Factor V Leiden deficiency also predisposes to cerebral vessel thrombosis.

Many children with cerebral arterial thrombosis are healthy before the vascular occlusion occurs and there is no apparent predisposing factor. A dissecting aneurysm due to a congenital defect of the arterial wall has been implicated in some of these idiopathic cases.

Signs and Symptoms

Depending on the predisposing factor, the child with arterial thrombosis has specific clinical signs of the underlying disorder plus neurologic signs of the occluded cerebral artery that are usually found in the anterior circulation. A previously healthy child usually has an acute hemiplegia that is preceded by focal or generalized convulsions, fever, and altered consciousness; less commonly, a series of transient ischemic attacks eventually results in a completed stroke. Acute hemiplegia is the typical neurologic finding, but hemisensory loss, visual field defects, and aphasia may be seen. The disorder maximally involves the hand; if it persists, the involved limbs are spastic, short, and atrophic. Seizures, focal or generalized, are often refractory to anticonvulsants.

The hemiplegia is usually an isolated episode. Bilateral carotid artery thrombosis with telangiectasia typically presents with headaches before the hemiplegia, and recurrences or alternating hemiplegia is characteristic.

Laboratory Data

Blood count, erythrocyte sedimentation rate (ESR), and urinalysis are normal at the time of thrombosis. The cerebrospinal fluid (CSF) is normal at first, and a mild leukocyte pleocytosis may occur a few weeks later. The electroencephalogram often reveals a slow-wave focus over the involved area. Although skull radiographs are normal when thrombosis occurs, after several years they may show signs of cerebral atrophy with thickening of calvarium, enlargement of the frontal and ethmoid sinuses, and elevation of the petrous pyramid of the temporal bone on the involved side.

CT supplies information about the site and age of the infarct. Within 24 hours there is a nonhomogeneous decreased-density lesion secondary to edema (Fig. 43.3). By the end of the first week, liquefaction necrosis develops, and the infarct becomes homogeneous with defined margins (Fig. 43.4). At 3 months, the necrotic infarct is replaced by a cystic fluid-containing cavity, and the lesion with sharp margins has the homogeneous density of CSF.

Sonography is invaluable in defining cerebral anatomy and hemorrhagic complications in the infant, especially the premature infant (Fig. 43.1). MRI has become an important diagnostic tool in the early diagnosis of ischemic lesions (Fig. 43.2). Magnetic resonance angiography is useful in defining the major portions of large- and medium-size vessels of the intracranial circulation. magnetic resonance venography is helpful in the diagnosis of venous sinus thrombosis if there are changes in vascular outflow. Diffusion-weighted MR imaging is gaining prominence in diagnostic evaluation. Echo-planar diffusion-weighted MR imaging reveals acute and hyperacute ischemia not seen on conventional spin-echo imaging.

Arteriography, when performed early, may demonstrate the thrombosed cerebral artery; later there may be a recanalized vessel or evidence of collateral circulation. Cerebral angiography can usually be performed safely in children of all ages. The patency of other cerebral arteries and the ample collateral circulation in children contrast with the status of the cerebral arteries and collateral circulation in adult stroke patients. Children with sickle cell disease are at greater risk if the level of hemoglobin S is not maintained at a level below 20% by exchange transfusion.

The following practical angiographic classification was formulated by Hilal et al. (1971) to supply diagnostic and prognostic information for the following patterns.

Extracranial Occlusion

Trauma is the most common cause of thrombosis of the cervical portion of the internal carotid artery. Blunt trauma in the paratonsillar area of the oropharynx or direct impact of the carotid artery against the transverse process of the second cervical segment can cause occlusion. Characteristically, about 24 hours lapse between the traumatic incident and clinical manifestations. Nontraumatic conditions are usually infectious in origin.

Basal Occlusion Disease Without Telangiectasia

The thrombotic lesion involves the arteries of the base of the brain: supraclinoid area of the internal carotid artery, proximal segments of anterior or middle cerebral artery, or basilar artery. The condition is unilateral and does not recur.

Basal Occlusive Disease with Telangiectasia (Moyamoya)

This condition involves the arteries at the base of the brain, is often bilateral, and is associated with prominent telangiectasia, especially in the region of the basal ganglia (Fig. 43.5). Of varied etiology, it may complicate sickle cell disease, bacterial or tuberculous meningitis, or neurofibromatosis; it may also complicate the treatment plans of radiotherapy. Recurrent episodes of thrombosis are common and may result in alternating hemiplegia, epilepsy, and learning disabilities. Neuropsychological testing has demonstrated the benefit of surgical intervention in preventing further deterioration of function.

Peripheral Leptomeningeal Artery Occlusions

Branch occlusions of the distal leptomeningeal arteries may occur with diabetes mellitus, sickle cell disease, trauma, infection, tumor encasement, or neurocutaneous syndromes. The excellent collateral circulation usually results in rapid recovery from the acute hemiplegia.

Perforating Artery Occlusion

Involvement of the small perforating arteries, most commonly the striate arteries, is seen in children with homocystinuria or periarteritis nodosa. Episodes recur, causing a progressive neurologic deficit with alternating hemiparesis or quadriparesis, subarachnoid hemorrhage, or death.

Treatment

Therapeutic measures may include parenteral fluids, antibiotics when indicated, anticonvulsants, anticoagulants to prevent extension of the thrombus, and variations of the agents to control increased intracranial pressure. Variations of the synangiosis procedure are used to enhance circulation to ischemic areas of the brain in moyamoya. Anastomoses of external carotid to internal carotid arteries are not feasible because the arteries of the child's brain are too small in diameter. Instead, the superficial temporal artery is attached to the surface of the brain, allowing the formation of a rich collateral network, which supplies parts of the brain that would otherwise be ischemic.

Anticoagulants are rarely indicated except when a stroke is in progress. Rarely does arterial thrombosis result in sufficient increased pressure to require intracranial pressure monitoring or measures to reduce intracranial pressure. Bilateral cervical sympathectomies to increase regional blood flow and anastomosis of the external and internal carotid arteries have been of dubious value.

Sickle cell disease is treated by repeated blood transfusions. The risk of future strokes is reduced by a long-term transfusion program to maintain hemoglobin S at a level below 20%. This has been demonstrated in clinical trials that have looked at accumulation of neurologic deficits and radiographic evidence of ischemic events.

CEREBRAL EMBOLISM

In cerebral embolism, an artery can be occluded by air, fat, tumor, bacteria, parasites, foreign body, or a fragment from an organized thrombus. The middle cerebral artery or its branches are most commonly involved.

Cerebral embolism in childhood is usually cardiogenic, especially after cardiac catheterization or open heart surgery but is also seen with cardiac arrhythmias due to cyanotic congenital heart disease or rheumatic valvular disease, bacterial endocarditis, or atrial myxoma. Septic embolism from pulmonary inflammatory disease or bacterial endocarditis may result in brain abscesses or mycotic aneurysms. Fat embolism is an unusual complication of long-bone fractures.

Signs and Symptoms

The focal neurologic signs vary according to the artery occluded; manifestations are complete within seconds or minutes. There are also signs and symptoms of the causal disorder: transient blindness with air embolism; petechiae and hematuria with septic emboli; cutaneous petechiae, urinary free fat, and fat in the retinal vessels with fat emboli due to long-bone fracture or intravenous fat infusions.

Fat embolism has a characteristic clinical picture. A lucid interval of 12 to 48 hours occurs after a long-bone fracture. The child then becomes febrile with pulmonary symptoms that include dyspnea, cyanosis, and blood-tinged sputum. Within a few hours, there is an acute encephalopathy that may include focal neurologic signs, diabetes insipidus, seizures, delirium, stupor, or coma.

Laboratory Data

Routine laboratory studies after cerebral embolism are often normal, but a moderate polymorphonuclear leukocytosis may be present. The CSF is usually normal, but there may be a mild elevation of the protein content. Septic embolism in bacterial endocarditis may cause an elevated CSF protein content and pleocytosis. Atrial myxomas commonly show peripheral blood leukocytosis, anemia, and an elevated ESR. The electroencephalogram characteristically shows a slow-wave abnormality in the areas supplied by the occluded vessel.

MRI is often characteristic in showing multiple infarcts, some of which are hemorrhagic (Fig. 43.6). The lesions become lucent with sharp margins 2 to 3 months later. Diffusion-weighted imaging and fluid attenuated inversion recovery FLAIR MRI studies assist the rapid detection of stroke events. Lesions that conform to a territorial distribution are the sequelae of embolic strokes. Cerebral angiography should be performed in all children with septic emboli. It delineates the occluded artery and may demonstrate mycotic aneurysm.

Treatment

Management of cerebral embolism is primarily symptomatic, including anticonvulsants for seizures. Anticoagulants are rarely used in children. Corticosteroids, in dosages used in the management of cerebral edema, are effective in reversing the pulmonary symptoms of fat embolism.

INTRACRANIAL HEMORRHAGE

Hemorrhagic stroke in children usually results from trauma or bleeding disorders. When these conditions are excluded, intracranial hemorrhage is caused by an arteriovenous malformation or aneurysm.

Signs and Symptoms

The child with subarachnoid hemorrhage usually presents with acute onset of headache, vomiting, stupor or coma, and convulsions. Findings include stiff neck and Brudzinski and Kernig signs. Extensor plantar responses and subhyaloid hemorrhages on funduscopic examination are often noted early. Fever and systemic hypertension are nonspecific findings. Ruptured cerebral aneurysm frequently presents with a catastrophic clinical picture. Bleeding from an arteriovenous malformation is less dramatic and is often associated with focal signs.

Laboratory Data

Blood dyscrasias are identified by appropriate blood studies. Children with bleeding from other causes have polymorphonuclear leukocytosis, normal or moderately elevated ESR, and transient albuminuria and glycosuria.

CSF analysis and CT document subarachnoid hemorrhage. Sonography in the infant with an open fontanel and CT at any age are invaluable in the diagnosis of intracranial hemorrhage and its complications. CT may demonstrate arteriovenous malformation (Fig. 43.7) or giant cerebral arterial aneurysm. Cerebral angiography is the definitive diagnostic technique for these conditions.

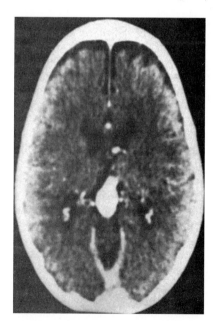

FIG. 43.7. Arteriovenous malformation. Computed tomography shows aneurysmal dilatation of vein of Galen due to large deep malformation. Note enlargement of draining sinuses and mild hydrocephalus with ventricular enlargement.

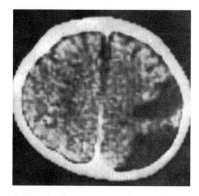

FIG. 43.6. Cerebral embolism. Computed tomography 3 months after cerebral embolism shows multiple infarcts. Sharp margins have density of CSF.

Treatment

The management of intracranial hemorrhage varies with the cause of the hemorrhage. Repeated lumbar punctures, mannitol, and corticosteroids are often used, but their effectiveness is controversial. Ruptured intracranial aneurysms require good nursing care, and unless the child is comatose or there is a medical contraindication, surgical extirpation offers the best prognosis. Except in cases of mycotic aneurysms, the occurrence of a second hemorrhage shortly after the initial hemorrhage is uncommon in children. Arteriovenous malformations should be surgically removed whenever possible. Embolization may be used preoperatively to reduce the size of the malformation or to treat inaccessible lesions. Traumatic arteriovenous fistulas are treated by ligation of the fistula, embolization, or the implantation of detachable balloons.

METABOLIC DISORDERS

MELAS is a mitochondrial disorder associated with two identifiable mitochondrial DNA mutations. MELAS is characterized by four criteria: a strokelike episode before age 40 years; encephalopathy characterized by seizures, dementia, or both; lactic acidosis; and ragged red fibers in the muscle biopsy (Chap. 96). Some patients with MELAS have features of other mitochondrial disorders.

Homocystinuria (cystathionine synthetase deficiency) is an autosomal recessive inherited disorder featuring elevated serum methionine and homocystine concentrations and excessive urinary excretion of homocystine. Cerebral arterial occlusive disease and venous thrombosis occur in this condition.

SUGGESTED READINGS

Adams RJ, McKie VC, Brambilla PhD, et al. Stroke prevention trial in sickle cell anemia. *Control Clin Trials* 1997;1:110–129.

Adams RJ, McKie VC, Hsu L, et al. Prevention of a first stroke by transfusions in children with sickle cell anemia and abnormal results on transcranial doppler ultrasonography. *N Engl J Med* 1998;339:5–11.

Allan WC, Volpe JJ. Periventricular-intraventricular hemorrhage. *Pediatr Clin North Am* 1986;36:47–63.

Carter S, Gold AP. Acute infantile hemiplegia. *Pediatr Clin North Am* 1964;14:851–864.

Devilat M, Toso M, Morales M. Childhood stroke associated with protein C or S deficiency and primary antiphospholipid syndrome. *Pediatr Neurol* 1993;9:67–70.

Eeg-Olofsson O, Ringheim Y. Stroke in children. Clinical characteristics and prognosis. *Acta Paediatr Scand* 1983;72:391–396.

Fisher M, Sotak CH, Minematsu K, et al. New magnetic resonance techniques for evaluating cerebrovascular disease. *Ann Neurol* 1992;32:115–122.

Ganesan V, Savvy L, Chong WK, et al. Conventional cerebral angiography in children with ischemic stroke. *Pediatr Neurol* 1999;20:38–42.

Gold AP, Challenor YB, Gilles FH, et al. IX Strokes in children. *Stroke* 1973;4:835–894, 1009–1052.

Gold AP, Ransohoff J, Carter S. Arteriovenous malformation of the vein of Galen in children. *Acta Neurol Scand* 1964;40[Suppl 11]:1–31.

Grossman R, Novak G, Patel M, et al. MRI in neonatal dural sinus thrombosis. *Pediatr Neurol* 1993;9:235–238.

Hilal SK, Solomon GE, Gold AP, et al. Primary cerebral arterial occlusive disease in children. II. Neurocutaneous syndromes. *Radiology* 1971;99:71–87.

Hirano M, Ricci E, Koenigsberger MR, et al. MELAS: an original case and clinical criteria for diagnosis. *Neuromusc Disord* 1992;2:125–135.

Humphreys RP. Complications of hemorrhagic stroke in children. *Pediatr Neurosurg* 1991;17:163–168.

Johnson AJ, Lee BCP, Lin W. Echoplanar diffusion-weighted imaging in neonates and infants with suspected hypoxic-ischemic injury: correlation with patient outcome. *AJR Am J Roentgenol* 1999;172:219–226.

Kamholz J, Tremblay G. Chickenpox with delayed contralateral hemiparesis caused by cerebral angiitis. *Ann Neurol* 1985;18:358–360.

Kinugasa K, Mandai S, Kamata I, et al. Surgical treatment of moyamoya disease. Operative technique for encephalo-duro-arterio-myo-synangiosis: follow-up, clinical results, and angiograms. *Neurosurgery* 1993;32:527–531.

Koo B, Becker LE, Chuang S, et al. Mitochondrial encephalomyopathy, lactic acidosis, stroke-like episodes (MELAS): clinical, radiological, pathological, and genetic observations. *Ann Neurol* 1993;34:25–32.

Lacey DJ, Terplan K. Intraventricular hemorrhage in full-term neonates. *Dev Med Child Neurol* 1982;14:332–337.

Laxer RM, Dunn HG, Flodmark O. Acute hemiplegia in Kawasaki disease and infantile polyarteritis nodosa. *Dev Med Child Neurol* 1984;26:814–821.

Limbord TG, Ruderman RJ. Fat embolism in children. *Clin Orthop* 1978;136:267–269.

Martinowitz U, Heim M, Tadmor R, et al. Intracranial hemorrhage in patients with hemophilia. *Neurosurgery* 1986;18:538–540.

Matsushima Y, Aoyagi M, Niimi Y, et al. Symptoms and their pattern of progression in childhood moyamoya disease. *Brain Dev* 1990;12:784–789.

Michiels JJ, Stibbe J, Bertina R, et al. Effectiveness of long term oral anticoagulation treatment in preventing venous thrombosis in hereditary protein S deficiency. *Br Med J* 1987;295:641–643.

Natowicz M, Kelley RI. Mendelian etiologies of stroke. *Ann Neurol* 1987;22:175–192.

Packer RJ, Rorke LB, Lange BJ, et al. Cerebrovascular accidents in children with cancer. *Pediatrics* 1985;76:194–201.

Paradis K, Bernstein ML, Adelson JW. Thrombosis as a complication of inflammatory bowel disease in children: a report of four cases. *J Pediatr Gastroenterol Nutr* 1985;4:659–662.

Pavlakis S, et al. Brain infarction in sickle cell anemia: MRI correlates. *Ann Neurol* 1988;23:125–130.

Sandok BA, von Estorff I, Giuliani ER. CNS embolism due to atrial myxoma—clinical features and diagnosis. *Arch Neurol* 1980;37:485–488.

Seibert JJ, Glasier CM, Kirby RS, et al. Transcranial Doppler, MRA, and MRI as a screening examination for cerebrovascular disease in patients with sickle cell anemia: an 8-year study. *Pediatr Radiol* 1998;28:138–142.

Shahar E, Gilday DL, Hwang PA, et al. Pediatric cerebrovascular disease: alterations of regional cerebral blood flow detected by Tc 99m-HMPAO SPECT. *Arch Neurol* 1990;47:578–584.

Shields WD, Manger MN. Ultrasound evaluation of neonatal intraventricular hemorrhage. I. Anatomy. *Perinatol Neonatol* 1983;75:19–25.

Shields WD, Manger MN. Ultrasound evaluation of neonatal intraventricular hemorrhage. I. Pathology. *Perinatol Neonatol* 1983;76:28–35.

Solomon GE, Hilal SK, Gold AP, et al. Natural history of acute hemiplegia of childhood. *Brain* 1970;93:107–120.

Stein BM, Wolpert SM. Arteriovenous malformations of the brain. Current concepts and treatment. *Arch Neurol* 1980;37:1–5, 69–75.

Thorarensen O, Ryan S, Hunter J, Younkin DP. Factor V Leiden mutation: an unrecognized cause of hemiplegic cerebral palsy, neonatal stroke, and placental thrombosis. *Ann Neurol* 1997;42:372–375.

Ueki K, Meyer FB, Mellinger JF. Moyamoya disease: the disorder and surgical treatment. *Mayo Clin Proc* 1994;69:749–759.

van Hoff J, Ritchey AK, Shaywitz BA. Intracranial hemorrhage in children with sickle cell disease. *Am J Dis Child* 1985;139:1120–1123.

Volpe JJ. Neonatal periventricular hemorrhage: past, present, and future. *J Pediatr* 1978;92:693–696.

Whitlock JA, Janco RL, Phillips JA. Inherited hypercoagulable states in children. *Am J Pediatr Hematol Oncol* 1989;11:170–173.

Wilimas J, Goff JR, Anderson HR, et al. Efficacy of transfusion therapy for one to two years in patients with sickle cell disease and cerebrovascular accidents. *J Pediatr* 1980;96:205–208.

Yoffe G, Buchanan GR. Intracranial hemorrhage in newborn and young infants with hemophilia. *J Pediatr* 1988;113:333–336.

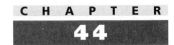

TREATMENT AND PREVENTION OF STROKE

FRANK M. YATSU

Medical therapies for stroke are designed to (1) minimize or prevent ischemic brain infarction, (2) optimize functional recovery, and (3) avert stroke recurrence. Specific therapies depend on the stroke syndrome, as discussed in this chapter.

Atherothrombotic brain infarction (ABI) and artery-to-artery thromboembolic strokes are the most common stroke syndromes and result from atherosclerosis. ABI represents a continuum from transient ischemic attacks (TIAs) to completed strokes with fixed neurologic deficits. Intermediate manifestations of ABI are progressing strokes or strokes in evolution.

TRANSIENT ISCHEMIC ATTACKS

TIAs are brief attacks of neurologic symptoms in either the carotid or vertebrobasilar circulations. In attacks involving the carotid circulation, focal neurolgic symptoms develop, such as amaurosis fugax or transient monocular blindness, hemiparesis, or aphasia; in the vertebrobasilar circulation, symptoms are more generalized, such as visual blurring, vertigo, ataxia, dysarthria, and diplopia. TIAs usually last for minutes to hours, but by convention symptoms and signs may persist for up to 24 hours. TIAs usually result from platelet aggregates forming on atheromatous plaques and embolizing to temporarily occlude a distal arteriole. The resulting ischemic symptoms of brain or retina correspond to the arteriole temporarily rendered ischemic. Because hemodynamic factors can cause similar symptoms of ischemia due to reduced cerebral or retinal blood flow and by compressive brain lesions, transient neurologic symptoms alone cannot definitively identify the underlying cause or pathology. For example, these symptoms may occur with emboli of cardiac origin, thrombocytosis, polycythemia vera, arteritis, or, rarely, mass lesions (e.g., meningioma and subdural hematoma) or seizures.

With vertebrobasilar TIAs or vertebrobasilar insufficiency, these symptoms may be simulated by hemodynamic causes of reduced blood flow, such as decreased cardiac output. Because cardiac arrhythmias may be etiologic, Holter monitoring may be required to establish a diagnosis.

For patients with carotid TIAs and greater than 70% carotid bifurcation stenosis, carotid endarterectomy (CEA), performed by demonstrably skilled surgeons, is the treatment of choice in medically suitable patients. Three prospective, randomized studies assessing the value of CEA in these patients were published in 1991, and each demonstrated the benefits of CEA. The three studies were the North American Symptomatic Carotid Endarterectomy Trial (NASCET), the MRC European Carotid Surgery Trial, and the Veterans Affairs Cooperative Study on Carotid Endarterectomy. In 1998, preliminary results of NASCET showed a 6.5% reduction in strokes following CEA in patients with 50% to 69% stenosis; there was no reduction in strokes for those with less than 50% stenosis. Because the actual cost-benefit of CEA is controversial, as is the use of CEA in asymptomatic subjects, clinicians must make their decisions on the basis of whether the stenosis is progressing, on factors related to operative risk, and on stroke-risk factors.

Extracranial–intracranial bypass surgery, or the anastomosis of the superficial temporal artery to the middle cerebral artery, does not prevent further strokes following TIAs or minor strokes in patients with inaccessible stenoses or occlusions in the carotid artery territory. However, this procedure may be beneficial in patients with hemodynamic causes of TIAs, although this has not been proven. A new and promising area of therapy is balloon angioplasty and stenting for both extracranial and intracranial occlusive disease. Although a steep learning curve indicates that experience conveys improved outcome, aggregate results are encouraging. For example, a review of over 2,000 cases of carotid angioplasty and stenting showed a success rate of nearly 98%, with death and stroke rates of approximately 2%. Despite these encouraging outcomes, it is too early to declare this procedure a standard. Nonetheless, for patients with occlusive disease who are not surgical candidates, angioplasty offers a reasonable alternative.

To prevent recurrence, medical therapy of TIAs or minor strokes due to occlusive vascular disease includes an anticoagulant and antiplatelet drugs such as aspirin, ticlopidine, clopidogrel, or dipyridamole in combination with aspirin. Aspirin reduces the incidence of stroke by about 25%, as determined by a large metaanalysis. The most effective dose of aspirin, whether ultralow at 30 to 75 mg per day or large at 1,300 mg per day, is controversial and will require a prospective study to resolve. Until those studies are undertaken, one or two adult aspirin tablets daily can be recommended, since this dose has less bleeding complications. Ticlopidine is more effective than aspirin, particularly in the elderly (greater than 75 years) and women, as well as for vertebrobasilar symptoms, small-vessel disease of brain, and aspirin failure. This drug is ineffective with high-grade carotid stenosis (greater than 70%). Clopidogrel, an analog of ticlopidine, has fewer side effects such as diarrhea, bruising, and leukopenia that require monitoring over the first several months of use, as with ticlopidine. The combination of dipyridamole and aspirin is controversial because of the design of the study in which it was tried, but certain patients may benefit. Short-term subcutaneous heparin does not avert stroke as effectively as aspirin according to the International Stroke Trial with nearly 20,000 subjects worldwide. Furthermore, the low-molecular-weight heparin study showed no benefit with this therapy. The value of aspirin was also demonstrated in the Chinese Acute Stroke Trial with over 20,000 patients. Anticoagulation with warfarin sodium (Coumadin) appears to reduce stroke recurrence with intracranial arterial stenoses, as shown in a retrospective study, but the true value of this treatment will await the prospective study. Until the results of that study, however, anticoagulation can be recommended in suitable patients with an international normalized ratio (INR) between 2.0 and 3.0.

PROGRESSING STROKES

A gradual or stuttering increase in neurologic deficits over hours suggests the diagnosis of progressing stroke, provided mass lesions (e.g., hematoma or edema) have been excluded. The progressive symptoms are attributed to an enlarging intraarterial thrombus.

Although thrombolytic agents such as alteplase (tissue plasminogen activator [t-PA]) or urokinase have not been systematically investigated under these circumstances, thrombolysis should be considered if the National Institutes of Health (NIH) guidelines (reviewed below) are met. However, in the posterior circulation, some authorities recommend intraarterial, catheter-delivered thrombolysis, even in patients who are stuporous and whose symptoms have progress beyond 12 hours. The objective benefits of this therapy will require prospective, randomized studies.

COMPLETED STROKES WITH FIXED NEUROLOGIC DEFICITS

The approach to acute ischemic stroke has been dramatically and convincingly altered since t-PA was shown to significantly improve neurologic recovery, provided treatment begins within 3 hours of stroke onset and computed tomography (CT) of the brain is normal or shows only minimal infarction. The protocol approved by the U.S. Food and Drug Administration and NIH for t-PA use is shown in Table 44.1. Despite approval of this guideline, controversy exists on the use of t-PA, particularly if specialized stroke units and teams are not available.

Similar benefits with t-PA were shown in the European Cooperative Acute Stroke Study when protocol violators were excluded. This same group in Europe will try to replicate the NIH study, and in North America, use of t-PA in the 3- to 5-hour poststroke period was being assessed, but the trial has been put on hold. In European and Australian studies of streptokinase, increased incidence of hemorrhage caused early termination of the trials.

The success with thrombolysis further stimulated the use of so-called neuroprotective agents to minimize ischemic brain damage resulting from both increased release of excitotoxins (e.g., glutamic acid) during ischemia and oxidative and other injuries during reperfusion with recanalization. Although experimental studies demonstrated the value of these agents, particularly those that blocked or inhibited the excitotoxins, calcium uptake, adhesion molecules, and free radical formation, clinical trials of these compounds have been disappointing.

TABLE 44.1. THROMBOLYSIS WITH TPA IN ACUTE ISCHEMIC STROKE

Duration	<3 h from onset
CT brain	No hemorrhage or clear infarction
Laboratory studies	Hematocrit, platelets, PT/PTT
If above are negative or normal, treat with intravenous tPA	
Administer tPA, 0.9 mg/kg: 10% in 1 min; remainder in 60 min	
Perform hourly neurologic examinations × 6, then every 2 h for first 24 h	
Repeat CT and blood studies at day 2	

These include *N*-methyl-D-aspartate (NMDA) receptor blockers such as selfotel, aptiganel (Cerestat), and MK-801; the glutamate secretion inhibitor lubeluzole; and the anti-ICAM (intercellular adhesion molecule) monoclonal antibody enlimomab. However, other compounds such as clomethiazole, citicoline, and still others show promise but must await further prospective studies.

Another area of current investigation is the use of mechanical devices either to physically extract or suction out the thrombus. These corkscrew, laser, or suction devices are promising, but it is too early to determine their proper clinical role.

EMBOLIC STROKE OF CARDIAC AND AORTIC ORIGIN

Therapy of cardiac emboli depends on the cardiac pathology: An infected prosthetic valve may require replacement, and myxomatous emboli necessitate surgical excision of the tumor. The most common cause (more than 50%) of embolic stroke of cardiac origin is atrial fibrillation with or without mitral pathology and recent myocardial infarction. Postinfarction emboli are likely to follow large anterior or septal infarcts or infarcts with akinetic segments detected by two-dimensional echocardiography. Before age 45 years, mitral valve prolapse may be a cause, but primarily in those with leaflet redundancy.

For emboli associated with atrial fibrillation or myocardial infarction, anticoagulation to reduce reembolization is warranted. In the Stroke Prevention in Atrial Fibrillation (SPAF) study, anticoagulation substantially reduced embolic stroke regardless of the subject's age, even after age 75 years. An increased incidence of embolization with atrial fibrillation was associated with the following factors: previous embolic strokes, left ventricular hypertrophy with reduced ejection fraction, hypertension, and congestive failure. Having no risk factors was associated with a 1.5% to 2.5% per year incidence of stroke, while two or more risk factors raised the incidence to more than 17%.

One common cardiac anatomic abnormality causing embolic stroke is patent foramen ovale (PFO). Implicating PFO as the cause of stroke requires certain criteria: absence of a likely cause of stroke, demonstration of right-to-left shunting (as shown by transthoracic echocardiography following intravenous saline bubbles), evidence of straining at the onset of the stroke (which raises intrathoracic pressure), and a PFO of sufficient size (e.g., greater than 2 mm in diameter). Although prospective studies on the treatment of PFO have not been performed, it is reasonable to treat symptomatic patients initially with aspirin or anticoagulation. However, recurrent stroke symptoms require either percutaneous, catheter-delivered clamshell closure or open heart surgery with foraminal closure, which is the more definitive option.

A newly recognized cause of embolic stroke is aortic atheromas. Significant atheromas measure greater than 4 mm in diameter and are usually not calcified. Whether anticoagulation will reduce emboli will be the subject of an international prospective study.

Anticoagulation is not recommended if an infarct is large either by CT or clinical signs. Lumbar puncture is unnecessary to exclude hemorrhage if CT studies are adequate.

INTRACEREBRAL HEMORRHAGE

Medical treatment of intracerebral hemorrhage is supportive. For large cerebellar hemorrhages, as with sizable infarcts, surgical decompression is required if vital structures of the medulla are at risk, as suggested by fourth ventricle displacement, lateral ventricular enlargement, cisternal obliteration, and declining levels of consciousness. Surgical evacuation of a hematoma is considered for lobar or cortical white matter hemorrhages if there are signs of declining sensorium or herniation in an operatively suitable candidate. However, ongoing studies should clarify precise criteria for surgery of polar or white matter hemorrhages. Surgery is not beneficial for hemorrhages in the other common sites, such as putamen, thalamus, and pons. Lumbar puncture in the presence of intracerebral hemorrhage may precipitate herniation and is contraindicated.

SUBARACHNOID HEMORRHAGE WITH CONGENITAL OR BERRY ANEURYSM

Surgical, balloon, or coagulative extirpation of an aneurysm is definitive therapy in subarachnoid hemorrhage (SAH). After SAH, sedation and a quiet environment are essential to prevent marked elevation of arterial pressure that may provoke rebleeding, a major complication of SAH. Use of antifibrinolytic agents to prevent rebleeding by preserving the thrombus around the bleeding site has not been successful. A second complication of SAH is vasospasm, which correlates with the amount of blood in the subarachnoid space. Nimodipine, a calcium channel blocker, has been shown in prospective, randomized studies to avert vasospasm or at least ischemic complications. A third complication is hydrocephalus due to the obstructive nature of subarachnoid blood to cerebrospinal fluid flow, and ventricular shunting may be required to relieve pressure. Other, less common complications that may require intervention include seizures, the syndrome of inappropriate antidiuretic hormone secretion, and cardiac arrhythmias.

STROKE REHABILITATION

Physical rehabilitative measures should begin as soon as possible after stroke onset to maximize functional recovery. These measures are directed toward improvement in activities of daily living, muscle strength, ambulation, transfer, dressing, and hygiene, as well as toward avoidance of contractures and psychologic factors such as depression and motivation. Depression can occur in cerebral lesions of both hemispheres and may respond well to antidepressants such as the tricyclics and the serotonin-reuptake inhibitors. Speech and occupational therapies should be utilized to optimize rehabilitation.

STROKE PREVENTION

Stroke prevention is directed to the underlying pathologic processes such as atherosclerosis, arteritis, cardiac disease, dissection, and so on.

Atherothrombotic Brain Infarction

Treatment of hypertension is the most powerful preventive measure to avoid ABI and has resulted in a greater than 25% reduction in stroke incidence over the last several decades. Control of hypertension also reduces stroke recurrence; the optimum blood pressure, as determined by an international study, is approximately 145/85 mm Hg. In African-American subjects, the optimum blood pressure control may be lower, at approximately 115 mm Hg systolic. Measures to intervene aggressively against other risk factors for atherosclerosis should be undertaken. These include tight (but not excessive) control of blood glucose in diabetics, dietary and drug control of blood cholesterol, and reduction of smoking, obesity, stress, and sedentary lifestyles. The total cholesterol level should be less than 240 mg/dL, but preferably less than 200 mg/dL; and the low-density lipoprotein fraction should be less than 130 mg/dL, preferably near 100 to 110 mg/dL. A metaanalysis of all forms of treatment aimed at reducing cholesterol following myocardial infarction, namely, a diet low in cholesterol and saturated fats, fibric acid derivatives, resins, and HMG-CoA reductase inhibitors (statins) show that statins are the most effective in both reducing cholesterol and preventing myocardial infarction and stroke. Whether or not statins prevent recurrent stroke following ABI has not been studied, but a statin is a reasonable therapeutic option if the cholesterol is elevated and cost is not an issue.

Prophylactic use of aspirin to prevent stroke in asymptomatic persons, based on the rationale of its benefit in TIA patients with extracranial occlusive disease, is controversial. A few studies suggest an increased incidence of hemorrhagic stroke in asymptomatic elderly individuals. However, until a definitive prospective, randomized study is performed, one adult aspirin tablet daily can be recommended, since the benefit of preventing myocardial infarction appears to outweigh the risk of stroke.

SUGGESTED READINGS

Adams HP Jr, Brott TG, Furlan AJ, et al. Guidelines for thrombolytic therapy for acute stroke: a supplement to the guidelines for the management of patients with acute ischemic stroke. A statement for healthcare professionals from a special writing group of the Stroke Council, American Heart Association. *Stroke* 1996;27:1711–1718.

Adams HP Jr, Woolson RF, Clarke WR, et al. Design of the trial of org 10172 in acute stroke treatment (TOAST). *Control Clin Trials* 1997;18:358–377.

Adjusted-dose warfarin versus low-intensity, fixed-dose warfarin plus aspirin for high-risk patients with atrial fibrillation. Stroke Prevention in Atrial Fibrillation III randomized clinical trial. *Lancet* 1996;348:633–638.

Barnett HJM, Gent M, Sackett DL, et al. A randomized trial of aspirin and sulfinpyrazone in threatened stroke: the Canadian Cooperative Study Group. *Circulation* 1980;62[Suppl V];V97–V105.

Bendixen BH, Adams HP. Ticlopidine or clopidogrel as alternatives to aspirin in prevention of ischemic stroke. *Eur Neurol* 1996;36:256–257.

Beneficial effect of carotid endarterectomy in symptomatic patients with high-grade carotid stenosis. North American Symptomatic Carotid Endarterectomy Trial Collaborators. *N Engl J Med* 1991;325:445–453.

Biller J, Feinberg WM, Castaldo JE, et al. Guidelines for carotid endarterectomy: a statement for healthcare professionals from a special writing group of the Stroke Council, American Heart Association. *Stroke* 1998;29:554–562.

Bucher HC, Griffith LE, Guyatt GH. Effect of HMG-CoA reductase inhibitors on stroke: a meta-analysis of randomized, controlled trials. *Ann Intern Med* 1998;128:89–95.

Caplan LR, Mohr, JP, Kistler JP, Korshetz W. Thrombolysis—not a panacea for ischemic stroke. *N Engl J Med* 1997;337;1309–1310.

CAST: randomised placebo-controlled trial of early aspirin use in 20,000 patients with acute ischaemic stroke. CAST (Chinese Acute Stroke Trial) Collaborative Group. *Lancet* 1997;349;1641–1649.

Chiu D, Krieger D, Villar-Cordova C, et al. Intravenous tissue plasminogen activator of acute ischemic stroke: feasibility, safety, and efficacy in the first year of clinical practice. *Stroke* 1998;29;18–22.

Del Zoppo GJ. Thrombolytic therapy in cerebrovascular disease. *Stroke* 1988;19:1174–1179.

Dietrich EB, Ndiave M, Reid DB. Stenting in the carotid artery: initial experience in 110 patients. *J Endovasc Surg* 1996;3;42–62.

Effect of intensive diabetes management on macrovascular events and risk factors in the Diabetes Control and Complication Trials. *Am J Cardiol* 1995;75;894–903.

Endarterectomy for asymptomatic carotid artery stenosis. Executive Committee for the Asymptomatic Carotid Atherosclerosis Study. *JAMA* 1995;273:1421–1428.

Failure of extracranial-intracranial arterial bypass to reduce the risk of ischemic stroke: results of an international randomized trial. The EC/IC Bypass Study Group. *N Engl J Med* 1985;33:1191–1200.

Grotta J. tPA—the best current option for most patients. *N Engl J Med* 1997;337;1311–1313.

Grotta JC, Yatsu FM, Pettigrew LC, et al. Prediction of carotid stenosis progression by lipid and hematologic measurements. *Neurology* 1989;39:1325–1331.

Hacke W, Kaste M, Fieschi C, et al. Intravenous thrombolysis with recombinant tissue plasminogen activator for acute hemispheric stroke. The European Cooperative Acute Stroke Study (ECASS). *JAMA* 1995;274;1017–1025.

Hachinski V, Graffagnino C, Beaudry M, et al. Lipids and stroke: a paradox resolved. *Arch Neurol* 1996;53;303–308.

Hansson L, Zanchetti A, Carruthers SG, et al. Effects of intensive blood-pressure lowering and low-dose aspirin in patients with hypertension: principal results of the Hypertension Optimal Treatment (HOT) randomised trial. *Lancet* 1998;351;1755–1762.

Haynes RB, Sandler RS, Larson EB, et al. A critical appraisal of ticlopidine, a new antiplatelet agent: effectiveness and clinical indications for prophylaxis of atherosclerotic events. *Arch Intern Med* 1992;152:1376–1380.

The International Stroke Trial (IST): a randomised trial of aspirin, subcutaneous heparin, both, or neither among 19,435 patients with acute ischaemic stroke. International Stroke Trial Collaborative Group. *Lancet* 1997;349;1569–1581.

Mayberg MR, Wilson SE, Yatsu FM, et al. Carotid endarterectomy and prevention of cerebral ischemia in symptomatic carotid stenosis. Veterans Affairs Cooperative Studies Program 309 Trialist Group. *JAMA* 1991;266:3289–3294.

Miller VT, Pearce LA, Feinberg WM, Rothrock JF, Anderson DC, Hart RG. Differential effect of aspirin versus warfarin on clinical stroke types in patients with atrial fibrillation. Stroke Prevention in Atrial Fibrillation Investigators. *Neurology* 1996;46;238–240.

Moore WS, Barnett HJ, Beebe HG, et al. Guidelines for carotid endarterectomy: a multidisciplinary consensus statement from the ad hoc committee, American Heart Association. *Stroke* 1995;26;188–201.

MRC European Carotid Surgery Trial: interim results for symptomatic patients with severe (70-99%) or with mild (0-29%) carotid stenosis. European Carotid Surgery Trialists' Collaborative Group. *Lancet* 1991;337:1235–1243.

Pessin MS, Adams HP Jr, Adams RJ, et al. American Heart Association prevention conference. IV. Prevention and rehabilitation of stroke acute intervention. *Stroke* 1997;28:1518–1521.

Robinson RG. Neuropsychiatric consequences of stroke. *Annu Rev Med* 1997;48:217–229.

Secondary prevention of vascular disease by prolonged antiplatelet treatment. Antiplatelet Trialists' Collaboration. *Br Med J (Clin Res Ed)* 1988;296;320–331.

Tissue plasminogen activator for acute ischemic stroke. The National Institute of Neurological Disorders and Stroke rt-PA Stroke Study Group. *N Engl J Med* 1995;333;1581–1587.

Yatsu FM, Villar-Cordova C. Atherosclerosis. In: Barnett HJM, Mohr JP, Stein B, Yatsu FM, eds. *Stroke: pathophysiology, diagnosis, and management.* Philadelphia: WB Saunders, 1998:29–39.

Zöller B, Hillurp A. Berntorp E, Dahlbäck B. Activated protein C resistance due to a common factor V gene mutation is a major risk for venous thrombosis. *Annu Rev Med* 1997;48:45–58.

Merritt's Neurology, 10th ed., edited by L.P. Rowland. Lippincott Williams & Wilkins, Philadelphia © 2000.

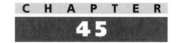

CHAPTER 45

SUBARACHNOID HEMORRHAGE

**STEPHAN A. MAYER
GARY L. BERNARDINI
JOHN C.M. BRUST
ROBERT A. SOLOMON**

Subarachnoid hemorrhage (SAH) accounts for 5% of all strokes; it affects nearly 30,000 individuals per year in the United States, with an annual incidence of 1 per 10,000. Saccular (or berry) aneurysms at the base of the brain cause 80% of all cases of SAH. Nonaneurysmal causes of SAH are listed in Table 45.1. SAH most frequently occurs between ages 40 and 60 years, and women are affected more often than men.

SAH due to the rupture of an intracranial aneurysm is a devastating event; approximately 12% of patients die before receiving medical attention, and another 20% die after admission to the hospital. Of the two-thirds of patients who survive, approximately one-half remain permanently disabled, primarily due to severe cognitive deficits. Advances in neurosurgery and intensive care, including an emphasis on early aneurysm clipping and aggressive therapy for vasospasm, have led to improved survival over the last three decades, with a reduction in overall case fatality from approximately 50% to 33%.

PATHOLOGY AND EPIDEMIOLOGY OF INTRACRANIAL ANEURYSMS

Saccular aneurysms most often occur at the circle of Willis or its major branches, especially at bifurcations. They arise where the arterial elastic lamina and tunica media are defective, and tend to enlarge with age. The typical aneurysm wall is composed only of intima and adventitia and can become paper-thin. Many aneurysms, particularly those that rupture, are irregular and multilobulated, and larger aneurysms may be partially or completely filled with an organized clot, which occasionally is calcified. The point of rupture is usually through the dome of the aneurysm.

Eighty-five to ninety percent of intracranial aneurysms are located in the anterior circulation, with the three most common

TABLE 45.1. NONANEURYSMAL CAUSES OF SAH

Trauma
Idiopathic perimesencephalic SAH
Arteriovenous malformation
Intracranial arterial dissection
Cocaine and amphetamine use
Mycotic aneurysm
Pituitary apoplexy
Moyamoya disease
Central nervous system vasculitis
Sickle cell disease
Coagulation disorders
Primary or metastatic neoplasm

sites being the junction of the posterior communicating and internal carotid artery (approximately 40%), the anterior communicating artery complex (approximately 30%), and the middle cerebral artery at the first major branch point in the sylvian fissure (approximately 20%). Posterior circulation aneurysms most often occur at the apex of the basilar artery or at the junction of the vertebral and posteroinferior cerebellar artery. Saccular aneurysms of the distal cerebral arterial tree are rare. Nearly 20% of patients have two or more aneurysms; many of these are "mirror" aneurysms on the same vessel contralaterally.

Intracranial aneurysms are uncommon in children but occur with a frequency of 2% in adults, suggesting that approximately 2 to 3 million Americans have an aneurysm. However, more than 90% of these are small (less than 10 mm) and remain asymptomatic throughout life.

The annual risk of rupture of an asymptomatic intracranial aneurysm is approximately 0.7%. By contrast, the annual risk of bleeding of a previously ruptured aneurysm after 6 months is substantially higher, between 2% and 4% per year.

The prevalence of aneurysms increases with age and is higher in patients with atherosclerosis, a family history of intracranial aneurysm, or autosomal-dominant polycystic kidney disease (PCKD). Intracranial aneurysms have also been associated with Ehlers-Danlos syndrome, Marfan syndrome, pseudoxanthoma elasticum, coarctation of the aorta, and sickle-cell disease. Screening for unruptured intracranial aneurysms with magnetic resonance angiography (MRA) is indicated in patients with PCKD and in family members who have two or more first-degree relatives with intracranial aneurysms; testing will be positive in 5% to 10% of these individuals.

Among patients who harbor an intracranial aneurysm, the strongest risk factors for bleeding are previous rupture, large size, and cigarette smoking. The risk of SAH is approximately five times higher for aneurysms greater than 10 mm in diameter than for smaller aneurysms, and 3 to 10 times higher among smokers than nonsmokers. Other risk factors for aneurysm rupture include hypertension, alcohol use, female sex, posterior circulation location, multiple aneurysms, and cocaine or amphetamine use.

CLINICAL MANIFESTATIONS

SAH usually commences with an explosive "thunderclap" headache followed by neck stiffness. The pain is often described as "the worst headache of my life." The headache is usually generalized, but focal pain may refer to the site of aneurysmal rupture (e.g., periorbital pain related to an ophthalmic artery aneurysm). Common associated symptoms include loss of consciousness, nausea and vomiting, back or leg pain, and photophobia. In patients who lose consciousness, tonic posturing may occur and may be difficult to differentiate from a seizure. Although aneurysmal rupture often occurs during periods of exercise or physical stress, SAH can occur at any time, including sleep.

More than one-third of patients give a history of suspicious symptoms days or weeks earlier, including headache, stiff neck, nausea and vomiting, syncope, or disturbed vision. These prodromal symptoms are often due to minor leaking of blood from the aneurysm, and are therefore referred to as "warning leaks" or "sentinel headaches." In 25% of patients, the initial manifestations of SAH are misdiagnosed, which can lead to delays in treatment and increased morbidity and mortality.

Neck stiffness and the Kernig sign are hallmarks of SAH. However, these signs are not invariably present, and low back pain is sometimes more prominent than headache. Preretinal or subhyaloid hemorrhages—large, smooth-bordered, and on the retinal surface—occur in up to 25% of patients and are practically pathognomonic of SAH.

The most important *determinant* of outcome after SAH is the patient's neurologic condition on arrival at the hospital. Alterations in mental status are the most common abnormality; some patients remain alert and lucid; others are confused, delirious, amnestic, lethargic, stuporous, or comatose. The modified Hunt and Hess grading scale serves as a means for risk stratification for SAH based on the first neurologic examination (Table 45.2). Patients classified as grade I or II SAH have a relatively good prognosis, grade III carries an intermediate prognosis, and grades IV and V have a poor prognosis. Focal neurologic signs occur in a minority of patients but may point to the site of bleeding; hemiparesis or aphasia suggests a middle cerebral artery aneurysm, and paraparesis or abulia suggests an aneurysm of the proximal anterior cerebral artery. These focal signs are sometimes due to a large focal hematoma, which may require emergency evacuation.

In 10% of patients with nontraumatic SAH and in two-thirds

TABLE 45.2. HUNT AND HESS GRADING SCALE FOR ANEURYSMAL SAH

Grade	Clinical Findings	Hospital Mortality (%)	
		1968	1997
I	Asymptomatic or mild headache	11	1
II	Moderate to severe headache or oculomotor palsy	26	5
III	Confused, drowsy, or mild focal signs	37	19
IV	Stupor (localizes to pain)	71	42
V	Coma (posturing or no motor response to pain)	100	77
Total		35	18

Data from 275 patients reported by Hunt and Hess in 1968, and 214 patients reported by Oshiro et al. 1997; mortality figures do not include out-of-hospital deaths. (Modified from Tamargo RJ, Walter KA, Oshiro EM. Aneurysmal subarachnoid hemorrhage: prognostic features and outcomes. *New Horiz* 1997, 5:364–375.)

of those with negative angiography, computed tomography (CT) reveals blood confined to the perimesencephalic cisterns, with the center of bleeding adjacent to the midbrain and pons. These patients with "perimesencephalic" SAH always have a normal neurologic examination and a benign clinical course; sentinel headaches, rebleeding and vasospasm almost never occur. The source of hemorrhage in these patients is unknown but is presumably venous.

Symptoms and signs of an unruptured intracranial aneurysm may result from compression of adjacent neural structures or thromboembolism. These aneurysms are often, but not always, large or giant (greater than 25 mm). Aneurysms of the posterior communicating artery frequently compress the oculomotor nerve (almost always affecting the pupil). Aneurysms of the intracavernous segment of the internal carotid artery may damage the third, fourth, fifth, or sixth cranial nerves, and their rupture can lead to formation of a carotid cavernous fistula. Less often, large aneurysms compress the cortex or brainstem, causing focal neurologic signs or seizures. Thrombosis within the aneurysmal sac occasionally sends emboli to the artery's distal territory, causing transient ischemic attacks or infarction. In the absence of SAH, some patients experience sudden, severe headache without nuchal rigidity, perhaps related to aneurysmal enlargement, thrombosis, or meningeal irritation; these symptoms can clear with aneurysm clipping.

DIAGNOSTIC STUDIES

Computed Tomography

CT should be the first diagnostic study for establishing the diagnosis of SAH. CT most commonly demonstrates diffuse blood in the basal cisterns (Fig. 45.1); with more severe hemorrhages, blood extends into the sylvian and interhemispheral fissures, ventricular system, and over the convexities. The distribution of blood can provide important clues regarding the location of the ruptured aneurysm. CT may also demonstrate a focal intraparenchymal or subdural hemorrhage, ventricular enlargement, a large thrombosed aneurysm, or infarction due to vasospasm. The sensitivity of CT for SAH is 90% to 95% within 24 hours, 80% at 3 days, and 50% at 1 week. Accordingly, a normal CT never rules out SAH, and a lumbar puncture should always be performed in patients with suspected SAH and negative CT. Magnetic resonance imaging (MRI) is most useful for evaluating patients with amalgram-negative SAH.

Lumbar Puncture

The cerebrospinal fluid (CSF) is usually grossly bloody. SAH can be differentiated from a traumatic tap by a xanthochromic (yellow-tinged) appearance of the centrifuged supernatant; however, xanthochromia may take up to 12 hours to appear. CSF pressure is nearly always high and the protein elevated. Initially, the proportion of CSF leukocytes to erythrocytes is that of the peripheral blood, with a usual ratio of 1:700; after several days a reactive pleocytosis and low glucose levels may develop due to a sterile chemical meningitis caused by the blood. Red blood cells and xanthochromia disappear in about 2 weeks, unless hemorrhage recurs.

Angiography

Cerebral angiography is the definitive diagnostic procedure for detecting intracranial aneurysms and defining their anatomy (Fig. 45.2). Because there is often more than one aneurysm, the entire cerebral arterial system must be studied. Vasospasm, local thrombosis, or poor technique can lead to a false-negative angiogram. For this reason, patients with a negative angiogram at first should have a follow-up study 1 to 2 weeks later; an aneurysm will be demonstrated in about 5% of these cases. The exception to this rule is patients with "perimesencephalic" SAH, who usually do not require follow-up angiography. At present, neither MRA nor CT angiography is sensitive enough to serve as the diagnostic test of choice for detecting intracranial aneurysms.

COMPLICATIONS OF ANEURYSMAL SUBARACHNOID HEMORRHAGE

Rebleeding

Aneurysmal rebleeding is a dreaded complication of SAH. The risk of rebleeding is highest within the first 24 hours after the initial aneurysmal rupture (4%), and remains elevated (approximately 1% to 2% per day) for the next 4 weeks (Fig. 45.3). The cumulative risk of rebleeding in untreated patients is 20% at 2 weeks, 30% at 1 month, and 40% at 6 months. After the first 6 months, the risk of rebleeding is 2% to 4% annually. The prognosis of patients who rebleed is poor; approximately 50% die immediately, while another 30% die from subsequent complications. Although rebleeding is often attributed to uncontrolled hypertension, endogenous fibrinolysis of clot around the rupture point of the aneurysm may be a more important causative mechanism.

Vasospasm

Delayed cerebral ischemia from vasospasm accounts for a large proportion of morbidity and mortality after SAH. Progressive arterial narrowing develops after SAH in approximately 70% of patients, but delayed ischemic deficits develop in only 20% to 30%. The process begins 3 to 5 days after the hemorrhage, becomes maximal at 5 to 14 days, and gradually resolves over 2 to 4 weeks. Accordingly, deterioration attributable to vasospasm never occurs before the third day after SAH, and occurs with peak frequency between 5 and 7 days (see Fig. 45.3). There is a strong relationship between the amount of cisternal blood seen on initial CT and the risk for the development of symptomatic ischemia. Symptoms usually include a change in level of consciousness, focal neurologic signs (e.g., hemiparesis), or both, and the process is usually most severe in the immediate vicinity of the aneurysm.

Although thick subarachnoid blood is the principal precipitating factor, the precise cause of arterial narrowing after SAH is poorly understood. Vasospasm is not simply due to vascular smooth muscle contraction; arteriopathic changes are seen in the vessel wall, including subintimal edema and infiltration of leukocytes. The prevailing view is that substances released from the blood clot interact with the vessel wall to cause inflammatory ar-

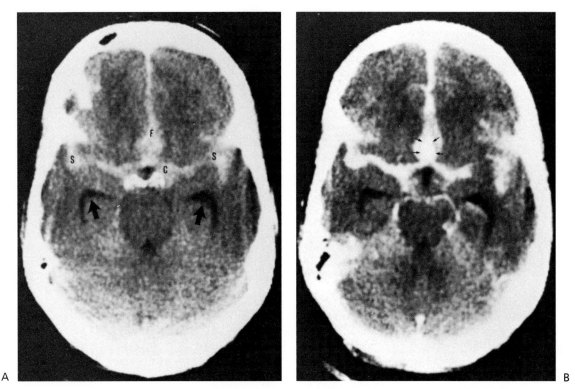

A

B

FIG. 45.1. A: Noncontrast CT demonstrates hyperdensity within the suprasellar cistern *(C)* and interhemispheral fissure *(F)*. Note the hyperdensity of subarachnoid blood within both sylvian fissures *(S)*. There is prominence of both temporal horns, indicative of mild communicating hydrocephalus. **B:** Contrast CT demonstrates enhancement of an anterior communicating artery aneurysm observed within the interhemispheral fissure *(arrows)*. (Courtesy of Dr. Richard S. Pinto.)

terial spasm. Putative mediators include oxyhemoglobin (with its intrinsic vasoconstrictive properties), hydroperoxides and leukotrienes, free radicals, prostaglandins, thromboxane A_2, serotonin, endothelin, platelet-derived growth factor, and other inflammatory mediators.

Hydrocephalus

Acute hydrocephalus occurs in 15% to 20% of patients with SAH and is primarily related to the volume of intraventricular and subarachnoid blood. In mild cases, hydrocephalus causes

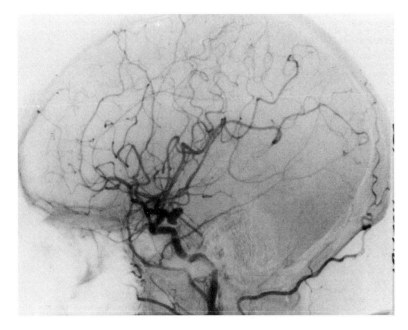

FIG. 45.2. Lateral view of a left common carotid angiogram demonstrates a bilobed aneurysm of the left internal carotid artery at the level of the posterior communicating artery. (Courtesy Dr. S. Chan.)

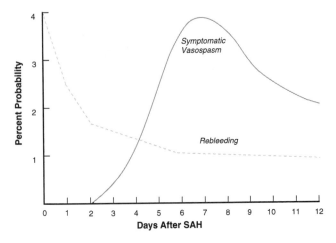

FIG. 45.3. The daily percentage probability for the development of symptomatic vasospasm *(solid line)* or rebleeding *(dashed line)* after SAH. Day 0 denotes day of onset of SAH.

lethargy, psychomotor slowing, and impaired short-term memory. Additional findings may include limitation of upward gaze, sixth cranial nerve palsies, and lower extremity hyperreflexia. In more severe cases, acute obstructive hydrocephalus leads to elevated intracranial pressure. Affected patients are stuporous or comatose, and progressive brainstem herniation eventually results from continued CSF production unless a ventricular catheter is inserted.

Delayed hydrocephalus may develop from 3 to 21 days after SAH. The clinical syndrome is identical to that of normal pressure hydrocephalus, with insidious onset of dementia, gait disturbance, and urinary incontinence. The clinical response to ventriculoperitoneal shunting is usually excellent. Overall, 20% of SAH patients require shunting for chronic hydrocephalus.

Seizures

Seizures occur in 5% to 10% of SAH patients. Two-thirds of seizures occur within the first month, and the remainder occur within the first year. Seizures after SAH are related primarily to large amounts of subarachnoid or parenchymal clot. Ictal events at the onset of bleeding do not portend an increased risk of late seizures.

Fluid and Electrolyte Disturbances

Hyponatremia and intravascular volume contraction frequently occur after SAH and reflect homeostatic derangements that favor excessive free-water retention and sodium loss. Hyponatremia occurs in to 5% to 30% of patients after SAH and is primarily related to inappropriate secretion of antidiuretic hormone and free-water retention. This process may be further exacerbated by excessive natriuresis that occurs after SAH ("cerebral salt-wasting"), related to elevations of atrial natriuretic factor and the glomerular filtration rate. Whereas hyponatremia after SAH is usually mild and asymptomatic, sodium loss and intravascular volume contraction increase the risk of ischemia in the presence of severe vasospasm. To minimize the development of hypovolemia and hyponatremia after SAH, patients should be given large volumes of isotonic crystalloid, with restriction of other potential sources of free water.

Neurogenic Cardiac and Pulmonary Disturbances

Severe SAH is typically associated with a surge in catecholamine levels and sympathetic tone, which in turn can lead to neurogenic cardiac dysfunction, neurogenic pulmonary edema, or both. Transient electrocardiographic abnormalities occur in at least 50% of patients with SAH but usually do not produce symptoms. In some poor-grade patients, however, cardiac enzyme release and a reversible form of neurogenic "stunned myocardium" can occur. Hypotension and reduction of cardiac output may result, leading to impaired cerebral perfusion in the face of increased intracranial pressure or vasospasm. Neurogenic pulmonary edema, characterized by increased permeability of the pulmonary vasculature, may occur in isolation or in combination with neurogenic cardiac injury.

TREATMENT OF ANEURYSMAL SUBARACHNOID HEMORRHAGE

The initial goal of treatment is to prevent rebleeding by excluding the aneurysmal sac from the intracranial circulation while preserving the parent artery and its branches. Once the aneurysm has been secured, the focus shifts toward monitoring and treating vasospasm and other secondary complications of SAH. This is best performed in an intensive care unit (ICU).

Surgical Management

Surgical clipping is the definitive treatment for aneurysms. In the 1980s, neurosurgeons began to abandon the traditional practice of delaying surgery until several weeks after aneurysmal rupture, in favor of early clipping within 48 to 72 hours. This change in practice became feasible with safer microsurgical techniques. Nonetheless, surgery still remains hazardous, with a 5% to 10% risk of major morbidity or mortality in most cases. Besides preventing early rebleeding, early surgery permits aggressive treatment of vasospasm with hypertensive hypervolemic therapy, which can be dangerous with an unclipped aneurysm. Although early surgery was first reserved for patients in good clinical condition (Hunt and Hess grades I to III), this approach has been extended to all but the most moribund patients. The advent of endovascular coil embolization has been a major advance because it is a treatment option for high-risk patients who are not good candidates for early surgery.

Very large aneurysms of the basilar artery, long deemed untreatable, can now be clipped in specialized centers that provide deep hypothermic circulatory arrest. This technique gives the surgeon the necessary exposure to identify and preserve penetrating arteries that supply the brainstem. Good neurologic outcomes can be attained in more than 80% of patients, despite total circulatory arrest for 20 to 40 minutes.

The management of asymptomatic unruptured aneurysms is controversial. Most neurosurgeons recommend surgery for

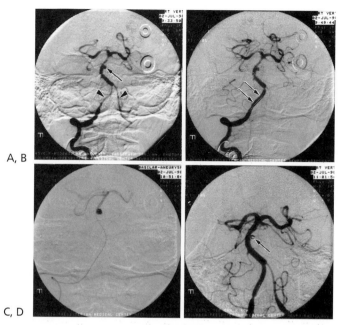

A, B

C, D

FIG. 45.4. A: Cerebral angiogram demonstrates a left-pointing, 3-mm, midbasilar aneurysm *(closed arrow)* and vasospasm of both vertebral arteries *(open arrows)*, the distal basilar artery, and the proximal right posterior cerebral artery. **B:** Significant increase in luminal diameter of the right vertebral artery after balloon angioplasty *(arrows)*. **C:** Microcatheter positioned at the neck of the midbasilar aneurysm. **D:** Midbasilar aneurysm *(arrow)* with no residual filling after packing with a single platinum detachable coil. (Courtesy of Dr. Huang Duong.)

highest for large aneurysms and for aneurysms of the basilar artery.

Endovascular Therapy

Endovascular therapy, introduced in the early 1990s, is a promising alternative for the treatment of aneurysms that are not amenable to surgical repair. Endovascular packing of aneurysms (Fig. 45.4) with soft, thrombogenic detachable platinum coils leads to at least short-term obliteration of small-necked aneurysms in 80% to 90% of cases, with an acceptable complication rate of approximately 9%. Aneurysms with wider necks are less amenable to treatment because it is more difficult to attain complete obliteration and the coils or thrombus may migrate. The main disadvantage of endovascular treatment is the potential for rebleeding after many years due to coil compaction and aneurysm regrowth at the residual neck. Until long-term follow-up studies define this risk more precisely, long-term serial angiography is recommended for patients with intracranial aneurysms treated with coils.

Large, expanding aneurysms of the intracavernous internal carotid artery can be treated with proximal endovascular occlusion. Before permanent occlusion, a trial balloon occlusion is performed to determine whether there is adequate collateral flow through the circle of Willis to prevent symptomatic ischemia in the ipsilateral hemisphere. If the test occlusion is negative, an extracranial–intracranial bypass procedure may be considered before permanent occlusion is attempted.

Intensive Care Management

A suggested algorithm for the postoperative management of SAH is outlined in Table 45.3. All patients with SAH should be

aneurysms larger than 5 mm, as long as the potential benefit of surgery (reduced lifetime risk of bleeding) outweighs the risks. In good hands, the risk of major morbidity or mortality from clipping of an unruptured aneurysm is 2% to 5%; the risk is

TABLE 45.3. COLUMBIA-PRESBYTERIAN MANAGEMENT PROTOCOL FOR ACUTE SAH

Blood pressure	Control elevated blood pressure (BP) during the preoperative phase (systolic BP >150 mm Hg) with intravenous labetolol or nicardipine to prevent rebleeding
Intravenous hydration	Preoperative: normal (0.9%) saline at 80–100 mL/h Postoperative (low risk[a]): normal (0.9%) saline at 80–100 mL/h, and 250 mL 5% albumin every 6 h Postoperative (high risk[b]): normal (0.9%) saline at 80–100 mL/h, and 250 mL 5% albumin every 2 h if the central venous pressure is ≤8 mm Hg or pulmonary artery diastolic pressure is ≤14 mm Hg
Laboratory testing	Periodically, check complete blood cell count; transfuse for hematocrit <24% in stable patients or <30% in patients with symptomatic vasospasm Periodically, check electrolytes to detect hyponatremia Obtain serial ECGs, and check admission creatine kinase MB to evaluate for cardiac injury; perform echocardiography in patients with abnormal ECG findings
Seizure prophylaxis	Fosphenytoin or phenytoin i.v. load (15–20 mg/kg); discontinue on postop day 2 unless patient is unstable
Vasospasm prophylaxis	Nimodipine, 60mg p.o. every 4 h for 21 d
Vasospasm diagnosis	Transcranial Doppler sonography every 1–3 days until day 8–14 after SAH
Therapy for symptomatic vasospasm	Place patient in Trendelenburg (head-down) position Infuse 500mL 5% albumin over 15 min If the deficit persists, raise the systolic BP with phenylephrine or dopamine until the deficit resolves, up to a maximum of 220mm Hg. Continue "high risk" IV hydration protocol, place pulmonary artery catheter, and add dobutamine to maintain cardiac index ≥4.0 L/min/m². Emergency angiogram for possible cerebral angioplasty if the patient has a severe deficit (e.g., two-point drop in Glasgow Coma Scale score or 2/5 limb paresis) of 2-hour duration despite antihypertensive therapy

[a]Low risk for symptomatic vasospasm: Hunt and Hess grades I or II, and minimal or diffuse thin cisternal blood on admission CT.
[b]High risk for symptomatic vasospasm: Hunt and Hess grades III, IV, or V, or thick cisternal blood (>5 mm) on admission CT.

monitored in an ICU, where neurologic examinations can be performed frequently. Although the efficacy of blood pressure reduction in preventing early rebleeding has not been established, it seems prudent to maintain systolic pressure at 150 mm Hg or less until the aneurysm has been secured. Similarly, a loading dose of an intravenous anticonvulsant, such as fosphenytoin, is given to prevent early rebleeding related to seizures, although this risk is small. Anticonvulsants may be discontinued on the second postoperative day if the patient has not had a seizure.

Most centers advocate the use of prophylactic volume expansion with isotonic crystalloid (with or without additional colloids) to prevent volume contraction, although this has not been proven to reduce the risk of symptomatic ischemia from vasospasm. A central venous or pulmonary artery catheter is used in high-risk patients to guide fluid administration on the basis of target cardiac filling pressures. The calcium channel blocker nimodipine has been shown to reduce the frequency of delayed ischemic deterioration by approximately 30% in several clinical trials; this effect is presumably mediated by reduction of calcium entry into ischemic neurons or by improvement in microcollateral flow, since no effect on angiographic spasm was demonstrated.

Use of dexamethasone in acute SAH is controversial; it is often used in the perioperative period for brain relaxation. There is no specific evidence to suggest that it is beneficial, although it may reduce the headache sometimes associated with vasospasm. Externalized ventricular drains are used to treat obstructive hydrocephalus in patients who are stuporous or comatose, but these devices carry a high risk of infection (15% overall) that increases beyond 5 days. Serial lumbar puncture is used to treat hydrocephalus in patients who are following commands.

Transcranial Doppler ultrasonography is widely used to diagnose vasospasm of the larger cerebral arteries after SAH. Accelerated blood flow velocities, which occur as flow is maintained through narrowed arteries, have a sensitivity and specificity of 90% for angiographic vasospasm of the proximal middle cerebral artery, but they are less sensitive for detecting spasm of the anterior cerebral or basilar arteries.

Treatment of acute symptomatic vasospasm relies on increasing blood volume, blood pressure, and cardiac output in an attempt to improve cerebral blood flow through arteries in spasm that have lost the capacity to autoregulate. Crystalloid or colloid solutions are given to maintain pulmonary artery diastolic pressure greater than 14 mm Hg or central venous pressure greater than 8 mm Hg. Pressors such as dopamine and phenylephrine are used to elevate systolic blood pressure to levels as high as 180 to 220 mm Hg. Hypertensive-hypervolemic hemodilution ("triple-H therapy") of this type results in clinical improvement in about 70% of patients; cerebral angioplasty can lead to dramatic improvement in patients with severe deficits that are refractory to hemodynamic augmentation (see Fig. 45.4).

Outcome after Subarachnoid Hemorrhage

In contrast to the severe physical handicaps that follow ischemic stroke, survivors of SAH are disabled primarily by cognitive impairment. Neuropsychologic testing reveals long-term problems in memory, concentration, psychomotor speed, visuospatial skills, or executive function in 60% to 80% of SAH patients. Depression and anxiety are also common. These disturbances do not lead to the outward appearance of disability but can affect work, relationships, and quality of life; about 50% of SAH patients do not return to their previous level of employment. Cognitive and physical rehabilitation are essential for maximizing recovery in severely affected patients.

OTHER KINDS OF MACROSCOPIC ANEURYSMS

Fusiform or Dolichoectatic Aneurysms

These circumferential vessel dilatations usually involve the carotid, basilar, or vertebral arteries. Atherosclerosis probably plays a role in their formation, but a developmental defect of the wall may be present in some. Fusiform aneurysms seldom become occluded with thrombus and rarely rupture. If bleeding occurs, treatment often requires proximal vessel occlusion.

Mycotic Aneurysm

Mycotic aneurysms are caused by septic emboli, which are most often formed by bacterial endocarditis. They are usually only a few millimeters in size and tend to occur on distal branches of pial vessels, especially those of the middle cerebral artery. Mycotic aneurysms have been reported in up to 10% of endocarditis patients, but arteriography is not routinely performed, and the incidence is probably underestimated. Pyogenic segmental arteritis from septic emboli in the absence of frank aneurysm formation can also lead to intracranial hemorrhage. Because rupture is fatal in 80% of patients with mycotic aneurysms, cerebral arteriography should be performed when endocarditis is accompanied by suspicious headaches, stiff neck, seizure, focal neurologic symptoms, or CSF pleocytosis. Although mycotic aneurysms occasionally disappear radiographically with antimicrobial therapy, the outcome cannot be predicted, and the aneurysm should be treated surgically as soon as possible.

Pseudoaneurysm

Dissection of an intracranial vessel, which usually results from trauma, can lead to extension of blood from the false lumen through the entire vessel wall. The extravasated blood is contained by either a thin layer of adventitia or the surrounding tissues and does not have a true aneurysmal wall, hence the designation *pseudoaneurysm*. If a vessel traversing the subarachnoid space is affected, SAH can result. Treatment may require endovascular or surgical vessel occlusion or trapping, or angioplasty and stenting of the involved segment.

Vascular (Arteriovenous) Malformations

Vascular malformations account for less than 5% of all cases of SAH. Intracranial and spinal vascular malformations can be classified into five main types: (1) arteriovenous malformations (AVMs), which are high-flow and most often symptomatic; (2) cavernous malformations; (3) capillary telangiectasias; (4) venous malformations; and (5) mixed malformations. More than

90% of vascular malformations are asymptomatic throughout life. Bleeding may occur in patients at any age but is most likely to occur in patients younger than 40 years. They are occasionally familial, and in 7% to 10% of cases AVMs coexist with saccular aneurysms.

AVMs are a conglomerate of abnormal arteries and veins with intervening gliotic brain tissue; they resemble a "bag of worms." When bleeding from an AVM occurs, reported initial mortality has ranged from 4% to 20%. Early rebleeding is far less likely than after aneurysm rupture, but recurrent hemorrhage occurs in 8% to 18% of patients annually over the next several years. For patients without hemorrhage, the risk of bleeding is 2% to 4% per year. Besides prior hemorrhage, reported risk factors for bleeding from an AVM include deep venous drainage, small size, a single draining vein, high feeding-artery pressure, male sex, and a diffuse nidus.

The diagnosis of an AVM is made by MRI and arteriography. Small or thrombosed AVMs, especially in the brainstem, are occasionally missed by arteriography but detected by MRI, which better demonstrates the relationship of the malformation to surrounding brain and identifies its nidus. MRI is the preferred screening procedure for detecting vascular malformations; if surgery is contemplated, conventional angiography is required to delineate the vascular supply. Dural and spinal cord AVM should be kept in mind in patients with radiographically unexplained SAH.

Treatment depends on the location of the AVM and the age and condition of the patient. Direct surgical resection, endovascular glue embolization, and directed-beam radiation therapy with a linear accelerator or gamma-knife are the main treatment modalities. The long-term value of these treatments is unclear. Embolization is most useful for shrinking the malformation before surgery or radiation; it is occasionally curative as a single mode of therapy.

SUGGESTED READINGS

Barnwell SL, Higasheda RT, Halbach VV, et al. Transluminal angioplasty of intracerebral vessels for cerebral arterial spasm: reversal of neurological deficits after delayed treatment. *Neurosurgery* 1989;25:424–429.

Brust JCM, Dickinson PCT, Hughes JEO, et al. The diagnosis and treatment of cerebral mycotic aneurysms. *Ann Neurol* 1990;27:238–246.

Feigin VL, Rinkel GJE, Algra A, et al. Calcium antagonists in patients with aneurysmal subarachnoid hemorrhage: a systematic review. *Neurology* 1998;50:876–883.

Fisher CM, Kistler JP, Davis JM. Relation of cerebral vasospasm to subarachnoid hemorrhage visualized by computerized tomographic scanning. *Neurosurgery* 1980;6:1–9.

Grosset DG, Straiton J, McDonald I, Cockburn M, Bullock R. Use of transcranial Doppler sonography to predict development of a delayed ischemic deficit after subarachnoid hemorrhage. *J Neurosurg* 1993;78:183–187.

Haley EC, Kassell NF, Torner JC, et al. The International Cooperative Study on the Timing of Aneurysm Surgery: the North American experience. *Stroke* 1992;23:205–214.

Hasan D, Schonck RSM, Avezaar CJJ, et al. Epileptic seizures after subarachnoid hemorrhage. *Ann Neurol* 1993;33:286–291.

Hop JW, Rinkel GJE, Algra A, van Gijn J. Case-fatality rates and functional outcome after subarachnoid hemorrhage: a systematic review. *Stroke* 1997;28:660–664.

Juvela S, Porras M, Heiskanen O. Natural history of unruptured intracranial aneurysms: a long-term follow-up study. *J Neurosurg* 1993;79:174–182.

Kassell NF, Torner JC, Haley EC Jr, et al. The International Cooperative Study on the Timing of Aneurysm Surgery. 1. Overall management results. *J Neurosurg* 1990;73:18–36.

Longstreth WT Jr, Nelson LM, Koepsell TD, et al. Clinical course of spontaneous subarachnoid hemorrhage: a population-based study in King County, Washington. *Neurology* 1993;43:712–718.

Mast H, Young WL, Koennecke HC, et al. Risk of spontaneous hemorrhage after diagnosis of cerebral arteriovenous malformation. *Lancet* 1997;350:1065–1068.

Mayberg MR, Batjer HH, Dacey R, et al. Guidelines for the management of subarachnoid hemorrhage: a statement for healthcare professionals from a special writing group of the Stroke Council, American Heart Association. *Circulation* 1994;90:2592–2605.

Mayer SA, Fink ME, Homma S, et al. Cardiac injury associated with neurogenic pulmonary edema following subarachnoid hemorrhage. *Neurology* 1994;44:815–820.

Mayer SA, Solomon RA, Fink ME, et al. Effect of 5% albumin solution on sodium balance and blood volume after subarachnoid hemorrhage. *Neurosurgery* 1998;42:759–768.

Raps EC, Solomon RA, Lennihan L, et al. The clinical spectrum of unruptured intracranial aneurysms. *Arch Neurol* 1993;50:265–278.

Rinkel GJE, Djibuti M, Algra A, et al. Prevalence and risk of rupture of intracranial aneurysms: a systematic review. *Stroke* 1998;29:251–256.

Rinkel GJE, van Gijn J, Wijdicks EFM. Subarachnoid hemorrhage without detectable aneurysm: a review of the causes. *Stroke* 1993;24:1403–1409.

Ronkainen A, Hernesniemi J, Puranen M, et al. Familial intracranial aneurysms. *Lancet* 1997;349:380–384.

Sahs AL, Nibbelink DW, Torner JC, eds. *Aneurysmal subarachnoid hemorrhage: report of the cooperative study.* Baltimore: Urban & Schwartzenberg, 1981.

Schievink WI. Intracranial aneurysms. *N Engl J Med* 1997;336:28–40.

Solomon RA, Fink ME, Pile-Spellman J. Surgical management of unruptured intracranial aneurysms. *J Neurosurg* 1994;80:440–446.

Teunissen LL, Rinkel GJ, Algra A. Risk factors for subarachnoid hemorrhage: a systematic review. *Stroke* 1996;27:544–549.

Vinuela G, Duckwiler G, Mawad M. Guglielmi detachable coil embolization of acute intracranial aneurysm: perioperative anatomical and clinical outcome in 403 patients. *J Neurosurg* 1997;86:475–482.

Merritt's Neurology, 10th ed., edited by L.P. Rowland. Lippincott Williams & Wilkins, Philadelphia © 2000.

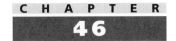

CEREBRAL VEINS AND SINUSES

ROBERT A. FISHMAN

Occlusion of the cerebral veins and sinuses occurs owing to thrombus, thrombophlebitis, or tumors. Occlusion of the cortical and subcortical veins may cause focal neurologic symptoms and signs. The dural sinuses that are most frequently thrombosed are the lateral, cavernous, and superior sagittal sinuses. Less frequently affected are the straight sinus and the vein of Galen. Factors predisposing to thrombosis and associated disorders include the following:

Primary idiopathic thrombosis
Secondary thrombosis
    Pregnancy
    Postpartum
    Birth control pills
    Trauma—after open or closed head injury
    Tumors
        Meningioma
        Metastatic tumors
    Malnutrition and dehydration (marantic thrombosis)
    Infection—sinus thrombophlebitis, bacterial, fungal
    Hematologic disorders
        Polycythemia
        Cryofibrinogenemia
        Sickle-cell anemia
        Leukemia
        Disseminated intravascular coagulation and other
           coagulopathies
    Behçet syndrome

LATERAL SINUS THROMBOSIS

Thrombosis of the lateral sinus is usually secondary to otitis media and mastoiditis. Infants and children are most commonly affected. Thrombosis may be coincident with the acute attack of otitis and mastoiditis, or it may occur in the chronic stage of infection.

Symptoms and Signs

Onset is usually heralded by fever and chills; however, fever may be absent. Septicemia most commonly occurs with hemolytic streptococci and is present in about 50% of patients. Petechiae in the skin and mucous membranes and septic embolism of the lungs, joints, and muscles are infrequent complications of the septicemia.

The classic symptoms of lateral sinus thrombosis are fever, headache, and nausea and vomiting. The latter signs are due to increased intracranial pressure and are most apt to occur when the right sinus is occluded; in most individuals, the right sinus drains the greater portion of blood from the brain. Local signs of thrombosis of the sinus are usually absent, but occasionally there is swelling over the mastoid region with distention of the superficial veins and tenderness over the jugular vein in the neck.

Papilledema develops in about 50% of patients. It is usually bilateral but is occasionally only on one side, possibly the result of asymmetric extension of the process to the cavernous sinuses. Increased intracranial pressure may cause separation of the sutures or bulging of the fontanels in infants.

Drowsiness and coma are not uncommon symptoms. Convulsive seizures may also occur. Jacksonian seizures followed by hemiplegia may reflect extension of infection into the veins draining the hemispheres. These signs, however, often indicate a brain abscess. Diplopia may result from injury to the sixth cranial nerve by increased intracranial pressure or from involvement of the nerve by extension of the infection in the petrous bone. The combination of sixth nerve palsy (lateral rectus weakness) and pain in the face as the result of damage to the fifth nerve is the Gradenigo syndrome. There may be signs of damage to the ninth, tenth, and eleventh cranial nerves. These are attributed to pressure on these nerves by the distended jugular vein, as they pass through the jugular foramen. It seems more probable that they are caused by extension of the infection into the bone (osteomyelitis) surrounding these structures.

Laboratory Data

Leukocytosis is present in the blood, and the organism may be recovered from the blood in 50% of cases. The cerebrospinal fluid (CSF) shows the changes characteristic of an aseptic meningeal reaction. The pressure is increased. The fluid is usually slightly turbid or cloudy and contains several to many hundred leukocytes per cubic millimeter. The glucose content of the fluid is normal, and cultures are sterile, unless bacterial meningitis has developed.

Diagnosis

The diagnosis of lateral sinus thrombosis is usually made, based on signs of increased intracranial pressure in a patient with an acute or chronic otitis and mastoiditis. The development of a hemiplegia, aphasia, or hemianopia favors the possibility of an intracerebral abscess, which should be excluded with imaging studies.

Course and Prognosis

The mortality rate is high in untreated lateral sinus thrombosis. Occasionally, the infected thrombus may heal by complete organization, but more commonly death results from septicemia, meningitis, extension of the infection to the cavernous or longitudinal sinus, or abscess of the brain. When patients recover, intracranial pressure may continue to be elevated for some months, especially if the jugular vein on the right side is ligated.

Treatment

The occurrence of a thrombosis of the lateral sinus should be prevented by the prompt treatment of infections of the middle ear. Treatment of a thrombosis involves antibiotics and surgical drainage. Infected bone should be removed, the sinus should be exposed and drained, and the jugular vein should be ligated if necessary. Nonseptic patients may be candidates for thrombolytic therapy.

CAVERNOUS SINUS THROMBOSIS

Cavernous sinus thrombosis usually originates in suppurative processes of the orbit, nasal sinuses, or upper one-half of the face. The infection commonly involves only one sinus at the onset but rapidly spreads through the circular sinus to the opposite side. One or both sides may be secondarily involved by extension of infection from the other dural sinuses. Nonseptic thrombosis of the cavernous sinus is rare. The sinus may be partially or totally occluded by tumor masses, trauma, or arteriovenous aneurysms.

Symptoms and Signs

The onset of a septic thrombosis is usually sudden and dramatic. The patient appears acutely ill, and there is a septic type of fever. There is pain in the eyes, and the orbits are painful to pressure. The globes are proptosed by orbital edema and chemosis of the conjunctivae and eyelids. Diplopia follows involvement of the oculomotor nerves. Ptosis may be present and obscured by the exophthalmos. The optic discs are swollen, and there are numerous small or large hemorrhages around the disc when the orbital veins are occluded. The corneas are cloudy and ulcers may develop. The pupils may be dilated or small. Pupillary reactions may be lost. Visual acuity may be normal or moderately impaired. The laboratory findings in patients with cavernous sinus thrombosis are similar to those in patients with lateral sinus thrombosis.

Diagnosis

Cavernous sinus thrombosis must be distinguished from other conditions that produce exophthalmos and congestion in the orbit. These include orbital tumors, meningiomas and other tumors in the region of the sphenoid, malignant exophthalmos, and arteriovenous fistulas. The evolution of symptoms is slow in the latter conditions, except arteriovenous fistulas. These can be differentiated by the presence of pulsating exophthalmos and an orbital bruit, and recession of the exophthalmos when the carotid artery is occluded by digital pressure. Computed tomography (CT), magnetic resonance imaging (MRI), and MR venography (MRV) are valuable in establishing the diagnosis.

Treatment

Septic thrombosis of the cavernous sinus was once almost invariably fatal because of the development of an acute meningitis. Cures now are possible with appropriate antibiotics, with or without anticoagulation.

SUPERIOR SAGITTAL SINUS THROMBOSIS

The superior sagittal sinus is less commonly the site of an infective thrombosis than either the lateral or cavernous sinuses. Infections may reach the superior sagittal sinus from the nasal cavities or as secondary extensions from the lateral or cavernous sinuses. The superior sagittal sinus may also be occluded by extension of infection from osteomyelitis or from epidural or subdural infection.

The superior sagittal sinus is the most common site of nonseptic sinus thrombosis associated with dehydration and marasmus in infancy. It may also be occluded by trauma or by tumors (meningiomas). Sagittal sinus thrombosis has also been associated with oral contraceptive use, pregnancy, hemolytic anemia, sickle-cell trait, thrombocytopenia, ulcerative colitis, diabetes mellitus, Behçet syndrome, and other diseases. Nonseptic thrombosis of the sinus occasionally occurs in adults without any known cause.

Symptoms and Signs

The general signs are prostration, fever, headache, and papilledema. Local signs include edema of the forehead and anterior part of the scalp and engorgement of the veins in the area of the anterior or posterior fontanels, with the formation of a caput medusae. Focal neurologic signs and symptoms may be entirely absent in nonseptic thrombosis, with increased intracranial pressure as the only presenting sign. However, extension of the clot into the larger cerebral veins is almost always accompanied by the onset of dramatic signs caused by hemorrhage into the cortical white and gray matter. Extension into these veins is common in septic thrombosis and in a high percentage of the nonseptic type. Convulsive seizures (often unilateral), hemiplegia, aphasia, or hemianopia may occur. The diagnosis of nonseptic thrombosis should be considered in all infants who show signs of increased intracranial pressure and cerebral symptoms during the course of severe nutritional disturbances and cachexia.

The laboratory findings with septic thrombosis of the superior sagittal sinus are similar to those in patients with lateral sinus thrombosis. Occasionally, the CSF is bloody or xanthochromic as the result of cortical and meningeal hemorrhage.

Diagnosis

The diagnosis can be established by radiography or MR angiography. CT and MRV may show multiple, often bilateral lesions, some hemorrhagic and others radiolucent (Figs. 46.1 and 46.2). The *cord sign* is a linear area of increased density that is related to clot in veins or sinus. The *empty delta sign* appears after injection of contrast material, which outlines the periphery of the sinus where blood still flows, leaving the central area of the clot dark; there may also be enhancement of the gyri or tentorium. Ventricles may be large or small. Cerebral angiography is definitive, showing the venous block or collateral flow. MRV, a noninvasive procedure, may graphically demonstrate the occlusion.

Prognosis

The prognosis is guarded in patients with a septic thrombosis. Death may result from meningitis or hemorrhagic lesions in the brain. Survivors may have focal neurologic deficits and recurrent convulsive seizures. The prognosis is less grave in patients with nonseptic thrombosis. Symptoms may recede several months af-

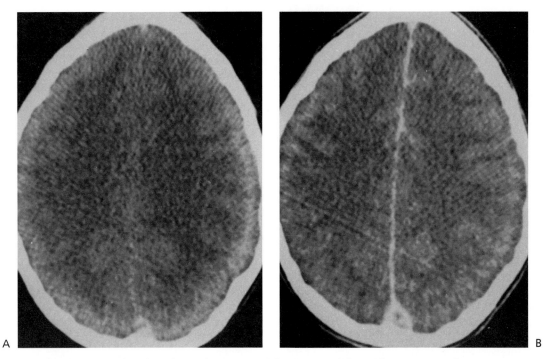

FIG. 46.1. Sinus thrombosis, hemorrhagic venous infarction. **A:** Axial CT without contrast enhancement demonstrates density in the sagittal sinus posteriorly. **B:** At the same level postcontrast, the empty delta sign is noted in the affected sinus. Thrombus density caused a central filling defect within the sinus. Triangular enhancement at the periphery is related to collateral venous channels within the dura. (Courtesy of Drs. S.K. Hilal and J.A. Bello.)

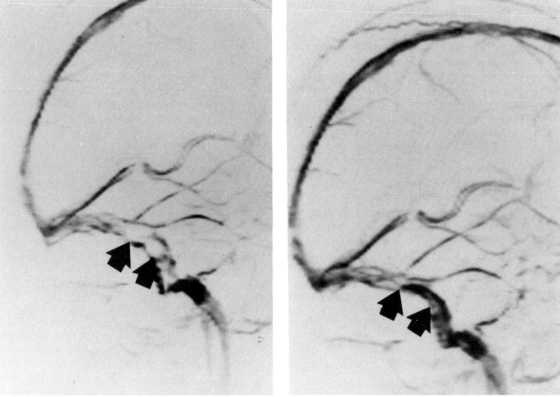

FIG. 46.2. A 34-year-old man with bilateral papilledema, increasing headache, and blurred vision. Routine spin-echo MR image was normal. **A:** Two-dimensional time-of-flight (TOF) MRV at time of symptoms shows filling defects at the junction of right transverse and sigmoid sinuses *(arrows)*. **B:** Two-dimensional TOF MRV after local infusion of urokinase shows near-total resolution of filling defects *(arrows)*. The patient's symptoms were markedly improved. (Courtesy of Drs. Phillip Baum and David Norman.)

ter recanalization of the sinus or development of collateral circulation.

Treatment

Antibiotics should be administered to patients with septic thrombosis. Craniotomy with evacuation of subdural or epidural abscess should be performed when these are present. Heparin or thrombolytic therapy has been beneficial in some patients despite the risks of hemorrhagic infarction. Acetazolamide may be useful in lowering intracranial pressure. The role of steroids has not been established.

THROMBOSIS OF OTHER DURAL SINUSES

Thrombosis of the inferior longitudinal sinus, the straight sinus, the petrosals, or the vein of Galen rarely occurs alone. These sites are usually involved by secondary extension of a septic or nonseptic thrombosis of the lateral, superior sagittal, or cavernous sinuses. Any signs or symptoms that may be produced by thrombosis of the inferior longitudinal, straight, or petrosal sinuses are usually masked by those resulting from involvement of the more important sinuses. Thrombosis of the great vein of Galen may cause hemorrhages in the central white matter of the hemispheres or in the basal ganglia and lateral ventricles.

DURAL ARTERIOVENOUS MALFORMATIONS

Dural arteriovenous malformations (AVMs) are more common in women than men, and occur more often in the posterior fossa than above the tentorium. They may cause peripheral cranial nerve involvement (most commonly, third, seventh, eighth, and twelfth) or central nervous system manifestations. The latter are attributed to intracranial venous hypertension, decreased CSF absorption, venous sinus thrombosis, or minimal subarachnoid bleeding. Seizures, motor weakness, and brainstem and cerebellar syndromes have been observed, depending on the region involved. Some patients experience subarachnoid hemorrhaging or papilledema and headache only, as in idiopathic pseudotumor. Diagnosis usually requires detailed cerebral angiography, including selective injection of the external carotid and both vertebral arteries. Therapy with selective embolization using silicone or other agents may be beneficial and may require direct surgical excision. Spontaneous thrombosis of a dural AVM with remission of symptoms is not unusual; many lesions have a benign prognosis. Dural AVMs also occur in the spinal cord, often presenting as an insidiously progressive paraparesis.

SUGGESTED READINGS

Bousser MG, Russell RR. *Cerebral venous thrombosis.* Philadelphia: WB Saunders, 1997:175.

Horowitz M, Purdy P, Unwin H, et al. Treatment of dural sinus thrombosis using selective catheterization and urokinase. *Ann Neurol* 1995;38:58–67.

Smith TP, Higashida RT, Barnwell SL, et al. Treatment of dural sinus thrombosis by urokinase infusion. *ANJR* 1994;15:801–807.

Southwick FS, Richardson EP, Swartz MN. Septic thrombosis of the dural venous sinuses. *Medicine* 1986;65:82–106.

Merritt's Neurology, 10th ed., edited by L.P. Rowland. Lippincott Williams & Wilkins, Philadelphia © 2000.

CHAPTER 47

VASCULAR DISEASE OF THE SPINAL CORD

LEON A. WEISBERG

Blood supply to the spinal cord and nerve roots originates in the vertebral, thyrocervical, costocervical, intercostal, and lumbar arteries, which give rise to radicular and medullary arteries. The segmental radicular arteries supply the nerve roots, originating near the vertebral foramina. Six to nine large medullary arteries originate from the vertebral, subclavian, or iliac arteries and the aorta (Fig. 47.1). Branches of the medullary arteries form a single anterior median spinal artery and two posterior spinal arteries, which perfuse the spinal cord. The anterior median spinal artery arises from the vertebral artery, and it runs along the entire length of the cord. The pial arteriolar plexus and posterior spinal arteries supply the dorsal aspect of the cord.

In the cervical region, the anterior median artery is collateralized at several levels by unpaired medullary arteries derived from the vertebral and subclavian arteries; this blood supply is rich in collateral branches. In the thoracic region, the anterior median spinal artery is joined by only a few branches of the thoracic aorta, and blood supply is relatively sparse, especially in the lower segments. The midthoracic spinal cord is supplied by terminal vessels descending from the subclavian and vertebral arteries or ascending from the abdominal aorta; this watershed is particularly vulnerable to vascular insufficiency, and spinal cord infarction is most likely to occur at T-4 to T-9. Because of its relative hypovascularity, the midthoracic region is particularly vulnerable to effects of hypotensive infarction. Midthoracic spinal syndrome (e.g., T-4 myelopathy) may be "false localizing," and apparent clinical dysfunction at this level may actually be due to impaired perfusion at higher or lower cord levels or to global ischemia. Lumbar and sacral spinal areas are supplied by the largest and most constant of medullary arteries, the "great anterior radicular artery" of Adamkiewicz. This is usually found at L-1 or L-2 (occasionally as high as T-12 or as low as L-4). This artery, paired or single, travels through the vertebral foramen and anastomoses with the anterior medial spinal artery; the largest branch supplies the lumbosacral spinal cord and conus

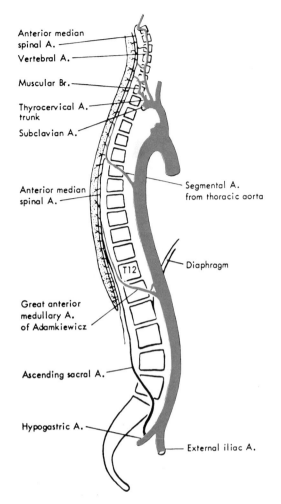

Anterior median spinal A.

Vertebral A.

Muscular Br.

Thyrocervical A. trunk

Subclavian A.

Anterior median spinal A.

Segmental A. from thoracic aorta

Diaphragm

T 12

Great anterior medullary A. of Adamkiewicz

Ascending sacral A.

Hypogastric A.

External iliac A.

FIG. 47.1. The anterior median spinal artery is joined at various levels by arteries arising from the vertebral and subclavian arteries, the aorta, and the iliac arteries.

medullaris. Conus and cauda equina are also supplied by sacral branches ascending from the iliac arteries.

The central (sulcal) arteries originate in the anterior spinal artery to supply the anterior two-thirds and central area of the spinal cord. Penetrating branches from the pial arterial plexus supply the periphery and posterior one-third of the cord. Within the spinal cord, these arterial feeders anastomose in their most distal parts, creating border zones similar to those in the brain. These vascular border zones may explain the development of incomplete or partial syndromes seen after some spinal cord infarctions (see Fig. 47.1).

The plexiform venous system interconnects freely with the radicular arteries within subarachnoid space. The radicular veins empty into the epidural venous plexus, which in turn communicates with the inferior vena cava and azygos system through the perivertebral plexus.

INFARCTION OF THE SPINAL CORD

Softening or infarction of the spinal cord (myelomalacia) results from occlusion of major vessels. Anterior spinal artery infarction

is much more common than the posterior spinal artery syndrome because of the difference in collateral supply between these two regions.

Etiology

Spinal cord infarction is most often caused by atheromas involving the aorta and results as a potential complication of thoracoabdominal aneurysm repair. In one series, spinal infarction represented 1.2% of stroke admissions. Less common causes of spinal cord infarction include collagen vascular disease (including systemic lupus and polyarteritis), syphilitic angiitis, dissecting aortic aneurysm, embolic infarction (bacterial endocarditis, nucleus pulposus), pregnancy, sickle-cell disease, neurotoxic effects of iodinated contrast material used in angiography, compression of spinal arteries by tumor, systemic arterial hypotension as a consequence of cardiac arrest, and decompression sickness. Paraplegia may follow surgical repair of an aortic aneurysm when cross-clamp time is longer than 25 minutes; the risk of neurologic deficit may be lessened by avoiding systemic arterial hypotension, placing the shunt around the cross-clamp, and using thiopental anesthesia. Spinal cord ischemia may occur as an early complication of spinal arteriovenous malformation (AVM) repair (surgery, embolization).

Symptoms and Signs

The symptoms of spinal stroke usually appear within a few minutes or hours of the onset of ischemia. The first symptom may be local or radicular back pain. This may be lancinating or burning and is usually transient. There may also be diffuse, deep, aching pain in both legs, or a burning, dysesthetic pain may start in the feet and rapidly ascend to calves, thighs, and abdomen. These sensory symptoms are followed by rapid onset of leg weakness; the patient is soon unable to walk, reaching a peak of disability within minutes. Occlusion of the cervical part of the anterior spinal artery causes tetraplegia, incontinence of urine and feces, and sensory impairment below the level of the lesion. Proprioception and vibration sensations are spared because the posterior columns are supplied by the posterior arterial plexus. If proprioception and vibration sensation are impaired, the lesion is most likely not an anterior spinal artery infarction, and alternative diagnoses should be considered. Spastic weakness in the legs results from lesions of the lateral corticospinal tract. Sometimes, signs are restricted to those of either upper or lower motor neurons (or both) in a pattern similar to that of amyotrophic lateral sclerosis (ALS), but with major differences in mode of onset and lack of progressive worsening in spinal stroke. If the spinal ischemia involves only the gray matter supplied by sulcal arterial branches, there may be only lower motor neuron deficit (amyotrophy). The sudden onset of the motor deficit is consistent with a vascular etiology; however, if the deficit develops more slowly and progressively, clinical differentiation from ALS or spinal cord tumor may be difficult.

The level of the deficit in spinal ischemia may involve high-cervical or low-sacral regions, with the mean level of deficit occurring at T-8. Most clinical spinal cord strokes affect the midthoracic region, where paraplegia, urinary incontinence, and loss of pain and temperature sensation, with sparing of proprioception and vibration, localize the level. The weakness is flaccid at first, but Babinski signs are seen, and spasticity and hyperreflexia usually develop in a few weeks.

Arterial insufficiency of the lumbar region causes paraplegia, sphincter symptoms, and loss of cutaneous sensation with sacral sparing. The weakness is more likely to remain flaccid because the anterior horn cells are affected.

Transient ischemic attacks of the spinal cord and cauda equina may occur, but there is no way to confirm this clinical impression. These attacks may precede spinal artery infarction, sometimes in association with lumbar spondylosis and stenosis. Symptoms may be precipitated by postural change in patients with lumbar stenosis. In cervical spondylosis, the role of arterial compression is uncertain in the subsequent development of myelopathy.

Diagnosis

Shadow spine radiography, myelography, computed tomography (CT), and magnetic resonance imaging (MRI) are needed to rule out spinal cord neoplasm or cervical spondylosis, which may simulate spinal cord stroke. Lumbar puncture excludes hemorrhagic or infectious disorders. In spinal cord infarction, cerebrospinal fluid (CSF) may show a slight protein content elevation, but gamma globulin content is normal. Two conditions that may simulate spinal infarction are multiple sclerosis (MS) and cord neoplasm. In MS or transverse myelitis, CSF frequently shows elevated gamma globulin content. Neoplasms are more likely to increase CSF protein content to values of several hundred milligrams per deciliter. In spinal cord infarction, myelography is usually normal; however, edema may cause signs of an intramedullary mass and subarachnoid block. Spinal angiography may cause cord infarction and is contraindicated unless spinal vascular malformation is considered likely. MRI may initially be normal in spinal ischemia but may later show focal swelling and abnormal (hyperintense) signal characteristics on T2-weighted sequences. Gadolinium-enhanced MRI would suggest an alternative etiology, such as MS, an infectious–inflammatory condition, neoplasm, vasculitis, or AVM. CT is unlikely to visualize an ischemic spinal lesion; however, it is likely to visualize spinal cord hemorrhage or vertebral abnormalities that may be the cause of the spinal syndrome.

Treatment and Prognosis

The general principles of care for patients with quadriplegia or paraplegia should be followed. Naloxone hydrochloride (Narcan) and calcium channel blockers have been used experimentally to treat spinal cord ischemia, but no studies have been undertaken in humans. There is no evidence to support utilization of antiplatelets or anticoagulants for spinal ischemia. The prognosis for recovery is varied. In one review, the following was reported: died (22%), unimproved (24%), minimally improved (9%), improved (25%), markedly improved (20%).

The major predisposing factor for spinal ischemia is surgical reconstruction of thoracoabdominal aortic aneurysm. The potential for spinal ischemia and resulting neurologic deficit depends on aneurysm extension and whether dissection has occurred. Despite utilization of hypothermia, intraoperative

somatosensory monitoring, reanastomosis of intercostal arteries, short clamp time, distal aortic perfusion, and CSF drainage techniques, spinal ischemia is a potential risk of aortic aneurysm repair.

VENOUS DISEASE

Venous disorders of the spinal cord are even less common than arterial lesions. Venous infarction may occur in patients with sepsis, systemic malignancy, or spinal vascular malformation. Patients experience sudden back pain, and motor, sensory, and autonomic dysfunctions develop. Sensory impairment does not necessarily spare the posterior columns (as is characteristic of anterior spinal artery ischemia). CSF examination is necessary to exclude infectious–inflammatory or neoplastic conditions in patients with spinal cord ischemia. CT or MRI is necessary to exclude alternative lesions, including vascular malformations.

Foix-Alajouanine syndrome (subacute or progressive necrotic myelopathy) is characterized by spinal cord necrosis and evidence of enlarged, tortuous, thrombosed veins. Although this necrotic myelitis is attributed to venous thrombosis, there is usually no angiographic evidence of venous thrombosis or vascular spinal cord malformation. There is pathologic evidence of vascular malformations that are believed to have undergone spontaneous vascular thrombosis. There are multiple small infarcts and hemorrhagic spinal lesions. Pathologically, the necrosis for the most part involves the corticospinal tract, sparing anterior horn cells, and the lesion is most prominent in the thoracolumbar region. Clinically, there is usually subacute or progressive worsening of the condition for several weeks. The prodrome may include back or leg pain. Symptoms include leg weakness, incontinence, and sensory loss. Findings usually include spastic paraparesis, hyperreflexia, bilateral Babinski signs, and sensory level below the lesion. CSF may show a markedly elevated protein content, leukocytic pleocytosis, and red blood cells. Treatment with anticoagulants or corticosteroids has not been effective. Because some venous infarctions of the spinal cord are hemorrhagic, anticoagulation is potentially dangerous in this condition.

SPINAL CORD HEMORRHAGE

Hemorrhage in the spinal cord is rare and may be epidural, subdural, subarachnoid, or intramedullary in location. Hematomyelia (hemorrhage into the substance of the spinal cord) usually immediately follows a spinal injury; however, it may be delayed for hours or days. Nontraumatic causes of spinal cord hemorrhage include blood disorders (e.g., leukemia), anticoagulation therapy, AVM, or venous spinal cord infarction.

Pathology

In intramedullary spinal cord hemorrhage, the spinal cord is swollen because of an intramedullary central blood clot. The blood dissects longitudinally for several segments below and above the hemorrhage, most severely affecting the gray matter and contiguous white matter. The clot is usually surrounded by a rim of normal nervous tissue. With time, the blood is liquefied and removed by phagocytes. Glial replacement is usually incomplete, resulting in a syrinxlike cavity that extends over several cord segments.

Signs and Symptoms

Localized back or radicular pain is sudden in onset. If hemorrhage is small, there may be only spastic weakness associated with hyperreflexia in the legs and bladder dysfunction. If hemorrhage is large, signs of cord transection include flaccid paralysis, complete sensory loss below the lesion, absent reflexes, Babinski signs, and loss of sphincter control. Autonomic disturbance and vasomotor instability may result in cardiovascular shock. If the patient survives, the hematoma is reabsorbed and symptoms may improve, but outcome is uncertain. Spinal subdural or epidural hemorrhage is usually due to trauma (including lumbar puncture) or coagulopathy. Initially, patients experience neck or back pain and radiculopathy, or myelopathy may subsequently develop.

Diagnosis

CSF is bloody or xanthochromic (especially if there is an associated subarachnoid hemorrhage), and protein content is increased. Myelography shows evidence of an intradural intramedullary mass with subarachnoid block. CT shows the hyperdense hematoma more clearly than MRI. Spinal angiography may be indicated in nontraumatic cases if spinal vascular malformation is suspected.

Spinal epidural or subdural hemorrhage may cause mass effect that rapidly compresses the cord. This may follow spinal trauma, even without evidence of bone fracture; other causes include anticoagulation and blood dyscrasias, and there are cases without obvious etiology. Epidural hemorrhage may follow lumbar puncture in patients with a coagulation disorder. The symptoms of epidural and subdural spinal hematoma are similar. Symptoms of epidural hemorrhage appear rapidly, with back pain, sensory loss, and sphincter impairment. The diagnosis is established by CT, which directly visualizes the hemorrhage, or myelography, which shows evidence of cord compression by an extradural mass. Spinal subarachnoid hemorrhage may be due to vascular malformation, spinal neoplasm (most commonly ependymoma), blood dyscrasia, or periarteritis nodosa, which is characterized by sudden, severe back pain at the level of the lesion. Symptoms may be due to blood in the subarachnoid space or to blood dissecting into the spinal cord or along the nerve root sheaths. CSF is bloody and xanthochromic. CT shows the hyperdense hemorrhage. Myelography and spinal angiography are necessary to establish the cause. Ruptured intracranial aneurysm occasionally causes severe back pain with clinical findings indicative of spinal hemorrhage; in these cases, cerebral angiography may be necessary to determine the etiology, especially if the patient also reports headache and has nuchal rigidity.

Treatment

Treatment of spinal cord hemorrhage depends on the cause and location of the hemorrhage. For subdural and epidural hemorrhage, surgery is necessary, but the prognosis is poor when paraplegia is present and there is delay in surgical intervention. Patients with spinal cord hematomas caused by anticoagulant therapy should receive fresh whole blood and vitamin K. Spinal cord decompression is carried out if effective hemostasis can be achieved, but should be avoided if bleeding impairment is not correctable.

SUGGESTED READINGS

Cheshire WP, Santos CC, Massey EW, Howard JF. Spinal cord infarction: etiology and outcome. *Neurology* 1996;47:321–330.

Crawford ES, Crawford JL, Safi HJ. Thoraco-abdominal aortic aneurysms: preoperative and intraoperative factors determining immediate and long-term results of operations in 605 patients. *J Vasc Surg* 1986;3:389–404.

Garland H, Greenberg J, Harriman DGF. Infarction of the spinal cord. *Brain* 1966;89:645–662.

Henson RA, Parson M. Ischemic lesions in the spinal cord: an illustrated review. *Q J Med* 1967;36:205–222.

Hogan EL, Romanul F. Spinal cord infarction occurring during insertion of aortic graft. *Neurology* 1966;16:67–74.

Hughes JT. Venous infarction of the spinal cord. *Neurology* 1971;21:794–800.

Kim RC, Smith HR, Henbest ML. Nonhemorrhagic venous infarction of the spinal cord. *Ann Neurol* 1984;15:379–385.

Kim SW, Kim RC, Choi BH, Gordon SK. Non-traumatic ischemic myelopathy: a review fo 25 cases. *Paraplegia* 1988;26:262–272.

Mair WCP, Folkerts JF. Necrosis of spinal cord due to thrombophlebitis (subacute necrotic myelitis). *Brain* 1953;76:536–572.

Maroon JC, Abla AA, Wilberger JI, Bailes JE, Sternau LL. Central cord syndrome. *Clin Neurosurg* 1991;37:612–621.

Nagashima C, Nagashima R, Morota N, Kobayashi S. Magnetic resonance imaging of human spinal cord infarction. *Surg Neurol* 1991;35:368–373.

Ross RT. Spinal cord infarction in disease and surgery of the aorta. *Can J Neurol Sci* 1985;12:289–295.

Russel NA, Benoit BG. Spinal subdural hematoma: a review. *Surg Neurol* 1983;20:133–137.

Sandson TA, Friedman JH. Spinal cord infarction: report of 8 cases and review of the literature. *Medicine* 1989;68:282–292.

Satran R. Spinal cord infarction. *Stroke* 1988;19:529–532.

Silver JR, Buxton PH. Spinal stroke. *Brain* 1974;97:539–550.

Sliwa JA, Maclean IC. Ischemic myelopathy: a review of spinal vasculature and related clinical syndromes. *Arch Phys Med Rehabil* 1992;73:365–372.

Zull D, Cydulka R. Acute paraplegia and aortic dissection. *Am J Med* 1988;84:765–770.

Merritt's Neurology, 10th ed., edited by L.P. Rowland. Lippincott Williams & Wilkins, Philadelphia © 2000.

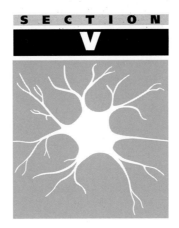

SECTION
V

DISORDERS OF CEREBROSPINAL AND BRAIN FLUIDS

CHAPTER 48

HYDROCEPHALUS

LEON D. PROCKOP

Hydrocephalus is characterized by increased cerebrospinal fluid (CSF) volume and dilation of the cerebral ventricles. It is classified according the following types:

Obstructive hydrocephalus
- Congenital malformations
- Postinflammatory or posthemorrhagic
- Mass lesions

Normal pressure hydrocephalus

Communicating hydrocephalus
- Overproduction of CSF
- Defective absorption of CSF
- Venous drainage insufficiency

Hydrocephalus *ex vacuo*

When there are no clinical signs or symptoms of intracranial hypertension, hydrocephalus is *occult*. It is *active* when the disease is progressive, and there is increased intracranial pressure; hydrocephalus is *arrested* when ventricular enlargement has ceased. Dandy and Blackfan introduced the terms *communicating* and *noncommunicating* hydrocephalus to describe the flow of CSF. They injected a tracer dye into one lateral ventricle. If the dye appeared in lumbar CSF, the hydrocephalus was termed *communicating;* if the dye did not appear in the lumbar CSF, the hydrocephalus was termed *noncommunicating.* This functional

classification was widely accepted because it proved useful in surgical shunt placement; however, by this definition, noncommunicating hydrocephalus refers only to that caused by obstruction within the ventricular system. The term *obstructive hydrocephalus* is used to describe conditions after obstruction of either intraventricular or extraventricular pathways. In communicating hydrocephalus, no obstruction can be demonstrated by standard tests. *Normal pressure hydrocephalus* (NPH) warrants separate classification and discussion. These forms of hydrocephalus are distinguished from *hydrocephalus ex vacuo*, in which CSF volume increases without change in CSF pressure, because brain tissue has been lost (e.g., Alzheimer disease) (Fig. 48.1).

OBSTRUCTIVE HYDROCEPHALUS

Obstructive hydrocephalus is the best characterized and most common form of hydrocephalus. To facilitate clinical diagnosis and management, obstructive hydrocephalus is further classified as intraventricular obstructive hydrocephalus (IVOH) and extraventricular obstructive hydrocephalus (EVOH). In IVOH, the obstruction site determines proximal dilatation, with preservation of normal ventricular size distal to the block. Obstruction may occur at the foramen of Monro, the third ventricle, the aqueduct of Sylvius, the fourth ventricle, or the outflow of the foramina of Luschka and Magendie. In obstruction of extraventricular CSF pathways (EVOH), absolute or relative reduction of flow may occur in the subarachnoid spaces at the base of the brain, at the tentorial level, and over the hemispheral convexities. Because of the limitations of the clinical tests discussed later, the precise location of the obstruction or absorptive block cannot always be determined.

Obstructive hydrocephalus is caused by congenital malfor-

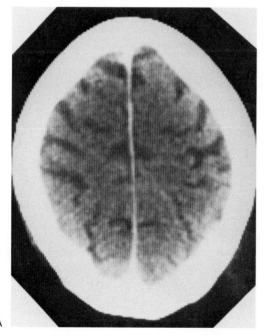
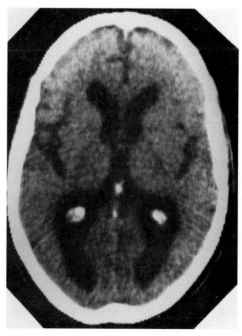

FIG. 48.1. Brain CT. Marked ventricular dilatation **(A)** and widening of cortical sulci **(B)** are indicative of hydrocephalus *ex vacuo* in a 64-year-old woman with dementia.

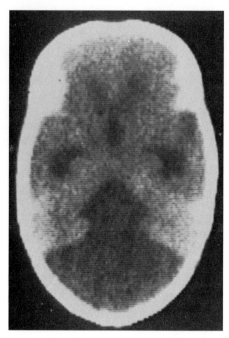

FIG. 48.2. Brain CT. Hydrocephalus associated with Dandy-Walker malformation in a 4-month-old child with increasing head circumference and bulging fontanels.

mations or developmental lesions, postinflammatory or posthemorrhagic fibrosis, or mass lesion.

Congenital Malformations or Developmental Lesions

Congenital hydrocephalus occurs with an incidence of 0.5 to 1.8 per 1,000 births and may result from either genetic or nongenetic causes. Common nongenetic causes include intrauterine infection, intracranial hemorrhage secondary to birth trauma or prematurity, and meningitis. Genetically, an X-linked hydrocephalus has been described. In most of these cases, aqueductal stenosis has been documented radiographically, by magnetic res-

onance imaging (MRI), or at postmortem examination. In some families, the occurrence of aqueductal stenosis, hydrocephalus of undetermined anatomic type, and the Dandy-Walker syndrome in siblings of both sexes has suggested alternate modes of inheritance. In the Dandy-Walker syndrome, there is expansion of the fourth ventricle and the posterior fossa, with obstruction of the foramina of Luschka and Magendie (Fig. 48.2). It is not clear whether aqueductal lesions (e.g., gliosis or fibrosis) occur developmentally or whether they are the residue of prior viral inflammatory disease contracted *in utero* or in early life (Fig. 48.3). The Arnold-Chiari malformation may be associated with hydrocephalus at birth, or it may develop later.

Postinflammatory or Posthemorrhagic Hydrocephalus

Posthemorrhagic hydrocephalus is a major complication of cerebral intraventricular hemorrhage in low-birthweight infants, with an incidence 26% to 70%, depending on the severity of the hemorrhage. Hydrocephalus results from obstruction of CSF flow by a clot within the ventricular system or by obliterative basilar or transcortical arachnoiditis. After subarachnoid hemorrhage, the arachnoid villi are distended with packed red cells, suggesting an absorptive defect. Consequently, fibrotic impairment of extraventricular CSF pathways after intracranial hemorrhage may be complicated by dysfunction of arachnoid villi.

Likewise, intramedullary or intraventricular hemorrhage in adults causes hydrocephalus, especially if there are clots in the ventricles (Fig. 48.4A). Hydrocephalus also occurs in adults after subarachnoid bleeding owing to head trauma or aneurysmal rupture (Fig. 48.4B). In some patients, the obstruction of CSF flow is transient; intracranial pressure increases, and hydrocephalus appears but then disappears spontaneously. Other patients exhibit progressive hydrocephalus. This form of obstructive hydrocephalus is due to extraventricular obstruction to CSF flow and may be a form of, or may cause, NPH (Fig. 48.5).

Among infectious diseases, tuberculous and luetic meningitis may cause hydrocephalus secondary to basal arachnoiditis. Com-

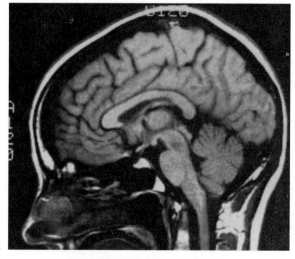
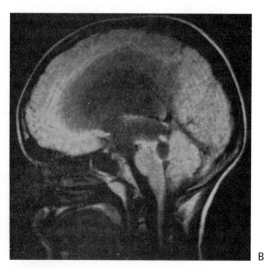

A   B

FIG. 48.3.   A: Normal midsagittal brain anatomy demonstrated by T1-weighted MRI. **B:** On a similar scan of a child, abnormal membranous structures within the fourth ventricle and aqueduct of Sylvius caused dilation of the upper fourth, third, and lateral ventricles. (Courtesy of Dr. Reed Murtagh.)

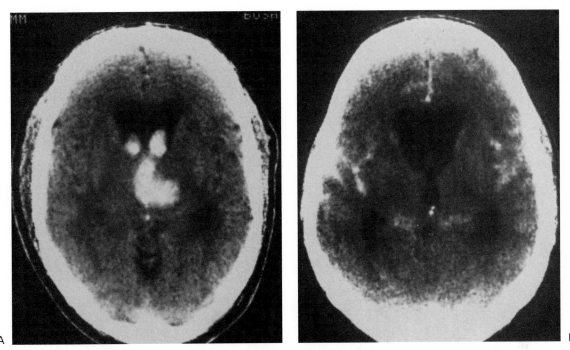

FIG. 48.4. **A:** Brain CT in a 58-year-old individual several hours after the sudden development of coma and right hemiparesis. Blood in the left thalamus and within the third and lateral ventricles is associated with hydrocephalus. **B:** Similar scan of adult 24 hours after the sudden onset of severe headache and meningism. Acute hydrocephalus with subarachnoid space blood is seen.

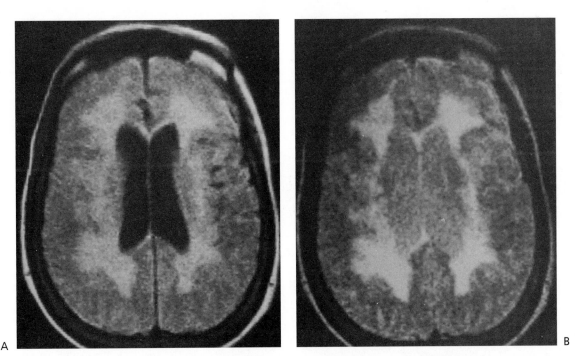

FIG. 48.5. **A:** Axial T1-weighted MR image of the brain shows lateral ventricular dilatation in a 42-year-old woman with dementia, ataxia, and urinary incontinence 3 months after subarachnoid hemorrhage. **B:** Axial, more T2-weighted image in this woman demonstrates periventricular increased signal intensity consistent with transependymal migration of CSF. Her condition improved after CSF shunting.

puted tomography (CT) has demonstrated that hydrocephalus may also follow other forms of meningitis (e.g., bacterial, fungal, viral, carcinomatous) (Fig. 48.6).

Mass Lesions

Intracranial neoplasms may cause obstructive hydrocephalus (Fig. 48.7). Other mass lesions, such as intraparenchymal cerebral hemorrhage and cerebellar infarction or hemorrhage, may

lead to acute hydrocephalus. Basilar artery ectasia and other vascular abnormalities (e.g., vein of Galen malformation) have been associated with hydrocephalus.

COMMUNICATING HYDROCEPHALUS

When impairment of neither intraventricular nor extraventricular CSF flow can be documented, three other mechanisms may

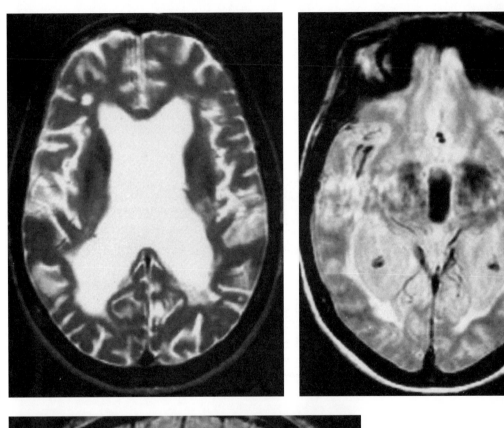

A   B

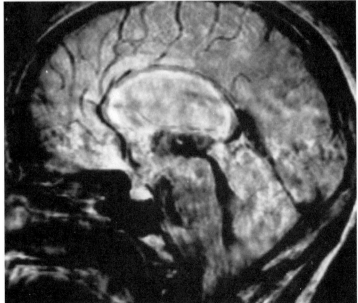

C

FIG. 48.6. Normal pressure hydrocephalus. **A:** Axial T2-weighted MR image shows dilated lateral ventricles with no evidence of sulcal effacement. **B,C:** Axial and sagittal proton-density MRI shows increased signal intensity around both lateral ventricles consistent with interstitial edema within the periventricular white matter. Pronounced flow void is seen within the third ventricle on the axial view; the sagittal view shows extension of the flow void down the aqueduct of Sylvius and into the fourth ventricle. This indicates abnormally increased CSF pulsations through these structures and may represent a prognostic marker for successful ventricular shunt placement for NPH. A ventricular shunt was placed, and this patient showed improvement in mental status and gait difficulty. (Courtesy of Dr. R. Muntagh.)

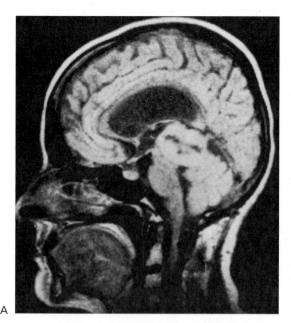
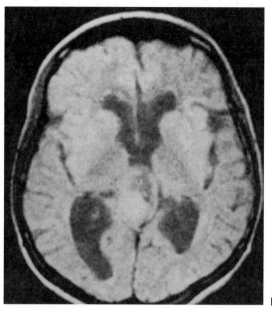

FIG. 48.7. A: Midsagittal T1-weighted MR image in a 42-year-old woman demonstrates a pinealoma causing lateral ventricular dilation with a normal fourth ventricle. **B:** Axial T1-weighted imaging demonstrates the pineal region tumor and dilation of the proximal third and lateral ventricles.

cause hydrocephalus: oversecretion of CSF, venous insufficiency, or impaired absorption of CSF by arachnoid villi.

When CSF *oversecretion* occurs, the absorptive capacity of the subarachnoid space is about three times the normal CSF formation rate of 0.35 mL per minute; formation rates greater than 1.0 mL per minute may produce hydrocephalus. Clinically, *choroid plexus papilloma* is the only known cause of oversecretion hydrocephalus.

Otitic hydrocephalus is a condition that occurs in children after chronic otitis media or mastoiditis with lateral sinus thrombosis; otherwise, impaired cerebral *venous drainage* (e.g., thrombosis of cortical veins or intracranial venous sinuses) rarely causes hydrocephalus. Hydrocephalus owing to extracranial venous drainage impairment only rarely follows radical neck dissection or obstruction of the superior vena cava.

Communicating hydrocephalus has been attributed to *congenital agenesis of the arachnoid villi* with consequent impairment of CSF absorption. Because detailed pathologic study of the number of villi and their structural characteristics is difficult and rarely performed, this defect may be more common than statistics indicate. Likewise, dysfunction of arachnoid villi without obstruction of basilar or transcortical CSF pathways cannot be assessed easily.

Hydrocephalus has also been described when CSF protein content exceeds 500 mg/dL in cases of polyneuritis or spinal cord tumor. The protein may interfere with CSF absorption. Ependymoma, the most common spinal cord tumor associated with hydrocephalus, may be due to tumor seeding of the arachnoid villi.

NORMAL PRESSURE HYDROCEPHALUS

As a potentially treatable cause of dementia, NPH has captured wide attention. The syndrome was first delineated in 1964 as an

occult form of hydrocephalus. The absence of papilledema with normal CSF pressure at lumbar puncture led to the term *normal pressure hydrocephalus;* however, intracranial hypertension probably occurs before diagnosis. Intermittent intracranial hypertension has been noted during monitoring of suspected cases. Often, the syndrome follows head trauma, subarachnoid hemorrhage, or meningitis, or is associated with an occult mass lesion.

There is much speculation about the pathophysiology of NPH. Obliteration or insufficiency of the transcortical subarachnoid space may occur alone or with an impaired absorption defect at the arachnoid villi, leading to reduced conductance to CSF outflow.

General Clinical Data

Signs and Symptoms

In children before the cranial sutures fuse, hydrocephalus causes skull enlargement and widened fontanels. The face, although of normal size, appears small relative to the enlarged head. Exophthalmos and scleral prominence result from downward displacement of the orbits. Severe intracranial hypertension produces sluggish pupillary reaction, absence of upward gaze, impaired lateral gaze, paralysis or spasm of conversion, nystagmus, retractions, and absence of visual fixation or response to visible threat. Untreated hydrocephalic infants fail to thrive and show retardation of motor and intellectual development. Limb movements, particularly of the legs, show progressive weakness and spasticity. Seizures are common. Prominent skull veins are evident, and a sound similar to that made by a cracked pot is noted on percussion. Wasting of trunk and limb muscles is apparent, with spasticity, increased tendon reflexes, and Babinski signs. With progression, the child is unable to lift the enlarged head. Visual loss is followed by optic atrophy. Scalp necrosis may lead to CSF leakage, infection, and death.

In otitic hydrocephalus, the child may be febrile and listless. Eardrum perforation and purulent otic discharge usually occur. Ipsilateral sixth nerve paralysis and papilledema are often noted.

In adults, symptoms include headache, lethargy, malaise, incoordination, and weakness. Seizures are uncommon. Findings may include dementia, altered consciousness, ocular nerve palsies, papilledema, ataxia, or corticospinal tract signs. Ventricular enlargement is not usually a uniform process and frequently occurs at the expense of periventricular white matter but with relative preservation of gray matter. Therefore, severe hydrocephalus may remain occult and, even though uncomplicated by brain tumor or other obvious causes, may be found by CT in adults with preserved mental state and signs limited to pyramidal tract or cerebellar dysfunction.

NPH is characterized by insidious onset and gradual development for weeks or months of the triad of dementia, ataxia of gait, and urinary incontinence. Headache and signs of increased intracranial pressure do not occur. Symptoms may begin weeks after head trauma or subarachnoid hemorrhage. In advanced disease, there may be frontal release signs, with hyperactive tendon reflexes and Babinski signs.

Laboratory Data

In infants, hydrocephalus must be distinguished from other forms of macrocephaly, such as subdural hematoma. Skull transillumination should be performed. Plain skull radiographs and skull measurements are useful to follow the course. Nonetheless, CT and MRI are the best diagnostic aids for all forms of hydrocephalus.

Lumbar puncture is sometimes indicated to measure CSF pressure and determine the presence of blood or signs of inflammatory or infectious disease. Continuous monitoring of intraventricular pressure may differentiate arrested from progressive disease when lumbar sac CSF pressure is normal and may not accurately reflect the intraventricular pressure. Likewise, CSF pulse-wave analysis may be more reliable than CSF pressure alone in diagnosis of hydrocephalus.

Ultrasonography is useful in evaluating subependymal and intraventricular hemorrhage in high-risk premature infants and in following the infants for possible later development of progressive hydrocephalus. Results correlate well with CT. As a bedside procedure, ultrasonography requires minimal manipulation of critically ill infants.

In adult-onset NPH, some clinicians believe that the best results from CSF shunting are achieved in patients who have the full clinical triad or who show improvement when 30 to 50 mL of CSF is removed by lumbar puncture. However, because brain NPH represents a potentially reversible form of dementia, other diagnostic techniques are used to improve the selection of patients likely to benefit from CSF shunting. The following tests are preferred by one or more groups, but none is universally accepted as reliably prognostic of a favorable outcome: CT or MRI evidence of transependymal diffusion of fluid; "isotope cisternography," a measure of the direction of CSF flow, showing CSF reflux from the subarachnoid space to the lateral ventricles

(reversing the normal flow) and delayed clearance or intraventricular transependymal penetration of the isotope; CSF compartment infusion or perfusion tests; intracranial pressure monitoring to assess high-pressure waves; measurement of CSF blood flow; and dynamic MRI studies to determine the direction and volume of CSF flow. Cerebral angiography is occasionally indicated in diagnostic problems of hydrocephalus owing to intracranial mass lesions.

Prognosis and Treatment

Prognosis is sometimes related to an underlying disease (e.g., cerebral neoplasm), and treatment of hydrocephalus is palliative if it is given. However, present-day management of conditions such as brain tumor and cerebrovascular disease can yield prolongation of quality of life. Therefore, relief of obstructive hydrocephalus by a shunting procedure is often indicated to prevent acute brain herniation and death. In other cases, there may be spontaneous arrest, as in benign communicating hydrocephalus of infants. A shunting procedure may allow the underlying condition to stabilize or arrest. The patient's prognosis is then related to the severity of that condition (e.g., Dandy-Walker syndrome or status after basal arachnoiditis). In some patients (e.g., adult aqueductal stenosis), shunting can produce an excellent outcome. In untreated progressive infantile hydrocephalus, the mortality rate is 50% at age 1 year and 75% at age 10 years. After intracranial hemorrhage in high-risk premature infants, the outcome in hydrocephalus is usually related to factors (e.g., asphyxia) other than shunt responsiveness.

The problem of selecting patients with idiopathic NPH (as opposed to those who have had prior subarachnoid hemorrhage or meningitis) for CSF shunting persists. In the series of Vanneste and colleagues (1992,1993), 36% of patients with idiopathic NPH improved (Table 48.1), and 28% suffered complications of the procedure, with death or persistent disability in 7%. Complications included cerebral infarction and hemorrhage, subdural hematoma or effusion, intracranial infection, seizures, and extracranial infections. Of 166 patients, 32 had shunt revisions.

Higher rates of improvement have been reported; however, favorable results are more likely to be reported. The best results are attained in patients who have no adverse risk factors, clear evidence of dementia and ataxia with or without urinary inconti-

TABLE 48.1. RESULTS OF CEREBROSPINAL FLUID SHUNTING FOR NORMAL PRESSURE HYDROCEPHALUS (NPH)

Cause of NP	Patients (n)	Grade of Improvement		
		None	Slight	Marked
Idiopathic	127	87	21	19 (15%)
Known cause				
Communicating	11	7	0	4 (36%)
Noncommunicating	14	3	2	9 (64%)
Total	152	97	23	32
Percent		64%	15%	21%

Modified from Vanneste et al., 1992.

nence, CT evidence of chronic hydrocephalus, and normal CSF at lumbar puncture.

Pharmacologic therapy is of limited value; there have been favorable reports of acetazolamide (Diamox), furosemide (Lasix), and isosorbide use, with or without repeated lumbar punctures. The major therapeutic choice is surgery, including choroid plexectomy for papilloma. Numerous CSF shunting procedures have been advocated to effect CSF removal from one portion of the craniospinal space to another (ventriculocisternal shunting) or from the craniospinal space to an extracranial reservoir (ventriculopleural shunt). Results vary with the procedures used, operative techniques, patient status, cause and duration of hydrocephalus, and incidence of complications, such as infection, subdural hematoma, shunt failure, or seizures.

Ventricular enlargement begins immediately and is grossly evident within 3 hours of experimental obstruction of the fourth ventricle in monkeys. After 3 weeks, damage is irreversible. If these experimental results apply to humans, early intervention is indicated. Even when management of progressive infantile hydrocephalus is optimal, the survival rate is 50% after age 15 years, with 15% incidence of mental retardation. In NPH, the success rate is best in patients with recent progression of mild dementia, gait disorder, and urinary incontinence. Under those circumstances, 60% of patients may show improvement, but a complication rate of 35% is not uncommon.

SUGGESTED READINGS

Bell WO. Cerebrospinal fluid reabsorption: a critical appraisal, 1990. *Pediatr Neurosurg* 1995;23:42–53.

Boon AJ, Tans JT, Delwel EJ, et al. Dutch normal-pressure hydrocephalus study: prediction of outcome after shunting by resistance to outflow of cerebrospinal fluid. *J Neurosurg* 1997;87:687–693.

Bradley WG Jr. Magnetic resonance imaging in the evaluation of cerebrospinal fluid flow abnormalities. *Magn Reson Q* 1992;8:169–196.

Bradley WG Jr, Scalzo D, Queralt J, Nitz WN, Atkinson DJ, Wong P. Normal-pressure hydrocephalus: evaluation with cerebrospinal fluid flow measurements at MR imaging. *Radiology* 1996;198:523–529.

Callen PW, Hashimoto BE, Newton TH. Sonographic evaluation of cerebral cortical mantle thickness in the fetus and neonate with hydrocephalus. *J Ultrasound Med* 1986;5:251–255.

Chervenak FA, Berkowitz RL, Tortora M, et al. The management of fetal hydrocephalus. *Am J Obstet Gynecol* 1985;151:933–942.

Choux M, Genitori L, Lang D, Lena G. Shunt implantation: reducing the incidence of shunt infection. *Neurosurgery* 1992;77:875–880.

Dippel DWJ, Habbema JDF. Probabilistic diagnosis of normal pressure hydrocephalus and other treatable cerebral lesions in dementia. *J Neurol Sci* 1993;119:123–133.

Fishman RA. *Cerebrospinal fluid in diseases of the nervous system*, 2nd ed. Philadelphia: WB Saunders, 1992.

Foltz EL, Blanks J, Meyer R. Hydrocephalus: the zero ICP ventricle shunt (ZIPS) to control gravity shunt flow: a clinical study in 56 patients. *Childs Nerv Syst* 1994;10:43–48.

Gideon P, Stahlberg F, Thomsen C, Gjerris F, Sorensen PS, Henriksen O. Cerebrospinal fluid flow and production in patients with normal pressure hydrocephalus studied by MRI. *Neuroradiology* 1994;36:210–215.

Go KG. The normal and pathological physiology of brain water. *Adv Tech Stand Neurosurg* 1997;23:47–142.

Goh D, Minns RA, Hendry GM, et al. Cerebrovascular resistive index assessed by duplex Doppler sonography and its relationship to intracranial pressure in infantile hydrocephalus. *Pediatr Radiol* 1992;22:246–250.

Gradin WC, Taylon C, Fruin AH. Choroid plexus papilloma of the third ventricle: case report and review of the literature. *Neurosurgery* 1983;12:217–220.

Greitz D, Hannerz J, Rahn T, Bolander H, Ericsson A. MR imaging of cerebrospinal fluid dynamics in health and disease: on the vascular pathogenesis of communicating hydrocephalus and benign intracranial hypertension. *Acta Radiol* 1994;35:204–211.

Hakim R, Black PM. Correlation between lumbo-ventricular perfusion and MRI-CSF flow studies in idiopathic normal pressure hydrocephalus. *Surg Neurol* 1998;49:14–19.

Hakim S, Adams RD. The special clinical problem of symptomatic hydrocephalus with normal cerebrospinal fluid pressure. *J Neurol Sci* 1965;2:307–327.

Jansen J, Jorgensen M. Prognostic significance of signs and symptoms in hydrocephalus: analysis of survival. *Acta Neurol Scand* 1986;73:55–65.

Klinge P, Fischer J, Heissler HE, et al. PET and CBF studies of chronic hydrocephalus: a contribution to surgical indication and prognosis. *J Neuroimaging* 1998;8:205–209.

Krauss JK, Regel JP. The predictive value of ventricular CSF removal in normal pressure hydrocephalus. *Neurol Res* 1997;19:357–360.

Malm J, Kristensen B, Karlsson T, Fagerlund M, Elfverson J, Ekstedt J. The predictive value of cerebrospinal fluid dynamic tests in patients with idiopathic adult hydrocephalus syndrome. *Arch Neurol* 1995;52:783–789.

Naidich TP, Altman NR, Gonzalez-Arias SM. Phase contrast cine magnetic resonance imaging: normal cerebrospinal fluid oscillation and applications to hydrocephalus. *Neurosurg Clin N Am* 1993;4:677–705.

Quencer RM. Intracranial CSF flow in pediatric hydrocephalus: evaluation with cine-MR imaging. *AJNR* 1992;13:601–608.

Rekate HL. Shunt revision: complications and their prevention. *Pediatr Neurosurg* 1991–1992;17:155–162.

Schurr PH, Polkey CE, eds. *Hydrocephalus.* Oxford: Oxford University Press, 1993.

Sgouros S, John P, Walsh AR, Hockley AD. The value of colour Doppler imaging in assessing flow through ventriculo-peritoneal shunts. *Childs Nerv Syst* 1996;12:454–459.

Skinner S, Gammon K, Bergman E, et al. Management of hydrocephalus in infancy: use of acetazolamide and furosemide to avoid cerebrospinal fluid shunts. *J Pediatr* 1985;107:31–37.

Spanu G, Karussos G, Adinolfi D, et al. An analysis of cerebrospinal fluid shunt infection in adults: a clinical experience of twelve years. *Acta Neurochir (Wien)* 1986;80:79–82.

Vanneste J, Augustijn P, Dirven C, et al. Shunting normal pressue hydrocephalus: do the benefits outweigh the risks? A multicenter study and literature review. *Neurology* 1992;43:54–59.

Vanneste J, Augustijn P, Tan WF, et al. Shunting normal pressure hydrocephalus: predictive value of combined clinical and CT data. *J Neurol Neurosurg Psychiatry* 1993;56:251–256.

Merritt's Neurology, 10th ed., edited by L.P. Rowland. Lippincott Williams & Wilkins, Philadelphia © 2000.

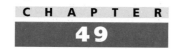

BRAIN EDEMA AND DISORDERS OF INTRACRANIAL PRESSURE

ROBERT A. FISHMAN

BRAIN EDEMA

Brain edema accompanies a wide variety of pathologic processes. It plays a major role in head injury, stroke, and brain tumor, as well as in cerebral infections, including brain abscess, encephalitis, and meningitis; lead encephalopathy; hypoxia; hypoosmolality; the dysequilibrium syndromes associated with dialysis and diabetic ketoacidosis; Reye syndrome; fulminant hepatic encephalopathy; and hydrocephalus. Brain edema occurs in several different forms; clearly it is not a single pathologic or clinical entity.

Brain edema is defined as an increase in brain volume due to an increase in water and sodium content. Brain edema, when well localized or mild in degree, is associated with little or no clinical evidence of brain dysfunction; however, when it is severe, it causes focal or generalized signs of brain dysfunction, including various forms of brain herniation and medullary failure of respiration and circulation. The major forms of herniation are uncal, cerebellar tonsillar, upward cerebellar, cingulate, and transcalvarial herniation.

Brain edema and brain engorgement are different processes. *Brain engorgement* is an increase in the blood volume of the brain caused by obstruction of the cerebral veins and venous sinuses or by arterial vasodilatation, such as that caused by hypercapnia. Focal or generalized brain edema results in intracranial hypertension when it is severe enough to exceed the compensatory mechanisms modulating intracranial pressure.

Brain edema is classified into three major categories: vasogenic, cellular (cytotoxic), and interstitial (hydrocephalic). The features of the three forms of cerebral edema are summarized in Table 49.1 in terms of pathogenesis, location and composition of the edema fluid, and changes in capillary permeability.

Vasogenic Edema

Vasogenic edema is characterized by increased permeability of brain capillary endothelial cells to macromolecules, such as the plasma proteins whose entry is limited by the capillary endothelial cells. The increase in permeability is visualized when contrast enhancement is observed with computed tomography (CT). Increased cerebrospinal fluid (CSF) protein levels are also indicative of increased endothelial permeability. Magnetic resonance imaging (MRI) is more sensitive than CT in demonstrating the increases in brain water and extracellular volume that characterize vasogenic edema.

Vasogenic edema is characteristic of clinical disorders in

TABLE 49.1. CLASSIFICATION OF BRAIN EDEMA

	Vasogenic	Cytotoxic	Interstitial (hydrocephalic)
Pathogenesis	Increased capillary permeability	Cellular swelling (glial, neuronal, endothelial)	Increased brain fluid due to block of CSF absorption
Location of edema	Chiefly, white matter	Gray and white matter	Chiefly, periventricular white matter in hydrocephalus
Edema fluid composition	Plasma filtrate including plasma proteins	Increased intracellular water and sodium	CSF
Extracellular fluid volume	Increased	Decreased	Increased
Capillary permeability to large molecules (radioindated serum albumin, inulin)	Increased	Normal	Normal
Clinical disorders			
Syndromes	Brain tumor, abscess, infarction, trauma, hemorrhage, lead encephalopathy	Hypoxia, hypoosmolality (e.g., water intoxication); eysequilibrium syndromes	Obstructive hydrocephalus, pseudotumor (benign intracranial hypertension)
	Ischemia	Ischemia	
	Purulent meningitis (granulocytic edema)	Purulent meningitis (granulocytic edema) fulminant hepatic encephalopathy	Purulent meningitis (granulocytic edema)
EEG changes	Focal slowing common	Generalized slowing	Often normal
Therapeutic effects			
Steroids	Beneficial in brain tumor, abscess	Not effective (? fulminant hepatic encephalopathy)	Uncertain effectiveness
Osmotherapy	Reduces volume of normal brain tissue only, *acutely*	Reduces brain volume *acutely*	Rarely useful

Modified from Fishman RA. Brain edema. In: *Cerebrospinal fluid in diseases of the nervous system.* Philadelphia: WB Saunders, 1992:116–137.

which contrast-enhanced CT is frequently positive or MRI shows increased signal intensity. These disorders include brain tumor, abscess, hemorrhage, infarction, and contusion. These radiologic changes are also seen with acute demyelinating lesions in multiple sclerosis. They also occur with lead encephalopathy or purulent meningitis. The functional manifestations of vasogenic edema include focal neurologic deficits, focal electroencephalogram (EEG) slowing, disturbances of consciousness, and severe intracranial hypertension. In patients with brain tumor, whether primary or metastatic, the clinical signs are often caused more by the surrounding edema than by the tumor mass itself.

Cellular (Cytotoxic) Edema

Cellular edema is characterized by swelling of all the cellular elements of the brain (neurons, glia, and endothelial cells), with a concomitant reduction in the volume of the extracellular fluid space of the brain. Capillary permeability is not usually affected in the various cellular edemas; patients so affected have a normal CSF protein and isotopic brain scan. CT does not reveal contrast enhancement, and MRI is usually normal.

There are several causes of cellular edema: hypoxia, acute hypoosmolality of the plasma, and osmotic dysequilibrium syndromes. *Hypoxia* after cardiac arrest or asphyxia results in cerebral energy depletion. The cellular swelling is determined by the appearance of increased intracellular osmoles (especially sodium, lactate, and hydrogen ions) that induce the rapid entry of water into cells. *Acute hypoosmolality of the plasma* and extracellular fluid is caused by acute dilutional hyponatremia, inappropriate secretion of antidiuretic hormone, or acute sodium depletion. *Osmotic dysequilibrium syndromes* occur with hemodialysis or diabetic ketoacidosis, in which excessive brain intracellular solutes result in excessive cellular hydration when the plasma osmolality is rapidly reduced with therapy. In uremia, the intracellular solutes presumably include a number of organic acids recovered in the dialysis bath. In diabetic ketoacidosis, the intracellular solutes include glucose and ketone bodies; however, there are also unidentified, osmotically active, intracellular solutes, termed *idiogenic osmoles,* that favor cellular swelling.

Major changes in cerebral function occur with the cellular edemas, including stupor, coma, EEG changes and asterixis, myoclonus, and focal or generalized seizures. The encephalopathy is often severe with acute hypoosmolality, but in more chronic states of hypoosmolality of the same severity, neurologic function may be spared. Acute hypoxia causes cellular edema, which is followed by vasogenic edema as infarction develops. Vasogenic edema increases progressively for several days after an acute arterial occlusion. The delay in obtaining contrast enhancement with CT following an ischemic stroke illustrates that time is needed for defects in endothelial cell function to develop.

Ischemic Brain Edema

Most patients with arterial occlusion have a combination of cellular edema first and then vasogenic edema, together termed *ischemic brain edema.* The cellular phase takes place after acute ischemia over minutes to hours and may be reversible. The vasogenic phase takes place over hours to days and results in in-farction, a largely irreversible process, although the increased endothelial cell permeability usually reverts to normal within weeks.

Fulminant Hepatic Encephalopathy

Acute hepatocellular failure occurs secondary to acute viral or toxic hepatitis and in Reye syndrome, a disorder affecting children. The resulting encephalopathy is characterized by progressive stupor and coma. Severe intracranial hypertension with brain edema is a major and often fatal complication. Imaging studies reveal a "tight" brain with normal permeability to contrast material.

Interstitial (Hydrocephalic) Edema

Interstitial edema is the third type of edema, best characterized in obstructive hydrocephalus, in which the water and sodium content of the periventricular white matter is increased because of the movement of CSF across the ventricular walls. Obstruction of the circulation of the CSF results in the transependymal movement of CSF and thereby an absolute increase in the volume of the extracellular fluid of the brain. This is observed in obstructive hydrocephalus with CT and MRI. Low-density changes are observed at the angles of the lateral ventricles. The chemical changes are those of edema, with one exception: The volume of periventricular white matter is reduced rather than increased. After successful shunting of CSF, interstitial edema is reduced, and the thickness of the mantle is restored.

Functional manifestations of interstitial edema are usually relatively minor in chronic hydrocephalus, unless the changes are advanced, when dementia and gait disorder become prominent. The EEG is often normal in interstitial edema. This finding indicates that the accumulation of CSF in the periventricular extracellular fluid space is much better tolerated than is the presence of plasma in the extracellular fluid space, as seen with vasogenic edema, which is characterized by focal neurologic signs and EEG slowing.

Granulocytic Brain Edema

Severe brain edema occurs with brain abscess and purulent meningitis due to collections of pus, which are often sterile as a result of antibiotic treatment. Such edema, associated with membranous products of granulocytes (pus), has been termed *granulocytic brain edema.* The features of cellular and vasogenic edema occur concurrently in purulent meningitis, and in severe cases hydrocephalic edema also develops, so that granulocytic brain edema may include the features of all three types of brain edema.

Therapeutic Considerations

The therapy of brain edema depends on the cause. Appropriate and early treatment of intracranial infection is essential. Surgical therapy is directed toward alleviating the cause by excision or decompression of intracranial mass lesions as well as by a variety of shunting procedures. A patent airway, maintenance of an adequate blood pressure, and the avoidance of hypoxia are fundamental requirements in the care of these patients.

The administration of appropriate parenteral fluids to meet the needs of patients is also essential. Administration of salt-free fluids should be avoided. In patients with cerebral edema, serum hypoosmolality has deleterious effects and should be avoided.

The pharmacologic treatment of brain edema is based on the use of glucocorticoids, osmotherapy, and drugs that reduce CSF formation. Hyperventilation, hypothermia, and barbiturate therapy have also been tested experimentally and in clinical practice; they are hardly ever used.

Glucocorticoids

The rationale for the use of steroids is largely empiric. Glucocorticoids dramatically and rapidly (in hours) begin to reduce the focal and general signs of brain edema around tumors. The major mechanism explaining their usefulness in vasogenic brain edema is a direct normalizing effect on endothelial cell function and permeability.

The biochemical basis of the changes in membrane integrity that underlie vasogenic and cellular edema is now under study. Attention has focused on the role of free radicals (i.e., superoxide ions, hydroxyl radicals, singlet oxygen, and nitric oxide) and on the effects of polyunsaturated fatty acids, most notably arachidonic acid, in the peroxidation of membrane phospholipids. The ability of adrenal glucocorticoids to inhibit the release of arachidonic acid from cell membranes may explain their beneficial effects in vasogenic edema; however, steroids have not been shown to be therapeutically useful in the brain edema of hypoxia or ischemia. Cellular damage is more important than brain edema in these conditions.

Long-acting, high-potency glucocorticoids are the most widely used. The usual dosage of dexamethasone is a starting dose of 10 mg followed by 4 mg administered four times a day thereafter—a dose equivalent in potency to 400 mg of cortisol daily. These large doses are about 20 times the normal rate of human endogenous cortisol production. Even larger dosages are sometimes used. Insufficient data are available to establish a formal dose–response curve for steroids in the treatment of brain edema; dosage schedules remain empiric.

Although any of the usual complications of steroid therapy are to be expected, gastric hemorrhage is usually the most troublesome. Fortunately, convulsive seizures apparently have not been increased in frequency by high dosages of the glucocorticoids. The risks of increased wound infection and impaired wound healing appear to be outweighed by the therapeutic effects in most patients receiving short-term therapy.

Although published data indicate that dexamethasone is valuable in the treatment of vasogenic edema associated with brain tumor and abscess, the literature recommending its use in stroke has, in general, been poorly documented and is controversial. Steroids may be useful in the treatment of intracerebral hematoma with extensive vasogenic edema due to the mass effect of the clot. In head injury, steroid therapy has frequently been used. Although some effectiveness following trauma has been documented, reductions in morbidity and mortality attributable to steroids are not great. The role of megadose steroids in the treatment of acute spinal cord injury is discussed elsewhere.

There are no convincing data, clinical or experimental, that glucocorticoids have beneficial effects in the cellular edema associated with hypoosmolality, asphyxia, or hypoxia in the absence of infarction with mass effects. There is little basis for recommending steroids in the treatment of the cerebral edema associated with cardiac arrest or asphyxia. The use of steroids in the management of fulminant hepatic encephalopathy is controversial. There are no controlled data regarding its effectiveness.

When intracranial hypertension and obstructive hydrocephalus occur because of inflammatory changes in the subarachnoid space or at the arachnoid villi, whether attributable to leukocytes or to blood, there is a reasonable rationale for the use of steroids. Despite the frequent use of steroids in purulent or tuberculous meningitis, however, few data are available to document the effectiveness of steroids against the acute disease. There are conflicting reports about the efficacy of steroids in acute bacterial meningitis or tuberculous meningitis. Use of steroids has not been shown to affect the subsequent incidence of chronic sequelae, such as obstructive hydrocephalus or seizures. Steroids do reduce the incidence of deafness in infants with bacterial meningitis. Steroids appear useful in the management of other conditions characterized by an inflammatory CSF, such as chemical meningitis following intrathecal radioiodinated serum albumin, meningeal sarcoidosis, or cysticercosis.

Osmotherapy

Hypertonic mannitol (Osmitrol) is the most widely used solute for the treatment of intracranial hypertension associated with brain edema. The effectiveness of osmotherapy depends on several factors. First, it is effective in reducing brain volume and elastance only as long as an osmotic gradient exists between blood and brain. Second, osmotic gradients obtained with hypertonic parenteral fluids are short-lived because the solute reaches an equilibrium concentration in the brain after a delay of only a few hours. Third, the parts of the brain most likely to "shrink" are normal areas; thus, with focal vasogenic edema, the normal regions of the hemisphere shrink, but edematous regions with increased capillary permeability do not. Fourth, a rebound in the severity of the edema may follow use of any hypertonic solution because the solute is not excluded from the edematous tissue; if tissue osmolality rises, the tissue water is increased. Finally, there is scant rationale for long-term use of hypertonic fluids, either orally or parenterally, because the brain adapts to sustained hyperosmolality with an increase in intracellular osmolality due to the solute and to idiogenic osmoles.

There is some uncertainty about the size of an increase in plasma osmolality that causes a therapeutically significant decrease in brain volume and intracranial pressure in humans. Acute increases as small as 10 mOsm/L may be therapeutically effective. It should be emphasized that accurate dose–response relationships in different clinical situations have not been well-defined with mannitol.

Other Therapeutic Measures

Hyperventilation, hypothermia, and barbiturates have been used in the management of intracranial hypertension, but none is established, and the extensive literature is not reviewed here. Acetazolamide (Diamox) and furosemide (Lasix) reduce CSF formation in animals and have limited usefulness in the management of interstitial edema.

IDIOPATHIC INTRACRANIAL HYPERTENSION

Idiopathic intracranial hypertension (IIH) describes a heterogeneous group of disorders characterized by increased intracranial pressure when intracranial mass lesions, obstructive hydrocephalus, intracranial infection, and hypertensive encephalopathy have been excluded. IIH is also termed *pseudotumor cerebri.* In the past, it has also been referred to as "serous meningitis" and "otitic hydrocephalus." The term *benign* has also been used because spontaneous recovery is characteristic, but serious threats to vision make accurate diagnosis and therapeutic intervention a necessity.

Various pathologic conditions are associated with IIH, although in most cases the pathogenesis of the intracranial hypertension is poorly understood:

Endocrine and metabolic disorders
  Obesity and menstrual irregularities
  Pregnancy and postpartum (without sinus thrombosis)
  Menarche
  Female sex hormones
  Addison disease
  Adrenal steroid withdrawal
  Hyperadrenalism
  Acromegaly
  Hypoparathyroidism
Intracranial venous-sinus thrombosis
  Mastoiditis and lateral sinus thrombosis
  After head trauma
  Pregnancy and postpartum
  Oral progestational drugs
  "Marantic" sinus thrombosis
  Cryofibrinogenemia
  Primary (idiopathic) sinus thrombosis
Drugs and toxins
  Vitamin A
  Retinoic acid
  Tetracycline
  Nalidixic acid (NegGram)
  Chlordecone (Kepone)
  Danazol (Danocrine)
  Amiodarone hydrochloride (Cordarone)
  Lithium carbonate
  Nitrofurantoin
Hematologic and connective tissue disorders
  Iron deficiency anemia
  Infectious mononucleosis
  Lupus erythematosus
High CSF protein content
  Spinal cord tumors
  Polyneuritis
"Meningism" with systemic bacterial or viral infections
Empty-sella syndrome
Miscellaneous
  Sydenham chorea
  Familial syndromes
  Rapid growth in infancy
Idiopathic conditions

Symptomatic intracranial hypertension without localizing signs may simulate IIH. Such conditions include obstructive hydrocephalus, chronic meningitis (sarcoid, fungal, or neoplastic), hypertensive encephalopathy, pulmonary encephalopathy due to paralytic hypoventilation, obstructive pulmonary disease, or the pickwickian syndrome (morbid obesity). High-altitude cerebral edema is an unusual manifestation of hypoxia.

Clinical Manifestations

The presenting symptoms are headache and impaired vision. The headache may be worse on awakening and aggravated by coughing and straining. It is often mild or may be entirely absent. The most common ocular complaint is visual blurring, a manifestation of papilledema. Some patients complain of brief, fleeting movements of dimming or complete loss of vision, occurring many times during the day (amaurosis fugax), at times accentuated or precipitated by coughing and straining. This ominous symptom indicates that vision is in jeopardy. Visual loss may be minimal despite severe chronic papilledema, including retinal hemorrhages; however, blindness occasionally develops rapidly (i.e., less than 24 hours). Visual fields characteristically show enlargement of the blind spots and may show constriction of the peripheral fields and central or paracentral scotoma. Diplopia caused by unilateral or bilateral sixth nerve palsy may develop as a result of increased intracranial pressure. The neurologic examination is otherwise normal. A major clinical point is that patients with IIH usually look well; their apparent well-being belies the ominous appearance of the papilledema. Although the disorder most often lasts for months, it may persist for years without serious sequelae. Remissions may be followed by one or more recurrences in 5% to 10% of cases. In some patients, IIH may be responsible for development of the *empty-sella syndrome,* in which radiographic enlargement of the sella turcica simulates a pituitary tumor. CT reveals that the enlarged sella is filled with CSF due to a defect of its diaphragm.

Pathophysiology

Several mechanisms have been considered as possible explanations for the pathophysiology of IIH. These include an increased rate of CSF formation, a sustained increase in intracranial venous pressure, a decreased rate of CSF absorption by arachnoid villi apart from venous occlusive disease, and an increase in brain volume due to an increase in blood volume or extravascular fluid volume, simulating a form of brain edema.

No data are available regarding the rate of CSF formation in IIH because the only reliable method for measurement (ventriculocisternal perfusion) is not applicable to these patients. The only condition in which increased CSF formation has been demonstrated is choroid plexus papilloma. Increased CSF production might explain the pathophysiology in some of the diverse conditions associated with IIH, but this mechanism remains unproven. A sustained increase in intracranial venous pressure associated with decreased CSF absorption readily explains the pathophysiology of IIH associated with venous-sinus thrombosis. Increased venous-sinus pressures are readily transmitted to the CSF and would also interfere with CSF absorption. Decreased CSF absorption (in the absence of venous occlusion) due to altered function of the arachnoid villi would explain the occurrence of IIH in some cases; this reasonable hypothesis is also unproven. The fact that IIH is associated with normal or small ventricles rather than hydrocephalus is consonant with such a mechanism. Abnormal spinal infusion tests do not differentiate between impairment of CSF absorption and decreased intracranial compliance. The occurrence of IIH in patients with polyneuritis or spinal cord tumors appears to support the hypothesis that defective CSF absorption may be the basis for the syndrome. This is not directly correlated with the degree of CSF protein elevation; it is presumed to depend on an alteration of the function of the arachnoid villi.

The hypothesis that IIH might be due to an increase in brain volume (a special form of brain edema) secondary to an increase in blood or extracellular fluid volume is supported by the presence of small ventricles, although this is an uncommon finding. An increase in brain volume would be expected if the extracellular space of the brain were expanded; this might occur if there were an excessive amount of CSF in the brain owing to either increased formation or decreased absorption.

Any theory of the pathogenesis of IIH must be consonant with the rapid therapeutic response of IIH to shunting of CSF by a lumbar peritoneal shunt. Impaired CSF absorption or increased CSF formation would explain the occurrence of IIH in most cases; however, the limited data available do not allow any firm conclusions.

Endocrine and Metabolic Disorders

IIH is most commonly seen in healthy women with a history of menstrual dysfunction. Frequently, the women are moderately or markedly overweight (without evidence of alveolar hypoventilation). Menstrual irregularity or amenorrhea is common. Galactorrhea is an unusual associated symptom. The histories often emphasize excessive premenstrual weight gain. Endocrine studies have not revealed specific abnormalities of urinary gonadotropins or estrogens, and the pathogenesis is unknown. IIH has a complex relationship to adrenal hormones. Rarely is IIH a complication of Addison disease or Cushing disease. Improvement occurs after restoration of a normal adrenal state; the mechanism in either circumstance is unknown.

IIH has also occurred in patients treated with adrenal corticosteroids for prolonged periods. Many of the patients had allergic skin disorders or asthma during childhood; IIH generally occurred when the steroid dosage was reduced, but evidence of hyperadrenalism persisted. Hypoparathyroidism may also present with increased intracranial pressure; hypocalcemic seizures or cerebral calcifications may further complicate the clinical picture. IIH has been reported in women taking oral progestational drugs when angiography has excluded sinus thrombosis.

Intracranial Venous-sinus Thrombosis

Intracranial hypertension occurs secondary to occlusion of the intracranial venous sinuses as a consequence of acute or chronic otitis media with extension of the infection into the petrous bone and lateral sinus. The sixth cranial nerve may also be involved, giving rise to diplopia on lateral gaze. Thrombosis of the superior longitudinal sinus may occur after mild closed head injury, giving rise to IIH. Occlusion of this sinus, which drains both cerebral hemispheres, is more likely to result in hemorrhagic infarction of the cerebrum as the thrombosis extends into the cere-

bral veins, giving rise to bilateral signs. In such cases, the course is frequently fulminant and the prognosis guarded, although complete recovery may occur. Aseptic or primary thrombosis of the superior longitudinal sinus may also be responsible for a pseudotumor syndrome, especially as a complication of pregnancy; it has been reported in the first 2 to 3 weeks postpartum, as well as at the end of the first trimester of pregnancy. Sinus thrombosis has been reported with the use of oral progestational drugs. A coagulopathy is suggested as the basis for these events, although rarely has this been substantiated. Sinus thrombosis occurs as a complication of dehydration and cachexia ("marantic" thrombosis), particularly in infancy.

Drugs and Toxins

IIH has been reported in otherwise healthy adolescents taking huge doses of vitamin A for the treatment of acne. Oral doses as low as 25,000 U daily may cause headache and papilledema, with rapid improvement after cessation of the therapy. The syndrome is said to have occurred in Arctic explorers who consumed polar bear liver, a great source of vitamin A. Some cases of IIH, manifested by bulging fontanel and papilledema, have been reported in children given tetracycline or nalidixic acid. The mechanisms involved are obscure. Spontaneous, rapid recovery occurs when the drugs are stopped. The insecticide chlordecone, as well as amiodarone and lithium carbonate, has also been reported to cause IIH.

Hematologic and Connective Tissue Disorders

Papilledema and increased intracranial pressure have been attributed to severe iron deficiency anemia, with striking improvement after treatment of the anemia. Presumably, the mechanism partly reflects the marked increase in cerebral blood flow that accompanies profound anemia. IIH has been reported with infectious mononucleosis, but the mechanism is not known. It has also been observed as manifestation of systemic lupus erythematosus.

Pulmonary Encephalopathy

IIH can be a major complication of chronic hypoxic hypercapnia caused by paralytic states, such as muscular dystrophy and cervical myelopathy; it may also be a major complication of obstructive pulmonary disease and the pickwickian syndrome. There is a chronic increase of cerebral blood flow because of the anoxemia and carbon dioxide retention. Patients usually appear mentally dull and encephalopathic, and thus differ from most patients with IIH.

Spinal Cord Diseases

IIH rarely occurs with tumors of the spinal cord or cauda equina, or with polyneuritis. Papilledema and headache disappear with treatment of the spinal lesion or regression of the polyneuropathy. The mechanism may involve the effects of an elevated CSF protein on CSF absorption at the arachnoid villi in both cranial and spinal subarachnoid spaces. Occurrence of this syndrome, however, does not correlate with the degree of protein elevation.

Meningism is an old term that is applied to patients with stiff neck, increased intracranial pressure (usually 200 to 300 mm Hg), but an otherwise normal CSF. This syndrome occurs in patients with acute systemic viral infections such as influenza. The mechanism of the intracranial hypertension is unknown.

One of the more common forms of IIH appears in otherwise healthy persons in the absence of any of the aforementioned etiologic factors. Both sexes are affected, and the occurrence is most often between ages 10 and 50 years.

Diagnosis

The patient with headache and papilledema without other neurologic signs must be considered to have symptomatic intracranial hypertension due to intracranial infection until proven otherwise. This is true in about 35% of cases. Although the diagnosis of IIH may be suspected by the appearance of well-being and a history of some of the associated etiologic features listed previously, the diagnosis is essentially one of exclusion and depends on ruling out the more common causes of increased intracranial pressure. Brain tumor, particularly when located in relatively silent areas such as the frontal lobes or right temporal lobe, or when obstructing the ventricular system, may be manifested only by headache and papilledema. Patients with chronic subdural hematoma, without a history of significant trauma, may have the same symptoms.

Diagnostic evaluation depends on CT or MRI, which have obviated conventional angiography in most cases. MR venography promises to be the procedure of choice to exclude venous occlusion. Lumbar puncture should be deferred until CT indicates that the ventricular system is normal in size and location. Diagnostic lumbar puncture is mandatory to establish the diagnosis of IIH. In obesity, the normal upper limit of CSF pressure is 250 mm Hg. In IIH, the CSF pressure is elevated, usually between 250 and 600 mm Hg, but the fluid is otherwise normal. The protein content is often in the lower range of normal, and lumbar CSF protein levels of 10 to 20 mg/dL are common. A CSF protein content greater than 50 mg/dL, decreased CSF glucose, or increased cell count throws doubt on the diagnosis of IIH and suggests another disease.

Pseudopapilledema may be a source of diagnostic confusion. In this developmental anomaly of the fundus, the ophthalmologic appearance may be indistinguishable from true papilledema; there is elevation of the optic disc, although exudates and hemorrhages are absent. Visual acuity is normal, but visual fields may show enlargement of the blind spots. The unchanging appearance of the fundus in subsequent examinations favors the diagnosis of pseudopapilledema, as does the finding of normal CSF pressure on lumbar puncture. Optic neuritis is differentiated from IIH by visual loss and normal CSF pressure.

Treatment

The common form of IIH in patients with menstrual disorders and obesity requires individualized management. This syndrome is self-limited in most cases, and after some weeks or months, spontaneous remissions occur, making evaluation of therapy difficult. Recurrent episodes have been noted in about 5% to 10%

of patients, and the illness seldom lasts for years. In the extremely obese, weight reduction is recommended. Daily lumbar puncture was used in the past to lower CSF pressure to normal levels by removing sufficient fluid; 15 to 30 mL of fluid may be removed, but the value of this procedure is dubious. A CSF shunting procedure, such as a lumboperitoneal shunt, is useful in patients with intractable headache and progressive visual impairment. It may dramatically relieve symptoms. Optic nerve decompression has its advocates as the procedure of choice to preserve vision.

Dexamethasone has been used empirically because it minimizes cerebral edema of diverse causes and seems effective in some patients. Steroids, however, should be avoided unless acetazolamide and furosemide fail because hyperadrenocorticism may precipitate IIH. Acetazolamide has been used because this carbonic anhydrase inhibitor reduces CSF formation. Furosemide also reduces CSF formation in animals and is useful. Hypertonic intravenous solutions (25% mannitol) to lower intracranial pressure can be used in acute situations when there is rapidly failing vision and surgical intervention is awaited; however, prolonged dehydration therapy is deleterious. Use of oral glycerol has the disadvantage of high caloric intake for obese patients. Subtemporal decompression was widely used in the past, but its efficacy has been questioned. Either lumboperitoneal shunts or optic nerve decompression is used to treat progressive visual loss. Their comparative risks and benefits should be assessed on an individual basis.

In patients with lateral sinus thrombosis caused by chronic infection in the petrous bone, surgical decompression may be indicated. When the pseudotumor syndrome is a manifestation of hypoadrenalism or hypoparathyroidism, replacement therapy is indicated. Vitamin A intoxication disappears when administration of the vitamin is stopped. Anticoagulation therapy is recommended for some patients with dural-sinus thrombosis; however, with extension of the clot into cerebral veins and hemorrhagic infarction of tissue, anticoagulation is useful despite its hazards. Thrombolytic therapy has been used successfully in recent reports.

SPONTANEOUS INTRACRANIAL HYPOTENSION

In 1938, Schaltenbrand described the occurrence of primary spontaneous intracranial hypotension (SIH), or "essential aliquorrhea." The symptoms were self-limited, resolving spontaneously within several weeks to several months. Decreased choroidal secretion and increased CSF reabsorption were suggested as possible mechanisms, but evidence for either was lacking.

Spontaneous cryptic CSF leaks via dural fistulas adjacent to the spinal roots have been identified with radionuclide cisternography and contrast myelography. The defects appear to reflect rupture of arachnoid (Tarlov) cysts that occurred without trauma. The rapid urinary excretion of radioisotope following intraspinal injection of the tracer reflects such spinal dural deficits. This diagnosis has been established with an intraspinal combined injection of technetium-albumin and myelographic contrast material. In some cases, one agent alone may identify the leak, which explains the advantage of the double injection. Cervical injection (C-2 or C-3) is often preferred over lumbar injection because it is less likely to result in a postlumbar-puncture headache and the cervical region is distant from the more common sites of leakage in the thoracolumbar region.

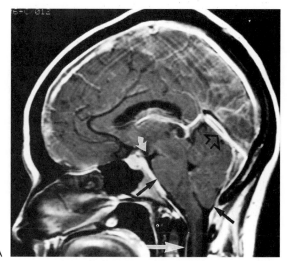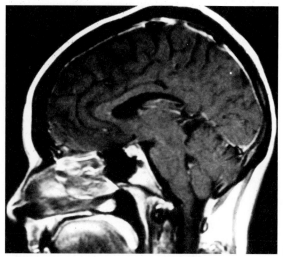

FIG. 49.1. Sagging brain in spontaneous intracranial hypotension. **A:** Gadolinium-enhanced T1-weighted sagittal MR image prior to lumbar epidural blood patch demonstrates enhancement of the dura, venous engorgement, displacement of the pons and cerebellum below the level of the prepontinal cistern *(arrow)*, and inferior displacement of the optic chiasm and third ventricle *(arrow)*. **B:** Gadolinium-enhanced T1-weighted images 5 days after large-volume (20 mL) lumbar epidural blood patch show resolution of dural enhancement and restoration of the cisterns, with elevation of the pons, tonsils, and optic chiasm. (From Fishman and Dillon, 1993; with permission.)

Gadolinium-enhanced MRI has revealed striking diffuse dural enhancement with CSF hypotension due to a CSF fistula associated with a "sagging" brain (i.e., flattening of the optic chiasm, displacement of the pons against the clivus, and the cerebellar tonsils below the foramen magnum simulating a Chiari malformation). Venous engorgement of the venous sinus is also observed. These changes rapidly resolve after closure of the CSF fistula. Figure 49.1 shows the characteristic MR findings in the sagging brain, together with their resolution 5 days after a successful epidural lumbar blood patch. The dural enhancement reflects the Monro-Kellie rule: Intracranial venous engorgement results from a reduced CSF volume.

SIH usually resolves spontaneously or with bedrest, analogous to postlumbar-puncture headache. For intractable cases, treatment with a large-volume lumbar epidural blood patch is usually preferred, with the head and spine then tilted downward (30 degrees) for 10 minutes to facilitate the movement of blood extradurally to the thoracic and cervical regions. In persistent cases, surgical closure of the fistula may be necessary.

Although postural headaches in the erect position are typical of SIH, some patients are headache-free despite characteristic radiologic changes. The occurrence of somnolence and stupor due to a sagging brain has been observed. SIH may simulate an acquired Chiari I malformation. Multiple cranial nerve signs have been noted, including binasal field defects, diplopia, tinnitus, and hearing loss.

SUGGESTED READINGS

Brain Edema

Fishman RA. Brain edema. In: *Cerebrospinal fluid in diseases of the nervous system,* 2nd ed. Philadelphia: WB Saunders, 1992:116–137.

Levine BD, Yoshimuri K, Kobayashi T, et al. Dexamethasone for the treatment of acute mountain sickness. *N Engl J Med* 1989;32:1707–1713.

Idiopathic Intracranial Hypertension

Duncan FJ, Corbett JJ, Wall M. The incidence of pseudotumor cerebri. *Arch Neurol* 1988;45:875–877.

Fishman RA. Pseudotumor cerebri. In: *Cerebrospinal fluid in diseases of the nervous system,* 2nd ed. Philadelphia: WB Saunders, 1992:138–151.

Knight RSG, Fielder AR, Firth JL. Benign intracranial hypertension: visual loss and optic nerve sheath fenestration. *J Neurol Neurosurg Psychiatry* 1986;49:243–250.

Ridsdale L, Moseley I. Thoracolumbar intraspinal tumors presenting features of raised intracranial pressure. *J Neurol Neurosurg Psychiatry* 1978;41:737–745.

Intracranial Hypotension

Atkinson JLD, Weinshenker BG, Miller GM, et al. Acquired Chiari I malformation secondary to spontaneous spinal cerebrospinal fluid leakage and chronic intracranial hypotension syndrome in seven cases. *J Neurosurg* 1998;88:237–242.

Bell WE, Joynt RJ, Sahs AL. Low spinal fluid pressure syndromes. *Neurology* 1960;10:512–521.

Fishman RA, Dillon WP. Dural enhancement and cerebral displacement secondary to intracranial hypotension. *Neurology* 1993;43:609–610.

Horton JC, Fishman RA. Neurovisual findings in the syndrome of spontaneous intracranial hypotension from dural cerebrospinal fluid leak. *Ophthalmology* 1994;101:244–251.

Mokri B, Piepgras DG, Miller GM. Syndrome of orthostatic headaches and diffuse pachymeningeal gadolinium enhancement. *Mayo Clin Proc* 1997;72:400–413.

Pleasure SJ, Abosch A, Friedman J, et al. Spontaneous intracranial hypotension resulting in stupor caused by diencephalic compression. *Neurology* 1998;50:1854–1857.

Rando TA, Fishman RA. Spontaneous intracranial hypotension: report of two cases and review of the literature. *Neurology* 1992;42:481–487.

Schaltenbrand VG. Normal and pathological physiology of the cerebrospinal fluid circulation. *Lancet* 1953;1:805–808.

Tarlov IM. Spinal perineurial and meningeal cysts. *J Neurol Neurosurg Psychiatry* 1970;33:833–843.

Merritt's Neurology, 10th ed., edited by L.P. Rowland. Lippincott Williams & Wilkins, Philadelphia © 2000.

C H A P T E R
50

SUPERFICIAL SIDEROSIS OF THE CENTRAL NERVOUS SYSTEM

ROBERT A. FISHMAN

Superficial siderosis is the deposition of hemosiderin over the pial surfaces and superficial neuropil of the brain and spinal cord. It is usually characterized by sequential development of sensorineural deafness and cerebellar ataxia followed by myelopathy, anosmia, and dementia. The condition usually evolves for many years as a consequence of chronic, intermittent, or persistent oozing of blood into the cerebrospinal fluid (CSF). The bleeding may be cryptic, that is, asymptomatic and unassociated with headache, backache, or signs of meningeal irritation. A common error is the faulty clinical diagnosis of a neurodegenerative disorder, cerebellar degeneration with deafness.

In the past, the condition was recognized chiefly at autopsy by the rust-colored appearance of the affected structures. Computed tomography (CT) and particularly magnetic resonance imaging (MRI) have shown that the condition is far more frequent than previously suspected. MRI has greater sensitivity because the strong paramagnetic effect of iron-containing compounds allows better visualization in T2-weighted images, which show striking rims of hypointensity over the surfaces of the cerebrum and particularly over the cerebellar vermis and adjacent cortical sulci. Hypointensities are observed rimming the brainstem and especially along the eighth cranial nerve, which is the most vulnerable cranial nerve because it is covered in the subarachnoid space by oligodendroglia, and not by the Schwann cells that cover the nerve roots and peripheral nerves. The first and second cranial nerves and spinal cord are similarly vulnerable. The Bergmann radial glia of the cerebellum are also susceptible to the deposition of iron pigments, perhaps because they can synthesize ferritin more readily than other neural cells. The presence of xanthochromic CSF, often without a cellular reaction, should alert the clinician that a patient with insidiously progressive ataxia and deafness may have superficial siderosis. T2-weighted MR imaging is more likely to establish the diagnosis than CT, which is less sensitive (Fig. 50.1).

The treatment of superficial siderosis requires identifying and

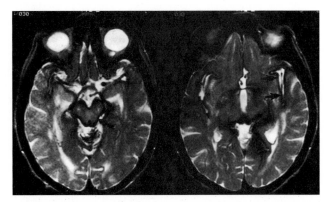

FIG. 50.1. Patient with 10-year history of progressive cerebellar ataxia, deafness, cognitive impairment, spasticity, and xanthochromic CSF. T2-weighted MR imges show deposition of low-signal hemosiderin on the surfaces of the midbrain, cerebellar folia, and cerebral cortex adjacent to the sylvian cisterns *(arrows)*. (Courtesy of Dr. William P. Dillon.)

treating the bleeding source, usually obvious in patients with aneurysms, vascular malformations, and tumors—especially ependymomas—of the brain or spinal cord. Siderosis may follow successful treatment of cerebellar tumors. Fearnley and colleagues (1995) reported identifying the precise source of bleeding in only about 50% of patients. Improvements in MRI should increase the success rate. There have been several reports of siderosis developing in patients with a variety of spinal dural defects, such as posttraumatic root avulsions, or with postoperative pseudomeningoceles following laminectomy. Closure of these dural defects arrests the progressive neurologic injury that results from chronic subarachnoid bleeding. Iron chelating agents have been ineffective in experimental animal models.

SUGGESTED READINGS

Anderson NE, Sheffield S, Hope JKA. Superficial siderosis of the central nervous system: a late complication of cerebellar tumors. *Neurology* 1999;52:163–169.

Fearnley JM, Stevens JM, Rudge P. Superficial siderosis of the central nervous system. *Brain* 1995;118:1051–1066.

Fishman RA. Superficial siderosis. *Ann Neurol* 1993;34:635–636.

Koeppen AH, Dickson AC, Chu RC, Thach RE. The pathogenesis of superficial siderosis of the central nervous system. *Ann Neurol* 1993;34:646–653.

Tapscott SJ, Askridge J, Kliot M. Surgical management of superficial siderosis following cervical nerve root avulsion. *Ann Neurol* 1996;40:936–949.

Merritt's Neurology, 10th ed., edited by L.P. Rowland. Lippincott Williams & Wilkins, Philadelphia © 2000.

HYPEROSMOLAR HYPERGLYCEMIC NONKETOTIC SYNDROME

LEON D. PROCKOP
STEPHAN A. MAYER

The hyperosmolar hyperglycemic nonketotic syndrome (HHNS) is characterized by an abnormally high serum glucose level, high osmolality, and a depressed level of consciousness in the absence of ketoacidosis. Modern awareness of the syndrome is ascribed to Sament and Schwartz, who in 1957 described diabetic stupor without ketosis. By 1968, the neurologic symptoms and signs of seizures and metabolic encephalopathy were well recognized. HHNS occurs in 10% to 20% of all patients with severe hyperglycemia; it is most common in elderly patients with mild adult-onset diabetes mellitus. Death ensues in 40% to 50%, usually related to medical comorbidity or neurologic complications.

HHNS is defined by serum osmolality greater than 350 mOsm/kg, plasma glucose content greater than 600 mg/dL, and no ketosis in a patient with depressed consciousness. Often, the patient is lethargic or confused; coma is unusual. The degree of lethargy correlates with the level of hyperosmolarity. Serum glucose levels are usually much higher than in diabetic ketoacidosis. Acidemia, Kussmaul respiration, and acetone on the breath are absent.

The average age of patients with HHNS is 60 years; men and women are affected equally. In most patients, the diabetes was not previously recognized, and only a few are insulin-dependent. Most patients with HHNS have some associated illness or medical therapy that precipitated the syndrome. Frequently associated illnesses include chronic renal insufficiency, gram-negative pneumonia or sepsis, gastrointestinal hemorrhage, myocardial infarction, pulmonary embolism, subdural hematoma, stroke, pancreatitis, and burns. Medications implicated in HHNS include diuretic agents (hydrochlorothiazide, furosemide [Lasix], ethacrynic acid [Edecrin]), corticosteroids, phenytoin sodium (Dilantin), propranolol, cimetidine, diazoxide, chlorpromazine hydrochloride (Thorazine), loxapine (Loxitane), asparaginase (Elspar), and immunosuppressive agents. Hyperalimentation, peritoneal dialysis or hemodialysis, and recent cardiac surgery have also been implicated.

Symptoms begin with several days or weeks of polyuria and polydipsia followed by dehydration and altered mental status. Depressed consciousness plays a key role in the development of the syndrome by preventing the patient from taking fluids in response to thirst. Confusion or unresponsiveness usually precipitates medical attention. Other neurologic findings include seizures (sometimes status epilepticus or epilepsia partialis continua), hemiparesis, aphasia, hemianopsia, visual loss, visual hal-

lucinations, nystagmus, pupillary reflex abnormalities, asymmetric caloric responses, dysphagia, hyperreflexia, myoclonus, Babinski signs, and urinary retention. Systemic signs of dehydration include orthostatic hypotension, poor skin turgor, dry mucous membranes, and reduced sweating. The differential diagnosis includes diabetic ketoacidosis, alcoholic ketoacidosis, lactic acidosis, hepatic failure, uremia, hypoglycemia, drug ingestion, and stroke.

The diagnosis of HHNS is made in the laboratory. The serum glucose level ranges from 600 to 2,700 mg/dL, and serum osmolality is in the range of 325 to 425 mOsm/kg. A difference between the measured and calculated osmolality (calculated osmolality (mOsm/L) = $2 \times$ [Na+] + [glucose]/18 + [BUN]/2.8) indicates the presence of an unmeasured solute, such as mannitol or ethylene glycol. Although ketones are absent, mild acidosis with an elevated anion gap is present in 50% of patients (pH range, 6.8 to 7.4). In some patients, an element of lactic acidosis can result from hypotension and poor tissue perfusion, although this never completely accounts for the anion gap. Mixed acid–base disturbances may be present in patients with a metabolic alkalosis due to diuretic use.

Plasma sodium concentrations vary over a wide range (120 to 180 mEq/L), although most patients are mildly hypernatremic. Elevated plasma glucose levels tend to depress the plasma sodium concentration (for every 100 mg/dL increment in glucose, sodium falls by 1.8 mEq/L). Therefore, a substantial free-water deficit may exist, even if the plasma sodium concentration is normal. Hypokalemia usually results from the sustained osmotic diuresis, and severe prerenal azotemia is the rule. In addition to laboratory studies, search for an underlying illness should include an electrocardiogram to rule out myocardial ischemia, blood and urine cultures and a chest x-ray to rule out infection, and brain computed tomography or magnetic resonance imaging if focal neurologic signs are present.

HHNS evolves when a physiologic stress and decreased insulin activity induce hyperglycemia. The hyperglycemia in turn induces an osmotic diuresis that continues until intravascular volume depletion reduces renal perfusion. The resulting free-water deficit and hyperosmolality cause cellular dehydration in both cerebral and extracerebral tissues, as water moves down the osmotic gradient from the intracellular to the extracellular compartment. Sodium and potassium losses occur as the osmotic diuresis interferes with normal tubular reabsorption, but water is always lost out of proportion to sodium, resulting in further extracellular hypertonicity. Cerebral dehydration is thought to be the primary cause of the neurologic changes of HHNS.

Treatment focuses on replacing volume deficits, correcting hyperosmolality, and managing any underlying illness. Patients in shock need immediate resuscitation with normal saline. The average total fluid deficit is 9 to 12 L. Central venous pressure monitoring may be useful in guiding therapy. Normal saline should be given until the blood pressure and urine output stabilize, at which point half-normal saline can be used. It is recommended that one-half of the estimated fluid deficit be replaced in the first 12 to 24 hours and the remainder replaced over the next few days.

Insulin may or may not be necessary in the initial management of HHNS. Serum glucose levels may drop by 25% with fluid replacement alone. Insulin is necessary if the patient is acidotic, hyperkalemic, or in renal failure. If insulin is used, a low-dose regimen should be given, that is, an initial intravenous bolus of 0.10 U/kg of regular insulin followed by a continuous intravenous infusion of 0.10 U/kg per hour. To avoid "overshoot" hypoglycemia, glucose levels should be monitored hourly; once they fall below 300 mg/dL, insulin is discontinued, and 5% dextrose is added to the infusion.

Most patients have total-body potassium deficits. Hydration and insulin administration further depress the serum potassium level. Therefore, potassium should be administered early in treatment.

If seizures develop, phenytoin should not be administered as initial therapy. It is ineffective in controlling seizures owing to hyperosmolarity and inhibits the release of endogenous insulin. Seizures may be controlled with intravenous benzodiazepines until the metabolic disturbance is corrected.

Because of the high mortality rate of patients with HHNS and the meticulous monitoring that treatment requires, these patients are best managed in an intensive care unit.

SUGGESTED READINGS

Arieff AI, Ayus JC. Strategies for diagnosing and managing hypernatremic encephalopathy. *J Crit Illness* 1996;11:720–727.

Arieff A, Carroll HJ. Non-ketotic hyperosmolar coma with hyperglycemia: clinical features, pathophysiology, renal function, acid–base balance, plasma-cerebrospinal fluid equilibrium and the effects of therapy on 37 cases. *Medicine* 1972;51:73–96.

Daugirdas JT, Knonfol NO, Tzamaloukas AH, et al. Hyperosmolar coma: cellular dehydration and the sodium concentration. *Ann Intern Med* 1989;110:855–857.

Genuth SM. Diabetic ketoacidosis and hyperglycemic hyperosmolar coma. *Curr Ther Endocrinol Metab* 1997;6:438–447.

Gonzalez-Campoy JM, Robertson RP. Diabetic ketoacidosis and hyperosmolar nonketotic state: gaining control over extreme hyperglycemic complications. *Postgrad Med* 1996;99:143–152.

Gullans SR, Verbalis JG. Control of brain volume during hyperosmolar and hyposmolar conditions. *Ann Rev Med* 1993;44:289–301.

Hennis A, Corbin D, Fraser H. Focal seizures and nonketotic hyperglycemia. *J Neurol Neurosurg Psychiatry* 1992;55:195–197.

Maccario M. Neurological dysfunction associated with nonketotic hyperglycemia. *Arch Neurol* 1968;19:525–534.

Prockop LD. Hyperglycemia, polyol accumulation and increased intracranial pressure. *Arch Neurol* 1971;25:126–140.

Prockop LD. Hyperglycemia: effects on the nervous system. In: Vinken PJ, Bruyn GW, eds. *Metabolic and deficiency diseases of the nervous system. Handbook of clinical neurology, vol 27.* Amsterdam: North-Holland, 1976:79–98.

Singh BM, Strobos RJ. Epilepsia partialis continua associated with non-ketotic hyperglycemia: clinical and biochemical profile of 21 patients. *Ann Neurol* 1980;8:155–160.

Umpierrez GE, Khajavi M, Kitabchi AE. Review: diabetic ketoacidosis and hyperosmolar nonketotic syndrome. *Am J Med Sci* 1996;311:225–233.

Vernon DD, Postellon DC. Non-ketotic hyperosmolar diabetic coma in a child: management with low-dose insulin infusion and intracranial pressure monitoring. *Pediatrics* 1986;77:770–777.

Merritt's Neurology, 10th ed., edited by L.P. Rowland. Lippincott Williams & Wilkins, Philadelphia © 2000.

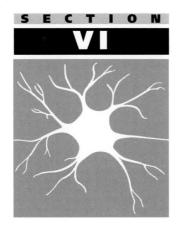

TUMORS

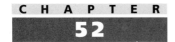

GENERAL CONSIDERATIONS

CASILDA M. BALMACEDA

EPIDEMIOLOGY

Nowhere else in oncology has there been a more vigorous explosion of research and therapy than in neurooncology. About 24,000 primary brain tumors are diagnosed each year in the United States alone. The estimated incidence for all ages, as determined from data largely collected before the era of computed tomography (CT), is 8.2 per 100,000 people (Table 52.1). Brain tumors are diagnosed more and more frequently, particularly in the growing number of elderly people. Brain tumors account for 20% of malignancies before age 15 years. There is a peak incidence in childhood, a steady rise from age 20 to age 70, and a decline thereafter (Fig. 52.1) Histologic type and location of tumors also vary by age and sex (Table 52.2). Rates in men are higher than in women for glioma, but the opposite occurs for meningioma. In children, medulloblastoma and asytrocytomas predominate. In adults, gliomas and meningiomas are the most common, constituting, respectively, about 60% and 20% of all primary brain tumors in this age group. In children, 70% of tumors are located beneath the tentorium, compared to 30% in adults. Survival differs by age group; central nervous system (CNS) tumors in children tend to have a better prognosis.

Epidemiologic reports of CNS tumors may be limited by several considerations: the histologic complexity of the tumors, lack of histologic verification in some cases, the retrospective nature of some studies, and the small number of patients in others. The possible effects of ethnicity, age, and sex may be distorted by unequal access to medical care or technology, as suggested by the

TABLE 52.1. PRIMARY INTRACRANIAL TUMORS: AVERAGE ANNUAL INCIDENCE RATES PER 100,000 POPULATION BY AGE AND SEX, UNITED STATES, 1973 TO 1974

Age group (yr)	Total (%)	Male (%)	Female (%)
All ages	8.2	8.2 (8.5[a])	8.1 (7.9[a])
<5	2.5	2.9	2.1
5–14	2.1	2.3	2.0
15–24	3.1	2.9	3.3
25–34	4.5	1.9	6.9
35–44	5.7	4.5	6.8
45–54	17.3	17.9	16.7
55–64	20.4	23.6	17.4
65–74	20.4	26.0	16.2
≥75	15.4	17.3	14.2

[a]Age-adjusted rates using the direct method. Modified from Walker et al., 1985.

variation in worldwide trends. It is possible that the increased incidence in the elderly may stem from the availability of CT in the 1970s and the introduction of stereotactic biopsy methods that are far less hazardous than diagnostic modalities employed earlier.

HISTORICAL PERSPECTIVE AND CLASSIFICATION

Although neurosurgical procedures were practiced as far back as the mesolithic period, it was Gallen (130 to 200 AD), Vesalius (1514 to 1564), and Willis (1621 to 1675) who laid the foundations for modern neuroanatomy. In the 19th century, neurology emerged as a discipline, cerebral localization was recognized, and the initial classifications of brain tumors appeared. In 1979, the World Health Organization formulated a classification of brain tumors that was based on the embryonal tissue of origin; this schema or its variations are currently used throughout the world. The current classification, based on conventional histologic features, is likely to be modified in the future by molecular and genetic markers. For the purposes of this volume, we have classified brain tumors as follows:

Primary brain tumors
    Glial tumors (see Chapter 55)
    Lymphomas (see Chapter 56)
    Pineal tumors (see Chapter 57)
Meningeal neoplasms (see Chapter 54)
    Meningioma
    Hemangiopericytoma
Tumors of the skull and cranial nerves (see Chapter 53)
Spinal tumors (see Chapter 62)
    Extramedullary tumors
    Intramedullary tumors
    Intradural tumors
    Vertebral tumors
Pituitary tumors (see Chapter 58)
Metastatic tumors (see Chapter 61)
    Parenchymal metastases
    Leptomeningeal metastases
    Spinal cord metastases
Vascular tumors and malformations (see Chapter 60)
Congenital and CNS tumors (see Chapter 59)

BRAIN TUMOR BIOLOGY AND GENETICS

The developmental diversity of brain tumors could lead to specific therapies on the basis of cell lineage, stage of differentiation, and specific behavior. Several progenitor cells are recognized. One is a pleuripotential cell that gives rise to both neuronal and microglial cell lines, as well as to tumors of either neuronal or glial types. Then, other forces play a role, including transcription and growth factors, matrix molecules, and proteases. Chromosomal aberrations in many primary brain tumors suggest a model of malignant progression. In this *multistep theory,* several genetic events are deemed necessary for the development of a brain tumor.

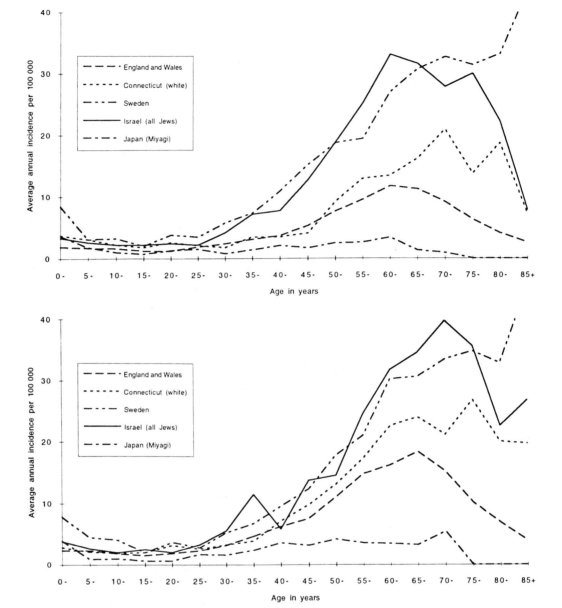

FIG. 52.1. Female (**top**) and male (**bottom**) age-specific incidence rates for malignant CNS tumors, 1978–1982. (From Muir et al.; with permission.)

RISK FACTORS

Host Factors

Menopause, stroke, and breast cancer are host factors that may increase the risk for primary brain tumors. Family clustering is rarely seen, except sometimes in Mendelian patterns of inheritance. The increased risk of some occupations (e.g., electronics, pharmaceutical, and manufacturing industries) could reflect common exposure to an environmental agent or better access to medical care.

Environmental Factors

Studies of environmental factors have been inconclusive; many are conflicting. The environment may contribute one of several steps in the development of a brain tumor. *Chemicals* and *viruses* have been implicated. Chemical induction of CNS tumors has been found in animals given nitrosoureas, hydrazines, triazines, or aromatic hydrocarbons. Astrocytomas have appeared in patients with progressive multifocal leukoencephalopathy, in which cells are infected by the papovavirus JC virus. The Epstein-Barr virus has been identified in cells of primary CNS lymphoma; both adenovirus and SV-40 can induce tumors in laboratory animals. Studies of exposure to *electromagnetic fields* have not confirmed an increased incidence of brain tumors.

Ionizing *radiation* is a recognized risk factor. Moderate-dose irradiation of the scalp for tinea capitis in children increases the later risk of CNS tumors, particularly meningioma, glioma, and nerve sheath tumor. In adults, radiation to the head and dental x-rays have been associated with an increased risk for menin-

TABLE 52.2. AVERAGE ANNUAL INCIDENCE OF PATHOLOGICALLY CONFIRMED INTRACRANIAL NEOPLASMS BY HISTOLOGIC DIAGNOSIS IN THE UNITED STATES, 1973 TO 1974

Histologic diagnosis	Patients	
	Number	%
Glioma	7,940	57.8
Glioblastoma	2,740	20.0
Medulloblastoma	300	2.2
Cerebellar astrocytoma	120	0.9
Other astrocytomas and gliomas	4,780	34.8
Meningiomas	2,680	19.5
Neurinoma	940	6.9
Adenoma[a]	1,970	14.4
Other	190	1.4

[a]Includes 1,110 unconfirmed cases of pituitary neoplasms that are assumed to be adenomas. Modified from Walker et al., 1985.

gioma. An association with *diet* remains speculative; consumption of *N*-nitrous compounds in cured meats has been implicated, while the ingestion of antioxidants may be protective.

CLINICAL DIAGNOSIS

Symptoms and signs may be due to direct tumor effects and compression of adjacent structures, or to *secondary effects* of edema, hydrocephalus, or increased intracranial pressure (ICP). *Negative* symptoms arise from loss of function (sensory loss, weakness); *positive* symptoms include seizures or headache. Specific symptoms are more related to tumor *location* than to histology. Since the introduction of CT and magnetic resonance imaging (MRI), it is unusual to find tumors that lead to clinical symptoms after attaining a larger size, unless the tumor is located in a relatively silent area, such as the anterior frontal lobe or the nondominant temporal lobe (Fig. 52.2). Clinical manifestations are affected by the *rapidity* of tumor growth; slowly growing tumors may not be symptomatic because the adjacent brain may accommodate to the mass. Surrounding edema suggests rapid growth and may cause symptoms, even when the tumor is small.

Headache is the first symptom in 35% of patients and occurs later in 70%. Supratentorial tumors usually produce frontal headaches, while those in the posterior fossa lead to neck and occipital pain. Some characteristics raise suspicion of a primary tumor: morning headaches or those that waken the patient from sleep, improving later in the day; headaches that increase in frequency and severity in weeks or months; headaches that differ from a person's pattern of chronic headaches; and, especially, headache associated with papilledema or focal cerebral signs. Pain is attributed to distortion of pain-sensitive structures in the intracranial compartment, such as the dura, venous sinuses, cerebral arteries, or the cranial nerves. Vomiting or nausea may be due to increased ICP or hydrocephalus. Involvement of the chemoreceptor trigger zone in the medulla may lead to *projectile* vomiting. Vomiting may terminate a headache because the hyperventilation that follows lowers ICP.

Facial pain may follow the distribution of the trigeminal

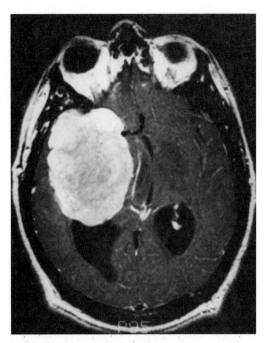

FIG. 52.2. Temporal meningioma (a large, slowly growing tumor affecting a "silent" area of the brain). This 38-year-old man had mild papilledema on routine eye examination. Gadolinium-enhanced MR image shows a 7-cm right temporal lobe meningioma.

nerve, with tumors at the base of the skull or nasopharynx. In contrast to trigeminal neuralgia, as tumor pain lasts longer, it is less likely to be lancinating and may be accompanied by sensory loss. *Temporal* or *auricular pain* may be seen with a thoracic malignancy, due to referred pain from irritation of the vagus nerve in the chest.

Plateau waves are periodic fluctuations of ICP. Typically, the elevation is abrupt, up to 100 mm Hg above baseline, and may be sustained for minutes or hours before quickly descending to normal. Clinically, the patient may have headache, nausea, vomiting, leg weakness, or other symptoms of incipient herniation. These waves arise with severely increased pressure and are ominous. They may be triggered by cerebral vasodilatation caused by events that lower arterial blood pressure, such as infections, anesthetics, or rapid eye movement sleep. With severely increased ICP, one may observe a *Cushing reflex*, consisting of rising blood pressure and bradycardia. *Dizziness, vertigo,* and *hearing loss* may be seen in posterior fossa tumors.

Seizures are the first symptom in 30% of brain tumors and are present in up to 70% of patients at some time. Brain tumors, however, account for only 5% of all patients with epilepsy. Slowly growing tumors and those in the rolandic fissure tend to be the most epileptogenic. The association between brain tumors and seizures increases with age; most seizures in children arise from developmental conditions or injuries, while up to 20% of adults with new-onset seizures harbor a brain tumor. In adults, a first seizure, particularly if focal, should be evaluated by MRI for an occult brain neoplasm. If the first MRI is normal, a follow-up study is recommended. Seizure frequency varies with histology; seizures are seen in 37% of patients with glioblastomas, 65% to 70% with low-grade astrocytomas, and 75% to 95% with oligodendrogliomas. Seizures occur in only about 18% of patients with brain metastases.

Alterations in consciousness may be evident in 20% of patients at the time of diagnosis and vary from subtle personality changes to confusion or coma. The changes are most common with frontal lobe tumors, but they are also seen with hydrocephalus, gliomatosis cerebri, or brainstem compression from incipient herniation.

Focal Symptoms and Signs

Signs of brain tumors are more related to tumor location than to histology. The *temporal* pattern, such as a steadily progressive hemiparesis or aphasia, strongly suggests a neoplasm.

Frontal lobe tumors are initially silent; with time there may be personality changes, impaired judgment, abulia, gait abnormalities, urinary incontinence, gaze preferences, or primitive reflexes. *Temporal lobe* tumors tend to cause seizures that range from simple olfactory hallucinations, feelings of fear (sometimes misdiagnosed as anxiety attacks), or complex partial seizures. Temporal field cuts or aphasia may be present. *Parietal* tumors cause cortical sensory loss, neglect, anosognosia, hemiparesis, and disturbances of visuospatial abilities. *Occipital* tumors cause visual-field changes or, less commonly, visual seizures. *Thalamic* tumors lead to contralateral sensory loss, cognitive changes, and, rarely, aphasia. *Brainstem* tumors can cause cranial nerve disturbances, hiccups, vomiting, vertigo, and hemiparesis. Hydrocephalus may accompany thalamic or brainstem tumors. *Pineal* tumors cause signs and symptoms of hydrocephalus, Parinaud syndrome, or precocious puberty. *Intraventricular* tumors usually produce hydrocephalus. Valsalva maneuvers or postural change may worsen cerebrospinal fluid (CSF) flow, leading to headaches, weakness, or syncope. There may also be symptoms of hypothalamic or autonomic dysfunction, as well as memory problems. *Cerebellar* tumors can lead to headaches and ataxia. One may also find neck stiffness, vertigo, nystagmus, hypotonia, and cranial nerve or corticospinal tract signs.

Skull base tumors commonly affect cranial nerves. Meningioma of the olfactory groove causes anosmia. Optic nerve involvement by glioma or meningioma cause unilateral visual loss. Pituitary tumor causes bitemporal hemianopia from chiasmal involvement. Extraocular abnormalities can occur with cavernous sinus or brainstem tumors. Hearing loss and, less commonly, facial weakness can be seen with acoustic neuroma. Multiple cranial nerve signs are seen with carcinomatous meningitis, which can lead to the *numb chin syndrome* from involvement of the mandibular nerve.

False localizing signs may arise from increased ICP. The most common is a sixth nerve palsy produced by compression of the abducens nerve as it passes over the petrous ridge. The nerve is particularly vulnerable because of its long course. *Ipsilateral hemiparesis* may occur as a herniating uncus compresses the contralateral cerebral peduncle against the tentorium. Hydrocephalus may lead to gait abnormalities, bitemporal hemianopsia from chiasmal compression or, rarely, endocrine deficiencies from hypothalamic compression.

Cranial nerve palsies include *third nerve palsy,* which is usually ipsilateral when there is uncal herniation, but is sometimes contralateral. The pupillomotor fibers are the most superficially located, and a dilated pupil may be the first manifestation, a sign suggesting a compressive lesion. *Fourth nerve palsies* are rare but are also attributed to the long intracranial course of the nerve. Involvement of the *eighth nerve* may cause hearing loss or vestibular signs, including vertigo or nystagmus.

Neuroophthalmologic Signs

Oculomotor problems are common with tumors of the pineal area. The *Parinaud syndrome* consists of light-near dissociation, as well as paralysis of convergence and of upgaze. It is common with pineal tumors that compress adjacent midbrain. Pineal tumors can also lead to other disorders of ocular motility, such as convergence-retraction nystagmus, ptosis, or lid retraction (*Collier sign*). In children, a setting-sun sign is characteristic, consisting of downward deviation of the eyes and lid retraction.

Papilledema is rare as the first sign of tumor, as it follows sustained ICP elevations for weeks or months; it is secondary to transmission of increased ICP along the optic nerve sheath and to blockade of axoplasmic transport. Papilledema related to increased ICP is bilateral. Unilateral papilledema is due to asymmetric swelling of the optic nerve either because of the location of the lesion or because of a congenital anomaly that prevents one of the nerves from developing edema, with the nerve becoming atrophic. On visual-field testing, characteristic findings are enlargement of the blind spot and constriction of the visual fields (Fig. 52.3). The *Foster Kennedy syndrome,* consisting of ipsilateral optic nerve atrophy and contralateral papilledema, is usually associated with orbital or skull base tumors that compress the optic nerves. Asymmetric herniation may also occlude the posterior cerebral artery, leading to *homonymous hemianopsia* or *cortical blindness.*

LABORATORY EXAMINATION

Plain Radiography

Skull x-rays are rarely obtained nowadays, but they may show calcification (oligodendroglioma, craniopharyngioma, and ependymoma), hyperostosis (meningioma), or bony erosion (pituitary tumors that erode the clinoid process). Spine radiography is rarely performed as a screening method for detecting metastatic disease or assessing the patency of a ventriculoperitoneal or ventriculothoracic shunt.

Computed Tomography

CT is widely used, better tolerated, less costly, and quicker to perform than MRI. CT is particularly useful in detecting calcification, the cranial bones, or intracerebral hemorrhage. Calcification is most common in slowly growing tumors. CT is less sensitive for small or posterior fossa tumors. Contrast administration is essential to visualize lesions hidden by an area of edema. CT is usually used to direct localization for a guided biopsy, but MRI technology for this is improving.

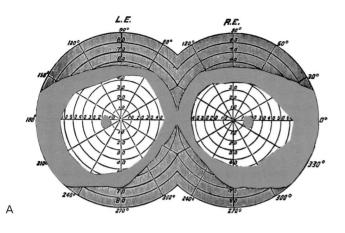

A

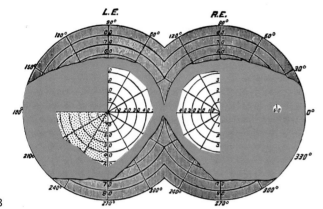

B

FIG. 52.3. Visual-field defects in intracranial tumors. **A:** Enlargement of blind spots and constriction of peripheral fields with increased ICP. **B:** Bitemporal hemianopia with pituitary adenoma. (From Merritt H, Mettler FA, Putnam TJ. *Fundamentals of clinical neurology.* New York: Blakiston Co, 1947; with permission.)

Magnetic Resonance Imaging

MRI is more sensitive than CT for delineating anatomic details and visualizing tumors in the brainstem or posterior fossa, as there is no bony artifact. MRI can detect solid and cystic components within a tumor and may show the relationship of the tumor to other intracranial structures. It allows visualization of the lesion in three planes (axial, coronal, and sagittal). Contrast administration detects defects in the blood–brain barrier (BBB) in many tumors and can be used for patients who are allergic to iodine or have renal failure. Furthermore, small lesions not seen on contrast-enhanced CT may be detected by MRI after the administration of gadolinium. Contrast studies are essential for some tumors, such as meningioma, which would otherwise not be visualized. Contrast enhancement on MRI performed within 48 hours of surgery is considered to be tumor, and not a postsurgical finding, which can be prominent and take several days to recede. MRI can be helpful in differentiating tumors from other intracerebral conditions, including brain abscess, which is characterized by a thin rim of enhancement, and cavernous angioma, which displays a characteristic target sign with a hypointense central area reflecting hemosiderin deposition. MRI of the spine has replaced myelography because it does not require a spinal tap, which may aggravate a spinal block in some metastatic cord tumors. Spine MRI with contrast can sometimes detect leptomeningeal tumor by enhancement.

Angiography

Angiography is used to define vascular anatomy before surgery (e.g., sphenoid-wing meningioma), to delineate the patency of the venous sinuses (e.g., falcine meningioma), to exclude an arteriovenous malformation in some patients with intracranial hemorrhage, and to embolize vascular tumors preoperatively to reduce the size and facilitate resection. *MR angiography* or *MR venography* may reveal prominent blood vessels or sinus obstruction caused by a tumor.

Positron-emission Tomography

Positron-emission tomography (PET) using fluorodeoxyglucose tagged with fluorine 18 (^{18}F-FDG) is used to measure tumor metabolism and to try to differentiate tumor from radiation necrosis. Rapidly growing tumors have an increased glycolysis and cause increased ^{18}F-FDG; in contrast, areas of radiation necrosis show decreased glycolytic activity. PET can also detect decreased metabolic activity as tumors respond to chemotherapy. This technique can also be used therapeutically to perform radiolabeling of drugs or antitumor antibodies.

Single-photon Emission Computed Tomography

Single-photon emission computed tomography (SPECT) involves the administration of radioactive tracers that can be taken up by tumor cells. It may be useful in differentiating low-grade from high-grade gliomas and radiation necrosis from recurrent glioma. SPECT and the facilities necessary for it are less expensive than for PET, and it is widely available. *MR spectroscopy* may differentiate tumor from radiation necrosis.

Electroencephalography

Unilateral sharp waves on the electroencephalogram (EEG) may be the first indication of a focal lesion requiring further evaluation with imaging. The EEG should not be used as a screening test. Intraoperative EEG monitoring may also be useful if both seizure ablation and tumor resection are goals. In all unresponsive patients, EEG can rule out subclinical seizures or status epilepticus.

Evoked Potentials

Brainstem auditory evoked potentials may be abnormal in up to 96% of patients with acoustic neuroma; and visual evoked responses may be abnormal in tumors affecting the anterior visual pathways. These tests are most helpful for intraoperative monitoring during surgical resection.

Cerebrospinal Fluid Analysis

CSF analysis is not routinely performed because of possible herniation. The main indications for spinal tap are to investigate the possibility of leptomeningeal tumor or to exclude an infection. Lumbar puncture is useful in primary CNS lymphoma because identification of neoplastic cells in the CSF may obviate a biopsy of the tumor. It is also recommended in patients with germ cell tumors, as the CSF tumor markers beta-human chorionic gonadotropin and alpha-fetoprotein are essential for future management. In medulloblastoma and other primitive neuroectodermal tumors, the possibly of leptomeningeal tumor must be determined before treatment.

PHENOMENA ASSOCIATED WITH BRAIN TUMORS

Blood–Brain Barrier Disruption

The concept of the BBB emerged in the 19th century. The anatomic site of this barrier is considered to be the capillary endothelial cells. Normal cerebral capillaries are nonfenestrated, closed by tight junctions, and lack pinocytic vesicles. In brain tumors, the BBB is disrupted, and the capillaries show defective tight junctions and fenestrations, increases in the pinocytic vesicles, endothelial proliferation, and wide gap junctions. Permeability is mainly determined by the characteristics of the solute; lipid-soluble, low-molecular-weight, and nonprotein-bound or nonpolar substances cross more readily. Manipulation of the BBB may be important in brain tumor therapy.

Brain Edema

Tumor-associated edema is considered *vasogenic edema,* whose underlying mechanism is increased capillary permeability secondary to focal disruption of the BBB. Edema contributes to signs and symptoms, and ultimately may lead to increased ICP. It may be difficult to determine whether clinical deterioration is due to the edema or the tumor itself, but improvement after increasing or starting corticosteroids is a rough measure of the contribution of the edema. Radiographically, edema appears as fingerlike projections into the white matter that are bright on T2-weighted MR images. Corticosteroids may reduce the permeability of the disrupted BBB, alleviating the neurologic disorders due to edema and, possibly, allowing a safer surgical resection. Response occurs within hours, and neurologic signs can be completely reversed. Dexamethasone is most commonly used. Side effects of steroids should not be underestimated, and the lowest possible dose should be used. Other agents studied for control of vasogenic edema are the nonsteroidal antiinflammatory drugs.

Increased Intracranial Pressure

Increased ICP may be an inevitable consequence of brain tumors. Several mechanisms play a role: (1) additional mass in the fixed intracranial vault, (2) peritumoral edema, (3) intratumoral hemorrhage, or (4) obstruction of CSF pathways. The increased tumor volume is initially compensated by CSF displacement, increased absorption, and, possibly, decreased CSF production. With tumor growth, compliance decreases, and ICP starts to increase exponentially. At this time, the patient is extremely vulnerable, and any increase in blood volume superimposed on a noncompliant brain will significantly alter ICP and precipitate clinical deterioration, sometimes attributed erroneously to an intratumoral hemorrhage. As ICP continues to increase, there is loss of cerebral autoregulation and perfusion, and brain herniation is the end result. Treatment includes corticosteroids, mannitol (Osmitrol), and hyperventilation. A ventricular drain or ventriculoperitoneal shunt may need to be placed unless tumor removal achieves decompression. Seizure control is important, as seizure may aggravate ICP.

Vascular Effects

Brain tumors are responsible for about 5% of all intracranial hemorrhages. Up to 15% of all brain tumors have associated bleeding, mostly subclinical. The tendency to bleed depends on histologic subtype; metastases (melanoma, choriocarcinoma, and renal cell carcinoma) tend to bleed more often than primary brain tumors, among which glioblastoma (6.3%), mixed glioma and oligodendroglioma (8.3%), and choroid plexus papilloma (16.6%) have the highest bleeding tendency. Hemorrhage is usually intraparenchymal, into the necrotic area of the tumor. Subdural hematoma and subarachnoid hemorrhage are seen with meningioma. Structural abnormalities in the brain tumor vasculature is the mechanism implicated. The onset may be apoplectic or subacute. Clues to an underlying tumor include a history of prior headaches, seizures, mental status changes, or focal signs. Another warning sign is a hemorrhage that is not in a typical location for amyloid, hypertensive, or subarachnoid hemorrhages. Up to 15.8% of pituitary tumors may be associated with intratumoral hemorrhage or hemorrhagic infarction, termed *pituitary apoplexy.* Embolic occlusion of cerebral vessels by tumor cells can lead to *hemorraghic infarction.* Less commonly, brain tumors may mimic an *ischemic infarct.* Transient ischemic attack–like or strokelike syndromes may be seen in about 3% of patients, especially those with meningioma or a skull base tumor. A possible mechanism is direct vascular occlusion, vessel thrombosis and distal embolization, or arterial steal. A postradiation arteriopathy may occur months to years after radiation.

Hematologic Problems

Thromboembolic complications may be a risk of intracranial surgery, or may be related to the presence of the tumor itself. Autopsy studies show an 8.4% incidence of pulmonary embolism and up to a 27% incidence of deep vein thrombosis (DVT) in brain tumor patients, compared to the 17% incidence found in general neurosurgery patients. Glioblastoma has the highest incidence of DVT (60%), followed by meningioma (72%) and metastases (20%). The basis for enhanced thrombogenicity is not clear, but tumors may induce a prothrombotic state through the release of thrombogenic substances. Alternatively, patients may have coagulation abnormalities. Treatment includes intravenous heparin or placement of an inferior vena cava filter. Prophylaxis against DVT is imperative in the perioperative period, and it is necessary to have a very high index of suspicion at any point during the course of the disease. Hemangioma, and less commonly, meningioma, can be associated with *polycythemia*.

DIFFERENTIAL DIAGNOSIS

Despite the appropriate clinical scenario, many other conditions can mimic intracranial tumors. These include inflammatory conditions (*sarcoidosis, multiple sclerosis*), infections (*brain abscess, toxoplasmosis, cystecercosis, syphilitic gumma*), and vascular conditions (*intraparenchymal hematoma, acute stroke*). Stroke usually has an apoplectic presentation, compared to tumors, but hemorrhage into a tumor may mimic amyloid angiopathy or a hypertensive hemorrhage. Infiltrative tumors can also appear radiographically as infarcts. Lesions from multiple sclerosis may have transient contrast enhancement if they are acute. If the only radiographic abnormality is a single, contrast-enhancing lesion, then a biopsy or surgical resection is crucial for diagnosis. In most circumstances in which a brain tumor is a strong consideration, a biopsy or surgical resection of the lesion will identify the pathology, if all other tests are nonconclusive. In other circumstances, close clinical and radiographic follow-up is imperative because, rarely, patients previously considered to have a stroke whose condition worsens with time may have an occult tumor.

SUGGESTED READINGS

Ahsan H, Neugut AI, Bruce JN. Trends in incidence of primary malignant brain tumors in the USA, 1981–1990. *Int J Epidemiol* 1995;24:1078–1085.

Archer GE, Sampson JH, Bigner DD. Viruses and oncogenes in brain tumors. *J Neurovirol* 1997;3[Suppl 1]:76–77.

Barrett JH, Parslow RC, McKinney PA, et al. Nitrate in drinking water and the incidence of gastric, esophageal, and brain cancer in Yorkshire, England. *Cancer Causes Control* 1998;9:153–159.

Bartolomei JC, Christopher S, Vives K, et al. Low-grade gliomas of chronic epilepsy: a distinct clinical and pathological entity. *J Neurooncol* 1997;34:79–84.

Bates MN. Extremely low frequency electromagnetic fields and cancer: the epidemiologic evidence. *Environ Health Perspect* 1991;95:147–156.

Bohnen NI, Kurland LT. Brain tumor and exposure to pesticides in humans: a review of the epidemiologic data. *J Neurol Sci* 1995;132:110–121.

Bongers KM, Willigers HM, Koehler PJ. Referred facial pain from lung carcinoma. *Neurology* 1992;42:1841–1842.

Broniscer A, Gajjar A, Bhargava R, et al. Brain stem involvement in children with neurofibromatosis type 1: role of magnetic resonance imaging and spectroscopy in the distinction from diffuse pontine glioma. *Neurosurgery* 1997;40:331–337.

Collier J. The false localizing signs of intracranial tumor. *Brain* 1904;27:490–508.

Counsell CE, Grant R. Incidence studies of primary and secondary intracranial tumors: a systematic review of their methodology and results. *J Neurooncol* 1998;37:241–250.

Forsyth P, Posner JB. Headaches in patients with brain tumors: a study of 111 patients. *Neurology* 1993;43:1678–1683.

Fried I. Management of low-grade gliomas: results of resections without electrocorticography. *Clin Neurosurg* 1995;42:453–463.

Gallia GL, Gordon J, Khalili K. Tumor pathogenesis of human neurotropic JC virus in the CNS. *J Neurovirol* 1998;4:175–181.

Gassel MM. False localizing signs: a review of the concept and analysis of the occurrence in 250 cases of intracranial meningioma. *Arch Neurol* 1961;4:526–554.

Giles GG. What do we know about risk factors for glioma? *Cancer Causes Control* 1997;8:3–4.

Girard N, Wang ZJ, Erbetta A, et al. Prognostic value of proton MR spectroscopy of cerebral hemisphere tumors in children. *Neuroradiology* 1998;40:121–125.

Greig NH, Ries LG, Yancik R, et al. Increasing annual incidence of primary malignant brain tumors in the elderly. *J Natl Cancer Inst* 1990;82:1621–1624.

Guenel P, Nicolau J, Imbernon E, et al. Exposure to 50-Hz electric field and incidence of leukemia, brain tumors, and other cancers among French electric utility workers. *Am J Epidemiol* 1996;144:1107–1121.

Gurney JG, Preston-Martin S, McDaniel AM, et al. Head injury as a risk factor for brain tumors in children: results from a multicenter case-control study. *Epidemiology* 1996;7:485–489.

Heesen M, Kemkes-Matthes B, Deinsberger W, et al. Coagulation alterations in patients undergoing elective craniotomy. *Surg Neurol* 1997;47:35–38.

Honing PJ, Charney EB. Children with brain tumor headaches: distinguishing features. *Am J Dis Child* 1982;136:121–124.

Isla A, Alvarez F, Gonzalez A, et al. Brain tumor and pregnancy. *Obstet Gynecol* 1997;8:19–23.

Johnson JD, Young B. Demographics of brain metastasis. *Neurosurg Clin N Am* 1996;7:337–344.

Kaplan S, Etlin S, Novikov I, Modan B. Occupational risks for the development of brain tumors. *Am J Ind Med* 1997;31:15–20.

Karlsson P, Holmberg E, Lundell M, et al. Intracranial tumors after exposure to ionizing radiation during infancy: a pooled analysis of two Swedish cohorts of 28,008 infants with skin hemangioma. *Radiat Res* 1998;15:357–364.

Knave B, Floderus B. Exposure to low-frequency electromagnetic fields—a health hazard? *Scand J Work Environ Health* 1988;14[Suppl 1]:46–48.

Koehler PJ. Use of corticosteroids in neuro-oncology. *Anticancer Drugs* 1995;6:19–33.

Krabbe K, Gideon P, Wagn P, et al. MR diffusion imaging of human intracranial tumours. *Neuroradiology* 1997;39:483–489.

Kroll RA, Neuwelt EA. Outwitting the blood–brain barrier for therapeutic purposes: osmotic opening and other means. *Neurosurgery* 1998;42:1083–1099.

Kumar PP, Good RR, Skultety M, et al. Radiation-induced neoplasms of the brain. *Cancer* 1987;59:1274–1282.

Kuratsu J, Ushio Y. Epidemiological study of primary intracranial tumours in elderly people. *J Neurol Neurosurg Psychiatry* 1997;63:116–118.

Listernick R, Louis DN, Packer RJ, Gutmann DH. Optic pathway gliomas in children with neurofibromatosis 1: consensus statement from the NF1 Optic Pathway Glioma Task Force. *Ann Neurol* 1997;41:143–149.

Lombardi D, Marsh R, de Tribolet N. Low grade glioma in intractable epilepsy: lesionectomy versus epilepsy surgery. *Arch Neurochir Suppl (Wien)* 1997;68:70–74.

Lote K, Stenwig AE, Skullerud K, Hirschberg H. Prevalence and prognostic significance of epilepsy in patients with gliomas. *Eur J Cancer* 1998;34:98–102.

Lowry JK, Snyder JJ, Lowry PW. Brain tumors in the elderly: recent trends in a Minnesota cohort study. *Arch Neurol* 1998;55:922–928.

Muir C, Waterhouse J, Mack T, Powell J, Whelan S, eds. *Cancer incidence in five continents, vol V.* IARC Scientific Publication No. 88. Lyon: International Agency for Research on Cancer.

Muroff LR, Runge VM. The use of MR contrast in neoplastic disease of the brain. *Top Magn Reson Imaging* 1995;7:137–157.

Non R, Modan B, Boice JDJ, et al. Tumors of the brain and nervous system after radiotherapy in childhood. *N Engl J Med* 1988;319:1033–1039.

Olivero WC, Dulebohn SC, Lister JR. The use of PET in evaluating patients with primary brain tumours: is it useful? *J Neurol Neurosurg Psychiatry* 1995;58:250–252.

Paraf F, Jothy S, Van Meir EG. Brain tumor-polyposis syndrome: two genetic diseases? *J Clin Oncol* 1997;15:2744–2758.

Pogoda JM, Preston-Martin S. Household pesticides and risk of pediatric brain tumors. *Environ Health Perspect* 1997;105:1214–1220.

Preston-Martin S. Epidemiology of primary CNS neoplasms. *Neurol Clin* 1996;14:273–290.

Preul MC, Leblanc R, Caramanos Z, et al. Magnetic resonance spectroscopy guided brain tumor resection: differentiation between recurrent glioma and radiation change in two diagnostically difficult cases. *Can J Neurol Sci* 1998;25:13–22.

Righini A, de Divitiis O, Prinster A, et al. Functional MRI: primary motor cortex localization in patients with brain tumors. *J Comput Assist Tomogr* 1996;20:702–708.

Rodvall Y, Ahlbom A, Spannare B, Nise G. Glioma and occupational exposure in Sweden: a case-control study. *Occup Environ Med* 1996;53:526–537.

Rudoltz MS, Regine WF, Langston JW, et al. Multiple causes of cerebrovascular events in children with tumors of the parasellar region. *J Neurooncol* 1998;37:251–261.

Sanderson WT, Talaska G, Zaebst D, et al. Pesticide prioritization for a brain cancer case-control study. *Environ Res* 1997;74:133–144.

Santarius T, Kirsch M, Rossi ML, Black PM. Molecular aspects of neurooncology. *Clin Neurol Neurosurg* 1997;9:184–195.

Schoenen J, De Leval L, Reznik M. Gliomatosis cerebri: clinical, radiological and pathological report of a case with a stroke-like onset. *Acta Neurol Belg* 1996;96:294–300.

Sedwick LA, Burde RM. Unilateral and asymmetric optic disk swelling with intracranial abnormalities. *Am J Ophthalmology* 1983;96:484–487.

Smith MA, Freidlin B, Ries LA, Simon R. Trends in reported incidence of primary malignant brain tumors in children in the United States. *J Natl Cancer Inst* 1998;90:1269–1277.

Soffer D, Pittaluga S, Feiner M, et al. Intracranial meningiomas following low-dose irradiation to the head. *J Neurosurg* 1983;59:1048–1053.

Thomas SV, Pradeep KS, Rajmohan SJ. First-ever seizures in the elderly: a seven-year follow-up study. *Seizure* 1997;6:107–110.

Villemure JG, de Tribolet N. Epilepsy in patients with central nervous system tumors. *Curr Opin Neurol* 1996;9:424–428.

Vukovich TC, Gabriel A, Schaeffer B, Veitl M, et al. Hemostasis activation in patients undergoing brain tumor surgery. *J Neurosurg* 1997;87:508–511.

Walker AE, Robins M, Weinfeld FD. Epidemiology of brain tumors: the National Survey of Intracranial Neoplasms. *Neurology* 1985;35:219–226.

Zingale A, Musumeci S, Nicoletti G, Zingale R, Albanese V. Thallium-201-SPECT and 99Tc-HM-PAO SPECT imaging to study functionally cerebral supratentorial neoplasms: the biological basis of the functional imaging interpretation. *J Neurosurg Sci* 1995;39:227–235.

Merritt's Neurology, 10th ed, edited by L.P. Rowland. Lippincott Williams & Wilkins, Philadelphia © 2000.AQ5AU: ref Muir et al ref: yr of pub?

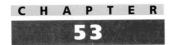

C H A P T E R 53

TUMORS OF THE SKULL AND CRANIAL NERVES

JEFFREY N. BRUCE
CASILDA M. BALMACEDA
MICHAEL R. FETELL

BENIGN TUMORS OF THE SKULL

Osteoma

Osteoma is a benign growth of mature dense cortical bone, arising from either the outer or inner table of the skull. It often arises in the paranasal sinuses but may be found in the cranial vault, mandible, or mastoid sinuses. It has been associated with Gardner syndrome, an autosomal-dominant disorder that includes colonic polyps and soft tissue fibromas.

In most cases, the tumor is asymptomatic because it is slow-growing. In the paranasal sinuses, it may cause local pain, headaches, or recurrent sinusitis. Proptosis may result from growth into the orbit, although dural erosion with cerebrospinal fluid (CSF) rhinorrhea or direct brain compression is rare (Fig. 53.1). Mucoceles may be associated with osteomas that obstruct the frontal sinuses. In the calvarium, tumors are hard but painless, localized masses without much intracranial extension.

Diagnosis is made on the characteristic radiographic appearance of a circumscribed homogeneous bone density best seen on computed tomography (CT) with bone windows. Symptomatic tumors are treated surgically, and reconstruction may be needed if the mass is extensive.

Chondroma

A chondroma is a rare, slow-growing benign tumor arising from the cartilaginous portion of bones formed by enchondral ossification. Since the bones of the cranial vault are formed by membranous ossification, chondromas are mainly limited to the skull base and paranasal sinuses. Lesions in the parasellar area or cerebellopontine angle often cause cranial nerve palsies. Radiographically, the tumors appear as lytic lesions with sharp margins and erosion of surrounding bone. Stippled calcification within the lesion helps distinguish it from a metastasis or chordoma. Treatment of symptomatic lesions is radical resection extending back to normal bone margins to prevent recurrence. Progression to a malignant chondrosarcoma is rare.

Hemangioma

Hemangioma is a benign vascular bone tumor comprising capillary or cavernous vascular channels. It is more common in the vertebral column than the cranial vault. Skull hemangioma varies from small, solitary lesions to huge lesions that receive blood from the scalp or meningeal vessels and may cause headache by periosteal involvement. Radiographically, a hemangioma creates an area of decreased density, often with a characteristic honeycomb or trabecular pattern. About 10% to 15% of lesions show the classic sunburst pattern of spicules radiating from a central point. On tangential views, the diploe is usually expanded, but the inner table is well preserved. Surgical resection is curative. Radiation therapy is sometimes recommended for incompletely resected or multiple tumors (particularly in the spine), but it is of uncertain efficacy.

Dermoid and Epidermoid Tumors

Dermoid and epidermoid tumors occur in the cranial vault, paranasal sinuses, orbit, and petrous bone. They are among the

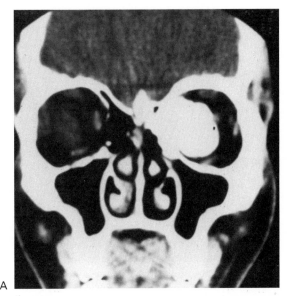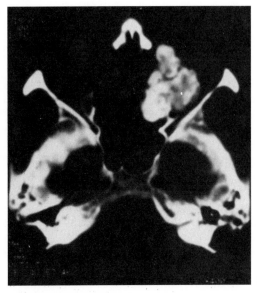

FIG. 53.1. Orbital osteoma. Coronal **(A)** and axial **(B)** CT with bone windows show an osteoma involving the orbit. The tumor, which had caused proptosis, was successfully resected.

most common benign skull lesions in children. Radiographically, they produce rounded or ovoid lytic lesions with sharp sclerotic margins that involve all three layers of bone. Treatment is rarely indicated.

Other Benign Tumors of the Skull

An *aneurysmal bone cyst* is a lytic lesion composed of large vascular spaces separated by trabeculae of connective tissue and bone. Although much more commonly found in the shaft of long bones, it can also cause painful swelling in the cranial vault. *Ossifying* and *nonossifying fibromas, osteoid osteoma,* and *osteoblastoma* are related tumors that contain varying degrees of fibrous tissue and mature bone. *Giant cell tumors* are composed of giant cells interspersed with indistinct stromal cells; they create in well demarcated areas of bony erosion. The clinical behavior of giant cell tumors varies; some are aggressive and malignant. As with most other benign tumors of the skull, these are best viewed on CT with bone windows. Magnetic resonance imaging (MRI) may help detail intracranial extension. Treatment is surgical resection.

MALIGNANT TUMORS INVOLVING THE SKULL AND SKULL BASE

Metastasis to the Skull Base

The cranial nerves exiting through the bony foramina are vulnerable to entrapment and compression by tumors that extend from osseous metastasis. This situation is most likely to be seen in patients with tumors of breast, lung, prostate, or the head and neck, or with lymphoma. Localized cranial or facial pain at the site of tumor invasion is attended by signs of cranial neuropathy. The pain is usually progressive, but the cranial neuropathy may appear during the course of a single day (Table 53.1).

Coronal- and axial-plane CT with appropriate adjustment of bone windows can visualize bony structure. MRI is becoming increasingly sensitive for small lesions. Erosion is not always seen on CT, and many metastatic tumors cannot be verified radiographically. When the clinical picture is clear and symptoms are progressive, it may be necessary to treat without radiographic documentation. Biopsy is difficult and hazardous, even with stereotactic approaches.

The most important differential diagnosis is meningeal carci-

TABLE 53.1. CLINICAL SYNDROMES ASSOCIATED WITH METASTASES TO THE BASE OF THE SKULL

Syndrome	Symptoms	Eponymic syndromes (cranial nerves affected)
Orbital	Proptosis, diplopia, facial numbness	Jacod-Rollet (orbital apex)
Parasellar	Diplopia, facial numbness	Foix (II, IV, VI), Jefferson
Petrous apex	Facial pain, diplopia	Gradenigo (V, VI)
Middle fossa or gasserian ganglion	Facial pain, trigeminal sensory loss, trigeminal neuralgia	Vernet (IX, X, XI)
Jugular foramen	Hoarseness, dysphagia, glossopharyngeal neuralgia	Collet-Sicard (IX, X, XI, XII)
Occipital condyle or hypoglossal canal	Dysarthria, hypoglossal, and accessory nerve palsies	Villaret (IX, X, XI, XII and Horner syndrome)
Mental nerve foramen	Numbness of chin with or without pain	Numb chin syndrome

nomatosis; therefore examination of CSF cytology is crucial. In meningeal carcinomatosis, pain is usually less prominent, and other sites are affected, especially spinal cord or nerve roots. Occasionally, meningeal carcinomatosis accompanies metastasis to the base of the brain.

Palliative treatment is recommended with radiotherapy dosages of at least 3,000 cGy given to the affected areas in 300-cGy fractions. Although palliation of symptoms is fairly good (86%), early treatment (within 1 month of onset of symptoms) is effective in 92% of patients; after 1 month, the figure drops to 78%.

Extension of Malignant Tumors to the Skull Base

Several malignant tumors involve the base of the skull by direct extension (Fig. 53.2). These include squamous cell carcinoma (nasal sinuses and temporal bone), adenoid cystic carcinoma (salivary glands), esthesioneuroblastoma (olfactory mucosa), and nasopharyngeal carcinoma. These tumors cause pain and involve the cranial nerves. Erosion of the skull base or the presence of a soft tissue mass may be seen on CT or MRI; biopsy is often diagnostic. Small tumors diagnosed before invasion of sensitive neural structures can sometimes be cured with wide surgical excision. Most tumors are more extensive when detected, and despite treatment with radical excision and radiation therapy, the prognosis is often poor.

Primary Malignant Tumors of the Skull

Chondrosarcoma is a malignant cartilage tumor originating in the enchondral bones of the skull base. It is most common in men during the fourth decade and often found in the parasellar

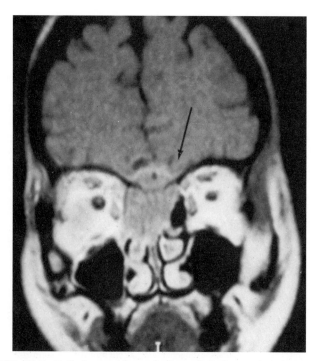

FIG. 53.2. Esthesioneuroblastoma. Coronal MR image demonstrates an esthesioneuroblastoma in the ethmoid sinus with intradural extension *(arrow)*. This tumor arises from the olfactory mucosa.

areas, cerebellopontine angle, and paranasal sinuses. Chordoma is a tumor derived from primitive notochordal tissue and tends to arise from either end of the vertebral column. Intracranial chordoma often extends from the clivus into the middle fossa or brainstem. It is a locally invasive tumor that destroys the surrounding skull base; however, it rarely metastasizes.

Osteogenic sarcoma (osteosarcoma) is the most common primary malignant bone tumor, most frequently seen in the second decade of life (Fig. 53.3). There may be an association between osteogenic sarcoma and prior radiation, Paget disease, fibrous dysplasia, or chronic osteomyelitis. This tumor has a particularly poor prognosis.

Fibrous sarcoma is a soft tissue tumor that arises from bone, periosteum, scalp, or dura. It is often accompanied by bony destruction, showing a regular but discrete lytic radiographic picture.

Treatment for all of these malignant tumors is radical surgical resection with extensive margins. Metastatic workup is routine in these patients. Surgery is often difficult for lesions at the base of the skull. Radiotherapy is usually given as adjunctive therapy, but it is of questionable value. Charged-particle irradiation, such as proton beam or helium, is particularly effective for chordoma or chondrosarcoma of the skull base.

Glomus Jugulare Tumors

Tumors of the glomus jugulare arise from chromaffin cells in the region of the jugular bulb and invade the neighboring temporal or occipital bones. They are locally invasive, although metastasis is rare. They may extend into the middle ear and posterior fossa to cause tinnitus, an audible bruit, deafness, and lower cranial neuropathies. Larger tumors may cause cerebellar and brainstem symptoms. Occasionally, they are discovered as small vascular masses protruding into the middle ear cavity. The differential diagnosis includes neurinoma, cholesteatoma, chondrosarcoma, carcinoma, metastatic tumor, and meningioma. The tumors are visualized by MRI or CT with contrast and confirmed angiographically. These tumors are highly vascular, and embolization may be palliative or used preoperatively to facilitate surgery. Surgery offers the best chance of cure or extended control of the disease. Radiation therapy may be beneficial, although responsiveness is difficult to evaluate.

NEOPLASTIC-LIKE LESIONS AFFECTING THE SKULL

Hyperostosis

Although local overgrowth of the skull bones may be secondary to intracranial tumors, such as meningioma, it may occur without any tumor. Hyperostosis of nonneoplastic etiology may involve either the outer or inner table of the skull. Outer-table involvement is insignificant, except for disfigurement from extensive growth. Hyperostosis of the inner table is rarely of sufficient size to compress intracranial contents. Hyperostosis of the inner table of the frontal bone (*hyperostosis frontalis interna*) is a common asymptomatic finding, particularly in routine radiographs of middle-aged or elderly women. Attempts have been made to associate these changes in the skull with headaches and other somatic symptoms common at the time of menopause, but

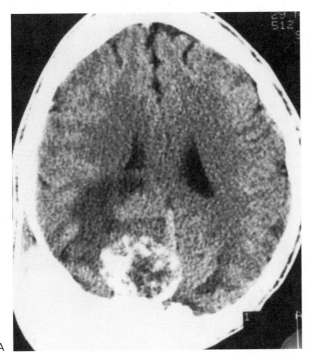
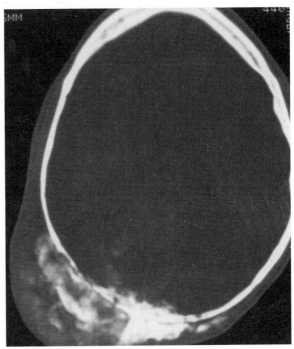

A   B

FIG. 53.3. Osteosarcoma. **A:** Noncontrast axial CT shows a calcified mass within the medial right parietooccipital lobes with massive extracranial soft tissue swelling. **B:** Corresponding bone window view shows thinning and erosive changes of calvarium with several large areas of calcification and ossification within extracranial soft tissues in the right parietooccipital region. These findings are classic for osteosarcoma, and the lesion was surgically proved.

this seems unlikely because hyperostosis is so often asymptomatic.

Fibrous Dysplasia

Fibrous dysplasia is more common in men and rarely occurs after age 40 years (Fig. 53.4). Localized involvement of the skull base and sphenoid wing, particularly by the sclerotic variety, may become symptomatic by compressing the contents of the foramina at the skull base. Nerve decompression is usually effective treatment because the process is rarely progressive. The etiology of fibrous dysplasia is unknown.

Paget Disease

Paget disease (*osteitis deformans*) is usually a multicentric disease that frequently involves the skull. Skull x-rays show a characteristic diffuse, mottled thickening of the cranial vaults and often

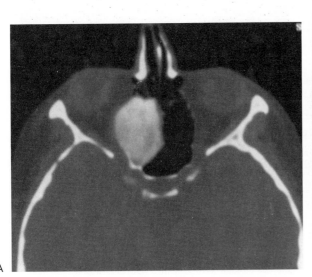
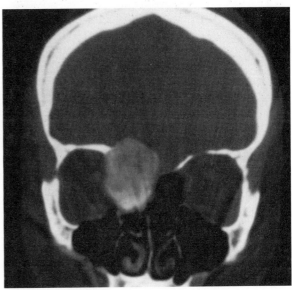

A   B

FIG. 53.4. Fibrous dysplasia. Axial **(A)** and coronal **(B)** CT with bone windows demonstrates fibrous dysplasia of the orbit and ethmoid sinus. This lesion was cured by surgical resection.

discrete lytic lesions. Pain is the most frequent symptom. Any of the neural foramina of the skull base may be compromised, but visual and hearing loss are the most common symptoms.

Mucocele

Obstruction of a nasal sinus ostium may result in an encapsulated thick fluid collection known as a mucocele (Fig. 53.5). Mucoceles may erode through the base of the skull and result in intracranial compression. Surgery with reconstruction is the treatment of choice.

Miscellaneous Diseases Involving the Skull

Systemic diseases may involve the skull. These include xanthomatosis (Hand-Schüller-Christian disease), multiple myeloma, and osteitis fibrosa cystica. The symptoms and signs of these conditions are considered in detail elsewhere.

Other disorders that simulate skull tumors include leptomeningeal cysts (growing skull fractures), sinus pericranii, metabolic diseases such as hyperparathyroidism and acromegaly, infections, sarcoidosis and histiocytosis X. Neuroectodermal dysplasia commonly involves the cranial bones, as well.

TUMORS OF THE CRANIAL NERVES

Neurinomas overwhelmingly involve sensory nerves; the eighth cranial nerve is the most common site and the fifth nerve a distant second. Among motor nerves, the seventh is most commonly affected. Ninth, tenth, and twelfth nerve neurinomas occur but are rare, except in von Recklinghausen disease. Neurinomas are generally firm, encapsulated, and circum-

scribed, well-suited for surgical resection if symptomatic. Surgical resection usually requires sacrifice of the involved nerve root.

Trigeminal Neurinoma

Trigeminal neurinomas are rare and originate along a root or ganglion or, less commonly, in a proximal division of the trigeminal nerve. Nearly all patients note numbness and pain in the trigeminal distribution. Fewer than 50% of patients note mild weakness in chewing. True trigeminal neuralgia is exceptional. Extension of the tumor into the posterior fossa is associated with seventh and eighth nerve dysfunction and cerebellar and pyramidal tract signs. About 50% of these tumors are limited to the middle fossa, while others extend into the posterior fossa. CT with bone windows may demonstrate erosion of the petrous apex, foramen ovale, or foramen rotundum (Fig. 53.6). The differential diagnosis includes meningioma, acoustic neuroma, epidermoid lesions, and primary bone tumors of the skull base. Surgical resection is highly successful in providing cure or long-term control of the tumor.

Acoustic Neuroma

Acoustic neuroma (acoustic neurinoma, acoustic neurofibroma) is a benign tumor arising from Schwann cells of the vestibular branch; it is actually a vestibular schwannoma. Acoustic neuroma accounts for 5% to 10% of all intracranial tumors and is the most common tumor of the cerebellopontine angle. It is found equally in men and women at an average age of around 50. Bilateral tumors occur in less than 5% of patients and are associated with neurofibromatosis in young patients (Fig. 53.7).

An acoustic neuroma grows off of the vestibular nerve, usually at the level of the porus acusticus, extending into both the

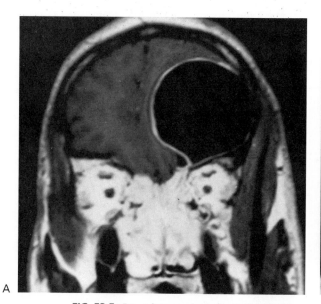

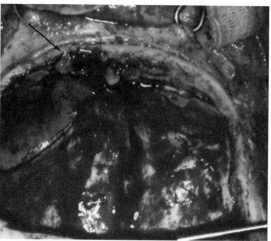

FIG. 53.5. Frontal mucocele. **A:** Coronal MRI with contrast enhancement shows a large mucocele compressing the frontal lobe, with chronic inflammation of the nasal mucosa obstructing the nasal sinuses. **B:** Intraoperative photograph shows the mucocele before its resection and subsequent reconstruction of the cranial base defect. The frontal sinus contains inflammatory tissue *(arrow)*, which had caused obstruction of the sinus.

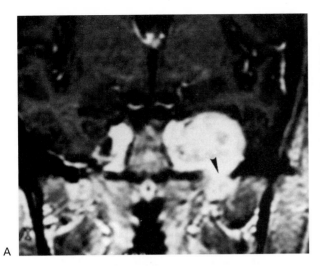
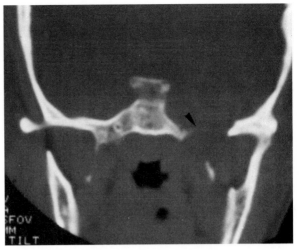

FIG. 53.6. Trigeminal neuroma. **A:** Coronal gadolinium-enhanced MRI shows a trigeminal neuroma that has extended through the foramen ovale *(arrowhead)*. **B:** Coronal CT with bone windows shows the widening of the foramen ovale by the tumor *(arrowhead)*.

internal auditory meatus and the cerebellopontine angle, where it displaces adjacent neural structures, cerebellum, pons, and cranial nerves VII and VIII. Although growth rates vary, most acoustic neuromas grow slowly at 2 to 10 mm per year; many are large and even cystic before they become symptomatic. The growth rate may increase during pregnancy.

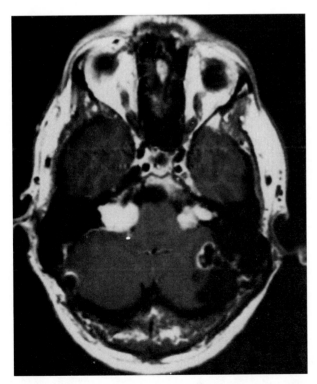

FIG. 53.7. Bilateral acoustic schwannomas. T1-weighted axial MR scan after gadolinium administration shows enhancing masses within both cerebellopontine angles and internal auditory canals, most consistent with bilateral acoustic schwannomas. (Courtesy of Dr. S. Chan, Columbia University College of Physicians and Surgeons, New York, NY.)

Macroscopically, a neuroma is usually yellowish, sometimes with areas of cystic degeneration. Microscopically, there are two main patterns: Antoni A type, with cells forming compact bands of elongated elements, often simulating a palisade effect; and Antoni B type, with a looser pattern of stellate cells with long irregular processes.

Increased clinical awareness and more sophisticated radiographic techniques, such as MRI, have allowed earlier detection, so that the clinical picture has changed in the last decade (Table 53.2). Gradually, progressive unilateral hearing loss occurs in nearly all patients. Actual hearing loss is often preceded by difficulty with speech discrimination, especially when the patient is talking on the telephone. Tinnitus (70%) and unsteady gait (70%) are common. Patients sometimes note true vertigo, but typical Meniere syndrome is rare. Further growth can cause facial numbness or, less often, facial weakness, loss of taste, and otalgia. Paroxysmal trigeminal pain is rare. Larger tumors may cause headache, nausea, vomiting, diplopia, and ataxia, or symptoms of increased intracranial pressure and hydrocephalus. Other signs include tinnitus, nystagmus, facial weakness, and decreased sensation in the trigeminal distribution with a decreased

TABLE 53.2. SYMPTOMS AND SIGNS IN 76 PATIENTS WITH SURGICALLY CONFIRMED ACOUSTIC NEUROMA

	%		%
Hearing loss	97	Decreased corneal reflex	37
Dysequilibrium	70	Nystagmus	34
Tinnitus	70	Facial hypesthesia	29
Headache	38	Abnormal eye movement	14
Facial numbness	33	Facial weakness	13
Nausea	13	Papilledema	12
Otalgia	11	Babinski sign	8
Diplopia	9		
Facial palsy	9		
Loss of taste	9		

From Harner SG, Laws ER Jr. Diagnosis of acoustic neuroma. *Neurosurgery* 1981;9:373–379; with permission.

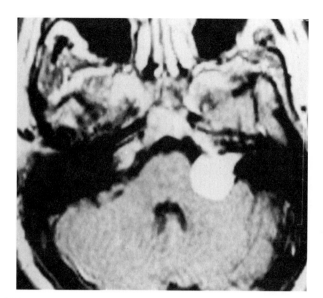

FIG. 53.8. Acoustic neuroma. T1-weighted axial MRI with gadolinium shows an acoustic neuroma with flaring of the internal auditory canal.

corneal reflex. Larger tumors may cause altered eye movements, cerebellar and pyramidal signs, and papilledema, or they may compromise the lower cranial nerves.

Gadolinium-enhanced MRI is the best way to demonstrate an acoustic neuroma (Fig. 53.8). CT with contrast demonstrates nearly all tumors greater than 1.5 cm. On rare occasions, installation of air or water-soluble dye with CT may demonstrate a tu-

mor that is only equivocal on MRI studies (Fig. 53.9). An acoustic neuroma growing in the internal auditory canal or meatus causes erosion of the superior margin of the canal or asymmetric widening of the canal, which can best be appreciated on CT with bone windows. Other radiographic signs include widening of the ipsilateral pontine cistern, deviation of the fourth ventricle, or hydrocephalus. Angiography is rarely necessary.

Brainstem auditory evoked potentials responses are abnormal in 98% of acoustic tumors. Caloric stimulation with electronystagmography is a sensitive test but is of limited usefulness because it does not discriminate between inner ear abnormalities and eighth nerve dysfunction and may be normal, even in the presence of a tumor. Nearly all patients have pure tone abnormalities on audiometry. Most commonly, there is high-frequency hearing loss with impaired speech discrimination.

The clinical picture of an acoustic neuroma can be simulated by any mass in the cerebellopontine angle, including neuromas of the fifth or other cranial nerves, meningioma, cholesteatoma, choroid plexus papilloma, glioma, cysts, and aneurysms.

Surgery using microsurgical techniques is usually curative. Facial nerve function can be preserved in more than 95% of patients with small tumors (less than 2 cm) and more than 80% of patients with medium tumors (2 to 3 cm), but in fewer with large tumors. If useful hearing was present preoperatively, hearing may be preserved in tumors smaller than 2 cm in diameter. Because of the relatively slow growth of these tumors, a subtotal resection or conservative treatment may be indicated in elderly patients with minimal symptoms. Radiosurgery may reduce or arrest the growth of acoustic neuromas, particularly in poor-risk

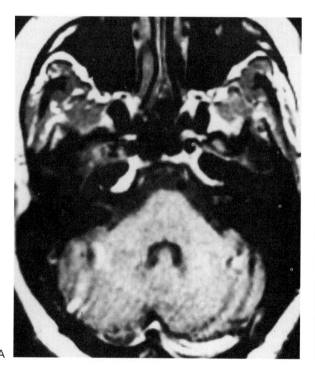
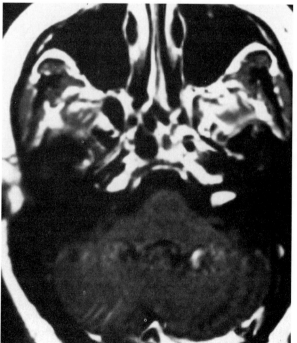

A   B

FIG. 53.9. Intracanalicular acoustic schwannoma. **A:** T1-weighted axial MR image before contrast administration shows no definite mass within the internal auditory canals. **B:** With gadolinium, there is clear-cut contrast enhancement within the left internal auditory canal, most consistent with intracanalicular acoustic schwannoma. (Courtesy of Dr. S. Chan, Columbia University College of Physicians and Surgeons, New York, NY.)

patients with tumors smaller than 3 cm in diameter. Long-term follow-up after radiosurgery has not been available, and careful microsurgical technique is currently the preferred treatment because of its low morbidity and nearly absent mortality rate.

SUGGESTED READINGS

Abramson M, Stein BM, Emerson RG, et al. Intraoperative BAER monitoring and hearing preservation in the treatment of acoustic neuromas. *Laryngoscope* 1985;95:1318–1322.

Al-Mefty O, Borba LAB. Skull base chordomas: a management challenge. *J Neurosurg* 1997;86:182–189.

Bederson JB, von Ammon K, Wichman WW, et al. Conservative treatment of patients with acoustic tumors. *Neurosurgery* 1991;28:646–651.

Calverley JR, Mohnac AM. Syndrome of the numb chin. *Arch Intern Med* 1963;112:819–821.

Castro JR, Linstadt DE, Bahary JP, et al. Experience in charged particle irradiation of tumors of the skull base: 1977–1992. *Int J Radiat Oncol Biol Phys* 1994;29:647–655.

Crossley GH, Dismukes WE. Central nervous system epidermoid cyst: a probable etiology of Mollaret's meningitis. *Am J Med* 1990;89:805–806.

Cushing H. *Tumors of the nervus acousticus and the syndrome of the cerebellopontine angle.* Philadelphia: WB Saunders, 1917.

Cushing H. *Intracranial tumors: notes upon a series of 2,000 verified cases with surgical mortality percentages pertaining thereto.* Springfield, IL: Charles C Thomas, 1932.

Dort JC, Fisch U. Facial nerve schwannomas. *Skull Base Surg* 1991;1:51–56.

Enzmann DR, O'Donohue J. Optimizing MR imaging for detecting small tumors in the cerebellopontine angle and internal auditory canal. *AJNR* 1987;8:99–106.

Glasscock ME, Hays JW, Minor LB, et al. Preservation of hearing in surgery for acoustic neuroma. *J Neurosurg* 1993;78:864–870.

Greenberg H, Deck MDF, Vikram B, et al. Metastases to the base of the skull: clinical findings in 43 cases. *Neurology* 1981;31:530–537.

Harner SG, Laws ER Jr. Clinical findings in patients with acoustic neurinoma. *Mayo Clin Proc* 1983;58:721–728.

Levinthal R, Bentson JR. Detection of small trigeminal neurinomas. *J Neurosurg* 1976;45:568–575.

Martuza RL, Ojemann RG. Bilateral acoustic neuromas: clinical aspects, pathogenesis and treatment. *Neurosurgery* 1982;10:1–12.

Massey EW, Moore J, Schold SC. Mental neuropathy from systemic cancer. *Neurology* 1981;31:1277–1281.

McCormick PC, Bello JA, Post KD. Trigeminal schwannoma: surgical series of 14 cases with review of the literature. *J Neurosurg* 1988;69:850–860.

Mikhael MA, Ciric IS, Wolff AP. MR diagnosis of acoustic neuromas. *J Comput Assist Tomogr* 1987;11:232–235.

Morita A, Ebersold MJ, Olsen KD, et al. Esthesioneuroblastoma: prognosis and management. *Neurosurgery* 1993;32:706–715.

Moskowitz N, Long DM. Acoustic neurinomas: historical review of a century of operative series. *Neurosurg Q* 1991;1:2–18.

O'Connell JX, Renard LG, Liebsch NJ, Efird JT, Munzenrider JE, Rosenberg AE. Base of skull chordoma: a correlative study of histological and clinical features of 62 cases. *Cancer* 1994;74:2261–2267.

Pereslegin IA, Ustinova VF, Podlyashok EL. Radiotherapy for eosinophilic granuloma of bone. *Int J Radiat Oncol Biol Phys* 1981;7:317–321.

Samii M, Matthies C. Management of 1000 vestibular schwannomas (acoustic neuromas): clinical presentation. *Neurosurgery* 1997;40:1–10.

Samii M, Matthies C. Management of 1000 vestibular schwannomas (acoustic neuromas): hearing function in 1000 tumor resections. *Neurosurgery* 1997;40:248–262.

Samii M, Matthies C. Management of 1000 vestibular schwannomas (acoustic neuromas): surgical management and results with emphasis on complications and how to avoid them. *Neurosurgery* 1997;40:11–23.

Sekhar LN, Janecka IP. *Surgery of cranial base tumors.* New York: Raven Press, 1993.

Storper IS, Glasscock ME 3rd, Jackson CG, Ishiyama A, Bruce JN. Management of nonacoustic cranial nerve neuroma. *Am J Otol* 1998;19:484–490.

Svien HJ, Baker HL, Rivers MH. Jugular foramen syndrome and allied syndromes. *Neurology* 1963;13:797–809.

Thomas JE, Yoss RE. The parasellar syndrome: problems in determining etiology. *Mayo Clin Proc* 1970;45:617–623.

Vikram B, Chu FCH. Radiation therapy for metastases to the base of the skull. *Radiology* 1979;130:465–468.

Merritt's Neurology, 10th ed., edited by L.P. Rowland. Lippincott Williams & Wilkins, Philadelphia © 2000.

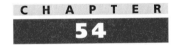

CHAPTER 54

TUMORS OF THE MENINGES

CASILDA M. BALMACEDA
MICHAEL B. SISTI
JEFFREY N. BRUCE

Meningiomas originate in the arachnoid coverings of the brain. They account for 20% of all intracranial tumors in men, and 38% of those in women, occurring in 2 per 100,000 people. These figures may be low because asymptomatic tumors are not included. Age at diagnosis is in the sixth or seventh decades. The frequency in women is twice that in men; spinal meningiomas occur 10 times more often in women. Meningiomas account for about 7% of all posterior cranial fossa tumors and 3% to 12% of cerebellopontine angle tumors. They are rare in children; in childhood there is a male predominance, and the tumors rarely have a dural attachment, are more common in the posterior fossa or at intraventricular sites, and commonly show sarcomatous changes that render surgical resection difficult. In children, meningiomas are frequently associated with neurofibromatosis. Multiple meningiomas occur in 5% to 15% of patients, especially those with neurofibromatosis. More than 90% of tumors are intracranial and 10% intraspinal.

ETIOLOGY

Some exogenous factors have been implicated in the etiology of meningiomas. Low-dose *radiation* was formerly used to treat children for tinea capitis of the scalp; 10 to 20 years later the incidence of meningiomas was four times higher in the irradiated group than in the nonirradiated group. Dental radiographs and radiation therapy for intracranial tumors have also been considered risk factors. After low-dose irradiation for nonneoplastic conditions, meningiomas may appear after an average latency of 36 years; after higher-dose irradiation for preexisting tumors, they appear as early as 5 years later (mean, 24 years; range, 5 to 40 years). Radiation-induced tumors tend to occur over the convexities, are more likely to be multiple and histologically malignant, and are more likely to recur. *Head trauma* has not been confirmed as a risk factor by epidemiologic studies.

Endogenous stimulation via *hormones* may play a role in etiology. Estrogen and progesterone have been implicated because of the higher rate for meningiomas in women, an apparent association with breast cancer, and the frequent increase in size of the tumor during pregnancy. Estrogen receptors are marginally present in meningiomas; binding occurs to a type II receptor that does not have as much affinity for estrogen as the receptor found in breast carcinomas. In contrast, the progesterone receptor is expressed in about 80% of women and 40% of men with meningiomas, and binding is seen in 50% to 100% of specimens. Binding sites for progesterone are less common in aggressive meningiomas. *In vitro* growth studies with progesterone are variable. Androgen receptor studies are still preliminary, but antiandrogens inhibit cultured meningioma growth. The relationship between the presence or absence of receptors and the effect of the ligand is not well understood, particularly because most receptors are located in the cytosol and not in the nucleus.

Viral antigens in meningiomas suggest a role in either tumor induction or maintenance, but not necessarily a causal relationship. Meningiomas are thought to arise through a multistep process involving both oncogene activation and loss of tumor suppressor genes. *Molecular genetics* has shown several alterations, most commonly loss of the long arm of chromosome 22 in 80% of all meningiomas. A tumor suppressor gene has been implicated because chromosome 22 also hosts the NF2 gene, absent in neurofibromatosis and mutated in many meningiomas. Almost all familial meningiomas occur with NF2; likewise, patients with type II neurofibromatosis (NF) are at increased risk for meningioma. The location of the c-sis protooncogene (a polypeptide homologous with platelet-derived growth factor [PDGF] receptor) on chromosome 22 strengthens the putative role of chromosome 22 in meningioma biology. Abnormalities have also been observed in other chromosomes, suggesting that there are several oncogenes or tumor suppressor genes.

BIOLOGY

With a paucity of animal models, most studies have used cell cultures. Several *growth factor* receptors expressed include those for epidermal growth factor (EGF), PDGF, insulin-like growth factors, transforming growth factor-β, and somatostatin, all of which increase meningioma cell proliferation. EGF is inhibited by interferon; clinical trials are in progress. *Angiogenesis* is of interest for potential therapy. Meningiomas contain vascular endothelial growth factor, but it seems to be confined to the stroma, not the meningioma cells themselves. PDGF and fibroblast growth factor are also angiogenic. *Proteolysis* may be involved. High levels of proteases are associated with more efficient invasion; a balance between the proteases and their inhibitors determines the infiltrative capacity.

PATHOLOGY

Meningiomas are thought to arise from the meningothelial cap cells that are normally distributed through the arachnoid trabeculations. The highest concentration of meningothelial cells are found in the arachnoid villi at dural sinuses, cranial nerve foramina, middle cranial fossa, and the cribriform plate. On *gross examination,* the tumors are nodular and compress adjacent structures. Occasionally, they are distributed in sheathlike formations (*meningioma en plaque*), especially at the sphenoid ridge. The tumors are encapsulated and attach to the dura, which provides blood supply; there may be adjacent hyperostosis. *Microscopically,* meningiomas appear histologically benign. There is no characteristic cytologic marker, and diagnosis is based on the typical features: whorls of arachnoid cells surrounding a central hyaline material that eventually calcifies to form psamomma bodies. Cells are arranged in sheaths separated by connective tissue trabeculae.

A widely used classification describes the tumors as meningotheliomatous (syncytial), fibrous, transitional, or psamommatous, but this division has little prognostic value. The World Health Organization grading system classifies tumors as *typical* or *benign, atypical,* or *malignant* on the basis of cellularity, mitosis, necrosis, and brain invasion. About 3% of "benign" meningiomas and 78% of the "atypical" tumors recur in 5 years. Median time to recurrence for benign lesions is 7.5 years and for malignant 3.5 years. *Malignant meningiomas* are rare, accounting for about 12% of such tumors. They invade both brain and dura, making surgical removal difficult. Systemic metastases occur in 24% of patients, usually to bone or lung. These tumors are not amenable to hormonal therapy. *Papillary* and *angioblastic* meningiomas are aggressive and have an increased incidence of metastases.

Hemangiopericytomas are meningothelial tumors that are derived not from meningothelial cells but from the pericytes, smooth muscle cells associated with small blood vessels. They were formerly considered angioblastic meningiomas, but ultrastructural studies revealed their distinct origin. They most often occur in the extremities, head and neck, and pelvis but may be found near the meninges. They account for up to 7% of all meningeal tumors and are highly aggressive, the incidence of recurrence varying from 26% to 80%. Survival rates of 44 to 68 months have been reported after surgery with or without postoperative radiotherapy, respectively. Up to 23% of hemangiopericytomas in the CNS metastasize, most often to bone, liver, or lung. Surgical excision is the most common therapy, and postoperative irradiation to doses greater than 55 Gy has led to a significantly improved relapse-free survival; however, recurrences are invariable despite irradiation.

CLINICAL MANIFESTATIONS

Meningiomas may be asymptomatic and found incidentally on magnetic resonance imaging (MRI). Neurologic disability is often due to tumor location rather than the histologic features. Local secondary effects include brain compression, edema, or destruction, or cerebral cortex invasion and hyperostosis. Symptoms include many years of seizures, visual problems, hemiparesis, cranial nerve dysfunction, or increased intracranial pressure.

IMAGING

Skull *x-rays* of a convexity meningioma may show calcification, hyperostosis, or enlargement of the vascular channels. On computed tomography (CT), the tumor appears isointense or slightly hyperdense, compared with the brain. The mass is smooth and sometimes lobulated, and may be calcified. Enhancement is strong and homogeneous. If calcification is dense, enhancement may not be evident. Margins are distinct, and the tumor seems to arise from the dura. Edema is common, appearing hypointense compared with the brain. Hyperostosis is seen in 25% of patients.

On *MRI,* the tumor is isointense (65%) or hypointense (35%), compared with the gray matter, on T1-weighted imaging, as well as on T2-weighted imaging. Enhancement with gadolinium is intense and homogeneous (Fig. 54.1). There may be a *dural tail* of attachment, which may also be seen in acoustic neuroma or dural metastasis. MRI shows the relationship of the tumor to the brainstem, cranial nerves, and blood vessels.

Angiography may show a relationship to blood vessels. The typical appearance is a mass with a blush. The venous phase can assess flow in the sinuses (which may be compressed or thrombosed by tumor), internal jugular vein, and the vein of Labbé. Angiography is not performed unless preoperative embolization is planned to reduce the risk of intraoperative bleeding, *MR angiography* may ultimately replace intraarterial injections.

Atypical radiographic features in about 15% of meningiomas include cysts, hemorrhage, and necrosis, which mimic gliomas. It may be difficult to distinguish intraaxial and extraaxial superficial lesions. CT or MRI may help identify the two types of intracranial lesions seen in patients with breast cancer: dural metastasis

and meningioma. Metastases are commonly associated with abundant surrounding edema and bone destruction; in contrast, hyperostosis and moderate edema suggest meningioma. Malignant meningiomas commonly show bone destruction, areas of necrosis, irregular enhancement, or projection toward the brain. Other imaging features, such as location or invasion of surrounding structures, are more likely to predict the clinical course.

TREATMENT
Surgery

Surgery can reverse most meningiomas, which are potentially curable. Factors that influence the type of surgery include location, preoperative cranial nerve deficits (for posterior fossa meningiomas), vascularity, invasion of venous sinuses, and encasement of arteries. Partial resection is an option if the patient is asymptomatic and total tumor removal may risk an unacceptable loss of function.

In convexity meningiomas, the dura is resected to decrease the chances of recurrence. If venous sinuses are totally occluded or thrombosed, the involved segment can be resected without influencing flow. Meningiomas of the medial sphenoid wing, orbit, sagittal sinus, cerebral ventricles, cerebellopontine angle, optic nerve sheath, or clivus may be difficult to remove entirely. For cavernous sinus meningiomas, the risk of injury to cranial nerves or internal carotid artery is a concern, and surgical cure may not be feasible.

Surgery can reverse most neurologic signs. Operative morbidity ranges from 1% to 14%. The extent of resection is the most important factor in determining recurrence. After complete resection, the estimated 10-year survival ranges from 43% to 77%. At 10 years, the recurrence rate for completely resected tumors is 9% and for subtotal resection 40%. New techniques include computerized virtual reality, a three-dimensional reconstruction of the brain that assists the surgeon in planning the procedure; it is an invaluable technique in establishing the rela-

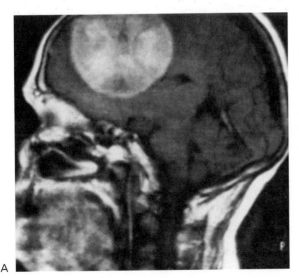
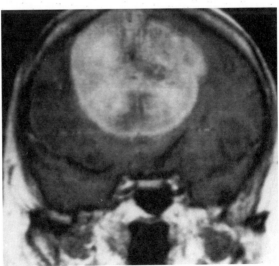

A   B

FIG. 54.1. Parasagittal falx meningioma. Sagittal **(A)** and coronal **(B)** T1-weighted contrast-enhanced MR images show an enormous tumor arising from the falx.

tionship of the tumor to brainstem, vessels, or cranial nerves. Intraoperative MRI shows real-time images during surgery.

Preoperative *embolization* is performed to decrease tumor vascularity, facilitate removal, and decrease blood loss. Embolization of the dural tail may decrease recurrences. The procedure is not routinely done either because most centers lack embolization personnel or because small lesions can be removed without much blood loss.

Radiation Therapy

Currently, accepted indications for radiation include residual tumor after surgery, particularly in a young patient; recurrent tumor; or malignant histology. Radiotherapy has rarely been used for primary therapy if the tumor is inaccessible or there is a medical contraindication to surgery. The 10-year local control rate for combined subtotal resection and radiation is 82% compared to 18% for subtotal resection alone. Time to recurrence was 125 months for irradiation and 66 months for resection without irradiation after subtotal resection. For malignant meningiomas, overall 5-year survival after surgery and radiation is 28%. The recurrence rate for malignant meningiomas is 90% after subtotal resection and 41% after resection plus radiation.

The *proton beam* delivers heavy charged particles; it may be more effective for deep therapy and may minimize damage to normal tissue in brainstem meningiomas. Because of the long survival of patients with benign meningiomas, radiation-induced secondary tumors are a concern. *Radiosurgery* involves focused radiation given in one large dose in an attempt to minimize damage to adjacent structures. Radiosurgery is done with a linear accelerator or gamma rays as sources of energy. Black and colleagues (1997) treated skull base meningiomas with radiosurgery; after 5 years, 41% of tumors had decreased in size, 54% remained stable, and 5% continued to grow. Reversible brainstem edema or permanent cranial nerve symptoms developed in 5 of 56 patients. Another approach is stereotactic radiotherapy, in which radiation is given in multiple small fractions for optic nerve tumors, cavernous sinus meningiomas, or tumors close to the brainstem in an effort to avoid the ill effects of single large doses. With this method, 71% of the patients survived for 5 years; 72% of symptomatic patients showed neurologic improvement, particularly those with cavernous sinus meningiomas. This supports the use subtotal resection plus radiation for these tumors.

Medical Treatment

Hormonal Treatment

Antiestrogen therapy has been ineffective. Mifepristone (RU-486), an antiprogesterone agent, has five times the affinity of progesterone, crosses the blood–brain barrier, and binds to androgen and antiglucocorticoid receptors. A size decrease in one-third of recurrent meningiomas with RU-486 has been reported, and the drug is now in clinical trial.

Chemotherapy

A last resort for patients with a recurrent meningioma who have undergone multiple resections and maximum irradiation is chemotherapy. Experience is limited, and no agent has been visibly effective. On the premise that meningiomas are of mesenchymal origin, agents such as ifosfamide (used for systemic sarcomas) are being studied for the treatment of malignant meningiomas.

Supportive Treatment

Because of side effects, corticosteroid therapy is avoided unless absolutely necessary. Prophylactic anticonvulsant therapy is also controversial. As with other brain tumors, thromboembolism is a hazard, warranting the use of antiembolic stockings, subcutaneous heparin, and early postoperative mobilization. Some experts advocate observation of tumors if they appear radiographically to be typical meningiomas and are small and asymptomatic, especially in patients older than 60 years. Among 57 patients with asymptomatic meningiomas, no patient experienced symptoms after being followed radiographically for an average of 32 months. The average growth rate was 0.24 cm per year.

Specific Tumor Locations

Convexity Meningiomas

Convexity meningiomas are the most amenable to surgical cure because wide dural margins can be resected (Fig. 54.2). If the tumor invades an eloquent area of the brain, complete resection may not be feasible. *Parasagittal* meningiomas tend to involve the superior sagittal sinus. If the sinus is patent, a subtotal resection may prevent occlusion and venous infarction. *Olfactory groove* meningiomas with invasion of the frontal sinuses usually require a bifrontal craniotomy. Piecemeal resection may preserve the optic nerves. *Tuberculum sellae* meningiomas usually cause visual loss, anosmia, headache, or hypopituitarism. Up to 42% of patients have visual improvement after surgery, 30% do not change, and 28% become worse. Meningiomas can occur within the sella region, originating from the diaphragma sellae. Radiographic evidence of sellar enlargement or calcification may help differentiate the tumor from a pituitary adenoma. *Optic sheath* meningiomas are difficult to resect, and surgery is reserved for patients with visual loss. Radiation may slow the growth of tumors that do not yet affect vision.

Posterior Fossa Meningiomas

Cerebellopontine angle meningiomas cause hearing loss and facial pain or numbness. Meningiomas are the second most common tumor of the posterior fossa after acoustic neuromas, and here they have a characteristic *en plaque* shape. Meningiomas recur more often than acoustic neuromas because they invade bone and cranial nerves; by the time that eight nerve dysfunction is evident, the tumor is large. CT with bone windows demonstrates the infratemporal components, and MRI shows the intracranial tumor. Abnormalities on electronystagmogram, audiogram, and brainstem auditory evoked potentials testing are less common than with acoustic neuromas. *Clivus* meningiomas grow from the dura anterior to the brainstem (Fig. 54.3). Lateral extension into the petrous bone may complicate surgery because cranial

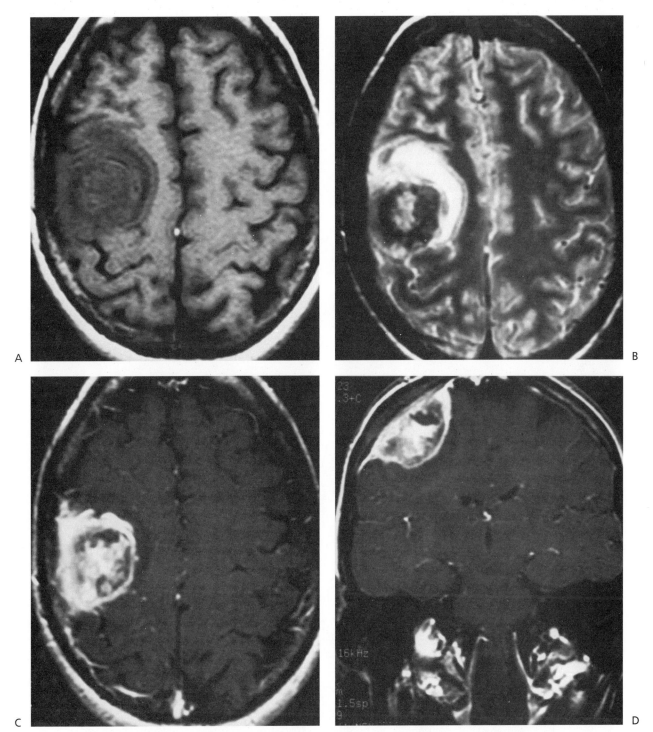

FIG. 54.2. Convexity meningioma. T1-weighted **(A)** and proton-density **(B)** axial MR images show a heterogeneous mass in the right parietal region. Surrounding edema is noted medial to the mass, and buckling of the cerebral white matter medially is also present. White matter buckling is considered a sign of extraaxial mass. T1-weighted axial **(C)** and coronal **(D)** MR images after gadolinium administration show marked enhancement within the lesion, with smaller nonenhancing areas correlating with known calcified portions. Coronal view shows dural enhancement and thickening both medially and laterally. The "dural tail" sign is most often seen with meningiomas but is occasionally seen with other tumors. (Courtesy of Dr. S. Chan, Columbia University College of Physicians and Surgeons, New York, NY.)

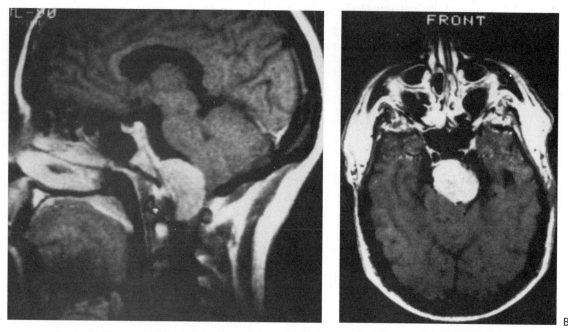

FIG. 54.3. Clivus meningioma. Contrast-enhanced sagittal **(A)** and axial **(B)** T1-weighted MR scans show a lower clivus–foramen magnum meningioma with marked compression of the medulla.

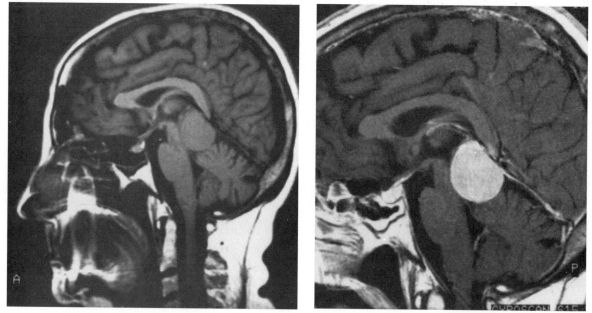

FIG. 54.4. Tentorial meningioma. **A:** T1-weighted sagittal MR image shows a large infratentorial mass that is isointense to brain and causing anterior displacement of the midbrain and inferior displacement of the superior vermis. T1-weighted sagittal **(B)** and coronal **(C)** MR scans after gadolinium administration demonstrate marked homogeneous enhancement of this mass, consistent with meningioma. The coronal view demonstrates the supratentorial component of the tumor. (Courtesy of Dr. S. Chan, Columbia University College of Physicians and Surgeons, New York, NY.)

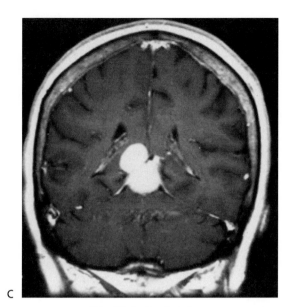

FIG. 54.4. *Continued*

nerves are affected. *Tentorial* meningiomas cause headache and cerebellar signs (Fig. 54.4). The major concern at surgery is the transverse sinus; if patent, it is not sacrificed. *Foramen magnum* meningiomas cause pain, gait difficulties, and hand muscle wasting. They are intimately entwined with the cranial nerves, making a complete resection difficult to achieve.

Cavernous Sinus Meningiomas

Therapy for cavernous sinus meningiomas presents a challenge because resection may damage the cranial nerves. In young patients with no ocular muscle palsy, some recommend subtotal resection and radiotherapy. *Intraventricular* meningiomas arise

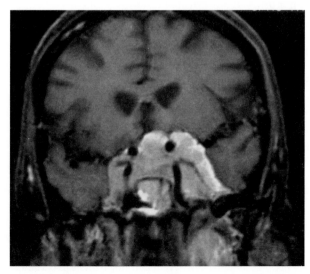

FIG. 54.5. Sphenoid ridge meningioma. Contrast-enhanced T1-weighted MR image shows an extensive sphenoid ridge meningioma with bilateral cavernous sinus invasion and encasement of both carotid arteries.

from the arachnoid cells in the choroid plexus and account for 1% of all intracranial meningiomas. Surgical approaches include cortical or transcallosal incisions. The callosal approach is contraindicated in patients with a right homonymous hemianopsia because it may cause the syndrome of alexia without agraphia. *Sphenoid wing* meningiomas include the *en plaque* meningiomas characterized by marked sphenoid hyperostosis, proptosis, visual loss, and third nerve palsy (Fig. 54.5). Surgery may include removal of the sphenoid wing itself. Some meningiomas here encase the middle cerebral artery.

Spinal Meningiomas

Spinal meningiomas account for 25% to 46% of primary spinal cord tumors. Clinical signs and symptoms include radicular pain (72%), paraparesis (76%), tendon reflex changes (77%), and sphincter dysfunction (37%). Symptoms usually antedate the diagnosis by months or years. Paraparesis or paraplegia is seen in 80% of patients at the time of diagnosis, but most patients (67%) are still walking. Pathologically, the meningothelial and psammomatous tumors are most common. Complete removal is possible for most patients, but tumors anterior to the spinal cord and those with calcification may be difficult. After surgical resection, 82% of patients show improvement, 13% are stable, and 2% become worse. Postoperative mortality is low; pia mater invasion or adhesion to the surface of the cord increases the risk. Attention is paid to the radiculomedullary artery of Adamkiewicz, which feeds the anterior spinal system, generating a risk of paraplegia.

SUGGESTED READINGS

Akeyson EW, McCutcheon IE. Management of benign and aggressive intracranial meningiomas. *Oncology* 1996;10:747–756.

Alexander MJ, DeSalles AA, Tomiyasu U. Multiple radiation-induced intracranial lesions after treatment for pituitary adenoma: case report. *J Neurosurg* 1998;88:111–115.

Berg SL, Poplack DG. Advances in the treatment of meningeal cancers. *Crit Rev Oncol Hematol* 1995;20:87–98.

Black PM. Benign brain tumors: meningiomas, pituitary tumors, and acoustic neuromas. *Neurol Clin* 1995;13:927–952.

Black PM. Hormones, radiosurgery and virtual reality: new aspects of meningioma management. *Can J Neurol Sci* 1997;24:302–306.

Bondy M, Ligon BL. Epidemiology and etiology of intracranial meningiomas: a review. *J Neurooncol* 1996;29:197–205.

Davis C. Surgical and non-surgical treatment of symptomatic intracranial meningiomas. *Br J Neurosurg* 1995;9:295–302.

De Monte F. Current management of meningiomas. *Oncology* 1995;9:83–91.

Erdincler P, Lena G, Sarioglu AC, et al. Intracranial meningiomas in children: review of 29 cases. *Surg Neurol* 1998;49:136–140.

Fahlbusch R. Hormonal dependency of cerebral meningiomas. *Acta Neurochir Suppl (Wien)* 1996;65:54–57.

Ginsberg LE. Radiology of meningiomas. *J Neurooncol* 1996;29:229–238.

Hart MJ, Lillehei KO. Management of posterior cranial fossa meningiomas. *Ann Otol Rhinol Laryngol* 1995;104:105–116.

Ing EB, Garrity JA, Cross SA, Ebersold MJ. Sarcoid masquerading as optic nerve sheath meningioma. *Mayo Clin Proc* 1997;72:38–43.

Kyritsis A. Chemotherapy for meningiomas. *J Neurooncol* 1996;29:269–272.

Langford LA. Pathology of meningiomas. *J Neurooncol* 1996;29:217–221.

Maxwell M, Shih SD, Galanopoulos T, Hedley-Whyte ET, Cosgrove GR.

Familial meningioma: analysis of expression of neurofibromatosis 2 protein Merlin. Report of two cases. *J Neurosurg* 1998;88:562–569.

McCutcheon IE. The biology of meningiomas. *J Neurooncol* 1996;29:207–216.

Nappi O, Ritter JH, Pettinato G, Wick MR. Hemangiopericytoma: histopathological pattern or clinicopathologic entity? *Semin Diagn Pathol* 1995;12:221–232.

Nozaki K, Nagata I, Oshida K, Kikuchi H. Intrasellar meningioma: case report and review of the literature. *Surg Neurol* 1997;47:447–452; discussion 452–454.

Roux FX, Nataf FM, Borne G, Devaux B, Meder JF. Intraspinal meningiomas: review of 54 cases with discussion of poor prognostic factors and modern therapeutic management. *Surg Neurol* 1996;46:458–463.

Salvati M, Cervoni L. Association of breast carcinoma and meningioma: report of nine new cases and review of the literature. *Tumori* 1996;82:491–493.

Salvati M, Cervoni L, Artico M. High-dose radiation-induced meningiomas following acute lymphoblastic leukemia in children. *Childs Nerv Syst* 1996;12:266–269.

Schrell UM, Nomikos P, Chrauzer T, et al. Jugular foramen meningioma: report of a case and review of the literature. *J Neurosurg Sci* 1997;41:283–292.

Merritt's Neurology, 10th ed., edited by L.P. Rowland. Lippincott Williams & Wilkins, Philadelphia © 2000.

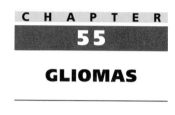

CHAPTER 55

GLIOMAS

CASILDA M. BALMACEDA
ROBERT L. FINE

EPIDEMIOLOGY

Brain tumors are the third most common cause of cancer-related death in middle-aged men, and second to stroke in all neurologic causes of death. Most brain tumors affect people in the productive years of their lives. Gliomas are the most common primary brain tumor, accounting for 60% of all cases.

PATHOLOGY

Gliomas

Derived from the neuroglia, gliomas include astrocytomas, oligodendroglioma, ependymoma, and primitive neuroectodermal tumors. *Astrocytomas* are classified by histology. Grading systems are for prognosis and for selection of patients for therapeutic trials. Several systems have been proposed. In 1949, Kernohan advocated a classification that would parallel biologic behavior. Tumors were separated into low or high grade. Grades 1 and 2 were low-grade, while grades 3 and 4 were malignant gliomas. By the 1980s, a three-tiered grading was adopted by the World Health Organization, consisting of *astrocytomas, anaplastic astrocytomas,* and *glioblastoma multiforme.*

Limitations of Histologic Classifications

Brain tumor neuropathology is no longer a static discipline, and both clinicians and neuropathologists complement each other. Tissue sampling, particularly after a biopsy, may be limited, and undergrading may result. A typical case is that of a "low-grade" astrocytoma found in an older patient. Such a scenario needs to be viewed with suspicion, as it is exceedingly unusual to find low-grade astrocytomas in patients older than 45 years. Even after a large resection, the full extent of the tumor is not delineated, as neoplastic cells infiltrate normal brain. The presence of necrosis on a specimen could be erroneously attributed to a glioblastoma, but it is crucial to consider that *radiation necrosis* could be present. *Brainstem gliomas* offer a particular challenge, as tumor location may render surgery impossible, and a tumor may be treated without a histologic diagnosis (Fig. 55.1). In other instances, the seemingly benign histologic nature of a tumor contradicts a rapid clinical deterioration.

Markers of Proliferation

Certain markers have been used to estimate the growth potential of astrocytic tumors; these include proliferating cell nuclear antigen (PCNA) and Ki-67 antigen. A labeling index (LI) can be determined by *in vitro* injection of bromodeoxyuridine, a thymidine analog, or ^{3}H-thymidine into the tumor specimens followed by monoclonal antibodies against it. Improved progression-free survival has been associated with an LI less than 4%. In the future, genetic characteristics may be determinants of tumor behavior more than of histology itself.

TUMORIGENESIS AND GENETIC CONDITIONS

Several factors are implicated in tumorigenesis: activation of *protooncogenes,* loss of *tumor suppressor genes,* and stimulation by *growth factors.* The end result is a disruption of the cell cycle. Low-grade astrocytomas contain few, if any, cytogenetic aberrations; evolution to anaplastic astrocytoma and later to glioblastoma is accompanied by more genetic mutations. The earliest alterations involve loss of 17p, 13q, and chromosome 22. Transition from a low-grade glioma to an anaplastic astrocytoma is thought to be mediated by loss of 9p. Later progression to glioblastoma is preceded by deletion of 10q and amplification of the epidermal growth factor receptor (EGFR) gene. Accordingly, deletions of 9p and 17p are seen in all grades of gliomas, suggesting that these are early events. Abnormalities in chromosome 10 were observed in no patients with low-grade astrocytomas, 23% of patients with anaplastic astrocytoma, and 61% of those with glioblastoma multiforme. Tumor progression has been as-

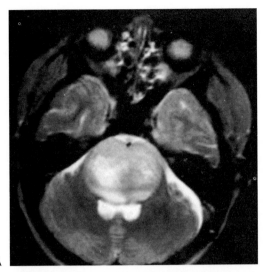

FIG. 55.1. Pontine glioma. Axial T2-weighted **(A)** and sagittal T1-weighted **(B)** MR images after gadolinium administration show massive enlargement of the pons by an intraaxial mass. There is no abnormal contrast enhancement. Pathology revealed a brainstem glioma. (Courtesy of Dr. S. Chan, Columbia University College of Physicians and Surgeons, New York, NY.) **C:** Brainstem glioma of medulla. T1-weighted MR scan in a patient with a subacutely progressing quadriparesis shows marked enlargement of the medulla *(arrow).* An exophytic component was biopsied and revealed low-grade astrocytoma.

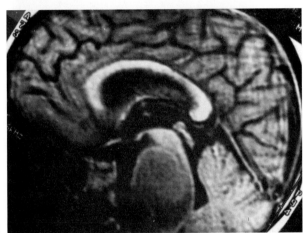

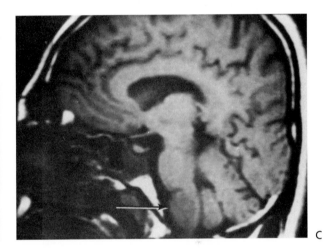

sociated with an increase in the proportion of cells showing mutant p53. Based on chromosomal aberrations in gliomas, a model of malignant progression has been proposed. The *multistep theory* stipulates that multiple events are considered necessary for tumor development.

Oncogenes

Oncogenes are a counterpart to normal cellular genes, the protooncogenes. Oncogenes promote growth by encoding growth factors, growth factor receptors, and proteins affecting cell proliferation. Tumor development is considered to be a result of overexpression of oncogenes, well recognized in central nervous system (CNS) tumors as c-erb-B1, c-myc, and ras. The most recognized oncogene product is EGFR, which is encoded by the c-erb-B1 protooncogene. Amplification of EGFR protooncogene was described in up to 50% of glioblastomas and 9% of astrocytomas. Other products are platelet-derived growth factor (PDGF) and PDGF receptor, as well as vascular endothelial growth factor (VEGF). Overactivation of one oncogene in itself may not be sufficient; multiple oncogenes may need to be activated, each one contributing to different aspects of cell growth. *Tumor suppressor genes* negatively regulate the activities of protooncogenes. Tumorgenesis results from activation of octogenes and inactivation of tumor supressor genes.

Retinoblastoma Gene

The first evidence of gene inactivation in tumor pathogenesis came from children with retinoblastoma, a childhood tumor. Retinoblastoma gene (rb) encodes a 105-kDa nuclear protein that may act as a tumor suppressor. Evidence for its role as a tumor suppressor comes from the fact that reintroduction of the normal rb gene into cultured retinoblastoma cells suppresses tumor growth. Retinoblastoma may be autosomal-dominant in inheritance, as well as sporadic. With autosomal-dominant disease, patients have bilateral retinoblastomas, osteosarcoma, or tumors of the pineal area (trilateral retinoblastoma). The disease has served as a model to explain how multiple genetic "hits" lead to tumorigenesis. About 5% of children with inherited retinoblastoma have a deletion at chromosome 13 in their normal cells; this is the first hit. Tumor development requires a second hit (a spontaneous mutation) in the other chromosome. The tumor cells then have loss of heterozygosity; that is, both alleles have lost the gene at 13q14. In the sporadic form of the disease, there are presumably two hits on the clones of retinal cells.

p53

Mutations at p53, the best characterized tumor suppressor gene, are the most common mutations in human cancers, commonly observed in colon and small cell lung carcinomas. Normal p53 gene and its gene product regulate cell proliferation by suppressing transition from cell phases G_1 to S and including apoptosis. Once the mutated p53 complexes with wild-type p53, it cannot exert its negative regulatory influence on cell growth. The gene is located at 17p13. p53 mutations are detected in 30% of gliomas (with earlier age at onset and longer survival), in 28% of glioblastomas and 36% of anaplastic astrocytomas; it is not detected in low-grade astrocytomas.

Role of Growth Factors

Many products of oncogenes resemble growth factors, and these regulate mitogenesis and gene transcription. Overexpression of a growth factor or its receptor may alter normal cellular proliferation. EGFR is found in 40% of gliomas; activation initiates cell cascades that lead to proliferation. The PDGF receptor has been localized to areas of proliferation, and it has been implicated in glioma development and transformation. *Insulin-like growth factor* is increased in human gliomas. *Angiogenic growth factors* and *transforming growth factor* are overexpressed in malignant gliomas but minimally expressed in normal brain.

FAMILIAL CONDITIONS

Although most gliomas occur sporadically, about 15% of patients have a family history of cancer, further strengthening the genetic theories of tumor development.

Li-Fraumeni Syndrome

Patients with the Li-Fraumeni syndrome have breast carcinomas (24%), bone sarcomas (13%), brain tumors (12%), and soft tissue sarcomas (12%). Affected individuals inherit a germ-line mutation of p53 that results in a 25-fold increase in the likelihood of cancer. Reintroduction of normal p53 gene into cells that lack the gene inhibits tumor growth.

Neurofibromatosis Type 1

Von Recklinghausen neurofibromatosis is associated with CNS and peripheral tumors; most common are optic nerve gliomas, seen in 15% of affected individuals. Low-grade gliomas of the hypothalamus, hemispheres, or spinal cord are less common. Peripheral neurofibromas arise from cutaneous nerves, peripheral nerves, plexus, or spinal roots. The disease is autosomal-dominant in transmission, but 50% of patients have new mutations. The NF1 gene, a tumor suppressor gene, was cloned and localized at 17q11.2 Affected individuals have one mutated gene and one normal copy. Mutation of the normal gene (a second hit) is a prerequisite for tumor development. The abnormal gene product, *neurofibromin,* cannot downregulate p21-*ras,* the product of the *ras* protooncogene, which results in unrestrained proliferation and tumor formation.

Neurofibromatosis Type 2

Neurofibromatosis type 2 is dominantly inherited, with 95% penetrance. Cranial and spinal meningiomas, bilateral vestibular schwannomas, astrocytomas, and ependymomas may develop. Meningiomas tend to be multiple, and astrocytomas favor an intraspinal location. The gene locus for this tumor suppressor gene was identified at 22q12, and individuals with neurofibromatosis type 2 have a mutation at 22q11.2. If a second event occurs at the other 22q11.2 allele, the affected cell is liberated from the tumor-suppressive capabilities and tumors result. The NF2 gene encodes *merlin* (a moesin-ezrin-radixin-like protein), which is similar to proteins that regulate signals between the cell cytoskeleton and the cell membrane.

Von Hippel-Landau Disease

Von Hippel-Landau disease may manifest with multiple hemangioblastomas along the neuraxis (cerebellum, brainstem, spinal cord) and retina, renal cysts, and renal cell carcinomas. A mutation at chromosome 3p has been described.

Familial Polyposis Syndromes

The familial polyposis syndromes associated with brain tumors may have a mutation of the tumor suppressor gene at the locus for adenomatous polyposis coli, 5q21. In Turcot syndrome, adenomatous polyposis coli is associated with neuroepithelial CNS tumors, including astrocytomas, glioblastoma, and medulloblastoma. There are two distinct genetic alterations. One involves a germ-line mutation in the adenomatous polyposis coli gene, probably a tumor suppressor gene. The other is a germ-line defect in a gene responsible for deoxyribonucleic acid (DNA) nucleotide mismatch repair. Patients with hereditary colon cancer and neurologic symptoms are suspect. Likewise, patients diagnosed with a CNS tumor and having a family history of adenomatous polyposis coli should undergo surveillance colonoscopy. *Gardner syndrome* is characterized by osteomas and soft tissue tumors. The two syndromes may occur in the same patient. Patients with familial polyposis should be examined for manifestations of Gardner syndrome. Likewise, if Gardner syndrome is suspected, brain computed tomography (CT) is recommended.

Multiple Endocrine Neoplasia

Multiple endocrine neoplasia (MEN) type 1 syndrome includes pituitary tumors, pancreas islet cell neoplasms, and parathyroid adenomas. An abnormality is described at 11q. In MEN type 2, patients have medullary thyroid carcinoma and pheochromocytoma. The abnormality maps to chromosome 10.

ASTROCYTOMAS
General

Astrocytomas constitute 25% of all brain tumors. The annual incidence of low-grade astrocytomas is about 0.9 per 100,000 population. Median age at diagnosis is 35 years, much younger than for malignant gliomas. There is a slight male predominance. The annual incidence of glioblastoma multiforme is 4.5 per 100,000 population, representing about 28% of all brain tumors in the United States; the incidence of anaplastic astrocytomas is 1.7 per 100,000, about 27% of all brain tumors. The probability that an astrocytoma is histologically malignant is 34% at ages of 3 to 34 years, and rises to 85% after age 60 years. Before age 25, 67% of astrocytomas are found in the posterior fossa; after age 25, 90% are supratentorial.

Pathology

Grossly, low-grade astrocytomas are superficial soft, gray expansions of cortex, with adjacent white matter involvement; borders are indistinct. Glioblastomas display a multiplicity of colors, textures, and consistencies. The surrounding white matter is edematous. Location is usually in the white matter, most commonly frontal (31%), temporal (32%), and frontoparietal (11%). Tumors may encompass different lobes. Spinal cord, brainstem, or cerebellar locations are rare. Ten percent of glioblastomas develop in the gray–white matter junction and may be confused with metastases.

Histopathology varies, depending on subtype. Low-grade astrocytomas show evenly distributed neoplastic cells; cytoplasm is abundant, and microcystic changes are characteristic. Mitosis is rare, and the nuclei are uniform. The infiltrated brain appears well preserved. *Protoplasmic* astrocytomas are aggressive and can transform into secondary glioblastoma. *Fibrillary* astrocytomas have a limited proliferative capacity; this category includes the pilocytic astrocytoma. *Gemistocytic* tumors have the worst prognosis. Before a tumor is determined to be "low-grade," all available tissue should be carefully examined. Foci of anaplasia have been observed in up to 50% of patients with "low-grade" astrocytomas at diagnosis. *Anaplastic* astrocytomas and glioblastoma are composed of cells with small, dark nuclei that vary in size and shape. Cytoplasm is scant, mitotic figures are present, and there is pseudopalisading (tumor cells arranged in picket-fence formation around a central area of necrosis). Endothelial hyperplasia is seen, but only glioblastomas have necrosis. There is variety of cell morphology and architecture, hence the name multiforme. Glial fibrillary acidic protein staining is seen in the cytoplasm of astrocytes and astrocytic tumors, but it is absent in highly undifferentiated tumors. *Giant cell glioblastoma* favors the temporal lobe; patients have a better prognosis. *Gliosarcomas* comprise both glial and sarcomatous elements.

Clinical Manifestations

Patients with low-grade astrocytomas may have years of seizures with nondiagnostic studies. Most typically for malignant gliomas, patients present with several months of progressive neurologic deficits; about 10% have symptoms for longer than 1 year. Memory and personality changes may be unnoticed until an ictal event leads to seeking medical attention.

Imaging

Typically, *low-grade astrocytomas* are nonenhancing lesions on magnetic resonance imaging (MRI), appearing hypointense to surrounding brain on T1-weighted imaging and usually homogeneous and well circumscribed. It may be difficult to distinguish tumor from edema, and there may be mass effect. Enhancement is faint, if present at all. *Anaplastic astrocytomas* and *glioblastoma* appear as contrast-enhancing, ring-shaped, white matter lesions on MRI and CT. Absence of enhancement should not exclude the diagnosis of a malignant astrocytoma, but once enhancement is observed, a low-grade histology should be doubted and may be due to sampling. There is surrounding edema, best appreciated on T2-weighted images, but less than with metastases. In contrast to metastases, fewer than 3% of malignant gliomas are multicentric. The central area of nonenhancement represents necrosis; enhancement reflects tumor and neovascularization. *Positron-emission tomography* shows hypermetabolic areas associated with malignant change.

Treatment

Defining Treatment Results

In the evaluation of new agents or comparison of their results to standard clinical treatments, there are three main measures: *response, time to progression,* and *survival. Response* is determined radiographically and clinically after two cycles of chemotherapy or after radiation. Measurements are taken along the largest diameter of the contrast-enhancing portions of the lesion, and then along the dimension perpendicular to it; these are then multiplied to obtain the cross-sectional area. *Complete response* means disappearance of all enhancing areas of tumor on MRI or CT, along with a stable or improving examination. *Partial response* is defined by a greater than 50% decrease in tumor size, with a stable or improving examination. A *minor response* corresponds to a 25% to 50% decrease in tumor size, *stable disease* to less than 25% change in tumor size, and *progressive disease* to tumor enlargement greater than 25%.

Specific problems in response evaluation include the following:

1. The tumor may enlarge along a third dimension that is not part of the conventional tumor measurement.
2. The dose of steroids at the time of MRI may affect the degree of enhancement, artificially altering tumor size; it is then preferable to have the patient on a stable dose of steroids when comparing studies.
3. Concurrent medications, such as anticonvulsants, affect performance and confound clinical response evaluation.
4. The standard response criteria apply to tumors that enhance, and there are no criteria for evaluating response for cystic or nonenhancing lesions.

Furthermore, response does not take into consideration changes observed in the periphery, which is known to be diffusely infiltrated by neoplastic cells. Recent studies have put into question the validity of response criteria as indicators of treatment benefit, and have found a lack of correlation between radiographic response and overall survival. Two other factors may be more clinically important: *time to progression,* defined as the time from treatment onset to radiographic progression of the tumor; and *survival,* the time from the onset of treatment to death.

From 13% to 45% of patients with gliomas return to work in the postoperative or postirradiation periods; up to 70% have a satisfactory level of functioning during an average of 8 months. Functional decompensation occurs late in the course of the disease and precedes terminal deterioration. This short window of opportunity is crucial in planning treatment.

Surgery

Surgery is controversial for low-grade astrocytomas. As imaging has become more sophisticated, tumors are being detected earlier, when the patient is neurologically intact. It is not clear whether earlier rather than delayed surgery will increase survival. Many delay surgery until there is progression. On the other hand, surgery provides tissue for histologic diagnosis, as MRI may not always predict grade. Absence of enhancement, typical of low-grade astrocytomas, is seen in up to 30% of patients with anaplastic astrocytomas and 4% of those with glioblastoma. The extent of surgery is also not agreed on. The goal is to remove as much tumor as possible without compromising function. Low-grade astrocytomas infiltrate the surrounding brain, and it is difficult to discern tissue planes; furthermore, invasion of functional cortex by tumor may limit a safe resection (Fig. 55.2).

For malignant gliomas, radical removal offers a survival advantage, compared to biopsy. *Surgery* can achieve several objectives: (1) alteration of cell kinetics, inducing entry of inactive cells into division and thus making them more susceptible to radiation and chemotherapy; (2) reduction of tumor burden and disturbance of the blood–brain barrier (BBB), potentiating the effect of chemotherapy; and (3) decreased intracranial hypertension and improvement in function. *Stereotactic biopsy* should be reserved for (1) poorly defined lesions in deep or inaccessible locations in patients who are neurologically intact and (2) patients too ill for large resections. Stereotactic biopsy has a less than 3% mortality, a less than 1% morbidity, and about a 3% incidence of hemorrhage. Open craniotomy can also benefit from image-directed stereotactic techniques.

Radiation Therapy

For low-grade astrocytomas, the benefit of adjuvant radiation is controversial. Most studies are retrospective, and they are not uniform with respect to patient selection, type of surgery, location, or radiation dosage. Although randomized trials have not been completed, there is a suggestion that radiation is effective. In 1975, Leibel and colleagues studied 147 patients with low-grade astrocytomas, excluding those who had a complete surgical resection. Radiation offered a distinct survival advantage; 5- and 10-year survivals of 46% and 35% for those who received radiation, compared to 19% and 10% for those who did not.

For anaplastic astrocytomas and glioblastomas, radiation remains the most effective treatment, as demonstrated by numerous trials. The value of postoperative radiation was most definitely shown in a cooperative trial (Walker, 1978). Median survival for patients undergoing surgery alone was 17 weeks compared with 37.5 weeks for those treated with radiation postoperatively ($p=0.001$). Radiation causes DNA breaks, and damage depends on the presence of oxygen. Brain tumors have a lower oxygen tension than the surrounding normal cortex, which helps explain their relative radioresistance. Survival correlates well with total dose of radiation; beyond 70-Gy, the benefits of treatment are outweighed by the toxic effects on the surrounding brain. Tumor growth during or immediately after irradiation or inability to decrease the steroid dose is an ominous sign. Because most recurrences are local, radiation is given to the tumor bed and 2 cm of surrounding brain, not to the whole brain (Fig. 55.3). Radiation is administered daily five times a week for 6 weeks, for a total dose of 6,000 cGy.

Chemotherapy

The introduction of the nitrosoureas has been the most important development in brain tumor chemotherapy. The 40% response rate to carmustine (BiCNU) for recurrent gliomas has not been surpassed to date. The limitations of chemotherapy stem

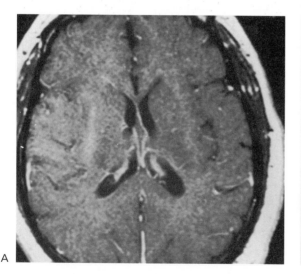
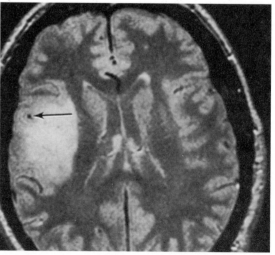

FIG. 55.2. Low-grade infiltrative astrocytoma. Contrast-enhanced T1-weighted **(A)** and T2-weighted **(B)** MR images show a right temporal low-grade infiltrative astrocytoma. There is faint contrast enhancement. The site of the stereotactic biopsy is visible *(arrow)*. The lesion is unchanged for 3 years without treatment.

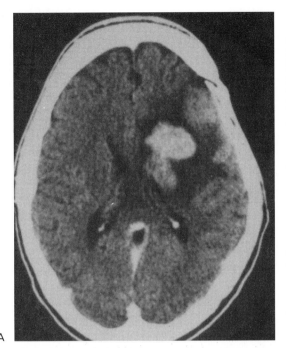
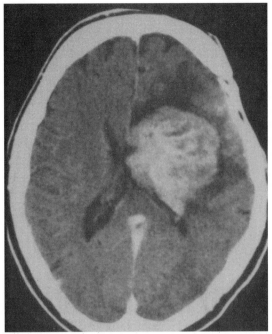

FIG. 55.3. Glioblastoma. **A,B:** Contrast-enhanced CT in a patient with an extremely rapidly recurring left frontotemporal glioblastoma shows a dramatic increase in tumor size in the intervening 8 weeks between the two scans.

from several factors, including inherent drug resistance and lack of penetration across the BBB. Some responses have been reported in low-grade astrocytomas after chemotherapy. For anaplastic astrocytomas and glioblastomas, median survival is not much improved when carmustine is given in addition to surgery and radiation (10 months), compared with survival after surgery and radiation alone (9.25 months). Further analysis showed that the only long-term survivors were in the carmustine arm. Tumor cells from patients younger than 40 years are more sensitive to carmustine than those of older patients. Carmustine is lipophilic and rapidly enters the cerebral circulation. The usual dose is 80 to 100 mg/m^2 per day for 3 days every 6 to 8 weeks, as allowed by blood cell recovery. Carmustine toxicity, particularly pulmonary, is cumulative and is seen at total doses greater than 1.2 g/m^2. Procarbazine hydrochloride (Matulane) may be used at a dose of 150 mg/m^2 per day for 28 days followed by a 28-day rest.

Novel Therapies

Exciting new areas of research for gliomas include restoration of lost tumor suppressor gene function, induced alterations in the cell cycle, inhibition of metastasis-inducing metalloproteinases, inhibition of angiogenesis, and inhibition of signal transduction pathways. The other major area of research relevant to experimental therapeutics for gliomas is the abrogation of the BBB. These are discussed below.

Novel Molecular/Biochemical Therapies

Gene Therapy. A gene encoding for a protein to which the host is deficient can be introduced via a viral vector and inhibit the expression of an abnormally expressed protein. In gliomas, gene

therapy has centered on herpes simplex–thymidine kinase (HSTK) gene. Glioma cells transfected with HSTK gene produce thymidine kinase and are targets for antiviral therapy with ganciclovir sodium (Cytovene). When exposed to ganciclovir, they accumulate phosphorylated ganciclovir, a toxic metabolite. There is a bystander effect, whereby neighboring cells not transfected also die. Clinical trials are in progress; one study reported regression in small lesions in 5 of 15 patients. p53 gene therapy is based on the finding that p53 is mutated or deleted in one-third of gliomas; tumor cells with wild-type p53 are more generally sensitive to chemotherapy and radiation. Glioma cells transfected *in vitro* with an adenovirus containing wild-type p53 undergo apoptosis or cell cycle arrest. *In vivo* experiments await the development of better viral vectors to increase transfection rates.

Alterations in Cell Cycle. Activity changes in cyclin and cyclin-dependent kinases (CDKs) can alter the cell cycle. Studies using CDK modulators such as flavopiridol, PDGF, or fibroblast growth factor are in progress. Metastasis-inhibitors include matrix metalloproteinase inhibitors, which block the effects of enzymes associated with metastasis. Antiangiogenesis therapies include antibodies to VEGF, thalidomide, and TNP-470. In the area of inhibition of signal transduction, studies have targeted protein kinase C (PKC) because of its importance for signal transduction and because of high concentrations in gliomas. PKC inhibitors such as UCN-01, tamoxifen citrate (Nolvadex), and bryostatin are in early clinical testing.

Alteration of the BBB. P-glycoprotein is partially responsible for the intact BBB, which acts like an efflux pump for natural-product drugs. High-dose tamoxifen inhibits P-glycoprotein efflux of natural-product chemotherapy drugs out of the cell. One preliminary study showed that pretreatment with tamoxifen in animals led to a threefold increase of intratumoral concentrations of paclitaxel (Taxol), an effective antiglioma agent *in vitro* (Fine, Bruce). These investigations may lead to the use of other anticancer agents typically not useful in the past because of the BBB (Fine, Balmaceda, and Bruce). New agents that by design are more lipophilic and may cross the BBB include temozolomide and topotecan hydrochloride (Hycamtin). Biodegradable polymers have attempted to bypass the BBB. These are impregnated with chemotherapy and surgically placed in the tumor bed. Chemotherapy is slowly released into the surrounding tissue. Studies with carmustine-impregnated polymers have shown a small but real survival benefit (31 weeks versus 23 weeks for patients with recurrent gliomas treated with carmustine wafers versus placebo wafers after surgery, respectively). This approach depends on passive diffusion of carmustine, usually less than 5 mm. Attempts to increase diffusion into the peritumoral region, the most common site for glioma relapse, have exciting but preliminary results. Studies by Bruce and Fine at Columbia in rodents have demonstrated cures in glioma implanted into rat brains when topotecan (a topo I inhibitor) was infused by high-flow interstitial microinfusion. Excellent drug penetration into distal areas of the brain was observed without toxicity. Brain tumors preferentially express Topo I in contrast to normal brain.

Neoadjuvant Chemotherapy.
Preirradiation chemotherapy allows new agents to be studied in their true neoadjuvant setting, prior to development of resistance. Several studies have concluded that irradiation can be safely delayed by several cycles of chemotherapy without compromising outcome in gliomas.

High-dose Chemotherapy.
Brain tumors are attractive to consider for high-dose chemotherapy. They may be sensitive to melphalan (Alkeran), thiotepa (Thioplex), or nitrosoureas, all of which have myelosuppression as their main toxicity. Drugs effective against brain tumors have dose–response relationships. Higher doses may better penetrate the BBB. Patients most likely to benefit are those with "responsive" tumors (oligodendrogliomas and primary CNS lymphoma) and minimal disease at treatment.

Novel Radiation Therapies
Short-course Radiotherapy.
This type of radiotherapy uses larger-than-conventional fractions over a shorter period of time (e.g., 37 Gy over 3 weeks instead of 60 Gy over 6 weeks). Studies suggest that for poor-prognosis patients this treatment may be a reasonable option, as it is easier to tolerate, and could offer patients more time off treatment, without compromising overall survival.

Brachytherapy.
Local implantation of radioactive seeds (iodine 125 or iridium 192) into the tumor bed allows delivery of radiation directly into the tumor while sparing the normal brain. Continuous low-dose radiation over several days allows neoplastic cells to reoxygenate and enter active cell division, making them more sensitive to treatment, especially when they are in G_2 phase. Brachytherapy requires surgical intervention, and there are limitations on size, geometry, and tumor location. Only about 20% of patients are eligible. Treatment is well tolerated, but radionecrosis requiring reoperation develops in 20% to 40% of patients. Improved survival for recurrent glioblastomas has been reported, but there is no clear advantage for anaplastic astrocytomas.

Superfractionation.
This approach consists of daily, multiple, low-dose fractions of radiation (e.g., three doses per day, total 5,000 cGy). In theory, the higher total dose will result in increased oxygenation, which lowers resistance to radiation. Furthermore, because of the increased number of fractions, the normal brain is relatively protected. Studies are not yet conclusive.

Radiation Sensitizers.
Metronidazole and misonidazole interfere with molecular repair mechanisms and sensitize hypoxic cells to the effects of radiation. Trials have failed to demonstrate an improved survival over radiation alone.

Boron Neutron Capture Therapy.
This form of therapy uses thermal neutrons generated by reactors. Neutron isotopes of boron 10 capture a neutron to become boron 11, which can dissipate energy in a localized fashion. Pathologic studies showed complete eradication of tumor in some patients.

Stereotactic Radiosurgery.
Delivery of a large single dose of radiation to a small target permits an increase in total dose at sites of greatest tumor cell density while sparing normal brain. Photon beams from both gamma-knife units and linear accelerators can be used. A national trial is studying the role of stereotactic radiosurgery (SRS) in newly diagnosed malignant gliomas. After surgery, patients are randomized to receive either SRS followed by conventional radiation and carmustine or conventional radiation and carmustine. Results are not yet available. Acute complications related to edema are transient in most patients. The best candidates are patients with small (less than 3 cm in diameter), radiographically distinct, and focally recurrent glioblastomas. Larger lesions and those adjacent to eloquent cortex must be evaluated with caution. There is a survival advantage with SRS for some patients, especially if it is appropriately used with surgery and other adjuvant therapies. Actuarial risk of reoperation can be as high as 48% and increases with larger target size.

Hyperthermia.
This technique induces apoptosis in poorly oxygenated, poorly vascularized, noncycling cells (i.e., cells resistant to radiation). The combination of hyperthermia with radiation is being explored.

Supportive Treatment

Increased intracranial pressure from edema may develop. Corticosteroids are the most effective agents for symptom relief. Side effects include truncal obesity, diabetes, psychosis, insomnia, excessive appetite, and stress fractures. Patients are usually placed on corticosteroids during radiation. The lowest possible dose is attempted. Failure to taper the steroid dose is an indication that that the tumor may be progressing. The rate of tapering depends on the duration of treatment. In the terminal stages of disease, steroids may be increased to as high as 40 to 80 mg per day as a comfort measure.

Overall Goals of Therapy

For patients with *low-grade* tumors, the benefit of treatment, compared to the neuropsychologic and cognitive impact of treatment itself, needs to be delicately balanced. For patients with *chemosensitive* tumors, treatment strategies may delay or attempt to avoid radiation altogether. If the tumor responds to chemotherapy, a smaller radiation field may minimize side effects without compromising outcome. One needs to consider potential long-term sequelae of chemotherapy (sterility, secondary malignancies) and compare them to potential toxicities of radiation and the behavior of the tumor itself. Above all, an attempt should be made to preserve a patient's *quality of life*. As gliomas usually affect middle-aged, productive individuals, supportive treatment also implies addressing the psychologic consequences of loss of control, alteration in family dynamics, and change in their roles as professionals or parents. Attention should be also provided to the *caregivers,* often forgotten players in the course of the disease.

Clinical Course

The frequency of dedifferentiation of low-grade astrocytomas is a matter of debate, but in about 50% of cases, there is a change to a more malignant form. More than 90% of recurrences occur within 2 cm of the original tumor. This observation supports the use of focal modalities of therapy, such as SRS. Conversely, a common pattern of spread is along white matter tracts, particularly the corpus callosum; and lesions distant from the original tumor site develop in 5% to 10% of patients. The observation of both the focal and infiltrative nature of tumor growth plays a key role in ultimately guiding therapy. Subependymal spread is rare but may be seen in young patients after intensive therapy. Cerebrospinal fluid (CSF) seeding develops in fewer than 2% of patients, who experience lumbosacral pain and leg weakness, and usually occurs late in the course of the disease (mean, 14.1 months after diagnosis, suggesting that most patients do not live long enough for this condition to develop). Extraneural metastases are seen in fewer than 0.5% of patients; gliosarcoma is most likely to cause such spread. Local dissemination to scalp or bone may be seen after multiple surgeries. Patients usually expire from local compression or microscopic invasion of vital areas.

Management of Recurrent Disease

Some advocate surgery at progression. If histology is "low-grade," then observation is recommended. If the histology shows anaplasia, then the patient should be treated for a more aggressive tumor. Others consider a tumor aggressive once it has progressed clinically or radiographically, and recommend treatment independent of histology at the time of recurrence. When possible, biopsy should be targeted to areas of enhancement.

Prognosis

For low-grade astrocytomas, 5-year survival is 40% to 65%; 10-year survival is about 20% to 40%. Median survival for patients with glioblastoma after surgery and radiation is 37 weeks, and less for patients older than 60 years. Over the last 20 years, the number of long-term survivors has increased without any significant change in overall survival. About 20% live more than 3 years after diagnosis. *Age* is the single most important determinant of prognosis; tumors in patients younger than 10 or older than 45 years fare worse. Tumor grade (anaplastic astrocytoma), good preoperative performance status, a complete surgical resection, and radiation greater than 6,000 cGy are prognosticators of better survival. *Histologic features* such as necrosis indicate a short survival. *Gene alterations,* such as p53 mutations or loss of heterozygosity on chromosomes 10 and 17, have been correlated with progression from astrocytoma to glioblastoma.

Astrocytic Variants

Pilocytic astrocytomas are the most common astrocytic variant. Peak incidence is in the second decade. The term is synonymous for what was called "juvenile pilocytic astrocytoma." The typical location is midline: cerebellum, third ventricle, or brainstem. Compared to diffusely infiltrating astrocytomas, pilocytic variants tend to be circumscribed and have a better prognosis. Microscopically, one sees bipolar cells with thin, hairlike processes, hence the term *pilocytic.* Macroscopically, they appear well circumscribed and have a cystic structure associated with a mural nodule. Histologic malignancy is rare. Behavior is indolent, and surgery offers the best outcome. Ten-year survival is 70%.

Pleomorphic xanthoastrocytomas are rare and occur in young adults. In up to 78% of cases, it is associated with seizures. Leptomeningeal infiltration is common, but the dura is spared. MRI shows a superficially located, cystic lesion with a mural nodule. Histologically, there is cellular pleomorphism; mitosis are rare. There are abundant lipid accumulations, hence the term *xantho* (yellow in Greek). Xanthoastrocytomas have a stronger potential for aggressive behavior than other circumscribed astrocytomas.

Subependymal giant cell astrocytoma occurs in the first two decades of life. The tumor is well demarcated, and calcifications are common. Favorite locations are the lateral ventricles and caudate nucleus. Five percent of patients with tuberous sclerosis have a subependymal giant cell astrocytoma arising in the foramen of Monro during adolescence. The tumors are slow-growing; surgical resection offers the best long-term outcome. Some advocate periodic MRI for patients with tuberous sclerosis. With surgery, 10-year survival is 80%.

Desmoplastic astrocytomas of infancy is seen exclusively in infants. Tumors are very large and superficially located in the frontal lobe, and tend to thin the overlying calvarium. Prognosis after surgery is good despite the large size and histologic pleomorphism.

Gliofibromas occur through the neuraxis. Median age at diagnosis is 7 years. Histologically, one finds neoplastic astrocytes and a second population of cells, possibly fibroblasts. Only 14 cases have been reported. The tumors can progress.

Unusual Growth Patterns

Gliomatosis cerebri is characterized by diffuse infiltration of neoplastic astrocytes throughout a large portion of a hemisphere Histologically, the tumor resembles a diffuse astrocytoma, but anaplastic foci may be found. T2-weighted MRI shows extensive areas of hyperintensity (Figs. 55.4 and 55.5). Contrast enhancement is usually absent, but it may be seen at a later stage of the disease. Clinical course varies from slowly to rapidly progressive.

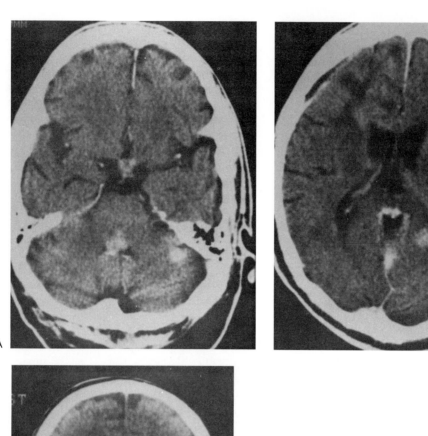

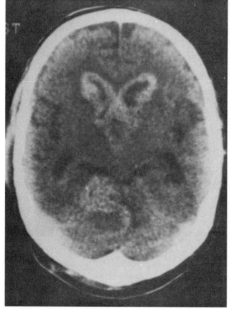

FIG. 55.4. Glioblastoma, ependymal and meningeal seeding (leptomeningeal gliomatosis). **A:** Axial contrast-enhanced CT demonstrates abnormal enhancement in the suprasellar cistern along the left tentorium and subependymal region of the fourth ventricle owing to CSF seeding of tumor. **B:** Higher scan section from the same examination demonstrates persistent abnormal enhancement and mild mass effect at the primary site (right frontal), where a chronic postoperative extraaxial collection is also seen. Abnormal enhancement in the periatrial regions, especially on the left, indicates further subependymal seeding. **C:** In another patient with a cerebellar glioblastoma, contrast enhancement outlining the frontal horns and the right tentorium indicates leptomeningeal gliomatosis.

Radiotherapy appears to stabilize or improve neurologic function in some patients.

Leptomeningeal gliomatosis can be seen in up to 25% of patients at autopsy; higher rates are seen in children. Symptoms include radiculopathy, myelopathy, or cranial nerve findings. CSF protein may be elevated.

OLIGODENDROGLIAL TUMORS

General

Oligodendrogliomas stand apart from other CNS malignancies. First, they are more indolent in behavior. Furthermore, they are exquisitely chemosensitive in contrast to other glial neoplasms.

This recognition may allow neurooncologists to develop treatment strategies that may eventually be applicable to other types of brain tumors.

Epidemiology

Oligodendrogliomas account for about 5% of all primary brain tumors and 30% of intracranial gliomas. Median age at diagnosis is 50 years; some studies suggest a male predominance. The tumors are exceedingly rare in children.

Clinical Manifestations

Because oligodendrogliomas are commonly cortical or subcortical, seizures are the initial presentation in up to 75% of patients.

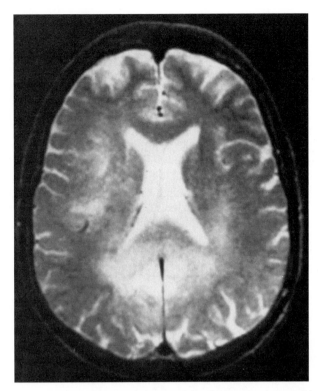

FIG. 55.5. Gliomatosis cerebri. T2-weighted MR scan shows widespread areas of increased signal in both cerebral hemispheres. Stereotactic biopsy revealed anaplastic astrocytoma.

Seizures are usually present for a median of 15 months but may be present for years (rarely, up to 10 to 20 years) before tumor diagnosis. The frontal lobe is the most common location, followed by the temporal and parietal lobes. About 25% of tumors cross the midline to the opposite hemisphere; posterior fossa or spinal cord location is unusual. Leptomeningeal dissemination is rare at presentation. On examination, tumors are remarkably silent despite their large size. This may be due to their slow-growing, infiltrative nature.

Pathology

Grossly, one observes calcification, cystic degeneration, necrosis, or hemorrhage. Tumor arises from a subcortical location and infiltrates the cortex. *Histologically,* tumor cells are homogeneous and have a characteristic "fried egg" appearance, showing a clear perinuclear halo surrounding a dense central nucleus as a result of a fixation artifact. This typical appearance is less common in anaplastic oligodendrogliomas. The neoplastic cells may be distributed into lobules separated by branching vessels, forming a "chicken wire" pattern. Microcyst formation from mucinous accumulation is common.

Histologically, oligodendrogliomas are tumors without anaplastic features. *Anaplastic* oligodendrogliomas have features of anaplasia: mitosis, endothelial proliferation, mitotic activity, and necrosis. Necrosis should not cause confusion with glioblastoma multiforme. *Mixed oligoastrocytomas* are composed of both oligodendroglial cells and astrocytes, which are believed to arise from a common precursor, the oligodendrocyte-type 2 astrocyte.

The exact proportion of astrocytic cells required to classify a tumor as mixed is a matter of debate; some require the minor component to be least 30% of the overall cell population. An astrocytic component has been associated with a worse prognosis. Growth may vary from that of a solid tumor that destroys the parenchyma to isolated tumor cells that infiltrate normal brain. The parenchyma-destructive pattern is more commonly associated with contrast enhancement, neurologic deficits, and more aggressive behavior.

There is no specific marker for oligodendroglial differentiation. The limitations of current histopathologic measures become apparent in the assessment of "progressive" oligodendrogliomas. By definition, these tumors lead to worsening symptoms and sometimes death. Despite their aggressive behavior, a second operation may reveal low-grade pathologic features identical to those of the original tumor. Researchers are turning to molecular genetics to explain and predict behavior. Allelic loss at chromosomes 1p and 19q have been implicated in oligodendroglioma development, and it has been postulated that 19q may contain a tumor suppressor gene. Anaplastic oligodendrogliomas may have further allelic losses on 9p and 10. Genetic changes in some oligodendrogliomas are being studied as markers of chemosensitivity.

Imaging

Certain features are suggestive of, but not specific for, oligodendrogliomas. On CT, the tumor is hypodense, well demarcated, and occasionally cystic. Calcification is common; intratumoral hemorrhage may be seen. On T1-weighted MR images, the tumor is hypo- to isointense and appears to infiltrate adjacent brain with no surrounding edema. With contrast, most "low-grade" oligodendrogliomas do not enhance; those that do are usually anaplastic oligodendrogliomas or "low-grade" oligodendrogliomas that have progressed.

Treatment

As oligodendrogliomas vary greatly in their behavior, treatment must be tailored to the specifics of the patient's tumor. For a patient with a "low-grade" oligodendroglioma and controlled symptoms, the best approach may be observation. A patient with a similar histology at diagnosis whose tumor has shown growth should be treated, usually with surgery, radiation, and/or chemotherapy. Newly diagnosed anaplastic oligodendrogliomas should receive therapy after surgery. Most authors recommend prophylactic use of anticonvulsants. This stands in contrast to practice in the treatment of other types of brain tumors, where use of anticonvulsants is debatable. Tumor resection and radiotherapy may facilitate seizure control.

Surgery

The extent of surgery varies with location, signs, symptoms, and proximity to eloquent areas. Biopsy is preferable for infiltrative lesions in an eloquent area that cause no mass effect, or for patients who have a normal examination. Resection is indicated if there is mass effect, the patient has progressive symptoms, and the tumor is not close to critical areas. Surgery with electroencephalograph monitoring may serve for both tissue diagnosis and seizure control.

Radiation Therapy

At most institutions, radiation is given to patients with anaplastic oligodendrogliomas at diagnosis, independent of the extent of surgery, or to patients with low-grade oligodendrogliomas at diagnosis whose tumors have mass effect or progress. The role of radiation in the treatment of low-grade, nonprogressive oligodendrogliomas is controversial. Infiltrative tumors may involve several lobes concurrently, and patients with such lesions, although seemingly normal, may have significant neuropsychologic deficits. Conversely, the main concern with administering radiation is the possible deterioration of neuropsychologic function when large areas of the brain are irradiated. Good local control is usually obtained with 60 Gy.

Chemotherapy

The realization that oligodendrogliomas are extremely chemosensitive has spurred new interest in the treatment of these tumors. As focal therapy becomes more effective, late relapses may involve the leptomeninges or distant organs, making the role of chemotherapy much more vital. In 1988, Cairncross and Macdonald found that oligodendrogliomas, unlike other glial tumors, had excellent response rates (75% to 100%) to the combination of procarbazine, CCNU, and vincristine (PCV). At recurrence, 100% of PCV-naive patients may respond to PCV (Fig. 55.6). Many institutions administer chemotherapy, in addition to radiation, to anaplastic oligodendrogliomas at diagnosis or to tumors for which radiation has failed. Response may be better for contrast-enhancing than for nonenhancing masses. There are many unanswered questions:

1. The benefit of chemotherapy for newly diagnosed low-grade oligodendrogliomas is not clear. One study showed responses

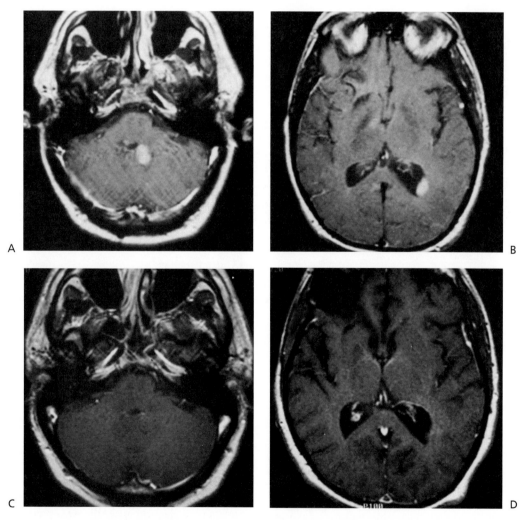

FIG. 55.6. Disseminated oligodendroglioma. Contrast-enhanced MRI in a patient with recurrent anaplastic oligodendroglioma shows ependymal seeding of the left lateral **(A)** and fourth **(B)** ventricles. **C,D:** In the same patient 4 months later, there is complete response of both intraventricular lesions after two cycles of PCV chemotherapy.

to PCV in seven of seven patients; the responses were sustained without radiotherapy for a median of 35 months.

2. The role of PCV as adjuvant treatment for newly diagnosed anaplastic oligodendrogliomas, in addition to radiation, is not known; and this is the basis for an ongoing multicenter trial.

3. It is uncertain whether mixed oligoastrocytomas are as sensitive to PCV as pure oligodendrogliomas. The difference may be due to the genetic constitution of the tumor; that is, some tumors may be more of an "oligodendroglioma" genotype with genetic losses at 1p and 19q, while other, less chemosensitive tumors may have more "astrocytic" features, such as p53 mutation.

4. It is not known whether PCV given as sole treatment can avoid radiation therapy. The PCV regimen is not curative, and the tumor recurs in all patients. Furthermore, PCV may cause prolonged myelosuppression, which may limit the use of chemotherapy in the future.

The biochemical basis for this exquisite *chemosensitivity* is unknown. The tumors are sensitive to carmustine and procarbazine hydrochloride (Matulane), both of which alkylate DNA at O6-guanine. Repair is mediated by the DNA-repair enzyme O6-methylguanine methyl transferase (MGMT). Sensitivity appears dependent on the level of MGMT in tumor cells. MGMT-positive cells become resistant to nitrosoureas, whereas depleted cells are sensitive. Low levels of MGMT have been found in both rat oligodendrocytes and PCV-responsive human oligodendrogliomas.

Prognosis

The limitations of standard measures as prognosticators of tumor behavior are well known. Age, extent of resection, performance status, and labeling indexes have been statistically associated with survival. Median survival for low-grade oligodendrogliomas after subtotal resection alone is reported at 2 years, and that after complete resection and radiotherapy at 7.9 years. Shaw (1995) reported a median survival and 5- and 10-year survival rates of 4.3 years, 45%, and 23% for anaplastic oligoastrocytomas versus 4.6 years, 46%, and 26% for anaplastic oligodendrogliomas, respectively. Disease recurrence beyond 5 years is common, so patients need frequent monitoring. The excellent survival for some patients with low-grade oligodendrogliomas without radiation or chemotherapy obliges clinicians to put in perspective any treatment strategy designed for this subgroup of patients.

EPENDYMAL TUMORS

These tumors arise from ependymal cells that line the ventricles or the central canal of the spinal cord. The median age at diagnosis is between 3 and 5 years of age. Radiographically, they often enhance with gadolinium and sometimes extend through the foramen magnum. Symptoms are related to location; for example, tumors in the fourth ventricle may cause hydrocephalus and those in the area postrema may cause vomiting. There is no

agreement with respect to grading. Variants include a *well differentiated ependymoma* and a more aggressive *malignant ependymoma*. In the past, the *ependymoblastoma* was classified as a malignant ependymoma but is now classified as a primitive neuroectodermal tumor (PNET).

The mainstay of treatment is surgery. If the tumor has leptomeningeal dissemination at diagnosis, surgery is palliative. Extent of resection is one of the most important predictors of outcome. Focal radiation is standard treatment after surgery, although some are studying whether radiation can be eliminated for patients with a complete resection. Chemotherapy is being investigated; responses have been seen to platinum agents. Most recurrences are focal. Two types have a better prognosis: *myxopapillary ependymoma,* arising from the filum terminale; and *subependymomas,* originating in the walls of the fourth or lateral ventricles. Histologically, subependymomas have features of both astrocytic and ependymal differentiation.

NEURONAL TUMORS AND MIXED NEURONAL-GLIAL TUMORS

Ganglioglioma

The most common mixed neuronal-glial tumor, gangliogliomas are usually slow-growing lesions in children and young adults; the most common location is the temporal lobe. Presentation is usually a progressive seizure disorder. Histologically, one finds both astrocytic and neuronal components; the glial component is usually astrocytic, and anaplastic degeneration is usually found in this component of the tumor. Surgery is the preferred treatment. Results of radiotherapy are not conclusive. Long-term survival after gross surgical resection is excellent. Malignant transformation is rare.

Desmoplastic Infantile Ganglioglioma

These tumors are rare and occur mostly in infancy. Patients experience seizures or show an increase in head circumference. Tumors are large, cystic, and located in the frontal and parietal lobes; they also have a cortical component that enhances intensely on MRI. There is moderate edema. Prognosis is excellent after surgery.

Gangliocytoma

Gangliocytomas are slow-growing and well-circumscribed. A variant is the *dysplastic gangliocytoma of the cerebellum* (Lhermitte-Duclos disease). The age at diagnosis is in the third decade. Most patients show signs of increased intracranial pressure or cerebellar dysfunction. Histologically, there is disruption of normal architecture, and it is often difficult to determine tissue planes. Prognosis is good if the tumor can be resected.

Ganglioglioneurocytomas

These tumors consist of small mature neoplastic neurons (neurocytes), large mature neoplastic neurons (gangliocytes), and astrocytes. In all of these, small cells are surrounded by clear cytoplasm and may be mistaken for oligodendrogliomas. Immuno-histochemistry and electron microscopy show that these two tumors are separate entities. Electron microscopy confirms the neuronal origin of ganglioglioneurocytomas, showing cells with neuronal processes, neurosecretory vesicles, and microtubular cytoskeletons. All subtypes have an indolent behavior, but recurrences can occur, especially with the white matter variants. Treatment is surgery.

Neurocytomas

Composed of mature neurons, neurocytomas are typically located within the ventricles (Fig. 55.7). Central neurocytomas are located outside the ventricles and are usually found in young adults. Tumors are well demarcated and may calcify. Histologically, there is a homogenous arrangement of uniform cells in a fibrillary matrix analogous to that of oligodendrogliomas. Prognosis is favorable after surgery. Actuarial 5-year survival is 81%. There may be malignant variants. The role of radiotherapy remains controversial and may be considered in cases of subtotal excision. Chemotherapy may be of benefit in recurrent tumors.

Dysembryogenic Neuroepithelial Tumors

These rare tumors usually develop in children or young adults with a long history of seizures. They arise from a cortical location in the temporal lobe and only rarely require therapy other than surgical resection.

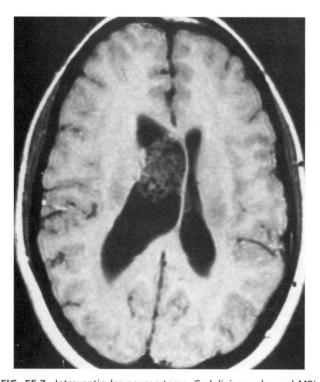

FIG. 55.7. Intraventicular neurocytoma. Gadolinium-enhanced MRI scan of 24-year-old woman with a 1-year history of headaches owing to a right lateral ventricular neurocytoma producing obstruction of the foramen of Monro. The tumor was completely resected.

Primitive Neuroectodermal Tumor

PNET is a term used to designate tumors derived from primitive progenitor cells. These are aggressive neoplasms, usually occurring in children. Common histologic features are a high mitotic rate, high cellularity, and a tendency for leptomeningeal dissemination. Radiographically, PNETs appear aggressive and infiltrate the adjacent brain; contrast enhancement is common. *Medulloblastomas* are the most common type. Most are located in the cerebellar vermis but may also be observed in the hemispheres, particularly in adults. Leptomeningeal involvement is common. Treatment is usually a combination of surgery, craniospinal radiation, and chemotherapy. *Neuroblastomas* are rare, occur in children, and favor the frontoparietal lobes. They are large and cystic, and appear separate from adjacent brain. *Olfactory neuroblastoma (esthesioneuroblastoma)* is thought to arise from the olfactory neuroepithelial cells in the nasal cavity. Patients experience epistaxis or nasal obstruction. Surgery alone is the treatment for low-grade tumors, but higher grade requires multimodality treatment. High-grade lesions can benefit from cisplatin-based chemotherapy, but prognosis is dismal even with radiation, surgery, and chemotherapy. Long-term follow-up is mandatory.

SUGGESTED READINGS

General

Azizi SA, Miyamoto C. Principles of treatment of malignant gliomas in adults: an overview. *J Neurovirol* 1998;4:204–216.

Barker FG II, Chang SM, Huhn SL, et al. Age and the risk of anaplasia in magnetic resonance-nonenhancing supratentorial cerebral tumors. *Cancer* 1997;80:936–941.

Forsyth PA, Cairncross JG. Treatment of malignant glioma in adults. *Curr Opin Neurol* 1995;8:414–418.

Frankel SA, German WI. Glioblastoma multiforme: review of 219 cases with regard to natural history, pathology, diagnostic methods and treatment. *J Neurosurg* 1958;15:489–503.

Greig NH, Ries LG, Yancik R, Rapoport SI. Increasing annual incidence of primary malignant brain tumors in the elderly. *J Natl Cancer Inst* 1990;82:1621–1624.

Kaplan RS. Complexities, pitfalls and strategies for evaluating brain tumor therapies. *Curr Opin Oncol* 1998;10:175–178.

Moots PL. Pitfalls in the management of patients with malignant gliomas. *Semin Neurol* 1998;18:257–265.

Pollak L, Gur R, Walach N, et al. Clinical determinants of long-term survival in patients with glioblastoma multiforme. *Tumori* 1997;83:613–617.

Preston-Martin S. Epidemiology of primary CNS neoplasms. *Neurol Clin* 1996;14:273–290.

Pathology

Bishop M, de la Monte SM. Dual lineage of astrocytomas. *Am J Pathol* 1989;135:517–527.

Liberski PP, Kordek R. Ultrastructural pathology of glial brain tumors revisited: a review. *Ultrastruct Pathol* 1997;21:1–31.

Rees JH, Smirniotopoulos JG, Jones RV, Wong K. Glioblastoma multiforme: radiologic-pathologic correlation. *Radiographics* 1996;16:1413–1438.

Ringertz N. Grading of gliomas. *Acta Pathol Microbiol* 1950;27:51–64.

Surgery

Laws ER Jr. Radical resection for the treatment of glioma. *Clin Neurosurg* 1995;42:480–487.

Ojemann JG, Miller JW, Silbergeld DL. Preserved function in brain invaded by tumor. *Neurosurgery* 1996;39:253–258.

Winger MJ, Macdonald DR, Cairncross JG. Supratentorial anaplastic glioma in adults: the prognostic importance of extent of resection and prior low-grade glioma. *J Neurosurg* 1989;71:487–493.

Radiation

Delattre JY, Uchuya M. Radiotherapy and chemotherapy for gliomas. *Curr Opin Oncol* 1996;8:196–203.

Larson DA, Wara WM. Radiotherapy of primary malignant brain tumors. *Semin Surg Oncol* 1998;14:34–42.

Liang BC, Weil M. Locoregional approaches to therapy with gliomas as the paradigm. *Curr Opin Oncol* 1998;10;201–206.

Liebel SA, Sheline GE, Wara WM, Bouldrey EB, Nielsen SL. The role of radiation therapy in the treatment of astrocymas. *Cancer* 1975;35:1551–1557.

Lunsford LD, Somaza S, Kondziolka D, Flickinger JC. Brain astrocytomas: biopsy, then irradiation. *Clin Neurosurg* 1995;42:464–479.

Roman DD, Sperduto PW. Neuropsychological effects of cranial radiation: current knowledge and future directions. *Int J Radiat Oncol Biol Phys* 1995;31:983–998.

Piepmeier JM, Gunel M. Management of low-grade gliomas: radiation therapy at time of recurrence. *Clin Neurosurg* 1995;42:495–507.

Shaw EG. The low-grade glioma debate: evidence defending the position of early radiation therapy. *Clin Neurosurg* 1995;42:488–494.

Shrieve DC, Loeffler JS. Advances in radiation therapy for brain tumors. *Neurol Clin* 1995;13:773–793.

Vigliani MC, Sichez N, Poisson M, Delattre JY. A prospective study of cognitive functions following conventional radiotherapy for supratentorial gliomas in young adults: 4-year results. *Int J Radiat Oncol Biol Phys* 1996;35:527–533.

Walker MD, Alexander E Jr, Hunt WE, et al. Evaluation of BCNU and/or radiotherapy in the treatment of anaplastic gliomas. A cooperative clinical trial. *J Neurosurg* 1978;49:333–343.

Chemotherapy

Balmaceda C. Advances in brain tumor chemosensitivity. *Curr Opin Oncol* 1998;10:194–200.

Brandes A, Fiorentino M. The role of chemotherapy in recurrent malignant gliomas: an overview. *Cancer Invest* 1997;14:551–559.

Brandes A, Rigon A, Zampieri P, et al. Early chemotherapy and concurrent radio-chemotherapy in high-grade glioma. *J Neurooncol* 1996;30:247–255.

DeAngelis LM, Burger PC, Green SB, et al. Adjuvant chemotherapy for malignant glioma: who benefits? *Ann Neurol* 1996;40:491–492.

Fine H, Dear K, Loeffler J, et al. Meta-analysis of radiation therapy for malignant gliomas in adults. *Cancer* 1993;71:2585–2597.

Fulton D, Urtasun R, Forsyth P. Phase II study of prolonged oral therapy with etoposide (VP16) for patients with recurrent malignant gliomas. *J Neurooncol* 1996;27:149–155.

Grant R, Liang BC, Page MA, et al. Age influences chemotherapy response in astrocytomas. *Neurology* 1995;45:929–933.

Grant R, Liang BC, Slattery J, et al. Chemotherapy response criteria in malignant glioma. *Neurology* 1997;48:1336–1340.

Kirby S, Macdonald D, Fisher B, Gaspar L, Cairncross G. Pre-radiation chemotherapy for malignant glioma in adults. *Can J Neurol Sci* 1996;23:123–127.

Lunardi P, Farah JO, Mastronardi L, et al. Intravenous administration of high doses of carboplatin in multimodal treatment of high-grade gliomas: a phase II study. *Acta Neurochir (Wien)* 1996;138:215–220.

Macdonald D, Cairncross G, Stewart D, et al. Phase II study of topotecan in patients with recurrent malignant gliomas. *Ann Oncol* 1996;7:205–207.

Mason W, Louis DN, Cairncross JG. Chemosensitive gliomas in adults: which ones and why? *J Clin Oncol* 1997;15:3423–3426.

Prados M, Warnick RE, Mack EE, et al. Intravenous carboplatin for recurrent gliomas: a dose-escalating phase II trial. *Am J Clin Oncol* 1996;19:609–612.

Rabinowicz AL. Hinton DR, Dyck P, Couldwell WT. High-dose tamoxifen in treatment of brain tumors: interaction with antiepileptic drugs. *Epilepsia* 1995;36:513–515.

Walker MD, Alexander E, Hunt WE et al. Evaluation of BCNU and/or radiotherapy in the treatment of anaplastic gliomas. *J Neurosurg* 1978;49;333–343.

Walker MD, Hurwitz BS. BCNU (1,3-bis(2-chloroethyl)-1-nitrosourea; NSC-409962) in the treatment of malignant brain tumor: a preliminary report. *Cancer Chemother Rep* 1970;54:263–271.

Wilson CB, Bladrey EB, Know KJ. 1,3-bis (2-chloroethyl)-1-nitrosourea (NSC-409962) in the treatment of brain tumors. *Cancer Chemother Rep* 1970;54:273–281.

Novel Therapies

Alexander E 3rd, Loeffler JS. Radiosurgery for primary malignant brain tumors. *Semin Surg Oncol* 1998;14:43–52.

Brem H, Piantadosi S, Burger PC, et al. Placebo-controlled trial of safety and efficacy of intraoperative controlled delivery by biodegradable polymers of chemotherapy for recurrent gliomas. The Polymer–Brain Tumor Treatment Group. *Lancet* 1995;345:1008–1012.

Buchholz TA, Laramore GE, Stelzer KJ, Risler R. Boron neutron capture enhanced fast neutron radiotherapy for malignant gliomas and other tumors. *J Neurooncol* 1997;33:171–178.

Finlay JL. The role of high-dose chemotherapy and stem cell rescue in the treatment of malignant brain tumors. *Bone Marrow Transplant* 1996;18[Suppl 3]:S1–S5.

Flickinger JC, Kondziolka D, Lunsford LD. Clinical applications of stereotactic radiosurgery. *Cancer Treat Res* 1998;93:283–297.

Hall JS, Kaiser MG, Chakrabarti I, et al. Local delivery of topotecan by intracerebral clysis improves efficacy and increases drug levels in the C6 RAT rat glioma model. *Cancer Research* (in press).

Iwadate Y, Fujimoto S, Tagawa M, et al. Association of p53 gene mutation with decreased chemosensitivity in human malignant gliomas. *Int J Cancer* 1996;69:236–240.

Kirby S, Macdonald D, Fisher B, Gaspar L, Cairncross G. Pre-radiation chemotherapy for malignant glioma in adults. *Can J Neurol Sci* 1996;23:123–127.

Kleinberg L, Slick T, Enger C, et al. Short-course radiotherapy is an appropriate option for most malignant glioma patients. *Int J Radiat Oncol Biol Phys* 1997;38:31–36.

Ram Z, Culver KW, Oshiro EM, et al. Therapy of malignant brain tumors by intratumoral implantation of retroviral vector-producing cells. *Nat Med* 1997;3:1354–1361.

Sneed PK, McDermott MW, Gutin PH. Interstitial brachytherapy procedures for brain tumors. *Semin Surg Oncol* 1997;13:157–166.

Tamiya T, Ono Y, Wei M, Mroz P, Moolten FL, Chiocca A. *Escherichia coli* gpt gene sensitizes rat glioma cells to killing by 6-thioxanthine or 6-thioguanine. *Cancer Gene Ther* 1996;3:155–162.

Teicher BA, Holden SA, Northey D, Dewhirst MW, Herman TS. Therapeutic effect of infused Fluosol-DA/carbogen with ephedrine, flunarizine, or nitroprusside. *Int J Radiat Oncol Biol Phys* 1993;26:103–109.

Walter KA, Tamargo RJ, Olivi A, et al. Intratumoral chemotherapy. *Neurosurgery* 1995;37:1128–1145.

Zhang W, Hinton D, Surnock A, Couldwell W. Malignant gliomas' sensitivity to radiotherapy, high-dose tamoxifen, and hypericin: corroborating clinical response *in vitro*: case report. *Neurosurgery* 1996;38:587–591.

Molecular Genetics

Belanich M, Pastor M, Randall T, et al. Retrospective study of the correlation between DNA repair protein alkyltransferase and survival of brain tumor patients treated with carmustine. *Cancer Res* 1996;56:783–788.

Bogler O, Huang HJ, Kleihues P, Cavenee WK. The p53 gene and its role in human brain tumors. *Glia* 199515:308–327.

Li YJ, Sanson M, Hoang-Xuan K, et al. Incidence of germ-line p53 mutations in patients with gliomas. *Int J Cancer* 1995;64:383–387.

Louis DN, Gusella JF. A tiger behind many doors: multiple genetic pathways to malignant glioma. *Trends Genet* 1995;11:412–415.

Maintz D, Fiedler K, Koopman J, et al. Molecular genetic evidence of subsets of oligoastrocytomas. *J Neuropathol Exp Neurol* 1997;56:1098–1104.

Rempel SA. Molecular biology of central nervous system tumors. *Curr Opin Oncol* 1998;10:179–185.

Familial Syndromes

Cervoni L, Celli P, Tarantino R, Fortuna A. Turcot's syndrome: case report and review of the classification. *J Neurooncol* 1995;23:63–66.

Evans SC, Lozano G. The Li-Fraumeni syndrome: an inherited susceptibility to cancer. *Mol Med Today* 1997;3:390–395.

Hamilton SR, Liu B, Parsons RE, et al. The molecular basis of Turcot's syndrome. *N Engl J Med* 1995;332:839–847.

Kleihues P, Schauble B, zur Hausen A, et al. Tumors associated with p53 germ-line mutations: a synopsis of 91 families. *Am J Pathol* 1997;150: 1–13.

Koot RW, Hulsebos TJ, van Overbeeke JJ. Polyposis coli, craniofacial exostosis and astrocytoma: the concomitant occurrence of the Gardner's and Turcot syndromes. *Surg Neurol* 1996;45:213–218.

Louis DN, von Deimling A. Hereditary tumor syndromes of the nervous system: overview and rare syndromes. *Brain Pathol* 1995;5:145–151.

Mullins KJ, Rubio A, Myers SP, et al. Malignant ependymomas in a patient with Turcot's syndrome: case report and management guidelines. *Surg Neurol* 1998;49:290–294.

Suzui M, Yoshimi N, Hara A, et al. Genetic alterations in a patient with Turcot's syndrome. *Pathol Int* 1998;48:126–133.

Varley JM, Evans DG, Birch JM. Li-Fraumeni syndrome—a molecular and clinical review. *Br J Cancer* 1997;76:1–14.

Ependymal Tumors

Merchant TE, Haida T, Wang M-H, et al. Anaplastic ependymoma: treatment of pediatric patients with or without craniospinal radiation therapy. *J Neurosurg* 1997;86:943–949.

Oligodendroglioma

Allison RR, Schulsinger A, Vongtama V, Barry T, Shin KH. Radiation and chemotherapy improve outcome in oligodendroglioma. *Int J Radiat Oncol Biol Phys* 1997;37:399–403.

Balmaceda C, Goldman J, Sisti M, Bruce J, Fetell MR. Long-term survivors of malignant astrocytomas: are they really oligodendrogliomas? *Neurology* 1996;46:451.

Burger PC, Rawlings CE, Cox EB, et al. Clinicopathologic correlations in the oligodendroglioma. *Cancer* 1987;59:1345–1352.

Cairncross JG, Eisenhauer EA. Response and control: lessons from oligodendroglioma. *Clin Oncol* 1995;13:2475–2476.

Caincross JG, Mcdonald DR, Ramsay DA. Aggressive oligodendrogliomas: a chemosensitive tumor. *Neurosurgery* 1992;31:78–82.

Chamberlain MC, Kormanik PA. Salvage chemotherapy with paclitaxel for recurrent oligodendroglioma *J Clin Oncol* 1997;15:3427–3432.

Chen R, Chir B, Macdonald DR, Ramsay DA. Primary diffuse leptomeningeal oligodendroglioma. *J Neurosurg* 1995;83:724–728.

Daumas-Duport C, Varlet P, Tucker ML, et al. Oligodendrogliomas. Part I: patterns of growth, histological diagnosis, clinical and imaging correlations: a study of 153 cases. *J Neurooncol* 1997;34:37–59.

Kim L, Hochberg FH, Thornton AF, et al. Procarbazine, lomustine, and vincristine (PCV) chemotherapy for grade III and grade IV oligoastrocytomas. *J Neurosurg* 1996;85:602–607.

Kros JM, de Jong AA, van der Kwast, et al. Ultrastructural characterization of transitional cells in oligodendrogliomas. *J Neuropathol Exp Neurol* 1992;51:186–193.

Levin VA. Controversies in the treatment of low-grade astrocytomas and oligodendrogliomas. *Curr Opin Oncol* 1996;8:175–177.

Lindegaard K, Mork SJ, Eide JE, et al. Statistical analysis of clinicopathological features, radiotherapy and survival in 170 cases of oligodendroglioma. *J Neurosurg* 1987;67:224–230.

Macdonald DR. Low-grade gliomas, mixed gliomas, and oligodendrogliomas. *Semin Oncol* 1994;21:236–248.

Macdonald DR. New therapies of primary CNS lymphomas and oligodendrogliomas. *J Neurooncol* 1995;24:97–101.

Margain D, Peretti-Viton P, Perez-Castillo AM, et al. Oligodendrogliomas. *J Neuroradiol* 1991;18:153–160.

Mason WP, Krol GS, DeAngelis LM. Low-grade oligodendroglioma responds to chemotherapy. *Neurology* 1996;46:203–207.

Mork SJ, Lindegaard K, Halvorsen TB, et al. Oligodendroglioma: incidence and biological behavior in a defined population. *J Neurosurg* 1985; 63:881–889.

Nijjar TS, Simpson WJ, Gadalla T, et al. Oligodendroglioma: the Princess Margaret Hospital experience (1958–1984). *Cancer* 1993;71:4002–4006.

Nutt CL, Costello JF, Bambrick LL, et al. O6-methylguanine-DNA methyltransferase in tumors and cells of the oligodendrocyte lineage. *Can J Neurol Sci* 1995;22:111–115.

Peterson K, Cairncross G. Oligodendroglioma. *Cancer Invest* 1996;14: 243–251.

Peterson K, Paleologos N, Forsyth P, Macdonald D, Cairncross G. Salvage chemotherapy for oligodendroglioma. *J Neurosurg* 1996;85:597–601.

Reifenberger J, Reifenberger G, Ichimura K, et al. Epidermal growth factor receptor expression in oligodendroglial tumors. *Am J Pathol* 1996; 49:29–35.

Saarinen UM, Pihko H, Makipernaa A. High-dose thiotepa with autologous bone marrow rescue in recurrent malignant oligodendroglioma: a case report. *J Neurooncol* 1990;9:57–61.

Schiffer D, Dutto A, Cavalla P, et al. Prognostic factors in oligodendroglioma. *Can J Neurol Sci* 1997;24:313–319.

Shaw EG. In search of better prognostic indicators for patients with oligodendrogliomas. *Cancer Invest* 1996;14:288–289.

Shaw EG, Scheithauer BW, O'Fallon JR, et al. Oligodendrogliomas: the Mayo Clinic experience. *J Neurosurg* 1992;76:428–434.

Shaw EG, Scheithauer BW, O'Fallon JR, et al. Mixed oligoastrocytomas: a survival and prognostic factor analysis. *Neurosurgery* 1994;34:577–582.

Westergaard L, Gjerris F, Klinken L. Prognostic factors in oligodendrogliomas. *Acta Neurochir (Wien)* 1997;139:600–605.

Whittle IR, Beaumont A. Seizures in patients with supratentorial oligodendroglial tumors: features and management considerations. *Acta Neurochir (Wien)* 1995;135:19–24.

Wu JK, Folkerth RD, Ye Z, et al. Aggressive oligodendroglioma predicted by chromosome 10 restriction fragment length polymorphism analysis: case study. *J Neurooncol* 1992;15:29–35.

Astrocytic Variants

Al-Sarraj ST, Bridges LR. Desmoplastic cerebral glioblastoma of infancy. *Br J Neurosurg* 1996;10:215–219.

Dirven CM, Mooij JJ, Molenaar WM. Cerebellar pilocytic astrocytoma: a treatment protocol based upon analysis of 73 cases and a review of the literature. *Childs Nerv Syst* 1997;13:17–23.

Hirose T, Scheithauer BW, Lopes MB, et al. Tuber and subependymal giant cell astrocytoma associated with tuberous sclerosis: an immunohistochemical, ultrastructural, and immunoelectron and microscopic study. *Acta Neuropathol (Berl)* 1995;90:387–399.

Kayama T, Tominaga T, Yoshimoto T. Management of pilocytic astrocytoma. *Neurosurg Rev* 1996;19:217–220.

Kordek R, Biernat W, Sapieja W, Alwasiak J. Pleomorphic xanthoastrocytoma with a gangliomatous component: an immunohistochemical and ultrastructural study. *Acta Neuropathol (Berl)* 1995;89:194–197.

Krieger MD, Gonzalez-Gomez I, Levy ML, McComb JG. Recurrence patterns and anaplastic change in a long-term study of pilocytic astrocytomas. *Pediatr Neurosurg* 1997;27:1–11.

Langford LA. Central nervous system neoplasms: indications for electron microscopy. *Ultrastruct Pathol* 1996;20:35–46.

Lopes MB, Altermatt HJ, Scheithauer BW, Shepherd CW. Immunohistochemical characterization of subependymal giant cell astrocytomas. *Acta Neuropathol (Berl)* 1996;91:368–375.

Olas E, Kordek R, Biernat W, et al. Desmoplastic cerebral astrocytoma of infancy: a case report. *Folia Neuropathol* 1998;36:45–51.

Patt S, Gries H, Giraldo M, et al. p53 Gene mutations in human astrocytic brain tumors including pilocytic astrocytomas. *Hum Pathol* 1996;27: 586–589.

Prayson RA. Gliofibroma: a distinct entity or a subtype of desmoplastic astrocytoma? *Hum Pathol* 1996;27:610–613.

Rothman S, Sharon N, Shiffer J, et al. Desmoplastic infantile ganglioglioma. *Acta Oncol* 1997;36:655–657.

Taraszewska A, Kroh H, Majchrowski A. Subependymal giant cell astrocytoma: clinical, histologic and immunohistochemical characteristic of 3 cases. *Folia Neuropathol* 1997;35:181–186.

Tenreiro-Picon OR, Kamath SV, Knorr JR, et al. Desmoplastic infantile ganglioglioma: CT and MRI features. *Pediatr Radiol* 1995;25:540–543.

Torres OA, Roach ES, Delgado MR, et al. Early diagnosis of subependymal giant cell astrocytoma in patients with tuberous sclerosis. *J Child Neurol* 1998;13:173–177.

Turgut M, Akalan N, Ozgen T, et al. Subependymal giant cell astrocytoma associated with tuberous sclerosis: diagnostic and surgical characteristics of five cases with unusual features. *Clin Neurol Neurosurg* 1996;98:217–221.

Neuronal and Mixed Neuronal–Glial Tumors

Balter-Seri J, Mor C, Shuper A, et al. Cure of recurrent medulloblastoma. *Cancer* 1997;79:1241–1257.

Chintagumpala MM, Armstrong D, Miki S, et al. Mixed neuronal-glial tumors (gangliogliomas) in children. *Pediatr Neurosurg* 1996;24:306–313.

Dodds D, Nonis J, Mehta M, Rampling R. Central neurocytoma: a clinical study of response to chemotherapy. *J Neurooncol* 1997;34:279–283.

Hakim R, Loeffler JS, Anthony DC, Black PM. Gangliogliomas in adults. *Cancer* 1997;79:127–131.

Hirose T, Schneithauer BW, Lopes MB, et al. Ganglioglioma: an ultrastructural and immunohistochemical study. *Cancer* 1997;79:989–1003.

Ishiuchi S, Tamura M. Central neurocytoma: an immunohistochemical, ultrastructural and cell culture study. *Acta Neuropathol (Berl)* 1997;94:425–435.

Kim DG, Paek SH, Kim IH, et al. Central neurocytoma: the role of radiation therapy and long-term outcome. *Cancer* 1997;79:1995–2002.

Kroh H, Matyja E, Bidzinski J. Cerebral ganglioglomas: morphological and immunohistochemical study. *Folia Neuropathol* 1996;34:107–113.

Langford LA. Central nervous system neoplasms: indications for electron microscopy. *Ultrastruct Pathol* 1996;20:35–46.

McElroy EA Jr, Buckner JC, Lewis JE. Chemotherapy for advanced esthesioneuroblastoma: the Mayo Clinic experience. *Neurosurgery* 1998;42:1023–1027.

Min KW, Cashman RE, Brumback RA. Glioneurocytoma: tumor with glial and neuronal differentiation. *J Child Neurol* 1995;10:219–226.

Morris HH, Matkovic Z, Estes ML, Prayson RA. Ganglioglioma and intractable epilepsy: clinical and neurophysiologic features and predictors of outcome after surgery. *Epilepsia* 1998;39:307–313.

Norenberg MD. Gangliogliomas: issues of prognosis and treatment [Comment]. *AJNR* 1998;19:810.

Packer RK, Suton LN, Elterman R, et al. Outcome for children with medulloblastoma treated with radiation and cisplatin, CCNU and vincristine chemotherapy. *J Neurosurg* 1994;81:690–698.

Quinn B. Diagnosis of ganglioglioma. *J Neurosurg* 1998;88:935–937.

Rothman S, Sharon N, Shiffer J, et al. Desmoplastic infantile ganglioglioma. *Acta Oncol* 1997;36:655–657.

Salvati M, Cervoni L, Caruso R, Gagliardi FM. Central neurocytoma: clinical features of 8 cases. *Neurosurg Rev* 1997;20:39–43.

Schild SE, Scheithauer BW, Haddock MG, et al. Central neurocytomas. *Cancer* 1997;79:790–795.

Schweitzer JB, Davies KG. Differentiating central neurocytoma: case report. *J Neurosurg* 1997;86:543–546.

Sgouros S, Carey M, Aluwihare N, et al. Central neurocytoma: a correlative clinicopathologic and radiologic analysis. *Surg Neurol* 1998;49:197–204.

Slevin NJ, Irwin CJ, Banerjee SS, Gupta NK. Olfactory neural tumours—the role of external beam radiotherapy. *J Laryngol Otol* 1996;110: 1012–1016.

Tacconi L, Thom M, Symon L. Central neurocytoma: a clinico-pathological study of five cases. *Br J Neurosurg* 1997;11:286–291.

Tatagiba M, Samii M, Dankoweit-Timpe E, Aguiar PH. Esthesioneuroblastomas with intracranial extension: proliferative potential and management. *Arq Neuropsiquiatr* 1995;53:577–586.

Tenreiro-Picon OR, Kamath SV, Knorr JR, et al. Desmoplastic infantile ganglioglioma: CT and MRI features. *Pediatr Radiol* 1995;25:540–543.

Unusual Glioma Growth Patterns

Beauchesne P, Pialat J, Duthel R, et al. Aggressive treatment with complete remission in primary diffuse leptomeningeal gliomatosis—a case report. *J Neurooncol* 1998;37:161–167.

Cozad SC, Townsend P, Morantz RA, et al. Gliomatosis cerebri: results with radiation therapy. *Cancer* 1996;78:1789–1793.

Del Carpio-O'Donovan R, Korah I, Salazar A. Gliomatosis cerebri. *Radiology* 1996;198:831–835.

Fallentin E, Skriver E, Herning M, Broholm H. Gliomatosis cerebri—an appropriate diagnosis? Case reports. *Acta Radiol* 1997;38:381–390.

Kannuki S, Hondo H, Ii K, et al. Gliomatosis cerebri with good prognosis. *Brain Tumor Pathol* 1997;14:53–57.

Nishioka H, Ito H, Miki T. Difficulties in the antemortem diagnosis of gliomatosis cerebri: report of a case with diffuse increase of gemistocyte-like cells, mimicking reactive gliosis. *Br J Neurosurg* 1996;10:103–107.

Rogers LR, Estes ML, Rosemblum SA, et al. Primary leptomeningeal oligodendroglioma: case report. *Neurosurgery* 1995;36:166–169.

Vajtai I. Meningeal gliomatosis. *Neurology* 1997;48:788–789.

Merritt's Neurology, 10th ed., edited by L.P. Rowland. Lippincott Williams & Wilkins, Philadelphia © 2000.

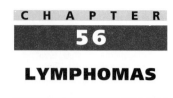

C H A P T E R
56

LYMPHOMAS

CASILDA M. BALMACEDA

SYSTEMIC LYMPHOMA

Lymphoma secondarily involves the central nervous system (CNS) in up to 10% of patients and in 1% of those at the time of diagnosis. The leptomeninges (76%), nerve roots (36%), CNS parenchyma (31%), and dura (14%) are commonly affected. The primary tumor is usually non-Hodgkin lymphoma (NHL), including diffuse poorly differentiated lymphocytic lymphoma in the original Rappaport classification or, in the modified version, lymphoblastic lymphoma and Burkitt lymphoma; nodular types usually convert to diffuse types before involving the CNS. For *Hodgkin disease*, the pattern differs with leptomeningeal disease or epidural cord compression; intracerebral lesions are rare.

A typical scenario is one of a progressive systemic lymphoma that does not respond to therapy. The median survival is 9 weeks; 1-year survival is 12%. The cause of death is usually progressive systemic disease. Prognosticators of decreased risk for CNS relapse are age less than 30 years, stable systemic disease, and lack of bone marrow involvement. Some authors recommend CNS prophylaxis for high-risk groups, including T-cell lymphomas and Burkitt lymphomas. NHL has been rarely associated with primary angiitis of the CNS; remission may accompany treatment for the lymphoma.

Meningeal involvement is seen in 4% to 8% or higher for some histologic subtypes. Symptoms include visual disturbances (39%), headache (29%), weakness (29%), drowsiness or confusion (21%), nausea and vomiting (18%), numbness (8%), or back pain (2%); 5% have no symptoms. Sixty percent of patients have cranial nerve palsies, 34% spinal nerve or root signs, and 24% behavioral changes. The oculomotor, abducens, and facial nerves are most commonly affected. Seventy-nine percent of the cerebrospinal fluid (CSF) examinations show tumor cells on the first spinal tap. A completely normal CSF is rare. Lymphoblastic or small noncleaved cell histology, age under 40 years, and stage IV disease are all associated with a high probability of leptomeningeal disease. Patients with three risk factors have an estimated probability of involvement of 50% at 12 months. At the time of leptomeningeal disease, up to 84% of patients have progressive systemic NHL or concomitant systemic relapse, 60% have bone marrow involvement, and 86% of patients can achieve a complete remission with irradiation and chemotherapy but median survival is 71 days.

Spinal cord involvement occurs in 6% of patients and appears as epidural disease. Magnetic resonance imaging (MRI) shows single, homogeneous, and isointense lesions that affect one to four vertebral segments. Paravertebral soft tissue masses communicate with the epidural lesions through the neural foramina. En-

hancement is nonspecific. Diffuse marrow replacement is common, but not vertebral collapse. Predilection for the thoracic cord is well known. Extension from the periaortic lymph nodes may be a mechanism of spread. Patients have backache with signs of spinal cord or radicular compression.

Dural involvement is rare; 38 cases have been reported. The most common site is the thoracic spine, followed by the cervical spine and brain. CSF can be abnormal even with negative cytology. Twenty percent are low-grade lymphomas and 80% high-grade lymphomas, most of B-cell lineage. The systemic lymphoma is usually in remission at the time of dural symptoms. Treatment is with local radiation. Median survival is 26 months after diagnosis for patients treated with both surgery and radiation.

PRIMARY CENTRAL NERVOUS SYSTEM LYMPHOMA

Epidemiology

Primary central nervous system lymphoma (PCNSL) accounts for less than 2% of all CNS neoplasms and 7% of all malignant lymphomas. The incidence is on the rise, both in the immunocompromised and the immunocompetent populations, more than what can be attributed to improved diagnosis by better imaging. A threefold increase has been observed in immunocompetent people. The peak incidence is the fifth to seventh decade, with a male to female ratio of 3:2. A peak in the first decade of life is a measure of children with acquired immunodeficiency syndrome (AIDS).

Clinical Manifestations

These are nonspecific. The most common symptoms are those related to an intracranial mass; an encephalitic-like picture; strokelike presentation, resembling demyelination disease; or cranial nerve palsies. Patients with PCNSL and AIDS tend to have more constitutional signs.

Pathology

The tumor was first described at the beginning of the century and called *perivascular sarcoma* or *reticulum cell sarcoma*. In 1974, the cells were recognized as transformed lymphocytes and the term PCNSL was introduced. The neoplastic cells of PCNSL and NHL have the same origin. Theories on pathogenesis include migration of lymphocytes to the CNS secondary to infection or inflammation or activation of lymphocytes that have a specific CNS predilection.

Many classifications have been proposed. PCNSL is classified as extranodal diffuse histiocytic lymphoma in the Rappaport classification or as large cell or immunoblastic lymphoma in the Working Formulation. Most are large B-cell variants; 5% are T cell in origin. The tumors contain pleomorphic B cells mixed with reactive T cells, recruited as a host response to the tumor. Up to 60% of the non-human immunodeficiency virus (HIV) PCNSL are diffuse large cell forms, but about 20% are small to medium sized. Polymerase chain reaction analysis of gene rearrangement may help determine monoclonality, although up to 16% of both AIDS and non-AIDS PCNSL display biclonal immunoglobulins light chains.

There are four pathologic manifestations. Intraaxial masses, commonly hemispheric, are the most common. Diffuse meningeal or periventricular involvement is seen in 24% of cases. The tumor can have a purely meningeal distribution, or primary leptomeningeal lymphoma. Uveal or vitreous lesions may be the first site of disease, as are intradural spinal metastases. A rare manifestation is the primary intramedullary lymphoma of the spinal cord. The tumors are firm and nodular, surrounded by edema and spread to the leptomeninges or subpial region. PCNSL is multifocal in 50% of cases. Histologically, the cells are closely packed, infiltrate surrounding brain, and have a characteristic perivascular concentration. Necrosis and hemorrhage are most common in tumors of immunocompromised patients. The pathogenesis is obscure. Epstein-Barr virus (EBV) may induce B-cell clone transformation. EBV genome has been found in the tumor of up to 100% of immunocompromised patients, in contrast to 16% of PCNSL in immunocompetent individuals, where EBV may not play an important role in pathogenesis.

Diagnosis

Diagnosis usually requires tissue, CSF, or aqueous humor (by vitreous examination). Corticosteroids induce a temporary resolution of the lesion in up to 60% of patients. Multiple contrast-enhancing lesions that recur rapidly after tapering the corticosteroid dosage should be suspicious. The incidence of leptomeningeal disease at diagnosis varies from 12% to 66%. CSF shows malignant cells in up to 43% of patients. Extent of disease workup includes neuroophthalmologic examination, contrast MRI of the spine, and lumbar puncture. Twenty percent of patients have ocular lesions at diagnosis. Both infectious and lymphomatous meningitis may coexist. The CSF shows a reactive pleocytosis in infectious meningitis, whereas monoclonal B lymphocytes are seen in lymphomatous meningitis.

Imaging

The lesions may be single or multiple and are often periventricular. The most common location is supratentorial; the posterior fossa is less favored. Fifty-five percent appear in the white matter or corpus callosum; 17% in the deep gray matter, basal ganglia, or hypothalamus; 11% in the posterior fossa; and 1% in the spinal cord. Lesions are hypodense but may be iso- or hyperintense on computed tomography (Fig. 56.1A). On MRI the lesions are round, oval, or gyral, usually hypointense relative to the gray matter on T1 images. On T2, they appear hypointense to isointense to the gray matter, a pattern attributed to an increased nuclear-to-cytoplasmic ratio. T2 changes help to differentiate PCNSL from gliomas or demyelination, which appear hyperintense (Fig. 56.2C). Contrast enhancement is dense and homogeneous in immunocompetent patients (Figs. 56.1, B and C, and 56.2, A and B).

The borders are not well demarcated. Mirror-image bilateral-enhancing lesions in the basal ganglia are pathognomonic but rare. MRI can show diffuse ependymal spread that is not appre-

ciated on computed tomography (Fig. 56.3, A and B). Ring enhancement, calcification, and hemorrhage are uncommon. The differential diagnosis includes high-grade gliomas, abscess, sarcoid, tuberculosis, or active areas of demyelination. Edema on MRI is moderate to severe in abscesses or metastases and mild to moderate in PCNSL, a difference that aids diagnosis.

Treatment

Corticosteroids

Response is dramatic, with a decrease in edema and a cytotoxic effect on lymphoma cells. Up to 10% of lesions disappear, sometimes lasting months after steroids have been discontinued. A biopsy taken after corticosteroid therapy has started may yield falsely negative results. Corticosteroid treatment for a suspected lesion is strongly contraindicated. Response to steroids is not pathognomonic because demyelinating conditions or sarcoidosis may behave similarly.

Surgery

Because the tumors are infiltrative and sometimes bilateral, surgical resection is not the mainstay of treatment. The goal of surgery is to provide tissue diagnosis; it does not prolong survival.

Radiation

PCNSL is characterized by high responses to radiation. Patients receive 180 cGy per fraction, for a total of 60 Gy. The median survival is 10 to 18 months; only 3% to 4% live 5 years with this treatment alone. Age less than 60 years and Karnofsky performance better than 70 are prognosticators of better outcome.

Chemotherapy

PCNSL is a chemosensitive tumor. The malignant lymphocytes infiltrate the intact brain and agents must reach all areas at risk. Up to 100% of patients have leptomeningeal disease at autopsy, so chemotherapy addressing this compartment is an important component of treatment. Methotrexate crosses the blood–brain barrier, and therapeutic CSF concentrations are seen after intravenous administration. Methotrexate-based regimens are more effective than cyclophosphamide, vincristine, adriamycin, and prednisone (CHOP), which is the traditional treatment for systemic lymphoma. Glass et al. (1996) treated 25 patients with high-dose maintenance intravenous methotrexate alone (more than 3.5 g/m^2 for one to six cycles). Eighty-two percent had a complete response, and the median survival of 42 months for the responding group compared favorably with regimens using multiple agents, with less toxicity; the Karnofsky performance improved.

Elderly patients are particularly prone to the neurotoxic effects of irradiation and may benefit from these chemotherapy-only regimens. Cytosine arabinoside in high doses achieves therapeutic levels in both brain parenchyma and CSF; it has also been used to treat ocular disease. Excellent responses have been observed to a regimen consisting of carmustine, methotrexate,

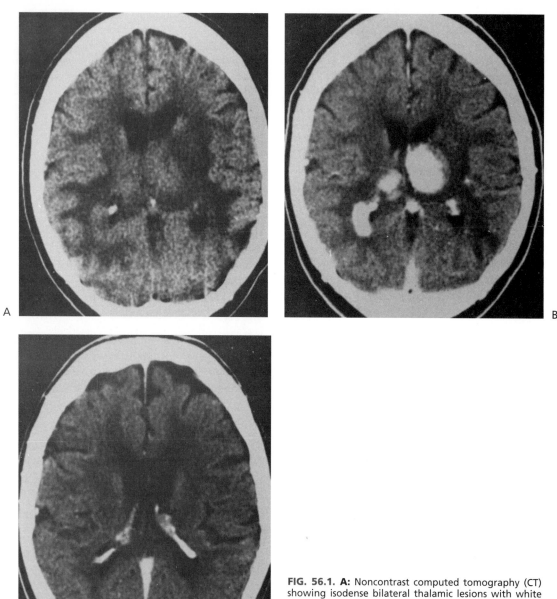

FIG. 56.1. A: Noncontrast computed tomography (CT) showing isodense bilateral thalamic lesions with white matter edema. **B:** Contrast-enhanced CT showing marked enhancement of diffuse lymphoma. Intraventricular tumor is also present. **C:** Contrast-enhanced CT 2 months after radiation therapy (with 5,000 cGy to the whole brain) is normal except for persistence of white matter lucency.

procarbazine, and dexamethasone. Chemotherapy alone, using a combination of agents, can lead to remission of intraocular lymphoma without radiotherapy.

Disruption of the blood–brain barrier followed by chemotherapy has led to prolonged survival. Newelt et al. (1991) administered methotrexate, cyclophosphamide, and procarbazine, achieving a median survival of 44 months without radiotherapy. High-dose chemotherapy followed by bone marrow/stem cell support is an accepted treatment for relapsed systemic NHL. The regimen of BCNU, etoposide, cytarabine, melphalan, followed by bone marrow reconstitution, is widely used for non-NHL and may be used for PCNSL in the future.

Combination Therapy

Several reports suggest that the combination of chemotherapy and radiation improves outcome over radiation alone, but this has not been observed in all series. DeAngelis and associates (1992) achieved a 41-month median survival with intravenous (1 g/m^2) and intrathecal methotrexate, radiotherapy, followed by intravenous cytosine arabinoside. Acute toxicity was minimal. Similar results have been observed with radiotherapy followed by intraventricular methotrexate and CHOP; procarbazine, CCNU, and vincristine; or vincristine, cyclophosphamide, prednisolone, and doxorubicin.

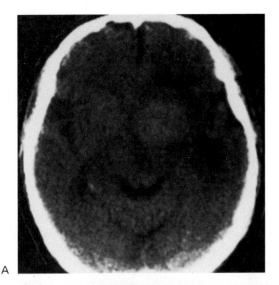

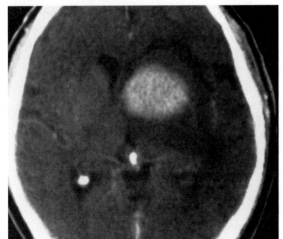

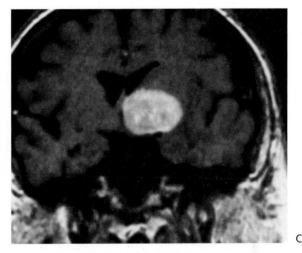

FIG. 56.2. Primary central nervous system lymphoma. Noncontrast-enhanced **(A)** and contrast-enhanced **(B)** axial computed tomographies and contrast-enhanced coronal magnetic resonance image **(C)** show large left basal ganglionic primary central nervous system lymphoma.

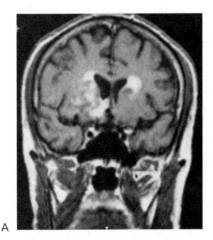

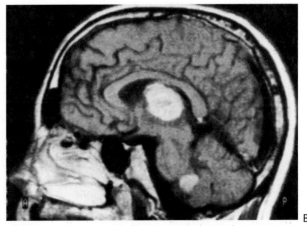

FIG. 56.3. Primary central nervous system lymphoma (PCNSL): ependymal spread. **A:** Contrast-enhanced coronal magnetic resonance image of a patient with progressive cognitive impairment and diabetes insipidus shows bilateral periventricular and hypothalamic lesions that enhance markedly after contrast administration. **B:** Sagittal contrast-enhanced magnetic resonance image of a different patient with gait ataxia caused by fourth ventricular spread of a thalamic PCNSL.

Prognosis

PCNSL is still a therapeutic challenge. The median survival for patients treated with combination regimens is 42 months, whereas for those treated solely with irradiation it is 12 to 18 months. Fifty percent of patients relapse, usually within 2 years of diagnosis and mostly at distant sites. Leptomeningeal or spinal cord recurrence occurs in 60%. Extraneural spread is rare but can involve the lymph nodes, heart, gastrointestinal tract, and bone marrow. About one-third of patients treated with chemotherapy and radiation have a syndrome of progressive ataxia, dementia, and urinary incontinence, which appears after a median of 13.2 months from diagnosis. A ventriculoperitoneal shunt may provide benefit. Other patients develop cerebrovascular disease, which may be related to treatment or to the disease itself. Delayed leukoencephalopathy is seen in 80% of patients older than 60 years who survive 1 year.

PRIMARY CENTRAL NERVOUS SYSTEM LYMPHOMA IN THE IMMUNOCOMPROMISED PATIENT

Epidemiology

The immunocompromised states associated with PCNSL include renal transplantation, Wiskott-Aldrich syndrome, ataxia telangiectasia, IgA deficiency, rheumatoid arthritis, progressive multifocal leukoencephalopathy, and IgM paraproteinemic neuropathy. PCNSL is the most common brain tumor in patients with AIDS, developing in 1% to 3% of all patients. Typically, patients have profound immunosuppression and marked T4 cell depletion (median CD4 counts are less than $50/\mu L$). At autopsy, 75% of patients with AIDS harbor PCNSL. In immunosuppressed subjects, lymphoma is symptomatic in the third or fourth decades. About 2% of renal transplant patients develop PCNSL, 100 times more than the general population.

Pathology and Pathogenesis

Transplant and HIV-related lymphomas are generally polyclonal high-grade B-cell lymphomas, whereas in the immunocompetent population they are intermediate grade. EBV may play a role in the induction of PCNSL, and molecular analysis has helped in understanding the steps to lymphocytic transformation. About 100% of HIV-related PCNSL are positive for EBV markers, whereas PCNSL in nonimmunocompromised patients are rarely positive for EBV. In the African Burkitt lymphoma, EBV genes are expressed in all the tumor cells. An immunosuppressed host has little immunity to EBV infection. A portion of the host's lymphocytes then become chronically infected, and the B-lymphocytic cell line becomes immortalized. The infected cells undergo expansion into clones of lymphocytes that eventually produce a lymphoma. The CNS may be a site of predilection. The more profound the immunosuppression, the greater the likelihood that a chronic EBV infection will result in a lymphoma. The EBV infection, or the chronic stimulation of B cells, then leads to oncogene activation, which further allows the proliferation of the lymphoma. Coinfection of the CNS with CMV has been observed, further suggesting a role for infection in AIDS-related PCNSL.

Some lymphomas in immunocompromised patients follow polyclonal proliferation of B cells. The *lymphoproliferative disorders*, although possibly fatal, are not monoclonal and thus do not fit the strict definition of lymphoma. When immunosuppression is decreased, the tumor may recede.

Diagnosis

The time from seroconversion to PCNSL is about 2 years. In 10% of patients, the symptoms of PCNSL led to the diagnosis of AIDS. About 56% of patients have focal signs or symptoms compared with 27% of patients with PCNSL and no HIV disease; this may be due to more rapid progression in people with AIDS. Many patients have concurrent opportunistic infections. The standard of practice for an HIV-positive patient and a cerebral mass is treatment with antitoxoplasmosis medication. If there is no clinical or radiographic response after 2 weeks, tissue diagnosis is considered, via brain biopsy, lumbar puncture, or vitreous examination. Immunocompromised patients with a single lesion are more likely to have PCNSL, and early biopsy is advocated. PCNSL may coexist with cerebral toxoplasmosis, and radiographic improvement may follow antitoxoplasmosis treatment even in patients who are later found to have a PCNSL. Positron emission tomography may help differentiate neoplastic from nonneoplastic conditions. CSF can be analyzed for EBV by polymerase chain reaction studies. The gold standard for diagnosis is still tissue histology.

Radiography

The tumor may have irregular ringlike contrast enhancement (corresponding to necrosis), and it may be difficult to distinguish the lesion from toxoplasmosis. An irregular type of enhancement is more commonly associated with PCNSL, whereas smooth enhancement is associated with toxoplasmosis. Cytomegalovirus ependymitis can mimic PCNSL.

Treatment

The standard treatment is whole brain radiation. Some report prolonged survival in selected patients treated with both chemotherapy and radiation. The best candidates are those with limited disease (i.e., no leptomeningeal metastases), good performance status, no coexisting medical conditions, and a CD4 count greater than $200/mm^3$. The optimal dose of radiation is not known. A regimen of 150 cGy per fraction to a total dose of 40 Gy and a boost of 20 Gy to the tumor bed has been recommended for patients with no other AIDS-related illnesses. For those with other AIDS-related illnesses, 200 cGy per fraction to a total dose of 54 Gy has been recommended. Most patients have a clinical response to radiotherapy. All patients should have a CSF examination to determine spinal seeding. If so, MRI of the spine can detect bulky disease that may need radiotherapy. Combined regimens of chemotherapy and radiation have shown mixed results because of the limited bone marrow reserve. Some new regimens have attempted to use low-dose chemotherapy and radiation, and these have better results than more aggressive regimens with higher doses of chemotherapy. Treatment also includes an attempt to reduce the immunosuppressive state.

Prognosis

The median survival after diagnosis is 1 to 2 months with supportive care alone and 2 to 6 months with radiation. Survival correlates closely with Karnofsky performance before treatment, length of time since seroconversion, and the presence of more than one risk factor for HIV. Patients who have radiation therapy commonly die of opportunistic infections, whereas patients who do not receive radiation usually die of the tumor.

A View of the Future

There are several unanswered questions. How can a tumor of neoplastic lymphocytes occur in an organ without endogenous lymphoid tissue? Why is the tumor so exquisitely radio- and chemosensitive, only to recur months after a complete response to treatment has been observed? Why does PCNSL fail at distant sites even if the initial site of disease is free of tumor? The optimal drugs, best treatment reschedule, or ways to minimize long-term treatment-related sequelae still need to be determined. Because of the long-term sequelae of whole brain irradiation, new treatment regimens may attempt to achieve durable responses, delaying radiation until recurrence, or eliminating it altogether. It is not clear whether high-dose intravenous chemotherapy alone could treat leptomeningeal disease or how much treatment can prevent leptomeningeal failures.

INTRAVASCULAR LYMPHOMA

This rare condition was first described in 1959 by Pfleger and Tappeiner; it is characterized by angiotropic growth, with predilection for the skin and CNS. The disease is considered a form of B-cell NHL and is also called *neoplastic angioendotheliomatosis* or *angiotropic lymphoma*. There are three main forms: a mild cutaneous form, a progressive form with both skin and visceral organ involvement, and an aggressive form with multiorgan involvement.

Diagnosis usually requires a brain biopsy. Pathologically, neoplastic cells are seen within and occlude the lumen of the capillaries, venues, arterioles, and small arteries. Only rarely do neoplastic cells extend beyond the vessel wall. Blood vessels in the subarachnoid space, cortex, white matter, and deep gray matter are involved. Immunoperoxidase staining is positive for B-cell markers. The cells may have surface properties that favor attachment to the blood vessels, skin, CNS, and peripheral nerves, differing from sites of involvement of lymphoma. White matter changes are characterized by axonal degeneration, loss of myelin, and macrophage infiltration. Bone marrow is spared. Because of the nonspecific clinical features and nonspecific imaging characteristics, the disease is often found only at autopsy, with dissemination to skin, adrenals, and brain. Polymerase chain reaction assay for rearrangement of immunoglobulin heavy chain genes can confirm the presence of a monoclonal B-cell population.

Clinically, the symptoms are nonspecific and usually develop over weeks or months. A strokelike syndrome can occur, but progressive encephalopathy is the most common manifestation, present in up to 82% at some time. Superimposed focal signs include hemiparesis (39%), myelopathy (34%), and aphasia (9%). Typically, a patient with multiple transient ischemic attacks or embolic strokes develops progressive dementia. Unexplained fever is seen in 25% of patients. Weight loss is common. The median age at onset is 60 years (range, 12 to 87 years). Systemic signs are rare. The condition may mimic systemic necrotizing vasculitis. Skin lesions include telangiectasias, hemorrhagic nodules, and leg lymphedema. The syndrome often occurs during the sixth or seventh decade of life, and the male to female ratio is usually 2:1. Average survival ranges from 9 to 12 months.

Laboratory results are mostly normal. Anemia is seen in up to 73% of patients, elevated erythrocyte sedimentation rate in 83%, and elevated lactate dehydrogenase in 89%. CSF protein is increased in 90% of patients, with 10 white blood cells/mm^3 in 57% and oligoclonal bands in 77%. Neoplastic cells in the CSF are rare (3%).

Imaging is nonspecific. Abnormalities are multifocal, reflecting diffuse brain involvement. The most common abnormality is a masslike lesion with increased signal on T2-weighted images, which correlates with areas of gliosis and edema pathologically. The white matter is most commonly affected, but lesions can also be seen in the gray matter. Infarctlike lesions are multifocal with gyriform enhancement. There may be enhancement along the corpus callosum. Meningeal enhancement results from direct infiltration of vessels, meningeal microinfarcts, or sluggish flow through that area. Angiography may show multifocal vessel stenosis or occlusion, as in vasculitis. Other conditions that may mimic this disease include multiinfarct dementia, vasculitis, Creutzfelt-Jakob disease, progressive multifocal leukoencephalopathy, or gliomatosis cerebri.

Treatment has included corticosteroids, cyclophosphamide, a combination of chemotherapy (CHOP-like regimens) and radiation, plasmapheresis, and intrathecal chemotherapy. Although complete responses have been observed, median survival is only 6 months. Spontaneous remission is rare.

CEREBRAL LYMPHOID GRANULOMATOSIS

This is an angiocentric lymphoproliferative process that preferentially involves the lungs. It was first described in 1972 by Liebow. The diagnostic triad includes a lymphoid infiltrate, angiitis (blood vessel infiltration), and granulomatosis (lesion necrosis). Extrathoracic manifestations include the skin (37%) and the CNS (30%). Neurologic complications lead to CNS symptoms in 65% of the patients: headache, altered consciousness, and cranial nerve palsies or a multiinfarct dementia. Peripheral neuropathy affects 25%. Radiographically, lesions are seen in the gray and white matter, accompanied by edema. Meningeal thickening and linear punctate enhancement in the brainstem can be seen. Pathologically, there is a lymphoid infiltrate (plasma cells, histiocytes, and lymphoreticular cells), with vascular proliferation and necrosis. The perivascular spaces are infiltrated with neoplastic cells, differing from the angiotrophic lymphoma, where the neoplastic cells are within the vessel lumen. Lung findings are similar. Prognosis is poor; median survival is about 2 years. Ultimately, many patients develop lymphoma, and some investigators consider this an angiocentric T-cell malignancy. A classification has been developed for purposes of treatment: Grade I lesions may not develop into aggressive malignancies, and grades II and III lesions warrant intensive chemotherapy. The EBV genome has been found in most grade II lesions, suggesting that EBV, contrary to earlier views, can transform and infect T cells.

SUGGESTED READINGS

Systemic Lymphoma

Ersboll J, Schultz HB, Thomsen BLR, et al. Meningeal involvement in non-Hodgkin's lymphoma: symptoms, incidence, risk factors and treatment. *Scand J Haematol* 1985;35:487–496.

Mackintosh FR, Colby TV, Podolsky WJ, et al. Central nervous system involvement in non-Hodgkin's lymphoma: an analysis of 105 cases. *Cancer* 1982;49:586–595.

Miranda RN, Glantz LK, Myint MA, et al. Stage IE non-Hodgkin's lymphoma involving the dura. A clinicopathologic study of five cases. *Arch Pathol Lab Med* 1996;120:254–260.

Primary Central Nervous System Lymphoma

Abrey LE, DeAngelis L, Yahalom J. Long-term survival in primary CNS lymphoma. *J Clin Oncol* 1998;16:859–863.

Balmaceda CM, Gaynor JJ, Sun M, et al. Leptomeningeal involvement in primary central nervous system lymphoma: recognition, significance and implications. *Ann Neurol* 1995;38:202–209.

Bashir R, Luka J, Cheloha K, Chamberlain M, Hochberg F. Expression of Epstein-Barr virus proteins in primary CNS lymphoma in AIDS patients. *Neurology* 1993;43:2358–2362.

Corn BW, Trock BJ, Curran WJ. Management of primary central nervous system lymphoma for the patient with acquired immunodeficiency syndrome. Confronting a clinical catch 22. *Cancer* 1995;76:163–166.

DeAngelis LM. Current management of primary central nervous system lymphoma. *Oncology* 1995;9:63–71.

DeAngelis LM, Yahalom J, Thaler HT, Kher U. Combined modality therapy for primary CNS lymphoma. *J Clin Oncol* 1992;10:635–643.

Forsyth P, Yahalom J, DeAngelis LM. Combined modality therapy in the treatment of primary central nervous system lymphoma in AIDS. *Neurology* 1994;44;1473–1479.

Glass J, Shustik C, Hochberg FG, Cher L, Gruber ML. Therapy of primary central nervous system lymphoma with pre-irradiation methotrexate, cyclophosphamide, doxorubicin, vincristine and dexamethasone (MCHOD). *J Neurooncol* 1996;30:257–265.

Herrlinger U, Schabet M, Clemens M, et al. Clinical presentation and therapeutic outcome in 26 patients with primary CNS lymphoma. *Acta Neurol Scand* 1998;97:257–264.

Herrlinger U, Schabet M, Eichhorn M, et al. Prolonged corticosteroid-induced remission in primary central nervous system lymphoma: report of a case and review of the literature. *Eur Neurol* 1996;36:241–243.

Johnson BA, Fram EK, Johnson PC, Jacobwitz R. The variable MR appearance of primary lymphoma of the central nervous system: comparison with histopathologic features. *AJNR* 1997;18:563–572.

Khalfallah S, Stamatoullas A, Fruchart C, Proust F, Delangre T, Tilly H. Durable remission of a relapsing primary central nervous system lymphoma after autologous bone marrow transplantation. *Bone Marrow Transplant* 1998;18:1021–1023.

Koeller KK, Smirniotopoulos JG, Jones RV. Primary central nervous system lymphoma: radiologic-pathologic correlation. *Radiographics* 1997;17:1497–1526.

Korfel A, Thiel E. Successful treatment of non-Hodgkin's lymphoma of the central nervous system with BMPD chemotherapy followed by radiotherapy. *Leuk Lymph* 1998;30:609–617.

Ling SM, Roach MI, Larson DA, Wara WM. Radiotherapy of primary central nervous system lymphoma in patients with and without human immunodeficiency virus. *Cancer* 1994;73:2570–2582.

Newelt EA, Goldman DL, Dahlborg SA, et al. Primary CNS lymphoma treated with osmotic blood-brain barrier disruption: prolonged survival and preservation of cognitive function. *J Clin Oncol* 1991;9:1580–1590.

O'Brien PC, Roos DE, Liew KH, et al. Preliminary results of combined chemotherapy and radiotherapy for non-AIDS primary central nervous system lymphoma. *Med J Austral* 1996;165:424–427.

O'Neill BP, O'Fallon JR, Earle JD, Colgan JP, Brown LD, Kriegel RL. Primary central nervous system non-Hodgkin's lymphoma: survival advantages with combined initial therapy? *Int J Radiat Oncol Biol Phys* 1995;33:663–673.

Peterson K, Gordon KB, Heinemann MH, DeAngelis LM. The clinical spectrum of ocular lymphoma. *Cancer* 1993;72:843–849.

Sandor V, Stark-Vancs V, Pearson D, et al. Phase II trial of chemotherapy alone for primary CNS and intraocular lymphoma. *J Clin Oncol* 1998;16:3000–3006.

Schiff D, Suman VJ, Yang P, et al. Risk factors for primary central nervous system lymphoma: a case-control study. *Cancer* 1998;82:975–982.

Schultz C, Scott C, Sherman W, et al. Preirradiation chemotherapy with cyclophosphamide, doxorubicin, vincristine, and dexamethasone for primary CNS lymphomas: initial report of radiation therapy oncology group protocol 88-06. *J Clin Oncol* 1996;14:556–564.

Villringer K, Jager H, Dichgans M, et al. Differential diagnosis of CNS lesions in AIDS patients by FDG-PET. *J Comput Assist Tomogr* 1995;19:532–536.

Intravascular Lymphoma

Ansell J, Bhawan J, Cohen S, et al. Histiocytic lymphoma and malignant angioendotheliomatosis. *Cancer* 1982;50:1506–1512.

Bhawan J, Wolff SM, Ucci AA, Bhan AK. Malignant lymphoma and malignant angioendotheliomatosis: one disease. *Cancer* 1985;3:570–576.

Chapin JE, Davis LE, Kornfeld M, Mandler RN. Neurologic manifestations of intravascular lymphomatosis. *Acta Neurol Scand* 1995;91:494–499.

Sanna P, Bertoni F, Roggero E, et al. Angiotropic (intravascular) large cell lymphoma: case report and short discussion of the literature. *Tumori* 1997;83:772–775.

Takagi Y, Kikuchi H. MR imaging of multiple cerebral infarctions in angiotropic lymphoma. *Acta Neurochir (Wien)* 1997;139:478–479.

Wick MR, Mills SE. Intravascular lymphomatosis: clinicopathologic features and differential diagnosis. *Semin Diagn Pathol* 1991;8:91–101.

Williams RL, Meltzer CC, Smirniotopoulos JG, et al. Cerebral MR imaging in intravascular lymphomatosis. *Am J Neuroradiol* 1998;19:427–431.

Cerebral lymphomatoid Granulomatosis

Bhagavatula K, Scott TF. Magnetic resonance appearance of cerebral lymphomatoid granulomatosis. *J Neuroimag* 1997;7:120–121.

Merritt's Neurology, 10th ed., edited by L.P. Rowland. Lippincott Williams & Wilkins, Philadelphia © 2000.

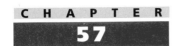

PINEAL REGION TUMORS

JEFFREY N. BRUCE
CASILDA M. BALMACEDA
BENNETT M. STEIN
MICHAEL R. FETELL

Among central nervous system (CNS) tumors, the widest variety of pathologic types occurs in the region of the pineal gland and posterior third ventricle (Table 57.1). The numerous cell types that make up the normal gland and surrounding periventricular region contribute to these diverse histologic subtypes. The pineal gland is composed of glandular tissue, glia, endothelial cells, and sympathetic nerve terminals. Pineal cell tumors and pineoblastomas arise from pineal glandular elements, astrocytomas and oligodendrogliomas from glial cells, hemangioblastomas from endothelial cells, and chemodectomas from sympathetic nerve cells. Arachnoid cells in the reflections of the tela choroidea adjacent to the pineal gland give rise to meningiomas. Ependymomas arise from ependymal cells that line the third ventricle. Germ cell tumors (GCTs) derive from primitive germ cell rests that are retained in the pineal and other midline structures after embryologic migration courses.

Pineal tumors account for approximately 1% of all intracranial tumors in the United States. In Asia, where GCTs are endemic, pineal cell tumors constitute 4% to 7% of all intracranial tumors.

GERM CELL TUMORS

GCTs account for approximately one-third of all pineal tumors and are histologically identical to gonadal GCTs with a predominance in men and younger age groups. Extragonadal GCTs (including pineal region) have a poorer prognosis than gonadal GCTs. GCTs range along a spectrum from benign (as in teratomas, dermoids, epidermoids, and lipomas) to highly malignant (as in choriocarcinomas, embryonal cell carcinomas, teratocarcinomas, and endodermal sinus tumors).

Germinomas are tumors of an intermediate degree of malignancy arising from primordial germ cells that can occur in the gonads or in midline sites in the nervous system (pineal and suprasellar region) or body (mediastinum and sacrococcygeal region). Although histologically identical in all sites of origin, by conventional nomenclature germinomas in the testes are called *seminomas*, those in the ovaries are *dysgerminomas*, and those in the CNS are *germinomas* (previously called atypical teratomas).

Unlike suprasellar GCTs, which show no sexual predisposition, GCTs of the pineal region occur predominantly in males. Germinomas are most common in boys in the first or second decade and have a propensity to seed the cerebrospinal fluid (CSF) pathways. Despite their malignant characteristics, germinomas are exquisitely sensitive to radiotherapy and chemotherapy; they can be cured in many patients. The presence of beta human chorionic gonadotropin (β-hCG) in a germinoma implies a slightly worse prognosis.

Embryonal cell carcinomas, choriocarcinomas, and endodermal sinus tumors are rare but highly malignant GCTs that may metastasize to the CSF. Choriocarcinoma contains cyto- and syncytiotrophoblastic cells that produce β-hCG. Endodermal sinus tumors contain yolk sac elements that produce alpha-fetoprotein (AFP). High levels of β-hCG or AFP in the CSF or serum indicate the presence of malignant germ cell elements, and histologic confirmation is not necessary for treatment with radiation, chemotherapy, or both (Table 57.2). GCTs in general are difficult to classify because 25% are of a mixed type, containing both malignant and benign elements or several different malignant elements (Table 57.3). Extensive specimen sampling is necessary for accurate histologic determination. High AFP or β-hCG levels in the CSF trigger an extensive search for malignant germ cell elements even if the pathologic specimens suggest otherwise. Benign GCTs such as teratomas, dermoids, and epidermoids are generally curable with surgery alone. Teratomas are composed of tissues from three germ cell lines (endo-, ecto-, and mesoderm). Immature teratomas are a variant of this tumor that may grow quickly and behave in a malignant fashion, including CSF seeding.

PINEAL CELL TUMORS

Pineal cell tumors arise from pineocytes and range from histologically primitive pineoblastomas to well-differentiated pineocytomas. Attempts to correlate prognosis and survival with either variant have been inconclusive because both may behave in a ma-

TABLE 57.1. SUMMARY OF PATHOLOGICALLY VERIFIED PINEAL TUMORS AT THE NEW YORK NEUROLOGICAL INSTITUTE (1978–1998)

Type	Benign	Malignant	Male : female	Average age (yr)
Germ cell	13	51	58/6	20.2
Pineal cell	9	41	25/25	36.2
Glial cell	19	34	27/26	25.6
Meningioma	10	0	6/4	50.8
Pineal cyst	10	0	3/7	33.8
Miscellaneous	3	5	4/4	50.6
Total	64	131	123/72	29.3

TABLE 57.2. BIOLOGIC MARKERS IN GERM CELL TUMORS

Tumors	βhCG	AFP
Benign germ cell	−	−
Immature teratoma	?	+/−
Germinoma	−	−
Germinoma with syncytiotrophoblastic cells	+	−
Embryonal cell carcinoma	+/−	+/−
Choriocarcinoma	++	−
Endodermal sinus tumor	−	++

β-hCG; beta human chorionic gonaditropin; AFP, alpha-fetoprotein.

TABLE 57.3. PURE VS. MIXED GERM CELL TUMORS AT THE NEW YORK NEUROLOGICAL INSTITUTE (1978–1998)

Tumor type	Number
Pure germ cell tumors	
Germinoma	30
Teratoma	9
Epidermoid	2
Immature teratoma	2
Embryonal carcinomas	2
Lipoma	2
Total	47
Mixed germ cell tumors	
Germinoma/teratoma	4
Germinoma/embryonal carcinomas	3
Immature teratoma/germinoma/EST	2
Germinoma/dermoid	1
Germinoma/immature teratoma	1
Choriocarcinoma/teratoma	1
Choriocarcinoma/immature teratoma	1
Embryonal carcinomas/EST	1
EST/embryonal carcinomas/ germinoma	1
Nonspecified mixed	2
Total	17

EST, endodermal sinus tumor.

lignant fashion, with recurring at the primary site and spreading through the CSF. Pineal cell tumors occur in children and young adults before age 40 with no sex predominance. They are occasionally found concurrently with retinoblastomas and may contain mixed cell types. The pineoblastomas are considered a variant of primitive neuroectodermal tumors. Pineal cell tumors are radiosensitive, but experience with chemotherapy is limited.

GLIOMAS

Gliomas, like GCTs, account for one-third of pineal tumors. Most are invasive and have a prognosis comparable with astrocy-tomas of the brainstem. About one-third of gliomas are low grade, cystic, and surgically curable. Anaplastic astrocytomas and glioblastomas are less common. Oligodendrogliomas and ependymomas may also occur. Treatment of these tumors is identical to the treatment of gliomas in other areas of the CNS.

MENINGIOMAS

Meningiomas can arise from the velum interpositum or from the tentorial edge with a higher incidence in middle age and the elderly. They are amenable to surgical resection.

METASTASIS AND OTHER MISCELLANEOUS TUMORS

The pineal gland does not have a blood–brain barrier and, like the pituitary gland, may be underrecognized as a possible site for CNS metastasis of systemic tumors. Miscellaneous tumors include sarcoma, hemangioblastoma, choroid plexus papilloma, lymphoma, and chemodectoma.

PINEAL CYSTS

Benign cysts of the pineal gland are often found incidentally on radiographic studies, and it is important to distinguish them from cystic tumors. They are normal variants of the pineal gland and consist of a cystic structure surrounded by normal pineal parenchymal tissue (Fig. 57.1). Radiographically they are up to 2 cm in diameter and often have some degree of peripheral enhancement that may be a compressed normal pineal gland. Pineal cysts may be found in 4% of all magnetic resonance images. These cysts are static anatomic variants and need no treatment unless they become symptomatic. In one series of 53 pineal cysts, fewer than 10% developed hydrocephalus requiring surgical intervention.

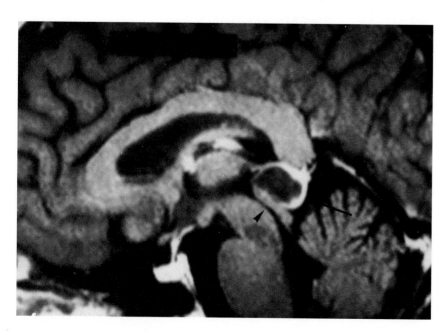

FIG. 57.1. Sagittal T1-weighted magnetic resonance image with gadolinium of a pineal cyst. These cysts can have rim enhancement (*arrow*) and can be up to 3 cm in diameter. They rarely cause compression of the Sylvian aqueduct (*arrowhead* on patent aqueduct) and are rarely symptomatic. Histologically, they are normal variants of the pineal gland and must be distinguished from cystic tumors and require no treatment. Growth of the cyst on serial magnetic resonance images or the development of hydrocephalus is sufficient cause to doubt the diagnosis, and surgical resection should be considered.

SYMPTOMS

Pineal region tumors can become symptomatic by three mechanisms: increased intracranial pressure from hydrocephalus, direct brainstem and cerebellar compression, or endocrine dysfunction. Headache, associated with hydrocephalus, is the most common symptom at onset and is caused by obstruction of third ventricle outflow at the aqueduct of Sylvius (Table 57.4). More advanced hydrocephalus can result in papilledema, gait disorder, nausea, vomiting, lethargy, and memory disturbance. Direct midbrain compression can cause disorders of ocular movements such as Parinaud syndrome (paralysis of upgaze, convergence or retraction, nystagmus, and light-near pupillary dissociation) or the Sylvian aqueduct syndrome (paralysis of downgaze or horizontal gaze superimposed upon a Parinaud syndrome). Either lid retraction (Collier sign) or ptosis may follow dorsal midbrain compression or infiltration. Fourth nerve palsies with diplopia and head tilt may be seen. Reversibility is a clue to pathogenesis; eye signs due to hydrocephalus recede promptly after ventricular shunting. Ataxia and dysmetria can result from direct cerebellar compression.

Endocrine dysfunction is rare, usually arising from secondary effects of hydrocephalus or tumor spread to the hypothalamic region. Diabetes insipidus occurs in less than 5% of pineal tumors, usually with a germinoma (Fig. 57.2). The symptoms may occur early, before any radiographic documentation of hypothalamic seeding. Although precocious puberty has been linked historically with pineal masses, documented cases are rare. Precocious puberty is actually precocious pseudopuberty because the hypothalamic-gonadal axis is not mature. It occurs strictly in boys with choriocarcinomas or germinomas with syncytiotrophoblastic cells and ectopic secretion of β-hCG. In boys, the luteinizing hormonelike effects of β-hCG can stimulate Leydig cells to produce androgens that induce development of secondary sexual

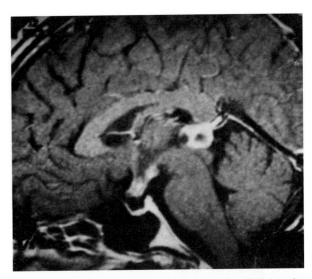

FIG. 57.2. Sagittal magnetic resonance image with gadolinium showing multicentric germinoma involving the pineal region and infiltrating the mammillary bodies, optic chiasm, and pituitary stalk. This patient presented with diminished visual fields and diabetes insipidus.

characteristics and pseudopuberty. This phenomenon does not occur in girls with pineal region tumors because GCTs are rare in females; also, and more important, both luteinizing hormone and follicle-stimulating hormone are necessary to trigger ovarian estrogen production.

DIAGNOSIS

Magnetic resonance imaging (MRI) is the principal diagnostic test for pineal region tumors. MRI with gadolinium enhancement is mandatory for all pineal tumors to determine the presence of hydrocephalus and to evaluate tumor size, vascularity, and homogeneity. In particular, sagittal MRI reveals the relationship of the tumor to surrounding structures as well as possible ventricular seeding (Fig. 57.3). Computed tomography is complementary but does not provide as much information as MRI. Angiography is not performed unless a vascular anomaly is suspected. Measurement of AFP and β-hCG in serum and CSF is routine in the preoperative workup. If β-hCG or AFP levels are elevated, malignant germ cell elements are present even if histologic examination gives a benign impression, because a small island of these cells in a large tumor may be overlooked. Despite improved imaging and CSF markers, a definite histologic diagnosis cannot be made without pathologic examination of tumor tissue.

SURGERY

Because of the wide variety of pineal region tumor subtypes, a histologic diagnosis is mandatory for optimal patient management (Fig. 57.4). The pineal region may be approached surgically from one of several variations, above or below the tentorium. Nearly one-third of pineal tumors are benign and curable with surgery alone. With malignant tumors, aggressive tumor resection provides the best opportunity for accurate histologic diagnosis and may increase the effectiveness of adjuvant radiother-

TABLE 57.4. PRESENTING SYMPTOMS AND SIGNS IN 100 CONSECUTIVE PATIENTS WITH PINEAL REGION TUMORS AT THE NEW YORK NEUROLOGICAL INSTITUTE

Symptoms	Number	Signs	Number
Headache	87	Parinauds' syndrome	75
Nausea/vomiting	32		
Gait unsteadiness	32	Ataxia	39
Diplopia	31	Papilledema	36
Blurred vision	19	Normal exam	12
Memory impairment	16	4th nerve palsy	5
Lethargy	11	Obtundation	4
Altered consciousness	9	6th nerve palsy	3
Personality change	9	Spasticity	3
Visual obscurations	4	Visual field deficit	1
Syncope	3		
Polyuria/polydipsia	3	Psychomotor retardation	1
Seizures	3		
Tremor	3		
Neck stiffness	2		
Numbness	2		
Developmental delay	2		
Incontinence	2		
Precocious puberty	1		
Rigidity	1		
Amenorrhea	1		
Subarachnoid hemorrhage	1		

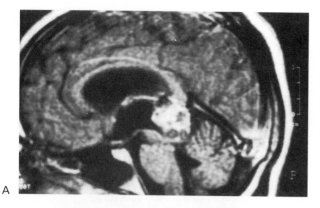

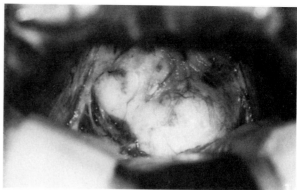

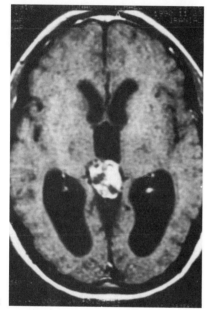

FIG. 57.3. Sagittal **(A)** and axial **(B)** magnetic resonance images with gadolinium of a mixed dermoid/germinoma causing hydrocephalus. **C:** Intraoperative photograph shows the tumor, which was completely resected through a supracerebellar-infratentorial approach without neurologic deficits (cerebellum is at the bottom of the photograph covered by a retractor). **D and E:** Histologic analysis revealed a mixed dermoid/germinoma.

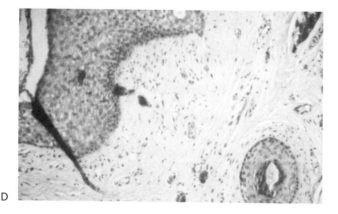

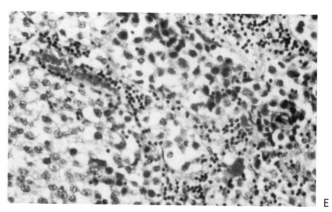

apy or chemotherapy. The overall operative mortality is about 4%, with an additional 3% permanent major morbidity. The most serious complication of surgery is hemorrhage into a partially resected malignant tumor. The most common postoperative complications are ocular palsies, altered mental status, and ataxia; all are usually transient. For patients with obviously disseminated tumor or those with medical problems that pose excessive surgical risks, stereotactic biopsy is a reasonable alternative for obtaining diagnostic tissue. Although gaining in popularity, stereotactic biopsy is not performed routinely for

these reasons: increased sampling error through insufficient tissue analysis, increased risk of hemorrhage from adjacent deep venous system and highly vascular pineal tumors, and the better prognosis that follows aggressive resection.

POSTOPERATIVE STAGING

All patients with pineal cell tumors, malignant GCTs, and ependymomas are thoroughly evaluated for CSF seeding even

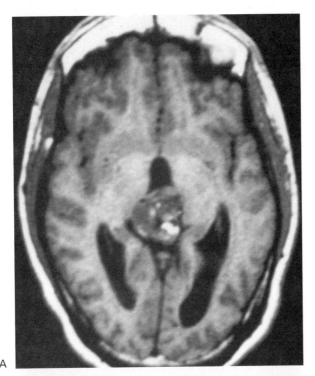

A

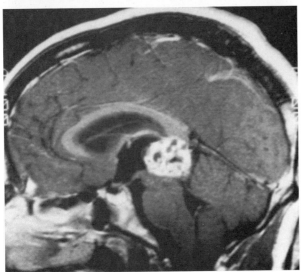

B

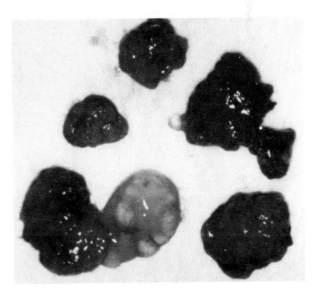

C

FIG. 57.4. Axial **(A)** and sagittal **(B)** magnetic resonance images with gadolinium of a heterogeneously enhancing pineal region tumor. The tumor comprised several germ cell elements, including immature teratoma, germinoma, endodermal sinus tumor, and embryonal cell carcinoma **(C)**. Pineal region tumors can be extremely heterogeneous, and extensive tumor sampling is necessary to avoid diagnostic errors.

though this is a rare occurrence (Fig. 57.5). High-resolution MRI is more sensitive than computed tomography myelography. CSF cytology is not reliable in predicting seeding.

RADIATION THERAPY

Radiation therapy consists of 4,000 cGy to the whole brain with an additional 1,500 cGy to the pineal region; it is recommended for all patients with malignant pineal region tumors. Spinal radiation is not recommended unless there is radiographic documentation of spinal seeding.

Radiosurgery for pineal tumors is promising, but experience is limited. It could be most useful for malignant pineal cell tumors and other small malignant tumors (less than 3 cm in diam-

eter), particularly if combined with fractionated radiation. It may also be helpful for tumors that recur after radiation therapy. Germinomas historically have had an excellent response to external fractionated radiotherapy, and radiosurgery seems unlikely to improve upon those results.

CHEMOTHERAPY

Chemotherapy has been of most benefit with nongerminomatous malignant GCTs. The most commonly used regimens are combinations of cisplatin, vinblastine, and bleomycin or cisplatin and VP-16 (etoposide), which are usually given before radiation therapy. The results of chemotherapy alone may be comparable with those of radiation therapy for pure germino-

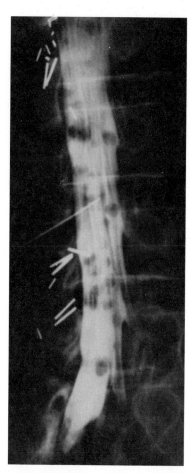

FIG. 57.5. Intradural seeding from a pineal tumor. Lumbar myelography, oblique view, demonstrates intradural filling defects studding the lumbar nerve roots. These represent "drop" metastases. (Courtesy of Drs. J.A. Bello and S.K. Hilal.)

mas. There has been a trend to reduce radiation dosage because of long-term neurotoxicity by combining it with chemotherapy.

LONG-TERM OUTCOME

Generally, benign pineal tumors are curable with surgery alone. Among malignant tumors, the prognosis depends on the tumor histology (Table 57.1). Germinomas have a 75% to 80% 5-year survival with combined surgery and radiotherapy. Patients with a nongerminomatous malignant GCT rarely survive beyond 2 years, but this may improve with better chemotherapy. About one-third of astrocytomas are cystic tumors and are cured by surgery alone. Solid astrocytomas behave clinically like other brainstem gliomas and have a 67% 5-year survival rate. Radiation therapy is usually recommended for these tumors, but any effect on survival is difficult to evaluate. Among pineal cell tumors, a few are discrete, histologically benign, and completely resectable. Most malignant pineal cell tumors, however, are not resectable and have a 55% 5-year survival rate with surgery and radiation.

SUGGESTED READINGS

Allen JC, Nisselbaum J, Epstein F, Rosen G, Schwartz MK. Alphafetoprotein and human chorionic gonadotropin determination in cerebrospinal fluid. *J Neurosurg* 1979;51:368–374.

Bjornsson J, Scheithauer BW, Okazaki H, Leech RW. Intracranial germ cell tumors: pathobiological and immunohistological aspects of 70 cases. *J Neuropathol Exp Neurol* 1985;44:32–46.

Bruce J. Management of pineal region tumors. *Neurosurg Q* 1993;3:103–119.

Bruce JN, Connolly ES, Stein BM. Pineal and germ cell tumors. In: Kaye AH, Laws ER, ed. *Brain tumors*. London: Churchill Livingstone, 1995:725–755.

Bruce JN, Fetell MR, Balmaceda CM, Stein BM. Tumors of the pineal region. In: Black PM, Loeffler JS, ed. *Cancer of the nervous system*. Malden, MA: Blackwell Science, 1996:576–592.

Bruce JN, Stein BM. Surgical management of pineal region tumors. *Acta Neurochir (Wien)* 1995;134:130–135.

Choi JU, Kim DS, Chung SS, Kim TS. Treatment of germ cell tumors in the pineal region. *Childs Nerv Syst* 1998;14:41–48.

Dandy WE. Operative experience of cases of pineal tumor. *Arch Surg* 1936;33:19–46.

Dattoli MJ, Newall J. Radiation therapy for intracranial germinoma: the case for limited volume treatment. *Int J Radiat Oncol Biol Phys* 1990;19:429–433.

Edwards MSB, Hudgins RJ, Wilson CB, Levin VA, Wara WM. Pineal region tumors in children. *J Neurosurg* 1988;68:689–697.

Fetell MR, Bruce JN, Burke AM, et al. Nonneoplastic pineal cysts. *Neurology* 1991;41:1034–1040.

Fetell MR, Stein BM. Neuroendocrine aspects of pineal tumors. *Neurol Clin* 1986;4:877–905.

Herrick MK, Rubinstein LJ. The cytological differentiating potential of pineal parenchymal neoplasms (true pinealomas). *Brain* 1979;102:289–320.

Herrmann HD, Westphal M, Winkler K, Laas RW, Schulte FJ. Treatment of nongerminomatous germ cell tumors of the pineal region. *Neurosurgery* 1994;34:524–529.

Hoffman HJ, Otsubo H, Hendrick EB, et al. Intracranial germ cell tumors in children. *J Neurosurg* 1991;74:545–551.

Jennings MT, Gelman R, Hochberg F. Intracranial germ cell tumors: natural history and pathogenesis. *J Neurosurg* 1985;63:155–167.

Kersh CR, Constable WC, Eisert DR, et al. Primary central nervous system germ cell tumors: effect of histologic confirmation on radiotherapy. *Cancer* 1988;61:2148–2152.

Kobayashi T, Yoshida J, Ishiyama J, Satoshi N, Kito A, Kida Y. Combination chemotherapy with cisplatin and etoposide for malignant intracranial germ cell tumors. *J Neurosurg* 1989;70:676–681.

Kreth F, Schatz C, Pagenstecher A, Faist M, Volk B, Ostertag C. Stereotactic management of lesions of the pineal region. *Neurosurgery* 1996;39:280–291.

Linstadt D, Wara WM, Edwards MS, Hudgins RJ, Sheline GE. Radiotherapy of primary intracranial germinomas: the case against routine craniospinal irradiation. *Int J Radiat Oncol Biol Phys* 1988;15:291–297.

Matsutani M, Sano K, Takakura K, et al. Primary intracranial germ cell tumors: a clinical analysis of 153 histologically verified cases. *J Neurosurg* 1997;86:446–455.

Patel SR, Buckner JC, Smithson WA, Scheithauer BW, Groover RV. Cisplatin-based chemotherapy in primary central nervous system germ cell tumors. *J Neurooncol* 1992;12:47–52.

Regis J, Bouillot P, Rouby-Volot F, Figarella-Branger D, Dufour H, Peragut J. Pineal region tumors and the role of stereotactic biopsy: review of the mortality, morbidity, and diagnostic rates in 370 cases. *Neurosurgery* 1996;39:907–914.

Robertson PL, DaRosso RC, Allen JC. Improved prognosis of intracranial nongerminoma germ cell tumors with multimodality therapy. *J Neurooncol* 1997; 32:71–80.

Rubinstein LJ. Cytogenesis and differentiation of pineal neoplasms. *Hum Pathol* 1980;12:441–448.

Sawamura Y, de Tribolet N, Ishii N, Abe H. Management of primary intracranial germinomas: diagnostic surgery or radical resection? *J Neurosurg* 1997;87:262–266.

Schild SE, Scheithauer BW, Schomberg PJ, et al. Pineal parenchymal tumors. Clinical, pathologic, and therapeutic aspects. *Cancer* 1993;72:870–880.

Stein BM, Bruce JN. Pineal region tumors. *Clin Neurosurg* 1992;39:509–532.

Sung D, Harisiadis L, Chang CH. Midline pineal tumors and suprasellar germinomas: highly curable by irradiation. *Radiology* 1978;128:745–751.

Tien RD, Barkovich AJ, Edwards MSB. MR imaging of pineal tumors. *AJNR* 1990;11:557–565.

Wolden SL, Wara WM, Larson DA, Prados MD, Edwards MS, Sneed PK. Radiation therapy for primary intracranial germ cell tumors. *Int J Radiat Oncol Biol Phys* 1995;32:943–949.

Yoshida J, Sugita K, Kobayashi T, et al. Prognosis of intracranial germ cell tumours: effectiveness of chemotherapy with cisplatin and etoposide (CDDP and VP-16). *Acta Neurochir* 1993;120:111–117.

Merritt's Neurology, 10th ed., edited by L.P. Rowland. Lippincott Williams & Wilkins, Philadelphia © 2000.

CHAPTER 58

TUMORS OF THE PITUITARY GLAND

JEFFREY N. BRUCE
MICHAEL R. FETELL
PAMELA U. FREDA

The true incidence of pituitary adenomas is difficult to ascertain because they are often asymptomatic; autopsy estimates range from 2.7% to 27%. There is no sexual predilection, but the tumors are most common in adults, peaking in the third and fourth decades; children and adolescents account for about 10%. These tumors are not hereditary except for rare families with multiple endocrine neoplasia, an autosomal dominant trait, manifested by a high incidence of pituitary adenomas and tumors of other endocrine glands.

PATHOLOGY

In the past, pituitary adenomas were classified by a now-obsolete system that identified them as acidophilic, basophilic, or chromophobic as determined by staining characteristics with hematoxylin and eosin. Growth hormone-secreting tumors were acidophilic adenomas, adrenocorticotropic hormone-secreting tumors were basophilic adenomas, and chromophobic adenomas were thought to be nonsecretory. With improved immunohistochemistry, pituitary hormone secretion was detected within an adenoma, making it clear that the traditional histologic dyes are unreliable guides. The modern functional classification is based on endocrinologic activity, dividing tumors into secreting and nonsecreting types. Secreting tumors are less common and produce one or more anterior pituitary hormones, including prolactin (the most common endocrinologically active tumor), growth hormone, adrenocorticotropic hormone, follicle-stimulating hormone, or luteinizing hormone. Mixed secretory tumors account for 10% of adenomas, and secretion of more than one hormone has implications for medical therapy. Some tumors secrete the alpha subunit of the large precursor molecules that

form one of the polypeptide chains of glycoprotein hormones, even if the tumor is nonfunctional. "Null cell" adenomas or nonsecreting adenomas demonstrate no clinical or immunohistochemical evidence of hormone secretion.

For clinical purposes, pituitary adenomas are arbitrarily divided by size into *microadenomas* (less than 1.0 cm in diameter) or *macroadenomas* (more than 1.0 cm in diameter). When tumors erode the dura or bone, they are considered invasive and may infiltrate surrounding structures such as the cavernous sinus, cranial nerves, blood vessels, sphenoid bone, and sinus or brain. Locally invasive pituitary adenomas are nearly always histologically benign. Different staging systems have been based on degrees of invasion or extent, characteristics that are useful for prognosis and treatment (Table 58.1).

Pituitary carcinomas are extremely rare. They are highly invasive, rapidly growing, and anaplastic, but unequivocal diagnosis relies on the presence of distant metastases. Histologic appearance of pleomorphism and mitotic figures is insufficient to justify the diagnosis of carcinoma.

The posterior pituitary, which contains the terminal processes of hypothalamic neurons and supporting glial cells, is a rare site of neoplasia. *Infundibulomas* are rare tumors of the neurohypophysis; they are variants of pilocytic astrocytomas. *Granular cell tumors* (*myoblastomas* or *choristomas*), also rare tumors of the neurohypophysis, are of uncertain origin.

TABLE 58.1. SUMMARY OF STAGING SYSTEMS FOR PITUITARY ADENOMAS

Grading system (Hardy and Vezina) based on radiologic characteristics
    Grade I—microadenoma, remaining completely within the sella
    Grade II—adenoma greater than 1cm, with expansion of the sellar floor but without perforating the floor
    Grade III—perforation through the dura, with extension into the sphenoid sinus
    Grade IV—diffuse infiltration of the sphenoid sinus and bone
    Grade V—spread through the *cerebrospinal fluid* pathways
Grading system (Wilson) based on extrasellar extension
    Stage 0—no suprasellar extension
    Stage A—extension into suprasellar cistern only
    Stage B—extension into anterior recess of third ventricle
    Stage C—obliteration of anterior recess and deformation of floor of third ventricle
    Stage D—intradural extension into anterior, middle, or posterior fossa
    Stage E—extradural invasion into cavernous sinus

From Hardy J, Vezina JL. Transphenoidal neurosurgery of intracranial neoplasm. *Adv Neurol* 1976; 15:261–274; and Wilson CB, 1984.

Histologically, adenomas lose the typical acinar structure of the normal gland and may contain follicular, trabecular, or cystic portions or components growing as a diffuse sheet. Microscopically, the cells are arranged in a syncytial or sinusoidal pattern. Tumors often show small foci of hemorrhage or necrosis but usually no mitotic activity. Pituitary adenomas lack a discrete capsule, but the presence of a pseudocapsule facilitates surgical separation from adjacent normal glands.

CLINICAL FEATURES

Clinical manifestations stem from either endocrine dysfunction or mass effect with invasion or compression of surrounding neural and vascular structures. The manifestations and management of hormonally active tumors are discussed in Chapter 146. Here, we limit discussion to nonsecretory tumors. Mass effects include headache, hypopituitarism, and visual loss. Headaches result from stretching of the diaphragm sella and adjacent dural structures that transmit sensation through the first branch of the trigeminal nerve. Visual loss may be accompanied by optic disc pallor, loss of central visual acuity, and visual field defects, but papilledema is rare. Visual field abnormalities are caused by compression of the crossing fibers in the optic chiasm, first affecting the superior temporal quadrants and then the inferior temporal quadrants. Further expansion compromises the noncrossing fibers and affects the lower nasal quadrants and finally the upper nasal quadrants (Fig. 58.1). Patients usually note blurring or dimming of vision. Formal visual field testing is important because some tumors affect only the macular fibers to cause central hemianopic scotomas that may be missed on routine screening. Although bitemporal hemianopia is most common, any pattern of visual loss is possible, including unilateral or homonymous hemianopia.

Lateral extension of the tumor with compression or invasion of the cavernous sinus can compromise III, IV, or VI cranial nerve functions, manifesting as diplopia. The third cranial nerve is most commonly affected. There may be numbness in the V1 or V2 distribution. Overall, however, cranial nerve dysfunction is not a common feature of adenomas and may be more suggestive of other neoplasms of the cavernous sinus.

Adenomas may become enormous. Suprasellar extension may compress the foramen of Monro to cause hydrocephalus and symptoms of increased intracranial pressure. Hypothalamic dysfunction may be expressed as diabetes insipidus, although diabetes insipidus is relatively rare with adenomas and, if present, is more suggestive of conditions associated with inflammation or tumor invasion of the pituitary stalk. Extensive subfrontal extension with compression of both frontal lobes may cause personality changes or dementia. There may be seizures or motor and sensory dysfunction. Erosion of the skull base may cause cerebrospinal fluid (CSF) rhinorrhea.

Complete endocrine evaluation is necessary for all patients with pituitary tumors, not only to make the diagnosis of a secreting adenoma but also to determine the presence of hypopituitarism. Hypopituitarism may result from compression of the normal pituitary gland or blood supply; adequate replacement and long-term follow-up are then needed. Hormonal replacement most commonly includes thyroid and adrenal hormones. Nonsecreting tumors may be associated with slight elevations of serum prolactin levels to 100 mg/mL, which is attributed to compression of the pituitary stalk, interrupting dopaminergic fibers that inhibit prolactin release. Mild elevations are common and must be distinguished from prolactin-secreting tumors because bromocriptine has little or no effect on nonsecretory tumors.

In about 5% of pituitary tumors, the first symptoms are those of "pituitary apoplexy" due to hemorrhage or infarction of the adenoma. Symptoms include sudden onset of severe headache, oculomotor palsies, nausea, vomiting, altered mental state, diplopia, and rapidly progressive visual loss. Apoplexy is diagnosed by computed tomography or magnetic resonance imaging (MRI) and is usually an indication for emergency surgery (Fig. 58.2). Histologically, hematoxylin and eosin stains show massive necrosis of the adenoma.

Pituitary adenomas may enlarge during pregnancy. Sometimes pregnancy is induced in a woman treated for infertility problems with an unrecognized pituitary adenoma.

RADIOGRAPHIC FEATURES

MRI is the best way to evaluate pituitary pathology, because soft tissue is identified without interference from the bony surround-

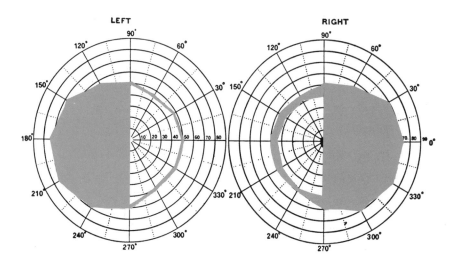

FIG. 58.1. Pituitary macroadenoma. Bitemporal hemianopia; visual acuity O.D. 15/200, O.S. 15/30. The blind half-fields are black. (Courtesy of Dr. Max Chamlin.)

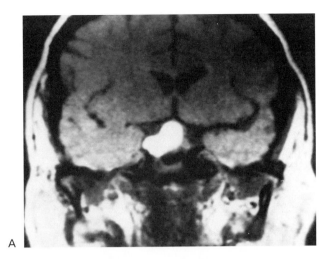 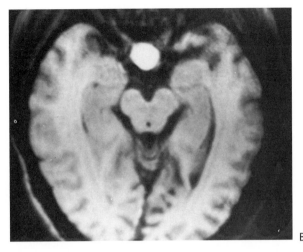

FIG. 58.2. Coronal **(A)** and axial **(B)** magnetic resonance images demonstrating a high signal pituitary mass that turned out to be a hemorrhage in a patient with apoplexy. This patient underwent a successful tumor resection through a standard transsphenoidal approach.

ings of the sella; MRI also produces images in any plane. Vascular structures such as the adjacent carotid artery are easily visualized by signal void. Normally, the anterior lobe of the pituitary gland has the same signal as white matter on T1-weighted imaging. With gadolinium, the normal gland enhances homogeneously. Small punctate areas of heterogeneity may be due to local variations in vascularity, microcyst formation, or granularity within the gland. The posterior lobe shows increased signal on T1-weighted images, probably representing neurosecretory granules in the antidiuretic hormone (ADH)–containing axons. The cavernous sinuses also enhance.

Microadenomas are sometimes difficult to see directly on MRI but may be inferred by glandular asymmetry, focal sellar erosion, asymmetric convexity of the upper margin of the gland, or displacement of the infundibulum (Fig. 58.3). The normal gland usually shows more enhancement than the microadenoma (Fig. 58.4). In the presence of a macroadenoma, the normal gland may not be visualized and the bright signal of the posterior lobe may be absent. Areas of increased signal on the T1-weighted image may be due to hemorrhage; areas of low signal may represent cystic degeneration. Although the cavernous sinus often appears expanded in the presence of a macroadenoma, it is difficult to distinguish invasion or compression from stretching of the cavernous sinus.

MRI alone is usually sufficient, but computed tomography may show the bony anatomy in better detail. MRI can usually exclude an aneurysm, but an angiogram is indicated if uncertainty exists.

DIFFERENTIAL DIAGNOSIS

Most lesions in the differential diagnosis have characteristic radiographic or clinical syndromes that distinguish them from pituitary adenoma. Craniopharyngiomas have a predilection for children, are calcified, and usually contain cystic areas that contain highly proteinaceous fluid with cholesterol crystals. Rathke

cleft cysts are similar to craniopharyngiomas but have a cystic appearance without any solid component. Meningiomas are commonly found in the diaphragm sella, planum sphenoidale, and tuberculum sella and may be difficult to distinguish from a macroadenoma. Distinguishing characteristics of meningiomas include enhancement, visualization of a cleavage plane between the mass and the sellar contents, normally sized sella, and the presence of a dural "tail" of enhancement. Optic glioma, hypothalamic glioma, germinoma, dermoid tumor, metastasis, and nasopharyngeal carcinoma are less common entities to be considered. Chordomas characteristically show extensive clival bony destruction. Mucoceles of the sphenoid sinus may simulate pituitary adenoma. Visual symptoms and sellar enlargement may also result from chronic increased intracranial pressure of any origin. Characteristic signal voids on MRI usually distinguish an aneurysm. Differential diagnosis also includes sarcoidosis, lymphoma, lymphocytic hypophysitis, and other granulomatous diseases.

Herniation of the subarachnoid space into the sella through an incompetent diaphragm sella may produce the empty-sella syndrome with enlargement of the sella and flattening of the pituitary gland on the floor (Fig. 58.5). This syndrome may be associated with pseudotumor cerebri or CSF rhinorrhea. Although most are not symptomatic, an empty sella may be associated with headaches and, occasionally, mild hypopituitarism, but the visual fields are usually normal. The condition is readily seen on MRI and may follow previous transsphenoidal surgery.

TREATMENT

Treatment of pituitary adenomas begins with the correction of electrolyte dysfunction and replacement of pituitary hormones, if necessary, immediately after diagnostic blood specimens have been sent. Replacement of thyroid or adrenal hormones is of particular importance. Steroid replacement must be adequate for stressful situations, including the perioperative period.

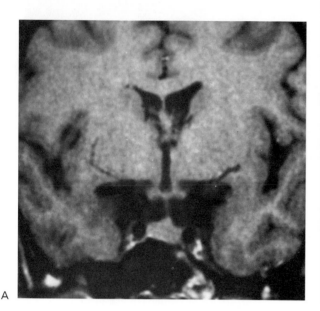

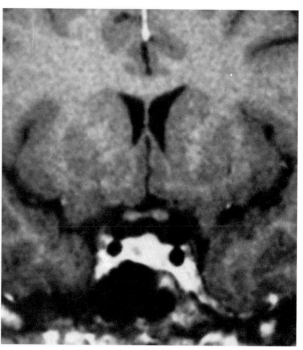

FIG. 58.3. Pituitary microadenoma. **A:** T1-weighted coronal magnetic resonance (MR) scan shows slight tilting of the pituitary stalk to the left, with questionable fullness of the right pituitary gland. These are secondary signs of pituitary microadenoma but are not sufficient to clinch the diagnosis radiographically. **B:** T1-weighted coronal MR scan after gadolinium enhancement demonstrates a tiny focus of relative hypointensity within the right pituitary gland. This is consistent with right-sided pituitary microadenoma. (Courtesy of Dr. S. Chan.)

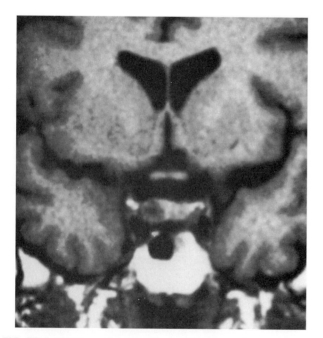

FIG. 58.4. Pituitary adenoma. T1-weighted coronal magnetic resonance scan after gadolinium enhancement demonstrates a discrete focus of hypointensity in the right pituitary gland, most consistent with pituitary adenoma. (Courtesy of Dr. S. Chan.)

The goals of treatment differ according to the functional activity of the tumor. For endocrinologically active tumors, an aggressive approach toward reversing hypersecretion is essential while preserving normal pituitary function. This can usually be achieved by surgical excision, although prolactinomas are better controlled medically by giving dopamine agonists that achieve tumor shrinkage in 75% to 80% of patients (Fig. 58.6). Candidates for surgical treatment include patients with prolactinomas that fail to respond medically or those who cannot tolerate the side effects of medication. The treatment strategies for secretory adenomas are covered in detail in Chapter 146.

Nonsecreting tumors are best treated by surgical reduction of the mass but maintaining pituitary function. Although complete surgical resection is desired, the radiosensitivity of these tumors invites subtotal debulking followed by radiation therapy to reduce the risk of recurrence or progression.

Incidentally discovered asymptomatic adenomas require no intervention but should be followed with periodic visual field examination and MRI. Onset of symptoms or MRI documentation of growth are indications for treatment.

Surgery

The efficacy and safety of the transsphenoidal approach make it the procedure of choice for the removal of adenomas. Most tumors are soft and friable; transsphenoidal access, although limited, permits complete removal even if there is suprasellar extension or the sella is not enlarged. Transsphenoidal surgery was originally developed by Cushing and popularized by others, es-

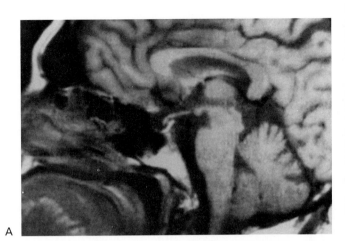

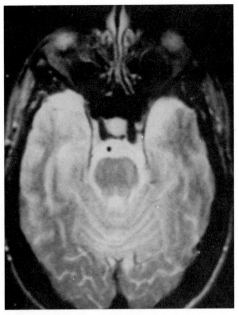

FIG. 58.5. Empty sella. **A:** Sagittal T1-weighted magnetic resonance (MR) scan demonstrates low-intensity intrasellar signal representing cerebrospinal fluid (CSF; compare with signal within the fourth ventricle). **B:** Axial T2-weighted MR scan on a different patient shows increased signal within the sella representing CSF on this pulse sequence (compare with signal from incidentally noted anterior temporal arachnoid cysts). (Courtesy of Drs. J.A. Bello and S.K. Hilal.)

pecially Hardy (1971). Refinements in microsurgery and the availability of steroid replacement and antibiotics have dramatically improved the results. Mortality rates are less than 1%. Major morbidity is less than 3.5%, including stroke, visual loss, meningitis, CSF leak, or cranial nerve palsy. Permanent diabetes insipidus appears after surgery in 25% of patients and is treated by replacement.

A transcranial approach may be preferred for tumors extending into the middle fossa or if there is suprasellar growth through an intact diaphragm sella, with a waistband constriction of the

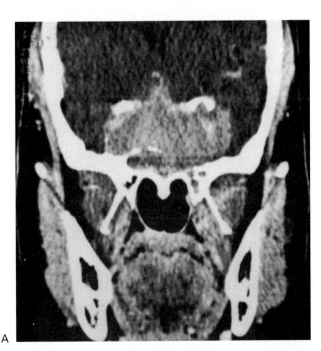

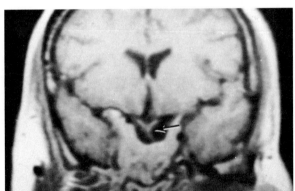

FIG. 58.6. **A:** Coronal computed tomography with contrast from a 40-year-old man with bitemporal hemianopsia and a markedly elevated serum prolactin level. A large pituitary adenoma with suprasellar and parasellar extension can be easily seen. **B:** Coronal magnetic resonance scan with contrast after bromocriptine therapy shows marked decrease in the tumor size such that the infundibulum and optic chiasm are decompressed (*arrow*).

tumor (Fig. 58.7). A transcranial approach may be necessary to decompress the optic structures before radiation when a transsphenoidal approach fails to adequately debulk the tumor and there is persistent major visual loss.

Radiation Therapy

Radiation therapy is complementary to surgery in preventing progression or recurrence. Standard radiation uses three fields (parallel opposed fields with a coronal field) or rotational techniques to avoid unnecessary dosage of the temporal lobes. Dosages of 4,500 to 5,000 cGy delivered in 180-cGy fractions are recommended. Radiation may be the only treatment for patients who are poor operative risks, but histologic confirmation is generally desired. Radiation therapy is usually not the initial

treatment for hormonally active tumors because it rarely lowers hormone levels to normal and then only after a delay of months or years.

In general, patients with subtotally resected tumors are given radiation therapy. Although radiation reduces the risk of recurrence or delays recurrence of gross total resection, we follow these patients with serial MR images and visual field examination and withhold radiation unless there is documented tumor regrowth.

Early complications of radiation therapy are transient and involve minor inconvenience such as epilation, dry mouth, and altered taste or smell. The most common and important delayed complication is hypopituitarism, which may occur any time from 6 months to 10 years after treatment. Some degree of hypopituitarism occurs in 30% to 50% of patients. Annual endocrine evaluation is necessary to treat this appropriately. Other

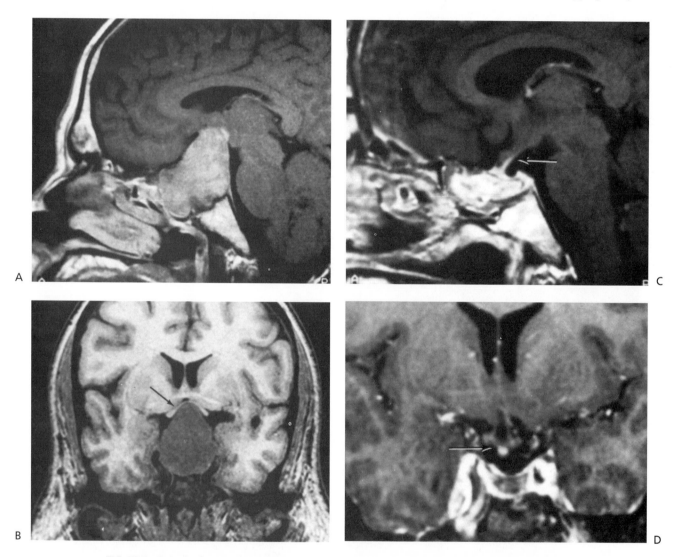

FIG. 58.7. A: Sagittal magnetic resonance (MR) scan showing a large pituitary adenoma filling the sphenoid sinus and extending into the floor of the third ventricle. **B:** On the coronal view, the suprasellar component can be seen compressing the optic chiasm (*arrow*). A large tumor such as this often requires a craniotomy to decompress the optic structures adequately. **C:** Sagittal MR scan after a gross total resection of the pituitary adenoma through an extended frontal craniotomy. There are postoperative changes in the sella and sphenoid sinus, and the infundibulum is well decompressed (*arrow*). **D:** On the coronal view, there is no residual tumor, and the optic chiasm and a portion of the infundibulum can be clearly seen (*arrow*).

rare complications include visual loss, radiation necrosis of the temporal lobes, and radiation-induced tumors. To minimize risk of visual loss, optic structures should be decompressed before radiation therapy.

New techniques such as focused beam therapy with proton beams, gamma knife, or linear accelerator are being investigated. In these methods, a single high-dose fraction is directed to a limited volume, giving a biologic effect that differs from fractionated radiotherapy. Although these methods may produce adequate tumor control, there is concern about damage to critical structures in the optic chiasm or even cranial nerves; there may be a higher incidence of hypopituitarism. Intrasellar implantation of radioactive isotopes is also being evaluated.

Recurrent Tumors

Patients with recurrent tumors are management challenges. Treatment must be individualized. If the patient has not had prior radiation, then radiation would be the treatment of choice. Otherwise, repeat transsphenoidal surgery is usually indicated. Other treatment options include additional salvage radiation or some form of stereotactic radiation.

SUGGESTED READINGS

Arafa BM. Reversible hypopituitarism in patients with large nonfunctioning pituitary adenomas. *J Clin Endocrinol Metab* 1986;62:1173–1179.

Barrow DL, Mizuno J, Tindall GT. Management of prolactinomas associated with very high serum prolactin levels. *J Neurosurg* 1988;68:554–559.

Bills DC, Meyer FB, Laws ER Jr, et al. A retrospective analysis of pituitary apoplexy. *Neurosurgery* 1993;33:602–609.

Black PM, Hsu DW, Klibanski A, et al. Hormone production in clinically nonfunctioning pituitary adenomas. *J Neurosurg* 1987;66:244–250.

Bradley KM, Adams CBT, Potter CPS, Wheeler DW, Anslow PJ, Burke CW. An audit of selected patients with nonfunctioning pituitary adenoma treated by transsphenoidal surgery without irradiation. *Clin Endocrinol* 1994;41:655–659.

Breen P, Flickinger JC, Kondziolka D, Martinez AJ. Radiotherapy for nonfunctional pituitary adenoma: analysis of long-term tumor control. *J Neurosurg* 1998;89:933–938.

Ciric I, Mikhael M, Stafford T, et al. Transsphenoidal microsurgery of pituitary macroadenomas with long-term follow-up results. *J Neurosurg* 1984;59:395–401.

Cohen AR, Cooper PR, Kupersmith MJ, Flamm ES, Ransohoff J. Visual recovery after transsphenoidal removal of pituitary adenomas. *Neurosurgery* 1985;17:446–452.

Ebersold MJ, Laws ER, Scheithauer BW, Randall RV. Pituitary apoplexy treated by transsphenoidal surgery. A clinicopathological and immunocytochemical study. *J Neurosurg* 1983;58:315–320.

Hall WA, Luciano MG, Doppman JL, Patronas NJ, Oldfield EH. Pituitary magnetic resonance imaging in normal human volunteers: occult adenomas in the general population. *Ann Intern Med* 1994;120:817–820.

Hardy J. Transsphenoidal hypophysectomy. *J Neurosurg* 1971;34:582–594.

Harris JR, Levene MB. Visual complications following irradiation for pituitary adenomas and craniopharyngiomas. *Radiology* 1976;120:167–171.

Laws ERJ, Trautman JC, Hollenhorst RWJ. Transsphenoidal decompression of the optic nerve and chiasm: visual results in 62 patients. *J Neurosurg* 1977;46:717–722.

McDonald WI. The symptomatology of tumors of the anterior visual pathways. *Can J Neurol Sci* 1982;9:381–390.

Mukai K. Pituitary adenomas: immunocytochemical study of 150 tumors with clinicopathologic correlation. *Cancer* 1983;52:648–653.

Newton DR, Dillon WP, Norman D, et al. Gd-DTPA-enhanced MR imaging of pituitary adenomas. *AJNR* 1989;10:949–954.

Nichols DA, Laws ERJ, Houser OW, et al. Comparison of magnetic resonance imaging and computed tomography in the preoperative evaluation of pituitary adenomas. *Neurosurgery* 1988;22:380–385.

Nishizawa S, Ohta S, Yokoyama T, Uemura K. Therapeutic strategy for incidentally found pituitary tumors ("pituitary incidentalomas"). *Neurosurgery* 1998;43:1344–1350.

Ober KP, Kelly DL. Return of gonadal function with resection of nonfunctioning pituitary adenoma. *Neurosurgery* 1988;22:386–387.

Scheithauer BW, Kovacs KT, Laws EWJ, et al. Pathology of invasive pituitary tumors with special reference to functional classification. *J Neurosurg* 1986;65:733–744.

Steiner E, Imhof H, Knosp E. Gd-DTPA-enhanced high resolution MR imaging of pituitary adenomas. *Radiographics* 1989;9:587–598.

Symon L, Logue V, Mohanty S. Recurrence of pituitary adenomas after transcranial operation. *J Neurol Neurosurg Psychiatry* 1982;45:780–785.

Tsang RW, Brierley JD, Panzarella T, Gospodarowicz MK, Sutcliffe SB, Simpson WJ. Radiation therapy for pituitary adenoma: treatment outcome and prognostic factors. *Int J Radiat Oncol Biol Phys* 1994;30:557–565.

Wilson CB. A decade of pituitary microsurgery. The Herbert Olivecrona Lecture. *J Neurosurg* 1984;61:814–833.

Wray SH. Neuroophthalmologic manifestations of pituitary and parasellar lesion. *Clin Neurosurg* 1977;24:86–117.

Merritt's Neurology, 10th ed., edited by L.P. Rowland. Lippincott Williams & Wilkins, Philadelphia © 2000.

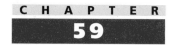

CONGENITAL AND CHILDHOOD CENTRAL NERVOUS SYSTEM TUMORS

JAMES H. GARVIN, JR.
NEIL A. FELDSTEIN

EPIDEMIOLOGY

Malignant and benign tumors of the central nervous system (CNS) may occur at any time in infancy and childhood. Astrocytomas are the largest group, mostly of low-grade histology. Next are medulloblastomas, the most frequent malignant tumor. After these are congenital and acquired lesions, a diverse group that includes craniopharyngiomas, ependymomas, choroid plexus tumors, teratomas, and other germ cell tumors. Apart from occasional high-grade astrocytomas, the usual tumors of adults (glioblastoma multiforme, anaplastic astrocytoma, meningioma, oligodendroglioma, pituitary adenoma) are rarely seen. CNS metastases from solid tumors are also uncommon in children compared with adults.

Primary CNS tumors account for 20% of all childhood cancers, second only to leukemia. Approximately 2,200 cases are diagnosed annually in the United States in children under age 15 years, an incidence of 2.8 per 100,000. The reported incidence of childhood brain tumors in the United States increased by 35% between 1973 and 1994, due mainly to increased numbers of supratentorial low-grade gliomas and brainstem tumors diagnosed annually starting in the mid-1980s. This is probably related to the introduction and rapid dissemination of magnetic resonance imaging (MRI) at that time and the fact that MRI is considerably more sensitive than computed tomography (CT) for detection of focal low-grade tumors of the cerebrum and brainstem.

The causes of congenital and childhood CNS tumors remain unknown. There is a slight male preponderance. Most CNS tumors are sporadic, but some are seen in association with inherited genetic disorders. Children with neurocutaneous syndromes are at increased risk. For example, individuals with *neurofibromatosis type 1* (NF-1) have a 10% chance of developing an intracranial tumor, and in childhood these may include optic pathway gliomas and astrocytomas elsewhere in the brain and spinal cord. The *NF1* gene maps to chromosome 17q11.2, so it is of interest that allelic loss on chromosome 17q occurs in one-fourth of pilocytic astrocytomas, suggesting the presence of a tumor suppressor gene. In the less common *neurofibromatosis type 2*, there is a predisposition to bilateral vestibular schwannomas, which exhibit chromosome 22q deletion and *NF2* gene mutations in at least half of cases. *NF2* also predisposes to ependymomas, which commonly show chromosome 22q deletion, but analysis of the *NF2* gene in ependymomas has revealed only a single mutation in a tumor that had lost the remaining wild-type allele.

Children with *tuberous sclerosis* may develop subependymal giant cell astrocytoma or occasionally ependymoma. Linkage studies have identified tuberous sclerosis genes on chromosomes 9q and 16p; allelic loss of 9q and 16p loci has been demonstrated in some subendymal giant cell astrocytomas, suggesting a tumor suppressor function. In the *epidermal nevus syndrome*, there is an increased risk of astrocytomas and primitive neuroectodermal tumors (PNETs). Hemangioblastomas of the cerebellum, medulla, and spinal cord are associated with *von Hippel-Lindau disease*, and choroid plexus tumors have occasionally been reported. Loss of chromosome 3p sequences has been described in one choroid plexus tumor, suggesting involvement of the VHL gene.

Combined cytogenetic and molecular studies of the common sporadic childhood brain tumors have identified certain genomic alterations that may also lead to the identification of genes contributing to tumorigenesis. For example, isochromosome 17q is found in approximately half of medulloblastomas (PNETs), suggesting the presence of a tumor suppressor gene.

Environmental risk factors for the development of CNS tumors include exposure to ionizing radiation. In children treated for acute lymphoblastic leukemia, there was a 1.39% cumulative incidence of secondary brain tumors (gliomas and meningiomas) at 20 years, and cranial irradiation was a dose-dependent predisposing factor. There is inconclusive evidence for any risk associated with electromagnetic fields (from electric blankets or other residential exposure). Several studies have shown an association between farm and animal exposures and childhood brain tumors, but dietary exposure to N-nitroso compounds, implicated in animal studies of brain tumor causation, was not a risk factor in young children. Maternal intake of folic acid in pregnancy may be protective against the development of PNETs, and a study in England found that the incidence of medulloblastoma declined after 1984, when multivitamin supplementation in pregnancy became widespread after reports that multivitamins with folate reduced the risk of neural tube defects.

SYMPTOMS

Children with brain tumors most often present with symptoms and signs of increased intracranial pressure. This results from obstruction of normal cerebrospinal fluid (CSF) pathways, leading to ventriculomegaly, and secondarily from direct mass effect of bulky tumors. Characteristic signs are headache, vomiting, and diplopia, but the onset may be gradual and nonfocal. Fatigue, personality change, or worsening school performance may be described. Symptoms in infants are particularly nonspecific and may include irritability, anorexia, persistent vomiting, and developmental delay or regression, with macrocephaly and seemingly forced downward deviation of the eyes ("sunsetting sign"). Persistent vomiting, recurrent headache (awakening the child from sleep), neurologic findings (ataxia, head tilt, vision loss, papilledema), endocrine disturbance (growth deceleration, diabetes insipidus), and stigmata of neurofibromatosis should all prompt further evaluation for the presence of a CNS tumor.

Symptoms and signs reflect tumor location, and in children (unlike adults), CNS tumors are divided about equally between supratentorial and infratentorial sites (Table 59.1). *Supratentorial tumors*, which predominate in infants and toddlers and also occur in older children, cause headache, motor weakness, sensory loss, and occasionally seizures, deteriorating school performance, or personality change. Frontal lobe tumors affect personality and movement. Temporal lobe tumors may cause partial complex seizures or fluent aphasias. The incidence of underlying neoplasm in children with intractable epilepsy approaches 20%, and the increased risk of having a brain tumor is noted even 10 or more years after a diagnosis of epilepsy. Parietal lobe tumors affect reading ability and awareness of contralateral extremities (hemineglect). Occipital lobe tumors cause visual field disturbance and occasionally hallucinations. Suprasellar lesions may cause both visual field defects and endocrine dysfunction. Parinaud syndrome (upgaze paresis and mild pupil dilatation with better reaction to accommodation than light, retraction or convergence nystagmus, and lid retraction) is specifically found in patients with pineal region tumors.

Infratentorial tumors, which predominate from ages 4 to 11 years, typically present with headache, vomiting, diplopia, and imbalance. Bilateral sixth cranial nerve palsy is a frequent sign of increased intracranial pressure. Brainstem tumors present with facial and extraocular muscle palsies, ataxia, and hemiparesis. Leptomeningeal spread occurs at diagnosis or recurrence in up to 15% of children with CNS tumors (more often in medulloblastoma/PNET) and may be asymptomatic or cause pain, irritability, weakness, or bowel and bladder dysfunction.

DIAGNOSIS AND MANAGEMENT

MRI is the preferred modality for imaging CNS tumors in the pediatric age group. Compared with CT, MRI is more sensitive (especially for nonenhancing infiltrative tumors and leptomeningeal involvement), can generate images in any plane (axial, coronal, sagittal), and is not compromised in the posterior fossa by bone artifact. Nonetheless, it can be difficult to distinguish tumor from surrounding edema or residual tumor from postoperative changes. MRI of the spine has replaced myelography as the standard procedure for evaluation of spinal cord le-

sions and leptomeningeal disease in cases of medulloblastoma, ependymoma, and pineal region tumors. Lumbar puncture for CSF cytology and tumor markers should be done in children with these diagnoses. Recommended baseline and surveillance studies, based on tumor aggressiveness and patterns of recurrence, are shown in Table 59.2. *Positron emission tomography* is potentially useful in characterizing metabolic abnormalities that could distinguish residual or recurrent tumor from cerebral necrosis. Thallium-201 single-photon emission CT may be more sensitive for recurrent tumors. Proton magnetic resonance spectroscopy offers similar capability and is more widely available.

The mainstay of therapy is *surgery*, which can be curative by itself in congenital and benign tumors. Gross total resection is generally also attempted in malignant tumors, with the exception of intrinsic brainstem tumors and lesions deep in diencephalic structures such as the thalamus. The introduction of the operating microscope and ultrasonic aspirator has improved both the safety and effectiveness of surgery. Stereotactic (CT or MRI guided) techniques are used increasingly for biopsy or subtotal resection in difficult areas such as the basal ganglia. However, even a 99% resection of a lesion that is 10 cm^3 in size will leave 10^8 tumor cells behind, and additional postoperative treatment will be necessary to prevent the lesion from regrowing. Surgery is important for establishing a tissue diagnosis and relieving obstructive hydrocephalus. With placement of an external drain or endoscopic third ventriculostomy followed by tumor resection, it may be possible to avoid the need for a permanent ventriculoperitoneal shunt in most patients. Operative mortality is generally not more than 1%, but morbidity varies according to the extent of surgery and condition of the child. Surgery may be facilitated by intraoperative monitoring of sensory and other evoked potentials. Adjunctive measures include the use of corticosteroids, which counteract tumor edema and are often used in the perioperative period but should be tapered within 1 to 2 weeks if possible. Patients undergoing surgery for supratentorial tumors are placed on anticonvulsants if they have had seizures or if the surgical approach is likely to cause seizures. Prophylactic anticonvulsants are generally continued for 3 to 12 months.

Radiation therapy is an important treatment for nearly all malignant CNS tumors and certain benign lesions as well. Standard

TABLE 59.1. LOCATION OF CENTRAL NERVOUS SYSTEMS TUMORS IN INFANTS, CHILDREN, AND ADOLESCENTS

Location	Infants	Children	Adolescents
Supratentorial	Teratoma	Cerebral astrocytoma	Cerebral astrocytoma
	Cerebral astrocytoma	Optic pathway or diencephalic glioma	Glioblastoma multiforme
	Choroid plexus tumor	Craniopharyngioma	Pineal germ cell tumor
	PNET (primitive neuroectodermal tumor)	Suprasellar germ cell tumor	Craniopharyngioma
	Craniopharyngioma	Ependymoma	Oligodendroglioma
	Optic glioma	Ganglioglioma	Meningioma
	Dermoid		Lymphoma
			Colloid cyst
Infratentorial	Medulloblastoma	Medulloblastoma	Medulloblastoma
	Ependymoma	Brainstem glioma	Cerebellar astrocytoma
	Astrocytoma	Ependymoma	Ependymoma
		Cerebellar astrocytoma	Epidermoid

TABLE 59.2. STAGING AND SURVEILLANCE OF CHILDREN WITH CENTRAL NERVIOUS SYSTEM TUMORS (21 MONTHS FROM END OF TREATMENT)

Tumor category	Baseline evaluation	Survelliance (mo)
Medulloblastoma/PNET High-grade astrocytoma Posterior fossa ependymoma Germ cell tumor/pineocytoma	Head/spine MR w/Gd CSF exam including cytology	Head 3, 6, 9, 12, 16, 20, 24, 30, 36, 48, 60, 84, 120 Spine 12, 24*, 36, 48* (*if residual or dissemination)
Brainstem glioma Supratentorial ependymoma Oligodendroglioma	Head/spine MR w/Gd CSF exam for ependymoma	Head 4, 8, 12, 16, 20, 24, 30*, 36, 48, 60, 84, 120 Spine 18*, 48* (*if residual or dissemination)
Cerebellar astrocytoma Supratentorial astrocytoma Hypothalamic/chiasmatic glioma Craniopharyngioma Choroid plexus papilloma	Head MR w/Gd CSF exam optional	Head 6, 12, 18*, 24, 36*, 48*, 60, 84, 120 (*if residual, and all craniopharyngioma)

PNET, primitive neuroectodermal tumor; MR, magnetic resonance; Gd, gadolinium; CSF, cerebrospinal fluid.
From Kramer ED, Vezine LG, Packer RJ, et al. Staging and surveillance of children with central nervous system neoplasms; recommendations of the Neurology and Tumor Imaging Committees of the Children's Cancer Group. *Pediatr Neurosurg* 1994;20:254–263.

doses used to achieve local control range from 45 to 55 Gy, in divided fractions of 150 to 200 cGy, to the tumor as localized on MR scan plus 1- to 2-cm margin. Higher doses can be given, often in smaller twice-daily doses ("hyperfractionated technique"), but with very high total doses there is increased risk of toxicity to the surrounding normal brain. The volume irradiated depends on tumor histology and may include an involved field or whole brain and spine. Presymptomatic craniospinal irradiation is almost always given for medulloblastoma, because of its propensity to disseminate throughout the neuraxis. Doses of 36 Gy have been used conventionally, but lower doses may be adequate if adjuvant chemotherapy is given.

Newer radiotherapy techniques may increase the effective tumor dose and limit toxicity to the surrounding brain. Stereotactic irradiation techniques in conjunction with rigid head fixation systems include single high-dose delivery ("radiosurgery"), fractionated convergence therapy, and three-dimensional conformal therapy. Interstitial radioactive implants (brachytherapy) may be appropriate in some cases. Alternative radiation sources such as neutron beam and the use of radiation sensitizers are also under study. Acute side effects of radiation therapy include headache, nausea, alopecia, skin hyperpigmentation and desquamation, and a transient "somnolence syndrome" occurring 4 to 8 weeks after treatment.

Chemotherapy is used increasingly as an adjunct to radiotherapy, as primary postsurgical treatment in infants, and in recurrent tumors. There is evidence that chemotherapy increases survival for children with medulloblastoma and high-grade astrocytoma (see below) and may be effective in delaying the need for radiotherapy in infants and young children with malignant CNS tumors. Effective agents include the nitrosoureas (carmustine, lomustine), vincristine, cisplatin, carboplatin, etoposide, and cyclophosphamide. Newer agents such as temozolomide appear promising. Chemotherapy is generally given systemically and in combination because of complementary mechanisms of action of different agents and to subvert potential tumor resistance. Regional delivery of drugs (intraarterial, intrathecal, intratumor), although potentially affording higher concentration within the tumor, has not yet been shown to be ef-

fective in childhood CNS tumors. The dose intensity of conventional systemic chemotherapy can be increased with the use of hematopoietic growth factors, which shorten the period of myelosuppression and permit use of higher doses and/or shorter intervals between treatments. A related approach is the use of extremely high doses of chemotherapy supported by autologous hematopoietic stem cell rescue for recurrent tumors or as an intensive consolidation therapy for infants.

CONGENITAL TUMORS

Craniopharyngiomas originate from rests of embryonic tissue located in the Rathke pouch, which later forms the anterior pituitary gland. They may appear clinically at any age, even later adulthood, and constitute 6% to 10% of intracranial tumors in children. They vary from small, well-circumscribed, solid nodules to huge multilocular cysts invading the sella turcica. The cysts are filled with turbid fluid that may contain cholesterin crystals. Craniopharyngiomas are histologically benign and may be categorized as mucoid epithelial cysts, squamous epitheliomas, or adamantinomas. Total surgical removal may be difficult because the tumor may invade the hypothalamus or third ventricle and adhere to optic nerves or blood vessels. Presenting signs may include short stature, hypothyroidism, and diabetes insipidus, with vision loss and signs of increased intracranial pressure. Although CT is useful for demonstrating calcification and bony expansion of the sella, MRI is preferred because of better definition of the tumor's relationship to vessels, optic chiasm and nerves, and the hypothalamus (Fig. 59.1). A conservative approach is to drain the cyst and resect nonadherent tumor and then administer radiation therapy to the involved area. Alternatively, gross total resection can be attempted, avoiding irradiation. Recurrence rates are similar (20% to 25%), and radical surgery is likely to be accompanied by panhypopituitarism necessitating lifelong hormonal replacement therapy, whereas irradiation has lesser hormonal sequelae but causes cognitive deficits, especially in younger children. Focused treatment by stereotactic radiosurgery ("gamma knife") may be advantageous in this regard.

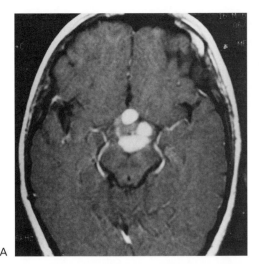 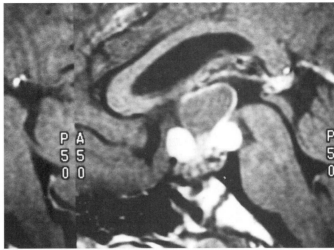

FIG. 59.1. Axial **(A)** and sagittal **(B)** magnetic resonance images of a craniopharyngioma.

Epidermoids (*cholesteatomas*) are the most common embryonal CNS tumors and account for about 2% of all intracranial tumors. They arise within skull tables or adjacent to the dura, usually in the suprasellar region, skull base, brainstem or cerebellopontine angle, or within a ventricle. They are encapsulated, have a pearly appearance, and may contain cyst fluid with cholesterol crystals. Clinical onset is usually in young adulthood, with variable rate of progression depending on location. MRI demonstrates a lesion with low T1-weighted signal intensity and high T2-weighted signal intensity (Fig. 59.2). Diffusion imaging can be helpful. Treatment is surgical resection.

Dermoid tumors are also cystic, and sebaceous gland secretions impart a dark yellow color to the cyst fluid. Intracranial dermoids are associated with Goldenhar syndrome (oculo-auriculo-vertebral dysplasia). Treatment is surgical resection.

Teratomas occur in infants and young children. Prenatal diagnosis of an intracranial teratoma has been reported. Mature teratomas are generally lobulated and cystic, often containing differentiated tissues such as bone, cartilage, teeth, hair, or intestine. Immature and malignant teratomas are less common. Teratomas tend to occur in the pineal region, presenting with Parinaud syndrome and hydrocephalus. They comprise about 4% of childhood intracranial tumors and also occur in the spine. Treatment is surgical resection.

Chordomas develop from remnants of the embryonic notochord. Half are in the sacrococcygeal region, one-third at the sphenoid-occipital junction, and the remainder elsewhere along the spinal column. They are rare, accounting for less than 1% of CNS tumors, and usually remain asymptomatic until adulthood. These tumors are locally invasive and cause vision loss or cranial nerve dysfunction. They can invade the nasopharynx or intracranial sinuses and may extend into the neck, causing torticollis. Chordomas have a smooth nodular surface that resembles cartilage; the characteristic histologic feature is the presence of large masses of physaliferous cells, round or polygonal cells arranged in cords and having large cytoplasmic vacuoles containing mucin. Chordomas grow slowly but may recur after excision. A chondroid variant contains prominent cartilage. A malignant variant is distinguished by mitotic spindle cells and may metastasize to the lung. Chordoma should be suspected in a patient

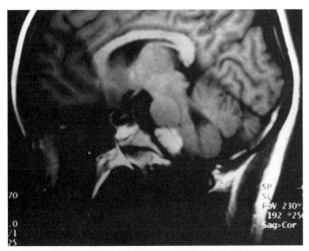 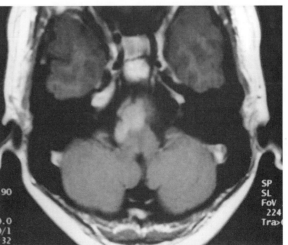

FIG. 59.2. Saggital **(A)** and axial **(B)** magnetic resonance images of a pontomedullary epidermoid.

presenting with multiple cranial nerve palsies or erosion of the skull base. Treatment is surgical resection, occasionally with postoperative irradiation.

Choroid plexus tumors are rare congenital tumors found in or near a lateral ventricle. They may cause symptoms shortly after birth, and most are diagnosed before age 2 years. About two-thirds are benign papillomas, and the remainder are carcinomas. The first manifestation is likely to be macrocephaly due to hydrocephalus, with bulging fontanelle and split sutures noted in infants. Excess CSF production due to tumor may approach 2,000 mL/day. Papillomas usually grow into the ventricle and tend not to be invasive. Carcinomas typically invade the parenchyma and cause hydrocephalus (Fig. 59.3). Surgical resection is curative and stops the excessive production of CSF. Carcinomas are invasive and nearly half disseminate in the CSF. Total excision of localized lesions can be curative, whereas cisplatin-based chemotherapy appears to be effective in patients with residual tumor.

Colloid cysts of the third ventricle presumably arise from the anlage of the paraphysis. These lesions grow in the anterior superior portion of the third ventricle as small white cysts filled with homogeneous gelatinous material. They do not usually cause symptoms until adulthood, when there may be intermittent hydrocephalus. Disturbance of the limbic system may cause emotional and behavioral changes in some instances. Treatment is surgical excision.

ASTROCYTOMAS

Cerebellar astrocytomas constitute approximately 12% of childhood brain tumors and 30% to 40% of posterior fossa tumors. The peak incidence is early in the second decade. These tumors arise most often in the lateral cerebellar hemispheres rather than in the vermis. Symptoms of clumsiness and unsteadiness may be present for months and eventually are accompanied by intermittent morning headache and vomiting. Midline lesions have a shorter symptom interval. Truncal ataxia, dysmetria, and pa-

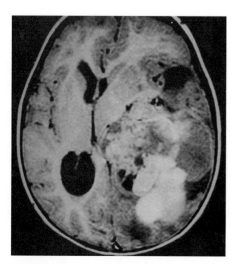

FIG. 59.3. Magnetic resonance image of a choroid plexus carcinoma of the lateral ventricle, with parenchymal invasion.

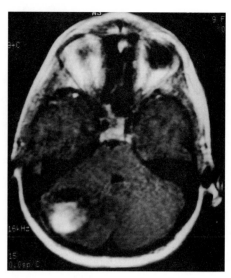

FIG. 59.4. Magnetic resonance image showing lateral location of a partly cystic, partly solid cerebellar astrocytoma.

pilledema are usually present at diagnosis. Head tilt may be present, but other cranial nerve palsies or long tract signs are infrequent and suggest brainstem invasion. Cerebellar astrocytomas may be primarily cystic or solid, and cystic lesions may have a nodule (Fig. 59.4). Most are histologically benign. The typical juvenile pilocytic astrocytoma contains areas of compact fibrillated cells with microcysts and eosinophilic structures called Rosenthal fibers. These lesions have greater than 90% survival with surgery alone. The tumor and associated cyst should be removed completely. If there is residual tumor, re-resection should be considered; focal radiotherapy may be offered if there is disease progression. Some patients have infiltrating tumors with hypercellularity or frank anaplasia; these have been considered diffuse or anaplastic astrocytomas, are harder to resect because of brainstem invasion, and have approximately 30% recurrence-free survival. Local radiotherapy does not appear to improve survival, and the value of craniospinal irradiation or chemotherapy is unclear.

Brainstem gliomas carry the worst prognosis of any childhood brain tumor. Brainstem tumors constitute 10% to 20% of posterior fossa tumors, with a peak age of 5 to 8 years. Most arise in the pons, and there may be contiguous spread to the medulla or midbrain. Despite the clinical aggressiveness of these tumors, the histologic appearance at initial diagnosis is quite variable, but at autopsy a substantial portion shows anaplastic features. This may reflect sampling error at initial biopsy or subsequent malignant transformation. These tumors infiltrate the brainstem and compress normal structures, while extending superiorly and inferiorly to produce diffuse enlargement of the brainstem. Diffuse intrinsic pontine lesions are nearly uniformly fatal within 18 to 24 months. Some tumors extend ventrally, laterally, or posteriorly, and the primarily exophytic tumors tend to be more accessible to surgical resection and carry a better prognosis, as do focal midbrain lesions.

The course is insidious, with slowly progressive cranial neuropathy, motor symptoms, and disturbance of gait, swallowing, and speech. Vomiting and headache indicate the presence of hydrocephalus, generally a late finding. Children with dorsal exophytic lesions may have more unsteadiness and less evidence of cranial nerve dysfunction. CT shows a low-density lesion in the brainstem with compression and obliteration of surrounding cisterns but little if any contrast enhancement. Uncommonly, brainstem tumors may be isodense or hyperdense with cystic areas. MRI is preferred because of the detail appreciated on sagittal images, typically revealing more extensive disease than appreciated on CT. The MR appearance is of decreased signal intensity on T1-weighted images (Fig. 59.5A) and increased T2-weighted signal. MRI may also demonstrate infiltration of the medulla (Fig. 59.5B) or thalamus.

Given the accuracy of MR diagnosis, the morbidity of surgery, and the variable prognostic impact of biopsy, it has been accepted that surgery is not warranted for the 70% of patients with diffuse intrinsic pontine lesions, in whom major resection when attempted has not improved survival. Patients with exophytic cervicomedullary tumors are more likely to benefit from surgery, as are patients with atypical clinical course or MR findings (symptom duration exceeding 6 months, absence of cranial nerve findings, primarily exophytic or focal ring-enhancing lesions). Standard treatment has involved field radiation therapy, except in the case of completely resected focal lesions. Most children with brainstem gliomas benefit at least transiently from radiation therapy to a dose of 54 to 56 Gy. Hyperfractionated irradiation to a dose of 72 to 78 Gy in smaller twice-daily fractions did not alter survival for patients with diffuse pontine lesions, nor did accelerated radiotherapy in standard fractions given twice daily. Although leptomeningeal dissemination can occur, the main risk is for local recurrence. Chemotherapy and immunotherapy have been unsuccessful in this condition, although new agents continue to be studied.

Diencephalic and optic pathway gliomas constitute up to 5% of childhood CNS tumors. Unilateral optic nerve tumors are generally diagnosed in the first decade of life, and optic chiasm tumors tend to present either in infancy or the second decade. An association with NF-1 is present in 50% to 70% of patients with isolated optic nerve tumors and 10% to 20% of patients with optic chiasm tumors. Adolescents are more likely to complain of slowly progressive vision loss. Infants are more likely to be evaluated because of strabismus, nystagmus, or developmental delay. Patients with contiguous optic nerve involvement usually present with proptosis and optic pallor or atrophy. Intraorbital lesions usually cause decrease in central vision, whereas chiasmatic tumors produce bitemporal hemianoptic field deficits. Nystagmus may be present in the more involved eye, and amblyopia is common. With routine MRI of NF-1 patients, lesions may be detected before onset of any symptoms. There may be associated endocrine disturbances such as growth deceleration, precocious puberty, and diencephalic emaciation. Thalamic lesions present with hemiparesis or hemisensory loss. Hypothalamic tumors have insidious onset and may be associated with altered mental status, endocrine dysfunction, and focal neurologic deficits.

CT or MRI appearance of diencephalic gliomas is of hypo- or isodense lesions with variable contrast enhancement. Larger lesions may be cystic (Fig.59.6, A and B). Visual pathway tumors may be confined to the optic chiasm (Fig. 59.7, A and B) or may show abnormal enhancement along the optic tracts and radiations. This streaking phenomenon is best appreciated on MRI, particularly with FLAIR sequence. Most diencephalic tumors are low-grade fibrillary or pilocytic astrocytomas. The natural history of these lesions is unpredictable. Visual pathway tumors have a particular tendency to spread to contiguous structures. The role of surgery is unclear. In patients with diffusely infiltrating lesions, especially with NF-1, diagnosis may be confirmed with near certainty on neuroimaging alone, and surgery may be deemed of little benefit. In patients with unilateral blindness, surgery may be recommended for treatment of a severely proptotic eye. However, if some vision persists, local radiotherapy may be recommended. Radiotherapy at doses of 45 to 55 Gy generally reverses tumor progression in nearly all patients and stabilizes or improves vision in most. There may be apparent tumor enlargement at 6 to 12 weeks as a transient effect of the radiation. Patients with very large lesions may benefit from preliminary surgical debulking. The major disadvantage of radiotherapy is potential adverse endocrine and neurocognitive

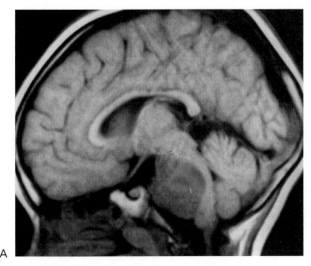
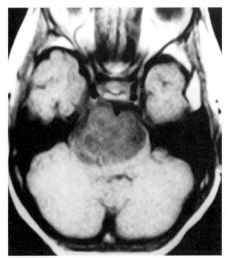

FIG. 59.5. A: Sagittal magnetic resonance image of a diffuse brainstem glioma. **B:** Axial image showing infiltration of the medulla.

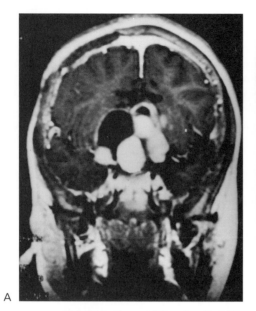
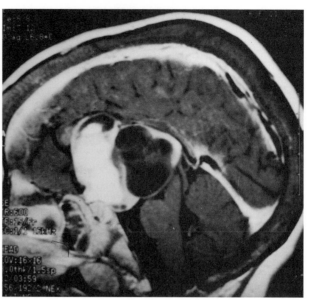

FIG. 59.6. Coronal **(A)** and sagittal **(B)** magnetic resonance images of a large hypothalamic glioma.

effects, especially in younger children. Chemotherapy (vincristine and carboplatin) has been beneficial as initial treatment in children under 5 years of age with progressive optic pathway and hypothalamic/chiasmatic gliomas, delaying the need for radiotherapy by a median of 4 years; most eventually relapse, however, except for NF-1 patients who tend to have indolent disease. The same chemotherapy regimen has been advocated as initial treatment for infants with tumor-associated diencephalic syndrome of emaciation.

Cerebral hemispheric low-grade gliomas appear with a peak incidence between ages 2 and 4 years and again in early adolescence. In toddlers there may be symptoms of increased intracranial pressure, developmental delay, and growth retardation and specific signs such as weakness, sensory loss, or vision deficit. These slow-growing pediatric tumors are far less likely than adult gliomas to undergo malignant degeneration. They are infiltrating, however, and may cause seizures, either generalized or focal,

the latter particularly suggestive of an occult brain tumor such as a ganglioglioma. CT most often reveals a relatively homogeneous low-density variably enhancing lesion with indistinct margins. MRI is more sensitive, showing decreased T1-weighted signal and increased T2-weighted signal and providing better resolution of tumor and peritumoral edema. Gross total resection often affords long-term disease control but may not be curative. Radiation therapy at doses of 50 to 55 Gy is commonly given postoperatively, at least in older children with less than radical resection, and 5-year survival rates are 75% to 85%. For younger children with residual or recurrent tumor, chemotherapy (vincristine and carboplatin) has been used in an attempt to defer radiotherapy, and prospective trials evaluating this approach are in progress.

Cerebral hemispheric high-grade astrocytomas account for about 11% of childhood brain tumors. High-grade astrocytomas can be classified according to cytologic appearance (as fibrillary,

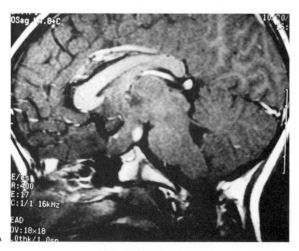
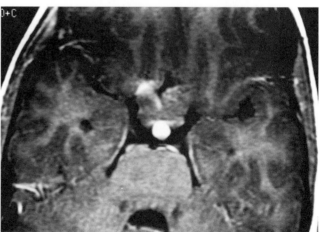

FIG. 59.7. Sagittal **(A)** and coronal **(B)** magnetic resonance images of an optic pathway tumor.

pilocytic, gemistocytic, xanthomatous, or protoplasmic) and by degree of anaplasia. Kernohan's classification grades astrocytomas on a scale of 1 to 4, with grade 3 (*anaplastic astrocytoma*) and grade 4 (*glioblastoma multiforme*) representing high-grade lesions. The World Health Organization classification emphasizes degree of cellularity, nuclear and cellular pleomorphism, mitosis, endothelial proliferation, and necrosis and identifies three gradations: astrocytomas, anaplastic astrocytomas, and glioblastoma multiforme. In general, anaplastic astrocytomas are composed of astrocytes with increased cellularity, pleomorphism, and numbers of mitoses. There may be focal necrosis, but not so extensive as to form pseudopalisades. Glioblastoma multiforme has prominent vascular proliferation and a pseudopalisading pattern of necrosis. Cytogenetic analyses (mainly of tumors from adults) has shown consistent chromosomal abnormalities in all tumor grades, but one aberration, the loss of part or all of chromosome 10, has been specifically associated with glioblastoma multiforme, and amplification and rearrangement of the epidermal growth factor receptor gene have also been associated with malignant histology.

Common symptoms include headache, vomiting, seizures, motor weakness, and behavioral abnormalities. Symptom duration is generally less than 3 months. Diagnosis is best made by contrast-enhanced CT or preferably MRI. Surgery is important for establishing a diagnosis and removing tumor, and major resection is associated with improved survival. However, because these are infiltrative tumors that may also disseminate in the CSF, they will almost certainly recur without further therapy. Postoperative involved field irradiation (59 to 60 Gy) and adjuvant chemotherapy both increase survival. Adjuvant vincristine plus lomustine was effective in a prospective randomized trial, but survival in recent studies remains below 35%. Survival is clearly influenced by extent of tumor resection, and there may be a benefit of consolidative high-dose chemotherapy with hematopoietic stem cell rescue in patients rendered free of detectable tumor after surgery and radiotherapy, based on experience with this approach in patients with recurrent high-grade astrocytomas.

Spinal cord astrocytomas are rare, accounting for only about 4% of childhood CNS neoplasms. They may occur in any part of the cord, with the solid component extending an average of five spinal segments and additional cystic component within or at either end of the lesion. Most have benign histologic appearance and grow slowly. Symptoms and signs may include pain (either localized or radicular), weakness or spasticity, gait disturbance, and bowel or bladder dysfunction. Gadolinium-enhanced MRI is the preferred modality for demonstrating the location of the solid tumor, associated cyst, and edema. Intramedullary tumors may be missed altogether on myelography unless CT is done. Treatment may be attempted gross total or near total resection or partial resection with decompression of cysts and postoperative radiotherapy. The degree of neurologic recovery depends on the preoperative condition of the patient. A potential complication is spinal deformity, due to laminectomy, radiotherapy, or both. For children with low-grade tumors, survival rates of 55% at 10 years have been reported after partial resection and radiotherapy. Chemotherapy has been substituted for radiotherapy in very young children. The prognosis for children with high-grade tumors is worse, although 5-year progression-free

survival of 46% was reported in a study using combined radiation therapy and chemotherapy.

MEDULLOBLASTOMAS/PRIMITIVE NEUROECTODERMAL TUMORS

Medulloblastoma and related PNETs outside the posterior fossa collectively represent the most common malignant CNS tumors of childhood. The presumed cell of origin is derived from remnants of fetal external granular cells of the cerebellum or rests in the posterior medullary velum. Most PNETs arise in the posterior fossa and are specifically called medulloblastomas. These tumors account for about 30% of infratentorial tumors in children but are extremely uncommon in adults. Medulloblastomas typically involve the cerebellar vermis and grow to fill the fourth ventricle and infiltrate the floor of the ventricle and adjacent structures. The tumor may arise more laterally, especially in older patients. The histologic appearance is of a small round cell tumor with glial or other types of differentiation in some cases. There may be staining for both neurofilament protein and glial fibrillary acidic protein but also for synaptophysin, which is more specific for PNET. In infants, medulloblastoma must be distinguished from the atypical teratoid/rhabdoid tumor, which has a small cell component resembling medulloblastoma but also cords of cells in a mucinous background (simulating chordoma), with "rhabdoid" appearance of the cytoplasm of the larger cells.

A specific chromosome abnormality, isochromosome 17q (duplication of the long arm or deletion of the short arm of chromosome 17), may be seen in one-third of cases. This could result in inactivation of a tumor suppressor gene located on chromosome 17 but apparently distinct from p53. It is unclear whether chromosome 17p deletions impart poor prognosis, but analysis of DNA content indicates that diploid tumors have worse outcome than aneuploid or hyperdiploid tumors. Relatively less is known about the cytogenetic and molecular features of supratentorial PNETs. An animal model of medulloblastoma has been produced by intracisternal injection of human medulloblastoma cells into nude rats.

Children with medulloblastoma typically present with symptoms of increased intracranial pressure (vomiting, lethargy, morning headache), unsteadiness, and diplopia. The median age is 5 years. Symptom duration is generally less than 3 months. There may be recent onset of head tilt due to ophthalmoparesis or incipient cerebellar herniation. Laterally situated lesions present slightly differently, with symptoms of cerebellopontine angle disturbance or appendicular ataxia. These tumors appear isodense or hyperdense on noncontrast CT and usually enhance homogeneously with contrast. Evidence of hydrocephalus is present in more than 80% of patients. Other features on CT may include small cysts, calcification, and hemorrhage. MRI may give a better indication of tumor extent (Fig. 59.8A) and possible leptomeningeal dissemination (Fig. 59.8, B and C). MRI is also the preferred study for evaluation of the spine for disseminated tumor, which may be present in up to one-third of patients.

Modern neurosurgical techniques permit complete or near complete resection of medulloblastomas in most cases, limited

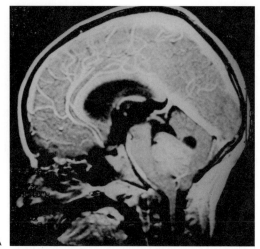

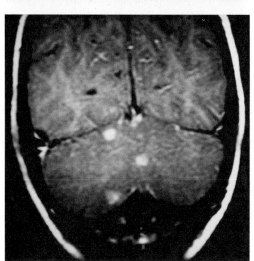

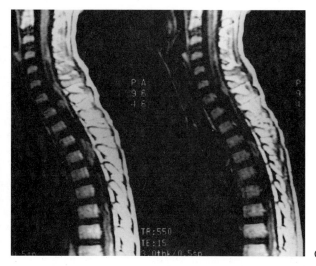

FIG. 59.8. (A) Sagittal magnetic resonance image of a medulloblastoma in the posterior fossa, with (B) coronal image showing parenchymal nodules and (C) spine images showing seeding of the cord.

mainly by infiltration of the fourth ventricle, the brainstem, or one of the cerebellar peduncles. Neurologic morbidity may include the "posterior fossa syndrome" of aseptic meningitis or, less commonly, mutism, pharyngeal dysfunction, and ataxia. Preoperative ventriculoperitoneal shunting is not done routinely because of the risk of upward herniation and because hydrocephalus will be relieved by tumor removal in most patients. About 30% to 40% will require permanent shunting. Postoperative CT or MRI is indicated to confirm the extent of resection, and this study should be done within 72 hours when there is less edema than later. The overall 5-year disease-free survival is approximately 50%. Children with completely resected localized tumors have up to 70% disease-free survival. The presence of residual tumor (more than 1.5 cm³), brainstem invasion, or leptomeningeal spread portends a worse prognosis. It has also been suggested that boys may have an inferior outcome. Radiation therapy is the standard postoperative treatment for this disease, and craniospinal irradiation is given because the entire neuraxis is at risk for recurrence. Conventional doses are 36 Gy to the brain and spine, with an 18- to 20-Gy boost to the local tumor site.

Adjuvant chemotherapy with vincristine and lomustine has

been shown to improve survival in advanced stages of medulloblastoma, and with the addition of cisplatin progression-free survival of 85% at 5 years has been reported. This result suggests that chemotherapy could improve results even in patients with localized tumors, who are conventionally treated with radiation therapy alone. Chemotherapy can potentially allow for reduction in the dose of radiation to the brain and spine in such patients, and this approach is currently under study. Chemotherapy has also been used as primary postoperative treatment in infants, with the goal of deferring or avoiding radiotherapy. Current protocols for infants up to age 3 years use this approach, with increasingly intensive regimens to enhance the response rate to chemotherapy and improve the control of leptomeningeal disease. Finally, high-dose chemotherapy with hematopoietic stem cell rescue is an effective salvage therapy for selected patients with recurrent medulloblastoma.

Supratentorial PNETs are histologically equivalent to medulloblastoma and treated with the same approach of resection, craniospinal irradiation, and chemotherapy. Prognosis is also similar, about 50% survival at 5 years. Pineal region PNETs (pineoblastomas) must be distinguished from pineal germ cell tumors (see below) and pineocytomas, which are considered benign and treated by surgery with or without radiotherapy. Pineoblastomas are treated like medulloblastoma, with craniospinal irradiation and adjuvant chemotherapy, and 60% 3-year progression-free survival has been reported.

EPENDYMOMAS

Ependymomas usually arise within or adjacent to the ependymal lining of the ventricular system, with 60% to 75% in the posterior fossa. They constitute 5% to 10% of all primary childhood brain tumors. Ependymomas are glial neoplasms derived from ependymal cells, and most appear to be histologically mature. Variants include anaplastic ependymoma, which may or may not have a worse outcome, and subependymoma, a lower grade lesion in which the fibrillary subependymal astrocyte predominates. Ependymoblastoma, a primitive tumor, is better categorized as a type of PNET. Simian virus 40-related DNA sequences have been demonstrated in ependymomas and choroid plexus carcinomas, suggesting a potential viral etiology. Cytogenetic and molecular studies of childhood ependymomas have revealed rearrangements or deletions of chromosome 6 and of chromosomes 22 and 17.

Clinical symptoms depend on tumor location. Children with ependymoma filling or compressing the fourth ventricle present with nausea, vomiting, and morning headache due to obstructive hydrocephalus. Tumors arising low in the fourth ventricle and extending into the lower medulla may cause neck pain, whereas cranial nerve palsies may result from brainstem invasion or compression of cranial nerves. In patients with supratentorial lesions, seizures and focal deficits are seen. Features on CT include calcification and variable enhancement. MRI may better demonstrate invasion of posterior fossa lesions into the brainstem (Fig. 59.9) or upper cervical spinal cord. The most important predictor of outcome is the extent of surgical resection. In posterior fossa lesions, this can be limited by infiltration of the brainstem, extension into the cerebellar pontine angle, or involvement of

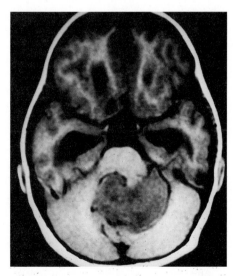

FIG. 59.9. Magnetic resonance appearance of an ependynoma, showing tumor extension through the foramen of Luschka and invasion of the brainstem.

cranial nerve nuclei. Supratentorial lesions may also be quite infiltrative and difficult to remove. Total resection of ependymomas affords 60% or greater survival at 5 years, whereas two-thirds recur after subtotal resection. Postoperative imaging has been considered more accurate than surgeons's estimate of presence of residual tumor.

Postoperative radiation therapy seems to increase overall survival, and treatment to an involved field (at a dose of 55 Gy) is generally considered sufficient because relapses are overwhelmingly local. The need for larger volumes of radiation therapy to anaplastic lesions or presymptomatic irradiation to the neuraxis for posterior fossa lesions is not definitely established. Adjuvant chemotherapy may improve outcome, based on response of recurrent ependymoma to cisplatin and other agents, and preirradiation chemotherapy is being evaluated in patients with postoperative residual tumor based on responses seen in infants with ependymoma. Recurrent ependymomas are managed by re-resection and chemotherapy or stereotactic radiosurgery.

GERM CELL TUMORS

Germ cell tumors tend to arise in the pineal and suprasellar regions. They account for about half of pineal tumors and 5% to 10% of parasellar lesions. Pineal germ cell tumors have a male preponderance and usually present in adolescence, whereas suprasellar germ cell tumors predominate in younger females. About 50% to 65% of germ cell tumors are germinomas, histologically primitive lesions resembling gonadal germ cell tumors and presumably derived from embryonic migration of totipotent germ cells. Teratomas and mixed germ cell tumors are variously comprised of mature, immature, and malignant elements. Choriocarcinomas are rare but highly malignant.

Symptoms and signs of pineal region germ cell tumors most often include headache and Parinaud syndrome of upgaze paresis. With extension to the overlying thalamus there may be hemiparesis, incoordination, vision disturbance, or movement disorder. Suprasellar germ cell tumors produce pituitary and hypothalamic dysfunction but usually not vision loss. CT appearance is of an irregular lesion of mixed density, occasionally with calcification and with variable contrast enhancement. MRI may be preferred as it is more sensitive for purposes of follow-up evaluation. Because of its sensitivity, MRI may reveal the presence of a pineal cyst in otherwise healthy children being evaluated for headache; lack of hydrocephalus and Parinaud syndrome should lead one away from the diagnosis of a pineal tumor. Diagnosis can be aided by measurement of alpha-fetoprotein and beta subunit of human chorionic gonadotropin, which are secreted by germ cell tumors (but not pineal parenchymal cell tumors or cysts) and detectable in serum and CSF. Alpha-fetoprotein is elevated in endodermal sinus tumors and some immature teratomas; human chorionic gonadotropin is elevated in choriocarcinoma and embryonal carcinomas. Elevation of both indicates the presence of mixed malignant elements. Even with marker elevation, however, histologic confirmation is recommended.

Surgery for pineal region tumors is technically difficult, but major resections can be achieved with acceptable morbidity by a supratentorial suboccipital or infratentorial supracerebellar approach. There may be transient visual migraine due to occipital lobe contusion. Teratomas may be encapsulated and easier to remove. Germ cell tumors may disseminate throughout the neuraxis in up to 10% of cases. Radiotherapy is the standard treatment for pure germinomas, typically 35 to 45 Gy to the brain and spine with a 10- to 15-Gy boost to the area of the tumor, affording 90% survival at 5 years. Survival rates for mixed malignant germ cell tumors are considerably lower, less than 30% with radiotherapy alone, but about 50% with the addition of chemotherapy. Current protocols are based on cisplatin-containing regimens active in gonadal germ cell tumors.

LYMPHOMAS

Primary CNS lymphomas are rare, constituting less than 1% of intracranial tumors. They may occur at any age. They are generally of B-lymphocyte origin, including Burkitt type. They are associations with congenital and acquired immunodeficiency, including immunosuppressive therapy for autoimmune disease and organ transplant. The incidence has increased in both immunodeficient and immunocompetent individuals. The most common location is the cerebral cortex. CT appearance is of an isodense or hyperdense lesion with moderate to marked contrast enhancement. MRI shows an iso- to hypointense lesion on T1-weighted images and iso-, hypo-, or slightly hyperintense lesion on T2-weighted images, with variable gadolinium enhancement. Survival rates in adults of 20% to 30% have been reported with combined radiation and chemotherapy or intensive chemotherapy alone.

MENINGIOMAS

Meningiomas are rare in childhood. There is an association with neurofibromatosis. They usually arise on the meningeal surface but (in contrast to adults) may grow as parenchymal lesions, presumably from meningeal cell rests. CT and MRI show an isointense or hyperintense lesion enhancing with contrast (Fig. 59.10). Most lesions are clinically benign, although pediatric tumors may show evidence of anaplasia. Surgery is the primary treatment modality. Radiotherapy is of uncertain value but has been used in patients with recurrent tumor, especially after unsuccessful attempts at re-resection. Meningioma may occasionally involve primarily the leptomeninges, and these tumors, also called meningeal sarcomas, tend to behave aggressively. Treatment has most often been with combined radiation and chemotherapy.

LATE EFFECTS OF TREATMENT AND QUALITY OF LIFE

Radiation therapy may be followed at 4 to 8 weeks by a transient "somnolence syndrome" of sleepiness, irritability, anorexia, and headache, lasting about a week. A much more serious complication is radiation necrosis, which develops in 0.1% to 5.0% of pa-

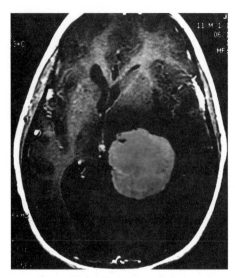

FIG. 59.10. Axial magnetic resonance image of a meningioma.

tients after conventional treatment at 50 to 60 Gy in daily fractions of 180 to 200 cGy. The onset may be within 3 months and usually by 3 years, although occasionally much later, and symptoms and signs are those of a recurrent intracranial mass, with possible seizures and progressive neuropsychological impairment. Surgical resection should be attempted; unresectable lesions may be treated with corticosteroids, but subsequent taper may be difficult. Children younger than 2 to 3 years are particularly susceptible to radiation injury because of incomplete development of the CNS. Large-vessel thrombosis is a rare complication of radiation therapy, occurring between 2 and 30 years after cranial irradiation. Treatment is symptomatic.

Endocrine dysfunction may follow irradiation to the hypothalamus and pituitary. Doses as low as 18 Gy may produce growth hormone deficiency, and doses above 36 Gy may cause hypothyroidism and gonadal dysfunction in more than half of patients receiving conventional whole brain irradiation. Precocious puberty was noted in nearly one-fourth of girls. The incidence of hypothyroidism appears to be considerably lower in children receiving hyperfractionated irradiation. Frank adrenal insufficiency is uncommon, but subtle abnormalities in adrenal function may be present. Children should be followed for measurement of linear growth, periodic thyroid function studies, and additional endocrine evaluation if there is precocious or delayed onset of puberty.

Radiation therapy may contribute to neurocognitive disorders in children with CNS tumors. Other factors include acute or chronic increased intracranial pressure, tumor mass effect, poorly controlled seizure disorders, and complications of surgery and chemotherapy. All these factors may have a negative impact on overall quality of life. Neurocognitive problems are more likely in children treated at a young age or with high doses of radiation, especially to cerebral cortical areas associated with higher functions. The effects may be progressive over several years and include attention deficit, impairment of short-term memory, and lowering of IQ. The anticipated decline in IQ can be estimated based on initial IQ, radiation dose, and age at time of irradiation. These children will generally require formal psychologic intervention and special education programs.

Chronic neurotoxicity of chemotherapy used in treating CNS tumors may include hearing loss (relatively common after cisplatin) and peripheral neuropathy (seen with vincristine and to a lesser extent cisplatin and etoposide). Restrictive lung disease and cardiac dysfunction may occur after spinal irradiation, and the risk could be increased by chemotherapy. Osteopenia was found in half of children surviving brain tumors, and bone pain may limit physical activity in these individuals; the cause is probably multifactorial. Chemotherapy may potentiate the deleterious effect of craniospinal irradiation on growth. There is an increased risk (approximately 3% to 5%) of second tumors after cranial irradiation, including meningiomas and sarcomas, arising 10 to 20 years after treatment. Secondary leukemia has been reported after chemotherapy with alkylating agents and etoposide.

SUGGESTED READINGS

Albright AL, Packer RJ, Zimmerman R, Rorke LB, Boyett J, Hammond GD. Magnetic resonance scans should replace biopsies for the diagnosis of diffuse brain stem gliomas: A report from the Children's Cancer Group. *Neurosurgery* 1993;33:1026–1029.

Allen J, Wissof J, Helson L, Pearce J, Arenson E. Choroid plexus carcinoma: responses to chemotherapy alone in newly diagnosed young children. *J Neurooncol* 1992;12:69–74.

Allen JC, Aviner S, Yates AJ, et al. Treatment of high-grade spinal cord astrocytoma of childhood with "8-in-1" chemotherapy and radiotherapy: a pilot study of CCG-945. Children's Cancer Group. *J Neurosurg* 1998;88:215–220.

Allen JC, Kim JH, Packer RJ. Neoadjuvant chemotherapy for newly diagnosed germ-cell tumors of the central nervous system. *J Neurosurg* 1987;67:65–70.

arr RD, Simpson T, Webber CE, et al. Osteopenia in children surviving brain tumors. *Eur J Cancer* 1998;34:873–877.

Backlund EO, Axelsson B, Bergstrand CG, et al. Treatment of craniopharyngiomas: the stereotactic approach in a ten to twenty-three years' perspective. I. Surgical, radiological and ophthalmological aspects. *Acta Neurochir* 1989;99:11–19.

Bergsagel DJ, Finegold MJ, Butel JS, Kupsky WJ, Garcea RL. DNA sequences similar to those of simian virus 40 in ependymomas and choroid plexus tumors of childhood. *N Engl J Med* 1992;326:988–993.

Biegel JA. Genetics of pediatric central nervous system tumors. *J Pediatr Hematol Oncol* 1997;19:492–501.

Biegel JA, Janss AJ, Raffel C, et al. Prognostic significance of chromosome 17p deletions in childhood primitive neuroectodermal tumors (medulloblastomas) of the central nervous system. *Clin Cancer Res* 1997;3:473–478.

Blamires TL, Maher ER. Choroid plexus papilloma. A new presentation of von Hippel-Lindau (VHL) disease. *Eye* 1992;6:90–92.

Bunin GR, Buckley JD, Boesel CP, Rorke LB, Meadows AT. Risk factors for astrocytic glioma and primitive neuroectodermal tumor of the brain in young children: a report from the Children's Cancer Group. *Cancer Epidemiol Biomarkers Prev* 1994;3:197–204.

Bunin GR, Kuijten RR, Buckley JD, Rorke LB, Meadows AT. Relation between maternal diet and subsequent primitive neuroectodermal brain tumors in young children. *N Engl J Med* 1993;329:536–541.

Burger PC, Yu IT, Tihan T, et al. Atypical teratoid/rhabdoid tumor of the central nervous system: a highly malignant tumor of infancy and childhood frequently mistaken for medulloblastoma. A Pediatric Oncology Group study. *Am J Surg Pathol* 1998;22:1083–1092.

Camacho A, Abernathy CD, Kelly PJ, Laws ER Jr. Colloid cysts: experience with the management of 84 cases since the introduction of computed tomography. *Neurosurgery* 1989;4:693–700.

Carlson-Green B, Morris RD, Krawiecki N. Family and illness predictors of outcome in pediatric brain tumors. *J Pediatr Psychol* 1995;20:769–784.

Cheng AL, Yeh KH, Uen WC, Hung RL, Liu MY, Wang CH. Systemic chemotherapy alone for patients with non-acquired immunodeficiency syndrome-related central nervous system lymphoma. A pilot study of the BOMES protocol. *Cancer* 1998;82:1946–1951.

Cochrane DD, Gustavsson B, Poskitt KP, Steinbok P, Kestle JR. The surgical and natural morbidity of aggressive resection for posterior fossa tumors in childhood. *Pediatr Neurosurg* 1994;20:19–29.

Cogen PH, Daneshvar L, Metzger AK, Edwards MS. Deletion mapping of the medulloblastoma locus on chromosome 17p. *Genomics* 1990;8:279–285.

Cohen BH, Bury E, Packer RJ, Sutton LN, Bilaniuk LT, Zimmerman RA. Gadolinium-DPTA-enhanced magnetic resonance imaging in childhood brain tumors. *Neurology* 1989;39:1178–1183.

Cohen BH, Rothner AD. Incidence, types, and management of cancer in patients with neurofibromatosis. *Oncology* 1989;3:23–30.

Cohen M, Duffner P, Heffner RR, Lacey DJ, Brecher M. Prognostic factors in brain stem gliomas. *Neurology* 1986;36:602–605.

Constine LS, Woolf PD, Cann D, et al. Hypothalamic-pituitary dysfunction after radiation for brain tumors. *N Engl J Med* 1993;328:87–94.

D'Andrea AD, Packer RJ, Rorke LB, et al. Pineocytomas of childhood: a reappraisal of natural history and response to therapy. *Cancer* 1987;59:1353–1357.

Danoff BF, Cowchock S, Marquette C, Mulgrew L, Kramer S. Assessment of the long-term effects of primary brain tumors in children. *Cancer* 1982;49:1580–1586.

DeAngelis LM, Yahalom J, Thaler HT, Kher U. Combined modality therapy for primary CNS lymphoma. *J Clin Oncol* 1992;10:635–643.

Dias MS, Albright AL. Management of hydrocephalus complicating childhood posterior fossa tumors. *Pediatr Neurosci* 1989;15:283–289.

Duffner PK, Cohen ME, Anderson SW, et al. Long-term effects of treatment on endocrine function in children with brain tumors. *Ann Neurol* 1983;14:528–532.

Duffner PK, Horowitz ME, Krischer JP, et al. Postoperative chemotherapy and delayed radiation in children less than three years of age with malignant brain tumors. *N Engl J Med* 1993;328:1725–1731.

Dunkel IJ, Boyett JM, Yates A, et al. High-dose carboplatin, thiotepa, and etoposide with autologous stem-cell rescue for patients with recurrent medulloblastoma. *J Clin Oncol* 1998;16:222–228.

Eby NL, Grufferman S, Flannelly CM, Schold SC Jr, Vogel FS, Burger PC. Increasing incidence of primary brain lymphoma in the US. *Cancer* 1988;62:2461–2465.

Edwards MS, Hudgins RJ, Wilson CB, Levin VA, Wara WM. Pineal region tumors in children. *J Neurosurg* 1988;68:689–697.

Epstein F, Epstein N. Surgical treatment of spinal cord astrocytomas of childhood. *J Neurosurg* 1982;57:685–689.

Erdincler P, Lena G, Sarioglu AC, Kuday C, Choux M. Intracranial meningiomas in children: review of 29 cases. *Surg Neurol* 1998;49:136–140.

Evans AE, Jenkin RDT, Sposto R, et al. The treatment of medulloblastoma. Results of a prospective randomized trial of radiation therapy with and without CCNU, vincristine, and prednisone. *J Neurosurg* 1990;72:572–582.

Ferreira J, Eviatar L, Schneider S, Grossman R. Prenatal diagnosis of intracranial teratoma. Prolonged survival after resection of a malignant teratoma diagnosed prenatally by ultrasound: a case report and literature review. *Pediatr Neurosurg* 1993;19:84–88.

Finlay JF, Goldman S, Wong MC, et al. Pilot study of high-dose thiotepa and etoposide with autologous bone marrow rescue in children and young adults with recurrent CNS tumors. *J Clin Oncol* 1996;14:2495–2503.

Finlay JL, August C, Packer R, et al. High-dose multi-agent chemotherapy followed by bone marrow "rescue" for malignant astrocytomas of childhood and adolescence. *J Neurooncol* 1990;9:239–248.

Finlay JL, Boyett JM, Yates AJ, et al. Randomized phase III tiral in childhood high-grade astrocytoma comparing vincristine, lomustine, and prednisone with the eight-drugs-in-1-day regimen. *J Clin Oncol* 1995;13:112–123.

Fischer EG, Welch K, Shillito J Jr, Winston KA, Tarbell NJ. Craniopharyngiomas in children. Long-term effects of conservative surgical procedures combined with radiation therapy. *J Neurosurg* 1990;73:534–540.

Gajjar A, Heideman RL, Kovnar EH, et al. Response of pediatric low-grade gliomas to chemotherapy. *Pediatr Neurosurg* 1993;19:113–120.

Gajjar AJ, Heideman RL, Douglass EC, et al. Relation of tumor-cell ploidy to survival in children with medulloblastoma. *J Clin Oncol* 1993;11:2211–2217.

Gilles F. Cerebellar tumors in children. *Clin Neurosurg* 1983;30:181–188.

Gjerris F, Klinken L. Long-term prognosis in children with benign cerebellar astrocytoma. *J Neurosurg* 1978;49:179–184.

Goldwein JW, Leahy JM, Packer RJ, et al. Intracranial ependymomas in children. *Int J Radiat Oncol Biol Phys* 1990;99:1497–1502.

Goldwein JW, Radcliffe J, Packer RJ, et al. Results of a pilot study of low-dose craniospinal radiation therapy plus chemotherapy for children younger than 5 years with primitive neuroectodermal tumors. *Cancer* 1993;71:2647–2652.

Green AJ, Smith M, Yates JR. Loss of heterozygosity on chromosome 16p13.3 in hamartomas from tuberous sclerosis patients. *Nat Genet* 1994;6:193–196.

Greenberg SB, Schneck MJ, Faerber EN, Kanev PM. Malignant meningioma in a child: CT and MR findings. *AJR* 1993;160:1111–1112.

Gropman AL, Packer RJ, Nicholson HS, et al. Treatment of diencephalic syndrome with chemotherapy: growth, tumor response, and long term control. *Cancer* 1998;83:166–172.

Gurney JG, Mueller BA, Preston-Martin S, et al. A study of pediatric brain tumors and their association with epilepsy and anticonvulsant use. *Neuroepidemiology* 1997;16:248–255.

Gurney JG, Severson RK, Davis S, Robison LL. Incidence of cancer in children in the United States. Sex-, race-, and 1-year age-specific rates by histologic type. *Cancer* 1995;75:2186–2195.

Hardison HH, Packer RJ, Rorke LB, Schut L, Sutton LN, Bruce DA. Outcome of children with primary intramedullary spinal cord tumors. *Childs Nerv Syst* 1987;3:89–92.

Healey JH, Lane JM. Chordoma: a critical review of diagnosis and treatment. *Orthop Clin North Am* 1989;20:417–426.

Heidemen RL, Kuttesch J Jr, Gajjar AJ, et al. Supratentorial malignant gliomas in childhood. A single institution perspective. *Cancer* 1997;80:497–504.

Hoffman HJ, DeSilva M, Humphreys RP, Drake JM, Smith ML, Blaser SI. Aggressive surgical management of craniopharyngiomas in children. *J Neurosurg* 1992;76:47–52.

Holly EA, Bracci PM, Mueller BA, Preston-Martin S. Farm and animal exposures and pediatric brain tumors: results from the United States West Coast Childhood Brain Tumor Study. *Cancer Epidemiol Biomark Prev* 1998;7:797–802.

Honig PJ, Charney EB. Children with brain tumor headaches. Distinguishing features. *Am J Dis Child* 1982;136:121–124.

Jakacki RI, Goldwein JW, Larsen RL, Barber G, Silber J. Cardiac dysfunction following spinal irradiation during childhood. *J Clin Oncol* 1993;11:1033–1038.

Jakacki RI, Schramm CM, Donahue BR, Haas F, Allen JC. Restrictive lung disease following treatment for malignant brain tumors: a potential late effect of craniospinal irradiation. *J Clin Oncol* 1995;13:1478–1485.

Jakacki RI, Zeltzer PM, Boyett JM, et al. Survival and prognostic factors following radiation and/or chemotherapy for primitive neuroectodermal tumors of the pineal region in infants and children: a report of the Children's Cancer Group. *J Clin Oncol* 1995;13:1377–1383.

James CD, Carlbom E, Dumanski JP, et al. Clonal genomic alterations in glioma malignancy stages. *Cancer Res* 1988;48:5546–5551.

Janss AJ, Grundy R, Cnaan A, et al. Optic pathway and hypothalamic/chiasmatic gliomas in children younger than age 5 years with a 6-year follow-up. *Cancer* 1995;75:1051–1059.

Jennings MT, Gelman R, Hochberg F. Intracranial germ-cell tumors: natural history and pathogenesis. *J Neurosurg* 1985;63:155–167.

Kernohan JW, Mabon RF, Svien H, Adson AW. A simplified classification of the gliomas. *Mayo Clin Proc* 1949;24:71–75.

Kheifets LI, Sussman SS, Preston-Martin S. Childhood brain tumors and residential electromagnetic fields (EMF). *Rev Environ Contam Toxicol* 1999;159:111–129.

Kleihues P, Burger PC, Scheithauer BW. The new WHO classification of brain tumours. *Brain Pathol* 1993;3:255–268.

Kortmann RD, Timmermann B, Becker G, Kuhl J, Bamberg M. Advances in treatment techniques and time/dose schedules in external radiation therapy of brain tumors in childhood. *Klin Pediatr* 1998;210:220–226.

Kramer DL, Parmiter AH, Rorke LB, Sutton LN, Biegel JA. Molecular cytogenetic studies of pediatric ependymomas. *J Neurooncol* 1998;37:25–33.

Kramer ED, Vezine LG, Packer RJ, Fitz CR, Zimmerman RA, Cohen MD. Staging and surveillance of children with central nervous system neoplasms: recommendations of the Neurology and Tumor Imaging Committees of the Children's Cancer Group. *Pediatr Neurosurg* 1994;20:254–263.

Kun LE, Constine LS. Medulloblastoma: caution regarding new treatment approaches. *Int J Radiat Oncol Biol Phys* 1991;20:897–899.

Lashford LS, Campbell RH, Gattamaneni HR, Robinson K, Walker D, Bailey C. An intensive multiagent chemotherapy regimen for brain tumours occurring in very young children. *Arch Dis Child* 1996;74:219–223.

Lewis J, Lucraft H, Gholkar A. UKCCSG study of accelerated radiotherapy for pediatric brain stem gliomas. United Kingdom Childhood Cancer Study Group. *Int J Radiat Oncol Biol Phys* 1997;38:925–929.

Linstadt DE, Wara WM, Leibel SA, Gutin PH, Wilson CB, Sheline GE. Postoperative radiotherapy of primary spinal cord tumors. *Int J Radiat Oncol Biol Phys* 1989;16:1397–1403.

Louis DN, Ramesh V, Gusella JF. Neuropathology and molecular genetics of neurofibromatosis 2 and related tumors. *Brain Pathol* 1995;5:163–172.

Lowis SP, Pizer BL, Coakham H, Nelson RJ, Bouffet E. Chemotherapy for spinal cord astrocytoma: Can natural history be modified? *Childs Nerv Syst* 1998;14:317–321.

Lunardi P, Missori P. Supratentorial dermoid cysts. *J Neurosurg* 1991;75:262–266.

Maria BL, Drane WE, Mastin ST, Jiminez LA. Comparative value of thallium and glucose SPECT imaging in childhood brain tumors. *Pediatr Neurol* 1998;19:351–357.

Mason WP, Grovas A, Halpern S, et al. Intensive chemotherapy and bone marrow rescue for young children with newly diagnosed malignant brain tumors. *J Clin Oncol* 1998;16:210–221.

McGirr SJ, Ebersold MJ, Scheithauer BW, Quast LM, Shaw EG. Choroid plexus papillomas: long-term follow-up results in a surgically treated series. *J Neurosurg* 1988;69:843–849.

Needle MN, Goldwein JW, Grass J, et al. Adjuvant chemotherapy for the treatment of intracranial ependymoma of childhood. *Cancer* 1997;80:341–347.

Netsky MG. Epidermoid tumors: review of the literature. *Surg Neurol* 1988;29:477–483.

North CA, North RB, Epstein JA, Piantadosi S, Wharam MD. Low-grade cerebral astrocytomas. Survival and quality of life after radiation therapy. *Cancer* 1990;66:6–14.

Oberfield SE, Allen JC, Pollack J, New MI, Levine LS. Long-term endocrine sequelae after treatment of medulloblastoma: prospective study of growth and thyroid function. *J Pediatr* 1986;108:219–223.

Oberfield SE, Chin D, Uli N, David R, Sklar C. Endocrine late effects of childhood cancers. *J Pediatr* 1997;131(Pt 2):S37–S41.

Olshan JS, Gubernick J, Packer RJ, et al. The effects of adjuvant chemotherapy on growth in children with medulloblastoma. *Cancer* 1992;70:2013–2017.

Packer RJ, Bilaniuk LT, Cohen BH, et al. Intracranial visual pathway gliomas in children with neurofibromatosis. *Neurofibromatosis* 1988;1:212–222.

Packer RJ, Boyett JM, Zimmerman RA, et al. Hyperfractionated radiation therapy (72 Gy) for children with brain stem gliomas: a Children's Cancer Group phase I/II trial. *Cancer* 1993;72:1414–1421.

Packer RJ, Prados M, Phillips P, et al. Treatment of children with newly diagnosed brain stem gliomas with intravenous recombinant beta-interferon and hyperfractionated radiation therapy: a Children's Cancer Group phase I/II study. *Cancer* 1996;77:2150–2152.

Packer RJ, Savino PJ, Bilaniuk K, et al. Chiasmatic gliomas of childhood: A reappraisal of natural history and effectiveness of cranial irradiation. *Childs Brain* 1983;10:393–403.

Packer RJ, Sutton LN, Atkins TE, et al. A prospective study of cognitive deficits in children receiving whole brain radiotherapy: 2 year results. *J Neurosurg* 1989;70:707–713.

Packer RJ, Sutton LN, Elterman R, et al. Outcome for children with medulloblastoma treated with radiation and cisplatin, CCNU, and vincristine chemotherapy. *J Neurosurg* 1994;81:690–698.

Pigott TJ, Punt JA, Lowe JS, Henderson MJ, Beck A, Gray T. The clinical, radiological and histopathological features of cerebral primitive neuroectodermal tumours. *Br J Neurosurg* 1990;4:287–297.

Ransom DT, Ritland SR, Kimmel PJ, et al. Cytogenetic and loss of heterozygosity studies in ependymomas, pilocytic astrocytomas, and oligodendrogliomas. *Genes Chromosomes Cancer* 1992;5:348–356.

Rubio MP, Correa KM, Ramesh V, et al. Analysis of the neurofibromatosis 2 gene in human ependymomas and astrocytomas. *Cancer Res* 1994;54:45–47.

Salazar OM, Casto-Vita M, Van Houtte P, Rubin P, Aygun C. Improved survival in cases of intracranial ependymoma after radiation therapy: late report and recommendations. *J Neurosurg* 1983;59:652–659.

Schabet M, Martos J, Buchholz R, Pietsch T. Animal model of human medulloblastoma: clinical, magnetic resonance imaging, and histopathological findings after intra-cisternal injection of MHH-MED-1 cells into nude rats. *Med Pediatr Oncol* 1997;29:92–97.

Sheline GE, Wara WM, Smith V. Therapeutic irradiation and brain injury. *Int J Radiat Oncol Biol Phys* 1980;6:1215–1228.

Silber JH, Radcliffe J, Peckham V, et al. Whole-brain irradiation and decline in intelligence: the influence of dose and age on IQ score. *J Clin Oncol* 1992;10:1390–1396.

Smith MA, Freidlin B, Ries LA, Simon R. Trends in reported incidence of primary malignant brain tumors in children in the United States. *J Natl Cancer Inst* 1998;90:1269–1277.

Spencer DD, Spencer SS, Matson RH, Williamson PD. Intracerebral masses in patients with intractable partial epilepsy. *Neurology* 1984;34:432–436.

Sposto R, Ertel IH, Jenkin RD, et al. The effectiveness of chemotherapy for treatment of high grade astrocytoma in children: results of a randomized trial. A report from the Children's Cancer Study Group. *J Neurooncol* 1989;7:165–177.

Sutton LN, Goldwein J, Perilongo G, et al. Prognostic factors in childhood ependymomas. *Pediatr Neurosurg* 1990;16:57–65.

Tait DM, Thornton-Jones H, Bloom HJ, Lemerle J, Morris-Jones P. Adjuvant chemotherapy for medulloblastoma: the first multi-centre control trial of the International Society of Pediatric Oncology (SIOP I). *Eur J Cancer* 1990;26:464–469.

Tao ML, Barnes PD, Billett AL, et al. Childhood optic chiasm gliomas: Radiographic response following radiotherapy and long-term clinical outcome. *Int J Radiat Oncol Biol Phys* 1997;39:579–587.

Taylor JS, Langston JW, Reddick WE, et al. Clinical value of proton magnetic resonance spectroscopy for differentiating recurrent or residual brain tumor from delayed cerebral necrosis. *Int J Radiat Oncol Biol Phys* 1996;36:1251–1261.

Thorne RN, Pearson AD, Nicoll JA, et al. Decline in incidence of medulloblastoma in children. *Cancer* 1994;74:3240–3244.

Valk PE, Budinger TF, Levin VA, Silver P, Gutin PH, Doyle WK. PET of malignant cerebral tumors after interstitial brachytherapy: demonstration of metabolic activity and correlation with clinical outcome. *J Neurosurg* 1988;69:830–838.

von Deimling A, Louis DN, Menon AG, Ellison D, Wiestler OD, Seizinger BR. Deletions on the long arm of chromosome 17 in pilocytic astrocytoma. *Acta Neuropathol* 1993;86:81–85.

Walter AW, Hancock ML, Pui CH, et al. Secondary brain tumors in children treated for acute lymphoblastic leukemia at St Jude Children's Research Hospital. *J Clin Oncol* 1998;16:3761–3767.

Weil MD, Lamborn K, Edwards MS, Wara WM. Influence of a child's sex on medulloblastoma outcome. *JAMA* 1998;279:1474–1476.

Whittle IR, Simpson DA. Surgical treatment of neonatal intracranial teratoma. *Surg Neurol* 1981;15:268–273.

Wisoff JH, Abbott R, Epstein F. Surgical management of exophytic chiasmatic-hypothalamic tumors of childhood. *J Neurosurg* 1990;73:661–667.

Wisoff JH, Boyett JM, Berger MS, et al. Current neurosurgical management and the impact of the extent of resection in the treatment of malignant gliomas of childhood: a report of the Children's Cancer Group Trial No. CCG-945. *J Neurosurg* 1998;89:52–59.

Merritt's Neurology, 10th ed., edited by L.P. Rowland. Lippincott Williams & Wilkins, Philadelphia © 2000.

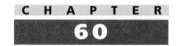

CHAPTER 60

VASCULAR TUMORS AND MALFORMATIONS

ROBERT A. SOLOMON
JOHN PILE-SPELLMAN
J. P. MOHR

The heterogeneous group of vascular lesions reviewed in this brief chapter includes a group of anomalies, some true vascular malformations, some acquired fistulas, and a few belonging to a category of neoplasms.

Vascular malformations
    Arteriovenous malformations
    Venous malformations
    Cavernous malformations
    Telangiectases
    Sturge-Weber disorder
    Sinus pericranii
Vascular tumors
    Angioblastic meningiomas

    Hemangiopericytomas
    Hemangioblastomas

VASCULAR MALFORMATIONS

Vascular lesions referred to as malformations (arteriovenous malformations, AVMs) of the brain have been confused with vascular neoplasms because the clinical course may be progressive and the angiographic picture is sometimes indistinguishable from a neoplasm of blood vessels. However, none are true neoplasms, at least showing no capacity for metastasis and the limited histologic data showing no signs of mitotic figures. Most are inferred to be congenital lesions, but some are arteriovenous fistulae acquired from trauma and arterial or venous occlusions.

Arteriovenous Malformations

AVMs, whether congenital or acquired, are limited to the brain, dura, or both. Those confined to the brain are the more common. Histologically, at the main site of linkage between the arteries and veins, there are no capillaries, the nidus consisting of a tangle of abnormal arteries and veins with interposed sinuses of irregularly sized vascular channels lacking a media and identifiable neither as arteries nor veins. Most are congenital, thought to grow with and displacing adjacent brain tissue. They may be limited to the brain surface, have their major focus in the subsurface white matter, be confined to the deep structures (e.g., basal ganglia, thalamus), lie in the cerebellum or the brainstem, and a few affect the arteries to the choroid plexus alone. Those on the brain surface lying in the borderzone between the major cerebral arteries typically draw supply from more than one of the adjacent cerebral arterial branches. Collateral from the adjacent dura may occur. Those that penetrate to the ventricular wall often draw collaterals from the deep vasculature supplying the basal ganglia. Venous draining may be by superficial or deep venous systems. The threat to health is hemorrhage. The risk of bleeding approximates that of cerebral aneurysms but the morbidity differs, being less. Usually arising from the nidus, hemorrhage may displace adjacent brain with varying degrees of damage, vent into the ventricular system causing mainly a hemo- or hydrocephalus, or spread into the subarachnoid space. Typical subarachnoid hemorrhage may also occur from aneurysms commonly found along the path of intracranial vessels feeding the malformation. Hemorrhage occurs most commonly in the middle decades of life. Separately, AVMs may be associated with seizures or headaches. No distinctive features separate either the seizures or the types of headache (including migraine) from non-AVM causes (Figs. 60.1 through 60.3).

Computed tomography (CT) or magnetic resonance imaging detects acute hemorrhage; magnetic resonance imaging and magnetic resonance angiogram document the AVM, any prior major hemorrhage, intranidal aneurysms, and the main sources

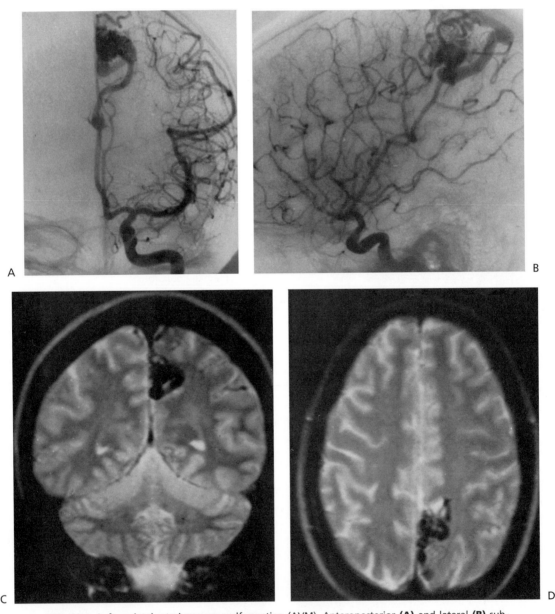

FIG. 60.1. Left parietal arteriovenous malformation (AVM). Anteroposterior **(A)** and lateral **(B)** subtraction films in the arterial phase of a left internal carotid injection show the anterior cerebral artery (ACA) supply and early superficial venous drainage of a left parietal AVM. Coronal **(C)** and axial **(D)** T2-weighted magnetic resonance images of the same patient show a serpiginous pattern of signal void representing flow in vascular structures. (Courtesy of Drs. J. A. Bello and S. K. Hilal.)

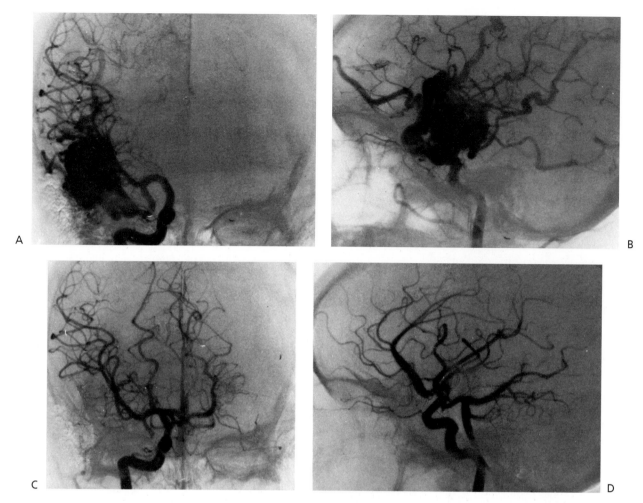

FIG. 60.2. Right temporal arteriovenous malformation (AVM). **A:** Anteroposterior view from arterial phase of right internal carotid arteriogram shows a large enhancing vascular lesion in right temporal region supplied by enlarged branches of right middle cerebral artery. **B:** Lateral view demonstrates prominent early draining cortical veins emanating from AVM. Postembolization anteroposterior **(C)** and lateral **(D)** views of right internal carotid arteriogram show interval disappearance of right temporal AVM with multiple metallic coils seen within right middle cerebral arterial feeders. Note normal filling of both anterior and both posterior cerebral arteries, thereby confirming increase in blood flow to normal brain structures. Patient did well after embolization with no complications. Follow-up definitive surgery found no evidence of flow within AVM, and the nidus was removed to prevent recurrence. (Courtesy of Drs. S. Chan and S. K. Hilal, Columbia University College of Physicians and Surgeons, New York, NY.)

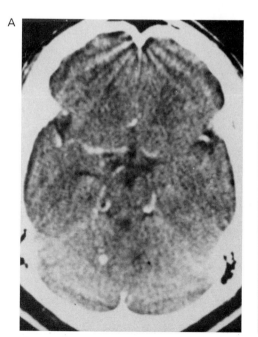 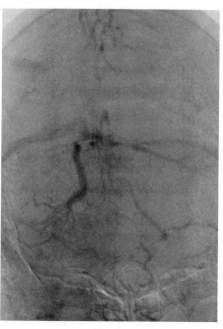

FIG. 60.3. Venous angioma. **A:** Postcontrast computed tomography (CT) demonstrates a round enhancing structure in the right cerebellar hemisphere, seen on contiguous axial sections as well, and therefore consistent with a single prominent vessel, "end-on." This is the typical CT appearance of a venous angioma. **B:** An anteroposterior subtraction film in the venous phase of a vertebral angiogram shows medullary veins in the right cerebellar hemisphere converging toward a single vertically oriented draining vein, which corresponds to the vessel seen in cross section on CT. (The arterial phase was typically normal.) (Courtesy of Drs. J. A. Bello and S.K. Hilal.)

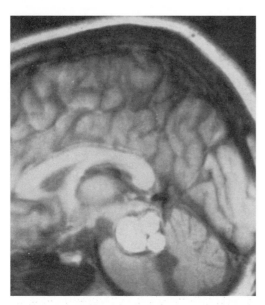

FIG. 60.4. Cavernous malformation, brainstem. Sagittal T1-weighted magnetic resonance imaging demonstrates a loculated-appearing midbrain lesion of increased signal intensity surrounded by ring of decreased signal intensity, which is characteristic of a subacute hemorrhage surrounded by a ring of hemosiderin. Cavernous vascular malformations typically show evidence of previous hemorrhage. (Courtesy of Drs. J. A. Bello and S. K. Hilal.)

of supply. The vascular anatomy in cases intended for treatment is best defined by angiography, which should be reserved for such times (Figs. 60.4 and 60.5).

Because of the threat of disability from hemorrhage, AVMs should be approached with a plan for treatment. Intravascular occlusive therapy using fast-acting glues and other agents may occasionally obliterate some AVMs but more commonly lowers the operative risk by reducing the size and pressure within the malformation before surgery. Surgery is the most effective means of eliminating AVMs. For the smaller (less than 2.5 cm) deeply lying lesions not suitable for embolization or surgery, focused-beam radiotherapy (radiosurgery) is an alternative therapy, and experts currently debate the general applicability for larger lesions.

The vein of Galen malformation is a special AVM associated with the deep venous system, often with marked aneurysmal dilatation of the vein of Galen region. The arterial supply may be complex and difficult to occlude by intravascular or surgical techniques. These lesions are symptomatic in neonates or young children; severe shunting leads to cardiac failure and compression of the midbrain, which causes hydrocephalus. The currently accepted treatment of these lesions is embolization, occasionally followed by surgery.

Venous Malformations

Venous malformations (also deep venous anomalies) exist and have no apparent arterial supply. They may cause headaches, seizures, or, rarely, hemorrhage. Large venous channels may be seen on a prolonged high-volume contrast angiogram (Fig. 60.6). They are easily recognized using CT because of their contrast enhancement. They generally lie in the deep white matter and portions of the brainstem and cerebellum and are often diffuse, ill-defined, do not allow obliteration of arterial supply as the lesion is entirely venous, and are thus not amenable to safe surgical resection. They generally follow a benign course. The symptoms produced by the lesion are treated individually. Only under extenuating circumstances is surgical resection considered.

Cavernous Malformation

Cavernous malformations are highly focal usually small anomalies, and the histologically distinct cluster of tiny vessels of uniform size is the basis of the name "cavernous." The vessels are too small and the shunt is too limited for them to be seen on angiogram. They may cause a limited local hemorrhage, and it may recur, but major bleeding is uncommon. Multiple lesions have been documented in families. They may occur anywhere in the brain. Because of calcium content from inferred prior asymptomatic hemorrhage, the lesion may be visible on CT without contrast or enhance moderately with contrast. It may be mistaken for a vascular tumor, however, without displacement of the surrounding structure. Magnetic resonance imaging is characterized by a "target" appearance (Fig. 60.7). Seizures, headaches, or vague neurologic symptoms may occur. If hemorrhage has

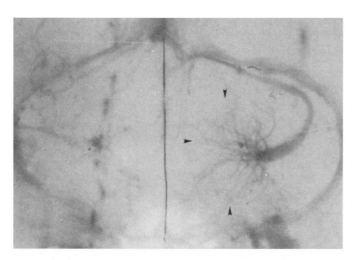

FIG. 60.5. Subtraction posterior fossa angiogram, venous phase. In this anteroposterior view, the characteristic venous malformation is demonstrated (*arrows*).

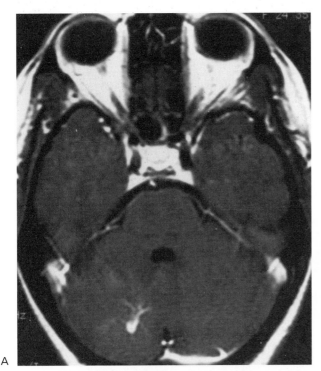

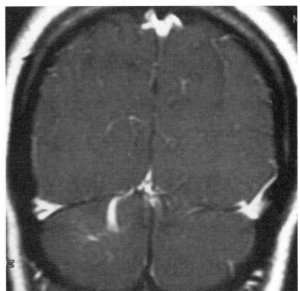

A

B

FIG. 60.6. Venous angioma. T1-weighted gadolinium-enhanced axial **(A)** and coronal **(B)** magnetic resonance scans demonstrate prominent vascular enhancement within the right cerebellar hemisphere with prominent venous radicles draining into an enlarged draining vein. This configuration is characteristic of venous angioma. (Courtesy of Dr. S. Chan, Columbia University College of Physicians and Surgeons, New York, NY.)

occurred and the lesion is readily accessible, surgery is usually recommended.

Telangiectasia

Telangiectases are collections of engorged capillaries or cavernous spaces separated by relatively normal brain tissue. They are usually small and poorly circumscribed and may be found in any portion of the central nervous system. Telangiectases have a propensity for the white matter. They may be associated with telangiectasia of the skin; mucous membranes; and the respiratory, gastrointestinal, and genitourinary tracts, as in the *Rendu-Osler-Weber syndrome*. The associated pulmonary shunts may provide a path for septic material for brain abscess formation. These lesions infrequently lead to gross hemorrhage and fatality. For the most part, these are neurologic curiosities; they cannot be identified on angiography or CT and have no surgical significance. They are usually recognized only at autopsy.

Sturge-Weber Disease (Krabbe-Weber-Dimitri Disease)

The two cardinal features of Sturge-Weber disease (discussed elsewhere) are a localized atrophy and calcification of the cerebral cortex associated with an ipsilateral port wine-colored facial nevus, usually in the distribution of the first division of the trigeminal nerve. Angiomatous malformation in the meninges, ipsilateral exophthalmos, glaucoma, buphthalmos, angiomas of

the retina, optic atrophy, and dilated vessels in the sclera may also be present. Any portion of the cerebral cortex may be affected by the atrophic process, but the occipital and parietal regions are most commonly involved.

In the atrophic cortical areas there is a loss of nerve cells and axons and a proliferation of the fibrous glia. The small vessels are thickened and calcified, particularly in the second and third cortical layers. Small calcium deposits are also present in the cerebral substance (Fig. 60.8), and rarely are there large calcified nodules. When an angioma is present, it is limited to the meninges overlying the area of shrunken cortex. It is now generally agreed that the atrophy and calcification of the cortex are not secondary to the angiomatous malformations of the leptomeninges.

It is possible for the combination of a port wine facial nevus and localized cortical atrophy to exist without clinical symptoms, but in most patients, convulsive seizures are present from infancy. Mental retardation, glaucoma, contralateral hemiplegia (Fig. 60.9), and hemianopia are also present in most cases.

Sturge-Weber disease can be diagnosed without difficulty from the clinical syndrome. The presence of the cortical lesion can be demonstrated in most cases by the appearance of characteristic shadows in the radiographs (Fig. 60.10). The calcified area in the cortex appears as a sinuous shadow with a double contour, showing both the gyri and sulci of the affected cerebral convolutions. The lesions in the occipital or parietal lobes are usually more definitely calcified than are those that occur in the frontal lobe.

The treatment of Sturge-Weber disease is essentially symp-

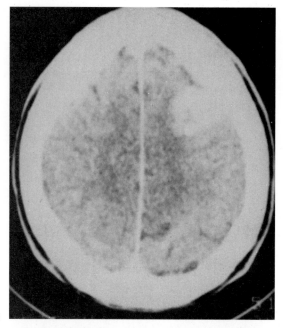

A

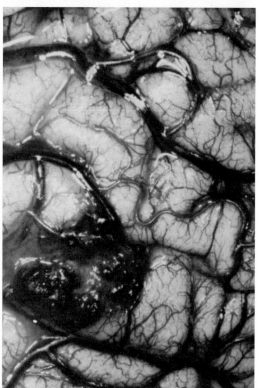

B

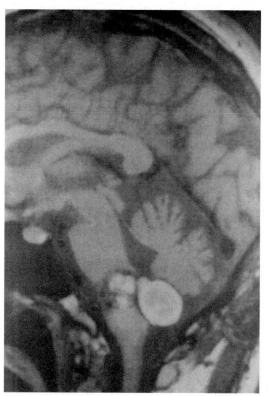

C

FIG. 60.7. A: Axial computed tomography demonstrates a cavernous malformation extending deep from the cortical surface. **B:** Operative exposure of cavernous malformation shows the cortical component of this lesion. **C:** Magnetic resonance imaging shows the characteristic variegated appearance of a cavernous malformation of the brainstem in a different patient.

tomatic. Anticonvulsive drugs are given for the seizures. Radiation therapy has been recommended, but there is no evidence that it is of any benefit. Hemispherectomy may control the convulsive seizures but is avoided because of a high complication rate.

Sinus Pericranii

Sinus pericranii is composed of thin-walled vascular spaces interconnected by numerous anastomoses that protrude from the skull and communicate with the superior longitudinal sinus. The malformation appears early in life and is soft and compressible; it increases in size when the venous pressure in the head is raised by coughing, straining, or lowering the head. It may enlarge slowly over a period of years. The external protuberance may be seen at any portion of the midline of the skull, including the occiput, but is most often found in the midportion of the forehead. Except for the external swelling, there are usually no symptoms. There may be occasionally a pulsating tinnitus, increased intracranial pressure, or a variety of cerebral symptoms. Radio-

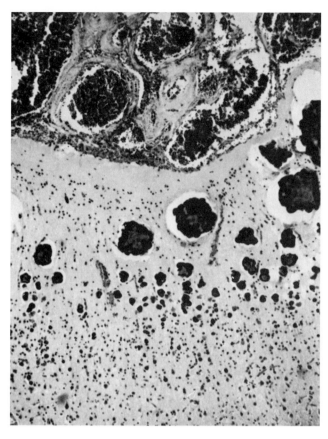

FIG. 60.8. Sturge-Weber syndrome. Angiomatous malformation in meninges and calcification in cortex. Hemotoxylin and eosin stain. (Courtesy of Dr. P. Duffy.)

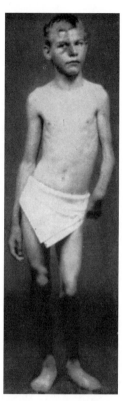

FIG. 60.9. Sturge-Weber disease. Right facial nevus in patient with convulsions and left hemiparesis. (Courtesy of Dr. P.I. Yakovlev.)

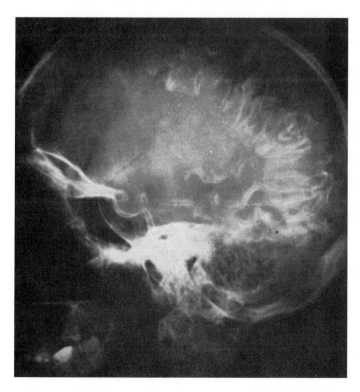

FIG. 60.10. Radiograph shows the intracerebral calcification in Sturge-Weber disease. (Courtesy of Dr. P.I. Yakovlev.)

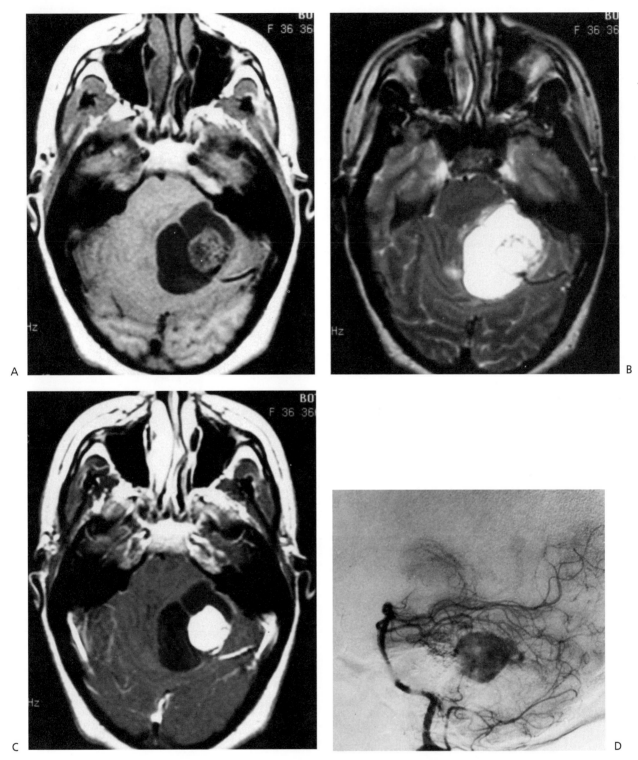

FIG. 60.11. Cerebellar hemangioblastoma. T1-weighted **(A)** and T2-weighted **(B)** axial magnetic resonance scans demonstrate a large fluid-filled cyst in the left cerebellar hemisphere that appears dark on T1 scan and bright on T2 scan. A mass of heterogeneous signal intensity present within the left posterior aspect of the cyst appears attached to the wall of the cyst. Note prominent blood vessel projecting to the left from the posterior aspect of this mural nodule, probably representing draining vein. **C:** T1-weighted axial magnetic resonance scan with gadolinium enhancement shows marked enhancement of mural nodule and no enhancement of the cyst. Note prominent enhancement of enlarged draining vein. **D:** Lateral view from late arterial phase of conventional vertebral arteriogram shows densely enhancing mass in posterior fossa with posterior draining vein. (Courtesy of Drs. S. Chan and A. G. Khandji, Columbia University College of Physicians and Surgeons, New York, NY.)

graphs show a defect of the underlying bone, through which the lesion communicates with the longitudinal sinus.

VASCULAR TUMORS

The three forms of the neoplastic lesions may be variations of the same tumor. By light microscopy they are indistinguishable; however, the hemangioblastoma is confined to the posterior fossa and has no dural attachment. The angioblastic meningioma is grossly identical to other meningiomas but has a significant dural attachment and is located either above or below the tentorium. The hemangiopericytoma originates in other areas of the body, presumably from blood vessel elements.

Angioblastic Meningiomas

These tumors are included here because they are histologically similar to the other tumors reviewed in this section.

Hemangiopericytomas

The hemangiopericytoma arises from the endothelial elements of blood vessels and is recognized elsewhere in the body. It is histologically similar to the angioblastic meningioma and the hemangioblastoma, especially when the vascular spaces are separated more widely and the stroma cells are collected about the vascular spaces. It may be that the pial and endothelial cells are interconvertible.

Hemangioblastomas

Hemangioblastomas are composed of primitive vascular elements and are rare, accounting for 1% to 2% of all intracranial neoplasms. They occur at all ages, but young and middle-aged adults are more frequently afflicted. In children, they are almost as common in the posterior fossa as are meningiomas (Fig. 60.11). Symptoms are generally present for approximately a year before the diagnosis is made. Male incidence predominates. *Von Hippel-Lindau disease* is defined by the coexistence of hemangioblastoma and multiple angiomatoses of the retina, cysts of the kidney and pancreas, and, occasionally, renal cell carcinomas and capillary nevi of the skin. There is a familial incidence in 20% of cases. Only 10% to 20% of the hemangioblastomas, however, are associated with the systemic signs known as the Lindau syndrome. All gradations of clinical expression between the full syndrome and incomplete manifestations may be seen in the same family. Pheochromocytoma and syringomyelia may occur, especially when the hemangioblastoma is in the spinal cord. Polycythemia disappears after resection of the neoplasm, but returns with recurrence; an erythropoietic substance from the cystic fluid has been identified.

These tumors are predominantly in the cerebellum and are often associated with large cysts that are surrounded by a glial wall containing yellow proteinaceous fluid, the result of secretion and hemorrhage from the tumor. It resembles the cyst and mural nodule of the cystic cerebellar astrocytoma but has a distinctive vascular appearance on an angiogram. They may be multi-

ple, in which case difficulty in achieving a cure or total removal of the lesion may be encountered. They have no dural attachment and rarely occur in the supratentorial area, where they may be confused with angioblastic meningiomas.

The most common site of the hemangioblastoma is in the paramedian cerebellar hemispheric area; the second most common site is the spinal cord. Hemangioblastomas also occur in the medulla in the area postrema.

Clinical features of the hemangioblastoma of the cerebellum are symptoms typical of any cerebellar mass, such as headache, papilledema, and ataxia. When the tumor is multiple, lesions may involve the brainstem and upper cervical cord as well. Hemangioblastoma of the cerebellum can be diagnosed without difficulty from the CT and posterior fossa angiogram. The diagnosis is even more certain when the tumor is associated with angiomas of the retina and polycythemia.

Treatment is surgical, with evacuation of the cyst and removal of the mural nodule; 85% of all patients who undergo this treatment are alive and well 5 to 20 years after surgery. There is a high incidence of recurrence, however, if the tumor is partially removed or is associated with multiple tumors.

SUGGESTED READINGS

Atuk NO, McDonald T, Wood T, et al. Familial pheochromocytoma, hypercalcemia, and von Hippel-Lindau disease. A ten year study of a large family. *Medicine (Baltimore)* 1979;58:209–218.

Challa VR, Moody DM, Brown WR. Vascular malformations of the central nervous system. *J Neuropath Exp Neurol* 1995;54:609–621.

Crawford PM, West CR, Chadwick DW, Shaw MDM. Arteriovenous malformations of the brain: natural history in unoperated patients. *J Neurol Neurosurg Psychiatry* 1986;49:1–10.

Cushing H, Bailey P. *Tumors arising from the blood vessels of the brain.* Springfield, IL: Charles C Thomas, 1928.

Farrell DF, Forno LS. Symptomatic capillary telangiectasis of the brainstem without hemorrhage. Report of an unusual case. *Neurology* 1970;20:341–346.

Fischbein NJ, Barkovich AJ, Wu Y, et al. Surge-Weber syndrome with no leptomeningeal enhancement on MRI. *Neuroradiology* 1998;40:177–180.

Gold AP, Ransohoff J, Carter S. Vein of Galen malformation. *Acta Neurol Scand* 1964;40(suppl 2).

Guttmacher AE, Marchuk DA, White RI. Hereditary hemorrhagic telangiectasia. *N Engl J Med* 1995;333:918–924.

Hartmann A, Mast H, Mohr JP, et al. Morbidity of intracranial hemorrhage in patients with cerebral arteriovenous malformation. *Stroke* 1998;29:931–934.

Horton JC, Chambers WA, Lyons SL, et al. Pregnancy and the risk of hemorrhage from cerebral arteriovenous malformations. *Neurosurgery* 1990;27:867–871.

Jeffreys RV, Napier JA, Reynolds SH. Erythropoietin levels in posterior fossa haemangioblastoma. *J Neurol Neurosurg Psychiatry* 1982;45:264–266.

Kruse F Jr. Hemangiopericytomas of the meninges (angioblastic meningioma of Cushing and Eisenhardt). Clinicopathologic aspects and follow-up studies in 8 cases. *Neurology* 1961;11:771–777.

Lasjaunias P. *Vascular diseases in neonates, infants and children. Interventional neuroradiology management.* Berlin, Germany: Springer-Verlag, 1997.

Mast H, Young WL, Koennecke HC, et al. Risk of spontaneous hemorrhage after diagnosis of cerebral arteriovenous malformations. *Lancet* 1997;350:1065–1068.

McLaughlin, MR, Kondziolka D, Flickinger JC, Lunsford S, Lunsford LD. The prospective natural history of cerebral venous malformations. *Neurosurgery* 1998;43:195–200.

Mohr JP, Stein BM, Pile-Spellman J. Arteriovenous malformations. In: Barnett JM, Mohr JP, Stein BM, Yatsu FM, eds. *Stroke. Pathophysiology, diagnosis and management.* Philadelphia, PA: Churchill Livingstone, 1998:725–750.

Moritake K, Handa H, Mori K, et al. Venous angiomas of the brain. *Surg Neurol* 1980;14:95–105.

Naff NJ, Wemmer J, Hoenig-Rigamonti K, Rigamonti DR. A longitudinal study of venous malformations: documentation of a negligible risk and benign natural history. *Neurology* 1998;50:1709–1714.

Neumann HP, Lips CJ, Hsia YE, Zbar B. Von Hippel-Lindau syndrome. *Brain Pathol* 1995;5:181–193.

Ondra SL, Troupp H, George ED, Schwab K. The natural history of symptomatic arteriovenous malformations of the brain: a 24 year follow up assessment. *J Neurosurg* 1990;73:387–391.

Petty GW, Massaro AR, Tatemichi TK, et al. Transcranial Doppler ultrasonographic changes after treatment for arteriovenous malformations. *Stroke* 1990;21:260–266.

Rigamonti D, et al. Cerebral cavernous malformations: incidence and familial occurrence. *N Engl J Med* 1988;319:343–347.

Romanowski CW, Cavallin LI. Tuberous sclerosis, von Hippel-Lindau disease, Sturge-Weber syndrome. *Hosp Med* 1998;59:226–231.

Sarwar M, McCormick WF. Intracerebral venous angioma. *Arch Neurol* 1978;35:323–325.

Schaller C, Pavlidis C, Schramm J. Differential therapy of cerebral arteriovenous malformations. An analysis with reference to personal microsurgery experience. *Nervenarzt* 1996;67:860–869.

Seeger JF, Burke DP, Knake JE, Gabrielsen TO. Computed tomographic and angiographic evaluation of hemangioblastomas. *Radiology* 1981;138:65–73.

Statham P, Macpherson P, Johnston R, et al. Cerebral radiation necrosis complicating stereotactic radiosurgery for arteriovenous malformation. *J Neurol Neurosurg Psychiatry* 1990;53:476–479.

Stein BM, Wolpert SM. Arteriovenous malformations of the brain I and II: current concepts and treatment. *Arch Neurol* 1980;37:1–5, 69–75.

Sujansky E, Conradi S. Outcome of Sturge-Weber syndrome in 52 adults. *Am J Med Genet* 1995;57:35–45.

Sung DI, Thang CH, Harisiadis L. Cerebellar hemangioblastomas. *Cancer* 1982;49:553–555.

Merritt's Neurology, 10th ed., edited by L.P. Rowland. Lippincott Williams & Wilkins, Philadelphia © 2000.

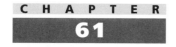

METASTATIC TUMORS

CASILDA M. BALMACEDA

EPIDEMIOLOGY

Up to 35% of all patients with systemic cancer have central nervous system (CNS) metastases. The incidence may be increasing because longer survival may permit a tumor to grow in sanctuary sites such as the brain. Brain metastases are 10 times more common than primary brain tumors; 12,000 people die with primary brain tumors and 130,000 die with brain metastases each year.

DISTRIBUTION

About 66% of CNS metastases affect the parenchyma; spread to leptomeninges, calvarium, or dura is less common. In the spine, the vertebrae are most frequently affected. Some systemic tumors rarely metastasize to the brain. For instance, prostate carcinoma affects the vertebrae and compresses the spinal cord but rarely spreads to the brain or cord parenchyma. Dural metastases arise from prostate or breast carcinoma, and sarcomas.

In *parenchymal metastases* on computed tomography (CT), 49% of patients with brain metastasis have a single lesion, 21% have two, and 30%, three or more. Therefore, 70% of brain metastases can be treated by focal therapy. The tumor distribution parallels blood flow to the brain; about 3% affect the brainstem, 15% the cerebellum, and the others are supratentorial. Some primary tumors show a predilection for particular areas. Pelvic tumors (uterus, colon, or prostate) tend to metastasize to the cerebellum and breast tumors to the pituitary. Breast tumors or melanoma metastasize early to the lungs and enter the systemic circulation. They have the highest incidence of parenchymal brain metastases and tend to be multiple.

Pituitary metastases are uncommon; breast carcinoma accounts for 50%. They are often found incidentally at autopsy in 1.8% of all cancer patients and 15% of patients with breast cancer. One percent of patients undergoing transsphenoidal surgery for a symptomatic pituitary tumor have metastatic carcinoma, and 80% of pituitary metastases affect the posterior pituitary gland or infundibulum. Incidental pituitary metastases are microscopic; symptomatic cases show a characteristic triad of diabetes insipidus, headache, and visual loss. A pituitary mass in a patient with diabetes insipidus and known carcinoma should be considered metastatic until proven otherwise. In contrast to the slow progression of symptoms from pituitary adenoma, manifestations of a metastasis evolve in days or weeks. Pineal spread is usually discovered at autopsy in patients with extensive systemic malignancy. Leptomeningeal seeding frequently accompanies pineal metastases because the tumor sits in the suprasellar cistern and sheds cells into the subarachnoid space.

Dural and subdural metastases are most common in breast or prostate cancer, melanoma, leukemia, neuroblastoma, or lymphoma. Symptoms are produced by compression of the superior sagittal sinus or cranial nerves. Leptomeningeal metastases are most common in patients with leukemia, lymphoma, or carcinoma (breast, lung, melanoma). Perineural metastases usually affect the trigeminal nerve, facial nerve, greater auricular nerve, or oculomotor nerve. Squamous carcinoma, basal cell carcinoma, and carcinoma of the minor salivary glands are most commonly responsible.

In *calvarial and base of the skull metastases*, the most common tumor that metastasizes to the skull base is breast carcinoma, followed by lung and prostate. About 44% of these patients have had bone metastases somewhere else. Five syndromes are recognized. For the clinician, any of these syndromes should raise concern about metastases, even if a primary cancer is thought to have been cured. The *orbital syndrome* comprises supraorbital pain, blurred vision, and diplopia. Examination reveals proptosis, ophthalmoplegia, or decreased opthalmic trigeminal sensation. In the *parasellar syndrome*, cavernous sinus metastases cause frontal headache and ophthalmoparesis. Papilledema is present in a third of the patients; visual loss is less frequent. Primary neoplasms, Tolosa-Hunt syndrome, and carotid artery aneurysms are in the differential diagnosis. In the *middle fossa syndrome*, involvement of the Gasserion ganglion or branches of the trigeminal nerve leads to sensory loss, paresthesias, or pain in the V2 and V3 distribution; lancinating pain is atypical. In the *jugular foramen syndrome*, unilateral occipital, postauricular, or glosopharyngeal pain is followed by hoarseness, dysphagia, and sometimes syncope. By the time of diagnosis, most patients have glosopharyngeal, vagus, and accessory nerve dysfunction, including paresis of the palate, vocal cords, and the sternocleidomastoid. Decreased hearing and facial paralysis indicate extension into the petrous bone. *Occipital condyle syndrome* consists of occipital pain worse on flexion of the neck, with or without a twelfth cranial nerve palsy.

Spinal metastases are described below.

PRIMARY TUMORS LEADING TO CENTRAL NERVOUS SYSTEM METASTASES

Systemic neoplasms vary in propensity to metastasize to the brain. The most common primary neoplasms are melanoma, lung carcinoma, breast carcinoma, and leukemia (Table 61.1). Prostate, genitourinary malignancies, some sarcomas, and malignancies from the endocrine glands or digestive tract rarely spread to the brain.

Melanoma

About 46% of patients develop brain metastases, 96% have systemic disease, 75% of the brain metastases are multiple, and 33% to 50% show hemorrhage (Fig. 61.1). The risk of brain

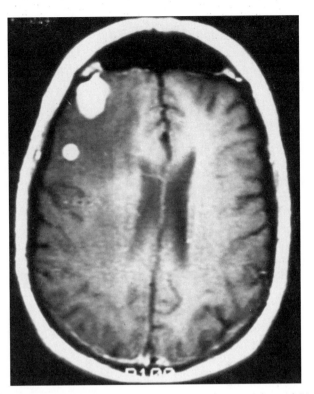

FIG. 61.1. Melanoma brain metastases. Noncontrast-enhanced T1-weighted magnetic resonance image of patient with recurrent melanoma. The metastases are high signal because of either the presence of melanin within the tumor or hemorrhage. Note the extensive surrounding edema.

metastasis is higher with deeper primary lesions or head, neck, or shoulder tumors.

Lung Cancer

At the time of diagnosis, 10% of patients have brain metastases, which may be asymptomatic; 20% develop brain metastases dur-

TABLE 61.1. FREQUENCY AND NUMBER OF ESTIMATED CASES OF INTRACRANIAL AND BRAIN METASTASES (USA)

Type of malignancy	No. of expected deaths (1993)	Intracranial metastases		Brain metastases	
		Frequency (%)	n^a	Frequency (%)	n^a
Lung	149,000	41	61,000	35	52,150
Colon, rectum	57,000	8	4,500	6	3,400
Breast	46,300	51	23,500	21	9,600
Liver, pancreas	37,600	6	2,200	1	400
Prostate	35,000	17	6,000	6	2,100
Female genital	24,400	7	1,700	2	500
Esophageal, stomach	24,000	8	1,900	6	1,400
Urinary tract	20,800	21	4,400	17	3,500
Lymphoma	20,500	22	4,500	5	1,000
Leukemia	18,600	48	8,900	8	1,500
Head and neck	11,500	18	2,000	7	800
Melanoma	6,800	65	4,400	49	3,300
Sarcoma	4,150	10	400	5	225
Thyroid	1,050	25	25	15	15
Others	69,300	5	3,500	25	1,750
Total	526,000	25	128,925	15	81,240

^{a}Derived by multiplying frequency by number of expected deaths.
From Galicich et al., 1996, with permission.

ing treatment; and 50% of those who survive 2 years develop them. Forty percent of patients with small cell lung carcinoma develop brain metastases, as do 28% of those with adenocarcinoma of the lung. About 50% of patients with lung cancer have brain metastases at autopsy.

Breast Carcinoma

This is the most common source of brain metastases in women, seen in 20% of women with this tumor. In contrast to brain metastases from other solid tumors, two-thirds of these patients die of the intracranial disease. Several intracranial compartments may be affected simultaneously: parenchyma, dura, leptomeninges, or a combination. Benign meningiomas are disproportionately frequent in women with breast carcinoma, so a dural-based mass in such a patient may require a biopsy or serial imaging to clarify the diagnosis.

Gynecological malignancies uncommonly metastasize to the CNS. The most characteristic is the rare choriocarcinoma.

Colon Cancer

An infrequent cause of brain metastases, colon cancer affects 4% of patients. Most patients have extensive systemic disease; 85% have pulmonary metastases. Posterior fossa lesions are overrepresented, affecting 35% of patients. In patients with liver metastases, the incidence of brain metastases is lower, possibly related to a filtering effect. CT may show a hyperdense lesion, hypointense on T2-weighted magnetic resonance images, perhaps caused by coagulative tumor necrosis.

Carcinoma of an Unknown Primary

This represents 8% of patients with brain metastasis. The site of origin is eventually identified in 25% of the cases, and in half of these, the primary tumor is lung carcinoma. In contrast to clinically evident systemic tumors, morbidity and mortality are related to the brain metastasis, and aggressive treatment of the brain lesion is indicated.

DIAGNOSIS

Clinical Diagnosis

Symptoms are similar to those of any space-occupying lesion, including motor impairment (66%), headache (53%), mental changes (31%), papilledema (26%), ataxia (20%), and seizures (15%). Multiple brain metastases can mimic encephalopathy or dementia. Headache may be caused by the tumor, edema, hydrocephalus, sinus thrombosis from dural metastases, or leptomeningeal metastasis. Pain-sensitive structures vulnerable to distortion include the dura, tentorium, and cranial nerves. Seizures are the first symptom in 15% to 20% of patients, but up to 10% of additional patients develop seizures later. Seizures occur more frequently with multiple, frontal, or temporal metastases. Tumor histology does not correlate with epileptogenicity. It is debatable whether all patients with metastases should be

treated prophylactically. In a double-blind, prospective, randomized trial of patients with brain metastases with no prior seizure, there was no significant difference in seizure frequency of those who received valproic acid or placebo. Anticonvulsant therapy is not without risk, including a 4% incidence of drug allergy with phenytoin, elevation of hepatic enzymes, alteration of metabolism of dexamethasone and chemotherapy, and the risk of Stevens-Johnson syndrome when combined with radiotherapy. Other metastatic symptoms include strokelike episodes in 10% of patients with cerebral metastases and attributed to intratumor hemorrhage or sudden obstruction of cerebrospinal fluid (CSF) flow. Hemorrhage occurs most commonly in choriocarcinoma, melanoma, and lung and renal cell carcinoma.

Radiographic Diagnosis

Magnetic resonance imaging (MRI) with contrast administration of gadolinium is the most sensitive diagnostic method for detection of either intraparenchymal or leptomeningeal brain metastases, particularly for posterior fossa lesions. It is also best for differentiating intraparenchymal and dural-based lesions. MRI may identify multiple lesions when CT shows only single lesions that might be considered candidates for surgical therapy. CT is better in detecting lytic bony lesions.

Most brain metastases appear as round well-circumscribed lesions, hypointense on T1-weighted images and hyperintense on T2.

Up to 90% enhance after gadolinium. Lesions as small as 3 mm can be detected on contrast-enhanced images but may be invisible on precontrast. T2-weighted images are useful for identifying hemorrhagic metastases and surrounding edema that might be mistaken for an infarct. Enhancement may be heterogeneous. Ringlike enhancement is also seen in brain abscess, but abscesses typically have thinner rims and may show a target-type sign.

Histology cannot be determined by MRI alone. Malignant melanoma is an exception: The lesions are isointense to hyperintense on T1-weighted images and hypointense on T2-weighted images. Colon carcinoma metastases may display a characteristic hypointensity on T2-weighted images. Some tumors spread to the brain with little reaction in surrounding tissue, so-called miliary brain metastases, seen with neuroectodermal tumors (Fig. 61.2). The MRI pattern is caused by the perivascular distribution of lesions with multiple tumor nodules, which may not be evident on contrast T1-weighted MRI, appearing only as T2-weighted changes.

About 14% of brain metastases are hemorrhagic, mimicking a stroke. The hemorrhage is usually intraparenchymal but may be subarachnoid, intraventricular, or subdural. Multiple sites of intracerebral hemorrhage argue strongly in favor of metastatic disease. Metastases are more likely to bleed than primary brain tumors. Hemorrhage may be spontaneous or due to thrombocytopenia from chemotherapy or a coagulopathy. If the platelet count is less than 20,000, hemorrhage may occur in areas of the brain unaffected by tumor spread. Calcification of the metastasis may be seen with colon, lung, or breast carcinoma. Magnetic resonance angiography may show the relationship of the tumor to major blood vessels before surgery or distinguish hemorrhagic

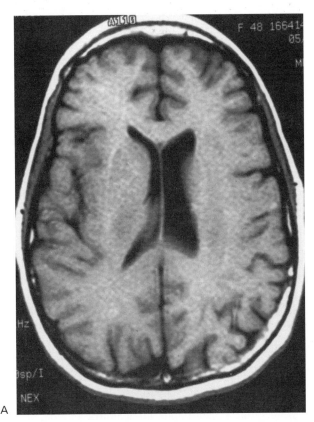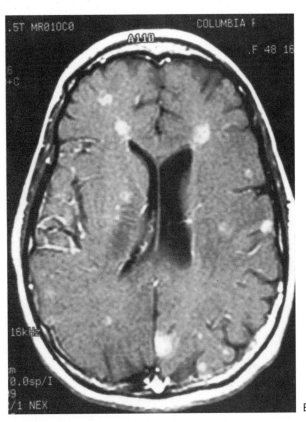

FIG. 61.2. Miliary brain metastases. Noncontrast-enhanced **(A)** and contrast-enhanced **(B)** magnetic resonance images of a patient with breast cancer. Note that the nonenhanced scan appears almost normal. The contrast-enhanced scan shows greater than 20 separate metastatic lesions with no significant surrounding edema. This patient was neurologically normal at the time of this scan, which was performed after a cervical spine magnetic resonance image showed a cerebellar metastasis.

metastases from vascular malformations. Positron emission tomography with fluorine-18 fluorodeoxyglucose may distinguish recurrent tumors from radiation necrosis.

Clinical Evaluation

In the patient without a known primary tumor and suspected brain metastases, a focused screening workup is appropriate. Attention is directed to a chest radiogram or chest CT, followed by abdominal or pelvic CT or endoscopy if gastrointestinal symptoms are evident. Physical examination should address possible breast, testicle, prostate, or rectal lesions. Stool should be examined for occult blood. If imaging suggests a melanoma, consider acral lentiginous melanoma on palms or soles, melanoma of the uveal tract, or subungual tumor. If screening is unrevealing and a single lesion is surgically accessible, resection is performed for diagnosis and treatment. If multiple brain lesions are present, a stereotactic brain biopsy is preferred.

Differential Diagnosis

When a patient with a primary neoplasm develops neurologic symptoms, other conditions may mimic metastases. In patients immunosuppressed by chemotherapy, pulmonary infections may lead to septic emboli and *brain abscess.* The diagnosis may be suspected when location is atypical for a metastases, such as

the basal ganglia. Multiple small contrast-enhancing lesions may be seen in *tuberculosis* or *fungal abscesses.* On MRI, abscesses have thin-walled rings of contrast enhancement, different from the thicker nodular enhancement with metastases. Multifocal gliomas may mimic brain metastases.

Demyelinating disease can occasionally appear on CT or MRI as large contrast-enhancing lesions with mass effect. The clinical disorder may be acute and monophasic rather than the typical relapsing and remitting pattern of multiple sclerosis. Histologically, large reactive astrocytes seen in active demyelinating lesions may be misinterpreted as neoplastic.

Delayed *radiation necrosis* can cause a contrast-enhancing mass, which may enlarge on subsequent scans. *Stroke* may mimic metastases clinically and radiographically, with discrete lesions and contrast enhancement. With time, the infarct improves radiographically. Dural metastases of prostate or breast carcinoma may mimic *meningiomas.* An unusual phenomena is "tumore-in-tumori," a systemic malignancy metastasizing to already existing primary intracranial tumor, favored by the high blood flow to the recipient tumor.

Pathophysiology

In 1889, Paget proposed the "soil-seed" hypothesis, that tumors metastasize preferentially to organs that provide a favorable environment. In 1928, Ewing speculated that metastases are directly related to the vascular supply of the target organ. The pattern is not random, and organs similar in developmental origin have a similar propensity for metastasis. In the CNS, metastases to cortex and white matter correlate with metastases to leptomeninges, another neuroectodermally derived tissue, but not with metastases to dura, which originates from mesoderm. In animal models, some tumors show predilection for specific organs, providing evidence against a purely hemodynamic theory.

Spread to the brain occurs when the primary tumor sheds tumor emboli into the circulation. The lung effectively filters larger tumor emboli, and a pulmonary lesion is present before a brain metastasis. An embolic mechanism is also suggested by higher incidence of brain metastases in watershed vascular regions than in other areas of the brain. Metastases may bypass the lungs via a patent foramen ovale or with pelvic and abdominal tumors, when cells pass through the Batson plexus to the paravertebral and intracranial venous plexi. Contiguous spread to adjacent bony structures is another mechanism with tumors expanding locally and invading the CNS secondarily.

Metastasis is a multistep process that includes passage of malignant cells to the target organ, thrombosis in capillaries, adherence to endothelial cells, invasion of the subendothelial matrix, digestion of the basement membrane by proteolytic enzymes, and passage of tumor cells into the interstitial space. The first step involves cell attachment to the endothelium at the target site. For invasion to proceed, proteolytic enzymes then degrade the extracellular matrix and permit migration into surrounding tissues. Host cellular inhibitors of invasion (metalloprotease inhibitors) control extracellular matrix degradation. Direct cell–cell interactions or interactions between tumor cells and basement membrane may influence the organ specificity of metastases. In the early stages, tumor metastasis probably depends on paracrine growth factors, but as the malignancy advances, it develops autocrine means of growth stimulation. This parallels the clinical observation that in the early metastatic stage, tumors may show restricted organ distribution, but in the latter stages tumors may metastasize freely to multiple organs.

TREATMENT

Among patients with brain metastases, the lesions are lethal in less than half. In most, survival is determined by responsiveness of systemic tumor. Therapy is evaluated by local control and by overall survival. Corticosteroids were first used in the 1960s to decrease the permeability in the abnormal blood vessels surrounding metastases, reducing tumor edema or radiation-related edema. Corticosteroids often reverse neurologic symptoms within 24 hours in 80% of patients. Dexamethasone is used most often because of its low mineralocorticoid activity. Steroids are usually given during the course of radiation, at the lowest dose that controls neurologic symptoms. Twenty percent of patients take steroids chronically to reverse or stabilize neurologic symptoms. Even when therapy has failed and patients are moribund, steroids may relieve the headaches or vomiting of increased intracranial pressure.

Radiotherapy improves neurologic symptoms in 49% to 93% of patients. The degree of neurologic recovery is inversely proportional to the severity of symptoms before irradiation. External whole brain irradiation is given for either multiple brain metastases or single surgically inaccessible lesions. The goal of whole brain radiotherapy is to eradicate microscopic foci of tumor. Radiotherapy is palliative, prolonging survival from an average of 1 month without treatment (2 months with corticosteroids) to 4 to 6 months or more. Response is best in patients with breast carcinoma, those with a long interval between diagnosis of systemic tumor and brain metastases, or those with limited extracranial disease. A dose of 30 Gy is usually administered in 10 daily fractions of 0.3 Gy; higher doses are not more effective. Even with radiotherapy, fewer than 10% of patients survive 2 years; metastasis causes death in about 50%. It is uncertain whether radiotherapy improves the ultimate prognosis for single brain metastases that have been surgically resected. Radiosensitive tumors include germ cell tumors, lymphoma, and small cell lung cancer. Radioresistant tumors include melanoma, renal cell carcinoma, colon, and thyroid.

Brain metastases are usually well demarcated from the parenchyma, allowing complete removal and local control. Surgery may also provide a diagnosis when histology is not known. In a few patients, a single brain metastasis is the only evidence of spread from lung cancer. In this situation, surgery is elected for both the pulmonary lesion and the brain metastasis. Survival up to 7 years has been reported. Among 231 patients with non-small cell lung carcinoma who underwent resection for brain metastases, survival was shorter with incomplete resection of the primary brain tumor, infratentorial location, presence of systemic metastases, or age older than 60 years. Patients with single brain metastases who are treated with both surgery and radiotherapy remain functionally independent longer (median 38 versus 8 weeks), have a longer time to recurrence (more than 59 versus 21 weeks), and have a longer survival (40 versus 15 weeks) compared with those treated with radiation alone.

Chemotherapy has a limited role in treating brain metastases, which may be related to lack of chemosensitivity. Also, brain metastases often appear after primary chemotherapy has failed and the tumor has become resistant to effective agents. Nevertheless, brain metastases of breast, small cell carcinoma of the lung, or choriocarcinoma may respond.

With improved survival of patients with small cell lung cancer, more of them develop brain metastases. In 17% of patients, the CNS is the first site of failure. Prophylactic cranial irradiation is controversial, although studies abound in favor or against it. In one study, the 2-year cumulative incidence of brain metastases dropped from 47% to 10%, but there was no improvement in overall survival. In adenocarcinoma or large cell carcinoma of the lung, prophylactic cranial irradiation did not alter overall survival, but it delayed the onset of brain metastases. Long-term survivors may develop a syndrome of leukoencephalopathy.

Radiosurgery was developed by Leskell in 1951 in an attempt to deliver high doses of radiotherapy to a confined region of brain. The spherical nature and defined borders of brain metastases make them ideal candidates. Also, multiple lesions can be treated with minimal dose overlap. Radiosurgery is administered using a gamma knife or linear accelerator. Radiosurgery has been used for either single or multiple brain metastases before whole brain radiotherapy, at diagnosis, or at the time of progression after conventional radiation. Radiosurgery may reduce the incidence of treatment-related leukoencephalopathy, particularly for patients with no evidence of active systemic disease. The local control rate with radiosurgery is 88%, about twice as much as the 45% local control rates with whole brain radiation. Melanoma and renal cell carcinoma, traditionally resistant to whole brain radiotherapy, are paradoxically among the tumors that respond most favorably to radiosurgery (Fig 61.3). Interstitial radiation allows treatment of defined lesions, sparing the surrounding brain. Radioactive seeds are placed in the tumor bed, which then receives local continuous radiation. Iodine-125 is used most often to treat either recurrent or newly diagnosed brain metastases.

CARCINOMATOUS MENINGITIS

Leptomeningeal metastasis develops in 4% to 15% of all patients with cancer. The increased incidence is attributed to improved

survival of patients with cancer. Solid tumors are most commonly associated; breast cancer accounts for 12% to 34% of all patients, followed by lung cancer (10% to 26%), melanoma (17% to 25%), gastrointestinal cancer (4% to 14%), non-Hodgkin lymphoma, and acute lymphocytic leukemia. The primary site is unknown in 7% of cases. Patients usually have systemic disease at the same time; otherwise, the systemic tumor reoccurs within weeks of diagnosis of the carcinomatous meningitis.

Pathogenesis

Metastatic cells may reach the leptomeninges by various routes: hematogenous dissemination, spread from bone metastases, dissemination via the perivascular space, or along perineural spaces. There is a good correlation, with most systemic malignancies, between the development of osseous metastases and carcinoma-

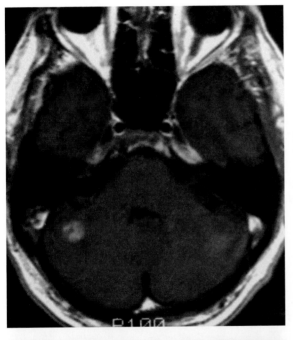

A

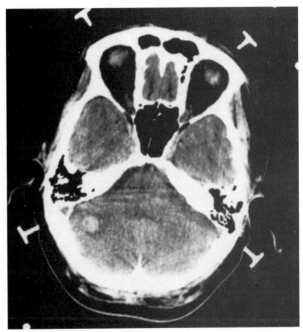

B

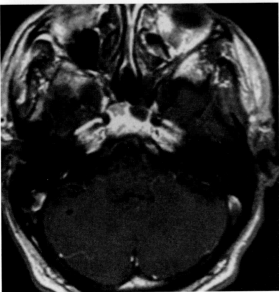

C

FIG. 61.3. Successful radiosurgical treatment of renal cell carcinoma. **A:** Contrast-enhanced magnetic resonance image shows a 1-cm right cerebellar hemisphere metastasis. **B:** Contrast-enhanced computed tomography in stereotactic frame for radiosurgery treatment planning. **C:** Contrast-enhanced magnetic resonance image 8 months after radiosurgery shows complete disappearance of the previous metastasis. All that remains is a focal area of atrophy.

tous meningitis. Spread can develop via transgression of the dura through a primary extension from a vertebral, paravertebral, or calvarial lesion (Fig. 61.4). Tumor cells bind to the endothelial cells, extravasate or form a thrombus inside the lumen, and eventually disrupt the endothelium. Cells in the subarachnoid space spread along the leptomeninges to form perivascular cuffs, enter the Virchow-Robin spaces, and may penetrate the pia to involve the brain. Pathologically, the disease is characterized by diffuse infiltration of the leptomeninges. Hydrocephalus arises if tumor nodules obstruct the ventricles or basal cisterns. In the spinal

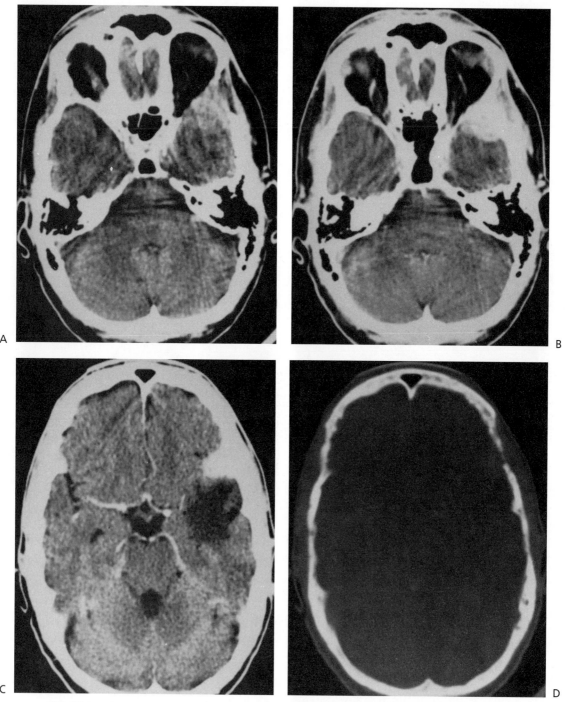

FIG. 61.4. Calvarial and epidural metastases. Precontrast **(A)** and postcontrast **(B)** axial computed tomographies demonstrate that the anterior wall of the middle cranial fossa is missing; it is replaced by an enhancing metastasis from breast carcinoma with an epidural component anterior to the left temporal lobe. The patient had left V1 sensory loss. Higher postcontrast cut **(C)** and bone window **(D)** at the same level demonstrate extension of the epidural metastasis. Transdural involvement is suggested by the prominent white matter edema in the underlying temporal lobe, with effacement of the left sylvian fissure due to mass effect. Note the extensive calvarial involvement in **D**. Malignant cells were recovered from cerebrospinal fluid, thus indicating coexistent meningeal carcinomatosis. (Courtesy of Drs. J.A. Bello and S.K. Hilal.)

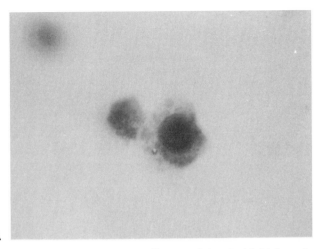

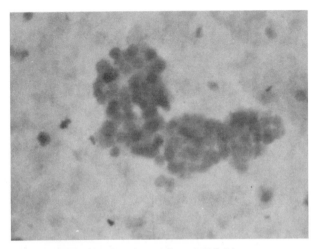

A B

FIG. 61.5. Malignant cells in spinal fluid. Formalin-fixed millipore filtrates of lumbar cerebrospinal fluid in two patients with meningeal spread of neoplasm. **A:** Isolated large cells with increased nuclear-to-cytoplasm ratio and fine clumps of cytoplasmic pigment in a patient with meningeal carcinomatosis due to malignant melanoma (hematoxylin stain, ×450). **B:** A clump of cohesive cells in patient with a primitive neuroectodermal tumor and extensive meningeal seeding (hematoxylin stain, ×180).

cord, tumor infiltration is most prominent over the dorsal cord or cauda equina.

Diagnosis

Symptoms and signs vary because the disease affects all levels of the CNS. Cerebral symptoms include headache (75%), mental status changes (65%), difficulty walking (27%), nausea and vomiting (22%), and seizures (11%). Cranial nerve symptoms include diplopia (30%), facial weakness (27%), hearing loss (12%), optic neuropathy (8%), and trigeminal neuropathy (8%). Spinal findings comprise reflex asymmetry (86%), limb weakness (73%), paresthesias (42%), radicular pain (26%), and sphincter dysfunction (16%).

CSF abnormalities include elevated pressure (42% to 72%), pleocytosis (64% to 77%), elevated protein (79% to 91%), and low glucose (41% to 77%). Proof of diagnosis is the demonstration of neoplastic cells in the CSF (Fig. 61.5). Repeated spinal punctures are often needed. In about 5% of patients, CSF cytology is positive when fluid is sampled from the ventricles or cisterna magna but not from the lumbar compartment. The first lumbar CSF examination shows neoplastic cells in 55%, rising to 80% after a second tap. Twenty-nine percent of patients with abnormal cytology have no CSF pleocytosis. Normal cytology does not exclude the disease; 41% of patients with carcinomatous meningitis at autopsy had a normal antemortem CSF.

Cranial CT findings include sulcal enhancement (21%), ependymal enhancement (75%), subarachnoid enhancing nodules (29%), intraventricular nodules (10%), and hydrocephalus (10%) (Fig. 61.6). Coexistent CNS metastases include parenchymal lesions (25% to 40%), dural metastases (16% to 37%), epidural cord compression (1% to 5%), and nodular leptomeningeal disease (10% to 15%). Head MRI with contrast can detect meningeal tumor in about 50% of patients with negative CSF cytology and no spinal symptoms and in up to 92% of those with positive CSF cytology. Head MRI is more sensitive than CT but both are often false negative (30% by MRI and 58% by CT).

CT myelography findings include thickened nerve roots,

nerve root filling defects, block of CSF flow, and subarachnoid nodules (Fig. 61.7). Spinal MRI shows pial enhancement along the cord. CT myelogram is better in detecting cord enlargement; spinal MRI with contrast shows subarachnoid nodules, intraparenchymal cord tumor, or epidural cord compression.

Radionuclide CSF flow studies with ^{111}In-DTPA injected into either the ventricles or lumbar CSF compartment is abnormal in 40% of patients. It can determine whether there is homogeneous distribution of intrathecal chemotherapy.

The following are recommended for patients with documented carcinomatous meningitis: head CT or MRI to show areas of bulky disease and the presence or absence of hydrocephalus, CT myelogram or spine MRI, and radionuclide flow

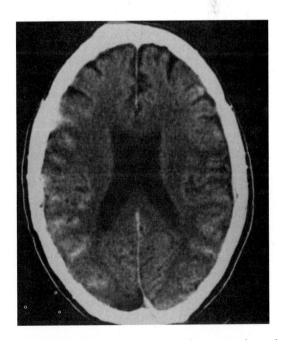

FIG. 61.6. Meningeal carcinomatosis. An axial contrast-enhanced computed tomography demonstrates abnormal sulcal enhancement causing sulcal effacement in a patient with metastatic breast carcinoma.

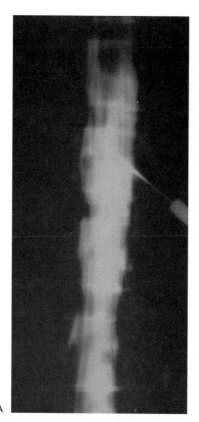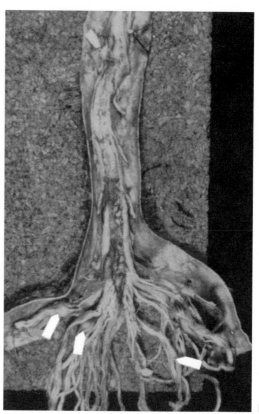

A   B

FIG. 61.7. Meningeal carcinomatosis. Myelogram and autopsy specimen of spinal cord from same patient with meningeal carcinomatosis. Note the intradural filling defects in the myelogram **(A)** that correspond to tumor nodules (*arrows*) seen on multiple nerve roots and thoracic spinal cord in pathologic specimen **(B)**.

study is performed in some institutions. Suspected cases should have at least two lumbar punctures. If negative, sampling can be done from the cisternal or intraventricular compartments.

Treatment

Meningeal carcinomatosis affects the entire neuraxis, and treatment must encompasses all CSF compartments. Treatment is palliative. Radiotherapy is given to subarachnoid tumor nodules or intraparenchymal metastases, but craniospinal radiotherapy is not given routinely because of myelosuppression. Radiotherapy can be given to sites of CSF obstruction to provide homogeneous distribution of intrathecal chemotherapy.

Systemic chemotherapy is not routine, because of the limited CSF penetration of most agents. Meningeal lymphoma, breast, or lung cancer can be treated with systemic chemotherapy and radiation to the focal areas of disease. Patients with symptomatic hydrocephalus that does not respond to focal radiation require CSF shunting. Frequently, an intraventricular catheter and a subgaleal reservoir are installed for intrathecal chemotherapy. Intrathecal chemotherapy is limited to three agents (methotrexate, cytosine arabinoside, and thiotepa). Cytologic responses are seen in 60% of patients to first-line intrathecal therapy, in 29% to second, and in 13% to third-line treatment. The ventricular route achieves more uniform drug distribution than lumbar injections. Triple-agent therapy may give better responses and improved survival than single agents. Most complications of intraventricular treatment are transient and characterized by aseptic meningitis (43%). Patients may experience myelosuppression, particularly if they are given concurrent systemic therapy. A dreaded complication is chemotherapy-related leukoencephalopathy. Novel therapies include gene therapy with the herpes virus thymidine kinase gene, which increases survival in experimental neoplastic meningitis in rats. Intrathecal application of cytokines has been tested for interleukin-2, interferon-alfa, and lymphocyte-activated killer cells, and clearance of neoplastic cells have been observed in humans. Median survival of meningeal carcinomatosis is 6 months, but treatment may prevent neurologic deterioration. Prognosis is worse with widespread systemic disease, CSF block, and coexistent bulky CNS metastases. Sixty percent of patients die of progression of the systemic cancer, and 10% of treatment-related complications.

SPINAL METASTASES

Spinal involvement is seen at autopsy in 60% of patients with breast cancer and in 67% of living patients with prostate cancer. Small cell carcinoma of the lung spreads to the spine in 40% of all cases. Vertebral metastases cause epidural cord compression in 5% of patients, usually with widespread malignancy; in about 3% cord compression is the first sign of metastatic disease. The most common site of compression is thoracic (70%); lumbar compression occurs in 20% and cervical in 10%. In prostate carcinoma, compression involves one vertebral body in 26%, two in 42%, and three or more in 32%.

Pathogenesis

The vertebral column is the most common site of skeletal metastases. Several theories are proposed. First, bone marrow has a high concentration of factors that stimulate neoplastic growth. Second, the Batson vertebral venous plexus is a preferred site of drainage for pelvic, abdominal, and thoracic organs. Third, the lymphatic system, which anastomoses with the vertebral plexus, may also play a role. Concentration of blood vessels in the vertebral body exceeds other parts of the vertebra and makes it most vulnerable. Epidural cord compression usually results from direct extension of tumor from the vertebral column or metastases in the paravertebral spaces that grow through the neural foramina without affecting the bone. The mechanism of cord injury includes vertebral venous plexus compression with resultant cord edema and ischemia.

Clinical

Vertebral metastases may be completely asymptomatic. Pain is the first symptom in 95% of the patients with cord compression. Pain can be local or radicular and may be aggravated by movement, similar to arthritic pain. Several clinical features may help differentiate; pain from metastases may arise at any level, whereas degenerative arthritic pain is usually lumbar or cervical. Lying supine usually alleviates arthritic pain but aggravates metastatic pain. Limb weakness (76%), autonomic disturbances (57%), and sensory dysfunction (51%) are also observed. Urinary incontinence is a late symptom. Bandlike pain across the chest or abdomen may be misinterpreted as arising from abdominal viscera. The location of cord compression is usually indicated by a sensory level.

Diagnostic Evaluation

Plain spine radiographs reveal metastases in 85% of patients with cord compression; loss of vertebral pedicles is the first sign, but it occurs after there is extensive bone destruction. Radiographic abnormalities are common in patients with breast, lung, or prostate carcinoma but rare in patients with lymphoma. Prostate carcinoma produces osteoblastic lesions, whereas breast cancer leads to lytic ones. In patients with pain and abnormal radiographs, cord compression is documented on myelography in 86%, but in those with symptoms and normal radiographs, compression is found in 8%. Noncontrast MRI is the preferred test for epidural tumor. About 27% of patients with focal signs show multiple sites of compression, so MRI should include the entire spine to identify areas of unrecognized epidural tumor that might benefit from early irradiation. A diagnostic protocol has been proposed by Portenoy (1987). If the only symptom is pain, with no neurologic signs but radiographs are abnormal, many would irradiate the symptomatic vertebra without further imaging. If the patient has mild signs or symptoms, MRI or myelo-

gram may be performed the next day; patients with severe or rapidly progressive symptoms must have an emergency MRI or myelogram.

Therapy

The most important aspects of management are preservation of neurologic function and alleviation of pain. Pain without cord compression may be treated with analgesics or radiation if analgesics are ineffective. Early recognition and treatment are crucial. Corticosteroids alleviate pain and improve the neurologic disorder. Many centers start dexamethasone at 4 mg four times a day, others give an intravenous bolus of 100 mg, followed by 24 mg four times a day, and a tapering schedule with the radiation.

A common radiation program is 3,000 to 4,000 cGy over 2 to 4 weeks. Radiation usually includes two vertebral bodies above and two below the lesion. In some studies, surgery and radiotherapy were not better than radiation alone. Posterior tumors are best approached by laminectomy, whereas anterior ones may require thoracotomy, vertebral body resection, and spinal stabilization. Surgery is considered in the following circumstances: cord compression and unknown primary tumor, worsening symptoms and signs referable to a previously irradiated level, spinal instability, neurologic deterioration despite radiotherapy and steroids, and radioresistant tumors. In patients with prostate cancer, the use of orchiectomy as the sole therapy to reduce the testosterone level, may lead to improvement. The most important prognostic factor is the neurologic status at the time of treatment: Up to 80% of ambulatory patients remained ambulatory, whereas only 50% of those with leg weakness and 10% of those with paralysis walked again. Pain can be relieved in 96% of patients treated with corticosteroids and radiation. Patients with compression fractures are less likely to have a favorable response to external radiotherapy, and early surgery should be considered. Survival depends mostly on control of the underlying malignancy.

GRANULOMAS

CNS granulomas may mimic metastatic or primary brain tumors and are discussed in Chapters 24, 25, and 26. The lesions have histologic signs of chronic inflammation and are seen with sarcoidosis, syphilis, tuberculosis, fungi, or parasites.

Intracranial tuberculomas constitute one-third of all intracranial space-occupying lesions in developing countries but are rare in the United States and Europe, even in patients with acquired immunodeficiency syndrome and tuberculosis. Parenchymal disease can occur with or without meningitis. *Miliary pulmonary tuberculosis* commonly affects the brain; the patient may be asymptomatic despite multiple, small, contrast-enhancing lesions in the gray–white matter junction. Symptoms are related to location. Children favor the infratentorial compartment, whereas lesions in adults are mostly in the frontal and parietal lobes.

Pathologically, at first, the lesion is noncaseating. Eventually, a central zone of necrosis is surrounded by a capsule composed of epitheloid cells, multinucleated giant cells, collagen, and mononuclear inflammatory cells. Tuberculosis organisms are rarely seen. CT and MRI show lobular masses with irregular enhancement. A target sign is helpful in diagnosis. Thirty-four percent of the lesions are multiple, mainly at the corticomedullary junction. MRI features depend on the stage of the granuloma. An "en plaque" tuberculoma may mimic a meningeal neoplasm.

Tuberculous abscess is also rare. Compared with granulomas, it is larger, composed of pus and tubercle bacilli, accompanied by edema, and with a more rapid course. On CT, it may seem to be a pyogenic abscess. The walls are thin, and enhancement is smooth. Surgical treatment is considered if a lesion suspected of being a tuberculoma does not respond to antibiotic treatment.

Calvarial tuberculosis results from hematogenous or lymphatic dissemination or from direct extension from sinuses, nasal cavity, or orbit. Radiographically there is a single circumscribed calvarial defect. *Tuberculous otomastoiditis* causes otorrhea, facial paralysis, and multiple tympanic membrane perforations.

The first account of *spinal tuberculosis* was done by Sir Percival Pott in 1779, and the condition was named after him. Location is commonly the thoracolumbar junction, usually involving two adjoining vertebrae. Focal destruction of a vertebral body is the most common lesion, spreading to the intervertebral discs, epidural space, or paraspinal soft tissues. The route of infection is hematogenous, and the mycobacteria lodge in the vascular marrow. In children, disks may be affected without vertebral body disease. The course is indolent, with persistent pain, local tenderness, or limitation of mobility. Myelopathic signs may be seen if there is associated epidural infection or if bony fragments enter the spinal canal. About 40% of patients have paraparesis. Fever is seen late in the course. The erythrocyte sedimentation rate is high and skin tuberculosis tests are positive. CT-guided biopsy confirms the diagnosis. Spinal radiculomyelitis occurs if the exudates encompass the cord and spinal roots. Treatment consists of an antituberculosis regimen in addition to surgical drainage, removal of necrotic tissue, and decompression of the epidural spine or spinal fusion.

SUGGESTED READINGS

Alexander E 3rd, Loeffler JS. Recurrent brain metastases. *Neurosurg Clin North Am* 1996;7:517–526.

Das A, Hochberg FH. Clinical presentation of intracranial metastases. *Neurosurg Clin North Am* 1996;7:377–391.

Galicich J, Arbit E, Wronski M. Metastatic brain tumors. In: Wilkins R, Rengachary S, eds. *Neurosurgery*. New York: McGraw-Hill, 1996:807–821.

Hiraki A, Tabata M, Ueoka H, et al. Direct intracerebral invasion from skull metastasis of large cell lung cancer. *Intern Med* 1997;36:720–723.

Johnson JD, Young B. Demographics of brain metastasis. *Neurosurg Clin North Am* 1996;7:337–344.

Oneschuk D, Bruera E. Palliative management of brain metastases. *Support Care Cancer* 1998;6:365–372.

Patchell RA. The treatment of brain metastases. *Cancer Invest* 1996;14:169–177.

Posner JB. Brain metastases: 1995. A brief review. *J Neurooncol* 1996 27:287–293.

Roberts WS, Sell JJ, Orrison WW Jr. Multiple ischemic infarcts versus metastatic disease. *Acad Radiol* 1994;1:75–77.

Vecht CJ. Clinical management of brain metastasis. *J Neurol* 1998;245:127–131.

Pathogenesis

Hwang TL, Close TP, Grego JM, et al. Predilection of brain metastasis in gray and white matter junction and vascular border zones. *Cancer* 1996;77:1551–1555.

Nicolson GL, Menter DG, Herrmann JL, et al. Brain metastasis: role of trophic, autocrine, and paracrine factors in tumor invasion and colonization of the central nervous system. *Curr Top Microbiol Immunol* 1996;213:89–115.

Pilkington GJ, Bjerkvig R, De Ridder L, Kaaijk P. In vitro and in vivo models for the study of brain tumour invasion. *Anticancer Res* 1997;17:4107–4109.

Takahashi JA, Llena JF, Hirano A. Pathology of cerebral metastases. *Neurosurg Clin North Am* 1996;7:345–367.

Walsh JW. Biology of a brain metastasis. *Neurosurg Clin North Am* 1996;7:369–376.

Imaging

Akeson P, Larsson EM, Kristoffersen DT, et al. Brain metastases—comparison of gadodiamide injection-enhanced MR imaging at standard and high dose, contrast-enhanced CT and non-contrast-enhanced MR imaging. *Acta Radiol* 1995;36:300–306.

Ginsberg LE, Lang FF. Neuroradiologic screening for brain metastases—can quadruple dose gadolinium be far behind? *AJNR* 1998;19:829–830.

Schaefer PW, Budzik RF Jr, Gonzalez RG. Imaging of cerebral metastases. *Neurosurg Clin North Am* 1996;7:393–423.

Shirai H, Imai S, Kajihara Y, et al. MRI in carcinomatous encephalitis. *Neuroradiology* 1997;39:437–440.

Surgery

Bindal AK, Bindal RK, Hess KR, et al. Surgery versus radiosurgery in the treatment of brain metastasis. *J Neurosurg* 1996;84:748–754.

Lang FF, Sawaya R. Surgical treatment of metastatic brain tumors. *Semin Surg Oncol* 1998;14:53–63.

Ludwig HC, Behnke J, Markakis E. Brain metastases in neurosurgery: indications, surgical procedures and outcome. *Anticancer Res* 1998;18:2215–2218.

Mintz AH, Kestle J, Rathbone MP, et al. A randomized trial to assess the efficacy of surgery in addition to radiotherapy in patients with a single cerebral metastasis. *Cancer* 1996;78:1470–1476.

Patchell RA, Tibbs PA, Walsh JW, et al. A randomized trial of surgery in the treatment of single metastases to the brain. *N Engl J Med* 1990;322:494–500.

Wronski M, Arbit E, Burt M, Galicich JH. Survival after surgical treatment of brain metastases from lung cancer: a follow-up study of 231 patients treated between 1976 and 1991. *J Neurosurg* 1995;83:605–616.

Radiation

Flickinger JC, Kondziolka D. Radiosurgery instead of resection for solitary brain metastasis: the gold standard redefined. *Int J Radiat Oncol Biol Phys* 1996;35:185–186.

Gregor A. Prophylactic cranial irradiation in small-cell lung cancer: is it ever indicated? *Oncology* 1998;12(1 suppl 2):19–24.

Larson DA, Wara WM. Radiotherapy for cerebral metastases. *Neurosurg Clin North Am* 1996;7:505–515.

McDermott MW, Cosgrove GR, Larson DA, et al. Interstitial brachytherapy for intracranial metastases. *Neurosurg Clin North Am* 1996;7:485–495.

Nieder C, Berberich W, Schnabel K. Tumor-related prognostic factors for remission of brain metastases after radiotherapy. *Int J Radiat Oncol Biol Phys* 1997;39:25–30.

Shirato H, Takamura A, Tomita M, et al. Stereotactic irradiation without whole-brain irradiation for single brain metastasis. *Int J Radiat Oncol Biol Phys* 1997;37:385–391.

Vermeulen SS. Whole brain radiotherapy in the treatment of metastatic brain tumors. *Semin Surg Oncol* 1998;14:64–69.

Young RF. Radiosurgery for the treatment of brain metastases. *Semin Surg Oncol* 1998;14:70–77.

Chemotherapy

Batchelor T, DeAngelis LM. Medical management of cerebral metastases. *Neurosurg Clin North Am* 1996;7:435–446.

Cormio G, Gabriele A, Maneo A, et al. Complete remission of brain metastases from ovarian carcinoma with carboplatin. *Eur J Obstet Gynecol Reprod Biol* 1998;78:91–93.

Lee JS, Pisters KM, Komaki R, et al. Paclitaxel/carboplatin chemotherapy as primary treatment of brain metastases in non-small cell lung cancer: a preliminary report. *Semin Oncol* 1997;24:S12–S55.

Lesser GJ. Chemotherapy of cerebral metastases from solid tumors. *Neurosurg Clin North Am* 1996;7:527–536.

Orhan B, Yalcin S, Evrensel T, et al. Successful treatment of cranial metastases of extrapulmonary small cell carcinoma with chemotherapy alone. *Med Oncol* 1998;15:66–69.

Spinal Metastases

Cook AM, Lau TN, Tomlinson MJ, et al. Magnetic resonance imaging of the whole spine in suspected malignant spinal cord compression: impact on management. *Clin Oncol R Coll Radiol* 1998;10:39–43.

Faul CM, Flickinger JC. The use of radiation in the management of spinal metastases. *J Neurooncol* 1995;23:149–161.

Harris JK, Sutcliffe JC, Robinson NE. The role of emergency surgery in malignant spinal extradural compression: assessment of functional outcome. *Br J Neurosurg* 1996;10:27–33.

Helweg-Larsen S, Johnsen A, Boesen J, Sorensen PS. Radiologic features compared to clinical findings in a prospective study of 153 patients with metastatic spinal cord compression treated by radiotherapy. *Acta Neurochir (Wien)* 1997;139:105–111.

Hirano A. Neuropathology of tumors of the spinal cord: the Montefiore experience. *Brain Tumor Pathol* 1997;14:1–4.

Koehler PJ. Use of corticosteroids in neuro-oncology. *Anticancer Drugs* 1995;6:19–33.

Janjan NA. Radiation for bone metastases: conventional techniques and the role of systemic radiopharmaceuticals. *Cancer* 1997;80:1628–1645.

Loblaw DA, Laperriere NJ. Emergency treatment of malignant extradural spinal cord compression: an evidence-based guideline. *J Clin Oncol* 1998;16:1613–1614.

Schiff D, O'Neill BP. Intramedullary spinal cord metastases: clinical features and treatment outcome. *Neurology* 1996;47:906–912.

Carcinomatous Meningitis

Bokstein F, Lossos A, Siegal T. Leptomeningeal metastases from solid tumors: a comparison of two prospective series treated with and without intra-cerebrospinal chemotherapy. *Cancer* 1998;82:1756–1763.

Chamberlain MC. Leptomeningeal metastases: a review of evaluation and treatment. *Neurooncology* 1998;37:271–284.

Chamberlain MC, Kormanik PR. Carcinomatous meningitis secondary to breast cancer: predictors of response to combined modality therapy. *J Neurooncol* 1997;35:55–64.

Chamberlain MC, Kormanik PA, Barba D. Complications associated with intraventricular chemotherapy in patients with leptomeningeal metastases. *J Neurosurg* 1997;87:694–699.

Elliott P, Ku NN, Werner MH. Neoplastic meningitis with normal neurological findings. Magnetic resonance imaging results. *J Neuroimaging* 1995;5:233–266.

Freilich RJ, Krol D, DeAngelis LM. Neuroimaging and cerebrospinal fluid cytology in the diagnosis of leptomeningeal metastasis. Ann Neurol 1995;38:51–57.

Gomori JM, Heching N, Siegal T. Leptomeningeal metastases: evaluation by gadolinium enhanced spinal magnetic resonance imaging. *J Neurooncol* 1998;36:55–60.

Herrlinger U, Weller M, Schabet M. New aspects of immunotherapy of leptomeningeal metastases. *J Neurooncol* 1998;38:233–239.

Mareel M, Leroy A. Bracke M. Cellular and molecular mechanisms of metastasis as applied to carcinomatous meningitis. *J Neurooncol* 1998;38:97–102.

Moots PL, Harrison MB, Vandenberg SR. Prolonged survival in carcinomatous meningitis associated with breast cancer. *South Med J* 1995;88:357–362.

Norris LK, Grossman SA, Olivi A. Neoplastic meningitis following surgical resection of isolated cerebellar metastasis: a potentially preventable complication. *J Neurooncol* 1997;32:215–223.

Portenoy RK, Lipton RE, Foley KM. Back pain in the cancer patient: an algorithm for evaluation and management. *Neurology* 1987;37:134–138.

Schiff D, O'Neill BP. Intramedullary spinal cord metastases: clinical features and treatment outcome. *Neurology* 1996;47:906–912.

Siegal T. Leptomeningeal metastases: rationale for systemic chemotherapy or what is the role of intra-CSF-chemotherapy? *J Neurooncol* 1998;38:151–157.

Wasserstrom W, Glass J, Posner J. Diagnosis and treatment of leptomeningeal metastases from solid tumors experience with 90 patients. *Cancer* 1982;49:759–772.

Granulomas

Awada A, Daif AK, Pirani M, et al. Evolution of brain tuberculomas under standard antituberculous treatment. *J Neurol Sci* 1998;156:47–52.

Brismar J, Hugosson C, Larsson SG, et al. Imaging of tuberculosis. III. Tuberculosis as a mimicker of brain tumour. *Acta Radiol* 1996;37:496–505.

Dastur DK, Manghani DK, Udani PM. Pathology and pathogenetic mechanisms in neurotuberculosis. *Radiol Clin North Am* 1995;33:733–752.

el-Sonbaty MR, Abdul-Ghaffar NU, Marafy AA. Multiple intracranial tuberculomas mimicking brain metastases. *Tuber Lung Dis* 1995;76:271–272.

Goyal M, Sharma A, Mishra NK, et al. Imaging appearance of pachymeningeal tuberculosis. *AJR* 1997;169:1421–1424.

Gupta RK, Kohli A, Gaur V, et al. MRI of the brain in patients with miliary pulmonary tuberculosis without symptoms or signs of central nervous system involvement. *Neuroradiology* 1997;39:699–704.

Isenmann S, Zimmermann DR, Wichmann W, Moll C. Tuberculoma mimicking meningioma of the falx cerebri. PCR diagnosis of mycobacterial DNA from formalin-fixed tissue. *Clin Neuropathol* 1996;15:155–158.

Jamieson DH. Imaging intracranial tuberculosis in childhood. *Pediatr Radiol* 1995;25:165–170.

Jinkins JR, Gupta R, Chang KH, Rodriguez-Carbajal J. MR imaging of central nervous system tuberculosis. *Radiol Clin North Am* 1995;33:771–776.

Lesprit P, Zagdanski AM, de La Blanchardiere A, et al. Cerebral tuberculosis in patients with the acquired immunodeficiency syndrome (AIDS). Report of 6 cases and review. *Medicine (Baltimore)* 1997;76:423–431.

Reiser M, Fatkenheuer G, Diehl V. Paradoxical expansion of intracranial tuberculomas during chemotherapy. *J Infect* 1997;35:88–90.

Whiteman ML. Neuroimaging of central nervous system tuberculosis in HIV-infected patients. *Neuroimag Clin North Am* 1997;7:199–214.

Merritt's Neurology, 10th ed., edited by L.P. Rowland. Lippincott Williams & Wilkins, Philadelphia © 2000.

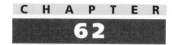

CHAPTER
62

SPINAL TUMORS

PAUL C. MCCORMICK
MICHAEL R. FETELL
LEWIS P. ROWLAND

TABLE 62.1. RELATIVE FREQUENCY OF VARIOUS TYPES OF SPINAL TUMOR

Type	Percent
Neurofibromas	29
Meningiomas	26
Ependymomas	13
Miscellaneous	12
Astrocytomas	7
Metastatic and other	13
Total	100

Tumors of the spinal cord or nerve roots are similar to intracranial tumors in cellular type. They may arise from the parenchyma of the cord, nerve roots, meninges, intraspinal blood vessels, sympathetic nerves, or vertebrae. Metastases may arise from remote tumors.

Spinal tumors are divided by location into three groups: intramedullary, intradural, or extradural. Occasionally, an extradural tumor extends through an intervertebral foramen to be partially within and partially outside the spinal canal (dumbbell or hourglass tumors).

PATHOLOGY

The histologic characteristics (Table 62.1) of primary and secondary tumors are similar to those of intracranial tumors. Intramedullary tumors are rare, accounting for about 10% of all spinal tumors. In contrast, benign encapsulated tumors (Figs. 62.1 and 62.2), meningiomas, and neurofibromas comprise

about 65% of all primary spinal tumors. Intramedullary tumors are more common in children, and extramedullary tumors are more common in adults.

The primary sites of metastatic tumors to the spine in order of frequency are lung, breast, and prostate. Other origins include gastrointestinal tract, lymphoma, melanoma, kidney, sarcoma, thyroid, and myeloma.

FREQUENCY

Spinal cord tumors are much less prevalent than intracranial tumors in a ratio of 1:4, but this varies by histology. The intracranial-to-spinal ratio of astrocytoma is 10:1, and the ratio for ependymomas varies from 3:1 to 20:1. Men and women are affected equally often, except that meningiomas are more common in women and ependymomas are more common in men. Spinal tumors occur predominantly in young or middle-aged adults

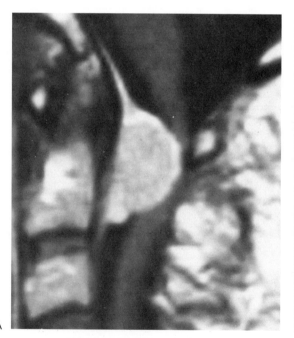
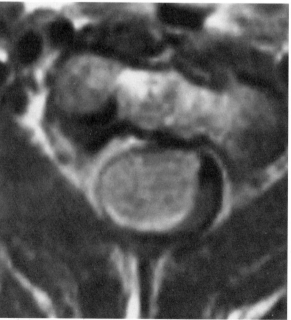

FIG. 62.1. Cervical meningioma. **A:** T1-weighted contrast-enhanced sagittal magnetic resonance image demonstrates a large intradural mass at C1-2. **B:** Axial magnetic resonance image demonstrates the large size of this lesion, probably a meningioma. Despite marked spinal cord compression, the patient had no abnormality on neurologic examination.

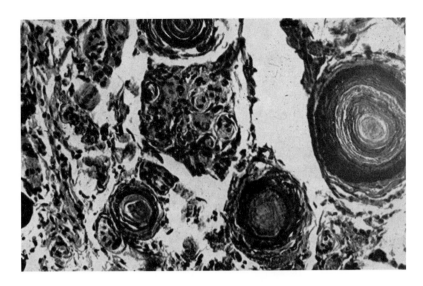

FIG. 62.2. Meningioma of the spinal cord with whorls.

and are less common in childhood or after age 60 (Table 62.2). Spinal tumors appear most often in the thoracic region, but if the relative lengths of the divisions of the spinal cord are considered, the distribution is relatively equal. Ependymomas may be either intramedullary or extramedullary; at the conus, an ependymoma may be wholly or partially extramedullary.

SYMPTOMS

Extramedullary tumors cause symptoms by compressing nerve roots or spinal cord or by occluding the spinal blood vessels. The symptoms of intramedullary tumors result from direct interference with the intrinsic structures of the spinal cord from mass effect, edema, or development of syringomyelia. Descriptions of special syndromes follow.

EXTRAMEDULLARY TUMORS

These tumors may be either intradural or extradural. They usually involve a few cord segments and cause focal signs by compressing nerve roots, especially the dorsal roots. Extramedullary tumors may ultimately affect the spinal cord, with complete loss of function below the level of the lesion. The first symptoms are focal pain and paresthesias, arising from pressure on the dorsal

TABLE 62.2. AGE INCIDENCE OF SPINAL TUMORS OF ALL TYPES[a]

Age (yr)	No. of cases	Percent
0–9	19	2
10–19	98	10
20–29	156	16
30–39	177	18
40–49	238	25
50–59	186	19
Over 60	101	10
Total	975	100

[a]Data compiled from the literature.

nerve roots, and neurofibromas originate from these structures. This symptom pattern is soon followed by sensory loss, weakness, and muscular wasting in the distribution of the affected roots. Compression of the spinal cord first interrupts the functions of the pathways that lie at the periphery of the spinal cord. The early signs of cord compression include spastic weakness below the lesion; impairment of cutaneous and proprioceptive sensation below the lesion; impaired control of the bladder and, less often, the rectum; and increased tendon reflexes, Babinski signs, and loss of superficial abdominal reflexes. If untreated, this syndrome may lead to signs and symptoms of complete transection of spinal cord, with wasting and atrophy of muscles at the level of the root lesion and, below the lesion, paraplegia or quadriplegia in flexion.

The severity and distribution of weakness and sensory loss varies, depending in part on the location of the tumor in relation to the anterior, lateral, or posterior portion of the spinal cord. Eccentrically placed tumors may cause a typical Brown-Séquard syndrome: ipsilateral signs of posterior column and pyramidal tract dysfunction, with contralateral loss of pain and temperature due to involvement of the lateral spinothalamic tract. Usually, however, the Brown-Séquard features are incomplete.

Spinal vessels may be occluded by extradural tumors, particularly metastatic carcinoma, lymphoma, or abscess. When the arteries destined for the spinal cord are occluded, the resulting myelomalacia causes signs and symptoms similar to those of severe intradural compression and necrosis of the spinal cord. Occlusion of major components of the anterior spinal artery, however, results in segmental lower motor neuron signs at the appropriate level, bilateral loss of pain and temperature sensation, and upper motor neuron signs below the lesion. The posterior columns are generally spared.

SPINAL METASTASES

Epidural Spinal Cord Compression

Epidural spinal metastases can be considered a disorder of the vertebral column; the neurologic consequences result from extension of tumor into the spinal canal. Patients with primary malignant tumors now survive longer, and the incidence of epidural spinal cord compression has increased to about 5% to 10% of all cancer patients. Treatment of cord compression does not prolong survival but may relieve pain and may prevent neurologic disability.

Signs and symptoms of epidural spinal cord compression are easily overlooked in a patient with cancer who is often wracked by asthenia and diffuse pain. The physician, however, must respond to neck or back pain that is relentless and persists when the patient lies in bed, even if the pain is relieved by analgesics. Limb weakness, paresthesias in the distribution of a nerve root, and bowel or bladder dysfunction create a neurooncologic emergency that commands prompt evaluation and treatment. Rarely, the only manifestation of cord compression is a gait disorder, often due to sensory ataxia, without overt evidence of weakness or cutaneous sensory loss. It may even be difficult to demonstrate impaired proprioception. The ataxia may be caused by compression of spinocerebellar pathways. The tumor in more than 50% of cases of epidural cord compression arises from lung or breast; more than 80% of cases arise from primary tumors in lung, breast, gastrointestinal system, prostate, melanoma, or lymphoma.

These tumors spread to the epidural space by direct centripetal invasion from a paravertebral focus through a nerve root foramen, hematogenous metastasis to the vertebrae with extension from bone into the epidural space, or retrograde spread along the venous plexus of Batson. Hematogenous spread is the most common, and computed tomography (CT) shows lytic or blastic changes in 85% of patients. Osteoblastic changes are common with myeloma, prostate carcinoma, and Hodgkin disease and are occasionally seen with breast cancer. CT and magnetic resonance imaging (MRI) are sensitive techniques for the detection of spinal osseous metastases, and MRI has largely replaced myelography (Figs. 62.3 and 62.4).

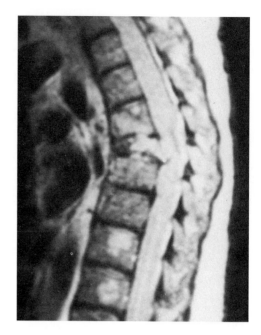

FIG. 62.4. Epidural spinal metastases. T1-weighted sagittal magnetic resonance image demonstrates destruction and collapse of the T6 vertebra in a patient with multiple myeloma. In addition to spinal cord compression from epidural extension of the neoplasm, there is a kyphotic deformity of the spine, indicating instability. Note the hyperintense marrow signal in the bodies of T9 and T10, indicating additional metastatic deposits.

Treatment of Epidural Metastatic Disease

Treatment of epidural metastasis is palliative in nearly all patients. Management must be individually tailored to consider the patient's age, clinical state, extent of systemic disease, life ex-

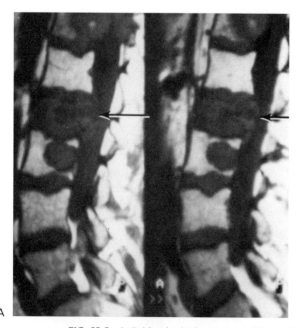

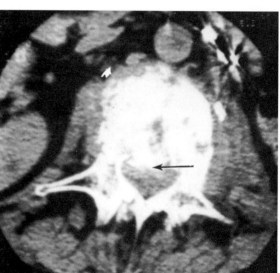

FIG. 62.3. A: Epidural spinal metastases. T1-weighted sagittal magnetic resonance image demonstrates multiple levels of spinal involvement from metastatic renal carcinoma. The L2 vertebra (*arrow*) is collapsed, and there is epidural extension of tumor and bone at this level. **B:** Axial computed tomography demonstrates the degree of bone destruction at the L2 level. Note the retropulsion of bone fragments into the epidural space (*arrow*).

pectancy, tumor pathology (if known), and extent of spinal lesions. The keys to successful management are timely diagnosis and prompt treatment. Persistent back or neck pain in a patient with known cancer is presumed to indicate metastatic spinal disease until proved otherwise. Emergency treatment of the patient with rapidly progressive paraparesis rarely reverses the neurologic signs. Loss of bowel or bladder function is an ominous prognostic sign and is usually irreversible. Among patients diagnosed and treated early (while they can still walk), 94% remain ambulatory until they die.

Radiation (3,000 cGy in 10 fractions of 300 cGy each) is the treatment of choice for most patients with spinal metastases. It is tolerated well even by patients who are seriously ill, and in most cases, palliation is achieved with relief of pain, local tumor control, and prevention or reversal of neurologic impairment. Indications for surgery include tumors such as melanoma and other radioresistant tumors, recurrent tumor at a site of prior radiation therapy, spinal instability, unknown tissue diagnosis, or rapid progression of neurologic disorder. Patients with advanced systemic disease are poor surgical candidates. The choice of operative approach is debated; some surgeons advocate an anterior approach over radiation therapy or posterior laminectomy. The attendant surgical risks of anterior decompression have to be considered.

INTRAMEDULLARY METASTASES

The most common tumors that cause intramedullary metastases are lung cancer or breast cancer (Fig. 62.5). Intramedullary metastases occur with advanced metastatic disease, and 61% of patients with intramedullary metastases have had multiple sites

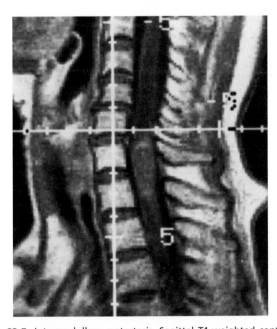

FIG. 62.5. Intramedullary metastasis. Sagittal T1-weighted contrast-enhanced magnetic resonance image shows a faintly contrast-enhancing tumor at C6-7 expanding the cervical cord in a patient with widely metastatic small cell lung cancer. Biopsy was not performed, and the tumor receded with radiation therapy.

of cerebral or spinal lesions at autopsy. MRI is the preferred diagnostic method for detection of intramedullary metastases. Reversal or stabilization of neurologic signs depends on early diagnosis, but survival is poor; 80% of patients in one series died within 3 months of diagnosis.

PRIMARY INTRAMEDULLARY TUMORS

Primary intramedullary tumors usually extend over many segments, sometimes involving the whole length of the spinal cord. For this reason, the signs and symptoms of intramedullary tumors are more variable than those of extramedullary tumors (Fig. 62.6). If the tumor is restricted to one or two segments, the syndrome is similar to that of an extramedullary tumor. Commonly, however, the tumor involves several segments. Pain may be an early manifestation if the dorsal root entry zone is affected. Compression of the crossing pain fibers in the central cord may cause loss of pain and temperature only in the affected segments. As the tumor spreads peripherally, the spinothalamic tracts may be affected; in the thoracic and cervical areas, pain and temperature fibers from the sacral area lie near the external surface of the cord and may be spared (sacral sparing). Involvement of the central gray matter destroys the anterior horn cells, with local weakness and atrophy. However, pyramidal fibers may be spared. The clinical picture may be identical to that of syringomyelia.

INTRADURAL TUMORS

Neurofibromas, schwannomas, and *meningiomas* are the most common primary intradural tumors of the spinal cord. On MRI after the administration of gadolinium, the lesions enhance brightly (Fig. 62.7). Meningiomas may be identified by the presence of a "dural tail," where the tumor attaches to the dura. *Leptomeningeal metastasis* and *drop metastases* of intracranial tumors also involve the intradural space but typically appear as small nodules attached to the surface of the cord or cauda equina nerve roots (Fig. 62.8).

REGIONAL SYNDROMES
Foramen Magnum Tumors

Tumors in the region of the foramen magnum may extend up into the posterior fossa or down into the cervical region. The syndrome is typified by signs and symptoms of dysfunction of the lower cranial nerves—primarily the eleventh, twelfth, and, rarely, the ninth and tenth. The most characteristic foramen magnum tumor, the ventrolateral meningioma, compresses the spinal cord at the cervicomedullary junction to cause posterior column signs: loss of position, vibratory, and light touch perception, more prominent in the arms than in the legs. Upper motor neuron signs are seen in all four limbs. There may be cutaneous sensory loss in distribution of C2 or the occiput, with posterior cranial headache and high cervical pain. Progression of sensory and motor symptoms may involve the limbs asymmetrically.

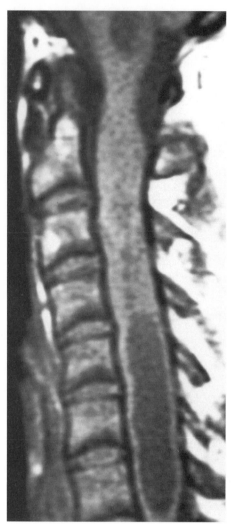
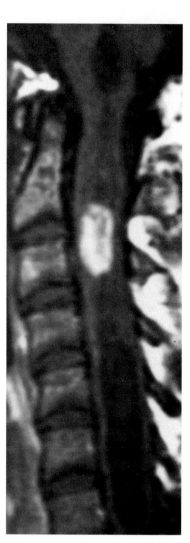

A, B

FIG. 62.6. Intramedullary astrocytoma. **A:** T1-weighted sagittal magnetic resonance image demonstrates a large cyst in the lower cervical spinal cord and a smaller cyst extending up into the medulla. The intervening spinal cord is slightly enlarged but demonstrates no signal abnormality. **B:** T1-weighted magnetic resonance image shows a contrast-enhancing intramedullary tumor at the C2-3 level. At operation, a well-circumscribed pilocytic astrocytoma was removed.

Cervical Tumors

Tumors of the upper cervical segments cause pain or paresthesias in the occipital or cervical region and stiff neck, with weakness and wasting of neck muscles. Below the lesion, there may be a spastic tetraplegia or hemiplegia. Cutaneous sensation may be affected below the lesion, and the descending trigeminal nucleus may be involved. Characteristic findings make it possible to localize the upper level of spinal tumors in the middle and lower cervical segments or T1 as follows:

C4: Paralysis of the diaphragm.

C5: Atrophy and paralysis of the deltoid, biceps, supinator longus, rhomboid, and spinati muscles. The upper arms hang limp at the side. The sensory level extends to the outer surface of the arm. The biceps and supinator reflexes are lost.

C6: Paralysis of triceps and wrist extensors. The forearm is held semiflexed and there is a partial wristdrop. The triceps reflex is lost. Sensory impairment extends to a line running down the middle of the arm slightly to the radial side.

C7: Paralysis of the flexors of the wrist and of the flexors and extensors of the fingers. Efforts to close the hands result in extension of the wrist and slight flexion of the fingers (preacher's

hand). The sensory level is similar to that of the sixth cervical segment but slightly more to the ulnar side of the arm.

C8: Atrophy and paralysis of the small muscles of the hand with resulting clawhand (main-en-griffe). *Horner syndrome*, unilateral or bilateral, results from lesions at this level and is characterized by the triad of ptosis, small pupil (miosis), and loss of sweating on the face. Sensory loss extends to the inner aspect of the arm and involves the fourth and fifth fingers and the ulnar aspect of the middle finger.

T1: Lesions rarely cause motor symptoms because the T1 nerve root normally provides little functional innervation of the small hand muscles.

Other signs of cervical tumors include nystagmus, which is attributed to involvement of the descending portion of the median longitudinal fasciculus. A Horner syndrome may be found with intramedullary lesions in any portion of the cervical cord if the descending sympathetic pathways are affected.

Thoracic Tumors

Clinical localization of tumors in the thoracic region of the cord is best made by the sensory level. It is not possible to determine the

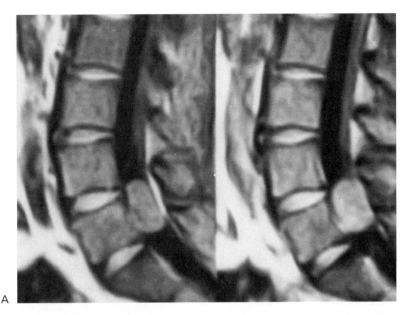

A

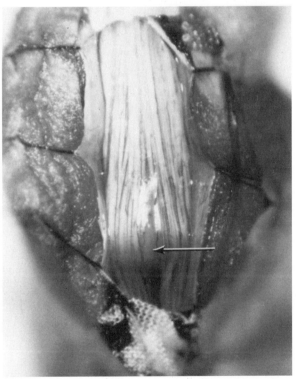

B

FIG. 62.7. Schwannoma. **A:** Gadolinium-enhanced T1-weighted sagittal magnetic resonance image demonstrates large intradural tumor at the L5 level. Differential diagnosis includes nerve sheath tumor, meningioma, filum terminale ependymoma, and intradural ("drop") metastases. **B:** Intraoperative photograph demonstrates a large intradural schwannoma (*arrow*) that displaces the cauda equina dorsally.

location of a lesion in the upper half of the thoracic cord by testing the strength of intercostal muscles. Lesions that affect the abdominal muscles below T10 but spare the upper ones can be localized by the Beevor sign: the umbilicus moves upward when the patient, lying in the supine position, attempts to flex the neck against resistance. Abdominal skin reflexes are absent below the lesion.

Lumbar Tumors

Lesions in the lumbar region can be localized by the level of the sensory loss and motor weakness. Tumors that compress only the

L1 and L2 segments cause loss of the cremasteric reflexes. The abdominal reflexes are preserved, as are the knee and ankle jerks.

If the tumor affects the L3 and L4 segments and does not involve the cauda equina, the signs are weakness of the quadriceps, loss of the patellar reflexes, and hyperactive Achilles reflexes. More commonly, lesions at this level also involve the cauda equina to cause flaccid paralysis of the legs with loss of knee and ankle reflexes. If both the spinal cord and cauda equina are affected, there may be spastic paralysis of one leg with an overactive ankle reflex on that side and flaccid paralysis with loss of reflexes on the other side.

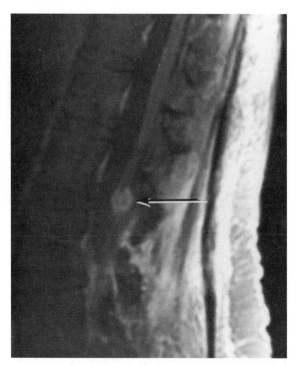

FIG. 62.8. "Drop metastases." Sagittal T1-weighted contrast-enhanced magnetic resonance image shows an intradural module (*arrow*) of a fourth ventricular choroid plexus papilloma that has seeded the cauda equina.

Tumors of the Conus and Cauda Equina

The first symptom of a tumor that involves the conus or cauda equina is pain in the back, rectal area, or both lower legs, often leading to the diagnosis of sciatica. Loss of bladder function and impotence are seen early. As the tumor grows, there may be flaccid paralysis of the legs, with atrophy of leg muscles and foot drop. Fasciculation may be evident. Sensory loss may affect the perianal or saddle area and the remaining sacral and lumbar dermatomes. This loss may be slight or so severe that a trophic ulcer develops over the lumbosacral region, buttocks, hips, or heels.

Signs of raised intracranial pressure may be seen with ependymomas of this region if the cerebrospinal fluid (CSF) protein content is over 100 mg/dL.

DIAGNOSIS OF SPINAL TUMORS

Tumors compressing the spinal cord or the cauda equina cause radicular pain and the slow evolution of signs of an incomplete transverse lesion of the cord or signs of compression of the cauda equina. Extradural tumors that do not compress the spinal cord may obstruct the blood supply to the cord; if this occurs, the symptoms are often of sudden onset, and the tumor is either metastatic or a granuloma of the Hodgkin type. In a patient with Von Recklinghausen disease, the skin lesions may suggest the presence of a neurofibroma, glioma, or ependymoma.

The diagnosis of an intraspinal tumor can be established be-

fore operation with absolute certainty by CT, MRI, or myelography. Vascular malformations or vascular tumors may be visualized by spinal angiography. Examination of the CSF may also be helpful.

Radiography

CT and MRI have largely replaced plain films but are not available everywhere. In about 15% of spinal neoplasms, one or more of the following abnormalities are seen in plain radiographs.

1. Localized destruction of the vertebrae is manifested by scalloping of the posterior margin of the vertebral body or lucency of a portion of the vertebra or pedicle.
2. Changes occur in the contour of or separation of the pedicles (the interpediculate distance can be measured and compared with normal values). Localized enlargement of foramina is seen in the dumbbell neurofibroma. Localized enlargement of the spinal canal is usually diagnostic of an intraspinal tumor, but enlargement of many segments may be a developmental anomaly.
3. Paraspinal tissues are distorted by tumors (frequently neurofibromas) that extend through the intervertebral foramen or by tumors that originate in the paraspinal structures.
4. Proliferation of bone, which is rare except in osteomas and sarcomas, is also occasionally seen in hemangiomas of bone and meninges.
5. Calcium deposits are occasionally present in meningiomas or congenital tumors.

Diagnostic Imaging

MRI has largely supplanted myelography. In patients with partial spinal block, myelography may alter CSF pressure relationships, causing complete spinal block and neurologic deterioration. MRI is the most useful test for evaluating spinal tumors. The vertebral bodies, spinal canal, and spinal cord itself are clearly delineated. Injection of gadolinium assists because most spinal neoplasms display contrast enhancement. When a metastatic tumor is demonstrated, it is advisable to image the entire cord because more than one lesion may be present.

CT is more limited than MRI. Without the intrathecal instillation of a contrast agent, CT cannot be relied on to demonstrate the soft tissue changes of intraspinal tumors. However, the extraspinal aspects, such as metastatic cancer, may be identified. With intrathecal injection of contrast agents, intraspinal tumors are usually seen. The contrast material may leach into the cavity to establish the diagnosis of syringomyelia or cystic tumor.

Cerebrospinal Fluid

When there is a complete subarachnoid block, the CSF is xanthochromic as a result of the high protein content. It may be only slightly yellow or colorless if the subarachnoid block is incomplete. The cell count is usually normal, but a slight pleocytosis is found in about 30% of patients. Cell counts between 25 and 100/mm^3 are found in about 15% of the patients. The protein content is increased in more than 95%. Values over 100 mg/dL are present in 60% of the patients and values over 1,000 mg/dL are present in 5% and may, in rare cases, lead to communicating hydrocephalus. The glucose content is normal unless there is meningeal spread. Cytologic evaluation of the CSF is useful when malignant tumors are suspected.

Differential Diagnosis

Spinal tumors must be differentiated from other disorders of the spinal cord, including transverse myelitis, multiple sclerosis, syringomyelia, combined system disease, syphilis, amyotrophic lateral sclerosis, anomalies of the cervical spine and base of the skull, spondylosis, adhesive arachnoiditis, radiculitis of the cauda equina, hypertrophic arthritis, ruptured intervertebral discs, and vascular anomalies. *Epidural lipomatosis* is a complication of prolonged steroid therapy but sometimes occurs without apparent cause; the fat accumulations act as an intraspinal mass lesion, causing low back pain and compression of the spinal cord or cauda equina.

Multiple sclerosis, with a complete or incomplete transverse lesion of the cord, can usually be differentiated from spinal cord tumors by the remitting course, signs and symptoms or more than one lesion, evoked potential studies, cranial MRI, and presence of CSF oligoclonal bands. Acute transverse myelitis may occasionally enlarge the cord to simulate an intramedullary tumor.

The differential diagnosis between syringomyelia and intramedullary tumors is complicated because intramedullary cysts are commonly associated with these tumors. Extramedullary tumors in the cervical region may give rise to localized pains and muscular atrophy in conjunction with a Brown-Séquard syndrome, producing a clinical picture similar to that of syringomyelia. The diagnosis of syringomyelia is likely when trophic disturbances are present. The differential diagnosis can often be made by contrast-enhanced MRI that reveals a tumor nodule (Fig. 62.6).

The combination of atrophy of hand muscles and spastic weakness in the legs in amyotrophic lateral sclerosis may suggest the diagnosis of a cervical cord tumor. Tumor is excluded by the lack of paresthesias and normal sensation on examination and the presence of fasciculation or atrophy in leg muscles.

Cervical spondylosis, with or without rupture of the intervertebral disks, may cause symptoms and signs of root irritation and compression of the spinal cord. The osteoarthritis can be diagnosed by findings in plain radiographs, but this is so common in asymptomatic people that MRI may be necessary to determine whether there is spondylotic myelopathy or an extramedullary tumor. Even MRI may show spondylosis in asymtomatic people.

Anomalies in the cervical region or at the base of the skull, such as *platybasia* or *Klippel-Feil syndrome*, are diagnosed by CT or MRI. Occasionally, arachnoiditis may interfere with the circulation in the cord, causing signs and symptoms of a transverse lesion. The CSF protein content is elevated. Diagnosis is made by complete or partial arrest of the contrast column on myelography or by fragmentation of the material at the site of the lesion. Separation of the adhesions and removal of the thickened arachnoid by surgery have been of little benefit; steroid therapy is no better.

COURSE AND PROGNOSIS

Benign tumors of the spinal cord are characterized by slow progression for years. If a neurofibroma arises from a dorsal root, there may be years of radicular pain before the tumor is evident from other manifestations of growth. Intramedullary tumors are generally benign and slow growing; they may attain enormous size (over the course of 6 to 8 years) before they are discovered.

Conversely, the sudden onset of a severe neurologic disorder, with or without pain, is usually indicative of a malignant extradural tumor, such as metastatic carcinoma or lymphoma.

TREATMENT OF PRIMARY SPINAL TUMORS

Once the diagnosis of an intraspinal tumor has been made, the treatment is surgical removal of the tumor whenever possible. When the neurologic disorder is severe or rapidly progressing, emergency surgery is indicated. With microneurosurgery, the best results are obtained when the signs and symptoms are due solely to compression of the spinal cord by a meningioma, neurofibroma, or other benign encapsulated tumor. Some of these tumors, especially meningiomas, may lie anterior to the spinal cord and require the most delicate expertise of the neurosurgeon. Function may be completely restored even when severe spastic weakness has been present for years. The postoperative results, however, are often predicated on the severity of preoperative neurologic disability, which is a strong point in favor of early diagnosis and surgery for these tumors. Radiotherapy is not indicated for most intradural extramedullary tumors, even when removal has been incomplete, because these tumors are usually benign.

The most common intramedullary tumors are ependymomas and astrocytomas. In almost all ependymomas, the tumor can be resected by myelotomy and microsurgery (Fig. 62.9). Radiotherapy is not indicated after total removal and is rarely indicated after partial removal; the patient should be observed for recurrence. Additional operative procedures should be considered if they are indicated. Perhaps half of all intramedullary astrocytomas are resectable by microsurgery; again, postoperative radiotherapy is not indicated. When radiotherapy is given after incomplete removal of an astrocytoma, the results are discouraging. In the uncommon presence of other intramedullary tumors, such as hemangioblastomas, teratomas, or dermoids, complete removal without adjuvant radiotherapy is the rule.

After radical and extensive surgery for these tumors, spinal deformities (which may have been present preoperatively) may appear or increase, requiring fixation. These deformities, if allowed to progress, may in turn create neurologic syndromes due to spinal cord compression. This condition is especially pertinent in children. Some surgeons have advocated replacement of the lamina after definitive surgery rather than the standard laminectomy. The additional use of radiotherapy for intraspinal tumors in children may affect the growth of the spine, leading to or increasing preexisting deformities of the spine.

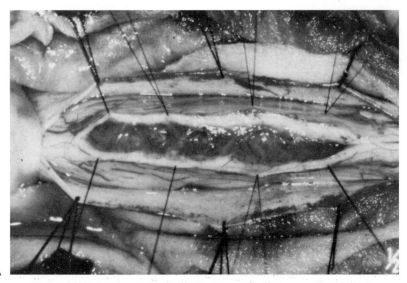

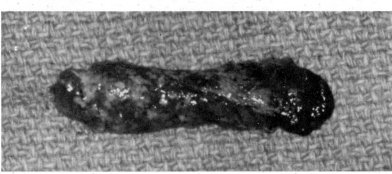

FIG. 62.9. Intramedullary ependymoma. **A:** Operative photograph. Myelotomy exposes the dorsal surface of the tumor. Note the clear demarcation of the tumor from the surrounding spinal cord. **B:** Operative photograph of the tumor specimen that has been completely removed.

SUGGESTED READINGS

Ammerman BJ, Smith DR. Papilledema and spinal cord tumors. *Surg Neurol* 1975;3:55–57.

Cook AM, Lau TN, Tomlinson MJ, Valdya M, Wakeley CJ, Goddard P. MRI of the whole spine in suspected malignant spinal cord compression: impact on management. *Clin Oncol R Coll Radiol* 1998;10:39–43.

Doppman JL, DiChiro G, Dwyer AJ, et al. MRI of spinal arteriovenous malformations. *J Neurosurg* 1987;66:830–834.

Elsberg CA. *Surgical diseases of the spinal cord, membranes and nerve roots.* New York: Paul B Hoeber, 1941.

George B, Lot G, Boissonnet H. Meningioma of the foramen magnum: a series of 40 cases. *Surg Neurol* 1997;47:371–379.

Goel A, Bhatjiwale M, Desai K. Basilar invagination: a study based on 190 surgically treated patients. *J Neurosurg* 1998;88:962–968.

Goh KY, Velasquez L, Epstein FJ. Pediatric intramedullary spinal cord tumors: is surgery alone enough? *Pediatr Neurosurg* 1997;27:334–339.

Greenberg HS, Kim JH, Posner JB. Epidural spinal cord compression from metastatic tumor: results with a new treatment protocol. *Ann Neurol* 1980;8:361–366.

Grem JL, Burgess J, Trump DL. Clinical features and natural history of intramedullary spinal cord metastasis. *Cancer* 1985;56:2305–2314.

Hainline B, Tuszynski MH, Posner JB. Ataxia in epidural spinal cord compression. *Neurology* 1992;42:2193–2195.

Harrison SK, Ditchfield MR, Waters K. Correlation of MRI and CSF cytology in the diagnosis of medulloblastoma spinal metastases. *Pediatr Radiol* 1998;28:571–574.

Hirano A. Neuropathology of tumors of the spinal cord: the Montefiore experience. *Brain Tumor Pathol* 1997;14:1–4.

Jenis LG, Dunn EJ, An HS. Metastatic disease of the cervical spine. A review. *Clin Orthop* 1999;359:89–103.

Katzman H, Waugh T, Berdon W. Skeletal changes following irradiation of childhood tumors. *J Bone Joint Surg* 1969;51A:825–843.

King AT, Sharr MM, Gullan RW, Bartlett JR. Spinal meningiomas: a 20 year review. *Br J Neurosurg* 1998;12:521–526.

Lee M, Epstein FJ, Rezai AR, Zagzag D. Nonneoplastic intramedullary spinal cord lesions mimicking tumors. *Neurosurgery* 1998;43:788–794.

Lee TT, Gromelski EB, Green BA. Surgical treatment of spinal ependymoma and postoperative radiotherapy. *Acta Neurochir* 1998;140:309–313.

Lefton DR, Pinto RS, Martin SW. MRI features of intracranial and spinal ependymomas. *Pediatr Neurosurg* 1998;28:97–105.

Mathew P, Todd NV. Intradural conus and cauda equina tumours: a retrospective review of presentation, diagnosis and early outcome. *J Neurol Neurosurg Psychiatry* 1993;56:69–74.

Matson DD. *Neurosurgery of infancy and childhood,* 2nd ed. Springfield, IL: Charles C Thomas, 1969.

McCormick PC, Stein BM. Intramedullary tumors in adults. *Neurosurg Clin North Am* 1990;1:609–630.

McCormick PC, Torres R, Post K, et al. Intramedullary ependymoma of the spinal cord. *J Neurosurg* 1990;72:523–532.

McLain RF, Bell GR. Newer management options in patients with spinal metastasis. *Cleve Clin J Med* 1998;65:359–366.

Nadkami TD, Rekate HL. Pediatric intramedullary spinal cord tumors. Critical review of the literature. *Childs Nerv Syst* 1999;15:17–28.

Robertson SC, Traynelis VC, Follett KA, Meunezes AH. Idiopathic spinal epidural lipomatosis. *Neurosurgery* 1997;41:68–74.

Schiffer D, Gordana MT. Prognosis of ependymoma. *Childs Nerv Syst* 1998;14:357–361.

Schild SE, Nisi K, Scheithauer BW, et al. The results of radiotherapy for ependymomas: the Mayo Clinic experience. *Int J Radiat Oncol* 1998;42:953–958.

Stein BM, Leeds NE, Taveras JM, et al. Meningiomas of the foramen magnum. *J Neurosurg* 1963;20:740–751.

Takacs I, Hamilton AJ. Extracranial stereotactic radiosurgery: applications for the spine and beyond. *Neurosurg Clin North Am* 1999;10:257–270.

Turner S, Marosszeky B, Timms I, et al. Malignant spinal cord compression: a prospective evaluation. *Int J Radiat Oncol Biol Phys* 1993;26:141–146.

Vindlacheeruvu RR, McEvoy AW, Kitchen ND. Intramedullary thoracic cord metastasis managed effectively without surgery. *Clin Oncol R Coll Radiol* 1997;9:343–345.

Williams AL, Haughton VM, Pojunas KW, et al. Differentiation of intramedullary neoplasms and cysts by MR. *AJR* 1987;149:159–164.

Winkleman MD, Adelstein DJ, Karlins NL. Intramedullary spinal cord metastasis. Diagnostic and therapeutic considerations. *Arch Neurol* 1987;44:526–531.

Merritt's Neurology, 10th ed., edited by L.P. Rowland. Lippincott Williams & Wilkins, Philadelphia © 2000.

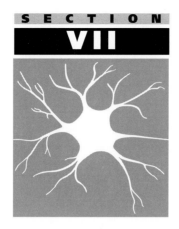

TRAUMA

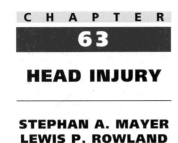

CHAPTER
63

HEAD INJURY

STEPHAN A. MAYER
LEWIS P. ROWLAND

EPIDEMIOLOGY

Head injury is a modern scourge of industrialized society. It is a major cause of death, especially in young adults, and a major cause of disability. The costs in human misery and dollars are exceeded by few other conditions.

More than 2 million patients with head injuries are seen annually in U.S. emergency rooms, and 25% of these patients are hospitalized. Almost 10% of all deaths in the United States are caused by injury, and about half of traumatic deaths involve the brain. In the United States, a head injury occurs every 7 seconds and a death every 5 minutes. About 200,000 people are killed or permanently disabled annually as a result.

Brain injuries occur at all ages, but the peak is in young adults between the ages of 15 and 24. Head injury is the leading cause of death among people under the age of 24 years. Men are affected three or four times as often as women. The major causes of brain injury differ in different parts of the United States; in all areas, motor vehicle accidents are prominent, and in metropolitan areas, personal violence is particularly prevalent. Between 1979 and 1992, firearms surpassed vehicular trauma as the most common cause of fatal brain injury.

PATHOLOGY AND PATHOPHYSIOLOGY OF CRANIOCEREBRAL TRAUMA

Skull Fractures

Skull fractures can be divided into linear, depressed, or comminuted types. If the scalp is lacerated over the fracture, it is considered an open or *compound fracture*. Skull fractures are important markers of potentially serious injury but rarely cause problems by themselves; prognosis depends more on the nature and severity of injury to the brain than on the severity of injury to the skull.

About 80% of fractures are linear. They occur most commonly in the temporoparietal region, where the skull is thinnest. Detection of a linear fracture often raises the suspicion of serious brain injury, but computed tomography (CT) in most patients is otherwise normal. Nondisplaced linear skull fractures generally do not require surgical intervention and can be managed conservatively.

In *depressed fracture* of the skull, one or more fragments of bone are displaced inward, compressing the underlying brain. In comminuted fracture there are multiple shattered bone fragments, which may or may not be displaced. In 85% of cases, depressed fractures are open (or compound) and liable to become infected or leak cerebrospinal fluid (CSF). Even when closed, most depressed or comminuted fractures require surgical exploration for debridement, elevation of bone fragments, and repair of dural lacerations. The underlying brain is injured in many cases. In some patients, depressed skull fractures are associated with tearing, compression, or thrombosis of underlying venous dural sinuses.

Basilar skull fractures may be linear, depressed, or comminuted. They are frequently missed by plain skull x-rays and are best identified by CT with "bone windows." There may be associated cranial nerve injury or a dural tear adjacent to the fracture site, which can lead to delayed meningitis if bacteria enter the subarachnoid space. Signs that lead the physician to suspect a fracture of the petrous portion of the temporal bone include hemotympanum or tympanic perforation, hearing loss, CSF otorrhea, peripheral facial nerve weakness, or ecchymosis of the scalp overlying the mastoid process (Battle sign). Anosmia, bilateral periorbital ecchymosis, and CSF rhinorrhea suggest possible fracture of the spenoid, frontal, or ethmoid bones.

Cerebral Concussion and Axonal Shearing Injury

Loss of consciousness at the moment of impact is caused by acceleration-deceleration movements of the head, which result in the stretching and shearing of axons. When the alteration of consciousness is brief (less than 6 hours), the term *concussion* is used. These patients may be completely unconscious or remain awake but "dazed"; most recover within seconds to minutes (rather than hours) and have retrograde and anterograde amnesia surrounding the event.

The mechanism by which concussion leads to loss of consciousness is believed to be transient functional disruption of the reticular activating system caused by rotational forces on the upper brainstem. Experimentally, violent head rotation can produce concussion without impact to the head. Most patients with concussion have normal CT or magnetic resonance (MR) findings, because concussion results from physiologic, rather than structural, injury to the brain. Only 5% of patients who have sustained a concussion and are otherwise intact have an intracranial hemorrhage on CT.

The term *diffuse axonal injury* (DAI) is applied to traumatic coma lasting more than 6 hours. In these cases, when no other cause of coma is identified by CT or MR imaging (MRI), it is presumed that widespread microscopic and macroscopic axonal shearing injury has occurred. Coma of 6 to 24 hours in duration is deemed mild DAI; coma lasting more than 24 hours is referred to as moderate or severe DAI, depending on the absence or presence of brainstem signs such as decorticate or decerebrate posturing (Table 63.1). Autonomic dysfunction (e.g., hypertension, hyperhidrosis, hyperpyrexia) is common in patients with acute severe DAI and may reflect brainstem or hypothalamic injury. Patients may remain unconscious for days, months, or years, and those who recover may be left with severe cognitive and motor impairment, including spasticity and ataxia. DAI is considered the single most important cause of persistent disability after traumatic brain damage.

Axonal shearing injury tends to be most severe in specific brain regions that are anatomically predisposed to maximal stress

TABLE 63.1. CLINICAL CHARACTERISTICS AND OUTCOME OF DIFFUSE BRAIN INJURIES

	Mild concussion	Cerebral contusion	Diffuse axonal injury		
			Mild	Moderate	Severe
Loss of consciousness	None	Immediate	Immediate	Immediate	Immediate
Length of unconsciousness	None	<6hr	6–24	>24hr	Days–weeks
Decerebrate posturing	None	None	Rare	Occasionally	Present
Posttraumatic amnesia	Minutes	Minutes-hours	Hours	Days	Weeks
Memory deficit	None	Mild	Mild-mod	Mild-mod	Severe
Motor deficits	None	None	None	Mild	Severe
Outcome at 3 months (%)					
Good recovery	100	95	63	38	15
Moderate deficit	0	5	15	21	13
Severe deficit	0	0	6	12	14
Vegetative	0	0	1	5	7
Death	0	0	15	24	51

Adapted from Gennarelli TA. Cerebral concussion and diffuse brain injuries. In: Cooper PR, ed. *Head injury*, 3rd ed. Baltimore: Williams & Wilkins, 1993:140.

from rotational forces. At the time of injury, microscopic damage occurs diffusely, as manifest by axonal retraction bulbs throughout the white matter of the cerebral hemispheres. Macroscopic tissue tears, best visualized by MRI, tend to occur in midline structures, including the dorsolateral midbrain and pons, posterior corpus callosum, parasagittal white matter, periventricular regions, and internal capsule. Prolonged loss of consciousness from DAI tends to be associated with bilateral asymmetric focal lesions of the midbrain tegmentum, a region densely populated with reticular activating system neurons. Small hemorrhages, known as "gliding contusions," are sometimes associated with focal shearing lesions.

Axonal shearing is thought to initiate a dynamic sequence of pathologic events that evolve over days to weeks. Initially, injury causes physical transection of some neurons and internal axonal damage to many others. In both cases, the process of axoplasmic transport continues, and materials flow from the cell body to the site of damage. These materials accumulate and can lead to secondary axonal transection with formation of a "retraction ball" from 12 hours to several days after the injury. Membrane channels may open to admit toxic levels of calcium. If the patient survives, there may be later evidence of Wallerian degeneration and gliosis.

Brain Swelling and Cerebral Edema

Brain swelling after head injury is a poorly understood phenomenon that can result from several different mechanisms. Posttraumatic brain swelling may result from *cerebral edema* (defined as an increase in the content of extravascular brain water), an increase in *cerebral blood volume* due to abnormal vasodilation, or both. Cerebral edema can be further classified as cytotoxic, vasogenic, or interstitial (see Chapter 49). The swelling may be diffuse or focal, adjacent to a parenchymal or extradural hemorrhage.

Brain swelling can follow any type of head injury. Curiously, the magnitude of swelling does not always correlate well with the severity of injury. In some cases, particularly in young people, severe diffuse brain swelling, which may be fatal, occurs minutes to hours after a minor concussion. Abnormal dilation of the cerebral blood vessels is thought to lead to increased cerebral blood

volume, hyperperfusion, and increased vascular permeability, resulting in secondary leakage of plasma and vasogenic cerebral edema. Cerebral blood flow studies indicate that some degree of hyperemia occurs in nearly all patients 1 to 3 days after severe head injury. Severe brain swelling may be related to this phenomenon or may result from damage to cerebral vasomotor regulatory centers in the brainstem.

Parenchymal Contusion and Hemorrhage

Cerebral *contusions* are focal parenchymal hemorrhages that result from "scraping" and "bruising" of the brain as it moves across the inner surface of the skull. The inferior frontal and temporal lobes, where brain tissue comes in contact with irregular protuberances at the base of the skull, are the most common sites of traumatic contusion (Fig. 63.1). Tearing of the meninges or cerebral tissue, usually a result of cuts from the sharp edges of depressed skull fragments, is called a *laceration*.

Contusions may occur at the site of a skull fracture but more

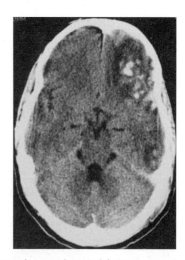

FIG. 63.1. Traumatic contusions. Axial noncontrast view demonstrates areas of contusion with small focal hemorrhages involving the lower poles of the left frontal and temporal lobes adjacent to the rough cranial vault. (Courtesy of Drs. S.K. Hilal, J.A. Bello, and T.L. Chi.)

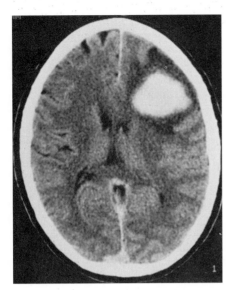

FIG. 63.2. Traumatic intracerebral hemorrhage, frontal lobe. Axial noncontrast computed tomography demonstrates left frontal lobe density (hemorrhage), surrounding lucency (edema), and mass effect (sulcal and ventricular effacement). (Courtesy of Drs. S.K. Hilal and J.A. Bello.)

often occur without a fracture and with the overlying pia and arachnoid left intact. In most patients, contusions are small and multiple. With lateral forces, contusions can occur at the site of the blow to the head ("coup lesions") or at the opposite pole as the brain impacts on the inner table of the skull ("contrecoup lesions"). Contusions frequently enlarge over 12 to 24 hours; in some cases, contusions develop 1 or more days after injury.

When rotational forces lead to tearing of a small- or medium-sized vessel within the parenchyma, a intracerebral *hematoma* may occur (Fig. 63.2). Hematomas are focal collections of blood clot that displace the brain, in contrast to contusions, which resemble bruised and bloodied brain tissue (Fig. 63.3). Most parenchymal hematomas are located in the deep white matter, in contrast to contusions, which tend to be cortical.

If there is no DAI, brain swelling, or secondary hemorrhage, recovery from one or more small contusions may be excellent. Healed contusions are often found at autopsy of people with no clinical evidence of permanent brain damage. Large parenchymal hematomas with mass effect may require surgical evacuation.

Subdural Hematoma

Subdural hematomas usually arise from a venous source, with blood filling the potential space between the dural and arachnoid membranes. In most cases, the bleeding is caused by movements of the brain within the skull, which can lead to stretching and tearing of veins that drain from the surface of the brain to the dural sinuses. Less often, the source of the hematoma is a small pial artery.

Most subdural hematomas are located over the lateral cerebral convexities, but subdural blood can also collect along the medial surface of the hemisphere, between the tentorium and occipital lobe, between the temporal lobe and the base of the skull, or in the posterior fossa. CT usually reveals a high-density crescentic collection across the entire hemispheric convexity (Fig. 63.4). Elderly or alcoholic patients with cerebral atrophy are particularly prone to subdural bleeding; in these patients, large hematomas can result from trivial impact or even from pure acceleration-deceleration injuries such as whiplash.

Acute subdural hematoma, by definition, is symptomatic within 72 hours of injury, but most patients have neurologic symptoms from the moment of impact. They can occur after any type of head injury but seem to be less common after vehicular trauma and relatively more common after falls or assaults. Half of patients with an acute subdural hematoma lose consciousness at the time of injury; 25% are in coma when they arrive at the hospital, and half of those who awaken lose consciousness for a second time after a "lucid interval" of minutes to hours, as the subdural hematoma grows in size. Hemiparesis and pupillary abnormalities are the most common focal neurologic signs; each occur in one-half to two-thirds of patients; the usual picture is

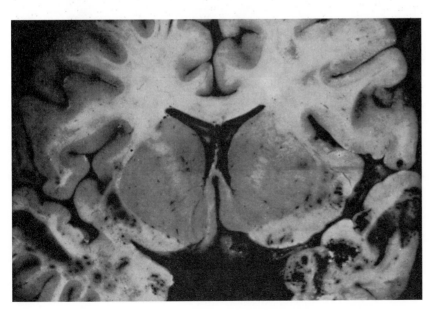

FIG. 63.3. Pathologic specimen demonstrating traumatic contusions in the temporal lobes.

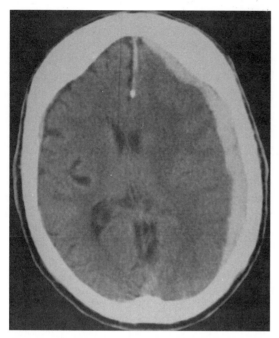

FIG. 63.4. Acute subdural hematoma. Noncontrast axial computed tomography demonstrates a hyperdense, crescent-shaped, extraaxial collection showing mass effect (sulcal and ventricular effacement) and midline shift from left to right. (Courtesy of Drs. J.A. Bello and S.K. Hilal.)

ipsilateral pupillary dilation and contralateral hemiparesis. However, so-called false localizing signs are common with acute subdural hematoma, because uncal herniation can lead to compression of the contralateral cerebral peduncle or third cranial nerve against the tentorial edge (*Kernohan notch*).

Chronic subdural hematoma becomes symptomatic after 21 days or later. It is more likely to occur after age 50. In 25% to 50% of cases, there is no recognized head trauma. Almost half have a history of alcoholism or epilepsy and the trauma may have been forgotten. Other risk factors for chronic subdural hematoma include shunts and bleeding disorders, including anticoagulant medication.

In most cases of chronic subdural hematoma, the bleeding results from trivial trauma with little or no brain compression because of coexisting cerebral atrophy. After 1 week, fibroblasts on the inner surface of the dura form a thick outer membrane, and after 2 weeks a thin inner membrane develops, resulting in encapsulation of the clot, which begins to liquify. Enlargement of the hematoma may then result from recurrent bleeding ("acute-on-chronic" subdural hematoma) or because of osmotic effects related to a high protein content of the fluid. Symptoms may be restricted to altered mental status, a syndrome sometimes mistaken for dementia. CT typically shows an isodense or hypodense crescent-shaped mass that deforms the surface of the brain, and the membranes may enhance with intravenous contrast (Fig. 63.5). Long-standing chronic subdural hematomas eventually liquify and form a *hygroma*, and, in some cases, the membranes may calcify.

Acute and chronic subdural hematoma with significant mass effect should be evacuated. Reoperation for acute subdural hematomas is needed in about 15%. Small lesions, however, need not be treated surgically, and there is room for decision making, depending on the clinical condition of the patient.

Epidural Hematoma

Epidural hematoma is a rare complication of head injury. It occurs in less than 1% of all cases but is found in 5% to 15% of autopsy series, attesting to the potential seriousness of this complication.

Bleeding into the epidural space is generally caused by a tear

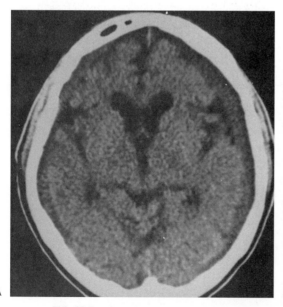
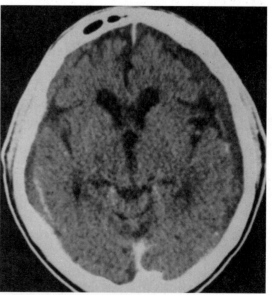

FIG. 63.5. Bilateral chronic subdural hematoma. **A:** Noncontrast axial computed tomography shows bilateral isodense extraaxial collections, larger on the left. **B:** These are better demonstrated on the postcontrast scan, in which enhancing membranes, typical of the subacute phase, can be seen. (Courtesy of Drs. J.A. Bello and S.K. Hilal.)

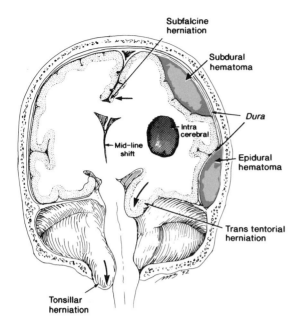

FIG. 63.6. Patterns of traumatic intracranial hemorrhage and brain herniation. [From White RJ, Likavei MJ, 1992.)

travasated blood, and the size of the clot increases until the ruptured vessel is compressed or occluded by the hematoma.

Most epidural hematomas are located over the convexity of the hemisphere in the middle cranial fossa, but occasionally the hemorrhage may be confined to the anterior fossa, possibly as a result of tearing of an anterior meningeal artery. Extradural hemorrhage in the posterior fossa may occur when the torcula Herophili is torn. In most cases, the hematoma is ipsilateral to the site of impact.

Epidural hematoma is primarily a problem of young adults; it is rarely seen in the elderly because the dura becomes increasingly adherent to the skull with age. The clinical course in one-third of patients proceeds from an immediate loss of consciousness due to concussion, to a lucid interval, and then a relapse into coma with hemiplegia as the epidural hematoma expands. The ipsilateral pupil becomes fixed and dilated because the third cranial nerve is compressed by the hippocampal gyrus as it herniates over the free edge of the tentorium; the pupillary change signals impending brainstem compression (Fig. 63.6). As with acute subdural hematoma, false localizing signs may occur. The presence of cerebellar signs, nuchal rigidity, and drowsiness, together with a fracture of the occipital bone, should lead to the suspicion of a clot in the posterior fossa.

Epidural blood takes on a "bulging" convex pattern on CT (Fig. 63.7) because the collection is limited by firm attachments of the dura to the cranial sutures. Progression to herniation and death can occur rapidly because the bleeding is arterial. The mortality rate approaches 100% in untreated patients and ranges from 5% to 30% in treated patients. As the interval between in-

in the wall of one of the meningeal arteries, usually the middle meningeal artery, but in 15% of patients the bleeding is from one of the dural sinuses. Seventy-five percent are associated with a skull fracture. The dura is separated from the skull by the ex-

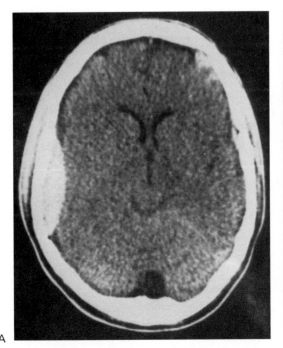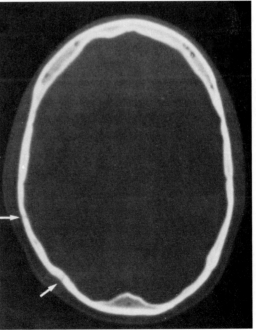

FIG. 63.7. A: Epidural hematoma is evident on computed tomography (CT). **B:** CT with bone windows shows two adjacent fractures (*arrows*); the anterior fracture is at the site of the groove for the middle meningeal artery.

jury and surgical intervention decreases, survival improves. If there is little coexisting brain damage, functional recovery may be excellent.

Subarachnoid Hemorrhage

Some extravasation of blood into the subarachnoid spaces is to be expected in any head injury. In most cases, subarachnoid blood is detected only by CSF examination and is of little clinical importance. With more serious injuries, when larger vessels traversing the subarachnoid space are torn, focal or diffuse *subarachnoid hemorrhage* can be detected by CT. In these cases, blood is often distributed over the convexities; in contrast, aneurysmal bleeding results in collections of blood that are restricted to the basal cisterns. Although a large amount of subarachnoid blood is a poor prognostic sign, delayed complications of aneurysmal subarachnoid hemorrhage, such as hydrocephalus and ischemia from vasospasm, are rare after traumatic subarachnoid hemorrhage.

INITIAL ASSESSMENT AND STABILIZATION

On admission to the emergency room, resuscitation measures, history taking, and examination should begin simultaneously. The immediate goals of management are to assess and stabilize the airway, breathing, and circulation; to judge the severity of the head injury as low, moderate, or high risk; to rule out a fracture of the cervical spine; and to identify any extracranial injuries. All moderate- and high-risk patients require a CT to rule out a fracture or intracranial bleeding.

Hypoxia and *hypotension* can have devastating effects in head-injured patients. If the patient is hypoxic or in respiratory distress, endotracheal intubation is performed, ensuring that the spine remains immobilized. Hypotension should be corrected with intravenous boluses of isotonic fluids such as normal saline or lactated Ringer solution, blood transfusions, or pressors. Systolic blood pressure during the stabilization phase should be maintained above 90 mm Hg to ensure adequate cerebral blood flow. If the patient is hypotensive, bleeding into the abdomen, thorax, retroperitoneal space, or tissues surrounding a long bone fracture should be excluded. Hypotension may also reflect *spinal shock* related to a coexisting spinal cord injury (see Chapter 64). Hypertension associated with a wide pulse pressure and bradycardia (Cushing reflex) may reflect increased intracranial pressure (ICP) or focal brainstem injury.

A baseline neurologic evaluation should be performed immediately, while airway, breathing, and circulation are assessed. Injuries can be ranked as low, moderate, or high risk according to risk factors and a rapid initial neurologic assessment (Table 63.2). The Glasgow Coma Scale (Table 63.3) is based on eye opening and the patient's best verbal and motor responses. It is widely used as a semiquantitative clinical measure of the severity of brain injury; it also provides a guide to prognosis (Table 63.4).

Except for asymptomatic patients in the low-risk group, all should have CT. In all patients, a lateral cervical spine x-ray should be performed to rule out an unstable fracture. Before a

TABLE 63.2. RISK STRATIFICATION OF PATIENTS WITH HEAD INJURY

Risk category	Characteristics
Mild	Normal neurologic examination
	No concussion
	No drug or alcohol intoxication
	May complain of headache and dizziness
	May have scalp abrasion, laceration, or hematoma
	Absence of moderate or severe injury criteria
Moderate	Glasgow coma score of 9–14 (confused, lethargic, stuporous)
	Concussion
	Posttraumatic amnesia
	Vomiting
	Seizure
	Signs of possible basilar or depressed skull fracture or serious facial injury
	Alcohol or drug intoxication
	Unreliable or no history of injury
	Age <2 years, or possible child abuse
Severe	Glasgow coma scale score of 3–8 (comatose)
	Progressive decline in level of consciousness ("talked and deteriorated")
	Focal neurologic signs
	Penetrating skull injury or palpable depressed skull fracture

Adapted from Masters SJ, McClean PM, Arcanese MS, et al. 1987.

cervical collar can be removed, the cervical spine must be cleared completely from C1 to C7.

Even before CT is performed, patients who are comatose (Glasgow Coma Scale Score ≤8) or who show clinical signs of herniation require emergency measures to reduce ICP, including head elevation, hyperventilation, and mannitol (Table 63.5).

TABLE 63.3. GLASGOW COMA SCALE

Activity/Response	Score[a]
Eye opening	
Spontaneous	4
To voice	3
To pain	2
None	1
Best motor response	
Obeys commands	6
Localizes to pain	5
Withdraws to pain	4
Flexor posturing	3
Extensor posturing	2
None	1
Best verbal response	
Conversant and oriented	5
Conversant and disorientes	4
Inappropriate words	3
Incomprehensible sounds	2
None	1

[a]Total score = sum of the score for each of the three components.
From Teasdale G, Jennett B, 1974.

TABLE 63.4. ESTIMATED MORTALITY BASED ON VARIOUS FEATURES OF HEAD INJURY

	Mortality (%)
Glasgow Coma Scale score	
15	<1
11–14	3
8–10	15
6–7	20
4–5	50
3	80
Age, among comatose patients	
16–35	30
36–45	40
46–55	50
≥56	80
CT abnormalities, among comatose patients	
None	10
Intracranial pathology without diffuse swelling or midline shift	15
Intracranial pathology with diffuse swelling (cisterns compressed or absent)	35
Intracranial pathology with midline shift (>5 mm)	55
Intracranial pressure, among comatose patients	
<20 mm Hg	15
>20 mm Hg, reducible	45
>20 mm Hg, not reducible	90
Pathologic entity	
Epidural hematoma	5–15
Gunshot wound	55
Acute subdural hematoma	
Simple	20–25
Complicated	40–75
Bilateral	75–100

Percentages are adapted from several sources and have been rounded.
From Greenberg J, Brawanaki A. Cranial trauma. In: Hacke W, *Neurocritical care*. New York: Springer-Verlag; 1994: 705; Vollmer DG, Torner JC, Jane LA, et al. *J Neurosurg* 1991; 75 [Suppl 1]: S37–S49; Marshall LF, Gautille T, Klauber MR, et al. *J Neurosurg* 1991; 75 [Suppl 1]: S28–S36; Miller JD, Becker DP, Ward JD, et al. *J Neurosurg* 1977; 47: 503–516.

DIAGNOSIS

History

The circumstances of the accident and the clinical condition of the patient before admission to the emergency room should be ascertained from emergency medical services records, the patient (if possible), and eyewitnesses. The force and location of head impact should be determined as precisely as possible. Specific inquiry should be made regarding concussion; because patients are amnestic during concussion, only an eyewitness can accurately gauge the duration of loss of consciousness.

Patients who have "talked and deteriorated" should be assumed to have an expanding intracranial hematoma until proven otherwise. Reports of headache, nausea, vomiting, confusion, or seizure activity must be noted. A medical history, including medications and drug and alcohol use, should be obtained. Recent drug and alcohol use occurs in a large percentage of trauma patients, and intoxication can confound assessments of mental status.

Examination

After the initial neurologic assessment, a more detailed physical and neurologic examination should be performed. The skull should be palpated for fractures, hematomas, and lacerations. A "step off," or palpable bony shelf, is presumed to represent a depressed skull fracture. The patient should be thoroughly examined for external signs of trauma to the neck, chest, back, abdomen, and limbs. A bloody discharge from the nose or ear may indicate leakage of CSF; bloody CSF can be differentiated from blood by a positive halo test (a "halo" of CSF forms around the blood when dropped on a white cloth sheet). If there is no admixture of blood, CSF can be distinguished from nasal secretions because the CSF glucose concentration is 30 mg/dL or more, whereas lacrimal secretions and nasal mucus usually contain less than 5 mg/dL.

After determining the patient's level of consciousness (alert, lethargic, stuporous, or comatose), a focused mental status examination should be performed if the patient is conversant. Particular attention should be paid to attention, concentration (counting backward from 20 to 1 or reciting the months in reverse), orientation, and memory, including assessment for retrograde and anterograde amnesia.

Eye movements and pupillary size, shape, and reactivity to light should be noted. A sluggishly reactive or dilated pupil suggests transtentorial herniation with compression of the third nerve. A midposition, poorly reactive, irregular pupil may result from injury to the oculomotor nucleus in the midbrain tegmentum. Nystagmus often follows a concussion. In comatose patients, the oculocephalic and oculovestibular reflexes should be tested (see Chapter 4).

Motor examination should focus on identifying asymmetric weakness or posturing. Spontaneous movements should be assessed for preferential use of the limbs on one side. If the patient is not fully cooperative, lateralized weakness can be detected by an asymmetry in tone or tendon reflexes, or by the presence of an arm drift, preferential localizing response to sternal rub, or extensor plantar reflex. Noxious stimuli, such as pinching the medial arm or applying nailbed pressure, may reveal subtle motor posturing in a limb that otherwise moves normally. *Decorticate posturing* (flexion of arms, extension of legs) results from injury to the corticospinal pathways at the level of the diencephalon or upper midbrain. *Decerebrate posturing* (extension of legs and arms) implies injury to the motor pathways at the level of the lower midbrain, pons, or medulla.

TABLE 63.5. EMERGENCY MEASURES FOR ICP REDUCTION IN AN UNMONITORED PATIENT WITH CLINICAL SIGNS OF HERNIATION

1. Elevate head of bed 15–30 degrees
2. Normal saline (0.9%) at 80–100mL/hr (avoid hypotonic fluids)
3. Intubate and hyperventilate (target Pco_2 = 28–32 mm Hg)
4. Mannitol 20% 1–1.5 g/kg via rapid i.v. infusion
5. Foley catheter
6. Neurosurgical consulation

ICP, intracranial pressure.
From Mayer SA, Dennis L, 1998.

Gait is particularly important to check in low-risk patients who are treated and released without CT. Balance and equilibrium, tested by tandem heel-to-toe walking, are frequently impaired after a concussion.

Radiography and Imaging

In the United States, CT has become the imaging method of choice for head injury. CT is more informative than plain skull films for detecting skull fractures and provides unsurpassed sensitivity for detecting intracranial blood. MRI is better for detecting subtle injury to the brain, particularly focal lesions related to DAI, but is generally not suitable for emergency evaluations because of the time and expense.

There has been intense debate about guidelines for taking skull films or CT after mild head injury. In 1987, guidelines were published for skull radiography after head injury, but the widespread availability of CT since then has made skull films obsolete, and these criteria have now been adopted for CT. In general, all patients with head injury should have CT, except for those who are low risk—without concussion, with no neurologic abnormalities on examination, and with no evidence or suspicion of a skull fracture, alcohol or drug intoxication, or other moderate-risk criteria (Table 63.2). The likelihood of detecting intracranial hemorrhage by CT in these patients is only 1 in 10,000.

CTs of head-injured patients should be assessed for the presence of epidural or subdural hematoma, subarachnoid or intraventricular blood, parenchymal contusions and hemorrhages, cerebral edema, and "gliding contusions" related to DAI. With bone-window settings, fractures, sinus opacification, and pneumocephalus can be identified. CT evidence of mass effect and brain tissue displacement—compression or obliteration of the mesencephalic cisterns or midline shift—correlates with increased ICP and decreased chances of survival.

MANAGEMENT

Admission to the Hospital

Low-Risk Group

Low-risk patients, who meet all criteria described in Table 63.2, can generally be discharged from the emergency room without CT, as long as a responsible person is available to observe the patient for the next 24 hours. In general, these are patients who did not sustain a concussion and have normal findings on neurologic examination. Patients are given a checklist of symptoms (e.g., headache, vomiting, confusion) and instructed to return immediately to the emergency room if any occur.

Moderate-Risk Group

Among patients who have experienced a concussion, a normal Glasgow Coma Scale score of 15 (alert, fully oriented, and following commands) and normal CT eliminate the need for hospital admission. These patients can be discharged to home for observation with a warning card, even in the presence of

headache, nausea, vomiting, dizziness, or retrograde amnesia, because the risk of a significant intracranial lesion developing thereafter is minimal. Criteria for hospital admission for patients with head injury are listed in Table 63.6.

Patients with mild-to-moderate neurologic deficits (generally corresponding to Glasgow Coma Scale scores of 9 to 14) and CT findings that do not require neurosurgical intervention should be admitted to an intermediate or intensive care unit (ICU) for observation. A follow-up CT at 24 hours is often helpful to check for progression of bleeding.

High-Risk Group

All patients with a serious head injury are admitted to the hospital. An early neurosurgical consultation is crucial, because once the patient has been stabilized, assessed, and imaged, the immediate consideration is whether an indication exists for emergent surgical intervention. If the decision is made to operate, surgery should proceed immediately, because delays can only increase the likelihood of further brain damage during the waiting period. Medical management of severe injury patients should take place in an ICU. Although little can be done about brain damage that occurs on impact, ICU care can play a major role in reducing secondary brain injury that develops over hours to days.

Surgical Intervention

Simple wounds of the scalp should be thoroughly cleaned and sutured. Compound fractures of the skull should be completely debrided. Operative treatment of compound fractures should be performed as soon as possible but may be delayed for 24 hours until the patient is transported to a hospital equipped for this purpose or until the patient is hemodynamically stable. Elevation of small depressed fractures need not be performed immediately, but the depressed fragments should be elevated before the patient is discharged from the hospital, particularly if the inner table of the skull is involved.

The treatment of acute subdural, epidural, or parenchymal hematoma with mass effect is *craniotomy* and surgical removal of the clot. The bleeding point should be identified and either ligated or clipped. The operative results depend to a great extent on the degree of associated brain damage. In the absence of coexisting brain injury, remarkable improvement can occur after evacuation of a subdural or epidural hematoma, with disappearance of the hemiplegia or other focal neurologic signs.

Burr hole evacuation is insufficient for acute subdural and epidural hematomas, but for liquified chronic subdural

TABLE 63.6. CRITERIA FOR HOSPITAL ADMISSION AFTER HEAD INJURY

- Intracranial blood or fracture identified on head computed tomography (CT)
- Confusion, agitation, or depressed level of consciousness
- Focal neurologic signs or symptoms
- Posttraumatic seizure
- Alcohol or drug intoxication
- Significant comorbid medical illness
- Lack of a reliable home environment for observation

hematomas, one or more burr holes can be placed to allow drainage of the collection over several days. A plastic catheter (Jackson-Pratt drain) is usually placed in the subural space for several days until the drainage subsides.

Intracranial Pressure Management

As a general rule, an ICP monitor should be placed in all head-injured patients who are comatose (Glasgow Coma Scale score 8) after resuscitation, unless the prognosis is sufficiently dismal that aggressive care in unwarranted. Intracranial hypertension occurs in over 50% of comatose patients with CT evidence of mass effect from intracranial hemorrhage or cerebral edema and in 10% to 15% of patients with normal scans. A ventricular catheter or fiberoptic parenchymal monitor may be used. Ventriculostomy has the advantage of allowing CSF drainage to reduce ICP but has a high risk of infection (approximately 15%), which increases sharply if a catheter is in place for more than 5 days. The risk of infection or hemorrhage is substantially lower with parenchymal ICP monitors (approximately 1% to 2%).

Normal ICP is less than 15 mm Hg, or 20 cm H_2O. Cerebral perfusion pressure (CPP) is routinely monitored in conjunction with ICP because it is an important determinant of cerebral blood flow; CPP is defined as mean arterial blood pressure minus ICP. The goal of ICP management after head injury is to maintain ICP less than 20 mm Hg and CPP greater than 70 mm Hg.

Contemporary ICP management has changed in two important aspects: CPP manipulation has become increasingly emphasized, and the potential for overzealous hyperventilation to aggravate ischemia by causing excessive vasoconstriction has become increasingly appreciated. A stepwise management protocol (Table 63.7) is followed for treating ICP elevations greater than 20 mm Hg for more than 10 minutes.

An acute severe increase in ICP always prompts a repeat CT to assess the need for a definitive neurosurgical procedure. If the patient is agitated or "fighting" the ventilator, an intravenous sedative agent such as propofol or fentanyl should be given to attain a quiet motionless state. Thereafter, if CPP is less than 70 mm Hg, vasopressors such as dopamine or phenylephrine can lead to reduction of ICP by decreasing cerebral vasodilation that occurs in response to inadequate perfusion. Alternately, if CPP is

more than 120 mm Hg, blood pressure reduction with intravenous labetolol or nicardipine can sometimes lead to a parallel decrease of ICP.

Mannitol and hyperventilation are used only after sedation and CPP management fail to normalize ICP. Mannitol, an osmotic diuretic, lowers ICP via its cerebral dehydrating effects. The initial dose of mannitol 20% solution is 1 to 1.5 g/kg, followed by doses of 0.25 to 1.0 g/kg as needed. Further doses should be given on the basis of ICP measurements rather than on a standing basis. The effect of mannitol is maximal when given rapidly; ICP reduction occurs within 10 to 20 minutes and can last for 2 to 6 hours. Serum osmolality should be monitored closely, with a secondary goal of attaining levels of 300–320 mOsm/kg. Urinary losses should be replaced with normal saline to avoid secondary hypovolemia.

Hyperventilation lowers ICP by inducing cerebral alkalosis and reflex vasoconstriction, with a concomitant reduction of cerebral blood volume. Hyperventilation to Pco_2 levels of 28 to 32 mm Hg can lower ICP within minutes, although the effect gradually diminishes over 1 to 3 hours as acid-base buffering mechanisms correct the alkylosis within the central nervous system. Overly aggressive hyperventilation to Pco_2 levels less than 25 mm Hg may exacerbate cerebral ischemia and should be avoided.

High-dose barbiturate therapy with pentobarbital, given in doses equivalent to those used for general anesthesia, effectively lowers ICP in most patients who are refractory to the steps outlined above. The effect of pentobarbital is multifactorial but most likely stems from a coupled decrease in cerebral metabolism, blood flow, and blood volume. Pentobarbital can cause profound hypotension and usually requires the use of vasopressors to maintain CPP $\geq$70 mHg. Systemic hypothermia (32 to 33°C) is used in some centers to treat increased ICP refractory to pentobarbital, but experience with this technique is limited. The mortality of head-injured patients with increased ICP refractory to pentobarbital exceeds 90%.

Intensive Care Unit Management of Severe Head Injury

Severely head injured patients are best treated in an ICU. In some hospitals, head injuries are treated in a special neurologic or neurosurgical ICU. A time-coded flow sheet is helpful to allow for continuous updating of the patient's clinical, neurologic, and physiologic status.

Serial Neurologic Evaluation

The patient should be examined repeatedly to evaluate level of consciousness and the presence or absence of signs of injury to the brain or cranial nerves. Variations in level of consciousness, reflected by changes in the Glasgow Coma Scale score, or the appearance of hemiplegia or other focal neurologic signs should prompt repeat CT.

Airway and Ventilation

In general, patients who are unable to protect their airway due to depressed level of consciousness should be intubated with an en-

TABLE 63.7. STEPWISE TREATMENT PROTOCOL FOR ELEVATED ICP (> 20 mm Hg FOR MORE THAN 10 MIN) IN A MONITORED PATIENT

1. Consider repeat computed tomography and surgical removal of an intracranial mass lesion or ventricular drainage.
2. i.v. sedation to attain a motionless quiet state.
3. Pressor infusion if CPP <70 mm Hg, or reduction of blood pressure if CPP remains >120mm Hg.
4. Mannitol 0.25–1 g/kg i.v. every 2–6 h as needed.
5. Hyperventilation to Pco_2 levels of 28–32 mm Hg
6. High-dose pentobarbital therapy (load with 5–20 mg/kg, maintain with 1–4 mg/k/h).
7. Systemic hypothermia.

See text for details.
CPP, cerebral perfusion pressure.
From Mayer SA, Dennis L, 1998.

dotracheal tube. Routine hyperventilation is not recommended: in the absence of increased ICP, ventilatory parameters should be set to maintain Pco_2 at 35 to 40 mm Hg and Po_2 at 90 to 100 mm Hg.

Blood Pressure Management

If the patient shows signs of hemodynamic instability, a radial artery catheter should be placed to monitor blood pressure. Because cerebral blood flow autoregulation is frequently impaired in acute head injury, mean blood pressure (or CPP if ICP is being monitored) must be carefully regulated to avoid hypotension, which can lead to cerebral ischemia, or hypertension, which can exacerbate cerebral edema.

Fluid Management

Only *isotonic fluids*, such as 0.9% (normal) saline or lactated Ringer solution, should be administered to head-injured patients, because the extra free water in half-normal saline or D5W can exacerbate cerebral edema. Colloid solutions (5% or 25% albumin) or hypertonic (3% or 9%) saline may also be used in patients with increased ICP, but their benefit remains unclear. Central venous pressure monitoring may be helpful to guide fluid management in hypotensive or hyporolemic patients.

Nutrition

Severe head injury leads to a generalized hypermetabolic and catabolic response, with caloric requirements that are 50% to 100% higher than normal. Enteral feedings via a nasogastric or nasoduodenal tube should be instituted as soon as possible (usually after 24 to 48 hours). Parenteral nutrition carries significant risks (primarily infection and electrolyte derangements) and should be used only if enteral feeding cannot be tolerated.

Sedation

Patients may be agitated or delirious, which can lead to self-injury, removal of monitoring devices, systemic and cerebral hypermetabolism, and increased ICP. Intubated patients can be sedated using a continuous intravenous infusion of a rapidly acting sedative agent such as propofol or fentanyl, which can be turned off periodically to allow neurologic assessments. Nonintubated patients can be treated with haloperidol 2 to 10 mg intramuscularly every 4 hours as needed.

Temperature Management

Fever (greater than 101°F) exacerbates traumatic and ischemic brain injury and should be aggressively treated with acetaminophen or cooling blankets. A single randomized trial in 82 patients with Glasgow Coma Scale scores of 3 to 7 showed that initial 24-hour management with hypothermia (32 to 33°C) and vecuronium and fentanyl to prevent shivering improved outcome. More studies are under way to determine whether systemic hypothermia should become standard care in comatose patients with traumatic brain injury.

Anticonvulsants

Phenytoin or fosphenytoin (15 to 20 mg/kg loading dose, then 300 mg/day) reduced the frequency of early (i.e., first week) posttraumatic seizures from 14% to 4% in a clinical trial of patients with intracranial hemorrhage but did not prevent later seizures. Carbamazepine or valproic acid are acceptable alternatives. If the patient has not experienced a seizure, prophylactic anticonvulsants should be discontinued after 7 days. Anticonvulsant levels should be monitored closely, because subtherapeutic levels frequently result from drug hypermetabolism.

Nimodipine for Subarachnoid Hemorrhage

In a clinical trial, nimodipine 60 mg orally every 6 hours was associated with improved outcome in head injury patients with evidence of subarachnoid hemorrhage on admission CT. Nimodipine may increase neuronal ischemic tolerance at the cellular level or improve collateral blood flow. Hypotension was the most common adverse event.

Steroids

Glucocorticoids have been used to treat cerebral edema for years, but have not been shown to favorably alter outcome or lower ICP in head-injured patients and may lead to increased risk of infection, hyperglycemia, or other complications. For these reasons, dexamethasone and other steroids are not recommended for use in patients with head injury.

Deep Vein Thrombosis Prophylaxis

Patients with head injury who are immobilized are at high risk for lower extremity deep vein thrombosis and pulmonary thromboembolism. Pneumatic compression boots should be routinely used to protect against this risk, and subcutaneous heparin 5,000 U every 12 hours can be safely added 72 hours after injury, even in the presence of intracranial hemorrhage.

Gastric Stress Ulcer Prophylaxis

Patients on mechanical ventilation or with coagulopathy are at increased risk of gastric stress ulceration and should receive ranitidine 50 mg intravenously every 8 hours, famotidine 20 mg intravenously every 12 hours, or sucralfate 1 g orally every 6 hours.

Antibiotics

The routine use of prophylactic antibiotics in patients with open skull injuries is controversial, and opinions are sharply divided. Prophylactic antibiotics with gram-positive activity, such as oxacillin, are often used to reduce the risk of meningitis in patients with CSF otorrhea, rhinorrhea, or intracranial air; however, these agents may increase the risk of infection with more virulent or resistant organisms.

ACUTE COMPLICATIONS OF HEAD INJURY

Cerebrospinal Fluid Fistula

CSF fistulas result from tearing of the dura and arachnoid membranes. They occur in 3% of patients with closed head injury and in 5% to 10% of those with basilar skull fractures. They are usually associated with fractures of the ethmoid, sphenoid, or orbital plate of the frontal bone.

CSF leakage ceases after head elevation alone for a few days in 85% of cases. If it persists, a lumbar drain may lower CSF pressure, reduce flow through the fistula, and hasten spontaneous closure of the dural tear. Patients with dural leaks are at increased risk for meningitis, and although the use of prophylactic antibiotics is controversial, most physicians use them. Persistent CSF otorrhea or rhinorrhea for more than 2 weeks calls for surgical repair, as does recurrent meningitis. If there is a leak and the site of the fracture is not evident, a metrizamide CT study is the diagnostic method of choice.

Pneumocephalus

Pneumocephalus is a collection of air in the intracranial cavity, usually in the subarachnoid space. It usually occurs with a fracture of a frontal sinus. The air may not appear for several days after injury and then only after the patient sneezes or blows his or her nose. The presence of intracranial air has the same implications as a CSF fistula. Most pneumoceles are asymptomatic, but headaches or mental symptoms may result from intracranial hypotension. The diagnosis is made by CT, and the site of the dural defect can be identified by CT-metrizamide studies. If spontaneous resorption of the air does not occur, the opening in the frontal sinus should be surgically repaired through a transfrontal craniotomy.

Carotid-Cavernous Fistula

A *carotid-cavernous fistula* is characterized by the clinical triad of pulsating exophthalmos, ocular chemosis, and orbital bruit. They result from traumatic laceration of the internal carotid artery as it passes through the cavernous sinus; approximately 20% of cases are nontraumatic, and most of these are related to spontaneous rupture of an intracavernous internal carotid artery aneurysm. Other symptoms may include distended orbital and periorbital veins and paralysis of the cranial nerves (III, IV, V, and VI) that pass through or within the wall of the cavernous sinus.

Traumatic carotid-cavernous fistulae may develop immediately or days after injury. Angiography is required to confirm the diagnosis (Fig. 63.8). Endovascular treatment, with a balloon placed through the defect in the arterial wall into the venous side of the fistula, is the most effective means of repair and can prevent permanent visual loss due to venous retinal infarction if performed quickly.

Vascular Injury and Thrombosis

Traumatic injuries may be associated with dissections of the extracranial or intracranial internal carotid or vertebral arteries, which can lead to thrombosis at the site of the intimal flap and stroke due to distal thromboembolism. The diagnosis is established by conventional or MR angiography, and anticoagulation should be used to prevent thrombosis and infarction, although this may be relatively contraindicated if there is coexisting intracranial hemorrhage.

Basilar skull fractures are sometimes associated with thrombosis of adjacent dural sinuses. In most cases, *dural sinus thrombosis* takes several days to develop; the sigmoid and transverse sinuses are most commonly involved. Symptoms are related to increased ICP or associated venous infarction and may include headache, vomiting, seizures, depressed level of consciousness, or hemiparesis. The diagnosis is established by angiography or MR venography, and anticoagulation is the treatment of choice (see Chapter 46).

In patients with large epidural or subdural hematomas and subfalcine herniation, secondary cerebral infarction can sometimes result from compression of the ipsilateral anterior cerebral artery against the falx or contralateral posterior cerebral artery against the tentorium.

Cranial Nerve Injury

Injury to the cranial nerves is a frequent complication of fracture at the base of the skull (see Chapter 68). The facial nerve is the most commonly injured nerve, complicating 0.3% to 5% of all head injuries. Occasionally, the paralysis may not develop until several days after the injury. Partial or complete recovery of function is the rule with traumatic injuries to the cranial nerves, with the exception of the first or second nerves.

Infections

Infections within the intracranial cavity after injury to the head may be extradural (osteomyelitis), subdural (empyema), subarachnoid (meningitis), or intracerebral (abscess). For more information, refer to Chapter 21.

Extradural infections are usually accompanied by, and are secondary to, infection of the external wound or osteomyelitis of the skull. *Subdural empyema* is a closed-space infection between the dura and arachnoid. *Intracerebral abscess* may follow compound fractures of the skull or penetrating injuries to the brain. All these infections usually develop in the first few weeks after injury but may be delayed. Diagnosis is suggested by CT and MRI and confirmed by culture of the infected tissue. Treatment includes surgical debridement and administration of antibiotics.

Meningitis may follow any type of open fracture associated with tearing of the dura, including compound fractures, penetrating missiles, or linear fractures that extend into the nasal sinuses or the middle ear. Within the past decade, there have been reports of meningitis in as few as 2% and as many as 22% of patients with basilar skull fractures. Meningitis commonly develops 2 to 8 days after injury but may be delayed for several or

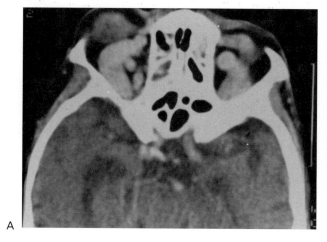

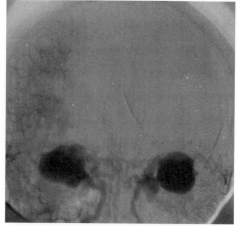

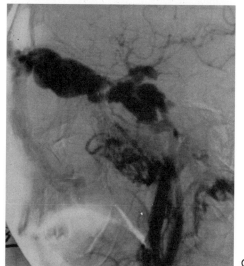

FIG. 63.8. Carotid cavernous fistula. **A:** Axial contrast-enhanced computed tomography demonstrates prominent superior ophthalmic veins bilaterally. Anteroposterior **(B)** and lateral subtraction **(C)** films from a right carotid arteriogram demonstrate bilateral carotid cavernous fistulae with drainage anterior into the superior ophthalmic veins. (Courtesy of Drs. T.L. Chi, J.A. Bello, and S.K. Hilal.)

many months, particularly in patients with fractures through the mastoid or nasal sinuses. Cases that develop within a few days after injury are almost always due to pneumococcus or other gram-positive bacteria, but any pathogenic organism may be the cause. Diagnosis depends on the CSF findings after lumbar puncture. The principles of treatment are those recommended for meningitis in general. The presence of a persistent CSF fistula with rhinorrhea or otorrhea favors the recurrence of meningitis; as many as seven or eight attacks have been reported. Treatment in such cases must include surgical closure of the fistula.

OUTCOME

The outcome that can be expected after head injury is often a matter of great concern, particularly in those with serious injuries. *Depth of coma*, *CT findings*, and *age* are the medical and demographic variables most predictive of late outcome. Other factors of prognostic importance include pupillary responses, hypotension or hypoxemia on admission, and persistently elevated ICP. In the Traumatic Coma Data Bank, an observational study of 746 patients, 33% died, 14% became vegetative, 28% remained dependent with severe disability, 19% regained independence with moderate disability, and only 7% made a full or near-complete recovery.

Severity of coma can be quantified using the admission Glasgow Coma Scale score (Table 63.3), which has substantial prognostic value: Patients scoring 3 or 4 (deep coma) have an 85% chance of dying or remaining vegetative, whereas these outcomes occur in only 5% to 10% of patients scoring 12 or more. In general, elderly patients do very poorly. In one series of comatose patients older than 65, only 10% survived and only 4% regained functional independence. Death may result from the direct effect of the injury or from the complications that ensue. Attempts to make a firm prognosis in severe head injuries, especially in the early stages, are hazardous because the outcome depends on so many variables. Some indices, however, are valuable as prognostic indicators (Table 63.4).

Persistent vegetative state is a much-feared potential outcome of traumatic coma. In general, the prospects of recovery from traumatic coma is better than from coma of other causes. Fifty percent of adults and 60% of children who are comatose for 30 days will recover consciousness within 1 year, compared with 15% of patients in coma from nontraumatic causes. Recovery of consciousness is operationally defined as the ability to follow commands convincingly and consistently.

Almost every patient with severe brain injury shows mental changes after recovery of consciousness from prolonged coma; disorientation and agitation are particularly common. With time, there is usually considerable improvement in the signs and symptoms of brain damage, but permanent sequelae are common. In addition to cognitive and motor deficits, headache, dizziness, or vertigo may be present in the immediate posttraumatic period. These symptoms usually disappear in a few weeks but may be prolonged for months.

Disabling cognitive problems include impaired memory, attention, and concentration; slowing of psychomotor speed and mental processing; and changes in personality. There may be loss of memory for the events that occurred in the immediate period after recovery of consciousness (*posttraumatic amnesia*) and a similar amnesia for the events immediately preceding the injury (*pretraumatic amnesia*). These periods of amnesia may encompass days, weeks, or years.

Early cognitive, physical, and occupational therapy is an important part of optimizing recovery after traumatic brain injury. Physical therapy, including range of motion exercises to prevent limb contractures, can begin even while patients are still in the ICU. Once the patient is stabilized, they should be transferred to an acute or subacute rehabilitation facility. Whether cognitive rehabilitative measures truly improve neuropsychological outcome remains to be established.

In a study of patients with moderate or severe injuries, only 46% returned to work 2 years later, and most of those who did return to work did not go back to their preinjury positions. Only 18% were financially independent, inducing considerable stress on the family. Vocational training can play a key role in helping patients reintegrate into the workplace.

Postconcussion Syndrome

Approximately 40% of patients who have sustained minor or severe injuries to the head complain of headache, dizziness, fatigue, insomnia, irritability, restlessness, and inability to concentrate. Often, there is overlap with symptoms of anxiety and depression. This group of symptoms, which may be present for only a few weeks or may persist for years, is known as *postconcussion syndrome*.

Postconcussion syndrome is somewhat misleadingly named, because affected individuals need not have suffered loss of consciousness. There are no criteria that make it possible to define the role of either physiologic or psychologic factors in the etiology of postconcussion syndrome. Patients may be severely disabled yet have a normal finding on neurologic examination and no MR evidence of brain injury. The correlation between the severity of the original injury and the severity and duration of later symptoms is poor. For instance, the incidence of postconcussion syndrome is not related to the duration of retrograde amnesia, coma, or the posttraumatic amnesia. In some patients, the symptoms may be related to the brain damage; in others, they seem to be entirely psychogenic. In practice, it is often difficult to sort out the complicated origins of this disorder.

Posttraumatic symptoms may develop in patients who had previously shown normal adjustment but are more likely to occur in patients who had psychiatric symptoms before the injury.

Factors such as domestic or financial difficulties, unrewarding occupations, and the desire to obtain compensation, financial or otherwise, tend to produce and may prolong the symptoms once they have developed.

The prognosis of the postconcussion syndrome is uncertain. In general, progressive improvement may be expected. The duration of symptoms is not related to the severity of the injury. In some patients with only a mild injury, symptoms continue for a long period, whereas patients with severe injuries may have only mild or transient symptoms. By and large, however, it is a matter of 2 to 6 months before the headache and dizziness and the more definite mental changes show much improvement. Treatment for postconcussion syndrome is based on psychotherapy, cognitive and occupational therapy, vocational rehabilitation, and treatment with antidepressant or antianxiety agents.

Seizures and Posttraumatic Epilepsy

Posttraumatic seizures may be immediate (within 24 hours), early (within the first week), or late (occurring after the first week).

The exact incidence of seizures after head injury is unknown, but figures in the literature vary from 2.5% to 40%. As a rule, the more severe the injury, the greater the likelihood that seizures will develop. The overall incidence of seizures is about 25% in those with brain contusion or hematoma and as high as 50% in those with penetrating head injury.

Immediate seizures are infrequent; they are a risk factor for further early seizures but not for late seizures. Early seizures occur in 3% to 6% of patients with head injury who are admitted to the hospital. Risk factors include depressed skull fracture, penetrating head injury, intracranial hemorrhage (epidural, subdural, or intraparenchymal), prolonged unconsciousness (more than 24 hours), and immediate seizures; the risk of early seizures in a patient with any of these risk factors is 20% to 30%. Children are more likely to develop early posttraumatic seizures than are adults. Patients who experience early seizures remain at risk for late seizures and should be maintained on anticonvulsants after discharge from the hospital.

The overall incidence of late seizures (posttraumatic epilepsy) after closed head injury is 5%, but the risk is as high as 30% among patients with intracranial hemorrhage or a depressed skull fracture and 50% among patients who have experienced early seizures. About 60% of patients experience their initial seizure during the first year, but the risk of seizures remains increased for up to 15 years after a severe head injury. Because 25% of patients have only a single late seizure, many practitioners begin anticonvulsants only after a second seizure occurs. Therapy of posttraumatic epilepsy is discussed in Chapter 140.

Posttraumatic Movement Disorders

Movement disorders are a rare sequelae of head injury. Action tremor is most common, although its pathogenesis remains obscure. Cerebellar ataxia, rubral tremor, and palatal myoclonus have been described in patients with focal shearing injuries of the superior cerebellar peduncle, midbrain, and dentatorubroolivary triangle, respectively. Parkinsonism and other basal ganglia syndromes have been reported after a single episode of head trauma. The treatment of movement disorders is discussed in Section XV.

PEDIATRIC TRAUMA

Injuries are the leading cause of death in children, and brain injury is the most common cause of pediatric traumatic death. Motor vehicle accidents account for the largest number of severe injuries in children, but children are also prone to unique forms of injury, such as birth injury and child abuse. Children are more likely than adults to experience brain swelling and seizures after head injury and in general make better recoveries.

Birth Injuries

The common neurosurgical lesions of neonates are skull fractures; subarachnoid hemorrhage; and epidural, subdural, and intracerebral hematomas. Extracranial subgaleal and subperiosteal hematomas due to trauma at the time of delivery are fairly common and rarely need treatment. Acute subdural hematoma was once considered the most common intracranial birth injury, but this syndrome seems to be disappearing with improved obstetric care. Diagnosis by subdural taps has been supplanted by the use of CT. Surgical evacuation is accomplished through a craniotomy rather than a burr hole.

Leptomeningeal Cysts

A rare complication of head injury is the formation of a leptomeningeal cyst in the space between the pia mater and the arachnoidal membrane. This complication is most common in infants and children less than 2 years of age; the clinical hallmark is a palpable nontender swelling that is getting larger in the area of a previous fracture. Also known as a "growing fracture," leptomeningeal cysts may develop when a linear fracture of the skull is associated with laceration of the dura; pulsation of the brain forces CSF into a cyst formed between the edges of the fracture, producing erosion of the skull. The diagnosis is made from radiographic evidence of a circular or oval area of erosion of the skull in a patient who has had a previous fracture of the skull. Treatment consists of excision of the cyst and repair of the dural defect.

Child Abuse

Child abuse is an important problem encountered in the care of children with head trauma. Certain characteristics may enable the physician to identify an abused child. There is often a delay in seeking medical care, and there may be a history of multiple previous injuries. Details of the history may be sketchy or may be inconsistent with the severity of the child's injury. Examination may reveal bruises or injuries that do not normally result from the day-to-day activities of a child, including injuries between the shoulder blades, circumferentially around the arm, or behind the legs. A skeletal survey may reveal multiple healed fractures.

The "shaken baby syndrome" should be suspected in children with significant neurologic injury with little evidence of external trauma. Retinal hemorrhages occur frequently and may be

pathognomonic for this syndrome, and subdural hematoma is also common. MRI can play a pivotal role in the diagnosis by identifying intracranial lesions of varying ages. Established protocols should be followed once there is a suspicion of child abuse to ensure that the child will not be subjected to further injury.

NEUROLOGY OF PROFESSIONAL BOXING

The term "punch drunk" is ascribed to a 1928 paper by Martland; another term is dementia pugilistica. The current nonprejorative term is *chronic traumatic encephalopathy*. Whatever the name, there seems to be little doubt that professional boxers are especially at risk for a syndrome that is dominated by parkinsonism and other extrapyramidal features—tremor, ataxia, cerebellar signs, and, in some, dementia. The disorder is attributed to the cumulative effects of repetitive subconcussive blows to the head. Pathologic studies show hypothalamic abnormalities, degeneration of substantia nigra, widespread neurofibrillary changes, and scarring of cerebellar folia.

Although the syndrome is well known, few prospective studies have been done to determine precise risk factors, whether signs can be seen early enough to prevent the severe late syndrome, whether the syndrome could be prevented by offering protective guidelines for boxing matches (e.g., neurologic examination, including CT and MRI, better head protection, different gloves), and whether it is a progressive disorder after the boxer has ceased to fight. According to the early study of Critchley (1957), manifestations begin from 6 to 40 years after starting a boxing career, with an average of 16 years.

Other sports involve the risk of serious injury, but only boxing includes the goal of deliberately injuring the brain of an opponent. Knockout is the prized achievement. Many neurologists have therefore urged the abolition of boxing, but this has not yet been achieved, and it may never be; many powerful social forces promote the sport in the United States and elsewhere. If boxing is not to be banned, physicians and other health care workers must take every opportunity to regulate the profession. Physicians must stop matches when there is evidence of brain injury. Better protection for boxers must be available during training and in the ring. Appropriate prospective epidemiologic studies are needed. Once the symptoms of chronic traumatic encephalopathy have become evident, no therapy is effective.

SUGGESTED READINGS

Head Injury, General Considerations

Adams JH, Graham DI, Gennarelli TA, et al. Diffuse axonal injury in nonmissile head injury. *J Neurol Neurosurg Psychiatry* 1991;54:481–483.
Àlvarez-Sabín J, Turon A, Lozano-Sánchez M, et al. Delayed posttraumatic hemorrhage: spat-apoplexie. *Stroke* 1995;26:1531–1535.
Bullock MR, Chestnut RM, Clifton G, et al. Guidelines for the management of severe head injury. *J Neurotrauma* 1996;13:639–734.
Cooper PR. *Head injury*, 3rd ed. Baltimore: Williams & Wilkins, 1993.
Dacey RG Jr, Alves WM, Rimel RW, et al. Neurosurgical complications after apparently minor head injury. *J Neurosurg* 1987;65:203–210.
Eisenberg HM, Frankowski RF, Contant CF, et al. High-dose barbiturate control of elevated intracranial pressure in patients with severe head injury. *J Neurosurg* 1988;69:15–23.

Frankowski RF, Annegers JF, Whitman S. Epidemiological and descriptive studies. Part 1. The descriptive epidemiology of head trauma in the United States. In: Becker DP, Povlishock JT, eds. *Central nervous system trauma status report—1985.* Bethesda: National Institutes of Health, NINCDS, 1985:33–43.

Gentleman D, Jennett B. Audit of transfer of unconscious head-injured patients to a neurosurgical unit. *Lancet* 1990;335:330–334.

Gruen P, Liu C. Current trends in the management of head injury. *Emerg Med Clin North Am* 1998;16:63–83.

Harders A, Kakarieka A, Braakman R, et al. Traumatic subarachnoid hemorrhage and its treatment with nimodpine. *J Neurosurg* 1996;85:82–89.

Jane JA, Anderson DK, Torner JC, Young W. *Central nervous system trauma status report—1991.* New York: Mary Ann Liebert, 1992.

Levi I, Guiliburd JN, Lemberger A, et al. Diffuse axonal injury: Analysis of 100 patients with radiological signs. *Neurosurgery* 1990;27:208–213.

Marion DW, Penrod LE, Kelsey SF, et al. Treatment of traumatic brain injury with moderate hypothermia. *N Engl J Med* 1997;336:540–546.

Marshall LF, Marshall SB, Klauber MR, et al. A new classification of head injury based on computerized tomography. *J Neurosurg* 1991;75(suppl 1):S14–S20.

Martin NA, Patwardhan RV, Alexander MJ, et al. Characterization of cerebral hemodynamic phases following severe head trauma: hypoperfusion, hyperemia, and vasospasm. *J Neurosurg* 1997;87:9–19.

Masters SJ, McClean PM, Arcanese MS, et al. Skull x-ray examinations after head injury: recommendations by a multidisciplinary panel and validation study. *N Engl J Med* 1987;316:84–91.

Mayer SA, Dennis LJ. Management of increased intracranial pressure. *The Neurologist* 1998;4:2–12.

Merritt HH. Head injury. *War Med* 1943;4:61–82.

Muizelaar JP, Marmarou A, Ward JD, et al. Adverse effects of prolonged hyperventilation in patients with head injury: a randomized clinical trial. *J Neurosurg* 1991;75:731–739.

Pearl GS. Traumatic neuropathology. *Clin Lab Med* 1998;18:39–64.

Rosner MJ, Rosner SD, Johnson AH. Cerebral perfusion pressure: management protocol and clinical results. *J Neurosurg* 1995;83:949–962.

Symonds C. Concussion and its sequelae. *Lancet* 1962;1:1–5.

Teasdale G, Jennett B. Assessment of coma and impaired consciousness. A practical scale. *Lancet* 1974;2:81–83.

Teasdale GM. Head injury. *J Neurol Neurosurg Psychiatry* 1995;58:526–539.

Teasdale GM, Murray G, Anderson E, et al. Risks of acute traumatic intracranial hematoma in children and adults: implications for management of head injuries. *BMJ* 1990;300:363–367.

Temkin NR, Dikman SS, Wilensky AJ, et al. A randomized, double-blind study of phenytoin for the prevention of posttraumatic seizures. *N Engl J Med* 1990;323:497–502.

Temkin NR, Haglund MM, Winn HR. Causes, prevention and treatment of post-traumatic epilepsy. *New Horizons* 1995;3:518–522.

White RJ, Likavec MJ. The diagnosis and management of head injury. *N Engl J Med* 1992;327:1507–1511.

Imaging

Gentry LR, Godersky JC, Thompson B. MR imaging of head trauma: review of the distribution and radiopathologic features of traumatic lesions. *AJR* 1988;150:663–672.

Hans JH, Kaufman B, Alfidi RJ, et al. Head injury evaluated by MRI and CT: a comparison. *Radiology* 1984;150:71–77.

Jeret JS, Mandell M, Anziska B, et al. Clinical predictors of abnormality disclosed by computed tomography after mild head trauma. *Neurosurgery* 1993;32:9–16.

Zee CS, Go JL. CT of head trauma. *Neuroimag Clin North Am* 1998;8:525–539.

Epidural Hematoma

Borzone M, Rivano C, Altomonte M, Baldini M. Acute traumatic posterior fossa haematomas. *Acta Neurochir* 1995;135:32–37.

Bricolo AP, Pasut LM. Extradural hematoma: Toward zero mortality. *Neurosurgery* 1984;14:8–12.

Bullock R, Smith RM, van Dellen JR. Nonoperative management of extradural hematoma. *Neurosurgery* 1985;16:602–606.

Dhellemmes P, Lejeune JP, Christiaens JL, et al. Traumatic extradural hematomas in infancy and childhood. *J Neurosurg* 1985;62:861–865.

Ingraham FD, Campbell JB, Cohen J. Extradural hematoma in infancy and childhood. *JAMA* 1949;140:1010–1013.

Subdural Hematoma

Bender MB. Recovery from subdural hematoma without surgery. *Mt Sinai J Med* 1960;26:52–58.

Gutman MB, Noulton RJ, Sullivan I, et al. Risk factors predicting operable intracranial hematomas in head injury. *J Neurosurg* 1992;77:9–14.

Howard MA, Gross AB, Dacey RG Jr, et al. Acute subdural hematoma: an age-dependent clinical entity. *J Neurosurg* 1989;71:858–863.

Klun B, Fettich M. Factors influencing the outcome in acute subdural hematoma: 330 cases. *Acta Neurochir* 1984;71:171–178.

Lee KS. The pathogenesis and clinical significance of traumatic subdural hygroma. *Brain Injury* 1998;12:595–603.

Munro D, Merritt HH. Surgical pathology of subdural hematoma. *Arch Neurol Psychiatry* 1936;35:64–78.

Complications of Head Injury

Davis JM, Zimmerman RA. Injury to the carotid and vertebral arteries. *Neuroradiology* 1983;25:55–70.

Dott NM. Carotid-cavernous arteriovenous fistula. *Clin Neurosurg* 1969;16:17–21.

Elijamel MSM, Foy PM. Post-traumatic CSF fistulae: the case for surgical repair. *Br J Neurosurg* 1990;4:479–483.

Friedman AP, Merritt HH. Damage to cranial nerves resulting from head injury. *Bull Los Angel Neurol Soc* 1944;9:135–139.

Kupersmith MJ, Berenstein A, Flamm E, et al. Neuro-opthalmologic abnormalities and intravascular therapy of traumatic carotid cavernous fistulas. *Ophthalmology* 1986;93:906–912.

Manelfe C, Cellerier P, Sobel D, et al. Cerebrospinal fluid rhinorrhea: Evaluation with metrizamide cisternography. *AJR* 1982;138:471–476.

Morgan MK, Besser M, Johnston I, et al. Intracranial carotid artery injury in closed head trauma. *J Neurosurg* 1987;66:192–197.

Scott BL, Jancovic J. Delayed-onset progressive movement disorders after static brain lesions. *Neurology* 1996;46:68–74.

Pediatric Trauma

Adelson PD, Kochanek PM. Head injury in children. *J Child Neurol* 1998;13:2–15.

Bruce DA, Alavi A, Bilaniuk L, et al. Diffuse cerebral swelling following head injuries in children. *J Neurosurg* 1981;54:170–178.

Duhaime AC, Christian CW, Rorke LB, Zimmerman RA. Nonaccidental head injury in infants—the "shaken baby syndrome." *N Engl J Med* 1998;338:1822–1829.

Ward JD. Pediatric issues in head trauma. *New Horizons* 1995;3:539–545.

Outcome

Annegers JF, Grabow JD, Groover RV, et al. Seizures after head trauma: a population study. *Neurology* 1980;30:683–689.

Brooke OG. Delayed effects of head injuries in children. *BMJ* 1988;296:948.

Dikman S, Machamer J, Temkin N. Psychosocial outcome in patients with moderate to severe head injury: 2-year follow-up. *Brain Injury* 1993;7:113–124.

Dikman S, Reitan RM, Temkin NR. Neuropsychological recovery in head injury. *Arch Neurol* 1983;40:333–338.

Dodwell D. The heterogeneity of social outcome following head injury. *J Neurol Neurosurg Psychiatry* 1988;51:833–838.

Gordon E, von Holst H, Rudehill A. Outcome of head injury in 2298 patients treated in a single clinic during a 21-year period. *J Neurosurg Anesth* 1995;7:235–247.

Klonoff H, Clark C, Klonoff PS. Long-term outcome of head injuries: 23-year follow-up of children. *J Neurol Neurosurg Psychiatry* 1993;56:410–415.

Levin HS, Amparo E, Eisenberg HM, et al. MRI and CT in relation to the neurobehavioral sequelae of mild and moderate head injuries. *J Neurosurg* 1987;66:706–713.

Levin HS, Gary HS Jr, Eisenberg MM, et al. Neurobehavioral outcome one year after severe head injury: experience of the Traumatic Coma Data Bank. *J Neurosurg* 1990;73:699–709.

Levin HS, High WM, Goethe KE, et al. The neurobehavioral rating scale: assessment of behavioral sequelae of head injury by the clinician. *J Neurol Neurosurg Psychiatry* 1987;50:183–193.

Lishman WA. Physiogenesis and psychogenesis in the "postconcussional" syndrome. *Br J Psychiatry* 1988;153:460.

Macciocchi SN, Barth JT, Littlefield LM. Outcome after mild head injury. *Clin Sports Med* 1998;17:27–36.

McMillan TM, Glucksman EE. The neuropsychology of moderate head injury. *J Neurol Neurosurg Psychiatry* 1987;50:393–397.

Sakas DE, Bullock MR, Teasdale GM. One-year outcome following craniotomy for traumatic hematoma in patients with fixed dilated pupils. *J Neurosurg* 1995;82:961–965.

Stambrook M, Moore AD, Peters LC, et al. Effects of mild, moderate, and severe closed head injury on long term vocational status. *Brain Injury* 1990;4:183–190.

Temkin NR, Holubkov R, Machamer JE, et al. Classification and regression trees (CART) for prediction of function 1 year following head trauma. *J Neurosurg* 1995;82:764–771.

Neurology of Boxing

Cantu RC. Return to play guidelines after a head injury. *Clin Sports Med* 1998;17:45–60.

Council Report. Brain injury in boxing. *JAMA* 1983;249:254–257.

Critchley M. Medical aspects of boxing, particularly from a neurological standpoint. *Br Med J* 1957;1:351–357.

Holzgraefe M, Lemme W, Funke W, et al. The significance of diagnostic imaging in acute and chronic brain damage in boxing. A prospective study in amateur boxing using MRI. *Int J Sports Med* 1992;13:616–620.

Jordan BD. Neurologic aspects of boxing. *Arch Neurol* 1987;44:453–459.

Jordan BD, Lahre C, Hauser WA, et al. CT of 338 professional boxers. *Radiology* 1992;185:509–512.

Kelly JP, Nichols JS, Filley CM, et al. Concussion in sports. Guidelines for the prevention of catastrophic outcome. *JAMA* 1991;266:2867–2869.

Martland HS. Punch drunk. *JAMA* 1928;91:1103–1107.

Richards NG. Ban boxing. *Neurology* 1984;34:1485–1486.

Ross RJ, Cole M, Thompson JS, et al. Boxers—computed tomography, EEG, and neurological examination. *JAMA* 1983;249:211–213.

Merritt's Neurology, 10th ed., edited by L.P. Rowland. Lippincott Williams & Wilkins, Philadelphia © 2000.

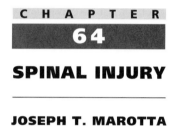

CHAPTER 64

SPINAL INJURY

JOSEPH T. MAROTTA

Trauma to the vertebral column may irreversibly damage the spinal cord and accompanying nerve roots. Spinal cord injury is acute and unexpected, dramatically changing the course of an individual's life. The social and economic consequences to patient, family, and society may be catastrophic.

The annual incidence of spinal cord injury is estimated at 30 to 40 per 1,000,000 persons, with about 8,000 to 10,000 new cases per year. The prevalence is approximately 900 to 950 per 1,000,000, with approximately 250,000 patients now in the United States. The mortality rate is estimated at 48%; approximately 80% of deaths occur at the scene of the accident. After hospital admission, mortality is estimated at 4% to 17%.

The most common level of injury is C-5 followed by C-4 and C-6. The most common lower level is T-12 followed by L-1 and T-10.

ETIOLOGY

Of those suffering spinal cord trauma, 65% are younger than 35 years. The greatest incidence occurs between 20 to 24 years. After age 35, there is a slightly increased incidence of spinal cord injury in those between 55 and 59 years. The male-to-female ratio is at least 3:1 to 4:1. The incidence of injury is highest during the summer months and on weekends.

Road accidents are the most common cause of traumatic paraplegia and tetraplegia. Patients in this group, which encompasses single and multiple motor vehicle accidents, motorcycle accidents, and injuries to pedestrians, account for approximately 48% of all new cases of spinal cord injury. Other causes include falls (21%), sports injuries (hockey, football, diving, and water sports) (13%), industrial accidents (12%), and acts of violence such as stabbing and gunshot wounds (16%). There are regional differences in frequency of injury (i.e., in large cities, gunshot wounds and stabbing are frequent causes). In the elderly, falls are an increasingly common cause of spinal injury. The relative frequency of these causes differs in different societies (Table 64.1). Birth injuries, particularly in breech deliveries, may result in a stretched or compressed spinal cord due to traction and hyperextension of the cervical spine.

MECHANISM OF INJURY

Indirect severe force applied to the vertebral column is the most frequent mechanism of spinal cord injury. Such a force, generated during sudden flexion, hyperextension, vertebral compression, or rotation of the vertebral column, may result in dislocation of facet joints, fracture of vertebral bodies, misalignment of the vertebral canal, herniation of disc material, and bone splintering. The spinal cord may consequently be contused, stretched, lacerated, or crushed. When there is preexisting cervical spondylosis or spinal stenosis, a trivial injury may cause major neurologic damage, even without fracture or dislocation. With the advent of magnetic resonance imaging (MRI), it is recognized that disc herniation is a more common cause of spinal contusion than was previously appreciated. Both direct and indirect injury to the cord from comminuted bone may occur when bullets and high-velocity missiles are responsible for the injury.

TABLE 64.1. CAUSES OF SPINAL CORD INJURY: NEW ADMISSIONS TO DUKE OF CORNWALL SPINAL TREATMENT CENTER 1989–1991

Causes	%
Motor vehicle accidents	51.5
Car, truck	27
Motorcycle	21
Bicycle	3
Pedestrian	1
Domestic and industrial accidents	27
Domestic	
Falls in house; stairs, ladders, trees	16
Industrial	
Falls from scaffolds, ladders; crush injuries	11
Athletic injuries	16
Diving in shallow water	7
Rugby	3
Horse riding	1
Gymnastics, skiing, others	5.5
Personal injury	5
Self-harm	4.5
Criminal assault	0.5
Major catastrophe	
Air crash	0.5

Modified from Grundy D, Swain A, eds. *ABC of spinal cord injury*, 2nd ed. London: BMJ Publishing Group, 1993.

Direct injury to the spinal cord results from stabbing with a sharp object such as a knife. With stabbing, the protection usually afforded by the laminae is bypassed when the sharp object is directed away from the midline in an angular direction.

Appreciation of the mechanism of injury provides insight into the potential stability or instability of spinal injury. Sudden, violent flexion, particularly in the cervical and thoracic regions, may cause anterior compression fractures of vertebral bodies and unilateral or bilateral facet joint dislocation. Rupture of longitudinal or interspinous ligaments may occur. As a result of severe compression injuries, bursting of a vertebral body may occur, with bone splinters and disc material being pushed into the spinal canal. Rotational injuries may result in unilateral fracture–dislocation with variable trauma to the cord. Hyperextension injuries, caused by a fall forward, result in fracture of the posterior elements of the vertebral bodies. Any combination of forces may occur in a single case. It is therefore important to recognize the mechanism of injury in the assessment. This understanding permits assessment not only of the nature, level, and extent of underlying cord injury but also of the stability of the spinal column at the site of injury.

In summary, an appreciation of the biomechanics of an injury is based on the most prominently recognized applied force. The common mechanisms include flexion, extension, axial compression, or any combination of these forces.

PATHOLOGY

The type and severity of spinal column injury determine the nature and extent of the underlying cord damage. There may be extensive contusion and compression of the cord with partial or complete laceration and gross spinal cord injury. With stab wounds, the pathology may be a discrete hemisection of the cord.

The extent of spinal cord injury results from a direct mechanical blow causing cord disruption of varying degree. This is acute and immediate. Macroscopic examination in acute spinal cord injury reveals a swollen, reddish, soft, and mushy cord. Contusion, extradural hemorrhages of modest size, subdural hemorrhages, and subarachnoid hemorrhage may be seen. Complete transection is rare.

Hyperemia is obvious within 12 to 24 hours. The vascular changes are likely due to the presence of vasoactive agents triggered by prostaglandins and catecholamines. Cross-sections of the swollen cord reveal centrally placed hemorrhages, softening, or necrosis. Microscopic investigation reveals fragmented myelin sheaths, splayed myelin lamellae, broken axons, and eosinophilic neurons. The exudate consists of red cells, polymorphonuclear leukocytes, lymphocytes, and plasma cells. These changes extend several segments above and below the level of injury. The edema and acute reaction subside within several weeks; hemorrhages are absorbed, and the acute exudate is replaced by macrophages, with the most prominent cell being a lipid phagocyte. This reparative stage may persist for 2 years, resulting in cavitation, gliosis, and fibrosis. In 5 years or more postinjury, the damaged area shrinks, and the cord is replaced by fibrous tissue. There is progressive proliferation of acellular connective tissue, resulting in dense and chronic adhesive arachnoiditis. The chronic results of spinal cord injury may include traumatic neuroma from injured nerve roots, posttraumatic syringomyelia, or spinal stenosis secondary to disc protrusion and associated osteophyte formation.

In traumatic hematomyelia, hemorrhage occurs within the central gray matter. It is limited in extent and is eventually absorbed, leaving a centrally placed, smooth-walled cyst. This differs from the much more common central hemorrhagic softening and necrosis that occur.

On rare occasions, after several years of neurologic stability, residual intramedullary cysts may become distended, leading to a progressive neurologic deterioration. There is no explanation for this delayed myelopathy, referred to as traumatic syringomyelia. The neurologic deterioration that occurs is invariably rostral to the original injury. Traumatic syringomyelia most frequently occurs in the cervical region.

NEUROLOGIC ASSESSMENT AND CLASSIFICATION

A comprehensive, thorough neurologic assessment is pivotal in determining the level, type, and severity of cord injury. Many attempts have been made over the years to standardize the clinical neurologic assessment. A standard assessment would permit comparison of different observations in different centers. One of the original scales was that of Frankel, a global scale devised in 1969; it consists of five groups: (1) no motor or sensory function, (2) no motor but some sensory preservation, (3) useless motor function preserved, (4) useful motor function preserved, and (5) normal function with or without minor neurologic deficit.

The American Spinal Injury Association (ASIA) and the International Medical Society of Paraplegia (IMSOP) jointly published the "International Standards for Neurological and Func-

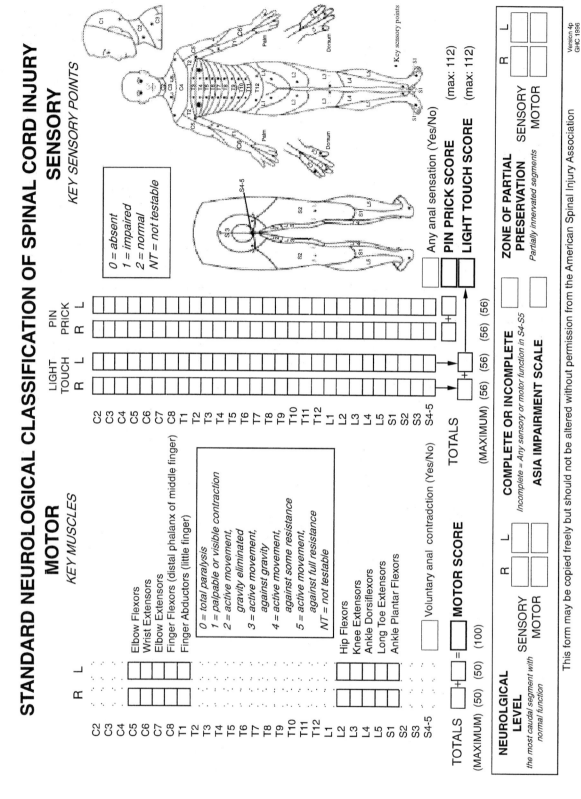

FIG. 64.1. ASIA neurologic examination form for spinal cord injury.

tional Classification of Spinal Cord Injury" (Maynard et al., 1997). This is an excellent method of clinical neurologic assessment, allowing comparison of findings from center to center and investigator to investigator (Fig. 64.1). The ASIA/IMSOP have also published a new impairment scale that improves on the Frankel scale. This ASIA/IMSOP scale has reduced the number of criteria for the category of incomplete cord transection.

The ASIA/IMSOP impairment scale consists of the following categories:

Complete: no motor or sensory function is preserved in the sacral segments S-4 and S-5.

Incomplete: sensory but not motor function is preserved below the neurologic level and extends through to the sacral segments S-4 and S-5.

Incomplete: motor function is preserved below the neurologic level, and the majority of key muscles below the neurologic level have a muscle grade less than 3.

Incomplete: motor function is preserved below the neurologic level, and the majority of key muscles have a muscle grade of 3 or greater.

Normal: motor and sensory function is normal.

The following definitions are noted:

Incomplete spinal cord injury: if partial preservation of sensory and/or motor functions is found below the neurologic level and includes the lowest sacral segment, the injury is defined as incomplete. Sacral sensation also includes deep anal sensation. Voluntary contraction of the anal sphincter muscle is used to demonstrate preserved muscle function.

Complete spinal cord injury: this term is used when there is no sensory or motor function in the lowest sacral segment. The neurologic level is given as the lowest level where there is still some evidence of muscle function or sensation but no preservation in the sacral area.

Zone of Partial Preservation: this refers to dermatomes and myotomes below the neurologic level that remain partially innervated. When some impaired sensory or motor function is found below the lowest normal segment, the exact number of segments so affected constitute the zone of partial preservation. This term is used only with incomplete injuries.

The clinical patterns seen in spinal injury are the following:

- Cauda equina lesions
- Conus medullaris lesions
- Mixed cauda–conus lesions
- Spinal cord injuries
  - Spinal cord concussion
  - Spinal shock
  - Complete cord transection
  - Incomplete cord transection
- Brown-Séquard syndrome
- Central cervical cord syndrome
- Anterior cord syndrome
- Posterior cord syndrome

Damage to the roots of the cauda equina causes flaccid, areflexic paralysis and sensory loss in the area supplied by the affected roots, with paralysis of bladder and rectum. The findings may be symmetric or asymmetric. If only the conus is damaged, there is urinary and fecal incontinence, failure of erection and ejaculation in men, paralysis of the pelvic floor muscles, and sensory impairment, which is frequently dissociated in the saddle region. In a pure conus lesion, tendon reflexes are frequently preserved, but occasionally the ankle jerks are lost. A mixture of anatomically appropriate clinical signs is seen because conus and cauda injuries commonly occur together.

Spinal cord concussion is the term for transient neurologic symptoms with recovery in minutes or hours. Symptoms develop below the level of the blow. *Spinal shock* occurs after an abrupt, complete, or incomplete lesion of the spinal cord. There is immediate complete paralysis and anesthesia below the lesion with hypotonia and areflexia. The plantar responses may be absent, extensor, or equivocal. The areflexic hypotonic state is gradually replaced by pyramidal signs, usually within 3 or 4 weeks. The evolution from an areflexic to hyperreflexic state may be delayed by urinary tract infection, infected bed sores, anemia, or malnutrition.

Chronic and complete transection of the cord after the period of spinal shock results in permanent motor, sensory, and autonomic paralysis below the level of the lesion. Chronic and incomplete transverse section results in different clinical pictures, depending on the pathways involved. In the *Brown-Séquard syndrome* after hemisection of the spinal cord, the following signs are found, usually with the upper level one or two segments below that of the lesion: ipsilateral paresis, ipsilateral corticospinal signs, contralateral loss of pain and temperature sensation, and ipsilateral impairment of vibration and joint position sense. There is usually little loss of tactile sensation. There may be ipsilateral segmental loss of sensation or weakness appropriate to the level of the lesion.

The *central cervical cord syndrome* is characterized by weakness that is more marked in the arms than the legs, urinary retention, and patchy sensory loss below the level of the lesion. The arms or hands may be paralyzed or moderately weak; in the legs there may be severe paresis or only minimal weakness, with overactive tendon reflexes and Babinski signs. Micturition may be normal. Complete cord transection may be diagnosed at first because there seems to be no cord function below the level of the lesion. Careful testing, however, may reveal sacral sparing and therefore an incomplete lesion. If so, the potential for recovery without operative intervention is better and depends on the degree of central hemorrhage.

In the *anterior cervical cord syndrome,* immediate complete paralysis is associated with mild to moderate impairment of pinprick response and light touch below the injury with preservation of position and vibration sense. This syndrome may be caused by an acutely ruptured disc with or without fracture or fracture–dislocation in the cervical region.

The *posterior cord syndrome* is characterized by pain and paresthesia in the neck, upper arms, and trunk. Paresthesia is usually symmetric and has a burning quality. The sensory manifestations may be combined with mild paresis of the arms and hands, but the long tracts are only slightly affected. The symptoms of both the anterior and posterior cord syndromes are reversible.

Clear demarcation between incomplete and complete spinal cord syndromes may be clinically difficult at the time of injury. An accurate neurologic examination may be feasible only 24 to

48 hours after the injury. This period permits any interference from alcohol, drugs, or multiple trauma to be dealt with, resulting in a more alert and cooperative patient.

DIAGNOSIS

After clinical neurologic assessment and stabilization, diagnosis of the injury is enhanced by diagnostic imaging and neurophysiologic studies. It is essential to obtain accurate and complete plain radiographs of the spinal column at the time of injury. This is done to rule out unsuspected other spinal column pathology.

Anteroposterior (AP) and lateral plain-film x-rays must be taken at the appropriate level as directed by the clinical evaluation. Some observers advise AP and lateral films of the entire spine to rule out clinically unsuspected lesions. Lateral x-rays of the cervical spine encompassing the lower cervical region are mandatory. Open-mouth odontoid views should form part of the initial examination. In thoracic and lumbar injuries, AP, lateral, oblique, and extension views may be required.

Computed tomography (CT) is the best procedure for evaluating uncertain findings on plain x-rays, as well as detecting bone pathology. High-resolution CT with sagittal reconstruction enhances radiologic diagnosis to 95%.

In general, magnetic resonance imaging (MRI) is the best technique for soft tissue imaging and CT is best for detecting bone pathology. Recent advances in MRI technology have overcome technical problems such as slow scanning speed and poor resolution, improving the MR images. Multiplanar high-resolution MRI with T1-weighted and gradient-echo or T2-weighted imaging is the most specific and sensitive technique for soft tissue paraspinal lesions, disc herniation, spinal cord hemorrhage, spinal cord edema, and intra- and extradural hemorrhage. Monitoring of severely injured patients during MRI procedures, although improved, is still inadequate in many institutions. The ability to monitor the critically injured must be a priority when MRI is considered. If MRI is not available, intrathecally enhanced CT is the current best alternative. Standard myelography is seldom done under acute circumstances.

Neurophysiologic assessment of spinal cord function is feasible with the use of sensory and motor evoked responses. Mixed nerve evoked potentials may be useful in determining the integrity of certain spinal cord pathways (e.g., dorsal columns). These procedures are used at times in intensive care units or intraoperatively for monitoring spinal cord function and identifying spinal conduction block.

COURSE AND PROGNOSIS

It is estimated that 48% of patients with a spinal cord injury die within 24 hours of sustaining the injury, the majority at the site of the accident or on arrival at the hospital. Long-term survival depends on the level and extent of the lesion, patient age, and the availability of special treatment units in which multidisciplinary personnel are available.

A long-term follow-up of survival in 1,501 patients with spinal cord injury was presented by a Toronto group in a series

of reports (Geisler & Jousse, 1992). The follow-up extended from January 1, 1945, to December 31, 1980, and revealed the following:

1. Spinal-cord-injured patients had a higher mortality rate than those in the general population.
2. The mortality rate was highest for those with complete lesions, particularly tetraplegia.
3. The mortality rate was significantly reduced over the length of the follow-up, especially in complete lesions.
4. The mortality rate of incomplete lesions was closer to that of the general population.
5. There was a marked decrease in the number of deaths caused by renal disease in those with spinal cord injury.
6. Deaths from suicide remained high.

De Vivo and colleagues (1987) studied the 7-year survival following spinal cord injury. This was a retrospective study of 5,131 persons with acute spinal cord injury between 1973 and 1980. All study subjects were treated in one of seven federally designated "model regional spinal cord injury care systems." Each had survived at least 24 hours after injury. The older group fared less well than the younger. Complete lesions predictably did less well than incomplete lesions. The cumulative 7-year survival rate among neurologically complete quadriplegics who were at least 50 years old when injured was only 22.7%. The cumulative 7-year survival rate for all groups was 86.7%.

De Vivo and associates (1990) also studied the influence of age at the time of spinal cord injury on the course of rehabilitation. Data were collected from 866 patients admitted between 1973 and 1985. Compared with patients 16 to 30 years old, patients who were at least 61 years old were (1) 2.1 times more likely to have developed pneumonia, (2) 2.7 times more likely to experience a gastrointestinal hemorrhage, (3) 5.6 times more likely to develop pulmonary emboli, (4) 16.8 times more likely to have renal stones, (5) 3.9 times more likely to have been readmitted to the hospital during the second postinjury year, (6) 2.1 times more likely to have required artificial ventilatory support before discharge, (7) 22.7 times more likely to have been discharged to a nursing home, (8) 71.8 times more likely to be in a nursing home 2 years after injury, and (9) 7.3 times more likely to have used hired attendants during the second postinjury year. Two-year survival rates were 59% for patients ages 61 to 86 years and 95% for those 16 to 30 years. The leading causes of death in patients with spinal cord injury were pneumonia, unintentional injuries, and suicide. Pneumonia was the leading cause of death among tetraplegics in individuals at least 55 years old. In paraplegics and persons younger than 55 years, unintentional injuries and suicides were the leading causes of death.

The prognosis for neurologic recovery is assessed by changes in the ASIA impairment scale grade and by a change in spinal cord level. Recovery of neurologic function depends on the nature and severity of the original injury, associated injuries, age, general health, emergency treatment, appropriate surgery, and complications. Knowledge of the site and severity of the injury and the degree of loss of neurologic function are critical in predicting the recovery of function. It is important to differentiate between neurologic recovery and functional recovery.

On review of a number of studies, certain observations become apparent:

1. Complete loss of cord function below the level of the injury is seen in the largest number of spinal cord injuries.
2. Patients with the most severe injuries have the worst prognosis for any neurologic recovery, as well as the longest hospital stays, the highest mortality, and the most complications.
3. The majority of patients with complete lesions do not show improvement from a functional point of view.

Any recovery after an apparent complete transection is rare. It may be the result of an inappropriate assessment at the time of injury. Incomplete lesions of the spinal cord (anterior, central, Brown-Séquard, and concussion of the spinal cord) carry a better prognosis in terms of return of function.

Recovery rates related to operative or nonoperative care indicate no significant difference in neurologic outcome between the two groups. Dolan and colleagues (1980) detected a decrease in mortality in the surgical group (6.1%) compared to nonsurgical patients (15.2%). The difference in mortality rates may indicate that nonsurgical patients were significantly sicker than operative patients. The value of surgical decompression immediately after injury was studied. Their analysis failed to find any correlation between the outcome and the amount of vertebral body displacement or timing of surgical intervention.

In summary, neurologic assessment within the first 24 to 48 hours after spinal cord injury offers the best method of predicting the eventual outcome. The initial assessment must be done in an alert, cooperative patient, without alcohol or drugs interfering with the assessment. In both complete and incomplete lesions, predictors for return of neurologic function are inconsistent. A serious sign is failure of return of any function within 48 hours of the accident.

TREATMENT

Treatment of the spinal-cord-injured patient encompasses five phases: (1) emergency treatment with attention to circulation, breathing, patent airway, appropriate immobilization of the spine, and transfer to a specialized center; (2) treatment of general medical problems (e.g., hypotension, hypoxia, poikilothermy, ileus); (3) spinal alignment; (4) surgical decompression of the spinal cord, if indicated; and (5) a well structured rehabilitation program.

Prehospital management is critical in preventing further complications. Treatment at the site cannot change the primary spinal cord injury, but it does have a significant effect on preventing secondary damage. Secondary injury of the spinal cord may result from hypotension, hypoxia, lack of immobilization of the spine, poor methods of extrication, inexact monitoring of the patient in transit to hospital, and inability to communicate with the physicians at the accepting trauma center.

Cervical traction must be delayed until adequate radiologic studies can be done.

At the trauma center, the ABC's are reviewed: airway, breathing, and circulation. In addition, D and E have been added, representing "disability" and "exposure." Disability refers to the assessment of neurologic status, and exposure indicates that removal of all clothing is necessary for a complete examination.

Clinical signs of shock require the insertion of an arterial line and a Swan-Ganz catheter. Meticulous attention must be paid to cardiac output and mean blood pressure to prevent the cardiopulmonary complications that frequently accompany cord injuries.

Because cord injury may result in loss of sympathetic tone with peripheral vasodilation, bradycardia, and hypotension, secondary ischemic damage may aggravate the spinal cord injury resulting from mechanical causes. Treatment of this potential hazard includes judicious administration of intravenous fluids to prevent fluid overload, alpha-agonists, and, occasionally, intravenous atropine sulfate to counter unopposed parasympathetic activity. Vasomotor paralysis may also cause loss of thermal control and lead to poikilothermy, which can usually be treated by the appropriate use of blankets.

Extrication of the patient from an automobile must be attempted only after the patient's head and back have been strapped in a neutral position on a firm base. There must be similar concern for head and neck stability in diving accidents. Rapid evacuation to a hospital is essential. It is estimated that 10% of patients suffer progressive cord or root damage between the time of diagnosis at the site of the accident and the beginning of appropriate treatment by trained personnel in the hospital.

In the acute phase, intermittent bladder catheterization must be instituted to prevent permanent bladder atony that may result from urinary retention. The insertion of a nasogastric tube will control abdominal distention, reducing the risk of secondary respiratory impairment.

In the acute phase and before imaging, methylprednisolone therapy is indicated. The National Acute Spinal Cord Injury Study demonstrated the benefit of high-dose methylprednisolone in reducing the severity of neurologic damage (Bracken and Holford, 1993). Methylprednisolone is thought to improve spinal cord function by inhibiting lipid peroxidase. Other pharmacologic agents being studied include a 21-aminosteroid, a synthetic nonglucocorticoid steroid that acts as an antioxidant. Gangliosides (acidic glycosphingolipids) are also being evaluated. These agents are thought to become part of the lipid bilayer of the plasma membrane and simulate formation of endogenous gangliosides. GM_1 gangliosides are started within 72 hours of injury and continued for 18 to 32 doses over 3 to 4 weeks. Combination therapy of methylprednisolone followed by gangliosides is being tested. Methylprednisolone is administered by bolus injection of 30 mg/kg followed by 5.4 mg/kg per hour for 23 hours. Benefit was found for both complete and incomplete lesions. Medical complications and mortality rates were unchanged. This treatment must be started within 8 hours of the injury.

With control of systemic functions, attention is directed toward correcting malalignment or instability of the vertebral column. In cervical fracture–dislocation, this is usually done by external skeletal traction (e.g., with Crutchfield tongs, Gardner-Wells tongs, or halo fixation). Thoracolumbar injuries do not lend themselves to external traction, and accordingly surgical stabilization is attempted with devices such as Harrington rods or Weiss springs.

Formerly, it was customary to operate on most patients with acute spinal cord injury to decompress the damaged cord. It has become apparent that surgery has little effect on the neurologic outcome. When cord compression is certain or the neurologic disorder progresses, benefit may be seen following immediate decompression (1 to 2 hours). (Comprehensive reviews of this controversial topic are given in the suggested readings.) There are no set rules for early or late surgical intervention. Clinical judgment and experience direct the appropriate surgical timing in each case.

Patients with spinal cord injury need the facilities of a special spinal care unit. After the acute treatment phase, specialized and continuing therapy is required. Mechanical devices for turning patients are unnecessary; when skilled nursing is available, regular hospital beds may be used. Frequent turning of patients and the use of pillows or pads prevent pressure sores. Antiembolic stockings reduce the incidence of venous thrombosis, and administration of low-dose heparin reduces the risk of pulmonary embolus. Intermittent catheterization of the bladder has replaced use of an indwelling catheter and suprapubic cystostomy. Rehabilitation therapy should be started as soon as possible.

COMPLICATIONS

Bladder

Restoration of a balanced bladder implies a balance between storage and evacuation of urine. A balanced bladder shows no outlet obstruction, a sterile urine, low residual volume (less than 100 mL), and low voiding pressures. Failure to attain this requires further urodynamic studies to determine whether the problem is an obstruction (i.e., bladder neck hypertrophy, prostatism, sphincter-detrusor dyssynergia) or a disturbance of storage (i.e., uninhibited bladder contractions, outflow incontinence, decreased outlet resistance). Intermittent catheterization (no-touch technique) is superior to the use of indwelling catheters in reducing complications and developing bladder training.

Urinary tract complications are the result of high residual urine volume and infection. Cystitis and pyelitis respond to antibiotics. Complications occurring months or years after injury include renal and bladder stones, hydronephrosis, pyonephrosis, bladder diverticula, and ureteral reflux. The incidence of these complications has been markedly reduced in the past few decades.

Bowel Training

For several weeks after acute spinal injury, laxatives and digital removal of feces are necessary. Glycerin suppositories are useful at this time. Stretching of the anus must be avoided. Subsequent training for regular defecation includes the use of laxatives on alternate days and the judicious use of glycerin suppositories, which are inserted approximately 20 minutes before the desired time of evacuation. The goal is a consistent schedule of bowel evacuation.

Pressure Sores

Decubitus ulcers develop in almost all patients with complete transection unless preventive measures are vigorously pursued. These ulcers develop wherever bony prominences are covered by skin; the sacrum, trochanters, heels, ischium, knees, and anterosuperior iliac spine are the most common sites. Preventive measures include eliminating pressure points by padding, frequent changing of patient position, and keeping the bed scrupulously clean. Sheepskin, alternating pressure mattresses, gel pads, and waterbeds are also commonly used for prevention. Mechanical aids (e.g., Foster or Stryker frame or Circolectric beds) are rarely necessary in well organized and well staffed nursing units.

Once pressure sores have developed, repeated changes of dressings, topical agents, and systemic antibiotics may be used, but these are not always successful. The most effective treatment is repositioning the patient so that pressure is continuously removed. Conservative therapy may be beneficial, but surgical debridement and early closure are usually required.

Nutritional Deficiency

Attention to general nutrition is paramount in the treatment of patients with spinal cord injury. Early loss of weight occurs in many patients because of anorexia. In addition, protein may be lost through bedsores. A diet high in protein, calories, and vitamins is advised. If the patient cannot eat sufficient quantities by mouth, parenteral hyperalimentation may be recommended. Anemia may be treated with iron and, when severe, by blood transfusion.

Muscle Spasms

Flexor or extensor spasms require treatment when they are painful, interfere with rehabilitation, or delay healing of bedsores. The aims are reduction in the number of painful and disabling flexor spasms and a decrease in muscle tone when it interferes with function, nursing care, or rehabilitation. The most useful drugs are dantrolene sodium (Dantrium), diazepam, and baclofen (Lioresal). Intrathecal administration of baclofen has become increasingly popular. It is most effective in relieving flexor spasms, may relieve other adverse effects of spasticity and hypertonia, and can be given safely with appropriate precautions. Physical therapy for leg spasticity includes longitudinal myelotomy and percutaneous radiofrequency rhizotomies of the lower lumbar and upper sacral roots. Obturator neurectomy in the pelvis, myotomy of the iliopsoas at the hip, lengthening of the hamstring at the knee, and percutaneous heel cord lengthening are peripheral methods that are safe but have not been carefully evaluated. Intrathecal injections of phenol or absolute alcohol should be used only by those experienced in the treatment of spinal cord injuries.

Sexual Function

Various forms of treatment are available for neurogenic erectile dysfunction. These include a vacuum device that fits over the penis and is kept in place by a constricting ring around the base of the penis; injection of vasoactive agents such as phentolamine mesylate (Regitine), papaverine, or prostaglandin E_1 into the corpora cavernosa; and use of an implantable prosthesis. Sildenafil (Viagra) has been reported to be useful in erectile dysfunction secondary to traumatic spinal cord disease.

Pain

Pain may affect anesthetic areas after complete transverse lesions. There may be sharp shooting pains in the distribution of one or more roots; burning pain may be poorly localized; or deep pain may be localized in the viscera. Treatment includes placebos, spinal anesthesia, posterior rhizotomy, sympathectomy, cordotomy, and posterior column tractotomy. None has been uniformly successful. Narcotic analgesic medication should be avoided, and analgesics generally should not routinely be prescribed. Transcutaneous electrical neurostimulation has been reported to be effective.

Rehabilitation

The ultimate aim for all patients with spinal cord injury is ambulation and economic independence. This can be accomplished in many patients who have injuries below the cervical area and is best done in a rehabilitation center with trained personnel and adequate equipment. Diligent cooperation of the patient with the physiatrist and the application of supportive braces are of major importance. When the arms are paralyzed, the therapeutic goal is more limited, but devices controlled by intact muscles and appropriate surgery may permit useful motion of paralyzed arms. Implantation of diaphragmatic stimulators has permitted survival of high-level-cervical-cord-injured patients.

The development of spinal cord units specializing in the care of tetraplegia and paraplegia is important. An increase in life expectancy, reduction in the frequency of complications, elevation of patient morale, and development of new techniques are some of the benefits.

Finally, the best mode of treatment must be prevention. Nationwide educational programs should be concerned with motor vehicle and water safety, speed limits should be lowered, and the use of seatbelts should be mandatory to reduce the incidence of these injuries.

SUGGESTED READINGS

Baskin DS. Spinal cord injury. In: Evans RW, ed. *Neurology and trauma.* Philadelphia: WB Saunders, 1996:276–299.

Bracken MB, Holford TR. Effects of timing of methylprednisolone or naloxone administration on recovery of segmental and long-tract neurological function in NASCIS 2. *J Neurosurg* 1993;79:500–507.

Bracken MB, Shepard MJ, Collins WF, et al. A randomized, controlled trial of methylprednisolone or naloxone in the treatment of acute spinal-cord injury: results of Second Naloxone Acute Spinal Cord Injury Study. *N Engl J Med* 1990;322:1405–1411.

Bracken MB, Shepard MJ, Collins WF, et al. Methylprednisolone or naloxone treatment after acute spinal cord injury: 1 year follow-up data: results of the Second National Acute Spinal Cord Injury Study. *J Neurosurg* 1992;76:23–31.

Bracken MB, Shepard MJ, Holford TR, et al. Administration of methylprednisolone for 24 or 48 hours or tirilazad mesylate for 48 hours in the treatment of acute spinal cord injury: results of the Third National Acute Spinal Cord Injury Randomized Controlled Trial. National Acute Spinal Cord Injury Study. *JAMA* 1997;277:1597–1604.

Burney RE, Maio RF, Maynard F, Karunas R. Incidence, characteristics, and outcome of spinal cord injury at trauma centers in North America. *Arch Surg* 1993;128:596–599.

Derry F. Sildenafil (Viagra): a double-blind, placebo controlled, single-dose, two-way crossover study in men with erectile dysfunction caused by traumatic spinal cord injury; American Urological Association 92nd annual meeting 1997, April 12–17. *J Urol* 1997;157[Suppl]:181(abst 702).

De Vivo MJ, Kartus PL, Rutt RD, Stover SL, Fine PR. The influence of age at time of spinal cord injury on rehabilitation outcome. *Arch Neurol* 1990;47:687–691.

De Vivo MJ, Kartus PL, Stover SL, Rutt RD, Fine PR. Seven-year survival following spinal cord injury. *Arch Neurol* 1987;44:872–875.

De Vivo MJ, Kartus PL, Stover SL, Rutt RD, Fine PR. Cause of death for patients with spinal cord injuries. *Arch Intern Med* 1989;149:1761–1766.

Dolan EJ, Tator CH, Endrenyi L. The value of decompression for acute experimental cord compression injury. *J Neurosurg* 1980;53:749–755.

Donovan WH. Rehabilitation treatment of complications of spinal cord injury. In: Evans RW, ed. *Neurology and trauma.* Philadelphia: WB Saunders, 1996:300–322.

Duh MS, Shephard MJ, Wilberger JE, Bracken MB. The effectiveness of surgery on the treatment of acute spinal cord injury and its relation to pharmacological treatment. *Neurosurgery* 1994;35:240–248; discussion 248–249.

Formal CS, Ditunno JF Jr. Rehabilitation of patients with traumatic spinal cord injury. In: Frymoyer JW, Ducker TB, Hadler NM, et al., eds. *The adult spine: principles and practice*, 2nd ed. Philadelphia: Lippincott–Raven Publishers, 1997;1:931–947.

Geisler FH. GM-1 ganglioside and motor recovery following human spinal cord injury. *J Emerg Med* 1993;11[Suppl 1]:49–55.

Geisler FH, Dorsey FC, Coleman WP. Recovery of motor function after spinal cord injury: a randomized, placebo-controlled trial with GM-1 ganglioside. *N Engl J Med* 1991;324:1829–1838. Erratum: *N Engl J Med* 1991;325:1659–1660.

Geisler WO, Jousse AT. Life expectancy following traumatic spinal cord injury. In: Vinken PJ, Bruyn GW, Klawans HL, Frankel HL, eds. *Spinal cord trauma. Handbook of clinical neurology, vol 61.* Amsterdam: Elsevier, 1992:499–513.

George ER, Scholten DJ, Buechler CM, et al. Failure of methylprednisolone to improve outcome of spinal cord injuries. *Am Surg* 1995;61:659–663; discussion 663–664.

Gerrelts BD, Petersen EU, Mabray J. Delayed diagnosis of cervical spine injuries. *J Trauma* 1991;31:1622–1626.

Kakulas BA, Taylor JR. Pathology of injuries of vertebral column and spinal cord. *Spinal cord trauma. Handbook of clinical neurology, vol 61.* Amsterdam: Elsevier, 1992:21–51.

Kraus JF, Franti CE, Riggins RS, Richards D, Borhani NO. Incidence of traumatic spinal cord lesions. *J Chronic Dis* 1975;28:471–492.

Lee TT, Arias JM, Andrus HL, et al. Progressive post-traumatic myelomalacic myelopathy: treatment with untethering and expansive duraplasty. *J Neurosurg* 1997;86:624–628.

Lewis KS, Mueller WM. Intrathecal baclofen for severe spasticity secondary to spinal cord injury. *Ann Pharmacother* 1993;27:767–774.

Maynard FM Jr, Bracken MB, Creasey G, et al. International standards for neurological and functional classification of spinal cord injury. American Spinal Injury Association. *Spinal Cord* 1997;35:266–274.

Piepmeier JM, Collins WF. Recovery of function following spinal cord injury. In: Vinken PJ, Bruyn GW, Klawans HL, Frankel HL, eds. *Spinal cord trauma. Handbook of clinical neurology, vol 61.* Amsterdam: Elsevier, 1992:421–433.

Smith EM, Bodner DR. Sexual dysfunction after spinal cord injury. *Urol Clin North Am* 1993;20:535–542.

Sonntag VKH, Francis PM. *Patient selection and timing of surgery in contemporary management of spinal cord injury.* Park Ridge, IL: AANS Publication Committee, 1995:97–107.

Stringer WA, Andersen BJ. Imaging after spine trauma. In: Evans RW, ed. *Neurology and trauma.* Philadelphia: WB Saunders, 1996;251–275.

Merritt's Neurology, 10th ed., edited by L.P. Rowland. Lippincott Williams & Wilkins, Philadelphia © 2000.

C H A P T E R
65

INTERVERTEBRAL DISCS AND RADICULOPATHY

PAUL C. MCCORMICK

Rupture of an intervertebral disc into the body of a vertebra was first described by Schmorl in 1927. Earlier, in a 1909 text on neurologic surgery, Krause described operating on an iceman who had been diagnosed by Oppenheimer as suffering from a lesion localized to L-4. Krause found an extradural mass that was described pathologically as a chondroma; the operation apparently effected a cure. There were other reports of "chondromas" removed at explorations of the intervertebral area. It remained for Mixter and Barr in 1934 to point out that these lesions were actually fragments of intervertebral discs and that they were responsible for sciatica.

PATHOGENESIS

Displaced disc material may create signs and symptoms by bulging or protruding beneath an attenuated annulus fibrosus, or the material may extrude through a tear in the annulus and project directly into the spinal canal. In either case, the encroaching disc material may irritate or compress nerve roots that are coursing to foramina of exit. In the cervical or thoracic regions, the problem is more complex neurologically because the spinal cord itself, as well as the adjacent nerve roots, may be involved. There, signs and symptoms are caused by either cord compression or a combination of cord and root compression. In the lumbar region, signs and symptoms relate to an individual root lesion (compressed laterally) or to compression of the cauda equina if the disc is large enough to crowd the entire spinal canal.

In the cervical region, the levels most commonly affected are in the C-5 to C-7 segments (Table 65.1). In the lumbar, area

most disc protrusions occur at L4-5 and L5-S1. This pattern suggests that the dynamics of pathologic change are partly related to the trauma of motion and wear and tear. Thoracic disc protrusion, except at the lower thoracic levels, differs from cervical and lumbar disorders in genesis and histopathology. Motion plays no role there because the thoracic vertebrae are designed for stability rather than motion, and the heavy rib cage contributes to the rigidity of this structure. One must therefore look elsewhere for the cause of thoracic disc rupture. On gross and microscopic examination, the lesion is unique, markedly degenerated, and characterized by gritty calcified deposits; it almost never has the consistency of cervical and lumbar ruptured discs; thoracic disc protrusion is more granular and yellowish.

Although trauma has been accepted as the prime cause of disc herniation, it is not the only cause. There seems to be a genetic predisposition in many patients. Trauma may aggravate this propensity and ultimately cause rupture. In the most florid preordained syndrome, there may be multiple levels of severe disc degeneration throughout the spine with progressive clinical involvement in different areas. This syndrome may explain why fusion often fails to prevent recurrent symptoms.

Spinal stenosis, which is an abnormally narrow spinal canal, is an example of an inherited anomaly, as are the spinal abnormalities of achondroplastic dwarfism. These abnormal spinal configurations, along with spondylosis, are major contributors to compression syndromes of the spinal cord and cauda equina. When disc protrusion occurs in a patient with spinal stenosis, it further compromises an already limited canal, as do changes caused by arthritic proliferation or ligamentous degeneration.

The signs and symptoms of herniated discs relate not only to the size and strategic location of the disc fragments but also to the size and configuration of the canal. The anteroposterior and lateral dimensions of the canal, particularly the foramina, play a key role. Spinal stenosis and osteoarthritic changes may compress roots, even with small protrusions. In a canal of normal dimensions, the severity of compression depends more on the site of rupture and the volume of the extruded material. There may be single-root compression or cauda equina compression. A laterally placed lesion in the cervical region may involve a single root, but if it is large enough, it may compress the cord. This is also true in the thoracic region. Although single-root syndromes in the lumbar region are usual, truly ventral or large lesions can

TABLE 65.1. COMMON ROOT SYNDROMES OF INTERVERTEBRAL DISC DISEASE

Disc space	L3-4	L4-5	L5-S1	C4-5	C5-6	C6-7	C7-T1
Root affected	L-4	L-5	S-1	C-5	C-6	C-7	C-8
Muscles affected	Quadriceps	Peroneals, anterior tibial, extensor hallucis longus	Gluteus maximus, gastrocnemius, plantar flexors of toes	Deltoid, biceps		Triceps, wrist extensors	Intrinsic hand muscles
Area of pain and sensory loss	Anterior thigh, medial shin	Great toe, dorsum of foot	Lateral foot, small toe	Shoulder, anterior arm, radial forearm		Thumb, middle fingers	Index, fourth, fifth fingers
Reflex affected	Knee jerk	Posterior tibial	Ankle jerk	Biceps		Triceps	Triceps
Straight leg raising	May not increase pain	Aggravates root pain	Aggravates root pain	—		—	—

lead to less easily recognized clinical pictures. For instance, scoliosis may be the major feature, with severe back pain and muscle splinting but without signs of mechanical root compression in the straight leg-raising test.

INCIDENCE

Rupture of an intervertebral disc is common, especially in the fourth to sixth decades of life. It is rare before age 25 years and uncommon after age 60. About 80% of patients are men. Many patients have a history of earlier trauma.

LUMBAR INTERVERTEBRAL DISC RUPTURE

Root syndromes of intervertebral disc disease are often episodic, so that remissions are characteristic. Pain may be aggravated by Valsalva maneuvers (coughing, sneezing, or straining at defecation). The pain may be restricted to the back or follow a radicular distribution in one or both legs. Lumbar pain may increase after heavy lifting or twisting of the spine. No matter how severe the pain is when the patient is erect, characteristically it is promptly relieved when the patient lies down. Some patients, however, are more comfortable sitting, and some can find no comfortable position. Relief of pain on bedrest is useful in diagnosing disc disease from intraspinal tumor, in which pain is often not relieved or may be worsened.

Examination reveals loss of lumbar lordosis or flattening of the lumbar spine, with splinting and asymmetric prominence of the long erector muscles. A list or tilt may be present, with one iliac crest elevated. This asymmetry is responsible for the commonly diagnosed "longer leg on one side" and the erroneous assignment of the back pain to asymmetry of leg length. (This asymmetry often causes a patient to raise the heel on the shoe of the "short" leg to level of the pelvis.) Range of motion of the lumbar spine is reduced by the protective splinting of paraspinal muscles, and attempted movement in some planes induces severe back pain. There may be tenderness of the adjacent vertebrae. When the patient is erect, one gluteal fold may hang down and show added skin creases because the gluteus is wasted, evidence of involvement of the S-1 root. Passive straight leg raising is reduced in range and increases back and leg pain. Muscle atrophy and weakness or sciatic tenderness and discomfort may occur on direct pressure at some point along the nerve from the sciatic notch to the calf. This is particularly true in older patients. Paresthesia in the realm of the involved root is common; fasciculation is rare.

The typical syndromes of root compression at lumbar levels are given in Table 65.2, although the signs may not be as distinct in actual practice as the table implies. More than 80% of syndromes affect L-5 or S-1 (Figs. 65.1 and 65.2). When the lesion affects L-4 or higher roots, straight leg raising does not stretch the roots above L-5. The affected roots may be tensed, however, by extension of the limb with the knee flexed when the patient is prone, thus reproducing the typical radicular spread of pain.

About 10% of lumbar disc herniations occur lateral to the spinal canal and root sleeve. Myelography is unrevealing in these

TABLE 65.2. SIGNS OF LUMBAR DISC HERNIATION IN 97 PATIENTS

Disc Space	L2-3	L3-4	L4-5	L5-S1
Patients (n)	1	9	45	42
Weak muscles				
Anterior tibial, extensor hallucis	0	3	13	3
Gastrocnemius, plantar responses of foot	0	0	2	3
Quadriceps	0	3	0	0
Reflex affected				
Knee jerk	1	6	4	0
Ankle jerk	0	1	12	23

Data from Hardy RW Jr, Plank NM. Clinical diagnosis of herniated lumbar disc. In: Hardy RW, ed. *Lumbar disc disease.* New York: Raven Press, 1982.

cases. These far lateral disc herniations compress the rostral lumbar nerve root at the affected level. A far lateral L3-4 lumbar disc herniation, for example, may compress the L-3 nerve root either within the foramen or more distally as the root passes over the disc space (Fig. 65.3). These herniations often affect higher lumbar (e.g., L3-4) levels and are likely to cause objective neurologic deficit. A far lateral disc herniation should be suspected with acute onset of an isolated upper lumbar radiculopathy, one that affects L-2, L-3, or L-4. Diagnosis of far lateral lumbar disc herniation is made by computed tomography (CT) or magnetic resonance imaging (MRI).

THORACIC INTERVERTEBRAL DISC RUPTURE

Because the thoracic spine is designed for rigidity rather than excursion, wear and tear from motion and stress cannot cause thoracic disc protrusion, and clinical disorders are rare. Thoracic disc disease may result from chronic vertebral changes incident to Scheuermann disease or juvenile osteochondritis with later trauma. The radiographic changes of Scheuermann disease, when seen with thoracic cord compression, should raise the possibility of disc protrusion (Fig. 65.4). Calcific changes in the intervertebral disc and the typical vertebral changes of that disease are diagnostic markers.

The small capacity of the thoracic canal makes clinical syndromes of cord compression more critical than at other levels. By the same token, decompressive operations are more precarious and require meticulous care to avoid damaging the spinal cord. The lower thoracic levels, however, are more capacious, and although the conus medullaris or cauda equina may be damaged by disc protrusions, surgical approaches are less hazardous than at higher levels.

CERVICAL DISC DISEASE

Cervical disc herniation may involve both the root and the spinal cord, depending on the volume of the canal and the size of the lesion. Cord compression is uncommon, except with spinal stenosis or massive rupture of a disc. The sites of the most fre-

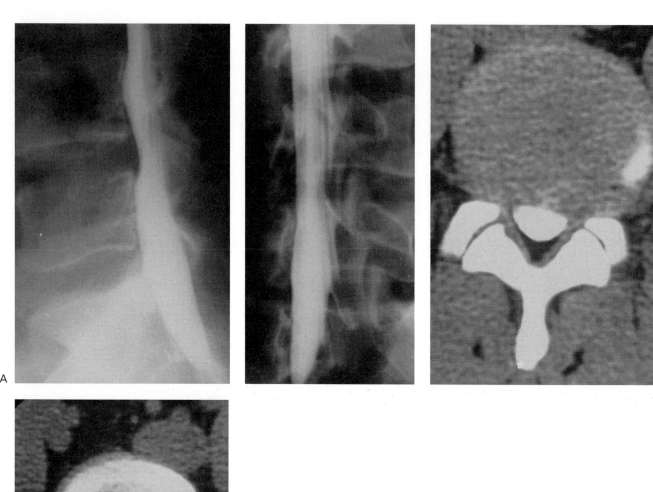

FIG. 65.1. Lumbar disc herniation. **A:** Lateral film from a lumbar myelogram demonstrates a large ventral defect at L4-5. The L5-S1 level is unremarkable. **B:** Left posterior oblique projection demonstrates swelling and amputation of the left L-5 root and possible compression of the left S-1 root with subtle thinning of the contrast. **C:** Postmyelogram axial CT at the L4-5 level confirms a large herniated nucleus pulposus obliterating the neural foramina bilaterally with eccentric deformity of the sac on the left. **D:** At the L5-S1 level, CT is more sensitive than myelography in diagnosing lateral disc herniation into the left foramen. Compare its appearance with that of the preserved lucent fat in the right foramen. Minimal deformity of the sac ventrally accounts for the unimpressive myelogram at this level. (Courtesy of Dr. J.A. Bello, Dr. T.L. Chi, and Dr. S.K. Hilal.)

quent disc herniations are C5-6 (Fig. 65.5) and C6-7; C4-5 and C7-T1 are less frequently affected, and other levels are rarely involved (Table 65.3). Because movement of the cervical spine is normally incremental, any process contributing to focal stress at individual levels adds to local wear and tear and to progressive pathologic changes in the disc and in joint mechanics. Development of a new fulcrum of motion above a fusion or congenital block vertebrae increases susceptibility to these changes.

The signs and symptoms of cervical disc disease usually begin with stiff neck, reactive splinting of the erector capital muscles,

and discomfort at the medial order of the scapula. Radicular paresthesia and pain supervene when the root is more severely compromised. These symptoms are worsened by movements of the head and neck and, often, by stretching of the dependent arm. For relief, the patient often adopts a position with the arm elevated and flexed behind the head, unlike the patient with shoulder disease who maintains the arm in a dependent position, avoiding elevation or abduction at the shoulder joint.

As compression proceeds, discrete root syndromes appear (see Tables 65.1 and 65.2). C-5 lesions cause pain in the shoulder

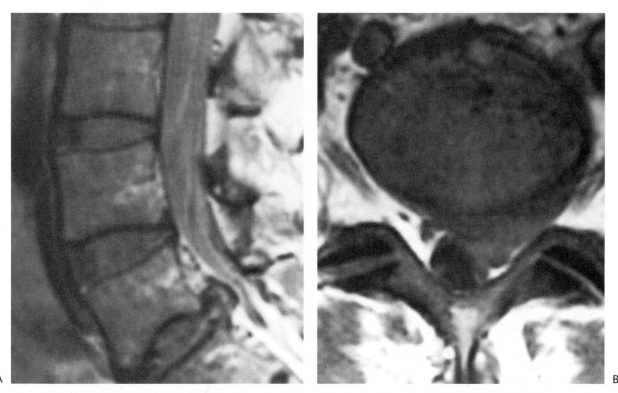

A   B

FIG. 65.2. Lumbosacral disc herniation. Sagittal proton-density **(A)** and axial T1-weighted **(B)** MRI demonstrate a large L5-S1 disc herniation on the left side. Clinically, this patient had an S-1 radiculopathy that did not respond to conservative therapy. Complete relief of symptoms followed lumbar discectomy.

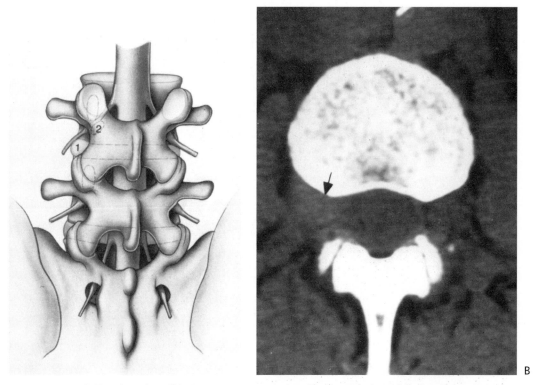

A   B

FIG. 65.3. **A:** Two sites of possible upper nerve root compression from a far lateral disc herniation. Root compression may occur at the level of the disc space *(1)* or from a rostrally migrated fragment into the foramen of the upper nerve root *(2)*. **B:** CT demonstrates a large far lateral disc herniation *(arrow)*.

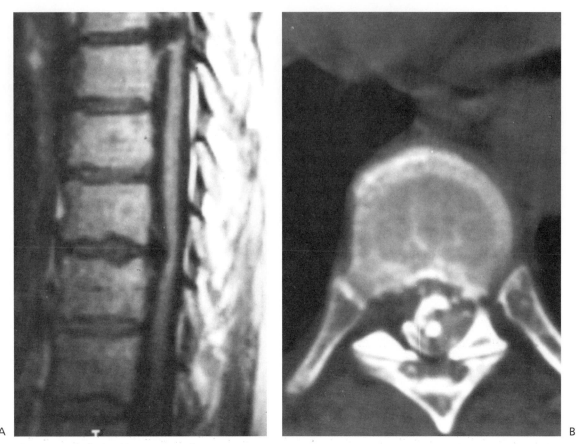

FIG. 65.4. A: Sagittal T1-weighted MRI demonstrates two large thoracic discs in a patient with a subacute myelopathy. **B:** Postmyelographic CT in the same patient demonstrates a large calcified thoracic disc at T-6 compressing the spinal cord.

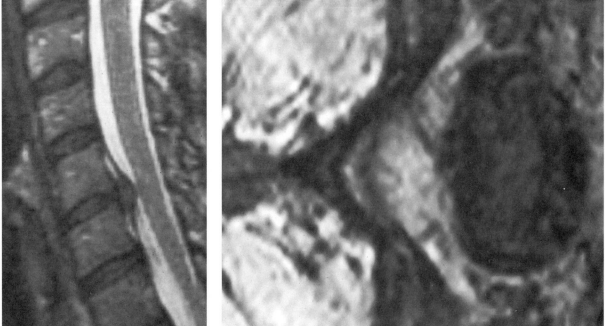

FIG. 65.5. A: Sagittal T2-weighted MRI shows C5-6 disc herniation. **B:** Axial MRI demonstrates foraminal disc herniation in a patient with radiculopathy.

TABLE 65.3. FREQUENCY OF COMPRESSION OF THE CERVICAL ROOTS BY RUPTURED INTERVERTEBRAL DISC

Root	%
C-5	2
C-6	19
C-7	69
C-8	10

Modified from Yoss et al., 1957.

and dermatomic sensory diminution with weakness and atrophy of the deltoid. C-6 lesions cause paresthesia of the thumb and depression of the biceps reflex with weakness and atrophy of that muscle. In C-7 lesions, paresthesia may involve the index and middle fingers, and even the thumb, with atrophy and weakness in the triceps muscles, wrist extensors, and pectoral muscles, as well as a parallel reflex depression. C-8 subserves important intrinsic muscle functions in the hand and sensation in the fourth and fifth fingers. Because these are important in discriminatory and fine finger maneuvers, C-8 damage can be disabling. Large disc protrusions, particularly with spinal stenosis, can cause clinical syndromes of cord compression.

Lesions such as supraspinatus tendinitis, arthritic changes in the acromioclavicular joint, and rotator cuff tears may be difficult to differentiate from cervical root compression, especially because prolonged pain and lack of range of motion lead to atrophy and frozen shoulder in these syndromes. C-8 and T1 lesions commonly cause a partial Horner syndrome. A diagnostic workup for syndromes of these levels must include apical lordotic views of the chest, and special care must be taken to rule out sulcus neoplasms or abnormal cervical ribs.

OTHER DIAGNOSTIC FEATURES

Because many disc syndromes are genetic, abnormal skeletal features throughout the spine should be sought on radiographs. These include spinal stenosis, spondylolisthesis, widespread disc disease, or Marfan syndrome. Acquired disorders, such as osteochondritis juvenilis, and metabolic states such as osteoporosis, may contribute to pathologic changes in the disc and adjacent joints, as do several forms of arthritis.

MRI is the imaging procedure of choice for the evaluation of disc disorders. MRI identifies spinal cord or root compression and also shows the degree of degenerative change within the disc. It clearly delineates both intra- and extradural structure and is the ideal screening procedure for the differential diagnosis of structural disorders affecting the spinal cord and nerve roots.

Myelography has largely been replaced by MRI in the evaluation of disc disease. However, myelography does allow scrutiny of the entire spinal canal and can identify dynamic changes of spinal canal size that may occur with standing and flexion or extension of the spine. Postmyelography CT is useful as an adjunct to MRI if equivocal or multilevel disc disease is present; it is particularly useful in evaluating foraminal nerve root compression.

Electromyography and evoked potentials studies can be helpful in localizing root involvement but are not essential. The cerebrospinal fluid protein level is only rarely higher than 100 mg/dL; higher values are more characteristic of tumors.

Disc syndromes can be duplicated by tumors (primary or metastatic), infections (e.g., epidural abscess), and arachnoiditis. Epidural lipomatosis, a rare cause of low-back syndromes, is a complication of steroid therapy.

TREATMENT

Conservative treatment should continue as long as the patient shows improvement. Most acute attacks subside spontaneously, with analgesics and bedrest for lumbar disc disorders and immobilization of the neck by a collar for cervical disc disorders. Surgery for a lumbar disc disorder is indicated when there is no improvement over a reasonable period of strict bedrest or when a severe neurologic disorder is found on examination.

Discectomy of a herniated lumbar disc fragment almost always results in long-term satisfactory relief of symptoms. Lumbar fusion is rarely required for treatment of radiculopathy from a herniated lumbar disc.

Excessively prolonged physiotherapy and bedrest may cause emotional exhaustion, muscle loss, or drug dependence. Use of chymopapain (Chymodiactin) or collagenase to digest the disc material is controversial.

Cord compression requires consideration of decompressive measures as soon as it is recognized. Root syndromes of the cervical spine can be separated into those that require careful supervision and early operation and those that tolerate and may respond to conservative care. The muscles served by C-5 may rapidly atrophy, leaving abduction paresis, poor prognosis for restoration of function, and a painful frozen shoulder. C-8 is also vulnerable, and unrelieved compression may lead to irreversible atrophy with complex shoulder-arm-hand disorders that include circulatory and sweating abnormalities.

C-6 and C-7 subserve large muscles and tolerate pressure more benignly, even for long periods, and with good functional return. Cervical root syndromes are less likely to recur than lumbar disorders, and conservative therapy is worthwhile within the outlines described.

Removal of a cervical herniated disc may be performed through either a posterior laminotomy or an anterior approach. Excellent results may be anticipated in appropriately selected patients. Success in disc surgery also includes adequate evaluation of psychologic patterns and motivation.

SUGGESTED READINGS

Awwad EE, Martin DS, Smith KR Jr, Baker BK. Asymptomatic versus symptomatic herniated thoracic discs: frequency and characteristics as detected by computed tomography after myelography. *Neurosurgery* 1991;28:180–186.

Borenstein D. Epidemiology, etiology, diagnostic evaluation, and treatment of low back pain. *Curr Opin Rheumatol* 1992;4:226–232.

Cavanagh S, Stevens J, Johnson JR. High-resolution MRI in the investigation of recurrent pain after lumbar discectomy. *J Bone Joint Surg Br* 1993;75:524–528.

Charlesworth CH, Savy LE, Stevens J, et al. MRI demonstration of arachnoiditis in cauda equina syndrome of ankylosing spondylitis. *Neuroradiology* 1996;38:462–465.

Conforti R, Scuotto A, Muras I, et al. Herniated disk in adolescents. *J Neuroradiol* 1993;20:60–69.

Deyo RA. Conservative therapy for low back pain: distinguishing useful from useless therapy. *JAMA* 1983;250:1057–1062.

Deyo RA, Cherkin DC, Loeser JD, et al. Morbidity and mortality in association with operations on the lumbar spine. *J Bone Joint Surg Am* 1992;74:536–543.

Esses SI, Morley TP. Spinal arachnoiditis. *Can J Neurol Sci* 1983;10:2–10.

Fessler RG, Johnson DL, Brown FD, et al. Epidural lipomatosis in steroid-treated patients. *Spine* 1992;17:183–188.

Fiirgaard B, Marsden FH. Spinal epidural lipomatosis: case report and review of the literature. *Scand J Med Sci Sports* 1997;7:354–357.

Francavilla TL, Powers A, Dina T, Rizzoli HV. Case report: MR imaging of thoracic disk herniations. *J Comput Assist Tomogr* 1987;2:1062–1065.

Hansen FR, Bendix T, Skov P, et al. Intensive, dynamic back muscle exercises, conventional physiotherapy, or placebo-control treatment of low back pain: a randomized, observer-blind trial. *Spine* 1993;18:98–108.

Hardy RW Jr, ed. *Lumbar disc disease.* New York: Raven Press, 1982.

Koenigsberg RA, Klahr J, Zito JL, et al. Magnetic resonance imaging of cauda equina syndrome in ankylosing spondylitis: a case report. *J Neuroimaging* 1995;5:46–48.

Maroon JC, Kupitnik TA, Schulhuf LA. Diagnosis and microsurgical approach to far lateral disc herniations in the lumbar spine. *J Neurosurg* 1990;72:378–382.

Martin DS, Awwad EE, Pittman T, et al. Current imaging concepts of thoracic intervertebral disks. *Crit Rev Diagn Imaging* 1992;33:109–181.

Milamed DR, Warfield CA, Hedley-Whyte J, Mosteller F. Laminectomy and the treatment of lower back pain in Massachusetts. *Int J Technol Assess Health Care* 1993;9:426–439.

Mixter WJ, Barr JS. Rupture of the intervertebral disc with involvement of the spinal canal. *N Engl J Med* 1934;211:210.

Mohanty S, Sutter B, Mokry M, Ascher PW. Herniation of calcified cervical intervertebral disk in children. *Surg Neurol* 1992;38:407–410.

Noel P, Pepersack T, Vanbinst A, Alle JL. Spinal epidural lipomatosis in Cushing's syndrome secondary to an adrenal tumor. *Neurology* 1992;42:1250–1251.

Onel D, Sari H, Donmez C. Lumbar spinal stenosis: clinical/radiologic therapeutic evaluation in 145 patients: conservative treatment or surgical intervention? *Spine* 1993;18:291–298.

Pyeritz RE, Sack GH Jr, Udvarhelyi GB. Thoracolumbosacral laminectomy in achondroplasia: long-term results in 22 patients. *Am J Med Genet* 1987;28:433–444.

Robertson SC, Traynelis VC, Follett KA, et al. Idiopathic spinal epidural lipomatosis. *Neurosurgery* 1997;41:68–74.

Ross JS, Ruggieri P, Tkach J, et al. Lumbar degenerative disk disease: prospective comparison of conventional T2-weighted spin-echo imaging and T2-weighted rapid acquisition relaxation-enhanced imaging. *AJNR* 1993;14:1215–1223.

Shapiro S. Cauda equina syndrome secondary to lumbar disc herniation. *Neurosurgery* 1993;332:743–747.

Shaw MDM, Russell JA, Grossart KW. Changing pattern of spinal arachnoiditis. *J Neurol Neurosurg Psychiatry* 1978;41:97–107.

Thornbury JR, Fryback DG, Turski PA, et al. Disk-caused nerve compression in patients with acute low-back pain: diagnosis with MR, CT myelography, and plain CT. *Radiology* 1993;186:731–738.

Turner JA, Ersek M, Hernon L, et al. Patient outcomes after lumbar spinal fusions. *JAMA* 1992;268:907–911.

Yoss RE, Corbin KB, MacCarty CS, Love JG. Significance of symptoms and signs in localization of involved root in cervical disc protrusion. *Neurology* 1957;7:673–683.

Merritt's Neurology, 10th ed., edited by L.P. Rowland. Lippincott Williams & Wilkins, Philadelphia © 2000.

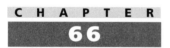

CHAPTER 66

CERVICAL SPONDYLOTIC MYELOPATHY

LEWIS P. ROWLAND
PAUL C. MCCORMICK

Cervical spondylosis is a condition in which progressive degeneration of the intervertebral discs leads to proliferative changes of surrounding structures, especially the bones, meninges, and supporting tissues of the spine. Damage to the spinal cord can be demonstrated at autopsy. The myelopathy is attributed to one or more of three possible mechanisms: (1) direct compression of the spinal cord by bony or fibrocalcific tissues, (2) ischemia caused by compromise of the vascular supply to the cord, and (3) repeated trauma in the course of normal flexion and extension of the neck. It is difficult, however, to be precise in identifying this type of myelopathy in living patients. The very concept may be one of the persistent myths of clinical neurology, and the situation begs for critical review.

INCIDENCE

Radiographic evidence of cervical spondylosis increases with each decade of life. It is seen in 5% to 10% of people between 20 and 30 years of age and increases to more than 50% by 45 years and to more than 90% after age 60 years. Signs of cervical myelopathy of unknown cause appear in only a few patients. Victims of myelopathy do not usually have a history of repeated single-root syndromes; that is, radiculopathy caused by cervical disc herniation and myelopathy seem to be distinct syndromes affecting different populations.

PATHOLOGY

The water content of the intervertebral disc and annulus fibrosus declines progressively with advancing age. Concomitantly, there are degenerative changes in the disc. The intervertebral space narrows and may be obliterated, and the annulus fibrosus protrudes into the spinal canal. Osteophytes form at the margins of the vertebral body, converge on the protruded annulus, and may convert it into a bony ridge or bar. The bar may extend laterally into the intervertebral foramen; there is also fibrosis of the dural sleeves of the nerve roots. All these changes narrow the canal, a process that may be aggravated by fibrosis and hypertrophy of the ligamenta flava. The likelihood of cord compression or vascular compromise increases in direct relation to the decrease in the original diameter of the spinal canal.

Spondylotic bars may leave deep indentations (visible at autopsy) on the ventral surface of the spinal cord. At the level of the lesion (there may be several levels), there is degeneration of the gray matter, sometimes with necrosis and cavitation. Above the compression, there is degeneration of the posterior columns; below the compression corticospinal tracts are demyelinated.

Dense ossification of the posterior longitudinal ligament is a variant of cervical spondylosis that may also cause progressive myelopathy. The condition may be focal or diffuse and seems to be most common in Asians.

One theory of pathogenesis holds that the cord is damaged by tensile stresses transmitted from the dura via the dentate ligaments. The spondylotic bar increases dentate tension by displacing the cord dorsally while the ligaments are anchored.

SYMPTOMS AND SIGNS

Neck pain may be prominent. Root pain is uncommon, but paresthesias may indicate the most affected root. The most common symptom is spastic gait disorder (Table 66.1). Weakness and wasting of the hands may be seen. Fasciculations may also be noted. Urinary sphincter symptoms occur in a minority of patients. Overt sensory loss is uncommon, but the diagnosis is facilitated if there is a sensory level or if there is sensory loss that occurs in the distribution of a cervical dermatome. The course of the

TABLE 66.1. CLINICAL MANIFESTATIONS OF CERVICAL SPONDYLOTIC MYELOPATHY

Symptom or sign	% of patients
Reflexes	
Hyperreflexia	87
Babinski sign	51
Hoffmann sign	13
Spastic gait disorder	49
Bladder symptoms	49
Sensation	
Vague sensory level	41
Proprioceptive sensory loss	39
Cervical dermatome sensory loss	33
Motor functions	
Arm weakness	31
Paraparesis	21
Hemiparesis	18
Quadriparesis	10
Brown-Séquard syndrome	18
Hand atrophy	13
Fasciculation	13
Pain	
Radicular arm	41
Radicular leg	13
Neck	8

Data from Lunsford et al., 1980.

disorder is slowly progressive, but the natural history is not well delineated. Study of patients who were not treated surgically indicates that the condition may become arrested or even improve spontaneously. In one report, 39 of 45 patients were unchanged or better without surgery many years after the original diagnosis.

LABORATORY DATA

Formerly, the most important diagnostic tests were plain radiographs of the cervical spine and myelography. Plain radiographs show narrowing of the disc spaces and the presence of osteophytes, especially at C5-6 and C6-7. Posterior osteophytes tend to be smaller than anterior projections and may not be seen without tomography. The disc bodies may be normal or show sclerosis. Changes in the zygapophyseal joints account for the designation "osteoarthritis" and may encroach on the intervertebral foramen; the changes may cause subluxation of the articular surfaces or compression of vertebral arteries.

Computed tomography (CT) has supplanted plain radiographic examination because it can show evidence of disc degeneration and protrusion of bars into the spinal canal. Combining CT with intrathecal injection of water-soluble contrast agents (*CT–iohexol myelography*) shows where and how severely the spinal cord is compressed and distorted. Spinal cord "atrophy" has become a new diagnosis.

Myelography in patients with spinal cord compression is associated with a slight risk that the existing myelopathy may worsen and become permanent. Magnetic resonance imaging (MRI) is therefore the procedure of choice; it is noninvasive and provides exquisite resolution of spinal cord structures (Figs. 66.1 and 66.2). MRI allows evaluation of spondylosis and the alternative possibilities: Chiari malformation, arteriovenous malfor-

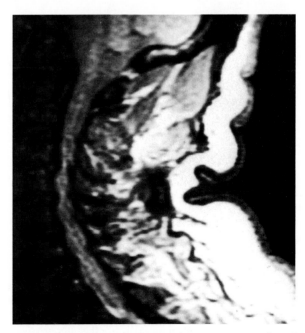

FIG. 66.1. Sagittal proton-density MRI demonstrates extensive spinal cord compression caused by a combination of ventral bone spurs and preexisting (congenital) canal stenosis.

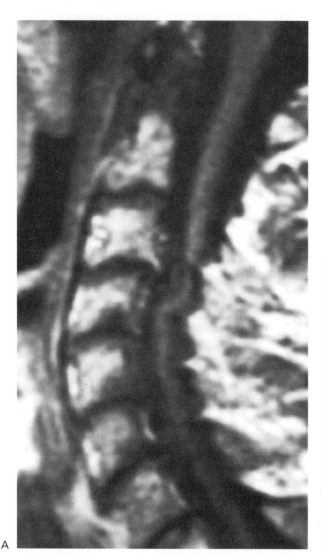

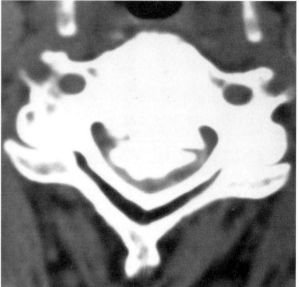

FIG. 66.2. A: Sagittal T1-weighted MRI shows focal spinal cord compression from a single osteophyte at the C3-4 level. This dense calcification is typical of segmental ossification of the posterior longitudinal ligament. **B:** Axial CT scan in same patient.

mation, extramedullary tumor, syringomyelia, or multiple sclerosis (MS). In time, the technical advances in MRI may make myelography obsolete.

Somatosensory evoked responses have been used to aid in diagnosis but are not crucial. The cerebrospinal fluid (CSF) is usually normal or has a protein concentration of 50 to 100 mg/dL. Higher protein levels or CSF pleocytosis should raise the question of MS or tumor, including meningeal carcinomatosis. The role of transcranial magnetic stimulation in diagnosis remains to be ascertained.

DIFFERENTIAL DIAGNOSIS

There are two types of problems in the differential diagnosis. In one group, there is compression of the cervical spinal cord, but not by spondylosis (or at least not by spondylosis alone). Cervical spinal tumors are the best example of this category of problem. Such lesions are revealed by MRI. In other compressive lesions, the primary bony changes are congenital (anomalies of the

craniocervical junction) or acquired (rheumatoid arthritis or basilar impression) and may be further complicated by spondylosis. These disorders are recognized by CT or MRI. Arteriovenous malformations may also be found.

Another group of myelopathies presents more of a diagnostic problem. Cervical spondylosis is so common in the general population that it may be present by chance and harmless in a person with another disease of the spinal cord. The ultimate test of the pathogenic significance of spondylosis would be complete relief of symptoms after decompressive surgery, but this is rarely seen. Among the other diseases that can cause clinical syndromes similar to those attributed to spondylosis are MS, amyotrophic lateral sclerosis (ALS), neurosyphilis, and possibly subacute combined system disease. In 12% of patients diagnosed with spondylotic myelopathy, some other diagnosis was ultimately made.

MS is probably the most common cause of spastic paraplegia in middle life and is probably the actual cause of the disorder in some people who have had cervical laminectomies. Therefore, before laminectomy it is imperative to test for MS by use of visual, somatosensory, and brainstem evoked responses; CSF gamma globulin and oligoclonal bands; and MRI examination of the cerebral white matter, foramen magnum, brainstem, and cervical spinal cord. Proper use and interpretation of the test results often remove diagnostic uncertainty.

ALS must be considered whenever wasting and fasciculations are seen in arm and hand muscles, and especially when there are fasciculations in the legs. The presence of overt fasciculation makes it unlikely that spondylotic myelopathy is the cause of symptoms; in such cases caution is warranted when laminectomy is being considered. There is no diagnostic test for ALS, however, and the distinction may be difficult.

Rare causes of spastic paraplegia in middle life are tropical myelopathy caused by human T-cell lymphotropic virus type I and adult-onset adrenoleukodystrophy. The diagnosis of exclusion, when no other cause is identified, is primary lateral sclerosis, which is almost as common a diagnosis as MS.

In northern England, a prospective survey of 585 patients with nontraumatic spastic paraparesis gave the following order of frequency of diagnosis: cervical spondylotic myelopathy, 24%; tumor, 16%; MS, 18%; diagnosis uncertain, 19%; and ALS, 4%. The absence of primary lateral sclerosis from this list suggests regional differences in making a diagnosis. Of course, the problem is ascertaining the diagnosis of spondylotic myelopathy.

An old adage: Be wary of the diagnosis of cervical spondylotic myelopathy if there is no sensory loss.

TREATMENT

The natural history of cervical spondylotic myelopathy varies greatly and is unpredictable in individual patients. Moreover, no controlled trials of surgical therapy have been undertaken, and several different operations have been advocated. Therefore, uniform recommendations for treatment have been difficult to establish. Decompressive operations include posterior laminectomy, anterior discectomy, or vertebrectomy; these procedures are widely used but are associated with a high failure rate. Although contemporary surgical series report a 70% to 80% rate of improvement, only about 50% of patients show satisfactory functional improvement or complete reversal of symptoms that is maintained for a long time. The efficacy of surgical decompression seems to have been established in these improved patients. The others show little or no improvement, and their condition may even become worse as a result of surgery. Sometimes, symptoms return and progress after immediate postoperative improvement.

Sooner or later, an attempt will be made to standardize the collection of data to evaluate the outcome of these operations, and there might even be a therapeutic trial. Surgeons still contend that a controlled trial is neither feasible nor necessary. However, one randomized trial of corpectomy for single-level disc disease found that fusion added nothing to decompression alone. Commenting on the trial, orthopedist Jeremy Fairbank noted all the problems to be faced but nevertheless reaffirmed the need to document the advantages of surgery over nonsurgical management.

In the absence of clear guidelines, management is tailored to the specific circumstances of individual patients and to the experiences of the treating physicians and surgeons. Conservative treatment with physical therapy for gait training and with neck immobilization with a firm collar is appropriate for patients with mild myelopathy. Surgery should be considered if the myelopathy progresses despite conservative treatment.

SUGGESTED READINGS

Adams CBT, Logue V. Movement and contour of spine in relation to neural complications of cervical spondylosis. *Brain* 1971;94:569–586.

Adams CBT, Logue V. Some functional effects of operations for cervical spondylotic myelopathy. *Brain* 1971;94:587–594.

Arlien-Soborg P, Kjaer L, Praestholm J. Myelography, CT, and MRI of the spinal canal in patients with myelopathy: a prospective study. *Acta Neurol Scand* 1993;87:95–102.

Barnes MP, Saunders M. The effect of cervical mobility on the natural history of cervical spondylotic myelopathy. *J Neurol Neurosurg Psychiatry* 1984;47:17–20.

Bednarik J, Kadanka Z, Vohanka S, et al. The value of somatosensory and motor evoked potentials in spondylotic cervical cord compression. *Eur Spine J* 1998;493–500.

Braakman R. Management of cervical spondylotic myelopathy and radiculopathy. *J Neurol Neurosurg Psychiatry* 1994;57:257–263.

Caruso PA, Patel MR, Joseph J, Rachlin J. Primary intramedullary lymphoma of the spinal cord mimicking cervical spondylotic myelopathy. *AJR* 1998;171:526–527.

Cooper PR, ed. *Degenerative diseases of the cervical spine.* Park Ridge, IL: AANS Publications, 1993.

Crockard HA, Heilman AE, Stevens JM. Progressive myelopathy secondary to odontoid fractures: clinical, radiological and surgical features. *J Neurosurg* 1993;78:579–586.

Ebara S, Yonenobu K, Fujiwara K, et al. Myelopathy hand characterized by muscle wasting: a different type of myelopathy hand in patients with cervical spondylosis. *Spine* 1988;13:785–791.

Emery SE, Bohlman HH, Bolesta MJ, Jones PK. Anterior cervical decompression and arthrodesis for the treatment of cervical spondylotic myelopathy. Two- to seventeen-year follow-up. *J Bone Joint Surg Am* 1998;80:941–951.

Fessler RG, Steck JC, Giovanni MA. Anterior cervical corpectomy for cervical spondylotic myelopathy. *Neurosurgery* 1998;43:257–265.

Hirose G, Kadoya S. Cervical spondylotic radiculo-myelopathy in patients with athetoid-dystonic cerebral palsy: clinical evaluation and surgical treatment. *J Neurol Neurosurg Psychiatry* 1984;47:775–780.

Kardon D. Cervical spondylotic myelopathy with reversible fasciculations in the lower extremities. *Arch Neurol* 1977;34:774–776.

Lees F, Turner JWA. Natural history and prognosis of cervical spondylosis. *BMJ* 1963;2:1607–1610.

Levine DN. Pathogenesis of cervical spondylotic myelopathy. *J Neurol Neurosurg Psychiatry* 1997;62:334–340.

Lunsford LD, Bissonette DJ, Zorub DS. Anterior surgery for cervical disc disease. Part 2: treatment of cervical spondylotic myelopathy in 32 cases. *J Neurosurg* 1980;53:12–19.

Moore AP, Blumhardt LD. A prospective survey of the causes of non-traumatic spastic paraparesis and tetraparesis in 585 patients. *Spinal Cord* 1997;5:361–367.

Nakamura K, Kurokawa T, Hoshino Y, et al. Conservative treatment for cervical spondylotic myelopathy: achievement and sustainability of a level of "no disability". *J Spinal Disord* 1998;11:175–179.

Nurick S. The pathogenesis of the spinal cord disorder associated with cervical spondylosis. *Brain* 1972;95:87–100.

Nurick S. The natural history and results of surgical treatment of the spinal cord disorder associated with cervical spondylosis. *Brain* 1972;95:101–108.

Olive PM, Whitecloud TS 3rd, Bennett JT. Lower cervical spondylosis and myelopathy in adults with Down's syndrome. *Spine* 1988;13:781–784.

Restuccia D, DiLazzaro V, Valeriani M, et al. Segmental dysfunction of the cervical cord revealed by abnormalities of the spinal N13 potential in cervical spondylotic myelopathy. *Neurology* 1992;42:1054–1063.

Rowland LP. Surgical treatment of cervical spondylotic myelopathy: time for a controlled trial. *Neurology* 1992;42:5–13.

Saunders RL, Bernini PM, eds. *Cervical spondylotic myelopathy.* Oxford: Blackwell Science, 1992.

Saunders RL, Bernini PM, Shirreffs TG, Reeves AG. Central corpectomy for cervical spondylotic myelopathy: a consecutive series with long-term follow-up evaluation. *J Neurosurg* 1991;74:163–170.

Tavy DLJ, Wagner GL, Keunen RWM, et al. Transcranial magnetic stimulation in patients with cervical spondylotic myelopathy: clinical and radiological correlations. *Muscle Nerve* 1994;17:235–241.

Wilkinson H, ed. *Cervical spondylosis: its early diagnosis and treatment.* Philadelphia: WB Saunders, 1971.

Yu YL, Moseley IF. Syringomyelia and cervical spondylosis: a clinicoradiological investigation. *Neuroradiology* 1987;29:143–151.

Merritt's Neurology, 10th ed., edited by L.P. Rowland. Lippincott Williams & Wilkins, Philadelphia © 2000.

C H A P T E R
67

LUMBAR SPONDYLOSIS

LEWIS P. ROWLAND
PAUL C. McCORMICK

The same pathologic changes that define cervical spondylosis may affect the lower spine. Here, however, the roots of the cauda equina are affected rather than the spinal cord. The spinal cord becomes narrow because of age-related degenerative changes that affect the vertebral column articulations, including disc bulging and spur formation, facet joint enlargement, and hypertrophy of the ligamenta flava and facet capsule. Encroachment is usually maximal at the disc spaces. *Spinal stenosis* is the term for this narrowing. Congenital stenosis makes a person more vulnerable to these changes.

The stenosis caused by spondylosis may be diffuse, but it is usually confined to one or two lumbar levels. Isolated L4-5 disorder with unilateral or bilateral L-5 radiculopathy is the most common syndrome (Fig. 67.1). The L3-4 segment is less often affected either alone or in combination with L4-5 stenosis. Disorders at other levels are rare.

The resulting syndrome differs from acute herniation in many respects. Most patients are older than 40 years, and many are older than 60. Progression of symptoms is likely to be gradual rather than acute. Twisting of the back, lifting, or falling are precipitating factors in fewer than one-third of cases, and back pain is not the dominant symptom but may be reported by more than 50% of patients. Leg pain, when present, is as often bilateral as unilateral. Weakness of the legs and urinary incontinence are symptoms in a minority of patients, but many show weakness of isolated muscles and loss of reflexes on examination. Straight leg raising is limited in a few patients.

The characteristic symptom is *pseudoclaudication,* seen in almost all patients, and is defined as unilateral or bilateral discomfort in buttock, thigh, or leg on standing or walking that is relieved by rest. Patients use the words "pain," "numbness," or "weakness" to describe the discomfort, but there is often no objective sensory loss or focal muscle weakness. The discomfort is relieved by lying down, sitting, or flexing at the waist. Sometimes, pain persists in recumbency until the spine is flexed. Unlike vascular claudication, the pain persists if the patient stops walking without flexing the spine, and sometimes the discomfort is brought on by prolonged standing without walking.

The pathogenesis of pseudoclaudication is uncertain. Sometimes, myelography shows that hyperextension of the spine increases the protrusion of intervertebral discs, with relief of nerve root compression in flexed postures. In addition, blood flow to the lumbar spinal cord may increase when leg muscles are exercised. As a result, vessels on nerve roots dilate, but are then confined by the bony changes and thus compress the nerve roots. This is relieved by cessation of activity.

The diagnosis is made from the characteristic history, clinical findings, and radiography. Formerly, the syndrome was defined by changes in plain spine radiographs and by evidence of partial or complete subarachnoid block found by contrast myelography. Diagnosis was facilitated by the advent of computed tomography (CT), alone or with intrathecal contrast agents (see Fig. 67.1). Now, however, magnetic resonance imaging alone usually suffices to show the specific patterns and extent of compression. Electromyography can reveal that denervation is restricted to muscles innervated by lumbosacral roots. The cerebrospinal fluid protein level may be normal if the tap is performed above the level of the block, but values greater than 100 mg/dL may be found if there are multiple blocks.

The differential diagnosis includes intermittent claudication caused by peripheral arterial occlusive disease, which is recognized by the loss of pulses and characteristic trophic changes in the skin of the feet. Aortoiliac occlusive disease may spare peripheral pulses, but the femoral pulse is usually affected; it may cause claudication and wasting of leg muscles but does not cause postural claudication. The pain of aortoiliac disease is localized to exercising muscles. The radicular pattern of spinal claudication is not seen. The pain of aortoiliac disease persists as long as exercise is continued, regardless of body position. Vascular sonography may be in order.

Osteoarthritis of the hip joint may also cause activity-induced leg pain that is relieved by rest. The pain originates in the hip and usually radiates into the groin or anterior thigh, but does not extend below the knee. Pain and limitation of hip rotation are the usual findings. The diagnosis is confirmed radiographically.

The treatment of lumbar stenosis varies according to the severity of the symptoms. Mild symptoms often respond to nonsteroidal antiinflammatory drugs and physical therapy. The symptoms of lumbar stenosis may be episodic; even severe pain

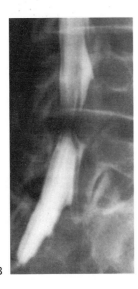 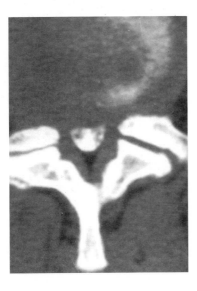

A, B

FIG. 67.1. A: Lumbar myelogram demonstrates focal high-grade stenosis at L4-5. **B:** Postmyelographic CT at the L4-5 interspace demonstrates circumferential stenosis caused by disc bulging, enlarged facets, and hypertrophy of the ligamenta flava.

should be treated conservatively because a prolonged remission may ensue. Surgical treatment consists of decompressive laminectomy with medial facetectomy and resection of the ligamenta flava at the stenosed levels. Epidural injection of steroids does not relieve the pain of spinal claudication.

Surgery is reserved for patients who have pain and claudication severe enough to affect the quality of life and who do not respond to conservative therapy. Surgery is usually well tolerated and is highly effective; about two-thirds of the patients report considerable improvement that is sustained for years after surgery. In one study, the following features indicated a favorable prognosis for patients with weak legs: disc herniation, stenosis at one level, duration of leg weakness of less than 6 weeks, and age younger than 65. In another study, the radiographic severity of stenosis was the best predictor of long-term outcome regardless of therapy, surgical or nonsurgical. There have been no controlled trials of surgical treatment.

SUGGESTED READINGS

Bischoff RJ, Rodriguez RP, Gupta K, et al. Comparison of CT, MRI and myelography in the diagnosis of herniated nucleus pulposus and spinal stenosis. *J Spinal Disord* 1993;6:289–295.

Caputy AJ, Lessenhup AJ. Long-term evaluation of decompressive surgery for degenerative lumbar stenosis. *J Neurosurg* 1992;77:669–678.

DeVilliers JC. Combined neurogenic and vascular claudication. *S Afr Med J* 1980;57:650–654.

Epstein NE, Maldonado VC, Cusick JF. Symptomatic lumbar spinal stenosis. *Surg Neurol* 1998;50:3–10.

Fukusaki M, Kobayashi I, Hara T, Sumikawa K. Symptoms of spinal stenosis do not improve after epidural steroid injection. *Clin J Pain* 1998; 14:148–151.

Giugui P, Benoist M, Delecourt C, Delhoume J, Deburge A. Motor deficit in lumbar spinal stenosis: a retrospective study of a series of 50 patients. *J Spinal Disorder* 1998;11:283–288.

Hall S, Bartelson JD, Onofrio BM, et al. Lumbar spinal stenosis: clinical features, diagnostic procedures, and results of surgical treatment in 68 patients. *Ann Intern Med* 1985;103:271–275.

Hurri H, Slatis P, Soini J, et al. Lumbar spinal stenosis: assessment of long-term outcome 12 years after operative and conservative treatment. *J Spinal Disord* 1998;11:110–115.

Javid MJ, Hadar EJ. Long-term follow-up review of patients who underwent laminectomy for lumbar stenosis. *J Neurosurg* 1998;89:1–7.

Lange M, Hamburger C, Waldhauser E, Beck OJ. Surgical treatment and results in patients with lumbar spinal stenosis. *Neurosurg Rev* 1993;16:27–33.

Onel D, Sari H, Donmez C. Lumbar spinal stenosis: clinical-radiologic therapeutic evaluation in 145 patients: conservative treatment or surgery? *Spine* 1993;18:291–298.

Sanderson PL, Wood PL. Surgery for lumbar spinal stenosis in old people. *J Bone Joint Surg Br* 1993;75:393–397.

Silvers HR, Lewis PJ, Asch HL. Decompressive lumbar laminectomy for spinal stenosis. *J Neurosurg* 1993;78:695–701.

Spivak JM. Degenerative lumbar spinal stenosis. *J Bone Joint Surg Am* 1998;80:1053–1066.

Merritt's Neurology, 10th ed., edited by L.P. Rowland. Lippincott Williams & Wilkins, Philadelphia © 2000.

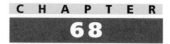

PERIPHERAL AND CRANIAL NERVE LESIONS

DALE J. LANGE
WERNER TROJABORG
LEWIS P. ROWLAND

INJURY TO CRANIAL AND PERIPHERAL NERVES

The peripheral and cranial nerves are subject to trauma, infections, tumors, toxic agents, and vascular or metabolic disorders. Trauma is the most common cause of localized injury to a single nerve (mononeuropathy). Toxic and metabolic disorders usually affect many nerves (mononeuropathy multiplex or symmetric polyneuropathy).

Pathology

After nerve damage, the pathologic changes depend on the nature of the injury, which also affects the regenerative response and the prognosis for recovery. According to Seddon (1954), mechanical nerve injuries are classified as follows: (1) complete severing of a nerve (*neurotmesis*), (2) axonal interruption with distal degeneration but an intact endoneurium (*axonotmesis*), or (3) conduction block at the site of the lesion but normal distal conduction without degeneration of distal fibers (*neurapraxia*).

Within the first 24 hours of injury, focal swelling occurs adjacent to the damaged site with fragmentation of endoplasmic reticulum, neurotubules, and neurofilaments, and accumulation of organelles. The axolemma becomes discontinuous; axons swell at some sites and narrow at others to give a beaded appearance. This process begins between the nodes of Ranvier and appears first in smaller fibers. Changes in myelin sheaths lag behind those in axons but progress in a similar way along the entire distal stump, again affecting small fibers first. The myelin surrounding the fragmented axons breaks up to form rows of elliptoids. Finally, Schwann cells and macrophages degrade the axon and myelin debris. In addition to these distal nerve changes, a *retrograde axon reaction* or *chromatolysis* is seen, with retraction of axons proximal to the lesion and alterations in the somata of neurons, such as cell body swelling, disruption of Nissl substance, migration of the cell nucleus, and increase in the size of the nucleolus. Presynaptic terminals gradually withdraw from the soma and dendrites; synaptic transmission is reduced until dorsal root stimulation fails to excite the motor neuron and evoke a reflex discharge in the ventral root. The pathologic distal changes of degeneration and retrograde axon reaction are similar in crush injury or complete nerve transection.

If a nerve has been completely severed, the orderly process just described is interfered with in proportion to the length of the discontinuity between proximal and distal ends. If this distance is great, regeneration is not possible, unless the ends are apposed at operation. If the distance is small, the fine processes of the axon penetrate the fibrin and connective tissue in the scar and enter the distal end of the nerve. Some of these may be deflected from the proper path by the scar and become entangled to form a *neuroma*.

Clinical Manifestations

The symptoms and signs of nerve injury depend on the type of nerve affected. If the nerve is mainly motor, the result is flaccid paralysis with wasting of the muscles innervated by the nerve. If the nerve contains sensory fibers, the result is loss of sensation in an area that is usually smaller than the anatomic distribution of the nerve. Vasomotor disorders and "trophic disturbances" are more common when a sensory or mixed type of nerve is injured than when a motor nerve is damaged. Partial injury or incomplete division of a nerve may be accompanied by pain that may be stabbing in character, by dysesthesia in the form of a pins-and-needles sensation, or, rarely, by severe burning pain (*causalgia*). Complete or incomplete interruption of a nerve may be followed by changes in the skin, mucous membranes, bones, and nails (trophic changes).

Diagnosis

The diagnosis of injury to one or more peripheral nerves can usually be made clinically by the distribution of the motor and sensory abnormalities. These patterns are considered later in connection with the description of isolated peripheral nerve lesions. The differentiation between lesions of the spinal roots and one or more peripheral nerves can be made by determining whether the muscular weakness and sensory loss are segmental rather than in the pattern of a nerve distribution. Electromyography (EMG) can be used to study the patterns of denervation and later reinnervation; nerve conduction studies can ascertain the site and the nature of the injury.

The differential diagnosis between polyneuropathy and other causes of generalized weakness is reviewed in Chapter 105.

Prognosis

The prognosis after injury of peripheral nerves is related to the degree of axonal injury and, to some extent, to the site of the injury. As a rule, the nearer the injury is to the central nervous system (CNS), the lower the probability will be that a completely severed nerve will regenerate, particularly cranial nerves, which are part of the CNS.

When injury to a peripheral nerve involves no loss of axons (i.e., conduction block) or little axonal loss, recovery is complete within a few days or weeks. If axonal loss is severe, recovery is slow, because axonal regeneration is required for recovery of function. If the nerve is severed or the damage is so great that axons regrow along appropriate tubules, recovery may not be complete or may fail to occur at all. In this circumstance, the neuronal dysfunction is permanent.

Treatment

When a peripheral nerve is severed by trauma, the ends should be surgically anastomosed. There is no agreement about the best time to explore and repair lesions of peripheral nerves if it cannot be determined whether there has been anatomic or physiologic interruption of the nerve. Most clinicians believe that surgery should be performed as soon as possible if there is any doubt about the state of the nerve.

After surgical therapy, or in patients who do not need operative therapy, rehabilitation measures should commence immediately with passive range-of-motion exercises for paralyzed muscles and reeducative exercises for weak muscles. Electrical stimulation is of unproven value in preventing permanent weakness. Splints, braces, and other corrective devices should be used when the lesion produces a deformity, but should be removable for the regular application of physiotherapy.

CRANIAL NEUROPATHIES

Olfactory Nerve and Tract

The ability to smell is a special quality relegated to the olfactory cells in the nasal mucosa. The molecular biology of smell is uncertain, but transcription-activating factors, such as Olf-1, found exclusively in neurons with olfactory receptors, probably direct cellular differentiation. Smell may be impaired after injury of the nasal mucosa, the olfactory bulb or its filaments, or CNS connections. Lesions of the nerve cause diminution or loss of the sense of smell. Injury to the CNS connections usually is not accompanied by any detectable loss of olfactory sense. Occasionally, olfactory hallucinations of a transient and paroxysmal nature may occur with lesions in the temporal lobe. Loss of the sense of smell is often accompanied by impaired taste, depending on the volatile substances in the food and beverages.

The sense of smell may be temporarily impaired in connection with the common cold. Inflammatory or neuritic lesions of the bulb or tract are uncommon, but these structures are sometimes affected in meningitis or in multiple peripheral neuritis. Patients with diabetes mellitus may have impaired sensation of smell. Hyposmia or anosmia is common early in Refsum disease. The olfactory bulb or tract may be compressed by meningiomas, metastatic tumors, or aneurysms in the anterior fossa or by infiltrating tumors of the frontal lobe. The filaments of the olfactory nerve may be torn from the cribriform plate, or the olfactory bulb may be contused or lacerated in head injuries. Leigh and Zee (1991) reported altered olfactory sense in 7.2% of 1,000 patients with head injuries observed at a military hospital. The loss was complete in 4.1% and partial in 3.1%. Recovery of smell occurred in only 6 of 72 patients. *Parosmia* (perversion of sense of smell) was present in 12 patients. In a study of head injuries in civilians, Friedman and Merritt (1944) found that the olfactory nerve was damaged in 11 (2.6%) of 430 patients. In all patients, the anosmia was bilateral. In three, the loss was transient and disappeared within 2 weeks of injury.

Parosmia is not accompanied by impairment of olfactory acuity and is most commonly caused by lesions of the temporal lobe, although it has been reported when the injury was probably in the olfactory bulb or tract. Hallucinations of smell may occur in psychotic persons or may be an aura in patients with convulsive seizures (hippocampal or uncinate gyrus fits). The aura in such cases is usually an unpleasant odor that is described with difficulty.

Increased sensitivity to olfactory stimuli is rare, but cases have been reported in which the sense of smell is so acute that it is a source of discomfort. Such a symptom is usually psychogenic.

Optic Nerve and Tract

The retina, optic nerve, and optic tract are subject to injury from many causes with resulting loss of vision, impairment of pupillary light reflexes, and abnormalities in pupil size (Table 68.1).

Changes in the retina or optic nerve may result from direct trauma, damage by toxins, systemic diseases (e.g., chronic renal failure, diabetes mellitus, leukemia, anemia, polycythemia, nutritional deficiencies, syphilis, tuberculosis, the lipodystrophies,

TABLE 68.1. EFFECTS OF LESIONS OF THE OPTIC, OCULOMOTOR, AND SYMPATHETIC PATHWAYS ON THE PUPILS

Site of lesion on right side	Size of pupil		Reaction of homolateral pupil to stimulation by light directed into		Consensual reaction of contralateral pupil to stimulation by light directed into		Accommodation–convergence reaction
	Right	Left	Right	Left	Right	Left	
Retina	Normal	Normal	Impaired	Normal	Impaired	Normal	Normal
Optic nerve	Normal	Normal	Lost	Normal	Lost	Normal	Normal
Optic chiasm	Normal	Normal	Normal[a]	Normal[a]	Normal[a]	Normal[a]	Normal
Optic tract	Normal	Normal	Normal[a]	Normal[a]	Normal[a]	Normal[a]	Normal
Optic radiation	Normal	Normal	Normal	Normal	Normal	Normal	Normal
Periaqueductal region[b]	Contracted	Normal	Lost	Normal	Normal	Lost	Normal
Ocutomotor nuclear complex or nerve	Dilated	Normal	Lost	Normal	Normal	Lost	Lost on right
Sympathetic pathways	Contracted	Normal	Normal	Normal	Normal	Normal	Normal

[a]No reaction of the pupils if the beam of light is focused sharply on the amblyopic portions of the retina.
[b]Argyll-Robertson pupil.

giant cell arteritis, or generalized arteriosclerosis), demyelinating hereditary diseases, local conditions (e.g., chorioretinitis, glaucoma, tumors, congenital anomalies, or thrombosis or embolism of the veins or arteries of the retina), infiltration or compression of the nerve (e.g., by glioma, meningioma, pituitary tumor, craniopharyngioma, metastatic tumor, or aneurysm), or increased intracranial pressure. Most of these conditions are considered elsewhere in this volume. Disorders of vision are also discussed in Chapter 7.

Optic neuritis is a term used loosely to describe lesions of the optic nerve accompanied by diminution in visual acuity with or without changes in the peripheral fields of vision and caused by inflammatory, degenerative, demyelinating, or toxic disorders (Fig. 68.1). On ophthalmoscopic examination, the disc may appear normal at first, or swelling and congestion of the nerve may be apparent. Later, the disc is pale and smaller than normal.

The optic nerve or retina may be injured by many toxic substances, including methyl alcohol, ethyl alcohol, tobacco, quinine, pentavalent arsenicals, thallium, lead, or mercury.

Alcohol–Tobacco Amblyopia

This term is used to describe the optic neuritis that is attributed to long and continued use of both tobacco and ethyl alcohol. The lesion could be an interstitial neuritis with destruction of the papillomacular bundle. A more reasonable hypothesis, however, is that the ganglion cells in the macular region of the retina are damaged. The neuritis is most common in middle-aged men who smoke a pipe and drink alcohol in large quantities. It usually affects both eyes. At the onset, a central or paracentral scotoma for colors exists that progresses to a complete central scotoma. The peripheral fields of vision are normal. Alcohol–tobacco amblyopia has been noted in association with pernicious anemia; malabsorption of vitamin B_{12} may be a factor in causing alcohol–tobacco amblyopia. Many authorities believe that the condition is primarily a nutritional disorder in alcoholic persons who are not eating properly. Absolute withdrawal of all forms of alcohol and tobacco may improve vision, unless the disease has progressed to the point of complete atrophy of the retinal cells of the optic nerve.

Oculomotor, Trochlear, and Abducens Nerves

Injury to the nerves or nuclei that innervate the ocular muscles causes diplopia, deviation of the eyeball, and impairment of ocular movements (Table 68.2).

Complete lesions of the third nerve or its nucleus produce paralysis of the extrinsic muscles of the eye supplied by this nerve (medial rectus, superior rectus, inferior rectus, inferior oblique, and levator palpebrae superior), as well as the constrictor of the ciliary muscles. There is ptosis of the lid with loss of the ability to open the eye; the eyeball is deviated outward and slightly downward; the pupil is dilated, does not react to light, and loses the power of accommodation. Partial lesions of the third nerve or its nucleus produce fragments of the above picture according to the extent of involvement of the nerve fibers or neurons.

Lesions of the fourth nerve or nucleus cause paralysis of the superior oblique muscle with impairment of the ability to turn the eye downward and inward. Deviation of the eyeball is slight, and diplopia is prevented by inclination of the head forward and to the side of the normal eye.

Injury to the sixth nerve causes paralysis of the lateral rectus muscle. The eyeball is deviated inward, and diplopia is present in almost all ranges of movement of the eye, except on gaze to the side opposite the lesion. Lesions in the brainstem that involve the sixth nerve nucleus are accompanied by a paralysis of lateral gaze. On attempts to look toward the affected side, neither eyeball moves beyond the midline. An intact third nerve on the opposite side can be demonstrated by the ability of the patient to move the internal rectus muscle of that eye in accommodation–convergence movements.

Paralysis of the ocular muscles may result from injury to the corresponding motor nerves or cells of origin by many conditions, including trauma, neurosyphilis, multiple sclerosis (MS) and other demyelinating diseases, tumors or aneurysms at the base of the skull, acute or subacute meningitis, thrombosis of intracranial venous sinuses, encephalitis, acute anterior poliomyelitis, diphtheria, diabetes mellitus, syringobulbia, vascular accidents in the brainstem, lead poisoning, botulism, alcoholic polioencephalitis (Wernicke encephalitis), osteomyelitis of the skull, and following spinal anesthesia or sim-

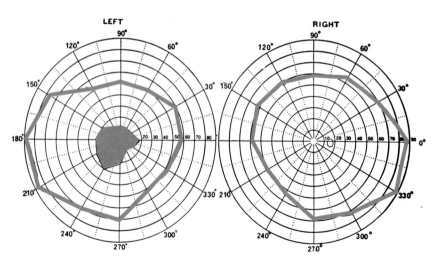

FIG. 68.1. Chart of visual fields in a patient with retrobulbar neuritis indicates large central scotoma in left eye. Visual acuity: OD 15/15, OS 1/400. (Courtesy of Dr. M. Chamlin.)

TABLE 68.2. CAUSES OF THIRD AND SIXTH CRANIAL NERVE PALSIES

	Third nerve		Sixth nerve	
	Cases (n)	%	Cases (n)	%
Total	290	100	419	100
Undetermined	67	23.1	124	29.6
Head trauma	47	16.2	70	16.7
Neoplasm	34	11.7	61	14.6
Vascular	60[a]	20.7	74[b]	17.7
Aneurysm	40[c]	13.8	15[d]	3.6
Other	42	14.5	75	17.9

[a]25 had diabetes mellitus
[b]24 had diabetes mellitus
[c]8 had subarachnoid hemorrhage
[d]11 had subarachnoid hemorrhage
From Rush and Younge, 1981; with permission.

ple lumbar puncture. Intraorbital lesions may cause ophthalmoplegia, proptosis, and local pain; retroorbital lesions may cause similar symptoms.

Intracavernous inflammation is held to be responsible for a form of painful ophthalmoplegia known as the *Tolosa-Hunt syndrome,* but the pathology has been documented in few cases; most would also be considered examples of *orbital myositis* or *orbital pseudotumor,* in which swelling of the muscles within the orbit can be demonstrated by computed tomography (CT). Ocular palsies are frequently seen in myasthenia gravis, ocular myopathy, and, rarely, polyneuropathy. Discussion in this section is restricted to the disturbance of eye movements in patients with increased intracranial pressure.

Paralysis of Eye Muscles Associated with Increased Intracranial Pressure

The sixth nerve has a long course from its point of emergence from the brainstem to the lateral rectus muscle in the orbit. Although it lies in a fluid-cushioned channel for a portion of this course, it is peculiarly subject to injury by compression against the floor of the skull when intracranial pressure is increased from any cause. Thus, unilateral or bilateral paralysis of the lateral rectus muscle may develop in patients with increased intracranial pressure. In these patients, the paralysis is of no value in localizing the site of the lesion (see Table 68.2).

Rarely, the third nerve is injured by increased intracranial pressure. The nerve may be damaged when the increase in pressure develops slowly, as with tumors of the brain, but it is more likely to be injured when the increased pressure is of sudden onset, with herniation of the uncinate gyrus through the tentorial notch and compression of the nerve. It is most commonly seen in patients with massive intracerebral hemorrhage or with extradural or subdural hematomas. Patients are usually comatose, and thus it is impossible to test eye movements, except by doll's eye or caloric tests, which may not suffice to show paresis of muscles innervated by the third cranial nerve. However, compression of the third nerve may be manifest by a dilated pupil nonresponsive to light ipsilateral to the herniation.

Fifth (Trigeminal) Nerve

Injury to the fifth cranial nerve causes paralysis of the muscles of mastication with deviation of the jaw toward the side of the lesion; loss of ability to appreciate soft tactile, thermal, or painful sensations in the face; and loss of the corneal and sneezing (*sternutatory*) reflexes.

The dorsal root ganglion for sensory fibers in the trigeminal nerve is the trigeminal (gasserian) ganglion in the middle cranial fossa. Sensory fibers pass into the brainstem at the midpons level and either ascend to terminate in the main sensory nucleus (subserving light touch) or descend to terminate in the nucleus of the spinal tract (pain and temperature sensation) or in the mesencephalic nucleus (subserving proprioception for jaw muscles). Lesions in the pons usually involve the motor and main sensory nuclei, causing paralysis of the muscles of mastication and loss of sensation of light touch in the face. Lesions in the medulla affect only the descending tract and cause loss of the sensation of light touch in the face.

The fifth nerve may be injured by trauma, neoplasms, aneurysm, or meningeal infections. Occasionally, it may be involved in poliomyelitis and generalized polyneuropathy. The sensory and motor nuclei in the pons and medulla may be destroyed by intramedullary tumors or vascular lesions. In addition, an isolated lesion of the descending tract may occur in syringobulbia or MS.

If no accompanying neurologic signs facilitate localization, isolated facial numbness (*idiopathic trigeminal neuropathy*) may be a difficult problem to solve. Common causes of facial numbness are dental trauma, herpes zoster, cranial trauma, head and neck tumors, intracranial tumors, and idiopathic trigeminal neuropathy. Systemic sclerosis, mixed connective tissue diseases, amyloidosis, MS, and sarcoidosis are less common causes of facial numbness. Although restricted loss of sensation over the chin (*numb-chin syndrome*) may result from dental trauma or even poorly fitting dentures, it may be the only manifestation of systemic malignancy, such as lymphoma, metastatic breast carcinoma, melanoma, or prostatic cancer. Magnetic resonance imaging (MRI) or CT of the mandible often identifies the disorder.

Painful facial numbness may herald the presence of nasopharyngeal carcinoma or metastatic carcinoma. Severe facial pain in the absence of numbness or other objective findings (tic douloureux) is caused by fifth nerve dysfunction.

Trigeminal Neuralgia (Tic Douloureux)

This disorder of the sensory division of the trigeminal nerve is characterized by recurrent paroxysms of sharp, stabbing pains in the distribution of one or more branches of the nerve. The cause is unknown. In most cases, no organic disease of the fifth nerve or CNS can be identified. Degenerative or fibrotic changes in the gasserian ganglion have been found but are too variable to be considered causal. Some investigators believe that most patients with idiopathic trigeminal neuralgia have anomalous blood vessels that compress the nerve.

Pain typical of trigeminal neuralgia occasionally affects patients with lesions in the brainstem as a result of MS or with vascular lesions that involve the descending root of the fifth nerve. Usually, trigeminal neuralgia follows other symptoms of MS. Of all patients with MS, however, 10% have facial pain first, and other symptoms of MS may not appear for 6 years.

The attacks of facial pain in trigeminal neuralgia are attributed to discharges in the descending nucleus of the nerve, presumably because of excessive inflow of impulses to the nucleus. In support of this hypothesis is evidence that typical attacks of trigeminal neuralgia may be relieved by section of the greater auricular or occipital nerves or that an episode of trigeminal neuralgia can be interrupted by intravenous injection of phenytoin sodium (Dilantin).

Trigeminal neuralgia is the most common of all neuralgias. Onset is usually in middle or late life but may occur at any age. Typical trigeminal neuralgia occasionally affects children but rarely occurs before age 35. The incidence is slightly greater in women than in men.

The pain occurs in paroxysms. Between attacks, the patient is free of symptoms, except for fear of an impending attack. The pain is searing or burning, coming in lightning like jabs. A paroxysm may last 15 minutes or more. The frequency of attacks varies from many times a day to a few times a month. The patient ceases to talk when the pain strikes and may rub or pinch the face; movements of the face and jaw may accompany the pain. Sometimes, ipsilateral lacrimation is prominent. No objective loss of cutaneous sensation is found during or after the paroxysms, but the patient may complain of facial hyperesthesia.

A characteristic feature is the *trigger zone,* stimulation of which sets off a typical paroxysm of pain. This zone is a small area on the cheek, lip, or nose that may be stimulated by facial movement, chewing, or touch. The patient may avoid making facial expressions during conversation, may go without eating for days, or may avoid the slightest breeze to prevent an attack. The pain is limited strictly to one or more branches of the fifth nerve and does not spread beyond the distribution of that nerve. The second division is involved more frequently than the third. The first division is primarily affected in less than 5% of patients. Pain may spread to one or both of the other divisions. In cases of long duration, all three divisions are affected in 15%. The pain is occasionally bilateral (5%) but rarely occurs at the same time. Bilateral trigeminal neuralgia is encountered most often in patients with MS.

The physical findings in patients with trigeminal neuralgia are normal. Hemifacial spasm, however, may accompany trigeminal neuralgia. The patient may be undernourished or emaciated if attacks are provoked by eating. There is no objective sensory loss, and motor functions are normal. The results of laboratory examinations are normal.

The diagnosis of trigeminal neuralgia is usually made from the history without difficulty. Also characteristic is the method patients use to demonstrate the site of origin and mode of spread of the pain. They do not touch the area but hold the tip of the index finger a short distance from the face to point to areas of origin and spread.

Trigeminal neuralgia must be differentiated from other types of pain that occur in the face or head, particularly from infections of the teeth and nasal sinus. The pains of dental and nasal sinus disease differ from those of trigeminal neuralgia in that they are usually steady and throbbing and persist for many hours. Nevertheless, many patients with trigeminal neuralgia have had numerous operations on the sinuses, and most of their teeth have been removed before the diagnosis is established. Conversely, many patients with diseased teeth are referred to neurologists with the diagnosis of trigeminal neuralgia. In these patients, the role of the diseased tooth in the production of pain can be demonstrated by syringing it and the surrounding gum with ice water. Patients with temporomandibular joint disease may have symptoms similar to those of trigeminal neuralgia, but the pain is not paroxysmal, is exacerbated by eating, and has no trigger point. Cluster headaches may be confused with trigeminal neuralgia, especially when the ipsilateral eye is red and watery. The pain of cluster headaches, however, is not paroxysmal, does not conform to the trigeminal distribution, and is accompanied by nasal stuffiness with Horner syndrome on the affected side.

Atypical facial pain occurs in the territory of the trigeminal nerve, but the characteristics are different from those of trigeminal neuralgia. The pain may be as excruciating, but the individual paroxysm always last longer than a few seconds—usually minutes or even continuously. The pain itself is dull, aching, crushing, or burning. Surgical treatment is not effective in atypical facial pain, which may sometimes be a manifestation of depression.

Treatment of trigeminal neuralgia with carbamazepine (Tegretol) is often successful. The effective dose is usually 200 mg four times daily. Larger doses may be needed, with monitoring of serum levels and clinical signs of toxicity. Toxicity is manifested as drowsiness, dizziness, unsteady gait, and nausea. A rare but serious complication is aplastic anemia. Unfortunately, tolerance to this medication frequently develops. Baclofen (Lioresal), 50 to 60 mg daily, also relieves symptoms. Phenytoin in a dose of 300 to 400 mg per day may help some patients unresponsive to carbamazepine or baclofen, but it is more commonly used as an adjunct to these medications.

Surgical procedures to control pain are used in common practice. Techniques include microvascular decompression, radiofrequency and chemical gangliolysis using stereotactic techniques, and rhizotomy. One of the more popular procedures is radiofrequency surgery, which selectively interferes with pain-conducting small fibers but spares the large-diameter motor fibers. Some studies report 90% to 97% partial or complete relief. The rate of recurrence is uncertain.

Increasing evidence indicates that many patients with trigeminal neuralgia have compression of the trigeminal nerve by arterial loops. Posterior fossa exploration is therefore recommended for patients whose symptoms are difficult to control. Other chronic masses, such as arteriovenous malformation, aneurysm, and cholesteatoma, may be found.

Seventh (Facial) Nerve

As the facial nerve leaves the brainstem, it has two divisions: the motor root and the nervus intermedius. The functions of the intermedius are much like those of the glossopharyngeal nerve. It conducts taste sensation from the anterior two-thirds of the tongue and supplies autonomic fibers to the submaxillary and sphenopalatine ganglia that innervate the salivary and lacrimal glands. Whether the seventh nerve has any somatic sensory function is debatable. It is thought to carry proprioceptive impulses from the facial muscles and cutaneous sensation from a small strip of skin on the posteromedial surface of the pinna and around the external auditory canal. In fact, however, sensory loss is only rarely detected in patients with lesions of the seventh nerve. Similarly, hearing is seldom impaired, although the ear may become more sensitive to low tones when the stapedius is paralyzed.

Injuries to the facial nerve cause paralysis of the facial muscles with or without loss of taste on the anterior two-thirds of the tongue or altered secretion of the lacrimal and salivary glands, depending on the portion of the nerve involved. Lesions near the origin or in the region of the geniculate ganglion are accompanied by a paralysis of the motor, gustatory, and autonomic functions. Lesions between the geniculate ganglion and the origin of the chorda tympani produce the same dysfunction as that resulting from injury in the region of the geniculate ganglion, except that lacrimal secretion is not affected. Lesions near the stylomastoid foramen result only in facial paralysis.

Lesions of the facial nucleus in the brainstem cause paralysis of all facial muscles. Lesions of the motor cortex or the connections between the cortex and the facial nucleus are accompanied by partial paralysis, usually most severe in muscles of the lower half of the face (supranuclear palsy). Asymmetric facial movements may follow voluntary or emotional stimuli.

Because they are superficial, the peripheral branches of the seventh nerve are subject to injury by stab and gunshot wounds, cuts, and birth trauma. The nerve is occasionally injured in operations on the mastoid and parotid gland and in acoustic neuromas or trigeminal neuralgia. Damage to the seventh nerve is often found with fracture of the temporal bone and is usually evident immediately after injury. Occasionally, however, facial paralysis is delayed for several days after the accident. The mechanism of this delayed paralysis is not clear. Improvement is the rule when the nerve damage is associated with head trauma, but recovery may not be complete.

Within the skull, the nerve may be affected by tumors, aneurysms, meningeal infections, leukemia, osteomyelitis, herpes zoster, Paget disease, and sarcomas or other tumors of bone. Occasionally, it is affected in the course of generalized polyneuritis, which is common in leprosy, Guillain-Barré syndrome, or diphtheritic polyneuropathy, but seldom in diabetic or alcoholic neuropathy. The peripheral portion of the nerve may be compressed by tumors of the parotid gland. Facial palsy is rare in mumps but is common in sarcoidosis. Bilateral facial palsy may be caused by many of the conditions that produce unilateral paralysis, but is most often seen in sarcoidosis, Guillain-Barré syndrome, leprosy, leukemia, and meningococcal meningitis. The facial nucleus may be damaged by tumors, inflammatory lesions, vascular lesions, acute poliomyelitis, and MS.

Bell Palsy

Paralysis of the seventh nerve may occur without any known cause. Bell palsy often follows exposure to cold (e.g., riding in an open car) and is thought to be caused by swelling of the nerve within the facial (fallopian) canal. It occurs at all ages but is slightly more common in the third to fifth decades. The frequency of involvement on the two sides is approximately equal. Paralysis occasionally recurs either on the same or on the opposite side. Familial occurrence of Bell palsy is occasionally seen.

The onset of facial paralysis may be accompanied by a feeling of stiffness of the muscles. Pain is rare, however, except in the *Ramsay Hunt syndrome,* which is caused by herpes zoster and includes pain in the ear ipsilateral to the facial paralysis.

The signs of complete paralysis of the seventh nerve can be divided into motor, secretory, and sensory. When the damage is severe, facial paralysis is obvious, even when the face is at rest. Muscles of the lower half of the face sag. The normal folds and lines around the lips, nose, and forehead are ironed out, and the palpebral fissure is wider than normal. Absence of voluntary and associated movements of the facial and platysmal muscles is complete. When the patient attempts to smile, the lower facial muscles are pulled to the opposite side. This distortion of the facial muscles may give the false appearance of deviation of the protruded tongue or the open jaw. Saliva and food are likely to collect on the paralyzed side. The patient cannot close the eye, and with attempts to do so, the eyeball can be seen to divert upward and slightly inward (the Bell phenomenon). When the lesion is peripheral to the ganglion, the lacrimal fibers are spared and the collection of tears in the conjunctival sac is excessive because the tears are not expressed into the lacrimal duct by lid movements. The corneal reflex is absent as a result of paralysis of the upper lid; preservation of corneal sensation and the afferent portion of the reflex is manifested by blinking of the other lid. Secretion of tears is diminished only if the lesion is proximal to the geniculate ganglion. Decrease in salivary secretion and loss of taste in the anterior two-thirds of the tongue are found when the chorda tympani is affected.

Although the seventh nerve presumably transmits proprioceptive sense from the facial muscles and cutaneous sensation from a small area of the pinna and the external auditory canal, loss of these sensations is rarely detected.

Partial injury to the facial nerve causes weakness of the upper and lower halves of the face. Occasionally, however, the lower half is more severely affected than the upper half; rarely, the opposite is seen. Recovery from facial paralysis depends on the severity of the lesion. If the nerve is anatomically sectioned, the chances of complete or even partial recovery are remote. In most patients, especially those with Bell palsy, partial or complete recovery occurs. With complete recovery, no apparent difference can be detected between the two sides of the face at rest or in motion. When recovery is partial, "contractures" may develop on the paralyzed side; superficial inspection seems to reveal weakness of muscles on the normal side. The inaccuracy of this impression becomes obvious as soon as the patient smiles or attempts to move the facial muscles.

Abnormal movement of facial muscles and lacrimation may follow facial palsy. A slight twitch of the labial muscles may occur whenever the patient blinks (*synkinesis*), or an excess secretion of tears may result when the salivary glands are activated during eating. Paroxysmal clonic contractions of all facial muscles may simulate focal jacksonian seizures. These spasms are occasionally seen in patients who have never had any obvious lesion of the facial nerve. The cause of these sequelae is not known.

They are attributed by some researchers to misdirection of the regenerated fibers or to the spread of impulses between fibers within the nerve (*ephaptic conduction*).

The differential diagnosis between facial paralysis caused by a cortical lesion and that resulting from a lesion of the nucleus or nerve can be made without difficulty, except when weakness is barely evident. Other signs of supranuclear cortical involvement include sparing of the muscles of the forehead and upper lid and preservation of electrical reactions. In addition, the weakness of a peripheral lesion is equal for all movements, whereas in supranuclear lesions volitional contractions may be greater or less than those in the emotional responses of smiling or laughing.

The differentiation between lesions of the nucleus and those of the nerve is made by associated findings. Lesions in the tegmentum of the brainstem are accompanied by paralysis of lateral gaze because of concomitant injury to the sixth nerve nucleus and parapontine gaze center. Lesions in the basal part of the brainstem are accompanied by corticospinal signs. Lesions of the nerve as it emerges from the brainstem may be caused by tumors, meningitis, or other infections, resulting in concomitant paralysis of the facial nerve with abnormalities of the eighth, sixth, and, possibly, the fifth nerves.

Attempts should be made to remove the lesion that causes the facial paralysis. Without formal therapeutic trials, some clinicians recommend massage or electrical stimulation of the paralyzed muscles to preserve tone. Surgical procedures may help when spontaneous recovery does not occur. Neurolysis or end-to-end suture may be indicated in extracranial lesions of the nerve or its branches. When the nerve is damaged proximal to the stylomastoid foramen, end-to-end suture is not possible, and innervation of the facial muscles can be restored only by suturing the distal portion of the seventh nerve to the central portion of the eleventh or the twelfth nerves. If the eleventh nerve is used, paralysis of the sternocleidomastoid and upper fibers of the trapezius is permanent. The resultant deformity is slight, but the facial muscles contract whenever the patient attempts to turn the head or elevate the shoulder. Sooner or later, a new motor pattern develops in the cerebral cortex, and movements of the facial muscles are dissociated from those of the shoulder. Conversely, anastomosis of the twelfth nerve with the seventh nerve is followed by atrophy and paralysis of one-half of the tongue. This outcome causes little discomfort, and control of the facial muscles returns without adventitious movement of other muscles.

Anastomosis of the facial nerve with either the eleventh or the twelfth nerve should be performed as soon as possible if the nerve is cut in mastoid surgery or in removal of an acoustic neuroma. In other types of peripheral facial paralysis, surgery should be delayed for 6 months or more to determine whether spontaneous regeneration occurs.

Steroid therapy has been recommended for Bell palsy to relieve edema in the nerve. Reports of this therapy have not been convincing; therapeutic trials have not been adequately controlled, because improvement is seen spontaneously in almost all cases. Acyclovir (Zovirax) therapy is also unproven. Decompression of the nerve in the canal is recommended by some otologists to expedite and enhance return of function in Bell palsy. No available evidence suggests that this treatment changes the course of the disorder, and the surgery itself is not without risk. Therefore, many surgeons have stopped performing this operation.

Surgery may be necessary to alleviate the facial spasm that occurs spontaneously or after partial regeneration of the injured nerve. The nerve or one of its branches can be injected with alcohol or partially sectioned when the spasms are localized. These operations occasionally give permanent relief from the spasms, but the spasms usually recur when the nerve regenerates. Permanent relief can be obtained by anastomosing the seventh nerve with the eleventh or twelfth cranial nerve.

Blepharospasm, Myokymia, and Hemifacial Spasm

Blepharospasm is a state of forceful closure of the eye. Unilateral and repeated brief blepharospasm is a focal dystonia and may be part of hemifacial spasm. Bilateral blepharospasm may be seen in basal ganglia disorders, especially parkinsonism. The combination of blepharospasm and oromandibular dyskinesia is the Meige syndrome. Injections of botulinum toxin are effective and safe in treating of blepharospasm.

Facial myokymia is characterized by fine rippling movements of facial muscles. EMG shows bursts of rapidly firing motor units that tend to recur in a regular fashion. Persistent facial myokymia is sometimes a manifestation of MS, brainstem glioma, or some other disorder of the brainstem. These CNS lesions presumably interrupt descending inhibitory impulses that act on motor neurons in the facial nucleus, thereby releasing the involuntary activity. Myokymia also can arise peripherally, especially in the acute phase of the Guillain-Barré syndrome.

Hemifacial spasm is characterized by clonic spasms of the facial muscles, usually starting around the eye and often spreading to other muscles of one side of the face. It increases in intensity during stress and may occur in sleep. The characteristic EMG findings include bursts of muscle action potentials that occur either regularly or irregularly at 5 to 20 per second. Synkinetic motor responses in muscles innervated by the facial nerve follow stimulation of the ipsilateral fifth nerve (blink reflex). Hemifacial spasm does not have the ominous implications of myokymia, but the cosmetic effects may be distressing. The cause is usually obscure, but it may follow facial nerve trauma. Treatment with anticonvulsant medication, such as carbamazepine, may be effective. Jannetta (1977) reported relief of the involuntary movements by exposing the facial nerve in the posterior fossa and decompressing vessels at the root entry zone. Botulinum toxin is also effective.

Eighth (Acoustic) Nerve

Eighth nerve disorders are described in Chapter 6.

Ninth (Glossopharyngeal) Nerve

The ninth cranial nerve contains both motor and sensory fibers. The motor fibers supply the stylopharyngeus muscle and the constrictors of the pharynx. Other efferent fibers innervate secretory glands in the pharyngeal mucosa. The sensory fibers carry general sensation from the upper part of the pharynx and the special sensation of taste from the posterior one-third of the tongue.

Isolated lesions of the nerve or its nuclei are rare and are not accompanied by perceptible disability. Taste is lost on the posterior one-third of the tongue, and the gag reflex is absent on the side of the lesion. Injuries of the ninth nerve by infections or tumors are usually accompanied by signs of involvement of the neighboring nerves. The tractus solitarius receives taste fibers from both the seventh and the ninth nerves and may be destroyed by vascular or neoplastic lesions in the brainstem. Because the ninth, tenth, and eleventh nerves exit the jugular foramen together, tumors here produce multiple cranial nerve palsies (*jugular foramen syndrome*). The territory of the ninth nerve is the distribution also affected in glossopharyngeal neuralgia.

Glossopharyngeal neuralgia (tic douloureux of the ninth nerve) is characterized by paroxysms of excruciating pain in the region of the tonsils, posterior pharynx, back of the tongue, and middle ear. The cause of glossopharyngeal neuralgia is unknown, and no significant pathologic changes occur in most cases. Pain in the distribution of the nerve occasionally follows injury of the nerve in the neck by tumors.

Glossopharyngeal neuralgia is rare, with a frequency about 5% that of trigeminal neuralgia. The paroxysms are burning or stabbing in nature. They may occur spontaneously but are often precipitated by swallowing, talking, or touching the tonsils or posterior pharynx. The attacks last only a few seconds but sometimes last several minutes. The frequency of attacks varies from many times daily to once in several weeks.

The diagnosis of glossopharyngeal neuralgia can be made from the description of the pain. The only differential diagnosis of any importance is neuralgia of the mandibular branch of the fifth nerve. The diagnosis of glossopharyngeal neuralgia is established when an attack of pain can be precipitated by stimulation of the tonsils, posterior pharynx, or base of the tongue or when the pain is relieved by spraying the affected area with local anesthetic. When the membrane becomes anesthetized, the pains disappear and cannot be precipitated by stimulation with an applicator. During this period, the patient can swallow food and talk without discomfort.

There may be long remissions. During a remission the trigger zone disappears. The pains almost always recur, unless they are prevented by medical therapy or the nerve is surgically sectioned. The disease does not shorten life, but affected patients may become emaciated because of the fear that each morsel of food will precipitate a pain paroxysm.

Carbamazepine, alone or in combination with phenytoin, is usually effective in producing a remission. If medical therapy is not effective, the nerve can be sectioned intracranially; the results of the operation are satisfactory. The patient is relieved of the pain, and there are no serious sequelae. The mucous membrane supplied by the ninth nerve is permanently anesthetized with loss of the gag reflex on that side. Taste is lost on the posterior one-third of the tongue. There are no motor symptoms, such as dysphagia or dysarthria, unless the tenth nerve is injured during surgery.

Tenth (Vagus) Nerve

The motor fibers of the tenth nerve arise from the nucleus ambiguus (to innervate the somatic muscles of the pharynx and larynx) and from the dorsal motor nucleus (to supply the autonomic innervation of the heart, lungs, esophagus, and stomach). The vagus nerve also carries sensory (visceral afferent) fibers from the mucosa in the oropharynx and upper part of the gastrointestinal tract; sensory fibers from the thoracic and abdominal organs send information into the tractus solitarius.

Unilateral lesions of the nucleus ambiguus in the medulla cause dysarthria and dysphagia. Because the nucleus has a considerable longitudinal extent in the medulla, lesions in the brainstem may produce dysarthria without dysphagia, or vice versa, according to the site of the lesion. Lesions confined to the lower portion of the nucleus cause dysphagia, whereas lesions of the upper portions produce dysarthria.

The dysphagia or dysarthria that follows unilateral lesions of the nucleus ambiguus is rarely severe. The voice may be hoarse, but speech is intelligible. Difficulty in swallowing solid food is usually only slight, but occasionally a transient aphagia necessitates the administration of food by tube for a few days or weeks. On examination, the palate on the affected side is lax, and the uvula deviates to the opposite side on phonation. The palatal reflex is absent on the affected side. Lesions of the nucleus ambiguus on both sides cause complete aphonia and aphagia. Bilateral destruction of this nucleus is rare, except in the terminal stages of amyotrophic lateral sclerosis (ALS). Selective destruction of cells in the nucleus ambiguus may occur in syringobulbia or intramedullary tumors, consequently causing paralysis of the vocal cords in adduction. The patient can talk and swallow without difficulty, but inspiratory stridor and dyspnea may be severe enough to require tracheotomy.

Unilateral lesions of the dorsal motor nucleus are not accompanied by any symptoms of autonomic dysfunction. Bilateral lesions may be life-threatening. The nucleus of the tenth nerve may also be damaged by infections (especially acute poliomyelitis), intramedullary tumors, and vascular lesions. It may be involved in polyneuropathy, especially in the diphtheritic and Guillain-Barré forms.

Injury to the pharyngeal branches of the nerve results in dysphagia. Lesions of the superior laryngeal nerve produce anesthesia of the upper part of the larynx and paralysis of the cricothyroid muscle. The voice is weak and easily tires. Involvement of the recurrent laryngeal nerve, which is frequent with aneurysms of the aorta and occasionally occurs after operations in the neck, causes hoarseness and dysphonia as a result of paralysis of the vocal cords. Complete paralysis of both recurrent laryngeal nerves produces aphonia and inspiratory stridor. Partial bilateral paralysis may produce a paralysis of both abductors with severe dyspnea and inspiratory stridor; it does not cause any alteration in the voice, however.

Unilateral lesions of the vagus nerve do not produce any constant disturbance of the autonomic functions of the nerve. The heart rate may be unchanged, slowed, or accelerated. The respiratory rhythm is not affected, and no significant disturbance in the action of the gastrointestinal tract results.

Involuntary spasm of the vocal cords (*spastic dysphonia* or *laryngeal dystonia*) is of uncertain cause, but it interferes with speech. Injection of botulinum toxin is an effective treatment.

Eleventh (Spinal Accessory) Nerve

The spinal portion of the eleventh nerve innervates the sternocleidomastoid and part or all of the trapezius muscles. The fibers from the accessory portion of the nerve originate in the nucleus ambiguus, travel with the tenth nerve through the jugular foramen, and eventually merge with the axons from motor fibers from the upper four cervical levels. Fibers from the nucleus ambiguus portion innervate the larynx. Fibers from the spinal portion pass along the carotid artery, penetrate and innervate the sternocleidomastoid muscle, and emerge in the middle of that muscle at its posterior border, crossing the posterior triangle of the neck to innervate the upper portion of the trapezius. Lesions of the spinal portion produce weakness and atrophy of the trapezius muscle, impairing rotary movements of the neck and chin to the opposite side and weakness of shrugging movements of the shoulder. Weakness of the upper portion of the trapezius results in winging of the scapula, which must be differentiated from that produced by weakness of the serratus anterior. Scapular winging from weakness of the trapezius is present at rest (arms at side) and becomes worse on abduction of the shoulder. Scapular winging from weakness of the serratus anterior is negligible at rest and worsens during flexion of the shoulder.

The nucleus of the eleventh nerve may be destroyed by infections and degenerative disorders in the medulla, such as syringobulbia or ALS; the peripheral portion of the nerve may be involved in polyneuropathy, meningeal infection, extramedullary tumor (e.g., meningioma and neurinoma), or destructive processes in the occipital bone. Because of its passage through the posterior triangle of the neck, the nerve is susceptible to damage during lymph node biopsy, cannulation of the internal jugular vein, or carotid endarterectomy. The muscles supplied by this nerve are frequently involved in myotonic muscular dystrophy, polymyositis, and myasthenia gravis.

Twelfth (Hypoglossal) Nerve

The hypoglossal nerve is the motor nerve to the tongue. The nucleus in the medulla or the peripheral nerve portion may be injured by all the disorders mentioned in connection with the tenth and eleventh nuclei. Occlusions of the short branches of the basilar artery that nourish the paramedian area of the medulla cause paralysis of the tongue on one side and of the arm and leg on the opposite side (*alternating hemiplegia*).

Unilateral injury to the nucleus results in atrophy and paralysis of the muscles of one-half of the tongue. When the tongue is protruded, it deviates toward the paralyzed side, and while it is protruded, movement toward the normal side is absent or weakly performed. When the tongue lies on the floor of the mouth, it deviates slightly toward the healthy side, and movement of the tongue toward the back of the mouth on this side is impaired. Fibrillation of the muscles is seen in chronic processes involving the hypoglossal nucleus (e.g., syringobulbia, ALS). Bilateral paralysis of the nucleus or nerve produces atrophy of both sides of the tongue and paralysis of all movements, with severe dysarthria and resultant difficulty in manipulating food in the process of eating.

The tongue is only rarely affected by lesions in the cerebral hemispheres or corticobulbar connections. Homolateral weakness of the tongue may accompany severe hemiplegia. Such weakness appears as a slight deviation of the tongue to the paralyzed side when it is protruded. Moderate weakness of the tongue may accompany pseudobulbar palsy but is never as severe

as the weakness seen with destruction of both medullary nuclei. Tremor of the tongue is seen in chronic alcoholism. Apraxia of the tongue (i.e., inability to protrude the tongue on command but preservation of the associated movements in eating or licking of the lips) frequently accompanies motor aphasia.

PERIPHERAL NERVES

The peripheral nerves are subject to injury by pressure, constriction by fascial bands, or trauma associated with injection of drugs, perforating wounds, fractures of the bones, or stretching of the nerves. Isolated or multiple nerve paralysis may also be associated with a reaction to the injection of serum or to some toxic or metabolic disorders.

The radial, common peroneal, ulnar, and long thoracic nerves are subject to damage by external pressure. The median nerve is most frequently affected by constriction by fascial bands at the wrist. The axillary nerve is commonly affected in an allergic reaction to injections of serum. The sciatic nerve is affected by direct injection of drugs. Any peripheral nerve may be damaged by perforating wounds or fractures of the bones. The frequency of involvement of the peripheral nerves by trauma is shown in Table 68.3.

Nerves of the Arm

Radial Nerve

The radial nerve arises from the posterior secondary trunk of the brachial plexus (C-5 to C-8). It is predominantly a motor nerve and innervates the chief extensors of the forearm, wrist, and fingers (Table 68.4).

The radial nerve may be injured by cuts, gunshot wounds, callus formation after fracture of the humerus, pressure of crutches, or pressure against some hard surface, especially in sleep (*"Saturday night palsy"*). A complete lesion of the nerve in the axilla is characterized by paralysis of the triceps and abolition of the triceps reflex, in addition to the other signs of radial nerve palsy re-

TABLE 68.3. INCIDENCE OF PERIPHERAL NERVE LESIONS BY TRAUMA

Nerve	Cases (n)	%
Medial	707	19.3
Radial	516	14.1
Ulnar	1000	27.4
Musculocutaneous	44	1.2
Axillary	9	0.2
Sciatic-peroneal	404	11.1
Sciatic-tibial	394	10.8
Peroneal	341	9.3
Tibial	235	6.4
Femoral	6	0.2
	3656	100.0

Modified from Woodhall B, Beebe GW. *Peripheral nerve regeneration: a follow-up study of 3656 World War II injuries.* Washington DC: Veterans Administration Monographs, 1956.

TABLE 68.4. MUSCLES INNERVATED BY THE RADIAL NERVE

Triceps	Extensor digiti minimi
Anconeus	Extensor carpi ulnaris
Brachioradialis	Abductor pollicis longus
Extensor carpi radialis longus and brevis	Extensor pollicis longus and brevis
Supinator	Extensor indicis proprius
Extensor digitorum communis	

viewed in the following. Lesions of the radial nerve in the axilla are usually accompanied by evidence of injury to other nerves in this region. When the nerve is injured in the posteromedial surface of the arm, one or more of the branches to the triceps may be spared so that weakness of extension of the forearm is minimal.

The most common site of injury to the radial nerve is in the middle one-third of the arm proximal to the branch to the brachioradialis muscle. Lesions of the nerve at this level result in weakness of flexion of the forearm caused by paralysis of the brachioradialis muscle, which is a stronger flexor of the forearm than of the biceps, and paralysis of extension of the wrist, thumb, and fingers at the proximal joints. Extension at the distal phalanges is performed by the interosseus muscles. There is weakness of adduction of the hand as a result of loss of action of the extensor carpi ulnaris and loss of supination when the forearm is extended, because the supinating action of the biceps is evident only when the forearm is flexed. In addition, there is an apparent weakness of flexion of the fingers. This weakness is not real and is a result of faulty posture of the hand. When the wrist is passively extended, the fingers have normal power of flexion.

Sensory loss associated with lesions of the radial nerve is slight and is confined in most cases to a small area on the posterior radial surface of the hand and of the first and second metacarpals of the thumb and the index and middle fingers. Lesions of the nerve or its branches in the forearm or wrist are accompanied by fragments of the syndrome previously described, according to the site of the lesion.

Complete lesions of the radial nerve are followed by atrophy of the paralyzed muscles. Vasomotor or trophic disturbances are rare, unless there is an associated vascular lesion. Causalgia rarely follows partial injury to the nerve.

Median Nerve

The median nerve comprises fibers from the sixth, seventh, and eighth cervical nerves and first thoracic roots. It arises in two heads (lateral and medial cords), derived from the upper and lower trunks of the brachial plexus. It has important motor and sensory functions. The following movements are controlled by this nerve: pronation of the forearm by the pronator quadratus and pronator teres, flexion of the hand by the flexor carpi radialis and palmaris longus, flexion of the thumb and the index and middle fingers by the superficial and deep flexors, and opposition of the thumb (Table 68.5). The sensory region of the median nerve comprises the radial side of the palm of the hand, the volar surface of the thumb and the index and middle fingers, the radial one-half of the ring finger, the dorsal surface of the distal phalanx of the thumb, and the middle and terminal phalanges of the index and middle fingers.

Injury to the median nerve in the arm is characterized by loss of ability to pronate the forearm, weakness of flexion of the wrist, paralysis of flexion of the thumb and the index finger, weakness of flexion of the middle finger, paralysis of opposition of the thumb, atrophy of the muscles of the thenar eminence, and loss of sensation in an area somewhat smaller than that of the anatomic distribution of the nerve. Lesions of the median nerve at the wrist cause paralysis and atrophy of the thenar muscles and sensory loss in the characteristic distribution.

There is absolute paralysis of few movements of the wrist or fingers in isolated lesions of the median nerve because of the compensatory action of unparalyzed muscles. Pronation can be accomplished by the action of the deltoid in holding the arm outward when the forearm is flexed and by rotation of the arm inward by the subscapularis when the arm is extended. Flexion of the wrist can be performed by the action of the flexor carpi ulnaris with deviation of the hand toward the ulnar side of the arm. There is absence of flexion in the index and the middle fingers, although the middle finger is usually influenced by movements of the ring finger and its deep flexor may be supplied by the ulnar nerve. In addition, flexion of the proximal phalanx of the fingers, including the index finger in association with extension of the distal phalanges, is possible through the action of the interosseus muscles. Although the opponens pollicis is paralyzed, feeble movements of opposition can be made by energetic contraction of the adductors that causes the thumb to move to the ulnar edge of the hand by pressing against the base of the fingers.

Partial lesions of the median nerve are more frequent than complete interruption, with dissociation in the degree of involvement of the various muscles supplied by the nerve and with little or no sensory loss. Flexion of the index finger and opposition of the thumb are the movements that are usually most affected in partial lesions.

Vasomotor disturbances are common with median nerve lesions, probably because of associated lesions of blood vessels. The syndrome of causalgia is most commonly associated with lesions of the median nerve.

A slowly developing atrophy limited to the muscles of the outer radial side of the thenar eminence has been described by the term *partial thenar atrophy*. The atrophy is often bilateral and exceeds the motor weakness. Pain, paresthesia, and a mild degree of impairment of sensation in the distribution of the nerves with or without motor weakness are fairly common as a result of compression of the nerve by the transverse carpal segment (*carpal tunnel syndrome*). The pain is severe, often waking the patient

TABLE 68.5. MUSCLES INNERVATED BY THE MEDIAN NERVE

Pronator teres	Abductor pollicis brevis
Flexor carpi radialis	Opponens pollicis
Palmaris longus	Flexor pollicis brevis
Flexor digitorum sublimis	Lumbricales (digits one and two)
Flexor digitorum profundus	
Flexor pollicis longus	
Pronator quadratus	

from sleep. The pain is usually in the thumb and the index finger but may spread to other fingers or up the arm to the axilla. These symptoms most commonly occur in middle-aged persons and are often associated with arthritis or other changes in the tendons and connective tissues of the wrists in amyloid disease, myxedema, gout, or acromegaly. Surgical division of the transverse ligament results in relief of the pain and paresthesia and gradual decrease of the weakness.

Ulnar Nerve

The ulnar nerve is the main branch of the lower cord of the brachial plexus. The fibers arise from the eighth cervical and first thoracic segments. The motor fibers innervate the muscles listed in Table 68.6. The sensory portion of the nerve supplies the skin on the palmar and dorsal surfaces of the little finger, the inner one-half of the ring finger, and the ulnar side of the hand.

The ulnar nerve is frequently injured by gunshot wounds, stab wounds, and fractures of the lower end of the humerus, olecranon, or head of the radius. The nerve may be compressed in the axilla by a cervical rib. More frequently, it is compressed at the elbow in sleep or as an occupational neuritis in workers who rest their elbows on hard surfaces for prolonged periods.

Complete lesions of the ulnar nerve are characterized by weakness of flexion and adduction of the wrist and of flexion of the ring and the little fingers, paralysis of abduction and opposition of the little finger, paralysis of adduction of the thumb, and paralysis of adduction and abduction of the fingers. There is atrophy of the hypothenar muscles and the interossei. Atrophy of the first dorsal interosseous is especially obvious, seen on the dorsum of the hand between the thumb and the index finger. Sensory loss is greatest in the little finger and is present to a lesser extent on the inner side of the ring finger. There is clawing of the hand. Dissociated paralysis of the muscles supplied by the ulnar nerve may occur with partial lesions of the nerve in the arm or forearm.

Trophic and vasomotor symptoms are not prominent after complete lesions of the nerve. There may be some hyperkeratosis or changes in the palmar fascia. Irritative lesions may be accompanied by pain, but injuries to the ulnar nerve are only rarely accompanied by causalgia.

The diagnosis of ulnar palsy can usually be made without difficulty by the posture of the hand, which is always clawed, by atrophy of the hypothenar eminence and the first dorsal interosseous, and by the characteristic distribution of paralysis. One diagnostic sign of ulnar palsy, the Froment sign, is flexion of the terminal phalanx of the thumb when the patient attempts

to hold a sheet of paper between the thumb and the index finger (because the thumb cannot be adducted).

Musculocutaneous Nerve

The musculocutaneous nerve is the main branch of the upper trunk of the brachial plexus. Its fibers arise in the fifth and sixth cervical segments. The musculocutaneous nerve is a mixed nerve, innervating the coracobrachialis, biceps brachii, and brachialis muscles and transmitting cutaneous sensation from the anterior outer part and a small area on the posterior outer surface of the forearm. Isolated injuries of the nerve are rare. It may be involved in traumatic lesions of the brachial plexus.

Lesions of the musculocutaneous nerve produce weakness of flexion and supination of the forearm, a small area of hypesthesia or anesthesia on the anterior outer surface of the forearm, atrophy of the muscles on the anterior surface of the arm, and loss of the biceps reflex. Flexor movements of the forearm can still be vigorously performed by the brachioradialis muscle, which is innervated by the radial nerve. If flexion is performed against resistance, palpation reveals that the biceps muscle is inactive. If the forearm is kept in supination, forearm flexion is impossible. Because the biceps is the chief supinator of the forearm, this movement is paralyzed. Loss of function of the coracobrachialis muscle is compensated for by the action of other adductor muscles of the arm.

Axillary Nerve

The axillary nerve is the last branch of the posterior cord of the brachial plexus, including fibers from the fifth and sixth cervical segments. It innervates the deltoid muscle and transmits cutaneous sensation from a small area on the lateral surface of the shoulder.

Lesions of the axillary nerve caused by trauma or by fracture or dislocation of the head of the humerus are usually associated with injury to the brachial plexus. The axillary nerve may be involved alone or in combination with other nerves in the neuritis that follows serum (especially antitetanus) therapy. Lesions of the axillary nerve are characterized by loss of power in outward, backward, and forward movements of the arm because of paralysis of the deltoid muscle. The area of hypesthesia or anesthesia is inconstant and is much smaller than the anatomic distribution of the nerve.

Long Thoracic Nerve

The long thoracic nerve arises from the fifth, sixth, and seventh cervical roots. It is the motor nerve to the serratus anterior muscle.

Lesions of the long thoracic nerve are most common in men who do heavy labor. The nerve may be injured by continued muscular effort with the arm extended or by the carrying of heavy sharp-cornered objects on the shoulder ("hod carrier's palsy"). Injury of the nerve following acute or chronic trauma is characterized by weakness in elevation of the arm above the horizontal plane. Winging of the scapula is a constant sign when the arm is fully abducted or elevated anteriorly (Fig. 68.2). Winging is usually absent when the arm is held at the side.

TABLE 68.6. MUSCLES INNERVATED BY THE ULNAR NERVE

Flexor carpi ulnaris	All interossei
Flexor digitorum profundus (digits four and five)	Lumbricales (digits three and four)
Palmaris brevis	Flexor pollicis brevis
Abductor digiti minimi	
Opponens digiti minimi	
Flexor digiti minimi	

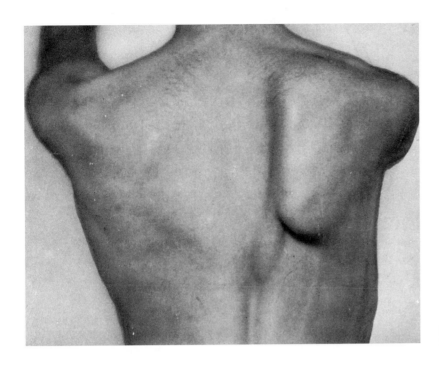

FIG. 68.2. Paralysis of the serratus magnus muscle with winging of the scapula.

Brachial Cutaneous and Antebrachial Cutaneous Nerves

The brachial and antebrachial cutaneous nerves, branches of the plexus (C8-T1), transmit sensory impulses from the inner surface of the arm and upper two-thirds of the forearm. These nerves are rarely affected, except in injuries of the medial cord of the brachial plexus. Lesions of these nerves produce hypesthesia on the inner surface of the arm and forearm.

Suprascapular Nerve

The suprascapular nerve arises from the upper trunk of the brachial plexus. Most of its fibers come from the fifth and sixth cervical roots. It is primarily motor and innervates the supraspinatus and infraspinatus muscles.

Isolated lesions of the nerve are rare. It may be wounded directly, injured in falls, or stretched by muscular overaction. It may be involved in association with the axillary nerve in serum reactions, or it may be injured in traumatic lesions of the brachial plexus. Lesions of the nerve produce an atrophic paralysis of the supraspinatus and infraspinatus muscles. Weakness of movements performed by these muscles (i.e., abduction and external rotation of the shoulder) is masked by the action of the deltoid and teres minor muscles.

Brachial Plexus

The fifth, sixth, seventh, and eighth cervical roots and the first thoracic root contribute to the formation of the brachial plexus (Fig. 68.3). The roots form three trunks: upper, middle, and lower. The upper is composed of fibers from C-5 and C-6, the middle receives fibers from C-7, and the lower receives fibers from C-8 and T-1. The redistribution of fibers from the trunks

results in the formation of the cords (lateral, posterior, and medial) that contribute to the formation of the peripheral nerves as follows: lateral cord, the musculocutaneous and the lateral head of the median nerve; posterior cord, the axillary and radial nerves; the medial cord, the brachial and antebrachial cutaneous nerves, the ulnar nerve, and the medial head of the median nerve.

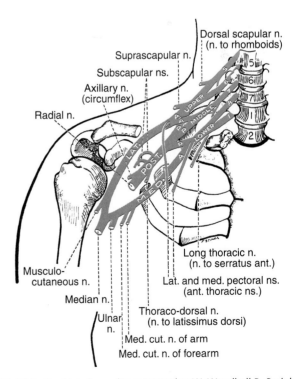

FIG. 68.3. Brachial plexus. (From Haymaker W, Woodhall B. *Peripheal nerve injuries.* Philadelphia: WB Saunders, 1945; with permission.)

In addition to these major nerves, which are formed by fibers in the secondary trunks, collateral branches from the roots and trunks form nerves that innervate the shoulder and scapular muscles and supply fibers to the interior cervical ganglion.

The roots or trunks of the brachial plexus may be damaged by cuts, gunshot wounds, or direct trauma (Fig. 68.4). They may be compressed by tumors or aneurysms or stretched and torn by violent movements of the shoulder in falls, dislocations of the shoulder, the carrying of heavy packs on the shoulder ("rucksack paralysis"), and traction in delivery at birth.

Unilateral or bilateral disorders of the brachial plexus may follow respiratory infections. The combination of local pain, weakness, and wasting of muscle had led to the popular terms *neuralgic amyotrophy* and *brachial plexopathy*. Weakness is maximal within a few days. The cerebrospinal fluid is normal. A similar disorder may affect the lumbosacral plexus. Myelography excludes intraspinal lesions. Nerve conduction studies may localize lesions of the brachial plexus. The condition remains stable for days or weeks and then improves. Some patients recover completely; others are left with moderate or severe disability.

Various complex syndromes result from injuries to the plexus. Only the trunk syndromes are reviewed here. A minute examination of muscular and sensory disability must be made and studied in connection with anatomic charts of the plexus to determine the site of the lesion and whether the fibers have been injured at their point of emergence from the spinal cord or after the formation of the primary or secondary trunks (Tables 68.7, 68.8, and 68.9).

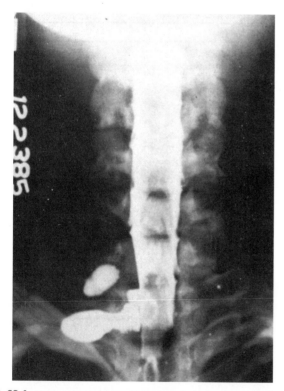

FIG. 68.4. Traumatic avulsion of lower cervical nerve roots. Iophendylate cervical myelogram (anteroposterior view) demonstrates contrast in avulsed right C-8 and T-1 root pouches. (Courtesy of Dr. S.K. Hilal and Dr. J.A. Bello.)

TABLE 68.7. INNERVATION OF THE MUSCLES OF THE SHOULDER GIRDLE

Muscle	Nerve	Spinal nerve roots
Sternocleidomastoid	Accessory	X-I, C-2, C-3
Trapezius	Accessory	C-3, C-4
Serratus anterior	Long thoracic	C-5, C-7
Levator scapulae	Dorsal scapular	C-5, C-6
Rhomboideus major	Dorsal scapular	C-5, C-6
Rhomboideus minor	Dorsal scapular	C-5, C-6
Subclavius	Subclavian	C-5, C-6
Supraspinatus	Suprascapular	C-5, C-6
Infraspinatus	Suprascapular	C-5, C-6
Pectoralis major	Medial and lateral pectoralis	C-5, C-6
Pectoralis minor	Medial pectoralis	C-5, C-6
Teres major	Subscapular	C-5, C-6
Latissimus dorsi	Thoracodorsal	C-6, C-7
Subscapularis	Subscapular	C-5, C-6
Deltoid	Axillaris	C-5, C-6
Teres minor	Axillaris	C-5, C-6

Radicular Syndromes (Roots and Primary Trunks)

The syndromes of the roots and primary trunks are essentially those of the roots involved, but partial paralysis and incomplete sensory loss are common because many muscles of the arm receive innervation from two or more roots and there are extensive substitutions among the various roots.

Upper Radicular (Erb-Duchenne) Syndrome

Lesions of the upper roots (fourth, fifth, and sixth cervical roots or upper trunk) are characterized by paralysis of the deltoid, biceps, brachialis anticus, brachioradialis, pectoralis major, supraspinatus, infraspinatus, subscapularis, and teres major muscles. If the lesion is near the roots, the serratus magnus, rhomboids, and levator anguli scapulae are also paralyzed.

TABLE 68.8. INNERVATION OF MUSCLES OF THE ARM AND FOREARM

Muscle	Nerve	Root
Biceps brachii / Brachialis	Musculocutaneous	C-5, C-6
Triceps	Radialis	C-7, C-8
Anconeus	Radialis	C-7, C-8
Brachioradialis	Radialis	C-5, C-6
Extensor carpi radialis	Radialis	C-6, C-7
Pronator teres	Medianus	C-6, C-7
Flexor carpi radialis	Medianus	C-7, C-8
Palmaris longus	Medianus	C-7, C-8
Flexor digitorum sublimis	Medianus	C-7, C-8
Flexor digitorum profundus	Medianus, ulnaris	C-7, C-8
Flexor carpi ulnaris	Ulnaris	C-7, C-8
Supinator	Radialis	C-7, C-8
Extensor digitorum communis	Radialis	C-7, C-8
Extensor digiti minimi	Radialis	C-7, C-8
Extensor carpi ulnaris	Radialis	C-7, C-8
Abductor pollicis longus and brevis	Radialis	C-7, C-8
Extensor indicis proprius	Radialis	C-7, C-8

TABLE 68.9. INNERVATION OF THE MUSCLES OF THE HAND

Muscle	Nerve	Root
Palmaris brevis	Ulnar	C-8, T-1
Abductor pollicis	Median	C-8, T-1
Opponens pollicis	Median	C-6, C-7
Flexor brevis pollicis	Median	C-6, C-7
Abductor digiti minimi	Ulnar	C-8, T-1
Opponens digiti minimi	Ulnar	C-8, T-1
Flexor brevis digiti minimi	Ulnar	C-8, T-1
Lumbricales	Median, ulnar	C-8, T-1
Abductor pollicis	Ulnar	C-8, T-1
Interossei palmaris	Ulnar	C-8, T-1
Interossei dorsales	Ulnar	C-8, T-1

The motor disability resulting from lesions of the upper radicular group is essentially paralysis of flexion of the forearm and of abduction and internal and external rotation of the arm. There is also weakness or paralysis of apposition of the scapula and backward-inward movements of the arm. Sensory loss is incomplete and consists of hypesthesia on the outer surface of the arm and forearm. The biceps reflex is absent, and percussion of the styloid process of the radius produces flexion of the fingers instead of the normal flexion of the forearm.

Middle Radicular Syndrome

Injury to the seventh cervical root or the middle trunk causes paralysis of the muscles supplied by the radial nerve with the exception of the brachioradialis, which is spared entirely. Weakness is essentially similar to that seen in paralysis of the radial nerve below the origin of the fibers to the brachioradialis or in lead palsy. Sensory loss is inconstant and, when present, is limited to hypesthesia over the dorsal surface of the forearm and the external part of the dorsal surface of the hand.

Lower Radicular (Klumpke) Syndrome

Injury to the lower primary trunk or eighth cervical and first thoracic root is characterized by paralysis of the flexor carpi ulnaris, the flexor digitorum, the interossei, and the thenar and hypothenar muscles. The motor disability is similar to that of a combined lesion of the median and ulnar nerves with a flattened or simian hand.

The sensory disturbance is hypesthesia on the inner side of the arm and forearm and on the ulnar side of the hand. The triceps reflex is abolished. If the communicating branch to the inferior cervical ganglion is injured, there is paralysis of the sympathetic nerves, with resulting Horner syndrome.

Cord Syndromes of the Brachial Plexus

Lesions of the cords of the brachial plexus produce motor and sensory disturbances that resemble those seen after injuries to two or more peripheral nerves. The syndrome of the *lateral cord* is a combination of the signs and symptoms caused by injury to the musculocutaneous nerve and the lateral head of the median nerve. These injuries are accompanied by a paralysis of the pronator teres, almost complete paralysis of the flexor carpi radialis, and weakness of the flexor pollicis and opponens. Injury to the *posterior cord* produces paralysis similar to that resulting from injury to the radial and axillary nerves. The syndrome of the *medial cord* is the same as that of the ulnar nerve combined with a paralysis of flexion of the fingers as a result of injury to the medial head of the median nerve.

Ischemic Paralysis of the Arm

Paralysis of arm muscles may follow injury to large arteries. Ischemic paralysis may follow ligation of the major vessels when the collateral circulation is inadequate, or it may follow prolonged constriction of the arm by plaster casts.

In the initial stages of ischemic paralysis, the distal part of the limb is cyanotic and edematous. Active movements of the finger and wrist muscles are possible but are of a limited range. There is diminution of cutaneous sensibility; all stimuli are poorly localized and have a painful quality. With the passage of time, the cyanosis and edema disappear, the skin becomes smooth and shiny, and the muscles undergo fibrotic changes; anesthesia extends in a glovelike distribution to the wrist or middle of the forearm. The hand is held extended, and the fingers are slightly flexed except when there are associated nerve lesions.

Ischemic paralysis can be differentiated from paralysis caused by lesions of the nerves by the absence of pulsations in the radial artery, the glovelike distribution of sensory loss, which does not correspond to that of any peripheral nerve, the fibrous consistency of the tissues, and, in some cases, persistence of feeble imperfect movements of some of the muscles.

Ischemic paralysis is frequently permanent. Improvement in some patients can be obtained by hot baths, massage, passive movements, and electrical stimulation.

NERVES OF THE LEG

Obturator Nerve

The obturator nerve is a mixed nerve that originates in the lumbar plexus from the second, third, and fourth lumbar roots. It transmits cutaneous sensation from a small area on the inner surface of the middle side of the hip, thigh, and knee joint. It innervates the obturator externus muscle, adductor longus, adductor brevis, gracilis, and adductor magnus muscles.

Lesions of the obturator nerve are uncommon. It may be injured by pressure within the pelvis by tumors, obturator hernias, or the fetal head in difficult labor. Injuries to the obturator nerve result in severe weakness of adduction and, to a lesser extent, internal and external rotation of the thigh. Pain in the knee joint is sometimes caused by pelvic involvement of the geniculate branch of the obturator.

Iliohypogastric Nerve

The iliohypogastric nerve is a mixed nerve that originates from the uppermost part of the lumbar plexus and is derived from the twelfth thoracic and first lumbar roots. It transmits cutaneous sensation from the outer and upper parts of the buttocks and the lower part of the abdomen and supplies partial innervation to the internal oblique and transversalis muscles. Lesions of the iliohypogastric nerve are rare. It may be divided by incisions in kidney operations or together with the ilioinguinal nerve in operations in the inguinal region. Lesions of these nerves do not produce any significant motor loss, and there is only a small area of cutaneous anesthesia.

Ilioinguinal Nerve

The ilioinguinal nerve, a branch of the lumbar plexus, arises from the twelfth thoracic and first lumbar roots. It transmits cutaneous sensation from the upper inner portion of the thigh, the pubic region, and the external genitalia. Motor filaments are given off to the transversalis, internal oblique, and external oblique muscles. The ilioinguinal nerve is usually injured in connection with the iliohypogastric nerve.

Genitofemoral Nerve

This nerve originates from the second lumbar root and is primarily a sensory nerve. It transmits cutaneous sensation from an oval area on the thigh in the region of the Scarpa triangle and from the scrotum and the contiguous area of the inner surface of the thigh. Lesions of the genitofemoral nerve are rare. Irritative lesions of the nerve in the abdominal wall are accompanied by painful hyperesthesia at the root of the thigh and the scrotum.

Lateral Cutaneous Nerve of Thigh

This nerve is formed by fibers from the second and third lumbar roots. It crosses beneath the fascia iliaca to emerge at the antero-superior iliac spine, descends in the thigh beneath the fascia lata, and divides into two branches. The posterior branch passes obliquely backward through the fascia lata and transmits cutaneous sensation from the superior external part of the buttocks. The anterior branch, which is more important clinically, pierces the fascia lata through a small fibrous canal about 10 cm below the ligament and transmits cutaneous fibrous sensation from the outer surface of the thigh.

The anterior portion of the nerve is occasionally the site of *meralgia paresthetica,* which is a sensory neuritis with dysesthesia in the nature of tingling, burning, prickling, or pins-and-needles sensations with or without sensory loss in the cutaneous distribution of the nerve. The long superficial course exposes it to various forms of trauma, but in most patients there is no history of trauma to explain the onset of symptoms. Various factors said to play a contributing role include pressure of tight belts or corsets and intermittent stretching by extensor movements of the thigh during walking. The involvement is unilateral in most cases. Men are affected about three times as frequently as women.

The diagnosis is not difficult when the dysesthesia is limited to the distribution of the anterior division of the nerve. Pains in the lateral surface of the thigh caused by spinal lesions or pelvic tumors must be excluded by appropriate diagnostic studies.

The course of meralgia paresthetica is variable. Occasionally, symptoms spontaneously disappear after a few weeks. In most patients, they clear up by the removal of tight belts and avoidance of excessive walking. It is rarely necessary to split the fascia

lata at the point of emergence of the nerve or correct the angulation of the nerve at the iliac spine.

Femoral Nerve

The femoral nerve arises from the second, third, and fourth lumbar nerves. It innervates the iliacus, psoas magnus, pectineus, sartorius, and quadriceps femoris muscles. It also transmits cutaneous sensation from the anterior surface of the thigh and, by its internal saphenous branch, from the entire inner surface of the leg and the anterior internal surface of the knee.

Traumatic lesions of the femoral nerve are uncommon. It may be compressed by tumors and other lesions in the pelvis, or it may be injured by fractures of the pubic ramus or femur. Often, there is no adequate explanation for the occurrence of an isolated femoral nerve palsy. In such cases, the nerve lesion is presumed to be a result of some toxic factor, such as diabetes, typhoid, or gout.

Injury to the femoral nerve produces paralysis of extension of the leg and weakness of flexion of the thigh. When the patient stands erect, the leg is held stiffly extended by contraction of the tensor fasciae femoris and the gracilis. Walking on level ground is possible as long as the leg can be kept extended, but if the slightest flexion occurs, the patient sinks down on the suddenly flexed knee. Climbing stairs or walking uphill is difficult or impossible. The quadriceps reflex is lost on the affected side, and cutaneous sensation is impaired in an area somewhat smaller than the anatomic distribution of the nerve.

Paralysis of the femoral nerve must be distinguished from hysterical paralysis and reflex muscular atrophies that follow fractures of the femur or lesions of the knee joint. Hysteric paralysis can be diagnosed by the presence of the knee jerk and by special tests. In hysteric paralysis, when the patient is in the recumbent position and attempts to elevate the "paralyzed" limb, there is an absence of the normal fixing movements (downward pressure of the heel) of the opposite leg (*Hoover sign*).

Orthopedic appliances that fix the knee joint in extension are of value in the treatment of femoral nerve paralysis. Transposition of tendons should be considered if paralysis persists.

Sciatic Nerve

The sciatic nerve is the largest nerve in the body. Its terminal branches consist of two distinct nerves, which are antagonists of each other: the common peroneal (external popliteal) and the tibial (internal popliteal) nerves. The common peroneal arises from the posterior and the tibial nerve from the anterior portion of the sacral plexus (i.e., L-4 to S-3). The main trunk of the sciatic nerve innervates the semitendinosus, the long and short heads of the biceps, the adductor magnus, and the semimembranosus muscles. The terminal branches of the nerve are considered separately in the following sections.

Total paralysis of muscles innervated by the sciatic nerve is rare; even with a lesion in the thigh, the common peroneal nerve is often more severely damaged than the tibial nerve. The sciatic nerve is frequently injured by gunshot, shrapnel, or stab wounds, although it is rarely injured in civilian life. Partial rupture may result from violent muscular contractions, or the nerve may be injured by fractures of the pelvis or femur, dislocations of the hip, pressure of the fetal head on the plexus in the mother's pelvis, or pelvic tumors. The nerve is sometimes inadvertently injured by intramuscular injection of drugs, especially in infants.

Total involvement of the sciatic nerve produces complete paralysis of all movements of the ankle and toes, as well as weakness or paralysis of flexion of the leg. The patient can stand, but the leg must be raised unduly high to correct for the footdrop when the patient walks (steppage gait). The ankle jerk is lost, and cutaneous sensation is lost on the outer surface of the leg, on the instep and sole of the foot, and over the toes. Vasomotor and trophic disturbances may also be present.

Sciatica is a term used to describe pain in the low back and in the leg along the course of the nerve. The symptoms may be caused by involvement of any portion of the nerve, including the intraspinal roots. In the older literature, the list of causes of sciatica was long and included alcohol, arsenic, lead, diabetes, gout, syphilis, gonorrhea, phlebitis, tuberculosis, arthritis of the sacroiliac joint or of the hip, fibrositis, gluteal bursitis, osteitis deformans, pelvic tumors, and inflammatory neuritis. Although pain in the low back that extends down the posterior surface of the leg may be associated with pathologic processes in the pelvis or lower spine, in most patients sciatic pain is caused by a ruptured intervertebral disc. The distinctive features of ruptured intervertebral discs are considered more fully in Chapter 65.

Sciatica is most common in the third to sixth decades of life and occurs about three times more frequently in men than in women. The pain of sciatica varies in severity. In some patients, there is a feeling of discomfort in the low back and down the posterior surface of the leg. In others, the pain may be so intense that it totally incapacitates the afflicted individual. The pain may be limited to the buttocks and sacroiliac region, it may extend only to the knee, or it may involve the calf and outer surface of the foot. There is usually no weakness, but the patient may keep the knee slightly flexed in walking to prevent stretching of the nerve. On examination, the nerve may be sensitive to pressure at any point along its course. Any movement of the leg that stretches the nerve is accompanied by pain and involuntary resistance to the movement. There is limitation of straight leg raising on the affected side, and complete extension of the leg is not possible when the hip is flexed. Similar movements of the unaffected limb can be performed more fully but may cause slight pain on the opposite side. Sensory loss and loss of the Achilles reflex are rarely found in sciatica associated with osteoarthritis of the spine or sacroiliac joint, and suggest involvement of the nerve roots in the spinal canal. The clinical course of sciatica depends on the nature of the underlying disorder. In most patients, the symptoms last for weeks or months and disappear, only to recur after a remission of months or years.

Diagnosis of sciatic and low back pain may be difficult. Diagnosis rests on the history, findings on examination, and CT or MRI of the spine. Contrast CT-myelography may be needed. The results of these studies can determine whether the symptoms are caused by a ruptured intervertebral disc, primary or metastatic tumor of the spine, osteoarthritic changes, or other causes.

The treatment of sciatica is essentially that of the underlying

cause. The criteria for the operative removal of ruptured intervertebral discs are reviewed in Chapter 65. The treatment of causalgic pain after trauma to the sciatic nerve is reviewed in Chapter 70.

Common Peroneal (External Popliteal) Nerve

The common peroneal is a mixed nerve that innervates the extensor muscles of the ankle and toes and the evertor (abductor) muscles of the foot. It transmits cutaneous sensation from the outer side of the leg, the front of its lower one-third, the instep, and the dorsal surface of the four inner toes over their proximal phalanges.

The common peroneal nerve is more frequently subjected to trauma than any other nerve of the body. It may be damaged by wounds near the knee or in the trunk of the sciatic nerve in the thigh. Because of its superficial position in close relation to the head and neck of the fibula, it is readily injured by pressure against hard objects while the patient is asleep, intoxicated, or under anesthesia. It may be stretched by prolonged squatting or compressed by crossing of the knees during sitting or by lying on a hard or uneven mattress during sleep, especially in acutely or chronically ill patients. Many cases of simple pressure neuropathy of the common peroneal nerve are falsely recorded as being caused by malarial, typhoid, or tuberculous neuritis. The nerve may be injured by ganglion cysts, which can usually be palpated at the head of the fibula. Compression of the nerve in this way leads to footdrop with burning pains on the lateral aspect of the leg and in the ankle or foot. Symptoms can be relieved by excision of the cyst.

Paralysis of the common peroneal nerve results in footdrop and inversion of the foot. The patient cannot dorsiflex the ankle, straighten or extend the toes, or evert the foot. The gait is characterized by overflexion of the knee in the steppage gait. Sensation is lost in an area less extensive than the anatomic distribution of the nerve, or it may be entirely absent when the injury is caused by pressure. Vasomotor and trophic disturbances consisting of swelling, local cyanosis, and anhidrosis may also be present.

Complete or partial recovery is the rule when the paralysis is caused by transient pressure. Treatment consists of physiotherapy and the use of a foot brace to overcome the footdrop.

Tibial (Internal Popliteal) Nerve

The tibial branch of the sciatic nerve innervates the muscles on the posterior surface of the leg and the plantar muscles. It transmits sensation from the entire sole of the foot, the back and lower part to the middle one-third of the leg, the outer dorsal surface of the foot, and the terminal phalanges of the toes.

Lesions of the tibial nerve are uncommon. It may be injured by gunshot wounds or fractures of the legs. A complete lesion of the nerve is characterized by paralysis of plantar flexion and adduction of the foot, flexion and separation of the toes, and sensory loss in an area less extensive than the anatomic distribution of the nerve. The ankle jerk and plantar reflex are lost. Causalgia is occasionally seen. Compression of the posterior tibial branch at the medial malleolus produces pain and paresthesia in the soles of the feet in a manner similar to compression of the median nerve at the wrist. Decompression results in the relief of symptoms.

SUGGESTED READINGS

General

Aminofff MJ. *Electromyography in clinical practice: clinical and electrodiagnostic aspects of neuromuscular disease,* 3rd ed. New York: Churchill Livingstone, 1998.

Dubuisson A, Kline DG. Indications for peripheral nerve and brachial plexus surgery. *Neurol Clin* 1992;10:935–951.

Dyck PJ, Thomas PK, Griffin JW, Low PA, Poduslo JF, eds. *Peripheral neuropathy,* 3rd ed. Philadelphia: WB Saunders, 1993.

Haymaker W, Woodhall B. *Peripheral nerve injuries,* 2nd ed. Philadelphia: WB Saunders, 1953.

Kimura J. *Electrodiagnosis in diseases of nerve and muscle: principles and practice,* 3rd ed. Philadelphia: FA Davis Co, 1992.

Liguori R, Krarup C, Trojaborg W. Determination of the segmental sensory and motor innervation of the lumbosacral spinal nerves. *Brain* 1992;115:915–934.

Parry GJ. Electrodiagnostic studies in the evaluation of peripheral nerve and brachial plexus injuries. *Neurol Clin* 1992;10:921–934.

Petrera J, Trojaborg W. Conduction studies of the long thoracic nerve in serratus anterior palsy of different etiology. *Neurology* 1984;34:1033–1037.

Stuart JD. *Focal peripheral neuropathies,* 2nd ed. New York: Raven Press, 1993.

Sunderland S. *Nerves and nerve injuries,* 2nd ed. Edinburgh: Churchill Livingstone, 1979.

Tinel J. *Nerve wounds: symptomatology of peripheral nerve lesions caused by war wounds.* London: Balliere, Tindall and Cox, 1917.

Cranial Nerves

Auger RG, Pipegras DG, Laws ER Jr. Hemifacial spasm: results of microvascular decompression of the facial nerve in 54 patients. *Mayo Clin Proc* 1986;61:640–644.

Boghen DR, Glaser JS. Ischemic optic neuropathy: the clinical profile and natural history. *Brain* 1975;98:689–708.

Brin MF, Blitzer A, Stewart C, Fahn S. Treatment of spasmodic dysphonia (laryngeal dystonia) with local injections of botulinum toxin: review and technical aspects. In: Blitzer A, Brin MF, Sasaki CT, Fahn S, Harris KS, eds. *Neurological disorders of the larynx.* New York: Thieme Medical Publishers, 1992.

Brisman R. Trigeminal neuralgia and multiple sclerosis. *Arch Neurol* 1987;44:379–381.

Carruthers J, Stubbs HA. Botulinum toxin for benign essential blepharospasm, hemifacial spasm and age-related lower eyelid entropion. *Can J Neurol Sci* 1987;14:4245–4248.

Ceylan S, Karakus A, Duru S, Koca O. Glossopharyngeal neuralgia: a study of 6 cases. *Neurosurg Rev* 1997;20:196–200.

Cohn DF, Carasso R, Steifler M. Painful ophthalmoplegia: the Tolosa-Hunt syndrome. *Eur Neurol* 1979;18:373–381.

De Diego JI, Prim MP, De Sarria MJ, et al. Idiopathic facial paralysis: a randomized, prospective, and controlled study using single-dose prednisone versus acyclovir three times daily. *Laryngoscope* 1998;108:573–575.

Dunphy EB. Alcohol-tobacco amblyopia: a historical survey. *Am J Ophthalmol* 1969;68:569–578.

Ehni G, Woltman HWW. Hemifacial spasm: review of 106 cases. *Arch Neurol Psychiatry* 1945;53:205–211.

Evidente VG, Adler CH. Hemifacial spasm and other craniofacial movement disorders. *Mayo Clin Proc* 1998;73:67–71.

Ford FR, Woodhall B. Phenomena due to misdirection of regenerating fibers of cranial, spinal and autonomic nerves: clinical observations. *Arch Surg* 1938;36:480–496.

Friedman AP, Merritt HH. Damage to cranial nerves resulting from head injury. *Bull Los Angeles Neurol Soc* 1944;9:135–139.

Furuta Y, Fukuda S, Chida E, et al. Reactivation of herpes simplex virus type 1 in patients with Bell's palsy. *J Med Virol* 1998;54:162–166.

Geller BD, Hallett M, Ravits J. Botulinum toxin therapy in hemifacial spasm: clinical and electrophysiologic studies. *Muscle Nerve* 1989;12:716–722.

Glocker FX, Krauss JK, Deuschl G, et al. Hemifacial spasm due to posterior fossa tumors: the impact of tumor location on electrophysiological findings. *Clin Neurol Neurosurg* 1998;100:104–111.

Gouda JJ, Brown JA. Atypical facial pain and other pain syndromes: differential diagnosis and treatment. *Neurosurg Clin N Am* 1997;8:87–100.

Jankovic J, Ford J. Blepharospasm and orofacial-cervical dystonia: clinical and pharmacological findings in 100 patients. *Ann Neurol* 1983;13:402–411.

Jannetta P. Observations on the etiology of trigeminal neuralgia, hemifacial spasm, acoustic nerve dysfunction and glossopharyngeal neuralgia: definitive microsurgical treatment and results in 11 patients. *Neurochirurgie* 1977;20:145–154.

Jitpimolmard S, Tiamkao S, Laopaiboon M. Long-term results of botulinum toxin type A (Dysport) in the treatment of hemifacial spasm: a report of 175 cases. *J Neurol Neurosurg Psychiatry* 1998;64:751–757.

Juncos JL, Beal MF. Idiopathic cranial polyneuropathy: a 5-year experience. *Brain* 1987;110:197–212.

Kalovidouris A, Mancuso AA, Dillon W. A CT-clinical approach to patients with symptoms related to the V, VII, IX–XII cranial nerves and cervical sympathetics. *Radiology* 1984;151:671–676.

Kondo A. Follow-up results of microvascular decompression in trigeminal neuralgia and hemifacial spasm. *Neurosurgery* 1997;40:46–51.

Kondziolka D, Perez B, Flickinger JC, et al. Gamma knife radiosurgery for trigeminal neuralgia: results and expectations. *Arch Neurol* 1998;55:1524–1529.

Lecky BRF, Hughes RAC, Murray NMF. Trigeminal sensory neuropathy. *Brain* 1987;110:1463–1486.

Leigh RJ, Zee DS. *The neurology of eye movements,* 2nd ed. Philadelphia: FA Davis Co, 1991.

Lossos A, Siegal T. Numb chin syndrome in cancer patients: etiology, response to treatment, and prognostic significance. *Neurology* 1992;42:1181–1184.

Ludlow CL, Naunton RF, Fujita M, et al. Effects of botulinum toxin injections on speech in adductor spasmodic dysphonia. *Neurology* 1988;38:1220–1225.

Majoie CB, Hulsmans FJ, Castelijns JA, et al. Symptoms and signs related to the trigeminal nerve: diagnostic yield of MR imaging. *Radiology* 1998;209:557–562.

Murakami S, Nakashiro Y, Mizobuchi M, et al. Varicella-zoster virus distribution in Ramsay Hunt syndrome revealed by polymerase chain reaction. *Acta Otolaryngol* 1998;118:145–149.

Nadeau SE, Trobe JD. Pupil sparing in oculomotor palsy: a brief review. *Ann Neurol* 1983;13:143–148.

Nielsen VK. Electrophysiology of the facial nerve in hemifacial spasm: ectopic/ephaptic excitation. *Muscle Nerve* 1985;8:545–555.

Pearce JM. Melkersson's syndrome. *J Neurol Neurosurg Psychiatry* 1995;58:340.

Pollock BE, Gorman DA, Schomberg PJ, Kline RW. The Mayo Clinic gamma knife experience: indications and initial results. *Mayo Clin Proc* 1999;74:5–13.

Portenoy RK, Duma C, Foley KM. Acute herpetic and postherpetic neuralgia: clinical review and current management. *Ann Neurol* 1986;20:651–664.

Rush JA, Younge BR. Paralysis of cranial nerves III, IV and VI: cause and prognosis in 1,000 cases. *Arch Ophthalmol* 1981;99:76–79.

Ryu H, Yamamoto S, Sugiyama K, et al. Hemifacial spasm caused by vascular compression of the distal portion of the facial nerve: report of seven cases. *J Neurosurg* 1998;88:605–609.

Searles RP, Mladinich K, Messner RP. Isolated trigeminal sensory neuropathy: early manifestations of mixed connective tissue disease. *Neurology* 1978;28:1286–1289.

Spillane JD, Wells CEC. Isolated trigeminal neuropathy. *Brain* 1959;82:391–416.

Stevens H. Melkersson's syndrome. *Neurology* 1965;15:263–266.

Tankere F, Maisonobe T, Lamas G, et al. Electrophysiological determination of the site involved in generating abnormal muscle responses in hemifacial spasm. *Muscle Nerve* 1998;21:1013–1018.

Taylor FH. Idiopathic Bell's facial palsy: natural history defies steroid and surgical treatment. *Laryngoscope* 1985;95:406–409.

Tenser RB. Trigeminal neuralgia: mechanisms of treatment. *Neurology* 1998;51:17–19.

Troost BT, Daroff RB. The ocular motor defects in progressive supranuclear palsy. *Ann Neurol* 1977;2:397–403.

Van Zandycke M, Martin JJ, Vande Gaer L, Van den Heyning P. Facial myokymia in the Guillain-Barré syndrome: a clinicopathologic study. *Neurology* 1982;32:744–748.

Victor M, Dreyfus PM. Tobacco-alcohol ambylopia: further comments on its pathology. *Arch Ophthalmol* 1965;74:649–657.

Wang A, Jankovic J. Hemifacial spasm: clinical findings and treatment. *Muscle Nerve* 1998;21:1740–1747.

Wartenberg R. *Hemifacial spasm: a clinical and pathological study.* London: Oxford University Press, 1952.

Willoughby EW, Anderson NE. Lower cranial nerve motor function in unilateral vascular lesions of the cerebral hemisphere. *BMJ* 1984;289:791–794.

Peripheral Nerves

Bowsher D. The management of postherpetic neuralgia. *Postgrad Med J* 1997;73:623–629.

Buchthal F, Rosenfalck A, Trojaborg W. Electrophysiological findings in entrapment of the median nerve at the wrist and elbow. *J Neurol Neurosurg Psychiatry* 1974;37:340–360.

Choi PD, Novak CB, Mackinnon SE, Kline DG. Quality of life and functional outcome following brachial plexus injury. *J Hand Surg [Am]* 1997;22:605–612.

D'Amour ML, Lebrun LH, Rabbat A, et al. Peripheral neurological complications of aortoiliac vascular disease. *Can J Neurol Sci* 1987;14:127–130.

Dawson DM. Entrapment neuropathies of the upper extremities. *N Engl J Med* 1993;329:2013–2018.

Dubuisson A, Kline DG. Indications for peripheral nerve and brachial plexus surgery. *Neurol Clin* 1992;10:935–951.

Friedman AH, Nashold BS Jr, Ovelmen-Levitt J. Dorsal root entry zone lesions for the treatment of postherpetic neuralgia. *J Neurosurg* 1984;60:1258–1262.

Gilliatt RW. Acute compression block. In: Sumner AJ, ed. *The physiology of peripheral nerve disease.* Philadelphia: WB Saunders, 1980.

Gilliatt RW, Willison RG, Dietz V, et al. Peripheral nerve conduction in patients with a cervical rib and band. *Ann Neurol* 1978;4:124–129.

Gossett JG, Chance PF. Is there a familial carpal tunnel syndrome? An evaluation and literature review. *Muscle Nerve* 1998;21:1533–1536.

Kline DG, Kim D, Midha R, et al. Management and results of sciatic nerve injuries: a 24-year experience. *J Neurosurg* 1998;89:13–23.

Kori SH, Foley KM, Posner JB. Brachial plexus lesions in patients with cancer: 100 cases. *Neurology* 1981;31:45–50.

Liguori R, Krarup C, Trojaborg W. Determination of the segmental sensory and motor innervation of the lumbosacral spinal nerves. *Brain* 1992;115:915–934.

Mastroianni PP, Roberts MP. Femoral neuropathy and retroperitoneal hemorrhage. *Neurosurgery* 1983;13:44–47.

Miller RG. Injury to peripheral nerves. *Muscle Nerve* 1987;10:698–710.

Morris HH, Peters PH. Pronator syndrome: clinical and electrophysiological features in seven cases. *J Neurol Neurosurg Psychiatry* 1976;39:461–464.

Nakano KK, Lundergan C, Okharo MM. Anterior interosseous syndromes:

diagnostic methods and alternative treatments. *Arch Neurol* 1977;34:477–480.

Oberle J, Kahamba J, Richter HP. Peripheral nerve schwannomas: an analysis of 16 patients. *Acta Neurochir (Wien)* 1997;139:949–953.

Petrera J, Trojaborg W. Conduction studies of the long thoracic nerve in serratus anterior palsy of different etiology. *Neurology* 1984;34:1033–1037.

Rempel D, Evanoff B, Amadio PC, et al. Consensus criteria for the classification of carpal tunnel syndrome in epidemiologic studies. *Am J Public Health* 1998;88:1447–1451.

Rowbotham M, Harden N, Stacey B, et al. Gabapentin for the treatment of postherpetic neuralgia: a randomized, controlled trial. *JAMA* 1998;280:1837–1842.

Seddon HJ. *Peripheral nerve injuries: Medical Research Council special report, series no. 282.* London: Her Majesty's Stationery Office, 1954.

Thomas JE, Pipegras DG, Scheithauer B, et al. Neurogenic tumors of the sciatic nerve: a clinicopathologic study of 35 cases. *Mayo Clin Proc* 1983;58:640–647.

Trojaborg W. Rate of recovery in motor and sensory fibres of the radial nerve. *J Neurol Neurosurg Psychiatry* 1970;33:625–638.

Trojaborg W. Early electrophysiological changes in conduction block. *Muscle Nerve* 1978;1:400–403.

Watson CP, Babul N. Efficacy of oxycodone in neuropathic pain: a randomized trial in postherpetic neuralgia. *Neurology* 1998;50:1837–1841.

Watson CP, Vernich L, Chipman M, et al. Nortriptyline versus amitriptyline in postherpetic neuralgia: a randomized trial. *Neurology* 1998;51:1166–1171.

Wiles CM, Whitehead S, Ward AB, Fletcher CDM. Not tarsal tunnel syndrome: a malignant "triton" tumour of the tibial nerve. *J Neurol Neurosurg Psychiatry* 1987;50:479–482.

Wulff CH, Hansen K, Strange P, Trojaborg W. Multiple mononeuritis and radiculitis with erythema, pain, elevated CSF protein and pleocytosis (Bannwarth's syndrome). *J Neurol Neurosurg Psychiatry* 1983;46:485–490.

Brachial Plexus and Lumbosacral Plexus

England JD, Sumner AJ. Neuralgic amyotrophy: an increasingly diverse entity. *Muscle Nerve* 1987;10:60–68.

Evans BA, Stevens JC, Dyck PJ. Lumbosacral plexus neuropathy. *Neurology* 1981;31:1327–1331.

Parry GJ. Electrodiagnosis studies in the evaluation of peripheral nerve and brachial plexus injuries. *Neurol Clin* 1992;10:921–934.

Pellegrino JE, George RA, Biegel J, et al. Hereditary neuralgic amyotrophy: evidence for genetic homogeneity and mapping to chromosome 17q25. *Hum Genet* 1997;101:277–283.

Shinder N, Polson A, Pringle E, O'Donnell DE. Neuralgic amyotrophy: a rare cause of bilateral diaphragmatic paralysis. *Can Respir J* 1998;5:139–142.

Subramony SH. Neuralgic amyotrophy (acute brachial neuropathy). *Muscle Nerve* 1988;11:39–44.

Swash M. Diagnosis of brachial root and plexus lesions. *J Neurol* 1986;233:131–135.

Thyagarajan D, Cascino T, Harms G. Magnetic resonance imaging in brachial plexopathy of cancer. *Neurology* 1995;45:421–427.

Trojaborg W. Electrophysiological finding in pressure palsy of the brachial plexus. *J Neurol Neurosurg Psychiatry* 1977;40:1160–1167.

Tsairis P, Dyck P, Mulder D. Natural history of brachial plexus neuropathy. *Arch Neurol* 1972;27:109–117.

Wouter van Es H, Engelen AM, Witkamp TD, et al. Radiation-induced brachial plexopathy: MR imaging. *Skeletal Radiol* 1997;26:284–288.

Merritt's Neurology, 10th ed., edited by L.P. Rowland. Lippincott Williams & Wilkins, Philadelphia © 2000.

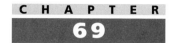

THORACIC OUTLET SYNDROME

LEWIS P. ROWLAND

The term *thoracic outlet syndrome* encompasses different syndromes that arise from compression of the nerves in the brachial plexus or blood vessels (subclavian or axillary arteries, or veins in the same area). The compressing lesions are also diverse.

How often these lesions are actually responsible for symptoms and how the symptoms should be treated are matters of intense debate. Studies done mainly by orthopedists, vascular surgeons, and neurosurgeons have included reports on several hundred patients who were treated surgically for this syndrome. When neurologists write about this neurologic disorder, however, the tone is always skeptical, and the syndrome is described as exceedingly rare, with an annual incidence of about 1 per 1 million persons. The debate warrants separate consideration, although this is actually another disorder of the peripheral nervous system.

PATHOLOGY

The T-1 and C-8 nerve roots and the lower trunk of the brachial plexus are exposed to compression and angulation by anatomic anomalies that include cervical ribs and fibrous bands of uncertain origin. Among the more imaginative lesions are those ascribed to hypertrophy of the scalenus muscles. Cervical ribs are commonly found in asymptomatic people, and it is difficult to assume that the mere presence of a cervical rib automatically explains local symptoms. In addition to the neural syndromes, the same anomalies may compress local blood vessels and cause vascular syndromes.

SYMPTOMS AND SIGNS

Patients have pain in the shoulder, arm, or hand, or in all three locations. The hand pain is often most severe in the fourth and fifth fingers. The pain is aggravated by use of the arm, and "fatigue" of the arm is often prominent. There may or may not be hypesthesia in the affected area.

Critics have divided cases into two groups: those with the "true" neurogenic thoracic outlet syndrome and those with the "disputed" syndrome. In the *true* syndrome, there are definite clinical and electrodiagnostic abnormalities. This syndrome is rare but is almost always caused by a cervical band extending from a cervical rib and compressing the C-8 and T-1 roots or lower brachial plexus. There is unequivocal wasting and weakness of muscles in the hand that are innervated by these segments, and results of electromyography and nerve conduction studies are compatible with the site of the nerve lesion. In the

"disputed" form, there are no objective signs and no consistent laboratory abnormalities. Attempts to reproduce the syndrome by abduction of the arm (Adson test) or other maneuvers have repeatedly been cited, but the same "abnormalities" can be demonstrated in normal persons and have no diagnostic value.

Similarly, application of electrodiagnostic techniques has not been blinded or controlled, so different abnormalities have been reported, then refuted. The list includes low amplitude of the sensory evoked potential in the ulnar nerve, slowing of proximal conduction after stimulation at the Erb point, ulnar F-wave determination, and abnormality of somatosensory evoked potentials from the ulnar nerve. Magnetic resonance imaging (MRI) may show deviation or distortion of nerves or blood vessels, the presence of bands extending from the C-7 transverse process, or other causes of the syndrome. MR angiography and Doppler ultrasonography may help assess the possibility of vascular compression.

DIAGNOSIS AND MANAGEMENT

In cases of "true" thoracic outlet syndrome, diagnosis must exclude entrapment syndromes in the arm and compressive lesions in the cervical spine. Arteriography may be indicated if there is any suggestion of an aneurysm of the subclavian artery. Surgery is indicated when the diagnosis is unequivocal.

In the disputed form, when no objective findings are noted on neurologic examination, there is a problem. Each case must be evaluated separately, but in the absence of objective changes, it would seem reasonable to be cautious. Psychogenic factors should be considered. Conservative therapy should be given a trial; postural adjustments, manual therapy to increase mobility of the shoulder girdle, and an exercise program have all been advocated. The results of surgery are difficult to evaluate when there are no objective signs or diagnostic laboratory abnormalities; placebo effects are rarely considered in the evaluation of surgery. Success rates of 90% for a particular operation may be followed by equally enthusiastic reports for reoperation after the "failed operation." Surgery is not without hazard; complications include causalgia, injury of the long thoracic nerve, infection, and laceration of the subclavian artery.

SUGGESTED READINGS

Aligne C, Barral X. Rehabilitation of patients with thoracic outlet syndrome. *Ann Vasc Surg* 1992;6:381–389.

Campbell JN, Naff NJ, Dellon AL. Thoracic outlet syndrome: neurosurgical perspective. *Neurosurg Clin N Am* 1991;2:227–233.

Cherington M, Cherington C. Thoracic outlet syndrome: reimbursement patterns and patient profiles. *Neurology* 1992;42:943–945.

Cherington M, Harper I, Machanic B, Parry L. Surgery for thoracic outlet syndrome may be hazardous to your health. *Muscle Nerve* 1986;9:632–634.

Cuetter AC, Bartoszek DM. Thoracic outlet syndrome: controversies, overdiagnosis, overtreatment, and recommendations for management. *Muscle Nerve* 1989;12:410–419.

Gregoudis R, Barnes RW. Thoracic outlet arterial compression: prevalence in normal persons. *Angiology* 1980;31:538–541.

Huffman JD. Electrodiagnostic techniques for and conservative treatment of thoracic outlet syndrome. *Clin Orthop* 1986;207:21–23.

Kenny RA, Traynor GB, Withington D, Keegan DJ. Thoracic outlet syn-

drome: a useful exercise treatment option. *Am J Surg* 1993;
165:282–284.

LeForestier N, Moulonguet A, Maisonobe T, Leger JM, Bouche P. True
neurogenic thoracic outlet syndrome: electrophysiological diagnosis in six
cases. *Muscle Nerve* 1998;21:1129–1134.

Longley DG, Finlay DE, Letouorneau JG. Sonography of the upper extremity and jugular veins. *AJR* 1993;160:957–962.

Novack CB, Mackinnon SE, Patterson GA. Evaluation of patients with thoracic outlet syndrome. *J Hand Surg [Am]* 1993;18:292–299.

Ohkawa Y, Isoada H, Hasegawa S, et al. MR angiography of thoracic outlet
syndrome. *J Comput Assist Tomogr* 1992;16:475–477.

Panegyres PK, Moore N, Gibson R, Rushworth G, Donaghy M. Thoracic
outlet syndromes and magnetic resonance imaging. *Brain*
1993;116:823–841.

Roos DB. Thoracic outlet syndrome is underdiagnosed. *Muscle Nerve*
1999;22:126–129.

Smith T, Trojaborg W. Diagnosis of thoracic outlet syndrome. *Arch Neurol*
1987;44:1161–1166.

Veilleux M, Stevens JC, Campbell JK. Somatosensory evoked potentials:
lack of value for diagnosis of thoracic outlet syndrome. *Muscle Nerve*
1988;11:571–575.

Wilbourn AJ. Thoracic outlet syndrome: a plea for conservatism. *Neurosurg
Clin N Am* 1991;2:235–245.

Wilbourn AJ. Thoracic outlet syndrome is overdiagnosed. *Muscle Nerve*
1999;22:130–136.

Wilbourn AJ, Lederman RJ. Evidence for conduction delay in thoracic
outlet syndrome is challenged. *N Engl J Med* 1984;310:1052–1053.

Merritt's Neurology, 10th ed., edited by L.P. Rowland. Lippincott Williams & Wilkins, Philadelphia © 2000.

CHAPTER 70

NEUROPATHIC PAIN AND POSTTRAUMATIC PAIN SYNDROMES

JAMES H. HALSEY

The term *complex regional pain syndrome* (CRPS) has been
adopted by the International Association for the Study of Pain.
CRPS type I was previously called *reflex sympathetic dystrophy*
(RSD) when the syndrome was not associated with injury to a
major nerve trunk. CRPS type II was previously *causalgia* for
syndromes with a major nerve trunk injury.

These disorders are characterized by continuous pain with
combinations of aching, throbbing, burning, allodynia (pain in
response to a stimulus that usually is not painful, such as light
touch), sensitivity to cold, and temporal summation (increasing
pain by repeated mild stimulation). Lancinating pain, as in
trigeminal neuralgia, is rarely present. Sometimes, physical signs
suggest autonomic dysfunction, with sweating, dry skin, vasomotor instability (edema, erythema, blotching, or blanching), atrophy of muscle, other soft tissues, and bone (Sudeck atrophy),
and stiff joints. These signs occur in varying combinations.

In some patients, the physical signs and the pain are abolished
or greatly reduced by selective sympathetic blockade. However,
failure of sympathetic block does not alter the classification, even
if it excludes sympathetic activity in the pathogenesis of the particular case.

These disorders may follow injuries involving a major peripheral nerve trunk (CRPS type II), especially a partial nerve injury rather than a complete transection. The nerves most often
affected are the median nerve, the tibial division of the sciatic
nerve, and portions of the brachial and lumbar plexuses from
which these nerves originate. Often, more than one nerve is involved. The injury may follow stretch, missiles, injections, compression of roots or peripheral nerves, or inadvertent surgical
damage. CRPS type I may follow a local crush injury of a hand
or foot, without nerve trunk injury. However, it can also follow
a less severe or even trivial injury, or no recognized injury at all.

If untreated, the syndrome may progress and involve more
proximal parts of the same limb. Rarely, it spreads to homologous parts of the other side or other parts of the body. Apparent
progression may result from inappropriate immobilization
brought on in part by the patient's desire to protect the painful
area, a process that may be aggravated if the patient fears that
progression is the natural history of the disorder.

The same qualities of pain and sometimes the same physical
signs can result from spinal cord or brain lesions, including
hemiplegic cerebral infarction, or poliomyelitis. Rheumatoid
arthritis and other collagen diseases, as well as osteoarthritis and
traumatic arthritis, may produce similar physical signs and similar pain.

Partial lesions of the spinothalamic tract, postherpetic neuralgia, and peripheral neuropathies involving small-diameter pain
fibers but without complete loss of pain perception may result in
neuropathic pain. A patient recovering from complete analgesia
may pass through a phase of partial analgesia, with the appearance
of pain that becomes progressively worse. In the face of increasing
complaints, the physician must rely on quantitative documentation of reflexes, strength, and sensory perception thresholds to determine whether the condition is improving or getting worse. A
corollary of this point is that pain without neurologic abnormality is unlikely to be due to an organic neurologic disorder.

DIAGNOSIS

Neuropathic pain is defined by the clinical picture of continuous
pain with or without nerve injury, sometimes associated with
physical signs of sympathetic overactivity and relief by differential sympathetic block. The physiologic severity of the disorder is
a function of allodynia, temporal summation, and (less objectively) sleep disturbance caused by the pain. The functional component is judged in large degree by observing pain behavior and
signs of conversion reaction. If the pain is focal and involves one
limb, it meets the criteria of CRPS.

TREATMENT

Medical therapy of pain caused by damaged nerves, whether central or peripheral, trunk or terminal branches, is influenced more by the quality of the pain and the accompanying behavioral complications (e.g., insomnia, anxiety, agitation, or depression) than by the anatomic source or pathologic cause of the pain. In general, tricyclic antidepressants are most effective for burning and aching pain; phenytoin sodium (Dilantin) is intermediate, and carbamazepine (Tegretol) is least effective. For lancinating pain, as in trigeminal neuralgia but only rarely in the disorders described here, the reverse is usually true, and carbamazepine is favored. In individual patients, however, any of the three agents may be optimal. Gabapentin (Neurontin) may offer some additional opportunities for nonnarcotic pain control. Of the tricyclic agents, amitriptyline is particularly useful for its sedative effect in patients who cannot sleep because of the pain. Any of these drugs may be usefully supplemented in individual patients with benzodiazepines, other antidepressants, baclofen (Lioresal), or phenothiazines. Narcotics are sometimes appropriate and are underused in elderly patients, in whom the consequences of habituation are low.

Transcutaneous electric nerve stimulation is sometimes a helpful adjuvant. Physical therapy is aimed specifically at minimizing the pathologic immobilization that seems to be responsible for many cases of progressive disability. Differential sympathetic and somatic nerve blocks may have diagnostic value and, when repeated, sometimes have cumulative therapeutic benefit with progressively longer intervals free of pain. In carefully selected patients with severe pain, effective treatments include surgical sympathectomy, dorsal column stimulation, and intrathecal administration of morphine.

FUNCTIONAL COMPONENT OF PAIN

The chronic pain is debilitating and demoralizing, often leading to serious depression. Additionally, many patients guard the painful limb from tactile stimulation because they fear the pain. The behavioral pattern may suggest a conversion reaction with much "pain behavior"(grunting, panting, moaning, and tensing muscles) during an examination or even on simple observation.

There is a considerable lay literature on RSD conveying a frightening prognosis and often aggravating the functional component of the disorder. The physician may facilitate or restrain this process by assessing the disorder in the context of the patient's total reaction to it. Not every hand or foot that tingles, burns, or aches should be labeled RSD, even if it follows an injury and seems to fit the definition of CRPS type I. Every effort should be exerted to reach a specific neurologic, vascular, orthopedic, or rheumatologic diagnosis for a specific treatment, without introducing or increasing the functional consequences of the labels "RSD" or "CRPS."

Behavioral pain control aims to teach the patient how to decrease the outward expression of pain behavior, decreasing the aggravating effects of increased muscle tension, the patient's anger, and the resulting guilt of family members and friends, all of which may feed back on the behavioral components of the suffering.

Before a surgical sympathectomy or other permanently destructive or invasive procedure is undertaken, benefit may come from a multidisciplinary review of the problem, involving a physician interested in pain management, a physical therapist, and a psychotherapist. Some patients feel better when the physician acknowledges the severity of the pain without necessarily curing it. For a few, acknowledgment is even more important than cure, implying that the physician will stay with the patient while he or she continues to live with the pain. Many unsatisfactory outcomes of surgery for relief of pain result from failure to address the behavioral component.

SUGGESTED READINGS

Geertzen JH, Dijkstra PU, Groothoff JW, et al. Reflex sympathetic dystrophy of the upper extremity: a 5.5 year follow-up. Part I: impairments and perceived disability. *Acta Orthop Scand* 1998;279:12–18.

Kozin F. Reflex sympathetic dystrophy syndrome: a review. *Clin Exp Rheumatol* 1992;10:401–409.

Levine D. Burning pain in an extremity: breaking the destructive cycle of reflex sympathetic dystrophy. *Postgrad Med* 1991;90:175–185.

Rowbotham M, Fields H. The relationship of pain, allodynia and thermal sensation in postherpetic neuralgia. *Brain* 1996;119:347–354.

Schwartzman R. Reflex sympathetic dystrophy and causalgia. *Neurol Clin* 1992;10:953–973.

Stanton-Hicks M, Janig W, Hassenbusch S, Haddox J, Boas R, Wilson P. Reflex sympathetic dystrophy: changing concepts and taxonomy. *Pain* 1995;63:127–133.

Tsuruoka M, Willis WD. Descending modulation from the region of the locus coeruleus on nociceptive sensitivity in a rat model of inflammatory hyperalgesia. *Brain Res* 1996;743:86–92.

Veldman PH, Reynen HM, Arntz IE, Goris RJ. Signs and symptoms of reflex sympathetic dystrophy: prospective study of 829 patients. *Lancet* 1993;342:1012–1016.

Zyluk A. The natural history of post-traumatic reflex sympathetic dystrophy. *J Hand Surg [Br]* 1998;23:20–23.

Merritt's Neurology, 10th ed., edited by L.P. Rowland. Lippincott Williams & Wilkins, Philadelphia © 2000.

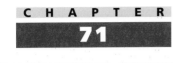

RADIATION INJURY

CASILDA M. BALMACEDA
STEVEN R. ISAACSON

Although irradiation is an essential treatment for many central nervous system (CNS) malignancies, injury to the brain or spinal cord is a feared complication. Healthy tissue may be exposed when the target of radiation is nearby in the brain or spinal cord or even after nonneural structures have been irradiated, if the peripheral or cranial nerves are within the field. Neurologic injury may follow scalp irradiation for tinea capitis, prophylactic whole-brain radiotherapy for small cell carcinoma of the lung or acute lymphocytic leukemia, or radiotherapy to the neck for systemic malignancy. There are three major categories: acute reactions (1 to 6 weeks after radiotherapy), early-delayed reactions (within 6 months afterward), and late-delayed reactions (months to years afterward).

EARLY (ACUTE) EFFECTS

Radiotherapy is usually well tolerated during the treatment period. The only acute CNS injury is edema days or weeks after the start of radiation therapy. Headache, nausea, and vomiting may occur with high daily dose fractions. Fractions of 750 cGy generate a complication rate of 49%, but daily doses of 200 cGy or less are seldom toxic. The acute lesions appear on magnetic resonance imaging (MRI) as localized swelling without enhancement. Steroids may reduce symptoms and are commonly given during radiotherapy to reduce the likelihood of this complication.

Tissues that have the fastest turnover rate are most often affected after CNS irradiation, causing alopecia and skin erythema. Otitis media or externa and pharyngitis may follow radiotherapy to the posterior fossa or brainstem because the eustachian tube is obstructed by swelling. Temporary hearing loss is seen, but deafness is rare. Marrow depression occurs with craniospinal radiotherapy, particularly in patients receiving concomitant chemotherapy, and may lead to infection or hemorrhage.

EARLY-DELAYED SYNDROMES

Reactions occurring 1 month to several years after treatment have been divided into early and late categories, but there are no clearly defined time boundaries. Two main clinical syndromes are seen. Somnolence and headache may occur in children receiving prophylactic whole-brain radiotherapy for acute lymphocytic leukemia or tinea capitis. The syndrome appears 24 to 66 days after radiotherapy; recovery is spontaneous. Fo-

cal signs are uncommon but may simulate tumor progression. Rhombencephaly with ataxia, dysarthria, and nystagmus may follow irradiation to the middle ear area for glomus jugulare tumors. Severe leukoencephalopathy can occur within the first 6 months. Early-delayed radiation myelopathy takes the form of the Lhermitte symptom, a sensation of electrical current radiating down the back or limbs induced by flexing the neck; it is seen in up to 15% of patients receiving mantle irradiation for Hodgkin lymphoma. This symptom can be distinguished from delayed radiation myelopathy because it is transient and appears within 6 months of the completion of treatment. Other causes of the symptom are multiple sclerosis, vitamin B_{12} deficiency, and cisplatin (Platinol) chemotherapy. Epidural cord compression by tumor may also cause Lhermitte sign but is usually painful.

The latent period for early-delayed effects is thought to correspond to the turnover time of myelin, and these syndromes are attributed to transient demyelination. Pathologic data are scarce because the syndrome is rarely lethal, but the few autopsies have showed areas of demyelination.

LATE-DELAYED SYNDROMES
Radiation Necrosis

It is not known how adverse effects relate to total dose of radiotherapy, fraction size, treatment time, volume of tissue irradiated, and host factors such as age. To standardize the biologic effects of different treatment regimens, Sheline and colleagues (1980) developed the concept of *neuroret* to specifically address brain tolerance to irradiation; the value is derived from a graph representing fractions (abscissa) and total dose (ordinate) to determine the threshold for necrosis. It occurs at doses greater than 1,000 to 1,100 neurorets (equivalent to 6,000 cGy given in 30 fractions for 6 weeks, a treatment commonly used for primary brain tumors).

Necrosis develops in about 5% of patients given total doses greater than 5,000 cGy with daily fraction sizes greater than 200 cGy. It may also follow irradiation of extracranial malignancies, such as squamous cell carcinoma, or stereotactic radiosurgery, proton beam irradiation, or brachytherapy (implantation of radioactive sources into the tumor bed). The median time for onset of symptoms is 14 months after radiotherapy, but symptoms may occur as early as 6 months afterward. In 75% of the patients, symptoms appear within 3 years of the treatment but may be seen as late as 7.5 years. The clinical manifestations may simulate those of the original tumor, with lateralizing signs, headache, or increased intracranial pressure. Patients irradiated for nasopharyngeal carcinoma may have lesions in the temporal lobe with or without hypothalamic dysfunction.

Radiation necrosis shows a predilection for the *white matter*. The underlying mechanisms are thought to be either loss of oligodendrocytes with demyelination and necrosis (*glial hypothesis*) or a *vasculopathy* with ischemia and infarction leading to necrosis. Contemporary views point to a vascular-mediated response resulting in delayed white matter necrosis. Glial cells, particularly oligodendrocytes, and the vascular endothelium are the major targets, not the neurons. Histologic changes include white matter necrosis, cystic cavitation with gliosis, and patchy demyelination. Vascular changes include endothelial proliferation, fibrinoid degeneration, perivascular lymphocytic infiltration, capillary occlusion, and intraluminal thrombosis of medium- and small-sized arteries. Vasogenic edema follows endothelial cell damage. The *immunologic hypothesis* speculates that irradiated glial cells release antigens that induce an autoimmune reaction. A *mineralizing microangiopathy* is seen at autopsy in up to 17% of patients who received cranial irradiation; it is usually asymptomatic. Radiographically, calcification may be seen at the gray–white matter junction, basal ganglia, or pons.

Neuroradiologic abnormalities are of two types. The first is a *mass lesion* located at the original tumor site or within the path of radiation. Enhancement is usually seen, mimicking the original neoplasm; it may be ringlike or heterogeneous. Angiography shows that the lesion is avascular. Computed tomography (CT) or MRI indicates that the lesion may resolve with time. Neuroimaging can often differentiate between early, transient and more progressive, later injury. Imaging differentiates mild edema from significant edema and frank necrosis. Early changes are confined to white matter, but after 6 months to 1 or 2 years gray matter lesions may be evident.

The second abnormality consists of diffuse *white matter changes,* appearing as areas of hypodensity on CT or increased signal intensity on MRI (Fig. 71.1). The imaging abnormalities vary from mild to severe and are usually irreversible. Mild changes (grade 1) lie adjacent to the frontal and occipital horns of the lateral ventricles. Grade 2 (intermediate) change affects the centrum semiovale, and grades 3 to 4 show diffuse white matter lesions with a characteristic scalloped configuration. Mass effect is rare. Accompanying changes include cortical atrophy or ventricular dilatation. MRI is more sensitive than CT in detecting these white matter abnormalities. Imaging abnormalities correlate poorly with symptoms; many patients with severe white matter changes are asymptomatic.

Distinguishing tumor recurrence from radiation necrosis may be difficult. Provided that steroid dosage is not increasing, radiation effect is suggested by clinical improvement accompanied by a decrease of mass effect on CT or MRI. Although positron-emission tomography (PET) may show hypometabolic areas of radiation necrosis, a tissue biopsy is usually needed to establish the diagnosis. Single-photon emission computed tomography and PET are complementary. *MR spectroscopy* may document metabolic changes in brain *N*-acetylaspartate, choline, creatine, and lactate that appear after radiation and later return to normal. The changes include a reduction in choline levels with radiation, indicating the transformation of tumor to necrotic tissue, as well as an increase in choline levels with tumor recurrence. Steroid therapy may lead to clinical stabilization, but when there is marked mass effect, surgical resection can improve neurologic function and may be life-saving. Radiation necrosis can be progressive and fatal.

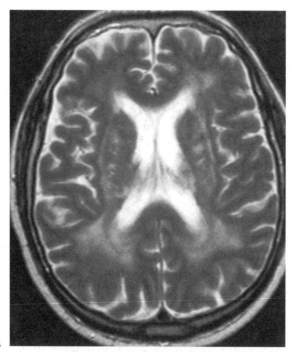
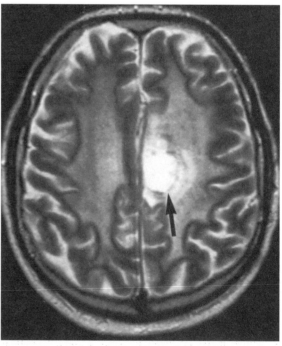

A B

FIG. 71.1. Radiation leukoencephalopathy. **A:** Axial T2-weighted MR scan shows diffuse increased signal intensity involving the periventricular white matter of both frontal lobes and parietal lobes, as well as the corona radiata and external capsules bilaterally. **B:** Axial T2-weighted MR scan at the level of the centrum semiovale demonstrates similar changes within the hemispheric white matter bilaterally. The known malignant glioma is identified in the posteromedial left frontal lobe *(arrow)*, for which the patient had received cranial radiation therapy. (Courtesy of Dr. S. Chan, Columbia University College of Physicians and Surgeons, New York, NY.)

Radiation Myelopathy

Delayed injury to the spinal cord, *radiation myelopathy*, develops 1 to 3 years after radiotherapy, with one peak at 12 to 14 months and another at 24 to 28 months. The average latent period is 12 months, and in 75% of the patients, radiation myelopathy occurs within 30 months. In patients with shorter intervals, the total dose of radiation and the average dose per fraction were higher. The incidence is about 5% when doses between 57 Gy and 61 Gy are given to the spinal cord. Latency periods are shorter in children, after a second course of radiation, or for lumbar lesions. The latency bimodality is attributed to dual mechanisms of injury. Higher doses cause white matter necrosis and early myelopathy; lower doses preferentially cause vascular damage and delayed manifestations. A case report describes syrinx formation after radiation to the spinal cord in a patient with a cervical astrocytoma.

The true incidence is not known. Wara and associates (1975) suggested a 5% risk in patients who received 4,500 cGy at fraction doses of 180 cGy, but the specifics of cord tolerance remain elusive. Symptoms are associated with increased fraction size, shorter treatment time, higher total dose, and cord exposure greater than 10 cm in length. Additional risk factors (e.g., diabetes mellitus, hypertension) may contribute to its development.

The clinical syndrome includes painless subacute numbness and paresthesia followed by progression of spastic gait, sphincter symptoms, and limb weakness. MRI may be normal or show cord swelling, atrophy, or complete subarachnoid block. Low signal intensity on T1-weighted imaging, high signal on T2-weighted imaging, and focal enhancement may be seen as early as 1 month after the clinical manifestations. Diagnosis must exclude extra- or intramedullary tumors, leptomeningeal metastases, or vertebral body abnormalities causing cord compression. As early as 10 months after the onset of symptoms, one can see cord atrophy or resolution of contrast enhancement. There is no effective treatment, although steroids may transiently improve symptoms. Pathologically, spinal cord infarction is associated with necrosis, hemorrhage, and demyelination. After experimental radiation, asymptomatic animals showed spongy vacuolation of the spinal cord white matter only, whereas those with paralysis had large areas of tissue destruction and vascular changes, particularly in the posterior and lateral columns. Other rare syndromes attributed to radiation-induced cord damage are an acute paraplegia that progresses for hours to days (thought to be induced by vascular damage to the cord with infarction), anterior horn cell damage, and a delayed clinical syndrome that simulates motor neuron disease but is arrested spontaneously after 1 to 2 years.

Radiation-induced Vasculopathy

Both intra- and extracranial circulation can be affected. Most patients have had neck irradiation for head and neck cancer or for optic nerve or suprasellar tumors. The latent period can be up to 23 years. Angiography reveals localized stenosis, an irregular contour of the vessel involved, or even complete occlusion of the portion of the artery in the radiation portal. Extracranially, internal and common carotid artery occlusion can be seen, with premature atherosclerosis and endothelial proliferation compromising vessel patency and leading to thrombosis and infarction. Intracranially, the supraclinoid carotid is most commonly affected, and a moyamoya pattern may develop. Autopsy studies reveal myointimal proliferation, hyalinization, and occlusion. Clinically, radiation-induced vasculopathy causes transient ischemic attacks or ischemic stroke. Cerebrovascular malformations have also been observed in the irradiated field. Aneurysm formation is rare.

Radiation-induced Plexopathy

Either brachial or lumbar plexus may be affected; most commonly the arm is affected after radiotherapy for breast carcinoma. Three different syndromes are observed. *Transient plexus injury* occurs in 1.4% of the patients treated with doses of 5,000 cGy to the area, with paresthesia or, less commonly, pain or weakness. Median onset is 4.5 months after radiotherapy. *Acute ischemic brachial neuropathy* follows subclavian artery occlusion owing to prior irradiation. The lesion is acute, nonprogressive, and painless. *Radiation fibrosis* appears about 4 years after radiotherapy, with paresthesia or swelling of the arm; the signs are sensorimotor, most commonly affecting the upper plexus. Pathologically, local fibrosis or scarring entraps the plexus or nerves. *Brachial plexopathy* was reported in the treatment of breast cancer when the fraction size was greater than 2 Gy. Patients may have symptoms of paresthesia, hypesthesia, and weak hands. *Lumbosacral plexopathy* is a rare occurrence in patients treated for cervical or endometrial carcinoma, even when total doses approach 70 to 80 Gy, by a combination of brachytherapy and external-beam radiation.

Clinically, the major difficulty lies in trying to differentiate radiation-induced plexopathy from tumor. Lymphedema, painless paresis and sensory loss, and upper plexus involvement suggest radiation plexopathy. Pain, lack of edema, and lower plexus involvement suggest recurrent tumor. *Myokymia*, when present on electromyography, strongly favors the diagnosis of radiation fibrosis. Typically, radiation fibrosis of the plexus appears on CT as diffuse involvement without a discrete mass. MRI may reveal radiation changes in the soft tissue or bone. Gadolinium enhancement of the irradiated area may occur and persist, even two decades after irradiation. Although the presence of enhancement is usually suggestive of recurrent tumor, the radiographic stability is more consistent with necrosis. When ancillary studies are ambiguous, surgical exploration of the plexus may be considered. Once the diagnosis of radiation plexopathy is established, attention should be given to preventing shoulder subluxation, treating lymphedema, and relieving pain. The plexopathy is usually irreversible.

Endocrine Dysfunction

Irradiation of the brain or neighboring sites can cause neuroendocrine disorders. These are primarily due to radiation effects on the hypothalamic–pituitary axis when this structure is included in the radiation field for treatment of primary brain tumors or head and neck cancer. For unknown reasons, the posterior pituitary is remarkably resistant to the effects of radiation. Several clinical syndromes may be evident. *Growth hormone* function is the most vulnerable. *Growth arrest* may occur in children treated with spinal radiotherapy because radiation impairs vertebral development and is exaggerated by endocrine deficiency. It is most visible in a growing child; the rate of growth slows and stature is short for age. Adults may exhibit a decrease in muscle mass and an increase in adipose tissue. These effects may become evident in children with doses of fractionated radiation as low as 18 Gy or single fractions of 9 to 10 Gy. Adults have a higher threshold. Among children treated for acute lymphoblastic leukemia with moderate doses of prophylactic cranial radiation (2,000 to 3,000 cGy), 65% have impaired growth hormone responses. Treatment includes growth hormone replacement. Modern treatment for chemosensitive tumors therefore emphasizes chemotherapy to reduce or avoid radiation.

Gonadotropin deficiency (luteinizing hormone and follicle-stimulating hormone) may develop, with failure to enter puberty and amenorrhea. Adults may demonstrate infertility, sexual dysfunction, and decreased libido. The tolerance dose appears to be between 40 and 50 Gy. *Thyrotropin deficiency* may be manifested as weight gain and lethargy. *Adrenocorticotropic hormone deficiency* is rarely seen, with lethargy, decreased stamina, fasting, hypoglycemia, and dilutional hyponatremia. *Hyperprolactinemia* may cause delay in puberty, galactorrhea, or amenorrhea. Men may experience decreased libido and impotence. These findings may be found in 20% to 50% of patients receiving greater than 50 Gy of radiation.

Neuropsychologic Sequelae

Cognitive impairment is a delayed complication of radiation, especially in long-term survivors who have been cured of the original disease. There has usually been concomitant use of intrathecal chemotherapy, but radiation itself may be the culprit. Children younger than 5 years are particularly susceptible to cognitive sequelae. In the treatment of *childhood* brain tumors, survivors demonstrate a 40% to 100% incidence of cognitive dysfunction on formal neuropsychologic testing. Cranial irradiation in children may be associated with mild delayed IQ decline, learning disability, and academic failure. There is considerable pediatric literature, but little is known about cognitive outcome in adults. However, in most studies, there were no controls, and often the most appropriate neuropsychologic procedures were not used. A syndrome of ataxia, cognitive disturbance, and urinary incontinence, sometimes ameliorated by ventriculoperitoneal shunting, has been described in adults treated with irradiation for brain tumors. Memory seems to be sensitive to radiotherapy. Local-field irradiation to the posterior fossa may also be accompanied by significant cognitive impairment. There have been few studies of the *quality of life* of patients surviving irradiation.

Other Complications of Radiation

Peripheral Nerves

Peripheral nerves are seldom damaged with fractionated doses of less than 6,000 cGy. Fraction size appears to play a significant role as a causative factor. There may be two phases of injury to nerves following radiation. First, direct effects may cause changes in electrophysiology and histochemistry. Fibrosis may occur later and surround the nerve. Vascular injury to nutrient vessels may also occur.

Radiation-induced Tumors

As the survival of cancer patients increases, secondary tumors become an important treatment complication. Radiation has been implicated in the development of secondary tumors. The association between radiation and CNS tumors is especially strong for *meningiomas,* which may follow irradiation for brain or spinal cord tumors or doses of less than 850 cGy to the scalp for tinea capitis. The mean latency is 37 years if low-dose irradiation was given and 18 months for doses greater than 2,000 cGy. Compared with spontaneously arising tumors, radiation-induced meningiomas are more likely to recur after surgical excision and to undergo malignant degeneration. Radiation-induced *sarcomas* are seen in the third, fourth, or fifth decades after radiation for pituitary adenomas or gliomas. The latency period is 8 to 11 years with doses greater than 5,000 cGy. The possible role of cranial irradiation in the pathogenesis of CNS *gliomas* is controversial. The main diagnostic problem is differentiation of radiation-induced malignancy from recurrence of the original tumor. *Peripheral nerve tumors,* benign or malignant, arising within the radiation port are seen in up to 9% of patients, especially those treated for breast cancer or lymphoma. Tumors are most frequently located in the brachial plexus followed by spinal roots or nerve. Clinically, an enlarging painful mass causes progressive motor and sensory signs of plexopathy. The mean interval between irradiation and diagnosis of these tumors is 16 years. Patients with neurofibromatosis are particularly prone to radiation-induced peripheral nerve tumors. Treatment is surgical resection, but the prognosis for malignant tumors is poor.

Radiation Optic Neuropathy

Radiation optic neuropathy follows treatment directed to the orbit, sinuses, pituitary, or intracranial tumors. There is painless visual loss, usually monocular, but both eyes may be affected. Symptoms develop within 3 years. Findings include decreased visual acuity, abnormal visual fields (especially altitudinal defects), papilledema (or optic atrophy later), and hemorrhagic exudates. About 50% of the patients experience improvement of the condition, but some become blind. Steroids are ineffective. Measures to shield the optic nerve from the radiation portals may reduce the incidence of this rare but devastating complication.

SUGGESTED READINGS

Radiation: CNS Effects

Al-Mefty O, Kersh JE, Routh A, et al. The long-term side effects of radiation therapy for benign brain tumors in adults. *J Neurosurg* 1990;73:502–512.

Archibald Y, Lunn D, Ruttan L, et al. Cognitive functioning in long-term survivors of high-grade gliomas. *J Neurosurg* 1994;80:247–253.

Armstrong C, Mollman J, Corn BW, et al. Effects of radiation therapy on adult brain behavior: evidence for a rebound phenomenon in a phase I trial. *Neurology* 1993;43:1961–1965.

Asai A, Matsutani M, Kohno T, et al. Subacute brain atrophy after radiation therapy for malignant brain tumor. *Cancer* 1989;63:1962–1974.

Ball WS, Prenger EC, Ballard ET. Neurotoxicity of radio/chemotherapy in children: pathologic and MR correlation. *AJNR* 1992;13:761–776.

Buchpiguel CA, Alavi JB, Alavi A, Kenyon L. PET versus SPECT in distinguishing radiation necrosis from tumor in the brain. *J Nucl Med* 1995;36:159–164.

Curnes J, Laster D, et al. MRI of radiation injury to the brain. *Am J Roentgenol* 1986;147:119–124.

DeAngelis LM, Delattre JY, Posner JB. Radiation-induced dementia in patients cured of brain metastases. *Neurology* 1989;39:789–796.

Donahue B. Short- and long-term complications of radiation therapy for pediatric brain tumors. *Pediatr Neurosurg* 1992;18:207–217.

Dooms GC, Hecht S, Brant-Zawadzki M, et al. Brain radiation lesions: MR imaging. *Radiology* 1986;158:149–155.

Doyle WK, Budinger TF, Valk PE, et al. Differentiation of cerebral radiation necrosis from tumor recurrence by [^{18}F]FDG and ^{82}RB PET scan. *J Comput Assist Tomogr* 1987;11:563–570.

Dropcho EJ. Central nervous system injury by therapeutic irradiation. *Neurol Clin* 1991;9:969–988.

Duffner PK, Cohen ME, Thomas PRM, et al. The long-term effects of cranial irradiation on the central nervous system. *Cancer* 1985;56: 1841–1846.

Eiser C. Intellectual abilities among survivors of childhood leukaemia as a function of CNS irradiation. *Arch Dis Child* 1978;53:391–395.

Esteve F, Rubin C, Grand S, et al. Transient metabolic changes observed with proton MR spectroscopy in normal human brain after radiation therapy. *Int J Radiat Oncol Biol Phys* 1998;40:279–286.

Glass JP, Hwang TL, Leavens ME, et al. Cerebral radiation necrosis following treatment of extracranial malignancies. *Cancer* 1984;54:1966–1972.

Grattan-Smith PJ, Morris JG, Langlands AO. Delayed radiation necrosis of the central nervous system in patients irradiated for pituitary tumours. *J Neurol Neurosurg Psychiatry* 1992;55:949–955.

Harris J, Levene M. Visual complications following irradiation for pituitary adenomas and craniopharyngiomas. *Radiology* 1976;120:167–171.

Johnson BE, Becker B, Goff WB, et al. Neurologic, neuropsychologic, and computed cranial tomography scan abnormalities in 2- to 10-year survivors of small-cell lung cancer. *J Clin Oncol* 1985;3:1659–1667.

Kaufman M, Swartz BE, Mandelkern M, et al. Diagnosis of delayed cerebral radiation necrosis following proton beam therapy. *Arch Neurol* 1990;47:474–476.

Landau K, Killer HE. Radiation damage [Letter]. *Neurology* 1996;46:889.

Loeffler JS, Siddon RL, Wen PY, et al. Stereotactic radiosurgery of the brain using a standard linear accelerator: a study of early and late effects. *Radiother Oncol* 1990;17:311–321.

Macdonald D, Rottenberg D, Schutz J, et al. Radiation-induced optic neuropathy. In: Rottenberg D, ed. *Neurological complications of cancer treatment*. Boston: Butterworth-Heinemann, 1991:37–61.

Marks JE, Baglan RJ, Prassad SC, et al. Cerebral radionecrosis: incidence and risk in relation to dose, time, fractionation and volume. *Int J Rad Oncol Biol Phys* 1981;7:243–252.

Meadows A, Massari D, Ferguson J, et al. Declines in IQ scores and cognitive dysfunctions in children with acute lymphocytic leukemia treated with cranial irradiation. *Lancet* 1981;2:1015–1018.

Mitomo M, Kawai R, Miura T, et al. Radiation necrosis of the brain and radiation-induced vasculopathy. *Acta Radiol* 1986;369[Suppl]:227–230.

Moss H, Nannis E. The effects of prophylactic treatment of the central nervous system on the intellectual functioning of children with acute lymphocytic leukemia. *Am J Med* 1981;71:47–52.

Mostow EN, Byrne J, Connelly RR, et al. Quality of life in long-term survivors of CNS tumors of childhood and adolescence. *J Clin Oncol* 1991;9:592–599.

Mulhern RK, Kovnar E, Langston J, et al. Long-term survivors of leukemia treated in infancy: factors associated with neuropsychologic status. *J Clin Oncol* 1992;10:1095–1102.

Nightingale S, Dawes PJDK, Cartlidge NEF. Early-delayed radiation rhombencephalopathy. *J Neurol Neurosurg Psychiatry* 1982;45:267–270.

Norris AM, Carrington BM, Slevin NJ. Late radiation change in the CNS: MR imaging following gadolinium enhancement. *Clin Radiol* 1997;52: 356–362.

Norris AM, Carrington BM. Late radiation change in the CNS: MR imaging following gadolinium enhancement. *Clin Radiol* 1997;52:356–362.

Packer RJ, Meadows AT, Rorke LB, et al. Long-term sequelae of cancer treatment on the central nervous system in childhood. *Med Pediatr Oncol* 1987;15:241–253.

Parsons J, Fitzgerald C, Hood C. The effects of irradiation on the eye and the optic nerve. *Int J Radiat Oncol Biol Phys* 1983;9:609–622.

Phuphanich S, Jacobs M, Murtagh FR, Gonzalvo A. MRI of spinal cord radiation necrosis simulating recurrent cervical cord astrocytoma and syringomyelia. *Surg Neurol* 1996;45:362–365.

Plowman PN. Haematologic toxicity during craniospinal irradiation—the impact of prior chemotherapy. *Med Pediatr Oncol* 1997;28:238–239.

Pomeranz HD, Henson JW, Lessell S. Radiation-associated cerebral blindness. *Am J Ophthalmol* 1998;126:609–611.

Schultheiss TE, Kun LE, Ang KK, Stephens LC. Radiation response of the central nervous system. *Int J Radiat Oncol Biol Phys* 1995;31:1093–1112.

Sheline GE, Wara WM, Smith V. Therapeutic irradiation and brain therapy. *Int J Radiat Oncol Biol Phys* 1980;6:1215–1228.

Sonoda Y, Kumabe T, Takahashi T, et al. Clinical usefulness of ^{11}C-MET PET and ^{201}Tl SPECT for differentiation of recurrent glioma from radiation necrosis. *Neurol Med Chir (Tokyo)* 1998;38:342–347.

Tada E, Matsumoto K, Nakagawa M, Tamiya T, Furuta T, Ohmoto T. Serial magnetic resonance imaging of delayed radiation necrosis treated with dexamethasone: case illustration. *Neurosurgery* 1997;86:1067.

Twijnstra A, Boon PJ, Lormans ACM, et al. Neurotoxicity of prophylactic cranial irradiation in patients with small cell carcinoma of the lung. *Eur J Cancer Clin Oncol* 1987;23:983–986.

Valk PE, Budinger TF, Levin VA, et al. PET of malignant cerebral tumors after interstitial brachytherapy. *J Neurosurg* 1988;69:830–838.

Wald LL, Nelson SJ, Day MR, et al. Serial proton magnetic resonance spectroscopy imaging of glioblastoma multiforme after brachytherapy. *J Neurosurg* 1997;87:525–534.

Radiation Myelopathy

Alfonso ED, De Gregorio MA, Mateo P, et al. Radiation myelopathy in over-irradiated patients: MR imaging findings. *Eur Radiol* 1997;7: 400–404.

Delattre JY, Rosenblum MK, Thaler HT, et al. A model of radiation myelopathy in the rat: pathology, regional capillary permeability changes and treatment with dexamethasone. *Brain* 1988;111:1319–1336.

Goldwein JW. Radiation myelopathy: a review. *Med Pediatr Oncol* 1987;15:89–95.

Grunewald R, Panayiotopoulos C, Enevoldson T. Late onset radiation-induced motor neuron syndrome. *J Neurol Neurosurg Psychiatry* 1992; 55:741–742.

Hopewell JW. Radiation injury to the central nervous system. *Med Pediatr Oncol* 1998;[Suppl 1]:1–9.

Jeremic B, Djuric L. Mijatovic L. Incidence of radiation myelitis of the cervical spinal cord at doses of 5,500 cGy or greater. *Cancer* 1991;68: 2138–2141.

Koehler PJ, Verbiest H, Jager J, Vecht CJ. Delayed radiation myelopathy: serial MR imaging and pathology. *Clin Neurol Neurosurg* 1996;98: 197–201.

Komachi H, Tsuchiya K, Ikeda M, et al. Radiation myelopathy: a clinico-pathological study with special reference to correlation between MRI findings and neuropathology. *J Neurol Sci* 1995;132:228–232.

Melki PS, Halimi P, Wibault P, et al. MRI in chronic progressive radiation myelopathy. *J Comput Assist Tomogr* 1994;18:1–6.

Phuphanich S, Jacobs M, Murtagh FR, Gonzalvo A. MRI of spinal cord recognition necrosis stimulating recurrent cervical cord astrocytoma and syringomyelia. *Surg Neurol* 1996;45:362–365.

Schultheiss TE, Higgins EM, El-Mahdi AM. The latent period in clinical radiation myelopathy. *Int J Radiat Oncol Biol Phys* 1984;10:1109–1115.

Tashima T, Morioka T, Nishio S, et al. Delayed cerebral radionecrosis with a high uptake of ^{11}C-methionine on positron emission tomography and ^{201}Tl-chloride on single-photon emission computed tomography. *Neuroradiology* 1998;40:435–438.

Thorton AF, Zimberg SH, Greenberg HS, et al. Protracted Lhermitte's sign following head and neck irradiation. *Arch Otolaryngol Head Neck Surg* 1991;117:1300–1303.

Van der Kogel AJ. Radiation tolerance of the rat spinal cord: time-dose relationships. *Radiology* 1977;122:505–509.

Wang PY, Shen WC, Jan JS. Serial MRI changes in radiation myelopathy. *Neuroradiology* 1995;37:374–377.

Wara W, Phillips T, Sheline G. Radiation tolerance of the spinal cord. *Cancer* 1975;35:1558–1562.

Radiation: Vascular Complications

Benson PJ, Sung JH. Cerebral aneurysms following radiotherapy for medulloblastoma. *J Neurosurg* 1989;70:545–550.

Chang SD, Vanefsky MA, Havton LA, et al. Bilateral cavernous malformations resulting from cranial irradiation of a choroid plexus papilloma. *Neurol Res* 1998;20:529–532.

Hirata Y, Matsukado Y, Mihara Y, et al. Occlusion of the internal carotid artery after radiation therapy for the chiasmal lesion. *Neurochirurgie* 1985;74:141–147.

McGuirt WF, Feehs RS, Strickland JL, et al. Irradiation-induced atherosclerosis: a factor in therapeutic planning. *Ann Otol Rhinol Laryngol* 1992;101:222–228.

Murros KE, Toole JF. The effect of radiation of carotid arteries: a review article. *Arch Neurol* 1989;46:449–455.

Pozzati E, Giangaspero F, Marliani F, Acciarri N. Occult cerebrovascular malformations after irradiation. *Neurosurgery* 1996;39:677–682.

Werner MH, Burger PC, Heinz ER, et al. Intracranial atherosclerosis following radiotherapy. *Neurology* 1988;38:1158–1160.

Radiation-induced Plexopathy

Bowen BC, Verma A, Brandon AH, Fiedler JA. Radiation-induced brachial plexopathy: MR and clinical findings. *AJNR* 1996;17:1932–1936.

Georgion A, Grigsby PW, Perez CA. Radiation-induced lumbosacral plexopathy in gynecologic tumors: clinical findings and dosimetric analysis. *Int J Radiat Oncol Biol Phys* 1993;26:479–482.

Harper CM, Thomas J, Cascino T, et al. Distinction between neoplastic and radiation-induced brachial plexopathy, with emphasis on the role of EMG. *Neurology* 1989;39:502–506.

Jaeckle KA, Young DF, Foley KM. The natural history of lumbosacral plexopathy in cancer. *Neurology* 1985;35:8–15.

Kori SH, Foley KM, Posner JB. Brachial plexus lesions in patients with cancer: 100 cases. *Neurology* 1981;31:45–50.

Olsen NK, Pfeiffer P, Johannsen L. Radiation-induced brachial plexopathy: neurological follow-up in 161 recurrence-free breast cancer patients. *Int J Radiat Oncol Biology Phys* 1993;26:43–49.

Thomas JE, Cascino TL, Earle JD. Differential diagnosis between radiation and tumor plexopathy of the pelvis. *Neurology* 1985;35:1–7.

Wouter van Es H, Engelen AM, Witkamp TD, et al. Radiation-induced brachial plexopathy: MR imaging. *Skeletal Radiol* 1997;26:284–288.

Endocrine Dysfunction

Burstein S. Poor growth after cranial irradiation. *Pediatr Rev* 1997;18:442–444.

Constine LS, Woolf PD, Cann D, et al. Hypothalamic-pituitary dysfunction after radiation for brain tumors. *N Engl J Med* 1993;328:87–94.

Duffner PK, Cohen ME, Voorhess ML, et al. Long-term effects of cranial irradiation on endocrine function in children with brain tumors: a prospective study. *Cancer* 1985;56:2189–2193.

Mechanik JI, Hochberg FH, LaRocque A. Hypothalamic dysfunction following whole-brain irradiation. *J Neurosurg* 1986;65:490–494.

Rappaport R, Brauner R. Growth and endocrine disorders secondary to cranial irradiation. *Pediatr Res* 1989;25:561–567.

Shalet SM. Radiation and pituitary dysfunction. *N Engl J Med* 1993;238:131–133.

Woo E, Lam K, Yu YL, Ma J, Wang C, Yeung RT. Temporal lobe and hypothalamic-pituitary dysfunctions after radiotherapy for nasopharyngeal carcinoma: a distinct clinical syndrome. *J Neurol Neurosurg Psychiatry* 1988;51:1302–1307.

Radiation: Neuropsychologic Effects

Anderson V, Godber T, Smibert E, Ekert H. Neurobehavioural sequelae following cranial irradiation and chemotherapy in children: an analysis of risk factors. *Pediatr Rehabil* 1997;1:63–76.

Armstrong C, Ruffer J, Corn B, De Vries K, Mollman J. Biphasic patterns of memory deficits following moderate-dose partial-brain irradiation: neuropsychologic outcome and proposed mechanisms. *J Clin Oncol* 1995;13:2263–2271.

Crossen JR, Garwood D, Glatstein E, et al. Neurobehavioral sequelae of cranial irradiation in adults: a review of radiation-induced encephalopathy. *J Clin Oncol* 1994;12:627–642.

Duffey P, Chari G, Cartlidge NEF, et al. Progressive deterioration of intellect and motor function occurring several decades after cranial irradiation. *Arch Neurol* 1996;53:814–818.

Glauser TA, Packer RJ. Cognitive deficits in long-term survivors of childhood brain tumors. *Childs Nerv Syst* 1991;7:2–12.

Roman DD, Sperduto PW. Neuropsychological effects of cranial radiation: current knowledge and future directions. *Int J Radiat Oncol Biol Phys* 1998;31:983–998.

Sklar CA, Copstine LS. Chronic neuropsychological sequela of radiation therapy. *Int J Radiat Oncol Biol Phys* 1995;31:1113–1121.

Radiation Damage to Peripheral Nerves

Giese WL, Kinsella TJ. Radiation injury to peripheral and cranial nerves. In: Gutin PH, Leibel SA, Sheline GE, eds. *Radiation injury to the nervous system.* New York: Raven Press, 1991:383–403.

Gillette EL, Mahler PA, Powers BE, Gillette SM, Vujaskovic Z. Late radiation injury to muscle and peripheral nerves. *Int J Radiat Oncol Biol Phys* 1995;31:1309–1318.

Radiation-induced Tumors

Dweik A, Maheut-Lourmiere J, Lioret E, Jan M. Radiation-induced meningioma. *Childs Nerv Syst* 1995;11:661–663.

Foley KM. Radiation-induced malignant and atypical peripheral nerve sheath tumors. *Ann Neurol* 1980;7:311–318.

Harrison MJ, Wolfe DE, Lau TS, et al. Radiation-induced meningiomas: experience at the Mount Sinai Hospital and review of the literature. *J Neurosurg* 1991;75:564–574.

Kumar PP, Good RR, Skultety FM, et al. Radiation-induced neoplasms of the brain. *Cancer* 1987;59:1274–1282.

Nadeem SQ, Feun LG, Bruce-Gregorios JH, et al. Post-radiation sarcoma (malignant fibrous histiocytoma) of the cervical spine following ependymoma: a case report. *J Neurooncol* 1991;11:263–268.

Ron E, Modan B, Boice JD Jr, et al. Tumors of the brain and nervous system after radiotherapy in childhood. *N Engl J Med* 1988;319:1033–1039.

Shapiro S, Mealey J, Sartorius C. Radiation-induced intracranial malignant gliomas. *J Neurosurg* 1989;71:77–82.

Radiation Optic Neuropathy

Piquemal R, Cottier JP, Arsene S, et al. Radiation-induced optic neuropathy 4 years after radiation: report of a case followed up with MRI. *Neuroradiology* 1998;40:439–441.

McClellan RL, el Gammal T, Kline LB. Early bilateral radiation-induced optic neuropathy with follow-up MRI. *Neuroradiology* 1995;37:131–133.

Merritt's Neurology, 10th ed., edited by L.P. Rowland. Lippincott Williams & Wilkins, Philadelphia © 2000.

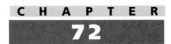

ELECTRICAL AND LIGHTNING INJURY

LEWIS P. ROWLAND

PATHOLOGY

High-voltage electric shock or lightning stroke may damage the central nervous system, motor neurons, or peripheral nerves. The lesions may involve either the brain or the spinal cord. In the spinal cord, myelomalacia may result without change in blood vessels, inflammation, or gliosis. Similarly, nonspecific lesions are found in the brain, and gray matter may be affected. In death from acute injury, cerebral lesions seem to be dominated by the effects of cardiac arrest and anoxia, with edema, perivascular hemorrhage, and neuronal loss.

Pathogenesis

The mechanism of injury is not clear. Investigators have stated that resistance to the flow of electric current is lower in neural tissue than in other organs and that the consequent syndromes result from the direct effects of high-voltage electricity on neural cells. Cerebellar injury has been attributed to heat injury as part of the insult. Demyelination does not seem to be the result of vascular injury, and it is not clear why symptoms are immediate in most patients but delayed in many. Nor is it clear why different parts of the nervous system are affected in different victims.

EPIDEMIOLOGY

In earlier times, electrocution was the result of accidents at work or in the home. With technologic advances, these causes have become less common but still account for about 1,000 deaths per year in the United States; lightning strikes account for about 100 deaths per year. Lightning strikes may be occupational (farming, ranching, roofing) or recreational (especially water sports, hiking, camping, or other outdoor activities).

SYMPTOMS AND SIGNS

Among survivors, the first signs occur immediately after the shock and may be transient. Unconsciousness and amnesia are common, and there may be transient limb paralysis or paresthesia. Cerebral infarction may result from cardiac arrhythmia and embolization. Days or weeks later, progressive disorders begin and resemble one or another of several syndromes, such as parkinsonism, cerebellar disorders, myelopathy, spinal muscular atrophy, or sensorimotor peripheral neuropathy. Because there are so few cases, it is not possible to determine whether all reported cases are consequences of the electric shock or are a coincidental occurrence of two conditions.

TREATMENT

Acutely, attention is directed to the cardiac disorder. The delayed-onset syndromes can only be managed symptomatically because no specific treatment exists.

SUGGESTED READINGS

Cherington M, Yarnell P, Hallmark D. MRI in lightning encephalopathy. *Neurology* 1993;43:1437–1438.

Cherington M, Yarnell P, Lammereste D. Lightning strikes: nature of neurological damage in patients evaluated in hospital emergency departments. Ann Emerg Med 1992;21:575–578.

Critchley M. Neurological effects of lightning and electricity. *Lancet* 1934;1:68–72.

Davidson GS, Deck JH. Delayed myelopathy following lightning strike: a demyelinating process. *Acta Neuropathol* 1988;77:104–108.

Gallagher JP, Talbert OR. Motor neuron syndrome after electric shock. *Acta Neurol Scand* 1991;83:79–82.

Fahmy FS, Brinsden MD, Smith J, Frame JD. Lightning: the multisystem group injuries. *J Trauma* 1999;46:937–940.

Hawke CH, Thorpe JW. Acute polyneuropathy due to lightning injury. *J Neurol Neurosurg Psychiatry* 1992;55:388–390.

Kleinschmidt-DeMasters DK. Neuropathology of lightning-strike injuries. *Semin Neurol* 1995;15:323–328.

Panse F. Electrical trauma. In: Vinken PJ, Bruyn GW, Braakman R, eds. *Injuries of the brain and skull. Handbook of clinical neurology, vol 23-24.* Amsterdam: North-Holland Publishing, 1975:683–729.

Sirdofsky MD, Hawley RJ, Manz H. Progressive motor neuron disease associated with electrical injury. *Muscle Nerve* 1991;14:977–980.

Stanley LD, Suss RA. Intracerebral hematoma secondary to lightning stroke: case report and review of the literature. *Neurosurgery* 1985;16:686–688.

Merritt's Neurology, 10th ed, edited by L.P. Rowland. Lippincott Williams & Wilkins, Philadelphia © 2000.

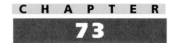

DECOMPRESSION SICKNESS

LEON D. PROCKOP

In scuba diving, caisson work, flying, and simulated altitude ascents, rapid reduction in ambient pressure may allow the formation of bubbles from inert gases (nitrogen in particular) that are normally dissolved in body tissues. Resultant lesions involve the limbs, cardiopulmonary system, and central nervous system. In divers, most neurologic lesions affect the spinal cord. In fliers, cerebral damage is most common.

The incidence of decompression sickness in divers is between 1% and 30%. Although the spinal cord is the most common site of neurologic lesions, encephalopathy is also well-described. Electrophysiologic studies, experimental models, and isolated postmortem examination of patients show predominant involvement of the posterolateral and posterior columns in the watershed areas of the thoracic, upper lumbar, and lower cervical cord. Ischemic perivascular lesions are usually confined to the white matter, but subsequent petechial hemorrhage may occur and extend into the gray matter. Lesions result from bubbles occluding vessels or directly disrupting tissue. Coincident intraarterial embolism may cause cerebral damage.

With cord damage, back pain is followed by leg paresthesia, paresis, and urinary retention. When the brain is affected, neurologic signs and symptoms include visual impairment, vertigo, hemiparesis, loss of consciousness, and seizures. Unless recompression is achieved promptly, the signs, including paralysis, may become permanent.

Serious manifestations of decompression sickness, including any neurologic signs, are a medical emergency. Current therapy consists of recompression in a hyperbaric chamber and the concurrent administration of high concentrations of inspired oxygen. Results of treatment vary, but the sooner recompression is begun, the better the outcome. For chamber locations, physicians should contact the local United States Coast Guard marine and air rescue centers listed in telephone directories in coastal areas.

SUGGESTED READINGS

Aharon-Peretz J, Adir Y, Gordon CR, et al. Spinal cord decompression sickness in sport diving. *Arch Neurol* 1993;50:753–756.

Bond JP, Kirschner DA. Spinal cord myelin is vulnerable to decompression. *Mol Chem Neuropathol* 1997;30:273–288.

Green RD, Leitch DR. Twenty years of treating decompression sickness. *Aviat Space Environ Med* 1987;58:362–366.

Haymaker W, Johnston AD. Pathology of decompression sickness: comparison of lesions in airmen with those in caisson workers and divers. *Mil Med* 1955;117:285–306.

James PB. Dysbarism: the medical problems from high and low atmospheric pressure. *J R Coll Phyicians Lond* 1993;27:367–374.

Lambersten CJ. Concepts for advances in the therapy of bends in undersea and aerospace activity. *Aerospace Med* 1968;39:1086–1093.

Leitch DR, Hallenbeck JM. Oxygen and pressure in the treatment of spinal cord decompression sickness. *Undersea Biomed Res* 1985;12:269–289.

Macleod MA, Houston AS, Kemp PM, Francis TJ. A voxel-by-voxel multivariate analysis of cerebral perfusion defects in divers with "bends." *Nucl Med Commun* 1996;17:795–798.

Palmer AC, Calder IM, Yates PO. Cerebral vasculopathy in divers. *Neuropathol Appl Neurobiol* 1992;18:113–124.

U.S. Navy diving manual, rev 3. Washington, DC: Naval Sea System Command, 1991.

Weiss LD, Van Meter KW. The applications of hyperbaric oxygen therapy in emergency medicine. *Am J Emerg Med* 1992;10:558–568.

Yiannikas C, Beran R. Somatosensory evoked potentials, electroencephalography and CT scans in the assessment of the neurological sequelae of decompression sickness. *Clin Exp Neurol* 1988;25:91–96.

Zorpette G. Flying and the bends. *Sci Am* 1997;277:22–24.

Merritt's Neurology, 10th ed, edited by L.P. Rowland. Lippincott Williams & Wilkins, Philadelphia © 2000.

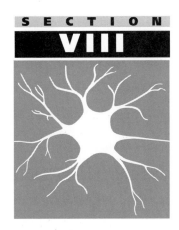

SECTION

VIII

BIRTH INJURIES AND DEVELOPMENTAL ABNORMALITIES

NEONATAL NEUROLOGY

**M. RICHARD KOENIGSBERGER
RAM KAIRAM**

INTRACRANIAL HEMORRHAGE

Gestational age is the best statistical indicator of the probable site of intracranial hemorrhage (ICH). *Supratentorial subdural hemorrhage* has become rare and occurs almost exclusively in full-term or large infants after difficult deliveries. *Parenchymal cerebral hemorrhage* originating in the periventricular area with or without secondary subarachnoid bleeding is common in infants of 32 weeks' gestation or less. *Primary subarachnoid supratentorial hemorrhage* of venous origin occurs in full-term newborns who have focal seizures and a benign clinical course. Subarachnoid hemorrhage may be found at autopsy in premature infants, but there is no recognized clinical syndrome. Posterior fossa hemorrhages are now more readily recognized in newborns, some needing only careful clinical observation, while others require surgical intervention.

PERIVENTRICULAR INTRAVENTRICULAR HEMORRHAGE

Incidence

With the advent of cranial ultrasonography, the incidence of parenchymal hemorrhage—more precisely, periventricular intraventricular hemorrhage (IVH)—used to be about 40% among newborns weighing less than 1,500 g. In the past few years, probably due to advances in pre- and perinatal care, the incidence is down to less than 20%, with very small premature infants (less than 900 g) still having a higher frequency.

Pathology and Pathophysiology

In most patients, the hemorrhage arises in the vascular germinal plate located in the region of the caudate near the foramen of Monro (Fig. 74.1). Bleeding may be confined to this friable matrix area (grade I), but more than 50% of such hemorrhages rupture into the lateral ventricles (grade II), and these sometimes progressively enlarge (grade III). Grade IV, formerly attributed to parenchymal extension of grade III hemorrhage, is now thought to originate in the brain parenchyma itself; its location and size are main contributors to neonatal mortality and neurologic morbidity.

It is not known whether IVH of grades I through III originates from an arterial source, the recurrent artery of Heubner, or from the thalamostriate veins. Proponents of the arterial theory cite hypotension followed by hypertension in an hypoxic brain that has lost autoregulation. The venous hypothesis suggests that

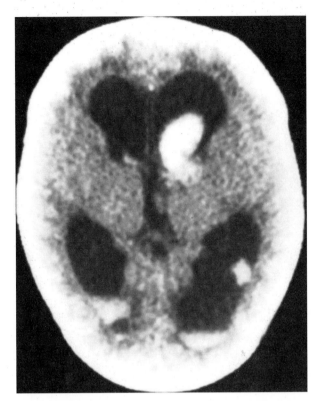

FIG. 74.1. Germinal matrix hemorrhage. Noncontrast axial CT shows small focal hemorrhage in the region of the left caudate head near the left thalamus with extension into the frontal horn of the left lateral ventricle. There is spread of hemorrhage into both occipital horns. This represents grade III germinal matrix hemorrhage. (Courtesy of Dr. S. Chan, Columbia University College of Physicians and Surgeons, New York, NY.)

increased venous pressure leads to stasis, thrombosis, and rupture of thin-walled vessels of the germinal plate. This mechanism of increased venous pressure is thought in some cases to produce a concurrent white matter parenchymal infarct, which may become bloody (grade IV).

Pneumothorax is frequently encountered in coexistent hyaline membrane disease and is often associated with IVH. This complication usually occurs in the first 48 hours of life but may occur several days after birth.

Signs and Symptoms

Grade I hemorrhage is usually asymptomatic. In grade II, there is nonspecific irritability or lethargy. Some grade III hemorrhages are clinically silent with asymptomatic ventriculomegaly, whereas others produce hydrocephalic symptoms of varying severity. When observed in combination with grade IV hemorrhage, deterioration may ensue soon after onset, with at least a 50% chance of mortality; signs include severe apnea, bradycardia, extensor posturing and opisthotonos, ocular conversion or diversion, and pupillary fixation, usually in midposition. Many neonates become flaccid and unresponsive and die within minutes or hours. Clonic limb movements may occur concurrently. The posturing and movements have been called "seizures," but there is little, if any, electroencephalographic (EEG) correlation. Less dramatic deterioration may occur over a few days.

Diagnosis

In preterm infants, gestation of less than 32 weeks places an infant at risk for periventricular IVH. A 20% or greater fall in the hematocrit suggests IVH. The cerebrospinal fluid (CSF) contains many red blood cells and has a protein content of 250 to 1,200 mg/dL. Lumbar puncture is not always diagnostic, because traumatic taps are common. Conversely, CSF may be normal, possibly because blood has not descended to the lumbar level. Days later, the CSF becomes xanthochromic with white and red blood cells and low glucose content; meningitis is ruled out by cultures.

Sonography has replaced computed tomography (CT) as the cornerstone of diagnosis. This portable cribside technique delineates the site of blood in the parenchyma and ventricles, ventricular size, and shifts of major structures. White matter infarctions and cystic periventricular leukomalacia can also be identified.

Prognosis and Therapy

In grades I and II IVH, prognosis is good, with an 80% to 90% survival rate without obvious neurologic abnormality. Many of these children, however, may show later disorders of learning and behavior. Morbidity is attributed to coexisting hypoxic damage, the result of susceptibility of the premature infant's brain to decreases in the partial pressure of oxygen. Grade III hemorrhage may develop into a static or reversible ventriculomegaly with normal pressure or may be followed by progressive hydrocephalus with at least a 40% incidence of cerebral palsy and mental retardation. Grade IV hemorrhage has a high mortality, particularly when large lesions occur. Morbidity can be predicted by the size of hemorrhage. Those with large, echodense parenchymal lesions have a universally poor outcome. Periventricular cysts develop in those with smaller lesions, with a high incidence of spastic diplegia.

No treatment is necessary for grades I and II hemorrhages. In grade III, serial lumbar punctures are most effective when large volumes can be drained (e.g., 10 mL) or when sonography after lumbar puncture shows diminished ventricular size. If sonographic evidence of ventricular enlargement and signs of intracranial pressure persist, external ventriculostomy is used for periods not exceeding 5 days (because of the danger of infection). Lastly, a ventriculoperitoneal shunt may be installed, but this procedure has a high complication rate in small infants. Every attempt should be made to delay shunting until the infant attains as much somatic growth as possible. Although medical therapy with acetazolamide (Diamox) to decrease production of CSF is only sometimes efficacious, it may postpone shunt placement.

Prevention

Many treatments for the prevention of germinal hemorrhage have been attempted. Pharmacologic agents administered to small preterm infants include phenobarbital, ethamsylate, vitamin E, and indomethacin (Indocin). Of these, indomethacin

appears to be most effective; however, late side effects remain to be delineated. Antenatal corticosteroids, primarily used to induce fetal lung maturation, clearly appear to reduce neonatal mortality, as well as the overall incidence and severity of IVH. Nursing techniques and pharmacotherapy that stabilizes systemic blood pressure with subsequent effects on cerebral blood flow may diminish the incidence of IVH and its spread. Among these, the technique of pancuronium bromide (Pavulon) paralysis while the infant is ventilated during the highest-risk first 48 hours of life has drawn much attention and controversy. The best prevention of ICH remains, when possible, the avoidance of premature birth.

HYPOXIC-ISCHEMIC ENCEPHALOPATHY

Incidence

After an era in which obstetric advances had lowered the frequency of asphyxia neonatorum, the incidence in the past decade has remained steady at 2 to 4 per 1,000 births; however, it is still a leading cause of static encephalopathy. Hypoxic-ischemic encephalopathy (HIE), the preferred term for asphyxia, probably occurs with equal frequency in pre- and full-term infants, but overt clinical patterns are seen mainly after 36 weeks' gestational age, often in the postmature baby.

Pathology and Pathophysiology

Hypoxic-ischemic insults had been thought to occur mainly during or immediately after labor. A majority of infants, however, suffer such insults *in utero,* and it is thought that congenital or metabolic abnormalities may increase susceptibility to peripartum stress. Therefore, neonatal HIE can occur despite optimal obstetric management. Concomitant anoxic cardiopulmonary and renal dysfunction may add to the cerebral insult. The resulting brain pathology depends on the maturity of the brain at the time of insult and its duration and location. The periventricular area is a vascular watershed region in premature infants and is especially vulnerable. Preterm infants experience periventricular leukomalacia in the centrum semiovale, which often affects the frontal myelinated fibers that project to the legs. This is the probable mechanism for spastic diplegia in these babies. After 36 weeks' gestation, lesions involve the cerebral gray matter, basal ganglia, brainstem, or cerebellar Purkinje cells. Acute neuronal necrosis is sometimes accompanied by edema and infarction. The chronic picture reveals neuronal loss and astrocytosis, along with ulegyria of the cortex, status marmoratus of the basal ganglia, or cerebellar atrophy (see Chapter 76).

Severe, brief, total HIE results in diffuse deep and superficial lesions that may be incompatible with life. Experimentally, similar lesions can be induced in monkeys by complete intrauterine asphyxia for less than 13 minutes. In humans, these lesions can be caused by abruptio placentae, uterine rupture, or umbilical cord infarction.

Partial HIE for minutes or hours results in predominantly supratentorial lesions, with generalized cerebral edema and laminar neuronal necrosis in the depths of the sulci. Some lesions have a parasagittal or watershed distribution, especially after fetal hypotension. These are the subacute variants most often recognized in the neonatal period. They are attributed to impaired placental exchange. Less severe episodes of hypoxic-ischemic insult of undetermined duration or timing may diffusely involve neurons or preferentially affect the hippocampal areas.

At the cellular level, magnetic resonance spectroscopy, positron-emission tomography, and experimental animal studies have added to knowledge about the pathophysiology of HIE. The data suggest that all brain cells do not die at once following anoxia and energy failure. After the anoxic insult, many cells go through a reoxygenation and reperfusion period. This leads to neuronal leakage from the altered membranes of the edematous cells in the form of excitatory amino acids, particularly glutamate. This substance in turn causes other cells with NMDA (*N*-methyl-d-aspartate) and AMPA (alpha-amino-3-hydroxy-5-methyl-4-isoxazolepropionate) receptors to be stimulated. The latter permit a large cytosolic accumulation of calcium, which in turn leads to a complex cascade of events resulting in secondary cell death. The excitotoxicity causes the release of nitric oxide, one of various free radicals that also contribute to further apoptotic cell death. This series of events caused by hypoxic-ischemic reperfusion takes place over 6 to 12 hours or longer after the original hypoxic-ischemic injury and leads to further neuronal destruction; however, it may also permit a therapeutic window in which pharmacologic therapy may limit the further injurious cascade set off by the original insult.

Signs and Symptoms

Infants who sustain hypoxic or ischemic insults weeks or months before birth may seem normal at birth but later show signs of static encephalopathy or seizures. Others, however, already exhibit signs of chronic cerebral disease at birth, with overt microcephaly and spasticity. In the perinatal period, HIE results in Apgar scores of less than 6 at 1 and 5 minutes. The infant may have poor color, reduced heart rate, and abnormal respiration, along with depressed muscle tone and reflexes. Low scores not only reflect HIE but also can be due to other causes, such as transplacental sedation or peripheral hypotonia due to lower motor neuron disease.

The clinical pattern in infants of less than 34 weeks' gestation differs from that of full-term infants because the findings are nonspecific. Unless there is concurrent IVH (grade III or IV), preterm infants may show only poor response to stimulation, frequent apnea, and bradycardia.

The more common clinical patterns of subacute HIE involving the cerebral cortex of infants of more than 36 weeks' gestation include three patterns: minimal lethargy and hypotonia; hyperalertness, often with hypertonia; or depression and severe hypotonia. Seizures are common in this last clinical pattern.

Some children gradually show improvement in alertness and tone. Others have a few seizures before showing improvement. Infants with severe encephalopathy become more stuporous in the first 24 hours and have seizures, respiratory depression, brainstem abnormalities, and intermittent decerebration. They lose Moro and sucking reflexes and become unresponsive. Even with vigorous anticonvulsant and supportive therapy, 20% to 30% die. If an infant survives the first 48 to 72 hours, seizures usually stop. The patients remain hypotonic and stuporous for a variable period, depending on the severity of brain damage and the amount of drugs given to control the seizures.

Laboratory Data

At the time of labor, fetal heart tone records indicating late and variable deceleration of heart rate relative to uterine contractions, fixed intrauterine heart rate, and persistent fetal bradycardia may be evidence of placental insufficiency and fetal distress, which can lead to HIE. Although providing a warning for appropriate action, such as cesarean section, abnormal fetal heart tones do not necessarily correlate with subsequent brain damage.

After birth, arterial blood gases show low partial pressure of oxygen, high partial pressure of carbon dioxide, and low pH. Serum glucose may be less than 40 μg/100 mL. Serum sodium may be decreased. Serum creatine kinase-BB isoenzyme activity may be elevated. CSF is usually normal, but the CSF lactic acid level is often increased. An EEG may reveal seizure activity that is clinically inapparent. In the interictal period, relatively inactive and burst-suppression patterns have been consistently correlated with poor outcome in infants of 36 weeks' gestational age or older. Impaired visual evoked responses and persistently abnormal brainstem auditory evoked responses may imply a poor prognosis. CT evidence of extensive areas of hypodensity of both gray and white matter suggests a guarded outlook. Magnetic resonance imaging (MRI), when not too risky to a patient's tenuous clinical state, may demonstrate early areas of hyperintensity, particularly in T2-weighted sequences, reflecting injury to the basal ganglia and other deep structures that is not evident on CT. Six months to 1 year later, the procedure may show delayed myelination, as well as gray and white matter changes in the infant's brain.

Treatment and Prognosis

Because the hypoxic-ischemic insult involves several body systems, attention must be directed to the respiratory, cardiovascular, and renal systems, as well as the brain. Measures include respiratory support and maintenance of normal blood pressure and renal output while specific treatment of seizures and brain edema is undertaken. The treatment of seizures is discussed later. Steroids and osmotic agents have been used to treat brain edema in this setting with little success. In addition, given the therapeutic window during hypoxic-ischemic reperfusion described above, animal and early clinical trials with antiexcitotoxic amino acids (NMDA receptor antagonists), antioxidative substances, and nitric oxide inhibitors are being attempted in order to reduce neuronal death due to hypoxic-ischemic reperfusion.

The prognosis is always guarded. The more rapid the recovery is from the initial depression, the better the outlook will be. Of infants with a benign neonatal course, 20% to 30% may still have neurologic sequelae ranging from intellectual impairment to spastic diplegia and seizures. At least 50% of those with neonatal seizures have serious morbidity. Prevention by rapid delivery (cesarean section) when there is evidence of intrauterine distress is still the best method of avoiding sequelae.

NEONATAL INFECTIONS

Bacterial infections are commonly acquired perinatally. Viral or protozoan infections may be acquired *in utero* from the first trimester until delivery. Infections constituting the TORCH syndrome (toxoplasmosis, other agents, rubella, cytomegalovirus, herpes simplex) are discussed in Section III, Infections of the Nervous System. Only some particular features of perinatally acquired herpes simplex virus (HSV) infection are dealt with here.

Neonatal Herpes Encephalitis

Estimates of the incidence of active neonatal HSV infection are 1 per 15,000 live births. HSV infection may be acquired *in utero* or during passage through the birth canal. Most neonatal HSV infections are caused by HSV type 2 rather than HSV type 1. Some infants have only skin-eye-mouth disease, but 70% have either systemic or CNS disease. Infants with CNS involvement usually present in the second or third weeks of life. At presentation, infants with HSV septicemia may have respiratory disease, jaundice, fever, and CNS symptoms without evidence of skin or mucous membrane vesicles, much like those with only CNS involvement, who present with fever, irritability, and seizures.

Laboratory investigation reveals lymphocytosis and increased protein in the CSF. Viral amplification with the polymerase chain reaction technique in the CSF has made diagnosis of HSV encephalitis quicker and more definite. Neuroimaging procedures, CT and MRI, may be normal but often show diffuse and, occasionally, focal abnormalities.

Infants with suspected HSV infection should be treated with acyclovir (Zovirax), 30 mg/kg intravenously for 21 days. Mortality is in the neighborhood of 33%. Serious neurologic sequelae are frequent, particularly when multicystic encephalomalacia develops.

Neonatal Meningitis

Bacterial meningitis is usually seen in association with sepsis. The incidence of sepsis neonatorum is about 0.51 per 1,000 live births. In about 30% of patients with neonatal sepsis, there is spread to the meninges. At present in the United States, the predominant organism causing neonatal septicemia and meningitis is group B streptococci followed by gram-negative organisms, the most common being *Escherichia coli, Proteus vulgaris,* and *Pseudomonas aeruginosa. Listeria monocytogenes* and other organisms are sometimes encountered. *Staphylococcus* is now rare. Susceptibility to these organisms is attributed to immaturity of immune responses or of the blood–brain barrier. Pathologic changes in the newborn brain are similar to those in older children or adults.

The clinical presentation of meningitis in the newborn is subtle. Meningeal signs are rarely elicited; lassitude and poor feeding may be the only abnormalities. Hypothermia, rather than fever, is a suggestive sign. Seizures may be the first sign. Only when the course is advanced does the fontanel bulge and the infant assumes a position of opisthotonos. Lumbar puncture shows CSF changes similar to those in older children, but CSF protein levels up to 150 μg/dL may be normal in newborns. The blood-to-CSF ratio is less valid, as newborns normally have blood glucose levels of 30 to 40 mg/dL. Cultures of the CSF may remain positive for 3 or 4 days, even after initiation of proper therapy.

Because the disease may be advanced when it is clinically manifest, both mortality and morbidity remain high. Appropriate intravenous antibiotic therapy should be given for 3 weeks. Intrathecal and intraventricular therapy have not been effective. Parenchymal invasion and clinically significant subdural effusions are rare at this age. Gram-negative organisms, particularly *Citrobacter,* are most frequently implicated in neonatal abscess, which is rare.

NEONATAL SEIZURES

Seizures in the neonatal period should always be considered symptomatic of serious underlying neurologic or systemic disease. Neonatal convulsions imply at least 17% mortality and 30% serious morbidity. The prognosis depends mainly on the cause of the seizures and on rapid establishment of the diagnosis and treatment; however, it is difficult to recognize the clinical expressions of abnormal cortical discharges, particularly in infants of less than 35 weeks' gestation in whom conventional clinical and EEG seizure patterns are infrequently seen.

Classification

Neonatal seizures occur in several forms. Focal and multifocal clonic seizures are the most frequent varieties that have clear electrical concomitants. They constitute 50% of neonatal convulsions and may begin as jerking of a limb, twitching on one side of the face, or rhythmic horizontal deviation of the eyes. More often than not, the convulsions become multifocal. Clonus or "jitteriness" may be misinterpreted as a seizure. The rhythm of a seizure is slow, three to four jerks per second; clonus or nonspecific tremor is about 6 to 12 jerks per second. Moreover, clonus or tremulousness can be started or stopped by altering the position of a limb.

Tonic postures are the next most common kind of neonatal seizure. An arm may be extended with or without horizontal eye deviation or head turning. These seizures may not be recognized by nursery personnel and may look like yawning or stretching. Total-body extension with arm flexion or opisthotonic postures and vertical eye movements may be overinterpreted as seizures. These decerebrate or decorticate postures have no electrographic correlation and are likely to occur in infants of less than 34 weeks' gestational age with IVH.

Classic grand mal seizures or infantile myoclonic seizures are rare in the newborn. Myoclonus is often stimulus-sensitive and suggests severe brain damage or drug withdrawal. Certain adventitious movements, frequently classified as "subtle seizures," in most cases do not show evidence of an electrical-cortical genesis on video/EEG studies. These abnormal movements include mouthing, tongue thrusting, "pedaling" and "bicycling" of limbs, and chaotic eye shifting. The movements are attributed to brainstem or frontal release phenomena. Often seen in severe encephalopathy, these movements then imply a grave prognosis. Until their genesis is established, calling them "seizures" is not advised because this term implies benefit from anticonvulsant drug therapy.

Apnea accompanied by bradycardia in the preterm infant is a frequent but poorly understood event. In infants of 36 weeks' gestation or older, apnea without bradycardia is often accompanied by other types of seizures and is an important type of convulsion to recognize. It responds to anticonvulsants, whereas depressant agents are contraindicated in the apnea of the premature.

Diagnosis

Once a seizure is identified, diagnostic evaluation should proceed as rapidly as possible. Family, pregnancy, delivery history, and physical examination may provide essential clues to etiology. The first laboratory tests should evaluate the common metabolic and infectious disorders that require specific treatment. A dipstick test for hypoglycemia and lumbar puncture to exclude meningitis or hemorrhage are essential. Then blood glucose, calcium, magnesium, sodium, and acid–base values should be obtained plus a blood culture. EEG studies must be promptly undertaken if abnormal movements are not clearly identified as seizures. Sonography provides information about large hemorrhages. CT will confirm these, other forms of ICH, calcifications, congenital anomalies, and ischemic damage. MRI is helpful for more subtle migration and myelinization defects. If a congenital infection is suspected, TORCH antibody titers should be drawn. If seizures do not respond to initial treatment, pyridoxine, 50 mg, should be given intravenously to rule out rare pyridoxine dependency. Blood, urine, and CSF should then be analyzed for errors of inborn metabolism that present in the neonatal period: phenylketonuria, maple syrup urine disease, lactic or organic acidemias, ammonia cycle abnormalities, and nonketotic hyperglycinemia.

Etiology and Prognosis

The outcome of neonatal seizures is linked to etiology (Table 74.1). In some metabolic disorders, prognosis is better the sooner treatment starts. Surveys of prognosis have given different estimates because some institutions see more neonatal seizures of benign etiology (e.g., late hypocalcemia), while others classify all adventitious movements as seizures.

The EEG, judiciously interpreted, may help determine the prognosis. The proper time for an EEG is 24 to 72 hours, as in newborns the EEG often becomes normal in a few days and may lose prognostic significance. Five types of interictal EEG patterns are observed in infants of 36 to 42 weeks' gestation: normal, unifocal spike with normal background, multifocal spike, burst-suppression, and inactive or flat. The first two types suggest a 70% chance of a good outcome. A poor prognostic cause, however, is more important than any EEG pattern. Multifocal spikes, especially with abnormal backgrounds, imply only a 20% chance of a good prognosis. The burst-suppression pattern, not to be confused with the normal deep-sleep pattern, invariably implies a bad outcome. The inactive or low-voltage EEG has the same poor prognosis, although it may be hard to interpret when anticonvulsant drug levels are high.

Treatment

Treatment of neonatal seizures is either specific or symptomatic. Metabolic encephalopathies require specific therapy. Documented neonatal hypoglycemia (defined as a blood glucose level of less than 40 mg/dL in a full-term infant and less than 30 mg/dL in a premature infant) is usually treated with an intravenous bolus of 25% to 50% glucose followed by a maintenance infusion of 10% dextrose.

Hypocalcemia (defined as a blood calcium level of less than 7 mg/dL) is of two varieties. The late-onset (after day 5) benign type is usually seen in full-term infants who are given high-phosphate formulas and who have multifocal seizures. When hypocalcemia is suspected, blood should be drawn for calcium levels. Treatment involves giving intravenous doses of calcium gluconate with electrocardiograph monitoring. When the blood calcium level does not rise in response to this therapy, it may respond to intramuscular therapy with magnesium sulfate. The seizures of infants with early-onset hypocalcemia may not re-

TABLE 74.1. RELATIONSHIP OF NEUROLOGIC DISEASE TO PROGNOSIS IN NEONATAL SEIZURES

Disease	Children who survive and become normal (%)	Comment
Perinatal asphyxia	50	—
Subarachnoid hemorrhage	90	—
Intraventricular hemorrhage	10	Seizures rare in prematures
Hypoglycemia	50	Outcome may be related to early-onset therapy
Late hypocalcemia	90	Presents day 5–10
Early hypocalcemia	50	Presents day 1–3 in conjunction with other encephalopathies
		A few with phenylketonuria or pyridoxine dependency may do well
Inborn metabolic errors	10	—
		Defects include lissencephaly, polymicrogyria, pachygyria
Bacterial meningitis	30	Good follow-up series unavailable; drugs include heroin and methadone
Congenital anomalies	0	10–20% of neonatal seizures, including benign familial seizure
Drug withdrawal	?	
Cause unknown	67	

Modified from Volpe JJ, Koenigsberger MR. *Neonatology: pathophysiology and management of the newborn.* Philadelphia: JB Lippincott Co, 1981.

spond to therapy because this type of hypocalcemia often accompanies severe ICH or HIE. Severe encephalopathy with inappropriate antidiuretic hormone secretion causes hyponatremia, which may also result from iatrogenic overhydration. It is controlled by fluid restriction. Other metabolic encephalopathies are difficult to treat and have a poor prognosis. General supportive care should not be forgotten; when possible, therapy should be carried out in a neonatal intensive care unit. An adequate airway should be ensured, and means for mechanical respiration should be available.

A single seizure is treated with an intravenous loading dose of phenobarbital, 20 mg/kg, over 10 minutes followed by a maintenance dose of 5 mg/kg per day in two 12-hour doses. Blood phenobarbital levels of 20 to 40 µg/dL should be established and maintained. In status epilepticus, the same loading dose is given over 2 minutes. If seizures persist, two more 10 mg/kg doses can be administered over 1 or 2 hours. A blood level of 40 to 60 mg/kg for 1 or 2 days is justified in the attempt to suppress continuous epileptic activity. If phenobarbital fails, phenytoin sodium (Dilantin), 20 mg/kg, can be given intravenously over 15 minutes with cardiac monitoring. If status epilepticus continues, a 4% paraldehyde intravenous drip is titrated against seizure activity. Intravenous diazepam and lorazepam (Ativan) have increasingly been employed. Awareness of severe respiratory depression when benzodiazepines are combined with barbiturates is essential.

In the newborn, maintenance dosage of phenobarbital is 3 to 5 mg/kg per day administered orally, intramuscularly, or intravenously in two 12-hour doses. Phenytoin should be given intravenously (because it has poor oral absorption) at 7 to 10 mg/kg per day in two 12-hour doses.

In infants with single or easily controlled seizures, an anticonvulsant may be tapered on discharge. Others remain on phenobarbital maintenance (5 µg/kg per day) for 1 to 3 months, allowing the infant to self-taper by not increasing the dose with weight gain.

SUGGESTED READINGS

Intracranial Hemorrhage

Allan WC. The IVH complex of lesions: cerebrovascular injury in the preterm infant. *Neurol Clin* 1990;8:529–551.

Bergman I, Bauer RE, Barmada MH. Intracerebral hemorrhage in the full-term neonatal infant. *Pediatrics* 1985;75:488–496.

Goddard-Finegold J, Mizrahi EM. Understanding and preventing perinatal peri- and intraventricular hemorrhage. *J Child Neurol* 1987;2:170–185.

Guzzetta F, Shackelford GD, Volpe S, et al. Periventricular intraparenchymal echodensities in the premature newborn: critical determinant of neurologic outcome. *Pediatrics* 1986;78:995–1006.

Horbar JD. Antenatal corticosteroid treatment and neonatal outcomes for infants 501 to 1500 gm in the Vernont-Oxford Trials Network. *Am J Obstet Gynecol* 1995;173:275–281.

Ment LR, Oh W, Ehrenkranz RA, et al. Low-dose indomethacin and prevention of intraventricular hemorrhage: a multicenter randomized trial. *Pediatrics* 1994;93:543–550.

Paneth N, Rudelli R, Monte W, et al. White matter necrosis in very low birth weight infants: neuropathologic and ultrasonographic findings in infants surviving six days or longer. *J Pediatr* 1990;116:975–984.

Pape KE, Wigglesworth JS. *Hemorrhage, ischemia and the perinatal brain.* Philadelphia: JB Lippincott Co, 1979.

Pearlman JM, Goodman S, Kreuser KL, et al. Reduction in intraventricular hemorrhage by elimination of fluctuating cerebral blood flow velocity in preterm infants with respiratory distress syndrome. *N Engl J Med* 1985;312:1353–1356.

Perrin RG, Rutha JT, Drake JM, et al. Management and outcome of posterior fossa subdural hematomas in neonates. *Neurosurgery* 1997;40:1190–1199.

Roland EH, Hill A. Intraventricular hemorrhage and posthemorrhagic hydrocephalus: current and potential future interventions. *Clin Perinatol* 1997;24:589–605.

Van de Bor M, den Ouden L, Guit GL. Value of cranial ultrasound and magnetic resonance imaging in predicting neurodevelopmental outcome in preterm infants. *Pediatrics* 1992;90:196–199.

Volpe JJ. *Neurology of the newborn,* 3rd ed. Philadelphia: WB Saunders, 1995.

Welch K, Strand R. Traumatic parturitional intracranial hemorrhage. *Dev Med Child Neurol* 1986;28:156–164.

Hypoxic-ischemic Encephalopathy

Adsett DB, Fitz CR, Hill A. Hypoxic-ischemic injury in the term newborn: correlation of CT findings with neurological outcome. *Dev Med Child Neurol* 1985;27:155–160.

Banker BA, Larroche JC. Periventricular leukomalacia of infancy. *Arch Neurol* 1962;7:386–410.

Du Plessis AJ, Johnston MV. Hypoxic-ischemic brain injury in the newborn: cellular mechanisms and potential strategies for neuroprotection. *Clin Perinatol* 1997;24:627–654.

Edwards AD, Yue X, Cox P, et al. Apoptosis in the brains of infants suffering intrauterine cerebral injury. *Pediatr Res* 1997;39:584–590.

Gluckman PD, Williams CE. When and why do brain cells die? *Dev Med Child Neurol* 1992;34:1010–1014.

Hanrahan JD, Sargentoni J, Azzopardi D, et al. Cerebral metabolism within 18 hours of birth asphyxia: a proton magnetic resonance spectroscopy study. *Pediatr Res* 1996;39:584–590.

Lupton BA, Hill A, Roland EH, Whitfield MF, Flodmark O. Brain swelling in the asphyxiated term newborn: pathogenesis and outcome. *Pediatrics* 1988;82:139–146.

Marin-Padilla M. Developmental neuropathology and impact of perinatal damage. I: hemorrhagic lesions of neocortex. *J Neuropathol Exp Neurol* 1996;55:758–773.

Myers RE. Experimental models of periventricular brain damage: relevance to human pathology. In: Gluck L, ed. *Intrauterine asphyxia and the developing brain.* Chicago: Year Book Medical Publishers, 1977:337–397.

Nelson KB, Ellenberg, JH. Antecedents of cerebral palsy. *N Engl J Med* 1986;315:81–86.

Painter MJ. Fetal heart rate patterns, perinatal asphyxia, and brain injury. *Pediatr Neurol* 1989;5:137–144.

Pasternak JF, Gorey MT. The syndrome of acute near-total intrauterine asphyxia in the term infant. *Pediatr Neurol* 1998;18:391–398.

Rivkin MJ. Hypoxic-ischemic brain injury in the term newborn: neuropathology, clinical aspects, and neuroimaging. *Clin Perinatol* 1997;24:607–626.

Roth SC, Edwards AD, Cady EB, et al. Relation of deranged neonatal cerebral oxidative metabolism asphyxia, with neurodevelopmental outcome and head circumference at 4 years. *Dev Med Child Neurol* 1997;39:758–773.

Infections

Bale JF Jr, Murph JR. Infections of the central nervous system in the newborn. *Clin Perinatol* 1997;24:787–806.

Bell WE, McCormick WF. *Neurologic infections in children,* 2nd ed. Philadelphia: WB Saunders, 1989.

Edwards MS, Rench MA, Haffer AA, et al. Long-term sequelae of group B streptococcal meningitis in infants. *J Pediatr* 1985;106:717–722.

Franco S, Cornelius V, Andrews B. Long-term outcome of neonatal meningitis. *Am J Dis Child* 1992;146:567–571.

Kline M. *Citrobacter* meningitis and brain abscess in infancy: epidemiology, pathogenesis and treatment. *J Pediatr* 1988;113:430–434.

Whitley R, Arvin A, Prober C, et al. A controlled trial comparing vidarabine with acyclovir in neonatal herpes simplex viral infection. *N Engl J Med* 1991;324:444–449.

Seizures

Clancy RR, Legido A. Postnatal epilepsy after EEG-confirmed neonatal seizures. *Epilepsia* 1991;32:69–76.

Holden KR, Mellitis ED, Freeman JM. Neonatal seizures I. Correlation of prenatal and perinatal events with outcome. *Pediatrics* 1982;70:165–176.

Koenigsberger MR. Abnormal neonatal movements, intracranial hemorrhage, asphyxia. *Pediatr Ann* 1983;12:798–804.

Koenigsberger MR, Caballar-Gonzaga FJ, Dierkes T. Neonatal seizures: initiation and discontinuation of therapy. *REV NEUROL* 1997;25:706–708.

Koivisto M, Blanco-Sequieros M, Krause U. Neonatal symptomatic hypoglycemia: a follow-up study of 151 children. *Dev Med Child Neurol* 1972;14:603–609.

Legido A, Clancy RR, Berman PH. Recent advances in the diagnosis, treatment, and prognosis of neonatal seizures. *Pediatr Neurol* 1988;4:79–86.

Lynch BJ, Rust RS. Natural history of neonatal hypocalcemic and hypomagnesemic seizures. *Pediatr Neurol* 1994;11:23–27.

Maytal J, Novak GP, King KC. Lorazepam in the treatment of refractory neonatal seizures. *J Child Neurol* 1991;6:319–323.

Mizrahi EM, Kellaway P. Characterization and classification of neonatal seizures. *Neurology* 1987;37:1837–1844.

Painter MJ, Gaus LM. Neonatal seizures: diagnosis and treatment. *J Child Neurol* 1991;6:101–108.

Rose AL, Lombroso CT. Neonatal seizures states: a study of clinical features in 137 full-term babies with long-term follow-up. *Pediatrics* 1970;45:404–425.

Ryan SG, Wizniter M, Hollman C, et al. Benign familial neonatal convulsion: evidence for clinical and genetic heterogeneity. *Ann Neurol* 1991;29:469–473.

Scher MS. Seizures in the newborn infant: diagnosis, outcome and treatment. *Clin Perinatol* 1997;24:736–772.

Volpe JJ. *Neurology of the newborn,* 3rd ed. Philadelphia: WB Saunders, 1995.

Merritt's Neurology, 10th ed., edited by L.P. Rowland. Lippincott Williams & Wilkins, Philadelphia

FLOPPY INFANT SYNDROME

THORNTON B.A. MASON II
DARRYL C. DE VIVO

When a normal infant is suspended in the prone position, the arms and legs move out, and the head is held in line with the body. In many different disorders, a child does not respond in this fashion. Rather, the limbs and head all hang limply—like a ragdoll. That is why the *floppy infant syndrome* has caught on as a popular term. In addition to children with these abnormal postures, some clinicians have extended the use of the term to include those with diminished resistance of limbs to passive movement and with abnormal extensibility of joints.

The number of conditions that sometimes cause these manifestations seems endless, including disorders of the brain, spinal cord, peripheral nerves, neuromuscular junction, muscles, and ligaments, as well as some disorders of unknown origin. The number of possible causes of floppy infant syndrome makes diagnosis of the primary disorder seem impossible. There are almost always clues of some kind, however, that narrow the list of possible causes to a few choices. An essential division separates conditions found in the newborn infant from those occurring later (Table 75.1). A second division separates conditions characterized by true limb weakness (often with no tendon reflexes) from those with clear neurologic signs or cerebral injury without true limb weakness. Among the latter, there are likely to be signs of mental retardation, dysmorphic physical evidence of chromosomal abnormality, or evidence of metabolic abnormality.

A third diagnostic consideration concerns illness in the mother and the perinatal history. If the mother is known to have myotonic muscular dystrophy or myasthenia gravis, depressed movement in the infant is immediately recognized. The correct diagnosis in the child may be the first clue to explain previously unrecognized manifestations of illness in the mother. Similarly, maternal narcotic drug abuse, alcoholism, or use of anticonvulsant medications may affect the infant. Perinatal events may lead to suspicion of asphyxia or cerebral hemorrhage.

A fourth consideration is the distribution of the abnormality. Are all four limbs, or only the legs, or one arm affected? Are sucking and swallowing impaired? The answers have different diagnostic implications.

The most common causes of hypotonia are perinatal insult to the brain or spinal cord, spinal muscular atrophy, and dysgenetic syndromes. About 75% of cases fall into these categories. Spinal muscular atrophy, however, is only rarely evident immediately after birth. The neonatologist considers common perinatal insults such as birth asphyxia, hypoxic-ischemic insults, intracranial hemorrhage, bacterial or viral infections, metabolic disturbances, and extreme prematurity as principal causes of hypotonia in the newborn nursery. Congenital hypoglycemia or hypothyroidism may be suggested by hypothermia. Spinal cord injuries usually follow intrauterine malpositioning or traumatic birth. Severe asphyxia may also affect the lower motor neurons of the spinal cord. Autopsy studies of fatally asphyxiated neonates with flaccid tone and areflexia demonstrate prominent ischemic necrosis of anterior spinal cord gray matter in a radially oriented, watershed distribution consistent with hypoperfusion between the anterior spinal artery and the paired dorsal spinal arteries. In these conditions, the perinatal history is informative, and the hypotonic infant has associated behavioral alterations, including decreased responsiveness or seizures. Dysmorphic features are absent, and tendon reflexes are present.

TABLE 75.1. FLOPPY INFANT SYNDROMES

	Neuromuscular disorders (weakness prominent)	Central disorders with abnormal neurologic signs or peripheral disorders (little or no weakness)
Neonatal	Infantile spinal muscular atrophy Congenital myotonic dystrophy Neonatal myasthenia gravis Congenital myopathies[a,b] Metabolic myopathies (Pompe disease)[c] Congenital muscular dystrophy (Fukuyama and Zellweger types)	Perinatal asphyxia or cerebral hemorrhage Sepsis Intoxication Spinal cord injury or malformation Failure-to-thrive syndromes Congenital hypothyroidism Dysgenetic syndromes (e.g., Down disease) Prader-Willi syndrome
Age 1–6mo (or later)	Infantile spinal muscular atrophy Infantile Guillain-Barré or other peripheral neuropathy Congenital myasthenia gravis[f] Botulism	Metabolic cerebral degenerations[d] Hypotonic cerebral palsy Connective tissue disorders[e] Metabolic and endocrine disease[g] Essential hypotonia
Failure to reach developmental stages but not really floppy	Congenital myopathies[b] Some Duchenne muscular dystrophy	— —

[a]Spinal muscular atrophy and congenital myopathies are more likely to cause symptoms *after* the neonatal period.
[b]Congenital myopathies include those characterized by specific histochemical abnormality (nemaline, central core, myotubular, and other structures).
[c]Metabolic myopathies include infantile acid maltase deficiency (Pompe disease), mitochondrial DNA depletion syndrome, and benign and fatal infantile cytochrome-C oxidase deficiency.
[d]Leukodystrophies, lipid storage diseases, peroxisomal diseases, mucopolysaccharidosis, aminoacidurias, Leigh syndrome.
[e]Congenital laxity of ligaments, Ehlers-Danlos syndrome, Marfan syndrome.
[f]Congenital myasthenia does not usually cause infantile symptoms other than ophthalmoplegia.
[g]Organic acidemia, hypocalcemia or hypercalcemia; hypothyroidism; renal tubular acidosis.

FOCAL NEONATAL HYPOTONIA

This disorder may be caused by trauma or developmental abnormality. A flaccid arm usually implies brachial plexus injury. Signs of injury to the upper brachial plexus may be associated with ipsilateral paralysis of the diaphragm; lower brachial plexus lesions may be accompanied by an ipsilateral Horner syndrome. Electromyography and spinal evoked potentials help define the severity of the nerve root injury. Spinal cord imaging may document nerve root avulsion.

Hypotonia and weakness of the legs indicate spinal cord pathology. Spinal dysraphism and the caudal regression syndrome are obvious on inspection of the back. An arthrogrypotic leg deformity or gross maldevelopment of the legs is associated with sacral agenesis. Fifteen percent of patients with sacral agenesis are infants of diabetic mothers.

DYSGENETIC SYNDROMES

These syndromes are often associated with distinctive dysmorphic physical features. The neurologic disorder may not be recognized until the infant fails to reach certain developmental stages. Common syndromes associated with hypotonia are Down syndrome, Prader-Willi syndrome, Lowe syndrome, Zellweger syndrome, Smith-Lemli-Opitz syndrome, and the Riley-Day (familial dysautonomia) syndrome. Environmental toxins may also produce hypotonia and dysmorphism. Common examples include fetal exposure to heroin, phenytoin sodium (Dilantin), trimethadione (Tridione), or alcohol. Strength is normal in these syndromes, but the tendon reflexes may vary from nondetectable to brisk.

NEUROMUSCULAR DISORDERS

Neuromuscular disorders that cause infantile hypotonia do not impair mental alertness but are characterized by decreased limb movement (because of muscle weakness) and decreased tendon reflexes. Dysmorphic features accompany many congenital myopathies. After the immediate neonatal period, spinal muscular atrophy is the most common cause of infantile hypotonia. This autosomal-recessive disorder (Werdnig-Hoffmann disease) may sometimes be evident at birth. The characteristic findings include limb weakness, areflexia, and fasciculations of the tongue. Although most affected infants die before age 2 years, some survive for decades.

Poliomyelitis is now uncommon as a cause of limb weakness. The neurologic findings are asymmetric and are accompanied by signs of meningeal irritation with cerebrospinal fluid (CSF) pleocytosis and elevated protein content.

Infantile neuropathies are uncommon causes of weakness, areflexia, and hypotonia. Examples include metachromatic leukodystrophy, globoid cell leukodystrophy, infantile neuroaxonal dystrophy, giant axonal neuropathy, neonatal adrenoleukodystrophy, hypertrophic interstitial polyneuropathy, and peroneal muscular atrophy. Important clues may include a family history, palpably enlarged peripheral nerves, upper motor neuron signs, elevated CSF protein concentration, and slowed nerve conduction velocities. Guillain-Barré syndrome rarely presents in infancy. Diphtheria, caused by *Corynebacterium diphtheriae,* produces a generalized demyelinating polyneuropathy clinically similar to Guillain-Barré syndrome. A protein exotoxin secreted by the organism inhibits myelin synthesis and may also activate cytotoxic mechanisms. Tick paralysis has a rapid onset, producing a hypotonic picture also similar to Guillain-Barré syndrome, and usually occurs in the spring and summer months. The paralysis is caused by a tick that is continuously attached and secreting toxin-laden saliva; removal of the tick is rapidly curative.

Disturbances at the myoneural junction may cause limb weakness. Fluctuating signs intensified by vigorous crying or limb activity are important observations. *Congenital myasthenia gravis* often affects siblings and is thought to be inherited as an autosomal-recessive disorder. This condition is considered nonimmunologic. Clinically, the infant may display external ophthalmoplegia and generalized weakness; sudden respiratory failure rarely occurs. Autoimmune forms of myasthenia gravis in infancy include the transient *neonatal form* in infants of myasthenic mothers. The *juvenile form* ordinarily does not cause symptoms before age 2 years. Acetylcholine receptor antibodies, sensitivity to curare, and responsiveness to plasmapheresis distinguish these myasthenic syndromes from the inherited nonimmunologic forms.

Another condition affecting neuromuscular transmission is *infantile botulism,* which results from ingestion of *Clostridium botulinum* spores that germinate in the intestinal tract. Manifestations include ileus, constipation, hypotonia, weakness, pupillary dilation, and apneic spells. The clinical picture is distinctive, and diagnosis can be confirmed by the recovery of the bacterium and the exotoxin in the feces. A facilitating response to repetitive stimulation (such as that of the Eaton-Lambert syndrome) can usually be demonstrated and may be an important diagnostic clue. Attention should be paid to avoiding any medications that might exacerbate the neuromuscular transmission deficit, in particular aminoglycoside antibiotics that are sometimes initiated empirically at presentation for possible sepsis. Complete recovery follows appropriate supportive care.

Myopathies that cause infantile limb weakness include the *congenital myopathies* with specific structural abnormalities, myotonic muscular dystrophy, and metabolic myopathies. Although the term *muscular dystrophy* usually implies progressive disease, the term has been applied to apparently static congenital disorders in which the changes in muscle biopsy are myopathic but have no specific features. In Japan, the Fukuyama type of *congenital muscular dystrophy* is characterized by severe mental retardation in all cases and seizures in about 50%. Symptoms may start soon after birth, with difficulty nursing and impoverished movement. The children never walk but may live for decades. The cerebral pathology is distinctive, with polymicrogyria of the occipital lobes in a pattern that can be recognized by magnetic resonance imaging. Similar cases have been seen in the United States and Europe.

The *histochemically defined myopathies* may be inherited as autosomal-dominant or autosomal-recessive traits or as a sex-linked recessive trait. These disorders share many phenotypic features that overlap with other syndromes. Examples include central core disease, multicore disease, nemaline myopathy, myotubular (centronuclear) myopathy, congenital fiber-type disproportion, sarcotubular myopathy, fingerprint-body myopathy, and reducing-body myopathy. Muscular weakness, decreased tendon reflexes, dysmorphic physical features, a predisposition to congenital hip dislocation, and later development of scoliosis characterize most of the histochemically defined myopathies. The similarities often outweigh the differences.

Infantile acid maltase deficiency (Pompe disease) is the classic example of a metabolic myopathy and motor neuron disease that causes infantile hypotonia. The affected infant is mentally alert but weak and areflexic. As associated findings, the tongue and heart are enlarged; congestive heart failure is the cause of death before age 6 months. Other *metabolic myopathies* that may cause infantile hypotonia and weakness include cytochrome-*c*-oxidase deficiency (benign reversible and fatal forms), the mitochondrial DNA depletion syndrome, glycogenosis type IV (debrancher enzyme deficiency), and glycogenosis type V (myophosphorylase deficiency). Cytochrome-*c*-oxidase deficiency and mitochondrial DNA depletion syndrome are associated with lactic acidosis.

A few hypotonic infants eventually develop normally after several years. The term *essential hypotonia* should be reserved to describe an otherwise healthy infant with unexplained hypotonia and normal strength, tendon reflexes, and general physical features.

SUGGESTED READINGS

Brooke MH, Carroll JE, Ringel SP. Congenital hypotonia revisited. *Muscle Nerve* 1979;2:84–100.

DiMauro S, Hartlage PL. Fatal infantile form of muscle phosphorylase deficiency. *Neurology* 1978;28:1124–1129.

DiMauro S, Mendell JR, Sahenk Z, et al. Fatal infantile mitochondrial myopathy and renal dysfunction due to cytochrome-c-oxidase deficiency. *Neurology* 1980;30:795–804.

DiMauro S, Nicholson JF, Hays AP, et al. Mitochondrial myopathy due to reversible cytochrome-c-oxidase deficiency. *Ann Neurol* 1983;14:226–234.

Dubowitz V. *The floppy infant.* London: Spastics International Medical Publications, 1969.

Dubowitz V. *Muscle disorders in childhood.* Philadelphia: WB Saunders, 1978.

Engel AG. *Myasthenia gravis and myasthenic syndromes.* Philadelphia: FA Davis, 1999.

Gillessen-Kaesbach G, Gross S, Kaya-Westerloh S, et al. DNA methylation based testing of 450 patients suspected of having Prader-Willi syndrome. *J Med Genet* 1995;32:88–92.

Hagberg B, Sanner G, Steen M. The dysequilibrium syndrome in cerebral palsy: clinical aspects and treatment. *Acta Paediatr Scand Suppl* 1972;226:1–63.

Helbling-Leclerc A, Zhang X, Topaloglu H, et al. Mutations of the laminin α2-chain gene (LAMA2) cause merosin-deficient congenital muscular dystrophy. *Nat Genet* 1995;11:216–218.

Osawa M, Shishikura K. Werdnig-Hoffmann disease and variants. In: Vinken PJ, Bruyn GW, Klawans HL, De Jong JMBV, ed. *Diseases of the motor system. Handbook of clinical neurology, vol 59.* New York: Elsevier Science, 1991:51–80.

Pickett J, Berg B, Chaplin E, Brunstetter-Shaffer MA. Syndrome of botulism in infancy: clinical and electrophysiological study. *N Engl J Med* 1976;295:770–772.

Sarnat HB. Neuromuscular disorders in the neonatal period. In: Korobkin R, Guilleminault C, eds. *Advances in perinatal neurology.* New York: SP Medical & Scientific Books, 1979;1.

Schaumburg HH, Kaplan JG. Toxic peripheral neuropathies. In: Asbury AK, Thomas PK, eds. *Peripheral nerve disorders 2.* Oxford: Butterworth-Heinemann, 1995:238–261.

Toda T, Segawa M, Nomura Y, et al. Localization of a gene for Fukuyama type congenital muscular dystrophy to chromosome 9q31-33. *Nat Genet* 1993;5:283–286.

Vu TH, Sciacco M, Tanji K, et al. Clinical manifestations of mitochondrial DNA depletion. *Neurology* 1998;50:1783–1790.

Merritt's Neurology, 10th ed., edited by L.P. Rowland. Lippincott Williams & Wilkins, Philadelphia © 2000.

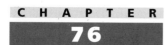

STATIC DISORDERS OF BRAIN DEVELOPMENT

ISABELLE RAPIN

TABLE 76.1. CLINICAL VARIANTS OF CEREBRAL PALSY (CP)

Spastic hemiparesis (hemiplegia)
Spastic diparesis (diplegia), Little disease
Spastic quadriparesis (quadriplegia)
Hypotonic CP
Dyskinetic CP (athetosis, choreoathetosis)
Ataxic CP
Mixed CP

The immature brain can be adversely affected at any time from fertilization to maturity because genetic or acquired disorders may disrupt developmental programs or inflict physical damage. Among the causes are cerebral malformations, intrauterine or extrauterine infections or strokes, and perinatal trauma or ischemic-anoxic insults that may or may not lead to gross motor impairments (cerebral palsy) or learning disorders. Genetic factors play a major etiologic role in developmental disabilities unassociated with detectable lesions or overt sensorimotor abnormalities.

DEVELOPMENTAL DISORDERS OF MOTOR FUNCTION

Minor Motor Disability

This term refers to subtle impairments of motor coordination, such as clumsiness, maladroitness, or developmental dyspraxia. Some of these impairments, such as reflex asymmetry or hyperactivity and minor dysmetria, are mild or "pastel" classic neurologic signs; others may be due to delayed acquisition of independent coordination of the two hands and maintenance of posture without adventitious movements. The neurologic basis of these "soft" signs is rarely known. They may occur in isolation but are often seen in children with specific learning disabilities or mild mental deficiency.

Cerebral Palsy

The term *cerebral palsy* (CP) has no etiologic specificity and refers to any nonprogressive motor disorder of cerebral or cerebellar origin. (CP does not apply to disorders of the spinal cord, peripheral nerves, or muscles.) The signs are present from early life and are evident on a standard neurologic examination. CP is often, though not invariably, an acquired lesion that is evident on neuroimaging (Table 76.1). The type of CP depends on the location of the lesion.

Spastic Hemiparesis (Hemiplegia)

Spastic hemiparesis (hemiplegia) arises from a lesion of the corticospinal system of one cerebral hemisphere. A common cause is an intrauterine stroke that results in congenital porencephaly in the territory of the trunk or a branch of the middle cerebral artery. Strokes can also occur during the birth process and in infancy (acute infantile hemiplegia). Another common cause of

hemiplegic CP is intraventricular hemorrhage complicated by intraparenchymal hemorrhage, which occurs in small, premature infants and starts as a germinal matrix hemorrhage. In late childhood, neuroimaging may reveal smallness of the entire hemisphere and an old infarct; the skull is thicker on the affected side, the sphenoid wing and petrous bone are elevated, and the frontal sinuses and mastoid air cells are larger. These changes are called the *Davidoff-Dyke-Masson syndrome.*

Typically, the hemiparesis affects the arm and hand more than the leg. All children with hemiplegic CP walk, albeit often later and on the toes of the affected foot because of a tight heel cord that may necessitate surgical lengthening. Growth "arrest" of the arm and leg is frequent in lesions that involve the parietal lobe; the arm and leg are shorter and thinner, and there may be a compensatory scoliosis. In mild cases, decreased associated movements of the arm may be seen only in running or walking on the heels. Comparing fingernails on the two sides may demonstrate minor growth arrest.

A purely motor hemiparesis may be due to a frontal lesion or one that affects the head of the caudate nucleus and adjacent internal capsule. Larger lesions are associated with cortical sensory loss involving position sense, stereognosis, neglect, and lack of use of the affected hand except as a prop. Tone in the hand may be decreased rather than increased, and there may be severe laxity of hand and finger ligaments, sometimes with joint deformities. Prognosis for habilitation of the hand is poor. Posterior lesions are associated with contralateral hemianopsia or spatial neglect.

Hemiparesis may not be evident until the child starts to grab for objects and shows precocious handedness or failure of hand use; this delay does not imply that the lesion was acquired postnatally. Spasticity tends to increase in the first and second years and is more evident when the child is erect than supine.

Seizures are frequent when the lesion affects the cortex. Children with large unilateral lesions, intractable seizures, and severe behavior disorders may be candidates for hemispherectomy or other excisional surgery.

Speech may be delayed but competent in children with hemiplegic CP and a strictly unilateral lesion in either hemisphere. Intelligence may be spared despite subtle neuropsychologic differences between right and left lesions; children with right lesions tend to pay more attention to details of a visual display than to the overall pattern, whereas those with left lesions attend to the overall pattern but overlook details. Drawings of young children with right-sided lesions are more disorganized than those of children with left-sided lesions. As infants, children with right-sided lesions tend to be more irritable and cry more than those with left-sided lesions.

Spastic Diplegia or Diparesis

In spastic diplegia or diparesis, or Little disease, spasticity predominates in the legs and less severely affects the hands and face. Tendon reflexes are hyperactive and the toes upturning. The most common causes are prematurity with bilateral germinal matrix hemorrhage with or without intraventricular hemorrhage and hydrocephalus, and perinatal ischemia in the watershed parasagittal zone between the territories of the anterior and posterior cerebral arteries. Adductor spasm is responsible for "scissoring" of the legs, and marked spasticity may preclude ambulation without a walker and long-leg braces. Intelligence and language are often unimpaired, but there may be variable clumsiness of the hands.

Spastic Quadriplegia

Spastic quadriplegia is the most severe variant of CP, often associated with moderate to severe mental deficiency. It denotes diffuse malformation of or damage to the brain such as multicystic leukomalacia following severe ischemia, or lissencephaly. In some cases, bilateral porencephalies cause a double hemiplegia, with the hands more severely affected than the legs. Severe limb spasticity may be associated with axial and neck hypotonia. Children with quadriparesis are rarely able to walk, and most are totally dependent and require wheelchairs, with neck and trunk supports. Pseudobulbar manifestations often preclude speech and severe dysphagia may lead to feeding gastrostomy. Seizures are frequent and difficult to control.

Poor hand use almost always prevents the acquisition of sign language, making the assessment of cognition very difficult. Every effort must be made to provide an alternate means of expression, such as pointing. A child who understands that pointing means "I want" may learn to use a communication board and, potentially, a computer with voice. Even such a rudimentary means for communication greatly enhances the quality of life of these children and their caretakers.

To relieve spasticity, dantrolene sodium (Dantrium) produces weakness, diazepam induces drowsiness, and oral baclofen (Lioresal) has a modest effect. Baclofen is more effective in spastic quadriplegia when administered by continuous intrathecal infusion. Injection of botulinum toxin into spastic muscles decreases spasticity for a number of months but requires reinjection. Selective dorsal rhizotomy relieves spasticity without causing weakness and may significantly enhance function. In most patients, ongoing physical therapy, orthoses, and orthopedic procedures are still needed.

Hypotonic Cerebral Palsy

Children with hypotonic CP are floppy, but most have hyperactive tendon reflexes, in contrast to those with lower motor neuron or primary muscle diseases. The pathophysiology of this syndrome is not understood, but there is usually severe mental deficiency with evidence of diffuse brain involvement, for example, a major malformation.

Dyskinetic Cerebral Palsy

In children with *dyskinetic CP*, basal ganglia lesions lead to abnormal involuntary movements, including athetosis, choreoathetosis, or dystonia. Most dyskinetic CP follows neonatal hyperbilirubinemia (kernicterus) and severe anoxia. The main cause of hyperbilirubinemia is neonatal blood group incompatibility, a preventable cause of CP that has become rare in the United States. Unconjugated bilirubin selectively damages the basal ganglia, central auditory and vestibular pathways, and the deep cerebellar nuclei, sparing the cortex. As a result, these children with dyskinetic CP, who may be unable to speak because of facial dyskinesia and hearing loss and have little or no hand use, may have normal intelligence. In contrast, children with dyskinetic CP following anoxia are likely to have both cortical and subcortical damage (status marmoratus of the basal ganglia) with intellectual as well as motor handicaps. It is crucial to test the hearing of all children with dyskinetic CP. The hearing loss of kernicterus is typically a high-tone loss; the children are not deaf but cannot discriminate the consonants that convey most of the meaning of speech. Assessment of cognitive skills is difficult because of the motor handicap and hearing loss, but it is crucial; it may have to rely on interest in the environment, development of nonverbal communication, and the views of parents.

Athetosis is not present at birth; the movements emerge after age 1 year. In early infancy, the children are hypotonic with poor head and trunk control and little or no use of the hands. The first sign of athetosis may be tongue thrusting that makes spoon-feeding difficult. Severely affected children are helpless and unable to walk. Some gain sufficient control of a fist, a foot, or the head to manipulate a wand and communicate with a computer or a communication board. Some children walk but assume grotesque postures and have stigmatizing facial grimaces, dysarthria, and dysphagia.

Many drugs have been tried in athetosis, but none is adequately effective. High doses of trihexyphenidyl pushed to tolerance may have a modest effect on dystonia; carbidopa is sometimes effective; chlorpromazine hydrochloride (Thorazine) is sedative and may have long-term side effects. The danger of irreversible anarthria following bilateral stereotactic surgery on the basal ganglia or thalamus has decreased with higher-resolution magnetic resonance imaging (MRI) and the making of smaller, better-targeted lesions.

Ataxic Cerebral Palsy

Ataxic CP is rare and usually denotes maldevelopment of the cerebellum or its pathways, which, if severe, may be associated with significant cognitive impairment. The differential diagnosis includes benign familial tremor, which may be seen in the preschool years, as well as a slowly progressive genetic metabolic disease rather than a static condition. Truncal and gait ataxia are more striking than limb ataxia, but some children take a long time to learn to feed themselves and have severe difficulty in writing. The children eventually learn to walk but fall frequently. Nystagmus is uncommon. Speech may be slow and scanning. Ataxic CP does not respond well to physical therapy or to any drug but may improve with age.

Mixed Cerebral Palsy

Mixed CP refers to the combination of dyskinetic and spastic CP, or ataxia and athetosis. It is also used for children who do not meet strict criteria for one of the major forms.

Management of Cerebral Palsy

Children with CP should be referred to a specialized assessment center as soon as they are identified. In the 1990s, most children with significant CP undergo neuroimaging to determine the basis of the motor disorder and to be sure that there is no remediable condition, such as hydrocephalus. Hearing must be tested early, with the use of brainstem evoked responses or cochlear emissions in children who cannot cooperate for audiometry. Vision must be assessed: Many children with CP have strabismus or a refractive error; myopia is particularly frequent in children born prematurely. Early evaluations of communication and cognitive skills, although essential, are descriptive and not necessarily predictive; response to intervention is a more reliable gauge of abilities than a one-shot test.

Early intervention programs typically provide all required therapies in one center. Physical therapy is essential to train ambulation, stretch spastic muscles, and prevent deformities; it may not avoid the need for surgical procedures such as tendon releases or transplants, as well as for those described earlier. Occupational therapy focuses on self-help skills and language therapy on interpersonal communication. These centers teach parents to foster independence and help them get needed appliances and services, provide support groups for parents, and are often a source for baby-sitting and respite care. In severely affected children with CP and cognitive impairment, the thrust is to foster feeding, toileting, and dressing; most end up in a nursing home when their parents can no longer care for them.

Less affected school-age children need an education tailored to their intellectual abilities. Sooner or later, they require counseling for adapting to the fact that they will always remain different from other people. Educated adults with CP provide excellent role models who can spur the child with CP to fight for independence and achievement.

DEVELOPMENTAL DISORDERS OF HIGHER CEREBRAL FUNCTIONS

All of these disorders are defined behaviorally. Their severity varies greatly. Comorbidity (more than one developmental disorder in a given child, for example, dyslexia and Tourette syndrome) is frequent and may result from lack of selectivity of the underlying pathology, genetic linkage, or fuzzy boundaries because diagnostic criteria are quantitative rather than dichotomous.

If general intelligence (cognition) is affected (mental deficiency), there is generally a diffuse disorder of neocortical (or cortical/subcortical) development and function, or multiple widespread lesions. Disorders selectively affecting cognitive abilities are considered specific developmental disorders and are generally classified according to their main functional consequence (Table 76.2). Progress in functional brain imaging and electrophysiology, which are rapidly identifying brain regions selectively activated by particular cognitive tasks, indicates that the responsible circuits are both modular and distributed. A particularly striking discovery is the unanticipated participation of the cerebellum in many cognitive tasks.

TABLE 76.2. DEVELOPMENTAL DISORDERS OF HIGHER CEREBRAL FUNCTION

Disorder	Function affected	Location of brain dysfunction
Mental deficiency (mental retardation)	Cognition	Diffuse or multifocal (nonspecific?)
Developmental language disorders (dysphasias)	Oral language	Language systems
Dyslexias (reading disability)	Written language	Language systems (usually), especially phonology
Dyscalculias (several variants)	Mathematics	Specific systems?
Attention deficit disorder with or without hyperactivity	Focused attention	Cingulate gyrus, striatum, others
Autistic disorders (pervasive developmental disorder)	Sociability, language, range of activities and interests	Undefined systems

Etiology

The label *minimal brain damage* (MBD), later replaced by *minimal brain dysfunction* (also MBD), was applied to clumsy, hyperkinetic, inattentive children with school problems when MBD was viewed as a global disorder with perinatal traumatic or ischemic-anoxic insult as its most common etiology. The Collaborative Perinatal Study of the 1960s and 1970s showed that, in contrast to severe prematurity, isolated perinatal insults account for fewer than 10% of the cases of CP and severe mental deficiency and play a minor role in milder cognitive impairments, such as learning disability. Mild mental subnormality is to a large degree attributable to environmental factors, such as poverty, social deprivation, inadequate nutrition or substance abuse during gestation, and low level of maternal education.

Genetics rather than exogenous factors plays a major causal role in the developmental disorders. Some disorders, such as autism, are polygenic, with several genes required to produce the full phenotype. Polygenic causation provides an explanation for overlapping and borderline phenotypes. Some families with many dyslexic members have linkage to different chromosomes, which suggests that dyslexia is not linked to a single gene defect. The effects of genes responsible for developmental disorders on brain development are unknown. Perhaps some exert their effect by enhancing susceptibility to generally well tolerated environmental exposures.

Mental Deficiency

The term *mental deficiency* is preferred to the term *mental retardation* because it implies that it is unrealistic to expect catch-up and the achievement of normalcy. The best definition of mental deficiency is not a low score on an intelligence test but inability to function independently due to general incompetence. Before general incompetence is assumed, it is necessary to exclude specific impairments in sensorimotor, visual, auditory, language, and other specific cognitive and social skills that might account for failure to perform at a level commensurate with chronologic age and cultural opportunity. These impairments may make valid assessment difficult because there are few standardized tests for children with CP, deafness, blindness, or autism.

Measurement of Intelligence and Neuropsychologic Skills

A modular view of brain function negates the concept of a single construct, "intelligence;" it posits that intelligence or cognitive competence depends on the functional integrity of many discrete brain circuits whose coordinated activity gives rise to adaptive responses to unpredictable endogenous and exogenous conditions. Intelligence test batteries are used to predict likely success in school or in a particular vocation. These tests are generally well standardized for normal people of a particular culture and sample a range of verbal and nonverbal abilities, but the scores must be applied cautiously whenever they are used in other cultures or with handicapped persons. Brief screening tests, such as the Peabody Picture Vocabulary Test or the Raven Progressive Matrices, may be adequate for some limited purposes.

For the practical purpose of assessing and predicting ability to function in real life, the Revised Vineland Adaptive Behavior Scales provide measures of communication, sociability, motor skills, and adaptive function. The data are derived from an interview with the parents or caretaker. These scales do not require the participation of the person being assessed and provide less culturally biased data than test data.

The Revised Wechsler scales—Wechsler Preschool and Primary Scale of Intelligence, Wechsler Intelligence Scale for Children, and Wechsler Adult Intelligence Scale—and the Revised Stanford-Binet scale provide verbal and nonverbal summary scores, as well as an overall IQ score, and extend from preschool children to adults. The most commonly used test-based criterion for mental deficiency is departure from the mean score of 100 (standard deviation ± 16) in the general population. Likely functional outcomes as a function of IQ score are listed in Table 76.3. IQ scores must be used cautiously: Tests in preschool and young school-age children may provide valid comparisons with peers and have satisfactory predictive validity when applied to groups, but they are not necessarily valid for long-term prediction in the individual child, especially in the face of a handicap.

In addition to associated handicaps, what determines the functional level of a mentally deficient person with a particular IQ level are motivation, efficacy of habilitation, and a supportive environment. Adequate self-help and social skills, rather than academic skills, may determine outcome. Severe behavior disorders that worsen functional outcome increase with the severity of the mental deficiency.

A quite different use of psychologic test data from the measure of "intelligence" is the identification of specific cognitive impairments. Neuropsychologic batteries incorporate tests to detect inadequacies in language; memory and learning; attention; visual, auditory, and somatosensory perception and processing; intersensory integration; fine motor abilities; planning; and even affect recognition, mood, and social cognition. Neuropsychologic tests generate a useful profile of strengths and weaknesses for planning remediation. Appropriately designed neuropsychologic measures are required to identify the neurologic basis of cognitively demanding tasks with the use of functional brain imaging and electrophysiology.

Developmental Language Disorders (or Dysphasias)

There is considerable variation in the manner and age at which normal children acquire various aspects of language. This makes the definition of developmental language disorders (DLDs) controversial because it depends on departure from some expected language age or on a discrepancy between verbal and nonverbal cognitive skills. The term *developmental language delay* is widely

TABLE 76.3. FUNCTIONAL ABILITY AND LEVEL OF COGNITIVE COMPETENCE

IQ	Abilities				
	Mental	Language	Education	Work	Daily living
>115	Superior		Unrestricted		
85–115	Average		Unrestricted		
70–85	Borderline	Usually normal	Remediation needed	Employable	Independent ADL, may need some living help
55–70	Mild mental deficiency	Normal or impaired	Limited ability	Employable at selected tasks	Need variable amounts of living help
40–55	Moderate mental deficiency	Normal or impaired	Very limited	May be capable of simple tasks	Dependent for living, may need ADL help
25–40	Severe mental deficiency	Limited or absent	Minimal functional	None or minimal	Need ADL help
<25	Profound mental deficiency	Absent	—	—	Totally dependent, often nonambulatory and incontinent

The American Association on Mental Retardation recommends a new classification of persons with IQs below 70–75 based on limitations in two or more adaptive skills and on the kinds and intensities of needed supports.
ADL, activities of daily living.

used because most children with a DLD learn to speak before school age; the term is inappropriate for the many children who later have trouble learning to read or express themselves coherently orally or in writing.

Neurologic Basis of the Dysphasias

Focal brain lesions are rare, in part because unilateral focal lesions acquired in early life do not preclude the acquisition of language, which reflects the greater potential for reorganization in the immature than in the mature brain. Most people are genetically destined to develop language in the left hemisphere, regardless of handedness. Yet language can develop and be sustained in either hemisphere, as shown by adequate development of language in young children with large hemispheric lesions or following hemispherectomy, albeit with subtle but demonstrable differences in language and nonverbal skills in those with right and left pathology. Dysphasic children are therefore thought to have bilateral dysfunction in circuits critical to language development.

Subtypes of Developmental Language Disorders

There is no fully accepted classification of the dysphasias. Despite some similarities, models based on the acquired aphasias of adults do not fully apply to disorders of language acquisition, yet focal brain lesions in adults have provided crucial information on the localization of particular aspects of language.

Some dysphasias, such as Broca aphasia in adults, are predominantly expressive and affect phonology (the production of the sounds of speech) and syntax (the grammar of language), whereas semantics (the meaning of language) and pragmatics (the communicative use of language) are spared.

Receptive dysphasias preclude or severely jeopardize the processing of phonology and syntax and, consequently, semantics and the acquisition of expressive language; they are therefore always mixed (receptive and expressive), in contrast to Wernicke aphasia of adults, in which automatized speech continues unabated, albeit with abnormal content. The closest analogy between adult aphasia and childhood dysphasia is word deafness, or *verbal auditory agnosia* (VAA), the most severe variant of receptive DLD. The difference in this analogy is that adults with bilateral temporal lesions may speak quite normally and can read and write, whereas children with VAA are nonverbal because profound impairment of comprehension precludes all language skills, with the possible exception of nonverbal pragmatics (gestures). VAA is especially frequent in children with acquired epileptic aphasia (*Landau-Kleffner syndrome*), which consists of chronic loss of speech (or failure to develop speech in the case of developmental VAA) associated with a seizure disorder or a frankly paroxysmal electroencephalogram (EEG) without clinical seizures. Children with VAA are often autistic with no sparing of pragmatics.

A third type of DLD largely spares the development of receptive and expressive phonology and syntax but impairs semantic processing. Children with this type have difficulty understanding complex sentences, answering open-ended questions, retrieving vocabulary, and formulating coherent discourse. They may speak clearly but, when younger, often produced a fluent incomprehensible jargon with word approximations. Some have an excellent rote verbal memory and impaired pragmatic skills; they are likely to be chatterboxes who rely on overlearned scripts. They often perseverate and speak aloud to themselves without a conversational partner. This semantic-pragmatic syndrome is particularly frequent in verbal autistic children.

Etiology and Pathophysiology

DLD clearly does not have a single cause. Genetics plays a major but not exclusive role. A few known syndromes are associated with particular subtypes of dysphasia, such as hydrocephalus and Williams syndrome with the semantic-pragmatic syndrome. Dysphasia is significantly more frequent in boys than girls. Disorders of the acquisition of phonology may be linked to a more general impairment of rapid auditory processing that jeopardizes the detection of the brief acoustic stimuli that differentiate one consonant from another. VAA is linked to dysfunction in temporal auditory cortices. The pathophysiology of other dysphasic syndromes is not understood.

Reading Disability (Dyslexia)

Learning to read is learning to decode written (visually coded) language. It may be difficult to distinguish true dyslexia from poor reading attributable to impoverished language stimulation, poor teaching, lack of motivation, or borderline intellectual competence. As with dysphasia, there are subtypes of dyslexia. Visual perceptual problems play a minor pathophysiologic role in dyslexia, which is almost always the consequence of a language problem. The most prevalent subtype involves inadequate phonologic processing, such as difficulty in segmenting speech into component phonemes (speech sounds), sequencing them, learning the relationship between graphemes (letters) and phonemes, sounding out strings of letters (nonwords), and spelling. Occasionally, children have more difficulty learning to read whole words than analyzing them phonologically. Others have visual problems in association with phonologic deficits, making learning to read arduous or nearly impossible. Poor readers may be more generally learning disabled. Some are clumsy and have a poor handwriting, difficulty with mathematics, or an attention deficit with or without hyperactivity.

Specific reading disability is virtually never the consequence of a detectable structural brain lesion. Galaburda and colleagues (1985) described minor migration cell defects and tiny scars located selectively in the perisylvian areas of the left hemisphere in dyslexics; he and others pointed out that dyslexia is statistically linked to lack of the expected asymmetry of the two hemispheres, associated with an atypically large planum temporale on the right.

Genetics, including linkage to chromosomes 6 or 15 in some families, plays a major but not exclusive etiologic role. Outcome depends in part on the general intellectual level and adequacy of intervention. Most intelligent dyslexics eventually learn to read more or less efficiently, but they tend to be poor spellers, have difficulty reading nonwords, and may not read for pleasure.

Other Learning Disabilities

There are at least two clearly differentiable reasons for difficulty in writing (*dysgraphia*): dysorthographia (the consequence of dyslexia) and poor handwriting (due to a minor motor or visuomotor disability). There are also several variants of *dyscalculia*: lack of understanding of the rules for calculation, spatial problems resulting in place errors while setting up written calculations and difficulty with geometry, higher-order language deficits interfering with the solving of word problems, and inadequate attention impairing short-term memory essential for mental arithmetic.

Children with *nonverbal learning disabilities* have lower performance than verbal abilities and dyscalculia. Many have social deficits that place them on the autistic spectrum. *Memory disorders* for specific types of materials and tasks resemble those of adults. *Executive* and *planning disorders* have a profound impact on organizational and reasoning abilities, which, as in adults, depend on the integrity of prefrontal circuits.

Disorders of Attention

Attention deficit disorder (ADD) is reportedly more frequent in boys. This may be because it is actually more frequent in boys, because boys are more likely than girls to have attention deficit with hyperactivity disorder (ADHD), or because boys are generally more active and aggressive than girls and ADD is therefore more conspicuous and difficult to tolerate in boys. ADD may be evident in infancy by reduced need for sleep, later by difficulty in falling asleep, waking too early in the morning, or by multiple awakenings during the night. Children with ADD are restless, have a short attention span, go from one toy to another without getting engaged, and in school get up from their seat or wander in the classroom. They are impulsive, disorganized, and forgetful and may have a labile affect. Other features, such as clumsiness and learning disability, are associated rather than an intrinsic manifestations. Marked distractibility may interfere with the acquisition of reading and arithmetic, but most children of normal intelligence with ADHD are not learning disabled. ADD persists in adult life, but motor hyperactivity usually abates in adolescence. Prognosis varies: ADHD tends to abate with maturation, but distractibility, impulsivity, a disorganized lifestyle, accident-proneness, and a short temper may be lifelong liabilities; the high level of energy and curtailed need for sleep may be assets in otherwise well-functioning adults.

The most widely used criterion for diagnosing ADD and gauging the efficacy of medication is Conner's questionnaire, administered to parents or teachers. Assessment of ADHD may include written or computerized tests of attention or direct recording of amount of movement.

Management combines parental counseling, environmental manipulations such as removing distractions, providing the opportunity for frequent breaks and opportunities to move about, and, in some cases, medication. ADHD is disruptive because it affects family, peers, and teachers alike. Medication alone is rarely sufficient, and in severe cases counseling of the family, adjustments of school routines, and, in older children, teaching strategies to minimize the consequences of ADD are necessary.

Methylphenidate hydrochloride (Ritalin) is the safest and most frequently prescribed drug. Its short half-life is advantageous for gauging efficacy but requires divided doses. In a young child, one starts with a small dose given in the morning and at midday, progressively increasing the dose until the desired effect is achieved or sleeplessness, oversedation, increased hyperkinesia, or tics appear. A sustained-release form of methylphenidate is available, but release may be erratic and some children still require a short-acting tablet after school to avoid behavioral rebound. Drug holidays in the summer are reasonable to gauge whether the child can do without, but if the drug is truly effective, giving it only on school days risks committing the child to an emotional roller coaster.

Pemoline (Cylert) has a long half-life so that a single pill in the morning suffices, but it requires 2 to 3 weeks for full effect and has recently been associated with rare cases of fatal liver damage. Dextroamphetamine sulfate (Dexedrine), especially time-release capsules, can also be tried, in doses one-half those of methylphenidate. Sedatives should be avoided because some, notably phenobarbital, may precipitate ADHD. There is no evidence that avoidance of sugar, foods with red dye or rich in salicylates, and megadoses of vitamins help either ADD or the learning disabilities. Drugs such as thioridazine (Mellaril), chlorpromazine, and haloperidol are contraindicated because they are sedating and have potential long-term, irreversible side effects.

Autism Spectrum Disorders—Pervasive Developmental Disorders

The term *pervasive developmental disorder* (PDD) is used in the *Diagnostic and Statistical Manual* of the American Psychiatric Association as an umbrella term for persons with classically autistic symptomatology referred to as "autistic disorder," as well as for others with similar but fewer, less severe symptoms. Using PDD to avoid mentioning "autism," which is considered stigmatizing because of the discredited theory that poor parenting was responsible and because it was erroneously thought to be hopeless, is confusing.

Etiology

Autism is a developmental disorder of brain function, and as with others, there are several causes. On the basis of twin and family studies, polygenic inheritance accounts for most cases with unknown causes. In some cases, there may be an inherited susceptibility to some environmentally determined stress. A minority of individuals with autism have tuberous sclerosis, hypomelanosis of Ito, fragile X, Rett or Angelman syndrome, phenylketonuria, congenital rubella, neonatal herpes simplex, hydrocephalus, a brain malformation, or other static encephalopathy. Perinatal brain injury does not cause autism as an isolated deficit.

Symptoms

There is great variability in severity and range of symptoms. The core problems involve sociability, verbal and nonverbal communication, and range of interests and activities. Intelligence is not a defining feature but strongly influences prognosis. There may be profound mental deficiency or superior ability, often with areas of major impairment coupled to normal or even prodigious rote memory, calculation, or music ability.

Problems in sociability range from almost total lack of interest in others, inability to engage another person in play or conversation, and gaze aversion to inappropriate intrusiveness, failure to maintain appropriate interpersonal distance, and lack of empathy. Children with autism may not lack affection, but they may be selectively affectionate. They may be anxious or fearful, have a labile mood, and may laugh or cry without discernible cause. Temper tantrums and seemingly unprovoked aggressive outbursts create social problems.

The second core problem, communicative incompetence, regularly presents as failure to learn to speak and limited comprehension of language. Nonverbal communication is affected, as young autistic children may not point to request or shake the head "yes" or "no." The most severely affected preschoolers may understand little or nothing; they may remain nonverbal into adulthood, even when comprehension has improved. Others learn to speak after age 3 or 4 years, but with inadequate syntax and phonology. Still others, once they start to speak, progress rapidly to full, clearly articulated sentences. Echolalia, use of verbatim scripts, stilted or wooden prosody (melody of language), and a high-pitched or singsong voice are frequent. A large and inappropriately sophisticated vocabulary may mask impaired comprehension. Many autistic children have better verbal skills for written than oral language. Some preschool autistic children are fascinated with letters and numbers and may learn to read without instruction, albeit often with limited comprehension (hyperlexia).

The third core characteristic of autism is a narrow range of interests, unusual preoccupations and choice of activities, inadequate play, perseveration, rigidity, and resistance to change. Young children may look at the same video or book for hours, play with a string or spin wheels of a car, and prefer to line up or classify toys rather than play with them. Imaginative play is absent or minimal in early childhood. Older autistic children may become engrossed in studying timetables or collecting bottle caps or sports statistics.

Frequent motor problems in autistic children include toe-walking, hypotonia, stereotypies, and apraxia (failure to imitate gestures and inadequate mastery of complex motor tasks). Stereotypies may be ticlike; they are most blatant in low-functioning autistic persons but may persist in miniature even in high-functioning adults. Stereotypies may consist of flapping the hands when excited, wringing or licking the hands, fiddling with clothing or a lock of hair, or twisting the fingers or gazing at them. There are few facts about the neurologic basis for self-injury, head-banging, or self-biting; failure to respond to sound but intolerance of certain sounds; withdrawal from tactile contact but enjoyment of tickling; excessive sniffing and licking; a narrow range of food choices; and enjoyment of staring at rotating objects, running around in circles, and antigravity play. Sleep disorders, overfocused attention or distractibility, labile mood, destructiveness, self-injury, and unprovoked aggression are frequent and troublesome complaints.

Children with autism may have epileptic seizures of any type. The probability of epilepsy is highest in autistic children with mental deficiency or frank motor abnormality. It is high in infancy and early childhood and increases to a second peak in adolescence. Autism may follow infantile spasms or the Lennox-Gastaut syndrome.

Course and Prognosis

In retrospect, signs of autism may already have been present in infancy. In almost 50% of cases, signs of autism appear in the toddler or early preschool years, either in a perfectly normal or less severely developmentally affected child. Inadequate language is usually the presenting complaint. One-third of parents report language regression at a mean age of 21 months, together with regression of sociability and play, usually without regression of motor skills. Regression may be insidious or may follow an acute illness or environmental stress. Development resumes after a plateau lasting weeks or months, although complete recovery is exceptional. In some children, regression is associated with a paroxysmal EEG with or without clinical seizures and falls within the definition of acquired epileptic aphasia (Landau-Kleffner syndrome). "Disintegrative disorder" refers to autistic regression after age 2 years in completely normal, fully verbal children. The neurologic basis of autistic regression, including the potential role of subclinical epilepsy, is not known because autistic regression is often overlooked, precluding early investigation. No reliably effective medical treatment for autistic regression is known.

Like other developmental disorders, autism is a lifelong condition, although sociability and language tend to improve. Unless an early history is available, autistic adults are likely to be diagnosed as mentally retarded, obsessive-compulsive, schizophrenic, or manic-depressive, or as having an antisocial or inadequate personality. Some intelligent verbal persons with autism lead independent lives. In general, they remain single and are likely to be underemployed but remarkably faithful workers. Less intelligent and multiply handicapped autistic persons need supervision throughout life, and the most severely affected require institutionalization.

Pathology and Pathophysiology

Information is scanty. Except in cases with a known cause, there is no evidence for gross malformation or destructive or inflammatory pathology. There may be developmental cellular anomalies in the limbic system, parts of the cerebellar cortex, and the inferior olive. Even high-resolution MRI is usually normal; therefore MRI is not indicated clinically unless the neurologic examination mandates it. In some autistic adults, MRI shows minor dysgenetic lesions of the type reported in dyslexia, as well as dysgenesis in vermal lobules VI and VII of the cerebellum. MRI morphometry indicates that autistic children may have larger, rather than smaller, cerebral hemispheres. Standard EEG and evoked potential studies are generally normal unless there are seizures. Recent loss of language mandates a prolonged sleep EEG to detect subclinical epilepsy. Research tools such as event-related potentials and functional imaging studies may be abnormal during the performance of cognitive and language tasks.

Abnormalities in neurotransmitter metabolism, notably serotonin, may be present in some autistic persons. There is no unifying hypothesis about the neurochemical basis of autism.

Management

Early individualized education that addresses both the behavioral and the communication needs of children with autistic spectrum disorders is the backbone of management. Parents need instruction in behavior management. Neurologists should discourage the squandering of resources on the many well meaning but unproven behavioral and dietary treatments offered to desperate parents.

No drug cures autism, but psychotropic drugs can be targeted to specific behavioral problems. Serotonin-uptake inhibitors are widely used to decrease perseveration and, perhaps, enhance language acquisition. Aggressive outbursts may respond to large doses of propranolol given in progressive increments to tolerance and, in a crisis, to acute use of haloperidol or phenothiazines, which need to be avoided long-term because of their potentially irreversible side effects. Risperidone (Risperdal) and clonidine hydrochloride (Catapres) may mitigate prominent obsessive or self-injurious behaviors, for which naltrexone hydrochloride (ReVia) has been disappointing. Anxiolytic drugs and tricyclic antidepressants have their place, and methylphenidate may help in ADHD, although stimulants are generally contraindicated in autism. Anticonvulsants can be tried in children with a frankly paroxysmal EEG without clinical seizures and may also have mood stabilizing efficacy.

SUGGESTED READINGS

Developmental Disorders of Motor Function: Cerebral Palsy

Arens LJ, Leary PM, Goldschmidt RB. Experience with botulinum toxin in the treatment of cerebral palsy. *S Afr Med J* 1997;87:1001–1003.

Armstrong RW, Steinbok P, Cochrane DD, Kube SD, Fife SE, Farrell K. Intrathecally administered baclofen for treatment of children with spasticity of cerebral origin. *J Neurosurg* 1997;87:409–414.

Crothers B, Paine RS. *The natural history of cerebral palsy.* Cambridge, MA: Harvard University Press, 1959.

DeSalles AA. Role of stereotaxis in the treatment of cerebral palsy. *J Child Neurol* 1996;11[Suppl 1]:S43–S50.

Filloux FM. Neuropathophysiology of movement disorders in cerebral palsy. *J Child Neurol* 1996;11[Suppl 1]:S5–S12.

Hoon AH Jr, Reinhardt EM, Kelley RI, et al. Brain magnetic imaging in suspected extrapyramidal cerebral palsy: observations in distinguishing genetic-metabolic from acquired causes. *J Pediatr* 1997;131:240–245.

Johnston MV. Hypoxic and ischemic disorders of infants and children. *Brain Dev* 1997;19:235–239.

Little WJ. On the influence of abnormal parturition, difficult labor, premature birth, and asphyxia neonatorum on the mental and physical conditions of the child, especially in relation to deformities. *Trans Obstet Soc Lond* 1862;3:293–344.

Murphy KP, Molnar GE, Lankasky K. Medical and functional status of adults with cerebral palsy. *Dev Med Child Neurol* 1995;37:1075–1084.

Nelson KB, Dambrosia JM, Ting TY, Grether JK. Uncertain value of electronic fetal monitoring in predicting cerebral palsy. *N Engl J Med* 1996;334:613–618.

Okumura A, Kato T, Kuno K, Hayakawa F, Watanabe K. MRI findings in patients with spastic cerebral palsy. II: correlation with type of cerebral palsy. *Dev Med Child Neurol* 1997;39:369–372.

Pranzatelli MR. Oral pharmacotherapy for the movement disorders of cerebral palsy. *J Child Neurol* 1996;11[Suppl 1]:S13–S22.

Staudt LA, Nuwer MR, Peacock WJ. Intraoperative monitoring during selective posterior rhizotomy: technique and patient outcome. *Electroencephalogr Clin Neurophysiol* 1995;97:296–309.

Stevenson DK, Sunshine P, eds. *Fetal and neonatal brain injury: mechanisms, management, and risks.* New York: Oxford University Press, 1997.

Developmental Disorders of Higher Cerebral Functions

Bates E, Thal D, Janowsky JS. Early language development and its neural correlates. In: Segalowitz SJ, Rapin I, eds. *Child neuropsychology. Handbook of neuropsychology, vol 7.* Amsterdam: Elsevier Science, 1992:66–110.

Bishop DV, North T, Donlan C. Genetic basis of specific language impairment: evidence from a twin study. *Dev Med Child Neurol* 1995;37:56–71.

Broman S, Nichols PL, Shaughnessy P, et al. *Retardation in young children.* Hillsdale, NJ: Lawrence Erlbaum Associates, 1987.

Denckla MB, Roeltgen DP. Disorders of motor function and control. In: Rapin I, Segalowitz SJ, eds. *Child neuropsychology. Handbook of neuropsychology, vol 6.* Amsterdam: Elsevier Science, 1992:455–476.

Dugas M, Gerard CL, Franc S, et al. Natural history, course and prognosis of the Landau and Kleffner syndrome. In: Martins IP, Castro-Caldas A, van Dongen HR, et al, eds. *Acquired aphasia in children: acquisition and breakdown of language in the developing brain.* Dordrecht: Kluwer Academic Publishers, 1991:263–277.

Filipek PA, Kennedy DN, Caviness VS Jr. Neuroimaging in child neuropsychology. In: Rapin I, Segalowitz SJ, eds. *Child neuropsychology. Handbook of neuropsychology, vol 6.* Amsterdam: Elsevier Science, 1992:301–329.

Fisher SE, Vargha-Khadem F, Watkins KE, Monaco AP, Pembrey ME. Localisation of a gene implicated in a severe speech and language disorder. *Nat Genet* 1998;18:168–170. Erratum: *Nat Genet* 1998;18:298.

Galaburda AM, Sherman GF, Rosen GD, Aboitiz F, Gischwind N. Developmental dyslexia: Four consecutive cases with cortical anomalies. *Ann Neurol* 1985;18:222–233.

Gillberg C, Coleman M. *The biology of the autistic syndromes,* 2nd ed. Oxford: MacKeith Press, 1992.

Mattis S. Neuropsychological assessment of school-aged children. In: Rapin I, Segalowitz SJ, eds. *Child neuropsychology. Handbook of neuropsychology, vol 6.* Amsterdam: Elsevier Science, 1992:395–415.

Mental retardation: definition, classification, and systems of supports, 9th ed. Washington, DC: American Association on Mental Retardation, 1992.

Nordentoft M, Lou HC, Hansen D, et al. Intrauterine growth retardation and premature delivery: the influence of maternal smoking and psychosocial factors. *Am J Public Health* 1996;86:347–354.

Pennington BF, Smith SD. Genetic analysis of dyslexia and other complex behavioral phenotypes. *Curr Opin Pediatr* 1997;9:626–641.

Pugh KR, Shaywitz BA, Shaywitz SE, et al. Cerebral organization of component processes in reading. *Brain* 1996;119:1221–1238.

Rapin I. Developmental language disorders: a clinical update. *J Child Psychol Psychiatry* 1996;37:643–655.

Rapin I. Autism. *N Engl J Med* 1997;337:97–104.

Rutter M, Bailey A, Simonoff E, Pickles A. Genetic influences and autism. In: Cohen DJ, Volkmar FR, eds. *Handbook of autism and pervasive developmental disorders,* 2nd ed. New York: John Wiley and Sons: 370–387.

Schmahmann JD, ed. *The cerebellum and cognition.* San Diego, CA: Academic Press, 1997.

Shaywitz BA, Fletcher JM, Shaywitz SE. Attention-deficit/hyperactivity disorder. *Adv Pediatr* 1997;44:331–367.

Shaywitz BA, Shaywitz SE, Pugh KR, et al. Sex differences in the functional organization of the brain for language. *Nature* 1995;373:607–609.

Steinschneider M, Kurtzberg D, Vaughan GG Jr. Event-related potentials in developmental neuropsychology. In: Rapin I, Segalowitz SJ, eds. *Child neuropsychology. Handbook of neuropsychology, vol 6.* Amsterdam: Elsevier Science, 1992:239–299.

Temple CM. Developmental dyscalculia. In: Segalowitz SJ, Rapin I, eds.

Child neuropsychology. Handbook of neuropsychology, vol 7. Amsterdam: Elsevier Science, 1992:211–222.

Tuchman RF, Rapin I. Regression in pervasive developmental disorders: seizures and epileptiform electroencephalogram correlates. *Pediatrics* 1997;99:560–566.

Weiss G, Trockenberg-Hechtman L. *Hyperactive children grown up.* New York: Guilford Press, 1986.

Wilson BC. The neuropsychological assessment of the preschool child: a branching model. In: Rapin I, Segalowitz SJ, eds. *Child neuropsychology. Handbook of neuropsychology, vol 6.* Amsterdam: Elsevier Science, 1992:377–394.

Merritt's Neurology, 10th ed., edited by L.P. Rowland. Lippincott Williams & Wilkins, Philadelphia © 2000.

C H A P T E R 77

LAURENCE-MOON-BIEDL SYNDROME

MELVIN GREER

A variable group of clinical features manifested primarily by obesity and hypogonadism was described in 1866 by Laurence and Moon. Subsequent redefinition of the syndrome by Bardet and Biedl may have established a new entity, but the clustering of manifestations appears similar. In essence, the features include obesity (85% to 95%); mental retardation (70% to 85%); retinal dystrophy and coloboma (92% to 95%); hypogenitalism and hypogonadism (74% to 86% of males and 45% to 53% of females); and polydactyly, syndactyly, or both (75% to 80%). Added to this are renal dysfunction and hypertension and, with lesser frequency, cardiac and hepatic defects. Isolated case reports include cranial nerve palsy, diabetes mellitus, diabetes insipidus, spinocerebellar degeneration, spastic quadriparesis with severe cervical stenosis, hydrocephalus, and facial dysostosis.

The salient early characteristic is obesity (Fig. 77.1). During the first decade of life, impaired night vision is the hallmark of retinitis pigmentosa, which progresses, and by age 20, 73% of the patients are blind.

Testicular atrophy, decrease in the number of germinal cells, and spermatogenic arrest have been described, but no identifiable endocrine cause explains the gonadal dysfunction. Indeed, in adolescence, some patients improve spontaneously. Testosterone therapy is ineffective in treating hypogonadism or hypogenitalism.

The mode of inheritance is autosomal recessive. Although the condition is compatible with a normal lifespan, a shortened longevity may occur because of renal or cardiac defects. No specific neuropathologic changes have been described. Several hereditary syndromes associated with pigmentary retinopathy have been described, including syndromes that loosely fit the Laurence-Moon-Biedl syndrome. The Alström-Hallgren syndrome, transmitted as an autosomal recessive disorder, includes obesity, hypogonadism, nerve deafness, diabetes mellitus, and retinitis pigmentosa. The Biemond syndrome is characterized by hypogonadotropic hypogonadism, obesity, postaxial polydactyly, mental retardation, and coloboma of the iris rather than retinitis pigmentosa. The Prader-Willi syndrome is also manifested by obesity, hypogonadism, and mental retardation, but there are no visual problems. DNA samples from 29 families with such disorders have identified loci in chromosome regions 11q13, 15q22.3-q23, and 16q21.

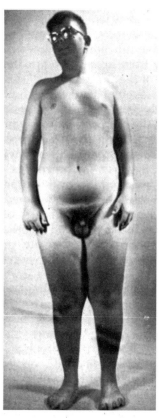

FIG. 77.1. Laurence-Moon-Biedl syndrome. A 19-year-old patient with obesity, hypogenitalism, polydactyly (toes), retinitis pigmentosa, and mental retardation.

SUGGESTED READINGS

Biedl A. Aduber das Laurence-Biedlsche Syndrome. *Med Klin* 1933;29:839–840.

Buford EA, Riise R, Teague PW, et al. Linkage mapping in 29 Bardet-Biedl syndrome families confirms loci in chromosomal regions 11q13, 15q22.3-q23 and 16q21. *Genomics* 1997;41:93–99.

Cantani A, Bellioni P, Bamonte G, et al. Seven hereditary syndromes with pigmentary retinopathy. *Clin Pediatr* 1985;24:578–583.

Koepp P. Laurence-Moon-Biedl syndrome associated with diabetes insipidus neurohormonalis. *Eur J Pediatr* 1975;121:59–62.

Mehrotra N, Taub S, Covert RF. Hydrometrocolpos as a neonatal manifestation of the Bardet-Biedl syndrome. *Am J Med Genet* 1997;69:220.

Pagon RA, Haas JE, Bunt AH, et al. Hepatic involvement in the Bardet-Biedl syndrome. *Am J Med Genet* 1982;13:373–381.

Soliman AT, Rajab A, Al Salmi I, et al. Empty sellae, impaired testosterone secretion, and defective hypothalamic-pituitary growth and gonadal axes in children with Bardet-Biedl syndrome. *Metabolism* 1996;45:1230–1234.

Verloes A, Temple IK, Bonnet S, Bottani A. Coloboma, mental retardation, hypogonadism, and obesity: critical review of the so-called Biemond syndrome type 2, updated nosology, and delineation of three "new" syndromes. *Am J Med Genet* 1997;69:370–379.

Merritt's Neurology, 10th ed., edited by L.P. Rowland. Lippincott Williams & Wilkins, Philadelphia © 2000.

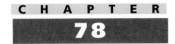

CHAPTER 78

STRUCTURAL MALFORMATIONS

MELVIN GREER

MALFORMATIONS OF CEREBRAL HEMISPHERES AND AGENESIS OF CORPUS CALLOSUM

Before day 23 of human gestation, failure of cleavage of the telencephalon and diencephalon results in a single-lobed structure with an undivided ventricle. This is *alobar holoprosencephaly* or *arhinencephaly*. It is commonly associated with defects and anomalies of the skull base, dura, face, eyes, and olfactory apparatus. Semilobar and lobar holoprosencephaly are variations wherein the hemispheres are partly or completely separated and are invariably associated with multiple deformities of cerebral architecture, ranging from absence or primitive appearance of gyri (*lissencephaly*) to heterotopias and migration defects.

Perisylvian polymicrogyria may be familial, and in some families, mothers and daughters have band heterotropia and their sons have lissencephaly. Linkage to xq21.3-24 has been reported.

Lissencephaly with malformations of muscle and eye have been identified in Fukuyama congenital muscular dystrophy and the Walker-Warburg syndrome. Common clinical manifestations noted early are facial dysmorphism, apneic episodes, seizures, and delayed psychomotor development. Causal mechanisms include chromosomal abnormalities and intrauterine acquired factors, such as maternal diabetes, toxoplasmosis, rubella, syphilis, or the fetal alcohol syndrome.

Endocrine disorders include pituitary, thyroid, and adrenal hypoplasia. Septooptic dysplasia, another midline developmental defect, includes hypoplasia of the optic nerve, lateral geniculate, hypothalamic, or posterior pituitary in addition to cerebral and cerebellar dysplasia.

Complete or partial agenesis of the corpus callosum is commonly noted in association with the holoprosencephalic brain. Callosal agenesis, unassociated with the major holoprosencephalic anomalies, is more common. This may be present in an otherwise clinically normal person and is attributed to impairment in development between gestation weeks 11 through 20. It may be partial or complete, familial or sporadic, and has been described as an autosomal dominant, autosomal recessive, or sex-limited recessive trait.

Computed tomography (CT) or magnetic resonance imaging (MRI) shows that the lateral ventricles are widely separated and angular (Fig. 78.1). The medial ventricular wall is convex, and the cavity is small. The septum pellucidum is superiorly displaced. When the agenesis is partial, the body and splenium are missing; the genu is present as a poorly formed anterior callosal rudiment. The third ventricle is wide and higher than normal.

Both microcephaly and macrocephaly in association with other cerebral malformations, including hydrocephalus, may be noted with agenesis of the corpus callosum. Seizures and mental retardation are seen in more than 50% of patients, and other anomalies seen with lesser frequency include defects of the skeleton, heart, craniofacial structures, gastrointestinal system, and genitourinary system. In some metabolic degenerative disorders, corpus callosum shrinkage may be postnatal in origin. This has been seen in the nonketotic hyperglycinemia, Menkes syndrome, Zellweger syndrome, adrenoleukodystrophy, pyruvate dehydrogenase deficiency, adenyl succinate deficiency, and glutaric aciduria type II.

Structural changes within the affected corpus callosum may include a lipoma or, more rarely, a midline meningioma, dermoid cyst, or hamartoma. Chromosome defects, including trisomy 8, 9, 13, and 18, may be seen with agenesis of the corpus callosum. Syndrome complexes that include agenesis of the corpus callosum are listed in Table 78.1.

The acallosal but clinically normal person has alternative pathways of information transfer, probably via intercollicular connections and posterior commissure. Myelination of the corpus callosum is accomplished in large measure by age 6 years but may not be complete before age 10. Callosotomy as a treatment of refractory seizures in children did not result in the same psychologic changes identified as the disconnection syndrome in the adult callosotomy patient. This difference implies plasticity of neuronal pathways.

MACROCEPHALY AND MEGALENCEPHALY

Head size enlargement greater than 2 standard deviations above the mean for age is *macrocephaly*. Progressive hydrocephalus and mass lesions are common causes of an enlarged head size in the infant and young child. Closure of the suture in the pubertal child prevents skull enlargement in the presence of these pressure-inducing disorders. Benign states of macrocephaly may be familial. Not infrequently, imaging studies reveal mildly dilated lateral ventricles and increase in subarachnoid fluid. Children

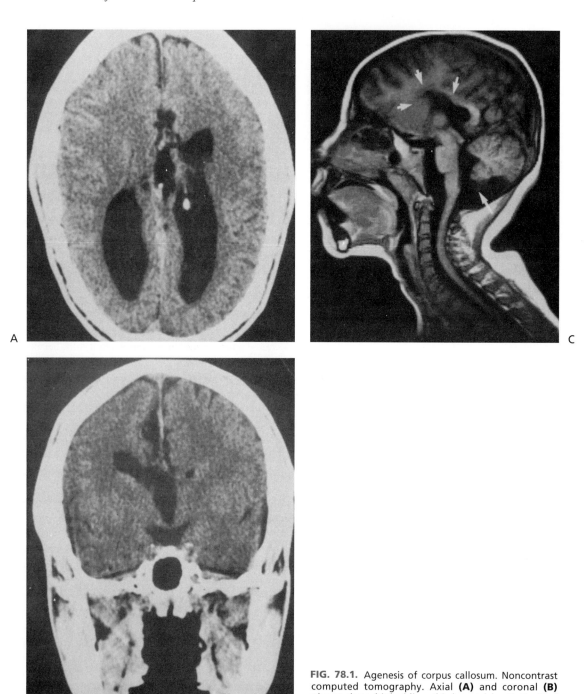

FIG. 78.1. Agenesis of corpus callosum. Noncontrast computed tomography. Axial **(A)** and coronal **(B)** planes show high-riding third ventricle. **C:** Sagittal magnetic resonance imaging showing agenesis of the anterior portion of the corpus callosum (*multiple arrows*). An associated anomaly, aplasia of the inferior portion of the cerebellat vermis, is indicated by the *single arrow*. (Courtesy of Dr. S.K. Hilal.)

who exhibit such features on CT or MRI have been identified as having *hydrocephalus ex vacuo*, but cerebrospinal fluid (CSF) shunts should be reserved for conditions in which there is progressive enlargement of the CSF spaces and, additionally, evidence of neurologic dysfunction.

Megalencephaly is an enlarged brain. Brain weight 2.5 standard deviations above the mean for sex and age or brain weight greater than 1,600 g qualifies for the diagnosis. Primarily, mega-

lencephaly may be an isolated finding. It has been described in families as an autosomal recessive trait and attributed to a disturbance of developmental cell proliferation.

Progressive enlargement of the brain with deterioration of neurologic function is seen in children with neurocutaneous syndromes, neuronal storage, or degenerative diseases such as mucopolysaccharidoses or leukodystrophies. Pathologic changes include new growths, such as the tubers of tuberous sclerosis,

TABLE 78.1. SYNDROMES ASSOCIATED WITH AGENESIS OF THE CORPUS CALLOSUM

Syndrome	Characteristics
Apert	Megalencephaly; anomalies of the skull base, hands, and feet; cerebral malformations including limbic system changes and polygyria
Aicardi	Females affected, mental retardation and seizures (infantile spasms), vertebral abnormalities, chorioretinopathy
Oral-facial digital	Mental retardation, midline oral and facial defects, hand and finger abnormalities, renal microcysts, cerebral migration defects
Miller-Dieker	Profound clinical cerebral dysfunction with death in first decade; chromosome 17 abnormality in most; anteverted nostrils, micrognathia, lissencephaly and other cerebral migration defects, cardiac anomalies
Neu-Laxova	Autosomal recessive; death in weeks; ocular abnormalities, everted lips, short neck, ichthyosis, edema, limb deformities, lissencephaly and cerebral, cerebellar, and brainstem atrophy
Fanconi anemia	Autosomal recessive, pancytopenia, skeletal anomalies including radial aplasia
Sensorimotor neuropathy and agenesis of corpus callosum	Autosomal recessive; sensorimotor agenesis of corpus callosum neuropathy, dysmorphism
Shapiro	Genitourinary and cardiac defects, mental retardation, hydrocephalus, holoprosencephaly, episodic hyperhidrosis, and hypothermia or hyperthermia
Osteochondrodysplasia	Nonlethal rhizomelic osteochondrodysplasia, hypertension, thrombocytopenia, hydrocephalus
XK syndrome	Aprosencephaly, congenital heart disease, preaxial limb malformation, abnormal genitalia, adrenohypoplasia. 13q32 deletions.

which may occlude ventricular fluid flow to cause hydrocephalus. The degenerative diseases are associated with a myriad of pathologic changes associated with megalencephaly, including cystic changes and extensive gliosis. Developmental brain defects causing macrocephaly and megalencephaly may be associated with other organ system defects and are often noted at birth (Table 78.2).

Unilateral megalencephaly is associated with unilateral hemisphere defects, such as an altered gyral pattern, including pachygyria and polymicrogyria, thickened cortex, and disorganization of gray matter. Such features are similar to the L'hermitte-Duclos syndrome, in which cerebellar granular cell hypertrophy and other cerebellar hamartomatous growths create a mass effect.

Children with hemimegalencephaly commonly have seizures, hemiparesis, and mental retardation. MRI depicts the structural changes and may also identify the asymptomatic hemimegalencephalic child with white matter low attenuation features early in life that later disappear.

MALFORMATIONS OF OCCIPITAL BONE AND CERVICAL SPINE

The defects in the development of the cervical spine and base of the skull may be divided into the following groups:

1. Basilar impression;
2. Malformation of the atlas and axis;
3. Malformation or fusion of other cervical vertebrae (Klippel-Feil anomaly) (Table 78.3).

Any of these malformations may occur singly or together; they also may be associated with developmental defects in the skull, spine, CNS, or other organs. These deformities can be present without clinical symptoms, but symptoms may appear because of mechanical compression of the neuraxis or due to an associated malformation of the nervous system.

Basilar Impression

Platybasia, basilar impression, and basilar invagination are names frequently used interchangeably for the skeletal malformation in which the base of the skull is flattened on the cervical spine. *Platybasia* (flat base skull) is present if the angle formed by a line connecting the nasion, tuberculum sella, and anterior margin of the foramen magnum is greater than 143 degrees (Fig. 78.2). *Basilar invagination* refers to an upward indentation of the base of the skull, which may be present in Paget disease, osteomalacia, or other forms of bone disease associated with softening of the bones of the skull. An upward displacement of the occipital bone and cervical spine with protrusion of the odontoid process into the foramen magnum constitutes *basilar impression*. Compression of the pons, medulla, cerebellum, and cervical cord and stretching of the cranial nerves may result from the upward ascent of the occipital bone and cervical spine and from narrowing of the foramen magnum.

Pathology and Pathogenesis

Minor degrees of platybasia and basilar invagination may not produce symptoms. In most symptomatic cases, the deformity is due to a congenital maldevelopment or hypoplasia of the basiocciput, which causes basilar impression, platybasia, partial or complete atlantooccipital fusion, atlantoaxial dislocation, and a narrowed foramen magnum. The pons, medulla, and cerebellum may be distorted and the cranial nerves stretched. Vertebral artery obstruction may be significant in the production of brain-

TABLE 78.2. MACROCEPHALY AND MEGALENCEPHALY

Developmental defects	Characteristics
Cerebral gigantism (Sotos syndrome)	Macrocephaly with mildly dilated ventricles; precocious increased size including enlarged hands and feet, dolichocephaly, hypertelorism, macroglossia, prognathism; often associated mental retardation, seizures, and clumsiness; frequent early respiratory and feeding problems; may be autosomal dominant
Trisomy 9p syndrome	Macrocephaly with somatic and genital growth delay; facial, hand, and feet deformities, periscapular muscle hypoplasia, delayed bone maturation; severe mental retardation
Robinow syndrome	Macrocephaly with macroglossia and other facial deformities; hemivertebrae and limb defects; genital hypoplasia; seizures may be present, variable degree of mental deficiency
FG syndrome	Megalencephaly with facial dysmorphism, imperforate anus, joint and hand deformities; occasional hydrocephalus, agenesis of corpus callosum, intestinal abnormalities, sensorineural deafness, cardiac and genitourinary defects
Achondroplasia	Macrocephaly with associated cranial defects; short cranial base, early sphenooccipital stenosis, depressed nasal bridge and facial hypoplasia. Skeletal deformities. May have hydrocephalus; spinal cord and foraminal narrowing with compression in about 46%, normal intelligence. Short stature. Frequency 1:26,000, autosomal dominant transmission
Greig cephalopolysyndactyly	Macrocephaly, frontal bossing and hypertelorism, broad thumbs and other hand deformities; autosomal dominant
Osteopetrosis	Macrocephaly with progressive compression of cranial foramina; multiple skeletal defects; increased alkaline phosphatase; autosomal recessive
Osteopathia striata with cranial sclerosis	Macrocephaly, linear striations of long bones, hypertelorism, palate anomalies, hearing deficits, mental retardation
Storage diseases/metabolic Tay-Sachs disease–infantile (GM$_2$ gangliosidosis)	Megalencephaly secondary to neuronal swelling and astrocytic hyperplasia; myoclonic seizures and rapidly progressive dementia, quadriparesis, hyperacusis with onset in first months of life; cherry-red spot in fundus; blindness; autosomal recessive
Hurler (mucopolysaccharidosis IH)	Macrocephaly with occasional hydrocephalus secondary to arachnoid mucopolysaccharide accumulation; growth retardation, mental retardation, coarse facial features, corneal and retinal changes, macroglossia, kyphosis and other skeletal deformities, deafness, hepatosplenomegaly, cardiac defects; autosomal recessive
Hurler-Scheie (mucopolysaccharidosis IH/S)	Macrocephaly with facial dysmorphism, corneal clouding; mild mental deficiency to normal; dysostosis multiplex, mild joint contractures, deafness, hepatosplenomegaly, cardiac defects
Maroteaux-Larny Mucopolysaccharidosis (mucopolysaccharidosis VI)	Occasional macrocephaly with coarse facial features, growth delay, joint and skeletal changes, hepatosplenomegaly, deafness; autosomal recessive
Mucopolysaccharidosis VII (Sly syndrome; glucuronidase deficiency)	Macrocephaly with mental deficiency; joint and skeletal deformities, hepatosplenomegaly, corneal clouding; autosomal recessive
Fucosidosis Mitochondrial respiratory chain	Megalencephaly with progressive psychomotor retardation; hepatosplenomegaly, dysostosis multiplex
Mitochondrial respiratory chain in complex I deficency	Fatal progressive macrocephaly and hypertrophic cardiomyopathy. Cerebral small vessel proliferation and gliosis
Leukodystrophies Spongy degeneration (Canavan)	Megalencephaly with progressive psychomotor retardation, seizures; vacuolation and Alzheimer type II astrocytes prominent
Alexander disease	Megalencephaly with progressive psychomotor retardation, seizures; Rosenthal fibers deep to internal and external brain surfaces
Neurocutaneous disorders Tuberous sclerosis	Megalencephic brain with cortical tubers, subependymal nodules, heterotopias; mental retardation, seizures, hypomelanotic macules, facial angiofibromas; ocular, cardiac, and renal defects; autosomal dominant
Klippel-Trenaunay-Weber	Macrocephaly with limb hypertrophy; hemangiomata, hyperpigmented nevi, and other skin lesions, ocular abnormalities, visceromegaly; may be mentally deficient; seizures
Ruvalcaba-Myhre syndrome	Macrocephaly and tan spots on penis; mental deficiency, intestinal hamartomas; macrosomia at birth; lipid storage myopathy
Proteus syndrome	Macrocephaly associated with hemihypertrophy thickened skin, hyperpigmented areas, hemangiomata and lipomata, bony defects, macrodactyly, mental deficiency
Cowden disease	Megalencephaly associated with Lhermitte-Duclos cerebellar dysplasia; facial, oral, and acral papules, tumors of breast and ovary; may see mental deficiency, seizures, tremor

TABLE 78.3. UNCOMMON SYNDROMES ASSOCIATED WITH CERVICOMEDULLARY AND CERVICAL SPINE MALFORMATIONS

Syndromes	Characteristics
Craniometaphyseal dysplasia	Hyperostosis and skull sclerosis, long bone metaphyseal widening, cranial nerve compression, foramen magnum narrowing causing hydrocephalus, cord and brainstem compression. Calcitrol treatment
MURCS (Müllerian duct aplasia, renal aplasia, cervicothoracic somite dysplasia)	Klippel-Feil anomaly with absence of vagina and uterus, absence or hypoplasia, renal agenesis or ectopy: other bony defects; hearing and gastrointestinal defects
Goldenhar	Cervical hemivertebrae or hypoplasia with associated facial bone, ear, and oral hypoplasias; deafness; occasional defects of heart, kidney, other bones; may be unilateral; mental deficiency in some
Escobar	Cervical vertebral fusion and other bony defects, ptosis, hypertelorism, pterygia of neck, axillae, and other joints; genital anomalies; small stature; autosomal recessive

stem symptoms (e.g., vertigo and drop attacks with head turning) in basilar impression.

Symptoms and Signs

Basilar impression is rare. Neurologic symptoms, when present, usually develop in childhood or early adult life. The head may appear to be elongated and its vertical diameter reduced. The neck appears shortened, and its movements may be limited by anomalies of the upper cervical vertebrae. Neurologic symptoms include spastic paraparesis, unsteady gait, cerebellar ataxia, nys-

tagmus, and paralyses of the lower cranial nerves. Papilledema and signs of increased pressure may occur if the deformity interferes with the circulation of the CSF. Partial or complete subarachnoid block is present at lumbar puncture in most cases. CSF protein levels are increased in 50% of patients.

Diagnosis

The diagnosis of basilar impression is usually obvious from the general appearance of the patient. It can be established with certainty by the characteristic radiographic or CT appearance of the

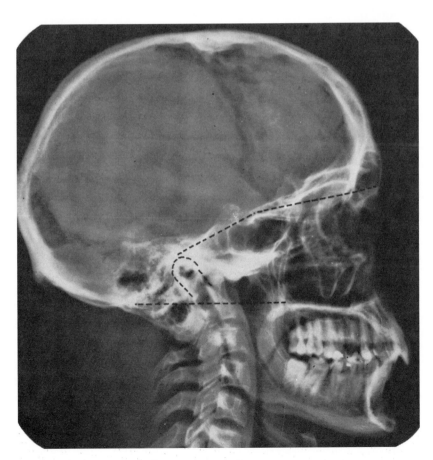

FIG. 78.2. Basilar impression with platybasia. The odontoid process is entirely above Chamberlain's line (hard palate to base of skull). Basal angle is flat. (Courtesy of Dr. Juan Taveras.)

base of the skull. The clinical syndromes produced by the anomaly can simulate those of multiple sclerosis, syringomyelia, the Arnold-Chiari malformation, and posterior fossa tumors. These diagnoses are readily excluded CT and MRI.

Treatment

The treatment is surgical decompression of the posterior fossa and the upper cervical cord.

Malformations of the Atlas and Axis

Maldevelopments of the atlas and axis may be found with basilar impression or may occur independently. Congenital defects resulting in weakness or absence of the structures maintaining stability of the atlantoaxial joints predispose to subluxation and dislocation. These include dens aplasia, a condition in which part of the odontoid process remains on the body of the second cervical vertebra, thereby reducing the stability of the joint. Neurologic symptoms may be produced by anterior dislocation of the atlas and compression of the cord between the protruding odontoid process and the posterior rim of the foramen magnum. There may be mild or severe spastic quadriparesis, with or without evidence of damage to the lower cranial nerves. Head movement causes pain. Sensory loss may be mild. Transitory signs or symptoms of a progressive myelopathy may occur, often after exaggerated movements of the neck. Respiratory embarrassment is prominent when the thoracic muscles are affected. The diagnosis is made by finding anterior dislocation of the atlas in CT. When the bony changes are slight, and especially when there is little or no posterior dislocation of the odontoid process, the symptoms may be due to other congenital defects, such as syringomyelia or Arnold-Chiari malformation.

Fusion of the Cervical Vertebrae

Fusion of the upper thoracic vertebrae and the entire cervical spine into a single bony mass was reported by Klippel and Feil in 1912. Since that time, numerous cases have been reported with variations of this deformity. In most, the abnormality consists of the fusion of the cervical vertebrae into one or more separate masses (Fig. 78.3). This vertebral fusion is the result of maldevelopment *in utero*, and there is evidence of both autosomal dominant and recessive transmission. This anomaly is associated with a short neck, low hairline, and limitation of neck movement, especially in the lateral direction. Fusion of the vertebrae is not in itself of any great clinical importance except for the resulting deformity in the appearance of the neck. Clinical symptoms are usually due to the presence of syringomyelia or other developmental defects of the spinal cord, brainstem, or cerebellum. Congenital cardiovascular defects have been reported in 4% and genitourinary anomalies in 2% of patients. Congenital deafness due to faulty development of the osseous inner ear was estimated to occur in up to 30% of patients.

More frequently, there may be fusion of only two adjacent cervical vertebrae causing only accentuation of symptoms in the presence of cervical osteoarthritis.

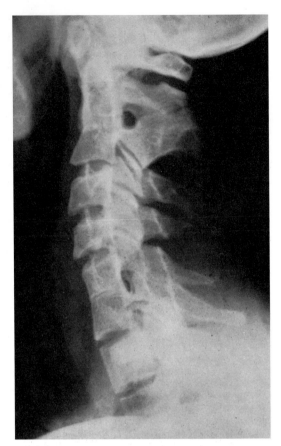

FIG. 78.3. Fusion of cervical vertebrae (Klippel-Feil syndrome).

PREMATURE CLOSURE OF CRANIAL SUTURES

Craniosynostosis or premature closure of cranial sutures occurs in childhood if cerebral growth is impaired. This is commonly manifested by a uniform closure of all sutures and microcephaly. True microcephaly is defined by a head circumference less than 3 standard deviations below the mean for age and sex. Rarely, early closure of the sutures may occur as a consequence of metabolic diseases, including rickets and hyperthyroidism.

Craniosynostosis is usually a primary congenital disturbance of skull growth with no neurologic disorder. The frequency is about 1 in 1,900 births. In 10% to 20%, there is a mendelian inheritance. Sixty-four mutations of six genes have been described in craniosynostosis syndromes commonly associated with limb malformations. Accompanying facial and other tissue deformities also may be seen in recognized syndromes (Table 78.4).

In essence, the skull deformity in primary craniosynostosis reflects the inhibition of growth perpendicular to the closed suture, with compensatory overgrowth in directions perpendicular to the unaffected sutures. Closure of a single suture is most common. Sagittal suture closure alone, seen in 55% of all patients with craniosynostosis, is clinically identified by a child with an oblong-shaped skull (*dolichocephalic* or *scaphocephalic*), often with visible ridging of the closed suture (Fig. 78.4).

TABLE 78.4. SYNDROMES ASSOCIATED WITH CRANIOSYNOSTOSIS

Syndromes	Characteristics
Apert (acrocephalosyndactyly) (Fig. 78.4)	Coronal suture closure, shallow orbits, hypertelorism, small nose, maxillary hypoplasia, narrow and occasional cleft palate; syndactyly and other skeletal deformities; occasional cardiac, gastrointestinal, and genitourinary malformations; autosomal dominant; mental deficiency often seen
Carpenter	Synostosis of coronal and often sagittal and lambdoid sutures, shallow supraorbital ridges, laterally displaced inner canthi; brachydactyly and other skeletal deformities; hypogenitalism, obesity; occasional cardiac and renal malformations; neurosensory and conductive hearing loss; probably autosomal recessive; may be mentally deficient
Crouzon (craniofacial dysostosis)	Coronal, lambdoid, and sagittal suture closure of variable degree, ocular proptosis and shallow orbits, hypertelorism, conductive hearing loss; autosomal dominant; may be mentally deficient and have agenesis of corpus callosum, optic atrophy, and seizures
Saethre-Chotzen	Coronal suture closure, maxillary hypoplasia, shallow orbits, hypertelorism, ptosis, small ears; cutaneous syndactyly and other skeletal deformities; short stature; may have renal and cardiac abnormalities; autosomal dominant; mental deficiency may be seen
Pfeiffer	Coronal and perhaps sagittal suture closure with hypertelorism, narrow maxilla. Broad distal phalanges, thumb, and hallux; other skeletal deformities including Arnold-Chiari malformation. Autosomal dominant
Autley-Bixler	Multiple suture closure, brachycephaly with midfacial hypoplasia, proptosis choanal stenosis, dysplastic ears; arachnodactyly, joint contractures, and other skeletal deformities; may have genitourinary anomalies, multiple hemangiomas; probable autosomal recessive
Baller-Gerold	One or more suture synostosis (usually metopic), radial hypoplasia, and other preaxial limb anomalies; other skeletal, genitourinary, and cardiac deformities; anal malformation; autosomal recessive; mental deficiency
Chromosome (9p monosomy)	Metopic suture closure, midfacial hypoplasia, poorly formed ears; long mid-phalanges of fingers with extra flexion creases, short distal phalanges with short nails; other skeletal anomalies, cardiac and genitourinary defects; deletion of distal portion of short arm chromosome 9

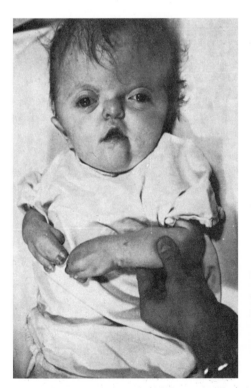 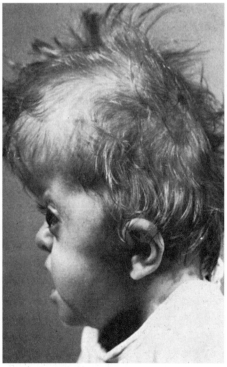

FIG. 78.4. Acrocephalosyndactyly (Apert syndrome). Head is shortened in anterioposterior dimension, forehead is prominent, and occiput flat. Typical facies showing shallow orbits and proptosis of eyes, downward slanting palpebral fissures, small nose, and low-set ears. Osseous and cutaneous syndactyly of hands and feet.

Unilateral closure of the coronal suture is seen in about 24% of all patients, appearing as a misshapen and unilaterally flattened head (plagiocephaly). Metopic suture closure occurs in about 5% of all craniosynostosis patients, with a prominent midforehead brow appearance (*trigonencephaly*).

Single suture closure does not lead to compression of intracranial tissues. Multiple suture closure occurs commonly with other skull and facial defects and may lead to increased intracranial pressure because of interference with intracranial CSF flow. The optic and acoustic nerves may be compressed, especially in infants with bilateral coronal suture closure (about 9% of all patients with craniosynostosis). These infants have a broad biparietal diameter skull (*brachycephaly*). Rarer forms of multiple suture disorder include some infants with closure of all sutures, resulting in a tower-shaped skull (oxycephaly) or a grossly distorted skull with an asymmetric, often bizarre clover-leaf shape (*Kleeblattschädel*).

Early diagnosis of primary craniosynostosis is essential because the best cosmetic results from surgery are accomplished before the infant is 3 months old. The longer the delay, the greater the compensatory deformity in other areas of the skull and the more complex the surgery. Three-dimensional CT identifies the overall craniofacial contours and guides the surgical procedures needed for the complicated deformities of infants with more than one closed suture. In these infants, the cosmetic benefits are less important than prevention of intracranial hypertension and cranial nerve compression.

Craniectomy to open up closed sutures is of no value in infants with craniostenosis and microcephaly in whom the injured brain has not grown adequately.

SPINA BIFIDA AND CRANIUM BIFIDUM

Both environmental factors and genetics may produce structural malformations of the developing nervous system. Moreover, the damaged fetal brain may be more vulnerable to hypoxic perinatal insults. Teratogenetic factors including certain anticonvulsants probably cause malformations in 1 of every 400 births; ge-

netic factors account for about a third of the malformations, and the cause is unknown in more than 50%.

Pathogenesis and Diagnosis

The neural tube begins to fuse on about day 27 and closes about day 28 of gestation. The primordium of the vertebrae forms from the mesoderm that, similar to the adjacent developing ectoderm, separates from the neural tube. Failure of closure of the neural tube and associated primitive mesodermal and ectodermal elements accounts for the appearance of congenital midline defects, termed dysraphism (Table 78.5).

Severe malformations may be detected *in utero* by ultrasonography and by finding elevated maternal serum levels of alpha-fetoprotein (AFP). AFP is the major circulating protein of early fetal life, synthesized in the fetal liver and yolk sac. Peak levels are found about 16 weeks after the last menstrual period, making that the optimum time for testing. The exposed fetal membranes and blood vessel surfaces increase the AFP levels in both maternal serum and amniotic fluid if there is an open neural tube. If results are ambiguous or in circumstances in which there is increased risk of a defect because of genetic factors, measurement of AFP and acetylcholinesterase by amniocentesis is warranted. Measurement of amniotic acetylcholinesterase activity helps to detect an open dysraphic state *in utero* because amniotic AFP levels may be high in gastroschisis, omphalocele, and nephrosis. Increased levels of amniotic AFP and acetylcholinesterase detect at least 90% of open spina bifida fetuses and almost all of the anencephalics, whereas maternal serum AFP levels detect 60% to 80% of open spina bifida fetuses and 90% of the anencephalics.

The use of folic acid or vitamin supplements containing folic acid during the periconceptional period significantly decreases the risk of neural tube closure defects in the offspring. The risk of another child born with a neural tube defect in a family with two unaffected parents is 3% to 5%. Although familial clustering of neural tube defects has been identified, the pattern best fits a polygenic model of inheritance.

The simplest defect, *spina bifida occulta*, is characterized by a

TABLE 78.5. NEURAL TUBE CLOSURE MALFORMATIONS

Malformation	Characteristics
Anencephaly	Absence of brain with associated defects in skull, meninges, and scalp; minimal hind brain structures may be present. Frequency 1:1,000 deliveries
Iniencephaly	Retroflexed head with defects of cervical spine; often combined with anencephaly or encephaloceles
Craniorachischisis	Brain and spinal cord necrosis secondary to exposure to amniotic fluid
Cephalocele	Partial brain protrusion through skull defect (cranium bifidum) with variable covering of meninges and skin; most common in occipital region but may be parietal or anterior skull
Meningocele	Skull or spine defect associated with meningeal protrusion
Dermal sinus tract	Incomplete separation of neural and epithelial ectoderm; may be associated with dermoid; marked externally by skin and hair changes; point of entry for bacteria with subsequent meningitis
Spina bifida	Varying degree of vertebral abnormality
Spina bifida occulta	Vertebral arch defect only. Up to 24% of population
Spina bifida cystica	Dura and arachnoid herniation through vertebral defect
Myelomeningocele	Herniation of spinal cord and meninges through defect

lack of vertebral arch closure without any other associated defect. It is usually localized to L5-S1 and does not seem to have an increased risk of neural tube closure malformations in that individual's progeny. This is in contrast to anencephaly and other forms of spina bifida in which there is a close genetic relationship and in which the recurrence risk is equally distributed.

Many severely affected fetuses are spontaneously aborted. Associated anomalies of other organ systems include congenital heart disorders, diaphragmatic defects, and esophageal atresia. Other central nervous system anomalies are common but may not be clinically apparent in the newborn infant with neural tube closure defect. Abnormalities of the basal ganglia, hippocampi, commissural pathways, brainstem, and cerebellum may be seen in infants born with occipital encephaloceles. Ventricular wall deformities, corpus callosum defects, and hydrocephalus may be noted with parietal encephaloceles. Basal ganglia and commissural anomalies may be seen with anterior encephaloceles that are most common in the frontoethmoidal junction.

Spina bifida deformities commonly include other nervous system abnormalities: tethering of the cord (Fig. 78.5), diastematomyelia, hydromyelia, and hydrocephalus usually associated with Arnold-Chiari type II malformation. Occult spinal dysraphic states reflect other defects of ectodermal and mesodermal origin, including pelvic meningoceles, hamartomas, lipomas, and dermoid tumors, and may be suspected if there are skin markers: skin tags, hair tufts, abnormal dimpling, or aplasia cutis congenita.

The congenital syndromes associated with defects of neural tube closure include the *Meckel-Gruber syndrome* (posterior encephalocele, microcephaly, cerebral and cerebellar hypoplasia, and associated defects of face, neck, limbs, kidney, liver, and genitalia) and the *Walker-Warburg syndrome* (occipital encephalo-

cele, Dandy-Walker cyst, hydrocephalus, cerebellar hypoplasia, and eye defects).

Treatment

MRI of the brain and spine has enhanced an understanding of the extent of the primary defect and the associated anomalies. MRI also guides treatment. Neurologic evaluation defines the level of function by evaluating anal reaction and sensory, reflex, and motor functions.

Surgical excision of the meningocele and the encephalocele must include meticulous protection of the neural elements underlying and sometimes adherent to the tissue to be excised. Postexcision assessment is vital to detect complications or the emergence of secondary or associated abnormalities (e.g., hydrocephalus after closure of a spinal meningocele or tethering of the spinal cord). Orthopedic and urologic approaches are essential for maximizing functional ability and preventing skin, bone, and renal problems. Concomitant or resultant bone and joint changes include the Klippel-Feil syndrome, foot deformities, scoliosis, and hip dysplasia, which may point to an associated disorder, such as cord tethering, hydromyelia, adhesive arachnoiditis, or a lipoma.

In a series of 286 patients who had surgical closure of a spinal defect within 48 hours of birth, 42% had a thoracic defect and 58% had a lumbar or sacral defect. With an average age at follow-up of 61.4 months, 11% had lost quadriceps function between birth and the most recent examination. This was attributed to the development of a tethered cord. Only 24% of the thoracic-level patients could walk, whereas 92% of the lumbosacral-level patients did so. Prevalence of quadriceps function was critical. Ninety-three percent of all patients had shunts placed for the treatment of clinically overt hydrocephalus; 74% had more than one shunt.

Psychologic development depends on the extent of cerebral pathology due to associated congenital defects or the sequelae of an open spina bifida such as neonatal meningitis, hydrocephalus, and shunting plus the emotional impact of the multiplicity of treatment regimens.

ARNOLD-CHIARI MALFORMATION

A congenital anomaly of the hindbrain characterized by a downward elongation of the brainstem and cerebellum into the cervical portion of the spinal cord was originally described by Arnold in 1894 and Chiari in 1895.

Pathology

Because of its common association with spina bifida occulta or the presence of a meningocele or meningomyelocele in the lumbosacral region, the downward displacement of the brainstem and cerebellum was attributed to fixation of the cord at the site of the spinal defect early in fetal life. This hypothesis is not applicable to the many cases in which there is no defect in the lower spine, and the theory fails to account for the other anomalies commonly associated with the hindbrain malformation (e.g., ab-

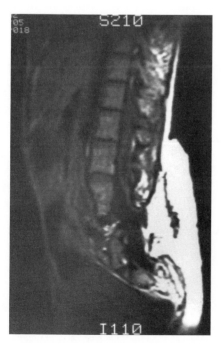

FIG. 78.5. Lumbosacral myelomeningocele. Sagittal magnetic resonance imaging shows spinal dysraphism and tethered cord.

sence of the septum pellucidum, fusion of the thalami, hypoplasia of the falx cerebri, fusion of the corporea quadrigemina and microgyri). Some type of developmental arrest and overgrowth of the neural tube in embryonic life is a more plausible explanation of the anomaly.

The gross description of the abnormality has been remarkably similar in all the reported cases. The inferior poles of the cerebellar hemispheres extend downward through the foramen magnum in two tonguelike processes and are often adherent to the adjacent medulla; more than half is usually below the level of the foramen magnum (Fig. 78.6). The medulla is elongated and flattened anteroposteriorly, and the lower cranial nerves are stretched.

Incidence

The Arnold-Chiari malformation is not as rare as would be expected from the small number of reported cases. Ingraham and Swan found 20 instances of this abnormality among 290 patients with myelomeningoceles. The defect is almost always, but not invariably, associated with a meningomyelocele or spina bifida occulta in the lumbosacral region. Hydrocephalus is present in most cases. Other associated defects of development include rounded defects in the bones of the skull (craniolacunia, Lückenschädel), defects in the spinal cord (hydromyelia, syringomyelia, double cord), and defects in the spinal column (basilar impression).

Symptoms and Signs

The neurologic signs and symptoms of the Arnold-Chiari malformation that appear in the first few months of life are usually due to hydrocephalus and other developmental defects in the nervous system. The prognosis is poor in these cases. The onset of symptoms may be delayed until adult life. There may be signs and symptoms of injury to the cerebellum, medulla, and the lower cranial nerves, with or without evidence of increased intracranial pressure. Progressive ataxia, leg weakness, and visual complaints are characteristic. Oscillopsia at rest and visual blurring of fixated targets are described. Downbeat nystagmus and seesaw nystagmus may be noted in lesions of the cervicomedullary region.

Diagnosis

The presence of an Arnold-Chiari malformation is probable when there is a coincidence of meningomyelocele, hydrocephalus, and craniolacunia in infancy. The diagnosis in adults should be considered whenever there are signs and symptoms of damage to the cerebellum, medulla, and lower cranial nerves. The signs and symptoms of the Arnold-Chiari malformation in adults may simulate the syndromes produced by tumors of the posterior fossa, multiple sclerosis, syringomyelia, or basilar impression. The diagnosis can be established by CT (Fig. 78.7) and MRI (Figs. 78.8, 78.9, and 78.10).

Treatment

Treatment of the malformation in infants includes excision of the sac in the spinal region and a ventriculoperitoneal shunt to relieve the hydrocephalus. Early hindbrain decompression is

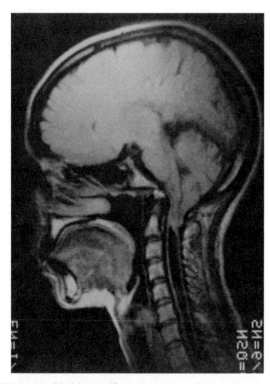

FIG. 78.6. Arnold-Chiari malformation. Magnetic resonance imaging T1-weighted image of midsagittal section of brain and cervical cord. Note small and elongated fourth ventricle, low position of obex of fourth ventricle below plane of foramen magnum, cerebellar tonsillar ectopia, short clivus, wide foramen magnum, kinked cervical medullary junction, and prominent superior vermis. Large hydromyelia in cervical cord.

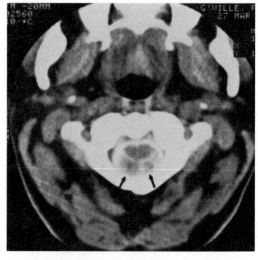

FIG. 78.7. Arnold-Chiari malformation. Postmyelography computed tomography. At level of odontoid in high cervical region, spinal cord is flattened by cerebellar tonsils (*arrows*). (Courtesy of Drs. S.K. Hilal and M. Mawad.)

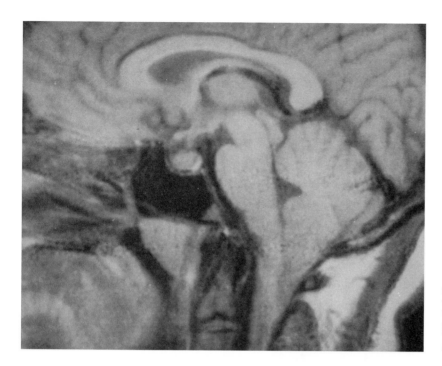

FIG. 78.8. Type I Arnold-Chiari malformation. Sagittal T1-weighted scan shows tonsillar herniation through foramen magnum. Fourth ventricle is of normal size and position as are aqueduct and brainstem. There is no hydrocephalus. (Courtesy of Drs. J.A. Bello and S.K. Hilal.)

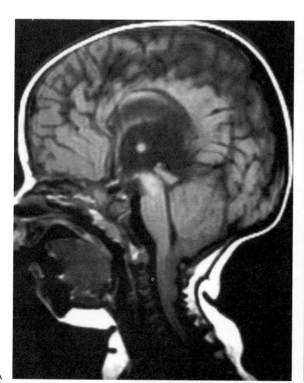

A

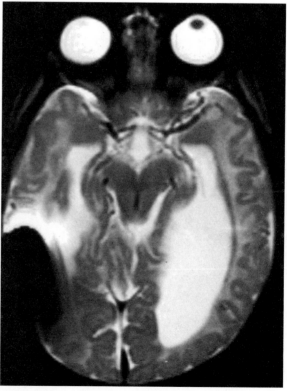

B

FIG. 78.9. Chiari II malformation. **A:** T1-weighted sagittal magnetic resonance (MR) image shows significant inferior displacement of cerebellar tonsil with tip located posterior to cervical cord at C3 level. The fourth ventricle is typically small. Also note agenesis of the corpus callosum. This is a separate congenital lesion but is often seen in association with Chiari malformation. **B and C:** T2-weighted axial MR image demonstrates "beaking" of dorsal midbrain, or tectum, characteristic of Chiari II malformation. There is enlargement of the occipital horns of both lateral ventricles (with ventricular shunt in right lateral ventricle), consistent with colpocephaly, which is often associated with agenesis of corpus callosum. (Courtesy of Dr. S. Chan, Columbia University College of Physicians and Surgeons, New York, NY.) figure *continues*

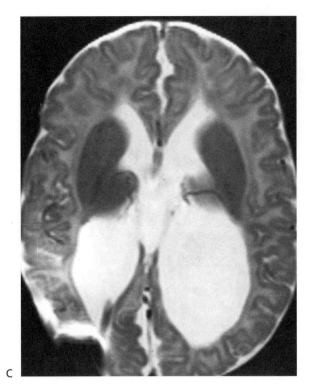

C   **FIG. 78.9.** *Continued.*

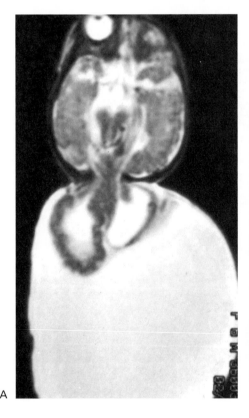

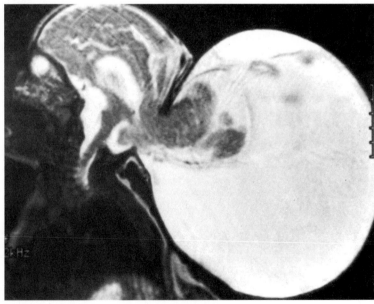

FIG. 78.10. Encephalocele with Chiari III malformation. **A and B:** T2-weighted sagittal and axial magnetic resonance images demonstrate a huge fluid-filled sac external to the skull posteriorly, with patent communication to intracranial structures. There is herniation of both cerebellar hemispheres into the extruded cerebrospinal fluid-filled sac, most consistent with occipital encephalocele. Distortion of the brainstem and absence of the corpus callosum are also apparent. (Courtesy of Dr. S. Chan, Columbia University College of Physicians and Surgeons, New York, NY.)

A   B needed in symptomatic neonates with vocal cord paralysis. In adults, the posterior fossa should be decompressed. The best results are obtained when there are few neurologic symptoms caused by the spinal defect or other congenital anomalies.

SUGGESTED READINGS

Agenesis of the Corpus Collosum

Berg MJ, Sohifitto G, Powers JM, et al. X-linked female band heterotropia-male lissencephaly syndrome. *Neurology* 1998;50:1143–1146.

Bertoni JM, von Loh S, Allen RJ. The Aicardi syndrome: report of 4 cases and review of the literature. *Ann Neurol* 1979;5:475–482.

Dobyns WB. Agenesis of the corpus callosum and gyral malformations are frequent manifestations of nonketotic hyperglycinemia. *Neurology* 1989;39:817–820.

Dobyns WB, Truwit CL. Lissencephaly and other malformations of cortical development. *Neuropediatrics* 1995;26:132–147.

Faye-Peterson OM, Ward K, Carey JC, Kinsley AS. Osteochondrodysplasia with rhizomelia, platyspondyly, callosal agenesis, thrombocytopenia, hydrocephalus and hypertension. *Am J Med Genet* 1991;40:183–187.

Guala A, Dellavecchia C, Mannarino S. Ring chromosome 13 with loss of the region D13S317-D13S285: phenotypic overlap with XK syndrome. *Am J Med Genet* 1997;72:319–323.

Haltia M, Leivo I, Samer H, et al. Muscle-eye-brain disease: a neuropathological study. *Ann Neurol* 1997;41:173–180.

Harding BN. Malformation of the nervous system. In: Adams JH, Duchen LW, eds. *Greenfield's neuropathology*, 5th ed. New York: Oxford University Press, 1992.

Jeret JS, Serur D, Wisniewski KE, et al. Clinicopathological findings associated with agenesis of the corpus callosum. *Brain Dev* 1987;9:255–264.

Jones KL. *Smith's recognizable patterns of human malformation,* 4th ed. Philadelphia: WB Saunders, 1988.

Loeser JD, Alvord EC. Agenesis of the corpus callosum. *Brain* 1968;91:553–570.

Pavlakis, SG, Frissora, CL, Giampietro PF, et al. Fanconi anemia a model for genetic causes of abnormal brain development. *Dev Med Child Neurol* 1992;34:1081–1084.

Macrocephaly and Megalencephaly

DeMeyer W. Megalencephaly: types, clinical syndromes, and management. *Pediatr Neurol* 1986;2:321–328.

Dionisi-Vici C, Ruitenbeek W, Fariello G, et al. New familial mitochondrial encephalopathy with macrocephaly, cardiomyopathy, and complex I deficiency. *Ann Neurol* 1997;42:661–665.

Fusco L, Ferracuti S, Fariello G, et al. Hemimegalencephaly and normal intellectual development. *J Neurol Neurosurg Psychiatry* 1992;55:720–722.

Gontieres F, Boulloche J, Bourgeois M, Aicardi J. Leucoencephalopathy, megalencephaly, and mild clinical course. A recently individualized familial lecodystrophy. *J Child Neurol* 1996;11:439–444.

Harding BN. Malformation of the nervous system. In: Adams JH, Duchen LW, eds. *Greenfield's neuropathology*, 5th ed. New York: Oxford University Press, 1992.

Laubscher B, Deonna T, Uske A, et al. Primitive megalencephaly in children: natural history, medium term prognosis with special reference to external hydrocephalus. *Eur J Pediatr* 1990;149:502–507.

Padberg GW, Schot JD, Vielvoye GJ, et al. L'hermitte-Duclos disease and Cowden disease: a single phakomatosis. *Ann Neurol* 1991;29:517–523.

Malformations of Occipital Bone and Cervical Spine

DeBarros MC, Farias W, Ataide L, et al. Basilar impression and Arnold-Chiari malformation. *J Neurol Neurosurg Psychiatry* 1968;31:596–605.

Dehaene I, Pattyn G, Calliauw L. Megadolicho-basilar anomaly, basilar impression and occipitovertebral anastomosis. *Clin Neurol Neurosurg* 1975;78:131–138.

Dunsker SB, Brown O, Thomson N. Craniovertebral anomalies. *Clin Neurosurg* 1980;27:430–439.

Gunderson CH, Greenspan RH, Glaser GH. The Klippel-Feil syndrome: genetic and clinical reevaluation of cervical fusion. *Medicine (Baltimore)* 1967;46:491–512.

Janeway R, Toole JF, Leinbach LB, et al. Vertebral artery obstruction with basilar impression. *Arch Neurol* 1966;15:211–214.

Jones KL. *Smith's recognizable patterns of human malformations*, 4th ed. Philadelphia: WB Saunders, 1988.

Kaplan JG, Rosenberg RS, DeSouza T, et al. Atlantoaxial subluxation in psoriatic arthropathy. *Ann Neurol* 1988;23:522–524.

Norot JC, Stauffer ES. Sequelae of atlanto-axial stabilization in two patients with Down's syndrome. *Spine* 1981;6:437–440.

Sakai M, Shinkawa A, Miyake H, et al. Klippel-Feil syndrome with conductive deafness: histological findings of removed stapes. *Ann Otol Rhinol Laryngol* 1983;92:202–206.

Stevens JM, Chong WK, Barber C, Kendall BE, Cockard HA. A new appraisal of abnormalities of the odontoid process associated with atlanto-axial subluxation and neurological disability. *Brain* 1994;117:133–148.

Vangilder JC, Menezes AH, Dlan KD. *The craniovertebral junction and its abnormalities*. Mt. Kisco, NY: Futura Publishing Co, 1987.

Premature Closure of Cranial Sutures

Carmel PW, Luken MG III, Ascherl GF. Craniosynostosis: computed tomographic evaluation of skull base and calvarial deformities and associated intracranial changes. *Neurosurgery* 1981;9:366–372.

Cohen MM. Craniosynostosis and syndromes with craniosynostosis: incidence, genetics, penetrance, variability, and new syndrome updating. *Birth Defects* 1979;15:13–63.

Crouzon Q. Dysostose cranio-faciale hereditaire. *Bull Mem Soc Med Hop Paris* 1912;33:545.

Gorlin RJ, Cohen MM Jr, Levin LS. *Syndromes of the head and neck*, 3rd ed. New York: Oxford University Press, 1990.

Gripp KW, McDonald-McGinn DM, Gaudenz K, et al. Identification of a genetic cause for isolated unilateral coronal synostosis: a unique mutation in the fibroblast growth factor receptor 3. *J Pediatr* 1998;132:714–716.

Hoffman HS, Epstein F. *Disorders of the developing nervous system: diagnosis and treatment*. Boston: Blackwell Scientific Publications, 1986.

Jones KL. *Smith's recognizable patterns of human malformation*, 4th ed. Philadelphia: WB Saunders, 1988.

Pellegrino JE, McDonald-McGinn DM, Schneider A. Further clinical delineation and increased morbidity in males with osteopathia striata with cranial sclerosis: an x-linked disorder? *Am J Med Genet* 1997;70:159–165.

Shillito J Jr. A plea for early operation for craniostenosis. *Surg Neurol* 1992;37:182–188.

Wilkie AOM. Craniosynostosis: genes and mechanisms. *Hum Mol Genet* 1997;6:1647–1656.

Spina Bifida and Cranium Bifidum

Czeizel AE, Duda I. Prevention of the first occurrence of neural tube defects by periconceptional vitamin supplementation. *N Engl J Med* 1992;327:1832–1835.

Gorlin RJ, Cohen MM Jr, Levin LS. *Syndromes of the head and neck,* 3rd ed. New York: Oxford University Press, 1990.

Harding BN. Malformation of the nervous system. In: Adams JH, Duchen LW, eds. *Greenfield's neuropathology*, 5th ed. New York: Oxford University Press, 1992.

Harper PS. *Practical genetic counselling*, 3rd ed. London: Wright, 1988.

Hoffman HS, Epstein F. *Disorders of the developing nervous system: diagnosis and treatment*. Boston: Blackwell Scientific Publications, 1986.

Patterson RS, Egelhoff JC, Crone KR, et al. Atretic parietal cephaloceles revisisted: an enlarging clinical and imaging spectrum. *Am J Neuroradiol* 1998;19:791–795.

Robert E, Guiband P. Maternal valproic acid and congenital neural tube defects. *Lancet* 1982;2:934.

Salonen R. The Meckel syndrome: clinicopathological findings in 67 patients. *Am J Med Genet* 1984;18:671–689.

Arnold-Chiari Malformation

Arnold J. Myelocyste. Transposition von Gewebskeimen und Sympodie. *Beitr Pathol Anat* 1894;16:1–28.

Balagura S, Kuo DC. Spontaneous retraction of cerebellar tonsils after surgery for Arnold-Chiari malformation and posterior fossa cyst. *Surg Neurol* 1988;29:137–140.

Banerji NK, Millar JHD. Chiari malformation presenting in adult life. Its relationship to syringomelia. *Brain* 1974;97:157–168.

Brill CB, Gutierrez J, Mishkin MM. Chiari I malformation: association with seizures and developmental disabilities. *J Child Neurol* 1997;12:101–106.

Caviness VS Jr. The Chiari malformations of the posterior fossa and their relation to hydrocephalus. *Dev Med Child Neurol* 1976;18:103–116.

Chiari H. Adüber Veränderungen des Kleinhirns, des Pons und der Medulla oblongata in Folge von congenitaler Hydrocephalie des Grosshirns. *Denkschr Akad Wiss Wien* 1896;63:71–116.

DeBarros MC, Farias W, Ataide L, et al. Basilar impression and Arnold-Chiari malformation. *J Neurol Neurosurg Psychiatry* 1968;31:596–605.

Dehaene I, Pattyn G, Calliauw L. Megadolicho-basilar anomaly, basilar impression and occipito-vertebral anastomosis. *Clin Neurol Neurosurg* 1975;78:131–138.

el Gammal T, Mark EK, Brooks BS. MR imaging of Chiari II malformation. *AJR* 1988;150:163–170.

Elster AD, Chen MY. Chiari I malformations: clinical and radiologic reappraisal. *Radiology* 1992;183:347–353.

Gilbert JN, Jones KL, Rorke LB, et al. Central nervous system anomalies associated with meningomyelocele hydrocephalus and the Arnold-Chiari malformation. *Neurosurgery* 1986;18:559–564.

Levy WJ, Mason L, Hahn JF. Chiari malformation presenting in adults: a surgical experience in 127 cases. *Neurosurgery* 1983;12:377–390.

Pollach IF, Dachling P, Albright AL, et al. Outcome following hindbrain decompression of symptomatic Chiari malformations in children previously treated with myelomeningocele closure and shunts. *J Neurosurg* 1992;77:881–888.

Salam MZ, Adams RD. The Arnold-Chiari malformation. In: Vinken P, Bruyn G, eds. *Handbook of clinical neurology.* Vol. 32. New York: American Elsevier-North Holland, 1978;99–110.

Merritt's Neurology, 10th ed., edited by L.P. Rowland. Lippincott Williams & Wilkins, Philadelphia © 2000.

MARCUS GUNN AND MÖBIUS SYNDROMES

LEWIS P. ROWLAND

MARCUS GUNN SYNDROME

Among the more bizarre and unexplained neurologic phenomena is *jaw winking.* The phenomenon was described by Marcus Gunn in 1863, and there have been many descriptions since then. The patient has congenital and unilateral ptosis. When the mouth is opened, the lid rises and there may even be retraction of the lid. Conversely, when the jaw closes, the lid comes down in a wink. Lateral movements of the jaw can substitute for opening. The patient can raise the lid voluntarily and on upward gaze, but the movements are exaggerated in response to movements of the jaw.

There is also an *inverted or reversed* Marcus Gunn phenomenon: The eye closes when the jaw opens. This is known as *Marin Amat* syndrome, which may follow Bell palsy.

How the Marcus Gunn syndrome arises is still not known; it is presumably a congenital error of neuronal wiring in the brainstem. In that respect, it is similar to the Duane retraction syndrome (retraction of the globe and narrowing of the palpebral fissure on attempted adduction). Another syndrome sometimes seen with the Marcus Gunn phenomenon and also attributed to neuronal miswiring is *synergistic divergence,* in which there is simultaneous abduction of both eyes on attempted gaze into the field of action of a paretic medial rectus; both eyes abduct on attempted lateral gaze. It is sometimes associated with other congenital anomalies that suggest an anomaly of tissues derived from

the neural crest, or there may be restriction of all ocular movements in a pattern suggesting congenital fibrosis of ocular muscles. The Marcus Gunn syndrome is sometimes an autosomal-dominant familial trait. The risk is increased in infants after a pregnant woman has used misoprotol as an abortifacent. Abnormal brainstem auditory evoked responses suggest that the problem is in the brainstem, but the levator muscle of the eyelid may show neurogenic changes, suggesting that the oculomotor nerve is affected. There have not been enough anatomic, imaging, or physiologic studies, however, to come to any conclusion.

The syndrome accounts for about 5% of all cases of congenital ptosis and may be so mild that it is of no functional consequence. The cosmetic distortion, however, has sometimes been sufficient to lead to surgical therapy in the form of operations on the levator or facial muscles.

The Marcus Gunn syndrome should not be confused with the Marcus Gunn pupil, for he also described what is now known as the *afferent pupillary defect.* Jaw winking is an abnormal *synkinesis,* simultaneous movements effected by muscles innervated by different nerves. Formally, this is a trigeminooculomotor synkinesis.

MÖBIUS SYNDROME

The usual definition of this syndrome is the combination of *congenital facial diplegia* and bilateral abducens palsies. Other cranial nerves, however, may be affected, with hearing loss, dysarthria, and dysphagia. Associated conditions include congenital anomalies of limbs or heart, Kallmann syndrome (hypogonadism and anosmia), or mental retardation.

The syndrome is often evident in the neonatal period because the children have difficulty sucking and they lack facial expression when they cry. Vertical gaze and convergence are preserved; there is usually a convergent squint. If facial paralysis is incomplete, as in almost half the cases, the syndrome may not be recognized until later in childhood. Then, in contrast to other supranuclear or lower motor neuron causes of facial paralysis, the weakness is more severe in the upper face than below; there is more of a problem with eye closure than in moving the lips. There may be complete ophthalmoplegia, ptosis, lingual hemiatrophy, and, in a few cases, mental retardation.

There is probably more than one mechanism in the pathogenesis of the facial paralysis. For instance, physiologic studies have shown cocontraction of the horizontal recti, but other cases have shown evidence of aplasia of ocular muscles or agenesis of motor neurons. In one autopsy, the facial muscles were absent but ocular muscles, nerves, and motor nerve cells were normal; there were, however, developmental anomalies of the brainstem, which may be evident on computed tomography or magnetic resonance imaging. In other autopsies, there was hypoplasia or degeneration of motor nuclei, but in some, no abnormality was seen in the central nervous system. Some cases later prove to be due to facioscapulohumeral muscular dystrophy. Congenital myotonic muscular dystrophy is another cause of facial diplegia.

SUGGESTED READINGS

Marcus Gunn Syndrome

Brodsky MC, Pollock SC, Buckley EG. Neural misdirection in congenital ocular fibrosis syndrome; implications and pathogenesis. *J Pediatr Ophthalmol Strabis* 1989;26:159–161.

Clausen N, Andersson P, Tommerup N. Familial occurrence of neuroblastoma, von Recklinghausen neurofibromatosis, Hirschsprung's agangliosis and jaw-winking syndrome. *Acta Paediatr Scand* 1989;78:736–741.

Creel DJ, Kivlin JD, Wolfley DE. Auditory brain stem responses in Marcus-Gunn ptosis. *Electroencephalogr Clin Neurophysiol* 1984;59:341–344.

Falls HF, Kruse WT, Cotterman CW. Three cases of Marcus Gunn phenomenon in two generations. *Am J Ophthalmol* 1949;32:53–59.

Grant FC. The Marcus Gunn phenomenon. *Arch Neurol Psychiatry* 1936;35:487–500.

Hamed LM, Dennehy PJ, Lingua RW. Synergistic divergence and jaw-winking phenomenon. *J Pediatr Ophthalmol Strabis* 1990;27:88–90.

Lewy FH, Groff RA, Grant FC. Autonomic innervation of the eyelids and the Marcus Gunn phenomenon. *Arch Neurol Psychiatry* 1937;37:1289–1297.

Lyness RW, Collin JR, Alexander RA, Garner A. Histologic appearances of the levator palpebral superioris muscle in the Marcus Gunn phenomenon. *Br J Ophthalmol* 1988;72:104–109.

Meirez F, Standaert L, Delaey JJ, Zeng LH. Waardenberg syndrome, Hirschsprung megacolon, and Marcus Gunn ptosis. *Am J Med Genet* 1987;27:683–686.

Pratt SG, Beyer CK, Johnson CC. The Marcus Gunn phenomenon. A review of 71 cases. *Ophthalmology* 1984;91:27–30.

Möbius Syndrome

Abid F, Hall R, Hudgson P, Weiser R. Möbius syndrome, peripheral neuropathy and hypogonadotrophic hypogonadism. *J Neurol Sci* 1978;35:309–315.

Bavinck JN, Weaver DD. Subclavian artery supply description sequence: hypothesis of a vascular etiology for Poland, Klippel-Feil, and Möbius anomalies. *Am J Med Genet* 1986;23:903–918.

Brackett LE, Demers LM, Mamourian AC, et al. Möbius syndrome in association with hypogonadotropic hypogonadism. *J Endocrinol Invest* 1991;14:599–607.

Hanson PA, Rowland LP. Möbius syndrome and facioscapulo-humeral muscular dystrophy. *Arch Neurol* 1971;24:31–39.

Henderson JL. The congenital facial diplegia syndrome. *Brain* 1939;62:381–403.

Hopper KD, Haas DK, Rice MM, et al. Poland-Möbius syndrome: evaluation by computerized tomography. *South Med J* 1985;78:523–527.

Kumar D. Möbius syndrome. *J Med Genet* 1990;27:122–126.

Olson WH, Bardin CW, Walsh GO, Engel WK. Möbius syndrome, lower motor neuron involvement and hypogonadotropic hypogonadism. *Neurology* 1970;20:1002–1008.

Pastuszak AL, Schuler L, Speck-Martins CE, et al. Use of misoprostol during pregnancy and Möbius syndrome in infants. *N Engl J Med* 1998;359:1553–1554.

Pitner SE, Edwards JE, McCormick WF. Observations on the pathology of the Möbius syndrome. *J Neurol Neurosurg Psychiatry* 1965;28:362–374.

Rojas-Martinez A, Garcia-Cruz D, Rodriguez-Garcia A, et al. Poland-Möbius syndrome in a boy and Poland syndrome in his mother. *Clin Genet* 1991;40:225–228.

Rubenstein AE, Lovelace RE, Behrens MM, Weisberg LA. Moebius syndrome in Kallmann syndrome. *Arch Neurol* 1975;32:480–482.

Slee JJ, Smart RD, Viljoen DL. Deletion of chromosome 13 in Möbius syndrome. *J Med Genet* 1991;28:413–414.

Towfighi J, Marks K, Palmer E, Vanucci R. Möbius syndrome. Neuropathologic observations. *Acta Neuropathol (Berl)* 1979;48:11–17.

Ziter FA, Wiser WC, Robinson A. Three generation pedigree of a Möbius syndrome variant with chromosome translocation. *Arch Neurol* 1977;34:437–442.

Merritt's Neurology, 10th ed., edited by L.P. Rowland. Lippincott Williams & Wilkins, Philadelphia © 2000.

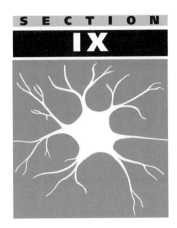

GENETIC DISEASES OF THE CENTRAL NERVOUS SYSTEM

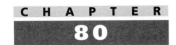

CHROMOSOMAL DISEASES

CHING H. WANG

Human chromosomal anomalies are manifest as change in the total number of chromosomes or as structural rearrangements. Examples of abnormal chromosome number (aneuploidy) are sex chromosomal aneuploidy such as 45,X (Turner syndrome) and autosomal aneuploidy such as 47,XX +21 (trisomy 21, Down syndrome). Structural abnormalities include regional deletions or insertions, segmental translocations (reciprocal or robertsonian) or inversions (pericentric or paracentric), duplications, and ring chromosomes. The chromosomal syndromes are many, but they primarily result from these chromosomal rearrangements, producing a functional monosomy or trisomy (one or three chromosomes instead of the normal two). The most common manifestation of these chromosomal anomalies is mental retardation. Congenital malformations are seen in variable frequencies and different severities. In the sex chromosome disorders, infertility is the most common feature. In this section, as examples, we discuss three chromosomal syndromes: trisomy 21, Prader-Willi, and Angelman syndromes.

TRISOMY 21 (DOWN SYNDROME)

Down syndrome was named after the English physician John Langdon Down, who described the clinical features in 1866. The chromosomal abnormality, the first described in humans, was identified only 3 years after the normal human chromosome number was established in 1956. Down syndrome is also named trisomy 21 because there is usually an extra copy of chromosome 21. The syndrome is encountered in about 1 in 800 live births, with a male-to-female ratio about 3:2. The risk of occurrence increases sharply with increased maternal age: 1 in 350 at age 35 and 1 in 110 at age 40. A 45-year-old woman is 60 times more likely to have an affected child than is a 20-year-old woman.

Clinical Features

The typical facial features include a round face and a short nose with flat nasal bridge. The eyes show upward slanting of the lateral palpebral fissures with epicanthal folds. Brushfield spots are often seen arranged in a circular ring around the outer third of the iris. The mouth is small and kept open by a large protruding tongue. The palate is high-arched or cleft. Structural anomalies of the middle and inner ear lead to frequent bouts of otitis. Skeletal anomalies include short stature, stubby fingers and toes, an increased space between the first and second toes, and clinodactyly (inward curvature) of the fifth finger. The pelvis is small with diminished iliac and acetabular angles. Atlantoaxial or at-

lantooccipital instability is found in 15% to 20% of patients. Unique dermatoglyphic features include the simian crease in the palm and unusual hand- and footprints.

There is an increased incidence of congenital heart diseases, such as septal and endocardial cushion defects. The genitalia are poorly developed in males, resulting in infertility. In women, ovarian defects and irregular menstruation commonly occur. Intestinal atresia, imperforate anus, and Hirschsprung disease are common. Hematologic abnormalities include an increased risk of leukemia. Infantile hypotonia and later mental retardation are the major neurologic signs. The IQ scores vary from 20 to 70 depending on the genetic background and environmental factors. Starting at ages 35 to 40, a further decline of cognitive function is attributed to dementia. Seizures are found more frequently in persons with Down syndrome, usually infantile spasms and tonic-clonic seizures with myoclonus in early life and partial simple or partial complex in the later years.

Neuropathology

The brain is spherical and small, with fewer secondary sulci than normal. The superior temporal lobes are hypoplastic, and the sylvian fissure is prominent. Microscopically, there is a reduction of neuronal density in diverse cortical areas. The pyramidal cells show a reduced number of apical dendrites and synapses. The cerebellum is small and includes an accumulation of undifferentiated fetal cells. There are striking microscopic similarities in the brains of those with Down syndrome and those with Alzheimer disease (AD), including degeneration of the cells in the nucleus basalis of Meynert with decreased choline acetyltransferase; pigmentary degeneration of neurons with accumulation of senile plaques and neurofibrillary tangles; and calcium deposits in hippocampus, basal ganglia, and cerebellar folia. Almost all Down syndrome adults over age 30 years have plaques and tangles, but because of the lifelong mental retardation, it is difficult to discern whether these neuropathologic findings contribute to clinical dementia.

Cytogenetics and Molecular Genetics

In 90% to 95% of cases, karyotype analysis showed trisomy 21, with a complete extra chromosome 21. In a few cases, trisomy is due to a translocation. Most free trisomy 21 results from meiotic nondisjunction in meiosis II, which correlates with advancing maternal age. Traditional cytogenetic techniques show maternal nondisjunction in about 80% and paternal in 20% of cases. With DNA analysis of polymorphisms, using highly informative markers and the polymerase chain reaction, the origin is paternal in only about 5% of cases. All of chromosome 21 need not be triplicated to produce the syndrome. In a few cases, the only extra chromosomal 21 material is the distal half of the long arm, specifically a region within bands q21.2 and q22.3. Many candidate genes have been isolated from this region. It is likely that multiple genes are responsible for the phenotypic variations in Down syndrome. The mosaic pattern (46/47, +21) occurs in 2% to 3%. The clinical features of these individuals range from virtually normal physical and intellectual characteristics to that of typical trisomy 21.

Down Syndrome and Familial Alzheimer Disease

In addition to the neuropathologic similarities of Down syndrome and AD, linkage studies indicate that one of the early-onset familial AD genes is linked to chromosome 21. In these families, a single base mutation in the amyloid precursor protein (APP) gene in 21q21.3 segregates with the disease. Mutations in the APP gene prevent the normal proteolytic breakdown of Ab core (a portion of APP) and result in accumulation of amyloid protein in the senile plaques. In one study, three copies of the amyloid gene were seen in three patients with AD and also in two patients with nontrisomy Down syndrome. This finding suggested a common genetic and pathophysiologic basis for the two diseases. There is genetic heterogeneity, however, in familial AD. Two other genes have been found to associate with early-onset AD: the presenilin 1 gene on chromosome 14 and the presenilin 2 gene on chromosome 1. The AD susceptibility locus apolipoprotein E (APOE4) allele on chromosome 19 and the recently identified a-2 M gene on chromosome 12 are associated with the late-onset AD. In Down syndrome, a triplicated region that includes the APP gene on chromosome 21 may be responsible for the increased APP production and the similar histopathology as seen in AD.

Management

There is no specific therapy for the neurologic or the cognitive impairment of Down syndrome. Several therapeutic trials using neurochemical (such as 5-hydroxytryptophan) or vitamin supplements have been unsuccessful. Management is addressed to the treatment of the medical and surgical conditions that accompany the syndrome. Computed tomography screening for atlantoaxial instability is indicated before a child participates in contact sports.

PRADER-WILLI AND ANGELMAN SYNDROMES

These clinically distinct syndromes are both associated with a DNA deletion within chromosome 15q11-13. The clinical differences are attributed to the derangements of the genes preferentially expressed on either the maternally or paternally derived chromosome, which is called genomic imprinting.

Prader-Willi Syndrome

First described by Prader in 1956, this syndrome is estimated to occur about 1 in 25,000 live births. It is usually sporadic, with an empiric risk of recurrence in siblings of less than 1:1,000. The clinical features can be divided into two stages. The first stage is characterized by neonatal hypotonia. A poor sucking reflex causes feeding problems that may lead to failure to thrive and requires tube feeding. The external genitalia are small. The hypotonia improves at ages 8 to 11 months. Electromyography, motor nerve conduction velocity, serum creatine kinase, and muscle biopsy are usually normal. The second stage, usually between ages 1 and 2 years, is characterized by delayed psychomotor de-

velopment and childhood obesity. As the hypotonia improves, the infant becomes more alert. Increased appetite causes excessive weight gain. Speech delay and cognitive dysfunction are mild or moderately severe. Other typical features include short stature, small hands and feet, almond-shaped eyes, strabismus, and poor dentition.

The syndrome is attributed to defective hypothalamic function. Thermoinstability, hyperphagia, hypogonadism, and growth hormone deficiency with short stature are clinical manifestations of hypothalamic dysfunction. However, no specific lesion of the hypothalamus has been identified at autopsy. Early death is occasionally caused by morbid obesity and cardiopulmonary complications.

Angelman Syndrome

In 1965, Angelman described three children with "flat heads, jerky movements, protruding tongues and bouts of laughter giving them a superficial resemblance to puppets." The prevalence was estimated at 1 in 12,000. Most Angelman syndrome (AS) cases occur sporadically, but some familial cases have also been reported. There is no association with advanced maternal or paternal age. The infants are usually normal at birth. Feeding difficulty is noted at ages 1 to 2 months, with a period of failure to thrive. Head circumference stays at less than fifth percentile. The children may not sit alone until age 1 year and may walk at 3 to 5 years. There is no development of speech. The child is usually happy and smiling. Hyperactivity is common. The gait is wide-based and ataxic with tremulous movements. The face is round with a large mouth and protruding tongue. Electroencephalogram abnormalities and seizure of various severities occur frequently in early infancy. The child is usually unable to perform activities of daily living. Pubertal development is delayed, and the adult height is less than the third percentile.

Molecular Basis

More than 50% of Prader-Willi syndrome (PWS) patients studied with high-resolution banding techniques showed some chromosome 15 anomalies. More than 90% of the abnormalities involve a deletion in band 15q11-13, and an equal proportion of AS patients have a similar deletion at 15q11-13. Using both cytogenetic techniques and DNA polymorphisms, it is possible to identify the parental origin of the deleted chromosome; all PWS patients inherit a deleted chromosome 15 from the father and all AS patients inherit a similar chromosome 15 deletion from the mother. In PWS, maternal heterodisomy (two different chromosome 15 derived from the mother) is found in some of those without a cytogenetic deletion. Therefore, loss of the expressed paternal allele, due to interstitial deletion or uniparental disomy, may be responsible for the specific PWS phenotype.

Six paternally expressed genes (SNRPN, IPW, ZNF127, PAR-1, PAR-5, and NDN) have been isolated from the PWS critical region. However, no mutation or deletion of any single gene can produce the full clinical phenotype of PWS. These findings suggest that PWS may be a contiguous gene syndrome. In AS, recent progress in the molecular genetics has led to the identification of a strong AS candidate gene UBE3A, located closely to but distal to the PWS critical region within chromosome 15q12. Mutations of UBE3A gene alone were sufficient to produce a full clinical AS phenotype. Using mouse model, the UBE3A gene is maternally expressed in the hippocampal and Purkinjie neurons. The other molecular causes of AS include *de novo* maternal deletions at 15q11-13 (about 70%), paternal uniparental disomy of chromosome 15 (about 2%), and mutations in the imprinting center (about 2% to 3%).

Genomic Imprinting

This epigenetic phenomenon illustrates an interesting non-Mendelian mode of inheritance in the mammalian genome. Several autosomal genes are inherited in a silent state on one parental allele and in an active state on the other parental allele. This parent-of-origin–specific gene expression is called genomic imprinting. The diseases that arise from these genes are mostly due to mutation of the active allele, duplication of the nonactive allele, or imprinting errors resulting in silencing of the active allele. Over 20 imprinted genes have now been identified in mouse genome; many of them have human homologues. For example, the insuline-like growth factor type 2 (IGF-2) gene is paternally active, and only when the gene defect is inherited from the father do the offspring express the dwarfing phenotype. In the cases of PWS and AS, deletions in the PWS critical region on the paternal chromosome or maternal uniparental disomy result in the silencing of the paternally active allele and the PWS phenotype, whereas deletion of the AS critical region on the maternal chromosome or paternal uniparental disomy result in the silencing of the maternal allele and the AS phenotype.

The PWS and AS critical regions are physically very close to each other on chromosome 15q12. Evidence of other human genomic imprinting includes the following. First, in germline tumors such as hydatidiform moles, there are paternally derived haploid sets of chromosomes. Ovarian teratomas have two sets of maternal chromosomes. In fetal triploids, diandric triploids (two paternal chromosomes) are found in large cystic placentas. Conversely, in digynic fetus (two maternal chromosomes), fetal development is severely retarded, and the placentas are small and usually nonmolar. Second, in somatic cell tumors (such as retinoblastoma and Wilms tumor), inactivation of one allele by imprinting and a second step of chromosomal loss or mutation result in "loss of heterozygosity" and tumorogenesis.

The molecular mechanism of genomic imprinting is largely unknown. The recent isolation of a *cis*-acting imprinting center located upstream to the promotor region of the SNRPN gene has helped us to understand the molecular basis of genomic imprinting. Deletions or mutations in this imprinting center have be shown to associate with PWS or AS depending on the origin of parental germlines. It is postulated that the imprinting center confers a male or female imprint by an "imprinting switch" during gametogenesis. In the female germline, the imprinting switch is needed to reset the male chromosome from the maternal grandfather to confer the charateristics of a female chromosome. In the male germline, the same process is needed to reset the female chromosome from the paternal grandmother to confer the

characteristics of a male chromosome. This epigenetic mark is thought to be achieved by DNA methylation. In the case of PWS, the inactive allele on the maternal chromosome is hypermethylated, which suppresses gene transcription. The hypermethylated cytosine residues on the DNA sequences may repel the transcription factors needed for the activation of gene transcription. In other imprinted genes like IGF-2 receptor, DNA methylation is associated with the active allele on the maternal chromosome. Therefore, other factors in addition to DNA methylation may be involved in genomic imprinting.

SUGGESTED READINGS

Down Syndrome

Antonarakis SE, Down syndrome collaborative group. Parental origin of the extra chromosome in trisomy 21 as indicated by analysis of DNA polymorphisms. *N Engl J Med* 1991;324:872–876.

Blacker D, Wilcox MA, Laird NM, et al. Alpha-2 macroglobulin is genetically associated with Alzheimer disease. *Nat Genet* 1998;19:357–360.

Epstein CJ. Down syndrome. In: Rosenberg RN, Prusiner SB, DiMauro S, et al., eds. *The molecular and genetic basis of neurological disease.* Boston: Butterworth-Heinemann, 1997.

Kallen B, Mastroiacovo P, and Robert E. Major congenital malformations in Down syndrome. *Am J Med Genet* 1996;65:160–166.

Karlinsky H, Vaula G, Haines L, et al. Molecular and prospective phenotypic characterization of a pedigree with familial Alzheimer disease and a missense mutation in codon 717 of the b-amyloid precursor protein (APP) gene. *Neurology* 1992;42:1445–1453.

St George-Hyslop P, Haines J, Rogaev E, et al. Genetic evidence for a novel familial Alzheimer's disease locus on chromosome 14. *Nat Genet* 1992;2:330–334.

Prader-Willi and Angelman Syndromes

Albrecht U, Sutcliffe JS, Cattanach BM, et al. Imprinted expression of the murine Angelman syndrome gene, Ube3a, in hippocampal and Purkinjie neurons. *Nat Genet* 1997;17:75–78.

Cassidy SB, Schwartz S. Prader-Willi and Angelman syndromes. Disorders of genomic imprinting. *Medicine (Baltimore)* 1998;77:140–151.

Glenn CC, Saitoh S, Jong MTC, et al. Gene structure, DNA methylation, and imprinting expression of the human SNRNP gene. *Am J Hum Genet* 1996;58:335–346.

Knoll JHM, Nicholls RD, Magenis RE, et al. Angelman and Prader-Willi syndromes share a common chromosome 15 deletion but differ in parental origin of deletion. *Am J Med Genet* 1989;32:285–290.

Genomic Imprinting

Bartolomei MS, Tilghman SM. Genomic imprinting in mammals. *Annu Rev Genet* 1997;31:493–525.

Buiting K, Saitoh S, Gross S, et al. Inherited microdeletions in the Angelman and Prader-Willi syndromes define an imprinting centre on human chromosome 15. *Nat Genet* 1995;9:395–400.

Dittrich B, Buiting K, Korn B, et al. Imprinting switch on human chromosome 15 may involve alternative transcripts of the SNRNP gene. *Nat Genet* 1996;14:163–170.

Feinberg AP. Genomic imprinting and gene activation in cancer. *Nat Genet* 1993;4:110–113.

Merritt's Neurology, 10th ed., edited by L.P. Rowland. Lippincott Williams & Wilkins, Philadelphia © 2000.

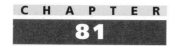

DISORDERS OF AMINO ACID METABOLISM

JOHN H. MENKES

There has been an exponential growth in our understanding of the multiplicity of genetic defects that underlie the various disorders of amino acid metabolism. Rather than elaborate on the molecular biology of these disorders, this chapter focuses on their neurologic aspects and their diagnosis and management.

Mass screening for disorders of amino acid metabolism has resulted in early biochemical diagnosis of phenylketonuria (PKU) and other aminoacidopathies. In one screening program, the incidence of PKU was 1:10,000 in New South Wales, Australia, the incidence of defects of amino acid transport was about 2:10,000, and the combined incidence of all other aminoacidopathies was less than 8:100,000. Although these conditions are rare, they are important because they provide information about the development and functions of the brain.

PHENYLKETONURIA (MIM 261600)

PKU (phenylalanine hydroxylase deficiency) is an inborn error of metabolism transmitted as an autosomal recessive disorder and manifested by an impairment in the hepatic hydroxylation of phenylalanine to tyrosine. Untreated, the disorder causes a clinical picture highlighted by mental retardation, seizures, and imperfect hair pigmentation. Inasmuch as PKU is the prototype for demonstrating the interrelation between genetic alterations in intermediary metabolism and neurologic dysfunction, it deserves more space than its frequency in the panoply of neurologic disorders would otherwise warrant.

The disease has been found in all parts of the world. The frequency in the general population of the United States, as determined by screening programs, is about 1:11,700.

Pathogenesis and Pathology

The hydroxylation of phenylalanine to tyrosine is an irreversible and complex reaction that requires phenylalanine hydroxylase and three other enzymes in addition to several nonprotein components. Phenylalanine hydroxylase is normally found in liver, kidney, and pancreas but not in brain or skin fibroblasts. In classic PKU, as a result of multiple and distinct mutations in the gene for phenylalanine hydroxylase, enzyme activity is completely or nearly completely abolished. Cloning of a full-length complementary DNA has enabled characterization of the normal and mutant genes. Over 300 different mutations have been identified to date, and the genetic heterogeneity of phenylalanine hydroxylase deficiency is immense. There is a broad continuum of phenotypes. In addition to classic PKU, less severe forms have

been recognized, and based on their serum phenylalanine levels while on a free diet, patients have been arbitrarily subdivided into moderate PKU, mild PKU, and mild hyperphenylalaninemia. The different forms of PKU are allelic, and a high proportion of patients are compound heterozygotes rather than homozygotes.

Dihydropteridine reductase, the second enzyme required for phenylalanine hydroxylation, is present in normal amounts in classic PKU but is absent or defective in a rare variant of the disease, which manifests itself by elevated serum phenylalanine levels and progressive neurologic dysfunction.

The hydroxylation of phenylalanine also requires oxygen and tetrahydrobiopterin. Defects in the synthesis of tetrahydrobiopterin account for 1% to 3% of infants with phenylalanine elevation. These conditions lead to a syndrome of progressive neurologic deterioration, accompanied by a variety of involuntary movements.

Children suffering from classic PKU are born with only slightly elevated phenylalanine blood levels, but because of the defect in phenylalanine hydroxylase, the amino acid derived from food proteins accumulates in serum and cerebrospinal fluid and is excreted in large quantities. In lieu of the normal degradative pathway, phenylalanine is converted to phenylpyruvic acid, phenylacetic acid, and phenylacetylglutamine.

The transamination of phenylalanine to phenylpyruvic acid is sometimes deficient for the first few days of life, and the age when phenylpyruvic acid may be first detected ranges from 2 to 34 days.

Alterations within the brain are nonspecific and diffuse and involve both gray and white matter. There are three types of alterations within the brain:

1. Interference with normal maturation of the brain. Brain growth is reduced; there is microscopic evidence of impaired cortical layering, delayed outward migration of neuroblasts, and heterotopic gray matter. These changes suggest a period of abnormal brain development during the last trimester of gestation.
2. Defective myelination. This may be generalized or limited to areas in which postnatal deposition of myelin is normal. Except in some older patients, products of myelin degeneration are not seen. Generally, there is relative pallor of myelin, sometimes with mild gliosis and irregular areas of vacuolation (i.e., status spongiosus). The vacuoles are usually seen in central white matter of the cerebral hemispheres and in the cerebellum.
3. Diminished or absent pigmentation of the substantia nigra and locus ceruleus.

Symptoms and Signs

Patients suffering from PKU exhibit a wide range of clinical and biochemical severity. In the classic form, caused by a virtual absence of phenylalanine hydroxylase activity, infants appear normal at birth. During the first 2 months, there is vomiting (sometimes projectile) and irritability. Delayed intellectual development is apparent by 4 to 9 months; mental retardation may be severe, precluding speech or toilet training. Seizures, common in more severely retarded infants, usually start before age 18 months and may cease spontaneously. In infants, seizures may appear as infantile spasms, later changing to grand mal attacks.

The typical affected child is blond and blue-eyed with normal and often pleasant features. The skin is rough and dry, sometimes with eczema. A peculiar musty odor, attributable to phenylacetic acid, may suggest the diagnosis. Significant focal neurologic abnormalities are rare. Microcephaly may be present, and there may be a mild increase in muscle tone, particularly in the legs. A fine irregular tremor of the hands is seen in about 35% of subjects. The plantar response is often variable or extensor. Electroencephalogram abnormalities include hypsarrhythmia, recorded even in the absence of seizures, and single or multiple foci of spike and polyspike discharges.

Magnetic resonance imaging (MRI) is almost invariably abnormal, even in early treated patients. On T2-weighted images, high signal areas are seen in white matter. These are mainly located in the posterior temporal and occipital periventricular regions, notably in the watershed between the posterior and middle cerebral arteries. They are probably caused by abnormalities of myelin formation and maintenance.

Diagnosis

Most PKU patients are identified through a newborn screening program. Although most infants whose blood phenylalanine levels are above the threshold value of 2 to 4 mg/dL do not have PKU, such patients will require prompt reevaluation by an appropriate laboratory to determine whether hyperphenylalaninemia is persistent and to determine whether it is due to phenylalanine hydroxylase deficiency. Because the urine of most newborns does not contain appreciable amounts of phenylpyruvic acid, the ferric chloride and 2,4- dinitrophenylhydrazine tests are inadequate during the neonatal period. If the diagnosis of a case of classic PKU is missed, the most likely reason is laboratory error rather than insufficient protein intake or too early testing of the infant.

A combination of haplotype and mutation analysis has facilitated carrier detection and the prenatal diagnosis of PKU in families with at least one previously affected child.

The widespread screening programs that detect newborns with blood phenylalanine concentrations higher than normal have also uncovered other conditions in which blood phenylalanine levels are increased in the neonatal period. Patients with moderate and mild PKU and mild hyperphenylalaninemia, as these entities are termed, have phenylalanine levels that tend to be lower than those seen in classic PKU and have a less severe mutation in the gene for phenylalanine hydroxylase.

Treatment

On referral of an infant with a positive screening test, the first step is quantitative determination of serum phenylalanine and tyrosine levels. All infants whose blood phenylalanine concentration is greater than 10 mg/dL (606 μM/L) and whose tyrosine concentration is low or normal (1 to 4 mg/dL) should be started on a low-phenylalanine diet immediately. Infants whose blood phenylalanine concentrations remain in the range of 6.6 to 10.0 mg/dL should also be treated.

The generally accepted therapy for classic PKU is restriction of the dietary intake of phenylalanine by placing the infant on one of several low-phenylalanine formulas. To avoid symptoms of phenylalanine deficiency, milk is added to the diet in amounts sufficient to maintain blood levels of the amino acid between 2 and 6 mg/dL (121 to 363 μM/l). Generally, patients tolerate this diet quite well, and within 1 to 2 weeks the serum concentration of phenylalanine becomes normal.

Weekly serum phenylalanine determinations are essential to ensure adequate regulation of diet. Strict dietary control should be maintained for as long as possible, and most centers strive to keep levels below 6.0 mg/dL (360 μM/L) even in patients with moderate and mild PKU. Dietary lapses are frequently accompanied by progressive white matter abnormalities on MRI. Some workers have suggested supplementation of the low-phenylalanine diet with tyrosine, but there is no statistical evidence that this regimen results in a better intellectual outcome. Failure to treat subjects with mild hyperphenylalaninemias does not appear to produce either intellectual deficits or MRI abnormalities. The use of implanted microencapsulated genetically engineered cells to remove phenylalanine is under investigation. Vectors for efficient gene transfer have yet to be developed.

Treatment of phenylalaninemia due to tetrahydrobiopterin deficiency involves administration of tetrahydrobiopterin or a synthetic pterin and replenishment of the neurotransmitters (levodopa, 5-hydroxytryptophan) because synthesis of these substances is also impaired.

Early detection and dietary control of PKU has increased the number of homozygous PKU women who are of childbearing age. The harmful effects of maternal hyperphenylalaninemia on the heterozygous offspring include mental retardation, microcephaly, seizures, and congenital heart defects. Women who conceive while their blood phenylalanine levels are 15 mg/dL or above (greater than 900 μM/L) are at high risk for these malformations and should be offered termination of pregnancy. During pregnancy, phenylalanine levels should be monitored as closely as during infancy because the fetus is exposed to even higher phenylalanine concentrations than the mother.

Prognosis

When the patient with classic PKU is maintained on a low-phenylalanine diet, seizures disappear and the electroencephalogram tends to revert to normal. Abnormally blond hair regains natural color.

The effects on mental ability are less clearcut. In most studies, some deficit in intellectual development has been found, even in infants who had been diagnosed and treated as neonates, and there appears to be no threshold below which phenylalanine has no effect on cognition. When the measured IQ is normal, children may exhibit impaired perceptual functions, and progress in school is poorer than expected from the IQ score. Neurologic deterioration during adult life has been seen in some patients. This is generally the consequence of dietary lapses.

Failure to prevent mild mental retardation or cognitive deficits, even with optimal control, may be a consequence of prenatal brain damage induced by high phenylalanine levels in the fetus.

MAPLE SYRUP URINE DISEASE (MIM 248600)

Maple syrup urine disease (MSUD) is a familial cerebral degenerative disease caused by a defect in branched-chain amino acid metabolism and marked by the passage of urine with a sweet maple syrup-like odor. Its incidence is 1:220,000 to 1:400,000 newborns. In the Mennonite population of Pennsylvania, the incidence of the classic form of the disease is 1:176 births. The disorder is characterized by accumulation of three branched-chain ketoacids: α-keto-isocaproic acid, α-keto-isovaleric acid, and α-keto-β-methylvaleric acid, which are the respective derivatives of leucine, valine, and isoleucine. Accumulation of these substances results from an autosomal recessively inherited deficiency in the mitochondrial branched-chain α-ketoacid dehydrogenase. This is a multienzyme complex comprising six proteins: $E_{1\alpha}$ and $E_{1\beta}$, which form the decarboxylase; E_2 and E_3; and a branched-chain specific kinase and phosphatase. Mutations in the genes for $E_{1\alpha}$, $E_{1\beta}$, E_2, and E_3 have been described. These induce a continuum of disease severity that ranges from the severe classic form of MSUD to mild and intermittent forms. Patients with the severe classic phenotype can be compound heterozygote or homozygotes for defects in the genes for $E_{1\alpha}$ or $E_{1\beta}$.

Plasma levels of the corresponding amino acids are also elevated because the ketoacids are transaminated. In some cases, the branched-chain α-hydroxyacids, most prominently α-hydroxyisovaleric acid, are also excreted, and a sotolone derivative of α-ketobutyric acid, whose decarboxylation is impaired by accumulation of α-keto-β-methylvaleric acid, is responsible for the characteristic odor of the urine and sweat.

Structural alterations in the brain are similar to, but more severe than, those in PKU. Also, the cytoarchitecture of the cortex is generally immature with fewer cortical layers, persistence of ectopic foci of neuroblasts, and abnormal dendritic development.

Manifestations of the untreated classic form of the condition include opisthotonos, intermittent increase of muscle tone, seizures, and rapid deterioration of all cerebral functions. Some patients have presented with pseudotumor cerebri or with fluctuating ophthalmoplegia. About half the infants develop hypoglycemia. In the acute stage of the disease, MRI demonstrates both diffuse edema and a characteristic severe edema localized to the cerebellar deep white matter, the posterior part of the brainstem, the cerebral peduncles, the posterior limb of the internal capsule, and the posterior part of the centrum semiovale. The condition is suggested by the characteristic odor of the patient's urine and perspiration. It is confirmed by quantitation of plasma amino acids.

Treatment is based on a commercially available diet that contains restricted amounts of leucine, isoleucine, and valine. For optimal results, dietary management must be initiated during the first few days of life. The regimen is complex and requires frequent quantitative measurement of serum amino acids. Children with the classic form of the disease who have been maintained on this regimen have achieved near-normal intellectual development.

A subset of MSUD patients exhibits intermittent periods of ataxia, drowsiness, behavior disturbances, and seizures that appear between 6 and 9 months of age. In some of these subjects there is a defect in the gene coding for the E_2 subunit. In other children, there is only mild or moderate mental retardation. In yet another group of MSUD patients, the biochemical abnormality can be corrected by the administration of thiamin.

DEFECTS IN THE METABOLISM OF SULFUR AMINO ACIDS

Of the several defects in the metabolism of sulfur-containing amino acids, the most common is homocystinuria (MIM 236200). This inborn error of methionine metabolism is manifested by multiple thromboembolic episodes, ectopia lentis, and mental retardation. It is transmitted by an autosomal recessive gene. The condition occurs in 1:45,000 newborns; it is second in frequency only to PKU among metabolic errors responsible for brain damage.

In the most common form of homocystinuria, the metabolic defect affects cystathionine β-synthase, the enzyme that catalyzes the formation of cystathionine from homocysteine and serine. In most homocystinuric subjects, activity of this enzyme is completely absent, but there is residual enzyme activity in members of a significant proportion of affected families. In the latter group, about 25% to 50% of patients with homocystinuria, addition of pyridoxine stimulates enzyme activity and partially or completely abolishes the excretion of homocystine, the oxidized derivative of homocysteine. Such patients tend to have a milder phenotype of the disease. As a result of the enzymatic block, increased amounts of homocystine and its precursor, methionine, are found in urine and plasma.

Primary structural alterations are noted in blood vessels of all calibers. In most vessels, there is intimal thickening and fibrosis; in the aorta and its major branches, fraying of elastic fibers may be found. Both arterial and venous thromboses are common in different organs. In the brain, there are usually multiple infarcts of varying age. Dural sinus thrombosis has been recorded. The relationships between the metabolic defect and the predisposition to vascular thrombosis are multiple. Homocysteine is toxic to vascular endothelium, inhibiting intracellular protein transport; it potentiates the autooxidation of low-density lipoprotein cholesterol and promotes thrombosis by inhibiting the activation of anticoagulant protein C.

Homocystinuric infants appear normal at birth, and early development is unremarkable until seizures, developmental slowing, or strokes occur between 5 and 9 months of age. Ectopia lentis has been recognized by age 18 months and is invariable in older children. The typical older homocystinuric child's hair is sparse, blond, and brittle. There are multiple erythematous blotches over the skin, particularly across the maxillary areas and cheeks. The gait is shuffling, the limbs and digits are long, and genu valgum is usually present.

In about half, major thromboembolic episodes occur once or more. These include fatal thrombosis of the pulmonary artery or vein. Multiple major strokes may result in hemiplegia and, ultimately, in pseudobulbar palsy. Minor and unrecognized cerebral thrombi may be the direct cause of the mental retardation that occurs in more than 50% of homocystinuric patients. The observation that homocysteine acts as an agonist at the glutamate binding site of the *N*-methyl-D-aspartate receptor suggest that overstimulation of this receptor contributes to the pathogenesis of neurologic symptoms.

The diagnosis of homocystinuria is suggested by the appearance of the patient and can be confirmed by a positive urinary cyanide-nitroprusside reaction, by the increased urinary excretion of homocystine, and by elevated levels of plasma homocystine and methionine. The diagnosis is further established by assays of cystathionine β-synthase in skin fibroblasts or liver.

Administration of a commercially available low-methionine diet supplemented with cysteine lowers plasma methionine content and eliminates the abnormally high homocystine excretion. In some centers, the diet is further supplemented with betaine to use alternative pathways for removal of homocysteine. Pyridoxine (50 to 500 mg/day combined with folic acid) reduces the homocystine excretion of pyridoxine-responsive patients. Although the biochemical picture can be improved by these means, the variable clinical picture, particularly the thromboembolic episodes and mental retardation, has up to now rendered useless any evidence for clinical benefit.

Heterozygotes for homocystinuria have an increased propensity to peripheral vascular disease and premature cerebrovascular accidents, and one-third of all patients with premature arterial thrombotic disease have elevated blood levels of homocysteine. The incidence of myocardial infarcts in this population, however, is no higher than normal.

Several other genetic entities manifest themselves by increased excretion of homocystine. In some, the conversion of homocysteine to methionine is impaired. The most important of these entities is $N^{5,10}$-methylenetetrahydrofolate reductase deficiency. Children with this disorder can present with ataxia, spastic paraparesis, and mental retardation. Several conditions result from a deficiency of methyl cobalamine, the active cofactor for the conversion of homocysteine to methionine. These entities can present in infancy with lethargy and failure to thrive. Older children suffer from mental retardation, seizures, and spasticity. The characteristic biochemical feature of these diseases is that the excretion of homocystinuria is accompanied by methylmalonic aciduria.

OTHER DEFECTS OF AMINO ACID METABOLISM

There have been numerous reports of a neurologic disorder apparently associated with some abnormality in the amino acid pattern of serum or urine. The frequency in the general population can be gauged by routine mass newborn screening, such as the one by Wilcken et al. (1980) (Table 81.1). Other screening programs have found similar incidences.

Neurologic complications are also common in disorders of the urea cycle. These are discussed in Chapter 86. The neurologic deficits reported in some of the other more common conditions (such as histidinemia, sarcosinemia, hyperprolinemia, and cystathioninuria) are considered to be unrelated to the metabolic defect, but the result of screening a selected population, namely mentally retarded individuals. Some of the less uncommon disorders are summarized in Table 81.2.

TABLE 81.1. AMINOACIDURIAS DETECTED BY NEWBORN-INFANT URINE SCREENING

Condition	Cases/100,000 6-week-old infants
Disorders of amino-acid metabolism	
Phenylketonuria	10
Histidinemia	5.2
Hyperprolinemia	1.0
Cystathioninuria	0.33
Tyrosinemia	0.33
Argininosuccinic aciduria	0.25
Hyperlysinemia	0.1
Nonketotic hyperglycinemia	0.1
Homocystinuria	0.1
α-Ketoadipic aciduria	0.1
Others	0
Disorders of amino-acid transport	
Iminoglycinuria	10
Cystinuria	5.8
Hartnup disease	4.0
Cystinosis	0.33

DISORDERS OF AMINO ACID TRANSPORT

Renal amino acid transport is handled by five specific systems that have nonoverlapping substrate preferences. The disorders that result from genetic defects in each of these systems are listed in Table 81.3.

Lowe Syndrome (MIM 309000)

Lowe syndrome (*oculocerebrorenal syndrome*) is a sex-linked recessive disorder characterized clinically by severe mental retardation, delayed physical development, myopathy, and congenital glaucoma or cataract. The gene has been mapped to the long arm of the X chromosome and encodes a protein similar to inositol polyphosphate-5-phosphatase. Biochemically, there is generalized aminoaciduria of the Fanconi type, with renal tubular acidosis and rickets. There are no consistent neuropathologic findings. MRI shows various patterns of white matter involvement. The fundamental biochemical defect is unknown but is believed to be a defect in membrane transport due to a disorder in inositol metabolism. The urinary levels of lysine are more elevated than those of the other amino acids, and defective uptake of lysine and arginine by the intestinal mucosa has been demonstrated in two patients.

Hartnup Disease (MIM 236200)

This rare familial condition is characterized by photosensitive dermatitis, intermittent cerebellar ataxia, mental disturbances, and renal aminoaciduria. The name is that of the family in which the disorder was first detected.

Symptoms are caused by an extensive disturbance in the transport of neutral amino acids. There are four main biochemical abnormalities: renal aminoaciduria, increased excretion of indican, increased excretion of nonhydroxylated indole metabolites, and increased fecal amino acids.

TABLE 81.2. SOME UNCOMMON ERRORS OF AMINO ACID METABOLISM

Disease[a]	Enzymatic defect	Clinical features	Diagnosis
Argininosuccinic aciduria (207900)	Argininosuccinase	Recurrent generalized convulsions, poorly pigmented hair, ataxia, hepatomegaly, mental retardation	CSF shows large amounts of argininosuccinic acid, elevated blood ammonia
Citrullinemia (215700)	Argininosuccinic acid synthetase	Mental retardation, vomiting, irritability, seizures	Serum and urine citrulline elevated, elevated blood ammonia
Hyperammonemia	Ornithine transcarbamylase (311250)	Seizures, recurrent changes in consciousness, hepatomegaly, males succumb early. Ataxia in older children	Elevated blood ammonia, assay of liver enzymes
	Carbamyl phosphate synthetase (237300)	Episodic vomiting, lethargy	Elevated blood ammonia, assay of liver enzymes
Hyperlysinemia (238700)	Lysine-α-ketoglutarate reductase	Severe retardation, hypotonia (some normal)	Elevated plasma lysine, elevated urine lysine, also seen in heterozygotes for cystinuria
Saccharopinuria (268700)	Aminoadipic semialdehydeglutamate reductase	Mental retardation, progressive spastic diplegia	Elevated urine, serum lysine, saccharopine in urine and serum
Aspartylglucosaminuria (208400)	Aspartylglucosaminidase	Mental retardation, hepatosplenomegaly, vacuolated lymphocytes in 75%, coarse facial features	Elevated urine aspartylglucosamine
Carnosinemia (212200)	Carnosinase	Mental retardation, mixed major and minor motor seizures	Elevated serum, urine carnosine, elevated CSF homocarnosine
Argininemia (207800)	Arginase	Spastic diplegia, seizures	Elevated plasma and CSF argininine, elevated blood ammonia
Valinemia (277100)	Valine transaminase	Vomiting, failure to thrive, nystagmus, mental retardation	Increased blood and urine valine; no increase in ketoacid excretion
Sarcosinemia (folic acid dependent) (268900)	Impaired sarcosine-glycine conversion	Emotional disturbance in some; normal intelligence in most others	Increased blood and urine sarcosine, ethanolamine
Hyper-beta-alaninemia (237400)	β-Alanine-α-ketoglutarate transaminase	Seizures commencing at birth, somnolence	Plasma, urine β-alanine and β-aminoisobutyric acid elevated, urinary γ-amino butyric acid elevated
β-Methylcrotonylglycinuria (210200)	β-Methylcrotonyl-CoA carboxylase	Similar to infantile spinal muscular atrophy, persistent vomiting, mental retardation, urine smells like that of cat	Increased urine β-hydroxyisovaleric acid, β-methylcrotonylglycine; some patients are biotin-responsive
α-Methylacetoacetic aciduria (203750)	3-Ketothiolase	Recurrent severe metabolic acidosis	α-Methyl acetoacetate and α-methyl-β–hydroxy-butyric acid in urine
Cytosol tyrosine aminotransferase deficiency (276600)	Soluble tyrosine amino transferase	Herpetiform corneal ulcers, palmoplanter keratoses, mental retardation	p-Hydroxyphenylpyruvic and p-hydroxyphenyl lactic acid excretion increased
Tryptophanuria with dwarfism (276100)	Tryptophan pyrrolase	Ataxia, spasticity, mental retardation, pellagra-like skin rash	Elevated serum tryptophan, diminished kynurenine
Glutathione synthetase deficiency (231900)	γ-Glutamylcysteine synthetase	Hemolytic anemia, spinocerebellar degeneration, peripheral neuropathy	Reduced erythrocyte glutathione, generalized aminoaciduria
Pipoglutamic aciduria (266130)	Glutathione synthetase	Mental retardation, metabolic acidosis	Elevated urinary 5-oxoproline

[a] The numbers in parentheses refer to McKusick's *Mandelian Inheritance in Man* (MIM), as explained in the preface.

TABLE 81.3. DEFECTS IN AMINO-ACID TRANSPORT

Transport system	Condition	Biochemical features	Clinical features
Basic amino acids	Cystinuria (three types) (220100)[a]	Impaired renal clearance, defective intestinal transport of lysine, arginine, ornithine, and cystine	Renal stones, no neurologic disease.
	Lowe syndrome (309000)	Impaired intestinal transport of lysine and arginine, impaired tubular transport of lysine	Severe mental retardation, congenital glaucoma, cataracts, myopathy
Acidic amino acids	Dicarboxylic aminoaciduria (222730)	Increased excretion of glutamic, aspartic acids	Severe mental retardation glaucoma, cataracts, myopathy, sex-linked transmission
Neutral amino acids	Hartnup disease (234500)	Defective intestinal and renal tubular transport of tryptophan and other neutral amino acids	Intermittent cerebellar ataxia, photosensitive rash
Proline, hydroxyproline, glycine	Iminoglycinuria (242600)	Impaired tubular transport of proline, hydroxyproline, and glycine	Harmless variant
β-Amino acids	None known	Excretion of β-aminoisobutyric acid and taurine in β-alaninemia is increased due to competition at the tubular level	Harmless variant

[a] Numbers are taken from *Mendelian Inheritance in Man*, as explained in the Preface.

Symptoms usually occur in mildly malnourished children. When present, they are intermittent and variable, tending to improve with age. They include a red scaly rash on the exposed areas of the body (resembling the dermatitis of pellagra), intermittent personality disorders, migrainelike headaches, photophobia, and bouts of cerebellar ataxia. Neuroimaging studies are nonspecific; MRI shows delayed myelination. There are no consistent neuropathologic findings.

The similarity of Hartnup disease to pellagra has prompted treatment with nicotinic acid. The tendency, however, for symptoms to remit spontaneously and for general improvement to occur with improved dietary intake and advancing age makes such therapy difficult to evaluate.

SUGGESTED READINGS

General

Cedarbaum SD, Scott CR, Wilcox WR. Amino acid metabolism. In: Rimoin DL, Connor JM, Pyeritz RE, eds. *Principles and practice of medical genetics*, 3rd ed. New York: Churchill Livingstone, 1996:1867–1895.

Menkes JH. Metabolic diseases of the nervous system. In: Menkes JH, ed. *Textbook of child neurology*, 6th ed. Baltimore: Lippincott Williams & Wilkins, 2000.

Phenylketonuria

Baumeister AA, Baumeister AA. Dietary treatment of destructive behavior associated with hyperphenylalaninemia. *Clin Neuropharmacol* 1998;21:18–27.

Green A. Neonatal screening: current trends and quality control in the United Kingdom. *Jpn J Clin Pathol* 1998;46:211–216.

Guldberg P, Rey F, Zschocke J, et al. A European multicenter study of phenylalanine hydroxylase deficiency: classification of 105 mutations and a general system for genotype-based prediction of metabolic phenotype. *Am J Hum Genet* 1998;63:71–79.

Holtzman NA, Kronmal RA, van Doorninck W, et al. Effect of age at loss of dietary control of intellectual performance and behavior of children with phenylketonuria. *N Engl J Med* 1986;314:593–598.

Kaufman S, Kapatos G, Rizzo WB, et al. Tetrahydropterin therapy for hyperphenylalaninemia caused by defective synthesis of tetrahydrobiopterin. *Ann Neurol* 1983;14:308–315.

Lenke RR, Levy HL. Maternal phenylketonuria and hyperphenylalaninemia. *N Engl J Med* 1980;302:1202–1208.

Lou HC, Toft PB, Andresen J, et al. An occipito-temporal syndrome in adolescents with optimally controlled hyperphenylalaninaemia. *J Inher Metab Dis* 1992;15:687–695.

Malamud N. Neuropathology of phenylketonuria. *J Neuropathol Exp Neurol* 1966;25:254–268.

MRC Working Party on Phenylketonuria. Recommendations on the dietary management of phenylketonuria. *Arch Dis Child* 1993;68:426–427.

MRC Working Party on Phenylketonuria. Phenylketonuria due to phenylalanine hydroxylase deficiency: an unfolding story. *BMJ* 1993;306:115–119.

Partington MW. The early symptoms of phenylketonuria. *Pediatrics* 1961;27:465–473.

Schneider AJ. Newborn phenylalanine tyrosine metabolism. Implications for screening for phenylketonuria. *Am J Dis Child* 1983;137:427–432.

Smith I, Leeming RJ, Cavanagh NPC, et al. Neurologic aspects of biopterin metabolism. *Arch Dis Child* 1986;61:130–137.

Smith ML, Hanley WB, Clarke JT, et al. Randomized controlled trial of tyrosine supplementation on neuropsychological performance in phenylketonuria. *Arch Dis Child* 1998;78:116–121.

Thompson AJ, Smith I, Brenton D, et al. Neurological deterioration in young adults with phenylketonuria. *Lancet* 1990;336:602–605.

Waisbren SE, Mahon BE, Schnell RR, et al. Predictors of intelligence quotient and intelligence quotient change in persons treated for phenylketonuria early in life. *Pediatrics* 1987;79:351–355.

Weglage J, Ullrich K, Pietsch M, et al. Intellectual, neurologic, and neuropsychologic outcome in untreated subjects with nonphenylketonuria hyperphenylalaninemia. German Collaborative Study on Phenylketonuria. *Pediatr Res* 1997;42:378–384.

Wilcken B, Smith A, Brown DA. Urine screening for amino acidopathies: Is it beneficial? *J Pediatr* 1980;97:492–497.

Maple Syrup Urine Disease

Brismar J, Aqeel A, Brismar G, et al. Maple syrup urine disease: findings on CT and MR scans of the brain in 10 infants. *AJNR* 1990;11:1219–1228.

Chuang DT. Maple syrup urine disease: it has come a long way. *J Pediatr* 1998;132:S17–S23.

Kamei A, Takashima S, Chan F, et al. Abnormal dendritic development in maple syrup urine disease. *Pediatr Neurol* 1992;8:145–147.

Mantovani JF, Naidich TP, Prensky AL, et al. MSUD: presentation with pseudotumor cerebri and CT abnormalities. *J Pediatr* 1980;96:279–281.

Menkes JH. Maple syrup disease: isolation and identification of organic acids in the urine. *Pediatrics* 1959;23:348–353.

Menkes JH, Hurst PL, Craig JM. A new syndrome: progressive familial infantile cerebral dysfunction associated with unusual urinary substance. *Pediatrics* 1954;14:462–466.

Podebrad F, Heil M, Reichart S, et al. 4,5-dimethyl-3-hydroxy-2[5H]-furanone (sotolone)-the odor of maple syrup urine disease. *J Inherit Metab Dis* 1999;22:107–114.

Schadewaldt P, Wendel U. Metabolism of branched-chain amino acids in maple syrup urine disease. *Eur J Pediatr* 1997;156[Suppl 1]:S62–S66.

Tsuruta M, Mitsubuchi H, Mardy S, et al. Molecular basis of intermitted maple syrup urine disease: novel mutations in the E2 gene of the branched-chain alpha-keto acid dehydrogenase complex. *J Hum Genet* 1998;43:91–100.

Wynn RM, Davie JR, Chuang JL, et al. Impaired assembly of E1 decarboxylase of the branched-chain alpha-ketoacid dehydrogenase complex in type IA maple syrup urine disease. *J Biol Chem* 1998;273:13110–13118.

Defects in the Metabolism of Sulfur Amino Acids

Boers GHJ. Heterozygosity for homocystinuria in premature peripheral and cerebral occlusive arterial disease. *N Engl J Med* 1985;313:709–715.

Dixon MA, Leonard JV. Intercurrent illness in inborn errors of intermediary metabolism. *Arch Dis Child* 1992;67:1387–1391.

Lentz SR, Sadler JE. Homocysteine inhibits von Willebrand factor processing and secretion by preventing transport from the endoplasmic reticulum. *Blood* 1993;81:683–689.

Lipton SA, Kim WK, Choi YB, et al. Neurotoxicity associated with dual actions of homocysteine at the *N*-methyl-D-aspartate receptor. *Proc Natl Acad Sci USA* 1997;94:5923–5928.

Mitchell GA, Watkins D, Melancon SB, et al. Clinical heterogeneity in cobalamin C variant of combined homocystinuria and methylmalonic aciduria. *J Pediatr* 1986;108:410–415.

Schimke RN, McKusick VA, Huang T. Homocystinuria: studies of 20 families with 38 affected members. *JAMA* 1965;193:711–719.

Walter JH, Wraith JE, White FJ, et al. Strategies for the treatment of cystathionine beta-synthase deficiency: the experience of the Willink Biochemical Genetics Unit over the past 30 years. *Eur J Pediatr* 1998;157[Suppl 2]:S71–S76.

Disorders of Amino Acid Transport

Lowe Syndrome

Charnas L, Bernar J, Pezeshkpour GH, et al. MRI findings and peripheral neuropathy in Lowe's syndrome. *Neuropediatrics* 1988;19:7–9.

Charnas LR, Gahl WA. The oculocerebrorenal syndrome of Lowe. *Adv Pediatr* 1991;38:75–107.

Demmer LA, Wippold FJ 2d, Dowton SB. Periventricular white matter cystic lesions in Lowe (oculocerebrorenal) syndrome. A new MR finding. *Pediatr Radiol* 1992;22:76–77.

Kornfeld M, Synder RD, MacGee J, et al. The oculo-cerebral-renal syndrome of Lowe. *Arch Neurol* 1975;32:103–107.

Lin T, Orrison BM, Leahey AM, et al. Spectrum of mutations in the OCR1 gene in the Lowe oculocerebrorenal syndrome. *Am J Hum Genet* 1997;60:1384–1388.

Lowe CU, Terrey M, MacLachlan EA. Organic aciduria, decreased renal ammonia production, hydrophthalmos, and mental retardation. *Am J Dis Child* 1952;83:164–184.

Martin MA, Sylvester PE. Clinico-pathological studies of oculo-cerebral-renal syndrome of Lowe, Terrey and MacLachlan. *J Ment Defic Res* 1980;24:1–16.

Hartnup Disease

Baron DN. Hereditary pellagra-like skin rash with temporary cerebellar ataxia, constant renal aminoaciduria, and other bizarre chemical features. *Lancet* 1956;2:421–428.

Erly W, Castillo M, Foosaner D, et al. Hartnup disease: MR findings. *AJNR* 1991;12:1026–1027.

Jepson JB. Hartnup disease. In: Stanbury JB, Wyngaarden JB, Fredrickson DS, eds. *The metabolic basis of inherited disease*, 4th ed. New York: McGraw-Hill, 1978:1563–1577.

Wilcken B, Yu JS, Brown DA. Natural history of Hartnup disease. *Arch Dis Child* 1977;52:38–40.

Merritt's Neurology, 10th ed., edited by L.P. Rowland. Lippincott Williams & Wilkins, Philadelphia © 2000.

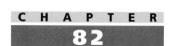

DISORDERS OF PURINE METABOLISM

LEWIS P. ROWLAND

LESCH-NYHAN SYNDROME (MIM 308000)

In 1964, Lesch and Nyhan described two brothers with hyperuricemia, mental retardation, choreoathetosis, and self-destructive biting of the lips and fingers. All known cases have affected boys; the trait is inherited as an X-linked recessive trait, and the gene has been localized to the long arm of the X chromosome. The basic defect is the lack of hypoxanthine-guanine phosphoribosyltransferase (HPRT) in all body fluids. The gene was one of the first human genes to be cloned. Because of the enzyme deficiency, the rate of purine biosynthesis is increased, and the content of the end product of purine metabolism, uric acid, reaches high values in blood, urine, and cerebrospinal fluid. Deposits of urate are found in the kidneys and joints and may result in debilitating nephropathy and gout.

The neurologic manifestations include severe mental retardation, spasticity, and choreoathetosis that start in the first year of life. The characteristic self-mutilating behavior appears in the second year. Death is usually due to renal failure and may occur in the second or third decade of life. The pathogenesis of the cerebral symptoms is not known. Although low levels of dopamine metabolites have been found in postmortem samples of tissue from the basal ganglia, it is not known how these abnormalities lead to the symptoms or how they relate to the enzyme disorder.

Diagnosis depends on recognition of the clinical manifestations and can be made precisely by biochemical assay of the enzyme in erythrocyte hemolysates or cultured fibroblasts. Hair root analysis of HPRT has become a convenient way to analyze activity. Prenatal enzymatic diagnosis is possible in the first trimester with chorionic villus sampling. DNA analysis can be used for prenatal diagnosis and carrier detection but not yet to diagnose all individual cases. The gene, however, has been mapped to Xq26.1, and numerous point mutations have been found.

Treatment is not satisfactory. Gout can be treated with allopurinol, but the neurologic disorder is daunting. Restraints may be needed to prevent the child from damaging himself or others; sometimes teeth must be removed. Enzyme replacement therapy with long-term erythrocyte transfusions in three patients gave only modest improvement of the neurologic symptoms, and drug therapy to modify dopamine metabolism has not yet been effective. Gene therapy is being evaluated in animals because the human gene has been introduced into transgenic mice and enzyme activity is expressed in the brain of the recipient animals.

There is evidence of both clinical and biochemical heterogeneity. Hyperuricemia and cerebellar ataxia have been noted in individuals with normal HPRT activity. Patients with partial enzyme deficiency may have gout without neurologic symptoms or there may be varying severity of mental retardation, movement disorders, spastic tetraplegia, or seizures. The self-mutilating behavior may be restricted to the classic form, which lacks all enzyme activity.

Neurologic abnormalities are also seen in patients without other enzymes of purine nucleoside metabolism. Adenosine deaminase deficiency (MIM 102700) causes severe combined immunodeficiency in infants; some patients have extrapyramidal or pyramidal signs and psychomotor development and may be retarded. Partial exchange transfusion may be clinically beneficial. Also, a few patients lacking purine nucleoside phosphorylase (MIM 164050), with impaired cellular immunity, have shown a form of spastic paraparesis in childhood.

SUGGESTED READINGS

Alford RL, Redman JB, O'Brien WE, Caskey CT. Lesch-Nyhan syndrome: carrier and prenatal diagnosis. *Prenatal Diag* 1995;15:329–338.

Coleman MS, Danton MJ, Philips A. Adenosine deaminase and immune dysfunction. *Ann N Y Acad Sci* 1985;451:54–65.

Edwards NL. Immunodeficiencies associated with errors in purine metabolism. *Med Clin North Am* 1985;69:505–518.

Edwards NL, Jeryc W, Fox IH. Enzyme replacement in the Lesch-Nyhan syndrome with long-term erythrocyte transfusions. *Adv Exp Med Biol* 1984;165:23–26.

Graham GW, Aitken DA, Connor JM. Prenatal diagnosis by enzyme analysis in 15 pregnancies at risk for the Lesch-Nyhan syndrome. *Prenatal Diag* 1996;16:647–651.

Harris JC, Lee BR, Jinah HA, Wong Df, Yaster M, Bryan RN. Craniocerebral magnetic resonance imaging measurement and findings in Lesch-Nyhan syndrome. *Arch Neurol* 1998;55:547–553.

Hirschhorn R. Complete and partial adenosine deaminase deficiency. *Ann N Y Acad Sci* 1985;451:20–25.

Hirschhorn R, Ellenbogen A. Genetic heterogeneity in adenosine deaminase (ADA) deficiency: five different mutations in five new patients with partial ADA deficiency. *Am J Hum Genet* 1986;38:13–25.

Jankovic J, Caskey TC, Stout JT, Butler IJ. Lesch-Nyhan syndrome: motor behavior and CSF neurotransmitters. *Ann Neurol* 1988;23:466–468.

Kuehn MR, Bradley A, Robertson EJ, Evans MJ. A potential animal model for Lesch-Nyhan syndrome through introduction of HPRT mutations into mice. *Nature* 1987;326:295–298.

Marcus S, Stern AM, Andersson B, et al. Mutation analysis and prenatal diagnosis in Lesch-Nyhan syndrome showing non-random C- inactivation interferes with carrier detection tests. *Hum Genet* 1992;89:395–400.

Markert ML. Purine nucleoside deficiency. *Immunodefic Rev* 1991;3:45–81.

Nyhan WL. The recognition of Lesch-Nyhan syndrome as an inborn error of purine metabolism. *J Inherit Metabol Dis* 1997;20:171–178.

Nyhan WL, Parkman R, Page T, et al. Bone marrow transplantation in Lesch-Nyhan disease. *Adv Exp Med Biol* 1986;195:167–170.

Rijksen G, Kuis W, Wadman SK, et al. A new case of purine nucleoside phosphorylase deficiency with neurologic disorder. *Pediatr Res* 1987;21:137–141.

Rossiter BJF, Edwards A, Casket CT. HPRT mutations in Lesch-Nyhan syndrome. In: Brosis J, Frenau B, eds. *Molecular genetic approach to neuropsychiatric diseases.* New York: Academic Press, 1991.

Scully DG, Dawson PA, Emerson BT, Gordon RS. Review of the molecular basis of HPRT deficiency. *Hum Genet* 1992;90:195–207.

Shapira J, Ziberman Y, Becker A. Lesch-Nyhan syndrome: a nonextracting approach to prevent mutilation. *Spec Care Dentist* 1985;5:210–212.

Silverstein FS, Johnson MV, Hutchinson RJ, Edwards NL. Lesch-Nyhan syndrome: CSF neurotransmitter abnormalities. *Neurology* 1985;35:907–911.

Stout JT, Chen HY, Brennand J, et al. Expression of human HPRT in the central nervous system of transgenic mice. *Nature* 1985;317:250–251.

Watson AR, Simmonds HA, Webster DR, et al. Purine nucleoside phosphorylase (PNP) deficiency: a therapeutic challenge. *Adv Exp Med Biol* 1984;165:53–59.

Watts RWE, Spellacy E, Gibbs DA, et al. Clinical, postmortem, biochemical and therapeutic observations on the Lesch-Nyhan syndrome with particular reference to the neurological manifestations. *Q J Med* 1982;201:43–78.

Wilson JM, Stout JT, Palella TD, et al. A molecular survey of hypoxanthine-guanine phosphoribosyltransferase deficiency in man. *J Clin Invest* 1986;77:188–195.

Wu CL, Melton DW. Production of model for Lesch-Nyhan syndrome in hypoxanthine phosphoribosyl transferase-deficient mice. *Nat Genet* 1993;3:235–239.

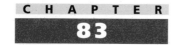

LYSOSOMAL AND OTHER STORAGE DISEASES

WILLIAM G. JOHNSON

In the lysosomal diseases, storage material accumulates within lysosomes because of genetically determined deficiency of a catabolic enzyme. The stored material is usually of a complex lipid or saccharide nature; the nervous system is usually affected. The inheritance pattern is recessive and usually autosomal but occasionally X-linked. Carrier detection and prenatal diagnosis have been accomplished in most of these disorders, but there is as yet no specific treatment for any of the lysosomal storage diseases except for enzyme replacement therapy for Gaucher disease. Bone marrow transplantation is being tried experimentally for the mucopolysaccharidoses.

LIPIDOSES

Lipid storage diseases involve all three major lipid classes: neutral lipids (i.e., cholesterol ester, fatty acid, and triglycerides), polar lipids (glycolipids and phospholipids), and very polar lipids (gangliosides). The largest group of stored lipids is the sphingolipids, based on sphingosine (Fig. 83.1A). When a long-chain fatty acid is attached to the 2-amino group of sphingosine, the resulting compounds are called ceramides. Further hydrophilic residues are attached at the 1-hydroxyl group to give the sphingolipids (Fig. 83.1, B to E).

GM2-GANGLIOSIDOSES

Hexosaminidase-deficiency diseases result from a genetically determined deficiency of the enzyme hexosaminidase (reaction 3, Figs. 83.1,B and C, 83.2, and 83.3), which causes accumulation in cells (especially in neurons) of GM2-ganglioside, certain other glycosphingolipids, and other compounds containing a terminal β-linked, *N*-acetylgalactosaminide or *N*-acetylglucosaminide moiety.

For full activity, hexosaminidase requires two different subunits: the α-subunit, coded for by the HEXA locus on chromosome 15, and the β-subunit, coded for by the HEXB locus on chromosome 5. Three isozymes of hexosaminidase have a defined subunit structure: hexosaminidase A ($\alpha\beta$), hexosaminidase B ($\beta\beta$), and hexosaminidase S ($\alpha\alpha$). Hexosaminidase A is required for cleavage of GM2-ganglioside, but the true substrate is the ganglioside bound to a protein activator whose deficiency also causes a GM2-gangliosidosis (the so-called AB variant). The GM2-gangliosidoses are classified according to the phenotype, the genetic locus, and the allele involved.

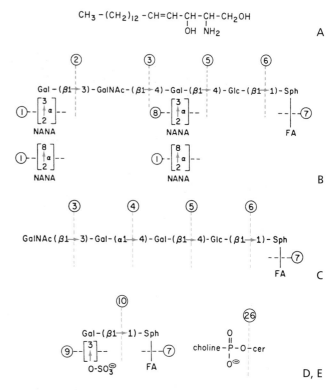

FIG. 83.1. A: Sphingosine. Addition of fatty acid in amide linkage gives ceramide (Cer). **B:** Structure of a ganglioside (here, a tetrasialoganglioside, GQ1a) containing sphingosine (Sph), fatty acid (FA), neutral hexoses (glucose, Glc; galactose, Gal), hexosamine (GalNAc, *N*-acetylgalactosamine), and sialic acid (NANA, *N*-acetylneuraminic acid). **C:** Structure of a glycolipid, globoside (GL4), containing sphingosine, fatty acid, neutral hexoses, and hexosamine. **D:** Structure of sulfatide (a major glycolipid of myelin) containing sphingosine, fatty acid, and galactose, which is sulfated on the 3-hydroxyl group. **E:** Structure of sphingomyelin or ceramide phosphorylcholine. Reactions 1-26 are illustrated in Figs. 83.1–83.3. *1,* Sialidase (sialidoses). *2,* Beta-galactosidase (GM1-gangliosidoses, Morquio syndrome type B, secondarily deficient in galactosialidosis). *3,* Hexosaminidase (GM2-gangliosidoses). *4,* Alpha-galactosidase (Fabry disease). *5,* Ceramide lactosidase. *6,* β-Glucosidase (Gaucher disease). *7,* Ceramidase (Farber disease). *8,* Ganglioside sialidase. *9,* Sulfatase A (metachromatic leukodystrophy, mucosulfatidosis, MSD). *10,* Galactocerebrosidase (Krabbe disease). *11,* α-L-Iduronidase (Hurler syndrome, Scheie syndrome, Hurler-Scheie compound). *12,* Iduronate-2-sulfate sulfatase (Hunter syndrome, MSD). *13,* Sulfamidase (Sanfilippo A, MSD). *14,* α-*N*-acetylglucosaminidase (Sanfilippo B). *15,* N-acetyl transferase (Sanfilippo D, MSD). *16,* Galactose-6-sulfate sulfatase or *N*-acetylgalactosamine-6-sulfate sulfatase (Morquio syndrome type A, MSD). *17,* N-acetylgalactosamine-4-sulfate sulfatase or sulfatase B (Maroteaux-Lamy syndrome, MSD). *18,* β-Glucuronidase (Sly syndrome). *19,* Acetylglucosamine-6-sulfate sulfatase (Sanfilippo D, MSD). *20,* Dermatan sulfate *N*-acetylgalactosamine-6-sulfate sulfatase. *21,* α-L-Fucosidase (fucosidosis). *22,* α-Mannosidase (α-mannosidosis). *23,* Mannosidase (β-mannosidosis). *24,* Endoglucosaminidase. *25,* Aspartylglucosaminidase (aspartylglucosaminuria). *26,* Sphingomyelinase (Niemann-Pick disease, types A, B, and F).

Progressive infantile encephalopathy was the most common clinical presentation in the past. The success of carrier screening among couples of Ashkenazi Jewish background dramatically reduced its incidence, and later onset variants are now seen more commonly. Hexosaminidase deficiencies present with a variety of phenotypes from infancy to adulthood. This diagnosis can reasonably be suspected with nearly any degenerative neurologic disorder except demyelinating neuropathy or myopathy. Sensory

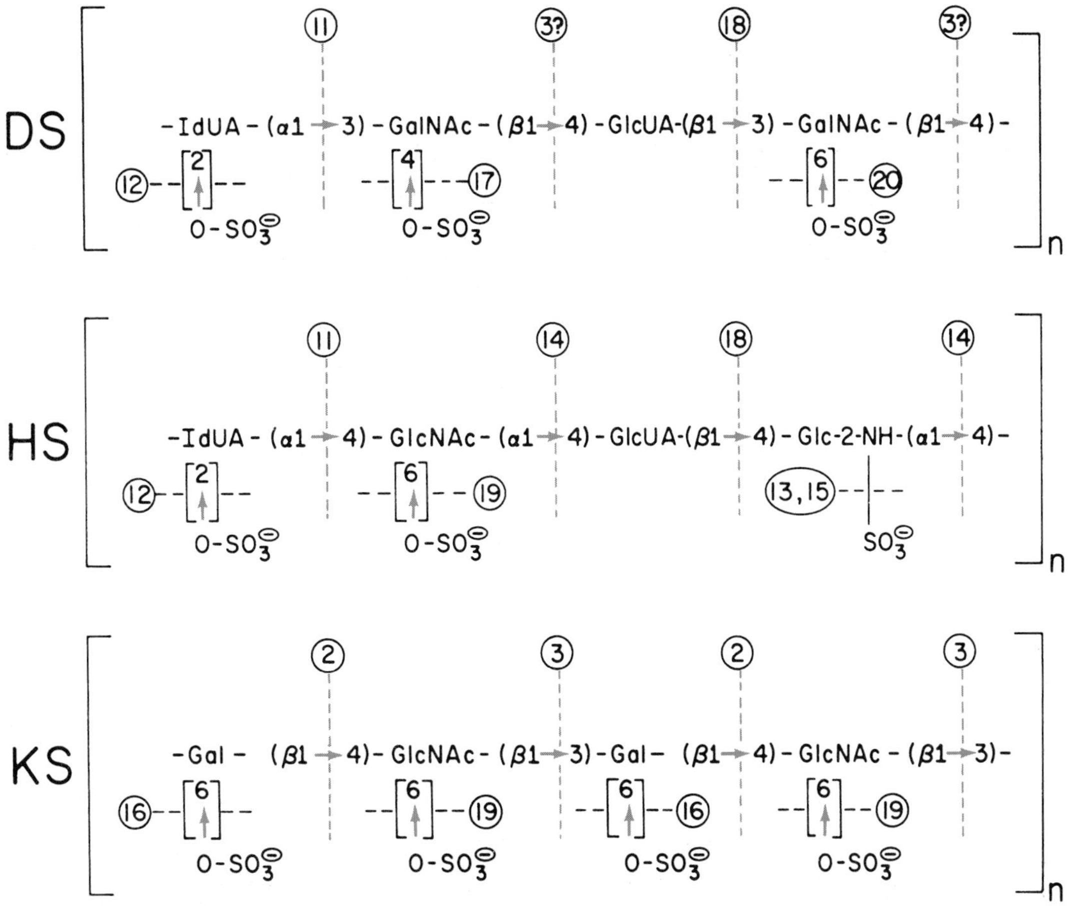

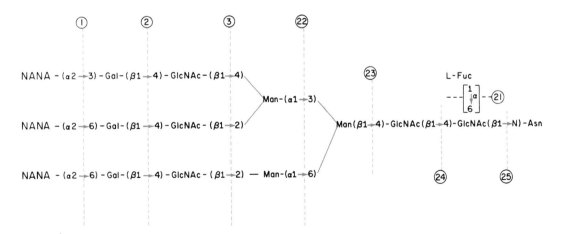

FIG. 83.2. Structure of three clinically important mucopolysaccharides: dermatan sulfate (DS), heparan sulfate (HS), and keratan sulfate (KS). Each consists of repeating dimers of uronic acid (IdUA, iduronic acid; GlcUA, glucuronic acid), hexosamine (GlcNAc, *N*-acetylglucosamine; GalNAc, *N*-acetylgalactosamine), and sulfate (OSO3). In DS, the hexosamine is GalNAc. In HS, the hexosamine is α-linked glucosamine, sometimes *N*-acetylated, sometimes *N*-sulfated. In KS, uronic acid is replaced by galactose (Gal). The glycan portion is bound to protein (not shown).

FIG. 83.3. Structure of an asparagine-linked glycoprotein consisting of asparagine (Asn), neutral sugars (Man, mannose; Gal, galactose; L-Fuc, L-fucose), hexosamine (GlcNAc, *N*-acetylglucosamine), and sialic acid (NANA, *N*-acetylneuraminic acid). The mannose-6-phosphate recognition marker is formed by transfer of GlcNAc1P to the 6-hydroxyl groups of the α-linked mannose residues and subsequent removal of the phosphate-linked GlcNAc residues.

dysfunction, ocular palsies, neurogenic bladder, and extraneural involvement are not prominent features.

The diagnosis is made by measuring the amount of hexosaminidase in blood serum and leukocytes. Rectal biopsy for electron microscopy of neurons is useful to confirm the diagnosis in variant phenotypes. DNA-based diagnosis is useful to specify the mutation involved.

Infantile Encephalopathy with Cherry-red Spots

Three disorders in this group are well known: classic infantile Tay-Sachs disease (α locus), infantile Sandhoff disease (β locus), and the so-called AB variant (activator locus). The α locus mutations occur with high frequency among people of Ashkenazi background (1 in 30 compared with 1 in 300 for the general population), accounting for the ethnic concentration of classic Tay-Sachs disease and genetic compounds containing α locus mutations.

In all three conditions, the infants appear normal until 4 to 6 months of age. They learn to smile and reach for objects but do not sit or crawl. A myoclonic jerk reaction to sound (hyperacusis) and the macular cherry-red spot (Fig. 83.4) are constant findings. The infants become floppy and weak but have hyperactive reflexes, clonus, and extensor plantar responses. Visual deterioration, apathy, and loss of developmental milestones lead to a vegetative state by the second year. Seizures and myoclonus are prominent for the first 2 years. The infants eventually become decorticate. They need tube feeding, have difficulty with secretions, and are blind. Head circumference enlarges progressively to about the 90th percentile from 1 to 3 years and then stabilizes.

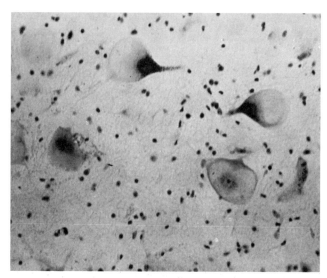

FIG. 83.5. Ballooned spinal cord ventral horn cells in Tay-Sachs disease. (Courtesy of Dr. Abner Wolf.)

Death is due to intercurrent infection, usually pneumonia. The disease is confined to the nervous system.

By light microscopy, grossly ballooned neurons (Fig. 83.5) are found throughout the brain, cerebellum, and spinal cord. The cytoplasm is filled with pale homogeneous-appearing material that pushes the nucleus and Nissl substrate to a corner of the cell. By electron microscopy, membranous cytoplasmic bodies (distended lysosomes) are seen with regularly spaced concentric dark and pale lamellae.

GM2-ganglioside (Fig. 83.1B) content is markedly increased in the brain and, to a much lesser degree, in the viscera. Other glycosphingolipids with a terminal β-linked N-acetylgalactosamine moiety, such as asialo-GM2 (Fig. 83.1B) and globoside (Fig. 83.1C), accumulate to a lesser degree.

The storage results from deficiency of hexosaminidase (reaction 3). In classic Tay-Sachs disease, hexosaminidase A is absent and hexosaminidase B increased. Heterozygous carriers have a partial decrease of hexosaminidase A.

In infantile Sandhoff disease, hexosaminidase A and B are deficient. Carriers have partially decreased hexosaminidase A and B. In one form of the AB variant, a hexosaminidase A activating protein is missing. Although levels of hexosaminidase A and B are increased, GM2-ganglioside cannot be cleaved. Diagnosis requires use of the radiolabeled natural substrate, M2-ganglioside, or direct testing for the activator or activator mutations. In a second form of the AB variant, the residual hexosaminidase A cleaves artificial but not sulfated artificial or natural substrate. Although this is detected as an AB variant, it is an α-locus disorder.

Late Infantile, Juvenile, and Adult GM2-Gangliosidoses

These present with dementia and ataxia with or without macular cherry-red spots. Spasticity, muscle wasting due to anterior

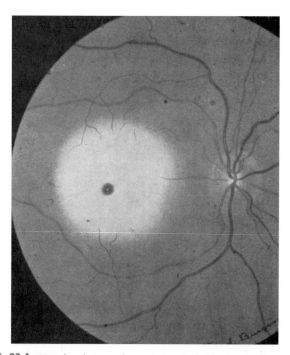

FIG. 83.4. Macular cherry-red spot in Tay-Sachs disease. (Courtesy of Dr. Arnold Gold.)

horn cell disease, and seizures are frequently seen. Hexosaminidase A deficiency or hexosaminidase A and B deficiency are found on biochemical study of serum, leukocytes, and cultured skin fibroblasts.

Other late-onset forms of GM2-gangliosidosis present as cerebellar ataxia or spinocerebellar ataxia. Hexosaminidase A or hexosaminidase A and B deficiency are found on biochemical study.

Motor neuron disease may be the presenting feature of late-onset GM2-gangliosidoses. Lower motor neuron disease may resemble Kugelberg-Welander or Aran-Duchenne syndrome. Upper motor neuron disease may be present, giving an amyotrophic lateral sclerosis-like phenotype.

Many, perhaps most, of these late-onset cases are genetic compounds. Rectal biopsy for electron microscopy of autonomic neurons, natural substrate hexosaminidase assays, and DNA-based diagnosis are important diagnostic tests for late onset GM2-gangliosidosis.

GM1-GANGLIOSIDOSIS

This group of disorders is characterized by deficiency of GM1-ganglioside β-galactosidase (reaction 2, Figs. 83.1B, 83.2, and 83.3) and storage of compounds that contain a terminal β-linked galactose moiety. These include GM1-ganglioside, asialo-M1, keratan sulfate-like oligosaccharides, and glycoproteins. Other β-galactosidases, such as those that cleave galactosylceramide (reaction 10, Fig. 83.1D) and lactosylceramide (reaction 5, Fig. 83.1B and C) are not deficient, and those compounds do not accumulate. There are at least three forms of deficiency of this enzyme: primary deficiency of β-galactosidase, causing infantile and late-infantile GM1-gangliosidosis and an adult form; combined neuraminidase and β-galactosidase deficiency, galactosialidosis; and combined deficiency of β-galactosidase and several other lysosomal enzymes in I-cell disease, mucolipidosis II. The latter two types are discussed under mucolipidoses.

Infantile GM1-Gangliosidosis

Infantile GM1-gangliosidosis is earlier in onset, more severe, and more rapidly progressive than infantile Tay-Sachs disease. Soon after birth, these infants become hypotonic, with poor sucking ability and slow weight gain. Their faces have frontal bossing, coarsened features, large low-set ears, and elongated philtrum. Gum hypertrophy, macroglossia, peripheral edema, and often faint corneal haze are noted. Strabismus and nystagmus may be seen. About half the patients develop macular cherry-red spots (Fig. 83.4). Development is slow, and they do not sit or crawl. By age 6 months, liver and spleen are enlarged; joint stiffness and claw-hand deformities may be seen, and the skin is coarse and thickened. Seizures may develop. The infants enter a vegetative state and die before age 2 of pneumonia or cardiac arrhythmias.

Bone radiographs after 6 to 12 months show changes similar to those of Hurler syndrome, with anterior beaking of vertebral bodies and J-shaped sella turcica. Lymphocytes from peripheral smear are vacuolated, and histiocytes in the bone marrow are foamy.

Diagnosis is made by the characteristic oligosaccharide pattern in urine, assay of GM1-ganglioside β-galactosidase (reaction 2, Figs. 83.1B and 83.2) in blood leukocytes or cultured skin fibroblasts, and demonstration of partially decreased enzyme levels in the obligate carrier parents. It is important to exclude sialidosis and to be prepared for prenatal diagnosis. Specific mutations can be detected by DNA-based diagnosis.

Late Infantile GM1-Gangliosidosis

Onset is usually between 1 and 3 years with gait ataxia, hypotonia, hyperreflexia, dysarthria, and speech regression. Seizures, dementia, and spastic quadriplegia lead to death, usually by pneumonia. Optic atrophy and evidence of anterior horn cell disease may be found. Corneas are clear, organomegaly is absent, and bone changes are scanty. Diagnosis is made in the same manner as for the infantile form.

FABRY DISEASE

Angiokeratoma corporis diffusum is an X-linked disorder affecting the skin, kidney, peripheral and autonomic nervous systems, and blood vessels with storage of trihexosylceramide, galactosyl galactosylglucosylceramide, a breakdown product of globoside (Fig. 83.1C). Trihexosylceramide accumulates because of a deficiency of trihexosylceramide β-galactosidase (reaction 4, Fig. 83.1C), also known as β-galactosidase A. Fabry disease is the only sphingolipidosis that is X-linked. It is incompletely recessive; that is, some female heterozygotes are clinically affected.

Symptoms usually begin in childhood or adolescence, with lancinating pains in the limbs, especially the feet and hands, often brought on by temperature changes, and accompanied by paresthesia or abdominal crises. Anhydrosis and unexplained fever are common.

The characteristic skin lesions, which become more numerous with age, are purple, macular and maculopapular, hyperkeratotic, 1 to 3 mm in size with a predilection for the groin, buttocks, scrotum, and umbilicus. Glycolipid storage in the renal glomeruli and tubules begins with asymptomatic proteinuria in children; it progresses to renal failure and hypertension in the third or fourth decade. Glycolipid storage in blood vessel walls may cause stroke. Edema of the limbs, faint haziness of the cornea visible by slit lamp, and myocardial involvement may occur. There is no specific treatment. Renal transplant is life-saving when renal failure supervenes. The lancinating pains may respond to phenytoin.

Heterozygous females may also be affected, but manifestations are less marked. Skin lesions are few or absent. Corneal opacity is more common. If renal or cardiac involvement occurs, they are later in onset and less severe. Diagnosis is by the finding of decreased β-galactosidase in plasma and leukocytes and by documentation of a specific mutation in the β-galactosidase gene.

GAUCHER DISEASE

Gaucher disease is an autosomal recessive sphingolipidosis in which glucocerebroside (Fig. 83.1B and C) is stored as a result of deficiency of glucocerebroside β-glucosidase (or glucocerebrosidase; reaction 6, Fig. 83.1, B and C). At least four forms are known (Table 83.1): the infantile neuronopathic form, the juvenile neuronopathic form, the adult neuronopathic form, and the adult nonneuronopathic form. The adult (nonneuropathic) form is more common in persons of Ashkenazi background. Diagnosis of all forms is made by the characteristic clinical picture, finding of Gaucher cells in bone marrow, finding of reduced glucocerebroside β-glucosidase in cultured skin fibroblasts or blood leukocytes, and documentation of a mutation in the β-glucosidase gene.

Infantile Neuronopathic Gaucher Disease

This disease occurs in the first year of life, often in the first 3 months. The course is rapid with developmental regression and death before age 2 years. Although the spleen and liver enlarge, the infants lose weight. They have stridor, difficulty in sucking and swallowing, strabismus, opisthotonic head retraction, spasticity, and hyperreflexia. Later, they enter a vegetative state, becoming flaccid and weak. Seizures may occur. Macular cherry-red spot and optic atrophy do not occur.

TABLE 83.1. LIPIDOSES

Disorder	Defective enzyme (reaction number)	Stored material	Clinical features
GM2-gangliosidoses	Hexosaminidase (3)	GM2, GA2, GL-4 globoside, OLS, ?GP, ?MPS	Infantile- to adult-onset phenotypes ranging from infantile encephalopathy with macular cherry-red spots to adult-onset spinal muscular atrophy
GM1-gangliosidoses	β-Galactosidase (2)	GM1, GA1, OLS, KS-like material	
Infantile form			Infantile encephalopathy, organomegaly, skeletal involvement, macular cherry-red spot (50%), corneal haze (occasionally)
Late-infantile form			Onset at age 1–3yr of dementia, seizures, ataxia, dysarthria, spastic quadriplegia
Fabry disease	α-Galactosidase (4)	Ceramide trihexoside, ? blood group substance type B	Purple skin lesions, painful hands and feet, renal disease, leg edema, stroke
Gaucher disease	β-Glucosidase (6)	Glucocerebroside	
Infantile neuronopathic form			Onset at age 3mo of dementia, organomegaly, poor suck and swallowing, opisthotonus, spasticity, seizures
Juvenile neuronopathic form			Variable onset of mental defect, splenomegaly, incoordination, seizures
Adult neuronopathic form			Splenomegaly (sometimes in infancy) and bony involvement; Ashkenazi Jewish predilection
Adult neuronopathic form			Splenomegaly, bony involvement, seizures, dementia
Nieman-Pick disease			
Infantile neuronopathic form, type A	Sphingomyelinase (26)	Sphingomyelin, cholesterol	Infantile encephalopathy, organomegaly, macular cherry-red spot (30%), lung infiltrates; Ashkenazi Jewish predilection
Juvenile nonneuronopathic form, type B	Sphingomyelinase (26)	Sphingomyelin, cholesterol	Hepatosplenomegaly
Juvenile neuronopathic form, type C	Cholesterol esterification induction (NCC1 gene)	Sphingomyelin, cholesterol	Onset at age 1–3yr of dementia, seizures, spasticity, ataxia; hepatosplenomegaly less prominent
Nova Scotia variant, type D	Cholesterol esterification induction (NPC1 gene)	Cholesterol, cholesterol ester, sphingomyelin, bis (monoacylglyceryl) phosphate	Infantile hepatosplenomegaly, onset age 2–5yr of dementia, seizures, ataxia, spasticity
Adult nonneuronopathic form, type E	?	Sphingomyelin	Adult hepatosplenomegaly
Juvenile nonneuronopathic form, type F	Sphingomyelinase (26)	Sphingomyelin	Resembles type B, juvenile hepatosplenomegaly, sea-blue histiocytes, heat-labile sphingomyelinase
Farber disease	Acid ceramidase (7)	Ceramide	Early infantile painful swollen joints, subcutaneous nodules, organomegaly, enlarged heart, dysphagia, vomiting, normal or impaired mentation

(continued)

TABLE 83.1. LIPIDOSES *(continued)*

Disorder	Defective enzyme (reaction number)	Stored material	Clinical features
Wolman disease	Acid lipase	Cholesterol ester, triglyceride	Early infantile organomegaly, vomiting, diarrhea, jaundice, variable nervous system involvement
Refsum disease	Phytanic acid α-hydroxylase	Phytanic acid	Night blindness, retinitis pigmentosa, ataxia, demyelinating neuropathy, ichthyosis
Cerebrotendinous xanthomatosis	?	Cholestanol, cholesterol	Static encephalopathy in first decade, adolescent or adult-onset cataracts, tendon xanthomas, ataxia, spasticity
Neuronal lipofuscinoses (Batten disease)	CLN1, CLN2, CLN3, CLN4, CLN5 gene products	Retinoic acid derivatives, dolichol derivatives (whether this storage is primary or secondary is unclear)	
Infantile (Finnish) form (Santavuori disease)	Palmitoyl-protein thioesterase enzyme (CNL1 gene)		Infantile onset of progressive visual loss, retinal degeneration, myoclonic jerks, microcephaly
Late-infantile form (Jansky-Bielschowsky)	CLN2 gene product		Onset at age 1–4yr of seizures, ataxia, dementia, then visual deterioration and retinal degeneration
Juvenile form (Spielmeyer-Sjögren)	CLN3 gene product		Onset at age 5–10yr of progressive visual loss and pigmentary retinal degeneration then seizures and dementia
Adult form (Kufs)			Adult onset of dementia, ataxia, seizures, and myoclonus

GM2, GM2-ganglioside; GA2, asialo-GM2-ganglioside; OLS, oligosaccharide; GP, glycoprotein; MPS, mucopolysaccharide; GM1, GM1-ganglioside; GA1, asialo-GM1-ganglioside; KS, keratan sulfate; DS, dermatan sulfate; HS, heparan sulfate; GM3, GM3-ganglioside; GD3, GD3-ganglioside.

Juvenile Neuronopathic Gaucher Disease

This form is characterized by splenomegaly, Gaucher cells in bone marrow, mental deficiency (retardation or dementia), seizures, incoordination, and tics. Neurologic signs develop in childhood or adolescence.

Adult Gaucher Disease

Characteristics are splenomegaly and bone lesions but not neurologic disorders. It is most common in individuals of Ashkenazi background. Despite the name, the disease may be found even in young children. Although thrombocytopenia may be a problem, splenectomy should be avoided if possible; however, severe and prolonged thrombocytopenia is an indication for splenectomy. Lesions of long bones, pelvis, or vertebral bodies may be painful. Liver, skin, lymph nodes, and lungs may be involved. Multiple myeloma may be a late complication. Purified modified β-glucosidase, alglucerase, or recombinant β-glucosidase, imiglucerase, infused into patients with Gaucher disease, causes dramatic reduction in splenomegaly and improvement in other symptoms.

Adult Neuronopathic Gaucher Disease

Although resembling adult-onset Gaucher disease, symptoms also include seizures and dementia.

NIEMANN-PICK DISEASE

This group of disorders is characterized by lysosomal storage of the glycosphingolipid sphingomyelin (ceramide phosphoryl-

choline) (Fig. 83.1E). Two basic types have been described. Type I consists of the earlier types A and B deficiency. In type II, consisting of the earlier type C and D, a defect of intracellular cholesterol transport has been found. In type I patients, deficiency of a sphingomyelin-cleaving enzyme, sphingomyelinase (reaction 26, Fig. 83.1E), has been found. Diagnosis is made by the clinical evidence of hepatosplenomegaly, with or without cerebral symptoms, by finding characteristic "mulberry" storage cells (which appear different from Gaucher cells) in bone marrow and by demonstrating decreased sphingomyelinase activity in cultured skin fibroblasts, leukocytes, or tissue.

Infantile Niemann-Pick Disease, Type A

This is the most common and most severe form of Niemann-Pick disease and occurs more commonly in individuals of Ashkenazi background. Transient neonatal jaundice is followed by progressive hepatosplenomegaly; developmental regression and weight loss lead to death by age 2. Dementia and hypotonia are noted. About one-third of patients develop macular cherry-red spots (Fig. 83.4). Seizures are uncommon. Bone involvement is mild. Skin often has a brownish-yellow tinge. Most patients have diffuse haziness or patchy infiltrates in the lungs.

Diagnosis is made by the characteristic clinical picture, by the finding of foam cells in the bone marrow, and by demonstration of nearly total sphingomyelinase (reaction 26, Fig. 83.1E) deficiency in leukocytes and cultured skin fibroblasts.

Juvenile Nonneuronopathic, Type B

This form presents with asymptomatic splenomegaly or hepatosplenomegaly without neurologic disorder in infants, children, or adults. Foam cells appear in the bone marrow, and sphingomyelinase (reaction 26, Fig. 83.1E) is reduced in cultured skin fibroblasts and leukocytes. These patients have more residual sphingomyelinase (15% to 20% of normal) than those with type A (up to 10%).

Niemann-Pick Disease Type C

Patients are normal in infancy but after 1 to 2 years develop progressive dementia, seizures, spasticity, vertical gaze paresis, and ataxia. Hepatosplenomegaly is less prominent than in other types. Diagnosis is by demonstration of foam cells (sea-blue histiocytes) in bone marrow and the demonstration in cultured skin fibroblasts of deficient induction of cholesterol esterification and of intravesicular storage of cholesterol after filipin staining. The abnormal gene, NPC1, is located in the short arm of chromosome 18.

In type D, found in Yarmouth County Acadians of Nova Scotia, the basic defect is also mutation in NPC1. Type E patients may simply be adult type B patients. Type F resembles type B except that sphingomyelinase is heat labile in type F.

FARBER LIPOGRANULOMATOSIS

In the first few months of life, as early as 2 weeks of age, infants with this disease have painful swollen joints, hoarseness, vomiting, respiratory difficulty, or limb edema.

Subcutaneous nodules are found near joints and tendon sheaths, especially on the hands, arms, and at pressure points such as the occiput or lumbosacral spine. Other findings include cardiac enlargement and murmurs, lymphadenopathy, hepatomegaly, splenomegaly, enlarged tongue, difficulty in swallowing, and pulmonary granulomata. Tendon reflexes may be hyperactive or hypoactive. Mental development may be normal or impaired. Seizures do not occur. Cerebrospinal fluid (CSF) protein may be elevated.

Ceramide (Fig. 83.1, B to E) and some related compounds accumulate in foam cells in affected tissues because of severe diminution of acid ceramidase (reaction 7, Fig. 83.1, B to E), an enzyme that catabolizes ceramide to sphingosine and fatty acid. Neutral ceramidase is not decreased. Diagnosis is made by the clinical picture and finding of deficiency of acid ceramidase in cultured skin fibroblasts or leukocytes. Prenatal diagnosis and carrier testing are possible. Most patients die of pulmonary disease before age 2 years, but some survive into adolescence.

WOLMAN DISEASE

Infants affected by Wolman disease are normal at birth but in the first few weeks of life have severe vomiting, abdominal distention, diarrhea, poor weight gain, jaundice, and unexplained fever. Hepatosplenomegaly may be massive, and there may be a papulovesiculopustular rash on face, neck, shoulders, and chest. The extent of neurologic disorder is not clear because the infants are so sick and die so early. Initially, they are active and alert, but activity decreases. Corticospinal signs have been found in some.

Laboratory findings include anemia and foam cells in bone marrow. A distinctive finding is calcification of the adrenals on radiographic examination. The course is usually rapidly progressive. Death usually occurs within 3 to 6 months, but some survive into the second year. The lipid storage consists primarily of cholesterol ester and smaller amounts of triglyceride because there is severe deficiency of a lysosomal fatty acid ester acid hydrolase (acid lipase, acid esterase, or acid cholesteryl ester hydrolase), which cleaves cholesterol ester, triglycerides, and artificial substrates. Nearly total deficiency of this acid lipase is found in tissues, leukocytes, and cultured fibroblasts from patients; carriers have been detected, and prenatal diagnosis is possible. The enzyme is coded for by a gene on the long arm of chromosome 10 (10q23.210q23).

A milder allelic form of Wolman disease with deficiency of the same enzyme is called cholesterol ester storage disease. These patients have hepatomegaly (with or without splenomegaly), hypercholesterolemia, and foam cells in the bone marrow.

CEREBROTENDINOUS XANTHOMATOSIS (CHOLESTANOL STORAGE DISEASE)

Although patients with cholestanol storage disease often have mental defect of early onset, the diagnosis is difficult in the first decade because cataracts, tendon xanthomas, and progressive spasticity, usually associated with ataxia, commonly do not begin before adolescence or young adulthood. The spasticity and ataxia are severe and progressive. Speech is affected. Neuropathy may appear with distal muscle wasting. Sensory deficits and Babinski signs are seen. Pseudobulbar palsy develops terminally. Death usually occurs in the fourth to sixth decade, caused by neurologic disease or myocardial infarction. Some patients have apparently normal mental function.

Tendon xanthomas are almost always seen on the Achilles tendon and may occur elsewhere. The cerebellar hemispheres contain large (up to 1.5 cm), yellowish, granulomatous, xanthomatous lesions with extensive demyelination of white matter. Microscopically, cystic areas of necrosis and clear needle-shaped clefts contain birefringent material surrounded by macrophages with foamy vacuolated cytoplasm and multinucleated giant cells. The brainstem and spinal cord may be involved.

Cholestanol is increased in plasma, brain, and tendon xanthomas. Cholesterol is increased in tendon xanthomas but is usually normal in plasma. Cholestanol is increased in bile, but chenodeoxycholic acid (a major component of normal bile) is virtually absent.

Diagnosis is by the characteristic clinical picture, and biochemical findings and demonstration of mutations in the sterol 27-hydroxylase gene (CYP27). Treatment with certain bile acids may be beneficial.

NEURONAL CEROID LIPOFUSCINOSES

The neuronal ceroid lipofuscinoses are defined by histologic and ultrastructural features. By light microscopy, neurons are engorged with periodic acid-Schiff–positive and autofluorescent material.

Ultrastructurally, abnormal lipopigments resembling ceroid and lipofuscin are found in distinctive abnormal cytosomes such as curvilinear and fingerprint bodies. Although the signs and symptoms are confined to the nervous system, the abnormal cytosomes are widely distributed in skin, muscle, peripheral nerves, leukocytes, urine sediment, and viscera. Dolichol is elevated in tissue and urine sediment. The gene (CLN1) for infantile neuronal ceroid lipofuscinosis and those for the late infantile (CLN2) and juvenile (CLN3) forms have been cloned. CLN1 codes for the palmitoylprotein thioesterase enzyme; mutations in this gene also cause a juvenile form of neuronal ceroid lipofuscinosis with granular osmiophilic deposits. CLN2 also codes for a lysosomal enzyme, but the function of the CLN3 protein is not yet known. CLN4 and CLN5 have been mapped. CLN5 codes for a putative transmembrane protein.

Diagnosis is made by the characteristic clinical picture, by abnormal electroretinogram (in the infantile, late-infantile, and juvenile forms), by electron microscopic examination of tissue (skin, nerve, muscle, or rectal biopsy for autonomic neurons) and by enzyme and mutation testing. Abnormal autofluorescence is seen on examination of frozen section of biopsied muscle, enabling rapid diagnosis. The neuronal ceroid lipofuscinoses are autosomal recessive.

Infantile (Finnish) Variant (Santavuori Disease)

This variant of neuronal ceroid lipofuscinosis begins at about 8 months with progressive visual loss, loss of developmental milestones, myoclonic jerks, and microcephaly. There is optic atrophy, macular and retinal degeneration, and no response in the electroretinogram. Progression is rapid, but infants may survive for several years.

Late-infantile Variant (Jansky-Bielschowsky Disease)

This begins between ages 1.5 and 4 years with seizures and ataxia. Seizures respond poorly to anticonvulsants. There is progressive visual deterioration with abolished electroretinogram and retinal deterioration. Progression is usually rapid to a vegetative state, but some affected children may survive several years.

Juvenile Variant (Spielmeyer-Sjögren Disease)

This variant of neuronal ceroid lipofuscinosis begins with progressive visual loss between the ages of 5 and 10 years, with pigmentary degeneration of the retina. Seizures, dementia, and motor abnormalities occur later and progress to death by the end of the second decade. The storage material contains large amounts of the ATP synthase subunit C protein.

Adult Variant (Kufs Disease)

This begins in the third or fourth decade with progressive dementia, seizures, myoclonus, and ataxia. Blindness and retinal degeneration are not features of the adult form.

LEUKODYSTROPHIES

The leukodystrophies are progressive genetic metabolic disorders affecting myelin metabolism (Table 83.2). Krabbe leukodystrophy (globoid cell leukodystrophy) was initially defined by the presence of globoid cells in demyelinated portions of the brain. Metachromatic leukodystrophy (MLD) was set apart by abnormal tissue metachromasia. Adrenoleukodystrophy was set apart by involvement of adrenal glands and by X-linked inheritance (see Chapter 87 for a discussion of adrenoleukodystrophy). Classic Pelizaeus-Merzbacher disease was set apart by X-linked inheritance, early onset, a long course, and islands of preserved myelin in the demyelinated areas. This leaves a heterogeneous group of unclassified leukodystrophies, sometimes called orthochromatic or sudanophilic leukodystrophies.

Metachromatic Leukodystrophy

MLD is a group of disorders with degeneration of central myelin (Fig. 83.6) and peripheral myelin, striking metachromasia of the stored substances, primarily sulfatides, and deficiency of the sulfatide-cleaving enzyme, sulfatase A (reaction 9, Fig. 83.1D), also called arylsulfatase A. At least four forms are known, the late-infantile form being the most common. All have autosomal recessive inheritance.

Alleles causing sulfatase A deficiency and MLD have either absent or low residual enzyme activity. Patients with two alleles giving absent enzyme activity have the severe late-infantile MLD. Patients with two alleles giving low residual enzyme activity have the mildest, adult type MLD. Compound heterozygotes with one allele of each type have the intermediate juvenile form of MLD.

The diagnosis of MLD is complicated by the existence of sulfatase A pseudodeficiency, an autosomal recessive condition in which sulfatase A activity is greatly diminished by the usual enzyme assays, but there is no neurologic disease. An additional complication is the requirement of sulfatase A for the sulfatide activator protein. Patients with genetic deficiency of sulfatide activator protein may have MLD, but the commonly used enzyme assays may fail to diagnosis this. Consequently, a high index of suspicion is required even if screening tests are apparently normal.

Late-Infantile Metachromatic Leukodystrophy

Affected infants have onset of difficulty in walking after the first year of life, usually between ages 12 and 30 months. Usually, flaccid paresis and diminished or absent tendon reflexes are seen. Occasionally, spastic paresis develops. Genu recurvatum may be noted. Mental functions deteriorate and dysarthria is noted.

Tendon reflexes decrease and disappear. Intermittent pain in arms and legs may be seen. Later, patients become bedridden and quadriplegic, with feeding difficulties, bulbar and pseudobulbar palsies, and optic atrophy. Finally, the children become blind, enter a vegetative stage, and die usually in the first decade. CSF protein is increased. Gallbladder function may be impaired. Metachromatic lipids are seen on sural nerve biopsy. Urinary sulfatide excretion is increased.

TABLE 83.2. LEUKODYSTROPHIES

Clinical disorder	Defective enzyme (reaction number)	Stored material	Clinical features
Krabbe leukodystrophy (GLD)			
Infantile form	Galactocerebrosidase (10)	Psychosine Galactocerebroside	Onset at age 3–6mo of irritability, spasticity, seizures, fevers. Progressive mental and motor loss to blind decerebrate vegetative state, with optic atrophy, decreased tendon reflexes, decreased nerve conduction velocities, increased CSF protein
Juvenile form	Galactocerebrosidase (10)	Galactocerebroside ? Psychosine	Juvenile onset of dementia, optic atrophy, pyramidal tract disorder
Adult form	? Galactocerebrosidase (10)	? Galactocerebroside ? Psychosine	Adult onset of slowly progressive dementia, optic atrophy, and pyramidal signs
Metachromatic leukodystrophy (MLD)			
Late-infantile form	Sulfatase A (9)	Sulfatide	Onset at age 1–2.5yr of walking difficulty with weakness, ataxia or spasticity; progressive dementia, optic atrophy, loss of deep tendon reflexes; slow nerve conduction velocities, increased CSF protein
Juvenile form	Sulfatase A (9)	Sulfatide	Onset at age 3–10yr of dementia, gait difficulty, neuropathy, elevated CSF protein; more slowly progressive
Adult form	Sulfatase A (9)	Sulfatide	Adult-onset dementia, often with ataxia and pyramidal findings; slowly progressive
MLD without sulfatase A deficiency	Sulfatase A (9) activator	Sulfatide	Same as late-infantile or juvenile form
Asymptomatic or presymptomatic adults with sulfatase A deficiency	Sulfatase A (9)	Sulfatide	Normal
Multiple sulfatase deficiency (mucosulfatidosis, MSD)	Sulfatase A (9) Sulfatase B (17) Sulfatase C Cholesterol sulfate sulfatase Dehydroepiandrosterone sulfate sulfatase Iduronate-2-sulfate sulfatase (12) Sulfamidase (13) N-acetylgalactosamine-6-sulfate sulfatase (16) N-acetylglucosamine-6-sulfate sulfatase (19) Basic defect presumed to be an enzyme affecting posttranslational modification of all sulfatases	Sulfatide MPS	Slowed early development. Onset at age 1–2yr of mental and motor deterioration and seizures; mildly coarsened facial features, ichthyosis, organomegaly, skeletal changes

Sulfatide accumulates in brain and peripheral nerves and in some extraneural tissues (e.g., kidney) and is seen histologically as brown metachromasia with acetic acid-cresyl violet staining in glial cells, Schwann cells, myelin lamellae, and neurons. The characteristic "tuffstone" bodies are seen by electron microscopy. Sulfatide consists primarily of galactosylsulfatide (Fig. 83.1D), although a smaller amount of lactosylsulfatide is found. The diagnosis is based on the clinical picture, demonstration of histologic and ultrastructural abnormalities in myelinated fibers of biopsied sural nerve or conjunctiva, the finding of severe defi-ciency of sulfatase A in leukocytes and cultured skin fibroblasts, and demonstration of a mutation in the sulfatase A gene.

Juvenile Metachromatic Leukodystrophy

These patients have later onset of symptoms (usually ages 3 to 10 years) and slower progression of the disease. The clinical features are similar to those late-infantile MLD. Juvenile MLD patients more frequently have emotional disturbance or dementia as the initial symptom, although they may present with gait disorder.

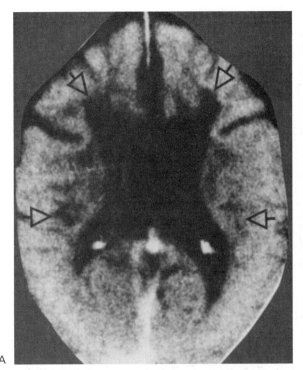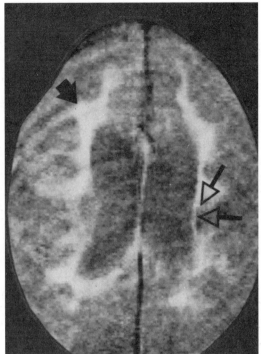

FIG. 83.6. **A:** Standard CT projection through the center cerebrum. Open arrows indicate symmetrical lesions of markedly decreased absorption in white matter. Adult MLD, age 36. **B:** A more T$_2$-weighted MRI scan of the same patient. Black arrow shows the confluent hyperintense signal in diseased white matter. So shrunken is this white matter that gyri now extend down next to the ventricle (open arrows).

Nystagmus and tremor may be noted. Nerve conduction velocities are slowed. CSF protein concentrations are elevated.

Adult Metachromatic Leukodystrophy

In adults, MLD commonly presents around age 30 years as a psychiatric disorder or progressive dementia. Other findings may include truncal ataxia, hyperactive reflexes, and seizures. CSF protein concentration is usually not elevated. The illness runs a protracted course, averaging 15 years.

Multiple Sulfatase Deficiency

This rare disorder, also known as sulfatidosis, Austin type or mucosulfatidosis, has clinical features of MLD and mucopolysaccharidosis, with excretion of both sulfatide and mucopolysaccharide in urine and deficiencies in at least nine sulfatases. Onset is usually earlier than with late-infantile MLD. Early development is slow. Patients do not achieve normal gait or speech, although they may walk or speak single words.

Neurologic deterioration is noted at 1 to 2 years, and the disease proceeds much like late-infantile MLD. However, patients develop mildly coarsened facial features, ichthyosis, and sometimes hepatosplenomegaly and dystosis multiplex. The histologic changes in brain and peripheral nerve resemble those of late-infantile MLD. Metachromatic material is found in liver, spleen, and kidney. The diagnosis is based on the characteristic clinical picture and the findings of deficiencies of sulfatase A and other sulfatases in cultured skin fibroblasts.

The biochemical basis for multiple sulfatase deficiency seems to be that all sulfatases require a posttranslational modification for sulfatase activity. This modification, conversion of a cysteine residue to 2-amino-3-oxopropionic acid, is believed to be defective in multiple sulfatase deficiency patients.

Krabbe Leukodystrophy (Globoid Cell)

Patients are normal at birth. Symptoms begin at ages 3 to 6 months with irritability, inexplicable crying, fevers, limb stiffness, seizures, feeding difficulty, vomiting, and slowing of mental and motor development. Later, mental and motor deterioration occur with marked hypertonia and extensor postures. Early tendon reflexes may be increased or already decreasing. Optic atrophy may be seen. Later, tendon reflexes decrease or disappear. Patients may develop flaccidity or flexor postures before death occurs at about age 2 years.

Important diagnostic features are increased CSF protein and decreased nerve conduction velocities. On electron microscopy, sural nerve biopsy specimens show needlelike inclusions in histiocytes and Schwann cells, also seen in globoid cells in demyelinated brain regions (Fig. 83.7).

Galactocerebrosidase (reaction 10, Fig. 83.1D) is deficient in serum, leukocytes, and cultured skin fibroblasts. Both galactosylcerebroside and galactosylsphingosine (psychosine) are substrates for that enzyme. Psychosine is increased at least 200-fold over levels in the normal brain, where it is barely detectable. Psychosine storage is probably the cause of the disease, because psychosine has been shown to be toxic to the brain.

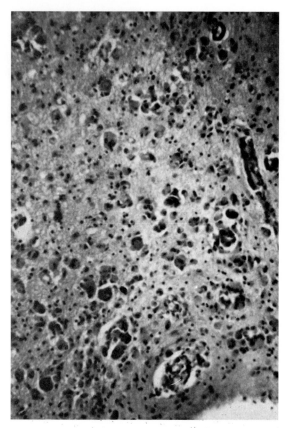

FIG. 83.7. Globoid cells in white matter, Krabbe leukodystrophy (H&E stain).

A few patients with juvenile onset and slower progression of dementia, optic atrophy, and pyramidal tract signs without neuropathy have had galactocerebrosidase deficiency. An adult-onset disorder with similar but more slowly progressive course has been described based on the pathologic findings of globoid cell leukodystrophy; however, the biochemical basis has not been established.

MUCOPOLYSACCHARIDOSES

The mucopolysaccharidoses are defined by a characteristic phenotype and by the tissue storage and urinary excretion of acid mucopolysaccharide (Table 83.3). They were originally regarded as a single disease, but eight clinical types and numerous subtypes are now known. Each is caused by deficiency of a lysosomal hydrolase enzyme required for degradation of one or more of three sulfated mucopolysaccharides: dermatan sulfate, heparan sulfate, and keratan sulfate (Fig. 83.2).

Diagnosis is based on the clinical picture, excessive amounts of one or more acid mucopolysaccharides in urine, and the presence of the enzyme defect. Urine screening tests for excess mucopolysaccharide are useful but show both false-positive and false-negative results. Positive screening tests require confirmation by quantitative and qualitative determination of urinary mucopolysaccharides, radiographic and histologic evidence of tissue storage, and demonstration of the enzyme defect. Screening tests may be falsely negative, especially in Sanfilippo and Morquio syndromes. If clinical suspicion of mucopolysaccharidosis is strong, diagnostic evaluation should be pursued even with a negative urine screening test. Prenatal diagnosis of these disorders is possible.

Hurler Syndrome

This is the most severe of the mucopolysaccharidoses, characterized by onset in infancy, progressive disability, and death usually occurring before 10 years of age. Nearly all the features found in other types are present in Hurler syndrome. Corneal clouding and lumbar gibbus are noted in the first year of life. Patients develop stiff joints with periarticular swelling, short stubby hands and feet, claw hands, lumbar lordosis, chest deformity, and dwarfing, which are usually apparent by 2 or 3 years of age. The facial features become coarsened and grotesque, with thickened eyelids and lips, frontal bossing, bushy eyebrows, depressed nasal bridge, hypertelorism, enlarged tongue, noisy breathing, rhinorrhea, and widely spaced peglike teeth. Mental retardation and deterioration, but not seizures, are noted. Deafness is frequent. Few patients develop speech. Leptomeningeal thickening, arachnoid cysts, and hydrocephalus may occur. Cardiac murmurs due to valvular heart disease, coronary occlusion, and cardiac enlargement may occur and cause death. Abdominal distention is commonly noted, with inguinal and umbilical hernias and hepatomegaly. Corneal clouding becomes progressively more severe and, with retinal degeneration, impairs vision. Cervical cord compression with quadriplegia may occur.

Radiographic changes are often helpful for the diagnosis of mucopolysaccharidosis but do not reliably distinguish the various types. These changes include ovoid or beaked lumbar vertebrae, peg-shaped metacarpals, a J-shaped sella turcica, and spatulate ribs. Peripheral leukocytes and bone marrow cells contain metachromatic granules. Clear vacuoles are seen in liver cells and cells of other tissues. Zebra bodies containing lipids occur in the brain. Both dermatan sulfate and heparan sulfate (Fig. 83.2) are stored. α-L-Iduronidase (reaction 11, Fig. 83.2), required for degradation of both, is deficient. The diagnosis is made by demonstrating severe deficiency of α-L-iduronidase in cultured skin fibroblasts and leukocytes. The α-L-iduronidase gene is located on the short arm of chromosome 4.

Scheie syndrome (MPS IS), a milder allelic variant of Hurler syndrome, is characterized by juvenile onset of stiff joints with the development of claw hands and deformed feet. Corneal clouding causes visual impairment; corneal grafts may become opacified. Other features are pigmentary degeneration of the retina, glaucoma, coarse facial features, genu valgus, carpal tunnel syndrome, and involvement of the aortic valve. Deafness may occur. Stature and intelligence are normal. Psychologic disturbances have been noted. Lifespan may be normal unless cardiac involvement becomes severe. A phenotype intermediate between that of the Hurler and Scheie syndromes is referred to as the Hurler-Scheie compound. Distinction from other α-L-iduronidase deficiency disorders is solely on clinical grounds.

TABLE 83.3. MUCOPOLYSACCHARIDOSES

Syndrome number	Syndrome name	Stored material	Deficient enzyme	Reaction number[a]	Mental defect	Cloudy corneas	Hearing loss	Coarse facial features	Dwarfing	Dysostosis multiplex	Heart disease	Organomegaly	Other features
MPS IH	Hurler	DS,HS	α-L-Iduronidase	11	3+	3+	2+	3+	3+	3+	3+	3+	Cord compression Pigmentary retinopathy
MPS IH/S	Hurler-Scheie compound	DS,HS	α-L-Iduronidase	11	±	3+		2+	1+	2+	1+	2+	Severe arachnoid cysts Pigmentary retinopathy
MPS IS	Scheie	DS	α-L-Iduronidase	11	0	3+	±	±	0	1+	1+	±	Carpal tunnel syndrome
MPS II A	Hunter (severe)	DS,HS	Iduronate-2-sulfate sulfatase	12	+	0	3+	2+	2+	2+	±	1+	Nodular skin lesions Pigmentary retinopathy
MPS II B	Hunter (mild)	DS,HS	Iduronate-2-sulfate sulfatase	12	0	0	2+	1+	1+	1+	±	±	Carpal tunnel syndrome Nodular skin lesions
MPS III A	Sanfilippo A	HS	Sulfamidase	13	3+	0	2+	1+	0	1+	1+	1+	Retinal degeneration May have seizures
MPS III B	Sanfilippo B	HS	α-N-acetylglucosaminidase	14	3+	0	2+	1+	0	1+	1+	1+	Retinal degeneration
MPS III C	Sanfilippo C	HS	N-acetyltransferase	15	3+	0	2+	1+	0	1+	1+	1+	
MPS III D	Sanfilippo D	HS,KS	N-acetylglucosamine-6-sulfate sulfatase	19	2+	0	1+	0	1+	1+	0	1+	Odontoid hypoplasia
MPS IV A	Morquio A	KS	Galactose-6-sulfate sulfatase	16	0	2+	2+	1+	3+	3+	2+	±	Cord compression Odontoid hypoplasia
MPS IV B	Morquio B	KS,OLS	β-Galactosidase	2	0	1+	0	0	0	2+	0	0	
MPS V	Category vacant	—											
MPS VI A	Maroteaux-Lamy (severe)	DS	Sulfatase B	17	0	2+	2+	2+	2+	2+	2+	±	Cord compression Carpal tunnel syndrome Hydrocephalus
MPS VI B	Maroteaux-Lamy (intermediate)	DS	Sulfatase B	17	0	2+		±	1+	2+	2+	0	Carpal tunnel syndrome
MPS VI C	Maroteaux-Lamy (mild)	DS	Sulfatase B	17	0	1+		±	1+	1+	1+	0	Cord compression Carpal tunnel syndrome
MPS VII	Sly	DS,HS	β-Glucuronidase	18	2+	±		1+	2+	2+	1+	1+	Hydrocephalus

[a]See Figs 83.1 through 83.3. OLS, oligosaccharide; MPS, mucopolysaccharide; KS, keratan sulfate; DS, dermatan sulfate; HS, heparan sulfate.

Hunter Syndrome (MPS II)

There are at least two forms, mild and severe. Both are X-linked recessive and show iduronate-2-sulfatase deficiency (reaction 12, Fig. 83.2). A Hunter-like phenotype in girls with iduronate-2-sulfatase deficiency is due to total sulfatase deficiency (MLD, Austin type).

Boys with the severe form have juvenile onset of joint stiffness, coarse facial features, dysostosis multiplex, hepatosplenomegaly, diarrhea, dwarfing, and mental deterioration. Progressive deafness is prominent. Pigmentary retinal deterioration, papilledema, and hydrocephalus may be seen. Nodular or pebbled skin change over the scapulae and absence of corneal clouding are important features distinguishing Hunter from Hurler syndrome. Patients usually die by age 15 years.

Patients with the mild form of Hunter syndrome may be asymptomatic. They have short stature, joint stiffness and limitation of motion, coarse features, and hepatosplenomegaly. They may have hernias and carpal tunnel syndrome. Intelligence is normal, but they may develop papilledema and neurologic deterioration late in the course. Lifespan may be normal.

Diagnosis is by finding excess urinary dermatan sulfate and heparan sulfate (Fig. 83.2) and demonstration of iduronate-2-sulfatase deficiency (reaction 12, Fig. 83.2) in serum or cultured skin fibroblasts.

Sanfilippo Syndrome (MPS III)

Patients with this syndrome have prominent mental involvement, mild somatic involvement, and urinary excretion of heparan sulfate alone. Four biochemically distinct forms reflect four metabolic steps required for the degradation of heparan sulfate but not that of dermatan sulfate or keratan sulfate. These patients have the juvenile onset of mental deterioration with delay or deterioration of speech or school performance. On evaluation for psychiatric disorder, mental retardation, or dementia, the examiner notes mild coarsening of facial features, hepatosplenomegaly, hirsutism, joint stiffness, and radiographic changes of dysostosis multiplex. These patients deteriorate neurologically with progressive dementia, spastic quadriparesis, tetraballism, athetosis, incontinence, and seizures. Cardiac involvement may occur. Corneal clouding is absent. Bone changes, dwarfing, and organ enlargement are slight. Patients may die in adolescence or survive into the third decade.

The diagnosis is made by the characteristic clinical picture, excess heparan sulfaturia, and demonstration of the enzyme defect. Urinary screening tests for mucopolysacchariduria may be negative in Sanfilippo syndrome.

In Sanfilippo syndrome type A, the enzyme heparan sulfate N-sulfatase (sulfamidase; reaction 13, Fig. 83.2) is deficient. In type B, α-N-acetylglucosaminidase (reaction 14, Fig. 83.2) is lacking. In type C, an N-acetyltransferase is deficient (reaction 15, Fig. 83.2); this enzyme acetylates the amino group from which sulfamidase removes the sulfate (reaction 13, Fig. 83.2), thus allowing the (N-acetylglucosaminidase (reaction 14, Fig. 83.2) to act. In type D, an N-acetylglucosamine-6-sulfatase is deficient (reaction 19, Fig. 83.2); this enzyme removes the 6-sulfate from N-acetylglucosamine in heparan sulfate and keratan sulfate. Type A is by far the most common.

Morquio Syndrome (MPS IV)

This mucopolysaccharidosis is characterized by a severe skeletal disorder, little neurologic abnormality, and the urinary excretion of keratan sulfate (Fig. 83.2). Two biochemically distinct forms are known, reflecting the two metabolic steps specifically required to degrade keratan sulfate.

Skeletal manifestations appear in the first year, as in Hurler syndrome, but corneal clouding is not prominent (corneas usually become mildly cloudy). Patients develop severe dwarfing, pectus carinatum joint laxity, knock knees, short neck, sensorineural deafness, abnormal facies, and hepatosplenomegaly. Intelligence is normal. Because of odontoid process hypoplasia and joint laxity, atlantoaxial subluxation may cause cervical cord compression even in young children; this may be prevented by posterior spinal fusion. Cardiac or respiratory disease may cause death in the third or fourth decade.

The diagnosis of type A is made by finding excess urinary keratan sulfate and that of type B by finding excess urinary oligosaccharides as well. Patients with type A Morquio syndrome lack an enzyme that cleaves 60 sulfate groups from galactose-6-sulfate (reaction 16, Fig. 83.2) and N-acetylgalactosamine-6-sulfate, causing the storage of keratan sulfate (which contains galactose-6-sulfate) and chondroitin-6-sulfate (which contains acetylgalactosamine-6-sulfate). The milder type B form of Morquio syndrome is caused by deficiency of β-galactosidase (reaction 2, Fig. 83.2), the same enzyme that is deficient in GM1-gangliosidosis. Presumably, the Morquio mutation severely affects the enzyme's ability to cleave the β-galactoside linkage in keratan sulfate but leaves sufficient activity against that linkage in GM1-ganglioside to prevent brain disease.

Maroteaux-Lamy Syndrome (MPS VI)

This syndrome resembles MPS type I syndrome because of the prominent skeletal disease, but intelligence is normal, and the predominant urinary mucopolysaccharide is dermatan sulfate. It is distinguished from Scheie syndrome by the affected patient's short stature.

At least three forms of Maroteaux-Lamy syndrome are known, all with deficiency of N-acetylgalactosamine-4-sulfate sulfatase or arylsulfatase B (reaction 17, Fig. 83.2). In the severe form, growth retardation is noted by 2 or 3 years of age. Coarse facial features, marked corneal clouding, and severe skeletal disease develop. Valvular heart disease and heart failure develop. Intelligence is normal, but neurologic complications include hydrocephalus and cervical cord compression resulting from hypoplasia of the odontoid process. Patients may survive into the second or third decade. In milder forms, cervical cord compression and carpal tunnel syndrome may occur.

MUCOLIPIDOSES

The mucolipidoses (Table 83.4) resemble the Hurler phenotype but lack excess urinary mucopolysaccharide, having instead excess urinary oligosaccharides or glycopeptides, most of which are fragments of more complex structures (Fig. 83.3). Urinary thin-

TABLE 83.4. MUCOLIPIDOSES

Clinical disorder	Defective enzyme (reaction number)[a]	Stored material	Clinical features
Sialidoses		GP, OLS, ? ganglioside	
Sialidoses with isolated sialidase deficiency			
Congenital sialidosis	Oligosaccharide sialidase (1)		Premature birth, congenital hydrops fetalis, organomegaly, severe mental and motor defect, death 0–5mo
Severe infantile sialidosis	Oligosaccharide sialidase (1)		Similar to congenital sialidosis, but with renal disease and survival until age 2
Nephrosialidosis	Oligosaccharide sialidase (1)		Onset age 4–6mo of organomegaly, facial dysmorphism and psychomotor retardation; progressive renal disease, macular cherry-red spot, and fine corneal opacities develop
Mucolipidosis I	Oligosaccharide sialidase (1)		Onset at age 6mo of mild Hurler-like facial and skeletal changes, corneal clouding, macular cherry-red spot, mental defect, myoclonic jerks, cerebellar syndrome, seizures, neuropathy
Macular cherry-red spot myoclonus syndrome	Oligosaccharide sialidase (1)		Onset around age 10yr of myoclonus, decreasing visual activity, and macular cherry-red spot; predilection for Italians
Sialidoses with additional β–galactosidase deficiency (galactosialidosis)			
Infantile sialidosis (GM$_1$-gangliosidosis phenotype)	Stabilizing protein for Oligosaccharide sialidase (1) and β-Galactosidase (2)		Same as GM$_1$-gangliosidosis
Goldberg syndrome	Stabilizing protein for Oligosaccharide sialidase (1) and β-galactosidase (2)		Similar to mucolipidosis I but juvenile or adolescent onset and slow progression, most common among Japanese
Salla disease	Sialic acid egress from lysosomes	Free sialic acid	Infantile onset of hypotonia, developmental delay; juvenile ataxia, mental and motor retardation, spasticity, athetosis, dysarthria, and sometimes convulsions; short stature
Fucosidosis	α-L-Fucosidase (21)	GP, OLS, fucolipids	Some resemble Hurler phenotype; some have coarse features and neurologic disorder resembling leukodystrophy
α-Mannosidosis	α-Mannosidase (22)	GP, OLS	Mild or severe disorder with mental defect, mild organomegaly, coarse features, and skeletal involvement; may have gingival hyperplasia, lenticular opacities, and survival into third decade
β-Mannosidosis	β-Mannosidase (23)	GP, OLS	Juvenile onset of mental retardation, speech delay, ± coarsened facial features, ± mild bony changes, ± angiokeratoma
Aspartylglycosaminuria	Aspartylglucosaminidase (25)	Aspartylglucosamine, OLS	Predilection for those of Finnish descent; characteristic facies, thickened skull, scoliosis, diarrhea, frequent respiratory infections, dementia, psychosis, and seizures
Mucolipidosis II (I-cell disease)	UDP-N-acetylgalactosamine-1-phosphate: glycoprotein N-acetylgalactosaminylphosphotransferase.	GP, OLS, MPS, ganglioside	Infantile onset of Hurler-like disorder, but corneas are usually clear
Mucolipidosis III (pseudopolydystrophy)	Same as mucolipidosis II	GP, OLS, MPS, ganglioside	Onset at age 2–4 of coarse facies, dwarfism, short neck, claw hands, shoulder stiffness; clear corneas, carpal tunnel syndrome, mental defect, and long survival
Mucolipidosis IV	?	GM3, GD3	Early infantile corneal clouding; juvenile mental and motor defect; Ashkenazi Jewish predilection

[a] See Figs. 82.1 through 82.3.
OLS, oligosaccharide; GP, glycoprotein; MPS, mucopolysaccharide; GM3, GM3-ganglioside; GD3, GD3-ganglioside.

layer chromatography for oligosaccharides is a useful screening test.

Sialidosis

Patients with sialidoses have deficiency of α-L-neuraminidase, also known as sialidase (reaction 1, Figs. 83.1B and 83.3). In most forms, sialic acid-containing glycoproteins, oligosaccharides, and glycolipids accumulate in tissue, and sialyloligosaccharides are excreted in urine.

The diagnosis is based on clinical findings; the presence of abnormal sialyloligosaccharides in the urine; and deficiency of the appropriate sialidase in cultured skin fibroblasts, tissue, or leukocytes. There are at least two distinct lysosomal sialidases, one that cleaves the (α2,3)-linked sialic acid in monosialoganglioside (reaction 8, Fig. 83.1B) and the other that cleaves (α2,3)-linked and (α2,6)-linked sialic acid in polysialogangliosides, oligosaccharides, and glycoproteins (reaction 1, Figs. 83.1B and 83.3). The latter enzyme is deficient in the other sialidoses. In addition to the isolated sialidase deficiencies, two other groups of mucolipidoses have sialidase deficiency. In one, galactosialidosis and both sialidase and β-galactosidase are deficient because a stabilizing protein they share is defective. In the second group, mucolipidosis II and III, sialidase, and several other lysosomal hydrolases are deficient.

Sialidoses with isolated sialidase deficiency have a highly variable clinical picture. Neonates with congenital sialidoses have hydrops fetalis, hepatosplenomegaly, and short survival times. They resemble infants with congenital lipidosis of Norman and Wood. Infants with nephrosialidosis resemble the Hurler phenotype and develop macular cherry-red spots and renal disease. Children with mucolipidosis I (lipomucopolysaccharidosis), a milder disorder, are similarly affected but develop ataxia, myoclonic jerks, and seizures. The mildest form is the cherry-red spot myoclonus disorder, in which adolescents, who are usually mentally normal, develop macular cherry-red spots, myoclonus, and myoclonic seizures. There is a predilection for individuals of Italian descent.

Galactosialidosis

Sialidosis with combined sialidase and β-galactosidase deficiency (galactosialidosis) includes two forms: an infantile disorder with the clinical phenotype of GM1-gangliosidosis and the Goldberg syndrome. The first disorder should be considered in any patient who is suspected of having GM1-gangliosidosis or is found to have β-galactosidase deficiency. Goldberg syndrome resembles mucolipidosis I but is milder with a predilection for those of Japanese origin; there is an adult form as well.

FREE SIALIC ACID STORAGE DISEASES

Onset of Salla disease is between ages 4 and 12 months with hypotonia, developmental delay, or both. Ataxia of trunk and limbs follows, and by age 2 years, there is mental and motor retardation. Patients are invariably severely mentally retarded and may never speak or walk. Usually, they develop spasticity, athetosis,

dysarthria, and sometimes convulsions. They are short, often with strabismus and with thickened calvaria. Ultrastructural analysis of blood lymphocytes, skin, and liver reveals abnormal lysosomal morphology. Free sialic acid is markedly increased in urine; defective sialic acid egress has been noted from isolated fibroblast lysosomes. There is a predilection for those of Finnish descent.

FUCOSIDOSIS

Some patients with fucosidosis have severe neurologic disease that resembles a leukodystrophy. Others with fucosidosis resemble the Hurler phenotype. Some have survived into the second or third decade. Fucose residues form part of the structure of oligosaccharides, glycoproteins, and glycolipids, including "fucogangliosides."

The diagnostic findings are excessive urinary abnormal oligosaccharides (Fig. 83.3) and by demonstrating severely decreased levels of α-L-fucosidase (reaction 21, Fig. 83.3) in serum, leukocytes, and cultured skin fibroblasts.

MANNOSIDOSES

α-Mannosidosis may be mild or severe. In severely affected patients, the diagnosis has been confused with mucolipidosis I. Other patients have slower progression of the disorder with greater dysmorphism, cataracts, and longer survival. Others have presented primarily with marked mental defect, striking gingival hyperplasia, and survival into the third decade or longer. Facial dysmorphism, skeletal involvement, and organ enlargement have been slight in these patients.

Diagnosis requires a high index of suspicion and findings of excessive abnormal urinary oligosaccharides and decreased α-mannosidase (reaction 22, Fig. 83.3) in leukocytes and cultured skin fibroblasts.

β-Mannosidosis, originally described in goats, was subsequently described in humans. One patient presented at 16 months with slowing of speech development and at 46 months had coarsened facial features, mild bone changes, speech delay, and mental retardation. Two brothers, aged 44 and 19 years, had angiokeratoma on the penis and scrotum; mental retardation from age 5 years or earlier; and no coarse features, organomegaly, or bone changes. Diagnosis was by lack of α-mannosidase in plasma, leukocytes, and fibroblasts and by presence of a mannose-containing disaccharide in urine. Interestingly, the first patient had absent sulfamidase, low sulfamidase in one parent, and urinary mucopolysaccharide excretion identical to that in Sanfilippo syndrome, type A, a clinically similar disorder.

ASPARTYLGLYCOSAMINURIA

Aspartylglycosaminuria occurs almost solely in Finland. Patients have juvenile onset of somatic and mental changes. Somatic changes include coarse facial features, anteverted nostrils, short neck, and scoliosis. Intellectual deterioration leads to severe mental defect in the adult. Episodic hyperactivity, psychotic behavior, and seizures may occur.

Patients excrete large amounts of aspartylglucosamine in their urine because of deficiency of N-aspartyl-β-glucosaminidase (reaction 25, Fig. 83.3). Diagnostic findings are aspartylglucosamine in the urine and deficiency of N-aspartyl-β-glucosaminidase (reaction 25, Fig. 83.3) in cultured skin fibroblasts.

MUCOLIPIDOSES II AND III

Mucolipidosis II (I-cell disease) is a severe disorder that resembles Hurler syndrome but the patient's corneas are clear. Cultured fibroblasts have coarse inclusions (I-cells). Diagnosis is made by finding excess sialo-oligosaccharides in the urine and deficiencies of multiple lysosomal enzymes in cultured skin fibroblasts with elevated levels of these enzymes in plasma. In brain and viscera, only β-galactosidase is consistently deficient. The basic defect is deficiency of the enzyme, UDP-N-acetylglucosamine: glycoprotein N-acetylglucosaminylphosphotransferase. This enzyme attaches the N-acetylglucosamine-1-phosphate of UDPGlcNAc1P to the 6-position of α-linked mannose residues of glycoproteins. The N-acetylglucosamine is subsequently removed to leave a mannose-6-phosphate residue, an important recognition marker for uptake of certain glycoproteins (including many lysosomal hydrolase enzymes) into the cell.

Mucolipidosis III (pseudo-Hurler polydystrophy) is a milder clinical disorder than mucolipidosis II but is caused by a deficiency of the same enzyme. Diagnosis is made as for mucolipidosis II.

MUCOLIPIDOSIS IV

Patients with mucolipidosis IV present with corneal clouding as early as 6 weeks of age. Mild retardation progresses to severe mental and motor defect. There is a predilection for those of Ashkenazi Jewish descent. Diagnosis is by the clinical picture, light microscopic findings (lipid-laden marrow histiocytes), and electron microscopic findings (vacuoles and membranous bodies in skin, conjunctiva, and cultured fibroblasts).

Gangliosides GM3 and GD3 (Fig. 83.1B) accumulate in fibroblasts. Soluble ganglioside sialidase (reaction 8, Fig. 83.1B) is reportedly deficient but the basic defect is unknown.

SUGGESTED READINGS

Lysosomal Diseases

Gieselmann V. Lysosomal storage diseases [Review]. *Biochim Biophys Acta* 1995;1270:103–136.

Lipidoses and Leukodystrophies

Berger J, Loschl B, Bernheimer H, et al. Occurrence, distribution, and phenotype of arylsulfatase A mutations in patients with metachromatic leukodystrophy. *Am J Med Genet* 1997;69:335–340.
Beutler E. Enzyme replacement therapy for Gaucher's disease [Review]. *Bailliere Clin Haematol* 1997;10:751–763.

Beutler E. Gaucher disease [Review]. *Curr Opin Hematol* 1997;4:19–23.
Brady RO. Gaucher's disease: past, present and future [Review]. *Bailliere Clin Haematol* 1997;10:621–634.
Chen W, Kubota S, Teramoto T, et al. Genetic analysis enables definite and rapid diagnosis of cerebrotendinous xanthomatosis. *Neurology* 1998;51:865–867.
Crutchfield KE, Patronas NJ, Dambrosia JM, et al. Quantitative analysis of cerebral vasculopathy in patients with Fabry disease. *Neurology* 1998;50:1746–1749.
Eng CM, Ashley GA, Burgert TS, et al. Fabry disease: thirty five mutations in the alpha-galactosidase A gene in patients with classic and variant phenotypes. *Mol Med* 1997;3:174–182.
Goebel HH, Sharp JD. The neuronal ceroid-lipofuscinoses. Recent advances. *Brain Pathol* 1998;8:151–162.
Grabowski GA, Horowitz M. Gaucher's disease: molecular, genetic and enzymological aspects [Review]. *Bailliere Clin Haematol* 1997;10:635–656.
Greer WL, Riddell DC, Gillan TL, et al. The Nova Scotia (type D) form of Niemann-Pick disease is caused by a G3097>T transversion in NPC1. *Am J Hum Genet* 1998;63:52–54.
Jan MM, Camfield PR. Nova Scotia Niemann-Pick disease (type D): clinical study of 20 cases. *J Child Neurol* 1998;13:758.
Kaye EM, Shalish C, Livermore J, et al. Beta-galactosidase gene mutations in patients with slowly progressive GM1 gangliosidosis [Review]. *J Child Neurol* 1997;12:24–27.
Koch J, Gartner S, Li CM, et al. Molecular cloning and characterization of a full-length complementary DNA encoding human acid ceramidase (Farber disease). *J Biol Chem* 1996;271:33110–33115.
Mitchison HM, Hofmann SL, Becerra CH, et al. Mutations in the palmitoylprotein thioesterase gene (PPT; CLN1) causing juvenile neuronal ceroid lipofuscinosis with granular osmiophilic deposits. *Hum Mol Genet* 1998;7:291–297.
Myerowitz R. Tay-Sachs disease-causing mutations and neutral polymorphisms in the Hex A gene [Review]. *Hum Mutat* 1997;9:195–208.
Nowaczyk MJ, Feigenbaum A, Silver MM, et al. Bone marrow involvement and obstructive jaundice in Farber lipogranulomatosis: clinical and autopsy report of a new case. *J Inherit Metab Dis* 1996;19:655–660.
Pagani F, Pariyarath R, Garcia R, et al. New lysosomal acid lipase gene mutants explain the phenotype of Wolman disease and cholesteryl ester storage disease. *J Lipid Res* 1998;39:1382–1388.
Schmidt B, Selmer T, Ingendoh A, et al. A novel amino acid modification in sulfatases that is defective in multiple sulfatase deficiency. *Cell* 1995;82:271–278.
Tylki-Szymanska AT, Czartoryska B, Lugowska A. Practical suggestions in diagnosing etachromatic leukodystrophy in probands and in testing family members. *Eur Neurol* 1998;40:67–70.
van Heijst AF, Verrips A, Wevers RA, et al. Treatment and follow-up of children with cerebrotendinous xanthomatosis. *Eur J Pediatr* 1998;157:31–36.
Wenger DA, Rafi MA, Luzi P. Molecular genetics of Krabbe disease (globoid cell leukodystrophy): diagnostic and clinical implications [Review]. *Hum Mutat* 1997;10:268–279.

Mucopolysaccharidoses and Mucolipidoses

Alkhayat AH, Kraemer SA, Leipprandt JR, et al. Human beta-mannosidase cDNA characterization and first identification of a mutation associated with human beta-mannosidosis. *Hum Mol Genet* 1998;7:75–83.
Beck M, Barone R, Hoffmann R, et al. Inter and intrafamilial variability in mucolipidosis II (I-cell disease). *Clin Genet* 1995;47:191–199.
Chen CS, Bach G, Pagano RE. Abnormal transport along the lysosomal pathway in mucolipidosis, type IV disease. *Proc Natl Acad Sci USA* 1998;95:637–638.
Leppanen P, Isosomppi J, Schleutker J, et al. A physical map of the 6q14q15 region harboring the locus for the lysosomal membrane sialic acid transport defect (Salla disease and infantile free sialic acid storage disease). *Genomics* 1996;37:62–67.
Nilssen O, Berg T, Riise HM, et al. Alpha-mannosidosis: functional cloning of the lysosomal alpha-mannosidase cDNA and identification of a mutation in two affected siblings. *Hum Mol Genet* 1997;6:717–726.
Peltola M, Tikkanen R, Peltonen L, et al. Ser72Pro active-site disease mu-

tation in human lysosomal aspartylglucosaminidase: abnormal intracellular processing and evidence for extracellular activation. *Hum Mol Genet* 1996;5:737–743.

Pshezhetsky AV, Richard C, Michaud L, et al. Cloning, expression and chromosomal mapping of human lysosomal sialidase and characterization of mutations in sialidosis. *Nat Genet* 1997;15:316–320.

Richard C, Tranchemontagne J, Elsliger MA, et al. Molecular pathology of galactosialidosis in a patient affected with two new frameshift mutations in the cathepsin A/protective protein gene. *Hum Mutat* 1998;11:461–469.

Umehara F, Matsumoto W, Kuriyama M, et al. Mucolipidosis III (pseudo-Hurler polydystrophy); clinical studies in aged patients in one family. *J Neurol Sci* 1997;146:167–172.

Wraith JE. The mucopolysaccharidoses: a clinical review and guide to management [Review]. *Arch Dis Child* 1995;72:26–37.

Merritt's Neurology, 10th ed., edited by L.P. Rowland. Lippincott Williams & Wilkins, Philadelphia © 2000.

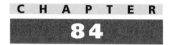

CHAPTER 84

DISORDERS OF CARBOHYDRATE METABOLISM

SALVATORE DIMAURO

GLYCOGEN STORAGE DISEASES

Abnormal metabolism of glycogen and glucose may occur in a series of genetically determined disorders, each representing a specific enzyme deficiency (Table 84.1). The signs and symptoms of each disease are largely determined by the tissues in which the enzyme defect is expressed. Virtually all enzymes of glycogen metabolism, including tissue-specific isoforms or subunits, have been assigned to chromosomal loci and the corresponding genes have been cloned and sequenced. Numerous mutations have been identified and a genotype-phenotype correlation is taking shape. The disorders affecting the neuromuscular system primarily are discussed in Section XVIII.

Severe fasting hypoglycemia may result in periodic episodes of lethargy, coma, convulsions, and anoxic brain damage in glucose-6-phosphatase deficiency (glycogenosis type I) or in glycogen synthetase deficiency. The liver is enlarged in both diseases. Clinical manifestations tend to become milder in patients who survive the first few years of life.

The nervous system is directly affected by the enzyme defect in generalized glycogen storage diseases, even though neurologic symptoms are lacking in some disorders and in others may be ascribed to liver rather than to brain dysfunction. The following enzyme defects seem to be generalized: acid maltase (type II), debrancher (type III), brancher (type IV), and phosphoglycerate kinase (type IX).

In the infantile form of acid maltase deficiency (Pompe disease), pathologic involvement of the central nervous system (CNS) has been documented, with accumulation of both free and intralysosomal glycogen in all cells, especially spinal motor neurons and neurons of the brainstem nuclei. Peripheral nerve biopsy specimens show accumulation of glycogen in Schwann cells. The profound generalized weakness of infants with Pompe disease is probably due to combined effects of glycogen storage in muscle, anterior horn cells, and peripheral nerves. In the childhood form of acid maltase deficiency, increased glycogen

deposition was seen in two children (one of whom was mentally retarded) but not in two other patients. No morphologic changes were seen in the CNS of a patient with adult-onset acid maltase deficiency despite marked decrease of enzyme activity.

Patients with debrancher deficiency (glycogenosis type III) have hepatomegaly, fasting hypoglycemia, and seizures in infancy and childhood, which usually remit around puberty. Although overt signs of peripheral neuropathy are rare, abnormal deposits of glycogen have been documented both in axons and in Schwann cells and may explain, in part at least, the distal wasting and mixed electromyographic pattern observed in adult patients with neuromuscular involvement.

In branching enzyme deficiency (glycogenosis type IV), the clinical picture is dominated by liver disease, with progressive cirrhosis and chronic hepatic failure causing death in childhood. Deposits of a basophilic intensely periodic acid-Schiff (PAS)-positive material that is partially resistant to β-amylase digestion have been found in all tissues; in the CNS, spheroids composed of branched filaments were present in astrocytic processes, particularly in the spinal cord and medulla. Ultrastructurally, the storage material was composed of aggregates of branched osmiophilic filaments, 6 nm in diameter, often surrounded by normal glycogen particles.

In phosphoglycerate kinase (PGK) deficiency (glycogenosis type IX), type and severity of clinical manifestations vary in different genetic variants of the disease and are probably related to the severity of the enzyme defect in different tissues. In several families, the clinical picture was characterized by the association of severe hemolytic anemia with mental retardation and seizures.

LAFORA DISEASE AND OTHER POLYGLUCOSAN STORAGE DISEASES

Myoclonus epilepsy with Lafora bodies (Lafora disease) is a hereditary neurologic disease transmitted as an autosomal recessive trait and affects both sexes equally. Clinically, the disease is characterized by the triad of epilepsy, myoclonus, and dementia. Inconstant other neurologic manifestations include ataxia, dysarthria, spasticity, and rigidity. Onset is in adolescence, and the course progresses rapidly to death, which in 90% of patients occurs between 17 and 24 years of age. Negative criteria or manifestations that imply some other disease include onset before 6 or after age 20, optic atrophy, macular degeneration, prolonged course, or normal intelligence. Epilepsy, with generalized seizures, is the first manifestation in most patients; status epilepticus is common in terminal stages. Myoclonus usually appears 2

TABLE 84.1 CLASSIFICATION OF GLYCOGEN STORAGE DISEASE

Type	Affected tissues	Clinical presentation	Glycogen structure	Enzyme defect	Mode of transmission
I	Liver and kidney	Severe hypoglycemia; hepatomegaly	Normal	Glucose-6-phosphatase	AR
II					
Infancy	Generalized	Cardiomegaly; weakness; hypotonia; death < age 1yr	Normal		
Childhood	Generalized	Myopathy simulating Duchenne dystrophy; respiratory insufficiency	Normal	Acid maltase	AR
Adult	Generalized	Myopathy simulating limb-girdle dystrophy or polymyositis; respiratory insufficiency	Normal		
III	Generalized	Hepatomegaly; fasting hypoglycemia; progressive weakness	PLD	Debrancher	AR
IV	Generalized	Hepatosplenomegaly; cirrhosis of liver; hepatic failure	Longer peripheral chains; fewer branching points	Brancher	AR
V	Skeletal muscle	Intolerance to intense exercise; cramps; myoglobinuria	Normal	Muscle phosphorylase	AR
VI	Liver; RBC	Mild hypoglycemia; hepatomegaly	Normal	Liver phosphorylase	AR
VII	Skeletal muscle; RBC	Intolerance to intense exercise; cramps; myoglobinuria	Normal (± longer peripheral chains)	Muscle phosphofructokinase (PFK-M)	AR
VIII	Liver	Asymptomatic hepatomegaly	Normal	Phosphorylase kinase	XR
	Liver and skeletal muscle	Hepatomegaly; growth retardation; hypotonia	Normal	Phosphorylase kinase	AR
	Skeletal muscle	Exercise intolerance; myoglobinuria	Normal	Phosphorylase kinase	AR
	Heart	Fatal infantile cardiomyopathy	Normal	Phosphorylase kinase	AR
IX	Generalized	Hemolytic anemia; seizures; mental retardation Intolerance to intense exercise; myoglobinuria	Normal (?)	Phosphoglycerate kinase (PGK)	XR
X	Skeletal muscle	Intolerance to intense exercise; myoglobinuria	Normal (?)	Muscle phosphoglycerate mutase (PGAM-M)	AR
XI	Skeletal muscle	Intolerance to intense exercise; myoglobinuria	Normal (?)	Muscle lactate dehydrogenase (LDH-M)	AR
	Liver	Severe hypoglycemia; hepatomegaly		Glycogen synthetase	AR (?)

AR, autosomal recessive; XR, X-linked recessive; PLD, phosphorylase-limit dextrin.

or 3 years after the onset of epilepsy, may affect any area of the body, is sensitive to startle, and is absent during sleep. Intellectual deterioration generally follows the appearance of seizures by 2 or 3 years and progresses rapidly to severe dementia. Therapy is symptomatic and is designed to suppress seizures and reduce the severity of myoclonus; some control of myoclonus is achieved with benzodiazepines.

Laboratory findings are normal except for electroencephalographic changes; bilaterally synchronous discharges of wave-and-spike formations are commonly seen in association with myoclonic jerks. Electroencephalographic abnormalities may be found in asymptomatic relatives. The pathologic hallmark of the disease is the presence in the CNS of the bodies first described by Lafora in 1911: round, basophilic, strongly PAS-positive intracellular inclusions that vary in size from "dustlike" bodies less than 3 nm in diameter to large bodies up to 30 nm in diameter.

The medium and large bodies often show a dense core and a lighter periphery. Lafora bodies are seen only in neuronal perikarya and processe and are most numerous in cerebral cortex, substantia nigra, thalamus, globus pallidus, and dentate nucleus.

Ultrastructurally, Lafora bodies are not limited by a membrane. They consist of two components in various proportions: amorphous electron-dense granules and irregular filaments. The filaments, which are about 6 nm in diameter, are often branched and frequently continuous with the granular material.

Irregular accumulations of a material similar to that of the Lafora bodies are found in liver, heart, skeletal muscle, skin, and retina, suggesting that Lafora disease is a generalized storage disease. Both histochemical and biochemical criteria indicate that the storage material is a branched polysaccharide composed of glucose (polyglucosan) similar to the amylopectin-like polysaccharide that accumulates in branching enzyme deficiency. The activity of branching enzyme, however, was normal in several tissues, including brain, of patients with Lafora disease. Linkage analysis in nine families has localized the gene responsible for Lafora's disease to chromosome 6q, and by positional cloning, the gene product has been identified as a tyrosine phosphatase. Six mutations have been found in the nine families.

A clinically distinct form of polyglucosan body disease (*adult polyglucosan body disease* [APBD]) was described in patients with a complex but stereotyped chronic neurologic disorder characterized by progressive upper and lower motor neuron involvement, sensory loss, sphincter problems, neurogenic bladder, and, in about half of the cases, dementia; there is no myoclonus or epilepsy. Onset is in the fifth or sixth decade of life, and the course ranges from 3 to 20 years. Electrophysiologic studies show axonal neuropathy. In some cases, the clinical picture simulates amyotrophic lateral sclerosis. Throughout the CNS, polyglucosan bodies are present in processes of neurons and astrocytes but not in perikarya. There are also polyglucosan accumulations in peripheral nerve and in other tissues, including liver, heart, skeletal, and smooth muscle. As in debranching enzyme deficiency and Lafora disease, the abnormal polysaccharide in APBD seems to have longer peripheral chains than normal glycogen. Branching enzyme activity was markedly decreased in leukocytes from Israeli patients, and this finding was confirmed in both leukocytes and peripheral nerve specimens from American Ashkenazi Jewish patients, whereas the activity was normal in both tissues from three non-Jewish white patients and from one African-American patient, suggesting genetic heterogeneity. A mutation in the gene encoding the branching enzyme has been found in five Ashkenazi Jewish families with APBD, confirming that APBD is a clinical variant of branching deficiency.

Another form of polyglucosan is represented by corpora amylacea, which accumulate progressively and nonspecifically with age. They are more commonly seen within astrocytic processes in the hippocampus and in subpial and subependymal regions; however, they also occur in intramuscular nerves in patients older than 40.

SUGGESTED READINGS

Bigio EH, Weiner MF, Bonte FJ, White CL. Familial dementia due to adult polyglucosan body disease. *Clin Neuropathol* 1997;16:227–234.

Bruno C, Servidei S, Shanske S, et al. Glycogen branching enzyme deficiency in adult polyglucosan body disease. *Ann Neurol* 1993;33:88–93.

Coleman DL, Gambetti PL, DiMauro S. Muscle in Lafora disease. *Arch Neurol* 1974;31:396–406.

DiMauro S, Servidei S, Tsujino S. Disorders of carbohydrate metabolism: Glycogen storage diseases. In: Rosenberg RN, Prusiner SB, DiMauro S, Barchi RL, eds. *The molecular and genetic basis of neurological disease.* Boston: Butterworth-Heinemann, 1997:1067–1097.

DiMauro S, Stern LZ, Mehler M, et al. Adult-onset acid maltase deficiency: a postmortem study. *Muscle Nerve* 1978;1:27–36.

DiMauro S, Tsujino S, Shanske S, Rowland LP. Biochemistry and molecular genetics of human glycogenoses: an overview. *Muscle Nerve* 1995;3:S10–S17.

Felice KJ, Grunnet ML, Rao KR, Wolfson LI. Childhood-onset spinocerebellar syndrome associated with massive polyglucosan body deposition. *Acta Neurol Scand* 1997;95:60–64.

Gambetti PL, DiMauro S, Baker L. Nervous system in Pompe's disease. *J Neuropath Exp Neurol* 1971;30:412–430.

Gambetti PL, DiMauro S, Hirt L, Blume RP. Myoclonic epilepsy with Lafora bodies. *Arch Neurol* 1971;25:483–493.

Lafora GR. Uber das Vorkommen amyloider Korperchen in Innern der Ganglienzellen. *Virchows Arch Pathol Anat* 1911;205:295–303.

Lossos A, Barash V, Soffer D, et al. Hereditary branching enzyme dysfunction in adult polyglucosan body disease: a possible cause in two patients. *Ann Neurol* 1991;30:655–662.

Lossos A, Meiner Z, Barash V, et al. Adult polyglucosan body disease in Ashkenazi Jewish patients carrying the Tyr329 mutation in the glycogen branching gene. *Ann Neurol* 1998;44:867–872.

McDonald ID, Faust PL, Bruno C, et al. Polyglucosan body disease simulating amyotrophic lateral sclerosis. *Neurology* 1993;43:785–790.

McMaster KR, Powers JM, Hennigar GR, et al. Nervous system involvement in type IV glycogenosis. *Arch Pathol Lab Med* 1979;103:105–111.

Minassian BA, Lee JR, Herbrick J-A, et al. Mutations in a gene encoding a novel protein tyrosine phosphatase cause progressive myoclonus epilepsy. *Nat Genet* 1998;20:171–174.

Peress NS, DiMauro S, Roxburgh VA. Adult polysaccharidosis. *Arch Neurol* 979;36:840–845.

Robitaille Y, Carpenter S, Karpati G, DiMauro S. A distinct form of adult polyglucosan body disease with massive involvement of central and peripheral neuronal processes and astrocytes. *Brain* 1980;103:315–336.

Sakai M, Austin J, Witmer F, Trueb L. Studies of corpora amylacea. *Arch Neurol* 1969;21:526–544.

Sakai M, Austin J, Witmer F, Trueb L. Studies in myoclonus epilepsy (Lafora body form). II. Polyglucosans in the systemic deposits of myoclonus epilepsy and in corpora amylacea. *Neurology* 1970;20:160–176.

Serratosa JM, Delgado-Escueta AV, Posada I, et al. The gene for progressive myoclonus epilepsy of the Lafora type maps to chromosome 6q. *Hum Mol Genet* 1995;4:1657–1663.

Spencer-Peet J, Norman ME, Lake BD, et al. Hepatic glycogen storage disease. *Q J Med* 1971;40:95–114.

Tarui S. Glycolytic defects in muscle: aspects of collaboration between basic science and clinical medicine. *Muscle Nerve* 1995;3:S2–S9.

Ugawa Y, Inoue K, Takemura T, Iwamasa T. Accumulation of glycogen in sural nerve axons in adult-onset type III glycogenosis. *Ann Neurol* 1986;19:294–297.

Merritt's Neurology, 10th ed., edited by L.P. Rowland. Lippincott Williams & Wilkins, Philadelphia © 2000.

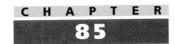

CHAPTER 85

GLUCOSE TRANSPORTER PROTEIN SYNDROME

DARRYL C. DE VIVO

CLINICAL SYNDROME

In 1991, De Vivo et al. described two children with infantile seizures, delayed motor and behavioral development, acquired microcephaly, ataxia, and hypotonia. Lumbar puncture revealed low cerebrospinal fluid glucose concentrations (hypoglycorrhachia) and low-normal to low cerebrospinal fluid lactate concentrations (Table 85.1). Since 1991, 26 additional patients have been identified. The dominant clinical features are shown in Table 85.2.

Seizures begin in early infancy, and the seizure types vary with age of the patient. In infancy, the dominant seizure types include behavioral arrest, pallor and cyanosis, and eye deviation. The electroencephalographic correlates are focal spikes, commonly originating in the temporal and posterior cerebral quadrants. In childhood, the seizures change in character and typically include astatic seizures, atypical absence seizures, and generalized tonic-clonic seizures. The electroencephalogram shows a generalized spike-wave pattern. The seizures are refractory to antiepileptic drugs but respond promptly and dramatically to a ketogenic diet.

LABORATORY DATA

Diagnosis requires awareness of the clinical manifestations and documentation of hypoglycorrhachia. A low or low-normal cerebrospinal fluid lactate concentration strengthens the presumptive diagnosis. Glucose uptake rates *in vitro* by intact washed erythrocytes are decreased by approximately 50% in patients. DNA studies may be diagnostic in 10% to 15% of cases.

MOLECULAR GENETICS AND PATHOGENESIS

D-Glucose is the obligate fuel for brain metabolism under virtually all circumstances. With acute or chronic fasting, the brain

TABLE 85.2. GLUCOSE TRANSPORTER PROTEIN SYNDROME: CLINICAL FEATURES

Symptoms	Frequency (%)
Seizures	100
Language delay	100
Motor delay	81
Microcephaly	75
Hypotonia	56
Ataxia	50
Spasticity	25
Hypoglycorrhachia	100

Seizures begin in early infancy.

adapts metabolically to use ketone bodies (β-hydroxybutyrate and acetoacetate) in partial lieu of glucose. However, glucose is necessary as a permissive substrate for brain ketone body utilization under these extreme physiologic conditions. The transport of D-glucose across the blood–brain barrier and into brain cells is selectively mediated by a sodium-independent facilitative mechanism. The protein that facilitates glucose transport across these tissue barriers is glucose transporter-1 (GLUT-1), a member of a multigene family of protein transporters that facilitate the diffusion of sugar molecules across tissue barriers. GLUT-1 is present in high abundance in brain capillaries, astroglial cells, and erythrocyte membranes.

The molecular basis of the syndrome is haploinsufficiency of the GLUT-1 protein. Haploinsufficiency has been determined in 18 patients by Wang and De Vivo (unpublished data). Three patients are hemizygous as determined by a positive fluorescent *in situ* hybridization study. The other 15 patients are heterozygous for nonsense mutations, missense mutations, frameshift mutations, or splice site mutations. These mutations are distributed throughout the gene, and each mutation is unique for the patient. The GLUT-1 cDNA is highly conserved across species, with 97% homology among humans, rats, mice, and rabbits. The highly conserved nature of the gene increases the likelihood of pathogenicity related to small-scale rearrangements.

The GLUT-1 protein is responsible for the transport of glucose across both luminal and abluminal sides of the brain capillary endothelial cell and across the astroglial plasma membrane. GLUT-1 haploinsufficiency may cause a severe decrease in the concentration of glucose in the brain interstitial space and in the astroglial cell. This syndrome is the first genetically determined defect involving the blood–brain barrier, but it was not familial in any of the first 24 patients studied. One German family transmitted the disease through three successive generations as an autosomal dominant trait. The molecular basis has not yet been determined.

DIAGNOSIS

The differential diagnosis includes cerebral palsy, Rett syndrome, hypoglycemia, infantile ataxia, and mitochondrial diseases. Seizures have been present in all cases, but this observation may represent an ascertainment bias. A lumbar puncture for

TABLE 85.1. CSF GLUCOSE AND LACTATE VALUES (MEAN + S.E.M)

		Glucose (mg/dl)		Lactate (mM/L)
	n	CSF	CSF/blood	CSF
Disease controls	318	62±0.96	0.65±0.01	1.3±0.07
GTPS	10	30.5±0.32	0.33±0.01	0.97±0.03

Values are mean ± SEM.
GTPS, glucose transporter protein syndrome; CSF, cerebrospinal fluid.

measurement of glucose and lactate is a critical test in establishing the diagnosis.

TREATMENT

Treatment is the ketogenic diet, which effectively controls the seizures but is less effective in improving cognition and behavior. Antiepileptic drugs have been uniformly ineffective. Thioctic acid may facilitate glucose transport and has been recommended as adjunctive therapy.

SUGGESTED READINGS

Bell IG, Burant CF, Takeda J, Gould GW. Structure and function of mammalian facilitative sugar transporters. *J Biol Chem* 1993; 268:19161–19164.

De Vivo DC, Garcia-Alvarez M, Roonen G, Trifiletti R. Glucose transport protein deficiency. An emerging syndrome with therapeutic implications. *Int Pediatr* 1995;10:51–56.

De Vivo DC, Garcia-Alvarez M, Tritschler HJ. Deficiency of glucose transporter protein type I: possible therapeutic role for alpha-lipoic acid (thioctic acid). *Diabetes Stoffwech* 1996;5:36–40.

De Vivo DC, Trifiletti RR, Jacobson RI, Ronen GM, Behmand RA, Harik SI. Defective glucose transport across the blood-brain barrier as a cause of persistent hypoglycorrhachia, seizures, and developmental delay. *N Engl J Med* 1991;325:703–709.

Pardridge WM, Boado RJ, Farrell CR. Brain-type glucose transporter (Glut-1) is selectively localized to the blood-brain barrier. *J Biol Chem* 1990;265:18035–18040.

Seidner G, Garcia-Alvarez M, Jeh J-I, et al. GLUT-1 deficiency syndrome caused by haploinsufficiency of the blood-brain barrier hexose carrier. *Nat Genet* 1998;18:188–191.

Vannucci SJ, Maher F, Simpson IA. Glucose transporter proteins in brain: delivery of glucose to neurons and glia. *Glia* 1997;21:2–21.

Merritt's Neurology, 10th ed., edited by L.P. Rowland. Lippincott Williams & Wilkins, Philadelphia © 2000.

C H A P T E R

86

HYPERAMMONEMIA

ROSARIO R. TRIFILETTI
DOUGLAS R. NORDLI, JR.

Hyperammonemia, an elevation in blood ammonia levels, has many causes (Table 86.1). The hepatic urea cycle is the major mammalian system for the detoxification of ammonia (Fig. 86.1), and defects have been described in all six urea cycle enzymes. An additional pathway from arginine to citrulline generates the putative second messenger and neurotransmitter, nitric oxide, catalyzed by nitric oxide synthetase. The enzyme is found in many tissues, including brain. The significance of this pathway is not yet clear, but it may be perturbed in urea cycle disorders.

The differential diagnosis of hyperammonemia differs considerably according to the age of the patient (Table 86.1).

HYPERAMMONEMIA IN THE NEONATAL PERIOD

Transient hyperammonemia of the newborn is occasionally seen in otherwise well premature infants and is attributed to metabolic immaturity, analogous to physiologic hyperbilirubinemia of the newborn. Transient hyperammonemia of the newborn is mild and reversible and rarely requires treatment. Hyperammonemia also may result from liver damage associated with birth asphyxia or congenital hepatic disease; the birth history may help to establish the diagnosis.

TABLE 86.1. MAJOR CAUSES OF HYPERAMMONEMIA

Newborn period
　Asymptomatic infant
　　Transient hyperammonemia of the newborn
　Asymptomatic at birth; symptomatic after 24–72h protein feeding
　　Organic acidurias
　　　Methylmalonic acidemia
　　　Propionic acidemia
　　　Isovaleric acidemia
　　　Multiple carboxylase (biotinidase) deficiency
　　　Others
　　Urea cycle enzymopathies other than arginase deficiency (see Fig. 86.1)
　Symptomatic at birth or within first day of life
　　Asphyxia
　　Congenital hepatic disease
　　Congenital lactic acidosis
　　　Pyruvate dehydrogenase deficiency
　　　Pyruvate carboxylase deficiency (type B)
　　Glutaric aciduria, type II
　　Short-chain acyl Co-A dehydrogenase deficiency

Older child and adult
　Primary metabolic disease
　　Urea cycle defects
　　　Incomplete blocks (i.e., ornithine carbamyl transferase deficiency heterozygotes)
　　　Arginase deficiency
　　Dibasic aminoacidurias
　　　Lysinuric protein intolerance
　　　Hyperornithinemic states
　　　　Partial defect of ornithine decarboxylase (hyperammonemia-hyperornithinemia-homocitrullinemia [HHH syndrome])
　　　　Deficiency of ornithine-ketoacid aminotransferase
　　　　Partial
　　　　Severe—associated with gyrate atrophy of the retina
　　Primary carnitine deficiency
　Drugs
　　Valproic acid
　　Salicylates
　　Others

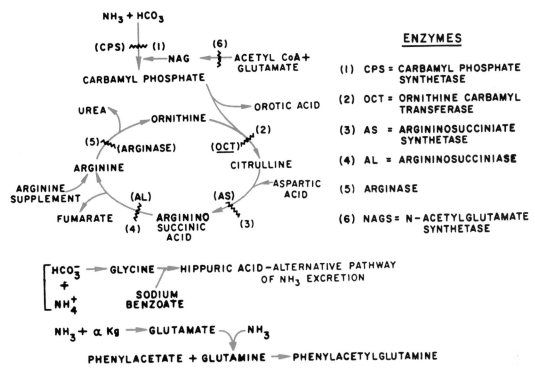

FIG. 86.1. The urea cycle.

The ill newborn child with hyperammonemia (especially marked hyperammonemia) without other explanation often has an inborn error of metabolism that, directly or indirectly, affects the urea cycle. The newborn infant with marked hyperammonemia, whatever the cause, has a constellation of symptoms, including progressive lethargy, vomiting, poor feeding, apneic episodes, and seizures. These symptoms are not specific for hyperammonemia, and other possible explanations should also be considered, for instance, sepsis. The age at onset of these symptoms is a useful differential diagnostic point. Infants with hyperammonemia due to urea cycle enzymopathies or organic acidurias typically are well for the first 24 hours of life but become symptomatic after 24 to 72 hours of protein feeding. In contrast, infants with hyperammonemia secondary to impaired pyruvate metabolism are symptomatic within the first 24 hours. Pyruvate dehydrogenase and (type B) pyruvate carboxylase deficiencies feature lactic acidosis, and these diagnoses can be confirmed by assay of enzyme activities in fibroblasts. Organic acidurias usually (but not invariably) lead to ketoacidosis, which distinguishes them from urea cycle enzymopathies. Specific diagnosis of organic acidurias requires study of the urine organic acid profile, usually by gas-liquid chromatography.

Lack of any one of the urea cycle enzymes listed in Figure 86.1, other than arginase, causes similar clinical syndromes. The affected child is well for the first 24 hours of life, but signs of hyperammonemia appear as protein feedings continue. There is no lactic acidosis or ketoacidosis, but there may be respiratory alkalosis with hyperventilation. Measurement of plasma citrulline and urinary orotic acid levels is most helpful in rapid determination of the site of block (Table 86.2). Confirmatory enzyme assays may then be performed; ornithine carbamyl transferase and carbamyl phosphate synthase activities can be measured only in liver, but other enzymes can be assayed in fibroblasts. All these enzymopathies are autosomal recessive diseases except for ornithine carbamyl transferase deficiency, which is X-linked. Prenatal screening is available for some of these disorders.

TABLE 86.2. PLASMA AMINO ACID AND URINARY OROTIC ACID FINDINGS IN UREA CYCLE DEFECTS

Enzymatic deficiency	Citrulline	Argininosuccinic acid	Orotic acid	Arginine
Carbamyl phosphate synthetase (CPS deficiency)	0 to trace	0	↓	↓
Ornithine carbamyl transferase (OTC deficiencies)	0 to trace	0	↑ ↑	↓
Argininosuccinate synthetase (citrullinuria)	↑ ↑	0	↑	↓
Argininosuccinase (argininosuccinic aciduria)	↑	↑ ↑	nl	↑ ↑
Arginase	nl	0	↑	↑ ↑
Transient hyperammonemia of newborn	nl or sl ↑	0	nl	nl

nl, normal in plasma and urine; ↑, increased in plasma and urine; ↓, decreased.
Modified from Batshaw ML, Brusilow SW, Waber L, et al. *N Engl J Med* 1982;306:1387–1392.

Management of Neonatal Hyperammonemia

It is not known how elevated ammonia levels damage the brain, but the outcome is worse the higher the ammonia level and the longer the exposure to elevated blood ammonia levels. For this reason, acute hyperammonemic coma in the newborn is a medical emergency, and rapid reduction in ammonia levels is necessary. Peritoneal dialysis is more effective than exchange transfusion; hemodialysis may also be effective. Useful adjuncts include intravenous administration of sodium benzoate (250 mg/kg body weight), followed by a constant infusion of 250 to 500 mg/kg body weight every 24 hours. The rationale for benzoate therapy is outlined in Figure 86.1. An important metabolic consequence of a block in the urea cycle (other than at arginase) is that arginine is rendered an essential amino acid. Therefore, patients with hyperammonemia due to urea cycle enzymopathies should be given supplemental arginine. A loading dose of 0.8 mg/kg body weight of arginine hydrochloride is administered as a loading dose, followed by 0.2 mg/kg/day (*N*-acetyl-glutamate synthetase, carbamyl phosphate synthetase, or ornithine transcarbamoylase [OTC] deficiencies) or 0.8 mg/kg/day (argininosuccinate synthetase or argininosuccinate lyase deficiencies). Protein catabolism should be minimized by temporarily deleting protein from the diet and by ensuring adequate caloric intake. Long-term management depends on the specific cause of the disorder.

OLDER CHILDREN AND ADULTS

As compared with the newborn, primary metabolic disease is much less likely a cause of hyperammonemia in an older child or adult. Incomplete urea cycle defects (as seen in female OTC-deficiency heterozygotes) may cause episodic hyperammonemia during periods of metabolic stress and should be considered, especially if there are affected relatives. Dibasic amino acidurias and primary systemic carnitine deficiency (Table 86.1) are rare. More likely, the older child or adult with hyperammonemia has severe liver disease or drug-induced hyperammonemia.

Valproate-associated Hyperammonemia

Valproate therapy is one of the most common causes of hyperammonemia in clinical neurologic practice. This silent dose-related side effect may occur without hepatic dysfunction. The pathogenesis is obscure but may involve increased renal production of ammonia and decreased function of carbamyl phosphate synthetase. Inhibition of this enzyme may be a direct effect of the drug or may be related to reduced amounts of *N*-acetylglutamate because valproate depresses fatty acid metabolism. It is unclear whether patients sometimes become symptomatic from the increased ammonia under these circumstances. Lethargy may be associated with elevated ammonia values, but the encephalopathy may be due to other substances, including known toxic metabolites of valproate or other organic acids.

Laboratory studies suggest that L-carnitine supplementation can prevent the development of hyperammonemia in animals receiving valproate and in cultured rat hepatocytes. Supplementation with carnitine also reduces the elevated levels of ammonia in patients treated with valproate. The clinical significance of this reduction is unclear. Some authorities routinely measure serum carnitine levels in patients with marked hyperammonemia. If there is evidence of carnitine deficiency, the patient is given supplementary L-carnitine.

SUGGESTED READINGS

Batshaw ML. Hyperammonemia. *Curr Probl Pediatr* 1984;14:1–69.

Batshaw ML, Brusilow SW. Asymptomatic hyperammonemia in low birth weight infants. *Pediatr Res* 1978;12:221–224.

Batshaw ML, Brusilow SW. Valproate-induced hyperammonemia. *Ann Neurol* 1982;11:319–321.

Brusilow SW, Batshaw ML, Waber L. Neonatal hyperammonemic coma. *Adv Pediatr* 1982;29:69–103.

Brusilow SW, Horwich AL. Urea cycle enzymes. In: Scriver CS, Beaudet AL, Sly WS, Valle D, eds. *The metabolic and molecular basis of inherited disease,* 7th ed. New York: McGraw-Hill, 1995:1187–1232.

Brusilow SW, Maestri NE. Urea cycle disorders: diagnosis, pathophysiology, and therapy. *Adv Pediatr* 1996;43:127–170.

Dawson TD, Dawson VL, Snyder SH. A novel neuronal messenger molecule in the brain: the free radical, nitric oxide. *Ann Neurol* 1992;32:297–311.

De Vivo DC, Bohan TP, Coulter DL, et al. L-carnitine supplementation in childhood epilepsy: current perspectives. *Epilepsia* 1998;39:1216–1225.

Stanley CA, Lieu YK, Hsu BY, et al. Hyperinsulinism and hyperammonemia in infants with regulatory mutations of the glutamate dehydrogenase gene. *N Engl J Med* 1998;338:1352–1357.

Merritt's Neurology, 10th ed., edited by L.P. Rowland. Lippincott Williams & Wilkins, Philadelphia © 2000.

PEROXISOMAL DISEASES: ADRENOLEUKODYSTROPHY, ZELLWEGER SYNDROME, AND REFSUM DISEASE

MIA MACCOLLIN
DARRYL C. DE VIVO

Peroxisomes are ubiquitous cellular organelles that participate in a variety of essential biochemical functions. Peroxisomes are contained by a single membrane and contain no DNA, implying that all peroxisomal-associated proteins are encoded by nuclear genes. A complex shuttle system transports peroxisomal enzymes and structural proteins from the cytosolic polyribosomes where they are made to the peroxisome. This system involves at least two recognition sequences (peroxisomal targeting sequences) that are embedded in the protein products themselves and several receptors or transporters; the system is ATP-dependent.

Peroxisomes participate in both anabolic and catabolic cellular functions, especially in the metabolism of lipids. For example, peroxisomes contain a complete series of enzymes for the beta oxidation of fatty acids. These enzymes are distinct from the mitochondrial enzymes of beta oxidation in both genetic coding and substrate specificity. Because mitochondrial enzymes of beta oxidation cannot metabolize carbon chain lengths greater than 24, the peroxisomal system is required for the degradation of endogenous and exogenous very-long-chain fatty acids (VLCFA). The peroxisome is also the site of the initial and rate-limiting steps of the synthesis of plasmalogens, ether-linked lipids that constitute the major portion of the myelin sheath. Other key functions include cholesterol and bile acid biosynthesis, degradation of pipecolic and phytanic acids, and transamination of glyoxalate.

Human diseases caused by disruption of peroxisome function are divided into two broad categories (Table 87.1). The first is characterized by abnormalities in more than one metabolic pathway, often accompanied by morphologic changes of the peroxisome. The prototype of this class is Zellweger syndrome discussed below, although patients with milder phenotypes have been described under various names such as neonatal adrenoleukodystrophy, infantile Refsum disease, and hyperpipecolic acidemia. This overlapping range of phenotypes is referred to as the Zellweger spectrum. A second phenotype, distinct from the Zellweger spectrum and termed rhizomelic chondrodysplasia punctata (RCDP), is associated with severe growth failure, profound developmental delay, cataracts, rhizomelia, epiphyseal calcifications, and ichthyosis. Patients with RCDP have decreased plasmalogens and elevated phytanic acid, but unlike the Zellweger spectrum patients, the beta oxidation pathway and VLCFA levels are normal. In recognition of the similar cellular pathophysiology in these phenotypes, *peroxisome biogenesis disorder* (PBD) is now the preferred term for all Zellweger spectrum and RCDP conditions.

TABLE 87.1. HUMAN GENETIC DISEASES DUE TO PEROXISOMAL DYSFUNCTION

Peroxisomal biogenesis disorders	Single peroxisomal enzyme disorders
Zellweger syndrome	X-linked adrenoleukodystrophy
Neonatal adrenoleukodystrophy	Oxidase deficiency (Pseudoneonatal adrenoleukodystrophy)
Infantile Refsum disease	Bifunctional enzyme deficiency
Hyperpipecolic acidemia	Thiolase deficiency (pseudo-Zellweger)
Rhizomelic chondrodysplasia punctata	DHAP acyl transferase deficiency
	Alky1 DHAP synthase deficiency
	Glutaric aciduria type III (1 case only)
	Refsum disease
	Hyperoxaluria type I
	Acatalasia

DHAP, dihydroxyacetone phosphate.

The second class of human peroxisomal diseases shows the genetic and biochemical features of single enzyme defects. In addition to X-linked adrenoleukodystrophy (ALD) and Refsum disease discussed below, this category includes defects in the beta oxidation pathway of VLCFA, which cause a Zellweger-like phenotype, and defects in plasmalogen synthesis, which result in an RCDP-like phenotype.

ZELLWEGER SYNDROME

The Zellweger syndrome (*cerebrohepatorenal syndrome*) is an autosomal recessive disease with no ethnic or racial predilection. Affected newborns are strikingly floppy and inactive; they lack the Moro, stepping, and placing reflexes. The characteristic facial appearance includes a high narrow forehead, round cheeks, flat root of the nose, wide-set eyes with shallow orbits, puffy eyelids, pursed lips, narrow high-arched palate, and small chin. The head circumference is normal, but the fontanels and sutures are widely open. Ophthalmologic findings include pigmentary retinopathy, retinal arteriolar attenuation, and optic atrophy. The pinnas may be abnormal and posteriorly rotated. Affected infants suck and swallow poorly and often require tube feeding. Some have congenital heart disease, notably patent ductus arteriosus or septal defects. The liver is cirrhotic and either enlarged or shrunken; some children are jaundiced, and some develop splenomegaly and a bleeding diathesis. Cystic dysplasia of the kidneys may be palpable and may cause mild renal failure. Genital anomalies include an enlarged clitoris, hypospadias, and cryptorchidism. Minor skeletal anomalies include contractures of large and small joints, polydactyly, low-set rotated thumbs, and clubfeet; there are also stippled calcifications of the patella and epiphyseal cartilage. The children are apathetic, poorly responsive to environmental stimuli, and limp. Tendon reflexes are absent or hypoactive. Many children have seizures and fail to thrive or develop; most succumb within the first few months of life.

Typical but nonspecific laboratory findings include elevated bilirubin levels, abnormal liver function tests, elevated serum iron, saturated iron binding capacity, and transferrin. The cerebrospinal fluid (CSF) protein content may be elevated. The electroencephalogram is abnormal, and magnetic resonance imaging (MRI) shows poor myelination, brain atrophy, pachygyria, polymicrogyria, and neuronal heterotopias.

The hallmark of Zellweger syndrome is dysfunction in multiple enzymatic pathways, including the following:

1. Levels of VLCFA—those with 24 or more carbons—are increased in plasma, fibroblasts, and chorionic villus;
2. In plasma and urine, increased content of intermediates of bile acid metabolism includes trihydroxycholestanoic acid and dihydroxycholestanoic acid;
3. Levels of pipecolic and phytanic acids increase;
4. Plasmalogen levels decrease.

In addition, levels of cholesterol and the fat-soluble vitamins may be low. PBD patients, including those with Zellweger syndrome, can be divided into at least 11 complementation groups, based on the ability of their cells to reconstitute peroxisomal structure and function in fusion experiments. These groups do not correspond to the clinical phenotypes but rather to the underlying molecular defect (Table 87.2).

Pathologically, the absence of functional peroxisomes in hepatocytes is a pathognomonic feature of Zellweger syndrome and one that helps distinguish it from other PBDs and from single enzyme disorders such as pseudo-Zellweger disease. Membrane proteins may assemble with membrane lipids to form rudimentary "ghosts" of peroxisomes that seem unable to import enzymes. For reasons not well understood, secondary abnormalities are seen in mitochondria that show an abnormally dense matrix and distorted cristae. Lipid leaflets resembling

those in adrenoleukodystrophy are found in several tissues, including the adrenal gland. The brain is dysgenic, with signs of disordered cell migration resulting in areas of pachygyria or micropolygyria and neuronal ectopias. The inferior olive is grossly disorganized. Myelination is severely affected. Neutral fat accumulates in fibrous astrocytes, hepatocytes, renal tubules and glomeruli, and muscle.

Therapy for Zellweger syndrome is primarily supportive and limited because of the multisystem impairment already present at birth. Therapeutic trials of the polyunsaturated fatty acid docohexaenate have shown some success in improving visual function of mildly affected patients. Other potential therapies, including the peroxisomal proliferator clofibrate and bile acids, are of less clear benefit. Reliable prenatal diagnosis is available by enzymatic assays in chorionic villus or amniotic fluid cells.

ADRENOLEUKODYSTROPHY (MIM 300100)

ALD is an X-linked incompletely recessive disorder with variable expressivity; it is well defined genetically, clinically, and pathologically. The most common phenotype is the childhood cerebral form, which appears in boys who have normal early development. Behavioral change is the most common initial feature, with abnormal withdrawal, aggression, poor memory, or difficulties in school. Ultimately, progressive dementia is evident. Visual loss with optic atrophy is a consistent feature due to demyelination along the entire visual pathway. The outer retina is notably spared. Progressive gait disturbance with pyramidal tract signs is an important feature. Dysphagia and deafness may occur. Seizures are common late in the disease but are occasionally the first manifestation. Some patients have overt signs of adrenal failure, including fatigue, vomiting, salt craving, and hyperpigmentation that is most prominent in skin folds. The course is relentlessly progressive. Patients enter a vegetative state and die from adrenal crisis or other causes 1 to 10 years after onset.

Several other clinical phenotypes have been described (Table 87.3). Adrenomyeloneuropathy (AMN) is the most common of the variant phenotypes. Typical features are spastic paraparesis, peripheral neuropathy, and adrenal insufficiency, beginning in the second decade. Hypogonadism, impotence, and sphincter disturbance are also seen. Cerebellar dysfunction and dementia have been reported. A similar syndrome is found in about 15% of women who are heterozygous for mutation at the *ALD* gene. MRI frequently reveals cortical demyelinating lesions in AMN patients, even in those without signs or symptoms of cortical involvement. Pathologic findings in AMN include demyelination and dying-back changes in the cord and lamellar cytoplasmic inclusions in brain, adrenal, and testis; the findings are similar to those of ALD.

A cerebral form of ALD is occasionally seen that is similar to the childhood form, but starts in adolescence. In adults, X-linked ALD may show symptoms of dementia, schizophrenia, or focal cerebral syndromes such as aphasia, Kluver-Bucy syndrome, or hemianopia; usually there is also evidence of adrenal insuffi-

TABLE 87.2. MOLECULAR BASIS OF PEROXISOMAL BIOGENESIS DISORDERS (PBD)

Complementation group	Percentage of patients[a]	Gene responsible	Function of gene product
1	45	PEX1	ATPase of the AAA protein family
2	1	PEX5	PTS1 receptor
3	2	PEX12	48-kDa peroxisomal membrane protein
4	7	PEX6	Cytoplasmic ATPase
6–9	11	—	—
10	1	PEX2	35-kDa peroxisomal membrane protein
11	32	PEX7	PTS2 receptor

[a] Approximated from Moser et al. (1995) who found that 20% of patients initially thought to have a PBD actually had a single enzyme defect of the beta oxidation or plasmalogen synthesis pathway. Complementation groups 1–10 cause Zellweger spectrum phenotypes; all RCDP-type patients are in complementation group 11.
PTS, peroxisomal transport signal.

TABLE 87.3. PHENOTYPES ASSOCIATED WITH MUTATION AT THE *ALD* LOCUS

Form	Percentage of patients	Age at onset (yr)	Major manifestations[a]
Childhood cerebral	50	5–9	Behavioral abnormalities, blindness, deafness, spasticity
Adolescent cerebral	5	10–21	Behavioral abnormalities, blindness, deafness, spasticity
Adrenomyelo neuropathy	25	18–36	Spastic paraparesis
Adrenal insufficiency only	10	1–14	Addison disease
Asymptomatic	10	—	Elevated VLCFA
Expressing carriers	(60% of obligate carriers)	20–50	Spastic paraparesis

[a]In all forms of ALD, radiographic abnormalities preceed clinical findings.

ciency. Adult ALD includes spastic paraparesis, cerebellar dysfunction, or olivopontocerebellar atrophy. Female heterozygotes may become symptomatic with adult ALD. Adrenal insufficiency can be seen without neurologic disorder; ALD should be considered in any boy with unexplained Addison disease. Finally, children and adults with the biochemical defect may be asymptomatic or presymptomatic. Phenotypic heterogeneity is the rule within families with multiple affected individuals; the disparate manifestations are probably the result of modifying genetic loci or environmental factors.

Laboratory evaluation of the patient with ALD reveals several abnormalities. The CSF protein content is often elevated. Computed tomography shows characteristic hyperdense and hypodense bandlike regions in parietooccipital white matter; if found, these are virtually diagnostic of ALD. MRI abnormalities are more diffuse and always predate clinical findings. Adrenal function tests, especially the corticotropin stimulation test, usually show adrenal insufficiency even in the absence of clinical signs. In the zona fasciculata and reticularis, adrenal biopsy shows many ballooned cortical cells and striated cytoplasm and microvacuoles, findings specific for ALD. Characteristic inclusions, accumulations of lamellar lipid profiles, may also be seen in the brain, sural nerve biopsy, or testis. The primary finding in the brain is extensive diffuse demyelination, sparing U-fibers in the centrum semiovale and elsewhere. In involved areas of white matter, perivascular infiltration of lymphocytes and plasma cells is prominent.

Diagnosis is suggested by the characteristic clinical findings of neurologic deterioration, demonstration of adrenal hypofunction, and MRI abnormalities. Definite diagnosis is made by finding elevated VLCFA levels in plasma and cultured skin fibroblasts without disruption of other peroxisomal functions. To date, elevated VLCFA levels in both tissues have been found only

in patients with ALD, PBDs, and single enzyme defects involving the VLCFA oxidation pathway. Unlike ALD patients, patients on the ketogenic diet may show elevated VLCFA levels in plasma but not cultured skin fibroblasts. Prenatal diagnosis of ALD is made by assay of VLCFA oxidation in amniotic fluid cells or chorionic villus sampling. Eighty-five percent of female carriers of ALD have elevated VLCFA levels in plasma and cultured skin fibroblasts.

The *ALD* gene has been cloned and encodes a member of the ATP binding cassette transporter class of proteins. Mutations at this locus have proven to be mostly private, limiting the usefulness of molecular analysis for diagnosis.

Several approaches have been taken to the rational treatment of ALD. Steroid replacement therapy is given during stressful periods, such as intercurrent illness, or if there is evidence of adrenal insufficiency. Dietary avoidance of VLCFA alone does not lead to biochemical change because of endogenous synthesis. Efforts to lower endogenous synthesis using glycerol trierucate oil and glycerol trioleate oil (Lorenzo oil) in conjunction with dietary restriction do produce a fall in VLCFA levels in both affected individuals and female carriers. Unfortunately, this striking biochemical change does not have an equally striking clinical correlate; its use is most likely limited to presymptomatic boys. Bone marrow transplantation cures the biochemical defect in ALD, but the morbidity and mortality are high, and neither neurologic defects nor radiologic abnormalities revert. In all cases, radiologic abnormalities and progression almost invariably precede neurologic progression; it is therfore imperative that every child whose family might consider bone marrow transplantation is closely followed radiographically. Immunotherapy has been considered in X-ALD because of the inflammatory component of the central lesions, but beta interferon and thalidomide have not been effective. Finally, the cloning and characterization of the *ALD* locus may lead to a gene or protein product replacement therapy.

REFSUM DISEASE (MIM-266510)

This autosomal recessive disease (also known as heredopathia atactica polyneuritiformis) is unique among the lipidoses because the stored lipid (phytanic acid) is not synthesized in the body but is exclusively dietary in origin. This has enabled successful therapy by dietary management. Symptoms begin in early childhood in some patients but may be delayed until the fifth decade in others. Progressive night blindness usually appears in the first or second decade, followed by limb weakness and gait ataxia. Symptoms are progressive, but abrupt exacerbations and gradual remissions may occur with intercurrent illness or pregnancy. There are no seizures, but some patients have psychiatric symptoms. Peripheral neuropathy is manifest by loss of tendon reflexes, weakness and wasting, and distal sensory loss. Ataxia may be seen. A granular pigmentary retinopathy is universally present. Other findings include ichthyosis, nerve deafness (often severe), cataracts, miosis and pupillary asymmetry, pes cavus, and bone deformities with shortening of the metatarsal bones, epiphyseal dysplasia, and, in some, kyphoscoliosis. CSF protein content is elevated. Nerve conduction velocities are slowed. Electrocardiographic changes may be seen, including conduction abnormalities. Peripheral nerves may feel thickened and, on histologic study, may show hypertrophic interstitial changes and onion-bulb formation. The course is generally progressive with exacerbations and remissions. Peripheral visual fields may ultimately be lost, with resulting telescopic vision. Sudden death may result from cardiac arrhythmia.

The biochemical defect in Refsum disease has been identified as phytanoyl-coenzyme A hydroxylase deficiency; the responsible gene has been cloned. Diagnosis is made by the characteristic clinical picture and elevation of phytanic acid levels in the plasma.

Therapy limits dietary phytanic acid and its precursor, phytol. When dairy products, ruminant fat, and chlorophyll-containing foods are eliminated, plasma phytanic acid levels are reduced and tissue stores are mobilized, with improvement of symptoms. Paradoxically, symptoms may worsen and plasma phytanic acid levels may rise shortly after institution of dietary therapy, especially if patients reduce caloric intake and lose weight. Increased plasma phytanic acid causes anorexia, increased weight loss, and still more severe symptoms. Adequate caloric intake helps prevent weight loss and abrupt fat mobilization. Plasmapheresis helps to prevent or treat exacerbations.

SUGGESTED READINGS

Peroxisomal Biogenesis and Biochemistry

Waterham H, Cregg J. Peroxisome biogenesis. *BioEssays* 1997;19:57–66.

Peroxisomal Biogenesis Disorders

Braverman N, Dodt G, Gould S, Valle D. Disorders of peroxisome biogenesis. *Human Mol Genet* 1996;4:1791–1798.

Martinez M, Vazquez E. MRI evidence that docosahexaenoic acid ethyl ester improves myelination in generalized peroxisomal disorders. *Neurology* 1998;51:26–32.

Moser A, Rasmussen M, Naidu S, et al. Phenotype of patients with peroxisomal disorders subdivided into sixteen complementation groups. *J Pediatr* 1995;127:13–22.

Reuber B, Germain-Lee E, Collins C, et al. Mutations in PEX1 are the most common cause of peroxisome biogenesis disorders. *Nat Genet* 1997;17:445–452.

Santos MJ, Imanaka T, Shio H, et al. Peroxisomal membrane ghosts in Zellweger syndrome—aberrant organelle assembly. *Science* 1988; 239:1536–1538.

Setchell K, Bragetti P, Zimmer-Nechemias L, et al. Oral bile acid treatment and the patient with Zellweger syndrome. *Hepatology* 1992;15:198–207.

Volpe JJ, Adams RD. Cerebro-hepato-renal syndrome of Zellweger: an inherited disorder of neuronal migration. *Acta Neuropathol (Berl)* 1972;20:175–198.

Adrenoleukodystrophy

Aubourg P, Adamsbaum C, Lavallard-Rousseau MC, et al. A two-year trial of oleic and erucic acids ("Lorenzo's oil") as treatment for adrenomyeloneuropathy. *N Engl J Med* 1993;329:745–752.

Aubourg P, Blanche S, Jambaque I, et al. Reversal of early neurologic and neuroradiologic manifestations of X-linked adrenoleukodystrophy by bone marrow transplantation. *N Engl J Med* 1990;322:1860–1866.

Bezman L, Moser H. Incidence of X-linked adrenoleukodystrophy and the relative frequency of its phenotypes. *Am J Med Genet* 1998;76:415–419.

Mosser J, Douar A, Sarde C, et al. Putative X-linked adrenoleukodystrophy gene shares unexpected homology with ABC transporters. *Nature* 1993;361:726–730.

Panegyres P, Goldswain P, Kakulas B. Adult-onset adrenoleukodystrophy manifesting as dementia. *Am J Med* 1989;87:481–482.

Sadeghi-Nejad A, Senior B. Adrenomyeloneuropathy presenting as Addison's disease in childhood. *N Engl J Med* 1990;322:13–16.

Shapiro E, Aubourg P, Lockman L et al. Bone marrow transplant for adrenoleukodystrophy: 5 year follow-up of 12 engrafted cases. *Ann Neurol* 1997;42:498.

Refsum Disease

Djupesland G, Flottorp G, Refsum S. Phytanic acid storage disease; hearing maintained after 15 years of dietary treatment. *Neurology* 1983;33:237–239.

Masters-Thomas A, Bailes J, Billimoria J, et al. Heredopathia atactica polyneuritiformis (Refsum's disease). 1. Clinical features and dietary management. *J Hum Nutr* 1980;34:245–250.

Mihalik S, Morrell J, Kim D, et al. Identification of PAHX, a Refsum disease gene. *Nat Genet* 1997;17:185–189.

Refsum S. Heredopathia atactica polyneuritiformis. *Acta Psychiatr Scand* (suppl) 1946;38:9–303.

Other Single Enzyme Defects

Schram AW, Goldfischer S, van Roermund CWT, et al. Human peroxisomal 3-oxoacyl-coenzyme A thiolase deficiency. *Proc Natl Acad Sci USA* 1987;84:2494–2496.

Wanders R, Schumacher H, Heikoop H, Schutgens R, Tager J. Human dihydroxyacetonephsphate acyltransferase deficiency: a new peroxisomal disorder. *J Inherit Metab Dis* 1992;15:389–391.

Watkins P, McGuinness M, Raymond G, et al. Distinction between peroxisomal bifunctional enzyme and acyl-CoA oxidase deficiencies. *Ann Neurol* 1995;38:472–477.

Merritt's Neurology, 10th ed., edited by L.P. Rowland. Lippincott Williams & Wilkins, Philadelphia © 2000.

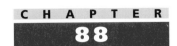

ORGANIC ACIDURIAS

STEFANO DI DONATO
GRAZIELLA UZIEL

The organic acidurias are inborn errors of metabolism that are characterized by abnormal accumulation of one or more organic acids in the urine. Although individually rare, these diseases comprise more than 50 specific disorders and collectively are the most frequent cause of acute encephalopathy in early infancy. They may appear later in life with more complex features of chronic brain disorder, including dystonia, seizures, or myopathy, sometimes with liver and heart pathology.

TABLE 88.1. ORGANIC ACIDURIAS

Disease	Enzyme
Amino acid metabolism	
Maple syrup urine disease	Branched-chain acyl-CoA dehydrogenase
Propionic acidemia	Propionyl-CoA carboxylase
Methylmalonic acidemia	Methylmalonyl-CoA mutase
Isovaleric acidemia	Isovalery-CoA dehydrogenase
Glutaric aciduria type I	Glutaryl-CoA dehydrogenase
3-Oxothiolase deficiency	2-methyl-acetoacetyl-CoA thiolase
3-Methylcrotonic aciduria	3-methylcrotonyl-CoA carboxylase
3-Methylglutaconic acidemia	3-methylglutaconyl-CoA hydratase
3-Hydroxy-3-methylglutaric aciduria[a]	3-hydroxy-3-methyl-glutaryl CoA lyase (HMG-CoA lyase)
Multiple carboxylase deficiency[b]	Holocarboxylase synthetase or biotinidase
4-Hydroxybutyric aciduria	Succinic semialdeide dehydrogenase
Krebs cycle	
Fumaric aciduria	Fumarase deficiency
Fatty acid metabolism	
Dicarboxylic aciduria (LCAD deficiency)	Long-chain fatty acyl-CoA dehydrogenase
Dicarboxylic aciduria (MCAD deficiency)	Medium-chain acyl-CoA dehydrogenase
Ethylmalonic aciduria (SCAD deficiency)	Short-chain acyl-CoA dehydrogenase
3-Hydroxydicarboxylic aciduria	Trifunctional protein or 3-hydroxyacyl CoA dehydrogenase
Glutaric aciduria type II (ETF), (ETFQR)[c]	Electron transfer flavoprotein or ETF-coenzyme-Q reductase

[a] HMG-CoA lyase deficiency also affects fatty acid (ketone bodies) metabolism.
[b] Holocarboxylase synthetase and biotinidase deficiencies also affect fatty acid (synthesis) and glucose (gluconeo-genesis) metabolism.
[c] ETF and ETF-QR deficiencies also affect amino acid metabolism (valine, leucine, isoleucine, and lysine).

The acute and frequently life-threatening manifestations in the newborn or young infant demand rapid differential diagnosis of the many acute encephalopathies of infancy, such as cerebral infection, hypoxia, space-occupying lesions, and ingestion of drugs or toxins. The issue is urgent because a few organic acidurias can be effectively cured, including multiple carboxylase deficiency responsive to biotin, methylmalonic aciduria responsive to vitamin B_{12}, and glutaric aciduria type II responsive to riboflavin. Early diagnosis is also important because treatment may prevent acute metabolic attacks and therefore mental retardation, epilepsy, severe brain damage, or death.

The most common inherited organic acidurias involve enzymes of two principal biochemical pathways. One is the stepwise degradation of amino acids, including methionine and threonine; the branched-chain amino acids valine, leucine, and isoleucine; tryptophan; and the basic amino acid lysine. The other is the β-oxidation of straight-chain fatty acid. Some of the final degradative pathways are the same in both amino acid and fatty acid catabolism, such as the funneling of flavin adenine dinucleotide-linked reducing equivalents to the respiratory chain through the electron transferring flavoproteins.

Lactic acidemia also results in an organic aciduria. Pyruvate dehydrogenase deficiency and respiratory chain defects, however, are the major causes of familial lactic acidosis of infancy, so lactic acidemia is discussed in Chapter 96. In fact, most organic acidurias are mitochondrial disorders, caused by genetic deficiencies of enzymes that catalyze the oxidative degradation of some amino acids and the β-oxidation of straight-chain fatty acids.

The organic acidurias that cause acute encephalopathy include multiple carboxylase deficiency, maple syrup urine disease, methylmalonic aciduria, propionic aciduria, isovaleric aciduria, fumaric aciduria, glutaric aciduria types I and II, methylcrotonic aciduria, hydroxymethylglutaric aciduria, dicarboxylic acidurias, and 3-hydroxydicarboxylic aciduria (Table 88.1).

CLINICAL MANIFESTATIONS AND DIAGNOSIS

The signs and symptoms of organic acidurias in the newborn or infant are usually nonspecific. Acute episodes of nausea and vomiting, hypotonia, drowsiness, and coma do not discriminate acquired from inherited conditions. The presence of hypoglycemia, however, with glucose blood concentrations less than 2.5 mmol/L or metabolic acidosis with blood pH less than 7.30 and, in some instances, such as in propionic and methylmalonic acidurias, hyperammonemia with plasma ammonia values of 100 mmol/L or more are suggestive of organic acidurias. Acute hypoglycemia, particularly with acidosis, may be fatal. Some infants with these diseases die abruptly without any evident prodromal or accompanying symptoms. Similar features are also part of two relatively common but pathogenetically ill-defined disorders of infancy: Reye hepatic encephalopathy and the sudden infant death syndrome. Both syndromes, currently viewed as nongenetic disorders, have much in common with inherited disorders of fatty acid metabolism because dicarboxylic aciduria has been reported in Reye syndrome and sudden infant death syndrome has been observed in a few patients with β-oxidation defects such as medium-chain acyl-CoA dehydrogenase deficiency.

Clinical manifestations seldom discriminate these diseases. The only conclusive way to reach a definite diagnosis is laboratory examination, including the analysis of body fluids for accumulating metabolites and study of the patients' cells for the specific enzymes listed in Table 88.1. Molecular genetic analysis of mutations of the corresponding genes usually follows biochemical diagnosis and is of less importance for early diagnosis. Together with analysis of amniotic fluid and enzyme assay in chorionic villi and amniocytes, however, DNA analysis is useful for prenatal diagnosis. Molecular diagnosis can be a first-choice diagnostic tool in case of prevalent mutations such as the A985G transition in medium-chain acyl-CoA dehydrogenase deficiency. Because most of these acids are effectively cleared from the blood by the kidneys, detection of abundant organic acids in urine is facilitated by gas chromatography mass spectrometry of a 24-hour urine specimen, which generally reveals the pattern of urinary metabolites characteristic of one disease.

Some infants with organic aciduria survive the acute metabolic attack but show poor growth, macrocephaly, and impaired psychomotor development. Dystonia, spastic tetraplegia, and intractable seizures may also mark the devastating effects of acidosis, acute energy shortage, and the accumulation of toxic metabolites on the developing brain. A few organic acidurias may not damage the human brain acutely but result in chronic neurologic disorder. In general, early-onset forms are devastatingly lethal, whereas late-onset forms are more benign. Different amounts of residual enzyme activity may account for the clinical heterogeneity.

Therefore, in addition to acute acidosis, chronic neurologic disorders of infancy or early childhood without evident etiology should lead to a search for metabolic disease. Mental retardation, ataxia, and behavioral changes suggest maple syrup urine disease but are also seen in 4-hydroxybutyric aciduria. Spasticity, ataxia, mental retardation, and seizures are present in L-2-hydroxyglutaric aciduria. Severe hypotonia, epilepsy, spastic tetraparesis, and early death are features of fumaric aciduria. Dystonia and spasticity, often with normal intellectual development, may underlie glutaric aciduria type I. Choreoathetosis and dystonic posture are signs of 3-hydroxy-3-methylglutaric aciduria. Seizures and ataxia are classically seen with alopecia and skin rash in late-onset multiple carboxylase deficiency. Ataxia, optic atrophy, and retinitis pigmentosa may be associated with 3-methylglutaconic aciduria. Some patients with mitochondrial trifunctional protein deficiency (type II) in addition to retinitis pigmentosa show peripheral neuropathy. Infantile spinal muscular atrophy with mental retardation can suggest 3-methylcrotonic aciduria. Lipid myopathy and cardiomyopathy develop in patients with the rare late-onset β-oxidation defects associated with dicarboxylic aciduria, such as carnitine translocase deficiency, mitochondrial trifunctional protein deficiency, very-long-chain acyl-CoA dehydrogenase deficiency, and the riboflavin-responsive form of glutaric aciduria type II.

NEUROIMAGING

Brain magnetic resonance imaging (MRI) and computed tomography (CT) help in the diagnosis of organic acidurias, al-though they often lack specificity. In maple syrup urine disease, CT and MRI show the leukoencephalopathic features of white matter, particularly involving the pallidum. In glutaric aciduria type I, CT shows dilated insular cisterns, temporal lobe shrinkage, and hypodensity of the lenticular nuclei. MRI demonstrates abnormal signal intensity in the white matter in glutaric aciduria type II. In methylmalonic aciduria, MRI shows symmetric abnormalities in the pallidum that may subsequently involve the whole basal ganglia. Progressive leukoencephalopathy starting in subcortical areas are characteristic of L-2-hydroxyglutaric aciduria.

THERAPY

Management of organic acidurias caused by defects in amino acid metabolism is based on accurate early dietary treatment with protein-modified diets that restrict the appropriate amino acids: leucine, valine, and isoleucine in maple syrup urine disease; leucine in 3-hydroxymethylglutaric aciduria; isoleucine, valine, threonine, and methionine in propionic and methylmalonic aciduria; and lysine and tryptophan in glutaric aciduria type I. Patients with methylmalonic aciduria and propionic acidemia may also benefit from oral carnitine supplementation, which increases urinary excretion of propionylcarnitine. Carnitine and medium-chain triglycerides have been also used to treat β-oxidation disorders such as long-chain acyl-CoA dehydrogenase deficiency, long-chain β-hydroxyacyl-CoA dehydrogenase deficiency, and trifunctional protein deficiency; the use of carnitine in these disorders has been questioned because of possible cardiotoxicity.

SUGGESTED READINGS

Barth PG, Hoffmann GF, Jaeken J, et al. L-2-Hydroxyglutaric acidemia: a novel inherited neurometabolic disease. *Ann Neurol* 1992;32:66–71.

Chalmers RA. Current research in the organic acidurias. *J Inherit Metab Dis* 1989;12:225–239.

DiDonato S. Diseases associated with defects of beta-oxidation. In: Rosenberg RN, Prusiner SB, DiMauro S, Barchi RL, eds. *The molecular and genetic basis of neurological disease*, 2nd ed. Boston: Butterworth-Heineman, 1997:939–956.

Gellera C, Uziel G, Rimoldi M, et al. Fumarase deficiency in an autosomal recessive encephalopathy affecting both mitochondrial and cytosolic enzymes. *Neurology* 1990;40:495–499.

Pollit RJ. Disorders of mitochondrial β-oxidation: prenatal and early postnatal diagnosis and their relevance to Reye syndrome and sudden infant death. *J Inherit Metab Dis* 1989;12:215–230.

Roe C, Coates P. AcylCoA dehydrogenase deficiency. In: Scriver CR, Beaudet AR, Sly WS, Valle D, eds. *The metabolic and molecular basis of inherited disease*, 7th ed. New York: McGraw-Hill, 1995.

Thomas E. Dietary management of inborn errors of amino acid metabolism with protein modified diets. *J Child Neurol* 1992;7:92–111.

Uziel G, Savoiardo M, Nardocci N. CT and MRI in maple syrup urine disease. *Neurology* 1988;38:486–488.

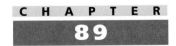

DISORDERS OF METAL METABOLISM

JOHN H. MENKES

HEPATOLENTICULAR DEGENERATION (WILSON DISEASE) (MIM 277900)

Wilson disease is an inborn error of copper metabolism that is associated with cirrhosis of the liver and degenerative changes in the basal ganglia.

During the second half of the 19th century, a condition termed pseudosclerosis was distinguished from multiple sclerosis by the lack of nystagmus and visual loss. In 1902, Kayser observed green corneal pigmentation in one such patient; Fleischer commented on the association of the corneal rings with pseudosclerosis in 1903 and fully required it in 1912. In 1912, Wilson gave the classic description of the disease and its pathologic anatomy. The worldwide prevalence of the disease is about 30 in 1 million, with a gene frequency of 1:180.

Pathogenesis and Pathology

Wilson disease is an autosomal recessive disorder with the gene being located on the long arm of chromosome 13. The gene has been cloned. It encodes a copper-transporting P-type ATPase that is expressed in liver and kidney. The protein is present in two forms: one is localized to the cellular trans-Golgi network and the other, probably representing a cleavage product, to mitochondria. A large number of mutations have been characterized. Some are large deletions that completely destroy function of the gene and result in an early onset of symptoms, whereas others that reduce but not eliminate copper transport are consistent with a late onset of symptoms. Most patients are compound heterozygotes.

The genetic mutation induces extensive changes in copper homeostasis. Normally, the amount of copper in the body is kept constant through excretion of copper from the liver into bile. In Wilson disease, the two fundamental defects are reduced biliary transport of copper and an impaired formation of plasma ceruloplasmin. Because ceruloplasmin is present in the liver of patients with Wilson disease, a posttranslational defect appears to be responsible for the absence of ceruloplasmin from both bile and serum.

In addition to these abnormalities, levels of nonceruloplasmin (free) copper in serum are increased and plasma iron-binding globulin is low to low normal. These abnormalities occur in asymptomatic carriers and suggest that Wilson disease may also encompass a disorder of iron metabolism. This may result from the deficiency of ceruloplasmin that is directly involved in the transfer of iron from tissue cells to plasma transferrin.

Another metabolic feature is a persistent aminoaciduria. This

is most marked during the later stages but may be noted in some asymptomatic patients. The presence of other tubular defects (e.g., impaired phosphate resorption in patients without aminoaciduria) suggests that a toxic action of the metal on renal tubules causes the aminoaciduria.

A defect in the gene encoding a different copper transporting P-type ATPase is responsible for Menkes disease. Although the gene for Menkes disease is located on the X chromosome, there is more than 60% identity between the two proteins. The similarities and differences between the two diseases are listed in Table 89.1.

The abnormalities in copper metabolism that occur in Wilson disease lead to accumulation of the metal in liver and consequently to progressive liver damage. Anatomically, the liver shows focal necrosis that leads to a coarsely nodular postnecrotic cirrhosis; the nodules vary in size and are separated by bands of fibrous tissue of different width. Some hepatic cells are enlarged and contain fat droplets, intranuclear glycogen, and clumped pigment granules; other cells are necrotic, and there are regenerative changes in the surrounding parenchyma.

Electron microscopic studies have shown that copper is sequestered by lysosomes that become more than normally sensitive to rupture and therefore lack normal alkaline phosphatase activity. Copper probably initiates and catalyzes oxidation of the lysosomal membrane lipids, resulting in lipofuscin accumulation. Subsequent overflow of copper from the liver produces ac-

TABLE 89.1. MOLECULAR BIOLOGY OF MENKES DISEASE AND WILSON DISEASE

	Menkes	Wilson
Gene locus	Xq13.3	13q14.3
Gene product	Copper-binding P-type ATPase	Copper-binding P-type ATPase, 60% identity with Menkes
Expression	All tissues except liver	Liver, kidney, placenta
Mutations	16% deletions	Point mutations, small deletions
Clinical		
Age of onset	Birth	Late childhood, adolescence
Symptomatic organs	Brain, hair, skin	Liver, CNS, Kayser-Fleischer rings
Duration	<3y	Decades
Laboratory		
Serum copper	Decreased	Decreased
Ceruloplasmin	Decreased	Decreased
Renal copper	Increased	Increased
Urinary copper	—	Increased
Liver copper	Decreased	Increased
Cultured cells	Copper accumulation Decreased copper release	Normal
Defect	Intestinal copper absorption Deficiency copper-dependent enzymes	Biliary copper excretion Incorporation copper into ceruloplasmin
Treatment	None effective	Penicillamine, zinc

aModified from Chelly J, Monaco AP. *Nat Genet* 1993;5:317–318.

cumulation in other organs, mainly brain, kidney, and cornea. Within the kidneys, the tubular epithelial cells may degenerate, and the cytoplasm may contain copper deposits.

In brain, the basal ganglia show the most striking alterations (Fig. 89.1). They have a brick-red pigmentation; spongy degeneration of the putamen frequently leads to the formation of small cavities. Microscopic studies reveal a loss of neurons, axonal degeneration, and large numbers of protoplasmic astrocytes, including giant forms known as *Alzheimer cells*. The cortex of the frontal lobe may also show spongy degeneration and astrocytosis. Copper is deposited in the pericapillary area and within astrocytes, where it is located in the subcellular soluble fraction and bound not only to cerebrocuprein but also to other cerebral proteins. Copper is uniformly absent from neurons and ground substance. Lesser degenerative changes are seen in the brainstem, the dentate nucleus, the substantia nigra, and the convolutional white matter. Copper is also found throughout the cornea, particularly the substantia propria.

In the cornea, the metal is deposited in the periphery where it appears in granular clumps close to the endothelial surface of the Descemet membrane. The deposits in this area are responsible for the appearance of the Kayser-Fleischer ring. The color of this ring varies from yellow to green to brown. Copper is deposited in two or more layers, with particle size and distance between layers influencing the ultimate appearance of the ring.

Symptoms and Signs

Wilson disease is a progressive condition with a tendency toward temporary clinical improvement and arrest. The condition occurs in all races, with a particularly high incidence among Eastern European Jews, Italians from southern Italy and Sicily, and people from some of the smaller islands of Japan—groups in which there is a high rate of inbreeding.

In most patients, symptoms begin between the ages of 11 and 25 years. Onset as early as age 3 and as late as the fifth decade has been recorded.

The signs and symptoms of hepatolenticular degeneration are generally those of damage to the liver and brain. Signs of liver damage, ascites, or jaundice may occur at any stage of the disease. They have been observed in some cases several or many years before the onset of neurologic symptoms.

The neurologic manifestations are so varied that it is impossible to describe a clinical picture that is characteristic. In the past, texts have distinguished between pseudosclerotic and dystonic forms of the disease: the former dominated by tremor, the latter by rigidity and contractures. In actuality, most patients, if untreated, ultimately develop both types of symptoms. In essence, Wilson disease is a disorder of motor function; despite often widespread cerebral atrophy, there are no sensory symptoms or reflex alterations. Symptoms at onset are shown in Table 89.2. Symptoms of basal ganglia damage usually predominate, but cerebellar symptoms may occasionally be in the foreground. Tremors and rigidity are the most common early signs. The tremor may be of the intention type or it may be the alternating tremor of Parkinson disease. More commonly, however, it is a bizarre tremor, localized to the arms and best described by the term "wing beating" (Fig. 89.2). This tremor is usually absent when the arms are at rest; it develops after a short latent period when the arms are extended. The beating movements may be confined to the muscles of the wrist, but it is more common for the arm to be thrown up and down in a wide arc. The movements increase in severity and may become so violent that the patient is thrown off balance. A change in the posture of the outstretched arms may alter the severity of the tremor. The tremor may affect both arms but is usually more severe in one. The tremor may occasionally be present even when the arm is at rest. Many patients have a fixed open-mouth smile.

Rigidity and spasms of the muscles are often present. In some cases, a typical parkinsonian rigidity may involve all muscles. Torticollis, tortipelvis, and other dystonic movements are not uncommon. Spasticity of the laryngeal and pharyngeal muscles may lead to dysarthria and dysphagia. Drooping of the lower jaw and excess salivation are common. Other symptoms include convulsions, transient periods of coma, and mental changes. Mental symptoms may dominate the clinical course for varying periods and simulate an affective disorder or a psychosis.

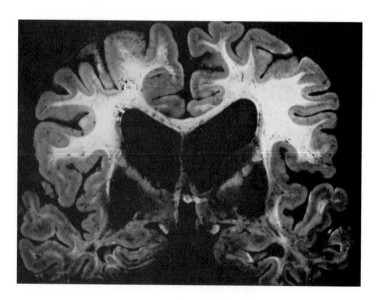

FIG. 89.1. Wilson disease. Ventricular dilation, atrophy of caudate nucleus. Cyst in lower half of putamen.

TABLE 89.2. CLINICAL MANIFESTATIONS AT ONSET OF WILSON DISEASE

Symptoms	Percentage
Hepatic or hematologic abnormalities	35
Behavioral abnormalities	25
Neurologic symptoms	40
Pseudosclerotic form–one or more of the following:	40
Tremor at rest or purposive	
Dysarthria or scanning speech	
Diminished dexterity or mild clumsiness	
Unsteady gait	
Tremor, alone	33
Dysarthria, alone	5
Dystonic form–one or more of the following:	60
Hypophonic speech or mutism	
Drooling	
Rigid mouth, arms, or legs	
Seizures	1
Chorea or small-amplitude twitches	<1

Prepared with Drs. I.H. Scheinberg and I Sternlieb, Department of Medicine, Albert Einstein College of Medicine, Bronx, New York.

Tendon reflexes are increased, but extensor plantar responses are exceptional. Somatosensory evoked potentials are abnormal in most patients with neurologic symptoms. The prevalence of epileptic seizures is 10 times higher in patients with Wilson disease than in the general population. Seizures can occur at any stage of the disease, but most begin after the initiation of treatment.

Behavioral or personality disorders were noted in the original description of the disease by Wilson. In the experience of Akil and Brewer (1995), the first symptoms of one-third of patients are psychiatric abnormalities. These include impaired school performance, depression, labile moods, and frank psychosis. In those patients who show primarily neurologic symptoms, about two-thirds have had psychiatric problems before the diagnosis was made. Symptoms in about one-half of patients were sufficiently severe to require treatment by a psychiatrist or a hospital admission.

The intracorneal ring-shaped pigmentation first noted by Kayser (1902) and Fleischer (1912) may be evident to the naked eye or may be seen only by slit-lamp examination. The ring may be complete or incomplete and is present in 75% of patients who present with hepatic symptoms and in all patients with cerebral symptoms alone or both cerebral and hepatic symptoms. The Kayser-Fleischer ring may antedate overt symptoms and has been detected even with normal liver functions. In the larger clinical series of Arima and colleagues (1977), it was never present before age 7 years.

Magnetic resonance imaging (MRI) usually reveals ventricular dilatation and diffuse atrophy of the cortex, cerebellum, and brainstem. The basal ganglia is usually abnormal with the putamen, thalamus, the head of the caudate, and the globus pallidus the most likely areas to be involved in patients presenting with neurologic symptoms (Fig. 89.3). Most patients with hepatic symptoms have increased signal in the basal ganglia on T1-weighted images. Abnormalities are also seen in the tegmentum of the midbrain, the substantia nigra, and pons. In a few subjects there are focal white matter lesions. On compured tomography (CT), increased density due to copper deposition is not observed. As a rule, MRI correlates better with the clinical symptoms than CT.

Diagnosis

The clinical picture of Wilson disease is fairly clearcut when the disease is advanced. The Kayser-Fleischer ring is the most im-

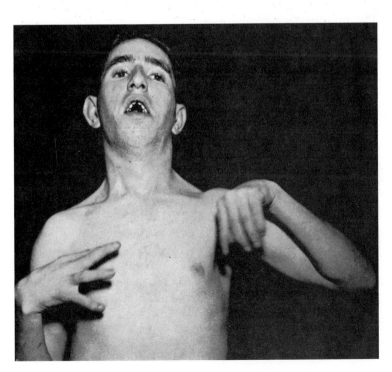

FIG. 89.2. Wilson disease. Open mouth, athetoid posture of arms, and wing-beating movements of left hand.

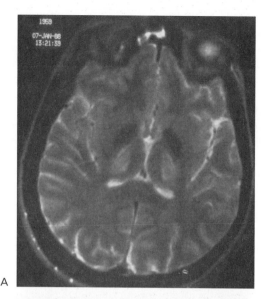

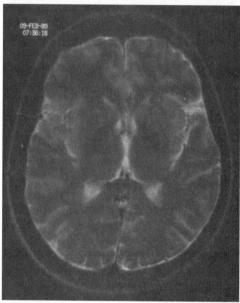

FIG. 89.3. Wilson disease. Coronal T2-weighted magnetic resonance images of a 22-year-old woman with Wilson disease. **A:** Three months after the disease has been diagnosed and at start of penicillamine therapy, there are bilateral hyperintense thalamic lesions that were hypointense on T1-weighted images. **B:** The same patient after 13 months of penicillamine therapy shows a significant regression of the thalamic lesions. Spin-echo sequences TR 2.5 ms, TE 90 ms, using Siemens Magneton 63 operating at 1.5 T. (Courtesy of Dr. I. Prayer, Zentral Institut fur Radiodiagnose und Ludwig Boltzmann Institut, University of Vienna, Austria; and Rosenberg RN, Prusiner SB, DiMauro S, Barchi RL. *Molecular and genetic basis of neurological disease.* Boston: Butterworth-Heinemann, 1997.)

portant diagnostic feature; absence of corneal pigmentation in untreated patients with neurologic symptoms rules out the diagnosis. The ring is not seen in most presymptomatic patients or in some children with hepatic symptoms. A low serum ceruloplasmin and elevated urinary copper support the diagnosis.

Although 96% of patients with Wilson disease have low or absent serum ceruloplasmin, some cases have been reported with normal ceruloplasmin levels. In affected families, the differential diagnosis between heterozygotes and presymptomatic homozygotes is of utmost importance because homozygotes should be treated preventively. Low ceruloplasmin levels in an asymptomatic patient suggest the presymptomatic stage of the disease. Because 6% of heterozygotes also have low ceruloplasmin levels, further studies are indicated. An elevation of urinary copper is diagnostic of a presymptomatic patient if the patient is 15 years or older. In children, urinary copper is not always elevated, and in such cases a liver biopsy to measure hepatic copper content is indicated to confirm the diagnosis. A screening test using penicillamine to stimulate urinary excretion of copper has not been standardized and is therefore of little value.

When a liver biopsy has been decided upon, both histologic studies with stains for copper and copper-associated proteins and chemical quantitation for copper are performed. In all confirmed cases of Wilson disease, hepatic copper is greater than 3.9 μmol/g dry weight (237.6 μg/g) compared with a normal range of 0.2 to 0.6 μmol/g. Because of the large number of mutations causing the disease, a combination of mutation and linkage analysis is required for prenatal diagnosis and as a rule is not useful in the diagnosis of an individual patient.

A variant of Wilson disease begins in adolescence and is marked by progressive tremor, dysarthria, disturbed eye movements, and dementia. Biochemically, it is characterized by low serum levels of copper and ceruloplasmin. Kayser-Fleischer rings are absent, and liver copper concentrations are low. Metabolic studies using labeled copper suggest a failure in copper absorption from the lower gut.

In familial apoceruloplasm deficiency, the clinical presentation is dementia, retinal degeneration, and a variety of movement disorders. MRI and neuropathologic examinations demonstrate iron deposition in the basal ganglia. The clinical and pathologic findings confirm the essential role of ceruloplasmin in iron metabolism and in brain iron homeostasis. The relationship between this condition and Hallervorden-Spatz syndrome is unclear.

Treatment

All patients with Wilson disease, whether symptomatic or asymptomatic, require treatment. The aims of treatment are initially to remove the toxic amounts of copper and secondarily to prevent tissue reaccumulation of the metal.

Treatment can be divided into two phases: the initial phase, when toxic copper levels are brought under control, and maintenance therapy. There is no currently agreed on regimen for the treatment of the new patient with neurologic or psychiatric symptoms. In the past, most centers recommended starting patients on penicillamine (600 mg to 3,000 mg/day). Although this drug is effective in promoting urinary excretion of copper, adverse reactions during both the initial and maintenance phases of treatment are seen in about 25% of patients. These include worsening of neurologic symptoms during the initial phases of treatment, seen in up to 50% of patients and frequently irreversible. Skin rashes, gastrointestinal discomfort, and hair loss are also encountered. During maintenance therapy, one may see polyneuropathy, polymyositis, and nephropathy. Some of these adverse effects can be prevented by giving pyridoxine (25 mg/day).

Because of these side effects, many institutions now advocate initial therapy with ammonium tetrathiomolybdate (60 to 300 mg/day, administered in six divided doses, three with meals and three between meals). Tetrathiomolybdate forms a complex with protein and copper and when given with food blocks the absorption of copper. The major drawback to using this drug is that it still has not been approved for general use in this country.

Triethylene tetramine dihydrochloride (trientine) (250 mg four times a day, given at least 1 hour before or 2 hours after meals) is also a chelator that increases urinary excretion of copper. Its effectiveness is less than that of penicillamine, but the incidence of toxicity and hypersensitivity reactions is lower.

Zinc acetate (50 mg of elemental zinc acetate three times a day) acts by inducing intestinal metallothionein, which has a high affinity for copper and prevents its entrance into blood. Zinc is far less toxic than penicillamine but is much slower acting. Diet does not play an important role in the management of Wilson disease, although Brewer (1995) recommended restriction of liver and shellfish during the first year of treatment.

Zinc is the optimum drug for maintenance therapy and for the treatment of the presymptomatic patient. Trientine in combination with zinc acetate has been suggested for patients who present in hepatic failure. Liver transplantation can be helpful in the patient who presents in end-stage liver disease. The procedure appears to correct the metabolic defect and can reverse neurologic symptoms.

Improvement of neurologic symptoms and signs and fading of the Kayser-Fleischer rings can be expected from therapy. As a rule, patients with the predominantly pseudosclerotic form of the disease fare better than those with dystonia as the main manifestation. Improvement of neurologic symptoms starts 5 to 6 months after therapy has begun and is generally complete in 24 months. Serial neuroimaging studies demonstrate progressive reduction of the abnormal areas in the basal ganglia (Fig. 89.3). Survival of patients who have completed the first few years of treatment is within the range of normal.

MENKES DISEASE (KINKY HAIR DISEASE) (MIM 309400)

Menkes disease (kinky hair disease [KHD]) is a focal degenerative disorder of gray matter that is transmitted by a gene mapped to the long arm of the X chromosome. The gene codes for a copper-transporting ATPase that has been localized to the Golgi complex. This transporter is required to mobilize copper from the intestinal mucosa cells and to transfer copper into apoenzymes. Numerous mutations have been documented. Partial gene deletions are seen in some 15% to 20% of patients. About half of the mutations lead to splicing abnormalities. Other mutations that have been encountered include small duplications, nonsense mutations, and missense mutations. To date, all mutations detected have been unique for each given family, and almost all have been associated with a decreased level of the mRNA for the copper-transporting ATPase. These observations explain the considerable variability in the severity of clinical manifestations.

The result of this gene defect is maldistribution of body copper. The metal accumulates to abnormal levels in a form or location that makes it inaccessible for the synthesis of various copper enzymes. These include cytochrome *c* oxidase, lysyl oxidase, superoxide dismutase, and tyrosinase. Cytochrome *c* oxidase (complex IV) is a copper-containing enzyme located in the mitochondrial inner membrane. It is the terminal oxidase of the respiratory chain. In KHD there is a marked reduction in the enzyme in all portions of the central nervous system. Lysyl oxidase normally deaminates lysine and hydoxylysine as the first step in collagen cross-link formation. Several groups of workers have found that lysyl oxidase activity is markedly reduced in children with KHD. Tyrosinase, an enzyme involved in melanin biosynthesis, is considered to be responsible for reduced pigmentation and hair and skin.

Copper levels are low in liver and all areas of the brain but are elevated in some other tissues, notably intestinal mucosa and kidney. Patients absorb little or no orally administered copper, but when the metal is given intravenously, there is a prompt rise in serum copper and ceruloplasmin. In fibroblasts, the copper content is markedly elevated as is metallothionein; synthesis of metallothionein is increased as a consequence of abnormally high intracellular copper levels.

As a consequence of tissue copper deficiency, a large number of pathologic changes is set into motion. Cerebral and systemic arteries are tortuous with irregular lumens and frayed and split intimal linings. In brain, there is extensive focal degeneration of cortical gray matter with neuronal loss and gliosis. Cellular loss is prominent in the cerebellum, where many Purkinje cells are lost; others show grotesque proliferation of the dendritic network. In the thalamus, there is primary cellular degeneration that spares the smaller inhibitory neurons.

The incidence is thought to be as high as 2 in 100,000 male live births. Symptoms appear in the neonatal period. Most commonly, hypothermia, poor feeding, and impaired weight gain are observed. Seizures soon become apparent with progressive deterioration of all neurologic functions. The most striking finding is the appearance of the hair, which is colorless and friable. On microscopic examination, a variety of abnormalities is evident, most often pili torti (twisted hair) and trichorrhexis nodosa (fractures of the hair shaft at regular intervals).

Radiographs of long bones reveal metaphyseal spurring and a diaphyseal periosteal reaction. On arteriography, the cerebral vessels are markedly elongated and tortuous. Similar changes are seen in systemic blood vessels. CT or MRI may reveal areas of cortical atrophy or tortuous and enlarged intracranial vessels. Subdural effusions are not unusual (Fig. 89.4).

The clinical history and appearance of the infant suggest the diagnosis. Serum ceruloplasmin and copper levels are normally low in the neonatal period and do not reach adult levels until age 1 month. Thus, these determinations must be performed serially to demonstrate that the expected rise does not occur. The increased copper content of fibroblasts permits intrauterine diagnosis. Even though copper infusions raise serum copper and ceruloplasmin, neurologic symptoms are neither alleviated nor prevented. Early treatment with copper-histidine could be beneficial in some instances. Several variants of Menkes syndrome have been recognized based on the low serum copper concentrations. Symptoms include ataxia, mild mental retardation, and

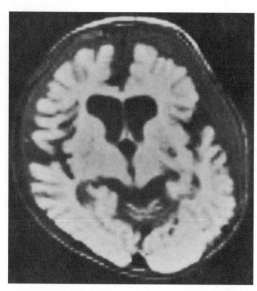

FIG. 89.4. Axial T1-weighted magnetic resonance image in patient with kinky hair disease. Patient was a 2-year-old girl with psychomotor retardation, seizures, and characteristic hair. No family history of neurologic disease. Chromosomal analysis revealed X/2 translocation. There is considerable periventricular and cortical atrophy. Fluid collection over left cortical margin represents and old subdural hematoma.

extrapyramidal movement disorders. In occipital horn syndrome, a condition allelic with KHD, the characteristic picture includes a hyperelastic and bruisable skin, hyperextensible joints, hernias, bladder diverticula or rupture, and multiple skeletal abnormalities, including wormian bones in the skull.

SUGGESTED READINGS

Aisen AM, Martel W, Gabrielsen TO, et al. Wilson disease of the brain. MR imaging. *Radiology* 1985;157:137–141.

Akil M, Brewer GJ. Psychiatric and behavioral abnormalities in Wilson's disease. *Adv Neurol* 1995;65:171–178.

Arima M, Takeshita K, Yoshino K, et al. Prognosis of Wilson's disease in childhood. *Eur J Pediatr* 1977;126:147–154.

Brewer GJ. Practical recommendations and new therapies for Wilson's disease. *Drugs* 1995;50:240–249.

Brewer GJ, Hill GM, Prasad AS, et al. Oral zinc for Wilson's disease. *Ann Intern Med* 1983;99:314–320.

Brewer GJ, Yuzbasian-Gurkan V. Wilson disease. *Medicine (Baltimore)* 1992;71:139–164.

Chelly J, Monaco AP. Cloning the Wilson disease gene. *Nat Genet* 1993;5:317–318.

Danks DM, Campbell PE, Stevens BJ, et al. Menkes' kinky hair syndrome: An inherited defect in copper absorption with widespread effects. *Pediatrics* 1972;50:188–201.

Davis W, Chowrimootoo GF, Seymour CA. Defective biliary copper exretion in Wilson's disease: the role of caeruloplasmin. *Eur J Clin Invest* 1996;26:893–901.

Fleischer, B. Über einer der "Pseudosklerose" nahestehende bisher unbekannte Krankheit (gekennzeichnet durch Tremor, psychische Störungen, bräunliche Pigmentierung bestimmter Gewebe, insbesondere auch der Hornhautperipherie, Lebercirrhose). *Deutsch Z Nervenheilk* 1912;44:179–201.

Francis MJ, Jones EE, Levy ER, et al. A Golgi localization signal identified in the Menkes recombinant protein. *Hum Mol Genet* 1998;7:1245–1252.

Gitlin J. Aceruloplasminemia. *Pediatr Res* 1998;44:271–276.

Glass JD, Reich SG, Delong MR. Wilson's disease. Development of neurologic disease after beginning penicillamine therapy. *Arch Neurol* 1990;47:595–596.

Grover WD, Johnson WC, Henkin RI. Clinical and biochemical aspects of trichopoliodystrophy. *Ann Neurol* 1979;5:65–71.

Heckmann J, Saffer D. Abnormal copper metabolism: another "non-Wilson's" case. *Neurology* 1988;38:1493–1496.

Hefter H, Rautenberg W, Kreuzpaintner G, et al. Does orthoptic liver transplantation heal Wilson's disease? Clinical follow-up of two liver-transplanted patients. *Acta Neurol Scand* 1991;84:192–196.

Kayser, B. Ueber einen Fall von angeborener grünlicher Verfärbung der Cornea. *Klin Monatsbl Augenheilkd* 1902;40:22–25.

Lutsenko S, Cooper MJ. Localization of the Wilson's disease protein product to mitochondria. *Proc Natl Acad Sci USA* 1998;95:6004–6009.

Menkes JH, Alter M, Steigleder GK, et al. A sex-linked recessive disorder with growth retardation, peculiar hair, and focal cerebral and cerebellar degeneration. *Pediatrics* 1962;29:764–779.

Royce PM, Camakaris J, Danks DM. Reduced lysyl oxidase activity in skin fibroblasts from patients with Menkes' syndrome. *Biochem J* 1980;192:579–586.

Scheinberg IH, Sternieb I. *Wilson's disease*, 2nd ed. Philadelphia: WB Saunders, 1999.

Shah AB, Chernov I, Zhang HT, et al. Identification and analysis of mutation in the Wilson disease gene ATP 7B. *Am J Hum Genet* 1997;61:317–339.

Starosta-Rubenstein S, Young AB, Kluin K, et al. Clinical assessment of 31 patients with Wilson's disease. *Arch Neurol* 1987;44:365–370.

Tanzi RE, Petrukhin K, Chernov I, et al. The Wilson disease gene is a copper-transporting ATPase with homology to the Menkes disease gene. *Nat Genet* 1993;5:344–350.

Thomas GR, Forbes JR, Roberts EA, et al. The Wilson disease gene: spectrum of mutations and their consequences. *Nat Genet* 1995;9:210–217.

Vulpe C, Levinson B, Whitney S, et al. Isolation of a candidate gene for Menkes disease and evidence that it encodes a copper-transporting ATPase. *Nat Genet* 1993;3:7–13.

Wilson SAK. Progressive lenticular degeneration: a familial nervous disease associated with cirrhosis of the liver. *Brain* 1912;34:295–509.

Merritt's Neurology, 10th ed., edited by L.P. Rowland. Lippincott Williams & Wilkins, Philadelphia © 2000.

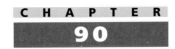

ACUTE INTERMITTENT PORPHYRIA

LEWIS P. ROWLAND

Excessive excretion of porphyrins makes the urine appear bright red. The change is so dramatic that one form of genetic porphyria was among the first inborn errors of metabolism when that class of disease was identified by Garrod. We now recognize both acquired and heritable forms; the genetic categories are further divided into hepatic and erythropoietic types, depending on the site of the enzymatic disorder. Neurologic manifestations are encountered in two classes of porphyria. *Acute intermittent porphyria* (AIP; MIM 176000) occurs worldwide; *variegate porphyria* (MIM 176200) occurs in Sweden and South Africa. These two forms differ primarily in that a rash occurs in the variegate form but not in AIP. Both are inherited as autosomal dominant traits, with low penetrance.

PATHOGENESIS

There are eight steps in the biosynthesis of heme. The crucial steps in understanding porphyria are as follows: delta *aminolevulinic acid* (ALA) is formed from succinyl CoA and glycine under the influence of ALA synthetase; two molecules of ALA are joined by ALA-dehydratase to form a monopyrrole, *porphobilinogen* (PBG); four molecules of PBG are linked to form a *porphyrin* by *uroporphyrinogen-1 synthase*—rearrangements of the side chains of this tetrapyrrole follow under the action of a series of other enzymes, including *protoporphyrinogen oxidase*; and the process culminates in the formation of heme by the addition of an iron molecule.

In AIP, there is excessive urinary excretion of ALA, PBG, and several porphyrins. Suggestions of a block in an alternate pathway of ALA metabolism have not been confirmed. It is still not certain how this pattern of metabolite excretion arises. The dominant theory is of a block in the activity of PBG deaminase in AIP and of protoporphyrinogen oxidase in the variegate form; this causes decreased amounts of heme to be formed downstream, and the lack of normal inhibitory feedback from heme on ALA synthetase releases that enzyme, accounting for the overproduction of ALA and PBG. However, there is no deficiency of heme compounds in blood or tissues, and the activity of PBG deaminase is about 50% of normal. This is the usual level of enzyme activity in asymptomatic heterozygote carriers of autosomal recessive diseases; it is not clear why the same level of activity should be linked to symptoms in AIP but not in so many other conditions. Moreover, the decreased activity of PBG deaminase has been demonstrated in liver biopsy specimens, cultured skin fibroblasts, amniotic cells, and erythrocytes.

Inexplicably, the enzyme activity is normal in some unequivocally affected individuals.

Neurologic symptoms do not appear in other genetic disorders of porphyrin synthesis. It has not been possible to attribute the characteristic neuropathy of AIP to the increased amounts of circulating ALA or PBG. Clinical symptoms of porphyria are similar to those of lead poisoning, in which ALA excretion also increases, but PBG excretion is normal in lead intoxication.

Whatever the abnormality, clinical symptoms seem to be caused by the interaction of genetic and environmental factors. Porphyric crises result most often from ingestion or administration of drugs that adversely affect porphyrin metabolism, especially barbiturates taken for sedation or for general anesthesia. Attacks are also attributed to menses, starvation, emotional stress, intercurrent infections, or other drugs.

MOLECULAR GENETICS

Genetic heterogeneity was evident even before DNA analysis was possible. For instance, using antibodies to PBG deaminase, 74% to 85% of families show cross-reacting immunologic material, whereas others do not. In most families, the enzyme in red blood cells has about half of normal activity; in others, the erythrocyte enzyme is normal.

The enzyme has been mapped to 11q24.1-q24.2. DNA studies have revealed 14 different mutations in the gene. In Sweden, about half of all families had the same point mutation. Fifteen of 49 Dutch families and 1 of 33 French families showed a single base mutation. There has been no convincing documentation of a homozygous individual, but one child was a "compound" of two different mutations at the same locus on the two chromosomes. DNA analysis is important in family studies, identifying people at risk more reliably than assays of erythrocyte PBG deaminase activity, which, in one study, missed 28% of those who carried the mutation and therefore might be susceptible to symptoms if exposed to responsible drugs.

PATHOLOGY

The functional disorder is not due to structural change. Even in fatal cases, it may be difficult to demonstrate any histologic lesions. Demyelinating lesions of central and peripheral nerves have been observed, but modern electrophysiologic studies show normal or nearly normal conduction velocities with signs of denervation in muscle, the pattern of an axonal neuropathy. This view has been supported by morphometric studies of peripheral nerves and nerve roots, with evidence also of a dying-back process. Large and small fibers are affected in peripheral nerves, and autonomic fibers are also attacked.

INCIDENCE

In South Africa, Dean and Barnes traced most current cases to a single colonist who arrived there in 1688. In Sweden, the prevalence varies from 1:1,000 in the north to 1:100,000 population in other parts. Prevalence figures for other countries are also about 1:100,000. In one psychiatric hospital, the prevalence was 2:1,000. Acute symptoms are rare, however, and in major academic medical centers in New York, new cases are seen less often than once a year. All races seem to be affected. In most series, women are more often affected than men. Symptoms are rare in childhood and are most likely to affect adolescents or young adults.

SYMPTOMS AND SIGNS

Asymptomatic individuals with acute porphyria or variegate porphyria are identified by biochemical tests. Symptoms of either disease occur in attacks that may be induced by commonly used drugs; these are described subsequently. The symptoms of an attack are most commonly gastrointestinal (attributed to autonomic neuropathy), psychiatric, and neurologic (Table 90.1). Abdominal pain is most common and may occur alone or with a neurologic or psychiatric disorder. There is usually no abdominal rigidity, but fever, leukocytosis, and diarrhea or constipation often lead to laparotomy. Patients with acute porphyria may actually have appendicitis or some other visceral emergency. The psychiatric disorder may suggest conversion reaction, acute delirium, mood change, or an acute or chronic psychosis. Symptoms of the neuropathy are like those of any peripheral neuropathy except that the signs may be purely motor and are almost always associated with abdominal pain. In one series, 18% of the cases with neuropathy were fatal, 25% recovered completely, and the others were left with some neurologic disability. Survivors may have recurrent attacks. Cerebral manifestations are unusual except for the syndrome of inappropriate secretion of antidiuretic hormone. Unexplained transient am-

blyopia has been reported. Autonomic abnormalities include hypertension and tachycardia.

LABORATORY DATA

Routine laboratory tests usually give normal results, including cerebrospinal fluid. Electromyogram shows signs of denervation, but motor and sensory nerve velocities are normal or only slightly slow.

Even between attacks, affected individuals can be identified by a qualitative test for PBG in the urine. The Watson-Schwartz test depends on the action of the monopyrrole with diaminobenzaldehyde to form a reddish compound that is soluble in chloroform. The test can be performed in a few minutes, and there are few false-positive or false-negative results. Quantitative measurement of urinary PBG and ALA can be achieved by column chromatography, now available in commercial laboratories in the United States. The most reliable test is assay of PBG-deaminase activity in red blood cell membranes, which is about 50% of control values in affected individuals with AIP, between and during attacks. The assay also identifies family members who are at risk even if they are asymptomatic, and DNA analysis is even more accurate.

Variegate porphyria cannot be distinguished from AIP clinically, unless there is a rash, which may be lacking in almost half of symptomatic individuals. The acute attacks are virtually identical to those of AIP. The difference is biochemical; excretion of PBG and ALA is increased during attacks but not between attacks. In contrast to AIP, there is increased fecal excretion of protoporphyrin, but even this may be normal, and measurement of the porphyrin in bile seems more accurate. The affected enzyme is protoporphyrinogen oxidase.

DIAGNOSIS

Clinical diagnosis is not difficult if there is a family history of the disease, but the condition is so rare in the United States that physicians often do not recognize the source of unexplained abdominal pain and personality disorder. If peripheral neuropathy is added to the syndrome, however, and the appropriate biochemical tests are made, the diagnosis is ascertained. These tests are more important than looking for red urine or measurement of porphyrins in urine. Neurologically, the major disorder to be considered is the Guillain-Barré syndrome, but the characteristic rise in cerebrospinal fluid protein content of that disease is not found in AIP; the cerebrospinal fluid protein rises so rarely in AIP that when the protein does rise, it may be a sign of Guillain-Barré syndrome in a person with porphyria.

TABLE 90.1. CLINICAL MANIFESTATIONS OF ACUTE INTERMITTENT PORPHYRIA

	% of Patients
Abdominal pain	85–95
Vomiting	52–75
Constipation	46–70
Diarrhea	9–11
Abdominal surgery	22–46
Paresis	42–72
Myalgia	53
Convulsions	10–16
Sensory loss	9–38
Transient amaurosis	4–6
Diplopia	3
Delirium	18–52
Mood change	28
Psychosis	12
Hypertension	40–55
Tachycardia	28–60
Fever	12–37
Azotemia	6–27

From 352 reported cases in three series cited by Rowland, 1961.

TREATMENT

The fundamental biochemical abnormality cannot be corrected, but the autonomic manifestations of an acute attack may be re-

TABLE 90.2. PORPHYROGENIC DRUGS IN ACUTE PORPHYRIA[a]

Drugs	Number of exposures	Only precipitant
Barbiturate	81	31
Analgesics	16	5
Sulfonamides	16	5
Nonbarbiturate hypnotics	15	4
Unidentified sedatives	14	10
Miscellaneous drugs	12	3
Anticonvulsants	10	5
Hormonal	6	5

[a]153 acute episodes in 138 patients.
From Eales, 1979.

versed by propanolol. Doses up to 100 mg every 4 hours may reverse tachycardia, abdominal pain, and anxiety.

The neuropathy and abdominal symptoms may respond dramatically to hematin given intravenously in amounts from 200 to 1,000 mg in attempts to suppress the activity of ALA dehydratase. The optimal dosage is uncertain; one recommendation is to use 4 mg hematin/kg body weight twice daily for 3 days. The wholesale price of hemin in 1996 was $120 to $475 daily. This may still be the most effective treatment, but some advocate the use of cimetidine orally, 800 mg daily.

Treatment of seizures is a problem because most commonly used anticonvulsants have been held responsible for porphyric attacks in human patients or they are porphyrogenic in experimental animals or cultured hepatic cells. In acute attacks of porphyria, seizures may be treated with diazepam or paraldehyde, whereas hematin and propanolol are used to abort the attacks. Between attacks, conventional anticonvulsants may be evaluated cautiously, monitoring urinary excretion of ALA and PBG. Gabapentin is said to be safe and effective.

Other drugs that are suitable for symptomatic relief include codeine and meperidine for pain, chlorpromazine and other psychoactive drugs, and almost all antibiotics. The major drugs to avoid are barbiturates in any form, including pentobarbital for general anesthesia (Table 90.2). Barbiturates may be especially hazardous when given for sedation or anesthesia in the early stages of an attack. It is otherwise difficult to prevent attacks, but some women have symptoms only and regularly in relation to menses; both suppression of ovulation and prophylactic use of hematin have been reported to be effective. In case of accident, patients should wear warning bracelets to identify the drug problem. Prophylactic care requires identification of gene carriers so that they can avoid drugs that precipitate attacks in susceptible people.

SUGGESTED READINGS

Becker DM, Kramer S. The neurological manifestations of porphyria: a review. *Medicine (Baltimore)* 1977;56:411–423.

Bottomley SS, Bonkowsky HL, Birnbaum MK. The diagnosis of acute intermittent porphyria. Usefulness and limitations of the erythrocyte uroporphyrinogen-1 synthase assay. *Am J Clin Pathol* 1981;76:133–139.

Brezis M, Ghanem J, Weiler-Ravell O, et al. Hematin and propanolol in acute intermittent porphyria. Full recovery from quadriplegic coma and respiratory failure. *Eur Neurol* 1979;18:289–294.

Dean G. *The porphyrias. A story of inheritance and the environment*, 2nd ed. London: Pitman, 1971.

Delfau MH, Picat C, DeRooij F, et al. Molecular heterogeneity of acute intermittent porphyria: identification of four additional mutations resulting in CRIM-negative subtype of the disease. *Am J Hum Genet* 1991;49:421–428.

Eales L. Porphyria and the dangerous life-threatening drugs. *S Afr Med J* 1979;2:914–917.

Flugel KA, Druschky KF. EMG and nerve conduction in patients with acute intermittent porphyria. *J Neurol* 1977;214:267–279.

Grandchamp B. Acute intermittent porphyria. *Semin Liver Dis* 1998;18:17–24.

Gu XF, deRooij F, Voortman G, et al. Detection of eleven mutations causing acute intermittent porphyria using denaturing gradient gel electrophoresis. *Hum Genet* 1994;93:47–52.

Herick AL, McColl KEL, Moore MR, Cook A. Controlled trial of haem arginate in acute hepatic porphyria. *Lancet* 1989;1:1295–1297.

Hindmarsh JT. Variable pheotypic expression of genotypic abnormalities in the porphyrias. *Clin Chim Acta* 1993;217:29–38.

King PH, Bragdon AC. MRI reveals multiple reversible lesions in an attack of acute intermittent porphyria. *Neurology* 1991;41:1300–1302.

Laiwah ACY, Moore MR, Goldberg A. Pathogenesis of acute porphyria. *Q J Med* 1987;63:377–392.

Lee JS, Anvret M. Identification of the most common mutation within the porphobilinogen deaminase gene in Swedish patients with acute intermittent porphyria. *Proc Natl Acad Sci USA* 1991;88:10912–10915.

Lee J-S, Anvret M, Lindsten J, et al. DNA polymorphisms within the porphobilinogen deaminase gene in acute intermittent porphyria. *Hum Genet* 1988;79:379–381.

Llewellyn DH, Smyth SJ, Elder GH, et al. Homozygous acute intermittent porphyria: compound heterozygosity for adjacent base transitions in the same codon of the porphobilinogen deaminase gene. *Hum Genet* 1992;89:97–98.

Loftus CS, Arnold WN. Vincent Van Gogh's illness: acute intermittent porphyria? *Br Med J* 1991;303:1585–1591.

McEneaney D, Hawkins S, Trimble E, Smye M. Porphyric neuropathy—a rare and often neglected differential diagnosis of Guillain-Barré syndrome. *J Neurol Sci* 1993;114:231–233.

Meyer UA, Schuurmans MM, Lindberg RL. Acute porphyrias: pathogenesis of neurological manifestations. *Semin Liv Dis* 1998;18:43–52.

Moore MR. The biochemistry of heme synthesis in porphyria and in the porphyrinurias. *Clin Dermatol* 1998;16:203–223.

Moore MR, Disler PB. Drug induction of the acute porphyrias. *Adverse Drug React Acute Poison Rev* 1983;2:149–189.

Mustajoki P, Desnick RJ. Genetic heterogeneity in acute intermittent porphyria: characterisation and frequency of porphobilinogen deaminase mutations in Finland. *Br Med J* 1985;291:505–509.

Muthane UB, Vengamma B, Bharathi KC, Mamatha P. Porphyric neuropathy: prevention of progression using haeme-arginate. *J Intern Med* 1993;234:611–613.

Pierach CA, Weimer MK, Cardinal RA, et al. Red blood cell porphobilinogen deaminase in the evaluation of acute intermittent porphyria. *JAMA* 1987;257:60–61.

Reynolds NC, Miska RM. Safety of anticonvulsants in hepatic porphyrias. *Neurology* 1981;31:480–484.

Ridley A. The neuropathy of acute intermittent porphyria. *Q J Med* 1969;38:307–333.

Rogers PD. Cimetidine in the treatment of acute intermittent porphyria. *Ann Pharmacother* 1997;31:365–367.

Rowland LP. Acute intermittent porphyria: search for an enzymatic defect with implications for neurology and psychiatry. *Dis Nerv Sys* 1961;22[Suppl]:1–12.

Sadeh H, Blatt I, Martonovits G, et al. Treatment of porphyric convulsions with magnesium sulfate. *Epilepsia* 1991;32:712–715.

Suarez JI, Cohen ML, Larkin J, Kernich CA, Hricik DE, Daroff RB. Acute intermittent porphyria: clinicopathologic correlation. Report of a case and review of the literature. *Neurology* 1997;48:1678–1683.

Suzuki A, Aso K, Ariyoshi C, Ishimaru N. Acute intermittent porphyria and epilepsy: safety of clonazepam. *Epilepsia* 1992;33:108–111.

Thorner PA, Bilbao JM, Sima AAF, Briggs S. Porphyric neuropathy: an ultrastructural and quantitative study. *Can J Neurol Sci* 1981;8:261–287.

Tishler PV, Woodward B, O'Connor J, et al. High prevalence of intermittent acute porphyria in a psychiatric patient population. *Am J Psychiatry* 1985;142:1430–1436.

Yamada M, Kondo M, Tanaka M, et al. An autopsy case of acute porphyria with a decrease of both uroporphyrinogen I synthetase and ferrochetalase activities. *Acta Neuropathol (Berl)* 1984;64:6–11.

Yeung AC, Moore MR, Goldberg A. Pathogenesis of acute porphyria. *Q J Med* 1987;163:377–392.

Merritt's Neurology, 10th ed., edited by L.P. Rowland. Lippincott Williams & Wilkins, Philadelphia © 2000.

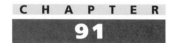

NEUROLOGICAL SYNDROMES WITH ACANTHOCYTES

TIMOTHY A. PEDLEY
LEWIS P. ROWLAND

Several neurologic syndromes are associated with abnormal erythrocytes that are called *acanthocytes* because of the spiny projections from the cell surface. *Acantho* is derived from a Greek word meaning thorns. Acanthocytes are seen in four neurologic disorders: abetalipoproteinemia, hypolipoproteinemia, neuroacanthocytosis, and McLeod syndrome.

ABETALIPOPROTEINEMIA

Abetalipoproteinemia, the *Bassen-Kornzweig syndrome*, is an autosomal recessive disease characterized by inability of the liver and intestine to secrete apolipoprotein B. It is caused by mutations in the microsomal triglyceride transfer protein gene, not the one for apolipoprotein B. Abetalipoproteinemia was originally defined clinically as a neurologic disorder resembling Friedreich ataxia in patients with chronic steatorrhea and acanthocytes.

There have been few autopsy examinations, but the neuropathologic findings account for the clinical syndrome. There is demyelination of the posterior columns, spinocerebellar tracts, and corticospinal tracts. Neuronal changes are seen in the Purkinje cells and molecular layer of the cerebellum and the anterior horn cells. Peripheral nerves show mainly axonal loss with focal areas of demyelination, especially in large myelinated nerves. There is no clear explanation, however, for the clinically evident ophthalmoplegia. Interstitial myocardial fibrosis may be seen. Muscle shows signs of denervation with accumulation of lipopigment.

Pathogenesis

Abetalipoproteinemia is caused by mutations in the microsomal triglyceride transfer protein, a heterodimer composed of a multifunctional protein, protein disulfide isomerase, and a unique 97-

kDa subunit. Mutations that functionally inactivate the 97-kDa subunit lead to defects in the assembly and secretion of apolipoprotein B-containing lipoproteins, probably because apolipoprotein B requires microsomal triglyceride transfer protein to enter the endoplasmic reticulum, where lipoproteins are assembled.

Neuropathologic findings and the clinical phenotype result from a nearly complete absence of apolipoprotein B-containing lipoproteins in the plasma. Beta-lipoproteins are an essential component of plasma chylomicrons and very-low-density lipoproteins. Apolipoprotein B is needed for the normal transport of lipids from intestinal mucosa to plasma, but in these patients, it is lacking from intestinal mucosa and plasma. As a result, there is intestinal malabsorption of lipids, and the serum content of lipids is drastically reduced, including cholesterol, triglycerides, and phospholipids. (Serum cholesterol levels, normally 135 to 335 mg/dL, are 25 to 61 mg/dL in affected individuals.) Low-density and very-low-density lipoproteins are also much reduced, as are chylomicrons. Levels of high-density lipoproteins are about 50% of normal.

As a consequence of the malabsorption, there is severe deficiency of the fat-soluble vitamins, A, D, E, and K. Vitamin A levels are 0 to 37 μg/dL (normal, 20 to 87), and this deficiency probably plays a role in the retinitis pigmentosa. Vitamin E levels are 0.06 to 0.1 μg/mL (normal, 0.5 to 1.5), a depletion held responsible for the neurologic disorder that resembles the spinocerebellar syndrome seen in other malabsorption states, including cholestatic liver disease and Crohn disease. The abnormal shape of the erythrocytes also seems to be secondary to the hypolipidemia; the red cell membranes show abnormal distribution of lipid constituents.

Symptoms and Signs

Fatty diarrhea is evident from infancy, with abdominal distention and retarded growth. The children are typically small and underweight, with delayed bone age. The first neurologic abnormality is loss of tendon jerks at about age 5 years. At about age 10, ataxic gait is noted, then limb ataxia, tremor of the head and hands, and evidence of sensorimotor neuropathy: distal limb weakness, distal paresthesias, and glove-stocking and proprioceptive sensory loss. There is also proximal limb weakness with scoliosis in 25% of patients and pedal abnormalities such as pes cavus. Babinski signs are inconsistent (Table 91.1).

Eye movements become progressively restricted, but before ophthalmoplegia is complete, nystagmus may be prominent. Concomitantly, as retinitis pigmentosa develops in adolescence, night-blindness (nyctalopia), with constriction of the visual

TABLE 91.1. NEUROLOGIC ABNORMALITIES IN A SERIES OF PATIENTS WITH ABETALIPOPROTEINEMIA

	Number of patients	% of patients
Mental retardation	4/16	25
Retinopathy	9/18	50
Abnormal eye movements	8/18	44
Lingual atrophy, fasciculation	7/18	39
Limb weakness	4/18	22
Areflexia	13/18	72
Sensory loss		
Cutaneous	3/18	17
Position, vibration	12/14	86
Romberg sign	5/10	50
Babinski sign	6/17	35

Adapted from Brin MF. Acanthocytosis. *Clin Neurol* 1993;19(Part 1):271–299.

fields and loss of visual acuity, occurs. The fundi show macular degeneration, with pigmentary degeneration in the midperiphery of the retina, arteriolar narrowing, bone spicules, and angioid streaks. The syndrome is fully developed by age 20.

Vitamin K deficiency may lead to subdural or retroperitoneal hemorrhage, or there may be excessive blood loss after surgery.

Laboratory Data

In addition to the plasma changes mentioned previously, the erythrocyte sedimentation rate is inordinately low, usually 1 mm/hr. Nerve conduction studies and electromyography indicate that the neuropathy is primarily axonal. Sensory evoked responses imply abnormality in the posterior columns; brainstem auditory responses are normal. Abnormalities of visual evoked potentials and electroretinography reflect the retinal degeneration and optic neuropathy. Electrocardiographic abnormalities, cardiac enlargement, and murmurs imply a cardiomyopathy, but heart block and symptomatic congestive heart failure are not part of the picture.

Diagnosis

The neurologic disorder resembles Friedreich ataxia, spinocerebellar degeneration, sensorimotor peripheral neuropathy, and progressive external ophthalmoplegia. The first clue to the diagnosis of abetalipoproteinemia is the finding of low values for serum cholesterol. Identifying acanthocytes usually requires a fresh blood smear (without ETDA) and even then may go unrecognized unless the technician has been asked to look for them specifically. Measurement of serum beta-lipoprotein and plasma lipids confirms the diagnosis.

Treatment

The essential element of treatment is dietary supplementation with vitamin E in doses of 10,000 to 25,000 units daily; blood levels should be monitored to avoid liver damage. In addition, adults should be given vitamin K, at least 5 mg daily. Supplemental corn oil has been recommended to correct or prevent deficiency of essential fatty acids.

With adequate tocopherol therapy, progression of the neurologic and retinal abnormalities ceases, and some patients even improve. Treatment is most effective when given early, preferably before neurologic signs are apparent. Under these circumstances, the neurologic syndrome may be prevented. Replacement therapy in adults with established symptoms is usually only partially successful.

Hypobetalipoproteinemia is an autosomal dominant disorder caused by different mutations in the gene for apolipoprotein B (apoB100), all of which seem to result in production of truncated forms of beta-lipoprotein that cannot be secreted by hepatocytes and enterocytes. In heterozygous patients, plasma levels of lipoproteins are about 50% of normal. An animal model has been created by gene targeting. Levels of low-density-lipoprotein cholesterol and triglycerides are also low. Heterozygous individuals usually have no neurologic symptoms. In contrast, homozygous patients usually have prominent steatorrhea, adult-onset ataxia, retinitis, and neuropathy with acanthocytosis, as in abetalipoproteinemia.

NEUROACANTHOCYTOSIS

Neuroacanthocytosis (Levine-Critchley syndrome or chorea-acanthocytosis) is a multisystem neurodegenerative disorder characterized by acanthocytes, normal plasma lipids and lipoproteins, and variable neurologic manifestations. Onset is usually in the fourth or fifth decade, but both juvenile and elderly forms are known. The most consistent clinical feature is a hyperkinetic movement disorder (chorea, orofacial dyskinesias, and dystonia). In many patients, dementia follows psychiatric features, including obsessive-compulsive disorder and personality changes. An axonal neuropathy with muscle wasting, weakness, and absent deep tendon reflexes occurs in most patients. About 40% of patients have epileptic seizures. The course is one of progressive disability, with a mean duration of illness of about 14 years. Only symptomatic therapy is available, but response of the involuntary movements to drug treatment is generally poor.

The clinical picture correlates with neuronal degeneration and astrocytic proliferation within the basal ganglia and substantia nigra. Despite the dementia and psychiatric symptoms, the cerebral cortex is histologically normal. The axonal neuropathy involves primarily large-diameter myelinated fibers, and muscle biopsy shows findings consistent with denervation. Magnetic resonance imaging findings are similar to those of Huntington chorea, including prominent atrophy of the caudate nuclei and increased T2 signal within the striatum.

Neuroacanthocytosis is typically familial, although sporadic cases occur. Most affected families exhibit an autosomal dominant pattern of inheritance; in others, however, autosomal recessive inheritance seems likely The disease has been linked to chromosome 9q21.

MCLEOD SYNDROME

The *McLeod syndrome* is an X-linked disorder defined by abnormal expression of the Kell blood group antigens and absence of the Kx erythrocyte surface antigen. The first cases were found in asymptomatic people who were donating blood and had blood typing carried out. When they were studied hematologically, the acanthocytes were recognized, and so were high serum levels of creatine kinase, high enough to suggest a true myopathy. Later, some people with the condition were found to have a symptomatic myopathy, amyotrophy, or involuntary movements, and a permanent hemolytic state. In some patients, the clinical features are similar to those of neuroacanthocytosis.

The McLeod syndrome results from a point mutation in the XK gene, which encodes a membrane transport protein. The XX protein corresponds to the Kx antigen and is associated with a marked reduction in all Kell antigens. Mutations in the XK gene result in premature termination of translation, so that the aberrant protein has only 128 amino acids instead of 444 and lacks 7 of the normal 10 transmembrane segments. Because several patients with a clinical diagnosis of McLeod syndrome have lacked any abnormality in the XK gene and because at least two point mutations have been found in normal subjects, it is unclear how often mutations in the McLeod gene lead to neurologic disease. The triad of creatine kinase myopathy, acanthocytosis, and neurologic disorder may be caused by mutations in contiguous genes.

SUGGESTED READINGS

Brin MF. Acanthocytosis. *Handb Clin Neurol* 1993;19(Part 1):271–299.

Du EZ, Wang SL, Kayden HJ, et al. Translocation of apolipoprotein B across the endoplasmic reticulum is blocked in abetalipoproteinemia. *J Lipid Res* 1996;37:1309–1315.

Feinberg TE, Cianci CD, Morrow JS, et al. Diagnostic tests for choreoacanthocytosis. *Neurology* 1991;41:1000–1006.

Hardie AE, Pullon HW, Harding AE, et al. Neuroacanthocytosis;a clinical, haematological, and pathological study of 19 cases. *Brain* 1991;114:13–49.

Harding AE. Vitamin E and the nervous system. *Crit Rev Neurobiol* 1987;3:89–103.

Higgins JJ, Patterson MC, Papadopoulos NM, et al. Hypobetalipoproteinemia, acanthocytosis, retinitis pigmentosa, and pallidal degeneration (HARP syndrome). *Neurology* 1992;42:194–198.

Ho MF, Chalmers RM, Davis MB, Harding AE, Monaco AP. A novel point mutation in the McLeod syndrome gene in neuroacanthocytosis. *Ann Neurol* 1996;39:672–675.

Kim E, Cham CM, Veniant MM, Ambroziak P, Young SG. Dual mechanisms for the low plasma levels of truncated apolipoprotein B proteins in familial hypobetalipoproteinemia. Analysis of a new mouse model with a nonsense mutation in the Apob gene. *J Clin Invest* 1998;101:1468–1477.

Levine IM, Estes JW, Looney JM. Hereditary neurological disease with acanthocytosis. A new syndrome. *Arch Neurol* 1968;19:403–409.

Levy E. The genetic basis of primary disorders of intestinal fat transport. *Clin Invest Med* 1996;19:317–324.

Lodi R, Rinaldi R, Gaddi A, et al. Brain and skeletal muscle bioenergetic failure in familial hypolipoproteinemia. *J Neurol Neurosurg Psychiatry* 1998;62:574–580.

MacGilchrist AJ, Mills PR, Noble M, et al. Abetalipoproteinemia in adults: role of vitamin therapy. *J Inherit Metab Dis* 1988;11:184–190.

Muller DPR, Lloyd JK, Wolff OH. The role of vitamin E in the treatment of the neurological features of abetalipoproteinemia and other disorders of fat absorption. *J Inherit Metab Dis* 1985;8[Suppl 1]:88–92.

Rader DJ, Brewer HB Jr. Abetalipoproteinemia. New insights into lipoprotein assembly and vitamin E metabolism from a rare genetic disease. *JAMA* 1993;270:865–869.

Rehberg EF, Samson-Bouma ME, Kienzle B, et al. A novel abetalipoproteinemia genotype. Identification of a missense mutation in the 97-kDa subunit of the microsomoal triglyceride transfer protein. *J Biol Chem* 1996;271:29945–29952.

Rinne J, Daniel SE, Scaravilli F, et al. The neuropathological features of neuroacanthocytosis. *Mov Disord* 1994;9:297–304.

Ross RS, Gregg RE, Law SW. Homozygous hypobetalipoproteinemia: a disease distinct from abetalipoproteinemia at the molecular level. *J Clin Invest* 1988;81:590–595.

Rubio JP, Danek A, Stone C, et al. Chorea-acanthocytosis: genetic linkage to chromosome 9q21. *Am J Hum Genet* 1997;61:899–908.

Runge P, Muller DP, McAllister J, et al. Oral vitamin E supplements can prevent the retinopathy of abetalipoproteinemia. *Br J Ophthalmol* 1986;70:166–173.

Sakai T, Iwashita H, Kakugawa M. Neuroacanthocytosis syndrome and choreoacanthocytosis (Levine-Critchley syndrome). *Neurology* 1985;35:1679.

Satya-Murti S, Howard L, Krohel G, Wolf B. The spectrum of neurologic disorder from vitamin E deficiency. *Neurology* 1986;36:917–921.

Schwartz JF, Rowland LP, Eder H, et al. Bassen-Kornzweig syndrome: deficiency of serum B-lipoprotein. *Arch Neurol* 1963;8:438–454.

Shizuka M, Watanabe M, Aoki M, et al. Analysis of the McLeod syndrome gene in three patients with neuroacanthocytosis. *J Neurol Sci* 1997;150:133–135.

Shoulders CC, Brett DJ, Bayliss JD, et al. Abetalipoproteinemia is caused by defects of the gene encoding the 97-kDa subunit of a microsomal triglyceride transfer protein. *Hum Mol Genet* 1993;2:2109–2116.

Sokol RJ. Vitamin E and neurologic deficits. *Adv Pediatr* 1990;37:119–148.

Vance JM, Pericak-Vance BA, Bowman MH, et al. Chorea-acanthocytosis: a report of three new families and implications for genetic counselling. *Am J Med Genet* 1987;28:403–410.

Welterau PJ, Aggerbeeli LP, Bouma ME, et al. Absence of microsomal triglyceride transfer protein in individuals with abetalipoproteinemia. *Science* 1992;258:999–1001.

Witt TN, Danek A, Reiter M, et al. McLeod syndrome: a distinct form of neuroacanthocytosis. Report of two cases and literature review with emphasis on neuromuscular manifestations. *J Neurol* 1992;349:302–306.

Merritt's Neurology, 10th ed., edited by L.P. Rowland. Lippincott Williams & Wilkins, Philadelphia © 2000.

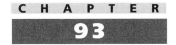

CHAPTER 92

XERODERMA PIGMENTOSUM

LEWIS P. ROWLAND

Xeroderma pigmentosum (MIM 278700) is a rare condition that is not a metabolic disorder in the conventional sense. Rather, cultured cells from affected patients are hypersensitive to being killed or to undergoing mutagenesis by ultraviolet light and chemical carcinogens. Autosomal-recessive inheritance results in lack of a gene product responsible for the excision of damaged deoxyribonucleic acid (DNA) or for replication past the damaged site of DNA. The mutations affect subunits of the transcription/repair factor TFIIH as modified by interaction with several tumor suppressor genes. Some patients have features of both xeroderma pigmentosum and Cockayne syndrome.

The syndrome was first described by Kaposi in 1874, but it is also known as the DeSanctis-Cacchione syndrome. Affected individuals show marked cutaneous hypersensitivity to sunlight beginning in early childhood. Erythema and blisters are followed by freckling, keratosis, and skin cancers. Dwarfism is common. Neurologic disorders include microcephaly, mental retardation, chorea, ataxia, corticospinal signs, and either motor neuron disorders or segmental demyelination of peripheral nerves. Hearing loss and supranuclear ophthalmoplegia have been prominent in some patients. In others, the neurologic disorder is more disabling than the cutaneous problems (see Chapter 107). In one autopsy case, the outstanding change was selective neuronal loss in the cerebral cortex, basal ganglia, olivary nuclei, and cerebellum. In another, the findings resembled olivopontocerebellar atrophy.

Management includes avoidance of sunlight. One patient with a spinal cord glioma was effectively treated with radiother-

apy, without evidence of abnormal responses to x-irradiation. Antenatal diagnosis is possible because cultured amniotic cells show the abnormal patterns of excision repair of DNA. There is no effective treatment for the neurologic disorders.

SUGGESTED READINGS

Coin F, Marinoni JC, Rodolfo C, Fribourg S, Pedrini AM, Egly JM. Mutations in the XPD helicase gene result in XP and TTD phenotypes, preventing interaction between XPD and the p44 subunit of TFIIH. *Nat Genet* 1998;20:184–188.

Ellison AR, Nouspikel T, Jaspers NG, Clarkson SG, Gruenert DC. Complementation of transformed fibroblasts from patients with combined xeroderma pigmentosum-Cockayne syndrome. *Exp Cell Res* 1998; 243:22–28.

Greenhaw GA, Hecht JT, Herbert AA, et al. Xeroderma pigmentosum with severe neurological involvement without significant DNA repair defect. *Am J Hum Genet* 1989;45:447.

Hakamada S, Watanbe K, Sobue G, et al. Xeroderma pigmentosum: neurological, neurophysiological and morphological studies. *Eur Neurol* 1982;21:69–76.

Hwang BJ, Ford JM, Hanawalt PC, Chu G. Expression of the p48 xeroderma pigmentosum gene is p53-dependent and is involved in global genomic repair. *Proc Natl Acad Sci U S A* 1999;96:424–428.

Kanda T, Oda M, Gonezawa M, et al. Peripheral neuropathy in xeroderma pigmentosum. *Brain* 1990;119:1025–1044.

Kenyon GS, Booth JB, Prasher DK, Rudge P. Neuro-otological abnormalities in xeroderma pigmentosum with particular reference to deafness. *Brain* 1985;108:771–784.

Kraemer KH, Lee MM, Scotto J. Xeroderma pigmentosum: cutaneous, ocular, and neurologic abnormalities in 830 published cases. *Arch Dermatol* 1987;123:241–250.

Roytta M, Amttinen A. Xeroderma pigmentosum with neurological abnormalities: clinical and neuropathological study. *Acta Neurol Scand* 1986;73:191–199.

Takeda N, Shibuya M, Maru Y. The BCR-ABL oncoprotein potentially interacts with the xeroderma pigmentosum group B protein. *Proc Nat Acad Sci U S A* 1999;96:203–207.

Woods CG. DNA repair disorders. *Arch Dis Child* 1998;78:178–184.

Merritt's Neurology, 10th ed., edited by L.P. Rowland. Lippincott Williams & Wilkins, Philadelphia © 2000.

CEREBRAL DEGENERATIONS OF CHILDHOOD

**EVELINE C. TRAEGER
ISABELLE RAPIN**

SPONGY DEGENERATION OF THE NERVOUS SYSTEM (CANAVAN DISEASE)

This autosomal-recessive illness (MIM 271900) is one of the more common cerebral degenerative diseases of infancy. Al-

though van Bogaert and Bertrand should be credited with the nosologic identification, it is often called Canavan disease in the United States. It affects all ethnic groups but is especially prevalent among Ashkenazi Jews from eastern Poland, Lithuania, and western Russia, and among Saudi Arabians. A characteristic feature that it shares with Alexander disease and classic Tay-Sachs disease is megalencephaly. The clinical picture is often sufficiently distinctive to suggest the diagnosis. It is prenatal in onset with variable progression; at least 50% of children are symptomatic by 4 months of age.

Extremely poor control of the enlarged head, lack of psychomotor development, spasticity, and optic atrophy are the main features. Affected children may achieve smiling, but they are characteristically quiet and apathetic. Few progress far enough to reach for objects or sit, and except for children with a rare protracted variant, none ever walks independently. Seizures occur in more than 50% of patients. By age 2 years, head growth plateaus as progressive parenchymal destruction leads to hydrocephalus *ex vacuo.* The children eventually become decerebrate and die of intercurrent illness; survival into the second or third decades is not uncommon.

Computed tomography (CT) and magnetic resonance imaging (MRI) show increased lucency of the white matter, poor demarcation of gray and white matter (Fig. 93.1), and, later, severe brain atrophy with ventricular enlargement and gaping sulci. Cerebrospinal fluid (CSF) and nerve conduction velocities are usually normal. The pathology includes two characteristic abnormalities: intramyelinic vacuolation of the deep layers of the cortex, and superficial layers of the white matter and gigantic abnormal mitochondria containing a dense filamentous granular matrix and distorted cristae in the watery cytoplasm of hypertrophied astrocytes. Sponginess eventually becomes diffuse and involves the centrum semiovale, brainstem, cerebellum, and spinal cord. As the disease progresses, the vacuoles enlarge and split the myelin sheath to form cysts that communicate with the extracellular space. This leads to extensive demyelination and tissue destruction with loss of neurons, axons, and oligodendroglia; extensive gliosis follows. Chemical analysis of the brain reveals markedly increased *N*-acetylaspartic acid (NAA) and water content, and nonspecific loss of myelin and other tissue constituents.

Deficiency of aspartoacylase in skin fibroblasts is diagnostic and is associated with elevated levels of NAA in blood and urine, as well as brain. Carrier detection based on aspartoacylase activity in cultured skin fibroblasts is possible; aspartoacylase activity in amniotic fluid, chorionic villi, or amniocytes is unreliable for prenatal diagnosis. The gene for Canavan disease has been cloned and is located on chromosome 17p. Two mutations account for 97% of the alleles in Ashkenazi-Jewish patients. In non-Jewish patients, the mutations are different and more diverse. Carrier detection and prenatal diagnosis by DNA analysis are available in most but not all high-risk families.

Spongy degeneration of the brain also occurs in other conditions, notably intoxication by triethyl tin or hexachlorophene, some neonatal acidurias, some mitochondrial disorders, and the Aicardi-Goutières syndrome (leukodystrophy with CSF lymphocytosis and basal ganglia calcification). In fact, prior to DNA analysis, some cases labeled juvenile spongy degeneration that started in childhood with external ophthalmoplegia and pigmentary degeneration of the retina, with or without other neurologic or systemic abnormalities, may have been Kearns-Sayre syndrome or some other mitochondrial disorder.

INFANTILE NEUROAXONAL DYSTROPHY

Infantile neuroaxonal dystrophy (Seitelberger disease) (MIM 256600) is an autosomal-recessive disease of unknown etiology that typically becomes manifest between 6 and 18 months of age and leads to death before the end of the first decade, usually after a variable period of purely vegetative existence. The first symptom is arrest of motor development, followed by loss of skills. The children may be floppy, spastic, or both. Most never achieve independent walking or speaking. In some, the motor disorder progresses from the legs, to the arms, and finally to the cranial muscles, causing severe dysphagia. There may be loss of sensation in the legs and urinary retention. Ataxia, nystagmus, and optic atrophy are common, but seizures are rare. The degree of dementia is difficult to ascertain because of anarthria; at first, affected children appear alert and seem to understand some language, but intellectual deterioration eventually becomes severe.

A newly described lysosomal storage disease due to alpha-*N*-acetylgalactosaminidase deficiency has been found in patients with a phenotype similar to that of infantile neuroaxonal dystrophy but differing by the presence of prominent generalized or myoclonic seizures. Atypical variants are seen. A few infants are symptomatic from birth, whereas others experience a later onset and more protracted course, some with prominent myoclonus, others with dystonic features.

The relationship of these more chronic cases to Hallervorden-Spatz disease is controversial. Some authorities consider neuroaxonal dystrophy and Hallervorden-Spatz disease to be the same nosologic entity because spheroid formation is seen in both and because there are clinical similarities. Spheroids, however, are not pathognomonic of either disease, and the distribution of these lesions differs in the two disorders; brown discoloration of the globus pallidus occurs only in Hallervorden-Spatz disease.

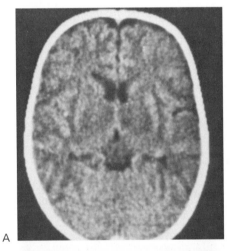

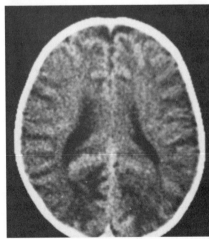

FIG. 93.1. A and B: Axial noncontrast CT in an 11-month-old boy with spongy degeneration. Note the diffuse low density of white matter with occipital preponderance and poor demarcation between gray and white matter. Sulci are mildly widened.

The linkage of Hallervorden-Spatz disease to chromosome 20 in 10 families will help resolve the question of the relationship of the two conditions.

The characteristic pathologic picture of neuroaxonal dystrophy is the profusion of axonal spheroids in the brain, spinal cord, and peripheral nerves. Spheroids are eosinophilic, argyrophilic ovoid inclusions that distend axons and myelin sheaths. They may be found anywhere along axons but are especially numerous in axon terminals, including those at the neuromuscular junction. Electron microscopy shows that they contain tubular structures, vesicles, and masses of smooth membranes arranged in stacks or, less often, in circular concentric arrays. The relation of these structures to synaptic vesicles or smooth endoplasmic reticulum is speculative. Spheroids also contain membrane-bound clefts and accumulations of mitochondria. Spheroids are particularly prevalent in the cerebellum, basal ganglia, thalamus, cuneate, gracile, and the brainstem nuclei. The cerebellum is strikingly atrophic because of loss of Purkinje and granular cells. The basal ganglia show neuronal loss and may appear spongy, with demyelinated axons and spheroid deposition. Although lipopigment granules are found in basal ganglia, there is no discoloration visible to the naked eye. The long tracts of the visual system, corticospinal system, spinocerebellar pathways, and posterior columns are degenerated, and there is pallor of the myelin. No characteristic lesions have been described in the viscera. Biochemical changes in the brain are viewed as nonspecific.

Laboratory tests are not helpful. The CSF is usually normal; electroencephalographic (EEG) changes are absent or nonspecific. Nerve conduction velocities may be normal or slow. Electromyography (EMG) usually suggests denervation. T2-weighted MRI shows diffuse cerebellar atrophy with hyperintensity of the cerebellar cortex. Definite diagnosis requires autopsy. Nerve, muscle, rectal, or conjunctival biopsy is confirmatory when spheroids are found in nerves or at the neuromuscular junction, but because of sampling problems normal peripheral nerve or even cortical biopsy does not exclude the diagnosis. There is no chemical or enzymatic test available; intrauterine diagnosis is not feasible. Treatment is limited to symptomatic measures and to support and genetic counseling for the child's family.

HALLERVORDEN-SPATZ DISEASE

Hallervorden-Spatz disease (MIM 234200) is an insidiously progressive, autosomal-recessive disease of childhood and adolescence in which motor symptoms predominate. It usually starts with stiffness of gait and is eventually associated with distal wasting, pes cavus or equinovarus, and toe-walking. The arms are held stiffly with hyperextended fingers; the hands may become useless when the child is still ambulatory. The children often have a characteristically frozen, pained expression with risus sardonicus and contracted platysma muscles. They speak through clenched teeth and have difficulty eating. Eventually, they become anarthric, although they continue to understand language. Muscle tone is both spastic and rigid, often with painful spasms, yet passive movement with the patient supine reveals an underlying hypotonia. Reflexes are hyperactive, including facial re-

flexes, and the toes are usually, but not always, upgoing. Some children become dystonic and assume bizarre postures that suggest dystonia musculorum deformans. Ataxia, tremor, nystagmus, and facial grimacing are seen in some patients, usually early in the illness. Pigmentary degeneration of the retina occurs in some families; in others the eyegrounds are normal or show primary optic atrophy. Assessing intellectual function is difficult; affected children remain alert, and if dementia occurs, it may not be severe. The course of the illness typically spans several decades. Therapy is limited to symptomatic measures.

Once the illness is full-blown, the clinical picture is sufficiently characteristic to suggest the diagnosis. T2-weighted MRI demonstrates striking hypointensity in the globus pallidus, so-called eye-of-the-tiger sign. Rare patients have osmiophilic deposits in lymphocytes and bone marrow macrophages resembling sea-blue histiocytes. Definite diagnosis requires autopsy because the biochemical basis of the illness is unknown. Linkage of Hallervorden-Spatz disease to chromosome 20p12.3-p13 has been reported in 10 families. Evidence for locus heterogeneity in other families does exist.

The pathology is so restricted in distribution that biopsy diagnosis is not practical. Olive or golden brown discoloration of the medial segment of the globus pallidus is the macroscopic hallmark of Hallervorden-Spatz disease. Less striking discoloration occurs in the red nucleus and zona reticulata of the substantia nigra. This appearance is due to granules of an iron-containing lipopigment (similar to neuromelanin) located inside and outside the neurons and hyperplastic astrocytes. Irregular mulberry concretions, some calcified, lie free in the tissue. Increased amounts of iron and other metals (e.g., zinc, copper) and calcium are found in the affected tissue, which contains axonal spheroids identical to those seen in neuroaxonal dystrophy. Neuronal loss and thinning of myelin sheaths are prominent in the globus pallidus, less severe in the rest of the basal ganglia, and uncommon elsewhere, although mild cerebellar atrophy does occur. In contrast to infantile neuroaxonal dystrophy, only small numbers of spheroids are found in the cortex and cerebral white matter.

Variants (Hallervorden-Spatz syndrome) include mid- or late-adult onset. Symptoms include acanthocytosis with or without hypoprebetalipoproteinemia.

PELIZAEUS-MERZBACHER DISEASE

The two clinical forms of Pelizaeus-Merzbacher disease (PMD) (MIM 312080) are both X-linked recessive and linked to the proteolipid protein (PLP) gene. One form is present at birth, the so-called connatal variant of Seitelberger, and the other is an infantile variant with a more protracted course, which is the classic form.

A prominent, irregular nystagmus and head tremor or head rolling from birth or the first few months of life are the most striking features of both forms. In the connatal form, these symptoms are associated with floppiness, head lag, grayness of the optic discs, and stridor. Meaningful development does not occur. Boys develop ataxia, severe spasticity, and optic atrophy. Seizures, microcephaly, and failure to thrive supervene, and most infants succumb in the first years of life. Others survive for 8 to 12 years but are mute with limited intellect, despite apparent alertness. In the classic form, slow motor development may enable the children to reach for objects, roll over, crawl, and say a few words. Independent walking is rarely achieved; even these few developmental milestones are lost as increasing ataxia, spasticity with hyperreflexia, and choreoathetotic movements develop. By school age, the affected boy is often mute and confined to a wheelchair.

Patients are likely to develop kyphoscoliosis and joint contractures; they become incontinent. Sensory loss does not occur. Dementia is difficult to assess but may not be profound. Optic atrophy is not severe. Hearing is preserved. Despite severe growth failure and small muscle mass, there is little further deterioration until the patient dies of an intercurrent illness, usually in late adolescence or early adulthood.

Normal nerve conduction velocities and usually normal CSF protein help differentiate the connatal variant from Krabbe disease and metachromatic leukodystrophy. Prominent nystagmus is the main differentiating symptom from infantile neuroaxonal dystrophy and early-onset Hallervorden-Spatz disease. EEG is normal or mildly slow. CT shows ventricular dilatation, decreased differentiation of gray and white matter, and cerebellar atrophy. T2-weighted MRI shows diffuse elongation in the white matter with atrophy, findings similar to those of other leukodystrophies.

At autopsy, the brain, cerebellum, brainstem, and spinal cord of children with the connatal variant are essentially devoid of myelin. In the late infantile variant, characteristic changes are limited to brainstem and cerebellar white matter. The hallmark of PMD is a tigroid appearance of the white matter on myelin stains because of perivascular islands of spared myelin against a nonmyelinated background. There is no sparing of U fibers. Axons are spared but are almost devoid of oligodendroglia. The cerebral cortex is preserved, although large pyramids in layer V of the motor cortex (Betz cells) may be lacking in the connatal form. Neuronal dropout is not severe, with the possible exception of granular cell loss in the cerebellum. Areas of cerebral dysgenesis and micropolygyria have been observed too often to be coincidental. Peripheral nerves are characteristically well myelinated.

Missense mutations of the X-linked PLP gene, a component of myelin, have been documented in 10% to 25% of patients with PMD. Tight linkage to the PLP gene has been documented in most others; recent studies suggest that duplications of the gene may be a frequent cause of the disease in this group. Differences in trafficking of the two PLP gene products, PLP and its smaller isoform DM20, correlate with the phenotypic variability of the connatal and classic forms of disease. A clinically distinct disease, X-linked spastic paraplegia type 2, in which demyelination spares most of the central white matter but selectively affects the spinal tracts, is also linked to PLP.

ALEXANDER DISEASE

Two main variants of Alexander disease (MIM 203450), which appears to affect astrocytes primarily, occur in children. The first is a rapidly progressive infantile variant that causes megalencephaly, severe motor and developmental deficits, and seizures. The large head is usually due to an enlarged brain, but some children develop hydrocephalus owing to an obstruction of the aqueduct of Sylvius by Rosenthal fibers. The children are usually but not invariably spastic. Most die in a vegetative state in infancy or during the preschool years. A few children survive into the second decade.

Neuroimaging suggests the diagnosis when there is marked demyelination with frontal predominance, especially if there are enlarged ventricles with a zone of increased density in the subependymal region (Fig. 93.2). Occasionally, the basal ganglia appear necrotic on CT, as in the infantile variant of Leigh disease. The main differential diagnosis is spongy degeneration, suggested by the enlarged head, early dementia, and decreased density of white matter, although optic atrophy is not characteristic of Alexander disease. Autosomal-recessive inheritance is suggested by some pedigrees.

The juvenile variant (or variants) has a more indolent, protracted course (usually without seizures), or it may present in adults with signs of bulbar palsy and ataxia with or without intellectual deterioration and spasticity. Few of these late-onset cases are familial.

Alexander disease is defined by the principal histologic characteristic, the so-called Rosenthal fibers, which are hyaline, eosinophilic, and argyrophilic inclusions found exclusively in astrocytic footplates. Rosenthal fibers contain small stress proteins: alpha B-crystallin and heat shock protein 27 (HSP27). The rela-

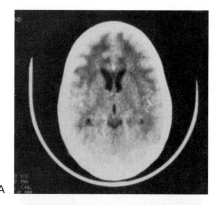

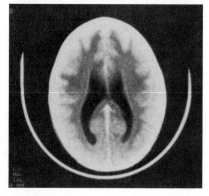

FIG. 93.2. A and B: Axial contrast CT in a 29-month-old girl with Alexander disease. Note the low density of the white matter with frontal-to-occipital gradient and increased periventricular density.

tionship of these proteins to the pathogenesis of the disease is not understood. Rosenthal fibers are characteristically distributed in subpial, subependymal, and perivascular locations. In some patients, especially infants, the fibers are found diffusely in the brain and spinal cord, especially the floor of the fourth ventricle. Rosenthal fibers are not pathognomonic of this illness; they occur in pilocytic astrocytomas, are rarely associated with multiple sclerosis plaques, and have been reported in adolescents and adults without known neurologic symptoms.

Demyelination with loss of oligodendroglia and sparing of axons occurs in regions rich in Rosenthal fibers. In infantile cases, demyelination of the centrum semiovale is so severe that it may lead to cavitation; loss of myelin is most severe frontally and has a characteristic frontal-to-occipital gradient. The myelin of peripheral nerves is spared. Neurons are also spared, with the exception of brainstem motor neurons in some juvenile and adult patients with bulbar symptoms, and of basal ganglia neurons in some infantile cases. No characteristic biochemical abnormality has been reported except for the loss of myelin constituents in patietns with severe demyelination. The fibers are proteinaceous, but whether they are derived from degraded glial filaments is not certain.

Presumptive diagnosis may be made clinically, aided by neuroimaging and elevated levels of alpha B-crystallin and HSP27 in the CSF. Prenatal diagnosis is not yet possible. Therapy remains purely symptomatic.

COCKAYNE SYNDROME

Cockayne syndrome (MIM 216400) is a progressive multisystem disease with autosomal-recessive inheritance characterized by extreme dwarfing, a characteristic cachectic appearance, and neurologic deterioration. The children are of normal size at birth. Failure to thrive with progressive decrease in height, weight, and head circumference becomes apparent before the child reaches age 2 years. These growth measures are many standard deviations below the mean by midchildhood or adolescence. Affected children have an arresting facies with large ears, long aquiline nose, deep-set eyes, thin lips, and jutting chin; the appearance is often accentuated by the loss of severely carious teeth. Some children have atrophic or hyperpigmented skin changes over exposed areas, especially the face. Body proportions, although miniature, are appropriate for the child's age. Signs of maturation, such as the shedding of deciduous teeth and puberty, occur on time, although testes and breasts are usually underdeveloped. The children may suffer from carbohydrate intolerance and anomalies of renal function. Most survive at least into the second decade.

Intellectual development is extremely limited, but affected children remain alert and have pleasant personalities. Most do not speak, and many do not walk independently because of progressive spasticity, widespread joint contractures, and deformities of the feet. Some have signs of a peripheral neuropathy and are ataxic. Many become deaf, and vision is impaired as the result of variable combinations of corneal opacity, cataract, pigmentary degeneration of the retina, and optic atrophy. The pupils are meiotic and respond poorly to mydriatics. Tearing is reduced or absent. Plain radiographs of the skull and CT typically show stippled calcification in the basal ganglia. Nerve conduction velocities are slow, and CSF protein may be elevated.

The diagnosis is suggested by the clinical features. The main differential diagnosis is Seckel (bird-headed) dwarfism, in which dwarfing is invariably present at birth, with extremely low weights for gestational age. The children do not suffer from progressive physical and neurologic deterioration; they learn to walk and speak, despite their extreme microcephaly; they are less retarded than children with Cockayne syndrome but share similar dysmorphic features. Children with progeria are usually of normal intelligence and have much more prominent signs of premature aging than children with Cockayne syndrome, who do not lose their hair, for example, even though mild, early graying may occur.

The brains of children with Cockayne syndrome (and of Seckel dwarfs) are tiny, weighing 500 to 700 g. A prominent feature is extreme thinness of the white matter, which has a tigroid appearance on myelin stains because of islands of myelinated fibers amid areas without myelin, a pattern reminiscent of that seen in PMD. Calcification of the basal ganglia and cerebellar atrophy are typical. Developmental anomalies include areas of deficient gyration of the neocortex and hippocampus, defective cell migration and cortical lamination, and evidence of diffuse neuronal and axonal loss. These findings indicate that the disease starts prenatally, despite allegedly normal head circumference and development in infancy. Other pathology features include grotesque dendrites of Purkinje cells and multinucleate astrocytes.

Cockayne fibroblasts and amniocytes are unable to recover their ribonucleic acid synthesis after ultraviolet irradiation. They are defective in the preferential repair of transcriptionally active genes. Cockayne syndrome is genetically heterogeneous, and so far two genes have been cloned. A few children suffer from both Cockayne syndrome and xeroderma pigmentosum (XP), another disease affecting DNA repair mechanisms resulting in extreme sensitivity to ultraviolet light. There are atypical Cockayne and Cockayne/XP cases, including both neonatal and adult variants. The complexities of the genetics of these related disorders and the pathophysiology of the Cockayne phenotype are not fully understood.

SUGGESTED READINGS

Spongy Degeneration of the Nervous System (Canavan Disease)

Banker BQ, Robertson JT, Victor M. Spongy degeneration of the central nervous system in infancy. *Neurology* 1964;14:981–1001.

Cardenas-Mera N, Campos-Castello J, Lucas F, et al. Progressive familial encephalopathy in infancy with calcification of the basal ganglia and cerebrospinal fluid lymphocytosis. *Acta Neuropediatr* 1995;1:207–213.

Gascon GG, Ozand PT, Mahdi A, et al. Infantile CNS spongy degeneration—14 cases: clinical update. *Neurology* 1990;40:1876–1882.

Matalon R, Michals-Matalon K. Molecular basis of Canavan disease. *Eur J Paediatr Neurol* 1998;2:69–76.

Matalon R, Michals K, Sebesta D, et al. Aspartoacylase deficiency and *N*-acetylaspartic aciduria in patients with Canavan disease. *Am J Med Genet* 1988;29:463–471.

McAdams H, Geyer C, Done S, et al. CT and MR imaging of Canavan disease. *AJNR* 1990;11:397–399.

Toft PB, Geiss-Holtorff R, Rolland MO, et al. Magnetic resonance imaging in juvenile Canavan disease. *Eur J Pediatr* 1993;152:750–753.

Traeger EC, Rapin I. The clinical course of Canavan disease. *Pediatr Neurol* 1998;18:207–212.

Van Bogaert L, Bertrand I. *Spongy degeneration of the brain in infancy.* Springfield, IL: Charles C Thomas, 1967.

Infantile Neuroaxonal Dystrophy

Dorfman LJ, Pedley TA, Tharp BR, Scheithauer BW. Juvenile neuroaxonal dystrophy: clinical, electrophysiological, and neuropathological features. *Ann Neurol* 1978;3:419–428.

Gilman S, Barrett RE. Hallervorden-Spatz disease and infantile neuroaxonal dystrophy. *J Neurol Sci* 1973;19:189–205.

Scheithauer BW, Forno LS, Dorfman LJ, Lane CA. Neuroaxonal dystrophy (Seitelberger's disease) with late onset, protracted course and myoclonic epilepsy. *J Neurol Sci* 1978;36:247–258.

Tanabe Y, Iai M, Ishii M, et al. The use of magnetic resonance imaging in diagnosing infantile neuroaxonal dystrophy. *Neurology* 1993; 43:110–113.

Taylor TD, Litt M, Kramer P, et al. Homozygosity mapping of Hallervorden-Spatz syndrome to chromosome 20p12.3-p13. *Nat Genet* 1996;14:479–481. Erratum: *Nat Genet* 1997;16:109.

Wolfe DE, Schindler D, Desnick RJ. Neuroaxonal dystrophy in infantile alpha-*N*-acetylgalactosaminidase deficiency. *J Neurol Sci* 1995;132:44–56.

Hallervorden-Spatz Disease

Jankovic J, Kirkpatrick JB, Blomqvist KA, et al. Late-onset Hallervorden-Spatz disease presenting as familial parkinsonism. *Neurology* 1985;35:227–234.

Orrell RW, Amrolia PJ, Heald A, et al. Acanthocytosis, retinitis pigmentosa, and pallidal degeneration: a report of three patients, including the second reported case with hypoprebetalipoproteinemia (HARP syndrome). *Neurology* 1995;45:487–492.

Porter-Grenn L, Silbergleit R, Mehta BA. Hallervorden-Spatz disease with bilateral involvement of globus pallidus and substantia nigra: MR demonstration. *J Comput Assist Tomogr* 1993;17:961–963.

Taylor TD, Litt M, Kramer P, et al. Homozygosity mapping of Hallervorden-Spatz syndrome to chromosome 20p12.3-p13. *Nat Genet* 1996;14:479–481. Erratum: *Nat Genet* 1997;16:109.

Wigboldus JM, Bruyn GW. Hallervorden-Spatz disease. In: Vinken PJ, Bruyn GW, eds. *Diseases of the basal ganglia. Handbook of clinical neurology, vol 6.* New York: Wiley Interscience, 1968:604–631.

Zupane M, Chun R, Gilbert-Barnes E. Osmiophilic deposits in cytosomes in Hallervorden-Spatz syndrome. *Pediatr Neurol* 1990;6:349–352.

Pelizaeus-Merzbacher Disease

Gow A, Lazzarini RA. A cellular mechanism governing the severity of Pelizaeus-Merzbacher disease. *Nat Genet* 1996;13:422–427.

Koepper AH, Ronca NA, Greenfield EA, Hans MB. Defective biosynthesis of proteolipid protein in Pelizaeus-Merzbacher disease. *Ann Neurol* 1987;21:159–170.

Saugier-Veber P, Munnich A, Bonneau D, et al. X-linked spastic paraplegia and Pelizaeus-Merzbacher disease are allelic disorders at the proteolipid protein locus. *Nat Genet* 1994;6:257–262.

Seitelberger F. Pelizaeus-Merzbacher disease. In: Vinken PJ, Bruyn GW, eds. *Handbook of clinical neurology, vol 10.* New York: Elsevier-North Holland, 1970:150–202.

Seitelberger F. Neuropathology and genetics of Pelizaeus-Merzbacher disease. *Brain Pathol* 1995;5:267–273.

Sistermans EA, de Coo R, De Wijs IJ, et al. Duplication of the proteolipid protein gene is the major cause of Pelizaeus-Merzbacher disease. *Neurology* 1998;50:1749–1754.

Takanashi J, Sugita K, Osaka H, Ishii M, Niimi H. Proton MR spectroscopy in Pelizaeus-Merzbacher disease. *AJNR* 1997;18:533–535.

Alexander Disease

Borrett D, Becker LE. Alexander disease: a disease of astrocytes. *Brain* 1985;108:367–385.

Head MW, Corbin E, Goldman JE. Overexpression and abnormal modification of the stress proteins alpha B-crystallin and HSP27 in Alexander disease. *Am J Pathol* 1993;143:1743–1753.

Holland IM, Kendall BE. Computed tomography in Alexander's disease. *Neuroradiology* 1980;20:103–106.

Shah M, Ross J. Infantile Alexander disease: MR appearance of a biopsy-proved case. *AJNR* 1990;11:1105–1106.

Takanashi J, Sugita K, Tanabe Y, Niimi H. Adolescent case of Alexander disease: MR imaging and MR spectroscopy. *Pediatr Neurol* 1998;18:67–70.

Cockayne Syndrome

Cockayne EA. Dwarfism with retinal atrophy and deafness. *Arch Dis Child* 1946;21:52–54.

Friedberg EC. Xeroderma pigmentosum, Cockayne syndrome, helicases and DNA repair. *Cell* 1992;128:1233–1237.

Goldstein S. Human genetic disorders which feature accelerated aging. In: Schneider EL, ed. *The genetics of aging.* New York: Plenum Publishing, 1978.

Kraemer KH, Lee MM, Scotto J. Xeroderma pigmentosum: cutaneous, ocular, and neurologic abnormalities in 830 published cases. *Arch Dermatol* 1987;123:241–250.

Lehmann AR, Francis AJ, Giannelli P. Prenatal diagnosis of Cockayne's syndrome. *Lancet* 1985;1:486–488.

Moriwaki S, Stefanini M, Lehmann A, et al. DNA repair and ultraviolet mutagenesis in cells from a new patient with xeroderma pigmentosum group G and Cockayne syndrome resemble xeroderma pigmentosum cells. *J Invest Dermatol* 1996;107:647–653.

Seckel HPG. *Birdheaded dwarfism.* Basel: Karger, 1960.

Sofer D, Grotsky HW, Rapin I, Suzuki K. Cockayne syndrome: unusual pathological findings and review of the literature. *Ann Neurol* 1979;6:340–348.

Venema J, Mullenders LH, Natarajan AT, et al. The genetic defect in Cockayne syndrome is associated with a defect in repair of UV- induced DNA damage in transcriptionally active DNA. *Proc Natl Acad Sci U S A* 1990;87:4707–4711.

Merritt's Neurology, 10th ed., edited by L.P. Rowland. Lippincott Williams & Wilkins, Philadelphia © 2000.

C H A P T E R
94

DIFFUSE SCLEROSIS

LEWIS P. ROWLAND

Some eponyms have lasted for more than 100 years; some come and go. Schilder disease has had its day and seems to be disappearing. Part of the problem was Schilder's genius for recognizing what were then new syndromes. In 1912, 1913, and 1924, he described three different patients with diffuse demyelination of the brain. Each of the cases was dramatic, and his contribution was recognized; diffuse sclerosis was called *Schilder disease.*

Unfortunately for the eponym, later advances identified the 1913 description as one of adrenoleukodystrophy, and the 1924 patient had subacute sclerosing panencephalitis. Nevertheless, the 1912 case delineated a clinical and pathologic syndrome that is still seen, even though cases of uncomplicated diffuse sclerosis are so few that each encounter results in a case report. In 1994, Afifi and colleagues counted 12 cases since 1912.

The situation was not helped by introduction of the term *myelinoclastic* as a tongue-twisting way of denoting demyelination in children; it was intended to distinguish the disorder from *dysmyelination* or loss of myelin because of an inherited biochemical abnormality in the myelin. Schilder disease was and is regarded as a variant of multiple sclerosis, but the etiology and pathogenesis are not known.

At autopsy, there are large areas of demyelination in the centrum ovale (Fig. 94.1), with relative preservation of axons. Subcortical U fibers are often spared. In acute lesions, there is perivascular infiltration by lymphocytes and giant cells. There may be actual necrosis. The lesions are similar to those of multiple sclerosis. In fact, in most cases that include large areas of demyelination, there are also smaller, more typical lesions of multiple sclerosis. For these cases, the term *transitional sclerosis* has been used. It is assumed that the small lesions coalesce to form the large ones.

The clinical syndrome is a leukoencephalopathy, with progressive dementia, psychosis, corticospinal signs, and loss of vision caused by either optic neuritis with papilledema or cerebral blindness. Brainstem signs may include nystagmus and internuclear ophthalmoplegia. The disease is relentlessly progressive, with average survival of about 6 years but sometimes as long as 45 years.

Diagnosis depends on imaging. Computed tomography shows large areas of ring-enhancing lucency. Magnetic resonance imaging shows gadolinium enhancement. There may be cerebrospinal fluid pleocytosis with evidence of intrathecal synthesis of gamma globulin and oligoclonal bands. Brain biopsy may be needed to identify the few cases that simulate mass lesions.

The differential diagnosis includes other childhood leukoencephalopathies (see Chapter 95). Most important is the exclusion of adrenoleukodystrophy, which is achieved by measurement of very-long-chain fatty acids. In areas where measles vaccination has not been practiced, subacute sclerosing panencephalitis must be considered. Steroid therapy is ineffective; management is therefore symptomatic.

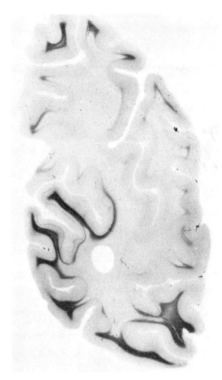

FIG. 94.1. Diffuse myelinoclastic sclerosis. On myelin sheath staining, there is almost complete loss of myelin in occipital white matter. U fibers are irregularly involved. (Courtesy of Dr. H. Shiraki, Tokyo.)

SUGGESTED READINGS

Afifi AK, Bell WE, Menezs AH, Moore SA. Myelinoclastic diffuse sclerosis (Schilder's disease): report of a case and review of the literature. *J Child Neurol* 1994;9:398–403.

Anselmi G, Masdeu JC, Macaluso C, Donnenfeld H. Disseminated-diffuse sclerosis: a variety of multiple sclerosis with characteristic clinical, neuroimaging, and pathological findings. *J Neuroimaging* 1993;3:143–145.

Bonsack TA, Robertson RL, Lacson A, Casadonte JA, Buonomo C. Pediatric case of the day: myelinoclastic diffuse sclerosis (MDS) (Schilder disease). *Radiographics* 1996;16:1509–1511.

Dresser LP, Tourian AY, Anthony DC. A case of myelinoclastic diffuse sclerosis in an adult. *Neurology* 1991;41:316–318.

Eblen F, Premba M, Grodd W, et al. Myelinoclastic diffuse sclerosis (Schilder's disease): cliniconeuroradiologic correlations. *Neurology* 1991;41:589–591.

Hainfellner JA, Schmidbauer M, Schmitahard E, et al. Devic's neuromyelitis optica and Schilder's myelinoclastic diffuse sclerosis. *J Neurol Neurosurg Psychiatry* 1992;55:1194–1196.

Poser CM, Foutieres F, Carpentier MA, Aicardi J. Schilder's myelinoclastic diffuse sclerosis. *Pediatrics* 1986;77:107–112.

Schilder P. Zur Kenntnis der sogennanten diffusen Sklerose. *Z Gesamte Neurol Psychiatrie* 1912;10:1–60.

Sewick LA, Lingele TG, Burde RM, et al. Schilder's (1912) disease: total cerebral blindness due to acute demyelination. *Arch Neurol* 1986;43:85–87.

Stachniak JB, Mickle JP, Ellis T, Quisling R, Rojiani AM. Myelinoclastic diffuse sclerosis presenting as a mass lesion in a child with Turner's syndrome. *Pediatr Neurosurg* 1995;22:266–269.

Merritt's Neurology, 10th ed., edited by L.P. Rowland. Lippincott Williams & Wilkins, Philadelphia © 2000.

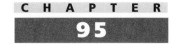

95

DIFFERENTIAL DIAGNOSIS

EVELINE C. TRAEGER
ISABELLE RAPIN

Although most of the degenerative diseases of infancy and childhood are not treatable today, neurologists are obligated to make as definite a diagnosis as possible. This allows them to provide the parents with a prognosis and genetic counseling. Of course, physicians are on the alert for the few treatable conditions, but there is also responsibility to advance knowledge, and precise diagnosis is the first step toward unraveling the chemical pathology of the illness and devising therapy. Clinicians' first concern is to determine that the illness is in fact progressive and to review the genetic evidence. Findings on physical and neurologic examination almost always narrow the diagnostic possibilities and guide the selection of laboratory tests. The most powerful diagnostic

resource is Online Mendelian Inheritance in Man (OMIM) (http://www.ncbi.nlm.nih.gov/Omin), which can be searched by phenotype and provides an extensive and up-to-date differential diagnosis of all currently identified genetic diseases. This database is authored and edited by Dr. Victor A. McKusick and his colleagues at Johns Hopkins University and elsewhere and was developed for the World Wide Web by the National Center for Biotechnology Information.

Deterioration is usually obvious when a disease affects an adult or adolescent, but in infancy and early childhood, the slope of the developmental curve is so steep that it can mask functional decay, as a child's symptoms represent the net difference between the two opposing trends (Fig. 95.1). An early sign of insidious dementia may be slowing of development rather than loss of milestones. As long as a child continues to acquire new skills, even too slowly, the illness is likely to be misinterpreted as a static condition. When the disease is already advanced at birth, dementia can masquerade as total failure to develop, suggesting an unrecognized intrauterine or perinatal catastrophe. In these situations, the correct diagnosis may not be contemplated until after the birth of an affected sibling.

A family history of similar disease or consanguinity is a strong clue, but neither is frequent. Most of these diseases are recessive,

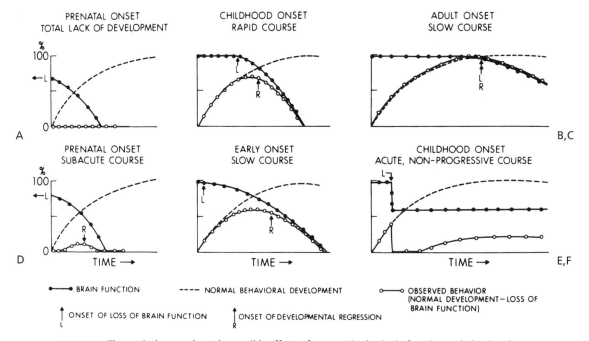

FIG. 95.1. Theoretical curves show the possible effects of progressive brain dysfunction on behavior, depending on time of onset and rapidity of course. The curve depicting observed behavior (o–o–o) is the difference between the curves indicating expected development (– – –) and brain function (•–•). **A:** Prenatal onset with damage at birth so advanced that no development is observed, suggesting a severe static encephalopathy. **B:** Prenatal onset with damage at birth somewhat less severe than in **A**. Development is minimal and markedly delayed but does appear to take place initially. **C,D:** Onset at birth with a less acute course. **E:** Onset in adulthood. Note that in **B**, **C**, and **D** loss of milestones may not appear until months or years after the onset of the illness, which therefore does not appear progressive unless it is realized that deceleration of development or developmental standstill implies deteriorating function. When a progressive disease starts after adolescence **(E)**, loss of function should be less delayed and the disease recognized as progressive virtually from its start. **F:** A severe static lesion acquired postnatally may produce total regression acutely, but development may be expected to resume until the time of puberty. (From Rapin I. Progressive genetic metabolic diseases. In: Rudolph AM, ed. *Pediatrics,* 16th ed. New York: Appleton-Century-Crofts, 1977; with permission.)

TABLE 95.1. UNUSUAL PATTERN OF INHERITANCE OTHER THAN AUTOSOMAL RECESSIVE

Some X-linked recessive diseases
Adrenoleukodystrophy
Pelizaeus-Merzbacher disease
Fabry disease
Hunter syndrome (mucopoly II saccharidosis)
Ornithine transcarbamylase deficiency
Lesch-Nyhan syndrome
Leber optic atrophy
Lowe oculocerebrorenial syndrome
Trichopoliodystrophy (Menkes syndrome)
Duchenne/Becker muscular dystrophy
Norrie disease
Fragile X syndrome
X-linked dysplosias
X-linked mental retardation syndromes

Some X-linked dominant diseases
Incontinentia pigmenti
Pseudo- and pseudopseudohypoparathyroidism
Rett syndrome
Aicardi syndrome

Some autosomal-dominant diseases
Neurofibromatosis
Tuberous sclerosis
Von Hippel-Lindau disease
Acute intermittent porphyria
Huntington disease
Tourette syndrome
Some dystonias
Dentatorubroluysial atrophy
Some multisystem atrophies (OPCA, etc.)

OPCA, olivopontocerebellar atrophy.

and the birth of the first affected child occurs as a sporadic event. It is important to detect X-linked diseases (Table 95.1) because even in the absence of a specific method for intrauterine diagnosis, sex identification of the fetus can limit the birth of affected children. Knowing that certain diseases are particularly frequent in children of particular ethnic backgrounds is also helpful (Table 95.2).

The age at onset may be a lead to the diagnosis (Table 95.3). Genetically homogeneous syndromes tend to run a predictable course and appear at about the same age, but what is considered to be genetically homogeneous today is likely to prove to be nonhomogeneous tomorrow because phenocopies are common. As a general rule, the younger a child is when the symptoms appear, the more rapid is the deterioration, but there are exceptions. For example, when Pelizaeus-Merzbacher disease is manifest before age 1 year, the patient may survive into the third decade. Two diseases of midchildhood or adolescence can progress rapidly to death from liver failure (Wilson disease) or adrenal insufficiency (adrenoleukodystrophy).

The general physical examination may provide helpful clues (Table 95.4). The neurologic symptoms and signs indicate which systems are most affected. Intractable seizures, abnormal involuntary movements, and myoclonus are more typical of diseases of gray matter than of white matter (Table 95.5), whereas spasticity appears early in diseases of white matter. Spasticity

may also be the result of diffuse neuronal dropout; it then occurs in later stages of the disease. Hypotonia suggests involvement of peripheral nerves, anterior horn cells, or cerebellum (Table 95.6). The combination of hypotonia and increased reflexes, seen in Tay-Sachs disease, suggests that both upper and lower motor neurons are affected. Ataxia and abnormal involuntary movements are particularly useful diagnostic signs. Sensory abnormalities are rarely detectable; lack of sensitivity to pain suggests dysautonomia and is reported in some cases of infantile neuroaxonal dystrophy.

The eyes are so likely to provide information of diagnostic importance that detailed examination is mandatory (Table 95.7). Dilating the pupil is required to afford an adequate view of the peripheral retina, macula, and disc. The mild corneal haze of some of the mucolipidoses and mucopolysaccharidoses and the detection of early Kayser-Fleischer rings call for slit-lamp examination. Electroretinography may disclose pigmentary degeneration of the retina before it is visible with the ophthalmoscope.

Repeated neuropsychologic testing may be needed to document progressive dementia. Lack of dementia, at least early, in the face of motor deterioration suggests a disease that spares the cortex and selectively affects the basal ganglia, brainstem, or cerebellar pathways.

In children with an undiagnosed disease, laboratory investigations are screening devices. How many are used depends partly on accessibility and cost (Table 95.8). "New" diseases are often discovered serendipitously rather than after a directed diagnostic endeavor.

Electrical studies may yield clues (Table 95.9). The plain electroencephalogram rarely provides decisive information. However, photomyoclonus suggests Lafora disease, and action myoclonus suggests sialidosis, ceroid lipofuscinosis, myoclonic

TABLE 95.2. PREDOMINANT ETHNIC BACKGROUND IN CERTAIN DISEASES

Ashkenazi Jews
Classic Tay-Sachs disease
Infantile Niemann-Pick disease
Juvenile Gaucher disease
Recessive dystonia musculorum deformans
Mucolipidosis IV
Canavan disease
Dysautonomia
Juvenile nonneuronopathic Gaucher disease

Saudi Arabia
Canavan disease

Nova Scotia
Type D Niemann-Pick disease

Japan
Sialidosis with chondrodystrophy

Scandinavia
Finnish ceroid lipofuscinos (types 1.5)
Juvenile neuronopathic Gaucher disease
Krabbe disease
Aspartylglucosaminuria
Baltic myoclonus epilepsy (Unverricht-Lundborg disease)

TABLE 95.3. TYPICAL AGE AT ONSET

Neonatal or early infantile onset
  Aminoacidurias and organic acidurias
  Urea cycle disorders
  Galactosemia
  Connatal Pelizaeus-Merzbacher disease
  Connatal Alexander disease
  Congenital sialidosis
  Early-onset mitochondrial diseases
  Spongy degeneration (Canavan)
  Aicardi-Goutières syndrome
  Infantile Gaucher disease
  Infantile adrenoleukodystrophy
  Zellweger syndrome
  Neonatal adrenoleukodystrophy
  Chondrodysplasia punctata
  Infantile Refsum disease
  GM_I gangliosidosis (infantile variant)
  I-cell disease (mucolipidosis II)
  Trichopoliodystrophy (Menkes)
  Neurocutaneous syndromes
  Progressive spinal muscular atrophy (Werdnig-Hoffmann disease)
  Seckel bird-headed dwarfs

Infantile onset
  Aminoacidurias, organic acidurias, urea cycle disorders with partial enzyme deficiency
  Many sphingolipidoses, mucopolysaccharidoses, mucolipidoses
  Infantile ceroid lipofuscinosis
  Leigh syndrome (early types)
  Other mitochondrial cytopathies
  Lesch-Nyhan syndrome
  Sjögren-Larson syndrome
  Spongy degeneration
  Wolman disease
  Alexander disease
  Pelizaeus-Merzbacher disease
  Neuraxonal dystrophy
  Alpha-*N*-acetylgalactosaminidose deficiency
  Infantile Hallervorden-Spatz disease
  Infantile fucosidosis
  Nephrosialidosis
  Sialidosis
  Pompe disease
  Xeroderma pigmentosum
  Cockayne disease
  Infantile galactosialidosis

  Progeria
  Rett syndrome

Onset in preschool years
  Aminoacidurias, organic acidurias, urea cycle disorders with partial enzyme deficiency
  Aspartylglucosaminuria
  Marinesco-Sjögren syndrome
  Alexander disease
  Ataxia telangiectasia
  Xeroderma pigmentosum
  Chédiak-Higashi disease
  Metachromatic leukodystrophy
  Late infantile gangliosidoses
  Niemann-Pick disease, Nova Scotia variant
  Late infantile ceroid lipofuscinoses
  Sanfilippo syndromes
  Maroteaux-Lamy disease
  Mild Hunter disease
  Leigh syndrome and other mitochondrial cytopathies
  Kearns-Sayre syndrome
  Disintegrative psychosis
  Other autistic regression

Onset in school age or adolescence
  Wilson disease
  Acute intermittent prophyria
  Juvenile ceroid lipofuscinosis
  Adrenoleukodystrophy
  Late variants of the gangliosidoses
  Niemann-Pick disease with vertical ophthalmoplegia
  Sialidosis with cherry-red spot myoclonus (variants with and without chondrodystrophy)
  Fabry disease
  Cerebrotendinous xanthomatosis
  Leigh syndrome (some variants)
  Other mitochondrial cytopathies (e.g., MERFF and MELAS syndromes)
  Refsum disease
  Friedreich ataxia
  Bassen-Kornzweig disease
  Other spinocerebellar degenerations
  Dystonia musculorum deformans
  Juvenile Huntington disease
  Juvenile parkinsonism
  Classic Hallervorden-Spatz disease
  Lafora disease
  Baltic myoclonus
  Subacute sclerosing panencephalitis

epilepsy with ragged-red fibers (MERRF) syndrome, Gaucher disease type III, and Baltic myoclonus.

Radiologic tests are crucial in some cases. Adrenal calcification is virtually pathognomonic of Wolman disease. The diagnostic yield of plain radiographs of the skull is extremely low, in contrast to the efficiency of computed tomography (CT) or magnetic resonance imaging (MRI). Even if CT or MRI shows only nonspecific atrophy, this is helpful if it is progressive. Adrenoleukodystrophy and Canavan, Alexander, and Krabbe diseases show characteristic patterns of lucency of white matter. A tiger's-eye pattern of the basal ganglia points to Hallervorden-Spatz disease, and lucency of the basal ganglia to acute mito-

chondrial encephalopathy. Lack of radioactive copper absorption into the liver can be shown in Menkes disease.

The need for a biopsy arises when noninvasive tests fail (Table 95.10). A skin biopsy specimen is examined under the electron microscope for abnormal inclusions and is also used for tissue culture. Cultured fibroblasts may yield an enzymatic or deoxyribonucleic acid (DNA) diagnosis. Equally important, the cultures can be kept viable indefinitely in the frozen state, and tissue will be available when new data suggest further study, especially as molecular techniques enable detection of additional mutations. Cell lines in federally funded repositories provide invaluable resources for such future studies. Conjunctival biopsies are helpful

TABLE 95.4. HELPFUL CLUES IN THE PHYSICAL EXAMINATION

Big head
Tay-Sachs disease
Alexander disease
Spongy degeneration (Canavan)
Hurler disease
Glutaric aciduria type 1
Other mucopolysaccharidoses with hydrocephalus

Small head
Krabbe disease
Infantile ceroid lipofuscinosis
Some infantile mitochondrial disorders
Neuraxonal dystrophy
Incontinentia pigmenti
Cockayne disease
Rett syndrome
Bird-headed dwarfs
Chromosomal abnormalities

Hair abnormalities
Stiff, wiry
Trichopoliodystrophy (Menkes)
Frizzy
Giant axonal neuropathy
Hirsutism
Infantile GM$_1$ gangliosidosis
Hurler, Hunter, Sanfilippo syndromes
I-cell disease
Gray
Ataxia telangiectasia
Cockayne disease
Chédiak-Higashi disease
Progeria

Skin abnormalities
Telangiectasia
Ataxia telangiectasia
Angiokeratoma
Fabry disease
Juvenile fucosidosis
Galactosialidosis
Adult-onset Alpha-*N*-acetylgalactosaminidase deficiency
Ichthyosis
Reisum disease
Sjögren-Larsson syndrome
Hypopigmentation
Trichopoliodystrophy (Menkes)
Chédiak-Higashi syndrome
Tuberous sclerosis (ash-leaf spots)
Hypomelanosis of Ito
Prader-Willi syndrome
Phenylketonuria
Hyperpigmentation
Niemann-Pick disease
Adrenoleukodystrophy
Farber disease
Neurofibromatosis (café-au-lait spots)
Xeroderma pigmentosum
Incontinentia pigmenti
Thin atrophic skin
Ataxia telangiectasia
Cockayne disease
Xeroderma pigmentosum
Progeria
Thick skin
I-cell disease
Mucopolysaccharidoses I, II, III

Infantile fucosidosis
Subcutaneous nodules
Farber disease
Neurofibromatosis
Cerebrotendinous xanthomatosis
Xanthomas
Neimann-Pick disease
Blotching
Dysautonomia

Enlarged nodes
Farber disease
Niemann-Pick disease
Juvenile Gaucher disease
Chédiak-Higashi disease
Ataxia telangiectasia (lymphoma)

Stridor, hoarseness
Infantile-onset peroxisomal disorders
Farber disease
Infantile Gaucher disease
Connatal Pelizaeus-Merzbacher disease

Enlarged orange tonsils
Tangier disease

Severe swallowing problems
(Present late in the course of all patients with severe bulbar, pseudobulbar, cerebellar, or basal ganglia pathology)
Infantile Gaucher disease
Dysautonomia
Hallervorden-Spatz disease
Dystonia musculorum deformans
Zellweger syndrome

Heart abnormalities
Pompe disease
Hurler disease and other mucopolysaccharidoses
Fabry disease
Infantile fucosidosis
Refsum disease
Friedreich ataxia
Abetalipoproteinemia (Bassen-Kornzweig disease)
Tuberous sclerosis
Progeria
Zellweger syndrome
Disorders of carnitine metabolism
Duchenne muscular dystrophy
Kearns-Sayre syndrome

Strokes
Fabry disease
Trichopoliodystrophy (Menkes)
Progeria
MELAS syndrome
Homocystinuria
Sickle-cell diseases

Organomegaly
Mucopolysaccharidoses (most types)
Infantile GM$_1$ gangliosidosis
Niemann-Pick disease
Gaucher disease
Generalized peroxisomal disorders
Galactosemia
Pompe disease
Mannosidosis

(continued)

TABLE 95.4. *(continued)*

Gastrointestinal problems
  Malabsorption
    Wolman disease
    Bassen-Kornzweig disease
  Nonfunctioning gallbladder
    Metachromatic leukodystrophy
    Infantile fucosidosis
  Jaundice
    Infantile Niemann-Pick disease
    Zellweger disease
    Galactosemia
    Niemann-Pick disease
  Vomiting
    Dysautonomia
    Urea cycle defects
  Diarrhea
    Hunter syndrome

Kidney problems
  Renal failure
    Fabry disease
    Nephrosialidosis
  Cysts
    Zellweger syndrome
    Von Hippel-Lindau disease
    Tuberous sclerosis
    Neonatal OPCA
    Joubert syndrome
  Stones
    Lesch-Nyhan disease
  Aminoacidurial
    Aminoacidurias
    Lowe syndrome
    Wilson disease

Bone and joint abnormalities
  Stiff joints
    Mucopolysaccharidoses (all but type I–S)
    Mucolipidoses (most types)
    Fucosidosis
    Farber disease
    Sialidoses (some forms)
    Zellweger syndrome
    Rhizometic chondrodysplasia punctata
    Cockayne disease
  Scoliosis

  Friedreich ataxia
  Ataxia telangiectasia
  Dystonia musculorum deformans
  All chronic diseases with muscle weakness, especially
    anterior horn cell involvement
  Rett syndrome
  Kyphosis
    Mucopolysaccharidoses

Endocrine dysfunction
  Adrenals
    Adrenoleukodystrophy
    Wolman disease
  Hypogonadism
    Xeroderma pigmentosum
    Ataxia telangiectasia
    Some spinocerebellar degenerations
  Diabetes
    Ataxia telangiectasia
  Dwarfing
    Morquio disease
    Other mucopolysaccharidoses
    Cockayne syndrome
    Progeria
    Diseases with severe malnutrition
  Hypothalamic dysfunction
    De Sanctis-Cacchione syndrome

Neoplasms
  Ataxia telangiectasia
  Xeroderma pigmentosum
  Neurofibromatosis
  Von Hipple-Lindau disease
  Tuberous sclerosis

Hearing loss
  Hunter disease
  Other mucopolysaccharidoses
  Generalized peroxisomal disorders
  Refsum disease
  Cockayne disease
  Kearns-Sayre and Leigh syndromes
  Other mitochondrial cytopathies
  Some spinocerebellar degenerations
  Usher syndrome

OPCA, olivopontocerebellar atrophy.

TABLE 95.5. DISEASES WITH PROMINENT SEIZURES OR MYOCLONUS

Acute intermittent porphyria
Gangliosidoses (infantile especially)
Ceroid lipofuscinoses (late infantile variant especially)
MERF and MELAS syndromes
Trichopoliodystrophy (Menkes)
Zellweger syndrome
Generalized peroxisomal disorders
Infantile Alexander disease
Krabbe disease
Lafora disease
Baltic myoclonus
Sanfilippo disease
Juvenile Huntington disease
Tuberous sclerosis
Juvenile neuropathic Gaucher disease
Subacute sclerosing panencephalitis

when storage in connective tissue is suspected and enzymatic diagnosis is unavailable (e.g., in mucolipidosis IV), or when axonal spheroids are being evaluated. Muscle biopsy to identify mitochondrial encephalomyopathies requires special histochemical, biochemical, and DNA studies.

Brain biopsy is rarely needed today and is reserved for patients in whom diagnosis remains elusive despite thorough peripheral investigation. It is imperative to sample the white matter, as well as the cortex. Routine histologic examination of the tissue is not sufficient because brain biopsy is reserved for disorders that are biochemical enigmas; therefore, brain biopsy should be carried out in a center that has the resources necessary for many avenues of investigation. Under these conditions, the informational yield of brain biopsy is sufficiently high and its morbidity sufficiently low to make it a rewarding procedure both clinically and scien-

TABLE 95.6. MOTOR SIGNS HELPFUL TO DIAGNOSIS

Floppiness in infancy
  Progressive spinal muscular atrophy
  Congenital myopathies
  Zellweger syndrome
  Pompe disease
  Trichopoliodystrophy
  Neuraxonal dystrophy
  Gangliosidoses (early variants)
  Fucosidosis (infantile variant)
  Infantile ceroid lipofuscinosis
  Spongy degeneration (early)
  Leigh syndrome (early variant)
  Neonatal OPCA

Peripheral neuropathy
  Acute intermittent porphyria
  Metachromatic leukodystrophy
  Fabry disease
  Krabbe disease
  Neuraxonal dystrophy
  Refsum disease
  Tangier disease
  Bassen-Kornzweig disease
  Sialidosis (some variants)
  Mucolipidosis III
  Cerebrotendinous xanthomatosis
  Ataxia telangiectasia
  Adrenomyeloneuropathy
  Mucopolysaccharidoses I, II, VI, VII
    (entrapment)
  Cockayne syndrome
  Some mitochondrial cytopathies
  Giant axonal neuropathy

Prominent cerebellar signs
  Wilson disease
  Late infantile ceroid lipofuscinosis
  Pelizaeus-Merzbacher disease
  Neuraxonal dystrophy

  Metachromatic leukodystrophy
  Ataxia telangiectasia
  Leigh syndrome
  Niemann-Pick disease type C
  Some late-onset gangliosidoses
  Some sialidoses
  Friedreich ataxia
  Bassen-Kornzweig disease
  Cerebrotendinous xanthomatosis
  Other spinocerebellar degenerations
  Lafora disease
  Baltic myoclonus
  Chédiak-Higashi disease
  Usher syndrome
  Neonatal OPCA
  De Sanctis-Cacchione syndrome

Abnormal posture or movements
  Wilson disease
  Lesch-Nyhan disease
  Hallervorden-Spatz syndrome
  Familial striatal necrosis
  Dystonia musculorum deformans
  Juvenile Niemann-Pick disease with
    ophthalmoplegia
  Chronic GM_1 and GM_2 gangliosidoses
  Pelizaeus-Merzbacher syndrome
  Crigler-Najjar disease
  Ataxia telangiectasia
  Juvenile ceroid lipofuscinosis
  Juvenile Huntington disease
  Juvenile parkinsonism
  Gilles de la Tourette syndrome
  De Sanctis-Cacchione syndrome (eroderma
    pigmentosum with endocrine
    dysfunction)
  Dentatorubroluysial atrophy
  Glutaric aciduria type 1

Spasticity is so common as to be nondiscriminating.

TABLE 95.7. EYE FINDINGS

Conjunctival telangiectasia
  Ataxia telangiectasia
  Fabry disease

Corneal opacity
  Wilson disease (Kayser-Fleischer ring)
  Mucopolysaccharidoses I, III, IV, VI
  Mucolipidoses III, IV
  Fabry disease
  Galactosialidosis
  Cockayne disease
  Xeroderma pigmentosum
  Zellweger syndrome (inconstant)

Lens opacity
  Wilson disease
  Galactosemia
  Marinesco-Sjögren syndrome
  Lowe disease
  Cerebrocutaneous xanthomatosis
  Sialidosis (rarely significant clinically)
  Mannosidosis
  Zellweger syndrome

Glaucoma
  Mucopolysaccharidosis I (Hurler-Scheie syndrome)
  Zellweger syndrome (infrequent)

Cherry-red Spot
  Tay-Sachs disease
  Sialidosis (usually)
  Infantile Niemann-Pick disease (50% of cases)
  Infantile GM_1 gangliosidosis (50% of cases)
  Farber disease (inconstant)
  Multiple sulfatase deficiency (metachromatic leukodystrophy variant)

Macular and retinal pigmentary degeneration
  Ceroid lipofuscinosis (most types)
    Mucopolysaccharidoses I-H and I-S, II, III
    Mucolipidosis IV
    Bassen-Kornzweig syndrome (abetalipoproteinemia)
    Peroxisomal disorders
    Olivoponlocerebellar variant
    Refsum disease (all types)
    Kearns-Sayre syndrome
    Leber congenital amaurosis
  Other mitochondrial cytopathies
    Hallervorden-Spatz syndrome (some types)
    Cockayne disease
    Sjögren-Larsson syndrome (not always)
    Usher syndrome
    Some other spinocerebellar syndromes
    Neurocutaneous syndromes

Optic atrophy
  Krabbe disease
  Metachromatic leukodystrophy

(continued)

TABLE 95.7. *(continued)*

Optic atrophy
Most sphingolipidoses late in their course
Adrenoleukodystrophy
Alexander disease
Spongy degeneration
Pelizaeus-Merzbacher disease
Neuraxonal dystrophy
Neonatal mitochondrial cytopathies
Leber congenital amaurosis
Leber hereditary optic neuropathy
Joubert syndrome
Some spinocerebellar degenerations
Diseases with retinal pigmentary degeneration

Nystagmus
Diseases with poor vision (searching nystagmus)
Pelizaeus-Merzbacher syndrome
Metachromatic leukodystrophy

Friedreich ataxia
Other spinocerebellar degenerations and cerebellar atrophies
Neuraxonal dystrophy
Ataxia telangiectasia
Joubert syndrome
Leigh syndrome (inconstant)
Marinesco-Sjögren syndrome
Opsoclonus-myoclonus syndrome
Chédiak-Higashi syndrome

Ophthalmoplegia
Leigh syndrome
Kearns-Sayre and Leigh syndromes
Niemann-Pick disease type C
Bassen-Kornzweig syndrome
Ataxia telangiectasia
Infantile Gaucher disease
Tangier disease

TABLE 95.8. **USEFUL LABORATORY TESTS**

Urine
Amino acids, organic acids
Galactose, other sugars
Mucopolysaccharides, sialidated oligosaccharides
N-Acetylaspartic acid
Copper excretion
Porphyrins
Metachromatic granules
Oxalate, cysteine crystals

Blood chemistry
Ammonia (urea cycle disorders, some mitochondrial encephalopathies)
Lactate-pyruvate ratio (Leigh syndrome, other mitochondrial cytopathies)
Amino acids, organic acids, and other special metabolites
C26/C22 very-long-chain fatty acid ratio (adrenoleukodystrophy, Zellweger disease, other peroxisomal diseases)
Phytanic acid
Pipecolic acid

White blood cells
Lysosomal enzymes and other enzymatic assays
DNA tests for genetic mutations
Lipid and other inclusions (ceroid lipofuscinoses, gangliosidoses)

Red blood cells
Enzymatic assays for galactosemia, porphyria

Cultured skin fibroblasts
Enzymatic assays for most diseases with known deficits
Lipid and other inclusions (in mucolipidosis IV, I-cell disease, mucopolysaccharidoses, Chédiak-Higashi syndrome)
DNA repair after ultraviolet or radiation exposure (ataxia telangiectasia, Cockayne disease, xeroderma pigmentosum)
DNA tests for genetic mutations

CSF protein increased
Metachromatic leukodystrophy, Krabbe disease, infantile adrenoleukodystrophy (not always in classic variant), Friedreich ataxia, and other spinocerebellar degenerations (inconstant), Zellweger disease (sometimes), Refsum disease, Cockayne disease

CSF lactate/pyruvate
Mitochondrial cytopathies

Amniotic cells
Enzymatic assays for disease of known enzymatic defect
Abnormal inclusion in mucolipidosis IV
Karyotype in X-linked disease
C26/C22 very-long-chain fatty acid ratio
DNA tests for genetic mutations

Intradermal histamine test
Dysautonomia

TABLE 95.9. ELECTRODIAGNOSIS

Electromyography and nerve conduction velocity	To detect neuropathy, anterior horn cell disease, or muscle involvement
Electroretinography	To detect retinal degeneration
Visual evoked responses	Giant potentials in late infantile ceroid lipofuscinosis; delayed latency and decreased amplitude in leukodystrophies or optic atrophy
Brainstem auditory evoked responses	Diagnosis of hearing loss; prolonged latency in leukodystrophies; delayed waves with decrease of amplitude in leukodystrophies and other disease of the brainstem
Somatosensory evoked responses	Giant potentials in sialidosis with cherry-red spot myoclonus; decreased amplitude in peripheral neuropathy; delayed waves with decreased amplitude in diseases of the white matter and peripheral nerves

TABLE 95.10. DISEASES IN WHICH BIOPSIES FOR HISTOLOGY ARE LIKELY TO HELP

Skin
 Ceroid lipofuscinosis
 Mucopolysaccharidoses
 Mucolipidosis IV
 Neuraxonal dystrophy
 Lafora disease

Conjunctiva
 Mucopolysaccharidoses
 Mucolipidoses
 Neuraxonal dystrophy

Bone marrow
 Niemann-Pick disease
 Gaucher disease
 Mucopolysaccharidoses

Muscle
 Glycogenoses
 Mitochondrial myopathies (Kearns-Sayre and Leigh syndromes)
 Other myopathies
 Neuraxonal dystrophy
 Lafora disease

Nerve
 Neuraxonal dystrophy
 Metachromatic leukodystrophy
 Other diseases with neuropathies

Brain
 (Rarely needed except possibly for the following)
 Alexander disease
 Neuraxonal dystrophy
 Undiagnosed disease with probable cortical involvement

tifically. Biopsy is not a substitute for autopsy because it may not be diagnostic and because some studies can be done only on biopsy tissue or only on autopsy tissue.

When all diagnostic methods have failed, the physician must broach the subject of an autopsy. This can be done when the parents are informed of the likelihood of a fatal outcome. Parents who understand how little is known about their child's illness are likely to want an autopsy; they will also be spared the unnecessary hurt of being pressed for an autopsy when the child actually dies and they are most distressed. A planned and speedy autopsy maximizes the probability of obtaining useful data. Viscera, peripheral nerves, muscle, and retina, as well as the brain, must be investigated. Tissue samples should be removed and frozen at −70°C for chemical analysis; other samples are fixed for electron microscopy before the organs are placed in formalin. If autopsy does not yield a diagnosis, brain tissue stored in federally funded brain banks remains available for later diagnosis or research. In the interim, the physician must explain to the parents that the child's illness may be one that is as yet unrecognized and that data of scientific importance may yet emerge from the study of their child, who will thus have made a unique contribution to other children and their families.

Merritt's Neurology, 10th ed., edited by L.P. Rowland. Lippincott Williams & Wilkins, Philadelphia © 2000.

SECTION

X

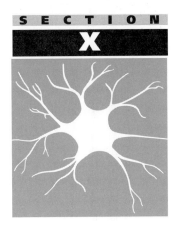

DISORDERS OF MITOCHONDRIAL DNA

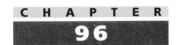

MITOCHONDRIAL ENCEPHALOMYOPATHIES: DISEASES OF MITOCHONDRIAL DNA

SALVATORE DIMAURO
ERIC A. SCHON
MICHIO HIRANO
LEWIS P. ROWLAND

Mitochondria are uniquely interesting organelles not only because they serve a variety of functions but also because they are under the control of two genomes: their own (mitochondrial deoxyribonucleic acid [mtDNA]) and that of the nucleus (nDNA). Therefore, mitochondrial diseases, that is, genetic diseases resulting in mitochondrial dysfunction, can be due to mutations in either genome (Table 96.1). Diseases caused by nDNA mutations are transmitted by mendelian inheritance (see Chapter 98). In this chapter, we consider diseases caused by mutations in mtDNA and also a group of disorders (defects of intergenomic signaling; see Table 96.1) characterized by mutations in nDNA that in turn alter mtDNA integrity or replication.

The ubiquitous nature of mtDNA and the peculiar rules of mitochondrial genetics (more akin to population genetics than to mendelian genetics) contribute to explaining the extraordinary clinical heterogeneity of mitochondrial disorders, which, due to the frequent involvement of brain and muscle tissues, are generally labeled *mitochondrial encephalomyopathies.*

The first human disease attributed to mitochondrial dysfunction was a hypermetabolic state in a patient with normal thyroid function and an excessive number of abnormally large mitochondria in skeletal muscle. Biochemical studies showed "loose coupling" of oxidative phosphorylation. The syndrome was

TABLE 96.1. GENETIC CLASSIFICATION OF MITOCHONDRIAL DISEASES

Defects of mtDNA
  Single deletions (sporadic)
  Duplications or duplications/deletions (maternal transmission)
  Point mutations (maternal transmission)
Defects of nuclear DNA (mendelian transmission)
  Mutations in genes encoding enzymes or translocases
    Defects of substrate transport
    Defect of substrate utilization
    Defects of the Krebs cycle
    Defects of the electron transport chain
    Defects of oxidation/phosphorylation coupling
  Defects of mitochondrial protein importation
  Defects of intergenomic signaling
    Multiple deletions of mtDNA
    Depletion of mtDNA

named after Rolf Luft, the endocrinologist who led the studies (Luft et al., 1962). In the 36 years since then, however, there has been only one other known case of Luft syndrome.

Mitochondrial diseases were brought to prominence by Shy and coworkers (1966) in the 1960s, when they set about assigning different myopathies to different organelles. They defined one category by the electron microscopic appearance of overabundant or enlarged mitochondria with paracrystalline inclusions. Soon, Olson and colleagues (1972) found that these abnormal mitochondria could be identified under the light microscope as *ragged-red fibers* (RRF) with a modified Gomori trichrome stain. For the next two decades, this observation was the basis for recognizing mitochondrial diseases, while biochemical tests were being developed and applied, eventually leading to a biochemical classification (see Table 96.1). Throughout this period, there were vigorous debates between those who thought that there were identifiable clinical syndromes and those who thought there was too much overlap of the clinical features (a foreshadowing of mitochondrial genetics). *Ophthalmoplegia plus* became a popular term for the lumpers. The splitters, however, recognized the constancy of clinical manifestations in the Kearns-Sayre syndrome (KSS) and noted that it was never familial, in contrast to the often familial nature of two other syndromes: *mitochondrial encephalomyopathy with lactic acidosis and stroke* (MELAS) and *myoclonic epilepsy with ragged-red fibers* (MERRF), both described in the early 1980s. The pattern of inheritance in these disorders was maternal, suggesting mtDNA involvement.

A revolution commenced in 1988 with the demonstration by Holt and colleagues (1990) of mtDNA single deletions in patients with mitochondrial myopathies, and with the simultaneous recognition by Wallace and associates (1988) of a point mutation in *Leber hereditary optic neuropathy* (see Chapter 97). Single deletions were found by Zeviani and associates (1988) to be characteristic of KSS and sporadic progressive external ophthalmoplegia (PEO), but not of familial PEO. In families with autosomal-dominant PEO (adPEO), they found multiple rather than single deletions of mtDNA. Demonstration soon followed that there were different point mutations of mtDNA in MELAS and MERRF syndromes. In the ensuing years, more than 50 pathogenic point mutations and myriad rearrangements in mtDNA have been associated with a bewildering array of clinical presentations (Fig. 96.1). A new lexicon was developed to encompass the new acronyms for multisystem diseases and for new concepts to deal with problems of pathogenesis.

PRINCIPLES OF MITOCHONDRIAL GENETICS AND PATHOGENESIS OF MITOCHONDRIAL DISEASES

Human mtDNA is a small (16.6 kilobase pairs [kbp]) circle of double-stranded DNA, comprising only 37 genes (see Fig. 96.1). Of these, 13 encode polypeptides, all subunits of the respiratory chain: seven subunits of complex I (NADH-ubiquinone oxidoreductase), one subunit of complex III (ubiquinone-cytochrome-*c* oxidoreductase), three subunits of complex IV (cytochrome-*c* oxidase [COX]), and two subunits of complex V (ATP synthetase). The other 24 genes encode 22 transfer ri-

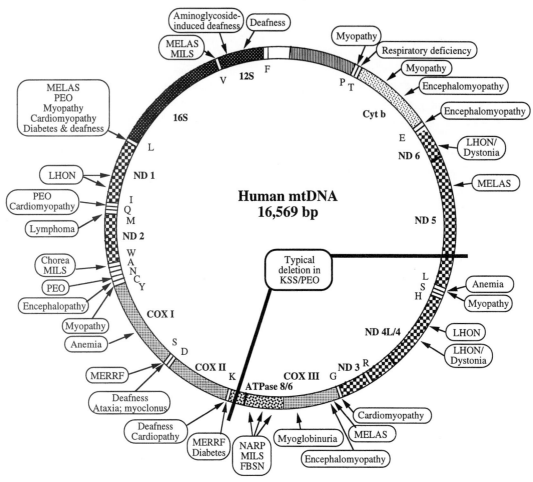

FIG. 96.1. Morbidity map of human mtDNA. The map of the 16.5-kbp mtDNA shows differently shaded areas representing the structural genes for the seven subunits of complex I (NADH-ubiquinone oxidoreductase [*ND*]), the three subunits of cytochrome-c oxidase *(COX)*, cytochrome *b* (*Cyt b*), the two subunits of ATP synthetase (*ATPase 6* and *8*), the 12S and 16S ribosomal RNAs (*rRNA*), and the 22 transfer RNAs (*tRNA*) identified by one-letter codes for the corresponding amino acids (FBSN, familial bilateral striatal necrosis; LHON, Leber hereditary optic neuropathy; MELAS, mitochondrial encephalomyopathy, lactic acidosis, and stroke; MERRF, myoclonus epilepsy with ragged-red fibers; MILS, maternally inherited Leigh syndrome; NARP, neuropathy, ataxia, retinitis pigmentosa; PEO, progressive external ophthalmoplegia). (Modified from DiMauro and Bonilla, 1997; with permission.)

bonucleic acids (tRNAs) and two ribosomal RNAs (rRNAs) that are required for translation of messenger RNAs on mitochondrial ribosomes. The subunits of complex II (succinate dehydrogenase-ubiquinone oxidoreductase) and two small electron carriers, coenzyme Q10 (ubiquinone) and cytochrome *c*, are encoded exclusively by nDNA.

Mendelian versus Mitochondrial Genetics

The following main principles distinguish mitochondrial genetics from mendelian genetics and help explain many of the clinical peculiarities of mtDNA-related disorders.

1. *Polyplasmy.* Most cells contain multiple mitochondria, and each mitochondrion contains multiple copies of mtDNA, so that there are hundreds or thousands of mitochondrial genomes in each cell.

2. *Heteroplasmy.* When an mtDNA mutation affects some but not all genomes, a cell, a tissue, indeed a whole individual

will harbor two populations of mtDNA, normal (or wild-type) and mutant, a condition known as heteroplasmy. In normal tissues, all mtDNAs are identical, a situation of homoplasmy. Usually, neutral mutations (or polymorphisms) are homoplasmic. In contrast, most (but not all) pathogenic mtDNA mutations are heteroplasmic.

3. *Threshold effect.* Functional impairment associated with a pathogenic mtDNA mutation is largely determined by the degree of heteroplasmy, and a minimum critical number of mutant genomes must be present before tissue dysfunction becomes evident (and related clinical signs become manifest), a concept aptly termed the *threshold effect*. However, this is a relative concept: Tissues with high metabolic demands, such as brain, heart, and muscle, tend to have lower tolerance for mtDNA mutations than metabolically less active tissues.

4. *Mitotic segregation.* Both organellar division and mtDNA replication are apparently stochastic events unrelated to cell division; thus, the number of mitochondria (and mtDNA) can vary

not just in space (i.e., among cells and tissues) but also in time (i.e., during development or aging). Moreover, at cell division, the proportion of mutant mtDNAs in daughter cells may drift, allowing relatively rapid changes in genotype that can translate into changes in phenotype, including the clinical picture, if and when the threshold is crossed.

5. *Maternal inheritance.* At fertilization, all mitochondria (and all mtDNA) are contributed to the zygote by the oocyte. Therefore, a mother carrying an mtDNA mutation will pass it on to all of her children, males and females, but only her daughters will transmit it to their progeny in a "vertical," matrilinear line. When maternal inheritance is evident in a clinical setting, it provides conclusive evidence that an mtDNA mutation must underlie the disease in question. However, the other features of mitochondrial genetics (e.g., heteroplasmy and the threshold effect) often mask maternal inheritance by causing striking intrafamilial clinical heterogeneity. Thus, when an mtDNA-related disorder is suspected, it is crucial to collect the family history meticulously, with special attention to "soft" signs (e.g., short stature, hearing loss, migrainous headache) in potentially oligosymptomatic maternal relatives.

Clinical Manifestations

Although specific syndromes can be identified by particular combinations of symptoms and signs (Table 96.2), several clinical manifestations seem to be prevalent among different syndromes, especially short stature, neurosensory hearing loss, and diabetes mellitus. Lactic acidosis, often detected in blood and cerebrospinal fluid (CSF), is the most common laboratory sign. Perhaps as a result of impaired respiration, mitochondria in muscle proliferate and enlarge, which is the basis for finding RRF (Fig. 96.2). Neuropathologic and neuroradiologic changes fall into five main patterns:

1. Microcephaly and ventricular dilatation, sometimes associated with agenesis of the corpus callosum, are seen in infants with severe congenital lactic acidosis.
2. Bilateral, symmetric lesions of basal ganglia, thalamus, brainstem, and cerebellar roof nuclei are the signature of Leigh syndrome.
3. Multifocal encephalomalacia, usually involving the cortex of the posterior cerebral hemispheres, corresponds to the "strokes" of the MELAS syndrome.
4. Spongy encephalopathy, predominantly in white matter, is characteristic of KSS.
5. Calcification of the basal ganglia can be seen in all of these disorders, but in a minority of patients with any syndrome.

Diagnosis of a mitochondrial disease is based on five crucial elements: (1) recognition of an appropriate clinical syndrome, (2) presence of lactic acidosis in blood or CSF, (3) demonstration of RRF in muscle biopsy, (4) documentation of impaired respiration in biochemical assays of muscle extracts or isolated mitochondria, or (5) identification of a pathogenic mutation in mtDNA. Not all of these criteria, however, are necessarily present in an individual syndrome. Unfortunately, there is no effective treatment for any of these diseases.

TABLE 96.2. CLASSIFICATION OF PROGRESSIVE EXTERNAL OPHTHALMOPLEGIA (PEO)

Mitochondrial
Sporadic PEO with single deletions of mtDNA
  PEO with proximal myopathy
  Kearns-Sayre syndrome
Maternally inherited PEO with mtDNA point mutations
  A3243G (MELAS syndrome)
  A8344G (MERRF syndrome)
  Other mutations
Autosomal-dominant PEO with multiple mtDNA deletions
Autosomal-recessive PEO with multiple mtDNA deletions
  With cardiomyopathy
  With gastrointestinal involvement (MNGIE)
Autosomal-recessive PEO with mtDNA depletion
Sporadic PEO and late-onset myopathy with multiple mtDNA deletions
Presumably myopathic
Oculopharyngeal muscular dystrophy, autosomal-dominant
Myotubular or centronuclear myopathy
Congenital myopathic ptosis or PEO, some with muscle fibrosis
PEO as part of other generalized myopathies
  Myotonic muscular dystrophy
  Myopathic myasthenia gravis
Presumably neurogenic
Congenital PEO and facial diplegia (Möbius syndrome)
PEO with myelopathy or encephalopathy
  Juvenile onset
  Hereditary ataxia
  Hereditary spastic paraplegia
  Hereditary multisystem disease, including Joseph disease
  Generalized dystonia
  Progressive supranuclear palsy
  Abetalipoproteinemia
PEO with motor neuron disease
  Infantile spinal muscular atrophy
  Juvenile spinal muscular atrophy
  Amyotrophic lateral sclerosis

PROGRESSIVE EXTERNAL OPHTHALMOPLEGIA

PEO is defined clinically as a slowly progressive limitation of eye movements until there is complete immobility (*ophthalmoplegia*). It is usually accompanied by eyelid droop (*ptosis*) because the eyelids cannot be held in the normal position by the levator palpebrae muscles. There may or may not be weakness of muscles of the face, oropharynx, neck, or limbs.

It is not known whether the ophthalmoplegia is myopathic, neurogenic, or both, because neither electromyography of ocular muscles nor autopsy findings suffice to make this determination. This condition is clearly heterogeneous, but several distinct syndromes can be recognized, some related to primary abnormalities of mtDNA (with sporadic single deletions or maternally inherited point mutations), others related to autosomal genes directly affecting mtDNA (defects of intergenomic signaling with multiple deletions of mtDNA). For convenience, a separation can be made into a mitochondrial group, a presumably myopathic group of PEO alone or with myopathic findings in limb muscles, and a third group, presumably neurogenic, associated with disease of the central nervous system or peripheral neuropathy (Table 96.2).

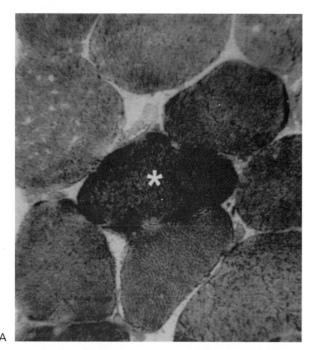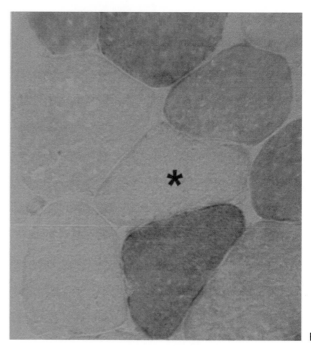

FIG. 96.2. Histochemistry detects ragged-red fibers in serial sections of human skeletal muscle. **A:** Succinate dehydrogenase enzyme activity shows an intensely staining ragged-red fiber (*white asterisk*). **B:** Cytochrome c oxidase shows that the ragged-red fiber (*black asterisk*) as well as other muscle fibers are deficient in this enzyme activity. (Courtesy of Dr. E. Bonilla, Columbia University College of Physicians and Surgeons, New York, N.Y.)

Sporadic PEO with Single mtDNA Deletions

PEO with or without Limb Weakness

This is a relatively benign condition, often compatible with a normal life span. Symptoms usually begin in childhood but may be delayed to adolescence or adult years. Ptosis is often the first symptom, followed by ophthalmoparesis. The disorder is bilateral and symmetric, so diplopia is exceptional. Some patients also have pharyngeal and limb weakness.

Kearns-Sayre Syndrome

This syndrome is identified by an invariant triad: onset before age 20 years, PEO, and pigmentary retinopathy. In addition, there must be one of the following: heart block (usually needing a pacemaker), cerebellar syndrome, or CSF protein content of 100 mg/dL or more. Seizures are distinctly infrequent and are usually associated with electrolyte disturbances, as may occur in hypoparathyroidism, one of several endocrine disorders sometimes associated with KSS. The course is relentlessly downhill, and patients rarely survive past the second decade.

Molecular Genetics

In both sporadic PEO and KSS, patients harbor a single deletion in their mtDNA that is identical in all tissues in any patient, although the number of deleted genomes varies from tissue to tissue (heteroplasmy). The single mtDNA deletions arise spontaneously early in oogenesis or embryogenesis. Although the molecular defect is the same in both conditions, intermediate cases are surprisingly few.

Laboratory Abnormalities

In both conditions, muscle biopsy shows RRFs that are devoid of histochemically demonstrable COX activity. Raised levels of lactate and pyruvate are usually found in blood in both sporadic PEO and KSS; increased lactate in the CSF is seen only in KSS. At postmortem examination, typical cases of KSS show spongy degeneration of the brain. Correspondingly, computed tomography or magnetic resonance imaging (MRI) shows evidence of leukoencephalopathy, and there may be calcification of basal ganglia.

Treatment

It is crucial to recognize KSS because sudden death as a result of the cardiac conduction disorder is a threat that can be prevented. Episodic coma may result from the combination of diabetes mellitus and encephalopathy. The cerebellar syndrome can be severe enough to be disabling. Because of their severe disabilities and hormonal problems, patients with KSS are not expected to have children, but the few women who have reproduced have had normal children. Treatment with coenzyme Q10 may reverse some electroencephalogram abnormalities but has not reversed heart block, ophthalmoplegia, or the neurologic syndrome.

Maternally Inherited PEO with Point Mutations of mtDNA

A substantial number of patients with mitochondrial PEO (i.e., PEO and RRF in the muscle biopsy) show maternal inheritance of their syndrome. PEO predominates in this syndrome but is often associated with various combinations of other symptoms, including hearing loss, endocrinopathy, heart block, cerebellar ataxia, or pigmentary retinopathy.

The most common mutation in these patients is the typical A3243G MELAS mutation, but other mutations have also been described, including the A8344G mutation typically seen in MERRF syndrome. The reason for the appearance of PEO in patients with the MELAS mutation is not known, but it may be related to a selective accumulation of mutant mtDNA in muscle.

There is usually lactic acidosis, and muscle biopsies show RRF.

Autosomal PEO with Multiple Deletions of mtDNA

PEO has been described in numerous families with autosomal-dominant (adPEO) or autosomal-recessive (arPEO) inheritance. Generally, adPEO syndromes are dominated by myopathic symptoms, while arPEO syndromes tend to be multisystemic.

Autosomal-dominant PEO

The clinical syndrome is characterized by ophthalmoplegia, although hearing loss, tremor, cataracts, and psychiatric disorders are variably present and suggest multisystemic involvement. Onset is usually in adult age, and there may be weakness of facial, pharyngeal, and respiratory muscles in addition to slowly progressive proximal limb weakness.

Autosomal-recessive PEO with Cardiomyopathy

Severe hypertrophic cardiomyopathy, proximal weakness, and PEO were the clinical hallmarks of two unrelated families from the eastern seaboard of the Arab peninsula. Onset was in childhood, and cardiac transplantation was needed to prevent early death.

Mitochondrial Neurogastrointestinal Encephalomyopathy

Mitochondrial neurogastrointestinal encephalomyopathy (MNGIE) starts in childhood or adolescence with chronic intractable diarrhea, loud borborygmi, and recurrent intestinal pseudoobstruction, causing severe emaciation. There is also PEO, both proximal and distal limb weakness, and sensory neuropathy. MRI shows diffuse leukodystrophy, although patients are rarely frankly demented. Death usually occurs in the fourth or fifth decade.

Laboratory Abnormalities

In all these conditions, muscle biopsy shows RRF and COX-negative fibers; these are more abundant in arPEO than in adPEO syndromes. Lactic acidosis is usually present but may not be very marked. In MNGIE, nerve conduction studies and nerve biopsies have shown features of both axonal and demyelinating neuropathy.

Molecular Genetics

Southern blot analyses of muscle mtDNA in these conditions show multiple bands representing species of mtDNA molecules harboring deletions of different sizes (more abundantly in arPEO than in adPEO patients). The autosomal nature of these disorders suggests that defects of nuclear genes either facilitate an intrinsic propensity of mtDNA to undergo rearrangements or cause a failure to eliminate spontaneously occurring rearrangements.

The heterogeneous nature of these disorders is exemplified by the different modes of transmission and the variety of clinical phenotypes, and has been confirmed by linkage analyses. Two distinct loci (one on chromosome 3, the other on chromosome 10) have been linked to adPEO in some but not all families, and a locus on chromosome 22 has been linked to MNGIE in four families of different ethnic origins. In MNGIE, several mutations have been identified in the gene encoding thymidine phosphorylase, and the diagnosis can be established by enzyme assay in leukocytes.

Other Forms of Mitochondrial PEO

Ophthalmoplegia is often seen in patients with the congenital or the infantile myopathic variants of *mtDNA depletion,* which are transmitted as autosomal-recessive traits (see below). Ptosis, PEO, or both can also accompany the late-onset mitochondrial myopathies, often associated with multiple mtDNA deletions, that have been described in sporadic elderly individuals and have been interpreted as an exaggerated manifestation of the normal aging process.

MULTISYSTEM NEUROLOGIC DISEASES WITHOUT OPHTHALMOPLEGIA

MELAS Syndrome

The distinguishing features of this syndrome are the strokes with hemiparesis, hemianopia, or cortical blindness that almost invariably occur before age 40 years, and often in childhood. Common additional features are focal or generalized seizures, recurrent migrainelike headaches and vomiting, and dementia. The course is one of gradual deterioration.

Laboratory abnormalities include elevated blood and CSF lactate and MRI evidence of encephalomalacic foci, usually involving the occipital cortex and not conforming to the distribution of major vessels. Muscle biopsy shows RRF, which are uncharacteristically COX-positive, rather than COX-negative as in most other mtDNA-related diseases.

In about 80% of patients, the molecular defect is a point mutation (A3243G) in the tRNA$^{Leu(UUR)}$ gene of mtDNA. In the remaining patients, a handful of mutations have been described, some of which affect protein-encoding genes rather than tRNA genes. A3243G is the most frequent pathogenic mtDNA mutation, and it has been associated not only with MELAS and maternally inherited PEO but also with diabetes mellitus alone or in combination with deafness.

MERRF Syndrome

Typical clinical features include myoclonus, generalized seizures, cerebellar ataxia, myopathy, and, in some families, multiple symmetric lipomas. Onset may occur in childhood or in adult life, and the course may be slowly progressive or rapidly downhill. As the acronym denotes, muscle biopsy shows RRF, which are COX-negative. Most patients with MERRF have a mutation (A8344G) in the tRNA^{Lys} gene of mtDNA.

Neuropathy, Ataxia, and Retinitis Pigmentosa

The combination of neuropathy, ataxia, and retinitis pigmentosa (NARP) is a maternally transmitted multisystem disorder of young adult life, comprising, in various combinations, sensory neuropathy, ataxia, seizures, dementia, and retinitis pigmentosa. Lactic acid in blood may be normal or slightly elevated, and muscle biopsy does not show RRF.

The molecular defect is a point mutation (T8993G) in the gene that encodes ATPase 6. When this mutation approaches homoplasmic levels, onset is in infancy, and the clinical and neuropathologic features are those of Leigh syndrome (maternally inherited Leigh syndrome [MILS]). A different mutation at the very same nucleotide (T8993C) causes a phenotype similar to MILS but generally milder. A few other mutations in the ATPase 6 gene have been associated with Leighlike syndromes or with familial bilateral striatal necrosis.

Leber hereditary optic neuropathy is discussed in Chapter 97.

DEPLETION OF mtDNA

Depletion of mtDNA is the other major defect of intergenomic signaling, together with multiple mtDNA deletions described above. As the name implies, this is a quantitative rather than qualitative mtDNA abnormality, consisting of markedly decreased levels of mtDNA in one or more tissues. The clinical spectrum of mtDNA depletion has been incompletely characterized and is probably more heterogeneous than was initially thought. Three syndromes stand out, all inherited as autosomal-recessive traits: congenital myopathy, infantile myopathy, and hepatopathy.

Congenital Myopathy

At or soon after birth, there is generalized weakness (sometimes including PEO) with lactic acidosis and markedly elevated serum creatine kinase. Some children also have renal involvement with Fanconi syndrome. Muscle biopsy shows abundant RRF that are COX-negative. Due to intractable respiratory failure, these children do not live more than a few months. Southern blot analysis shows a profound defect of mtDNA in muscle (less than 10% of normal).

Infantile Myopathy

In some children, weakness starts a little later but is usually evident by age 1 year and may cause PEO. Progression is rapid, leading to flaccid paralysis, respiratory insufficiency, and death within 1 or 2 more years. There is only partial mtDNA depletion in muscle (about 30% of normal), with some fibers virtually devoid of mtDNA while others look normal. Recognizing this en-

tity is especially difficult because the clinical presentation is nonspecific, lactic acidosis initially may not be present and is generally mild, and early biopsies may show nonspecific myopathic features rather than mitochondrial proliferation with RRF (which do appear in later biopsies).

Hepatopathy

Infants with severe mtDNA depletion in liver experience intractable liver failure soon after birth and die within months. Liver biopsy shows mitochondrial proliferation in hepatocytes, and biochemical analysis shows very low activities of all respiratory chain complexes containing mtDNA-encoded subunits.

It is likely that the genetic errors underlying the different variants of mtDNA depletion all involve one or more nDNA-encoded factors involved in the control of mtDNA replication. These factors, however, are unknown.

Acquired mtDNA Depletion

An iatrogenic form of mtDNA depletion has been recognized in patients with acquired immunodeficiency syndrome in whom a mitochondrial myopathy developed during treatment with zidovudine (Retrovir). The myopathy is reversible upon discontinuation of the drug.

SUGGESTED READINGS

Arnaudo E, Dalakas M, Shanske S, et al. Depletion of muscle mitochondrial DNA in AIDS patients with zidovudine-induced myopathy. *Lancet* 1991;337:508–510.

Berenberg RA, Pellock JM, DiMauro S, et al. Lumping or splitting? "ophthalmoplegia plus" or Kearns-Sayre syndrome? *Ann Neurol* 1977;1:37–54.

Bohlega S, Tanji K, Santorelli FM, et al. Multiple mtDNA deletions associated with autosomal recessive ophthalmoplegia and severe cardiomyopathy. *Neurology* 1996;46:1329–1334.

Carrozzo R, Hirano M, Fromenty B, et al. Multiple mtDNA deletions features in autosomal dominant and recessive diseases suggest distinct pathogeneses. *Neurology* 1998;50:99–106.

Ciafaloni E, Ricci E, Shanske S, et al. MELAS: clinical features, biochemistry, and molecular genetics. *Ann Neurol* 1992;31:391–398.

Dalakas M, Illa I, Pezeshkpour GH, et al. Mitochondrial myopathy caused by long-term zidovudine therapy. *N Engl J Med* 1990;322:1098–1105.

DiMauro S, Bonilla E. Mitochondrial encephalomyopathies. In: Rosenberg RN, Prusiner SB, DiMauro S, Barchi RL, eds. *The molecular and genetic basis of neurological disease.* Boston: Butterworth-Heinemann, 1997:201–235.

DiMauro S, Schon EA. Mitochondrial DNA and diseases of the nervous system: the spectrum. *Neuroscientist* 1998;4:53–63.

Engel WK, Cunningham CG. Rapid examination of muscle tissue: an improved trichrome stain method for fresh-frozen biopsy specimens. *Neurology* 1963;13:919–923.

Fukuhara N, Tokiguchi S, Shirakawa K, Tsubaki T. Myoclonus epilepsy associated with ragged red fibers (mitochondrial abnormalities): disease entity or syndrome? *J Neurol Sci* 1980;47:117–133.

Goto YI, Nonaka I, Horai S. A mutation in the tRNA$^{Leu(UUR)}$ gene associated with the MELAS subgroup of mitochondrial encephalomyopathies. *Nature* 1990;348:651–653.

Hirano M, Silvestri G, Blake DM, et al. Mitochondrial neurogastrointestinal encephalomyopathy (MNGIE): clinical, biochemical and genetic features of an autosomal-recessive disorder. *Neurology* 1994;44:721–727.

Hirano M, Yebenes J, Jones AC, et al. Mitochondrial neurogastrointestinal encephalomyopathy syndrome maps to chromosome 22q13.32qter. *Am J Hum Genet* 1998;63:526–533.

Holt IJ, Harding AE, Morgan-Hughes JA. Deletions of muscle mitochondrial DNA in patients with mitochondrial myopathy. *Nature* 1988;331:717–718.

Holt IJ, Harding AE, Morgan-Hughes JA. A new mitochondrial disease associated with mitochondrial DNA heteroplasmy. *Am J Hum Genet* 1990;46:428–433.

Johnston W, Karpati G, Carpenter S, Arnold D, Shoubridge EA. Late-onset mitochondrial myopathy. *Ann Neurol* 1995;37:16–23.

Kaukonen JA, Amati P, Suomalainen A, et al. An autosomal locus predisposing to multiple deletions of mtDNA on chromosome 3p. *Am J Hum Genet* 1996;58:763–769.

Kearns TP, Sayre G. Retinitis pigmentosa, external ophthalmoplegia, and complete heart block. *Arch Ophthalmol* 1958;60:280–289.

Luft R, Ikkos D, Palmieri G, et al. Severe hypermetabolism of nonthyroidal origin with a defect in the maintenance of mitochondrial respiratory control. *J Clin Invest* 1962;41:1776–1804.

Moraes CT, Ciacci F, Silvestri G, et al. Atypical presentation associated with the MELAS mutation at position 3243 of human mitochondrial DNA. *Neuromuscul Disord* 1993;3:43–50.

Moraes CT, DiMauro S, Zeviani M, et al. Mitochondrial DNA deletions in progressive external ophthalmoplegia and Kearns-Sayre syndrome. *N Engl J Med* 1989;320:1293–1299.

Moraes CT, Shanske S, Tritschler HJ, et al. mtDNA depletion with variable tissue expression: a novel genetic abnormality in mitochondrial diseases. *Am J Hum Genet* 1991;48:492–501.

Nishino I, Spinazzola A, Hirano M. Thymidine phosphorylase gene mutations in MNGIE, a human mitochondrial disorder. *Science* 1999;283:689–692.

Olson W, Engel WK, Einaugler R. Oculocraniosomatic neuromuscular disease with ragged red fibers. *Arch Neurol* 1972;26:193–211.

Pavlakis SG, Phillips PC, DiMauro S, et al. Mitochondrial myopathy, encephalopathy, lactic acidosis, and stroke-like episodes. *Ann Neurol* 1984;16:481–487.

Rowland LP. Progressive external ophthalmoplegia. In: Vinken PJ, Bruyn G, eds. *System disorders and atrophies. Handbook of clinical neurology, vol 22.* New York: American Elsevier, 1975.

Rowland LP, Blake DM, Hirano M, et al. Clinical syndromes associated with ragged red fibers. *Rev Neurol (Paris)* 1991;290:457–465.

Santorelli FM, Shanske S, Macaya A, et al. The mutation at nt 8993 of mitochondrial DNA is a common cause of Leigh's syndrome. *Ann Neurol* 1993;34:827–834.

Shy GM, Gonatas NK, Perez M. Childhood myopathies with abnormal mitochondria. I. Megaconial myopathy; II. Pleoconial myopathy. *Brain* 1966;89:133–158.

Silvestri G, Ciafaloni E, Santorelli FM, et al. Clinical features associated with the A→G transition at nucleotide 8344 of mtDNA ("MERRF mutation"). *Neurology* 1993;43:1200–1206.

Suomalainen A, Kaukonen JA, Amati P, et al. An autosomal locus predisposing to deletions of mitochondrial DNA. *Nat Genet* 1995;9:146–151.

Tatuch Y, Christodoulou J, Feigenbaum A, et al. Heteroplasmic mtDNA mutation (T→G) at 8993 can cause Leigh disease when the percentage of mtDNA is high. *Am J Hum Genet* 1992;50:852–858.

Vu TH, Sciacco M, Tanji K, et al. Clinical manifestations of mitochondrial DNA depletion. *Neurology* 1998;50:1783–1790.

Wallace DC, Singh G, Lott MT, et al. Mitochondrial DNA mutation associated with Leber's hereditary optic atrophy. *Science* 1988;242:1427–1430.

Wallace DC, Zhang X, Lott MT, et al. Familial mitochondrial encephalomyopathy (MERRF): genetic, pathophysiological, and biochemical characterization of a mitochondrial DNA disease. *Cell* 1988;55:601–610.

Zeviani M, Moraes CT, DiMauro S, et al. Deletions of mitochondrial DNA in Kearns-Sayre syndrome. *Neurology* 1988;38:1339–1346.

Zeviani M, Servidei S, Gellera C, et al. An autosomal-dominant disorder with multiple deletions of mitochondrial DNA starting at the D-loop region. *Nature* 1989;339:309–311.

Merritt's Neurology, 10th ed., edited by L.P. Rowland. Lippincott Williams & Wilkins, Philadelphia © 2000.

CHAPTER 97

LEBER HEREDITARY OPTIC NEUROPATHY

MYLES M. BEHRENS
MICHIO HIRANO

Leber hereditary optic neuropathy (LHON; MIM 535600) is a maternally inherited disorder characterized by loss of central vision and occurring more often in males. It was named for Leber because he reported 15 patients in four families in 1871, following von Graefe's initial description in 1858. Maternal inheritance was recognized by Wallace in 1970 in a large pedigree residing in Queensland, Australia, with LHON plus other neurologic manifestations. Nikoskelainen studied patients with more typical LHON and in 1984 proposed that mutations in mitochondrial DNA (mtDNA) might be responsible. A major breakthrough came in 1988 when Wallace, Nikoskelainen, and colleagues described the first mtDNA point mutation in a human disease. This accounted for the maternal inheritance, that is, transmission by women to all their progeny (male and female), but not by men.

CLINICAL MANIFESTATIONS

Onset usually occurs in adolescence or early-adult years but may occur from ages 5 to 80 years. Cloudiness of central vision progresses painlessly over weeks, usually first in one eye, to a larger, denser centrocecal scotoma, occasionally breaking out peripherally to a minor extent. Both eyes are usually affected within weeks or months, sometimes simultaneously; it is only rarely unilateral. Color vision is affected, and acuity drops to 20/200 or finger counting. Residual visual loss may be severe and generally remains stationary. Sometimes, there is later improvement, infrequently striking and occasionally sudden.

The fundus may appear normal until optic atrophy supervenes, but at onset, as first described by Smith, Hoyt, and Susac (1973), the disc often appears blurred and suggestive of edema, as in papillitis. However, the findings are due to swelling of the nerve fiber layer around the disc, with circumpapillary telangiectatic microangiopathy and without evidence of abnormal vascular permeability (leakage) on fluorescein angiography. The vascular abnormalities may be seen in presymptomatic and asymptomatic relatives and do not invariably predict imminent visual loss, which may never occur. As the acute stage approaches, vessels dilate and undulate in and out of the thickening peripapillary nerve fiber layer, with increased arteriovenous shunting. This subsides after a few weeks or months. Optic atrophy follows, starting in the temporal portion of the disc, then usually generalized.

In most patients with LHON, visual disturbance is the only symptom, but cardiac preexcitation is frequently associated. Neurologic examination, however, may reveal subtle neurologic abnormalities, including postural tremor, dystonia, motor tics, parkinsonism with dystonia, or peripheral neuropathy. Several patients (mostly women) with LHON have had multiple sclerosis–like manifestations. The Uhthoff symptom has been reported by a few patients with LHON itself. Two patients had ataxia and optic neuropathy with a mtDNA point mutation of LHON.

At least three Leber-plus syndromes have been reported: optic neuropathy and dystonia, optic neuropathy and spastic dystonia, and the Queensland variant with optic neuropathy, athetosis, tremor, corticospinal tract signs, posterior column dysfunction, psychiatric disturbances, and acute encephalopathy.

PATHOLOGY AND MOLECULAR GENETICS

Prior to the identification of molecular genetic defects, several autopsy studies of LHON patients revealed atrophy of the retinal ganglion cells and nerve fiber layers and optic nerve. The clinical manifestations of LHON are similar regardless of the specific genotype, but the molecular genetic features of LHON are complex and unique. First, there are mtDNA primary mutations that are thought to be pathogenic. Secondary mutations may be synergistically pathogenic in combination with each other or with primary mutations. Second, about 85% of patients with LHON harbor primary mutations that are usually homoplasmic, in contrast to the mitochondrial encephalomyopathies, which typically show heteroplasmic mutations.

The first and most common primary mtDNA mutation associated with LHON was found in the gene for subunit 4 of NADH-ubiquinone oxidoreductase, or complex I, of the mitochondrial respiratory chain. The A-to-G transition mutation at nucleotide 11778 (A11778G) in the mtDNA genome changes amino acid 340 in the ND4 gene from arginine to histidine. Two additional mtDNA mutations in complex I (ND) subunits have been identified: G3460A in ND1 and T14484C in ND6; both result in amino acid substitutions. Isolated LHON patients or individual families have had other mtDNA mutations thought to be pathogenic (Table 97.1). The penetrance rates of the LHON mutations are uncertain; however, some reports estimate that symptoms appear in 20% to 83% of men and 4% to 32% of women at risk. Sixty percent to 90% of LHON patients are men. The molecular basis for male predominance is not known. An unknown X-linked factor may interact with a LHON mtDNA mutation, but linkage studies have failed to identify such a locus.

Distinct mtDNA mutations have been associated with LHON-plus phenotypes. In the Queensland LHON-plus variant, two primary coexisting mutations were identified, T4160C

TABLE 97.1. MITOCHONDRIAL DNA MUTATIONS ASSOCIATED WITH LHON

Common LHON primary mutations

Mutation	Gene	Amino acid substitution	LHON patients with mutation (%)	Patients with visual recovery (%)
G11778A	ND4	Arg−>His	31–89	4
G3460A	ND1	Lys−>Pro	8–15	4–20
T14484C	ND6	Met−>Val	10–15	37–64

LHON-plus pathogenic mutations

Phenotype	Mutation	Gene	Amino acid substitution
LHON/dystonia	G14459A	ND6	Ala→Val
LHON/spastic dystonia	A11696G	ND4	Val→Ile
	T14596A	ND6	Ile→Met
Queensland LHON variant	T4160C	ND1	Leu→Pro

in ND1 and T14484C in ND6. Two distinct mitochondrial genotypes have been identified in pedigrees with LHON and dystonia, G14459A in ND6 and a combination of A11696G in ND1 plus T14596A in ND6.

DIFFERENTIAL DIAGNOSIS

The diagnosis of LHON is usually made when the typical course of visual loss occurs with an appropriate family history or with observation of the typical acute fundus appearance in a patient or compatible fundus changes in close maternal relatives. Now, it can be diagnosed, even without family history and even with optic neuropathy with less typical features, by genetic analysis of a blood sample.

Other forms of bilateral optic neuropathies with centrocecal scotomas include demyelinating, toxic-nutritional optic neuropathy (including tobacco—alcohol amblyopia), other types of hereditary optic atrophy, occasionally glaucoma or ischemic optic neuropathy, and only rarely compressive lesions. To help exclude tumors, computed tomography or magnetic resonance imaging includes axial and coronal orbital views with and without contrast to include the optic nerves and chiasm.

The dominant variety of hereditary optic atrophy as initially categorized by Kjer (1972) is the most common form of hereditary optic atrophy and must be distinguished from LHON. It is also characterized by centrocecal scotomas, dyschromatopsia, and temporal pallor but is generally milder, usually beginning insidiously between ages 4 and 8 years and slowly progressing with visual acuity from 20/30 to no worse than 20/200. It has been mapped to chromosome 3q27-3q28.

Other forms of hereditary optic atrophy may occur as part of complex neurologic disorders, including the lipidoses, spinocerebellar ataxias, and polyneuropathies, including Charcot-Marie-Tooth polyneuropathies. Autosomal-recessive *Behr complicated optic* atrophy may be a transitional form between the ataxias and isolated hereditary optic atrophy. Other autosomal-recessive forms of optic atrophy include the rare but severe simple optic atrophy beginning in early infancy and that associated with diabetes insipidus, diabetes mellitus, and hearing defect (DID-MOAD or Wolfram syndrome).

A source of confusion in nomenclature is the severe congenital visual loss known as *Leber congenital amaurosis*. This is an autosomal-recessive degeneration of the retina rather than of the optic nerve and is usually characterized by retinal arteriolar narrowing and retinal pigmentary degeneration. Occasionally, the fundus appears normal at first. The electroretinogram is extinguished, whereas it is normal with optic neuropathy.

TREATMENT

No treatment is of proven value, including corticosteroids, hydroxycobalamin (suggested because of evidence that cyanide toxicity might be a factor), optic nerve sheath fenestration, or craniotomy with lysis of optic nerve chiasm–arachnoidal adhesions. Given the usual sequential involvement of the two eyes, however, it may be possible to prevent loss of vision in the second eye. With the new insights into pathogenesis, it can be hoped that an effective therapy will be found, perhaps one that enhances or preserves mitochondrial respiratory enzyme function. Products that might enhance mitochondrial respiratory enzymes (coenzyme Q10, idebenone, and thiamine) have been used but are not of proven value. Antioxidants have also been used to reduce possible damage from free radicals generated by the impaired oxidative metabolism. According to consensus, tobacco and alcohol should be avoided in family members at risk.

SUGGESTED READINGS

Brown JJ, Fingert JH, Taylor CM, et al. Clinical and genetic analysis of a family affected with dominant optic atrophy (OPA1). *Arch Ophthalmol* 1997;115:95–99.

Chalmers RM, Harding AE. A case-control study of Leber's hereditary optic neuropathy. *Brain* 1996;119:1481–1486.

Harding AE, Sweeney MG, Miller DH, et al. Occurrence of a multiple sclerosis-like illness in women who have a Leber's hereditary optic atrophy mitochondrial DNA mutation. *Brain* 1992;115:979–989.

Howell N, Bogolin C, Jamieson R, et al. mtDNA mutations that cause optic neuropathy: how do we know? *Am J Hum Genet* 1998;62:196–202.

Huoponen K, Vilkki J, Aula P, et al. A new mtDNA mutation associated with Leber hereditary optic neuroretinopathy. *Am J Hum Genet* 1991;48:1147–1153.

Johns DR, Heher KL, Miller NR, Smith KH. Leber's hereditary optic neuropathy: clinical manifestations of the 14484 mutation. *Arch Ophthalmol* 1993;111:495–498.

Johns DR, Neufeld MJ, Park RD. An ND-6 mitochondrial DNA mutation associated with Leber hereditary optic neuropathy. *Biochem Biophys Res Comm* 1992;187:1551–1557.

Johns DR, Smith KH, Miller NR. Leber's hereditary optic neuropathy: clinical manifestations of the 3460 mutation. *Arch Ophthalmol* 1992;110:1577–1581.

Johnston RL, Burdon MA, Spalton DJ, et al. Dominant optic atrophy, Kjer type: linkage analysis and clinical features in a large British pedigree. *Arch Ophthalmol* 1997;115:100–103.

Kjer P. Infantile optic atrophy with dominant mode of inheritance. In: Vinken PJ, Bruyn GW, eds. *Neuroretinal degenerations. Handbook of clinical neurology, vol 13.* New York: American Elsevier Publishing, 1972:111–123.

Kline LB, Glaser JS. Dominant optic atrophy: the clinical profile. *Arch Ophthalmol* 1979;97:1680–1686.

Leber TH. Über hereditäre und congenital-angelegte Sehnervenleiden. *Graefes Archiv Ophthalmol* 1871;17:249–291.

McLeod JG, Low PA, Morgan JA. Charcot-Marie-Tooth disease with Leber optic atrophy. *Neurology* 1978;28:179–184.

Merritt HH. Hereditary optic atrophy (Leber's disease). *Arch Neurol Psychiatry* 1930;24:775–781.

Mojon DS, Herbert J, Sadiq SA, Miller JR, Madonna M, Hirano M. Leber's hereditary optic neuropathy mitochondrial DNA mutations at nucleotides 11778 and 3460 in multiple sclerosis. *Ophthalmologica* 1999;213:171–175.

Newman NJ. Leber's hereditary optic neuropathy: new genetic considerations. *Arch Neurol* 1993;50:540–548.

Newman NJ. Hereditary optic neuropathies. In: Miller NR, Newman NJ, eds. *Walsh and Hoyt's clinical neuro-ophthalmology,* 5th ed. Baltimore: Williams & Wilkins, 1998:741–773.

Nikoskelainen EK. New aspects of the genetic, etiologic, and clinical puzzle of Leber's disease. *Neurology* 1984;34:1482–1484.

Nikoskelainen EK, Hoyt WF, Nummelin KU. Ophthalmoscopic findings in Leber's hereditary optic neuropathy. I. Fundus findings in asymptomatic family members. *Arch Ophthalmol* 1982;100:1597–1602.

Nikoskelainen EK, Hoyt WF, Nummelin KU. Ophthalmoscopic findings in Leber's hereditary optic neuropathy. II. The fundus findings in the affected family members. *Arch Ophthalmol* 1983;101:1059–1068.

Nikoskelainen EK, Hoyt WF, Nummelin KU, Schatz H. Fundus findings in Leber's hereditary optic neuropathy. III. Fluorescein angiographic studies. *Arch Ophthalmol* 1984;102:981–989.

Nikoskelainen EK, Marttila RJ, Huoponen K, et al. Leber's "plus": neurological abnormalities in patients with Leber's hereditary optic neuropathy. *J Neurol Neurosurg Psychiatry* 1995;59:160–164.

Novotny EJ, Singh G, Wallace DC, et al. Leber's disease and dystonia: a mitochondrial disease. *Neurology* 1986;36:1053–1060.

Polymeropoulos MH, Swift RG, Swift M. Linkage of the gene for Wolfram syndrome to markers on the short arm of chromosome 4. *Nat Genet* 1994;8:95–97.

Scolding NJ, Keller-Wood HF, Shaw C, et al. Wolfram syndrome: hereditary diabetes mellitus with brainstem and optic atrophy. *Ann Neurol* 1996;39:352–360.

Shoffner JM, Brown MD, Stugard C, et al. Leber's hereditary optic neuropathy plus dystonia is caused by a mitochondrial DNA point mutation. *Ann Neurol* 1995;38:163–169.

Smith JL, Hoyt W, Susac JO. Ocular fundus in acute Leber optic neuropathy. *Arch Ophthalmol* 1973;90:349–354.

Von Graefe A. Ein ungewöhnlicher Fall von hereditären Amaurose. *Arch Ophthalmol* 1858;4:266–268.

Votruba M, Fitzke FW, Holder GE, Carter A, Bhattacharya SS, Moore AT. Clinical features in affected individuals from 21 pedigrees with dominant optic atrophy. *Arch Ophthalmol* 1998;116:351–358.

Wallace DC. A new manifestation of Leber's disease and a new explanation for the agency responsible for its unusual pattern of inheritance. *Brain* 1970;93:121–132.

Wallace DC, Singh G, Lott MT, et al. Mitochondrial DNA mutation associated with Leber's hereditary optic neuropathy. *Science* 1988;242:1427–1430.

Merritt's Neurology, 10th ed., edited by L.P. Rowland. Lippincott Williams & Wilkins, Philadelphia © 2000.

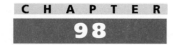

MITOCHONDRIAL DISEASES WITH MUTATIONS OF NUCLEAR DNA

DARRYL C. DE VIVO
MICHIO HIRANO

The vast majority of polypeptides in mitochondria are encoded in nuclear deoxyribonucleic acid (nDNA); therefore, nDNA mutations are likely to be the cause of many mitochondrial diseases. Most of these disorders are autosomal-recessive and lack ragged-red fibers (RRF) or other structural abnormalities of mitochondria. Exceptions are defects of intergenomic signaling (see Chapter 96) and an X-linked form of pyruvate dehydrogenase deficiency. These diseases can be classified biochemically (Table 98.1) and are beginning to be defined at the molecular genetic level. As a rule, symptoms begin in infancy or childhood, when the metabolic demands of growth and development are the greatest. Clinical manifestations may be tissue-specific or generalized. Diagnosis depends on the clinical syndrome plus biochemical and DNA analyses.

DISORDERS OF SUBSTRATE TRANSPORT AND UTILIZATION

Abnormalities of *fatty acid oxidation* provide examples of both substrate transport defects (e.g., carnitine disorders) and substrate utilization defects (e.g., abnormalities of *beta-oxidation*). These conditions are discussed in Chapter 88.

Impaired fatty acid oxidation leads to periods of metabolic decompensation during fasting. Liver, myocardium, and limb muscle are particularly vulnerable; the brain is affected secondarily, a result of nonketotic hypoglycemia and increased fatty acid levels in serum. In infants, the disorder may mimic Reye syndrome (see Chapter 32) and may cause sudden infant death.

The most common disorders of fatty acid metabolism are *medium-chain acyl-CoA dehydrogenase deficiency* (a Reye-like syndrome) and *carnitine palmityltransferase deficiency* (DiMauro syndrome), manifested by recurrent myoglobinuria.

Impaired substrate utilization is best illustrated by *pyruvate carboxylase deficiency,* which interferes with the synthesis of oxaloacetate. The syndrome includes congenital hypotonia, psychomotor retardation, failure to thrive, seizures, and metabolic acidosis. About 50% of all reported cases have what is called the French phenotype, with lactic acidosis, citrullinemia, hyperlysinemia, and hyperammonemia. Aspartate depletion impairs urea cycle activity, and oxaloacetate depletion limits Krebs cycle activity. Ketoacidosis, a prominent metabolic feature, results from the accumulation of acetyl-CoA. A North American phenotype may seem less severe at first but is ultimately fatal in late infancy or early childhood. The two phenotypes parallel the amount of residual enzyme activity.

Deficiencies of the *pyruvate dehydrogenase (PDH) complex* account for most cases of congenital lactic acidosis. The PDH complex comprises five enzymes encoded by at least nine nuclear genes. Most patients have an abnormality in the $E1\alpha$ subunit with a gene mutation on the short arm of the X-chromosome, with a male predominance. Female involvement is determined by the random pattern of inactivation of the X-chromosome. The disorder may be symptomatic in the newborn period with hypotonia, convulsions, episodic apnea, weak sucking, dysmorphic features, low birthweight, failure to thrive, and coma. The distinctive neuropathology includes cystic degeneration of subcortical white matter, basal ganglia, and brainstem. Less common features include agenesis of the corpus callosum, ectopic olivary nuclei, hydrocephalus, optic atrophy, spongy degeneration, and other nonspecific abnormalities. A similar phenotype may become symptomatic later in life. In addition, girls and women may manifest as carriers with mental retardation and ataxia. In these milder forms, lactic acidosis may be minimal.

DISORDERS OF THE CITRIC ACID CYCLE

Congenital lactic acidosis can be due to one of several enzymes of the Krebs cycle: dihydrolipoyl dehydrogenase, alpha-ketoglutarate dehydrogenase, or fumarase. Symptoms begin at birth or early infancy with failure to thrive, hypotonia, seizures, micro-

TABLE 98.1. CLASSIFICATION OF MITOCHONDRIAL DISEASES ASSOCIATED WITH MUTATIONS OF NUCLEAR DNA

Biochemical abnormality	Clinical example	MIM
Substrate transport	Carnitine deficiency	212140
Substrate utilization	Pyruvate dehydrogenase deficiency	312170
Citric acid cycle	Fumarase deficiency	136850
Respiratory chain	Cytochrome-c-oxidase deficiency	220110
Oxidation-phosphorylation	Luft disease (molecular basis not known)	238800
Protein importation	Methylmalonyl-CoA mutase deficiency	251000.0001
Intergenomic signaling	Depletion of mtDNA	251880

[a]MIM numbers are from McKusick VA. *Mendelian inheritance in man*, 12th ed. Baltimore: Johns Hopkins University Press, 1998.

cephaly, and optic atrophy. Diagnosis can be made by analysis of urinary organic acids, with patterns distinctive for each condition.

DISORDERS OF THE RESPIRATORY CHAIN

These conditions are another cause of congenital lactic acidosis. In contrast to the previously cited autosomal or X-linked conditions, respiratory enzyme disorders can result from mutations of either nDNA or mtDNA. Pathogenic mutations in two nDNA-encoded subunits of complex I have been identified. A homozygous five-base-pair duplication in the 18-kDa (AQDQ) subunit was found in an infant with recurrent vomiting, psychomotor retardation, seizures, hypotonia, and cardiopulmonary failure leading to death at 16 months. The second patient died of Leigh syndrome at age 11 weeks and harbored compound heterozygous mutations in the NDUFS8 (TYKY) subunit. Deficiency of succinate dehydrogenase, which functions as complex II of the respiratory chain, was attributed to a homozygous mutation in the flavoprotein subunit in two infants with Leigh syndrome. *Coenzyme Q_{10}* deficiency leads to an encephalomyopathy with recurrent myoglobinuria and RRF that responds to replacement therapy. *Cytochrome-c oxidase (COX) deficiency,* as mentioned previously, may be associated with a fatal infantile myopathy or a relatively benign condition.

LEIGH SYNDROME

The most common form of complex IV deficiency (COX) is *subacute necrotizing encephalomyelopathy (Leigh syndrome).* The condition was first described in 1951 in a 7-month-old infant who showed necrotizing lesions in the brainstem that resembled those of Wernicke encephalopathy. The lesions are found in the periaqueductal region of the midbrain and pons and in the medulla adjacent to the fourth ventricle (Table 98.2). Other parts of the central nervous system and peripheral nerves may also be affected. The lesions are a combination of cell necrosis, demyelination, and a vascular proliferation. The topology and vascular lesions are distinctive (Fig. 98.1). Pathologically, the condition

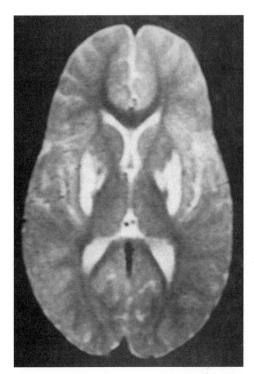

FIG. 98.1. A 2-year-old-girl with cytochrome-c-oxidase deficiency and Leigh syndrome. Heavily T2-weighted MRI shows prominent signal abnormality with bilaterally symmetric involvement of basal ganglia. Putaminal involvement is characteristic of Leigh syndrome.

differs from Wernicke disease because the hypothalamus and mammillary bodies are spared in Leigh syndrome.

The condition may be inherited in an autosomal-recessive, X-linked, or maternal pattern. In adults, it is usually sporadic. Infants may develop normally for months; others may show signs of encephalopathy in early infancy. Poor feeding, feeble crying, and respiratory difficulty may be early symptoms. This is followed by impaired vision and hearing, ataxia, limb weakness, intellectual deterioration, and seizures. Nystagmus is common. In patients with later onset, there may be progressive external ophthalmoplegia, dystonia, or ataxia. Once affected, the child may die in infancy or childhood; some live until the third decade.

Laboratory Abnormalities

Cerebrospinal fluid (CSF) protein content is mildly elevated in 25% of patients. Lactate and pyruvate levels are almost always increased in CSF and, to a lesser degree, in blood and urine. These findings and the histopathology lead to a search for an abnormality of pyruvate metabolism. Electroencephalogram changes and abnormal evoked responses are nonspecific. Computed tomography may show symmetric lucencies in basal ganglia and the thalamus; the ventricles may be enlarged. Magnetic resonance imaging (MRI) demonstrates the distinctive topography in detail (see Fig. 98.1).

Pathogenesis

The biochemical lesions are diverse but impair cerebral oxidative metabolism. Affected enzymes include PDH, biotinidase, or

TABLE 98.2. COMPARISON OF DISTRIBUTION OF BRAIN LESIONS IN SUBACUTE NECROTIZING ENCEPHALOMYELOPATHY (SNE) AND WERNICKE DISEASE (WD)

	SNE (%)	WD (%)
Brainstem	98	85
Midbrain	90	72
Tegmentum	78	—
Substantia nigra	62	5
Medulla	84	58
Spinal cord	74	33
Cerebellum	58	19
Cerebrum	92	97
Cortex	10	33
Basal ganglia	65	11
Thalamus	51	68
Hypothalamus	27	97

complex I, II, or IV (COX) of the respiratory chain. In most autosomally inherited cases, the mutations are in nDNA-encoded subunits of the enzymes; however, in COX-deficient Leigh syndrome, the first pathogenic mutations were identified in SURF1, a putative assembly or maintenance factor for COX. Point mutations of mtDNA, particularly the T8993G mutation in ATPase 6, have been associated with maternally inherited Leigh syndrome (see Chapter 96). There are no RRF in any of these conditions. Leigh syndrome is usually fatal before age 1 year when associated with the neuropathy, ataxia, and retinitis pigmentosa (NARP) mutation or PDH complex deficiency.

ALPERS SYNDROME

In 1931, Bernard Alpers described an infant girl with progressive poliodystrophy. The pathology had anoxic features, but in retrospect some authorities have ascribed the changes to status epilepticus and hypoxia-ischemia. Later, Huttenlocher described an autosomal-recessive condition with the same neuropathology and hepatic cirrhosis. The relation of this condition to mitochondrial dysfunction is at best uncertain.

IMPAIRED MITOCHONDRIAL TRANSPORT

In one patient with *methylmalonic aciduria,* a point mutation within the mitochondrial targeting sequence of methylmalonyl-CoA mutase led to failure of protein importation into mitochondria. One family with X-linked pyruvate dehydrogenase E1α deficiency harbored a point mutation that altered the structure of the polypeptide mitochondrial targeting sequence in affected individuals. The protein was not effectively transported across the mitochondrial membranes into the matrix. Finally, in *hyperoxaluria type I,* the enzyme is misdirected to the mitochondrial matrix rather than its normal location, the peroxisome.

Identification of gene mutations—frataxin in Friedreich ataxia (see Chapter 107) and a copper-transporting P-type ATPase in Wilson-Duchene (see Chapter 89) —has revealed defects in metal-transporting proteins located in mitochondria.

SUGGESTED READINGS

Alpers BJ. Diffuse progressive degeneration of the grey matter of the cerebrum. *Arch Neurol Psychiatry* 1931;25:469–505.

Atkin BM, Buist NR, Utter MF, et al. Pyruvate carboxylase deficiency and lactic acidosis in a retarded child without Leigh's disease. *Pediatr Res* 1979;13:109–116.

Babcock M, de Silva D, Oaks R, et al. Regulation of mitochondrial iron accumulation by Yfh1p, a putative homolog of frataxin. *Science* 1997;276:1709–1712.

Bourgeron T, Rustin P, Chretien D, et al. Mutation of a nuclear succinate dehydrogenase gene results in mitochondrial respiratory chain deficiency. *Nat Genet* 1995;11:144–149.

De Vivo DC. The expanding clinical spectrum of mitochondrial diseases. *Brain Dev* 1993;15:1–21.

De Vivo DC. Complexities of the pyruvate dehydrogenase complex. *Neurology* 1998;51:1247–1249.

De Vivo DC, Haymond MW, Leckie MP, Bussman YL. The clinical and biochemical implications of pyruvate carboxylase deficiency. *J Clin Endocrinol Metab* 1977;45:1281–1296.

De Vivo DC, Hirano M, DiMauro S. Mitochondrial disorders. In: Moser H, ed. *Neurodystrophies and neurolipidoses.* Amsterdam: Elsevier Science, 1997:389–446.

DiMauro S, Hirano M, Bonilla E, et al. *Cytochrome oxidase deficiency: progress and problems.* Oxford: Butterworth-Heinemann, 1994;1:91–115.

DiMauro S, Schon EA. Nuclear power and mitochondrial diseases. *Nat Genet* 1998;19:214–215.

Farrell DF, Clark AF, Scott CR, Wennberg RP. Absence of pyruvate decarboxylase activity in man: a cause of congenital lactic acidosis. *Science* 1975;187:1082–1084.

Feigin I, Wolf A. A disease in infants resembling chronic Wernicke's encephalopathy. *J Pediatr* 1954;45:243–263.

Gellera C, Uziel G, Rimoldi M, et al. Fumarase deficiency is an autosomal-recessive encephalopathy affecting both the mitochondrial and the cytosolic enzymes. *Neurology* 1990;40:495–499.

Hale DE. Fatty acid oxidation disorders: a new class of metabolic disorders. *J Pediatr* 1992;121:1–11.

Harding BN. Progressive neuronal degeneration of childhood with liver disease (Alpers-Huttenlocher syndrome): a personal review. *J Child Neurol* 1990;5:273–289.

Hommes FA, Polman HA, Reerink JD. Leigh's encephalomyelopathy: an inborn error of gluconeogenesis. *Arch Dis Child* 1968;43:423–426.

Huttenlocher PR, et al. *Arch Neurol* 1976;33:186–192.

Jellinger K, Zimprich H, Muller D. Relapsing form of subacute necrotizing encepalomyelopathy. *Neuropediatrics* 1973;4:314–321.

Ledley FD, Jansen R, Nham SU, et al. Mutations eliminating mitochondrial leader sequence of methylmalonyl-CoA cause mut⁰ methylmalonic acidemia. *Proc Natl Acad Sci U S A* 1990;87:3147–3150.

Leigh D. Subacute necrotizing encephalomyelopathy in an infant. *J Neurol Neurosurg Psychiatry* 1951;14:216–221.

Loeffen J, Smeitink J, Triepels R, et al. The first nuclear-encoded complex I mutation in a patient with Leigh syndrome. *Am J Hum Genet* 1998;63:1598–1608.

Lutsenko S, Cooper MJ. Localization of the Wilson's disease protein product to mitochondria. *Proc Natl Acad Sci U S A* 1998;95:6004–6009.

Rahman S, Blok RB, Dahl HH, et al. Leigh syndrome: clinical features and biochemical and DNA abnormalities. *Ann Neurol* 1996;39:343–351.

Santorelli FM, Shanske S, Macaya A, et al. The mutation at nt 8993 of mitochondrial DNA is a common cause of Leigh syndrome. *Ann Neurol* 1993;34:827–834.

Stanley CA, De Leeuw S, Coates PA, et al. Chronic cardiomyopathy and weakness or acute coma in children with a defect in carnitine uptake. *Ann Neurol* 1991;30:709–716.

Takakubo F, Cartwright P, Hoogenraad N, et al. An amino acid substitution in the pyruvate dehydrogenase E1 alpha gene, affecting mitochondrial import of the precursor protein. *Am J Hum Genet* 1995;57:772–780.

Tanzi RE, Petrukhin K, Chernov I, et al. The Wilson disease gene is a copper-transporting ATPase with homology to the Menkes disease gene. *Nat Genet* 1993;5:344–350.

Tiranti V, Hoertnagel K, Carrozzo R, et al. Mutations of SURF-1 in Leigh disease associated with cytochrome *c* oxidase deficiency. *Am J Hum Genet* 1998;63:1609–1621.

Van Coster R, Fernhoff PM, De Vivo DC. Pyruvate carboxylase deficiency: a benign variant with normal development. *Pediatr Res* 1991;30:1–4.

Van Coster R, Lombes A, De Vivo DC, et al. Cytochrome *c* oxidase-associated Leigh syndrome: phenotypic features and pathogenetic speculations. *J Neurol Sci* 1991;104:97–111.

van den Heuvel L, Ruitenbeek W, Smeets R, et al. Demonstration of a new pathogenic mutation in human complex I deficiency: a 5-bp duplication in the nuclear gene encoding the 18-kD (AQDQ) subunit. *Am J Hum Genet* 1998;62:262–268.

Zhu S, Yao J, Johns T, et al. SURF1, encoding a factor involved in the biogenesis of cytochrome *c* oxidase, is mutated in Leigh syndrome. *Nat Genet* 1998;20:337–343.

Zinn AB, Kerr DS, Hoppel CL. Fumarase deficiency: a new cause of mitochondrial encephalomyopathy. *N Engl J Med* 1986;315:469–475.

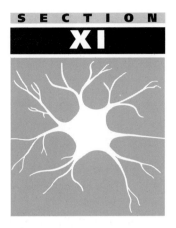

NEUROCUTANEOUS DISORDERS

Several genetic diseases involve both the skin and nervous system. These are called *neurocutaneous disorders* or *neuroectodermatoses*. In the past, they were referred to as the "phakomatoses" (*phakos* is the Greek word for lentil, flat plate, or spot). Retinal lesions are seen in tuberous sclerosis and sometimes in neurofibromatosis. Other distinct disorders are Sturge-Weber-Dimitri syndrome, linear nevus sebaceous, and incontinentia pigmenti.

Any portion of the central and peripheral nervous system may be affected by these heredodegenerative diseases, and different portions may be involved in various combinations. Some families breed true and show a remarkable consistency with regard to location and extent of the pathologic changes; other families demonstrate great discrepancies among individual members of the family. The clinical spectrum ranges from frequent abortive forms (*formes frustes*) to a severe, potentially lethal condition with highly protean clinical manifestations.

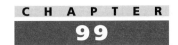

NEUROFIBROMATOSIS

ARNOLD P. GOLD

Neurofibromatosis (NF) was first described by von Recklinghausen in 1882; it is one of the most common single-gene disorders of the central nervous system (CNS). The two cardinal features are multiple hyperpigmented marks on the skin (*café-au-lait spots*) and multiple neurofibromas; other symptoms may result from lesions in bone, the CNS, the peripheral nervous system, or other organs. Two forms are recognized. Neurofibromatosis type 1 (NF-1) is also known as *von Recklinghausen disease* or *peripheral NF* (MIM 162200). It is one of the most common hereditary diseases, with a prevalence of 1 per 3,000 population. Neurofibromatosis type 2 (NF-2) is also known as *central NF* or *bilateral acoustic neuroma syndrome* (MIM 101000). The two conditions differ genetically, pathogenetically, and clinically.

Many of the clinical features, neurofibromas, and CNS lesions affect structures that originate in the neural crest. Other disorders include altered synthesis and secretion of melanin, disturbed cellular organization with hamartomatous collections, and abnormal production and distribution of nerve growth factors. In both syndromes, gene products seem to act as oncogenes.

GENETICS AND INCIDENCE

Both NF-1 and NF-2 are autosomal-dominant conditions; penetrance of NF-1 is almost 100%, but expressivity varies. Mutations are thought to account for 50% of new cases. Both sexes are affected equally, and the condition is found worldwide in all racial and ethnic groups. Incidence figures must be a minimal estimate because abortive cases are often unrecognized clinically.

MOLECULAR GENETICS AND PATHOGENESIS

The NF1 gene has been mapped to chromosome 17q11.2. The gene product is called neurofibromin. Since individuals with NF-1 are at increased risk for benign and malignant tumors, neurofibromin is considered a tumor-suppressor gene. Five different types of NF1 gene mutations are known: translocations, large megabase deletions, large internal deletions, small rearrangements, and point mutations. Although the genotypes differ, the phenotypes are indistinguishable. The marked clinical variability within families having an identical NF1 gene mutation equals the variability among families with different NF1 gene mutations. The only exception is the syndrome of large megabase deletions, where affected people are typically mentally retarded. Mutation inactivates the gene, and, by analogy with other oncogenes, loss of the allelic gene later in life could result in tumor formation. It is not known, however, how the other manifestations of the disease arise. Neurofibromin is expressed in neurons, but it is not known why some affected people have neurologic disorders and others do not. Modifying genes in other locations may play a role.

The NF2 gene maps to chromosome 22q12. The gene product is similar to that of moesin-, ezrin-, and radixin-like gene; for this reason, it is called *merlin*. Deletions of the gene have been found in schwannoma and meningioma cells, the major tumors in NF-2 patients.

NEUROPATHOLOGY

The neuropathologic changes result from changes in neural supporting tissue with resultant dysplasia, hyperplasia, and neoplasia. These pathologic changes may involve the central, peripheral, and autonomic nervous systems. Visceral manifestations result from hyperplasia of the autonomic ganglia and nerves within the organ. In addition to neural lesions, dysplastic and neoplastic changes affect skin, bone, endocrine glands, and blood vessels. Developmental anomalies include thoracic meningocele and syringomyelia. Patients affected by NF are more likely than others to have neoplastic disorders, including neuroblastoma, Wilms tumor, leukemia, pheochromocytoma, and sarcomas.

Neoplasms involving the peripheral nervous system and spinal nerve roots include schwannomas and neurofibromas. Intramedullary spinal cord tumors include ependymomas (especially of the conus medullaris and filum terminale) and, less often, astrocytomas. The most common intracranial tumors are hemispheral astrocytomas of any histologic grade from benign to highly malignant. Pilocytic astrocytic gliomas of the optic nerve and optic chiasm are also characteristic. Bilateral acoustic neuromas and solitary or multicentric menigiomas commonly occur in adults with NF-2.

SYMPTOMS AND SIGNS

There are at least four forms of NF. *Peripheral NF* (NF-1) as described by von Recklinghausen is most commonly encountered. *Central NF* (NF-2) is manifest by bilateral acoustic neuromas at about age 20 years. Cutaneous changes are mild, and there are only a few café-au-lait spots or neurofibromas. Antigenic activity of nerve growth factor is increased. *Segmental NF* probably arises from a somatic cell mutation; it is characterized by café-au-lait spots and neurofibromas that are limited, usually affecting an upper body segment. The lesions extend to the midline and include the ipsilateral arm but spare the head and neck. *Cutaneous NF* is limited to pigmentary changes; there are numerous café-au-lait spots but no other clinical manifestations.

NF-1 often presents with protean and progressive manifestations. Not uncommonly, once the diagnosis is established, a fate like that of the grotesque John Merrick (the Elephant Man) is anticipated by parents or physicians. In reality, many patients with this disease are functionally indistinguishable from normal. Often, they have only cutaneous lesions and are diagnosed when

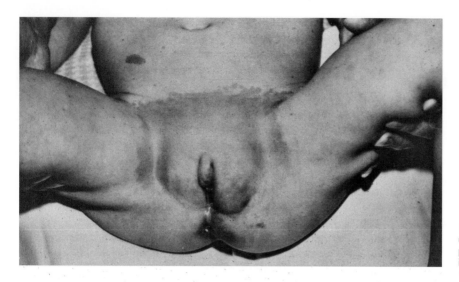

FIG. 99.1. Neurofibromatosis. Café-au-lait macule (abdomen) and larger pigmented lesion in the perineal area associated with an underlying plexiform neuroma and elephantiasis of the left labia.

they see a physician because of a learning disability, scoliosis, or another problem.

Cutaneous Symptoms

The café-au-lait macule is the pathognomonic lesion, being present in almost all patients (Fig. 99.1). Six or more café-au-lait spots larger than 5 mm in diameter before puberty and greater than 15 mm in diameter after puberty are diagnostic. The spots are usually present at birth but may not appear until age 1 or 2 years. Increasing in both size and number during the first decade of life, the macules tend to be less evident after the second decade because they blend into the surrounding hyperpigmented skin. These discrete, tan macules involve the trunk and limbs in a random fashion but tend to spare the face.

Other cutaneous manifestations may include freckles over the entire body, but freckles usually involve the axilla and other intertriginous areas. Larger, darker hyperpigmented lesions are often associated with an underlying plexiform neurofibroma (Fig. 99.2); if this involves the midline, it may indicate the presence of a spinal cord tumor.

Ocular Symptoms

Pigmented iris hamartomas (*Lisch nodules*), when present, are pathognomonic and consist of small translucent yellow or brown elevations on slit-lamp examination. The nodules increase in number with age and are present in almost all patients older than 20 years. They are observed only in NF-1 and are not seen in the normal eye.

Neurologic Symptoms

Neurofibromas are highly characteristic lesions and usually become clinically evident at ages 10 to 15 years. They always involve the skin, ultimately developing into sessile, pedunculated lesions. The nodules are found on deep peripheral nerves or nerve roots and on the autonomic nerves that innervate the viscera and blood vessels. The lesions increase in size and number during the second and third decades. There may be a few or

many thousands. These benign tumors consist of neurons, Schwann cells, fibroblasts, blood vessels, and mast cells. They rarely give rise to any symptoms other than pain as a result of pressure on nerves or nerve roots, but may undergo sarcomatous degeneration in the third and fourth decades of life (Fig. 99.3). Neurofibromas involving the terminal distribution of peripheral nerves form vascular plexiform neurofibromas that result in localized overgrowth of tissues or segmental hypertrophy of a limb (*elephantiasis neuromatosa*). Spinal root or cauda equina neurofi-

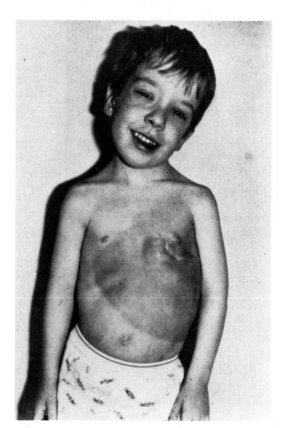

FIG. 99.2. Neurofibromatosis. Large pigmented lesion with associated progressive scoliosis.

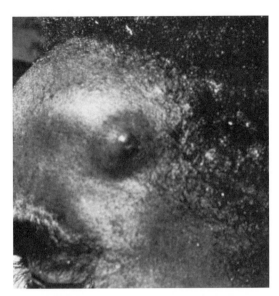

FIG. 99.3. Neurofibromatosis. Sarcomatous degeneration of a neurofibroma at 35 years.

bromas are often asymptomatic when they are small, but large tumors may compress the spinal cord, causing the appropriate clinical signs.

Optic gliomas, astrocytomas, acoustic neuromas, neurilemmomas, and meningiomas have a combined frequency of 5% to 10% in all patients with NF. Optic nerve gliomas and other intracranial neoplasms are often evident before age 10; acoustic neuromas become symptomatic at about age 20. When optic glioma is associated with NF, it commonly involves the optic nerve or is multicentric; less frequently, it involves the chiasm (Figs. 99.4 and 99.5). Optic nerve glioma must be distinguished from the commonly observed nonneoplastic optic nerve hyperplasia. The optic glioma of NF is slowly progressive and has a better prognosis than similar tumors without this association.

NF-2 is clinically evident at about age 20; symptoms include hearing loss, tinnitus, imbalance, and headache. Only a few café-au-lait spots and neurofibromas are seen. Intracranial and intraspinal neoplasms include meningiomas, schwannomas, and gliomas.

CNS involvement in NF is highly variable. Macrocephaly, a common clinical manifestation of postnatal origin, is an incidental finding with no correlation with academic performance, seizures, or neurologic function. Specific learning disabilities or attention deficit disorder, with or without impaired speech, is the most common neurologic complication of NF. Intellectual retardation or convulsive disorders each occur in about 5% of the patients. Brainstem tumors associated with NF-1 have a more indolent course than those without NF.

Occlusive cerebrovascular disease is rare but is sometimes seen in children, resulting in acute hemiplegia and convulsions. Magnetic resonance angiography or conventional angiography may demonstrate occlusion of the supraclinoid portion of the in-

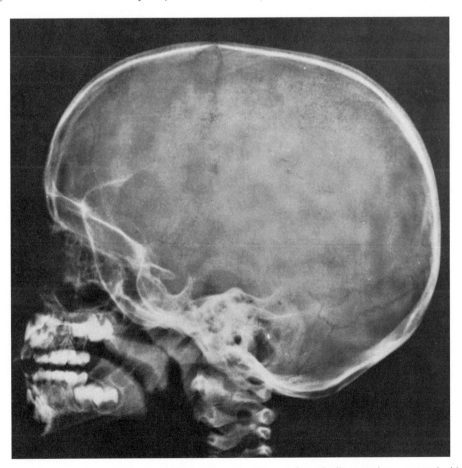

FIG. 99.4. Neurofibromatosis. Lateral skull radiograph shows a J-shaped sella secondary to an optic chiasm glioma.

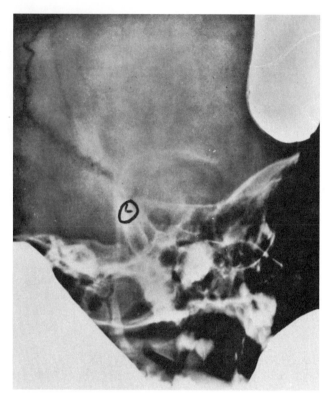

FIG. 99.5. Neurofibromatosis. Optic canal view shows an enlarged optic foramen secondary to an optic nerve glioma.

ternal carotid artery at the origin of the anterior and middle cerebral arteries with associated telangiectasia (moyamoya).

Symptoms of the Skull, Spine, and Limbs

Skeletal anomalies characteristic of NF include (1) unilateral defects in the posterosuperior wall of the orbit, with pulsating exophthalmos; (2) a defect in the lambdoid with underdevelopment of the ipsilateral mastoid; (3) dural ectasia with enlargement of the spinal canal and scalloping of the posterior portions of the vertebral bodies (also seen in connective tissue disorders such as Marfan and Ehlers-Danlos syndromes); (4) kyphoscoliosis, seen in 2% to 10% of patients with NF, most commonly involving the cervicothoracic vertebrae; unless corrected, it can be rapidly progressive, characterized by a short-segment angular scoliosis that typically involves the lower thoracic vertebrae; (5) pseudarthrosis, especially involving the tibia and radius; (6) "twisted ribbon" rib deformities; and (7) enlargement of long bones.

Miscellaneous Symptoms

Pheochromocytoma, an unusual complication of NF, is never seen in children. Hypertension may be due to a pheochromocytoma or a neurofibroma of a renal artery. Malignant tumors not uncommonly complicating NF include sarcoma, leukemia, Wilms tumor, ganglioglioma, and neuroblastoma. Medullary thyroid carcinoma and hyperparathyroidism rarely occur. Precocious puberty and, less commonly, sexual infantilism result from

involvement of the hypothalamus by glioma or hamartoma. Cystic lesions, malignancy, and interstitial pneumonia are pulmonary complications.

DIAGNOSIS

Diagnosis of NF-1 or NF-2 is based on clinical, radiologic, and pathologic findings, as well as the family history. Diagnostic criteria have been established by the National Institutes of Health Consensus Conference (Table 99.1).

LABORATORY DATA

Molecular genetic studies are now available but are not always specific or diagnostic. Therefore, all patients and those at risk should receive an extensive clinical evaluation aimed at diagnosis and identification of possible complications. Ancillary laboratory studies, however, should be individualized, determined by the clinical manifestations. Complete evaluation may include psychoeducational and psychometric testing; electroencephalogram; ophthalmologic and audiologic testing; cranial computed tomography (CT), including orbital views; CT of the spine and internal auditory foramina; magnetic resonance imaging of brain and spine; and quantitative measurement of 24-hour urinary catecholamines.

TREATMENT

There is no specific treatment for NF, but complications may be ameliorated with early recognition and prompt therapeutic intervention. Learning disabilities should be considered in all chil-

TABLE 99.1. DIAGNOSTIC CRITERIA FOR NEUROFIBROMATOSIS

Neurofibromatosis 1 (any two or more)
  Six or more café-au-lait macules
    Before puberty >5 mm diameter
    After puberty >15 mm diameter
  Freckling in the axillary or inguinal areas
  Two or more neurofibromas or one plexiform neurofibroma
  A first-degree relative with NF-1
  Two or more Lisch nodules (iris hamartomas)
  Bone lesion
    Sphenoid dysplasia
    Thinning of the cortex of long bones with or without pseudarthrosis

Neurofibromatosis 2
  Bilateral eighth nerve tumor (MRI, CT, or histologic confirmation)
  A first-degree relative with NF-2 and a unilateral eighth nerve tumor
  A first-degree relative with NF-2 and any two of the following:
    Neurofibroma, meningioma, schwannoma, glioma, or juvenile posterior subcapsular lenticular opacity

Modified from Conference statement, National Institutes of Health consensus development conference: neurofibromatosis. *Arch Neurol* 1988; 45:575–578.

dren with NF and may be complicated by behavioral problems (hyperkinesis or attention deficit disorder) that warrant educational therapy or behavioral modification, psychotherapy, and pharmacotherapy. Speech problems require a language evaluation and formal speech therapy, and seizures indicate the need for anticonvulsant medication. Progressive kyphoscoliosis usually requires surgical intervention. Surgery may be necessary for removal of pheochromocytomas and intracranial or spinal neoplasms; cutaneous neurofibromas require extirpation when they compromise function or are disfiguring. Radiation therapy is reserved for some CNS neoplasms, including optic glioma. Genetic counseling and psychotherapy with family counseling are important.

SUGGESTED READINGS

Neurofibromatosis. Conference Statement. National Institutes of Health Consensus Development Conference. *Arch Neurol* 1988;45:575–578.

Crowe FW, Schull WJ, Neel JV. *A clinical, pathological and genetic study of multiple neurofibromatosis.* Springfield, IL: Charles C Thomas, 1956.

Easton DF, Ponder MA, Huson SM, et al. Analysis of variation in expression of neurofibromatosis (NF1): evidence for modifying genes. *Am J Hum Genet* 1993;53:305–313.

Es SV, North KN, McHugh K, Silva MD. MRI findings in children with neurofibromatosis type I: a prospective study. *Pediatr Radiol* 1996:26;478–487.

Evans DGR, Huson SM, Donnai D, et al. A genetic study of type 2 neurofibromatosis in the United Kingdom. II. Guidelines for genetic counselling. *J Med Genet* 1992;29:847–852.

Gutmann DH. Recent insights into neurofibromatosis type 1: clear genetic progress. *Arch Neurol* 1998;55:778–780.

Gutmann DH, Collins FS. Recent progress toward understanding the molecular biology of von Recklinghausen neurofibromatosis. *Ann Neurol* 1992;31:555–561.

Gutmann DH, Collins FS. The neurofibromatosis type 1 gene and its protein product, neurofibromin. *Neuron* 1993;10:335–343.

Karmes PS. Neurofibromatosis: a common neurocutaneous disorder. *Mayo Clin Proc* 1998;73:1071–1076.

Korf BR. Neurocutaneous syndromes: neurofibromatosis 1, neurofibromatosis 2, and tuberous sclerosis. *Curr Opin Neurol* 1997;10:131–136.

Levinsohn PM, Mikahel MA, Rothman SM. Cerebrovascular changes in neurofibromatosis. *Dev Med Child Neurol* 1978;20:789–792.

Listernick R, Louis DN, Packer RJ, Gutmann DH. Optic pathway gliomas in neurofibromatosis I. Optic Pathway Glioma Taskforce. *Ann Neurol* 1997;41:143–149.

Martuza RL, Eldridge R. Neurofibromatosis 2 (bilateral acoustic neurofibromatosis). *N Engl J Med* 1988;318:684–688.

Mulvihill JJ, Pavory DM, Sherman JL, et al. Neurofibromatosis 1 (Recklinghausen disease) and neurofibromatosis 2 (bilateral acoustic neurofibromatosis): an update. *Ann Intern Med* 1990;113:39–52.

North K. *Neurofibromatosis type 1 in childhood.* London: MacKeith Press, 1997.

Pollack IF, Mulvihill JJ. Neurofibromatosis 1 and 2. *Brain Pathol* 1997;7:823–836.

Riccardi VM. *Neurofibromatosis: phenotype, natural history, and pathogenesis,* 2nd ed. Baltimore: Johns Hopkins University Press, 1992.

Romanowski CA, Cavallin LI. Neurofibromatosis types I and II: radiological appearance. *Hosp Med* 1998;59:134–139.

Rubenstein AE, Bunge RP, Housman DE, eds. Neurofibromatosis. *Ann N Y Acad Sci* 1986;486:1–414.

Smirniotopoulos JG, Murphy FM. The phakomatoses: neurofibromatosis. *AJNR* 1992;13:737–744.

Stern HJ, Saal HM, Lee JS, et al. Clinical variability of type 1 neurofibromatosis: is there a neurofibromatosis-Noonan syndrome? *J Med Genet* 1992;29:184–187.

Tibbles JAR, Cohen MM. The proteus syndrome: the Elephant Man diagnosed. *BMJ* 1986;293:683–685.

Trofatter JA, MacCollin MM, Rutter JL, et al. A novel moesin-, ezrin-, radixin-like gene is a candidate for neurofibromatosis 2 tumor suppressor. *Cell* 1993;72:1–20.

Upadhyaya M, Fryer A, MacMillan J, et al. Prenatal diagnosis and presymptomatic detection of neurofibromatosis type 1. *J Med Genet* 1992;29:180–183.

Merritt's Neurology, 10th ed., edited by L.P. Rowland. Lippincott Williams & Wilkins, Philadelphia © 2000.

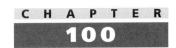

CHAPTER 100

ENCEPHALOTRIGEMINAL ANGIOMATOSIS

ARNOLD P. GOLD

Encephalotrigeminal angiomatosis (*Sturge-Weber-Dimitri syndrome*) (MIM 185300) is manifested by a cutaneous vascular port-wine nevus of the face, contralateral hemiparesis and hemiatrophy, glaucoma, seizures, and mental retardation. In 1847, Sturge described the clinical picture and attributed the neurologic manifestations to a nevoid lesion of the brain similar to the facial lesion. In 1923, Dimitri showed the gyriform pattern of calcification. Weber described the radiographic findings of intracranial calcification.

GENETICS

Most cases are sporadic, but affected siblings suggest autosomal-recessive inheritance in some families. Others cases suggest an autosomal-dominant pattern. As with other neurocutaneous disorders, there is incomplete penetrance with marked variability of the clinical manifestations. The gene locus has not yet been mapped.

NEUROPATHOLOGY

The occipital lobe is most often affected, but lesions may involve the temporal and parietal lobes or the entire cerebral hemisphere. Atrophy is characteristically unilateral and ipsilateral to the facial nevus. Leptomeningeal angiomatosis with small venules fills the subarachnoid space. Calcification of the arteries on the surface of the brain and intracerebral calcifications of small vessels are seen. The trolley-track or curvilinear calcifications seen on skull radiographs are due to calcification of the outer cortex rather than of blood vessels.

TABLE 100.1. ENCEPHALOFACIAL ANGIOMATOSIS

Type 1	Both facial and leptomeningeal angiomas; may have glaucoma (Sturge-Weber syndrome)
	Intracranial angioma should be documented histologically or by typical radiographic findings
	Epileptic seizures or EEG findings permit presumptive diagnosis in a child with typical nevus
Type 2	Facial angioma but no evidence of intracranial disease; may have glaucoma
Type 3	Leptomeningeal angioma but no facial nevus; may have glaucoma

Modified from Roach, 1992.

SYMPTOMS AND SIGNS

Facial nevus and a neurologic syndrome of seizures, hemiplegia, retardation, and glaucoma are characteristic. Typically, other than the facial nevus, the child has normal function for months or years. Subsequent clinical course is highly variable; a clinical classification has recently been proposed by Roach (1992) (Table 100.1).

Cutaneous Symptoms

The port-wine facial nevus flammeus is related to the cutaneous distribution of the trigeminal nerve (Fig. 100.1). Most com-

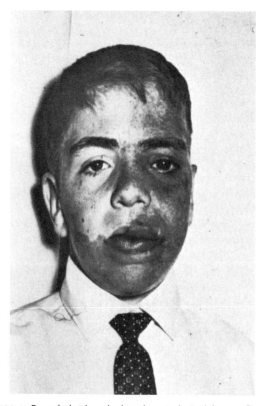

FIG. 100.1. Encephalotrigeminal angiomatosis. Facial nevus flammeus involves the cutaneous distribution of all three branches of the trigeminal nerve on one side and the mandibular branch on the contralateral side.

monly involving the forehead, the nevus may involve one-half of the face and may extend to the neck. The nevus may cross or fall short of the midline. Rarely, bilateral facial lesions are seen.

Only when the entire ophthalmic sensory area (forehead and upper eyelid) is covered by the nevus flammeus (with or without involvement of the maxillary and mandibular areas) is there a high risk of glaucoma or neurologic complications. Neuroocular disease is rare when only part of the ophthalmic area has a port-wine stain. There is little or no risk when the nevus is localized to the maxillary or mandibular trigeminal sensory areas without involving the ophthalmic area.

Neurologic Symptoms

Epilepsy is the most common neurologic manifestation, usually starting in the first year of life with focal motor, generalized major motor, or partial complex convulsions. Often refractory to anticonvulsants, the focal motor seizures, hemiparesis, and hemiatrophy are contralateral to the facial nevus. Onset of seizures before age 2 years and refractory epilepsy have prognostic significance; these patients are more likely to be intellectually impaired. Intellectual retardation often becomes more marked with age.

Ophthalmologic Symptoms

Raised intraocular pressure with glaucoma and buphthalmos occurs in approximately 30% of patients. Buphthalmos, which is more common than glaucoma, is due to antenatal intraocular hypertension. Homonymous hemianopia, a common visual-field complication, is invariable when the occipital lobe is affected. Other congenital anomalies include coloboma of the iris and deformity of the lens.

LABORATORY DATA

The highly characteristic calcifications are rarely seen on radiographs before age 2 years (Fig. 100.2). They appear as paired (trolley-track) curvilinear lines that follow the cerebral convolutions. Cerebral atrophy may be implied by asymmetry of the calvarium, with elevated petrous pyramid, thickening of the calvarial diploë, and enlargement of the paranasal sinuses and mastoid air cells on the side of the lesion. Computed tomography (CT) documents the intracranial calcification and unilateral cerebral atrophy (Fig. 100.3). Magnetic resonance imaging (MRI) with gadolinium defines the extent of the leptomeningeal angioma, whereas functional imaging with positron-emission tomography or single-photon emission computed tomography with underperfusion delineates the involved area of the brain. Combining these procedures enhances the effectiveness of precise functional neurosurgery. Cerebral angiography may demonstrate capillary and venous abnormalities. The capillaries over the affected hemisphere are homogeneously increased, the superficial cortical veins are markedly decreased, and the superior sagittal sinus may be diminished or not seen.

Electroencephalography shows a wide area of low potentials over the affected areas, and this electrical silence correlates with

FIG. 100.2. Encephalotrigeminal angiomatosis. **A:** Lateral skull radiograph shows characteristic calcifications consisting of paired curvilinear lines localized mostly to the occipital and parietal lobes. **B:** Posteroanterior view shows calcifications outlining an atrophic right cerebral hemisphere.

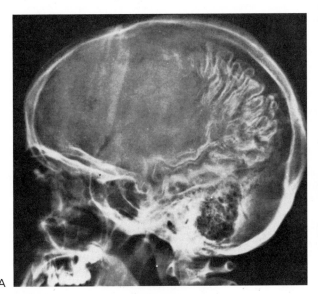

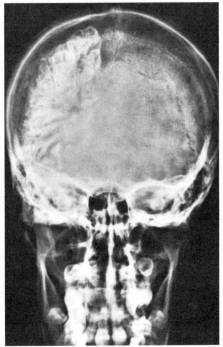

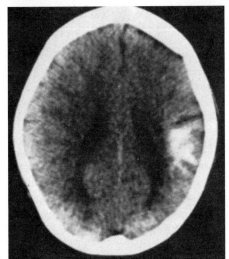

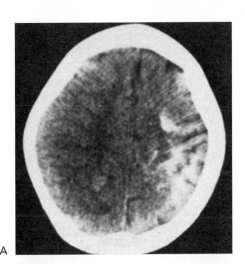

the degree of intracranial calcification. The remainder of the hemisphere may show epileptiform activity. Visual-field studies document the homonymous hemianopia.

DIAGNOSIS

The diagnosis is based on the facial vascular port-wine nevus flammeus and one or more of the following: seizures, contralateral hemiparesis and hemiatrophy, mental retardation, and ocular findings of glaucoma or buphthalmos. The appearance of calcifications on skull radiographs or CT reinforces the diagnosis. Rarely, Sturge-Weber-Dimitri syndrome may occur with the neurologic syndrome and the typical intracranial calcifications but without the facial nevus.

TREATMENT

The facial nevus rarely requires early cosmetic therapy. Later, this blemish can be covered with cosmetics or permanently treated with laser therapy. Seizures may be difficult to control with anticonvulsants; lobectomy or hemispherectomy may be efficacious. Physical and occupational therapy are indicated for the hemiparesis. Educational therapy and placement in a special school are important in the learning-disabled or intellectually impaired patient; vocational training is essential in affected older children and young adults. Behavioral problems are common

FIG. 100.3. Noncontrast CT shows subcortical calcification conforming to the gyral pattern of calcification in the Sturge-Weber-Dimitri syndrome. (Courtesy of Dr. S.K. Hilal and Dr. M. Mawad.)

and may include attention deficit disorder or overt psychopathology that warrants psychotropic drug therapy and psychotherapy. Prophylactic daily low-dose aspirin to prevent venous thrombosis is controversial but can be considered if there are recurrent transient ischemic attacks. Yearly monitoring for glaucoma is recommended for all patients and, if present, should be treated aggressively.

SUGGESTED READINGS

Aicardi J, Arzimanoglou A. Sturge-Weber syndrome. *Int Pediatr* 1991;6:129–134.

Alexander GL. Sturge-Weber syndrome. In: Vinken PJ, Bruyn GW, eds. *The phakomatoses. Handbook of clinical neurology, vol 14.* New York: American Elsevier Publishing, 1972:223–240.

Griffiths PD, Boodram MB, Blaser S, Armstrong D, Gilday DL, Harwood-Nash D. 99m Technetium HMPAO imaging in children with the Stuge-Weber syndrome: a study of nine cases with CT and MRI correlation. *Neuroradiology* 1997;39:219–224.

Poser CM, Taveras JM. Cerebral angiography in encephalotrigeminal angiomatosis. *Radiology* 1957;68:327–336.

Roach ES. Encephalofacial angiomatosis. *Pediatr Clin North Am* 1992;39:606–613.

Romanowski CA, Cavallin LI. Tuberous sclerosis, von Hippel-Lindau disease, Sturge-Weber syndrome. *Hosp Med* 1998;59:226–231.

Sturge WA. A case of partial epilepsy, apparently due to a lesion of one of the vaso-motor centres of the brain. *Trans Clin Soc Lond* 1879;12:162–167.

Sujansky E, Conradi S. Outcome of Sturge-Weber syndrome in 52 adults. *Am J Med Genet* 1995;57:35–45.

Sujansky E, Conradi S. Sturge-Weber syndrome: age of onset of seizures and glaucoma and the prognosis for affected children. *J Child Neurol* 1995;10:49–53.

Tallman B, Tan OT, Morelli JG, et al. Location of port-wine stains and the likelihood of ophthalmic and/or central nervous system complications. *Pediatrics* 1991;87:323–327.

Vogl J, Stemmler J, Bergman C, et al. MRI and MR angiography of Sturge-Weber syndrome. *AJNR* 1993;14:417–425.

Weber FP. Right-sided hemi-hypertrophy resulting from right-sided congenital spastic hemiplegia, with a morbid condition of the left side of the brain, revealed by radiograms. *J Neurol Psychopathol* 1922;3:134–139.

Merritt's Neurology, 10th ed., edited by L.P. Rowland. Lippincott Williams & Wilkins, Philadelphia © 2000.

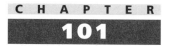

CHAPTER 101

INCONTINENTIA PIGMENTI

ARNOLD P. GOLD

INCONTINENTIA PIGMENTI

Incontinentia pigmenti (MIM 308300), described by Bloch and Sulzberger, is a genetic disorder affecting the skin in a characteristic manner and also involving the brain, eyes, nails, and hair.

Genetics

The disorder is thought to be an X-linked dominant condition that is lethal in males. The evidence includes high female-to-male ratio, female-to-female transmission, increased incidence of miscarriages, and affected males having a 47,XXY karyotype (Klinefelter syndrome). Incontinentia pigmenti has been mapped to Xq28 by linkage analysis, but some families show recombination with probes to this locus, so there must be other loci for the inherited form.

The disease has also appeared in girls with no family history of the disease. In these cases, there is a translocation with a breakpoint at Xp11.21; this is the sporadic form. Some patients and some families do not map to either site, so there must be *locus heterogeneity,* with still more gene loci to be discovered.

A related condition is *incontinentia pigmenti achromians* (hypomelanosis of Ito) (MIM 146150), which also maps to Xp11; this condition and sporadic incontinentia pigmenti may be different disorders (contiguous gene syndromes) or allelic forms of mutation in the same gene. A pregnant woman with incontinentia pigmenti runs a 25% risk of a spontaneous miscarriage (the affected male); 50% of her female children will be affected and will have the disease. Daughters are likely to be more severely affected than their mothers.

Neuropathology

The neuropathologic findings are nonspecific and include cerebral atrophy with microgyria, focal necrosis with formation of small cavities in the central white matter, and focal areas of neuronal loss in the cerebellar cortex.

Symptoms and Signs
Cutaneous Symptoms

One-half of affected infants have the initial linear vesicobullous lesions at birth, and most of the remaining children show the lesions in the first 2 weeks of life. About 10% are delayed, appearing as late as age 1 year. The skin lesions can recur and ultimately may undergo a characteristic change to linear verrucous and dyskeratotic growth, usually between the second and sixth weeks of life; pigmentary changes appear between 12 and 26 weeks. Some infants may show the pigmentary lesions at birth without further cutaneous progression. The pigmentation involves the trunk and extremities, is slate-gray blue or brown, and is distributed in irregular marbled or wavy lines. With age, the pigmentary lesions fade and become depigmented with atrophic skin changes.

Neurologic, Ophthalmic, and Other Symptoms

About 20% of affected children have a neurologic syndrome that may include slow motor development; pyramidal-tract dysfunction with spastic hemiparesis, quadriparesis, or diplegia; mental retardation; and convulsive disorders.

Strabismus, cataracts, and severe visual loss occur in about 20% of affected children. Retinal vascular changes may result in blindness with ectasia, microhemorrhages, avascularity, and, later, retinal pigmentation and atrophy.

Partial or total anodontia and peg-shaped teeth are characteristic of incontinentia pigmenti. Partial or complete diffuse alopecia with scarring and nail dystrophy may also occur.

Laboratory Data

Eosinophilia as high as 65% is often seen in infants younger than 1 year, together with an associated leukocytosis. Eosinophils are also found in the vesicobullous lesions and in affected dermis.

Treatment

There is no specific treatment for incontinentia pigmenti, and management is directed at complicating problems, such as anticonvulsants for seizures. Awareness of the ocular manifestations is essential because laser coagulation in retinal ectasia prevents blindness.

INCONTINENTIA PIGMENTI ACHROMIANS

This neurocutaneous entity was originally described by Ito (*hypomelanosis of Ito*) and is distinctive in both clinical manifestations and pathologic features.

Etiology

The pathogenesis of this disease is similar to that of other neurocutaneous disorders. Migration of neural cells to the brain and melanoblasts to the skin from the neural crest occurs between 3 and 6 months' gestational age. A disturbance of this migration results in both brain and cutaneous pigmentary disease.

Genetics

Incontinentia pigmenti achromians is found in all races and sexes and is inherited as an autosomal-dominant trait with variable penetrance. At least one form maps to Xp11, suggesting that different mutations at that locus give rise to the pigmented or hypomelanotic classes of incontinentia pigmenti.

Clinical Manifestations

In infancy, hypopigmented skin lesions appear as whorls or streaks on any part of the body (Fig. 101.1) and tend to progress onto uninvolved areas. This lesion is the negative image of incontinentia pigmenti. In later childhood, affected areas tend to return to normal skin color. The cutaneous lesion is often associated with developmental and neurologic abnormalities with hypotonia, pyramidal-tract dysfunction, mental retardation (approximately 80%), and seizures. Ophthalmologic disorders, including strabismus, optic atrophy, microophthalmia, tessellated fundus, eyelid ptosis, and heterochromia iridis, are also present. The hair, teeth, and musculoskeletal system may be affected.

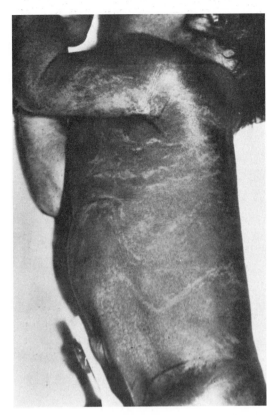

FIG. 101.1. Incontinentia pigmenti achromians. Hypopigmented skin lesions show streaks or whorls.

Pathology

The hypopigmented skin lesions are characterized by a decrease in the number of dopa-positive melanocytes and decreased pigment production in the basal layer of the epidermis.

Diagnosis and Laboratory Data

Because there is no pathognomonic laboratory test, diagnosis must be based solely on the characteristic hypomelanosis.

Treatment

The whorled, marble-cake hypopigmented skin lesions do not require any treatment. Therapy is directed toward the associated complications, such as anticonvulsants for seizures and specialized educational facilities for the learning-disabled or retarded child.

SUGGESTED READINGS

Aydingoz U, Midia M. Central nervous system involvement in incontinentia pigmenti: cranial MRI of two siblings. *Neuroradiology* 1998;40:364–366.

Donat JF, Walsworth DM, Turk LL. Focal cerebral atrophy in incontinentia pigmenti achromians. *Am J Dis Child* 1980;134:709–710.

Hyden-Gramskog C, Salonen R, von Koskull H. Three Finnish incontinentia pigmenti (IP) families with recombinations with the IP loci at Xq28 and Xp11. *Hum Genet* 1993;91:185–189.

Jelinek JE, Bart RS, Schiff GM. Hypomelanosis of Ito (incontinentia pigmenti achromians). *Arch Dermatol* 1973;107:596–601.

Koiffmann CP, deSouza DH, Diament A, et al. Incontinentia pigmenti achromians (hypomelanosis of Ito, MIM 146150): further evidence of localtization at Xp11. *Am J Med Genet* 1993;46:529–533.

Landy SJ, Domani D. Incontinentia pigmenti (Bloch-Sulzberger syndrome). *J Med Genet* 1993;30:53–59.

Larsen R, Ashwal S, Peckham N. Incontinentia pigmenti: association with anterior horn cell degeneration. *Neurology* 1987;37:446–450.

Lee AG, Goldberg MF, Gillard JH, Barker PB, Bryan RN. Intracranial assessment of incontinentia pigmenti using magnetic resonance imaging, angiography, and spectroscopic imaging. *Arch Pediatr Adolesc Med* 1995;149:573–580.

O'Brien JE, Feingold M. Incontinentia pigmenti: a longitudinal study. *Am J Dis Child* 1985;139:711–712.

Pascual-Castroviejo I, Roche C, Martinez-Bermejo A, et al. Hypomelanosis of Ito: a study of 76 infantile cases. *Brain Dev* 1998;20: 36–43.

Scheuerle AF. Male cases of incontinentia pigmenti: a case report and review. *Am J Med Genet* 1998;77:201–218.

Schwartz MF, Esterly NB, Fretzin DF, et al. Hypomelanosis of Ito (incontinentia pigmenti achromians): a neurocutaneous syndrome. *J Pediatr* 1977;90:236–240.

Sulzberger MB. Incontinentia pigmenti (Bloch-Sulzberger): report of an additional case, with comment on possible relation to a new syndrome of familial and congenital anomalies. *Arch Dermatol* 1938;38:57–69.

Wald KJ, Mehta MC, Katsumi O, et al. Retinal detachments in incontinentia pigmenti. *Arch Ophthalmol* 1993;111:614–617.

Merritt's Neurology, 10th ed., edited by L.P. Rowland. Lippincott Williams & Wilkins, Philadelphia © 2000.

C H A P T E R
102

TUBEROUS SCLEROSIS

ARNOLD P. GOLD

Tuberous sclerosis was first described by von Recklinghausen in 1863. In 1880, Bourneville coined the term *sclérose tubéreuse* for the potato-like lesions in the brain. In 1890, Pringle described the facial nevi, or *adenoma sebaceum*. Vogt later emphasized the classic triad of seizures, mental retardation, and adenoma sebaceum. Eponymically, tuberous sclerosis is called *Pringle disease* when there are only dermatologic findings, *Bourneville disease* when the nervous system is affected, and *West syndrome* when skin lesions are associated with infantile spasms, hypsarrhythmia, and mental retardation. Tuberous sclerosis (MIM 191100) is a hereditarily determined progressive disorder characterized by the development in early life of hamartomas, malformations, and congenital tumors of the nervous system, skin, and viscera.

GENETICS AND INCIDENCE

Tuberous sclerosis is inherited as an autosomal-dominant trait, with a high incidence of sporadic cases and protean clinical expressivity. These features are attributed to modifier genes, for which the homozygous condition results in a phenotypically normal individual despite the presence of the gene for tuberous sclerosis; when heterozygous, the modifier gene results in a mildly affected patient. The defective gene has been mapped to chromosome 9q34 (TSC1) in some families and to chromosome 16p13.3 (TSC2) in others. *Hamartin* is the gene product for TSC1, and *tuberin* is the gene product for TSC2. Both are involved in the regulation of cell growth and are considered tumor suppressor genes. As in other hereditary tumor syndromes, a second somatic mutation may be involved in pathogenesis.

Incidence figures must be considered minimal because milder varieties are often unrecognized. Autopsy data gave an incidence

of 1 in 10,000 people; clinical surveys gave a prevalence between 1 in 10,000 and 1 in 170,000. Although all races are affected, the disease is thought to be uncommon in blacks, and there may be a greater frequency in males.

PATHOLOGY AND PATHOGENESIS

The pathologic changes are widespread and include lesions in the nervous system, skin, bones, retina, kidney, lungs, and other viscera.

The brain is usually normal in size, but several or many hard nodules occur on the surface of the cortex. These nodules are smooth, round, or polygonal and project slightly above the surface of the neighboring cortex. They are white, firm to the touch, and of various sizes. Some involve only a small portion of one convolution; others encompass the convolutions of one whole lobe or a major portion of a hemisphere. In addition, there may be developmental anomalies of the cortical convolutions in the form of pachygyria or microgyria. On sectioning of the hemispheres, sclerotic nodules may be found in the subcortical gray matter, the white matter, and the basal ganglia. The lining of the lateral ventricles is frequently the site of numerous small nodules that project into the ventricular cavity (*candle gutterings*) (Fig. 102.1). Sclerotic nodules are less frequently found in the cerebellum. The brainstem and spinal cord are rarely involved.

Histologically, the nodules are characterized by a cluster of atypical glial cells in the center and giant cells in the periphery. Calcifications are relatively frequent. Other features include heterotopia, vascular hyperplasia (sometimes with actual angiomatous malformations), disturbances in the cortical architecture, and, occasionally, development of subependymal giant-cell astrocytomas. Intracranial giant aneurysm and arterial ectasia are uncommon findings.

The skin lesions are multiform and include the characteristic facial nevi (*adenoma sebaceum*) and patches of skin fibrosis. The facial lesions are not adenomas of the sebaceous glands but rather small hamartomas arising from nerve elements of the skin combined with hyperplasia of connective tissue and blood vessels (Fig. 102.2). In late childhood, lesions similar to those on the face are found around or underneath the fingernails and toenails (*ungual fibroma*). Circumscribed areas of hypomelanosis or

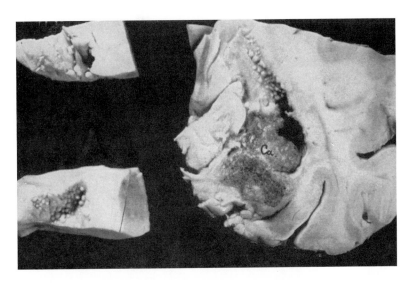

FIG. 102.1. Tuberous sclerosis. Nodules (candle gutterings) on the surface of ventricles. (Courtesy of Dr. Leon Roizin.)

white nevi are common in tuberous sclerosis and are often found in infants. Although these depigmented nevi are less specific than the sebaceous adenoma, they are of importance in raising suspicion for the diagnosis in infants with seizures. Histologically, the skin appears normal except for the loss of melanin, but ultrastructural studies show that melanosomes are small and have reduced content of melanin.

The retinal lesions are small congenital tumors (*phakomas*) composed of glia, ganglion cells, or fibroblasts. Glioma of the optic nerve has been reported.

Other lesions include cardiac rhabdomyoma; renal angiomyolipoma, renal cysts, and, rarely, renal carcinoma; cystic disease of the lungs and pulmonary lymphangioleiomyomatosis; hepatic angiomas and hamartomas; skeletal abnormalities with localized areas of osteosclerosis in the calvarium, spine, pelvis, and limbs;

cystic defects involving the phalanges; and periosteal new bone formation confined to the metacarpals and metatarsals.

SYMPTOMS AND SIGNS

The cardinal features of tuberous sclerosis are skin lesions, convulsive seizures, and mental retardation. The disease is characterized by variability and expressivity of the clinical manifestations.

CUTANEOUS SYMPTOMS

Depigmented or hypomelanotic macules are the earliest skin lesion (Fig. 102.3). They are present at birth, persist through life,

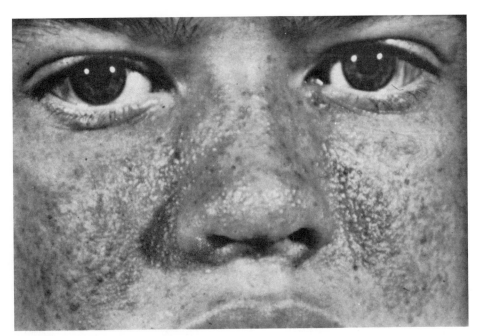

FIG. 102.2. Tuberous sclerosis. Facial adenoma sebaceum over the butterfly area of the face spares the upper lip.

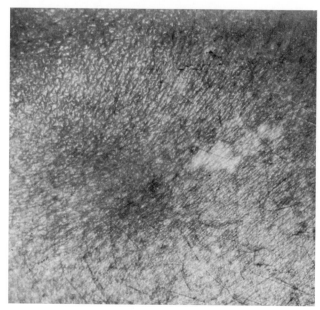

FIG. 102.3. Tuberous sclerosis. Hypomelanotic or ash leaf macules on the skin.

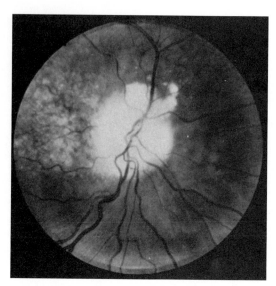

FIG. 102.4. Tuberous sclerosis. Central calcified hamartoma, or so-called "mulberry phakoma," at the optic nerve.

and may only be found with a Wood's-lamp examination. The diagnosis is suggested if there are three or more macules measuring 1 cm or more in length. Numerous small macules sometimes resemble confetti or depigmented freckles. Most macules are leaf-shaped, resembling the leaf of the European mountain ash tree and sometimes following a dermatomal distribution. Facial adenoma sebaceum (*facial angiofibroma*) is never present at birth but is clinically evident in more than 90% of affected children by age 4 years. At first, the facial lesion is the size of a pinhead and red because of the angiomatous component. It is distributed symmetrically on the nose and cheeks in a butterfly distribution. The lesions may involve the forehead and chin but rarely involve the upper lip. They gradually increase in size and become yellowish and glistening. *Shagreen patches,* a connective tissue hamartoma, are also characteristic. Rarely present in infancy, the patches become evident after age 10. Usually found in the lumbosacral region, shagreen plaques are yellowish-brown elevated plaques that have the texture of pig skin. Other skin lesions include *café-au-lait spots,* small fibromas that may be tiny and resemble coarse goose flesh, and ungual fibromas that appear after puberty.

Neurologic Symptoms

Seizures and mental retardation indicate a diffuse encephalopathy. Infantile myoclonic spasms with or without hypsarrhythmia are the characteristic seizures of young infants and, when associated with hypopigmented macules, are diagnostic of tuberous sclerosis. The older child or adult has generalized tonic-clonic or partial complex seizures. There is a close relationship between the onset of seizures at a young age and mental retardation. Mental retardation rarely occurs without clinical seizures, but intellect may be normal, despite seizures. Other than a delayed acquisition of developmental milestones, intellectual impairment, or nonspecific language or coordinative deficiencies, a formal neurologic examination is typically nonfocal.

Ophthalmic Symptoms

Hamartomas of the retina or optic nerve are observed in about 50% of patients. Two types of retinal lesions are seen on funduscopic examination: (1) the easily recognized calcified hamartoma near or at the disc with an elevated multinodular lesion that resembles mulberries, grains of tapioca, or salmon eggs (Fig. 102.4); and (2) the less distinct, relatively flat, smooth-surfaced, white or salmon-colored, circular or oval lesion located peripherally in the retina (Fig. 102.5). Nonretinal lesions may range from the specific depigmented lesion of the iris (Fig. 102.6) to nonspecific, nonparalytic strabismus, optic atrophy, visual-field defects, or cataracts.

Visceral Symptoms

Renal lesions include hamartomas (*angiomyolipomas*) and renal cysts. Typically, both are multiple, bilateral, and usually innocu-

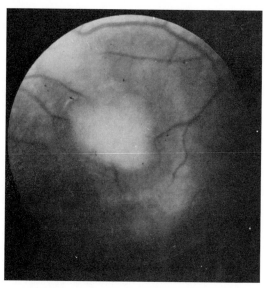

FIG. 102.5. Tuberous sclerosis. Phakoma or retinal hamartoma involves the peripheral retina.

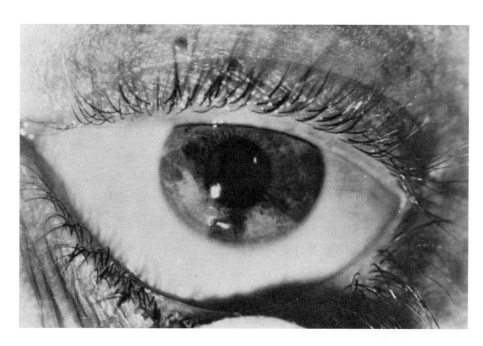

FIG. 102.6. Tuberous sclerosis. Depigmented or hypomelanotic lesions of the iris.

ous and silent. Renal cell carcinoma is a rare complication in the older child or adult. In one series, there was a 50% incidence of tuberous sclerosis in patients with cardiac rhabdomyoma. This cardiac tumor may be symptomatic at any age, even infancy, and can result in death.

Pulmonary hamartomatous lesions consisting of multifocal alveolar hyperplasia associated with cystic lymphangioleiomyomatosis occur in fewer than 1% of patients. These become symptomatic (often with a spontaneous pneumothorax) in the third or fourth decade and are progressive and often fatal. Sclerotic lesions of the calvaria and cystic lesions of the metacarpals and phalanges are asymptomatic. Hamartomatous hemangiomas of the spleen and racemose angiomas of the liver are rare and usually asymptomatic. Enamel pitting of the deciduous teeth may aid in diagnosis.

LABORATORY DATA

Unless renal lesions are present, routine laboratory studies are normal. Renal angiomyolipomas are usually asymptomatic and rarely cause gross hematuria, but they may show albuminuria and microscopic hematuria. Sonography (Fig. 102.7), angiography, and computed tomography (CT) are often diagnostic. Multiple or diffuse renal cysts may be associated with albuminuria or azotemia and hypertension. Intravenous pyelography is diagnostic.

Chest radiographs may reveal pulmonary lesions or rhabdomyoma with cardiomegaly. Electrocardiogram findings are variable, but the echocardiogram is diagnostic.

Skull radiographs usually reveal small calcifications within the substance of the cerebrum (Fig. 102.8). Cerebrospinal fluid is normal, except when a large intracerebral tumor is present. The electroencephalogram is often abnormal, especially in patients with clinical seizures. Abnormalities include slow-wave activity and epileptiform discharges such as hypsarrhythmia, focal or multifocal spike or sharp-wave discharges, and generalized spike-and-wave discharges. CT is diagnostic when calcified subependymal nodules encroach on the lateral ventricle (often in

the region of the foramen of Monro); there may also be calcified cortical or cerebellar nodules (Fig. 102.9). A few nodules appear isodense on CT and are better visualized on magnetic resonance imaging (MRI). Fluid-attenuated inversion recovery (FLAIR) MRI images allow more accurate delineation of cortical and subcortical tubers. Calcified paraventricular and cortical lesions have been visualized shortly after birth. The number of cortical tubers often correlates with the severity of cortical dysfunction. There is enough variation in clinical outcome that prognosis cannot be based on cortical tuber count alone.

DIAGNOSIS

Clinical diagnosis is possible at most ages. In infancy, three or more characteristic depigmented cutaneous lesions suggest the diagnosis, and this is reinforced in the presence of infantile myoclonic spasms. In the older child or adult, the diagnosis is made by the triad of tuberous sclerosis: facial adenoma sebaceum, epilepsy, and mental retardation. Retinal or visceral lesions may be diagnostic. The disease, however, is noted for protean manifestations, and a family history may be invaluable in establishing the diagnosis, which is often reinforced by CT or MRI evidence of calcified subependymal nodules.

The differential diagnosis includes other diseases that involve skin, nervous system, and retina. Neurofibromatous and encephalotrigeminal angiomatosis are differentiated by the characteristic skin lesions of those disorders.

Multisystem involvement may result in difficulties in establishing a diagnosis of tuberous sclerosis. The National Tuberous Sclerosis Association has developed a classification of diagnostic criteria (Table 102.1). Prenatal diagnosis is not currently available.

COURSE AND PROGNOSIS

Mild or solely cutaneous involvement often follows a static course, whereas patients with the full-blown syndrome have a

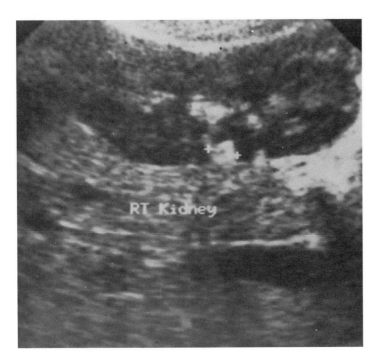

FIG. 102.7. Tuberous sclerosis. Renal sonogram demonstrates a renal angiomyolipoma.

progressive course with increasing seizures and dementia. The child with infantile myoclonic spasms is at great risk of later intellectual deficit. Brain tumor, status epilepticus, renal insufficiency, cardiac failure, or progressive pulmonary impairment can lead to death.

TREATMENT

There is no specific treatment. The cutaneous lesions do not compromise function, but cosmetic surgery may be indicated for facial adenoma sebaceum or large shagreen patches. Infantile myoclonic spasms previously responded to corticosteroid or corticotropin therapy, and currently vigabatrin is the drug of choice; focal and generalized seizures are treated with anticonvulsants. Progressive cystic renal disease often responds to surgical decompression, but with renal failure, dialysis or renal transplantation may be necessary. Intramural cardiac rhabdomyoma and complicating congestive heart failure are managed medically with cardiotonics, diuretics, and salt restriction. Whole obstructive intracavity tumors and congestive heart failure require surgical extirpation of the tumor. Progressive pulmonary involvement is an indication for respiratory therapy, but response is poor and most patients die a few years after the onset of this complication.

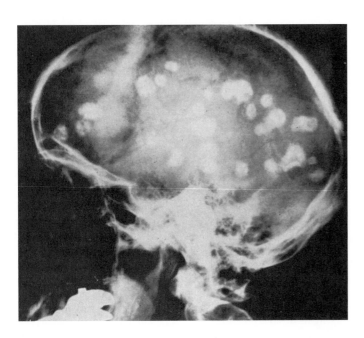

FIG. 102.8. Tuberous sclerosis. Calcified nodules in the cerebrum. (Courtesy of Dr. P.I. Yakovlev.)

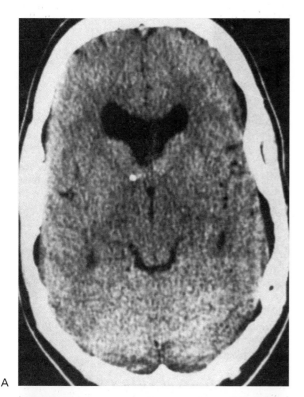

A

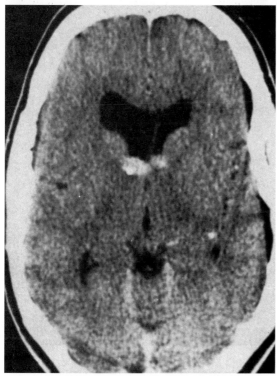

B

FIG. 102.9. Tuberous sclerosis. **A:** Noncontrast axial CT demonstrates a calcific density adjacent to the right foramen of Monro, a typical location for tubers. **B:** Postcontrast, this lesion enhances, as do additional noncalcified lesions on the contralateral side. (Courtesy of Dr. J.A. Bello and Dr. S.K. Hilal.)

TABLE 102.1. DIAGNOSTIC CRITERIA FOR TUBEROUS SCLEROSIS COMPLEX (TSC)

Primary features
  Facial angiofibromas[a]
  Multiple ungual fibromas[a]
  Cortical tuber (histologically confirmed)
  Subependymal nodule or giant cell astrocytoma (histologically confirmed)
  Multiple calcified subependymal nodules protruding into the ventricle (radiographic evidence)
  Multiple retinal astrocytomas[a]

Secondary features
  Affected first-degree relative
  Cardiac rhabdomyoma (histologic or radiographic confirmation)
  Other retinal hamartoma or achromic patch[a]
  Cerebral tubers (radiographic confirmation)
  Noncalcified subependymal nodules (radiographic confirmation)
  Shagreen patch[a]
  Forehead plaque[a]
  Pulmonary lymphangiomyomatosis (histologic confirmation)
  Renal angiomyolipoma (radiographic or histologic confirmation)
  Renal cysts (histologic confirmation)

Tertiary features
  Hypomelanotic macules[a]
  "Confetti" skin lesions[a]
  Renal cysts (radiographic evidence)
  Randomly distributed enamel pits in deciduous or permanent teeth
  Hamartomatous rectal polyps (histologic confirmation)
  Bone cysts (radiographic evidence)
  Pulmonary lymphangiomyomatosis (radiographic evidence)
  Cerebral white matter "migration tracts" or heterotopias (radiographic evidence)
  Gingival fibromas
  Hamartoma of other organs (histologic confirmation)
  Infantile spasms

Definite TSC	One primary feature, two secondary features; or one secondary plus two tertiary features
Probable TSC	Either one secondary plus one tertiary feature or three tertiary features
Suspect TSC	Either one secondary feature or two tertiary features

[a]Histologic confirmation is not required *if* the lesion is clinically obvious.
Developed by the National Tuberous Scelorosis Association Professional Advisory Board (Roach ES, Smith M, Huttenlocher P, Alcorn DN).

SUGGESTED READINGS

Bourneville DM. Sclerose tubereuse des circonvolutions cerebrales: idotie et epilepsie hemiplegique. *Arch Neurol* 1880;1:81–91.
Castro M, Shepherd CW, Gomez MR, Lie JT, Ryu JM. Pulmonary tuberous sclerosis. *Chest* 1995;107:189–195.
Gold AP, Freeman JM. Depigmented nevi: the earliest sign of tuberous sclerosis. *Pediatrics* 1965;35:1003–1005.
Goodman M, Lamm SH, Engle A, Shepherd CW, Houser OW, Gomez MR. Cortical tuber count: a biomarker indicating neurologic severity of tuberous sclerosis complex. *J Child Neurol* 1997;12:85–90.
Inoue Y, Nemoto Y, Murata R, et al. CT and MR imaging of cerebral tuberous sclerosis. *Brain Dev* 1998;20:209–221.
Johnson WG, Gomez MR, eds. Tuberous sclerosis and allied disorders: clinical, cellular and molecular studies. *Ann N Y Acad Sci* 1991;615:1–385.
Kandt RS, Gebarski SS, Geotting MG. Tuberous sclerosis with cardiogenic cerebral embolism: magnetic resonance imaging. *Neurology* 1985;35:1223–1225.
Korf BR. Neurocutaneous syndromes: neurofibromatosis 1, neurofibromatosis 2, and tuberous sclerosis. *Curr Opin Neurol* 1997;10:131–136.

Kwiatkowska J, Wigowska-Sowinska J, Napierala, D et al. Mosaicism in tuberous sclerosis as a potential cause of the failure of molecular diagnosis. *N Engl J Med* 1999;340:703–707.

Lucchese NJ, Goldberg MF. Iris and fundus pigmentary changes in tuberous sclerosis. *J Pediatr Ophthalmol Strabismus* 1981;18:45–46.

Nixon JR, Houser OW, Gomez MR, Okazaki H. Cerebral tuberous sclerosis: MR imaging. *Radiology* 1989;170:869–873.

Roach ES. Tuberous sclerosis. *Pediatr Clin North Am* 1992;39:591–620.

Roach ES, Smith M, Huttenlocher P, et al. Diagnostic criteria: tuberous sclerosis complex. Report of the diagnostic criteria committee of the National Tuberous Sclerosis Association. *J Child Neurol* 1992;7:221–224.

Romanowski CA, Cavallin LI. Tuberous sclerosis, von Hippel-Lindau disease, Sturge-Weber syndrome. *Hosp Med* 1998;59:226–231.

Smirniotopoulos JG, Murphy FM. The phakomatoses: tuberous sclerosis. *AJNR* 1992;13:732–737.

Weiner DM, Ewalt DH, Roach ES, et al. The tuberous sclerosis complex: a comprehensive review. *J Am Coll Surg* 1998;187:548–561.

Wielderhold WC, Gomez MR, Kurland LT. Incidence and prevalence of tuberous sclerosis in Rochester, Minnesota, 1950 through 1982. *Neurology* 1985;35:600–603.

Young J, Povey S. The genetic basis of tuberous sclerosis. *Mol Med Today* 1998;4:313–319.

Merritt's Neurology, 10th ed., edited by L.P. Rowland. Lippincott Williams & Wilkins, Philadelphia © 2000.

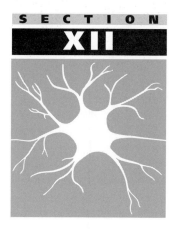

PERIPHERAL NEUROPATHIES

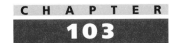

GENERAL CONSIDERATIONS

NORMAN LATOV

The peripheral nervous system is composed of multiple cell types and elements that subserve diverse motor, sensory, and autonomic functions. The clinical manifestations of neuropathies depend on the severity, distribution, and functions affected. *Peripheral neuropathy* and *polyneuropathy* are terms that describe syndromes resulting from diffuse lesions of peripheral nerves, usually manifested by weakness, sensory loss, and autonomic dysfunction. *Mononeuropathy* indicates a disorder of a single nerve and is often due to a local cause such as trauma or entrapment. *Mononeuropathy multiplex* signifies focal involvement of two or more nerves, usually as a result of a generalized disorder such as diabetes mellitus or vasculitis. *Neuritis* is typically reserved for inflammatory disorders of nerves resulting from infection or autoimmunity.

SYMPTOMS AND SIGNS

Polyneuropathy may occur at any age, although particular syndromes are more likely to occur in certain age groups. Charcot-Marie-Tooth (CMT) disease, for example, begins in childhood or adolescence, whereas neuropathy associated with paraproteinemia is seen in adults. The onset and progression differ; the Guillain-Barré syndrome (GBS), tick paralysis, and porphyria begin acutely and may remit. Others, such as vitamin B_{12} deficiency or carcinomatous neuropathy, begin insidiously and progress slowly. Still others, such as chronic inflammatory demyelinating polyneuropathy, may begin acutely or insidiously and then progress with remissions and exacerbations.

The myelin sheaths or the motor or sensory axons themselves may be predominantly affected, or the neuropathy may be mixed, axonal, or demyelinating. Most polyneuropathies, especially those with primary demyelination, affect both motor and sensory functions. A predominantly motor polyneuropathy is seen in lead toxicity, dapsone or hexane intoxication, tick paralysis, porphyria, in some cases of GBS, and in association with multifocal conduction block or anti-GM_1 antibodies. Sensory neuropathy, sometimes with concomitant autonomic dysfunction, is seen in thallium poisoning, acute idiopathic sensory neuronopathy or ganglioneuritis, pyridoxine (vitamin B_6) deficiency, inherited sensory neuropathies, primary biliary cirrhosis, and, occasionally, with diabetes mellitus, amyloidosis, carcinoma, or lepromatous leprosy. Predominant involvement of the autonomic system can be seen in acute or chronic autonomic neuropathy or in amyloidosis.

Symptoms of polyneuropathy include acral (distal) pain, paresthesia, weakness, and sensory loss. Pain may be spontaneous (parathesias) or elicited by stimulation of the skin (dysthesias) and may be sharp or burning. Paresthesia is usually described as numbness (a dead sensation), tingling, buzzing, stinging, burning, or a feeling of constriction. Lack of pain perception may result in repeated traumatic injuries with degeneration of joints (*arthropathy* or *Charcot joints*) and in chronic ulcerations.

Weakness is greatest in distal limb muscles in most neuropathies; there may be paralysis of the intrinsic foot and hand muscles with footdrop or wristdrop. Tendon reflexes are often lost, especially in demyelinating neuropathy. In severe polyneuropathy, the patient may become quadriplegic and respirator-dependent. The cranial nerves may be affected, particularly in GBS and diphtheritic neuropathy. Cutaneous sensory loss appears in a stocking-and-glove distribution. All modes of sensation may be affected, or there may be selective impairment of "large" myelinated fiber functions (position and vibratory sense) or "small" unmyelinated fiber functions (pain and temperature perception). Often, there is a rise in the threshold of perception of painful stimuli, but with a delayed and greater than normal reaction.

Involvement of autonomic nerves may cause miosis (small pupil), anhidrosis (impaired sweating), orthostatic hypotension, sphincter symptoms, impotence, and vasomotor abnormalities; these may occur without other evidence of neuropathy, but autonomic neuropathy is more commonly seen in association with symmetric distal polyneuropathy. The most common cause of predominantly autonomic neuropathy in the United States is diabetes mellitus. Amyloidosis is another cause. Tachycardia, rapid alterations in blood pressure, flushing and sweating, and abnormalities in gastrointestinal motility are sometimes prominent in thallium poisoning, porphyria, or GBS.

In *mononeuropathy* or *mononeuropathy multiplex,* focal motor, sensory, and reflex changes are restricted to areas innervated by specific nerves. When multiple distal subcutaneous nerves are affected in mononeuropathy multiplex, the stocking-and-glove pattern of symmetric distal sensory loss may suggest polyneuropathy. The most frequent causes of mononeuropathy multiplex are diabetes mellitus, periarteritis nodosa, human immunodeficiency virus type 1 infection, rheumatoid arthritis, brachial neuropathy, leprosy, nerve trauma, or sarcoid. Asymmetric motor neuropathy is also seen in multifocal neuropathy with motor conduction block, sometimes with increased titers of anti-GM_1 antibodies.

Superficial cutaneous nerves may be thickened and visibly enlarged secondary to Schwann cell proliferation and deposition of collagen as a result of repeated episodes of segmental demyelination and remyelination or to deposition of amyloid or polysaccharides in the nerves. Hypertrophic nerves may be observed in the demyelinating form of CMT disease (type I), Dejerine-Sottas neuropathy, Refsum disease, von Recklinghausen disease (neurofibromatosis), leprous neuritis, amyloidosis, chronic demyelinative polyneuritis, sarcoid, and acromegaly.

Fasciculations, or spontaneous contractions of individual motor units, are visible twitches of limb muscles under the skin and may be seen in the tongue. They are characteristic of anterior horn cell diseases but are also seen in motor neuropathy with multifocal motor conduction block and, occasionally, in chronic motor neuropathies involving axons.

TABLE 103.1. CLASSIFICATION AND EVALUATION OF POLYNEUROPATHIES

Disorder	Predominant presentation	Laboratory tests
Diabetes	Sensory, sensorimotor, motor, focal, and multifocal	Blood glucose
Nutritional and alcoholic		
Alcoholic	Sensorimotor	—
Vitamin B_1 deficiency	Sensorimotor and autonomic	Serum B_1
Vitamin B_{12} deficiency	Sensory or sensorimotor	CBC, serum B_{12}
Vitamin B_6 deficiency or excess	Sensory	Serum B_6
Vitamin E	Sensory	Serum E
Immune-mediated		
GBS and variants	Acute motor, sensorimotor, ophthalmoparesis (Miller-Fisher)	CSF, IgG anti-GM_1 antibodies (acute motor axonal neuropathy), IgG anti-GQ1b antibodies (Miller-Fisher)
CIDP	Chronic motor or sensorimotor, demyelinating	EMG, CSF
MNCB	Multifocal motor	EMG, anti-GM_1 antibodies
Sensory neuropathy or neuronopathy (ganglioneuritis)	Acute or chronic sensory	Antisulfatide, anti-SS-A-La, SS-B-Roab, and anti-Hu antibodies
Autonomic neuropathy	Acute or chronic autonomic	—
Vasculitic	Multifocal	ESR, EMG, nerve biopsy
Nonsystemic	Multifocal	ESR, EMG, nerve biopsy
Polyarteritis	Multifocal	HB, HC serology, HIV-1 serology, cryoglobulin
Sjögren	Multifocal, sensory	Anti-SS-A-La, SS-B-Ro antibodies
Wegener granulomatosis	Multifocal	ANCA
Rheumatoid arthritis	Multifocal	Rheumatoid factor
Cryoglobulinemia	Multifocal	Cryoglobulins
Paraproteinemia (IgG or IgA)		
Nonmaligant	Sensorimotor	Serum and urine IFE, quantitative Ig, bone marrow, skeletal survey, bone scan, cryoglobulin, nerve biopsy
Myeloma	Sensorimotor	
POEMS syndrome	Sensorimotor	
Amyloidosis	Sensorimotor, sensory, autonomic	
Cryoglobulinemia	Sensorimotor, vasculitic	
IgM autoantibodies (monoclonal or polyclonal)		IFE, IgM, bone marrow
Anti-MAG antibodies	Sensorimotor	Anti-MAG antibody, nerve biopsy
Anti-GM1 or GD1a antibodies	Motor	Anti-GM_1 and anti-GD1a antibodies
Antisulfatide or anti-GD1b and disialosyl ganglioside antibodies	Sensory or sensorimotor	Anti-sulfatide, anti-GD1b, and disialosyl ganglioside antibodies
Paraneoplastic		
Lung cancer	Sensory	Chest x-ray, anti-Hu antibodies
Lymphoma	Motor, sensorimotor	
Amyloidosis		Nerve biopsy
Primary	Sensory, autonomic, or sensorimotor	Serum and urine IFE
Familial		Transthyretin mutation
Infectious		
Herpes zoster	Sensory radiculopathy	Serum and CSF antibody titers, culture, nerve biopsy, PCR analysis for viral data
CMV	Acute sensorimotor	
HIV-1	Sensory or multifocal	
Diphtheria	Motor or sensorimotor	
Lyme disease	Sensorimotor or multifocal	
Leprosy	Sensory	
Trypanosomiasis	Sensorimotor, multifocal	
Granulomatous		
Sarcoid	Multifocal, sensorimotor	Biopsy, ACE
Metabolic and endocrine		
Renal failure	Sensory or sensorimotor	BUN, creatinine
Hepatic failure	Sensorimotor	Liver enzymes
Hypothyroidism	Sensory or sensorimotor	Thyroid functions
Acromegaly	Sensory or sensorimotor	Growth hormone

(continued)

TABLE 103.1. *(continued)*

Disorder	Predominant presentation	Laboratory tests
Toxic (selected)		
Metals		
Lead	Motor	Urine and tissue
Arsenic	Sensory	Metals
Mercury	Sensory or sensorimotor	Metals
Industrial agents	Sensory or sensorimotor	—
Drug-induced (selected)		
Chloroquine, dapsone, disulfiram, metronidizole, nitrofurantoin, vitamin B_6, vinca alkaloids		
Inherited (selected)	Sensory or sensorimotor	
CMT-1A	Sensorimotor	PMP22 duplication
CMT-1B	Sensorimotor	Po mutation
CMT-X	Sensorimotor	Connexin-32
HNPP	Multifocal	PMP22 deletion
FAP	Sensory, sensorimotor, autonomic	TTR mutation
Porphyria	Acute motor	Urine porphyrins

ACE, angiotensin-converting enzyme; ANCA, antineutrophil cytoplasmic antibody; CIDP, chronic inflammatory demyelinating neuropahty; CMT, Chareot-Marie-Tooth disease; CMV, cytomegalovirus; CSF, cerebrospinal fluid; EMG, electromyography and nerve conduction studies; FAP, familial amyloidotic polyneuropathy; GBS, Guillain-Barré syndrome; HB and CH, hepatitis B and C; HIV-1, human immunodeficiency virus 1; HNPP, hereditary neuropathy with predisposition to pressure palsy; IFE, immunofixation electrophoresis; Ig, immunoglobulins; MNMCB, motor neuropathy with multifocal conduction block; PPM22, peripheral myelin protein 22; Po, myelin Po glycoprotein; TTR, transthyretin.

ETIOLOGY AND DIAGNOSIS

Peripheral nerve disorders may be divided into hereditary and acquired forms. The most common hereditary disorder is CMT syndrome type 1A (peroneal muscular atrophy), associated with duplication of the peripheral myelin protein 22 (PMP22) gene region on chromosome 17. A deletion in the same region is seen in hereditary neuropathy with a liability to pressure palsies. The most common acquired neuropathies in the United States are associated with diabetes mellitus and alcoholism; other causes of polyneuropathy are listed in Table 103.1. Trauma and entrapment are considered in the differential diagnosis of mononeuropathies, particularly if the median nerve is affected at the wrist, the ulnar nerve at the elbow, or the peroneal nerve at the knee. Patients with any form of polyneuropathy seem to be more vulnerable to mechanical injury of nerves; in cachectic or immobile patients, neuropathy may result from pressure or trauma rather than from underlying disease.

In the evaluation of a patient with peripheral neuropathy, a detailed family, social, and medical history; neurologic examination; and electrodiagnostic, laboratory, and nerve biopsy studies are usually necessary for diagnosis. A classification of the most common acquired and hereditary polyneuropathies and their laboratory evaluation are presented in Table 103.1.

TREATMENT

Treatment of patients with peripheral nerve disorders can be divided into two phases: removal or treatment of the condition responsible for the disorder and symptomatic therapy. Specific treatments will be considered in discussions of the individual disorders.

Symptomatic treatment of polyneuropathy consists of general supportive measures, amelioration of pain, and physiotherapy. Tracheal intubation and respiratory support may be needed in GBS. The corneas are protected if there is weakness of eye closure. The bed is kept clean and the sheets are kept smooth to prevent injury to the anesthetic skin; a special mattress can be used to prevent pressure sores. Chronic compression of vulnerable nerves (ulnar at the elbow and common peroneal at the knee) is avoided. Paralyzed limbs are splinted to prevent contractures. Physical therapy includes massage of all weak muscles and passive movement of all joints. When voluntary movement begins to return, muscle training exercises are done daily. Patients should not attempt to walk before muscle testing indicates that they are ready. In chronic polyneuropathy with footdrop, an orthosis for the foot often helps the patient's gait. Patients with postural hypotension are instructed to rise gradually. Treatment includes the use of body stockings to minimize blood pooling in the legs and, if necessary, dietary salt supplementation or mineralocorticoid therapy to expand blood volume.

COURSE

The polyneuropathy may be progressive or remitting, and the prognosis is affected by the extent of destruction of nerves before treatment begins. With removal or treatment of the cause of the neuropathy, recovery is more rapid if macroscopic continuity of the nerves has not been interrupted. Conversely, recovery may be delayed for months if axons are destroyed. Axonal regeneration proceeds at a rate of 1 to 2 mm per day and may be delayed where the axons have to penetrate focally damaged segments of nerve. Aberrant growth of axonal sprouts may lead to formation of persistent neuromas. After severe wallerian degeneration, there may be permanent weakness, muscular wasting, diminution of reflexes, and sensory loss. In demyelinating neuropathies, recovery may sometimes be more rapid and complete.

SUGGESTED READINGS

Asbury AK, Thomas PK. *Peripheral nerve disorders 2.* London: Butterworths, 1995.

Dyck PJ, Thomas PK, Griffin JW, et al, eds. *Peripheral neuropathy,* 3rd ed. Philadelphia: WB Saunders, 1993.
Latov N, Wokke JHJ, Kelly JJ Jr, eds, *Immunological and infectious diseases of the peripheral nerves.* New York: Cambridge University Press, 1998.
Schaumberg HH, Berger AR, Thomas PK. *Disorders of peripheral nerves,* 2nd ed. Philadelphia: FA Davis Co, 1991.
Stewart JD. *Focal peripheral neuropathies,* 2nd ed. New York: Raven Press, 1993.

Merritt's Neurology, 10th ed., edited by L.P. Rowland. Lippincott Williams & Wilkins, Philadelphia © 2000.

C H A P T E R
104

HEREDITARY NEUROPATHIES

ROBERT E. LOVELACE
LEWIS P. ROWLAND

Hereditary diseases of peripheral nerves have been classified by different criteria through the years. At first, the distinctions were clinical, then by different combinations of histopathology, associated diseases, and patterns of inheritance (Table 104.1). In the 1960s, nerve conduction velocity became a major determinant (Table 104.2). Now, molecular genetics is a force, especially because the affected gene products are being identified (Table 104.3).

The most common of these hereditary peripheral nerve diseases are the ones originally called *Charcot-Marie-Tooth (CMT) disease* or *peroneal muscular atrophy.* Dyck introduced the term *hereditary motor and sensory neuropathy* as the formal designation, but the McKusick catalog still lists the diseases as CMT, which accounts for about 90% of all hereditary neuropathies. The prevalence of CMT in the United States is about 40 per 100,000 population, or about 125,000 affected people. This is more common than myasthenia gravis and twice the rate of Duchenne dystrophy.

A second important group of these diseases is formed by purely *sensory neuropathies,* some with autonomic disorders. A third group comprises the *familial amyloid polyneuropathies.* There are still others and new syndromes are still emerging. The focus of this chapter is on the major categories.

CHARCOT-MARIE-TOOTH DISEASES

Classification and Molecular Genetics

The most common form is type 1 (CMT-1), a demyelinating neuropathy with slow conduction velocity, histologic evidence of demyelination with remyelination in the form of "onion bulb" formations, and autosomal-dominant inheritance. CMT-1 was first linked to the Duffy blood group on chromosome 1, and the encoded gene product was identified as peripheral nerve protein (Po). This proved to be an uncommon form, however, because most families with type 1 features are linked to chromosome 17p12-p11.2, and the affected gene product is peripheral myelin protein 22 (PMP22). This became CMT type 1A; the disorder linked to chromosome 1 is type 1B (see Tables 104.2 and 104.3). Ionasescu and associates found that CMT-1A accounted for about 60% of hereditary neuropathies and CMT-1B was found in fewer than 2% (Table 104.4).

CMT-2 is clinically similar, including sensory loss. However, nerve conduction velocity is normal, and there is no histologic evidence of demyelination; therefore the disorder is considered neuronal. Some families show an autosomal-dominant pattern, others an autosomal-recessive. This category is therefore heterogeneous. Four types of the autosomal-dominant type have been mapped: 2A to chromosome 1, 2B at chromosome 3q, 2C (unmapped but includes vocal cord paralysis), and 2D to chromosome 7. Recessive infantile forms have also been described.

CMT type 3, the most severe form, is called the Dejerine-Sottas syndrome (DSS). Onset is usually in early childhood, and there is extreme disability from a hypertrophic demyelinating disorder, with extremely slow conduction velocity in the vicinity of 10 meters per second (mps). It was long thought to be autosomal recessive. In fact, deoxyribonucleic acid (DNA) analysis has shown that some patients are homozygous for the mutation,

TABLE 104.1. HEREDITARY PERIPHERAL NEUROPATHIES

Charcot-Marie-Tooth neuropathies
Hereditary sensory and autonomic neuropathies
Neuropathy with leukodystrophy
   Metachromatic leukodystrophies (infantile, juvenile, adult)
   Multiple sulfatase deficiency
   Krabbe disease
   Adrenoleukodystrophy, adrenoleukoneuropathy
   Cockayne syndrome
   Pelizaeus-Merzbacher disease
Friedreich ataxia
Acute intermittent porphyria
Familial amyloidotic polyneuropathy
Abetalipoproteinemia (Bassen-Kornzweig disease)
Analphalipoproteinemia (Tangier disease)
Fabry disease
Joseph disease
Lafora body disease; polyglucosan body disease
Leber hereditary optic neuropathy
Hereditary ataxias

TABLE 104.2. CHARCOT-MARIE-TOOTH DISEASES (CMT): HEREDITARY MOTOR AND SENSORY NEUROPATHIES (HMSN)

WFN No	McKusick no	Dyck no	Abbreviations	Name	Map position
III.A.1	118220	1	CMT-1A, HMSN-1 CMT-1B CMT-1C	AD, slow conduction	1q21.1-q23.3 17p12-p11.2 10q21
I.A.1.18	118210	2	CMT-2A, HMSN-2	AD normal conduction	1p36
	271120		CMT-2B	AD normal conduction	3q13-22
			CMT-2C	AD (infantile, vocal cords)	—
			CMT-2D	AD	7
	145900	3	CMT-3, HMSN-3	Hypertrophic, infantile (Dejerine-Sottas)	1q, 17p, Xq13 10q21
I.A.1.5	214400		CMT-4A	AR (McKusick: Tunisian, demyelinating severe proximal)	8q13-21-1
I.A.1.30	5 182700 275900		CMT-5, HMSN-5	Spastic paraplegia with amyotrophy AD (Silver syndrome) AR (Royer syndrome)	
		6	CMT-6, HMSN-6	CMT with optic atrophy	
		7	CMT-7, HMSN-7	CMT with retinitis pigmentosa	
	302801 302800		CMT-X	X-linked recessive CMT	Xp22.2 Xq26
	310490		CMT-X	X-linked dominant	Xq13
			CMT spinal	1. AR distal spinal muscular atrophy	12q-24
				2. AR Jarusch type (Jordanian)	9p21-12
			Others	Spinal muscular atrophy denoted by associated features of deafness Skin changes, ptosis, or tremor	

AD, autosomal dominant; AR, autosomal recessive.
Modified from Walton JN, Rowland LP, McLeod JG. In: Walton JN, ed. *Disorders of voluntary muscle,* 5th ed. London: Churchill Livingstone, 1994:333–360.

while the parents are consanguineous, heterozygous, and not affected clinically or subclinically because conduction velocity is normal in them. This pattern is consistent with recessive inheritance. Most patients, however, are heterozygous for the mutation, and the disorder must be autosomal-dominant. Remarkably, the affected gene may be myelin protein zero (MPZ), PMP22, or EGR2 (early growth response protein). It has become difficult to separate DSS from severe CMT-1A. Two forms have been mapped. There is at least one other version, and there

are perhaps more because some cases are not linked to any of the known genes. One child with abnormal Po had been previously identified as having *congenital hypomyelination.*

The McKusick catalog lists a severe autosomal-recessive form as CMT-4, which maps to chromosome 8q (see Table 104.2). CMT-5 comprises rare families with combinations of spastic paraplegia and amyotrophy, some autosomal dominant, others autosomal recessive. X-linked CMT syndromes, including some large families with X-dominant inheritance but only female

TABLE 104.3. GENETIC MAPPING OF CHARCOT-MARIE-TOOTH (CMT) AND RELATED NEUROPATHIES

Disease	Locus	Mutation	Gene/protein
CMT-1A	17p11.2p12	1.5 Mb tandem duplication	Duplication includes PMP22
CMT-1A	17p11.2p12	Missense point mutation	PMP22
HNPP	17p11.2p12	1.5 Mb deletion	Deleted region includes PMP22
DSS	17p11.2p12	Missense point mutation	PMP22
DSS	1q21.q23	Missense point mutation	MPZ (Po)
CMT-1B	1q21.q23	Missense point mutation	MPZ (Po)
CMT-IC	10q21	Missence point mutation	EGR2
CMT-X	Xq13	Missense point mutation	(connexin-32)
AR-CMT-1	8q13-q21	—	—
CMT-2A	1p35-36	—	—

AR, autosomal recessive, DSS, Dejerine-Sottas syndrome; EGR2, early growth response gene, 2; HNPP, hereditary neuropathy with liability to pressure palsies; MPZ, myelin protein zero (Po); PMP22, peripheral myelin protein 22

TABLE 104.4. RELATIVE FREQUENCY OF AUTOSOMAL-DOMINANT NEUROPATHIES IN 63 FAMILIES DETERMINED BY DNA ANALYSIS

Charcot-Marie-Tooth type	Families (n)	%
1A	38	60.3
1B	1	1.6
2	14	22.2
X-linked dominant	10	15.9

Adapted from Ionasescu et al., 1993.

TABLE 104.6. GENES IMPLICATED IN PERIPHERAL MYELINOPATHIES

	CMT-1	CMT-2	DSS	CH	HNPP
PMP22	X	—	X	—	X
MPZ	X	X	X	X	—
Cx32	X	X	—	—	—
EGR2	X	—	X	X	—

CH, congenital hypomyelination: CMT, Charcot-Marie-Tooth disease; Cx32, Connexion 32; DSS, Dejerine-Sottas syndrome; EGR2, early growth response gene; HNPP; hereditary neuropathy with liability to pressure palsies; MPZ, Myelin protein zero; PMP22, peripheral myelin protein 22.
Modified from Nelis et al., 1999.

transmission. CMT-X dominant is the second most common demyelinating CMT after CMT-1A. CMT-X results from point mutations in the connexin32 gene (Cx32) at Xq13; more than 200 mutations have been found in all domains of the protein.

Still other types of CMT are identified by companion disorders, such as pigmentary retinopathy, optic atrophy, hearing loss, or mental retardation.

Even before the advent of DNA analysis, this classification gave reasonably consistent results. Among 430 families studied by Lovelace and colleagues (Table 104.5), CMT-1 and CMT-2 were almost equally represented at first, but now CMT-1 is almost twice as prevalent. There were atypical manifestations in some families, however, and others showed features of more than one type (see Table 104.3). DNA analysis should resolve these unsettled diagnoses; direct DNA diagnosis is now reliable.

At first, it seemed that the only heterogeneity was *locus heterogeneity;* that is, CMT-1A and CMT-1B were linked to different chromosomes, and different gene products were involved. Moreover, the disorder in CMT-1A seemed to be related to *allelic heterogeneity* (mutations within the same gene) and also to gene dosage; if there are two copies of the PMP22 gene (normal state), there are no symptoms. If there is a duplication (triple dose), CMT-1A results. Remarkably, if there is a point mutation (one dose of the gene), a different peripheral nerve syndrome results, *hereditary neuropathy with liability to pressure palsies* (HNPP). How this comes about (the pathogenesis) is not known. The same gene product is implicated in the *trembler mouse.* Many sporadic cases prove to be new mutations of CMT1A, CMT1B, or CMTX.

The merits of the cinical classification have been demonstrated by the remarkable allelic heterogeneity (Table 104.6). The only

TABLE 104.5. RELATIVE FREQUENCY OF CHARCOT-MARIE-TOOTH (CMT) SYNDROMES

Syndrome	Propositi (n)
CMT-1	146
CMT-2	82
CMT-3	4
CMT spinal	25
Mixed	
CMT-1, CMT-2, spinal	34
Other (additional features)	129
Total	420

Data from Neuromuscular Database, Neurological Institute, Columbia University, New York

phenotype with a consistent genotype is HNPP, with mutations only in the PMP22 gene. In contrast, CMT-1A has been found with Po, PMP22, Cx32, and EGR2 mutations. Cx32 mutations have been found in both CMT-1 and CMT-2. Similarly, EGR2 mutations are found in CMT-1, DSS, and congenital hypomyelination. It is a continuing challenge to determine how these clinical differences arise from alterations of the same gene.

Clinical Features

Most forms of hereditary peripheral neuropathy begin in childhood or adolescence. The first signs may be skeletal, with pes cavus or other deformity of the feet, or with scoliosis. Disproportionate thinness of the lower legs ("stork legs") may be evident before there is footdrop and steppage gait. Weakness and wasting are usually symmetric, and progression is usually slow. Ultimately, the hands are also affected, and that may be more disabling than the gait disorder. The motor disorder is usually more impressive than any sensory loss. Cranial nerves are generally spared. Even within the same family, the severity varies; some of those who carry the mutant gene are asymptomatic but have abnormal feet or slow conduction velocities. Others may be totally without clinical manifestations, whereas some use crutches or wheelchairs.

Laboratory Studies

Nerve conduction studies are essential for classification. In CMT-1, conduction velocity is much reduced, from a normal value of about 50 mps to 20 mps or less. Conduction block is not seen. Nerve biopsy is useful in excluding other hereditary neuropathies in which there is deposition of metabolic products, as in Refsum disease, or in excluding lymphocytic infiltration or vasculitis seen in autoimmune neuropathies. DNA analysis is now also essential. Cerebrospinal fluid (CSF) is usually normal, except for modest increase in protein content. Antenatal diagnosis is increasingly reliable.

Diagnosis

Diagnosis is facilitated if there is a family history of CMT-1. Other familial neuropathies, such as familial amyloidotic polyneuropathy, can be distinguished clinically to some extent and also by DNA analysis.

In sporadic cases, the diagnosis is usually evident if the patient is a child or adolescent. In adults, however, it may be difficult to distinguish CMT from chronic inflammatory demyelinating polyneuropathy (CIDP), which differs in later onset, more rapid course, high CSF protein content, and therapeutic response to prednisone. This distinction may be difficult to make because some individuals in CMT families may show abrupt exacerbations, high CSF protein content, or even a therapeutic response to prednisone. People with CMT could be more susceptible to CIDP.

CMT-2, the neuronal form, can be identified if conduction velocities are normal and there is sensory loss in stocking distribution. If the disorder is purely motor, however, the condition could be considered a disease of the perikaryon of motor neurons, that is, distal spinal muscular atrophy.

HNPP was originally considered a different disease because the clinical manifestations are intermittent. In affected families, individuals suffer transient paralysis of muscles innervated by specific peripheral nerves (especially the median and ulnar nerves) or by components of the brachial plexus. The symptoms are usually transient, with complete or partial recovery from each bout. The condition is linked to CMT because nerve conduction velocities are often slow between attacks. In contrast to CMT, there may be conduction block. The hypertrophic component may be so dramatic that it was called *tomaculous neuropathy* (from the Latin word for sausage). DNA analysis established these conditions as allelic to CMT.

Treatment and Prognosis

There is not yet any specific drug or gene therapy. Treatment is therefore directed to mechanical assistance for leg weakness (orthoses), surgical correction of joint deformities and scoliosis, and physical therapy. The course of CMT-1 or CMT-2 is normally so slowly progressive that most affected people can enjoy a productive, satisfying life. Children with the DSS form, however, have serious problems and may never walk.

HEREDITARY SENSORY AND AUTONOMIC NEUROPATHY

Disorders in this category are defined by clinical, genetic, physiologic, and pathologic criteria. No DNA information is available yet. The dominant clinical disorder is sensory loss, which may be so profound that there are mutilating deformities of the hands and feet, a condition called *sensory neurogenic arthropathy* or *mu-tilating acropathy*. There may be weakness or skeletal changes similar to those in CMT disease.

Hereditary sensory and autonomic neuropathy type 1 (HSAN-1) is autosomal-dominant and begins in adolescence with pedal deformity and burning pain. HSAN types 2, 3, and 4 are all autosomal-recessive forms of *congenital indifference to pain.* HSAN-2 is similar to HSAN-1 in mutilation but begins earlier. HSAN-3 is the Riley-Day syndrome or familial dysautonomia. HSAN-4 is similar to HSAN-2, with the addition of anhidrosis to congenital pain insensitivity. As in CMT disease, there are sporadic forms and other forms identified by associated abnormalities of vision or hearing.

FAMILIAL AMYLOIDOTIC POLYNEUROPATHY

History and Molecular Genetics

In 1952, Andrade described an autosomal-dominant neuropathy characterized by deposition of amyloid in peripheral nerves. Identified first in Portugal, it was soon found in other countries visited by Portuguese sailors, especially former colonies, neighboring countries, and Japan. The disease has been found in non-Portuguese populations, including the United States. In 1979, Costa found immunologically that the amyloid contained a serum protein, then called prealbumin because of its electrophoretic characteristics and now known as *transthyretin.* More than 20 different mutations in the gene have been found by DNA analysis, with little correlation between different mutations and clinical manifestations. The number of mutations and the lack of evidence of a founder effect suggest that there is a high incidence of new mutations. The gene for transthyretin and familial amyloidotic polyneuropathy maps to 18q11.2-q12,1, and direct DNA diagnosis is feasible.

Clinical Manifestations

In Portugal, onset is between ages 20 and 35 years, with acral sensory loss, chronic diarrhea, and impotence (Table 104.7). Weakness follows the severe sensory symptoms by several years and becomes disabling. Neurogenic acropathy is common. The autonomic disorder may include sphincter symptoms and orthostatic hypotension. Cardiomyopathy may lead to heart block and pacemaker insertion. Nephrosis is a later manifestation. Inexorably progressive, the condition is fatal 7 to 15 years after onset. Similar patterns are seen in Majorca, Brazil, Sweden, and

TABLE 104.7. CLASSIFICATION OF FAMILIAL AMYLOIDOTIC POLYNEUROPATHIES (MIM 176300)

Gene product	Type	Name	Manifestations
Transthyretin	I	Portuguese	Sensorimotor neuropathy; trophic skin lesions; autonomic
	II	Appalachian–Irish	Late onset; severe motor neuropathy; cardiomyopathy
	III	Maryland–Indian German–Swiss	Carpal tunnel syndrome; sensorimotor neuropathy; fasciculations; bulbar; autonomic
Apoprotein A1	IV	Van Allen–Iowa	Similar to Portuguese form
Gelsonin	V	Finnish	Corneal lattice dystrophy; cranial neuropathy; sensory and autonomic neuropathy

Japan. In Sweden, onset is after age 40, and later onset also characterizes many sporadic cases.

Variants include forms that are primarily neuropathic, predominantly cardiomyopathic, or both. As in Huntington disease, there is no clinical difference between homozygous and heterozygous individuals.

Pathology and Pathogenesis

Amyloid is found in extracellular spaces of many organs, infiltrating blood vessels. The central nervous system is spared, but amyloid deposits are found in autonomic and myelinated or unmyelinated peripheral nerves. The disorder is both demyelinating and axonal.

Transthyretin is a serum protein involved in the transport of thyroid hormones and vitamin A. The main site of production is the liver, but the choroid plexus is also a source of the protein in CSF; it is also produced in the eye. It is not known how abnormalities of the protein lead to the clinical neuropathy. The abnormal gene has been introduced into transgenic mice; amyloid accumulates in serum and liver but not in peripheral nerves.

Treatment

The disease cannot be arrested. Symptomatic relief can ameliorate the gastrointestinal and cardiac symptoms, but little can be done about the sensorimotor neuropathy. Plasmapheresis has been used with limited success. Immunoabsorption of the abnormal protein may prove useful. Liver transplantation has been used to replace the abnormal transthyretin with the normal donor protein; in early trials, progression seemed to be arrested, but there was no functional improvement of the neuropathy. Antenatal diagnosis is feasible. The question of presymptomatic diagnosis is a problem for a disease that cannot be cured.

SUGGESTED READINGS

Charcot-Marie-Tooth Diseases

Ben Othmane K, Hentati F, Lennon F, et al. Linkage of a locus (CMT4A) for autosomal recessive Charcot-Marie-Tooth disease to chromosome 8q. *Hum Mol Genet* 1993;2:1625–1628.

Ben Othmane K, Middleton LT, Laprest LJ, et al. Localization of a gene (CMT2A) for autosomal dominant Charcot-Marie-Tooth disease type 2 to chromosome 1p and evidence of genetic heterogeneity. *Genomics* 1993;17:370–375.

Bone LJ, Deschenes SM, Balice-Gordon RJ, Fischbeck KH, Scherer SS. Connexin32 and X-linked Charcot-Marie-Tooth disease. *Neurobiol Dis* 1997;4:221–230.

Chance PF, Alderson MK, Lepig KA, et al. DNA deletion associated with hereditary neuropathy with liability to pressure palsies. *Cell* 1993;72:143–152.

Chance PF, Bird TD, Matsunami N, et al. Trisomy 17p associated with Charcot-Marie-Tooth neuropathy type 1A phenotype: evidence for gene dosage as a mechanism in CMT1A. *Neurology* 1992;42:2295–2299.

Chance PF, Dyck PJ. Hereditary neuropathy with liability to pressure palsies: a patient's point mutation in a mouse model. *Neurology* 1998;51:664–665.

DeJonghe P, Timmerman V, Van Broeckhoven C. Workshop report: classification and diagnostic guidelines for CMT2-HMSN II and distal hereditary motor neuropathy (distal HMN-spinal CMT). *Neuromuscul Disord* 1998;8:426–431.

Dyck PJ. Inherited neuronal degeneration and atrophy affecting peripheral motor, sensory and autonomic neurons. In: Dyck PJ, Thomas PK, Griffin JW, et al., eds. *Peripheral neuropathy,* 3rd ed. Philadelphia: WB Saunders, 1993.

Goebel HH. Hereditary metabolic neuropathies. *Zentralbl Allg Pathol* 1990;136:503–515.

Haites NE, Nelis E, Van Broeckhoven C. Workshop report: gentotype/phenotype correlations in CMT1 and HNNP. *Neuromuscul Disord* 1998;8:591–603.

Hannemann CO, Muller HW. Pathogenesis of CMT1A neuropathy. *Trends Neurosci* 1998;21:282–286.

Ionasescu VV, Ionasescu R, Searby C. Screening of dominantly inherited Charcot-Marie-Tooth neuropathies. *Muscle Nerve* 1993;16:1232–1238.

Ionasescu VV, Searby C, Ionasescu R. Point mutations of the connexin32 (GJB1) gene in X-linked dominant Charcot-Marie-Tooth neuropathy. *Hum Mol Genet* 1994;3:355–358.

Ionasescu VV, Searby CC, Ionasescu R, et al. Dejerine-Sottas neuropathy in mother and son with the same point mutation of PMP22 gene. *Muscle Nerve* 1997;20:97–99.

Lovelace RE. Charcot-Marie-Tooth disorders and other hereditary neuropathies. In: Younger DS, ed. *Textbook of motor disorders.* Philadelphia: Lippincott Williams & Wilkins, 1999:205–211.

Lovelace RE, Shapiro HK, eds. *Charcot-Marie-Tooth disorders: pathophysiology, molecular genetics and therapy.* New York: Wiley-Lee, 1990.

Lupski JR. Charcot-Marie-Tooth disease: lessons in genetic mechanisms. *Mol Med* 1998;4:3–11.

Malandrini A, Villanova M, Dotti MT, Federico A. Acute inflammatory neuropathy in Charcot-Marie-Tooth disease. *Neurology* 1999;52:859–861.

Nelis E, Haites N, Van Broeckhoven C. Mutations in peripheral myelin genes and associated genes in inherited peripheral neuropathies. *Hum Mutat* 1999;13:11–28.

Nicholson GA, Yeung L, Corbett A. Efficient neurophysiologic selection of X-linked Charcot-Marie-Tooth families: ten novel mutations. *Neurology* 1998;51:1412–1416.

Oda K, Miura H, Shibasaki H, et al. Hereditary pressure-sensitive neuropathy: demonstration of "tomacula" in motor nerve fibers. *J Neurol Sci* 1990;98:139–148.

Parman Y, Plante-Bordeneuve V, Guiochon-Mantel A, Eraksoy M, Said G. Recessive inheritance of a new point mutation of the PMP22 gene in Dejerine-Sottas diseae. *Ann Neurol* 1999;45:518–522.

Rouger H, LeGuerne, Birouk N, et al. CMT disease with intermediate motor nerve conduction velocities: characterization of 14 Cx32 mutations in 35 families. *Hum Mutat* 1997;10:443–452.

Saito M, Hayashi Y, Suzuki T, et al. Linkage mapping of the gene for Charcot-Marie-Tooth disease type 2 to chromosome 1p (CMT2A) and clinical features of CMT2A. *Neurology* 1997;49:1630–1635.

Sambuughin N, Sivakumar K, Selenge B, et al. Autosomal dominant distal spinal muscular atrophy type V (dSMA-V) and Charcot-Marie-Tooth disease type 2D (CMT2D) segregate within a single large kindred and map to a refined region on chromosome 7p15. *J Neurol Sci* 1998;161:23–28.

Sghirlanzoni A, Pareyson D, Balestrini MR, et al. HMSN III phenotype due to homozygous expression of a dominant HMSN II gene. *Neurology* 1992;42:2201–2203.

Shy ME, Arroyo E, Dladky J, et al. Heterozygous Po knockout mice develop a peripheral neuropathy that resembles chronic inflammataory demyelinating polyneuropathy. *J Neuropathol Exp Neurol* 1997;56:811–821.

Silander K, Meretoja P, Juvonen V, et al. Spectrum of mutations in Finnish patients with Charcot-Marie-Tooth and related neuropathies. *Hum Mutat* 1998;12:59–68.

Teunissen LL, Notermans NC, Franssen H, et al. Differences between hereditary motor and sensory neuropathy type 2 and chronic idiopathic axonal neuropathy: a clinical and electrophysiological study. *Brain* 1997;120:955–962.

Thomas PK, Ormerod JEC. Hereditary neuralgic amyotrophy associated with a relapsing multifocal sensory neuropathy. *J Neurol Neurosurg Psychiatry* 1993;56:107–109.

Verhagen WIM, Gabreels-Festen AAWM, van Wensen PJM, et al. Hereditary neuropathy with liability to pressure palsies: a clinical, electroneurophysiological and morphological study. *J Neurol Sci* 1993;116:176–184.

Warner LE, Garcia CA, Lupski JR. Hereditary peripheral neuropathies: clinical forms, genetics and molecular mechanisms. *Annu Rev Med* 1999;50:263–275.

Warner LE, Mancias P, Butler IJ, et al. Mutations in the early growth response 2 (EGR2) gene are associated with hereditary myelinopathies. *Nat Genet* 1998;18:382–384.

Wicklein EM, Orth U, Gal A, Kunze K. Missense mutation (R15W) of the connexin32 gene in a family with X chromosomal Charcot-Marie-Tooth neuropathy with only female members affected. *J Neurol Neurosurg Psychiatry* 1997;63:379–381.

Hereditary Sensory Neuropathies

Bejaoui K, McKenna-Yasek D, Hoisler BA, et al. Confirmation of linkage of type 1 hereditary sensory neuropathy to human chromosome 9q22. *Neurology* 1999;52:510–515.

DeJonghe P, Timmerman V, Fitzpatrick D, et al. Mutilating neuropathic ulcerations in a chromosome 3q13-q22 linked Charcot-Marie-Tooth disease type 2B family. *J Neurol Neurosurg Psychiatry* 1997;62:570–573.

Dyck PJ, Mellinger JF, Reagan TJ, et al. Not "indifference to pain" but varieties of hereditary sensory and autonomic neuropathy. *Brain* 1983;106:373–390.

Nicholson GA, Dawkins JL, Blair IP, et al. The gene for hereditary sensory neuropathy type 1 (HSN-1) maps to chromosome 9q22.1-q22.3. *Nat Genet* 1996;13:101–104.

Familial Amyloid Polyneuropathy

Andrade C. A peculiar form of peripheral neuropathy: familial atypical generalized amyloidosis with special involvement of the peripheral nerves. *Brain* 1952;75:408–427.

Coelho T. Familial amyloid polyneuropathy: new developments in genetics and treatment. *Curr Opin Neurol* 1996;9:355–359.

Costa PP, Figueira AS, Bravo FR. Amyloid fibril protein related to prealbumin in familial amyloidotic polyneuropathy. *Proc Natl Acad Sci U S A* 1978;75:4499–4503.

Plante-Bordeneuve V, Lalu T, Misrahi M, et al. Genotypic-phenotypic variations in a series of 65 patients with familial amyloidotic polyneuropathy. *Neurology* 1998;51:708–714.

Reilly MM, King RHM. Familial amyloid polyneuropathy. *Brain Pathol* 1993;3:165–176.

Saraiva MJM, Birken S, Costa PP, et al. Amyloid fibril protein in familial amyloid polyneuropathy, Portuguese type: definition of molecular abnormality in transthyretin (prealbumin). *J Clin Invest* 1984;74:104–119.

Suhr OB, Holmgren G, Ando Y. Improvement in the polyneuropathy associated with familial amyloid polyneuropathy after liver transplantation [Letter]. *Neurology* 1998;51:926–927.

Takaoka Y, Tashiro F, Yi S, et al. Comparison of amyloid deposition in two lines of transgenic mouse model of familial amyloidotic polyneuropathy type 1. *Transgenic Res* 1997;6:261–269.

Merritt's Neurology, 10th ed., edited by L.P. Rowland. Lippincott Williams & Wilkins, Philadelphia © 2000.

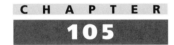

C H A P T E R 105

ACQUIRED NEUROPATHIES

DALE J. LANGE
NORMAN LATOV
WERNER TROJABORG

GUILLAIN-BARRÉ SYNDROME AND VARIANTS

The Guillain-Barré syndrome (GBS; acute inflammatory demyelinating neuropathy) is characterized by acute onset of peripheral and cranial nerve dysfunction. Viral respiratory or gastrointestinal infection, immunization, or surgery often precedes neurologic symptoms by 5 days to 3 weeks. Symptoms and signs include rapidly progressive symmetric weakness, loss of tendon reflexes, facial diplegia, oropharyngeal and respiratory paresis, and impaired sensation in the hands and feet. The condition worsens for several days to 3 weeks, followed by a period of stability and then gradual improvement to normal or nearly normal function. Early plasmapheresis or intravenous infusion of human gamma globulins accelerates recovery and diminishes the incidence of long-term neurologic disability.

Etiology

The cause of the GBS is unknown. It is thought to be immune-mediated because a disease with similar clinical features (i.e., similar pathologic, electrophysiologic, and cerebrospinal fluid [CSF] alterations) can be induced in experimental animals by immunization with whole peripheral nerve, peripheral nerve myelin, or, in some species, peripheral nerve myelin P2 basic protein or galactocerebroside. Although there is no evidence of sensitization to these antigens in humans with spontaneous GBS, activity of the disease seems to correlate with the appearance of serum antibodies to peripheral nerve myelin. When GBS is preceded by a viral infection, there is no evidence of direct viral infection of peripheral nerves or nerve roots.

Electrophysiology and Pathology

Nerve conduction velocities are reduced in GBS, but values may be normal early in the course. Distal sensory and motor latencies are prolonged. As a result of demyelination of nerve roots, F-wave conduction velocity is often slowed. Conduction slowing may persist for months or years after clinical recovery. In general, the severity of neurologic abnormality is not related to the degree of slowing of conduction but is related to the extent of conduction block. Long-standing weakness is most apt to occur when there is electromyographic (EMG) evidence of muscle denervation early in the course.

Histologically, GBS is characterized by focal segmental demyelination (Fig. 105.1) with perivascular and endoneurial infiltrates of lymphocytes and monocytes or macrophages (Fig. 105.2). These lesions are scattered throughout the nerves, nerve roots, and cranial nerves. In particularly severe lesions, there is both axonal degeneration and segmental demyelination. During recovery, remyelination occurs, but the lymphocytic infiltrates may persist.

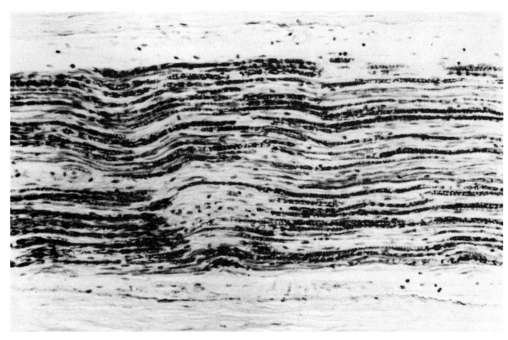

FIG. 105.1. Focal demyelination in acute GBS. (Courtesy of Dr. Arthur Asbury.)

Incidence

GBS is the most frequent acquired demyelinating neuropathy, with an incidence of 0.6 to 1.9 cases per 100,000 population. The incidence increases gradually with age, but the disease may occur at any age. Men and women are affected equally. The incidence increases in patients with Hodgkin disease, as well as with pregnancy or general surgery.

Symptoms and Signs

GBS often appears days to weeks after symptoms of a viral upper respiratory or gastrointestinal infection. Usually, the first neurologic symptoms are due to symmetric limb weakness, often with paresthesia. In contrast to most other neuropathies, proximal muscles are sometimes affected more often than distal muscles at first. Occasionally, facial, ocular, or oropharyngeal muscles may

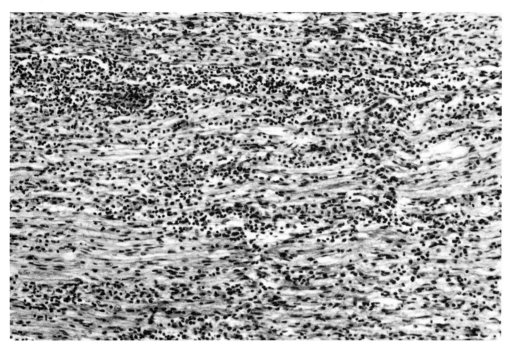

FIG. 105.2. Diffuse mononuclear infiltrate in peripheral nerve in GBS. (Courtesy of Dr. Arthur Asbury.)

be affected first; more than 50% of patients have facial diplegia, and dysphagia and dysarthria develop in a similar number. Some patients require mechanical ventilation. Tendon reflexes may be normal for the first few days but are then lost. The degree of sensory impairment varies. In some patients, all sensory modalities are preserved; others have marked diminution in perception of joint position, vibration, pain, and temperature in stocking-and-glove distribution. Patients occasionally exhibit papilledema, sensory ataxia, transient extensor plantar responses, or evidence of autonomic dysfunction (orthostatic hypotension, transient hypertension, or cardiac arrhythmia). Many have muscle tenderness, and the nerves may be sensitive to pressure, but there are no signs of meningeal irritation such as nuchal rigidity.

Variants

Acute motor axonal neuropathy (AMAN) is a variant of GBS. There is motor axonal degeneration and little or no demyelination or inflammation. AMAN may follow infection with *Campylobacter jejuni* or parenteral injection of gangliosides.

The *Miller-Fisher syndrome* is characterized by gait ataxia, areflexia, and ophthalmoparesis; pupillary abnormalities are sometimes present. It is considered a variant of GBS because it is often preceded by respiratory infection, it progresses for weeks and then improves, and CSF protein content is increased. There is no limb weakness, however, and nerve conductions are normal. Sometimes, magnetic resonance imaging shows brainstem lesions.

Other GBS variants include *acute motor and sensory axonal neuropathy*, *acute sensory neuropathy* or *neuronopathy*, and *acute autonomic neuropathy* or *pandysautonomia*.

Laboratory Data

The CSF protein content is elevated in most patients with GBS but may be normal in the first few days after onset. The CSF cell count is usually normal, but some patients with otherwise typical GBS have 10 to 100 mononuclear cells/μL of CSF. Antecedent infectious mononucleosis, cytomegalovirus (CMV) infection, viral hepatitis, human immunodeficiency virus (HIV) infection, or other viral diseases may be documented by serologic studies. Increased titers of immunoglobulin (Ig) G or IgA antibodies to GM_1 or GD_{1a} gangliosides may be found in the axonal form of GBS; anti-GQ_{1b} antibodies are closely associated with the Miller-Fisher syndrome.

Course and Prognosis

Symptoms are usually most severe within 1 week of onset but may progress for 3 weeks or more. Death is uncommon but may follow aspiration pneumonia, pulmonary embolism, intercurrent infection, or autonomic dysfunction. The rate of recovery varies. In some, it is rapid, with restoration to normal function within a few weeks. In most, recovery is slow and not complete for many months. Recovery is accelerated by early institution of plasmapheresis or intravenous immunoglobulin (IVIG) therapy. In untreated series, about 35% of patients have permanent residual hyporeflexia, atrophy, and weakness of distal muscles or fa-

cial paresis. A biphasic illness, with partial recovery followed by relapse, is present in fewer than 10% of patients. Recurrence after full recovery occurs in about 2%.

Diagnosis and Differential Diagnosis

The characteristic history of subacute development of symmetric motor or sensorimotor neuropathy after a viral illness, delivery, or surgery, together with slowing of conductions and a high CSF protein content with normal CSF cell count, define GBS.

In the past, the principal diseases to be differentiated from GBS were diphtheritic polyneuropathy and acute anterior poliomyelitis. Both are now rare in the United States. Diphtheritic polyneuropathy can usually be distinguished by the long latency period between the respiratory infection and onset of neuritis, the frequency of paralysis of accommodation, and the relatively slow evolution of symptoms. Acute anterior poliomyelitis was distinguished by asymmetry of paralysis, signs of meningeal irritation, fever, and CSF pleocytosis. Occasionally, patients with acquired immunodeficiency syndrome (AIDS) or AIDS-related complex have a disorder identical to GBS, sometimes but not always due to CMV infection. Porphyric neuropathy resembles GBS clinically but is differentiated by normal CSF protein, recurrent abdominal crisis, mental symptoms, onset after exposure to barbiturates or other drugs, and high urinary levels of δ-aminolevulinic acid and porphobilinogen. Development of a GBS-like syndrome during prolonged parenteral feeding should raise the possibility of hypophosphatemia-induced neural dysfunction. Toxic neuropathies caused by hexane inhalation or thallium or arsenic ingestion occasionally begin acutely or subacutely. These can be distinguished from GBS by history of toxin exposure or, in thallium or arsenic intoxication, by later alopecia. Botulism may be difficult to discriminate on clinical grounds from purely motor forms of GBS, but ocular muscles and the pupils are frequently affected. Electrophysiologic tests in botulism reveal normal nerve conduction velocities and a facilitating response to repetitive nerve stimulation. Tick paralysis should be excluded by careful examination of the scalp.

Treatment

Early plasmapheresis has proved useful in patients with GBS. IVIG therapy is also reported to be beneficial. Glucocorticoid administration does not shorten the course or affect the prognosis. Mechanically assisted ventilation is sometimes necessary, and precautions against aspiration of food or stomach contents must be taken if oropharyngeal muscles are affected. Exposure keratitis must be prevented in patients with facial diplegia.

CHRONIC INFLAMMATORY DEMYELINATING POLYNEUROPATHY

Chronic inflammatory demyelinating polyneuropathy (CIDP) may begin insidiously or acutely, as in GBS, and then follow a chronic progressive or relapsing course. As in GBS, it often follows nonspecific viral infections, segmental demyelination and lymphocytic infiltrates are present in peripheral nerves, and a similar disease can be induced in experimental animals by immunization with peripheral nerve myelin. The CSF protein content is often increased but less consistently than in GBS. An infantile form of CIDP begins with hypotonia and delayed motor development. Optic neuritis has been noted in some patients. Nerves may become enlarged because of Schwann cell proliferation and collagen deposition after recurrent segmental demyelination and remyelination.

In contrast to GBS, glucocorticoid therapy is often beneficial. CIDP is also responsive to plasmapheresis or IVIG therapy, and immunosuppressive drug therapy may be effective in resistant cases. Research criteria for the diagnosis of CIDP have been recommended, but there is no specific test, and the diagnosis is often made on clinical grounds. A predominantly sensory form of CIDP and an axonal form have been described; it is likely that CIDP is heterogeneous, including several different chronic immune-mediated diseases that affect peripheral nerves. Tests for HIV-1, monoclonal paraproteins, antibodies to myelin-associated glycoprotein (MAG) and, occasionally, Charcot-Marie-Tooth disease type 1 or hereditary neuropathy with liability to pressure palsy are carried out in suspected patients to evaluate possible causes of demyelinating neuropathy.

MULTIFOCAL MOTOR NEUROPATHY

Multifocal motor neuropathy (MMN) is manifested by a clinical syndrome restricted to signs of a lower motor neuron disorder. Typically, there is weakness, wasting, and fasciculation with active or absent tendon reflexes. The findings are often asymmetric and affect the arms and hands more than the legs. Electrophysiologic evidence of denervation is accompanied by the defining abnormality, physiologic evidence of multifocal motor conduction block. MMN is associated with increased titers of IgM anti-GM_1 in about one-third of the patients; less frequently, anti-GD_{1a} antibodies are found. It is important to recognize these patients and to distinguish them from patients with typical motor neuron disease because the weakness of MMN is reversible with IVIG or immunosuppressive drug therapy.

SENSORY NEURONOPATHY AND NEUROPATHY

Sensory neuropathy may result from primary involvement of the sensory root ganglia, as in ganglioneuritis or sensory neuronitis, or the nerve may be directly affected as in distal sensory neuropathy. *Ganglioneuritis* may be acute or subacute in onset and is characterized by numbness, paresthesia, and pain that can be distal or radicular or involve the entire body including the face. Ataxia and autonomic dysfunction may be evident. Small-fiber sensation alone or all sensory modalities may be affected to varying degrees. Tendon reflexes may be present or absent, and strength is normal. The disease may be self-limiting or chronic, with relapses or slow progression. Motor nerve conduction velocities are normal or near normal, but sensory potentials are reduced in amplitude or absent. Routine electrophysiologic studies may be normal if the disease is mild or if only small fibers are affected, but spinal somatosensory evoked responses and quanti-

tative sensory testing are usually abnormal. CSF protein content is normal or slightly elevated. Response to glucocorticoids or immunosuppressive therapy is variable. Pathologic studies of spinal root ganglia show inflammatory infiltrates with a predominance of T cells and macrophages. Some patients have sicca or Sjögren syndrome with anti-Ro and anti-La antibodies.

Several autoantibodies to peripheral nerve antigens have been reported to be associated with sensory neuropathy. Some patients with sensory axonal neuropathies have monoclonal or polyclonal IgM anti-sulfatide antibodies and monoclonal IgM autoantibodies with anti-GD_{1b} and disialosyl ganglioside antibody activity have been associated with large-fiber sensory neuropathy. Other causes of sensory neuropathy include HIV-1 infection, vitamin B_6 deficiency, paraneoplastic neuropathy, amyloidosis, and toxic neuropathy.

IDIOPATHIC AUTONOMIC NEUROPATHY

This condition is characterized by acute or subacute onset of hypofunction of sympathetic and parasympathetic nerve functions. Symptoms include postural syncope, diminished tear and sweat production, impaired bladder function, constipation, and diminished sexual potency. The autonomic preganglionic or postganglionic efferent neurons are thought to be affected. It may follow viral infection, as in GBS, and CSF protein concentration may be elevated. The disease is frequently self-limiting, and gradual partial or complete recovery occurs without specific therapy.

VASCULITIC AND CRYOGLOBULINEMIC NEUROPATHIES

Vasculitic neuropathy is manifested as mononeuritis multiplex or distal symmetric polyneuropathy. Nerve conduction studies may show electrical inexcitability of nerve segments distal to an infarct caused by vascular occlusion. If some fascicles in the nerves are spared, they conduct at a normal rate, but the amplitude of the evoked response is diminished. The diagnosis of peripheral nerve involvement may be established by nerve and muscle biopsies (Fig. 105.3), which typically show inflammatory cell infiltrates and necrosis of the walls of blood vessels. The biopsy specimen, however, may show only axonal degeneration if vasculitis has caused a nerve infarct that is proximal to the site of biopsy, or if no affected vessels are encountered in the specimen.

The vasculitis may be confined to the peripheral nerves or may be associated with systemic disease, such as polyarteritis or cryoglobulinemia. The most common systemic cause of vasculitic neuropathy is polyarteritis nodosa, which may cause purpuric skin lesions, renal failure, Raynaud phenomenon, constitutional symptoms, and, sometimes, mixed polyclonal cryoglobulinemia; hepatitis B or C virus (HBV or HCV) infection may be found. Cryoglobulins are immunoglobulins that precipitate in the cold and are classified as types I through III. Type I contains a monoclonal immunoglobulin only, type II contains both monoclonal and polyclonal immunoglobulins,

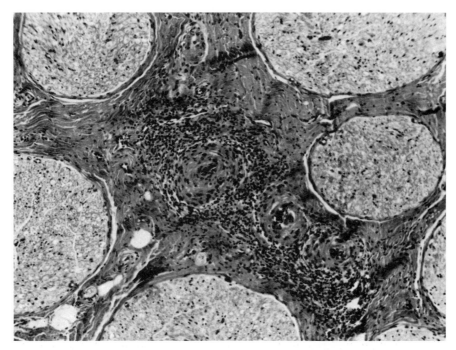

FIG. 105.3. Polyarteritis in large proximal nerve trunk. Three small epineurial arteries show inflammation in the vessel wall and adventitia, as well as luminal narrowing and fibrosis. Surrounding nerve fascicles are not involved in this section. (Courtesy of Dr. Arthur Asbury.)

and type III contains mixed polyclonal immunoglobulins. Types I and II are associated with plasma cell dyscrasia, and type III may be associated with polyarteritis nodosa and HBV or HCV infection.

Other causes of vasculitic neuropathy include the Churg-Strauss syndrome with asthma and eosinophilia; Sjögren syndrome with xerophthalmia, xerostomia, and anti-Ro and anti-La antibodies; and Wegener granulomatosis with necrotizing granulomatous lesions in the upper or lower respiratory tracts, glomerulonephritis, and antineutrophilic cytoplasmic antigen antibodies. Less commonly, vasculitic neuropathy is seen in rheumatoid arthritis, systemic lupus erythematosus, and systemic sclerosis. Vasculitis may respond to therapy with prednisone and cyclophosphamide. Plasmapheresis is also useful in the treatment of cryoglobulinemia.

NEUROPATHIES ASSOCIATED WITH MYELOMA AND NONMALIGNANT IgG OR IgA MONOCLONAL GAMMOPATHIES

Peripheral neuropathy is found in approximately 50% of patients with osteosclerotic myeloma and IgG or IgA monoclonal gammopathies. Some patients have the POEMS syndrome (polyneuropathy, organomegaly, endocrinopathy, myeloma, and skin changes) or Crow-Fukase syndrome with hyperpigmentation of skin, edema, excessive hair growth, hepatosplenomegaly, papilledema, elevated CSF protein content, hypogonadism, and hypothyroidism. POEMS syndrome is sometimes associated with nonosteosclerotic myeloma or with nonmalignant monoclonal gammopathy. The IgG or IgA light-chain type is almost always lambda. Electrophysiologic and pathologic abnormalities are consistent with demyelination and axonal degeneration; the patterns may resemble those of CIDP.

Malignant or nonmalignant IgG or IgA monoclonal gammopathy may also be associated with neuropathy in primary amyloidosis, in which fragments of the monoclonal light chains are deposited as amyloid in peripheral nerve, and in types I and II cryoglobulinemia, in which the monoclonal immunoglobulins are components of the cryoprecipitates.

The significance of IgG or IgA monoclonal gammopathies is uncertain in the absence of myeloma, POEMS syndrome, amyloidosis, or cryoglobulinemia. Nonmalignant monoclonal gammopathies are found more frequently in patients with neuropathy of otherwise unknown etiology; however, they are also present in approximately 1% of normal adults, and the frequency increases with age or in chronic infections or inflammatory diseases, so the association with neuropathy in some cases could be coincidental. Other causes of neuropathy, particularly inflammatory conditions such as CIDP, should be considered.

In cases of myeloma, irradiation, chemotherapy, or bone marrow transplantation may be beneficial.

NEUROPATHIES ASSOCIATED WITH IgM MONOCLONAL ANTIBODIES THAT REACT WITH PERIPHERAL NERVE GLYCOCONJUGATE ANTIGENS

In several syndromes, peripheral neuropathy is associated with polyclonal or monoclonal IgM autoantibodies that react with glycoconjugates in peripheral nerve. IgM antibodies that react with MAG are associated with a chronic demyelinating sensori-motor neuropathy. Pathologic studies show deposits of the monoclonal IgM and complement on affected myelin sheaths, and passive transfer of the autoantibodies in experimental animals reproduces the neuropathy. Treatment consisting of plasmapheresis and chemotherapy to reduce autoantibody concentrations, or IVIG, frequently results in clinical improvement.

Increased titers of polyclonal or monoclonal anti-GM$_1$ ganglioside antibodies are associated with a clinical syndrome of motor neuropathy or motor neuron disease. Typically, there is weakness, wasting, and fasciculation with active or absent tendon reflexes. The condition is associated with electrophysiologic evidence of denervation and conduction block. Conduction block is not always present, however, in patients with increased antibody titers. The same clinical syndrome may also occur in patients with normal titers of anti-GM$_1$ antibodies. It is important to recognize these patients and to distinguish them from patients with typical motor neuron disease because the weakness may be reversed by immunosuppressive chemotherapy or IVIG.

Other syndromes associated with monoclonal or polyclonal IgM autoantibodies include: multifocal motor neuropathy or lower motor neuron syndrome associated with anti-GM$_1$ or anti-GD$_{1a}$ ganglioside antibodies, large-fiber sensory neuropathy with anti-GD$_{1b}$ and disialosyl ganglioside antibodies, and axonal sensory neuropathy associated with antisulfatide antibodies.

AMYLOID NEUROPATHY

Amyloid is an insoluble extracellular aggregate of proteins that forms in nerve or other tissues when any of several proteins is produced in excess. The two principal forms of amyloid protein that cause neuropathy are immunoglobulin light chains in patients with primary amyloidosis and plasma cell dyscrasias, and transthyretin in hereditary amyloidosis. The syndrome is often that of a painful, small-fiber sensory neuropathy with progressive autonomic dysfunction, symmetric loss of pain and temperature sensations with spared position and vibratory senses, carpal tunnel syndrome, or some combination of these symptoms. The diagnosis of amyloid neuropathy can be established by histologic demonstration of amyloid in nerve (Fig. 105.4), followed by immunocytochemical characterization of the deposits with the use of antibodies to immunoglobulin light chains or transthyretin. Mutation of the transthyretin gene is detected by DNA analysis. Electrophoresis of serum and urine with immunofixation can assist in the diagnosis of primary amyloid neuropathy. Prognosis is generally poor. Liver transplantation has been reported to be beneficial for hereditary amyloidosis, and high-dose chemotherapy followed by bone marrow transplantation has been reported to help some patients with primary amyloidosis.

NEUROPATHY ASSOCIATED WITH CARCINOMA (PARANEOPLASTIC NEUROPATHY)

Both direct and indirect effects of malignant neoplasms on the peripheral nervous system are recognized. In some patients, the nerves or nerve roots are compressed or infiltrated by neoplastic cells. In others, there is no evidence of damage to the nerves by the neoplasm, and dietary deficiency or metabolic, toxic, or immunologic factors may be responsible.

The most characteristic paraneoplastic disorder is a sensory neuropathy of subacute onset, associated with small-cell carcinoma of the lung. Electrodiagnostic studies reveal loss of sensory

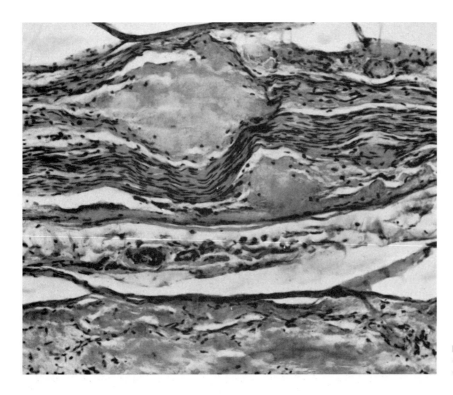

FIG. 105.4. Amyloid neuropathy. Massive deposits of endoneurial amyloid compress nerve fiber bundles. (Courtesy of Dr. Arthur Asbury.)

evoked responses. Autoantibodies against the Hu antigen in neuronal nuclei are characteristic, and postmortem studies show loss of neurons, deposition of antibodies, and inflammatory cells in dorsal root ganglia.

Less consistently associated with carcinoma is a distal sensorimotor polyneuropathy without specific features. Nerve biopsy may reveal infiltration by tumor cells, axonal degeneration, or demyelination. A primarily motor syndrome of subacute onset occurs in Hodgkin disease and other lymphomas. In these patients, the predominant lesion is degeneration of anterior horn cells, but demyelination, perivascular mononuclear cell infiltrates, and alterations in Schwann cell morphology in ventral roots are also observed. Some patients also have probable or definite upper motor neuron signs in life, and corticospinal tract degeneration is found at autopsy; that is, they have clinical and pathologic evidence of amyotrophic lateral sclerosis (ALS).

The diagnosis of malignancy should be suspected in a middle-aged or elderly patient with a subacute sensory neuropathy or polyradiculopathy of obscure cause, particularly with weight loss. The course is usually progressive until the primary malignancy is cured or until it causes death. CSF examination for malignant cells is valuable in the diagnosis of infiltration of the meninges by cancer. In some instances of meningeal infiltration, radiotherapy or intrathecal chemotherapy may be valuable.

HYPOTHYROID NEUROPATHY

Entrapment neuropathies are relatively common in patients with hypothyroidism, probably because acid mucopolysaccharide protein complexes (mucoid) are deposited in the nerve. Painful paresthesia in the hands and feet is the most common symptom of hypothyroidism. Weakness is not a feature. Tendon reflexes are reduced or absent, and, when present, may show the characteristic delayed or "hung-up" response. Direct percussion of muscle produces transient mounding of the underlying skin and muscle (myoedema). Nerve conduction studies show mild slowing of motor nerve conduction and decreased amplitude of the sensory evoked response. Morphologic studies show evidence of demyelination, axonal loss, and excessive glycogen within Schwann cells. CSF protein content is often more than 100 mg/dL. Rarely, dysfunction of cranial nerves IX, X, and XII causes hoarseness and dysarthria, probably as a result of local myxedematous infiltration of the nerves. Some hearing loss is reported in as many as 85% of hypothyroid patients. The peripheral neuropathy may occur before there is laboratory evidence of hypothyroidism. Once identified, thyroid replacement causes clinical, electrophysiologic, and morphologic improvement.

ACROMEGALIC NEUROPATHY

Entrapment neuropathy is also relatively common in patients with acromegaly. Rarely, acromegalic patients note distal paresthesia, but in contrast to myxedematous patients, weakness may be severe, and peripheral nerves may be palpable. There is a significant correlation between total exchangeable body sodium and the severity of the neuropathy. The nerves are enlarged because there is increased endoneurial and perineurial connective tissue, perhaps stimulated by increased levels of somatomedin C (insulin-like growth factor). Tendon reflexes are reduced. Nerve conduction velocities are mildly slow with low evoked response amplitudes. Morphologic changes suggest segmental demyelination.

HYPERTHYROID NEUROPATHY

Hyperthyroidism can produce a syndrome consisting of diffuse weakness and fasciculations with preserved or hyperactive tendon reflexes, resembling ALS. However, the symptoms and signs disappear with treatment of the toxic state. GBS is also seen with hyperthyroidism. No convincing pathologic studies have established the presence of chronic sensorimotor neuropathy with hyperthyroidism.

UREMIC NEUROPATHY

Peripheral neuropathy is only one of the neuromuscular syndromes associated with chronic renal failure. Restless legs, cramps, and muscle twitching may be early manifestations of peripheral nerve disease. Some 70% of patients with chronic renal failure have neuropathy, but most are subclinical and are identified by conduction studies. Symptoms include painful dysesthesia and glove-stocking loss of sensation, as well as weakness of distal muscles. Electrodiagnostic studies show a sensorimotor neuropathy with axonal features. Pathologic studies confirm the axonopathy. Segmental demyelination may result from axonal loss. Dialysis rarely reverses the neuropathy but may stabilize symptoms; peritoneal dialysis is more effective than hemodialysis. Serial nerve conduction studies can measure the effectiveness of hemodialysis. Renal transplantation often resolves the neuropathy shortly after surgery.

Mononeuropathy, particularly the carpal tunnel syndrome, often appears distal to an implanted arteriovenous fistula, suggesting ischemia as a possible mechanism. Distal ischemia from implanted bovine shunts may cause a more severe ischemic neuropathy in the median, ulnar, and radial nerves, possibly from excessive arteriovenous shunting. Chronic hemodialysis (more than 10 years) causes excessive accumulation of β_2-microglobulin (generalized amyloidosis), another possible cause of carpal tunnel syndrome and peripheral uremic neuropathy.

The cause of uremic neuropathy is uncertain. An accumulation of a toxic metabolite is most likely, but its identity is unknown. A 2- to 60-kDa molecular weight compound in the plasma of uremic patients induced an axonal neuropathy in experimental animals.

NEUROPATHY ASSOCIATED WITH HEPATIC DISEASE

Peripheral neuropathy is rarely associated with primary diseases of the liver. A chronic demyelinating neuropathy with chronic liver disease is usually subclinical. A painful sensory neuropathy is seen with primary biliary cirrhosis, probably caused by xanthoma formation in and around nerves. Electrodiagnostic studies may be normal, or the amplitude of the sensory evoked response may be low or absent. Nerve biopsy shows loss of small-diameter nerve fibers. Sudanophilic material is seen in cells of the perineurium. Treatment is directed at pain control. Tricyclic antidepressants or anticonvulsants may relieve paresthesia.

Infectious diseases of the liver may also be associated with peripheral neuropathy. Viral hepatitis (especially hepatitis C associated with cryoglobulinemia), HIV or CMV infection, and infectious mononucleosis may be associated with acute demyelinating neuropathy (GBS), chronic demyelinating neuropathy, or mononeuropathy multiplex. Immunologically mediated diseases such as polyarteritis and sarcoidosis may also cause liver abnormalities and mononeuropathy multiplex.

Peripheral neuropathy is often seen with toxic liver disease or hepatic metabolic diseases such as acute intermittent porphyria (see Chapter 90) and abetalipoproteinemia (see Chapter 91).

NEUROPATHIES ASSOCIATED WITH INFECTION

Neuropathy of Leprosy

Direct infiltration of small-diameter peripheral nerve fibers by *Mycobacterium leprae* causes the neuropathy of leprosy. It is the most common treatable neuropathy in the world. In the United States, the disease is less endemic but is seen in immigrants from India, Southeast Asia, and Central Africa.

Peripheral nerves are affected differently in tuberculoid and lepromatous forms. In tuberculoid leprosy, there are small hypopigmented areas with superficial sensory loss, and the underlying subcutaneous sensory nerves may be visibly or palpably enlarged. Large nerve trunks, such as the ulnar, peroneal, facial, and posterior auricular nerves, may be enmeshed in granulomas and scar tissue. Endoneurial caseation necrosis may occur. The clinical picture is one of mononeuritis or mononeuritis multiplex.

In lepromatous leprosy, Hansen bacilli proliferate in large numbers within Schwann cells and macrophages in the endoneurium and perineurium of subcutaneous nerve twigs (Fig. 105.5), particularly in cool areas of the body (pinnae of the ears and dorsum of the hands, forearms, and feet). Loss of cutaneous sensibility is observed in affected patches; these may later coalesce to cover large parts of the body. Position sense may be preserved in affected areas, whereas pain and temperature sensibility is lost, a dissociation similar to that in syringomyelia. Tendon reflexes are preserved.

Acute mononeuritis multiplex may appear during chemotherapy of lepromatous leprosy in conjunction with erythema nodosum. This complication is treated with thalidomide.

Treatment is designed to eradicate the bacterium using dapsone and to prevent secondary immune reactions that may damage nerves. Because of the dense sensory loss, painless and inadvertent traumatic injuries, such as self-inflicted burns, may occur without extreme caution to avoid trauma to the anesthetic areas.

Diphtheritic Neuropathy

Although diphtheria itself is rare, diphtheritic neuropathy is seen in approximately 20% of infected patients. *Corynebacterium diphtheriae* infects the larynx and pharynx, as well as cutaneous wounds. The organisms release an exotoxin that causes myocarditis and, later, symmetric neuropathy. The neuropathy of-

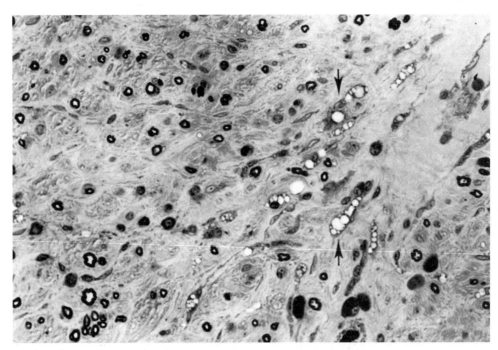

FIG. 105.5. Lepromatous leprous neuritis. Few myelinated fibers are scattered in fibrotic endoneurium. Abundant foam cells *(arrows)* contain *M. leprae* bacilli when viewed at higher magnification. (Courtesy of Dr. Arthur Asbury.)

ten begins with impaired visual accommodation and paresis of ocular and oropharyngeal muscles, and quadriparesis follows. Nerve conduction velocities are slow, reflecting the underlying demyelinating neuropathy. Diphtheria and its neuropathy may be prevented by immunization, and if infection occurs, antibiotic therapy may be used. Recovery may be slow, and physiologic measures resolve after the clinical syndrome.

HIV-related Neuropathies

Several neuropathies afflict patients infected with HIV, depending on the stage of the illness and the immunocompetence of the patient. An acute demyelinating neuropathy resembling GBS occurs early in the course of infection, often with no signs of immunodeficiency or at the time of seroconversion. This form of GBS with HIV infection differs from sporadic GBS in greater incidence of generalized lymphadenopathy, more frequent involvement of cranial nerves, and a higher frequency of other sexually transmitted diseases.

Subacute demyelinating neuropathy, clinically indistinguishable from idiopathic CIDP, is usually found in HIV-positive patients before there is evidence of immunodeficiency (AIDS). The CSF protein content is increased in both idiopathic CIDP and HIV-associated demyelinating neuropathy. The HIV syndrome, however, includes CSF pleocytosis, which is not seen in CIDP. Steroids, plasmapheresis, and IVIG therapy have been reported to be effective treatments.

Patients who fulfill diagnostic criteria for AIDS rarely have demyelinating neuropathy. Instead, there is a distal sensorimotor polyneuropathy with axonal features. The syndrome is dominated by severe painful paresthesia that affects the feet first and most intensely. This painful neuropathy can be the most functionally disabling manifestation of AIDS. The exact mechanism is uncertain, but one form is the diffuse infiltrating lymphocystosis syndrome, a hyperimmune reaction to HIV infection. No treatment reverses the symptoms, but carbamazepine (Tegretol) and amitriptyline may help.

Mononeuropathy multiplex occurs in HIV-infected patients at any stage of the disease, sometimes with hepatitis. When CD4 cells number less than $50/mm^3$, the likely cause of the mononeuropathy is CMV, and prompt treatment with ganciclovir sodium (Cytovene) may be life-saving. CMV infection is also associated with polyradiculopathy or GBS.

Neuropathy of Herpes Zoster

Varicella-zoster virus infection of the dorsal root ganglion produces radicular pain that may precede or follow the appearance of the characteristic skin eruption. Although primarily a sensory neuropathy, weakness from motor involvement occurs in 0.5% to 5% of infected patients, more often in elderly patients or those with a malignancy and usually in the same myotomal distribution as the dermatomal rash. Zoster infections are also associated with GBS and CSF pleocytosis. Because zoster infection often occurs in patients with HIV infection and CSF pleocytosis is seen in both conditions, the combination of herpes infection and focal weakness in a young person should alert the clinician to the possibility of HIV infection.

Herpes zoster may affect any level of the neuraxis, but it most often involves thoracic dermatomes and cranial nerves with sensory ganglia (V and VII). Ophthalmic herpes infection in the gasserian ganglion characteristically involves the first division of the trigeminal nerve. There may be weakness of ocular muscles and ptosis. Infection of the geniculate ganglion of the facial (VII) nerve causes a vesicular herpetic eruption in the external auditory meatus, vertigo, deafness, and facial weakness (Ramsay Hunt syndrome). Treatment with acyclovir (Zovirax), 4 g per day in five doses for 5 days, decreases the incidence of segmental motor neuritis and sensory axonopathy but does not reduce the incidence of postherpetic neuralgia.

SARCOID NEUROPATHY

Neurologic symptoms appear in 4% of patients with sarcoidosis. Most commonly, there are single or multiple cranial nerve palsies that fluctuate in intensity. Of the cranial nerves, the seventh is most commonly affected, and, as in diabetes mellitus, the facial nerve syndrome in sarcoidosis is indistinguishable from idiopathic Bell palsy. Some cranial neuropathies in sarcoidosis result from basilar meningitis. One distinguishing feature of sarcoid mononeuropathy is a large area of sensory loss on the trunk.

Patients with sarcoidosis occasionally experience symmetric polyneuropathy months or years after the diagnosis is established. The neuropathy may be the first manifestation before the diagnosis of sarcoidosis is made. The clinical syndromes may include GBS, lumbosacral plexopathy, mononeuritis multiplex, or pure sensory neuropathy. Almost all patients, however, have cranial nerve symptoms.

Nerve biopsy shows a mixture of wallerian degeneration and segmental demyelination with sarcoid granulomas in endoneurium and epineurium. Sarcoid neuropathy may respond to steroid therapy.

POLYNEUROPATHY ASSOCIATED WITH DIETARY STATES

The peripheral neuropathy of alcoholic abusers is well known, but the cause is still debated. No unequivocal evidence supports the concept that alcohol is toxic to peripheral nerve. A widely held belief is that the neuropathy of alcoholism is due to nutritional deficiency, particularly of vitamin B_1 (thiamine). *Thiamine deficiency* may cause two different clinical syndromes: *wet beriberi,* in which congestive heart failure is the predominant syndrome, and *dry beriberi,* in which peripheral neuropathy is the predominant symptom. The signs and symptoms of this neuropathy closely resemble those observed in alcoholics. Patients with thiamine deficiency have severe burning dysesthesia in the feet more than the hands, weakness and wasting of distal more than proximal muscles, trophic changes (shiny skin, hair loss), and sensory loss that is worse in distal portions of the legs. EMG and nerve conduction studies reveal the presence of a diffuse sensorimotor peripheral neuropathy that is axonal in nature. Axonal degeneration is also the principal finding seen on nerve biopsy specimens. Treatment of both beriberi and alcoholic neuropathy should be initiated with parenteral B-complex vitamins followed by oral thiamine. Recovery is slow; there may be residual muscular weakness and atrophy.

Niacin (nicotinic acid) deficiency causes pellagra characterized by hyperkeratotic skin lesions. Peripheral neuropathy is usually present in patients deficient in niacin, but the neuropathy does not improve with niacin supplementation. Symptoms improve only when thiamine and pyridoxine are added to the diet.

Vitamin B$_{12}$ deficiency causes the classic clinical syndrome of subacute combined degeneration of the spinal cord. Separation of the peripheral neuropathic symptoms from spinal cord involvement is difficult. Painful paresthesia accompanies vitamin B$_{12}$ deficiency, probably as a result of spinal cord involvement.

Vitamin B$_6$ (pyridoxine) deficiency produces a peripheral neuropathy, and the most common cause of pyridoxine deficiency is ingestion of the antituberculous drug, isoniazid. Isoniazid increases the excretion of pyridoxine. The resulting neuropathy affects sensory more than motor fibers and is caused by axonal loss. Treatment consists of administering excessive amounts of pyridoxine to compensate for the added excretion. The neuropathy can be prevented by prophylactic pyridoxine administration. Occasionally, isoniazid also elicits a vasculitic mononeuropathy multiplex.

Vitamin E deficiency contributes to neuropathy in fat malabsorption syndromes (e.g., chronic cholestasis). The clinical syndrome of vitamin E deficiency resembles spinocerebellar degeneration with ataxia, severe sensory loss of joint position and vibration, and hyporeflexia. Motor nerve conduction studies are normal, but sensory evoked responses are of low amplitude or absent. Somatosensory evoked responses show a delay in central conduction. EMG is usually normal. Vitamin E deficiency occurs in most fat malabsorption disorders including abetalipoproteinemia, congenital biliary atresia, pancreatic dysfunction, and surgical removal of large portions of the small intestine.

CRITICAL ILLNESS POLYNEUROPATHY

Severe sensorimotor peripheral neuropathy is seen in many patients who are critically ill, suffering from sepsis and multiple organ failure. Although this disorder may be suggested by other clinical manifestations, the diagnosis may arise when a patient experiences difficulty being weaned from a ventilator. Electrodiagnostic studies show a severe sensorimotor axonal neuropathy, but some pathologic studies have shown little axonal loss and extensive type 1 and 2 fiber atrophy disorder, a pattern attributed to pharmacologic denervation or treatment with drugs that interfere with neuromuscular transmission. A disorder of nerve terminals has been proposed.

Recovery of neuronal function may occur if the underlying cause of multiple organ failure is treated successfully. The cause is unknown, but dietary deficiency is not likely. Many respirator-dependent patients with critical illness neuropathy have received neuromuscular blocking agents, which may be the main cause.

Mononeuritis or mononeuritis multiplex occurs in 2% of patients with bacterial endocarditis because of septic emboli to peripheral nerves. Some patients with bacterial endocarditis may experience a severe axonal neuropathy, thought to be similar to the axonopathy seen in patients with critical illness polyneuropathy.

NEUROPATHIES CAUSED BY HEAVY METALS
Arsenic

Neuropathy may follow chronic exposure to small amounts of arsenic or ingestion or parenteral administration of a large amount. Chronic exposure may occur in industries in which arsenic is released as a byproduct, such as the copper smelting industry. Because of the prevalence of these byproducts, arsenic neuropathy is the most common of all heavy metal–induced neuropathies. Gastrointestinal symptoms, vomiting, and diarrhea occur when a toxic quantity of arsenic is ingested, but these symptoms may be absent if the arsenic is given parenterally or taken in small amounts over long periods. In acute arsenic poisoning, the onset of symptoms is delayed 4 to 8 weeks; once symptoms develop, they reach maximum intensity within a few days. The evolution of polyneuropathy is much slower in chronic arsenic poisoning. Sensory symptoms are prominent in the early stages. Pain and paresthesia in the legs may be present for several days or weeks before onset of weakness. The weakness progresses to complete flaccid paralysis of the legs and sometimes the arms. Cutaneous sensation is impaired in a stocking-and-glove distribution, with vibration and position sensation being most affected. Tendon reflexes are lost. Pigmentation and hyperkeratosis of the skin and changes in the nails (*Mees lines*) are frequently present. Arsenic is present in the urine in the acute stages of poisoning and, later, in the hair and nails. Nerve conduction velocities may be normal or mildly diminished; the amplitude of sensory evoked responses may be reduced. Pathologic examination of nerves shows axonal degeneration. Arsenic polyneuropathy should be treated with a chelating agent. Effectiveness of chelation therapy can be monitored by measuring arsenic excretion rates in 24-hour samples.

Lead

Most toxic neuropathies cause a symmetric weakness and loss of sensation in distal more than proximal regions, feet worse than legs. In contrast to most other toxic neuropathies, lead poisoning causes focal weakness of the extensor muscles of the fingers and wrist. Pure motor bilateral arm weakness and wasting may be caused by chronic lead intoxication.

Lead neuropathy occurs almost exclusively in adults. Infants poisoned with lead usually experience encephalopathy. Lead may enter the body through the lungs, skin, or gut. Occupational lead poisoning is encountered in battery workers, painters, and pottery glazers. Accidental lead poisoning follows ingestion of lead in food or beverages, or occurs in children who ingest lead paint. Lead poisoning may cause abdominal distress (lead colic). By its effect on renal tubules, lead poisoning often causes urate retention and gout. Weakness usually begins in distinct muscles innervated by the radial nerve, sparing the brachioradialis; it is often bilateral. Later, the weakness may extend to other muscles in the arms and, occasionally, to the legs. Sensory symptoms and signs are usually absent. Rarely, upper motor neuron signs occur with the lower motor neuron disorder and mimic ALS. Laboratory findings include anemia with basophilic stippling of the red cells, increased serum uric acid, and slight elevation of CSF protein content. Nerve conduction velocities are usually normal, raising the possibility that the disorder may be an anterior horn cell disorder rather than a neuropathy. Urinary lead excretion is elevated, particularly after administration of a chelating agent. Urinary porphobilinogen excretion is also elevated, but β-aminolevulinic acid is normal. Primary therapy is prevention of further exposure to lead. With termination of exposure and use of chelation therapy, recovery is gradual over several months.

Mercury

Mercury is used in the electrical and chemical industries. There are two forms of mercury: elemental and organic. The organic form of mercury (methyl and ethylmercury) is most toxic to the central nervous system (CNS), although distal paresthesia is a prominent symptom (presumably secondary to dorsal root ganglion degeneration). Ventral roots are spared.

Inorganic mercury may be absorbed through the gastrointestinal tract, and elemental mercury may be absorbed directly through the skin or lungs (it is volatile at room temperature). Elemental mercury exposure primarily causes weakness and wasting more than sensory symptoms. However, electrophysiologic studies reveal axonal affection of both motor and sensory fibers. Because of the prominent motor manifestations, confusion with ALS may occur.

Thallium

This element is used as a rodenticide and in other industrial processes. As with lead, children exposed to thallium are more likely to experience encephalopathy, whereas neuropathy develops in adults. In contrast to lead poisoning, however, thallium neuropathy is primarily sensory and autonomic. Severe disturbing dysesthesia appears acutely, and diffuse alopecia is a characteristic feature of thallium poisoning. Signs of cardiovascular autonomic neuropathy are sometimes delayed and recover slowly. Electrophysiologic findings are consistent with an axonal neuropathy.

Other Chemicals

Triorthocresyl phosphate (Jamaican ginger or "jake"), an adulterant used in illegal liquor (moonshine) and as a cooking oil contaminant, has been responsible for epidemics of neuropathy. A symmetric distal motor polyneuropathy progresses for 2 to 3 weeks and may be confused with ALS. In later stages, upper motor neuron findings appear. Electrophysiologic studies, however, show axonal loss in sensory nerves, as well as motor fibers. Nerve biopsy shows distal axonal fragmentation. As the neuropathy clears, evidence of previously unrecognized irreversible damage to corticospinal tracts may become apparent, and late spasticity becomes a problem.

Acrylamide monomer is used to prepare polyacrylamide. It is used in chemical laboratories and for the treatment of liquid sewerage. Exposure produces a distal sensorimotor neuropathy that

may be associated with trophic skin changes and a mild organic dementia. Nerve biopsy shows axonal degeneration with accumulations of neurofilaments in affected axons.

Many solvents used in manufacturing artificial materials or for polishing and dry cleaning are neurotoxic, as are many substances used in insecticides and rodenticides. The clinical and electrophysiologic features are similar to those of neuropathies caused by chemotherapeutics. Some, however, affect the CNS, as well as peripheral nerves, and some have certain specific features. For instance, *dimethylaminopropionitrile*, which is used to manufacture polyurethane foam, causes urologic dysfunction and sensory loss localized to sacral dermatomes. Exposure to *methylbromide*, an insecticide, results in a mixture of pyramidal tract, cerebellar, and peripheral nerve dysfunction. Accidental ingestion of *pyriminil*, a rat poison marketed under the name Vacor, gives rise to an acute severe distal axonopathy with prominent autonomic involvement accompanied by acute diabetes mellitus secondary to necrosis of pancreatic beta cells.

NEUROPATHIES CAUSED BY THERAPEUTIC DRUGS

A distal axonopathy is a common reaction to toxic chemicals, antineoplastic drugs, other medicaments, or industrial agents. Most of these neuropathies are dose-related, presenting with predominantly sensory symptoms and signs or with a combination of sensory and motor involvement. Numerous substances causing neuropathy have been described, and the interested reader should consult comprehensive reviews cited in the suggested readings. Here, we mention only a few to illustrate typical clinical features.

The most commonly used antineoplastic agents are *vincristine* and *cisplatin* (Platinol). Vincristine causes a symmetric progressive sensorimotor distal neuropathy that begins in the legs and is associated with areflexia. In contrast, cisplatin neuropathy is a pure sensory distal neuropathy with paresthesia, impaired vibration sense, and loss of ankle jerks. Motor and sensory conduction velocities are normal or mildly slowed in both conditions, but the most conspicuous finding is a marked reduction of the sensory action potential amplitude, implying loss of large myelinated fibers.

Paclitaxel (Taxol) is used to treat cancers of the breast, ovary, and lung. It causes a predominantly sensory neuropathy, but administration of a single high-dose may affect motor fibers, as well. Long-term administration of other therapeutic drugs, such as nitrofurantoin for treatment of pyelonephritis and amiodarone hydrochloride (Cordarone) for cardiac arrhythmias, may cause a severe symmetric distal sensorimotor neuropathy. Long-lasting therapy with phenytoin sodium (Dilantin) may give rise to distal sensory impairment and areflexia. A predominantly motor neuropathy has been related to disulfiram (Antabuse) used to treat alcoholism, or to dapsone for leprosy.

DIABETIC NEUROPATHY

The broad diversity of neurologic complications in patients with diabetes mellitus can be considered to consist of two distinct types. In one form, the symptoms and signs are transient; in the other, they progress steadily. The transient category includes acute painful neuropathies, mononeuropathies, and radiculopathies. The painful type starts abruptly with a disabling and continuous pain, often a burning sensation in a stocking distribution. Sometimes, the pain is localized to the thighs as a femoral neuropathy. The pain may last for months. Recovery from severe pain, however, is usually complete within 1 year, and the disorder does not necessarily progress to a conventional sensory polyneuropathy.

The progressive type comprises sensorimotor polyneuropathies with or without autonomic symptoms and signs. Although the actual cause of diabetic neuropathies is unknown, focal nerve involvement is considered to be vascular; and progressive symmetric polyneuropathy is probably due to a metabolic disorder. There may be as many causal factors as there are different clinical pictures. However, it seems that hyperglycemic hypoxia is mainly responsible for the conduction changes seen in damaged diabetic nerves. Dysfunction of ion conductances, especially voltage-gated ion channels, could contribute to abnormalities in the generation and conduction of action potentials.

A syndrome recognized by a triad of pain, severe asymmetric muscle weakness, and wasting of the iliopsoas, quadriceps, and adductor muscles is named *diabetic amyotrophy.* Onset is usually acute, but it may evolve over weeks. It occurs primarily in older noninsulin-dependent diabetics and is often accompanied by severe weight loss and cachexia. Knee jerks are absent, but there is little or no sensory loss. The condition resolves spontaneously but may last 1 to 3 years.

Mononeuropathies

It is generally believed but has never been proved that focal neuropathies are more frequent in diabetic patients than in the general population. The syndromes are usually localized to the common sites of nerve entrapment or external compression and may imply an increased liability to pressure palsies. This applies to the median nerve at the carpal tunnel, the ulnar at the elbow, and the peroneal at the fibular head. The electrophysiologic features are similar to those seen in nondiabetic patients with pressure palsies, except that abnormalities outside the clinically affected areas sometimes indicate that the palsies are superimposed on a generalized neuropathy. Cranial nerve palsies are most often localized to the third and sixth nerves. They start abruptly and usually spontaneously resolve completely within 6 months; relapses are rare.

Generalized Polyneuropathies

The most common diabetic neuropathy is a diffuse distal symmetric and predominantly sensory neuropathy with or without autonomic manifestations. Distal limb weakness is usually minor. The neuropathy develops slowly and is related to the duration of the diabetes, but not all patients are so afflicted. Once present, it never remits or recovers. Whether strict diabetic control or other measures can alter the course is still a matter of debate. Most evidence suggests that small nerve fibers, both myelinated and unmyelinated, are affected first. Thus, pain and

temperature sensation transmitted through the smallest fibers may be affected before the large-fiber modalities (vibration, light touch, position sense). Small-fiber function can be evaluated by determining thresholds for warming and cooling or by a pinprick threshold technique using weighted needles. Perception of cooling and pinprick is conveyed by small myelinated fibers; the sense of warming is carried by unmyelinated fibers.

The prevalence of diabetic autonomic neuropathy may be underestimated because nonspecific symptoms are undiagnosed or the condition may be asymptomatic. Symptoms appear insidiously, long after the onset of diabetes. They progress slowly and are usually irreversible. It is essential to screen for autonomic involvement in diabetics because those who have abnormal cardiovascular reflexes have an excess mortality risk of 56% compared with 11% for the general diabetic population, when followed up to 5 years. Autonomic function tests include determination of the heart rate at rest, during deep breathing, and during standing by measuring the electrocardiographic RR intervals (predominantly parasympathetic function); the change in mean arterial blood pressure from supine to standing position also tests the sympathetic function.

Slowing of motor and sensory conduction is a common finding in diabetics even among those without overt neuropathy. It is generally attributed to axonal degeneration with secondary demyelination. Therapeutic attempts, including continuous subcutaneous insulin infusion to correct hyperglycemia to prevent the diabetic complications, have been unsuccessful in most instances. Although combined pancreas and kidney transplantation may halt the progression of diabetic polyneuropathy, the long-term effect is still doubtful. Patients with burning pain may benefit from amitriptyline, but side effects often preclude treatment. Desipramine, which acts by blocking norepinephrine reuptake, may be a better choice.

BRACHIAL NEUROPATHY

This syndrome, also known as *neuralgic amyotrophy,* is characterized by acute onset of severe pain localized to the shoulder region and followed shortly by weakness of the shoulder girdle or arm muscles ipsilateral to the pain. It may be bilateral and asymmetric. Paresthesia and sensory loss may also be noted. In about 50% of patients, the clinical pattern is a mononeuropathy multiplex, followed by mononeuropathy in 33% and plexopathy in 20%. Autoimmune or infectious causes have been suggested, but the etiology is obscure. Some cases have occurred in small epidemics among military personnel, and the disorder may follow intravenous administration of heroin.

The typical EMG findings, including motor and sensory nerve studies, are consistent with a predominantly axonal neuropathy, but demyelination occasionally plays a role. The diversity of physiologic disorders in different nerves or even within the same nerve is attributed to involvement of the terminal nerve twigs or to patchy damage of discrete bundles of fibers within the cords or trunks of the brachial plexus or its branches. Recovery depends on the severity of the initial insult. It is considered good in about 66%, fair in 20%, and poor in 14%. Clinical recovery may take 2 months to 3 years.

RADIATION NEUROPATHY

Irradiation for carcinoma may damage nervous tissue, especially since the introduction of high-voltage therapy. Lesions of the brachial plexus are seen after radiotherapy for breast cancer; caudal roots and lumbosacral plexus are sometimes affected by radiation therapy for testicular cancer or Hodgkin disease. The first symptom is usually severe pain, followed by paresthesia and sensory loss. There may be a latent period of 12 to 20 months; in milder cases, several years may elapse before symptoms appear. Limb weakness peaks many months later. Latency intervals of up to 20 years have been reported. The damage may affect a single peripheral nerve initially and then progress slowly to involve others. Clinically, tendon reflexes disappear before weakness and atrophy become obvious; fasciculation and myokymia may be prominent. EMG and conduction studies reveal changes consistent with axonal damage; myokymic discharges are thought to be helpful in differentiating plexopathy caused by radiation from plexopathy caused by infiltration by malignancy.

LYME NEUROPATHY

Lyme disease is increasingly diagnosed in the United States and Europe. It is caused by a tick-borne spirochete, *Borrelia burgdorferi*. The most common clinical feature of neuroborreliosis is a painful sensory radiculitis, which may appear about 3 weeks after the erythema migrans. Pain intensity varies from day to day and is often severe, jumping from one area to another and often associated with patchy areas of unpleasant dysesthesia. Focal neurologic signs are common and may present as cranial neuropathy (61%), limb paresis (12%), or both (16%). The facial nerve is most frequently affected; involvement is unilateral twice as often as bilateral. Abducens and oculomotor paresis occasionally occurs. Myeloradiculitis and chronic progressive encephalomyelitis are rare. In some, the disorder is associated with dilated cardiomyopathy. Arthralgia is common among patients in the United States but rare among Europeans (6%). The triad of painful radiculitis, predominantly cranial mononeuritis multiplex, and lymphocytic pleocytosis in the CSF is known as *Bannwarth syndrome* in Europe. Peripheral nerve biopsy shows perineurial and epineurial vasculitis and axonal degeneration, consistent with the electrophysiologic findings. The diagnosis of neuroborreliosis is based on the presence of inflammatory CSF changes and specific intrathecal *B. burgdorferi* antibodies. In some infected patients, however, no free antibodies are detectable. Antigen detection in CSF could then be helpful. Polymerase chain reaction technique for detecting spirochetes or spirochetal DNA turned out to be less specific. The prognosis is good after high-dose penicillin treatment. Disabling sequelae are rare and occur mainly in patients with previous CNS lesions.

SUGGESTED READINGS

General

Dyck PJ, Thomas PK, Griffin JW, eds. *Peripheral neuropathy.* Philadelphia: WB Saunders, 1993.

Maravilla KR, Bowen BC. Imaging of the peripheral nervous system: evaluation of peripheral neuropathy and plexopathy. *AJNR* 1998;19:1011–1023.

Guillain-Barré Syndrome and Variants

Feasby TE, Gilbert JJ, Brown WP, et al. An acute axonal form of Guillain-Barré polyneuropathy. *Brain* 1986;109:1115–1126.

Feasby TE, Hughes RAC. *Campylobacter jejuni,* antiganglioside antibodies, and Guillain-Barré syndrome. *Neurology* 1998;51:340–342.

Gorson KC, Allam G, Ropper AH. Chronic inflammatory demyelinating polyneuropathy: clinical features and response to treatment in 67 consecutive patients with and without a monoclonal gammopathy. *Neurology* 1997;48:321–328.

Hadden RDM, Cornblath DR, Hughes RAC, et al. Electrophysiological classification of Guillain-Barré syndrome: clinical associations and outcome. *Ann Neurol* 1998;44:780–788.

Hainfellner JA, Kristoferitsch W, Lassman H, et al. T-cell mediated ganglioneuritis associated with acute sensory neuronopathy. *Ann Neurol* 1996;39:543–547.

Hartung HP, Pollard JD, Harvey GK, Tokya KV. Immunopathogenesis and treatment of the Guillain-Barré syndrome—part 1. *Muscle Nerve* 1995;18:137–153.

Hartung HP, Pollard JD, Harvey GK, Tokya KV. Immunopathogenesis and treatment of the Guillain-Barré syndrome—part 2. *Muscle Nerve* 1995;18:154–164.

Ho TW, Willison HJ, Nachamkin I, et al. Anti-GD1a antibody is associated with axonal but not demyelinating forms of Guillain-Barré syndrome. *Ann Neurol* 1999;45:168–173.

Latov N. Antibodies to glycoconjugates in neuropathy and motor neuron disease. *Prog Brain Res* 1993;101:295–303.

McKhann GM, Cornblath DR, Griffin JW, et al. Acute motor axonal neuropathy: a frequent cause of acute flaccid paralysis in China. *Ann Neurol* 1993;33:333–342.

Ogino M, Nobile-Orazio E, Latov N. IgG anti-GM1 antibodies from patients with acute motor axonal neuropathy are predominantly of the IgG1 and IgG3 subclass. *J Neuroimmunol* 1995;58:77–80.

Plomp JJ, Molenaar PC, O'Hanlon GM, et al. Miller Fisher anti-GQ1b antibodies: latrotoxin-like effects on motor end plates. *Ann Neurol* 1999;45:189–199.

Randomised trial of plasma exchange, intravenous immunoglobulin, and combined treatments in Guillain-Barré syndrome. Plasma Exchange/Sandoglobulin Guillain-Barré Trial Group. *Lancet* 1997;349:225–230.

Roper AH, Wijdicks EF, Truax BT. *Guillain-Barré syndrome.* Philadelphia: FA Davis Co, 1991.

Smit AA, Vermeulen M, Koelman JH, Wieling W. Unusual recovery from acute panautonomic neuropathy after immunoglobulin therapy. *Mayo Clin Proc* 1997;72:333–335.

Steck AJ, Schaeren-Wiemers N, Hartung HP. Demyelinating inflammatory neuropathies, including Guillain-Barré sydrome. *Curr Opin Neurol* 1998;11:311–316.

Trojaborg W. Acute and chronic neuropathies: new aspects of Guillain-Barré syndrome and chronic inflammatory demyelinating polyneuropathy, an overview and an update. *Electroencephalogr Clin Neurophysiol* 1998;107:303–316.

Chronic Inflammatory Demyelinating Polyneuropathy

Bouchard C, Lacroix C, Plante V, et al. Clinicopathologic findings and prognosis of chronic inflammatory demyelinating polyneuropathy. *Neurology* 1999;52:498–503.

Briani C, Brannagan TH, Trojaborg W, Latov N. Chronic inflammatory demyelinating polyneuropathy. *Neuromuscul Disord* 1996;6:311–325.

Case records of the Massachusetts General Hospital. Case 13-1998. Chronic inflammatory demyelinating polyneuropathy. *N Engl J Med* 1998;338:1212–1219.

Chroni E, Hall SM, Hughes RAC. Chronic relapsing axonal neuropathy: a first case report. *Ann Neurol* 1995;37:112–115.

Dyck PJ, Lais AC, Ohta M, et al. Chronic inflammatory polyradiculoneuropathy. *Mayo Clin Proc* 1975;50:621–637.

Good JL, Chehrenama M, Mayer RF, Koski CL. Pulse cyclophosphamide therapy in chronic inflammatory demyelinating polyneuropathy. *Neurology* 1998;51:1735–1738.

Hahn AF, Bolton CF, Zochodne D, et al. Intravenous gammaglobulin treatment in chronic inflammatory demyelinating polyneuropathy: a double blind, placebo-controlled, cross-over study. *Brain* 1996;119:1067–1077.

Moleneer DS, Vermeulen M, Haan R. Diagnostic value of sural nerve biopsy in chronic inflammatory demyelinating polyneuropathy. *J Neurol Neurosurg Psychiatry* 1998;64:84–89.

Research criteria for diagnosis of chronic inflammatory demyelinating polyneuropathy (CIDP). Report from an ad hoc subcommittee of the American Academy of Neurology AIDS Task Force. *Neurology* 1991;41:617–618.

Van Dijk GW, Notermans NC, Franssen H, Oey PL, Wokke JH. Response to intravenous immunoglobulin treatment in chronic inflammatory demyelinating polyneuropathy with only sensory symptoms. *J Neurol* 1996;243:318–322.

Multifocal Motor Neuropathy

Chaudhry V. Multifocal motor neuropathy. *Semin Neurol* 1998;18:73–81.

Chaudhry V, Corse AM, Cornblath DR, et al. Multifocal motor neuropathy: response to human immune globulin. *Ann Neurol* 1993;33:237–242.

Jaspert A, Claus D, Grehl H, Neundorfer B. Multifocal motor neuropathy: clinical and electrophysiological findings. *J Neurol* 1996;243:684–692.

Kinsella L, Lange D, Trojaborg T, Sadiq SA, Latov N. The clinical and electrophysiologic correlates of anti-GM1 antibodies. *Neurology* 1994;44:1278–1282.

Pestronk A. Motor neuropathies, motor neuron disorders, and anti-glycolipid antibodies. *Muscle Nerve* 1991;14:927–936.

Idiopathic Sensory Neuronopathy or Ganglioneuritis

Asahina N, Kuwabara S, Asahina M, et al. D-penicillamine treatment for chronic sensory ataxic neuropathy associated with Sjögrens syndrome. *Neurology* 1998;51:1451–1453.

Griffin JW, Cornblath DR, Alexander E, et al. Ataxic sensory neuropathy and dorsal root ganglioneuritis associated with Sjögren's syndrome. *Ann Neurol* 1990;27:304–315.

Quattrini A, Corbo M, Dhaliwal SK, et al. Anti-sulfatide antibodies in neurological disease: binding to rat dorsal root ganglia neurons. *J Neurol Sci* 1992;112:152–159.

Sobue G, Yasuda T, Kachi T, et al. Chronic progressive sensory ataxic neuropathy: clinicopathological features of idiopathic and Sjögren's syndrome associated cases. *J Neurol* 1993;240:1–7.

Windebank AJ, Blexrud MD, Dyck PJ, et al. The syndrome of acute sensory neuropathy. *Neurology* 1990;40:584–589.

Idiopathic Autonomic Neuropathy

Kurokawa K, Noda K, Mimori Y, et al. A case of pandysautonomia with associated sensory ganglionopathy. *J Neurol Neurosurg Psychiatry* 1998;65:278–279.

Mericle RA, Triggs WJ. Treatment of acute pandysautonomia with intravenous immunoglobulin. *J Neurol Neurosurg Psychiatry* 1997;62:529–531.

Miyazoe S, Matsuo H, Ohnishi A, et al. Acquired idiopathic generalized anhidrosis with isolated sudomotor neuropathy. *Ann Neurol* 1998;44:378–381.

Vasculitic and Cryoglobulinemic Neuropathies

Ferri C, La Civita L, Longombardo R, Zignego AL, Pasero G. Mixed cryoglobulinaemia: a cross-road between autoimmune and lymphoproliferative disorders. *Lupus* 1998;7:275–279.

Nemni R, Corbo M, Fazio R, et al. Cryoglobulinemic neuropathy: a clinical, morphological and immunocytochemical study of 8 cases. *Brain* 1988;111:541–552.

Said G, Lacroix-Ciaudo C, Fujimura H, et al. The peripheral neuropathy of necrotizing arteritis: a clinicopathological study. *Ann Neurol* 1988;23:461–466.

Neuropathies Associated with Myeloma and Nonmalignant IgG or IgA Monoclonal Gammopathies

Kelly JJ Jr, Kyle RA, Latov N. *Polyneuropathies associated with plasma cell dyscrasias.* Boston: Martinus-Nijhoff, 1987.

Latov N. Neuropathic syndromes associated with monoclonal gammopathies. In: Waksman BH, ed. *Immunologic mechanisms in neurologic and psychiatric disease.* New York: Raven Press, 1989.

Pedersen SF, Pullman SL, Latov N, et al. Physiological tremor analysis of patients with anti-myelin-associated glycoprotein associated neuropathy and tremor. *Muscle Nerve* 1997;20:38–44.

Motor, Sensory, and Sensorimotor Neuropathies Associated with IgM Monoclonal or Polyclonal Autoantibodies to Peripheral Nerve

Carpo M, Pedotti R, Lolli F, et al. Clinical correlates and fine specificity of anti-GQ1b antibodies in peripheral neuropathy. *J Neurol Sci* 1998;155:186–191.

Chassande B, Leger JM, Younes-Chennoufi AB, et al. Peripheral neuropathy associated with IgM monoclonal gammopathy: correlations between M-protein antibody activity and clinical/electrophysiological features in 40 cases. *Muscle Nerve* 1998;21:55–62.

Elle E, Vital A, Steck A, et al. Neuropathy associated with benign anti-myelin-associated glycoprotein IgM gammopathy: clinical immunological, neurophysiological, pathological findings and response to treatment in 33 cases. *J Neurol* 1996;243:34–43.

Latov N. Antibodies to glycoconjugates in neuropathy and motor neuron disease. *Prog Brain Res* 1993;101:295–302.

Quattrini A, Corbo M, Dhaliwal SK, et al. Anti-sulfatide antibodies in neurological disease: binding to rat dorsal root ganglia neurons. *J Neurol Sci* 1992;112:152–159.

Yuki N, Yamamoto T, Hirata K. Correlation between cytomegalovirus infection and IgM anti-MAG/SGPG antibody-associated neuropathy. *Ann Neurol* 1998;44:408–410.

Amyloid Neuropathy

Benson MD. Familial amyloidotic polyneuropathy. *Trends Neurosci* 1989;12:88–92.

Kelly JJ Jr, Kyle RA, O'Brien PC, et al. The natural history of peripheral neuropathy in primary systemic amyloidosis. *Ann Neurol* 1979;6:1–7.

Quattrini A, Nemni R, Sferrazza B, et al. Amyloid neuropathy simulating lower motor neuron disease. *Neurology* 1998;51:600–602.

Neuropathy Associated with Carcinoma (Paraneoplastic Neuropathy)

Dalmau J, Graus F, Rosenblum MK, et al. Anti-Hu associated paraneoplastic encephalomyelitis/sensory neuropathy: a clinical study of 71 patients. *Medicine* 1992;71:59–72.

Eggers C, Hagel C, Pfeiffer G. Anti-Hu-associated paraneoplastic sensory neuropathy with peripheral nerve demyelination and microvasculitis. *J Neurol Sci* 1998;155:178–181.

Rowland LP, Schneck S. Neuromuscular disorders associated with malignant neoplastic disease. *J Chronic Dis* 1963;16:777–795.

Schold SC, Cho ES, Somasundaram M, et al. Subacute motor neuronopathy: a remote effect of lymphoma. *Ann Neurol* 1979;5:271–287.

Hypothyroid Neuropathy

Dyck PJ, Lambert EH. Polyneuropathy associated with hypothyroidism. *J Neuropathol Exp Neurol* 1970;9:631–658.

Misiunas A, Niepomniszcze H, Ravera B, et al. Peripheral neuropathy in subclinical hypothyroidism. *Thyroid* 1995;5:283–286.

Nemni R, Bottacchi E, Fazio R, et al. Polyneuropathy in hypothyroidism: clinical, electrophysiological and morphological findings in four cases. *J Neurol Neurosurg Psychiatry* 1987;50:1454–1460.

Perkins AT, Morgenlander JC. Endocrinologic causes of peripheral neuropathy: pins and needles in a stocking-and-glove pattern and other symptoms. *Postgrad Med* 1997;102:81–82, 90–92, 102–106.

Rao SN, Katiuar BC, Nair KRP, et al. Neuromuscular status in hypothyroidism. *Acta Neurol Scand* 1980;61:167–173.

Torres CF, Moxley RT. Hypothyroid neuropathy and myopathy: clinical and electrodiagnostic longitudinal findings. *J Neurol* 1990;237:271–274.

Acromegalic Neuropathy

Jamal GA, Kerr DJ, McLellaan AR, et al. Generalized peripheral nerve dysfunction in acromegaly: a study by conventional and novel neurophysiological techniques. *J Neurol Neurosurg Psychiatry* 1987;50:885–894.

Khaleeli AA, Levy RD, Edwards RHT, et al. The neuromuscular features of acromegaly: a clinical and pathological study. *J Neurol Neurosurg Psychiatry* 1984;47:1009–1015.

Low PA, McLeod JG, Turtle JR, et al. Peripheral neuropathy in acromegaly. *Brain* 1974;97:139–152.

Pickett JBE III, Layzer RB, Levin SR, et al. Neuromuscular complications of acromegaly. *Neurology* 1975;25:638–645.

Stewart BM. The hypertrophic neuropathy of acromegaly: a rare neuropathy associated with acromegaly. *Arch Neurol* 1966;14:107–110.

Uremic Neuropathy

Bolton CF. Peripheral neuropathies associated with chronic renal failure. *Can J Neurol Sci* 1980;7:89–96.

Bolton CF, Young GB. *Neurological complications of renal disease.* Boston: Butterworths, 1990.

Cantaro S, Zara G, Battaggia C, et al. *In vivo* and *in vitro* neurotoxic action of plasma ultrafiltrate from uraemic patients. *Nephrol Dial Transplant* 1998;13:2288–2293.

Pirzada NA, Morgenlander JC. Peripheral neuropathy in patients with chronic renal failure: a treatable source of discomfort and disability. *Postgrad Med* 1997;102:249–250, 255–257, 261.

Neuropathy Associated with Hepatic Disease

Inoue A, Tsukada M, Koh CS, et al. Chronic relapsing demyelinating polyneuropathy associated with hepatitis B infection. *Neurology* 1987;37:1663–1666.

Taukada N, Koh CS, Inoue A, et al. Demyelinating neuropathy associated with hepatitis B virus infection: detection of immune complexes composed of hepatitis B virus antigen. *Neurol Sci* 1987;77:203–210.

Thomas PK, Walker JC. Xanthomatous neuropathy in primary biliary cirrhosis. *Brain* 1965;88:1079–1088.

Zaltron S, Puoti M, Liberini P, et al. High prevalence of peripheral neuropathy in hepatitis C virus infected patients with symptomatic and asymptomatic cryoglobulinaemia. *J Gastroenterol Hepatol* 1998;30:391–395.

Neuropathy of Leprosy

Nations SP, Katz JS, Lyde CB, et al. Leprous neuropathy: an American perspective. *Semin Neurol* 1998;18:113–124.

Pedley JC, Harman DJ, Waudby H, et al. Leprosy in peripheral nerves: histopathological findings in 119 untreated patients in Nepal. *J Neurol Neurosurg Psychiatry* 1980;43:198–204.

Rosenberg RN, Lovelace RE. Mononeuritis multiplex in lepromatous leprosy. *Arch Neurol* 1968;19:310–314.

Sunderland S. The internal anatomy of nerve trunks in relation to the neural lesions of leprosy: observations on pathology, symptomatology and treatment. *Brain* 1973;95:865–888.

Thomas PK. Tropical neuropathies. *J Neurol* 1997;244:475–482.

Diphtheritic Neuropathy

Kurdi A, Abdul-Kader M. Clinical and electrophysiological studies of diphtheritic neuritis in Jordan. *J Neurol Sci* 1979;42:243–250.

Solders G, Nennesmo I, Persson A. Diphtheritic neuropathy: an analysis based on muscle and nerve biopsy and repeated neurophysiological and autonomic function tests. *J Neurol Neurosurg Psychiatry* 1989;52:876–880.

HIV-related Neuropathies

Behar R, Wiley C, McCutchan JA. Cytomegalovirus polyradiculopathy in AIDS. *Neurology* 1987;37:557–561.

Bradley WG, Shapshak P, Delgado S, et al. Morphometric analysis of the peripheral neuropathy of AIDS. *Muscle Nerve* 1998;21:1188–1195.

Calore EE, Shulte G, Penalva De Oliveira AC, et al. Nerve biopsy in patients with AIDS. *Pathologica* 1998;90:31–35.

Cornblath DR, McArthur JC, Kennedy PGE, et al. Inflammatory demyelinating peripheral neuropathies associated with human T-cell lymphotropic virus type III infection. *Ann Neurol* 1987;21:32–40.

Eidelberg D, Sotrel A, Vogel H, et al. Progressive polyradiculopathy in acquired immunodeficiency syndrome. *Neurology* 1986;36:912–916.

Gherardi RK, Chretien F, Delfau-Larue MH, et al. Neuropathy in diffuse infiltrative lymphocytosis syndrome. *Neurology* 1998;50:1041–1044.

Ho DD, Rota TR, Schooley RT, et al. Isolation of HTLV-III from cerebrospinal fluid and neural tissues of patients with neurological syndromes related to the acquired immunodeficiency syndrome. *N Engl J Med* 1985;313:1493–1497.

Lange DJ. Neuromuscular diseases associated with HIV infection. *Muscle Nerve* 1994;17:16–30.

Said G, Lacroix C, Chemoulli P, et al. Cytomegalovirus neuropathy in acquired immunodeficiency syndrome: a clinical and pathological study. *Ann Neurol* 1991;29:139–195.

So YT, Holtzman DM, Abrams DI, et al. Peripheral neuropathy associated with AIDS: prevalence and clinical features from a population-based survey. *Arch Neurol* 1988;45:945–948.

Neuropathy of Herpes Zoster

Denny-Brown D, Adams RD, Brady PJ. Pathologic features of herpes zoster: a note on "geniculate herpes." *Arch Neurol Psychiatry* 1944;51:216–231.

Glynn C, Crockford G, Gavaghan D, et al. Epidemiology of shingles. *J R Soc Med* 1990;15:712–716.

Gottschau P, Trojaborg W. Abdominal muscle paralysis associated with herpes zoster. *Acta Neurol Scand* 1991;84:344–347.

Kendall D. Motor complications of herpes zoster. *BMJ* 1957;2:616–618.

Mondelli M, Romano C, Passero S, et al. Effects of acyclovir on sensory axonal neuropathy, segmental motor paresis and postherpetic neuralgia in herpes zoster patients. *Eur Neurol* 1996;36:288–292.

Nurmikko T, Bowsher D. Somatosensory findings in post-herpetic neuralgia. *J Neurol Neurosurg Psychiatry* 1990;53:135–141.

Schmader K. Postherpetic neuralgia in immunocompetent elderly people. *Vaccine* 1998;16:1768–1770.

Watson CP, Babul N. Efficacy of oxycodone in neuropathic pain: a randomized trial in postherpetic neuralgia. *Neurology* 1998;50:1837–1841.

Watson CP, Vermich L, Chipman M, et al. Nortriptyline versus amitriptyline in postherpetic neuralgia: a randomized trial. *Neurology* 1998;51:1166–1171.

Bacterial Endocarditis

Pruitt AA, Rubin RH, Karchmer AW, et al. Neurologic complications of bacterial endocarditis. *Medicine* 1978;57:329–343.

Tick Paralysis

Swift TR, Ignacio OJ. Tick paralysis: electrophysiologic signs. *Neurology* 1975;25:1130–1133.

Sarcoid Neuropathy

Luke RA, Stem BJ, Krumholz A, et al. Neurosarcoidosis: the long-term clinical course. *Neurology* 1987;37:461–463.

Matthews WB. Sarcoid neuropathy. In: Dyck PJ, Thomas PK, Griffin JW, et al., eds. *Peripheral neuropathy.* Philadelphia: WB Saunders, 1993.

Nemni R, Galassi G, Cohen M, et al. Symmetric sarcoid polyneuropathy: analysis of a sural nerve biopsy. *Neurology* 1981;31:1217–1223.

Zuniga G, Ropper AH, Frank J. Sarcoid peripheral neuropathy. *Neurology* 1991;41:1558–1561.

Polyneuropathy Associated with Dietary States

Cooke WT, Smith WE. Neurological disorders associated with adult coeliac disease. *Brain* 1966;89:683–722.

Hillbom M, Weinberg A. Prognosis of alcoholic peripheral neuropathy. *J Neurol Neurosurg Psychiatry* 1984;47:699–703.

Kaplan JG, Pack D, Horoupian D, et al. Distal axonopathy associated with chronic gluten enteropathy: a treatable disorder. *Neurology* 1988;38:642–645.

Lossos A, River Y, Eliakim A, et al. Neurologic aspects of inflammatory bowel disease. *Neurology* 1995;45:416–421.

Sokol RJ, Guggenheim MA, Iannaccone ST, et al. Improved neurologic function after long-term correction of vitamin E deficiency in children with chronic cholestasis. *N Engl J Med* 1985;313:1580–1586.

Tredici G, Minazzi M. Alcohol neuropathy: an electron-microscopic study. *J Neurol Sci* 1975;25:333–346.

Victor M, Adams RD, Collins GH. *The Wernicke-Korsakoff syndrome.* Philadelphia: FA Davis Co, 1971.

Critical Illness Polyneuropathy

Bolton CF, Laverty DA, Brown JD, et al. Critically ill polyneuropathy: electrophysiological studies and differentiation from Guillain-Barré syndrome. *J Neurol Neurosurg Psychiatry* 1986;49:563–573.

Gorson KC, Ropper AH. Acute respiratory failure neuropathy: a variant of critical illness polyneuropathy. *Crit Care Med* 1993;21:267–271.

Hirano M, Ott BR, Raps EC, et al. Acute quadriplegic myopathy: a complication of treatment with steroids, nondepolarizing blocking agents, or both. *Neurology* 1992;42:2082–2087.

Rich MM, Raps EC, Bird SJ. Distinction between acute myopathy syndrome and critical illness polyneuropathy. *Mayo Clin Proc* 1995;70:198–200.

Schwarz J, Planck J, Briegel J, Straube A. Single-fiber electromyography, nerve conduction studies, and conventional electromyography in patients with critical-illness polyneuropathy: evidence for a lesion of terminal motor axons. *Muscle Nerve* 1997;20:696–701.

Wokke JH, Jennekens FG, van den Ord CJ, et al. Histological investigations of muscle atrophy and end plates in two critically ill patients with generalized weakness. *J Neurol Sci* 1988;88:95–106.

Zifko UA, Zipko HT, Bolton CF. Clinical and electrophysiological findings in critical illness polyneuropathy. *J Neurol Sci* 1998;159:186–193.

Neuropathy Produced by Metals and Therapeutic Agents

Buchthal F, Behse F. Electromyography and nerve biopsy in men exposed to lead. *Br J Ind Med* 1979;36:135–147.

Chu CC, Huang CC, Ryu SJ, Wu TN. Chronic inorganic mercury-induced peripheral neuropathy. *Acta Neurol Scand* 1998;98:461–465.

Daugaard GK, Petrera J, Trojaborg W. Electrophysiological study of the peripheral and central neurotoxic effect of cis-platin. *Acta Neurol Scand* 1987;76:86–93.

Davis LE, Standefer JC, Kornfeld M, et al. Acute thallium poisoning: toxicological and morphological studies of the nervous system. *Ann Neurol* 1981;10:38–44.

Feldman RG, Niles CA, Kelly-Hayes M, et al. Peripheral neuropathy in arsenic smelter workers. *Neurology* 1979;29:939–944.

Gignoux L, Cortinovis-Tourniaire P, Grimaud J, Moreau T, Confavreux C. A brachial form of motor neuropathy caused by lead poisoning. *Rev Neurol (Paris)* 1998;154:771–773

Goebel HH, Schmidt PF, Bohl J, et al. Polyneuropathy due to acute arsenic intoxication: biopsy studies. *J Neuropathol Exp Neurol* 1990;49:137–149.

Hansen SW, Helweg-Larsen S, Trojaborg W. Long-term neurotoxicity in patients treated with cisplatin, vinblastine and bleomycin for metastatic germ cell cancer. *J Clin Oncol* 1989;7:457–461.

Iñiguez C, Larrodé P, Mayordomo JI, et al. Reversible peripheral neuropathy induced by a single administration of high-dose paclitaxel. *Neurology* 1998;51:868–870.

Laquery A, Ronnel A, Vignolly B, et al. Thalidomide neuropathy: an electrophysiologic study. *Muscle Nerve* 1986;9:837–844.

Lehning EJ, Persuad A, Dyer KR, et al. Biochemical and morphologic characterization of acrylamide peripheral neuropathy. *Toxicol Appl Pharmacol* 1998;151:211–221.

McFall TL, Richards JS, Matthews G. Rehabilitation in an individual with chronic arsenic poisoning: medical, psychological, and social implications. *J Spinal Cord Med* 1998;21:142–147.

Nordentoft T, Andersen EB, Mogensen PH. Initial sensorimotor and delayed autonomic neuropathy in acute thallium poisoning. *Neurotoxicology* 1998;19:421–426.

Ochoa J. Isoniazid neuropathy in man: quantitative electron microscope study. *Brain* 1970;93:831–850.

Oh S. Electrophysiological profile in arsenic neuropathy. *J Neurol Neurosurg Psychiatry* 1991;54:1103–1105.

Parry GJ, Bredeson DE. Sensory neuropathy with low-dose pyridoxine. *Neurology* 1985;35:1466–1468.

Ramirez JA, Mendell JR, Warmolts JR, Griggs RC. Phenytoin neuropathy: structural changes in the sural nerve. *Ann Neurol* 1986;19:162–167.

Sahenk Z, Barohn R, New P, Mendell JR. Taxol neuropathy: electrodiagnostic and sural nerve biopsy findings. *Arch Neurol* 1994;51:726–729.

Schaumberg HH, Berger AR. Human toxic neuropathy due to industrial agents. *Ann Neurol* 1978;3:1533–1548.

Schaumberg HH, Kaplan J, Windebank A, et al. Sensory neuropathy from pyridoxine abuse: a new megavitamin syndrome. *N Engl J Med* 1983;309:445–448.

Diabetic Neuropathy

Asbury AK. Proximal diabetic neuropathy. *Ann Neurol* 1977;2:179–180.

Asbury AK, Aldredge H, Hershberg R, et al. Oculomotor palsy in diabetes mellitus: a clinicopathological study. *Brain* 1970;93:555–566.

Behse F, Buchthal F, Carlsen F. Nerve biopsy and conduction studies in diabetic neuropathy. *J Neurol Neurosurg Psychiatry* 1977;10:1072–1082.

Dyck PJ, Giannini C. Pathologic alterations in the diabetic neuropathies of humans: a review. *J Neuropathol Exp Neurol* 1996;55:1181–1193.

Dyck PL, Thomas PK, Asbury AK, et al. *Diabetic neuropathy.* Philadelphia: WB Saunders, 1987.

Harati Y, Gooch C, Swenson M, et al. Double-blind randomized trial of tramadol for the treatment of the pain of diabetic neuropathy. *Neurology* 1998;50:1842–1846.

Lauria G, McArthur JC, Hauer PE, et al. Neuropathological alterations in diabetic truncal neuropathy: evaluation by skin biopsy. *J Neurol Neurosurg Psychiatry* 1998;65:762–766.

Llewelyn JG, Thomas PK, King RH. Epineurial microvasculitis in proximal diabetic neuropathy. *J Neurol* 1998;245:159–165.

Low PA, Walsh JC, Huang CY, et al. The sympathetic nervous system in diabetic neuropathy: a clinical and pathological study. *Brain* 1975;98:341–356.

Navarro X, Sutherland DE, Kennedy WR. Long-term effects of pancreatic transplantation on diabetic neuropathy. *Ann Neurol* 1998;44:149–150.

Quasthoff S. The role of axonal ion conductances in diabetic neuropathy: a review. *Muscle Nerve* 1998;21:1246–1255.

Report of the expert committee on the diagnosis and classification of diabetes mellitus. *Diabetes Care* 1997;20:1183–1197.

Said G, Elgrably F, Lacroix C, et al. Painful proximal diabetic neuropathy: inflammatory nerve lesions and spontaneous favorable outcome. *Ann Neurol* 1997;41:762–770.

Thomas PK. Diabetic neuropathy: models, mechanisms and mayhem. *Can J Neurol Sci* 1992;19:1–7.

Watkins PJ, Thomas PK. Diabetes mellitus and the nervous system. *J Neurol Neurosurg Psychiatry* 1998;65:620–632.

Brachial Neuropathy

Beghi E, Kurland LT, Mulder DW, et al. Brachial plexus neuropathy in the population of Rochester, Minnesota, 1970–1981. *Neurology* 1985;18:320–323.

Evans BA, Stevens JC, Dyck PJ. Lumbosacral plexus neuropathy. *Neurology* 1981;31:1327–1330.

Petrera JE. *Neuralgic amyotrophy: a clinical and electrophysiological study.* Thesis. Copenhagen: University of Copenhagen 1992:163.

Richter RW, Pearson J, Bruun B, Challenor YB, Brust JC, Baden MM. Neurological complications of addiction to heroin. *Bull N Y Acad Med* 1973;49:3–21.

Tsairis P, Dyck PJ, Mulder DW. Natural history of brachial plexus neuropathy: report on 99 patients. *Arch Neurol* 1972;27:109–117.

Radiation Neuropathy

Albers JW, Allen AA, Bastron JA, et al. Limb myokymia. *Muscle Nerve* 1981;4:494–504.

Foley KM, Woodruff JM, Ellis FT, Posner JB. Radiation-induced malignant and atypical peripheral nerve sheath tumors. *Ann Neurol* 1980;7:311–318.

Giese WL, Kinsella TJ. Radiation injury to peripheral and cranial nerves. In: Gulin PH, Leibel SH, eds. *Injury to the nervous system.* New York: Raven Press, 1991:383–406.

Lalu T, Mercier B, Birouk N, et al. Pure motor neuropathy after radiation therapy: 6 cases. *Rev Neurol (Paris)* 1998;154:40–44.

Lamy C, Mas JL, Varet B, et al. Postradiation lower motor neuron syndrome presenting as monomelic amyotrophy. *J Neurol Neurosurg Psychiatry* 1991;54:648–649.

Mollman JE. Neuromuscular toxicity of therapy. *Curr Opin Oncol* 1992;3:340–346.

Stoll BA, Andrews JT. Radiation-induced peripheral neuropathy. *BMJ* 1966;1:834–837.

Lyme Neuropathy

Coyle PK, Deng Z, Schutzer SE, et al. Detection of *Borrelia burgdorferi* antigens in cerebrospinal fluid. *Neurology* 1993;43:1093–1098.

Halperin J, Lul BJ, Volhnan DJ, et al. Lyme neuroborreliosis: peripheral nervous system manifestations. *Brain* 1990;11:1207–1221.

Hansen K, Lebech AM. The clinical and epidemiological profile of Lyme neuroborreliosis in Denmark 1985–1990: a prospective study of 187 patients with *Borrelia burgdorferi* specific intrathecal antibody production. *Brain* 1992;115:399–423.

Henriksson A, Link H, Cruz M, et al. Immunoglobulin abnormalities in cerebrospinal fluid and blood over the course of lymphocytic meningoradiculitis (Bannwarth's syndrome). *Ann Neurol* 1986;20:337–345.

Pachner AR, Steere AC. The triad of neurologic manifestations of Lyme disease: meningitis, cranial neuritis, and radiculoneuritis. *Neurology* 1985;35:47–53.

Reik L Jr, Burgdorfer W, Donaldson JO. Neurologic abnormalities in Lyme disease without chronicum migrans. *Am J Med* 1986;81:73–78.

Vailat JM, Hugon J, Lubeau M, et al. Tickbite meningoradiculoneuritis: clinical, electrophysiologic, and histologic findings in 10 cases. *Neurology* 1987;37:749–753.

Wulff CH, Hansen K, Strange P, Trojaborg W. Multiple mononeuritis and radiculitis with erythema, pain, elevated CSF protein and pleocytosis (Bannwarth's syndrome). *J Neurol Neurosurg Psychiatry* 1983;46:485–490.

Merritt's Neurology, 10th ed., edited by L.P. Rowland. Lippincott Williams & Wilkins, Philadelphia © 2000.

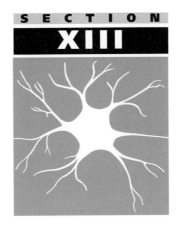

DEMENTIAS

CHAPTER 106

ALZHEIMER DISEASE AND RELATED DEMENTIAS

SCOTT A. SMALL
RICHARD MAYEUX

The defining features of dementia have evolved since the term was first introduced over 300 years ago. In this era of standardized criteria, those of the *Diagnostic and Statistical Manual of Mental Disorders*, 4th edition (DSM-IV) are most commonly used. According to DSM-IV, the diagnosis of dementia requires "the development of multiple cognitive deficits that are sufficiently severe to cause impairment in occupational or social functioning." The cognitive deficits must involve memory and other cognitive domains, must represent a decline from premorbid function, and cannot be attributed to delirium (see Chapter 1).

The cellular and molecular mechanisms underlying the pathogenesis of various forms of dementia have been elaborated in the last decade. Although there are many similarities, there are also important differences. Thus, the need for a classification system remains. Dementia can be grouped into four major categories: degenerative, vascular, infectious, and metabolic diseases.

DEGENERATIVE DISEASES

Alzheimer Disease

The most frequently encountered dementia was named after Alois Alzheimer by Kraeplin. Alzheimer described the clinical features and the pathologic manifestations of dementia in a 51-year-old woman at the turn of the century. For many years Alzheimer disease was considered a presenile form of dementia, limited to individuals with symptoms beginning before the age of 65. However, subsequent clinical, pathologic, ultrastructural, and biochemical analyses indicated that Alzheimer disease is identical to the more common senile dementia beginning after age 65.

Clinical Syndrome

The manifestations of Alzheimer disease evolve uniformly from the earliest signs of impaired memory to severe cognitive loss. The clinical course is progressive, terminating inevitably in complete incapacity and death. Plateaus sometimes occur; cognitive impairment does not change for a year or two, but progression then resumes.

Memory impairment for newly acquired information is the usual initial presenting complaint, whereas memory for remote events is relatively unimpaired at the beginning of the illness. As the disease progresses, deficits in language, abstract reasoning, and executive function can be elicited on specific probing. Ma-

jor depression with insomnia or anorexia occurs in 5% to 8% of patients with Alzheimer disease unrelated to severity. Delusions and psychotic behavior increase with progression of Alzheimer disease and remain persistent in 20%. Agitation may coexist in up to 20%, increasing with advanced disease. Hallucinations occur with similar frequency and may be either visual or auditory.

Except for the mental state, the neurologic examination is usually normal, but extrapyramidal features, including rigidity, bradykinesia, shuffling gait, and postural change, are relatively common in later stages of the disease. Primary motor and sensory functions are otherwise spared. Oculomotor, cerebellar, or peripheral nerve abnormalities on physical examination strongly raise the possibility of some other form of dementia.

Diagnosis

Criteria for the clinical diagnosis of Alzheimer disease were established by a joint effort of the National Institute of Neurological and Communicative Disorders and Stroke and the Alzheimer Disease and Related Disorders Association in 1984 and are referred to as the NINCDS-ADRDA criteria. These include a history of progressive deterioration in cognitive ability in the absence of other known neurologic or medical problems. Psychologic testing, brain imaging, and other criteria establish three levels of diagnostic certainty. The designation of "definite" Alzheimer disease is reserved for autopsy-confirmed disease. If there is no associated illness, the condition is called "probable" Alzheimer disease; "possible" refers to these who meet criteria for dementia but have another illness that may contribute, such as hypothyroidism or cerebrovascular disease. Comparing the clinical with the pathologic diagnosis, the NINCDS-ADRDA criteria provide 90% sensitivity for the diagnosis of probable or possible Alzheimer disease and 60% specificity. The designation of definite Alzheimer disease has been reserved only for autopsy-confirmed disease.

There are no specific changes in routine laboratory examinations. Cerebrospinal fluid (CSF) is normal, but there may be a slight increase in the protein content. Generalized slowing is seen regularly on the electroencephalogram (EEG). Neuropsychological testing can detect minimal or subtle cognitive impairment early in the disease, can document global impairment, or can follow the course of the disease.

Dilatation of the lateral ventricles and widening of the cortical sulci, particularly in the frontal and temporal regions, can be observed using either computed tomography or magnetic resonance imaging (MRI), especially late in the disease. Mild cortical atrophy, however, is seen in some older individuals who function normally by clinical and psychologic testing. Functional brain imaging studies, including positron emission tomography (PET), single-photon emission computed tomography (SPECT), or functional MRI, show hypometabolism in the temporal and parietal areas of patients with moderate to severe symptoms. Genetic tests may be useful in the diagnosis of Alzheimer disease in families with early-onset autosomal dominant forms of the disease. For sporadic or familial late-onset Alzheimer disease, the $\epsilon4$ polymorphism of the apolipoprotein E gene has been associated with a higher risk of the disease but does not provide sufficient sensitivity or specificity to be used for diagnosis and is not recommended.

Epidemiology

Before age 65, the prevalence, or proportion, of individuals with Alzheimer disease is less than 1%, but this rapidly increases to between 5% and 10% at age 65 years and to as high as 30% to 40% at age 85 and older. The age-specific incidence, or the number of new cases arising over a specific period of time, also rises steeply from less than 1% per year before age 65 years to 6.0% per year for individuals aged 85 and older. The average duration of symptoms until death may be 10 years, with a range of 4 to 16 years. Disease duration tends to be longer for women than for men. Rates of Alzheimer disease are slightly higher among women than in men, partly because affected women generally live longer than men do. However, the incidence rates for Alzheimer disease are also slightly higher in women, especially after age 85 years. In families with at least one affected individual, women who are first-degree relatives have a higher lifetime risk of developing Alzheimer disease than men.

Genetic Basis of Alzheimer Disease

Many families with autosomal dominant Alzheimer disease have been described. Siblings of patients have twice the expected lifetime risk of developing the disease. Also, monozygotic twins have significantly higher concordance of Alzheimer disease than do dizygotic twins. Mutations in three genes, the amyloid precursor protein (APP) gene on chromosome 21, the presenilin 1 (PS1) on chromosome 14, and the presenilin 2 (PS2) on chromosome 1, result in an autosomal dominant form of the disease beginning as early as the third decade of life. The existence of over 50 different mutations in PS1 suggests that this may be the most common form of familial early-onset Alzheimer disease. APP mutations can lead to enhanced generation or aggregation of amyloid-beta, indicating a pathogenic role. On the other hand, PS1 and PS2 are distinct from the immediate regulatory and coding regions of the APP gene, indicating that defects in molecules other than APP can also lead to cerebral amyloidogenesis and familial Alzheimer disease. Mutations in these genes may be considered deterministic because of nearly complete correspondence between the genotype and phenotype.

The $\epsilon4$ polymorphism of the apolipoprotein E (APOE) gene on chromosome 19 has been associated with the more typical sporadic and familial forms of Alzheimer disease, usually beginning after age 65. In contrast to the disease-causing mutations in the APP and PS1/2 genes, the $\epsilon4$ polymorphism of APOE is a normally occurring variant of the gene that appears to significantly increase susceptibility to the disease. In some families with late-onset Alzheimer disease, in a few families with mutations in the APP gene, and in patients with Down syndrome, each APOE $\epsilon4$ allele can lower the age at onset of dementia. The association between the APOE $\epsilon4$ polymorphism and Alzheimer disease is weaker among African-Americans and Caribbean Hispanics. Consistent with other genes involved in Alzheimer disease, apolipoprotein E may also act through a complex and poorly understood relationship with amyloid. The apolipoprotein E protein is an obligatory participant in amyloid accumulation, and different apolipoprotein E protein isoforms corresponding to polymorphisms exert at least some of their effects by controlling accumulation.

A genetic locus on chromosome 12 has pointed to the possibility of yet another susceptibility gene for Alzheimer disease. At least two polymorphisms in the gene encoding the α_2-macroglobulin protein have been associated with Alzheimer disease in these families. This candidate gene has also been implicated in amyloid clearance. Thus, mutations in at least three genes are associated with familial Alzheimer disease beginning before age 65, and polymorphisms in two genes are associated with susceptibility to Alzheimer disease after age 65 (Table 106.1).

Other Risk Factors

Though inconsistent, Alzheimer disease has also been associated with traumatic head injury, lower educational achievement, parental age at the time of birth, smoking, and Down syndrome in a first-degree relative. In several observational studies, the use of estrogen replacement therapy in postmenopausal women and the regular use of anti-inflammatory agents in both men and women have been associated with lower risks of Alzheimer disease and are currently being investigated in randomized clinical trials (Table 106.2).

Pathology

Alzheimer disease is characterized by atrophy of the cerebral cortex. At autopsy, the process is usually diffuse, but it may be more severe in the frontal, parietal, and temporal lobes (Fig. 106.1). On microscopic examination, there is loss of both neurons and

TABLE 106.1. GENETIC LOCI IN ALZHEIMER DISEASE

Location	Gene	Early onset	Late onset	Penetrance
Ch21pter-q21	Amyloid precursor protein	Ages 40–60	No	Complete
Ch14q24.3	Presenilin I	Ages 30–50	No	Complete
Ch 1q	Presenilin II	Ages 30–65	Rare	Incomplete
Ch19q13.2	Apolipoprotein±	Ages 40–60	Ages 60–75	Incomplete
Ch12p11-12[a]	Unknown (α-2-macroglobulin)	No	Late onset	Unknown

[a]Linkage only has been established and confirmed.

TABLE 106.2. RISK FACTORS MOST CONSISTENTLY ASSOCIATED WITH ALZHEIMER DISEASE

Risk factor or antecedent	Direction	Presumed mechanism
Head injury	Risk increased	A$ and APP in brain
Parental age	Risk increased	Advanced physiologic aging
Depression	Risk increased	Neurotransmitter alterations
Education	Risk decreased	"Cognitive reserve"
Anti-inflammatories	Risk decreased	Prevents complement activation
Estrogen	Risk decreased	Throphic; A$-APP metabolism
Smoking	Risk increased	Unknown

APP, amyloid precursor protein.

neuropil in the cortex; sometimes, secondary demyelination is seen in subcortical white matter. Quantitative morphometry suggests that the earliest cell loss occurs in the entorhinal region of the medial temporal lobe. The most characteristic histopathologic markers are the argentophilic senile plaques and neurofibrillary tangles.

The senile neuritic plaques are spherical microscopic lesions that are best seen with Bielschowsky stain; a core of extracellular amyloid is surrounded by enlarged axonal endings (neurites). The major protein in amyloid is beta-peptide, which is derived from APP—a transmembrane protein. This protein undergoes proteolysis, resulting in the accumulation of beta-amyloid peptide in brain, a key step in the pathogenesis of the disease. Amyloid is a generic description applied to a heterogeneous group of protein precipitates that may be deposited in a general manner throughout the body (systemic amyloids) or confined to a particular organ (e.g., cerebral amyloid, renal amyloid). In Alzheimer disease, amyloid is deposited around meningeal and cerebral vessels and in gray matter. The gray matter deposits are multifocal, coalescing into miliary structures known as plaques (Fig. 106.2). Parenchymal amyloid plaques are distributed in brain in a characteristic fashion, differentially affecting the various cerebral and cerebellar lobes and cortical laminae. A region of the APP molecule resides within an intramembranous domain of the neuron, and it is believed that proteases, termed γ-secretases, are responsible for cleavage of a site residing within a membranous domain. At least one of these γ-secretases may be under the control of PS1/2. The generation of highly aggregatable peptides is believed to initiate the accumulation of amyloid in all forms of the disease.

Neurofibrillary tangles are fibrillary intracytoplasmic structures within the neurons and are, like the plaques, also seen with the Bielschowsky stain. Electron microscopy shows paired helical filaments. Among the proteins within affected neurons are beta-amyloid and the tau protein, a microtubule protein. Although neurofibrillary tangles are not specific to Alzheimer dis-

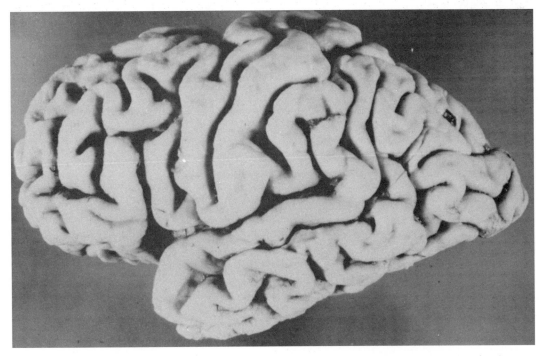

FIG. 106.1. Alzheimer disease. Diffuse atrophy of brain, especially severe in frontal, temporal, and parietal lobes with sparing of precentral and postcentral gyri. (Courtesy of Dr. Robert Terry.)

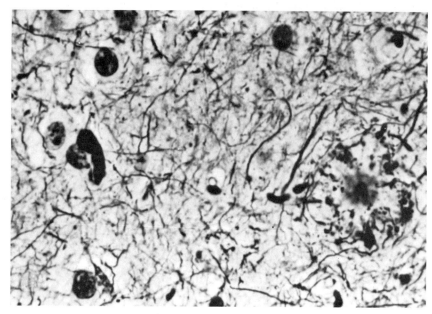

FIG. 106.2. Alzheimer disease. **Left:** Prominent senial plaques. **Right:** Several neurons with neurofibrillary tangles. Note also disruption of cortical organization. (Courtesy of Dr. Robert Terry.)

ease, they occur first in the hippocampal formation; later, neurofibrillary tangles may be seen throughout the cerebral cortex (Table 106.3).

Other features of Alzheimer disease include granulovacuolar degeneration of pyramidal cells of the hippocampus and amyloid angiopathy. The Hirano body, a rodlike body containing actin in a paracrystalline array, was first described in the Guam–parkinsonism–dementia complex; these neuronal inclusions are also found in Alzheimer disease. Some investigators believe that cognitive decline correlates, not with increased number of plaques but with a decrease in the density of presynaptic boutons from the pyramidal neurons in lamina III and IV, especially in the midfrontal neocortex. Arteriosclerotic changes are absent or inconspicuous in most cases.

Biochemically, the most consistent change is a 50% to 90% reduction of the activity of choline acetyltransferase, the biosynthetic enzyme for acetylcholine, in the cerebral cortex and hippocampus. This enzyme is found in cholinergic neurons, and there is a selective loss of cholinergic neurons, particularly of the cholinergic projection pathway, from deep nuclei in the septum

near the diagonal band of Broca to the hippocampus and from the nearby basal nucleus of Meynert to the cerebral cortex. Among the cholinergic receptor subtypes, M2—a presynaptic muscarinic receptor—displays decreased binding in the brains of Alzheimer patients. The severity of cognitive loss is roughly proportional to the loss of choline acetyltransferase. There is decreased content of corticotropin-releasing factor and somatostatin, both of which are found within degenerating neurites of the neuritic plaque. Glutaminergic neurons account for many large neurons lost in the cerebral cortex and hippocampus, and there is variable loss of ascending and descending serotoninergic and adrenergic systems.

Treatment

Anticholinesterases are currently the only U.S. Food and Drug Administration–approved treatments for Alzheimer disease and, at present, are considered palliative treatments. Anticholinesterases decrease the hydrolysis of acetylcholine released from the presynaptic neuron into the synaptic cleft by inhibiting acetylcholinesterase, resulting in stimulation of the cholinergic receptor. At the maximum dosages of the two approved drugs, tacrine improves cognitive test performance slightly more than donepezil. Donepezil scored slightly better in the clinicians' rating scales, had fewer side effects, did not alter liver transaminases, and could be given once a day. Though currently unavailable in the United States, rivastigmine and metrifonate compare with donepezil on cognitive performance, but adverse effects have been slightly more frequent.

Other drugs are also used. Both alpha tocopherol and selegiline are said to delay the later stages of Alzheimer disease. Unlike selegiline, alpha tocopherol does not interact with other medications, allowing it to be used in most patients without concern. Psychotropic drugs are frequently used to treat agitation, delu-

TABLE 106.3. PATHOLOGIC CHANGES IN ALZHEIMER DISEASE

Cell loss, plaques, and tangles occur regularly in
  Neocortex, especially association areas
  Hippocampus, including entorhinal cortex
  Amygdala
  Basal nucleus of Meynert
Sometimes in
  Medial nucleus of thalamus
  Dorsal tegmentum
  Locus coeruleus
  Paramedian reticular area
  Lateral hypothalamic nuclei

sions, and psychosis in Alzheimer disease. For depression, nearly all drugs are similar in efficacy, but there are only a handful of randomized controlled studies upon which to make therapeutic decisions.

Frontotemporal Dementias

Pick disease is a progressive form of dementia characterized by personality change, speech disturbance, inattentiveness, and sometimes extrapyramidal signs. In contrast to Alzheimer disease, Pick disease is rare. The disease can be familial. Atrophy of the frontal and temporal poles and argyrophilic round intraneuronal inclusions (Pick bodies) are the characteristic morphologic changes. Glial reaction is often pronounced in affected cerebral gray and white matter. Tau-immunoreactive glial inclusions and neuritic changes are recognized. Biochemical and immunocytochemical studies demonstrate that abnormal tau proteins are the major structural components of Pick bodies and differ from those seen in Alzheimer disease. As with other frontotemporal dementias, Pick disease shows filamentous tau pathology that has been associated with mutations in tau protein. Tau is a microtubule-associated protein found mainly in axons; it is involved in microtubule assembly and stabilization.

Frontotemporal dementias other than Pick disease are also rare and have been associated with mutations on chromosome 17 in the tau gene. Several different mutations account for a diverse array of clinical manifestations in addition to contributing to a characteristic pathologic change observed in Alzheimer disease: the neurofibrillary tangle. Table 106.4 lists the diseases associated with mutation in tau. Frontotemporal dementias are also characterized by personality change, deterioration of memory and executive functions, and stereotypical behavior. Extrapyramidal signs are usually prominent. Standard neuropsychologic tests and conventional brain imaging such as MRI and SPECT may not be sensitive to the early changes in the ventromedial frontal cortex. This suggests difficulty in distinguishing this form of dementia from other dementias early in the illness. Over time, however, there are abnormalities on SPECT, frontal atrophy on MRI, or a neuropsychologic profile more typical of frontotemporal dementia.

Although there is clinical and neuropathologic variability among and within families, the consistency of the syndrome led investigators to name the disease *frontotemporal dementia and parkinsonism linked to chromosome 17*. The pathologic changes include atrophy of frontal and temporal cortex and the basal ganglia and substantia nigra. In most cases, these features are accompanied by neuronal loss, gliosis, and deposits of microtubule-associated protein tau in both neurons and glial cells. The

TABLE 106.4. DEGENERATIVE DISEASES ASSOCIATED WITH DEMENTIA AND WITH SPECIFIC TAU MUTATIONS

Familial frontotemporal dementia and parkinsonism
Progressive supranuclear palsy
Familiar progressive subcortical gliosis
Corticobasal ganglionic degeneration
Familial multiple system tauopathy with presenile dementia

distribution and structural and biochemical characteristics of the tau deposits differentiate them from those of Alzheimer disease, corticobasal degeneration, progressive supranuclear palsy, and Pick disease. No beta-amyloid deposits are present.

Other degenerative diseases that may include dementia and are associated with tau mutations include progressive supranuclear palsy, familial progressive subcortical gliosis, and corticobasal ganglionic degeneration. Familial multiple-system tauopathy with presenile dementia shows abundant filamentous tau protein pathology.

Parkinson Disease and Lewy Body Dementia

As many as 40% of patients with Parkinson disease (see Chapter 114) can develop dementia. The risk of dementia with Parkinson disease is about four times that of other people of the same age. The risk of dementia increases with age at the time of the diagnosis of Parkinson disease and with depression or advanced motor disease. Neither computed tomography nor MRI reliably distinguishes demented from nondemented patients with Parkinson disease. Compared with patients with Parkinson disease who are not demented, those with dementia may show hypometabolism in the frontal lobes and the basal ganglia on PET or SPECT. Dementia associated with Parkinson disease is the third most common form of dementia overall. In addition, the presence of dementia limits the usefulness of nearly all forms of treatment for the motor manifestations because adverse effects such as delusions are more frequent.

Dementia is often superimposed on a mild degree of cognitive loss that is specific to Parkinson disease. Impairment in mental speed and visuospatial functions are impaired in most patients with Parkinson disease in the absence of dementia. With the onset of dementia, impaired memory, verbal fluency, and language compound these manifestations. New dementia occurs at the rate of 7% per year among patients with Parkinson disease. With increasing age, the cumulative risk of dementia by age 85 may be over 65%, suggesting that dementia is an inevitable consequence of Parkinson disease.

Three distinct neuropathologic changes are associated with dementia in Parkinson disease: coincident Alzheimer disease (senile plaques and neurofibrillary tangles), Lewy bodies (in cortical and subcortical structures), and primary nigral degeneration.

Dementia associated with Lewy bodies is considered clinically distinct from dementia associated with Parkinson disease and Alzheimer disease. Features include cognitive decline, visual hallucinations, parkinsonism, repeated falls, and sensitivity to neuroleptic medications. A "Lewy body variant" of Alzheimer disease characterized by a greater degree of impairment in attention, verbal fluency, and visuospatial function than typically seen in Alzheimer disease has been described in retrospective postmortem studies. Although criteria for dementia associated with cortical Lewy bodies have been proposed by the Nottingham Group for the Study of Neurodegenerative Diseases, they require the presence of parkinsonism, which is an inconsistent finding. Some patients with cortical Lewy bodies and dementia have no history or clinical evidence of rigidity, tremor, bradykinesia, or postural change. A fluctuating decline in cognitive function, characterized by episodes of confusion and lucid intervals, is believed by some to distinguish between senile dementia of the Lewy body type and Alzheimer disease. Depression, complex visual hallucinations, and delusions are also part of the clinical spectrum. Yet none of these clinical manifestations is specific for any single form of dementia.

The first described cases had only Lewy bodies on histologic analysis. Nevertheless, most subsequent cases showed both Lewy bodies and histologic markers of Alzheimer disease. Unique histologic findings include ubiquitin immunostaining in the CA2 subregion of the hippocampal formation.

Huntington Disease

This disorder is described in Chapter 108. In addition to chorea and other motor manifestations, memory loss and difficulty performing complex or sequential mental activities are seen early in the disease. After several years, chorea, postural instability, and frank dementia are evident, contributing to functional decline. In a mildly impaired patient, metabolic activity is reduced in the striatum and frontoparietal areas bilaterally. With progression, glucose metabolism is reduced at the junction of temporal and occipital regions. The severity of chorea correlates with subcortical metabolic activity, and the severity of dementia is linked to cortical metabolic rates.

The pathologic correlates of dementia in Huntington disease have not been established. There is atrophy of the caudate nucleus and putamen with extensive nerve cell loss and astrocytosis. Neurons containing gamma-aminobutyric acid, enkephalin, substance P, and dynorphin are reduced in number, with low brain concentrations of gamma-aminobutyric acid and glutamic acid decarboxylase.

VASCULAR DISEASES

Cerebrovascular Disease and Dementia

Dementia in association with stroke is the second most frequent cause of dementia overall. As many as 15% to 20% of patients with acute ischemic stroke over age 60 years have dementia at the time of the stroke, and 5% per year become demented thereafter. Risk factors include advancing age, diabetes, history of prior stroke, and the size and location of the stroke. There is a complex interaction between stroke, vascular risk factors, and Alzheimer disease, although the exact nature of this interaction remains unknown.

Dementia and intellectual impairment can result from brain injury caused by stroke, either hemorrhagic or ischemic. The manifestations of dementia after stroke include loss of memory and impairment in at least two other cognitive domains: orientation, attention, language-verbal skills, visuospatial abilities, calculation, executive functions, motor control, praxis, abstraction, and judgment. The impairment must be severe enough to impair "functioning in daily living" or "to interfere broadly with the conduct of the patient's customary affairs of life."

Although stroke increases the risk of dementia, the definition of vascular dementia remains unsettled despite numerous attempts at clarification. Dementia after stroke may be predominantly of the mixed type, a combination of Alzheimer disease

and stroke, and the etiology is likely to be multifactorial. High blood pressure is associated with both Alzheimer disease and dementia after stroke and can be associated with leukoaraiosis found on brain imaging. Severe leukoaraiosis, cerebral hypoperfusion, fluctuations in systemic blood pressure, hypotension induced by medication or systemic conditions, ischemia, carotid atherosclerosis, and diabetes may each increase the risk of dementia after stroke. Although APOE may influence the risk of Alzheimer disease, its role in dementia after stroke is unsettled.

Different clinical subtypes of cerebrovascular dementia are described. A cortical syndrome is generally characterized by repeated atherothrombotic or cardioembolic strokes, obvious focal sensorimotor signs, more severe aphasic disturbance when present, and an abrupt onset of cognitive failure. A subcortical syndrome accompanied by deep white matter lesions is characterized by pseudobulbar signs, isolated pyramidal signs, depression or emotional lability, "frontal" behavior, mildly impaired memory, disorientation, poor response to novelty, restricted field of interest, decreased ability to make associations, difficulty passing from one idea to another, inattention, and perseveration.

Cerebral autosomal dominant arteriopathy with subcortical infarcts and leukoencephalopathy is an autosomal dominant form of cerebrovascular dementia with onset in the third and forth decades of life and has been related to mutations in the notch3 gene on chromosome 19. In patients with multiple deep infarcts resulting in etat lacunaire, pseudobulbar palsy is often a central feature with emotional and urinary incontinence, dysarthria, bilateral pyramidal signs, and gait imbalance with marche a petit pas. Regardless of the clinical syndrome, the survival of patients with cerebrovascular dementia is less than that of other forms of dementia, including Alzheimer disease.

Control of hypertension reduces the risk of recurrent cerebral infarction and may secondarily reduce the risk of subsequent dementia. Any effective measure that prevents stroke recurrence could be applied to patients with vascular dementia: antiplatelet therapy, anticoagulants, carotid endarterectomy, and, for most patients, aspirin.

INFECTIOUS DISEASES

Prion-related Diseases

Dementia related to *prion disease* is rare. The worldwide incidence of sporadic Creutzfeldt-Jakob disease, the most common prion disease, is 0.5 to 1.5 per million population per year and less than 1 death per million per year. There are no established risk factors for contracting the disease. The *transmissible spongiform encephalopathies* are a group of disorders characterized by similar histopathology consisting of spongy degeneration, neuronal loss, and astrocytic proliferation. In all prion disorders, an abnormal protease-resistant prion protein accumulates in the brain (see Chapter 33).

There are several forms of prion diseases in humans (Table 106.5): Creutzfeldt-Jakob, Gerstmann-Sträussler-Scheinker, fatal familial insomnia, and Kuru. Prion disorders are inherited, acquired, or sporadic. The familial forms, which include Gerstmann-Sträussler-Scheinker and fatal familial insomnia, and 15% to 20% of patients with Creutzfeldt-Jakob disease are associated

TABLE 106.5. PRION-RELATED DEMENTIAS

Prion-related diseases	Markers on PrP gene, chromosome 20
Creutzfeldt-Jakob disease	Mutation in codon 200
Familial	88% homozygotes for polymorphism at codon 129[a]
Sporadic	100% homozygotes for polymorphism at codon 129[a]
New variant	
Gerstmann-Sträussler-Scheinker	Mutation in codon 102
Fatal familial insomnia	Mutation in codon 179

[a]Compared with 48% homozygotes among healthy control subjects.

with mutations in the prion protein (PrP). The most frequent mutations are at codons 178 and 200, both of which cause an alteration in the folding pattern of the protein to produce a beta-pleated configuration that polymerizes into amyloid fibrils.

The most common form is Creutzfeldt-Jakob disease. The diagnosis is usually made in individuals aged 50 to 70 years. A progressive dementia with myoclonus, pyramidal signs, periodic sharp waves on EEG, and cerebellar or extrapyramidal signs suffices for the diagnosis of probable Creutzfeldt-Jakob disease. Progression is subacute, with significant decline noted in weeks or months; most die within 1 year of onset.

"Variant Creutzfeldt-Jakob disease" begins before age 40 years and the course is more prolonged than the familial form. These patients are more likely to have psychiatric manifestations, to have paresthesias and sensory loss, and to develop cerebellar ataxia. They usually lack the periodic complexes on EEG and have no genetic mutations. These patients and cows with bovine spongiform encephalopathy share a unique glycosylation pattern of the PrP^res protein.

Fifteen percent to 20% of persons with Creutzfeldt-Jakob disease have an autosomal dominant inheritance pattern on family history. Point mutations, deletions, or insertions are found in the PRP gene on chromosome 20. In contrast to the sporadic form, these patients typically have a younger age at onset and a more protracted course; they are less likely to have the periodic EEG findings.

The Gerstmann-Sträussler-Scheinker disease is a familial form of prion disease with autosomal dominant ataxia, spastic paraplegia, and dementia. Multicentric prion plaques are found in the cerebellar and cerebral hemispheres. Deposition of PrP plaques is most marked in this form of prion disease. At least four distinct mutations in the PrP gene have been found.

Fatal familial insomnia is associated with mutations in the PrP gene at codon 178. The average age at onset varies from 20 to 60 years, and the duration is less that 2 years. Severe loss of weight, insomnia, autonomic dysfunction, and motor abnormalities can be present. The brain shows widespread cortical astrogliosis and brainstem degeneration. Deposition of the PrP in the form of plaques is found in the cerebellum and brainstem.

Kuru is sporadic prion disease that was associated with cannibalism among natives of New Guinea. The disease disappeared once cannibalism was halted.

The CFS in prion disease is typically normal, although the protein level can be mildly elevated. Immunoassays of CSF show the presence of a normal brain protein, "14-3-3." If recent stroke or viral menigoencephalitis can be ruled out, this assay is highly sensitive and specific for Creutzfeldt-Jakob disease. Early, EEG may be normal or show nonspecific slowing. Later, periodic bi- or triphasic complexes may be evident. With repeated recordings, most patients manifest these EEG findings and myoclonus occurs with the periodic complexes. Typically, neuroimaging studies are normal, but late in the disease generalized atrophy may be detected. Hyperintense signals in the basal ganglia have been described.

Human Immunodeficiency Virus Type 1-associated Dementia Complex

Human immunodeficiency virus type 1 dementia complex, a frequent sequela of acquired immunodeficiency syndrome is characterized by apathy, memory loss, and cognitive slowing often before there are other neurologic abnormalities. Diagnosis is established by clinical features and laboratory tests. The differential diagnosis includes cerebral toxoplasmosis, cerebral lymphoma, progressive multifocal leukoencephalopathy, neurosyphilis, cytomegalovirus encephalitis, and cryptococcal and tuberculous meningitis. Examination of the CSF and brain imaging are essential to rule out these treatable diseases. Subcortical hypermetabolism on PET characterizes the early stages of the dementia. There is predominantly frontotemporal atrophy; multinucleated giant cells, microglial nodules, and perivascular infiltrates are evident microscopically.

INHERITED METABOLIC DISEASES

These disorders rarely cause dementia in adults but are important because some are potentially treatable. Young onset of dementia or involvement of other areas of the nervous system (e.g., cerebellar, visual, peripheral nerve, muscle) and body (e.g., skin, skeletal, and visceral organs) should prompt and guide investigation into these disorders (Table 106.6). Most of these diseases are described elsewhere in this book. Wilson disease, Hallervorden-Spatz disease, and the Fahr syndrome are dementias associated with abnormal metal metabolism. X-linked adrenoleukodystrophy and adrenomyeloneuropathy are due to a defect in the peroxisomal enzyme, lignoceroyl-CoA ligase mapped to the gene Xq28. Dementia is one of several manifestations in late-onset forms of these diseases. Cerebrotendinous xanthomatosis, Kufs disease, and membranous lipodystrophy are disorders of lipid metabolism that can cause dementia in adults. Several mitochondrial disorders are associated with dementia, especially MELAS and MERRF (see Chapter 96).

Lysosomal disorders can cause dementia in adults. The most common lysosomal disease with adult-onset dementia is metachromatic leukodystrophy. Other rare lysosomal diseases include mucopolysaccharidosis III (Sanfilippo disease) with alpha-*N*-acetyl-glucosaminidase deficiency, Gaucher disease with glucocerebrosidase (glucosylceramide-beta-glucosidase) deficiency, Niemann-Pick disease type C with sphingomyelinase deficiency, Fabry disease with alpha-galactosidase deficiency, Krabbe disease (globoid cell leukodystrophy) with galactocere-

TABLE 106.6. LABORATORY INVESTIGATIONS OF INHERITED METABOLIC DEMENTIAS

Disease	Laboratory tests
Wilson disease	Serum ceruloplasmin, urinary copper
Adrenoleukodystrophy and adrenomyeloneuropathy	Very-long-chain fatty acids
Cerebrotendinous xanthomatosis	Serum cholestanol
Kuf disease	Urinary dolichols, skin or brain biopsy
Membranous lipodystrophy	Hand x-rays, bone biopsy
MERRF, MELAS	Lactic acid, muscle biopsy
Metachromatic leukodystrophy	Leukocyte arylsufatase A
Mucopolysaccaridosis III	Alpha-N-acteyl-glucosaminidase
Gaucher disease	Glucocerebrosidase
Niemann-Pick type C	Sphingomyelinase
Krabbe disease	Leukocyte galactocerebroside beta-galactosidase
GM_2-gangliosidosis	Leukocyte hexosaminidase A
GM_1-gangliosidosis	Leukocyte beta-galactosidase
Adult polyglucosan body disease	Sural nerve biopsy
Lafora disease	Muscle biopsy

brosidase deficiency, GM_2 gangliosidosis with hexosaminidase A deficiency, and GM_1 gangliosidosis with beta-galactosidase deficiency.

Adult polyglucosan body disease and Lafora disease are disorders of carbohydrate metabolism associated with dementia. Neuronal intranuclear hyaline inclusion disease, an autosomal dominant adult-onset leukodystrophy of unknown origin; Alexander disease; and Mast syndrome are rare causes of dementia.

SUGGESTED READINGS

American Psychiatric Association. *Diagnostic and statistical manual of mental disorders*, 4th ed. Washington, DC: American Psychiatric Association, 1994:143–147.

Backman L, Ahlbom A, Winblad B. Prevalence of Alzheimer's disease and other dementias in an elderly urban population,relationship with age, sex and education. *Neurology* 1991;41:1886–1892.

Baker M, Litvan I, Houlden H, et al. Association of an extended haplotype in the tau gene with progressive supranuclear palsy. *Hum Mol Genet* 1999;8:711–715.

Bales KR, Verina T, Dodel RC, et al. Lack of apolipoprotein E dramatically reduces amyloid beta-peptide deposition. *Nat Genet* 1997;17:263–264.

Beaudry P, Cohen P, Brandel JP, et al. Alpha-2-macroglobulin is genetically associated with Alzheimer disease. *Nat Genet* 1998;19:357–360.

Borchelt DR, Thinakaran G, Eckman CB, et al. Familial Alzheimer's disease-linked presenilin 1 variants elevate Abeta1-42/1-40 ratio in vitro and in vivo. *Neuron* 1996;17:1005–1013.

Borchelt DR, Thinakaran G, Eckman CB, et al. Incidence and distribution of parkinsonism in Olmsted County, Minnesota, 1976–1990. *Neurology* 1999;52:1214–1220.

Braak H, de Vos RA, Jansen EN, Bratzke H, Braak E. Neuropathological hallmarks of Alzheimer's and Parkinson's diseases. *Progr Brain Res* 1998;117:267–285.

Corder EH, Saunders AM, Strittmatter WJ, et al. Gene dose of apolipoprotein E type 4 allele and the risk of Alzheimer's disease in late onset families. *Science* 1993;261:828–829.

Corey-Bloom J, Anand R, Veach J. A randomized trial evaluating the efficacy and safety of ENA 713 (rivastigmine tartarate), a new acetylcholinesterase inhibitor, in patients with mild to moderately severe Alzheimer's disease. *J Geriatr Psychopharmacol* 1998;1:55–65.

Cummings JL, Cyrus F, Bieber J, et al. Metrifonate treatment of the cognitive deficits of Alzheimer's disease. *Neurology* 1998;50:1214–1221.

Dal Pan GJ, McArthur JC. Neuroepidemiology of HIV infection. *Neurol Clin* 1996;14:359–382.

Devanand D, Sano M, Tang M-X, et al. Depressed mood and the incidence of Alzheimer's disease in the community elderly. *Arch Gen Psychiatry* 1996;53:175–182.

Dickson DW. Pick's disease: a modern approach. *Brain Pathol* 1998;8:339–354.

Evans DA. Age-specific incidence of Alzheimer's disease in a community population. *JAMA* 1995;273:1354–1359.

Evans DA, Beckett LA, Field TS, et al. Apolipoprotein E4 and incidence of Alzheimer's disease in a community population of older persons. *JAMA* 1997;277:822–824.

Evans DA, Funkenstein HH, Albert MS, et al. APOE and Alzheimer's Disease Meta Analysis Consortium. Effects of age, gender and ethnicity on the association between apolipoprotein-E genotype and Alzheimer's disease. *JAMA* 1997;278:1349–1356.

Farrer LA, Cupples LA, van Duijn CM, et al. Processing of Aβ-amyloid precursor protein. Cell biology, regulation, and role in Alzheimer disease. *Int Rev Neurobiol* 1994;36:29–50.

Farrer LA, Cupples LA, van Duijn CM, et al. Apolipoprotein E genotype in patients with Alzheimer's disease, implications for the risk of dementia among relatives. *Ann Neurol* 1995;38:797–808.

Gearing M, Mirra SS, Hedreen JC, Sumi SM, Hansen LA, Hyman A. The consortium to establish a registry for Alzheimer's disease (CERAD). Part X. Neuropathology confirmation of the clinical diagnosis of Alzheimer's disease. *Neurology* 1995;45:461–566.

Goedert M, Spillantini MG, Crowther RA, et al. Tau gene mutation in familial progressive subcortical gliosis. *Nat Med* 1999;5:454–457.

Gracon SI, Knapp MJ, Berghoff WG, et al. Safety of tacrine: clinical trials, treatment IND, and postmarketing experience. *Alzheimer Dis Assoc Disord* 1998;12:93–101.

Halonen P, Kontula K. Apolipoprotein E, dementia, and cortical deposition of beta-amyloid protein. *N Engl J Med* 1995;333:1242–1247.

Hebert LE, Scherr PA, Beckett LA, et al. Prevalence of Alzheimer's disease in a community population of older persons. Higher than previously reported. *JAMA* 1989;262:2551–2556.

Iwatsubo T, Odaka A, Suzuki N, Mizusawa H, Nukina N, Ihara Y. Visualization of A beta 42(43) and A beta 40 in senile plaques with end-specific A beta monoclonals, evidence that an initially deposited species is A beta 42(43). *Neuron* 1994;12:45–53.

Johnson RT, Gibbs CJ. Creutzfeldt-Jakob disease and related transmissible spongiform encephalopathies. *N Engl J Med* 1998;339;1994–2004.

Laplanche JL. 14-3-3 protein, neuron-specific enolase, and S-100 protein in cerebrospinal fluid of patients with Creutzfeldt-Jakob disease. *Dement Geriatr Cogn Disord* 1999;10:40–46.

Levy-Lahad E, Bird TD. Genetic factors in Alzheimer's disease: a review of recent advances. *Ann Neurol* 1996;40:829–840.

Maestre G, Ottman R, Stern Y, et al. Apolipoprotein-+ and Alzheimer's disease: ethnic variation in genotypic risks. *Ann Neurol* 1995;37: 254–259.

Mayeux R, Ottman R, Tang M-X, et al. Genetic susceptibility and head injury as risk factors for Alzheimer's disease among community-dwelling elderly persons and their first-degree relatives. *Ann Neurol* 1993;33: 494–501.

Mayeux R, Sano M. Drug therapy: Treatment of Alzheimer's disease. *N. Eng J Med* 1999;341:1670–1679.

Mayeux R, Saunders AM, Shea S, et al. Utility of the APOE genotype in the diagnosis of Alzheimer's disease. *N Engl J Med* 1998;338:506–512.

McKeith IG, Ince P, Jaros EB, et al. What are the relations between Lewy body disease and AD? *J Neural Transm Suppl* 1998;54:107–116.

McKhann G, Drachman D, Folstein M, Katzman R, Price D, Stadlan EM. Clinical diagnosis of Alzheimer's disease: report of the NINCDS-ADRDA Work Group. *Neurology* 1984;34:939–944.

Merchant C, Tang M-X, Albert S, Manly J, Stern Y, Mayeux R. The influence of smoking on the risk of Alzheimer's disease. *Neurology* 1999;52:1408–1412.

Morris JC, Cyrus PA, Orazem J, et al. Metrifonate benefits cognitive, behavioral and global function in patients with Alzheimer's disease. *Neurology* 1998;50:1222–1230.

Ott A, Slooter AJC, Hofman A, et al. Smoking and risk of dementia and Alzheimer's disease in a population-based cohort study. *Lancet* 1998;351:1840–1843.

Paykel ES, Brayne C, Huppert FA, et al. Incidence of dementia in a population older than 75 years in the United Kingdom. *Arch Gen Psychiatry* 1994;51:325–332.

Paykel ES, Brayne C, Huppert FA, et al. Complete genomic screen in late-onset familial Alzheimer disease. Evidence for a new locus on chromosome 12. *JAMA* 1997;278:1237–1241.

Polvikoski T, Sulkava R, Haltia M, et al. Neuropathology of Alzheimer's disease and animal models. In: Markesbery WR, ed. *Neuropathology of dementing disorders*. London: Oxford University Press, 1998:121–141.

Rocca WA, Cha RH, Waring SC, Kokmen E. Incidence of dementia and Alzheimer's disease, A reanalysis of data from Rochester, Minnesota, 1975–1984. *Am J Epidemiol* 1998;148:51–62.

Rogaeva E, Premkumar S, Song Y, et al. Evidence for an Alzheimer disease susceptibility locus on chromosome 12 and for further locus heterogeneity. *JAMA* 1998;280:614–618.

Rogers SL, Farlow MR, Doody RS, Mohs R, Friedhoff LT and the Donepezil Study Group. A 24-week, double-blind, placebo-controlled trial of donepezil in patients with Alzheimer's disease. *Neurology* 1998;50:138–145.

Roman GC, Tatemichi TK, Erkinjuntti T, et al. Vascular dementia: diagnostic criteria for research studies. Report of the NINDS-AIREN international workshop. *Neurology* 1993;43:250–260.

Roses AD. Apolipoprotein E alleles as risk factors in Alzheimer's disease. *Annu Rev Med* 1996;47:387–400.

Sacktor N, McArthur J. Prospects for therapy of HIV-associated neurologic diseases. *Neurovirology* 1997;3:89–101.

Sano M, Ernesto C, Thomas RG, et al. A controlled trial of selegiline, alpha-tocopherol, or both as treatment for Alzheimer's disease. *N Engl J Med* 1997;336:1216–1222.

Scheuner D, Eckman C, Jensen M, et al. Secreted amyloid β-protein similar to that in senile plaques of Alzheimer's disease is increased in vivo by the presenilin 1 and 2 and APP mutations linked to familial Alzheimer's disease. *Nat Med* 1996;2:864–870.

Schupf N, Kapell D, Zigman W, Canto B, Tycko B, Mayeux R. Onset of dementia is associated with apolipoprotein ϵ4 in Down syndrome. *Ann Neurol* 1996;40:799–801.

Sergeant N, Wattez A, Delacourte A. Neurofibrillary degeneration in progressive supranuclear palsy and corticobasal degeneration: tau pathologies with exclusively "exon 10" isoforms. *J Neurochem* 1999;72:1243–1249.

Skoog I, Hesse C, Aevarsson O, et al. A population study of apoE genotype at the age of 85: relation to dementia, cerebrovascular disease, and mortality. *J Neurol Neurosurg Psychiatry* 1998;64:37–43.

Snowdon DA, Greiner LH, Mortimer JA, Riley KP, Greiner PA, Markesbery WR. Linguistic ability in early life and cognitive function and Alzheimer's disease in late life. *JAMA* 1996;275:528–532.

Snowdon DA, Greiner LH, Mortiner JA, Riley KP, Greiner PA, Markesbury WR. Brain infarction and the clinical expression of Alzheimer's disease. The Nun Study. *JAMA* 1997;277:813–817.

Spillantini MG, Goedert M. Tau protein pathology in neurodegenerative diseases. *Trends Neurosci* 1998;21:428–433.

Spillantini MG, Murrell JR, Goedert M, Farlow MR, Klug A, Ghetti B. Mutation in the tau gene in familial multiple system tauopathy with presenile dementia. *Proc Natl Acad Sci USA* 1998;95:7737–7741.

Stern Y, Gurland B, Tatemichi TK, Tang M-X, Wilder D, Mayeux R. Influence of education and occupation on the incidence of dementia. *JAMA* 1994;271:1004–1010.

Stewart W, Kawas C, Corrada M, Metter E. The risk of Alzheimer's disease and duration of NSAID use. *Neurology* 1997;48:626–632.

Strittmatter WJ, Saunders AM, Schmechel D, et al. Apolipoprotein E: high-avidity binding to beta-amyloid and increased frequency of type 4 allele in late-onset familial Alzheimer disease. *Proc Natl Acad Sci USA* 1993;90:1977–1981.

Tang M-X, Jacobs D, Stern Y, et al. Effect of oestrogen during menopause on risk and age-at-onset of Alzheimer's disease. *Lancet* 1996;348: 429–432.

Tang M-X, Stern Y, Marder K, et al. APOE risks and the frequency of Alzheimer's disease among African-Americans, Caucasians and Hispanics. *JAMA* 1998;279:751–755.

Tanzi RE, Kovacs DM, Kim TW, Moir RD, Guenette SY, Wasco W. The gene defects responsible for familial Alzheimer's disease. *Neurobiology Dis* 1996;3: 159–168.

Tatemichi TK, Desmond DW, Paik M, et al. Clinical determinants of dementia related to stroke. *Ann Neurol* 1993;33:568–575.

Tatemichi TK, Paik M, Bagiella E, et al. Risk of dementia after stroke in a hospitalized cohort: results of a longitudinal study. *Neurology* 1994;44:1885–1891.

Tranchant C, Geranton L, Guiraud-Chaumeil C, Mohr M, Warter JM. Basis of phenotypic variability in sporadic Creutzfeldt-Jakob disease. *Neurology* 1999;52:1244–1249.

Wolfe ME, Xia W, Ostaszewski B, Diehl TS, Kimberly WT, Selkoe DJ. Two transmembrane aspartates in presenilin-1 required for presenilin endoproteolysis and gamma-secretase activity. *Nature* 1999;398:513–517.

Wu WS, Holmans P, Wavrant-DeVrièze F, et al. Genetic studies on chromosome 12 in late onset Alzheimer disease. *JAMA* 1998;280:619–622.

Zakzanis KK. The subcortical dementia of Huntington's disease. *Clin Exp Neuropsychol* 1998;20:565–578.

Merritt's Neurology, 10th ed., edited by L.P. Rowland. Lippincott Williams & Wilkins, Philadelphia © 2000.

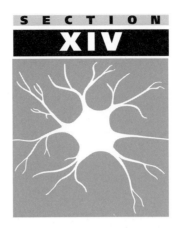

SECTION XIV

ATAXIAS

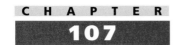

HEREDITARY ATAXIAS

SUSAN B. BRESSMAN
TIMOTHY LYNCH
ROGER N. ROSENBERG

CLASSIFICATION

The hereditary ataxias comprise heterogenous disorders that share three features: ataxia, an inherited genetic basis, and pathology involving the cerebellum or its connections. In most of these conditions, the pathology affects more than the cerebellum, especially the posterior columns, pyramidal tracts, pontine nuclei, and basal ganglia, and there are corresponding neurologic signs. Within a family, there may be a broad range of clinical and pathologic features; the heterogeneity has created problems for classification. In 1983 Harding proposed a scheme based on age at onset, mode of inheritance, and specific biochemical abnormality when known. Harding's classification has been widely adopted, especially for autosomal dominant cerebellar ataxia (ADCA) and its three subtypes. In the last decade loci for the ADCA subtypes have been mapped and assigned spinocerebellar ataxia (SCA) numbers (SCA1, 2, 3, etc.). In this chapter we concentrate on genetic causes of ataxia, excluding those due to inborn errors of metabolism, which are discussed in Sections IX and X.

EARLY-ONSET ATAXIAS

Friedreich Ataxia (MIM *2293000)

Friedreich ataxia (FRDA), described in 1863, is an autosomal recessive disorder and the most common early-onset ataxia. The essential clinical features are juvenile onset (between puberty and age 25) with progressive ataxia of gait and limbs, absent tendon reflexes, and extensor plantar responses. Other common features are dysarthria, corticospinal tract clumsiness, proprioceptive sensory loss in the legs, scoliosis, and cardiopathy. Onset before age 25 and absence of tendon reflexes in the legs separated FRDA from "FRDA-like" syndromes, including late-onset FRDA and other early-onset cerebellar ataxias such as FRDA with retained reflexes. Once the FRDA gene was cloned (see below), it became clear that some FRDA-like syndromes are also the result of FRDA mutations.

Epidemiology

The prevalence of FRDA in North America and Europe is about 2 per 100,000, with a carrier frequency of about 1:120. Boys and girls are equally affected. Because the disorder is autosomal recessive, parents are asymptomatic, and the rate of consanguinity is high, from 5.6% to 28% in different populations. The risk for siblings to be affected is 25%. In populations with small families, most patients are the only ones affected in the family.

Neuropathology

The spinal cord may be thinner than normal. Degeneration and sclerosis are seen in the posterior columns, spinocerebellar tracts, and corticospinal tracts. Nerve cells are lost in the dorsal root ganglia and Clarke column. Peripheral nerves are involved, with fewer large myelinated axons. The brainstem, cerebellum, and cerebrum are normal except for mild degenerative changes of the pontine and medullary nuclei, optic tracts, and Purkinje cells in the cerebellum. Cardiac muscle, nerves, and ganglia are also involved.

Genetics

The gene for FRDA (X25) maps to 9q and codes for a highly conserved protein, frataxin. More than 95% of FRDA patients are homozygous for an expansion of a GAA triplet repeat in the first intron of X25. A few FRDA patients harbor compound heterozygous mutations, with one GAA intronic expansion and a truncating or missense mutation in the other allele. Some, but not all, individuals who are compound heterozygotes have an atypical and milder disease.

Normal chromosomes have fewer than 42 triplets, and disease chromosomes have 66 to more than 1,700 repeats. Repeats in normal chromosomes are stable when transmitted from parent to child, but expanded GAA repeats show meiotic instability, usually contracting after paternal transmission and either expanding or contracting with maternal transmission. There is also mitotic instability of the expansion that varies in different tissues, including different brain regions.

FRDA is due to a deficiency of frataxin caused by the GAA intronic expansion, which interferes with the transcription of frataxin. As a result of the expansion, one DNA strand has a long segment of purines and the other has pyrimidines; these sequences adopt an abnormal helical structure that inhibits transcription. Larger repeats more profoundly inhibit frataxin transcription and cause earlier onset and more severe symptoms (see below).

Expression of the FRDA gene is tissue specific, highest in the sites most affected in FRDA such as heart, liver, skeletal muscle, and pancreas. In the central nervous system, the highest levels are found in the spinal cord, with lower levels in the cerebellum. Frataxin is localized to the inner mitochondrial membranes. Yeast cells deficient in the frataxin homologue accumulate iron in mitochondria and show increased sensitivity to oxidative stress. Iron deposits and iron-sulfur enzyme deficiencies have also been found in the hearts of FRDA patients. The pathogenesis of FRDA may be mitochondrial dysfunction and free radical toxicity.

Clinical Expression and Genotype-Phenotype Correlations

Symptoms usually begin between ages 8 and 15 years; it may start in infancy or after age 25, even in the fifth decade. Like other triplicate repeat disorders, there is a correlation between the GAA repeat size and clinical features, particularly age at onset and rate of progression. However, the age at onset correlates with the shorter of the two alleles because FRDA, unlike the other triplicate repeat disorders, is recessive (with expanded repeats in both alleles) and due to loss of frataxin function. The GAA size, however, does not entirely account for the variability in age at onset or clinical progressions; other factors, including somatic mosaicism and other genetic or environmental modifiers, play a role.

Ataxia of gait is the most common symptom and is usually the first. The gait disorder may be seen in children who have been walking normally; more commonly, children are slow in learning to walk, the gait is clumsy and awkward, and they are less agile than other children. Within a few years, ataxia appears in the arms and trunk, a combination of cerebellar asynergia and loss of proprioceptive sense. Movements are jerky, awkward, and poorly controlled. Intention tremor, most common in the arms, may affect the trunk (titubation). Frequent repositioning or pseudoathetosis and true generalized chorea may occur. Speech becomes explosive or slurred and finally unintelligible. Limb weakness is common, sometimes leading to paraplegia in flexion.

Loss of appreciation of vibration is an early sign. Frequently, position sense is impaired in the legs and later in the arms. Loss of two-point discrimination; partial astereognosis; and impaired appreciation of pain, temperature, or tactile sensation are occasionally seen. Loss of lower limb reflexes and the presence of Babinski signs were once considered necessary for diagnosis; they are characteristic, and almost all patients with typical recessive or sporadic early-onset ataxia with these features have the X25 hyperexpansion.

Ocular movements are usually abnormal; fixation instability and square wave jerks are the most common abnormalities. Also frequent are jerky pursuit, ocular dysmetria, and failure of fixation suppression of the vestibular ocular reflexes. Nystagmus and optic atrophy are each seen in about 25% of patients, but severely reduced visual acuity is rare. Deafness is also rare. Sphincter impairment occasionally occurs when patients are bedridden; dementia and psychosis are unusual, and the condition is not incompatible with a high degree of intellectual development.

Skeletal abnormalities are common. Scoliosis or kyphosis, usually in the upper thoracic region, affects more than 75%. Pes cavus and equinovarus deformities occur in more than 50%. Heart disease is found in more than 85%. The electrocardiogram most commonly shows ST segment changes and T-wave inversions. Ventricular hypertrophy, arrhythmia, and murmurs are less common. Congestive heart failure occurs late and may be precipitated by atrial fibrillation. Diabetes mellitus is found in 10% to 20%.

With the advent of FRDA testing in large ataxia populations, the spectrum of FRDA is wider than previously thought and includes late onset, retained reflexes, or absence of pyramidal signs. In one study of ataxic individuals thought on clinical grounds not to have FRDA, 10% of those with recessive disease and 5% with sporadic disease had homozygous GAA hyperexpansions. To some extent this variability, especially between families, is explained by the length of the GAA expansion. However, GAA expansion cannot explain all the variation, particularly with repeat sizes above 500. For example, Acadian FRDA patients descend from a single founder and have the typical homozygous hyperexpansion, with no other identified change in the gene. Nevertheless, they have milder symptoms and cardiopathy is rare. Other inherited factors, including possible differences in frataxin regulation, may play a role.

Laboratory findings include characteristic electrocardiogram changes and echocardiographic evidence of concentric ventricular hypertrophy or less commonly asymmetric septal hypertrophy. Normal peripheral nerve conduction studies with absent or markedly reduced sensory nerve action potentials distinguish FRDA from Charcot-Marie-Tooth disease. Other common abnormalities are reduced amplitude of visual evoked responses and small or absent somatosensory evoked potentials recorded over the clavicle and delayed dispersed potentials at the sensory cortex. Computed tomography and magnetic resonance imaging (MRI) of the brain are usually normal, but there may be mild cerebellar atrophy. Cervical spinal cord atrophy can often be detected on MRI. The cerebrospinal fluid is normal.

The course is progressive; most patients cannot walk 15 years after onset of symptoms, although variability rate of progression varies. The mean age at death is between 40 and 60 and results from infection or cardiac disease. No medical treatment influences the course, and treatment that modulates oxidative stress or directly affects frataxin expression may be expected.

Other Early-onset Ataxias

Another early-onset recessive ataxia is the *Marinesco-Sjögren syndrome* characterized by ataxia, bilateral cataracts, mental retardation, and short stature. Other rare autosomal recessive conditions include ataxia with pigmentary retinopathy, ataxia with deafness, and ataxia with hypogonadism. One rare infantile-onset autosomal recessive disorder in Finnish families was mapped to chromosome 10q23. These children develop ataxia, athetosis, and loss of tendon reflexes before age 2. This is followed by hypotonia, optic atrophy, ophthalmoplegia, deafness, and sensory neuropathy.

One early-onset ataxia, the *Ramsay Hunt syndrome*, is etiologically heterogeneous. The syndrome consists of myoclonus and progressive ataxia, which may be produced by several diseases, including MERRF (mitochondrial encephalomyopathy with ragged red fibers) and the autosomal recessive disorder Unverricht-Lundborg disease or progressive myoclonus epilepsy type 1, which maps to chromosome 2lq (MIM254800). The gene encodes cystatin B, which acts within cells to block the action of cathepsins, proteases that degrade other cell proteins. The Ramsay Hunt syndrome is most commonly caused by MERRF. Clinical features include ataxia, myoclonus, seizures, myopathy, and hearing loss. Maternal relatives may be asymptomatic or have partial syndromes, including a characteristic "horse collar" distribution of lipomas (see Chapter 96).

The pathogenesis of another autosomal recessive early-onset ataxia, *ataxia telangiectasia* (MIM208900), is defective DNA repair. Clinical symptoms and signs vary, but typically there is truncal ataxia in infancy, obvious when the child learns to walk, and motor development is delayed. Growth retardation, delayed sexual development, and mild mental retardation may be seen. Prominent oculomotor abnormalities include difficulty generating saccades, dependence on head thrusts to fixate, ocular dysmetria, and nystagmus. Facial hypomimia, drooling, dysarthria, dystonia, myoclonus, chorea, and peripheral neuropathy may appear around age 10 or in adolescence. Cutaneous telangiectases are characteristic but are not always present and generally do not appear in the first years of life. Telangiectases involve the conjunctivae, face, ears, and flexor creases (Fig. 107.1). Immune dysfunction is typical and includes recurrent respiratory and cutaneous infections, lymphopenia, and decreased concentrations of IgA and IgG. There may be progeria, including premature graying. About 20% of patients develop malignancies, most frequently acute lymphocytic leukemia or lymphoma. The rate of cancer in heterozygote carriers is also increased.

The disease is progressive with a median age at death at about 20 years. The two major causes of death are cancer and pulmonary disease. Rarely, the course is protracted and benign; ataxia telangiectasia may account for progressive ataxia of adult onset.

Pathologically, loss of Purkinje cells is seen in the cerebellum with less prominent changes in the granule cell layer, dentate and inferior olivary nuclei, ventral horns, and spinal ganglia. Aside from decreased serum concentrations of IgA and IgG, laboratory abnormalities include cytogenetic abnormalities, abnormal sensitivity to ionizing radiation, and an elevation in alpha-fetoprotein. Cultured cells from ataxia telangiectasia patients show an excess of chromosome breaks and rearrangements, and there is much greater cell death than expected after exposure to ionizing radiation. Almost all ataxia telangiectasia patients show high serum content of alpha-fetoprotein, which is positively correlated with age. A clinical picture consistent with ataxia telangiectasia and an elevated alpha-fetoprotein level suffice to make the diagnosis.

The gene maps to chromosome 11 and is named ATM (for "ataxia telangiectasia mutated") (Table 107.1). Coding sequence mutations include deletions leading to sequence changes with premature truncation and in-frame deletions. The ATM protein belongs to a family of protein kinases. ATM is a key regulator of multiple signaling cascades that respond to DNA strand breaks induced by damaging agents or by normal processes, such meiotic recombination. The altered responses involve activation of cell checkpoints, DNA repair, and apoptosis. Approximately 1% of the population is heterozygous for ATM; however, population screening for the mutation is difficult because the gene is large and there are many different mutations.

X-linked inherited ataxias are rare. Syndromes of pure ataxia and spastic paraparesis with ataxia beginning in childhood, adolescence, or early adulthood have been reported in several families with an X-linked recessive pattern. An infant-onset X-linked form includes ataxia, deafness, optic atrophy, and hypotonia.

The diagnostic workup of a patient with early-onset ataxia depends on the constellation of clinical features in the family. If FRDA genetic testing is not diagnostic, other causes of sporadic or recessive ataxia need to be considered. Evaluation includes blood lipids, vitamin E, alpha-fetoprotein, lysosomal analysis, very-long-chain fatty acids, lactate and pyruvate, ceruloplasmin, and thyroid function. Abetalipoproteinemia and isolated vitamin E deficiency, in particular, can mimic the spinocerebellar findings of FRDA.

If there is no FRDA mutation, the vitamin E level is measured because a treatment may improve or prevent progression of signs. In addition to abetalipoproteinemia and cholestatic liver disease, vitamin E deficiency may be an isolated abnormality, with no lipid malabsorption. This condition, known as isolated vitamin E deficiency or ataxia/vitamin E deficiency (MIM 277460), is autosomal recessive. Clinical features usually mimic FRDA, but late onset in the sixth decade has been reported, and prominent titubation may be more common with isolated vitamin E deficiency. The disease is due to frameshift or missense point mutations in the alpha-tocopherol transfer protein gene, which maps to chromosome 8q13. The result impairs incorpo-

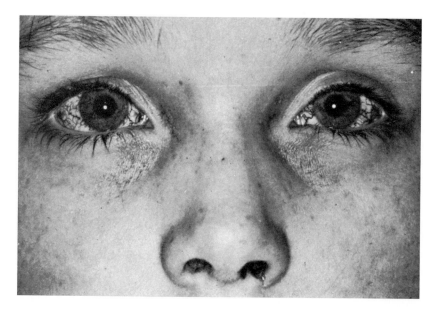

FIG. 107.1. Ataxia telangiectasia. Telangiectases in the bulbar conjunctiva. (Courtesy of Dr. G. Gaull.)

TABLE 107.1. GENETIC ASPECTS OF THE HEREDITARY ATAXIAS

Disorder	Inheritance	Chromosome	Gene	Trinucleotide	Protein
SCA-1	AD	6p	SCA1	CAG (exonic) $N < 39$ $A \geq 40$	Ataxin-1
SCA-2	AD	12q	SCA2	CAG (exonic) $N = 14–32$ $A \geq 35$	Ataxin-2
SCA-3/MJD	AD	14q	SCA3/MJD	CAG (exonic) $N < 42$ $A \geq 61$	Ataxin-3
SCA-4	AD	16q			
SCA-5	AD	11cent			
SCA-6	AD	19p	SCA6	CAG (exonic) $N < 20$ $A = 21–29$	CACNA1A
SCA-7	AD	3p	SCA7	CAG (exonic) $N < 36$ $A \geq 37$	Ataxin-7
SCA-8	AD	13q	SCA-8	CTG (untranslated) $N = 16–37$ $A > 80$	
SCA 10	AD	22q	SCA-10		
DRPLA	AD	12p	CTG-1337	CAG (exonic) $N < 36$ $A \geq 49$	Atrophin
EA-1	AD	12p	KCNA1	No	KCNA1
EA-2	AD	19p	CACNA1A	No	CACNA1A
FRDA	AR	9q	X25	GAA (intronic) $N < 42$ $A > 65$, up to 1700	Frataxin
Familial isolated vit E deficiency	AR	8q	AVED	No	Alpha-tocopherol transfer protein
AT	AR	11p	ATM	No	ATM protein (kinase)

SCA, spinocerebellar ataxia: MJD, Machado Joseph disease; DRPLA, dentato rubral pallidoluysian atrophy; AD, autosomal dominant; AR, autosomal recessive; cent, centromere; vit, vitamin; N, normal; A, affected; KCNAI, potassium voltage-gated channel; CACNAIA, alpha I A CA^{2+} channel; FRDA, Friedreich ataxia; AVED, ataxia/vitamin E deficiency; AT, ataxia telangiectasia; ATM, AT mutated; EA, episodic ataxia.

ration of alpha-tocopherol into very low density lipoprotein (VLDL), which is needed for the efficient recycling of vitamin E.

LATE-ONSET ATAXIAS

In 1893, Marie applied the term hereditary cerebellar ataxia to syndromes that differed from FRDA in later onset of symptoms, autosomal dominant inheritance, hyperactive tendon reflexes, and, frequently, ophthalmoplegia. Classification has been the subject of controversy because nosology was based on pathology, leading to eponyms named for Marie, Menzel, and Holmes, but with poor clinical-pathologic correlation, even within a single family. Harding challenged these confusing pathology-based schemes, lumping ADCA and then dividing them into clinical groups (Table 107.2). With the mapping and cloning of autosomal dominant ataxia genes, emphasis has shifted to a genetic classification, leading to a numbering system of autosomal spinocerebellar ataxia loci (SCA1, 2, 3, . . . 7). This classification has the advantage of defining causally related groups, but the numerous loci lack a connection to clinical or pathologic features. We try to bridge the clinical-genetic gap, incorporating both the ADCA and SCA classifications.

Autosomal Dominant Cerebellar Ataxia Type I

Many kindreds with ADCA I (SCA1–4, +SCA8) share clinical features, although clinical differences are still being defined. Symptoms usually begin in the third or fourth decade, but the age at onset varies from childhood to the seventh decade (Table 107.3). The first and generally most prominent sign is gait ataxia. Sudden falls may come first. Limb ataxia and dysarthria are early symptoms. Hyperreflexia may be present initially, but tendon reflexes may later be depressed and vibration and proprioception may be lost. Eye signs include nystagmus, slow saccades, and abnormal pursuit. Dementia, dystonia, facial fasciculations, and distal wasting may occur. Anticipation and potentiation, earlier onset, and more severe symptoms in succeeding generations are often observed. Most affected individuals are severely disabled 10 to 20 years after symptom onset (Table 107.3).

All cloned ADCA I except SCA8 genes share the same type of mutation, an unstable expansion of a CAG trinucleotide repeat in the protein-coding region of the gene. As in other dominant disorders with trinucleotide expansions (e.g., Huntington disease, dentatorubropallidoluysian atrophy), there is an inverse relation between repeat size and age at onset. Another feature of the trinucleotide expansion in ADCA I is meiotic instability. In

TABLE 107.2. INHERITED ATAXIAS

Early-onset ataxias (usually before 20 year) without a known biochemical defect
Autosomal recessive
 Friedreich ataxia
 Other recessive ataxias
  Resembling Friedreich but with retained tendon reflexes
  With hypogonadism
  With myoclonus
  With optic atrophy and mental retardation
  With deafness
  With cataracts and mental retardation (Marinesco-Sjögren)
X linked

Late-onset ataxias without a known biochemical defect
Autosomal dominant cerebellar ataxia (ADCA)
 With ophthalmoplegia/extrapyramidal features but without
  retinal degeneration (ADCA I)
  SCA-1
  SCA-2
  SCA-3/MJD
  SCA-4
  SCA-8
 With retinal degeneration (ADCA II)
  SCA-7
 "Pure" ADCA (ADCA III)
  SCA-5
  SCA-6
  SCA-10
  DRPLA
Paroxysmal ataxia
 with myokymia
 with nystagmus

Ataxias with identified biochemical defects
Ataxia/vitamin E deficiency
Abeta- and hypobetalipoproteinemia
Mitochondrial encephalomyopathies (MERRF, NARP, KSS)
Leigh syndrome
Carboxylase deficiencies
Urea cycle defects I
Aminoacidurias
Wilson disease
Sialidosis
Refsum
Ceroid lipofuscinosis
Leukodystrophies
Cholestanolosis (cerebrotendinous xanthomatosis)
Gangliosidosis (e.g., hexosaminidase deficiency)
Ataxia telangiectasia
Xeroderma pigmentosum
Cockayne syndrome

SCA, spinocerebellar ataxia; MJD, Machado-Joseph disease; DRPLA, dentato-rubral pallidoluysian atrophy; NARP, neurogenic weakness, ataxia, retinitis pigmentosa; KSS, Kearn Sayre syndrome.

a parent–child transmission, the size of the repeat changes. Also, paternal and maternal transmission differ, with a greater tendency for an increase in repeat size in paternally transmitted disease chromosomes. As a result, anticipation is greater in paternally transmitted disease.

The CAG expansions all result in an expanded polyglutamine tract, because CAG codes for glutamine. Unlike the FRDA triplet expansion, which causes a disease by inducing a loss of normal function (frataxin deficiency), the dominant SCA triplet expansions cause disease by altering the protein, which acquires a new activity that is toxic to the cell, a toxic gain of functions.

The pathogenic mechanism of the polyglutamine proteins is not yet clarified. However, each polyglutamine disorder has distinctive clinical-pathologic features, so some other feature of the protein, in addition to the polyglutamine, must play a role. Possible toxic mechanisms include nuclear targeting of protein fragments that contain the polyglutamine stretches and the formation of intranuclear filamentous inclusions.

SCA1 (MIM 164400)

Genetics
The first ADCA locus, SCA1, was mapped to the short arm of chromosome 6 in 1974, based on linkage to the human leukocyte antigen. In 1991, highly polymorphic DNA markers flanking the SCA1 gene were identified, and in 1993, the SCA1 mutation was identified. A trinucleotide expansion was specifically sought because of the known anticipation in SCA1 families and the earlier finding of expanded trinucleotide repeats and anticipation in Huntington disease.

Abnormal alleles have 40 or more repeats; normal alleles have fewer than 38. Normal alleles differ from abnormal repeats not only in size but also by the presence of one or more CAT repeats. The CAT repeats serve as anchors during replication and prevent slippage, which is presumably the mechanism reasonsible for repeat instability.

The protein coded by SCA1 is called *ataxin-1*, a novel protein of unknown function. It is expressed ubiquitously. Ataxin-1 is located in the nucleus in all cells except Purkinje cells where there is cytoplasmic and nuclear localization. In affected neurons of SCA1 patients and transgenic mice, mutant ataxin-1 aggregates and forms a ubiquitin-positive nuclear inclusion. However, studies in transgenic mice suggest that nuclear localization of mutant ataxin-1 may be necessary for the disease to occur, but nuclear aggregation is not.

Epidemiology
The prevalence of SCA1 (or any of the other ADCA genetic subtypes) is not known. However, the proportion of ADCA families with SCA1 (as determined by the CAG repeat) in different populations varies widely. In the United States and Germany, the proportion is low (1% to 9%), whereas in Italy and England the number is higher (30% to 35%), and even more so in some regions of Japan. In all series, SCA1 rarely if ever accounts for ataxia in singleton cases or those that seem to be recessive.

Clinical and Pathologic Features
Typically, SCA1 starts in the fourth decade, but the range of age at onset is 6 to 60 years. Gait ataxia always predominates and is often the first sign, accompanied by hypermetric saccades and nystagmus. Hyperreflexia, Babinski signs, ophthalmoparesis, (particularly upgaze), dysarthria, dysphagia, and sensory loss are common later (Table 107.3). Sphincter symptoms, optic atrophy, dementia, personality change, dystonia (torticollis), chorea, and fasciculations are less common.

The pathology includes neuronal loss in the cerebellum, brainstem, spinocerebellar tracts, and dorsal columns with rare involvement of the substantia nigra and basal ganglia. Purkinje cell loss and severe neuronal degeneration in the inferior olive are seen; degeneration is also seen in the cranial nerve nuclei, resti-

TABLE 107.3. CLINICAL FEATURES OF THE HEREDITARY ATAXIAS

Name	Inheritance	Onset average (range)	Phenotype	Gene
SCA-1	AD	30s (6–60)	Ataxia, dysarthria, pyramidal, extrapyramidal and bulbar signs, ophthalmoparesis	Yes
SCA-2	AD	30s (infant–67) slow saccades	Ataxia, dysarthria, neuropathy	Yes
SCA-3/MJD	AD	30s (6–70)	Ataxia, dysarthria ophthalmoparesis, pyramidal and extrapyramidal signs, amyotrophy	Yes
SCA-4	AD	30s (19–59)	Ataxia, dysarthria, sensory neuropathy, pyramidal signs	No
SCA-5	AD	30s (10–68)	Slowly progressive ataxia and dysarthria	No
SCA-6	AD	48 (24–75)	Slowly progressive ataxia, nystagmus dysarthria	Yes
SCA-7	AD	30s (infant–60)	Ataxia, pigmentary retinopathy ophthtalmoparesis, pyramidal extrapyramidal sign	Yes
SCA-8	AD	39 (18–65)	Ataxia, dysarthria, nystagmus Spasticity, decreased vibration	Yes
SCA-10	AD	35 (15–45)	Ataxia, dysarthria, nystagmus, seizures	No
DRPLA	AD	30s (child–70)	Ataxia, dementia, chorea, myoclonus, epilepsy	Yes
Episodic ataxia-1 EA-1/myokymia	AD	Child	Exercise- or startle-induced paroxysmal ataxia (min) myokymia	Yes
Episodic ataxia-2 EA-2/nystagmus	AD	Child	Stress- or fatigue-induced episodic ataxia (h) nystamus, acetazolamide-responsive	Yes
Friedreich ataxia	AR	13 (infant–50)	Ataxia, dysarthria, position sense loss, sensory loss, hyporeflexia Babinski sign, cardiomyopathy, scoliosis	Yes
Isolated vitamin E deficiency	AR	Child–adult	Friedreich-like phenotype	Yes
Ataxia telangiectasia	AR	Child	Ataxia, telangiectasia Immune deficiency Elevated alpha-fetoprotein	Yes

AD, autosomal dominant; AR, autosomal recessive.

form body, brachium conjunctivum, dorsal and ventral spinocerebellar tracts, posterior columns, and rarely the anterior horn cells.

SCA2 (MIM 183090)

This autosomal dominant locus was mapped to chromosome 12q23-24 in 1993. It was first localized in ataxic patients originating from the Holguin province of Cuba and descended from an Iberian founder. Subsequently, SCA2 families were found in Italy, Germany, French-Canada, Tunisia, and Japan. In 1996, three independent groups identified the SCA2 gene using different techniques: positional cloning, using antibody for polyglutamine repeats, and the direct identification of repeat and cloning technique.

Normal individuals have 14 to 32 CAG repeats (with most containing 22) interrupted by one to three CAAs within the CAG repeat. SCA2 patients have CAG expansions of 35 or more and no CAAs within the repeat. There is an inverse correlation between age at onset and CAG number. When the CAG expansion is large, manifestations are more likely to include dementia, chorea, myoclonus, and dystonia. The function of *ataxin-2*, the protein encoded by SCA2, is not known but it is localized in the cytoplasm of neurons, especially Purkinje cells.

Epidemiology

SCA2 is a relatively frequent cause of ADCA (excluding those with retinopathy) worldwide, varying from 10% in German families to 13% to 15% in U.S. families to 37% to 47% in Italian and English families. It is rarely a cause in families with apparent recessive inheritance or in sporadic cases.

Clinical and Pathologic Features

The disease usually begins in the fourth decade, but onset ranges from early childhood to the seventh decade. The most common clinical features are gait and limb ataxia and dysarthria. Other common features include depressed or absent tendon reflexes (especially in the arms), slow saccades, fasciculations, ophthalmoplegia, and vibratory and position sensory loss. Less common features are action tremor, cramps, staring gaze, dementia, leg hyperreflexia, and chorea. Nystagmus may be present at onset but tends to disappear as slow saccades emerge. Although there is considerable overlap among the different ADCA I subtypes, SCA2 patients are most likely to have slow saccades and hyporeflexia. Many show electrophysiologic evidence of axonal neuropathy, with severe involvement of sensory fibers. The highly variable phenotype occasionally seems to "breed true" in families (e.g., kindreds with dementia and extrapyramidal signs, or with moderate ataxia, facial fasciculations, and prominent eye signs that include lid lag).

Pathology, like clinical signs, varies. Usually there is olivopontocerebellar atrophy with severe neuronal loss in the inferior olive, pons, and cerebellum. However, there may also be degeneration of the substantia nigra, dorsal columns, and anterior horn cells. Rarely, degeneration is restricted to the cerebellum.

SCA3/Machado-Joseph Disease (MIM 109150)

Genetics and Clinical-Genetic Correlation

Machado-Joseph disease (MJD) was first described in families of Azorean Portuguese descent. Common signs, regardless of age at onset, include gait and limb ataxia, dysarthria, and progressive ophthalmoplegia. Findings more dependent on age at onset include pyramidal signs, dystonia and rigidity, amyotrophy, facial and lingual fasciculations, and lid retraction with bulging eyes. Four clinical subclasses were proposed:

1. Adolescent/young adult-onset: rapidly progressive, with spasticity, rigidity, bradykinesia, weakness, dystonia, and ataxia;
2. Mid-adult onset (ages 30 to 50): moderate progression of ataxia;
3. Late adult onset (ages 40 to 70): slower progression of ataxia, prominent peripheral nerve signs, and few extrapyramidal findings;
4. Adult onset: parkinsonism and peripheral neuropathy.

The pathology was considered distinct with primarily spinopontine atrophy and involvement of pontine nuclei, spinocerebellar tracts, Clarke column, anterior horn cells, substantia nigra, and basal ganglia; the inferior olives and cerebellar cortex were spared. With mutation screening, however, it is now evident that the olives and cerebellar cortex may be involved.

In addition to families of Portuguese descent, a similar disorder has been described in German, Dutch, African-American, and Japanese families. In 1993, Takiyama and colleagues mapped a gene in several Japanese families to chromosome 14q24.3-32. This locus then was confirmed in MJD families of Azorean descent. In 1994, linkage to the same region was found in French families that were not considered clinically different from SCA1 or 2 and the locus was numbered SCA3. Because these French families were not of Azorean descent and because of several clinical differences (lack of dystonia and facial fasciculation), it was uncertain whether MJD and SCA3 were due to different genes, different mutations in the same gene, or the varying phenotypic expressions of the same mutation in individuals with different ancestry. In 1994, an expanded and unstable CAG repeat was found in the coding region of the MJD gene. Subsequently, all 14q-linked families have been found to have the same unstable CAG repeat within the SCA3/MJD gene, so that SCA3 and MJD are a single genetic disorder with a wide clinical spectrum. As with the other ADCA genes, there may be intrafamilial genetic modifiers (including differences within the SCA3/MJD gene) that influence the phenotype.

Unlike SCA1 and SCA2, there is a wide gap between normal and disease repeat size, with normal ranging from 12 to 41 and disease alleles ranging from 61 to 89. As in all CAG repeat diseases, there is a strong inverse correlation between the length of the repeat and age at onset. Greater instability in paternal meioses seems to be true for SCA3, as in the other ADCA genes. Unlike Huntington disease and other dominant CAG repeat diseases, homozygous SCA3 individuals have early-onset severe disease, suggesting a gene-dosage effect.

The SCA3/MJD gene encodes *ataxin-3*, a protein of unknown function that is not related to ataxin-1 or -2. It is ubiquitously expressed in the cytoplasm of cell bodies and processes. In SCA3/MJD brain there is aberrant nuclear localization and accumulation of ubiquitinated nuclear inclusions.

Epidemiology

SCA3 is a common cause of ADCA in many but not all populations. In the United States, about 21% of families with ataxia have SCA3; in a study of mixed populations, 41% were SCA3, but this dropped to 17% when Portuguese families were excluded. SCA3 seems to be common in Germany (accounting for 50% of ADCA cases), India, and Japan but rare in Italy and uncommon in England.

SCA4 (MIM 600223)

This ADCA is based on linkage in a large U.S. family to chromosome 16q. The phenotype consists of late-onset (19 to 59 years) ataxia, prominent sensory axonal neuropathy, normal eye movements in most, and pyramidal tract signs. The gene is not yet identified. The earliest symptom is unsteadiness of gait. Dysarthria is present in 50%, absent ankle jerks in 100%, decreased sensation in 100%, extensor plantar responses in 20%, and saccadic pursuit eye movements in only 15%. Nerve conduction studies indicate an axonal sensory neuropathy.

SCA8

This is the most recently identified ADCA; it is based on the cloning of an untranslated CTG expansion as the mutation in eight families. This expansion maps to chromosome 13q, and the mechanism seems similar to that of myotonic dystrophy. There appears to be expansion of the CTG repeat in maternal transmission and deletion in paternal transmission; penetrance is reduced and depends on repeat size. Normal alleles have 16 to 37 repeats and affected alleles have 107 to 127 repeats.

Initial clinical features include dysarthria and gait instability. Age at onset averages 39 years (range, 18 to 65). In addition to limb and gait ataxia and dysarthria, the findings include nystagmus, limb spasticity, and diminished vibration sense. The course is slowly progressive, and the most severely affected are not able to walk by the fourth decade. SCA8 is estimated to account for 3% of ADCA families and 6% of those characterized as recessive.

Autosomal Dominant Cerebellar Ataxia Type III

Harding reserved this ADCA group for families with "pure" cerebellar features, usually of later onset and generally after age 50. It is unclear whether any genetically described families completely fulfill these criteria. Three mapped SCA genes, one cloned, differ from ADCA I in that the clinical picture is dominated by cerebellar features, with other signs contributing little to overall phenotype. Therefore, they are categorized separately from ADCA I. However, the clinical differences between ADCA I and III are not absolute, and an alternate classification may properly include all SCA subtypes without retinopathy under the SCA1 heading.

SCA5 (MIM 600224)

This locus was mapped to the pericentromeric region of chromosome 11q in a kindred descended from the paternal grandparents of President Abraham Lincoln. Symptoms of this relatively benign, slowly progressive, cerebellar syndrome appear at 10 to 68 years, with anticipation (Table 107.3). All four juvenile-onset patients (10 to 18 years) resulted from maternal transmission rather than the paternal pattern seen in the other SCA syndromes. The juvenile-onset patients showed cerebellar and pyramidal tract signs, as well as bulbar dysfunction. The gene is not yet identified.

SCA6 (MIM 183086)

Genetics

SCA6 was the designation for families excluded from linkage to previously identified loci. In 1996, SCA6 was mapped and the gene identified. The pathogenic mechanism of SCA6 may differ from the others, and mutations in this gene may underlie some sporadic cases.

The SCA6 gene maps to chromosome 19p13 and encodes for an alpha IA voltage-dependent calcium channel subunit (CACNA1A, previously named CACNLIA4). Different mutations have distinct phenotypes. The SCA6 symbol is reserved for a phenotype dominated by a late-onset progressive cerebellar syndrome associated with coding sequence CAG repeat expansions; the expansions are smaller than other SCA mutations. SCA6 CAG repeats are 21 to 29 (normal expansions are 4 to 18), in contrast to other SCA repeat expansions that range from 35 to 100 or more. Missense mutations in the same gene are found in familial hemiplegic migraine, and mutations causing premature termination of the coding sequence are found in families with episodic (or paroxysmal) ataxia type 2.

As with the other ADCA repeat disorders, there is a correlation between the number of SCA6 repeats and age at onset. However, unlike the other ADCA repeat disorders, the repeat is stable during transmission and anticipation is generally not observed. Like MJD, the phenotype is more severe in homozygous individuals. New mutations underlie some sporadic cases.

The molecular basis of disease in SCA6 may differ from the other repeat ataxias. First, the expansion in SCA6 is small; as few as 20 repeats can cause disease. Second, there is clinical overlap between episodic ataxia type 2 and SCA6; some family members with episodic ataxia have progressive ataxia and some SCA6 family members have episodic symptoms. This suggests a related pathogenesis despite the different mutations within CACNA1A. Third, homozygous individuals have a more severe phenotype, suggesting a dose effect. All three findings suggest loss of a normal function or a dominant negative effect in which a heterozygous mutation alters normal function. This contrasts with the "gain" or new toxic function that is intrinsic to the expanded CAG repeat in the SCA1, 2, 3, or 7.

Clinical and Pathologic Features

The clinical picture of SCA6 is fairly uniform. The average age at onset is about 45 years (range, 20 to 75). The first symptom is usually unsteady gait. Dysarthria, leg cramps, and diplopia can also be early symptoms. Occasionally, patients describe positional vertigo or nausea. Cerebellar signs include gait and limb ataxia (especially leg), cerebellar dysarthria, saccadic pursuit, and dysmetric saccades. Horizontal and downbeat nystagmus (most prominent on lateral gaze) are common eye signs. Noncerebellar

signs occur with less frequency and less clinical impact than other SCA disorders but include decreased vibration and position sense, peripheral neuropathy, and impaired upgaze. Long tract signs, parkinsonism, and chorea are rare. Onset of ataxia is occasionally episodic or apoplectic and may resemble episodic ataxia type 2 with attacks of unsteadiness, vertigo, and dysarthria that last for hours; between attacks there are few if any symptoms or signs. The attacks may occur for years before progressive cerebellar signs emerge.

The course is slowly progressive, but after 10 to 15 years most affected individuals are no longer able to walk without assistance. MRI shows cerebellar atrophy but little brainstem or cortical atrophy. Pathologically, there is cerebellar atrophy with loss of Purkinje and granule cells and limited involvement of the inferior olives.

Epidemiology

SCA6 accounts for 2% to 30% of dominantly inherited ataxia, depending on the population. In the United States and Germany, SCA6 accounts for 10% to 15% of ADCA families. It is more common in regions of Japan (30%) and is uncommon in France, where only 1% of ADCA families harbor the mutation. Five percent to 6% of sporadic ataxia patients demonstrate SCA6 expansions. Some are due to new mutations, but it is also likely that some appear sporadic because of the late age at onset and relatively indolent course.

SCA10

In 1999, two independent groups mapped this locus to chromosome 22q; the phenotype is marked by pure cerebellar signs and seizures. Both families are of Mexican ancestry and it is suspected that they descend from a common ancestor. Age at onset ranged from adolescence to 45 years with evidence of anticipation. There was gait and limb ataxia, dysarthria, and nystagmus in all affected individuals. Also, unlike the other SCA syndromes, partial complex and generalized motor seizures occurred in 20% of members of one family and 67% of the other.

Autosomal Dominant Cerebellar Ataxia type II

SCA7 (MIM 164500)

This type was first distinguished from other forms of ADCA in 1937 by the presence of retinal degeneration. The locus was mapped to chromosome 3p in 1995; the gene was cloned in 1997. As with most of the other ADCA genes, SCA7 is due to the expansion of a coding sequence CAG repeat. Normal alleles have 4 to 35 repeats. In affected individuals, the repeat contains 37 to more than 200. Dramatic examples of anticipation, especially with paternal transmission, were described before the gene was cloned and is due to repeat instability, which is greater in SCA7 than any other SCAs. There is a correlation between age at onset and repeat length. The rate of clinical progression and constellation of clinical signs also correlate with repeat size. *Ataxin-7* is expressed ubiquitously, is present in the nuclear fraction of lymphoblasts, and contains a nuclear localization signal, suggesting that it may be a transcription factor.

SCA7 age at onset ranges from infancy to the seventh decade and averages around 30 years. The clinical course varies with age at onset. A severe infantile form occurs with large expansions (more than 200) that are paternally inherited. These infants have hypotonia, dysphagia, visual loss, cerebellar and cerebral atrophy, and congestive heart failure with cardiac anomalies. This differs from childhood and adult forms that are marked by early visual loss, moderately progressive limb and gait ataxia, dysarthria, ophthalmoparesis (especially upgaze), and Babinski signs and rarely include dementia, peripheral neuropathy, hearing loss, dyskinesias, parkinsonism, or psychosis. In late-onset cases (fourth to sixth decade), ataxia may occur in isolation or it may precede visual symptoms (Table 107.3). Affected individuals all have abnormal yellow-blue color discrimination (which in the mildest forms may be asymptomatic) and clinically there is often optic disc pallor with granular and atrophic changes in the macula.

Pathology

Degeneration affects the cerebellum, basis pontis, inferior olive, and retinal ganglion cells. Neuronal intranuclear inclusions containing the expanded polyglutamine tract are found in many brain regions, most frequently in the inferior olive.

Epidemiology

SCA7 accounts for all or almost all families with both ADCA and retinal degeneration. Among 86 ADCA families of diverse ethnic background, 11.6% of the families were due to SCA7.

DRPLA

This condition, first described in 1946, is most common in Japan where it constitutes about 20% of ADCA families. Rare cases have been described in African-Americans, North American whites, and Europeans. The pathology involves the dentate, red nucleus, subthalamic nucleus, and the external globus pallidus; the posterior columns may be involved. The phenotype varies, even within a family, and depends to some extent on the age at onset. Early-onset cases tend to show severe and rapid progression of myoclonus, epilepsy, and cognitive decline (myoclonic epilepsy), whereas late-onset cases display ataxia, chorea, and dementia (resembling Huntington disease) (Table 107.3). Anticipation is evident, and paternal transmission is associated with more severe early-onset disease. One clinical variant, the *Haw River syndrome*, was described in an African-American family in North Carolina. This variant includes all the above symptoms except for myoclonic seizures, and additional features include basal ganglia calcification, neuroaxonal dystrophy, and demyelination of the central white matter. MRI may show atrophy of the cerebral cortex, cerebellum, and pontomesencephalic tegmentum, with increased signal in white matter of the cerebrum and brainstem.

The disorder is due to an expansion of a CAG repeat in the DRPLA gene, which maps to chromosome 12p. There is an inverse relationship between repeat size and age at onset; normal subjects have up to 35 repeats and disease alleles have 49 or more (Table 107.1). The gene is expressed in all tissues, including brain. The DRPLA gene product, *atrophin*, is found mainly in neuronal cytoplasm. Ubiquinated intranuclear inclusions are found in neurons and to a lesser extent in glia. The neuronal inclusions are concentrated in the striatum, pontine nuclei, inferior olive, cerebellar cortex, and dentate.

Other Unmapped Autosomal Dominant Cerebellar Ataxias

The mapped and cloned SCA genes account for most ADCAs, up to 90% in some series. Other loci for ADCA, however, remain to be identified. In several families, all known ADCA loci have been excluded.

EPISODIC OR PAROXYSMAL ATAXIAS

Episodes of ataxia can be the first manifestation of metabolic disorders such as multiple carboxylase deficiencies or amino acidurias. However, the term episodic or paroxysmal ataxia is generally applied to a condition in which the major expressions are self-limited episodes of cerebellar dysfunction with little fixed or progressive neurologic dysfunction. Two major clinical-genetic subtypes of this rare condition are described: *episodic ataxia with myokymia* (EA1/myokymia) and *episodic ataxia with nystagmus* (EA2/nystagmus). A third type is marked by *paroxysmal choreoathetosis with spasticity and episodic ataxia* (Table 107.3).

In EA1/myokymia, the attacks usually last a few minutes; they are provoked by startle, sudden movement, or change in posture and exercise (especially if the subject is excited or fatigued). Usually, these are one or a few attacks each day, but up to 15 may occur. Onset is in childhood or adolescence; the disorder is not associated with neurologic deterioration, but myokymia appears around the eyes and in the hands. The Achilles tendon may be shortened and there may be a tremor of the hands. The attacks are often heralded by an aura of weightlessness or weakness; an attack comprises ataxia, dysarthria, shaking tremor, and twitching. In some families, acetazolamide reduces the frequency of attacks; phenytoin and other anticonvulsants may reduce myokymia. This disorder is caused by missense point mutations in the potassium voltage-gated channel gene KCNAI on chromosome 12p (Table 107.1).

EA2/nystagmus attacks last longer, usually hours or even days. Attacks are provoked by stress, exercise, fatigue, and alcohol and do not generally occur more than once per day. Age at onset varies from infancy to 40 years. Unlike EA1/myokymia, the cerebellar syndrome may progress with increasing ataxia and dysarthria. Even when there is no progressive cerebellar syndrome, interictal nystagmus is often seen (Table 107.3). During an attack, associated symptoms include headache, diaphoresis, nausea, vertigo, ataxia, dysarthria, ptosis, and ocular palsy. Acetazolamide is usually effective in reducing attacks. The gene maps to chromosome 19p and encodes a brain-specific alpha 1A voltage-dependent calcium channel subunit (CACNAIA).

Different disease-causing point mutations result in premature termination of the coding sequence. CAG repeat expansion is responsible for SCA6.

A third form of episodic ataxia associated with spasticity and paroxysmal choreoathetosis maps to 1p.

SPORADIC CEREBELLAR ATAXIA OF LATE ONSET

Many patients with ataxia beginning after age 40 have no affected relatives. Some apparent sporadic cases with late-onset ataxia are due to SCA mutations. Compared with ADCA, sporadic cases begin later in life (in the sixth decade), have a more rapid course, and are less likely to have ophthalmoplegia, amyotrophy, retinal degeneration, or optic atrophy. However, many of these patients have parkinsonism and upper motor neuron signs. Some also have autonomic dysfunction and are classified as having multisystem atrophy of the olivopontocerebellar atrophy (OPCA) type; the cause of multisystem atrophy is not known, but a distinct pathologic finding of multisystem atrophy is the oligodendroglial cytoplasmic inclusion.

CONGENITAL AND ACQUIRED CEREBELLAR ATAXIAS

The cerebellum and spinocerebellar tracts are the primary sites involved in several developmental, metabolic, infectious, neoplastic, and vascular disorders (Table 107.2). Most of these syndromes are discussed elsewhere in this book. Two acquired cerebellar syndromes are common causes of subacute and chronic ataxia in adults, paraneoplastic (see Chapter 153) and alcohol-related cerebellar degeneration (see Chapter 157).

MANAGEMENT OF HEREDITARY ATAXIAS

No specific treatments influence the course of most hereditary ataxias. Vitamin E replacement can prevent or improve the ataxia of familial isolated vitamin E deficiency. In FRDA, orthopedic procedures are indicated for the relief of foot deformity. In the SCAs, especially MJD/SCA3, levodopa may bring symptomatic relief of rigidity or other parkinsonian features; baclofen or trizanidene may help spasticity. Acetazolamide controls the attacks of the episodic paroxysmal cerebellar ataxias (EA1 and EA2), and phenytoin ameliorates the facial and hand myokymia associated with EA1. Amantadine and buspirone may improve different forms of cerebellar ataxia, but any effect is moderate at best. Genetic counseling should be offered to patients and families with these disorders and should always accompany genetic testing. We can hope for novel specific therapies based on our increasing knowledge of the molecular mechanisms underlying the hereditary ataxias.

SUGGESTED READINGS

Early-Onset Inherited Ataxias

Friedreich Ataxia

Ackroyd RS, Finnegan JA, Green SH. Friedreich ataxia: a clinical review with neurophysiological and echocardiographic findings. *Arch Dis Child* 1984;59:217–221.

Campuzano V, Montermini L, Lutz Y, et al. Frataxin is reduced in Friedreich ataxia patients and is associated with mitochondrial membranes. *Hum Mol Genet* 1997;6:1771–1780.

Campuzano V, Montermini L, Molto MD, et al. Friedreich's ataxia: autosomal recessive disease caused by an intronic triplet repeat expansion. *Science* 1996;271:1374–1375.

Chamberlain S, Shaw S, Rowland S, et al. Mapping of the mutation causing Friedreich's ataxia to human chromosome 9. *Nature* 1988;334: 248–250.

Durr A, Cossee M, Agid Y, et al. Clinical and genetic abnormalities in patients with Friedreich's ataxia. *N Engl J Med* 1996;335:1222–1224.

Friedreich N. Uber Ataxic mit besonderer Berucksichtigung der hereditaren Formen. *Virchows Arch Pathol Anat* 1863;26:391–419, 433–459, 27:1–26.

Harding AE. Friedreich's ataxia: a clinical and genetic study of 90 families with an analysis of early diagnostic criteria and intrafamilial clustering of clinical features. *Brain* 1981;104:589–620.

Harding AE. Clinical features and classification of inherited ataxias. *Adv Neurol* 1993;61:1–14.

Lamont PJ, Davis MB, Wood NW. Identification and sizing of the GAA trinucleotide repeat expansion of Friedreich's ataxia in 56 patients. Clinical and genetic correlates. *Brain* 1997;120:673–680.

Montermini L, Richter A, Morgan K, et al. Phenotypic variability in Friedreich ataxia:role of the associated GAA triplet repeat expansion. *Ann Neurol* 1997;41:675–682.

Moseley ML, Benzow KA, Schut LJ, et al. Dominant cerebellar and Friedreich triplet repeats among 361 ataxia families. *Neurology* 1998;51: 1603–1607.

Pandolfo M, Montermini L. Molecular genetics of the hereditary ataxias. *Adv Genet* 1998;51:31–68.

Schols L, Amoiridis G, Przuntek H, et al. Friedreich ataxia: revision of the phenotype according to molecular genetics. *Brain* 1997;120:2131–2140.

Ragno M, De Michele G, Cavalcanti F, et al. Broadened Friedreich ataxia phenotype after gene cloning: minimal GAA expansion causes late-onset spastic ataxia. *Neurology* 1997;49:1617–1620.

Other Early-onset Ataxias

Ben Hamida C, Doerflinaer N, Belal S, et al. Localization of Friedreich ataxia phenotype with selective Vitamin E deficiency to chromosome 8q by homozygosity mapping. *Nat Genet* 1993;5:195–200.

Gatti RA, Berkel L, Boder E, et al. Localization of an ataxia-telangiectasia gene to chromosome I lq-22-23. *Nature* 1988;336:577–580.

Gotoda T, Arita M, Arai H, et al. Adult-onset spinocerebellar dysfunction caused by a mutation in the gene for the alpha tocopheral transfer protein. *N Engl J Med* 1995;333:1313–1318.

Pennacchio LA, Lehesjoki AE, Stone NE, et al. Mutations in the gene encoding cystatin B in progressive myoclonus epilepsy (EPMJ). *Science* 1996;27:1731–1734.

Yokota T, Shicjiri T, Gotoda T, et al. Friedreich-like ataxia with retinitis pigmentosa caused by the His101 Gln mutation of the alpha-tocopherol transfer protein gene. *Ann Neurol* 1997;41:826–832.

Late-Onset Autosomal Dominant Cerebellar Ataxia

Banfi S, Servadio A, Chung MY, et al. Identification and characterization of the gene causing type I spinocerebellar ataxia. *Nat Genet* 1994;7: 513–520.

Benomar A, Krols L, Stevanin G, et al. The gene for autosomal dominant cerebellar ataxia with pigmentary macular dystrophy maps to chromosome 3pl2-p2l.l. *Nat Genet* 1995;10:84–88.

Benton CS, de Silva R, Rutledge SL, Bohlega S, Ashizawa T, Zoghbi HY. Molecular/clinical studies in SCA 7 define a broad clinical spectrum and infantile phenotype. *Neurology* 1998;51:1081–1085.

Burke JR, Wingfield MS, Lewis KE, et al. The Haw River syndrome: dentatorubropallidoluysian atrophy in an African-American family. *Nat Genet* 1994;7:521–524.

David G, Abbas N, Stevanin G, et al. Cloning of the SCA7 gene reveals a highly unstable CAG repeat expansion. *Nat Genet* 1997;17:65–70.

Davies SW, Turmaine M, Cozens BA, et al. Formation of neuronal intranuclear inclusions underlies the neurological dysfunction in mice transgenic for the HD mutation. *Cell* 1997;90:537–548.

Flanigan K, Gardner K, Alderson K, et al. Autosomal dominant spinocerebellar ataxia with sensory axonal neuropathy (SCA4): clinical description and genetic localization to chromosome 16q22.1. *Am J Hum Genet* 1996;59:392–399.

Geshwind DH, Perlman S, Figueroa KP, Karrim J, Baloh RW, Pulst S. Spinocerebellar type 6: frequency of the mutation and genotype phenotype correlations. *Neurology* 1997;49:1247–1251.

Geshwind DS, Perlman H, Figueroa CP, Treiman J, Pulst SM. The prevalence and wide clinical spectrum of the spinocerebellar ataxia type 2 trinucleotide repeat in patients with autosomal dominant cerebellar ataxia. *Am J Hum Genet* 1997;60:842–850.

Giunti P, Sabbadini M, Sweeney MG, et al. The role of SCA2 trinucleotide repeat expansion in 89 autosomal dominant ataxia families. *Brain* 1998;121:459–467.

Grewel RP, Tayag E, Figueroa KP, et al. Clinical and genetic analysis of a distinct autosomal dominant spinocerebellar ataxia. *Neurology* 1998; 51:1423–1426.

Holmberg M, Duyckaerts C, Durr A, et al. Spinocerebellar ataxia type 7 (SCA7): a neurodegenerative disorder with neuronal intranuclear inclusions. *Hum Mol Genet* 1998;7:913–918.

Jodice C, Mantuano E, Veneziano L, et al. Episodic ataxia type 2 (EA2) and spinocerebellar ataxia type 6 (SCA6) due to CAG repeat expansion in the CACNA I A gene on chromosome l9p. *Hum Mol Genet* 1997;11: 1973–1978.

Johansson J, Forsgren L, Sandgren O, Brice A, Holmgren G, Holmberg M. Expanded CAG repeats in Swedish spinocerebellar ataxia type 7 (SCA7) patients: effect of CAG repeat length on the clinical manifestation. *Hum Mol Genet* 1998;7:171–176.

Koeppen AH. The hereditary ataxias. *J Neuropathol Exp Neurol* 1998; 57:531–543.

Koob MD, Moseley ML, Schut LJ, et al. An untranslated CTG expansion causes a novel form of spinocerebellar ataxia. *Nat Genet* 1999;4:379–384.

Matsuura T, Achari M, Khajavi M, Bachinski LL, Zoghbi HY, Ashizawa T. Mapping of the gene for a novel spinocerebellar ataxia with pure cerebellar signs and epilepsy. *Ann Neurol* 1999;45:407–411.

Nagafuchi S, Yanagisawa H, Ohsaki E, et al. Structure and expression of the gene responsible for the triplet repeat disorder, dentatorubral and pallidolysian atrophy (DRPLA). *Nat Genet* 1994;8:177–182.

Nakano K, Dawson D, Spence A. Machado disease: hereditary ataxia in Portuguese immigrants to Massachusetts. *Neurology* 1972;22:49–59.

Paulson HL, Perez MK, Trottier PY, et al. Intranuclear inclusions of expanded polyglutamine protein in spinocerebellar ataxia type 3. *Neuron* 1997;19:333–344.

Ranurn LP, Schut LJ, Lundgren JK, Orr HT, Livingston PM. Spinocerebellar ataxia type 5 in a family descended from the grandparents of President Lincoln maps to chromosome 11. *Nat Genet* 1994;8:280–284.

Rosenberg RN, Nyhan WL, Bay C, Shore P. Autosomal dominant striatonigral degeneration: a clinical, pathologic and biochemical study of a new genetic disorder. *Neurology* 1976;26:703–714.

Sanpei K, Takano H, Igarashi S, et al. Identification of the spinocerebellar ataxia type 2 gene using a direct identification of repeat expansion and cloning technique, DIRECT. *Nat Genet* 1996;14:277–284.

Stevanin G, Durr A, David G, et al. Clinical and molecular features of spinocerebellar type 6. *Neurology* 1997;49:1243–1246.

Tuite PJ, Rogaeva EA, St. George-Hyslop PH, Lang AE. Dopa-responsive parkinsonism phenotype of Machado-Joseph disease: confirmation of 14q CAG expansion. *Ann Neurol* 1995;38:684–687.

Woods BT, Schaumburg HH. Nigro-spinodentatal degeneration with nuclear ophthalmoplegia. A unique and partially treated clinico-pathologic entity. *J Neurol Sci* 1972;17:149–166.

Zhuchenko O, Bailey J, Bonnen P, et al. Autosomal dominant cerebellar ataxia (SCA6) associated with small polyglutamine expansions in the alpha IA-voltage-dependent calcium channel. *Nat Genet* 1997;15:62–69.

Zu L, Figueroa KP, Grewel R, Pulst SM. Mapping a new autosomal dominant spinocerebellar ataxia to chromosome 22. *Am J Hum Genet* 1999;64:594–599.

Episodic Ataxia

Auburger G, Ratzlaff T, Lunkes A, et al. A gene for autosomal dominant paroxysmal choreoathetosis/spasticity (CSE) maps to the vicinity of a potassium gene cluster on chromosome I p. probably within 2 cM between DIS443 and DIS197. *Genomics* 1996;31:90–94.

Baloh RW, Qing Y, Furman JM, Nelson SF. Familial episodic ataxia: clinical heterogeneity in four families linked to chromosome 19p. *Ann Neurol* 1997;41:8–16.

Baloh RW, Winder A. Acetazolamide-responsive vestibulocerebellar syndrome: clinical and oculographic features. *Neurology* 1991;41:429–432.

Browne DL, Gancher ST, Nutt JG, et al. Episodic ataxia-myokymia syndrome is associated with point mutations in the human potassium channel gene, KCNA 1. *Nat Genet* 1994;8:136–140.

Brunt EP, Van Weerden TW. Familial paroxysmal ataxia and continuous myokymia. *Brain* 1990;113:1361–1382.

Gancher ST, Nutt JG. Autosomal dominant episodic ataxia: a heterogenous syndrome. *Mov Dis* 1986;1:239–253.

Griggs RC, Moxley RT, Lafrance R-A, McQuillen J. Hereditary paroxysmal ataxia: responsive to acetazolamide. *Neurology* 1978;28:1259–1264.

Ophoff RA, Terwindt GM, Vergouwe MN, et al. Familial hemiplegic migraine and episodic ataxia type 2 are caused by mutations in the CA^{2+} channel gene CACNLIA4. *Cell* 1996;87:543–552.

Vahedi K, Joutel A, Van Bogaert P, et al. A gene for hereditary paroxysmal cerebellar ataxia maps to chromosome 19p. *Ann Neurol* 1995;7:289–293.

Treatment

Trouillas P, Jing X, Adeleine P, et al. Buspirone, a 5-hydroxy-tryptamine 1 A agonist, is active in cerebellar ataxia. *Arch Neurol* 1997;54:749–752.

Merritt's Neurology, 10th ed., edited by L.P. Rowland. Lippincott Williams & Wilkins, Philadelphia © 2000.

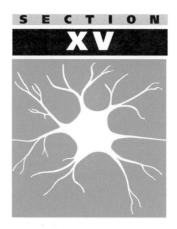

MOVEMENT DISORDERS

CHAPTER
108

HUNTINGTON DISEASE

STANLEY FAHN

Huntington disease (HD; MIM 143100) is a progressive hereditary disorder that usually appears in adult life. It is characterized by a movement disorder (usually chorea), dementia, and personality disorder. It was first recognized clinically by Waters in 1842 and became accepted as a clinical entity with the comprehensive description and interpretation of the mode of transmission by George Huntington in 1872.

PATHOLOGY

At postmortem examination, the brain is shrunken and atrophic; the caudate nucleus is the most affected structure (Fig. 108.1). Histologically, the cerebral cortex shows loss of neurons, especially in layer 3. The caudate nucleus and putamen are severely involved, with loss of neurons, particularly the medium-sized spiny neurons, and their GABAergic striatal efferents. Those lost earliest are the efferents (containing GABA and enkephalin) projecting to the lateral globus pallidus, which is thought to account for chorea. With progression of the disease, the striatal efferents projecting to the medial pallidum are lost; their loss is thought to account for the later developing rigidity and dystonia. Dementia is attributed to changes in both the cerebral cortex and deep nuclei (i.e., subcortical dementia).

Less marked changes occur in other structures, such as the thalamus and brainstem. A reactive gliosis is apparent in all affected areas. In advanced cases, the striatum may be completely devoid of cells and replaced by a gliotic process, at which time choreic movements abate and are replaced by dystonia and an akinetic-rigid state. Progressive striatal atrophy is the basis for staging the severity of the disease. The age at onset is inversely correlated to the severity of striatal degeneration.

BIOCHEMISTRY

There is loss of striatal and nigral GABA and its synthesizing enzyme glutamic acid decarboxylase, whereas the cholinergic and somatostatin striatal interneurons are relatively spared. The receptors for dopamine and acetylcholine are decreased in the striatum. *N*-methyl-D-aspartate receptors are reduced severely in the striatum and cerebral cortex. These defects can be duplicated experimentally in animals by striatal injection of excitotoxins, such as kainic acid, and an excitotoxic hypothesis has been proposed as the pathogenesis of the disease. The neurochemical changes have not been translated into effective therapy because trials with GABA and acetylcholine agonists have not been beneficial. A defect in mitochondrial energy metabolism is con-

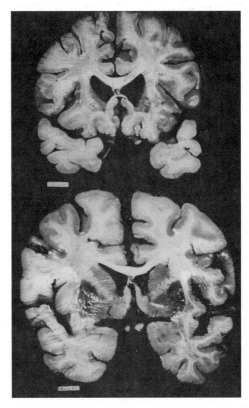

FIG. 108.1. Brain slices. **Top:** Huntington disease. Atrophy of caudate nucleus and lentiform nuclei with dilatation of lateral ventricle. **Bottom:** Normal brain.

sidered to be present in HD. This in turn can lead to oxidative stress, which has been measured in the vulnerable regions of brain of caudate and putamen.

PREVALENCE

HD occurs worldwide and in all ethnic groups, especially whites. The prevalence rate in the United States and Europe ranges from 4 to 8 per 100,000, whereas in Japan the rate is 10% of this figure. The highest incidence rates have been reported from geographically somewhat isolated regions where affected families have resided for many generations (e.g., the Lake Maracaibo region in Venezuela).

GENETICS

A major discovery was the identification and characterization of the HD gene near the tip of the short arm of chromosome 4 (4p16.3). Studies on HD families of different ethnic origins and countries found that despite the marked variability in phenotypic expression, there does not seem to be any genetic heterogeneity. The abnormal gene contains extra copies of trinucleotide repeats of CAG (cytosine-adenine-guanine). Normal individuals have 11 to 34 repeats; those with HD have 37 to 86 repeats. This trinucleotide repeat is unstable in gametes; change in the number of repeats is transmitted to the next generation, sometimes with a decrease in number but more often with an increase. Spontaneous mutations occur from expansion of repeats from parents who have repeat lengths of 34 to 38 units, which span the gap between the normal and HD distributions, the so-called intermediate alleles. Spontaneous mutations in HD previously were considered rare, but this concept has changed as more sporadic (simplex) cases are evaluated by DNA analysis.

Affected mothers tend to transmit the abnormal gene to offspring in approximately the same number of trinucleotide repeats, plus or minus about three repeats. Affected fathers often transmit a greater increase in the length of trinucleotide repeats to offspring, thus resulting in many more juvenile cases of HD when an individual inherits the gene from the father. The trinucleotide repeat is stable over time in lymphocyte DNA but is unstable in sperm DNA. This characteristic may account for the occasional marked increase in the number of trinucleotide repeats in offspring of affected fathers, leading to a 10:1 ratio of juvenile HD when the affected parent is the father. This is because an inverse correlation exists between the number of trinucleotide repeats and the age at onset of symptoms. Knowing the number of repeats in an at-risk offspring can fairly well predict the age at onset of symptoms. The rate of pathologic degeneration also correlates with the number of repeats.

HD is a true autosomal dominant disease in that homozygotes do not differ clinically from heterozygotes. Overexpression of the normal protein could explain why an individual with a double dose of the gene (i.e., the HD gene was transmitted to the offspring by each affected parent) does not differ phenotypically from heterozygotes with only one abnormal gene.

The protein product of the normal gene is called *huntingtin*. The trinu- cleotide CAG codes for glutamine, and the increase in polyglutamine appears to prevent the normal turnover of the protein, resulting in aggregation of the protein with accumulation in the cytoplasm and the nucleus. Other genetic disorders with expanded trinucleotide repeats of CAG include the Kennedy syndrome (X-linked spinal and bulbar muscular atrophy), myotonic dystrophy, many of the spinocerebellar atrophies, and dentatorubral-pallidoluysian atrophy. A similar pathogenesis for these disorders has been proposed.

One-third of individuals with HD share a common haplotype, thus implying a common ancestor. The other two-thirds appear to derive HD through a spontaneous mutation in the distant or near past. For the time being, without directly testing for the gene, lack of a positive family history raises questions of paternity or misdiagnosis. A diagnosis of HD can be established by testing for the gene in patients with adult-onset chorea without a clear positive family history. Preclinical and prenatal testing can also be carried out, but appropriate genetic counseling is required. Diagnosis is still uncertain in those with a borderline number of trinucleotide repeats (i.e., between 34 and 37); for them, the diagnosis is "inconclusive."

Disclosure of positive results of the HD gene in asymptomatic individuals often leads to transient symptoms of depression, but suicidal ideation has been rare. Because of the ethical and legal implications that arise with DNA identification of a gene carrier, predictive testing must be performed by a team of clinicians and geneticists who not only are knowledgeable about the disease and

the genetic techniques but also are sensitive to the psychosocial issues and counseling that precede and follow testing.

SIGNS AND SYMPTOMS

Symptoms usually appear between 35 and 40 years of age. The range of age at onset is broad, however, with cases recorded as early as age 5 and as late as age 70. The three characteristic manifestations of the disease are movement disorder, personality disorder, and mental deterioration. The three may occur together at onset or one may precede the others by a period of years. In general, the onset of symptoms is insidious, beginning with clumsiness, dropping of objects, fidgetiness, irritability, slovenliness, and neglect of duties, progressing to frank choreic movements and dementia. Overt psychotic episodes, depression, and irresponsible behavior may occur. The disease tends to run its course over a period of 15 years, more rapidly in those with an earlier age at onset.

CHOREIC MOVEMENTS

The most striking and diagnostic feature of the disease is the appearance of involuntary movements that seem purposeless and abrupt but less rapid and lightning-like than those seen in myoclonus. The somatic muscles are affected in a random manner, and choreic movements flow from one part of the body to another. Proximal, distal, and axial muscles are involved. In the early stages and in the less severe form, there is slight grimacing of the face, intermittent movements of the eyebrows and forehead, shrugging of the shoulders, and jerking movements of the limbs. Pseudopurposeful movements (*parakinesia*) are common in attempts to mask the involuntary jerking. As the disease progresses, walking is associated with more intense arm and leg movements, which cause a dancing, prancing, stuttering type of gait, an abnormality that is particularly characteristic of HD. Motor impersistence or inhibitory pauses during voluntary contraction probably account for "milkmaid grips," dropping of objects, and inability to keep the tongue steadily protruded. Ocular movements become impaired with reduced saccades and loss of smooth pursuit. The choreic movements are increased by emotional stimuli, disappear during sleep, and become superimposed on voluntary movements to the point that they make volitional activity difficult. With increased severity, the routine daily activities of living become difficult, as do speech and swallowing. Terminally, choreic movements may disappear and be replaced by muscular rigidity and dystonia.

MENTAL SYMPTOMS

Characteristically, there is an organic dementia with progressive impairment of memory, loss of intellectual capacity, apathy, and inattention to personal hygiene. Early in the disease, less profound abnormalities consist of irritability, impulsive behavior, and bouts of depression or fits of violence; these are not infrequent. In some patients, frank psychotic features that are schizophrenic predominate, and the underlying cause is not evident until choreic movements develop. The dementing and psychotic features of the disease usually lead to commitment to a mental institution.

OTHER NEUROLOGIC MANIFESTATIONS

Cranial nerves remain intact except for rapid eye movements, which are impaired in a large percentage of patients. Patients often blink during the execution of a saccadic eye movement. Sensation is usually unaffected. Tendon reflexes are usually normal but may be hyperactive; the plantar responses may be abnormal.

Muscle tone is hypotonic in most patients except for those with the so-called akinetic-rigid variety (*Westphal variant*). With childhood onset (approximately 10% of cases), the akinetic-rigid state usually occurs instead of chorea and in conjunction with mental abnormalities and convulsive seizures. This form of the disease is rapidly progressive with a fatal outcome in less than 10 years. The observation that 90% of all patients with childhood onset inherit the disease from their father stems from the greater likelihood of a large increase in the number of CAG repeats in sperm cells. In the terminal stages of the more classic form of HD, muscular rigidity and dystonia tend to replace chorea, and seizures are not unusual.

LABORATORY DATA

Routine studies of blood, urine, and cerebrospinal fluid show no abnormalities. Diffuse abnormalities are seen in the electroencephalogram. Radiographs of the skull are normal, but computed tomography and magnetic resonance imaging show enlarged ventricles with characteristic butterfly appearance of the lateral ventricles, a result of degeneration of the caudate nucleus (Fig. 108.2). Patients with the akinetic-rigid form of HD are likely to show striatal hyperintensity on T2-weighted magnetic resonance imaging. Positron emission tomography using fluorodeoxyglucose has shown hypometabolism in the caudate and the putamen in affected patients. Abnormalities in striatal metabolism may precede caudate atrophy, but positron emission tomography is not sufficiently sensitive to detect the disease in presymptomatic persons.

DIAGNOSIS AND DIFFERENTIAL DIAGNOSIS

HD can be diagnosed without difficulty in an adult with the clinical triad of chorea, dementia, and personality disorder and family history of the disease. Difficulties arise when the family history is lacking. The patient may be ignorant of the family history or may deny that history.

Other conditions in which choreic movements are a major manifestation can often be excluded on clinical grounds. The most common other adult-onset choreic disorder is neuroacanthocytosis. It is manifested by mild chorea, tics, tongue biting,

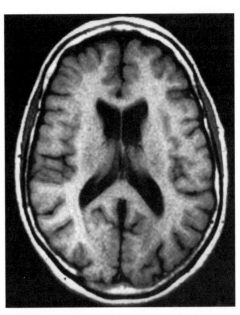

FIG. 108.2. T1-weighted magnetic resonance imaging of Huntington disease brain showing ventricular enlargement with atrophy of the head of the caudate nucleus.

peripheral neuropathy, feeding dystonia, increased serum creatine kinase, and red cell acanthocytes. It is also common for these patients to have had a few seizures. Dentatorubral-pallidoluysian atrophy can also mimic HD. Besides chorea, it can present with myoclonus, ataxia, seizures, and dementia. Differentiation is by gene testing. Sydenham chorea has an earlier age at onset, is self-limited, and lacks the characteristic mental disturbances. Chorea and mental disturbances occurring as manifestations of lupus erythematosus are usually more acute in onset, the chorea is more localized and often periodic, and there are characteristic serologic and clinical abnormalities. Involuntary movements occurring in psychiatric patients on long-term treatment with neuroleptic agents (the so-called *tardive dyskinesia*) occasionally pose a diagnostic problem. Such movements, however, are usually repetitive (stereotypy), in contrast to the nonrepetitive and random nature of chorea. Oral-lingual-buccal dyskinesia is the most common feature of tardive dyskinesia. Gait is usually normal in tardive dyskinesia and is abnormal in HD (see Table 116.1 for more distinguishing differences). The presenile dementias (Alzheimer and Pick diseases) are similar in the mental disorder, but language is more often involved; aphasic abnormalities are not seen early in HD. Myoclonus, rather than chorea, occasionally occurs. The peculiarities of the childhood disorder with rigidity, convulsive seizures, and mental retardation require differentiation from other heritable disorders, such as the leukodystrophies and gangliosidosis. Tics, particularly those of the Gilles de la Tourette syndrome, usually pose little problem in view of the complex nature of the involuntary movements, the characteristic vocalizations, and their suppressibility. Hereditary nonprogressive chorea begins in childhood, does not worsen, and is not associated with dementia or with personality disorder.

TREATMENT

There is at present no known means of altering the disease process or the fatal outcome. Attempts to replace the deficiency in GABA by using GABA-mimetic agents or inhibitors of GABA metabolism have been unsuccessful. Symptomatic treatment of depression and psychosis can be achieved with antidepressants and typical or atypical (i.e., clozapine and quetiapine) antipsychotic agents. The choreic movements can be controlled by the use of neuroleptic agents, including dopamine receptor blockers, such as haloperidol and perphenazine, and presynaptic dopamine depleters, such as reserpine and tetrabenazine. Using these drugs combined with supervision of the patient's daily activities allows management at home during the early stages of the disorder. As the disease advances, however, confinement to a psychiatric facility is often necessary.

SUGGESTED READINGS

Albin RL, Reiner A, Anderson KD, et al. Striatal and nigral neuron subpopulations in rigid Huntington's disease: implications for the functional anatomy of chorea and rigidity-akinesia. *Ann Neurol* 1990;27:357–365.

Alford RL, Ashizawa T, Jankovic J, Caskey CT, Richards CS. Molecular detection of new mutations, resolution of ambiguous results and complex genetic counseling issues in Huntington disease. *Am J Med Genet* 1996;66:281–286.

Bamford KA, Caine ED, Kido DK, Cox C, Shoulson I. A prospective evaluation of cognitive decline in early Huntington's disease: functional and radiographic correlates. *Neurology* 1995;45:1867–1873.

Brandt J, Bylsma FW, Gross R, Stine OC, Ranen N, Ross CA. Trinucleotide repeat length and clinical progression in Huntington's disease. *Neurology* 1996;46:527–531.

Brinkman RR, Mezei MM, Theilmann J, Almqvist E, Hayden MR. The likelihood of being affected with Huntington disease by a particular age, for a specific CAG size. *Am J Hum Genet* 1997;60:1202–1210.

Browne SE, Bowling AC, MacGarvey U, et al. Oxidative damage and metabolic dysfunction in Huntington's disease: selective vulnerability of the basal ganglia. *Ann Neurol* 1997;41:646–653.

Davies SW, Beardsall K, Turmaine M, DiFiglia M, Aronin N, Bates GP. Are neuronal intranuclear inclusions the common neuropathology of triple-repeat disorders with polyglutamine-repeat expansions? *Lancet* 1998;351:131–133.

Duyao M, Ambrose C, Myers R, et al. Trinucleotide repeat length instability and age of onset in Huntington's disease. *Nat Genet* 1993;4:387–392.

Feigin A, Kieburtz K, Bordwell K, et al. Functional decline in Huntington's disease. *Mov Disord* 1995;10:211–214.

Huntington's Disease Collaborative Research Group. A novel gene containing a trinucleotide repeat that is expanded and unstable on Huntington's disease chromosomes. *Cell* 1993;72:971–983.

Myers RH, MacDonald ME, Koroshetz WJ, et al. De novo expansion of a (CAG)(n) repeat in sporadic Huntington's disease. *Nat Genet* 1993;5:168–173.

Myers RH, Vonsattel JP, Stevens TJ, et al. Clinical and neuropathologic assessment of severity in Huntington's disease. *Neurology* 1988;38:341–347.

Penney JB, Vonsattel JP, MacDonald ME, Gusella JF, Myers RH. CAG repeat number governs the development rate of pathology in Huntington's disease. *Ann Neurol* 1997;41:689–692.

Penney JB, Young AB, Shoulson I, et al. Huntington's disease in Venezuela: 7 years of follow-up on symptomatic and asymptomatic individuals. *Mov Disord* 1990;5:93–99.

Thompson PD, Berardelli A, Rothwell JC, et al. The coexistence of bradykinesia and chorea in Huntington's disease and its implications for the theories of basal ganglia control of movement. *Brain* 1988;111:223–244.

Merritt's Neurology, 10th ed., edited by L.P. Rowland. Lippincott Williams & Wilkins, Philadelphia © 2000.

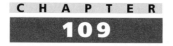

CHAPTER 109

SYDENHAM AND OTHER FORMS OF CHOREA

STANLEY FAHN

Choreic movements can be associated with many disorders; the most common are listed in Table 109.1.

SYDENHAM CHOREA

In 1686, Thomas Sydenham described the chorea now known by his name but originally called St. Vitus dance. His description was of children with a halting gait and jerky movements.

Sydenham chorea (acute chorea, St. Vitus dance, chorea minor, rheumatic chorea) is a disease of childhood characterized by rapid, irregular, aimless, involuntary movements of the muscles of the limbs, face, and trunk that resemble continuous restlessness. There is also muscular weakness, hypotonia, and emotional lability. Once fairly common, it now is encountered infrequently in developed countries. The course is self-limited and fatalities are rare except as a result of cardiac complications.

Etiology and Pathology

Sydenham chorea is considered an autoimmune disorder, a consequence of infection with group A beta-hemolytic streptococcus. Chorea may be delayed for 6 months or longer after the infection. The incidence of Sydenham chorea had fallen dramatically with the introduction of antibiotics and with better sanitary conditions. The streptococcus is thought to induce antibodies that cross-react with neuronal cytoplasmic antigens of caudate and subthalamic nuclei, which apparently account for the symptoms characteristic of rheumatic chorea. These antineuronal antibodies are found in nearly all patients with Sydenham chorea. Antibodies to cardiolipin, which have been found in chorea associated with lupus erythematosus, have not been found in Sydenham chorea. Pathologic studies are rare in this nonfatal disease. Postmortem changes in fatal cases can be attributed to embolic phenomena and terminal changes. A mild degree of inflammatory reaction has been found in a few patients.

Knowledge of the etiology and immunology of Sydenham chorea has spawned the concept of other pediatric autoimmune neuropsychiatric disorders associated with streptococcal infec-

TABLE 109.1. COMMON CAUSES OF CHOREA

Hereditary
   Hungtington disease
   Hereditary nonprogressive chorea
   Neuroacanthocytosis
   Dentatorubral-pallidoluysian atrophy
   Wilson disease
   Ataxia telangiectasia
   Lesch-Nyhan syndrome

Secondary
   Infections/immunologic
      Sydenham chorea
      Encephalitis
      Systemic lupus erythematosus
      Antiphospholipid syndrome
   Drug-induced
      Levodopa
      Anticonvulsants
      Anticholinergics
      Antipsychotics
   Metabolic and endocrine
      Chorea gravidarum
      Hyperthyroidism
      Birth control pills
      Hyperosmolar nonketotic hyperglycemic encephalopathy
   Vascular
      Hemichorea/hemiballism with subthalamic nucleus lesion
      Postpump choreoathetosis after cardiac surgery
      Periarteritis nodosa

Unknown etiology
   Senile chorea
   Essential chorea

For a complete listing of causes of chorea, see Shoulson I. *Clin Neuropharmacol* 1986;9[Suppl 2]:585–599.

tion. This diagnostic appellation is being applied to children or adolescents who develop tic disorders or obsessive-compulsive disorder after group A beta-hemolytic streptococcal infections.

Incidence

Acute chorea is almost exclusively a disease of childhood; over 80% of the cases occur in patients between the ages of 5 and 15. Onset before the age of 5 is rare, and the occurrence of the first attack after the age of 15 is uncommon, except during pregnancy or the use of oral contraceptives in the late teens and early twenties. All races are affected. Girls are affected more than twice as frequently as boys. The disease occurs at all times of the year but is less common in summer.

Symptoms and Signs

In addition to the choreic movements and accompanying motor impersistence, Sydenham chorea is associated with irritability, emotional lability, obsessive-compulsive symptoms, attention deficit, and anxiety. Neurologic manifestations other than chorea are speech impairment and, more rarely, encephalopathy, reflex changes, weakness, gait disturbance, headache, seizures, and cranial neuropathy. Chorea is generalized in about 80% and unilateral in 20% of cases.

The clinical features of the chorea in Sydenham chorea differ from those of Huntington chorea. In Sydenham chorea, the movements are usually more flowing, with a restless-appearing quality. In Huntington chorea, the movements tend to be more individualistic and jerky and become more flowing when the chorea worsens. Physiologic recordings in Sydenham chorea reveal the bursts of electromyographic activity to last more than 100 ms and to occur asynchronously in antagonistic muscles. These findings are in contrast to Huntington chorea, in which more frequent bursts of 10 to 30 ms and 50 to 100 ms occur.

Complications

Other manifestations of the rheumatic infection may occur during the course of the chorea or may precede or follow it. Cardiac complications, usually endocarditis, occur in approximately 20% of patients. Myocarditis and pericarditis are less common. Vegetative endocarditis and embolic phenomena may occur but are rare. A previous history of rheumatic polyarthritis is common, but involvement of the joints during the course of the chorea is rare. Other infrequent complications include subcutaneous rheumatic nodules, erythema nodosum, and purpura. Persistent mental and behavioral effects can also result from Sydenham chorea.

Diagnosis

The diagnosis is made without difficulty from the appearance of the characteristic choreic movements in a child. Helpful for diagnosis are the presence of behavioral changes and diffuse slowing on the electroencephalogram. Often, a history of prior streptococcal infection is not elicited, and tests for rheumatoid factor, antinuclear antibodies, antistreptolysin titers, and cerebrospinal fluid oligoclonal bands are often negative. Cerebrospinal fluid is usually normal, but pleocytosis has been reported in a few cases. Magnetic resonance imaging is usually normal except for selective enlargement of the caudate, putamen, and globus pallidus. In contrast to many other types of choreic disorders, positron emission tomography (PET) in Sydenham chorea reveals striatal hypermetabolism that returns to normal when the symptoms abate.

Some other causes of symptomatic chorea in childhood are presented in Table 109.2; some are reviewed here. The *withdrawal emergent syndrome*, occurring in children when neuroleptic agents are suddenly discontinued, closely resembles the type of chorea seen in Sydenham, but a history of having taken these drugs should enable this diagnosis to be made.

Other dyskinesias in childhood also could present a problem in differential diagnosis, but the distinctions between these and choreic movements should lead to the correct diagnosis. Tics may offer some difficulty, but these movements are stereotyped and localized always to the same muscle or groups of muscles.

Idiopathic torsion dystonia often begins in childhood, but the sustained and twisting movements are quite distinct from choreic movements. On the other hand, some dystonic movements are more rapid, but repetitive and twisting, and could be mistaken for chorea. Dystonic movements affect the same body parts repetitiously, so-called patterning, in contrast to chorea.

TABLE 109.2. OTHER CAUSES OF SYMPTOMATIC CHOREA IN CHILDHOOD

Systemic lupus erythematosus	Hypocalcemia, hypercalcemia
Antiphospholipid antibody	Adrenal insufficiency
Complication of cardiopulmonary bypass	Encephalitis, e.g., ECHO virus type 25, mononucleosis, HIV infection, bacterial endocarditis, tuberculosis, typhoid fever, Lyme disease
Anoxic encephalopathy	
Deep hypothermia	
	GM$_1$, gangliosidosis
Moyamoya disease	Juvenile Huntington disease
Benign hereditary chorea	Wilson disease
Withdrawal emergent syndrome (a form of tardive dyskinesia)	
Lesch-Nyhan syndrome	

HIV; Human immunodeficiency virus.

Also, childhood dystonia persists and does not have the self-limiting characteristic of Sydenham chorea. Essential hereditary myoclonus can begin in childhood and sometimes could be difficult to distinguish from chorea. Athetosis in childhood often is seen with static encephalopathy or some metabolic diseases and usually occurs in the first few years of life, not at the ages commonly encountered with Sydenham chorea.

Course and Prognosis

Sydenham chorea often is a benign disease, and complete recovery is the rule in uncomplicated cases. The mortality rate of approximately 2% is due to associated cardiac complications. The duration of the symptoms is quite variable. In the average case, they persist for 3 to 6 weeks. Occasionally, the course may be prolonged for several months, and it is not unusual for involuntary movements of a mild degree to persist for many months after recrudescence of the more severe movements. Recurrences after months or several years are reported in approximately 35% of the cases.

A rare patient may have persistent chorea throughout life. Residual behavioral and electroencephalographic changes are not uncommon in Sydenham chorea. Susceptibility to *chorea gravidarum*, chorea from oral contraceptives and topical vaginal creams containing estrogen, and even increased sensitivity to levodopa-induced chorea are sequelae of Sydenham chorea. The end of pregnancy and the discontinuation of oral contraceptives or estrogen provide relief from the involuntary movements. A postmortem examination of a case of chorea gravidarum revealed neuronal loss and astrocytosis in the striatum.

Treatment

There is no specific treatment for the disease. Symptomatic therapy may be of great value in the control of the movements. In the mild form, bedrest during the period of active movements is sufficient. The room should be quiet, and all external stimuli should be reduced to a minimum. When the severity of the movements interferes with proper rest, sedatives in the form of barbiturates, chloral hydrate, or paraldehyde may be needed. If further treatment is necessary, a benzodiazepine, valproate, or corticosteroids may be effective. Although antidopaminergic drugs can suppress choreic movements, a dopamine-receptor blocking agent, such as a phenothiazine, should not be administered because of its potential to produce tardive dyskinesia or tardive dystonia. A dopamine-depleting drug (e.g., reserpine) could be used if milder drugs are ineffective.

Prophylactic administration of penicillin for at least 10 years is recommended to prevent other manifestations of rheumatic fever, of which Sydenham chorea may be its sole manifestation.

OTHER IMMUNE CHOREAS

Chorea in *systemic lupus erythematosus* (SLE) has been associated with the presence of antiphospholipid antibodies (lupus anticoagulant), a heterogeneous group of antibodies that can cause platelet dysfunction and result in thrombosis. Chorea is intermittent in SLE. PET has not found caudate hypometabolism in SLE in contrast to many other choreas. Treatment with antidopaminergic agents has been successful.

The primary antiphospholipid antibody syndrome also causes chorea, particularly in young women. Systemically, patients have migraine, spontaneous abortions, venous and arterial thromboses, thickened cardiac valves, livedo reticularis, and Raynaud phenomenon. The central nervous system is involved with strokes, multiinfarct dementia, and chorea. Activated partial thromboplastin time is prolonged because of the presence of lupus anticoagulant, and high titers of anticardiolipin antibodies exist. Anticoagulation, immunosuppressive drugs, and plasmapheresis have had variable success; it is difficult to interpret the effectiveness of therapeutic interventions because spontaneous remission occurs frequently. Striatal hypermetabolism is seen in PET.

VASCULAR CHOREA AND BALLISM

Choreic movements confined to the arm and leg on one side of the body (hemichorea, hemiballism) may develop abruptly in middle-aged or elderly patients. Ballistic movements are a more violent form of chorea and are characterized by large amplitude uncoordinated activity of the proximal appendicular muscles, so vigorous that the limbs are forcefully and aimlessly thrown about. Padding of the limbs is necessary to prevent injury. The movements are present at rest and may be suppressed during voluntary limb movement.

The sudden onset suggests a vascular basis; indeed, it may be preceded by hemiplegia or hemiparesis. In such instances, the choreic or ballistic movements appear when return of motor function occurs. This type of movement disorder is the result of a destructive lesion of the contralateral subthalamic nucleus or its connections. It has also been seen with scattered encephalomalacic lesions involving the internal capsule and basal ganglia. Vascular lesions, hemorrhagic or occlusive in nature, are the most common cause, but hemiballism has been found in association with tumors and plaques from multiple sclerosis in the subthalamic nucleus and has occasionally followed attempted thalamotomy when the target was missed.

In general, the movements tend to diminish over time, but they may be persistent and require therapeutic intervention. The agents noted previously for the control of choreic movements in general have proved effective.

Chorea-ballism is a common feature of hyperosmolar hyperglycemic nonketotic syndrome, which appears related to hypoperfusion in the striatum (see Chapter 51).

Choreoathetosis as a sequela to surgery for congenital heart disease appears to be associated with prolonged time on pump, deep hypothermia, and circulatory arrest. In most cases of postpump syndrome, the chorea persists, and fewer than 25% improve with antidopaminergic therapy.

NEUROACANTHOCYTOSIS

Perhaps the most common hereditary chorea after Huntington disease is neuroacanthocytosis (MIM 100500), formerly called chorea-acanthocytosis, which is also described in Chapter 91. The chorea is typically less severe than that seen with Huntington disease but occasionally can be just as severe. In addition to chorea, patients with neuroacanthocytosis usually have tics, occasional seizures, amyotrophy, absent tendon reflexes, high serum creatine kinase, feeding dystonia (tongue pushes food out of the mouth), and self-mutilation with lip and tongue biting. Age at onset is typically in adolescence and young adulthood, but the range is wide (8 to 62 years). Like Huntington disease, a young age at onset is more likely to produce parkinsonism or dystonia rather than chorea. The diagnosis depends on finding more than 15% spiky erythrocytes (acanthocytes) in blood smears. Some authorities have proposed that detection of acanthocytes can be enhanced if a wet smear of blood is diluted 1:1 with normal saline.

The cerebral pathology is similar to that of Huntington disease, with striatal degeneration causing caudate atrophy and hypometabolism in the caudate nucleus in the PET. PET also reveals reduced fluorodopa uptake and decreased dopamine receptor binding in the striatum. Erythrocyte membrane lipids are altered. Tightly bound palmitic acid (C16:0) is increased, and stearic acid (C18:0) is decreased. Choline acetyltransferase and glutamic acid decarboxylase are normal in basal ganglia and cortex, substance P levels are low in the substantia nigra and striatum, and norepinephrine is elevated in the putamen and pallidum.

Both autosomal dominant and recessive transmission have been proposed for this condition, and the exact genetic mechanism is not known; recently, linkage in 11 families has been found on chromosome 9q21. A rare patient may have the McLeod phenotype, an X-linked (Xp21) form of acanthocytosis associated with chorea, seizures, neuropathy, liver disease, hemolysis, and elevated creatine kinase.

DENTATORUBRAL-PALLIDOLUYSIAN ATROPHY

Once thought to be found mainly in the Japanese population, this autosomal dominant disorder is now known to be more widespread thanks to discovery of an expanded CAG repeat on a gene on chromosome 12p12. Dentatorubral-pallidoluysian atrophy clinically overlaps with Huntington disease and manifests combinations of chorea, myoclonus, seizures, ataxia, and dementia. The phenotype varies according to repeat length, and anticipation and excess of paternal inheritance in younger onset cases with longer repeat lengths are seen. The neuropathologic spectrum is centered around the cerebellifugal and pallidofugal systems, but neurodegenerative changes can be found in many nuclei.

HEREDITARY NONPROGRESSIVE CHOREA (MIM 118700)

This rare disorder is not associated with dementia or other neurologic problems aside from chorea, which is nonprogressive and usually lessens in severity over time. It follows an autosomal dominant transmission pattern and usually begins in childhood. The glucose PET shows striatal hypometabolism.

In the absence of a family history, a benign nonprogressive chorea without other neurologic features can be rarely encountered, so-called essential chorea.

SENILE CHOREA

Senile chorea is characterized by the presence of late-onset generalized chorea with no family history and no dementia. As a rule, the movements begin insidiously, are mild, and usually involve the limbs. More complex movements of the lingual-facial-buccal regions, however, are on occasion encountered. Slow progression in the intensity and extent of the movements may occur. With molecular genetic testing, half the patients show the CAG expansion in the HD gene. Most other cases have been shown to have other diagnoses, such as the antiphospholipid antibody syndrome, hypocalcemia, tardive dyskinesia, and basal ganglia calcification. Still, a rare patient can remain undiagnosed despite extensive investigation and is left with the diagnosis of senile chorea. In such a case, pathologic changes are found in the caudate nucleus and putamen but not to the degree seen in Huntington disease. Significantly, degenerative changes in the cerebral cortex are absent. In general, the symptoms are mild and there is little need to resort to therapeutic measures. In those instances in which oral–facial and neck muscle involvement occurs, however, drugs used to control chorea as indicated previously may prove useful.

SUGGESTED READINGS

Aron AM, Freeman JM, Carter S. The natural history of Sydenham's chorea. *Am J Med* 1965;38:83–95.

Cardoso F, Eduardo C, Silva AP, Mota CCC. Chorea in fifty consecutive patients with rheumatic fever. *Mov Disord* 1997;12:701–703.

Emery ES, Vieco PT. Sydenham chorea: Magnetic resonance imaging reveals permanent basal ganglia injury. *Neurology* 1997;48:531–533.

Garvey MA, Giedd J, Swedo SE. PANDAS: The search for environmental triggers of pediatric neuropsychiatric disorders. Lessons from rheumatic fever. *J Child Neurol* 1998;13:413–423.

Gibb WRG, Lees AJ, Scadding JW. Persistent rheumatic chorea. *Neurology* 1985;35:101–102.

Giedd JN, Rapoport JL, Kruesi MJP, et al. Sydenham's chorea: magnetic resonance imaging of the basal ganglia. *Neurology* 1995;45:2199–2202.

Gledhill RF, Thompson PD. Standard neurodiagnostic tests in Sydenham chorea. *J Neurol Neurosurg Psychiatry* 1990;53:534–535.

Goldman S, Amrom D, Szliwowski HB, et al. Reversible striatal hypermetabolism in a case of Sydenham's chorea. *Mov Disord* 1993;8:355–358.

Hallett M, Kaufman C. Physiological observations in Sydenham's chorea. *J Neurol Neurosurg Psychiatry* 1981;44:829–832.

Husby G, Vande Rijn I, Zabriskie JB, et al. Antibodies reacting with cytoplasm of subthalamic and caudate nuclei neurons in chorea and acute rheumatic fever. *J Exp Med* 1976;144:1094–1110.

Ichikawa K, Kim RC, Givelber H, Collins GH. Chorea gravidarum. Report of a fatal case with neuropathological observations. *Arch Neurol* 1980;37:429–432.

Weindl A, Kuwert T, Leenders KL, et al. Increased striatal glucose consumption in Sydenham's chorea. *Mov Disord* 1993;8:437–444.

Other Immune Choreas

Cervera R, Asherson RA, Font J, et al. Chorea in the antiphospholipid syndrome: clinical, radiologic, and immunologic characteristics of 50 patients from our clinics and the recent literature. *Medicine (Baltimore)* 1997;76:203–212.

Furie R, Ishikawa T, Dhawan V, Eidelberg D. Alternating hemichorea in primary antiphospholipid syndrome: evidence for contralateral striatal hypermetabolism. *Neurology* 1994;44:2197–2199.

Vascular Chorea-Ballism

Holden KR, Sessions JC, Cure J, Whitcomb DS, Sade RM. Neurologic outcomes in children with postpump choreoathetosis. *J Pediatr* 1998;132:162–164.

Lai PH, Tien RD, Chang MH, et al. Choreaballismus with nonketotic hyperglycemia in primary diabetes mellitus. *Am J Neuroradiol* 1996;17:1057–1064.

Vidakovic A, Dragasevic N, Kostic VS. Hemiballism: report of 25 cases. *J Neurol Neurosurg Psychiatry* 1994;57:945–949.

Neuroacanthocytosis

Hardie RJ, Pullon HWH, Harding AE, et al. Neuroacanthocytosis—a clinical, haematological and pathological study of 19 cases. *Brain* 1991;114:13–49.

Rubio JP, Danek A, Stone C, et al. Chorea acanthocytosis: genetic linkage to chromosome 9q21. *Am J Hum Genet* 1997;61:899–908.

Sakai T, Antoku Y, Iwashita H, et al. Chorea-acanthocytosis: abnormal composition of covalently bound fatty acids of erythrocyte membrane proteins. *Ann Neurol* 1991;29:664–669.

Tanaka M, Hirai S, Kondo S, et al. Cerebral hypoperfusion and hypometabolism with altered striatal signal intensity in chorea-acanthocytosis: a combined PET and MRI study. *Mov Disord* 1998;13:100–107.

Dentatorubral-Pallidoluysian Atrophy

Becher MW, Rubinsztein DC, Leggo J, et al. Dentatorubral and pallidoluysian atrophy (DRPLA): clinical and neuropathological findings in genetically confirmed North American and European pedigrees. *Mov Disord* 1997;12:519–530.

Hereditary Nonprogressive Chorea

Kuwert T, Lange HW, Langen KJ, et al. Normal striatal glucose consumption in 2 patients with benign hereditary chorea as measured by positron emission tomography. *J Neurol* 1990;237:80–84.

Senile Chorea

Friedman JH, Ambler M. A case of senile chorea. *Mov Disord* 1990;5:251–253.

Ruiz PJG, Gomez-Tortosa E, Delbarrio A, et al. Senile chorea: a multicenter prospective study. *Acta Neurol Scand* 1997;95:180–183.

Warren JD, Firgaira F, Thompson EM, Kneebone CS, Blumbergs PC, Thompson PD. The causes of sporadic and "senile" chorea. *Aust N Z J Med* 1998;28:429–431.

Merritt's Neurology, 10th ed., edited by L.P. Rowland. Lippincott Williams & Wilkins, Philadelphia © 2000.

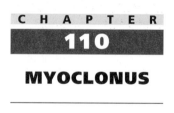

CHAPTER 110

MYOCLONUS

STANLEY FAHN

Myoclonus refers to brief lightning-like muscle jerks due to brief electromyographic bursts of 10 to 50 ms, rarely more than 100 ms in duration. The jerks are usually due to positive muscle contractions but can also be due to sudden brief lapses of contraction (i.e., so-called negative myoclonus) such as is seen in *asterixis*. Asterixis is a tremorlike phenomenon of the extended wrists due to brief lapses of muscle contraction. It is usually encountered in the metabolic encephalopathies that accompany severe hepatic, renal, and pulmonary disorders. Agonists and antagonists usually fire (or are inhibited in negative myoclonus) synchronously.

Clinically, there is a wide expression of myoclonus. The jerks may occur singly or repetitively. They may be focal, segmental, or generalized. The amplitude ranges from mild contractions that do not move a joint to gross contractions that move limbs, the head, or the trunk. Myoclonic jerks range in frequency from rare isolated events to many events each minute; they may occur at rest, with action, or with intention movements. Commonly, myoclonic jerks are stimulus sensitive (reflex myoclonus); they can be induced by sudden noise, movement, light, visual threat, or pinprick. Most often, myoclonic jerks occur irregularly and unpredictably. But some occur in bursts of oscillations, and some are very rhythmic, as in palatal myoclonus. They resemble tremor in this last situation.

Myoclonus arising from the cerebral cortex (cortical myoclonus) is usually focal and reflex-induced. *Epilepsia partialis continua* can be considered within the cortical myoclonus family. The cortical origin can be ascertained by enlarged somatosensory evoked potentials or by spikes in the electroencephalogram associated with electromyographic correlated jerks that are revealed by a back-averaging technique. *Rasmussen encephalitis* is a disorder of childhood and adolescence in which there is a unilateral focal seizure disorder, including epilepsia partialis continua, and a progressive hemiplegia due to focal cortical inflammation and destruction.

Myoclonus originating from the brainstem can be either generalized (reticular myoclonus) or segmental (e.g., *oculo-palatal-pharyngeal myoclonus*). Palatal myoclonus is rhythmical (approximately 2 Hz) and can be primary or secondary. The latter is more common and is the result of a lesion within the Guillain-Mollaret triangle encompassing the dentate, red, and inferior olivary nuclei. This results in an interuption of the dentatoolivary pathway, leading to denervation of the olives, which become hypertrophic. Vascular lesions and multiple sclerosis are common causes of secondary palatal myoclonus that persists during sleep. This disorder is commonly associated with vertical rhythmical ocular movements, also occurring at 2 Hz, so-called ocular myoclonus. Primary myoclonus is of unknown etiology and is often associated with annoying constant clicking sounds in the ear caused by contractions of the tensor veli palatini muscles, which open the eustachian tubes. Primary palatal myoclonus disappears during sleep.

Myoclonus arising from the spinal cord is of two clinical types. *Spinal segmental myoclonus* is rhythmic and persists during sleep, whereas *propriospinal myoclonus* causes truncal flexion jerks, usually triggered by a stimulus, such as when eliciting the knee jerk. In propriospinal myoclonus, the first muscles activated are usually from the thoracic cord, with slow upward and downward spread. Myoclonic jerks can sometimes arise from a peripheral nerve, plexus, or spinal root.

Myoclonus can be classified into the following etiologic categories: physiologic myoclonus, essential myoclonus, epileptic myoclonus, and symptomatic myoclonus. Examples of physiologic myoclonus include sleep jerks and hiccough. Essential myoclonus may be familial or sporadic, is not associated with other neurologic abnormalities, and does not have a progressive course. Some patients with essential myoclonus have features of dystonia, and it is uncertain whether essential myoclonus and the entity known as myoclonic dystonia are the same entity. Epileptic myoclonus occurs in patients whose main complaint is epilepsy but who also have myoclonus.

Symptomatic myoclonus is the largest etiologic group. In this category, myoclonus occurs as part of a more widespread encephalopathy, including storage diseases, spinocerebellar degenerations, dementias, infectious encephalopathies, metabolic encephalopathies, toxic encephalopathies, physical encephalopathies (e.g., posthypoxic and posttraumatic), and with focal brain damage. The infectious encephalopathy of Whipple disease features a facial myoclonus referred to as oculofacial-masticatory myorhythmia; other common features include a supranuclear vertical gaze palsy and cognitive changes. Among the toxic encephalopathies is the serotonin syndrome due to medications that produce excessive serotonergic stimulation; along with myoclonus there is diaphoresis, flushing, rigidity, hyperreflexia, shivering, confusion, agitation, restlessness, coma, and autonomic instability.

Thus, myoclonus is classified by three different approaches (Table 110.1). What was previously called "nocturnal myoclonus" is now referred to as periodic movements of sleep, which accompanies the restless-legs syndrome.

TABLE 110.1. CLASSIFICATION OF MYOCLONUS

Clinical	Anatomic	Etiology
1. At rest action reflex	1. Cortical Focal Multifocal Generalized Epilepsia partialis continua	1. Physiologic 2. Essential
2. Focal axial multifocal generalized	2. Thalamic	3. Epileptic 4. Symptomatic Storage diseases
3. Irregular oscillatory rhythmic	3. Brainstem Reticular Startle Palatal	Cerebellar degenerations Basal ganglia degenerations Dementias Infectious encephalopathy
	4. Spinal Segmental Propriospinal	Metabolic encephalopathy Toxic encephalopathy
	5. Peripheral	Hypoxia Focal damage

Myoclonus can be classified according to clinical features, by anatomic origin of the pathophysiology of the jerks, and by etiology.

An uncommon form of myoclonus is *polyminimyoclonus*, in which the jerks are of small amplitude, resembling irregular tremor that is continuous and generalized. The eyes are often involved with spontaneous, irregular, chaotic saccades. Because the dancing eyes are known as *opsoclonus*, the term *opsoclonus-myoclonus syndrome* is sometimes applied. First described as part of an encephalopathic picture in infants, particularly in association with a neuroblastoma, it also has been found in adults, usually as a paraneoplastic or postviral syndrome. The latter disorder is self-limiting after months or years. The paraneoplastic syndrome is associated with antineuronal antibodies and may remit on removal of the tumor.

Exaggerated startle syndromes, related to the myoclonias and of brainstem origin, consist of a sudden jump to an unexpected auditory, tactile, or visual stimulus. Included are a blink, contraction of the face, flexion of the neck and trunk, and abduction and flexion of the arms. The motor reaction can be either a short or a prolonged complex motor act; falling can result. Known as *hyperekplexia* (MIM 244100), this disorder can result from a brainstem disorder or can be primary and inherited as an autosomal dominant trait with mutations on chromosome 5q coding the α_1 subunit of the inhibitory glycine receptor. When hyperekplexia appears in infancy, it is sometimes called the stiff-baby syndrome because prolonged tonic spasms occur when the infant is handled. Apnea can occur during these spasms; the dibenzodiazepine, clobazam, has been reported to be an effective treatment. Certain excessive startle syndromes may be culturally related and also can manifest echolalia and automatic obedience. These syndromes are known by colorful regional names, such as *jumping Frenchmen of Maine* (Quebec), myriachit (Siberia), latah (Indonesia, Malaysia), and ragin' cajun (Louisiana). Myoclonus and hyperekplexia can sometimes be controlled with the anticonvulsants clonazepam and valproic acid and with the serotonin precursor 5-hydroxytryptophan.

Treatment of myoclonus usually requires polypharmacy. The most successful medications have been sodium valproate, clonazepam, primidone, and piracetam.

SUGGESTED READINGS

Antel JP, Rasmussen T. Rasmussen's encephalitis and the new hat. *Neurology* 1996;46:9–11.

Bodner RA, Lynch T, Lewis L, Kahn D. Serotonin syndrome. *Neurology* 1995;45:219–223.

Brown P. Myoclonus: a practical guide to drug therapy. *CNS Drugs* 1995;3:22–29.

Brown P, Rothwell JC, Thompson PD, et al. The hyperekplexias and their relationship to the normal startle reflex. *Brain* 1991;114:1903–1928.

Caviness JN. Myoclonus. *Mayo Clin Proc* 1996;71:679–688.

Caviness JN, Forsyth PA, Layton DD, McPhee TJ. The movement disorder of adult opsoclonus. *Mov Disord* 1995;10:22–27.

Cockerell OC, Rothwell J, Thompson PD, Marsden CD, Shovron SD. Clinical and physiological features of epilepsia partialis continua: Cases ascertained in the UK. *Brain* 1996;119:393–407.

Deuschl G, Toro C, Vallssole J, Zeffiro T, Zee DS, Hallett M. Symptomatic and essential palatal tremor. 1. Clinical, physiological and MRI analysis. *Brain* 1994;117:775–788.

Fahn S, Marsden CD, Van Woert NH, eds. Myoclonus. *Adv Neurol.* New York: Raven Press, 1986.

Fahn S, Sjaastad O. Hereditary essential myoclonus in a large Norwegian family. *Mov Disord* 1991; 6:237–247.

Hammer MS, Larsen MB, Stack CV. Outcome of children with opso-clonus-myoclonus regardless of etiology. *Pediatr Neurol* 1995;13:21–24.

Ikeda A, Shibasaki H, Tashiro K, et al. Clinical trial of piracetam in patients with myoclonus: nationwide multiinstitution study in Japan. *Mov Disord* 1996;11:691–700.

Koskiniemi M, Vanvleymen B, Hakamies L, Lamusuo S, Taalas J. Piracetam relieves symptoms in progressive myoclonus epilepsy: a multicentre, randomised, double blind, crossover study comparing the efficacy and safety of three dosages of oral piracetam with placebo. *J Neurol Neurosurg Psychiatry* 1998;64:344–348.

Lance JW, Adams RD. The syndrome of intention or action myoclonus as a sequel to hypoxic encephalopathy. *Brain* 1963;86:111–136.

Louis ED, Lynch T, Kaufmann P, Fahn S, Odel J. Diagnostic guidelines in central nervous system Whipple's disease. *Ann Neurol* 1996;40:561–568.

Marsden CD, Hallett M, Fahn S. The nosology and pathophysiology of myoclonus. In: Marsden CD, Fahn S, eds. *Movement disorders.* London: Butterworths, 1982:196–248.

Marsden CD, Harding AE, Obeso JA, Lu CS. Progressive myoclonic ataxia (the Ramsay Hunt syndrome). *Arch Neurol* 1990;47:1121–1125.

Obeso JA, Artieda J, Burleigh A. Clinical aspects of negative myoclonus. *Adv Neurol* 1995;67:1–7.

Quinn NP. Essential myoclonus and myoclonic dystonia. *Mov Disord* 1996;11:119–124.

Rio J, Montalban J, Pujadas F, Alvarez-Sabin J, Rovira A, Codina A. Asterixis associated with anatomic cerebral lesions: a study of 45 cases. *Acta Neurol Scand* 1995;91:377–381.

Scarcella A, Coppola G. Neonatal sporadic hyperekplexia: a rare and often unrecognized entity. *Brain Dev* 1997;19:226–228.

Shiang R, Ryan SG, Zhu YZ, et al. Mutations in the alpha 1 subunit of the inhibitory glycine receptor cause the dominant neurologic disorder, hyperekplexia. *Nat Genet* 1993;5:351–358.

Werhahn KJ, Brown P, Thompson PD, Marsden CD. The clinical features and prognosis of chronic posthypoxic myoclonus. *Mov Disord* 1997;12:216–220.

Merritt's Neurology, 10th ed., edited by L.P. Rowland. Lippincott Williams & Wilkins, Philadelphia © 2000.

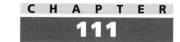

CHAPTER 111

GILLES DE LA TOURETTE SYNDROME

STANLEY FAHN

The Gilles de la Tourette syndrome (MIM 137580), commonly shortened to *Tourette syndrome*, is defined as a neurobehavioral disorder consisting of both multiple motor and phonic tics that change in character over time, onset before 21 years of age, and symptoms that wax and wane but last more than 1 year. Many patients have a behavioral component of obsessive-compulsive or attention deficit disorder. Although the definition is a useful criterion for research on the disorder, it excludes chronic motor tics or an onset beyond the age of 21 years. It is likely that these situations represent milder expressions of Tourette syndrome. Tourette syndrome is the most common cause of tics; other causes include neuroacanthocytosis, encephalitis, neuroleptics, and head trauma.

Tics range from intermittent simple brief jerks to a complex pattern of rapid, coordinated, involuntary movements, often preceded by an unpleasant sensation that is relieved by the movement. Although tics usually can be suppressed for short periods of time, the inner sensation builds up, consequently leading to a burst of tics when the patient stops suppressing them. Tics usually begin in the face (eye blinking, grimacing) and neck (head shaking). They may spread to involve the limbs and may be accompanied by sounds (sniffing, throat clearing, barking, words, or parts of words) and sometimes by foul utterances (coprolalia). Repeating sounds (echolalia) or movements (echopraxia) are sometimes seen. The speed of tics range from very fast (clonic tics) to sustained contractions (dystonic tics). Simple clonic tics resemble essential myoclonus, and the two conditions are difficult to distinguish. Dystonic tics need to be differentiated from primary torsion dystonia. Sydenham chorea is distinct in manifesting as a continuous restless type of movement pattern, and it is self-limited. Premonitory sensations, intermittency, and suppressibility help distinguish tics from most other movement disorders. On average, tics begin around age 5 years and increase in severity, reaching its most intense period around age 10. After the most severe period, there is usually a steady decline in tic severity. By age 18 years, nearly half of the patients are virtually free from tics.

Tourette syndrome is frequently associated with compulsive ideation and hyperactive behavior. Neuroimaging has shown inconsistent asymmetries in the basal ganglia. Serum antibodies against the putamen have been found. The genetic inheritance pattern of Tourette syndrome is controversial, but complex segregation analysis suggests that susceptibility is conveyed by a major locus in combination with a multifactorial background. The analysis does not support other models of inheritance, including polygenic models, single major locus models, and mixed models with dominant and recessive major loci. Genetic linkage has not yet been discovered, though most of the genome has been searched. The prevalence in adolescents is about 5 per 10,000 in males and 3 per 10,000 in females. In patients who have come to necropsy, no specific morphologic changes in the brain have been noted. Dopamine receptors are not increased in the striatum, but hyperinnervation with dopamine terminals has been suggested by increased mazindol binding.

When tics are mild and not socially disabling, no treatment is required. When more severe, motor and phonic tics can sometimes be reduced with clonidine or clonazepam. Dopamine antagonists and depletors are more effective but often have more adverse effects. The antagonists can cause the more serious complication of tardive dystonia and thus should be reserved as a last resort. Attention deficit and obsessive-compulsive disorders are usually a greater social problem than are the tics.

SUGGESTED READINGS

Chase TN, Friedhoff A, Cohen DJ, eds. Tourette's syndrome. *Adv Neurol.* New York: Raven Press, 1992.

Comings DE, Himes JA, Comings BG. An epidemiologic study of Tourette's syndrome in a single school district. *J Clin Psychiatry* 1990;51:463–469.

Fahn S. Motor and vocal tics. In: Kurlan R, ed. *Handbook of Tourette's syndrome and related tic and behavioral disorders.* New York: Marcel Dekker, 1993.

Kurlan R, ed. *Handbook of Tourette's syndrome and related tic and behavioral disorders.* New York: Marcel Dekker, 1993.

Leckman JF, Zhang HP, Vitale A, et al. Course of tic severity in Tourette syndrome: the first two decades. *Pediatrics* 1998;102:14–19.

Singer HS, Giuliano JD, Hansen BH, et al. Antibodies against human putamen in children with Tourette syndrome. *Neurology* 1998;50: 1618–1624.

Singer HS, Hahn IH, Moran TH. Abnormal dopamine uptake sites in postmortem striatum from patients with Tourette's syndrome. *Ann Neurol* 1991;30:558–562.

Tourette Syndrome Classification Study Group. Definitions and classification of tic disorders. *Arch Neurol* 1993;50:1013–1016.

Walkup JT, LaBuda MC, Singer HS, Brown J, Riddle MA, Hurko O. Family study and segregation analysis of Tourette syndrome: evidence for a mixed model of inheritance. *Am J Hum Genet* 1996;59:684–693.

Merritt's Neurology, 10th ed., edited by L.P. Rowland. Lippincott Williams & Wilkins, Philadelphia © 2000.

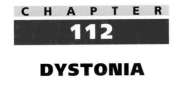

CHAPTER 112

DYSTONIA

STANLEY FAHN
SUSAN B. BRESSMAN

After parkinsonism, dystonia is the movement disorder most commonly encountered in movement disorder clinics. The term dystonia was coined by Oppenheim in 1911 to indicate that the disorder he was describing manifested hypotonia at one occasion and tonic muscle spasms at another, usually but not exclusively elicited upon volitional movements. Although the term dystonia has undergone various definitions since 1911, today it is defined as a syndrome of sustained muscle contractions, frequently causing twisting and repetitive movements or abnormal postures. Limb, axial, and cranial voluntary muscles can all be affected by dystonia. The involuntary movements are often exacerbated during voluntary movements, so-called *action dystonia*. If the dystonic contractions appear only with a specific action, it is referred to as *task-specific dystonia* (e.g., writer's cramp and musician's cramp). As the dystonic condition progresses, voluntary movements in parts of the body not affected with dystonia can induce dystonic movements of the involved body part, so-called overflow. Talking is the most common activity that causes overflow dystonia in other body parts. With still further worsening, the affected part can develop dystonic movements while at rest. Thus, dystonia at rest is usually more severe than pure action dystonia. Sustained abnormal postures of affected body parts may be the eventual outcome.

Dystonic movements tend to increase with fatigue, stress, and emotional states; they tend to be suppressed with relaxation, hypnosis, and sleep. Dystonia often disappears during deep sleep, unless the movements are extremely severe. A characteristic and almost unique feature of dystonic movements is that they can be diminished by tactile or proprioceptive "sensory tricks" (geste antagoniste). For example, patients with cervical dystonia (torticollis) often place a hand on the chin or side of the face to reduce nuchal contractions, and orolingual dystonia is often helped by touching the lips or placing an object in the mouth. Lying down may reduce truncal dystonia; walking backward or running may reduce leg dystonia.

Rapid muscle spasms that occur in a repetitive pattern may be present in torsion dystonia; when rhythmic, the term *dystonic tremor* is applied. Although rare, some children and adolescents with primary or secondary dystonia may experience a crisis, a sudden increase in the severity of dystonia, which has been called *dystonic storm* or *status dystonicus*. It can cause myoglobinuria, with a threat of death by renal failure. Placing the patient in an intensive care unit for barbiturate narcosis is usually necessary for relief.

CLASSIFICATION OF TORSION DYSTONIA

To emphasize the twisting quality of the abnormal movements and postures, the term *torsion* is often placed in front of the word dystonia. Torsion dystonia is classified in three ways: age at onset, body distribution of abnormal movements, and etiology (Table 112.1). Age at onset is the single most important factor related to prognosis of primary dystonia. As a general rule, the younger the age at onset, the more likely the dystonia will become severe and spread to multiple parts of the body. In contrast, the older the age at onset, the more likely dystonia will remain focal. Onset of dystonia in a leg is the second most important predictive factor for a more rapidly progressive course.

Because dystonia usually begins in a single body part and because dystonia either remains focal or spreads to other body parts, it is useful to classify dystonia according to anatomic distribution. *Focal dystonia* affects only a single area. Frequently seen types of focal dystonia tend to have specific labels: blepharospasm, torticollis, oromandibular dystonia, spastic dysphonia, writer's cramp, or occupational cramp. If dystonia spreads, it usually affects a contiguous body part. When dystonia affects two or more contiguous parts of the body, it is *segmental dystonia*. *Generalized dystonia* is a combination of leg involvement plus some other area. *Multifocal dystonia* fills a gap in the preceding designations, describing involvement of two or more noncontiguous parts. Dystonia affecting one half of the body is *hemidystonia*, which is usually symptomatic rather than primary. Adult-onset dystonia is much more often focal than generalized.

The most common focal dystonia is cervical dystonia (torticollis), followed by dystonias of cranial muscles: blepharospasm, spasmodic dysphonia, or oromandibular dystonia. Less common is arm dystonia, such as writer's cramp. The most common segmental dystonia involves the cranial muscles (Meige syndrome) or cranial and neck muscles (cranial-cervical dystonia).

The etiologic classification identifies four major categories: primary, dystonia-plus syndromes, secondary (environmental causes), and heredodegenerative diseases. *Primary dystonia* (familial or sporadic) is a pure dystonia (except that tremor may be present); primary excludes a symptomatic cause. *Dystonia-plus* syndromes are related to the primary dystonias in this classifica-

tion scheme because neither type is neurodegenerative; instead they are neurochemical disorders. Dystonia-plus syndromes include symptoms and signs in addition to dystonia; for instance, dopa-responsive dystonia includes parkinsonism and myoclonus-dystonia includes myoclonus. *Secondary dystonias* are due to environmental insult. *Heredodegenerative dystonias* are neurodegenerative diseases usually inherited; these conditions usually have other neurologic features in addition to dystonia.

PRIMARY TORSION DYSTONIAS

Primary torsion dystonia comprises familial and nonfamilial (sporadic) types. Neurologic abnormality is restricted to dystonic postures and movements except that there may be a tremor resembling essential tremor. Within the primary dystonias are several genetic disorders, some with genes already mapped (DYT1, DYT6, and DYT7). But most primary dystonias are sporadic and with an onset in adult years and a focal or segmental dystonia.

Openeheim Dystonia

The DYT1 gene has been cloned and causes the dystonia described by Oppenheim. The mean ($\pm$ SD) age at onset of symptoms in Oppenheim dystonia is 12.5 $\pm$ 8.2 years. Onset is rare after age 29 years. In about 95% of patients, symptoms begin in an arm or leg, and the disorder spreads to the neck or larynx. This gene is responsible for most cases of early and limbonset primary torsion dystonia.

When Oppenheim dystonia begins in a leg, the likelihood of eventual progression to generalized dystonia is about 90%. With onset in an arm, it is about 50%. With leg involvement, action dystonia results in a peculiar twisting of the leg when the child walks forward, even though walking backward, running, or dancing may still be normal. Bizarre stepping or a bowing gait may be noted when the dystonic movements affect proximal muscles of the leg. Difficulty in placing the heel on the ground is evident when distal muscles are affected (Fig. 112.1). As the disorder progresses, the movements may appear when the leg is at rest; the foot is often plantar flexed and turned inward, and the knee and hip often assume a flexed posture.

With arm involvement, action dystonia may interfere with writing; the fingers curl, the wrist flexes and pronates, the triceps contracts, and the elbow elevates. Dystonic tremor of the arm is common, with features of both postural and action tremors. With progression, other activities of the arm are impaired; the arm often moves backward behind the body when the patient walks. Later, dystonia may be present when the arm is at rest. With onset in the arm, spread is usually to the other arm or sometimes to the neighboring segments of neck and trunk.

As the dystonia becomes worse, the contractions become constant, so that instead of moving, the body part remains in a fixed twisted posture. Oppenheim dystonia also tends to spread to other parts of the body, particularly after onset in a leg, advancing from focal to segmental to generalized. The trunk may develop wiggling movements and fixed scoliosis, lordosis, and tortipelvis. The neck may become involved with torticollis,

TABLE 112.1. CLASSIFICATIONS OF TORSION DYSTONIA

By age at onset
Childhood onset, 0–12 yr
Adolescent onset, 13–20 yr
Adult onset, >20 yr

By distribution
Focal
Segmental
Multifocal
Generalized
Hemidystonia

By etiology
Primary (also known as idiopathic) dystonia
Dystonia plus
Secondary dystonia
Heredodegenerative diseases
(usually presents as dystonia plus)

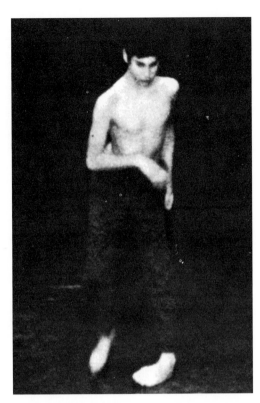

FIG. 112.1. Generalized dystonia with involvement of the legs, trunk, and arms. Patient is still able to walk.

Non-DYT1 Primary Dystonia

The DYT1 gene has been excluded in many families with primary torsion dystonia. The phenotype differs in that many begin in the cranial-cervical region, and most are focal and segmental. There is some clinical phenotypic overlap between Oppenheim dystonia and DYT6 dystonia, which has been mapped to 8p21q22. DYT6 dystonia has been found in the Mennonite population. It is an autosomal dominant dystonia with onset in either children or adults, involving limbs, cervical, and cranial regions. Dysphonia and dysarthria are often the most disabling features.

DYT7 dystonia is a predominantly cervical form in northwest Germany. It was originally mapped to chromosome 18p. Doubt has been raised about this locus in German and European populations. Some designations of DYT have been applied to other primary dystonias that have yet to be genetically mapped (Table 112.2). The primary dystonias are DYT1, DYT2, DYT4, DYT6, and DYT7. DYT5, DYT11, and DYT12 are dystonia-plus disorders, and DYT3 is a heredodegenerative dystonia. DYT8, DYT9, and DYT10 are paroxysmal dyskinesias.

Most primary dystonias are of adult onset and without a family history. Their precise prevalence is not known, but it is about 30 per 100,000 population in Rochester, Minnesota. These dystonias often remain in the site where the dystonia begins (i.e., a focal dystonia). Common sites are neck (cervical dystonia), face (blepharospasm), jaw (oromandibular dystonia), vocal cords (spastic dysphonia), and arm (writer's cramp). In some of these adult-onset cases, the disease spreads to neighboring segments.

anterocollis, retrocollis, or head tilt and shift. Facial grimacing and difficulties in speech may occur but are much less common. Although muscle tone and power seem normal, the involuntary movements interfere and make voluntary activity extremely difficult. In general, mental activity is normal, and there are no alterations in tendon reflexes or sensation. The rate of progression of this type is extremely variable; in most cases, it is most severe within the first 5 to 10 years, after which there may be a quiescent static phase. The continuous spasms result in marked distortion of the body to a degree rarely seen in any other disease (Fig. 112.2). With active treatment, it is now uncommon to encounter the severe deformities seen before the 1980s.

Oppenheim dystonia is an autosomal dominant disorder; the gene, DYT1, maps to chromosome 9q34.1. The penetrance rate of gene expression is between 30% and 40%. In all cases the only mutation is a deletion of one of a pair of GAG triplets in the ATP-binding protein, torsinA. TorsinA, previously unknown, is found in neurons in many parts of the brain; it is most abundantly expressed in the substantia nigra pars compacta, the hippocampus, and the cerebellum. There is moderate expression in striatal cholinergic neurons, which might explain some beneficial effect from anticholinergic agents. TorsinA is distantly related to the heat-shock protein family, which could explain why stress may induce the onset or worsening of Oppenheim dystonia.

Oppenheim dystonia affects most ethnic groups but is particularly prevalent in the Ashkenazi Jewish population, in which the disease occurs in about 1 per 6,000. The origin of the mutation has been traced to the northern part of the historic Jewish Pale of settlement in Lithuania and Byelorussia about 350 years ago.

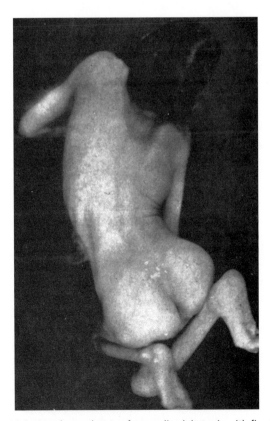

FIG. 112.2. An advanced state of generalized dystonia with fixed postures: torticollis, scoliosis, tortipelvis, and limb dystonia.

TABLE 112.2. GENE NOMENCLATURE FOR THE DYSTONIAS

DYT1 = 9q34, TorsinA, AD, young onset (Oppenheim)
DYT2 = unconfirmed, AR in Spanish gypsies
DYT3 = Xq13.1, lubag in Filipino males
DYT4 = a whispering dysphonia family, linkage unknown
DYT5 = 14q22.1, GCH-1, AD, DRD (Segawa) (tyrosine hydroxylase
          = 11p11.5, AR)
DYT6 = 8p21-q22, AD, mixed type, Mennonite/Amish
DYT7 = AD, familial torticollis, linkage unconfirmed
DYT8 = 2q33-q35, AD, PNKD (FDP1) (Mount-Rebak)
DYT9 = 1p, AD, paroxysmal dyskinesia with spasticity (CSE)
DYT10 = locus ?, AD, PKD
DYT11 = locus ?, AD, myoclonus-dystonia
DYT12 = chromosome 19q, AD, RDP

Genetic nomenclature is presented in the chronologic order named. DYT1 is the gene involved in Oppenheim dystonia, which is clinically marked by young- and limb-onset pure dystonia. The DYT1 gene has a deletion of one of a sequential pair of GAG triplets. DYT2 was set aside for any possible autosomal recessive forms, but none has as yet been firmly identified. DYT3 is the gene for X-linked dystonia-parkinsonism, known as lubag, and encountered in Filipino males. DYT4 was labeled for an Australian family with dystonia, including a whispering dysphonia. DYT5 is for the GCHI gene mutations causing DRD. DYT6 is the gene causing an adult- and childhood-onset dystonia of both limbs and cranial structures, so far seen in the Mennonite and Amish population. DYT7 is for familial torticollis in northwest Germany, but uncertainty has recently been raised about its reported linkage. DYT8–10 are for paroxysmal dyskinesias; 8 is for nonkinesigenic type, known as the Mount-Rebak syndrome; 9 is for a family with episodic choreoathetosis and spasticity; 10 is reserved for paroxysmal kinesigenic dyskinesia. DYT11 has been named the newly discovered gene mutation of the dopamine D2 receptor protein that causes myoclonus-dystonia. DYT12 is for a gene mapped to chromosome 19q causing rapid-onset dystonia-parkinsonism. AD; autosomal dominant; AR; autosomal recessive; DRD, dopa-responsive dystonia; PKND, paroxysmal nonkinesignic dyskinesia; FDP1, familial paroxysmal dyskinesia type 1; CSE, choreoathetosis/spasticity episodic; PKD, paroxysmal kinesigenic dyskinesia; RDP, rapid-onset dystonia parkinsonism.

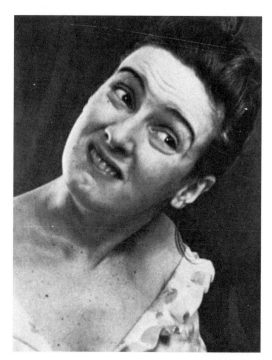

FIG. 112.3. Spasmodic torticollis with some dystonia of facial muscles (segmental dystonia).

Focal dystonia is the most common form (50%) of all primary dystonias, with segmental dystonia next (one-third) and generalized dystonia least (one-sixth).

Cervical dystonia, commonly known as *spasmodic torticollis* or *wry* neck, is the most common focal dystonia. It occurs at any age, usually beginning between ages 20 and 60. Any combination of neck muscles can be involved, especially the sternocleidomastoid, trapezius, splenius capitus, levator scapulae, and scalenus muscles. Sustained turning, tilting, flexing, or extending the neck or shifting the head laterally or anteriorly can result (Fig. 112.3). The shoulder is usually elevated and anteriorly displaced on the side to which the chin turns. Some neck muscles contract in compensation for the movements of the primary agonists, sometimes making it difficult to decide which muscles to inject with botulinum toxin. Instead of sustained deviation of the head, some patients have jerking movements of the head. Neck pain occurs in about two-thirds of patients with cervical dystonia and usually responds successfully to injections of botulinum toxin at the site of the pain. A common sensory trick to relieve cervical dystonia is the placement of one hand on the back of the head or on the chin. About 10% of patients with cervical dystonia have a remission, usually within a year of onset; most remissions are followed by a relapse years later. Some patients with torticollis have a horizontal head tremor that may be impossible to distinguish from essential tremor. Other considerations in the differential diagnosis of torticollis are congenital contracture of the sternocleidomastoid muscle, which can be treated with surgical release. In young boys after a full meal, extreme head tilt may be caused by gastroesophageal reflux (*Sandifer syndrome*) that can be treated by plication surgery. Other diagnostic considerations are trochlear nerve palsy; Arnold-Chiari malformation; malformations of the cervical spine, such as Klippel-Feil fusion or atlantoaxial subluxation; cervical infections; and spasms from cervical muscle shortening.

Blepharospasm is caused by contraction of the orbicularis oculi muscles. It usually begins with increased frequency of blinking, followed by closure of the eyelids and then more firm and prolonged closure of the lids. Sometimes lid closure is forceful. Untreated blepharospasm usually causes functional blindness. Blinking and lid closure can be intermittent and are often temporarily suppressed by talking, humming, singing, or looking down. The condition is worsened by walking and by bright light. A common sensory trick that relieves contractions is placing of a finger just lateral to the orbit. Blepharospasm is usually accompanied by cocontraction of lower facial muscles, such as the platysma and risorius. This type of focal dystonia sometimes becomes segmental by spreading to other cranial targets, such as the jaw, tongue, vocal cords, or cervical muscles. The combination of blepharospasm with other cranial dystonias is called *Meige syndrome*. Blepharospasm occurs more often in women than in men, usually beginning after age 50, although younger people may be affected. Abnormalities of the blink reflex have been found with blepharospasm and with other cranial or cervical dystonias.

The differential diagnosis of blepharospasm includes *hemifacial* spasm, which is unilateral. Rarely, hemifacial spasm is bilateral, but the contractions on the two sides of the face are not synchronous as they are in blepharospasm. *Blinking tics* can resemble blepharospasm, but tics almost always begin in childhood. *Sjögren syndrome* of dry eyes often causes the eyelids to close, but testing for tear production usually distinguishes this disorder. Injections of botulinum toxin are effective in more than 80% of patients with blepharospasm.

Writer's cramp of adult onset usually remains limited to one limb, usually the dominant side. In about 15% of cases, it spreads to the other arm. When it affects only writing, the patient may learn to write with the nondominant hand. For bilateral involvement or for dystonia that affects other activities (buttoning, shaving, or playing a musical instrument), carefully placed injections of botulinum toxin may be effective.

Dystonia of the vocal cords occurs in two forms. The more common type is *spastic (spasmodic) dysphonia* in which the vocalis muscles contract, bringing the vocal cords together and causing the voice to be restricted, strangled, and coarse, often broken up with pauses. *Breathy (whispering) dysphonia* is caused by contractions of the posterior cricoarytenoids (abductor muscles of the vocal cords), so that the patient cannot talk in a loud voice and tends to run out of air while trying to speak. Spastic dysphonia is often associated with tremor of the vocal cords. Essential tremor (with vocal cord tremor) is an important differential diagnosis; the presence of tremor in the hands or neck leads to such diagnosis. Injections of botulinum toxin can be dramatically effective for spastic dysphonia but are more uncertain for breathy dysphonia. For each type, a physician must be experienced with the procedure of injecting the correct muscle.

Pathology and Pathophysiology of Primary Dystonia

The pathology of the primary torsion dystonias is unknown. Gross examination of the brain and histologic studies by light microscopy do not reveal any consistent morphologic changes. These disorders are therefore considered neurochemical rather than neurodegenerative. Dystonic symptoms probably arise from dysfunction within the basal ganglia because, in those conditions with secondary and heredodegenerative dystonia, such as Wilson disease, encephalitis lethargica, and Hallervorden-Spatz disease, characteristic pathologic changes are found in this region. Furthermore, in traumatic hemidystonia, infarction of the contralateral caudate and putamen has been encountered. In support of a biochemical abnormality are the documented instances of dystonic reactions to pharmacologic agents, particularly those that affect striatal dopamine function, such as the dopamine receptor blocking agents and levodopa as used in treating Parkinson disease.

The electromyogram in the dystonias shows cocontraction of agonist and antagonist muscles with prolonged bursts and overflow to extraneous muscles. Spinal and brainstem reflex abnormalities, including reduced reciprocal inhibition and protracted blink reflex recovery, indicate a reduced presynaptic inhibition of muscle afferent input to the inhibitory interneurons as a result of defective descending motor control. The sensorimotor cerebral cortex shows an increased region of activation related to the affected body part. Positron emission tomography studies found increased metabolic activity in the lentiform nuclei. In DYT1 dystonia, two patterns of abnormal metabolic activity have been found. In nonmanifesting carriers and in affected carriers who are asleep, there is hypermetabolism of the lentiform, cerebellum, and supplementary motor cortex. On the other hand, in DYT1 patients having active muscle contractions, metabolic activity is increased in the thalamus, cerebellum, and midbrain.

DYSTONIA-PLUS SYNDROMES

This category includes nondegenerative disorders in which parkinsonism (dopa-responsive dystonia and rapid-onset dystonia-parkinsonism) or myoclonus (myoclonus-dystonia) coexists with the dystonia.

Dopa-responsive Dystonia

About 10% of patients with childhood-onset dystonia have the autosomal dominant disorder, *dopa-responsive dystonia* (DRD), sometimes called *Segawa disease*. Distinguishing DRD from primary torsion dystonia, usually Oppenheim dystonia, is important because DRD responds so well to treatment. It differs from other childhood dystonias by the presence of bradykinesia, cogwheel rigidity, and impaired postural reflexes; diurnal fluctuations with improvement after sleep and worsening as the day wears on; a peculiar "spastic" straight-legged gait, with a tendency to walk on the toes; hyperreflexia, particularly in the legs and sometimes with Babinski signs; and a remarkable therapeutic response to low doses of levodopa, dopamine agonists, or anticholinergic drugs.

DRD usually begins between ages 6 and 16 but can appear at any age. When it begins in infants, it resembles cerebral palsy. When it begins in adults, it usually manifests as pure parkinsonism, mimicking Parkinson disease, responding to levodopa, and with a generally benign course. DRD affects girls more often than boys (4:1 ratio), has a worldwide distribution, and is not known to have a higher prevalence in any specific ethnic group. Mutations of the gene for GTP cyclohydrolase I (GCHI) located at 14q22.1 are responsible. GCHI catalyzes the first step in the biosynthesis of tetrahydrobiopterin (BH4), the cofactor required for the enzymes tyrosine hydroxylase, phenylalanine hydroxylase, and tryptophan hydroxylase. These hydroxylase enzymes add an −OH group to the parent amino acid and are required for the synthesis of biogenic amines. The genetic label for DRD is DYT5.

Pathologic investigations of DRD revealed no loss of neurons within the substantia nigra pars compacta, but the cells are immature with little neuromelanin. Neuromelanin synthesis requires dopamine (or other monoamines) as the initial precursor. Biochemically, there is marked reduction of dopamine concentration within the striatum in DRD. These pathologic and biochemical findings demonstrate that the disorder is a neurochemical disease rather than a neurodegenerative disease.

Rare cases of DRD are found in an autosomal recessive disorder with mutations in the gene for tyrosine hydroxylase; the dystonia-parkinsonism begins in infancy or early childhood. Additionally, several autosomal recessive biopterin deficiency disorders show features of decreased norepinephrine and serotonin in addition to dystonia and parkinsonism. These clinical features include miosis, oculogyria, rigidity, hypokinesia, chorea, myoclonus, seizures, temperature disturbance, and hypersalivation; hyperphenylalaninemia is present, and the disorder may respond partially to levodopa. Another disorder of infants is the autosomal recessive deficiency of the enzyme aromatic L-amino acid decarboxylase, which catalyzes the transformation of levodopa to dopamine; levodopa is ineffective in this disorder, but patients respond to dopamine agonists coupled with a monoamine oxidase inhibitor.

In the differential diagnosis of DRD is juvenile parkinsonism, a progressive nigral degenerative disorder, in which dystonia often precedes the parkinsonian features that become the major clinical feature. One distinguishing laboratory test is fluorodopa positron emission tomography, which is normal in DRD; in juvenile parkinsonism, there is marked reduction of fluorodopa uptake in the striatum. A phenylalanine loading test has also been proposed; in DRD, there is a slower conversion to tyrosine. Other differential features of DRD from juvenile parkinsonism and Oppenheim dystonia are listed in Table 112.3.

One may also suspect DRD if a young patient with dystonia responds dramatically to low doses of anticholinergic agents. But the most effective agent is levodopa. The suggested starting dose of carbidopa/levodopa for DRD is 12.5/50 mg two or three times a day, a dose low enough to avoid dyskinesias. The usual maintenance dose is 25/100 mg two or three times a day.

Rapid-onset Dystonia-Parkinsonism

Rapid-onset dystonia-parkinsonism is an autosomal dominant disease; the gene has been mapped to 19q. Affected individuals develop dystonia and parkinsonism between ages 14 and 45 years, reaching maximum involvement of dystonia with parkinsonism in hours or days. Some affected members of the family may have a more gradual progression for 6–18 months. The cerebrospinal fluid homovanillic acid concentration is low, and there are no imaging abnormalities. There is no effective treatment.

Myoclonus-Dystonia

Although lightning-like movements occasionally occur in Oppenheim dystonia, they are a prominent feature in a distinct autosomal dominant disorder known as myoclonus-dystonia. The myoclonic jerks respond to alcohol. Myoclonus-dystonia may not be an entity separate from hereditary essential myoclonus, a problem to be resolved by genetic studies. The onset is in childhood or adolescence. The myoclonus and dystonia are located predominantly in the arms and neck, and the symptoms tend to plateau after a period of progression.

SECONDARY DYSTONIA

Secondary dystonia is defined as a dystonic disorder that develops mainly as the result of environmental factors that affect the brain. Spinal cord injury and peripheral injury are also recognized causes of dystonia. Examples include levodopa-induced dystonia in the treatment of parkinsonism; acute and tardive dystonia due to dopamine receptor blocking agents; and dystonias associated with cerebral palsy, cerebral hypoxia, cerebrovascular disease, cerebral infectious and postinfectious states, brain tumor, and toxicants such as manganese, cyanide, and 3-nitroproprionic acid. Other causes include psychogenic disorders, peripheral trauma followed by focal dystonia in the affected region, head injury, and delayed-onset dystonia after cerebral infarct or other cerebral insult. Prior history of one of these insults suggests the correct diagnosis, as does neuroimaging that shows a lesion in the basal ganglia or their connections.

A more complete listing of secondary dystonias is presented in Table 112.4. A number of disorders in this group, such as the infectious and toxicant-induced neurodegenerations, are not limited to pure dystonia but show a mixture of other neurologic

TABLE 112.3. DIFFERENTIAL FEATURES BETWEEN JUVENILE PARKINSON DISEASE (JPD), DOPA-RESPONSIVE DYSTONIA (DRD), AND PRIMARY TORSION DYSTONIA (PTD)

	JPD	DRD	Childhood PTD
Age at onset	Rare <8 yr	Infancy to 12 yr	Uncommon <6 yr
Gender	Predominantly male	Predominantly female	Equal
Initial sign	Foot dystonia or PD	Foot and leg dystonia, gait disorder	Arm or leg dystonia
Dystonia	At onset	Throughout	Throughout
Diurnal	No	Sometimes	No
Bradykinesia	Present	Present	No
Pull test	Abnormal	Abnormal	Normal
Gait	Abnormal	Abnormal	Abnormal if leg or trunk is affected
Anticholinergic response	Yes	Yes	Yes
Dopa responsive	Yes	Yes	No, or mild
Dopa dosage	Moderate to high	Very low	High
"Off" episodes	Fluctuations	Stable	Unknown
Dyskinesias	Prominent	Uncommon	Unknown
Fluorodopa PET	Decreased	Slight decrease	Normal
Prognosis	Progressive	Plateaus	Usually worsens

PET, positron emission tomography.

TABLE 112.4. CAUSES OF SECONDARY DYSTONIA

Secondary dystonia
1. Perinatal cerebral injury
   a. Athetoid cerebral palsy
   b. Delayed onset dystonia
   c. Pachygyria
2. Encephalitis, infections and postinfections
   a. Reye's syndrome
   b. Subacute sclerosing leukoencephalopathy
   c. Wasp sting
   d. Creutzfeldt-Jakob disease
   e. HIV infection
3. Head trauma
4. Thalamotomy
5. Primary antiphospholipid syndrome
6. Focal cerebral vascular injury
7. Arteriovenous malformation
8. Hypoxia
9. Brain tumor
10. Multiple sclerosis
11. Brainstem lesion, including pontine myelinolysis
12. Posterior fossa tumors
13. Cervical cord injury or lesion
14. Lumbar canal stenosis
15. Peripheral injury
16. Electrical injury
17. Drug induced
    a. Levodopa
    b. Dopamine D2 receptor blocking agents
       1. Acute dystonic reaction
       2. Tardive dystonia
    c. Ergotism
    d. Anticonvulsants
18. Toxins - Mn, CO, carbon disulfide, cyanide, methanol, disulfiram, 3-nitroproprionic acid
19. Metabolic - hypoparathyroidism
20. Psychogenic

HIV, human immunodeficiency virus.

features, often the parkinsonian features bradykinesia and rigidity. *Tardive dystonia*, a persistent complication of agents that block dopamine receptors, is the most common form of secondary dystonia. Tardive dystonia is usually focal or segmental, affecting the cranial structures in adults; in children, however, it can be generalized, involving the trunk and limbs. It often is associated with features of tardive dyskinesia, especially oral-buccal-lingual movements (see Chapter 116). Clues suggesting a secondary dystonia are listed in Table 112.5.

TABLE 112.5. CLUES SUGGESTIVE OF SYMPTOMATIC DYSTONIA

1. History of possible etiologic factor, e.g., head trauma, peripheral trauma, encephalitis, toxin exposure, drug exposure, perinatal anoxia
2. Presence of neurologic abnormality, e.g., dementia, seizures, ocular, ataxia, weakness, spasticity, amyotrophy, parkinsonism
3. Onset of rest, instead of action, dystonia
4. Early onset of speech involvement
5. Leg involvement in an adult
6. Hemidystonia
7. Abnormal brain imaging
8. Abnormal laboratory workup
9. Presence of false weakness or sensory exam, or other clues of psychogenic etiology (see Table 112.6)

Psychogenic dystonia can be considered within the secondary dystonia category. For many decades, Oppenheim dystonia was considered psychogenic because of the bizarre nature of the symptoms, exaggeration in periods of stress, variability, and suppression by sensory tricks. This misdiagnosis often led to a long delay in identification of the nature of the disorder and to prolonged periods of needless psychotherapy. Awareness of the capricious nature of the disorder and serial observation of patients can avoid this pitfall. On the other hand, psychogenic dystonia does occur but in less than 5% of patients who otherwise would be considered to have primary torsion dystonia. Clues suggestive of psychogenic dystonia are listed in Table 112.6.

HEREDODEGENERATIVE DYSTONIA

This is a category where neurodegenerations produce dystonia as a prominent feature. Usually other neurologic features, especially parkinsonism, are also present and can even predominate. In some patients with these disorders, dystonia may fail to appear, and other neurologic manifestations may be the presenting feature, for example, chorea in Huntington disease, in which dystonia may be a late-stage feature. Tremor or juvenile parkinsonism may be the mode of onset of Wilson disease, and dystonia may fail to appear in such patients. Because many of these neurodegenerations are due to genetic abnormalities, the term heredodegenerative is applied to this category. However, some of the diseases listed here are of unknown etiology, and it is not clear what the role of genetics might be. For convenience, we place all

TABLE 112.6. CLUES SUGGESTIVE OF PSYCHOGENIC DYSTONIA

Clues relating to the movements
1. Abrupt onset
2. Inconsistent movements (changing characteristics over time)
3. Incongruous movements and postures (movements do not fit with recognized patterns or with normal physiologic patterns)
4. Presence of additional types of abnormal movements that are not consistent with the basic abnormal movement pattern or are not congruous with a known movement disorder, particularly rhythmical shaking, bizarre gait, deliberate slowness carrying out requested voluntary movement, bursts of verbal gibberish, and excessive startle (bizarre movements in response to sudden unexpected noise or threatening movement)
5. Spontaneous remissions
6. Movements disappear with distraction
7. Response to placebo, suggestion, or psychotherapy
8. Present as a paroxysmal disorder
9. Dystonia beginning as a fixed posture
10. Twisting facial movements that move the mouth to one side or the other (note: organic dystonia of the facial muscles usually do not move the mouth sideways)

Clues relating to the other medical observations
1. False weakness
2. False sensory complaints
3. Multiple somatizations or undiagnosed conditions
4. Self-inflicted injuries
5. Obvious psychiatric disturbances
6. Employed in the health profession or in insurance claims field
7. Presence of secondary gain, including continuing care by a "devoted" spouse
8. Litigation or compensation pending

the neurodegenerations in this category. These are listed in Table 112.7 in which heredodegenerative disorders are organized by the nature of their genetics whenever the genes are known, followed by other neurodegenerations in which the etiology remains unknown.

An X-linked recessive disorder causing dystonia and parkinsonism affects young adult Filipino men. The Filipino name for the condition is *lubag*. It has been designated as DYT3. It can begin with dystonia in the feet or cranial structures; lingual and oromandibular dystonia are common, sometimes with stridor. With progression, generalized dystonia often develops. Many patients develop parkinsonism; in some patients, the sole manifestation may be progressive parkinsonism. The abnormal gene has been localized to the centromeric region of the X chromosome. Pathologic study reveals a mosaic pattern of gliosis in the striatum. Patients respond only partially to levodopa, anticholinergics, baclofen, or clonazepam.

TABLE 112.7. HEREDODEGENERATIVE DISEASES (TYPICALLY NOT PURE DYSTONIA)

1. **X-linked recessive**
   a. Lubag (X-linked dystonia-parkinsonism) (DYT3)
   b. Pelizaeus-Merzbacher disease
   c. Deafness, dystonia, retardation, blindness syndrome
2. **Autosomal dominant**
   a. Juvenile parkinsonism (presenting with dystonia) (can be autosomal dominant or recessive)
   b. Huntington's disease (usually presents as chorea)
   c. Machado-Joseph disease (SCA3)
   d. Dentatorubro-pallidoluysian atrophy
   e. Other spinocerebellar degenerations
   f. Familial basal ganglia calcification
3. **Autosomal recessive**
   a. Wilson disease
   b. Juvenile neuronal ceroid-lipofuscinosis (sea-blue histiocytosis, dystonic lipidosis; Batten disease)
   c. Gangliosidoses
   d. Metachromatic leukodystrophy
   e. Lesch-Nyhan syndrome
   f. Homocystinuria
   g. Glutaric acidemia
   h. Triosephosphate isomerase deficiency
   i. Methylmalonic aciduria
   j. Hartnup disease
   k. Ataxia telangiectasia
   l. Hallervorden-Spatz disease
   m. Neuroacanthocytosis
   n. Neuronal intranuclear hyaline inclusion disease
   o. Hereditary spastic paraplegia with dystonia
4. **Probable autosomal recessive**
   a. Progressive pallidal degeneration
   b. Rett syndrome
5. **Mitochondrial**
   a. Leigh disease
   b. Leber disease
   c. Other mitochondrial encephalopathies
6. **Associated with parkinsonian syndromes**
   a. Parkinson disease
   b. Progressive supranuclear palsy
   c. Multiple system atrophy
   d. Cortical-basal ganglionic degeneration

Adapted from Fahn et al. (1998).

TABLE 112.8. OTHER MOVEMENT DISORDERS IN WHICH DYSTONIA MAY BE PRESENT

Tic disorders with dystonic tics
Paroxysmal dyskinesias with dystonia
    Paroxysmal kinesigenic dyskinesia
    Paroxysmal nonkinesigenic dyskinesia
    Paroxysmal exertional dyskinesia
    Benign infantile paroxysmal dyskinesias
Hypnogenic dystonia
    (sometimes these are seizures)

OTHER DYSKINESIA SYNDROMES WITH DYSTONIA

Dystonia can appear in disorders not ordinarily considered to be a part of torsion dystonia (Table 112.8). These include dystonic tics that are more conveniently classified with tic disorders (see Chapter 111), paroxysmal dyskinesias more conveniently classified with paroxysmal dyskinesias (see Chapter 9), and hypnogenic dystonia that can be either paroxysmal dyskinesias or seizures (see Chapter 9).

PSEUDODYSTONIA

To complete the revised classification, Table 112.9 lists disorders that can mimic torsion dystonia but are not generally considered to be a true dystonia. These disorders typically manifest themselves as sustained muscle contractions or abnormal postures, which is why they are often mistaken for dystonia. But these contractions are secondary to either a peripheral or reflex mechanism

TABLE 112.9. PSEUDODYSTONIAS (NOT CLASSIFIED AS DYSTONIA BUT CAN BE MISTAKEN FOR DYSTONIA BECAUSE OF SUSTAINED POSTURES)

Sandifer syndrome
Stiff-man syndrome
Isaacs syndrome
Satoyoshi syndrome
Rotational atlantoaxial subluxation
Soft tissue nuchal mass
Bone disease
Ligamentous absence, laxity or damage
Congenital muscular torticollis
Congenital postural torticollis
Juvenile rheumatoid arthritis
Ocular postural torticollis
Congenital Klippel-Feil syndrome
Posterior fossa tumor
Syringomyelia
Arnold Chiari malformation
Trochlear nerve palsy
Vestibular torticollis
Seizures manifesting as sustained twisting postures
Inflammatory myopathy

or as a reaction to some other problem. For example, Sandifer syndrome is due to gastroesophageal reflux, with apparent reduction of the gastric contractions when the head is tilted to the side; Isaacs syndrome is due to continuous peripheral neural firing; orthopedic disease causes a number of postural changes; and seizures can result in sustained twisting postures.

TREATMENT

After levodopa therapy has been tested to be certain that DRD has not been overlooked, the following drugs that have been reported to be effective in dystonia should be tried: high-dose anticholinergics (e.g., trihexyphenidyl), high-dose baclofen, benzodiazepines (clonazepam, diazepam), and antidopaminergics (reserpine, dopamine receptor blockers). Stereotaxic thalamotomy may be useful in unilateral dystonia, but bilateral thalamotomy carries about a 30% risk of dysarthria. Posteroventral pallidotomy has been shown to be effective for some patients with Oppenheim dystonia; its comparison with thalamotomy still needs to be accomplished. For focal dystonias, such as blepharospasm, torticollis, oromandibular dystonia, and spastic dysphonia, local injections of botulinum toxin are beneficial. This agent also can be used to treat generalized dystonia, with injections limited to the most severely affected focal site. This muscle-weakening agent can be effective for about 3 months before a repeat injection is needed. About 5% of patients develop antibodies to botulinum toxin, thus rendering that particular strain of toxin ineffective. Local surgery also can be used for focal dystonias. Selective denervation of the affected muscles by section of extradural fibers of the anterior cervical root or the spinal accessory nerve has been successful is some patients in otherwise intractable cervical dystonia.

SUGGESTED READINGS

Almasy L, Bressman SB, Raymond D, et al. Idiopathic torsion dystonia linked to chromosome 8 in two Mennonite families. *Ann Neurol* 1997;42:670–673.

Augood SJ, Penney JB, Friberg IK, et al. Expression of the early-onset torsion dystonia gene (DYT1) in human brain. *Ann Neurol* 1998;43:669–673.

Bara-Jimenez W, Catalan MJ, Hallett M, Gerloff C. Abnormal somatosensory homunculus in dystonia of the hand. *Ann Neurol* 1998;44:828–831.

Berardelli A, Rothwell JC, Hallett M, Thompson PD, Manfredi M, Marsden CD. The pathophysiology of primary dystonia. *Brain* 1998;121:1195–1212.

Bhatia KP, Quinn NP, Marsden CD. Clinical features and natural history of axial predominant adult onset primary dystonia. *J Neurol Neurosurg Psychiatry* 1997;63:788–791.

Brashear A, de Leon D, Bressman SB, Thyagarajan D, Farlow MR, Dobyns WB. Rapid-onset dystonia-parkinsonism in a second family. *Neurology* 1997;48:1066–1069.

Bressman SB, de Leon D, Brin MF, et al. Idiopathic torsion dystonia among Ashkenazi Jews: Evidence for autosomal dominant inheritance. *Ann Neurol* 1989;26:612–620.

Burke RE, Fahn S, Marsden CD. Torsion dystonia: a double-blind, prospective trial of high-dosage trihexyphenidyl. *Neurology* 1986;36:160–164.

Dauer WT, Burke RE, Greene P, Fahn S. Current concepts on the clinical features, aetiology and management of idiopathic cervical dystonia. *Brain* 1998;121:547–560.

Eidelberg D, Moeller JR, Antonini A, et al. Functional brain networks in DYT1 dystonia. *Ann Neurol* 1998;44:303–312.

Fahn S. The varied clinical expressions of dystonia. *Neurol Clin* 1984;2:541–552.

Fahn S, Bressman SB, Marsden CD. Classification of dystonia. *Adv Neurol.* 1998;78:1–10.

Fahn S, Marsden CD, Calne DB, eds. Dystonia 2. *Adv Neurol* 1988;50.

Fahn S, Marsden CD, DeLong MR, eds. Dystonia 3. *Adv Neurol* 1998;78.

Ford B, Greene P, Louis ED, et al. Use of intrathecal baclofen in the treatment of patients with dystonia. *Arch Neurol* 1996;53:1241–1246.

Greene P, Kang UJ, Fahn S. Spread of symptoms in idiopathic torsion dystonia. *Mov Disord* 1995;10:143–152.

Hyland K, Fryburg JS, Wilson WG, et al. Oral phenylalanine loading in dopa-responsive dystonia: a possible diagnostic test. *Neurology* 1997;48:1290–1297.

Ichinose H, Ohye T, Takahashi E, et al. Hereditary progressive dystonia with marked diurnal fluctuation caused by mutations in the GTP cyclohydrolase I gene. *Nat Genet* 1994;8:236–242.

Jankovic J, Brin MF. Therapeutic uses of botulinum toxin. *N Engl J Med* 1991;324:1186–1194.

Knappskog PM, Flatmark T, Mallet J, Ludecke B, Bartholome K. Recessively inherited L-dopa-responsive dystonia caused by a point mutation (Q381K) in the tyrosine hydroxylase gene. *Hum Mol Genet* 1995;4:1209–1212.

Kupke KG, Graeber MB, Muller U. Dystonia-parkinsonism syndrome (XDP) locus—flanking markers in Xq12-q21.1. *Am J Hum Genet* 1992;50:808–815.

Lang AE. Psychogenic dystonia: a review of 18 cases. *Can J Neurol Sci* 1995;22:136–143.

Maller A, Hyland K, Milstien S, Biaggioni I, Butler IJ. Aromatic L-amino acid decarboxylase deficiency: clinical features, diagnosis, and treatment of a second family. *J Child Neurol* 1997;12:349–354.

Manji H, Howard RS, Miller DH, et al. Status dystonicus: the syndrome and its management. *Brain* 1998;121:243–252.

Marsden CD, Obeso JA, Zarranz JJ, Lang AE. The anatomical basis of symptomatic hemidystonia. *Brain* 1985;108:463–483.

Nutt JG, Muenter MD, Aronson A, et al. Epidemiology of focal and generalized dystonia in Rochester, Minnesota. *Mov Disord* 1988;3:188–194.

Nygaard TG, Trugman JM, de Yebenes JG, Fahn S. Dopa-responsive dystonia: the spectrum of clinical manifestations in a large North American family. *Neurology* 1990;40:66–69.

Oppenheim H. Uber eine eigenartige Krampfkrankheit des kindlichen und jugendlichen Alters (Dysbasia lordotica progressiva, Dystonia musculorum deformans). *Neurol Centrabl* 1911;30:1090–1107.

Ozelius LJ, Hewett JW, Page CE, et al. The early-onset torsion dystonia gene (DYT1) encodes an ATP binding protein. *Nat Genet* 1997;17:40–48.

Quinn NP. Essential myoclonus and myoclonic dystonia. *Mov Disord* 1996;11:119–124.

Rajput AH, Gibb WRG, Zhong XH, et al. DOPA-responsive dystonia: pathological and biochemical observations in a case. *Ann Neurol* 1994;35:396–402.

Saint-Hilaire M-H, Burke RE, Bressman SB, et al. Delayed-onset dystonia due to perinatal or early childhood asphyxia. *Neurology* 1991;41:216–222.

Sawle GV, Leenders KL, Brooks DJ, et al. Dopa-responsive dystonia: [F-18]dopa positron emission tomography. *Ann Neurol* 1991;30:24–30.

Thony B, Blau N. Mutations in the GTP cyclohydrolase I and 6-pyruvoyl-tetrahydropterin synthase genes. *Hum Mutat* 1997;10:11–20.

Zweig RM, Hedreen JC, Jankel WR, et al. Pathology in brainstem regions of individuals with primary dystonia. *Neurology* 1988;38:702–706.

Merritt's Neurology, 10th ed., edited by L.P. Rowland. Lippincott Williams & Wilkins, Philadelphia © 2000.

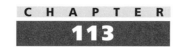

CHAPTER 113

ESSENTIAL TREMOR

ELAN D. LOUIS
PAUL E. GREENE

Essential tremor, the most common adult-onset movement disorder, is characterized by an 8- to 12-Hz postural and kinetic tremor of the arms. Tremor may also involve the head, the voice, and rarely the legs. The tremor is present with sustained posture (arms extended in front of the body) or during movement (touching finger-to-nose, writing, drinking water). The tremor is often mildly asymmetric. It is rarely present at rest, in contrast to the tremor of Parkinson disease. The crude prevalence of essential tremor in different populations has been estimated to be between 0.4% and 3.9%; among those over the age of 65 years, the prevalence is higher. The disorder is partly genetic. There are large kindreds with an autosomal dominant form of essential tremor, and in a small number, linkage has been demonstrated to regions on chromosomes 2p and 3q. However, the existence of sporadic cases of essential tremor and the variability in age at onset in familial cases argues for the presence of nongenetic environmental causes in some cases. The extent to which essential tremor is a genetic disorder or a sporadic disorder is unknown. In different studies, 17% to 100% of cases report at least one affected relative. There have been few published autopsy studies, and there are no pathognomonic pathologic abnormalities. Several positron emission tomography studies have revealed metabolic abnormalities in the cerebellum. It is not known whether the disease is the result of a progressive loss of selected neuronal populations or a static insult.

The onset occurs at any age, although incidence increases markedly with advancing age. Initially, the tremor may be mild, intermittent, and asymptomatic. In 90% to 99.5% of individuals with essential tremor, the tremor is mild and medical attention is never sought. The condition may remain static for years, even decades. However, patients often note a gradual increase in severity, confirming the finding in observational studies that older patients tend to have tremors of lower frequency and higher amplitude. The tremor may spread to involve the head in a rhythmic bobbing that may be either vertical or horizontal. It then may spread to the vocal cords or diaphragm, causing a characteristic vocal tremor. Many patients note that tremor is temporarily suppressed by drinking alcoholic beverages, but a rebound exacerbation sometimes follows.

TREATMENT

The tremor may be severe enough to result in embarrassment and functional disability. In up to 15% of those attending clinics, the tremor leads to early retirement. Beta-blockers and primidone, alone or in combination, are the most effective pharma-cologic therapies. Propranolol has been used in doses up to 240 mg daily; primidone may be effective in doses of 50 mg or less daily. Both drugs reduce the amplitude of tremor in some patients but do not abolish the tremor; benefit may disappear with time. Stereotactic thalamotomy can reduce essential tremor in the contralateral limbs, but the condition is rarely sufficiently disabling to warrant brain surgery. High-frequency thalamic stimulation has been effective in reducing tremor severity. Clonazepam, methazolamide, glutethimide, clozapine, and gabapentin have been reported to benefit some patients.

DIFFERENTIAL DIAGNOSIS

Essential tremor is frequently misdiagnosed as parkinsonism, especially in the elderly. Differentiation may readily be made, however, by the absence of parkinsonian features, such as rest tremor, muscular rigidity, bradykinesia, or loss of postural control. Handwriting is large, irregular, and tremulous in striking contrast to the tremulous micrographia of parkinsonism. Head tremor rarely occurs in parkinsonism; instead, tremor affects the lips, tongue, and jaw. Patients with a long history of tremor of both hands occasionally develop typical signs and symptoms of Parkinson disease. It is not known whether this development is a coincidence of common conditions or whether patients with essential tremor are at increased risk of parkinsonism. Absence of dysdiadochokinesia, dysmetria, exaggeration of the tremor with intention, and other cerebellar signs distinguishes essential tremor from cerebellar "intention" tremor. Hyperthyroidism or the use of lithium or valproate are usually excluded by clinical history. The most difficult differential is between a mild case of essential tremor and enhanced physiologic tremor. Task-specific tremors, such as tremors restricted to the act of writing, or tremor associated with a task-specific dystonic posturing, such as writer's cramp, are diagnostic gray areas between essential tremor and primary torsion dystonia.

SUGGESTED READINGS

Bain PG, Findley LJ, Thompson PD, et al. A study of heredity of essential tremor. *Brain* 1994;117:805–824.

Elble RJ. Central mechanisms of tremor. *J Clin Neurophysiol* 1996;13:133–144.

Findley LJ. The pharmacology of essential tremor. In: Marsden CD, Fahn S, eds. *Movement disorders II*. London: Butterworths, 1987.

Gulcher JR, Jonsson P, Kong A, et al. Mapping of a familial essential tremor gene, FET1, to chromosome 3q13. *Nat Genet* 1997;17:84–87.

Higgins JJ, Pho LT, Nee LE. A gene (ETM) for essential tremor maps to chromosome 2p22-p25. *Mov Disord* 1977;12:859–864.

Jenkins IH, Bain PG, Colebatch JG, et al. A positron emission tomography study of essential tremor: evidence for overactivity of cerebellar connections. *Ann Neurol* 1993;34:82–90.

Koller W, Pahwa R, Busenbark K, et al. High-frequency unilateral thalamic stimulation in the treatment of essential and Parkinsonian tremor. *Ann Neurol* 1997;42:292–299.

Larsson T, Sjögren T. Essential tremor: a clinical and genetic population study. *Acta Psychiatr Neurol Scand* 1960:36[Suppl 144]:1–176.

Louis ED, Ford B, Pullman S. Prevalence of asymptomatic tremor in relatives of patients with essential tremor. *Arch Neurol* 1997;54:197–200.

Louis ED, Ottman R. How familial is familial tremor? Genetic epidemiology of essential tremor. *Neurology* 1996;46:1200–1205.

Louis ED, Ottman R, Hauser WA. How common is the most common adult movement disorder? Estimates of the prevalence of essential tremor throughout the world. *Mov Disord* 1998;13:5–10.

Louis ED, Wendt KJ, Pullman SL, Ford B. Is essential tremor symmetric? Observational data from a community-based study of essential tremor. *Arch Neurol* 1998;55:1553–1559.

Rajput AH, Offord KP, Beard CM, Kurland LT. Essential tremor in

Rochester, Minnesota: a 45-year study. *J Neurol Neurosurg Psychiatry* 1984;47:466–470.

Rajput AH, Rozdilsky B, Ang L, Rajput A. Clinicopathological observations in essential tremor: report of six cases. *Neurology* 1991;41:1422–1424.

Merritt's Neurology, 10th ed., edited by L.P. Rowland. Lippincott Williams & Wilkins, Philadelphia © 2000.

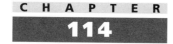

C H A P T E R 114

PARKINSONISM

STANLEY FAHN
SERGE PRZEDBORSKI

In 1817, James Parkinson described the major clinical features of what today is recognized as a symptom complex manifested by any combination of six cardinal features: tremor at rest, rigidity, bradykinesia-hypokinesia, flexed posture, loss of postural reflexes, and the freezing phenomenon. At least two of these features, with at least one being either tremor at rest or bradykinesia, must be present for a diagnosis of definite parkinsonism. The many causes of parkinsonism (Table 114.1) are divided into four categories—idiopathic, symptomatic, Parkinson-plus syndromes, and various heredodegenerative diseases in which parkinsonism is a manifestation.

The core biochemical pathology in parkinsonism is decreased dopaminergic neurotransmission in the basal ganglia. In most of the diseases in Table 114.1, degeneration of the nigrostriatal dopamine system results in marked loss of striatal dopamine content. In some, degeneration of the striatum with loss of dopamine receptors is characteristic. Drug-induced parkinsonism is the result of blockade of dopamine receptors or depletion of dopamine storage. It is not known how hydrocephalus or abnormal calcium metabolism produces parkinsonism. Physiologically, the decreased dopaminergic activity in the striatum leads to disinhibition of the subthalamic nucleus and the medial globus pallidus, which is the predominant efferent nucleus in the basal ganglia. Understanding the biochemical pathology led to dopamine replacement therapy; understanding the physiologic change led to surgical interventions, such as pallidotomy, thalamotomy, and subthalmic nucleus stimulation.

The clinical features of tremor, rigidity, and flexed posture are referred to as *positive phenomena* and are reviewed first; bradykinesia, loss of postural reflexes, and freezing are negative phenomena. In general, the negative phenomena are the more disabling. *Rest tremor* at a frequency of 4 to 5 Hz is present in the extremities, almost always distally; the classic "pill-rolling" tremor involves the thumb and forefinger. Rest tremor disappears with action but reemerges as the limbs maintain a posture. Rest tremor is also common in the lips, chin, and tongue. Rest tremor of the hands increases with walking and may be an early sign when others are not yet present. Stress worsens the tremor.

Rigidity is an increase of muscle tone that is elicited when the examiner moves the patient's limbs, neck, or trunk. This increased resistance to passive movement is equal in all directions and usually is manifest by a ratchety "give" during the movement. This so-called cogwheeling is caused by the underlying tremor even in the absence of visible tremor. Cogwheeling also occurs in patients with essential tremor. Rigidity of the passive limb increases while another limb is engaged in voluntary active movement.

The *flexed posture* commonly begins in the arms and spreads to involve the entire body (Fig. 114.1). The head is bowed, the trunk is bent forward, the back is kyphotic, the arms are held in front of the body, and the elbows, hips, and knees are flexed. De-

TABLE 114.1. CLASSIFICATION OF MAJOR PARKINSONIAN SYNDROMES

Primary parkinsonism
    Parkinson disease—sporadic and familial

Secondary parkinsonism
    Drug-induced: dopamine antagonists and depletors
    Hemiatrophy—hemiparkinsonism
    Hydrocephalus; normal pressure hydrocephalus
    Hypoxia
    Infectious; postencephalitic
    Metabolic; parathyroid dysfunction
    Toxin: Mn, CO, MPTP, cyanide
    Trauma
    Tumor
    Vascular; multiinfarct state

Parkinson-plus syndromes
    Cortical-basal ganglionic degeneration
    Dementia syndromes
        Alzheimer disease
        Diffuse Lewy body disease
        Frontotemporal dementia
    Lytico-Bodig (Guamanian parkinsonism-dementia-ALS)
    Multiple system atrophy syndromes
        Striatonigral degeneration
        Shy-Drager syndrome
        Sporadic olivopontocerebellar degeneration (OPCA)
        Motor neuron disease—parkinsonism
    Progressive pallidal atrophy
    Progressive supranuclear palsy

Heredodegenerative diseases
    Hallervorden-Spatz disease
    Huntington disease
    Lubag (X-linked dystonia-parkinsonism)
    Mitochondrial cytopathies with striatal necrosis
    Neuroacanthocytosis
    Wilson disease

MPTP,1-methyl-4-phenyl-1,2,3,6-tetrahydropyridine; ALS; amytrophic lateral sclerosis.

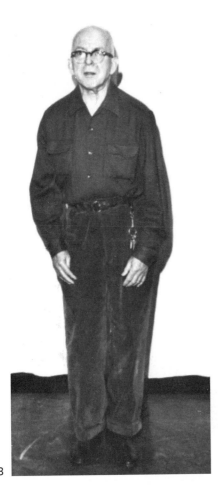 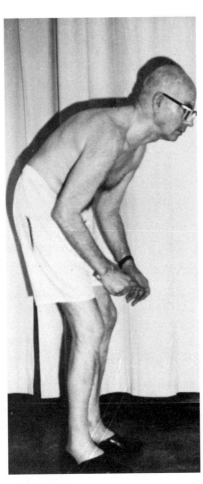

A,B

FIG. 114.1. Parkinson patient body posture. **A:** Front view. **B:** Side view.

formities of the hands include ulnar deviation of the hands, flexion of the metacarpal-phalangeal joints, and extension of the interphalangeal joints (striatal hand). Inversion of the feet is apparent, and the big toes may be dorsiflexed (striatal toe). Lateral tilting of the trunk is common.

Akinesia is a term used interchangeably with bradykinesia and hypokinesia. *Bradykinesia* (slowness of movement, difficulty initiating movement, and loss of automatic movement) and *hypokinesia* (reduction in amplitude of movement, particularly with repetitive movements, so-called decrementing) are the most common features of parkinsonism, although they may appear after the tremor. Bradykinesia has many facets, depending on the affected body parts. The face loses spontaneous expression (masked facies, *hypomimia*) with decreased frequency of blinking. Poverty of spontaneous movement is characterized by loss of gesturing and by the patient's tendency to sit motionless. Speech becomes soft (*hypophonia*), and the voice has a monotonous tone with a lack of inflection (*aprosody*). Some patients do not enunciate clearly (*dysarthria*) and do not separate syllables clearly, thus running the words together (*tachyphemia*). Bradykinesia of the dominant hand results in small and slow handwriting (*micrographia*) and in difficulty shaving, brushing teeth, combing hair, buttoning, or applying makeup. Playing musical instruments is impaired. Walking is slow, with a shortened stride length and a tendency to shuffle; arm swing decreases and eventually is lost. Difficulty rising from a deep chair, getting out of automobiles,

and turning in bed are symptoms of truncal bradykinesia. Drooling saliva results from failure to swallow spontaneously, a feature of bradykinesia, and is not caused by excessive production of saliva. The patients can swallow properly when asked to do so, but only constant reminders allow them to keep swallowing. Similarly, arm swing can be normal if the patient voluntarily and, with effort, wishes to have the arms swing on walking. Pronounced bradykinesia prevents a patient with parkinsonism from driving an automobile; foot movement from the accelerator to the brake pedal is too slow.

Bradykinesia is commonly misinterpreted by patients as weakness. Fatigue, a common complaint in parkinsonism, particularly in the mild stage of the disease before pronounced slowness appears, may be related to mild bradykinesia or rigidity. Subtle signs of bradykinesia can be detected even in the early stage of parkinsonism if one examines for slowness in shrugging the shoulders, lack of gesturing, decreased arm swing, and decrementing amplitude of rapid successive movements. With advancing bradykinesia, slowness and difficulty in the execution of activities of daily living increase. A meal normally consumed in 20 minutes may be only half eaten in an hour or more. Swallowing may become impaired with advancing disease, and choking and aspiration are concerns.

Loss of postural reflexes leads to falling and eventually to inability to stand unassisted. Postural reflexes are tested by the *pulltest*, which is performed by the examiner, who stands behind the patient, gives a sudden firm pull on the shoulders, and checks for retropulsion. With advance warning, a normal person can recover within one step. The examiner should always be prepared to catch the patient when this test is conducted; otherwise, a person who has lost postural reflexes could fall. As postural reflexes are impaired, the patient collapses into the chair on attempting to sit down (*sitting en bloc*). Walking is marked by festination, whereby the patient walks faster and faster, trying to move the feet forward to be under the flexed body's center of gravity and thus prevent falling.

The *freezing* phenomenon (motor block) is transient inability to perform active movements. It most often affects the legs when walking but also can involve eyelid opening (known as *apraxia of lid opening* or levator inhibition), speaking (palilalia), and writing. Freezing occurs suddenly and is transient, lasting usually no more than several seconds with each occurrence. The feet seem as if "glued to the ground" and then suddenly become "unstuck," allowing the patient to walk again. Freezing typically occurs when the patient begins to walk ("start-hesitation"), attempts to turn while walking, approaches a destination, such as a chair in which to sit (destination-hesitation), and is fearful about inability to deal with perceived barriers or time-restricted activities, such as entering revolving doors, elevator doors that may close, and crossing heavily trafficked streets (sudden transient freezing). Freezing is often overcome by visual clues, such as having the patient step over objects, and is much less frequent when the patient is going up steps than when walking on a level ground. The combination of freezing and loss of postural reflexes is particularly devastating. When the feet suddenly stop moving forward, the patient falls because the upper part of the body continues in motion as a result of the inability to recover an upright posture. Falling is responsible for the high incidence of hip fractures in parkinsonian patients. Likely related to the freezing phenomenon is the difficulty for parkinsonian patients to perform two motor acts simultaneously.

PARKINSON DISEASE (PRIMARY PARKINSONISM)

Pathology

The pathology of Parkinson disease (PD) is distinctive. Degeneration of the neuromelanin-containing neurons in the brainstem occurs, especially in the ventral tier of the pars compacta in the substantia nigra (Fig. 114.2) and in the locus ceruleus; many of the surviving neurons contain eosinophilic cytoplasmic inclusions known as *Lewy bodies*, the pathologic hallmark of the disease. By the time symptoms appear, the substantia nigra already has lost about 60% of dopaminergic neurons and the dopamine content in the striatum is about 80% less than normal.

Epidemiology

PD makes up approximately 80% of cases of parkinsonism listed in Table 114.1. The age at onset assumes a bell-shaped curve with a mean of 55 years in both sexes and a wide range in age from 20 to 80. Onset at younger than 20 years is known as *juvenile parkinsonism*; when primary, it is usually familial and without Lewy bodies in the degenerating substantia nigra. Juvenile parkinsonism is not always primary and can be due to heredodegenerative diseases such as Huntington disease and Wilson disease. Onset of primary parkinsonism between 20 and 40 years is known as young-onset PD. PD is more common in men, with a male-to-female ratio of 3:2. The prevalence of PD is approximately 160 per 100,000, and the incidence is about 20 per 100,000/yr. Prevalence and incidence increase with age. At age 70, the prevalence is approximately 550 per 100,000, and the incidence is 120 per 100,000/yr.

Symptoms and Signs

The clinical motor features of PD are the six cardinal features described for parkinsonism in general. The onset is insidious; tremor is the symptom first recognized in 70% (Table 114.2). Symptoms often begin unilaterally, but as the disease progresses, it becomes bilateral. The disease can remain confined to one side, although steadily worsening for several years before the other side becomes involved. The disease progresses slowly, and if untreated, the patient eventually becomes wheelchair-bound and bedridden. Despite severe bradykinesia with marked immobility, patients with PD may rise suddenly and move normally for a short burst of motor activity, so-called *kinesia paradoxica*.

In addition to the motor signs that are used to define parkinsonism, most patients with PD have behavioral signs as well. Attention span is reduced, and there is visuospatial impairment. The personality changes; the patient slowly becomes more dependent, fearful, indecisive, and passive. The spouse gradually makes more of the decisions and becomes the dominant partner.

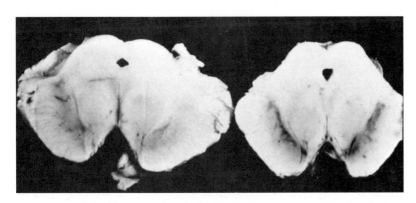

FIG. 114.2. Parkinson pathology. Depigmentation of substantia nigra of a Parkinson patient **(left)** in contrast to that of a normal patient **(right)**.

TABLE 114.2. INITIAL SYMPTOMS IN PARKINSON DISEASE

	No. of cases (*n* = 183)	Percent
Tremor	129.1	70.5
Stiffness or slowness of movement	36	19.7
Loss of dexterity and/or handwriting disturbance	23	12.6
Gait disturbance	21	11.5
Muscle pain, cramps, aching	15	8.2
Depression, nervousness, or other psychiatric disturbance	8	4.4
Speech disturbance	7	3.8
General fatigue, muscle weakness	5	2.7
Drooling	3	1.6
Loss of arm swing	3	1.6
Facial masking	3	1.6
Dysphagia	1	0.5
Paresthesia	1	0.5
Average number of initial symptoms per patient	1.4	

The patient speaks less spontaneously. The patient eventually sits much of the day and is inactive unless encouraged to exercise. Passivity and lack of motivation are common and are expressed by the patient's aversion for visiting friends. Depression is frequent in patients with PD, developing at a rate of about 2% per year.

Cognitive decline is another common feature but is usually not the severe type of dementia seen in Alzheimer disease. Memory impairment is not a feature of PD; rather the patient is just slow in responding to questions, so-called *bradyphrenia*. The correct answer can be obtained if the patient is given enough time. Subtle signs of bradyphrenia, such as the inability to change mental set rapidly, may be present early in the disease. Fifteen percent to 20% of patients with PD have a more profound dementia, similar to that in Alzheimer disease. These patients are usually elderly and have developed concurrent Alzheimer disease or diffuse Lewy body disease, in which Lewy bodies are present in cortical neurons. These disorders are not always distinguishable, but Lewy body disease is often characterized by fluctuating hallucinations.

Sensory symptoms are fairly common, but objective sensory impairment is not seen in PD. Symptoms of pain, burning, and tingling occur in the region of motor involvement. A patient may have dull pain in one shoulder as an early symptom of the disease, which often is misdiagnosed as arthritis or bursitis, and even before clearcut signs of bradykinesia appear in that same arm. *Akathisia* (inability to sit still, restlessness) and the *restless legs syndrome* occur in some patients with PD. In both syndromes, uncomfortable sensations disappear with movement, and sometimes the two conditions are difficult to distinguish. Akathisia is usually present most of the day; it may respond to levodopa but otherwise has not been treated successfully. The restless legs syndrome develops late in the day with crawling sensations in the legs and may be associated with periodic movements in sleep, thereby disturbing sleep. This problem can be treated successfully with opioids, such as propoxyphene, oxycodone, and codeine.

Autonomic disturbances also are encountered. The skin is cooler, constipation is a major complaint, bladder emptying is inadequate, erection may be difficult to achieve, and blood pressure may be low. A major diagnostic consideration is the Shy-Drager syndrome, also called multiple system atrophy (MSA). Seborrhea and seborrheic dermatitis are common but can be controlled with good hygiene.

Tendon reflexes are usually unimpaired in PD; an abnormal extensor plantar reflex suggests a Parkinson-plus syndrome. An uninhibited glabellar reflex (*Myerson sign*), snout reflex, and palmomental reflexes are common, even early in the disease.

Etiology, Pathogenesis, and Genetics

The cause of PD is unknown. Research has concentrated on genetics, exogenous toxins, and endogenous toxins from cellular oxidative reactions. Based on twin studies, onset of PD before age 50 has a higher likelihood of a genetic etiology.

Several genes have been identified, usually causing young-onset parkinsonism (Table 114.3). The first (PD1) is due to mutations in the gene for the protein, alpha-*synuclein*, located on chromosome 4q21-q22. This protein is present in synapses and cell nuclei, but its function is unclear. The resulting parkinsonism transmits in an autosomal dominant pattern. It is rare, being seen only in a few families in Greece, Italy, and Germany. After the discovery of this genetic defect, however, alpha-synuclein was found to be present in Lewy bodies (even in patients with PD without this genetic mutation). It is believed that the abnormal protein aggregates and accumulates in cells, causing neuronal death.

The most commonly occurring gene defect causing PD is PD2 on chromosome 6q25-q27, coding for a previously un-

TABLE 114.3. GENETIC FORMS OF PARKINSON DISEASE

Name of protein	Gene location	Transmission pattern
α-Synuclein	4q21-q22	Autosomal dominant
Parkin	6q25.2-q27	Autosomal recessive
Ubiquitin carbonyl-terminal hydrolase-L1	4p	Autosomal dominant
Iowa pedigree: PD/ET	4q	Autosomal dominant
tau; frontotemporal dementia	17q21	Autosomal dominant
Susceptibility gene	2p13	
GTP cyclo-hydrolase I (dopa-responsive dystonia)	14q22	Autosomal dominant
Maternal inheritance	mitochondrial DNA (suspected)	

known protein, named *parkin*. This protein is abundant in the substantia nigra and shares homology with ubiquitin and with other proteins involved in cell growth, differentiation, and development. Mutations in the parkin gene result in an autosomal recessive parkinsonism that is slowly progressive, with onset usually before the age of 40 years, and sleep benefit; rest tremor is not prominent. There is degeneration of substantia nigra neurons but no Lewy body inclusions.

Some affected members of the so-called Iowa pedigree have essential tremor in addition to parkinsonism. Rare families with PD seem to exhibit a maternal mode of inheritance, suggesting a mitochondrial DNA defect. Dopa-responsive dystonia may present during adulthood as PD. It tends to be benign, responding to relatively low doses of levodopa and not progressing. This disorder is discussed in Chapter 112.

The discovery that the chemical agent 1-methyl-4-phenyl-1,2,3,6-tetrahydropyridine (MPTP) can cause parkinsonism raised the possibility that PD might be caused by an environmental toxin. No single environmental factor has emerged as essential, but growing up in a rural environment was disproportionately frequent in some studies. Because aging is associated with a loss of catecholamine-containing neurons and an increase in monoamine oxidase (types A and B) activity, an endogenous toxin hypothesis has emerged. Cellular oxidation reactions (such as enzymatic oxidation and autooxidation of dopamine and other monoamines) result in the formation of hydrogen peroxide and free radicals (oxyradicals), and if not removed properly, these agents can damage the monoamine neurons. Substantia nigra in patients with PD shows severe depletion of reduced glutathione, the major substrate required for the elimination of hydrogen peroxide. This change is also seen in brains with incidental Lewy bodies and therefore could be the earliest biochemical abnormality of PD. It is not known, however, if this change causes oxidative stress (increasing oxyradicals) or is the result of oxidative stress (because reduced glutathione is oxidized under conditions of oxidative stress). Iron in the substantia nigra may also play a critical role because it can catalyze the formation of the highly reactive hydroxyl radical from hydrogen peroxide.

Postmortem biochemical observations showed that complex I activity of mitochondria is reduced in substantia nigra of patients with PD (MPP+ also affects complex I). This reduction could be the result of an exogenous toxin, oxidative stress, or a genetic defect stemming from the mitochondrial DNA. On the other hand, a primary defect of complex I would decrease the synthesis of ATP and also lead to the buildup of free electrons, thereby increasing oxyradicals and accentuating oxidative stress.

Differential Diagnosis

The diagnosis of PD is based on the clinical features of parkinsonism, insidious onset, slow progression, and the lack of other findings in the history, examination, or laboratory tests that would point to some other cause of parkinsonism. One of the most common disorders mistaken for PD is essential tremor (see Chapter 113), which is characterized by postural and kinetic tremor, not rest tremor.

Several clinical clues suggest that a patient with parkinsonism has some form of the syndrome other than PD itself (Table 114.4). In general, PD often appears with symptoms on only one side of the body, whereas patients with symptomatic parkinsonism or Parkinson-plus syndromes almost always have symmetric symptoms and signs (notable exceptions would be cortical-basal ganglionic degeneration and parkinsonism resulting from a focal brain injury, such as head trauma). Similarly, a rest tremor almost always indicates PD because it rarely is seen in symptomatic parkinsonism or Parkinson-plus syndromes, except in drug-induced and MPTP-induced parkinsonism, which do include rest tremor. The patient who does not have unilateral onset or rest tremor, however, still can have PD that begins symmetrically and without tremor. Perhaps the most important diagnostic aid is the response to levodopa. Patients with PD almost always have a satisfactory response to this drug. If a patient never responds to levodopa, the diagnosis of some other form of parkinsonism is likely. A response to levodopa, however, does not confirm the diagnosis of PD because many cases of symptomatic parkinsonism (e.g., MPTP, postencephalitic, reserpine-induced) and many forms of Parkinson-plus syndromes in their early stages (e.g., Shy-Drager syndrome, striatonigral degeneration, olivopontocerebellar atrophy) also respond to levodopa. Table 114.4 provides a list of some helpful clues.

DRUG-INDUCED PARKINSONISM

Drugs that block striatal dopamine D2 receptors (e.g., phenothiazines and butyrophenones) or deplete striatal dopamine (e.g., reserpine, tetrabenazine) can induce a parkinsonian state (see also Chapter 116). This condition is reversible when the offending agent is withdrawn, but it may require several weeks. Parkinsonism that persists longer than 6 months is attributed to underlying PD that becomes evident during exposure to these antidopaminergic drugs. Anticholinergic drugs can ameliorate the parkinsonian signs and symptoms. The atypical neuroleptic clonazapine is the least likely antipsychotic agent to induce or worsen parkinsonism.

HEMIPARKINSONISM-HEMIATROPHY SYNDROME

This relatively benign syndrome consists of hemiparkinsonism in association with ipsilateral body hemiatrophy or contralateral brain hemiatrophy. The parkinsonism usually begins in young adults and often remains as hemiparkinsonism, sometimes with hemidystonia. It tends to be nonprogressive or slowly progressive compared with PD. The disorder is thought to be the result of brain injury early in life, possibly even perinatally. It usually responds poorly to medications.

NORMAL PRESSURE HYDROCEPHALUS

The gait disorder in normal pressure hydrocephalus (see Chapter 48) resembles that of parkinsonism, with shuffling short steps and loss of postural reflexes and sometimes freezing. Features of urinary incontinence and dementia occur later. Tremor is rare.

TABLE 114.4. CLUES INDICATING THE LIKELY TYPE OF PARKINSONISM

Clinical
 Never responded to levodopa
  Other than PD
 Predominantly unilateral
  PD; HP-HA syndrome; CBGD
 Symmetric onset
  PD; most forms of parkinsonism
 Presence of rest tremor
  PD; secondary parkinsonism
 Lack of rest tremor
  Parkinson-plus syndromes
 History of encephalitis
  Postencephalitic parkinsonism
 History of toxin exposure
  Parkinsonism caused by the toxin
 Taking neuroleptics
  Drug-induced parkinsonism
 Severe unilateral rigidity
  CBGD
 Cortical sensory signs
  CBGD
 Unilateral cortical myoclonus
  CBGD
 Unilateral apraxia
  CBGD
 Alien limb
  CBGD
 Early dementia
  CBGD
 Psychotic sensitivity to levodopa
  Diffuse Lewy body disease; AD
 Early loss of postural reflexes
  Progressive supranuclear palsy
 Impaired downgaze
  Progressive supranuclear palsy
 Deep nasolabial folds
  Progressive supranuclear palsy
 Furrowed forehead and eyebrows
  Progressive supranuclear palsy
 Nuchal dystonia
  Progressive supranuclear palsy

Abducted arms when walking
 Progressive supranuclear palsy
Square wave jerks
 Progressive supranuclear palsy
Pure freezing
 Progressive supranuclear palsy
Meaningful orthostatic hypotension
 Shy-Drager syndrome
Urinary or fecal incontinence
 Shy-Drager syndrome
Cerebellar dysarthria and dysmetria
 Olivopontocerebellar degeneration
Laryngeal stridor (vocal cord paresis)
 Striatonigral degeneration
Lower motor neuron findings
 Multiple system atrophy
Upper motor neuron findings
 Multiple system atrophy
Laboratory
 Fresh blood smear: acanthocytes
  Neuroacanthocytosis
 Grossly elevated creatine kinase
  Neuroacanthocytosis
 MRI: many lacunes
  Vascular parkinsonism
 MRI: "tiger's eye" in pallidum
  Hallervorden-Spatz disease
 MRI: caudate atrophy
  HD; neuroacanthocytosis
 MRI: decreased T2 signal in striatum
  Multiple system atrophy
 MRI: midbrain atrophy
  Progressive supranuclear palsy
 MRI: huge ventricles
  Normal pressure hydrocephalus
 Abnormal autonomic function tests
  Shy-Drager syndrome
 Denervation on sphincter EMG
  Shy-Drager syndrome

CBGD, cortical-basal ganglionic degeneration; HP-HA, hemiparkinsonism-hemiatrophy syndrome; AD, Alzheimer disease; MRI, magnetic resonance imaging; HD, Huntington disease; EMG, electromyogram; PD, Parkinson disease.

The grossly enlarged ventricles lead to the correct diagnosis, with the symptoms improving on removal or shunting of cerebrospinal fluid. The gait disorder is in striking contrast to the lack of parkinsonism in the upper part of the body. The major differential diagnosis for *lower body parkinsonism* includes vascular parkinsonism and the idiopathic gait disorder of the elderly.

POSTENCEPHALITIC PARKINSONISM

Although rarely encountered today, postencephalitic parkinsonism was common in the first half of this century. Parkinsonism was the most prominent sequela of the pandemics of *encephalitis lethargica (von Economo encephalitis)* that occurred between 1919 and 1926. Although the causative agent was never established, it affected mainly the midbrain, thus destroying the substantia nigra. The pathology is distinctive because of the presence of neurofibrillary tangles in the remaining nigral neurons. In addition

to slowly progressive parkinsonism, with features similar to those of PD, oculogyric crises often occur in which the eyes deviate to a fixed position for minutes to hours. Dystonia, tics, behavioral disorders, and ocular palsies may be present. Patients with postencephalitic parkinsonism are more sensitive to levodopa, with limited tolerance because of the development of dyskinesias, mania or hypersexuality at low dosages. Anticholinergics are tolerated well, however.

1-METHYL-4-PHENYL-1,2,3,6-TETRAHYDROPYRIDINE-INDUCED PARKINSONISM

Although rare, this disorder is important because this toxin selectively destroys the dopamine nigrostriatal neurons, and its mechanism has been investigated intensively for possible clues to the pathoetiology of PD. MPTP is a protoxin, being converted to MPP+ by the action of the enzyme monoamine oxidase type B. MPP+ is taken up selectively by dopamine neurons and terminals via the dopamine transporter system. MPP+ inhibits complex I in the mitochondria, depletes ATP, and increases the content of superoxide ion radicals. Superoxide in turn can react with nitric oxide to form the oxyradical peroxynitrite. MPTP-induced parkinsonism has occurred in drug abusers who used it intravenously and possibly also in some laboratory workers exposed to the toxin. The clinical syndrome is indistinguishable from PD and responds to levodopa. Positron emission tomography (PET) indicates that a subclinical exposure to MPTP results in a reduction of fluorodopa uptake in the striatum, thereby making the person liable to future development of parkinsonism.

VASCULAR PARKINSONISM

Vascular parkinsonism resulting from lacunar disease is not common but can be diagnosed by neuroimaging with magnetic resonance imaging evidence of hyperintense T2-weighted signals compatible with small infarcts. Hypertension is usually required for the development of this disorder. The onset of symptoms, usually with a gait disorder, is insidious, and the course is progressive. A history of a major stroke preceding onset is rare, although a stepwise course is sometimes seen. Gait is profoundly affected (lower body parkinsonism), with freezing and loss of postural reflexes. Tremor is rare. Response to the typical antiparkinsonian agents is poor.

CORTICAL-BASAL GANGLIONIC DEGENERATION

Initially reported as *corticodentatonigral degeneration*, this disorder is characterized pathologically by enlarged achromatic neurons in cortical areas (particularly parietal and frontal lobes) along with nigral and striatal neuronal degeneration. The onset is insidious and typically unilateral, with marked rigidity-dystonia on the involved arm. Cortical signs of apraxia, *alien limb phenomena*, cortical sensory loss, and cortical reflex myoclonus of that limb are also seen. Speech is hesitant, gait is poor, and occasionally action tremor is evident. The disease usually spreads slowly to involve both sides of the body, and supranuclear gaze difficulties often occur late. Medications have been ineffective.

LYTICO-BODIG (PARKINSON–DEMENTIA–AMYOTROPHIC LATERAL SCLEROSIS COMPLEX OF GUAM)

A combination of parkinsonism, dementia, and motor neuron disease occurred among the Chamorro natives on Guam in the Western Pacific. The incidence has declined gradually. Epidemiologic evidence supports a probable environmental cause, with exposure occurring during adolescence or adulthood. One hypothesis is that environmental exposure to the neurotoxin found in the seed of the plant *Cycas circinalis* was responsible for the neuronal degeneration. Natives on Guam used this seed to make flour in World War II. But this hypothesis has been questioned. Besides parkinsonism, dementia, and motor neuron disease in various combinations, supranuclear gaze defects also appear. A characteristic pathologic finding is the presence of neurofibrillary tangles in the degenerating neurons, including the substantia nigra. Lewy bodies and senile plaques are absent.

OTHER PARKINSON-DEMENTIA SYNDROMES

Although bradyphrenia is common in PD, dementia also occurs in 15% to 20% of patients. The incidence of dementia increases with age, and those with dementia have a higher mortality rate. The two most common pathologic substrates for dementia in parkinsonism are the changes typical of Alzheimer disease and the presence of Lewy bodies diffusely in the cerebral cortex. It is not known if the Alzheimer changes are coincidental because of the elderly population of affected individuals or whether Alzheimer and PD are somehow related. Similarly, it is not known whether the spread of Lewy bodies into the cortex is a feature of progression of PD or a distinct entity. The presence of dementia limits the tolerance of antiparkinsonian agents because they tend to increase confusion and produce psychosis.

MULTIPLE SYSTEM ATROPHY

MSA has been applied to a tetrad of four syndromes previously considered as distinct and separate entities: striatonigral degeneration, Shy-Drager syndrome, olivopontocerebellar atrophy, and parkinsonism-amyotrophy syndrome (Table 114.5). The full pathologic spectrum consists of neuronal loss and gliosis in the neostriatum, substantia nigra, globus pallidus, cerebellum, inferior olives, basis pontine nuclei, intermediolateral horn cells, anterior horn cells, and corticospinal tracts. A common pathologic feature is the presence of widespread glial cytoplasmic inclusions, particularly in oligodendroglia. The presence of these argyophilic perinuclear structures, which are primarily composed of straight microtubules containing ubiquitin and tau protein, in this tetrad of syndromes supports the concept that these conditions are variations of the same disease process.

Patients with MSA have with parkinsonism one of the other clinical features listed in Table 114.5; each entity can be identified by its characteristic clinical feature. Corticospinal tract findings may be present as well. MSA may account for 10% of pa-

TABLE 114.5. DIFFERENT CLINICAL ENTITIES OF MULTIPLE SYSTEM ATROPHY

Characteristic feature	Nosology
Pure parkinsonism	Striatonigral degeneration
Autonomic dysfunction	Shy-Drager syndrome
Ataxia	Olivopontocerebellar atrophy
Amyotrophy	Amyotrophy-parkinsonism

tients with parkinsonism. In striatonigral degeneration, nerve cell loss and gliosis are found predominantly in the substantia nigra and neostriatum. The symptoms are those of parkinsonism, without tremor. Also, the beneficial response to levodopa is slight because striatal neurons containing dopamine receptors are lost. Dystonic reactions commonly follow low-dosage levodopa therapy. Laryngeal stridor may be caused by paresis of one or both vocal cords. Occasionally, degeneration is seen in the cerebellum, but the presence of cerebellar symptoms classifies the disorder as olivopontocerebellar atrophy.

In the Shy-Drager syndrome, the preganglionic sympathetic neurons in the intermediolateral horns are lost. In addition, other areas may be affected, particularly the substantia nigra (to produce parkinsonism), the cerebellum (to cause ataxia), and the striatum (to cause lack of response to levodopa). Less often, the anterior horn cells are involved (to cause amyotrophy). Because the postganglionic sympathetic neuron is intact in Shy-Drager syndrome, plasma norepinephrine is normal when the patient is supine but fails to rise when the patient stands. Orthostatic hypotension is a major disabling symptom, but other dysautonomic symptoms are also troublesome, including impotence and bladder and bowel dysfunction. Sometimes the striatum is spared, thus allowing a response to levodopa therapy. Levodopa, however, can exaggerate orthostatic hypotension. Measures to overcome this problem include wearing support hose, ingesting salt, and taking fludrocortisone or midodrine, but this approach can result in supine hypertension, which is partially offset if the patient sleeps at an incline instead of in a recumbent position. If the striatum becomes more involved, with presumed loss of dopamine receptors, the benefit of levodopa as an antibradykinetic drug diminishes.

Many disorders make up the complex known as olivopontocerebellar atrophy. Familial olivopontocerebellar atrophy appears as a cerebellar syndrome, whereas sporadic olivopontocerebellar atrophy is characterized by a mixture of parkinsonism and cerebellar syndrome. In addition to degeneration of the olives, pons, and cerebellum, neuronal loss in the striatum and substantia nigra occurs. Some patients respond to levodopa therapy if the striatum is not severely degenerated.

The least common part of the spectrum of MSA involves just the anterior horn cells (to cause amyotrophy) and the nigrostriatal complex (to cause parkinsonism). Only a few of these cases have been described.

Helpful in diagnosing MSA is fluorodeoxyglucose PET showing hypometabolism in the striatum and the frontal lobes.

Treatment of MSA, like other Parkinson-plus syndromes, requires testing levodopa to the maximum tolerated dose or up to 2 g/d (in the presence of carbidopa) to determine whether any therapeutic response can be obtained. In most situations, dopamine replacement therapy is of limited value. Anticholinergics may provide some mild benefit, however.

TREATMENT

Treatment of parkinsonism in general is based on the treatment of PD, which is the focus of this section. At present, treatment is aimed at controlling symptoms because no drug or surgical approach unequivocally prevents progression of the disease. Treatment is individualized because each patient has a unique set of symptoms, signs, response to medications, and a host of social, occupational, and emotional needs that must be considered. The goal is to keep the patient functioning independently as long as possible. Practical guides are the symptoms and degree of functional impairment and the expected benefits and risks of therapeutic agents.

Drug Therapy

Although pharmacotherapy is the basis of treatment, physiotherapy is also important. It involves patients in their own care, promotes exercise, keeps muscles active, and preserves mobility. This approach is especially beneficial as parkinsonism advances because many patients tend to remain sitting and inactive. Psychiatric assistance may be required to deal with depression and the social and familial problems that may develop with this chronic disabling illness. Electroconvulsive therapy may have a role in patients with severe intractable depression.

Table 114.6 lists the drugs useful in parkinsonism according to mechanisms of action. It also lists some of the surgical approaches available. Selection of the most suitable drugs for the individual patient and deciding when to use them in the course of the disease are challenges for the treating clinician. In many Parkinson-plus disorders, the response to treatment is not satisfactory, but the principles for treating PD are used in treating these disorders as well. Because PD is chronic and progressive,

TABLE 114.6. THERAPEUTIC CHOICES FOR PARKINSON DISEASE

Medications
  Dopamine precursor: levodopa ± carbidopa; standard and slow release
  Dopamine agonists: bromocriptine, pergolide, pramipexole, ropinirole, lisuride, apomorphine, cabergoline,
  Catecholamine-O-methyl transferase inhibitors: tolcapone and entacapone
  Dopamine releaser: amantadine
  Glutamate antagonist: amantadine
  Monoamine oxidase type B inhibitor: selegiline
  Anticholinergics: trihexyphenidyl, benztropine, ethopropazine, biperiden, cycrimine, procyclidine
  Anitihistaminics: diphenhydramine, orphenadrine, phenindamine, chlorphenoxamine
  Antidepressants: amitriptyline and other tricyclics, fluoxetine and other serotonin-uptake inhibitors
  Muscle relaxants: cyclobenzaprine, diazepam
  Peripheral antidopaminergic: domperidone
  Gut activator: cisapride
  Antipsychotic: clozapine, quetiapine

Surgery
  Ablative surgery
    Thalamotomy
    Pallidotomy
  Restorative surgery
    embryonic dopaminergic tissue transplantation
  Deep brain stimulation
    Thalamic stimulation
    Pallidal stimulation
    Subthalamic stimulation

treatment is lifelong. Medications and their doses change with time as adverse effects and new symptoms are encountered. Tactical strategy is based on the severity of symptoms.

In Table 114.6, *carbidopa* is listed as the peripheral dopa decarboxylase inhibitor, but in many countries *benserazide* is also available. These agents potentiate the effects of levodopa, thus allowing about a fourfold reduction in dosage to obtain the same benefit. Moreover, by preventing the formation of peripheral dopamine, which can act at the area postrema (vomiting center), they block the development of nausea and vomiting. *Domperidone* is a dopamine receptor antagonist that does not enter the central nervous system, it is used to prevent nausea, not only from levodopa but also from dopamine agonists. Domperidone is not available in the United States. Of the listed dopamine agonists, only bromocriptine, pergolide, pramipexole and ropinirole are available in the United States; they are reviewed in a following section. Because it is water soluble, apomorphine is used as an injectable, in countries where available, as a rapidly acting dopaminergic to overcome "off" states. Cabergoline has the longest half-life. Catecholamine-O-methyl transferase inhibitors extend the elimination half-life of levodopa.

Amantadine, selegiline, and the anticholinergics are reviewed in following sections. Because the anticholinergics can cause forgetfulness and even psychosis, they should be used cautiously in patients most susceptible (those older than 70 years). The antihistaminics, tricyclics, and cyclobenzaprine have milder anticholinergic properties that make them useful in PD, particularly in the older patient who should not take the stronger anticholinergics.

Antidepressants are needed for treating depression. Because of its anticholinergic and soporific effects, amitriptyline can be useful for these properties as well as for its antidepressant effect. The serotonin uptake inhibitors are also effective in treating depression of PD but may aggravate parkinsonism if antiparkinsonian drugs are not given concurrently. Diazepam is usually well tolerated without worsening parkinsonism and can help to lessen tremor by reducing the reaction to stress that worsens tremor. Cisapride can help to overcome constipation, a common complaint in patients with PD or the Shy-Drager syndrome. Clozapine, a selective dopamine D4 receptor antagonist, can ameliorate levodopa-induced psychosis without worsening parkinsonism, but weekly monitoring of white blood cells is necessary to prevent irreversible agranulocytosis. The drug is discontinued if the white blood cell count declines. Quetiapine, a related drug, does not need hematologic monitoring and therefore can be tried first to overcome psychosis.

Surgery

The surgical approaches listed in Table 114.6 are not considered in the early stages of PD but are reserved for patients who have failed to respond satisfactorily to drugs. *Thalamotomy and thalamic stimulation* (target for both is the ventral intermediate nucleus) are best for contralateral intractable tremor. Tremor can be relieved in at least 70% of cases. Although a unilateral lesion carries a small risk, bilateral operations result in dysarthria in 15% to 20% of patients. Thalamic stimulation seems to be safer and can be equally effective against tremor, but it runs the risks

TABLE 114.7. FIVE MAJOR OUTCOMES AFTER MORE THAN 5 YR OF LEVODOPA THERAPY (N = 330 PATIENTS)[a]

Smooth good response, *n* = 83 (25%)
Troublesome fluctuations, *n* = 142 (43%)
Troublesome dyskinesias, *n* = 67 (19%)
Toxicity at therapeutic or subtherapeutic dosages, *n* = 14 (4%)
Total or substantial loss of efficacy, *n* = 27 (8%)

[a]Thirty-six patients had both troublesome fluctuations and troublsome dykinesias.
From Fahn, S. Adverse effects of levodopa. In: Olanow CW, Lieberman AN, eds. *The scientific basis for the treatment of Parkinson's disease.* Carnforth, England: Parthenon Publishing Group, 1992.

associated with foreign bodies and thin electronic wires that can break. *Pallidotomy* (target is the posterolateral part of the globus pallidus interna) is most effective for treating contralateral dopa-induced dystonia and chorea but also has some benefit for bradykinesia and tremor. The target in the globus pallidus interna is believed to be the site of afferent excitatory glutamatergic fibers coming from the subthalamic nucleus, which is overactive in PD. *Lesions of the subthalamic nucleus,* although effective in relieving parkinsonism in animal models, are hazardous in humans because hemichorea or hemiballism may result. Instead, *stimulation of the subthalamic nucleus* is used and appears to be the most promising in reducing contralateral bradykinesia and tremor. Subthalamic nucleus stimulation in a patient appears to reduce symptoms of PD that respond to levodopa in that patient. It is not effective against symptoms that do not respond to levdodopa. This type of surgery often allows a marked reduction of levodopa dosage, thereby reducing dopa-induced dyskinesias and treating parkinsonian symptoms. *Fetal dopaminergic tissue implants* are being investigated. This surgical procedure may reduce bradykinesia and rigidity in younger patients but is less effective in those over age 60; it is not effective against tremor. Its long-term effect is not established, but in some patients it has replaced bradykinesia with persistent dyskinesia in the absence of levodopa. Until this problem can be solved, transplantation surgery is not a useful option.

Levodopa is uniformly accepted as the most effective drug available for symptomatic relief of PD. If it were uniformly and persistently successful and also free of complications, new strategies for other treatment would not be needed. Unfortunately, 75% of patients have serious complications after 5 years of levodopa therapy (Table 114.7).

STAGES OF PARKINSON DISEASE

Early Stage

It is debated whether early use of levodopa is responsible for later response fluctuations and other complications (Table 114.7). Authorities generally agree, however, that in the early stage of PD when symptoms are noticed but not troublesome, symptomatic treatment is not necessary. All symptomatic drugs can induce side effects, and if a patient is not troubled socially or occupationally by mild symptoms, drug therapy can be delayed until symptoms become more pronounced.

The major decision is when to introduce levodopa, the most effective drug. All patients are likely to develop complications associated with long-term use. Younger patients, in particular, are more likely to show response fluctuations, so other antiparkinsonian drugs should be used first to delay the introduction of levodopa; when deemed necessary, levodopa should be administered at the lowest effective dose. This approach is known as the *dopa-sparing strategy*. On the other hand, clinicians who doubt that levodopa is responsible for these complications might choose to use levodopa first because the therapeutic response is greater. No controlled clinical trials have been carried out to determine the role played by long-term use and high dosage of levodopa, and opinions differ about retrospective studies.

Selegiline delays the need for levodopa therapy by an average of 9 months. Although some protective effect from this monoamine oxidase type B inhibitor could have been a possible explanation, the 9-month delay can be explained entirely on its persistent mild symptomatic effect. Selegiline has few adverse effects when given without levodopa, but when given concurrently with levodopa, it can increase the dopaminergic effect, allows a lower dose of levodopa, and contributes to dopaminergic toxicity. Without proof that selegiline actually slows the progression of PD, no compelling reason exists for requiring its use for patients in the early stage of PD. It should be considered one of several symptomatic drugs that can be used in the early stage of the disease to delay the introduction of levodopa; the superiority of any of these drugs to the others is not known. The antioxidant *tocopherol* (vitamin E) was tested at a dose of 2,000 U/d in mild PD as part of a controlled clinical trial and had no effect in delaying the need for levodopa.

Stage When Symptoms and Signs Require Symptomatic Treatment

Eventually, PD progresses and symptomatic treatment must be used. The most common problems that clinicians consider important in deciding to use symptomatic agents are the following: threat to employment; threat to ability to handle domestic, financial, or social affairs; threat to handle activities of daily living; and appreciable worsening of gait or balance. In clinical practice, a global judgment for initiating such therapy is made in discussions between the patient and the treating physician.

The choice now is whether to introduce levodopa or some other antiparkinsonian drug, such as amantadine, an anticholinergic, or a dopamine agonist. Levodopa is superior in relieving symptoms. Patients and clinicians who prefer a dopa-sparing strategy, however, select other agents.

Amantadine

Amantadine is a mild indirect dopaminergic agent that acts by augmenting dopamine release for storage sites and possibly blocking reuptake of dopamine into the presynaptic terminals. It also has some anticholinergic and antiglutamatergic properties. In the early stages of PD, it is effective in about two-thirds of patients. A major advantage is that benefit, if it occurs, is seen in a couple of days. The effect can be substantial. Unfortunately, its benefit in more advanced PD is often short-lived, with patients reporting a fall-off effect after several months of treatment. After

dopamine stores are depleted, the effect of amantadine is exhausted. A common adverse effect is livedo reticularis (a reddish mottling of skin) around the knees; other adverse effects are ankle edema and visual hallucinosis. Sometimes, when the drug is discontinued, a gradual worsening of parkinsonian signs may follow, thus indicating that the drug has been helpful. The usual dose is 100 mg two times per day, but sometimes a higher dose (up to 200 mg two times per day) may be required. Amantadine can be useful not only in the early phases of symptomatic therapy by forestalling use of levodopa or reducing the required dosage of levodopa but also in the advanced stages as an adjunctive drug to levodopa and the dopamine agonists. It can also reduce the severity of dopa-induced dyskinesias, probably by its antiglutamatergic mechanism of action.

Anticholinergic (Antimuscarinic) Drugs

As a general rule, anticholinergic agents are less effective antiparkinsonian agents than are the dopamine agonists. The anticholinergic drugs are estimated to improve parkinsonism by about 20%. Many clinicians find that when tremor is not relieved by an agonist or levodopa, addition of an anticholinergic drug can be effective. Because the anticholinergic agent sometimes can lessen tremor severity even without levodopa, many clinicians use such an agent as monotherapy for tremor. If not helpful, continual use of the drug can be beneficial while a dopamine agonist or levodopa is added. Later, if tremor is relieved by the dopaminergic agent, the anticholinergic drug may be discontinued.

Trihexyphenidyl is a widely used anticholinergic agent. A common starting dose is 2 mg three times per day. It can be gradually increased to 20 mg or more per day.

Adverse effects from anticholinergic drugs are common, particularly in the age range of most patients with PD. Adverse cerebral effects are predominantly forgetfulness and decreased short-term memory. Occasionally, hallucinations and psychosis occur, particularly in the elderly patient; these drugs should be avoided in patients older than 70 years. If tremor is not relieved by dopaminergic drugs and one wishes to add an anticholinergic agent to the therapy for an elderly patient, amitriptyline, diphenhydramine, orphenadrine, or cyclobenzaprine are sometimes beneficial, without the central side effects of more potent agents. Diphenhydramine and amitriptyline can cause drowsiness and can be used as a hypnotic. For tremor control, the dose is increased gradually to 50 mg three times per day. A similar dose schedule is useful for orphenadrine. Cyclobenzaprine can be increased gradually until 20 mg three times per day is reached.

Peripheral side effects are common and are often the reason for discontinuing or limiting the dosage of anticholinergic drugs. These adverse effects, however, can usually be overcome by adding pilocarpine eye drops if blurred vision occurs or if glaucoma is present. Pyridostigmine, up to 60 mg three times per day, can help to overcome dry mouth and urinary difficulties.

Dopamine Agonists

Dopamine agonists can be used as conjunctive therapy with levodopa to potentiate an antiparkinsonian effect, to reduce the dosage needed for levodopa alone, and to overcome some of the adverse effects of long-term use of levodopa or as monotherapy in the early stage of the disease to delay introduction of levodopa. It is likely that early use of dopamine agonists, by delaying the introduction of levodopa, reduces the time to develop complications from chronic levodopa therapy.

The agonists are less effective than levodopa as antiparkinsonian agents, and most patients require the addition of levodopa within a couple of years. Bromocriptine, pergolide, lisuride, and cabergoline are ergot derivatives. As such, they could induce red inflamed skin (*St. Anthony's fire*), but this side effect is rare and is reversible on discontinuing the drug. Retroperitoneal fibrosis is a more serious adverse, but also rare, event. The nonergoline agonists, pramipexole and ropinirole, often are associated with drowsiness and ankle edema. Sleep attacks, including falling asleep when driving a vehicle, are infrequent problems with these two agents, but drivers need to be cautioned about such a serious possibility.

All agonists tend to induce orthostatic hypotension, particularly when the drug is first introduced. Afterward, this complication is much less common. Therefore, the best starting regimen is a small dose at bedtime for the first 3 days (bromocriptine 1.25 mg, pergolide 0.05 mg, pramipexole 0.125 mg, ropinirole 0.25 mg) and then switch from bedtime to daytime regimens at this dose for the next few days. The daily dose can be increased gradually at weekly intervals to avoid adverse effects (bromocriptine 1.25 mg, pergolide 0.25 mg, pramipexole 0.25 mg, ropinirole 0.75 mg) until a benefit or a plateau dosage is reached (bromocriptine 5 mg three times per day, pergolide and pramipexole 0.5 mg three times per day, ropinirole 1 mg three times per day). If this plateau is not satisfactory, the dose either can be increased gradually until it is quadrupled or can be held constant while beginning carbidopa/levodopa. If the agonists alone still are not effective, carbidopa/levodopa is needed.

Besides the adverse effects listed above, there are subtle differences among the dopamine agonists. Cabergoline has the longest pharmacologic half-life and theoretically could be taken in once-a-day dosing. Pergolide acts at both the D1 and D2 dopamine receptors (Table 114.8). Bromocriptine is a partial D1 antagonist. All act at the D2 receptor, which may account for most, if not all, of their anti-PD activity. Pergolide, pramipexole, and ropinirole also act at the D3 dopamine receptor, but it is not clear what effect this has clinically. All three appear to be equally effective against PD; bromocriptine appears to have the weakest anti-PD effect. It also seems to be more likely to induce psychosis and confusion, whereas the other three agonists are more likely to induce dyskinesias. As a general rule, however, dopamine agonists are less likely than levodopa to induce dyskinesias, and they have a half-life longer than that of levodopa, thus making them useful to reduce the severity of "off" states.

Levodopa

Some clinicians prefer to begin therapy with carbidopa/levodopa for early symptomatic treatment and to add an agonist after a small dose has been reached (e.g., 25/100 mg three times per day). This approach is particularly useful if a patient already has some disability. The advantage of using levodopa at this stage in preference to a dopamine agonist is that a therapeutic response is virtually guaranteed. Nearly all patients with PD respond to lev-

TABLE 114.8. EFFECT ON RECEPTORS BY DOPAMINE AGONISTS

Agonist	D1	D2	D3	D4	D5	5HT receptor
Bromocriptine	−	+	+ +	+	+	0
Pergolide	+	+ +	+ + +	?	+	?
Pramipexole	−	+ +	+ + + +	+ +	?	?
Ropinirole	−	+ +	+ + + +	+	−	?
Cabergoline	−	+ + +	?	?	?	?
Lisuride	+	+ +	?	?	?	+

+, activates; −, inhibits; 0, no effect; ?, uncertain.

odopa and do so quickly. In contrast, only some benefit adequately from a dopamine agonist alone, and it may take months to discover this because of a slower buildup of dosage. Therefore, if a definite response is needed quickly (e.g., to remain at work or to be self-sufficient), levodopa is preferable. On the other hand, if there is no particular urgency for a rapid clinical response and if the patient has no cognitive problems and is younger than 70 years of age, then beginning with a dopamine agonist allows one to use the dopa-sparing strategy.

Stage When Symptoms and Signs Require Treatment with Levodopa

When other antiparkinsonian medications are no longer bringing about a satisfactory response, levodopa is required to reduce the severity of parkinsonism. Levodopa is the most potent anti-PD drug. In treating patients with PD, the rule of thumb is to use the lowest dosage that can bring about adequate symptom reversal, not the highest dosage that the patient can tolerate. As previously mentioned, the longer the duration of levodopa therapy and the higher the dose, the greater the likelihood motor complications will occur. After 5 years of levodopa therapy, about 75% of patients with PD have some form of troublesome complication (Table 114.7).

Most clinicians prefer to use levodopa with a peripheral dopa decarboxylase inhibitor (e.g., carbidopa) to increase therapeutic potency and to avoid gastrointestinal adverse effects. Slow-release forms of carbidopa/levodopa (Sinemet CR) and benserazide/levodopa (Madopar HBS) provide a longer half-life and a lower peak plasma level of levodopa. In the early stage of levodopa therapy, when complications have not yet developed, use of slow-release carbidopa/levodopa has little proven advantage over use of the standard preparation; it does not delay motor fluctuations. However, it may be useful to start treatment with such a sustained release preparation in elderly patients to avoid too high a brain concentration of levodopa that might induce drowsiness.

Once response fluctuations have developed, the slow-release preparation could reduce mild wearing off. Also, a bedtime dose often allows more mobility during the night. Disadvantages are a delay in the response with each dose and the possibility of an excessive response that can be prolonged, thereby resulting in sustained severe dyskinesias. For a quick response on awakening, patients often take the standard preparation as the first morning dose in addition to the slow-release form. Some patients need a combination of standard and sustained-release preparations of levodopa throughout the day to obtain a smoother response and minimize their motor complications.

The slow-release tablets of carbidopa/levodopa are available in two strengths: scored (50/200 mg, which can be broken in half) and unscored (25/100 mg). Neither should be crushed because the matrix of the tablet that delays solubilization would no longer be effective. When added to a dopamine agonist, a dose of 25/100 mg three to four times per day often suffices. When used alone, a starting dose of 25/100 mg three times per day often is necessary and can be increased as needed to 50/200 mg three or four times per day. If greater relief is required, a dopamine agonist or standard carbidopa/levodopa should be added.

It should be noted that because all of the slow-release formulation is not absorbed before the tablet reaches the large intestine, a patient needs to consume an approximately 1.4 times greater dose to reach the comparable effectiveness of a dose of standard carbidopa/levodopa.

Inadequate Response to Levodopa Treatment

As a general rule, the single most important piece of information to help the differential diagnosis of PD and other forms of parkinsonism is the response to levodopa. If the response is nil or minor, the disorder probably is not PD. An adequate response, however, does not ensure the diagnosis of PD. All presynaptic disorders (e.g., reserpine-induced, MPTP-induced, postencephalitic parkinsonism) respond to levodopa. Also, a response to levodopa occurs in the early stages of MSA (including Shy-Drager syndrome, olivopontocerebellar atrophy, and even striatonigral degeneration); only later, when striatal dopamine receptors are lost, is the response lost.

Before concluding that levodopa is without effect on a given patient, an adequate dose must be tested. Not every symptom has to respond, but bradykinesia and rigidity respond best, whereas tremor can be resistant. Therefore, if rest tremor is the only symptom, lack of improvement does not exclude the diagnosis of PD. Tremor may never respond satisfactorily, even if adjunctive antiparkinsonian drugs are also used. Before concluding that carbidopa/levodopa is ineffective, a reasonable test dose of up to 2,000 mg levodopa/d should be given. If anorexia, nausea, or vomiting prevent attainment of a therapeutic dosage, the addition of extra carbidopa (additional 25 mg four times per day) or domperidone (10 to 20 mg before each levodopa dose) is usually effective in overcoming the adverse effect. If other adverse effects (drug-induced dystonia, psychosis, confusion, sleepiness, postural hypotension) prevent attainment of an effective dose, uncertainty about the diagnosis of PD will continue. In particular, dystonia induced by low doses of levodopa suggests a diagnosis of MSA. Similarly, drug-induced psychosis suggests diffuse Lewy body disease or accompanying Alzheimer disease. Using clozapine or quetiapine may suppress psychosis and allow the use of levodopa.

COMPLICATIONS OF LONG-TERM LEVODOPA THERAPY

Response fluctuations, dyskinesias, and behavioral effects are the major problems encountered with long-term levodopa therapy (Tables 114.9 and 114.10).

TABLE 114.9. MAJOR FLUCTUATIONS AND DYSKINESIAS AS COMPLICATIONS OF LEVODOPA

Fluctuations ("offs")	Dyskinesias
Slow "wearing-off"	Peak-dose chorea and dystonia
Sudden "off"	Diphasic chorea and dystonia
Random "off"	"Off" dystonia
Yoyoing	Myoclonus
Episodic failure to respond (dose failures)	
Delayed "on"	
Weak response at end of day	
Varied response in relationship to meals	
Sudden transient freezing	

Fluctuations

When levodopa therapy is initiated, the benefit from levodopa is usually sustained, with general improvement throughout the day and no dose-timing variations; this is the long-duration benefit. Skipping a dose is usually without loss of effect, and the response is evident on arising in the morning despite the lack of medication throughout the night. The pharmacokinetics of levodopa show a short initial distribution phase with a half-life of 5 to 10 minutes, a peak plasma concentration in about 30 minutes, and an elimination phase of about 90 minutes. Brain levels follow plasma levels. This long-duration benefit of levodopa is attributed to a combination of prolonged storage of dopamine from exogenous levodopa in residual nigrostriatal nerve terminals and a prolonged postsynaptic effect on dopamine receptors.

With chronic levodopa therapy, most patients, including all patients with onset before age 40, begin to experience fluctuations. At first, fluctuations take the form of *wearing off* (also known as end-of-dose deterioration), which is defined as a return of parkinsonian symptoms in less than 4 hours after the last dose. Gradually, the duration of benefit shortens further and the "off" state becomes more profound. Eventually, and possibly related to increasing frequency of dosing, these fluctuations become more abrupt in onset and random in timing; the condition is then the "on–off" effect and cannot be related to the timing of the levodopa intake. Motor "offs" are often accompanied by changes in mood (depression, dysphoria), anxiety, thought (more bradyphrenia), and sensory symptoms (pain).

Loss of striatal storage sites of dopamine by itself is not the sole cause of this problem. Treatment with direct-acting agonists does not eliminate the fluctuations but does make the depths of the "off" state less severe. It seems that both the central effects on dopamine receptors and the peripheral pharmacokinetics of lev-

TABLE 114.10. BEHAVIORAL ADVERSE EFFECTS WITH LEVODOPA

Drowsiness	Delusions
Reverse sleep-wake cycle	Paranoia
Vivid dreams	Confusion
Benign hallucinations	Dementia
Malignant hallucinations	
Behavioral "offs"	Depression, anxiety, panic, pain, akathisia, dysphoria

odopa are involved. The dopamine receptor becomes more sensitive to levodopa in patients with fluctuations, thus affecting both the antiparkinsonian and the dyskinetic effects. Simultaneously, the duration of response is shorter.

The brief peripheral half-life of levodopa, by itself, is not likely to be responsible for fluctuations. The half-life, present from the beginning of treatment, does not change. Also, no difference exists in the pharmacokinetics in patients with early disease who show a stable response and in those with advanced disease and fluctuations.

One hypothesis is that intermittent (compared with continuous) administration of levodopa contributes to the development of motor complications. These peaks and valleys of brain dopamine levels are thought to alter the striatal dopaminoceptive medium spiny neurons, with a potentiation of glutamate receptors (of the *N*-methyl-D-aspartate subtype) on these GABAergic striatal efferents. This increased glutamatergic activity then produces the motor complications. Another potential mechanism is that dopamine can lead to the formation of free radicals by autoxidation or by enzymatic oxidation, and these oxyradicals could be the culprits attacking and altering the dopamine receptors.

Once established, motor complications are seemingly irreversible. Substituting dopamine agonists for levodopa therapy or maintaining plasma concentrations at a constant therapeutic level by chronic infusion of levodopa diminishes the severity of the complications but does not eliminate them. In research centers, jejunal infusions of levodopa, subcutaneous infusions of apomorphine, and hourly oral administration of liquefied levodopa have been used. But these methods of treatment are often not practical. Selegiline is partially effective in treating mild wearing-off problems, probably by prolonging dopamine levels at the synapse. The addition of selegiline to patients taking levodopa, however, may lead to dopaminergic toxicity, including dyskinesias, confusion, and hallucinations. Another approach is to substitute the slow-release forms of carbidopa/levodopa (Sinemet CR) for the standard form. Again, this approach is effective mainly on wearing-off problems and not on complicated "on–off" fluctuations. Furthermore, the sustained-release formulation results in less predictable plasma levels of levodopa and often increases dyskinesias. Standard carbidopa/levodopa can be given alone by shortening the interval between doses. For the more severe state of "on–off" phenomenon, a more rapid and more predictable response sometimes can be achieved by dissolving the levodopa tablet in carbonated water or ascorbic acid solution because an acidic solvent is required to dissolve levodopa and to prevent autooxidation of the drug. Liquid levodopa enters the small intestine faster, is absorbed faster, and can be used to "fine-tune" dosing. Patients with fluctuations also usually have dose failures resulting from delayed entry of the tablet into the small intestine. Liquefying levodopa can help to resolve this problem.

Direct-acting dopamine agonists, with a biologic half-life longer than that of levodopa, can be used in combination with standard or slow-release forms of levodopa. The agonists are useful for treating both wearing-off and "on–off" by reducing both the frequency and the depth of the "off" states. In yet another approach to treating "on–offs," the patients inject themselves with apomorphine subcutaneously to quickly return the "on" state.

The peripheral dopamine receptor antagonist domperidone is used to block nausea and vomiting.

Catachol-O-methyl transferased inhibitors can extend the pharmokinetic half-life of levodopa, and thereby decrease the amount of "off" time. These drugs are added to levodopa therapy, but they can also increase dyskinesias, so the dose of levodopa may need to be reduced.

Some patients report that high-protein meals tend to produce "off" states. Levodopa is absorbed from the small intestine by the transport system for large neutral amino acids and thus competes with these other amino acids for this transport. Patients with this problem may benefit from special diets that contain little protein for the first two meals of the day, followed by a high-protein meal at the end of the day when they can afford to be "off."

Dyskinesias

Dyskinesias are commonly encountered with levodopa therapy but are often mild enough to be unnoticed by the patient. Severe forms, including chorea, ballism, dystonia, or combinations of these, can be disabling. The incidence and severity increase with duration and dosage of levodopa therapy, but they may appear early in patients with severe parkinsonism. Dyskinesias are divided into the following categories according to the timing of levodopa dosing:

1. Peak-dose dyskinesias appear at the height of antiparkinsonian benefit (20 minutes to 2 hours after a dose).
2. Diphasic dyskinesias, usually affecting the legs, appear at the beginning and end of the dosing interval.
3. "Off" dystonia, which can be painful sustained cramps, appear during "off" states and may be seen at first as early-morning dystonia presenting as foot cramps; these are relieved by the next dose of levodopa.

Dyskinesias are usually seen in patients who have fluctuations, and some patients may move rapidly from severe dyskinesias to severe "offs"; this process is known as *yo-yo–ing*. These patients may have only a brief "on" state. More commonly, they have good "ons" for parts of the day but are intermittently disabled by dyskinesias or "offs." These diurnal variations are major problems; patients with this combination have a narrow therapeutic window for levodopa. The mechanisms for dyskinesias and fluctuations are not thought to be identical or even linked. For example, sensitivity to dyskinesias is not altered by chronic infusion of levodopa, whereas fluctuations are suppressed. Because dopamine agonists are much less likely to cause dyskinesias (attributed to much less activation of the D1 receptor), increased sensitivity and response of the D1 receptor by dopamine derived from levodopa is thought to play a role in the production of dyskinesias.

Treatment of peak-dose dyskinesias includes reducing the size of each dose of levodopa. If doing so results in more wearing off, the drug is given more frequently, a switch is made to the slow-release form, or a dopamine agonist or selegiline is added with the reduced dose of levodopa. Diphasic dyskinesias are more difficult to treat. Increasing the dosage of levodopa can eliminate this type of dyskinesia, but peak-dose dyskinesia usually ensues. A switch to a dopamine agonist as the major antiparkinsonian drug is more effective; low doses of levodopa are used as an adjunctive agent. The principle of treating "off dystonia" is to try to keep the patient "on" most of the time. Here again, using a dopamine agonist as the major antiparkinsonian drug, with low doses of levodopa as an adjunct, can often be effective.

Freezing

The freezing phenomenon is often listed as a type of fluctuation because of transient difficulty in initiating movement. But this phenomenon should be considered as distinct from the other types of fluctuations. "Off-freezing" must be distinguished from "on-freezing." Off-freezing, best considered a feature of parkinsonism itself, was encountered before levodopa was discovered. The treatment goal of off-freezing is to keep the patient from getting "off." On-freezing remains an enigma; it tends to be aggravated by increasing the dosage of levodopa or by adding direct-acting dopamine agonists or selegiline without reducing the dosage of levodopa. Rather, it is lessened by reducing the dosage of levodopa. Both on- and off-freezing seem to correlate with both the duration of illness and the duration of levodopa therapy.

Patients with a combination of complicated fluctuations, dyskinesias, and off-freezing may respond to subthalamic nucleus stimulation.

MENTAL AND BEHAVIORAL CHANGES

The adverse effects of confusion, agitation, hallucinosis, hallucinations, delusions, depression, and mania are probably related to activation of dopamine receptors in nonstriatal regions, particularly cortical and limbic structures. Elderly patients and those with diffuse Lewy body disease or concomitant Alzheimer disease are sensitive to small doses of levodopa. But all patients with PD, regardless of age, can develop psychosis if they take excessive amounts of levodopa to overcome "off" periods. Psychosis can often be treated without worsening parkinsonism by adding quetiapine or clozapine, antipsychotic agents that block the dopamine D4 and serotonin receptors. These drugs easily induce drowsiness, and they should be given at bedtime, starting with a dose of 12.5 mg. The dose can be gradually increased if necessary. If quetapine is not effective, use clozapine instead. Because clozapine induces agranulocytosis in 1% to 2% of patients, patients must have blood counts monitored weekly, and the drug must be discontinued if leukopenia develops. If clozapine is not tolerated, other drugs, including small doses of olanzapine, molindone, pimozide, or other relatively weak antipsychotic drugs, can be used. If the antipsychotic drugs increase the parkinsonism, lowering the dosage of levodopa to avoid the psychosis is preferable to maintaining the antipsychotic agent at high dosage. Levodopa cannot be discontinued suddenly because the abrupt cessation may induce the neuroleptic malignant syndrome.

COURSE

The degenerative forms of parkinsonism, including PD, worsen with time. Before the introduction of levodopa, PD caused se-

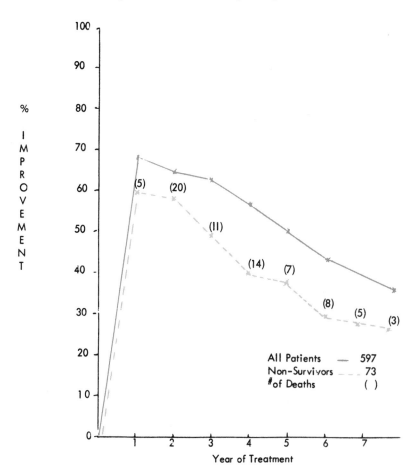

FIG. 114.3. Degree of improvement of Parkinson signs during each year of treatment with levodopa. Nonsurviving patients are compared with the total group treated.

vere disability or death in 25% of patients within 5 years of onset, in 65% in the next 5 years, and in 89% in those surviving 15 years. The mortality rate from PD was three times that of the general population matched for age, sex, and racial origin. Although no evidence indicates that levodopa alters the underlying pathologic process or stems the progressive nature of the disease, indications exist of a major impact on survival time and functional capacity. The mortality rate has dropped 50%, and longevity is extended by several years.

The hemiparkinsonism-hemiatrophy syndrome progresses more slowly and may never cause the severe disability seen with PD. In these patients, fluorodeoxyglucose PET studies reveal hypometabolism in the contralateral striatum and frontal cerebral cortex. Another relatively benign form of parkinsonism is adult-onset dopa-responsive dystonia (see Chapter 112). In that disorder, features of PD appear, but the patients continue to respond to low-dosage levodopa treatment and never develop the complications encountered so frequently with PD.

A debated point in the treatment of PD is the cause of declining efficacy from continuing treatment with levodopa seen in many patients (Fig. 114.3). End-stage PD is denoted when the response to levodopa is inadequate to allow patient-assisted activities of daily living. Progression of the illness with further loss of dopamine storage sites in the presynaptic terminals cannot be the explanation for this outcome because loss of these structures in postencephalitic parkinsonism results in greater, not lower, sensitivity to levodopa. Perhaps as PD progresses it is associated with loss of striatal dopamine receptors and loss of the presynaptic dopaminergic neuron.

SUGGESTED READINGS

Bergman H, Wichmann T, DeLong MR. Reversal of experimental parkinsonism by lesions of the subthalamic nucleus. *Science* 1990;249:1436–1438.

Chase TN. The significance of continuous dopaminergic stimulation in the treatment of Parkinson's disease. *Drugs* 1998;55:1–9.

Dooneief G, Chen J, Mirabello E, et al. An estimate of the incidence of depression in idiopathic Parkinson's disease. *Arch Neurol* 1992;49:305–307.

Dwork AJ, Balmaceda C, Fazzini EA, et al. Dominantly inherited, early-onset parkinsonism: neuropathology of a new form. *Neurology* 1993;43:69–74.

Eidelberg D, Takikawa S, Moeller JR, et al. Striatal hypometabolism distinguishes striatonigral degeneration from Parkinson's disease. *Ann Neurol* 1993;33:518–527.

Elble RJ, Hughes L, Higgins C. The syndrome of senile gait. *J Neurol* 1992;239:71–75.

Fahn S. Adverse effects of levodopa. In: Olanow CW, Lieberman AN, eds. *The scientific basis for the treatment of Parkinson's disease.* Carnforth, England: Parthenon Publishing Group, 1992.

Fahn S, Cohen G. The oxidant stress hypothesis in Parkinson's disease: evidence supporting it. *Ann Neurol* 1992;32:804–812.

FitzGerald PM, Jankovic J. Lower body parkinsonism: Evidence for vascular etiology. *Mov Disord* 1989;4:249–260.

Friedman J, Lannon M, Comella C, et al. Low-dose clozapine for the treatment of drug-induced psychosis in Parkinson's disease. *N Engl J Med* 1999;340:757–763.

Friedman JH, Feinberg SS, Feldman RG. A neuroleptic malignant-like syndrome due to levodopa therapy withdrawal. *JAMA* 1985;254:2792–2795.

Gibb WRG, Luthert PJ, Janota I, Lantos PL. Cortical Lewy body dementia: clinical features and classification. *J Neurol Neurosurg Psychiatry* 1989;52:185–192.

Gibb WRG, Luthert PJ, Marsden CD. Corticobasal degeneration. *Brain* 1989;112:1171–1192.

Giladi N, Burke RE, Kostic V, et al. Hemiparkinsonism-hemiatrophy syndrome: clinical and neuroradiological features. *Neurology* 1990;40:1731–1734.

Giladi N, McMahon D, Przedborski S, et al. Motor blocks in Parkinson's disease. *Neurology* 1992;42:333–339.

Hughes AJ, Daniel SE, Kilford L, Lees AJ. Accuracy of clinical diagnosis of idiopathic Parkinson's disease—a clinicopathological study of 100 cases. *J Neurol Neurosurg Psychiatry* 1992;55:181–184.

Jenner P, Schapira AHV, Marsden CD. New insights into the cause of Parkinson's disease. *Neurology* 1992;42:2241–2250.

Kitada T, Asakawa S, Hattori N, et al. Mutations in the parkin gene cause autosomal recessive juvenile parkinsonism. *Nature* 1998;392:605–608.

Laitinen LV, Bergenheim AT, Hariz MI. Leksell's posteroventral pallidotomy in the treatment of Parkinson's disease. *J Neurosurg* 1992;76:53–61.

Limousin P, Krack P, Pollak P, et al. Electrical stimulation of the subthalamic nucleus in advanced Parkinson's disease. *N Engl J Med* 1998;339:1105–1111.

Mayeux R, Denaro J, Hemenegildo N, et al. A population-based investigation of Parkinson's disease with and without dementia: relationship to age and gender. *Arch Neurol* 1992;49:492–497.

Metman LV, Deldotto P, van den Munckhof P, Fang J, Mouradian MM, Chase TN. Amantadine as treatment for dyskinesias and motor fluctuations in Parkinson's disease. *Neurology* 1998;50:1323–1326.

Metman LV, Locatelli ER, Bravi D, Mouradian MM, Chase TN. Apomorphine responses in Parkinson's disease and the pathogenesis of motor complications. *Neurology* 1997;48:369–372.

Polymeropoulos MH, Lavedan C, Leroy E, et al. Mutation in the alpha-synuclein gene identified in families with Parkinson's disease. *Science* 1997;276:2045–2047.

Przedborski S, Giladi N, Takikawa S, et al. The metabolic topography of the hemiparkinsonism-hemiatrophy syndrome. *Neurology* 1994;44:1622–1628.

Przedborski S, Jackson-Lewis V. Mechanisms of MPTP toxicity. *Mov Disord* 1998;13[Suppl 1]:35–38.

Quinn N. Multiple system atrophy—the nature of the beast. *J Neurol Neurosurg Psychiatry* 1989;[Suppl]:78–89.

Rajput AH, Rozdilsky B, Rajput A. Accuracy of clinical diagnosis in parkinsonism—a prospective study. *Can J Neurol Sci* 1991;18:275–278.

Tanner CM, Goldman SM. Epidemiology of Parkinson's disease. *Neuroepidemiology* 1996;14:317–335.

Tanner CM, Ottman R, Goldman SM, et al. Parkinson disease in twins: An etiologic study. *JAMA* 1999;281:341–346.

Wooten GF, Currie LJ, Bennett JP, Harrison MB, Trugman JM, Parker WD. Maternal inheritance in Parkinson's disease. *Ann Neurol* 1997;41:265–268.

Merritt's Neurology, 10th ed., edited by L.P. Rowland. Lippincott Williams & Wilkins, Philadelphia © 2000.

PROGRESSIVE SUPRANUCLEAR PALSY

PAUL E. GREENE

Olszewski, Steele, and Richardson reviewed autopsies of patients who had a syndrome of pseudobulbar palsy, supranuclear ocular palsy (chiefly affecting vertical gaze), extrapyramidal rigidity, gait ataxia, and dementia. They found a consistent pattern of neuronal degeneration and neurofibrillary tangles, chiefly affecting the pons and midbrain. This condition became known as *progressive supranuclear palsy* (PSP), or Steele-Richardson-Olszewski syndrome.

PATHOLOGY

Atrophy of the dorsal midbrain, globus pallidus, and subthalamic nucleus; depigmentation of the substantia nigra; and mild dilatation of the third and fourth ventricles and aqueduct are seen on gross visual inspection of the postmortem brain in typical PSP. Light microscopy shows neuronal loss with gliosis, numerous neurofibrillary tangles (NFTs), and neuropil threads in many subcortical structures, including the subthalamic nucleus, pallidum, substantia nigra, locus ceruleus, periaqueductal gray matter, superior colliculi, nucleus basalis, and vestibular, red, and oculomotor nuclei. Less severe neuronal loss, gliosis, and deposition of NFTs are usually found in the cerebral cortex, especially the prefrontal and precentral cortices.

The NFTs are argyrophilic and appear as skeins of fine fibrils, globose in shape in the brainstem and coil-shaped in the cortex. Ultrastructurally, they are composed of short straight 12- to 15-nm tubules arranged in circling and interlacing bundles. They react with antisera to several antigens on neurofilaments and the neurotubule-associated protein tau; the pattern of immunoreactivity differs from that of NFTs in Alzheimer disease (AD). The histologic features in typical PSP are similar to those found in postencephalitic (von Economo) parkinsonism and Guamanian amyotrophic lateral sclerosis–Parkinson–dementia syndrome (Lytico-Bodig). New histologic techniques have demonstrated overlap in pathology between some cases of clinicaly diagnosed PSP and AD, corticobasal ganglionic degeneration, and Parkinson disease (PD). The significance of this overlap is not known.

SYMPTOMS AND SIGNS

Patients with PSP have an akinetic rigid parkinson-like syndrome; rest tremor is uncommon. Balance difficulty and falling are early symptoms. Unlike PD, axial rigidity exceeds limb rigidity, and the posture may be erect. Patients have marked facial dystonia with deep nasolabial folds and furrowed brow, an appearance of surprise or concern (Fig. 115.1). When the patient walks, the neck may be extended; the arms are abducted at the shoulders and flexed at the elbows. Dysphagia and dysarthria are usually severe. The voice is slurred and hoarse, and some patients become anarthric as the disease progresses. "Freezing" may be prominent; transient arrest of motor activity interrupts walking, speaking, or other actions.

The first visual symptoms are failure to maintain eye contact in social interactions and difficulty with tasks requiring downgaze, such as reading, eating, or descending stairs. The patients often complain of diplopia, blurred vision, or difficulty reading. Disturbances of eyelid motility are common, including blepharospasm and apraxia of eyelid opening or closing.

The cognitive impairment of PSP has been considered the archetype of *subcortical dementia.* The striking features are severe bradyphrenia, impaired verbal fluency, and difficulty with sequential actions or shifting from one task to another. Cognitive tests that depend on visual performance are especially affected. Dementia is less severe than might be suggested by the dysarthria, bradyphrenia, poor eye contact, and loss of facial expression. Emotional incontinence is dominated by inappropriate weeping or, less frequently, laughing.

The course is aggressive; at 3 to 4 years after onset, patients cannot walk without assistance, and a median of 5 years after onset they are confined to bed and chair. They succumb to infection (from aspiration or pressure ulcers) or the sequelae of falls. The course is one of inexorable deterioration, culminating in death in 6 to 10 years.

LABORATORY DATA

Routine laboratory investigations are normal. The electroencephalogram may show some slowing and disorganization without localizing features. Atrophy of the pons, midbrain, and anterior temporal lobes may be noted on computed tomography or magnetic resonance imaging. Positron-emission tomography (PET) with [^{18}F]fluoro-l-dopa shows equal loss of uptake in caudate and putamen; PET using [^{18}F]fluorodeoxyglucose shows global reduction in metabolism, most severe in the frontal lobes. Neither of these PET findings is specific for PSP. Cerebrospinal fluid is unremarkable.

DIAGNOSIS

Levodopa-unresponsive parkinsonism with abnormal gait, loss of postural reflexes, and supranuclear ophthalmoplegia suggest the diagnosis of PSP. Clinical criteria for possible, probable, and definite PSP have been proposed by the National Institute of Neurological Disorders and Stroke (Table 115.1). These criteria are specific but will exclude some patients with PSP who are mild or have unusual clinical features. The chief differential diagnoses are PD, corticobasal ganglionic degeneration, cerebral multiinfarct disease, and diffuse Lewy body disease. Differentiation from olivopontocerebellar atrophy (OPCA) with ophthalmoplegia may also be difficult; but the ocular palsy in OPCA prefer-

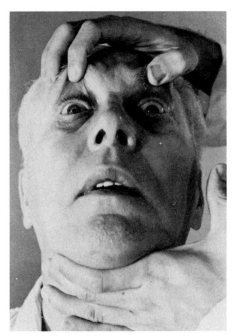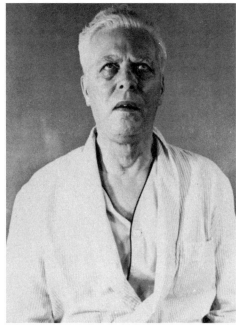

FIG. 115.1. Progressive supranuclear palsy. Oculocephalic maneuver demonstrates intact reflex downgaze in a patient unable to look down voluntarily.

TABLE 115.1. DIAGNOSTIC CRITERIA FOR PROGRESSIVE SUPRANUCLEAR PALSY (PSP)

Possible PSP

Gradually progressive parkinsonism

Onset after age 40 yr

Vertical supranuclear palsy or slow vertical saccades with early falling

Absence of each of these: history of encephalitis; focal cortical deficits (e.g., alien limb syndrome, cortical sensory deficits, focal cortical myoclonus); cortical dementia of the Alzheimer type; prominent, early cerebellar symptoms; unexplained dysautonomia (e.g., hypotension, urinary disturbances); severe, asymmetric parkinsonian signs; neuroradiologic evidence of relevant structural abnormality (e.g., lobar atrophy, basal ganglia or brainstem infarcts); evidence of Whipple disease (confirmed by polymerase chain reaction, if indicated)

Probable PSP

Possible PSP, but vertical supranuclear palsy is mandatory

Definite PSP

Possible PSP, or *probable PSP* and histopathologic evidence of typical PSP

Supportive criteria

Symmetric akinesia or rigidity, proximal more than distal

Abnormal neck posture, especially retrocollis

Poor or absent response of parkinsonian symptoms to levodopa therapy

Early dysphagia and dysarthria

Early onset of cognitive impairment, including at least two of the following:

Apathy

Impairment in abstract thought

Decreased verbal fluency utilization or imitation behavior

Frontal release signs

(Modified from Litvan et al., 1996.)

entially affects horizontal movements. In the absence of the characteristic ocular palsy, diagnosis is difficult.

Examination of ocular and eyelid motility is crucial to the clinical diagnosis of PSP. Eyelid opening and closing apraxias are far more common in PSP than in any other extrapyramidal disorder. Fixation instability with coarse square wave jerks and faulty suppression of the vestibuloocular reflex are helpful features. Hesitation on voluntary downgaze is one of the earliest signs. Loss of vertical optokinetic nystagmus on downward movement of the target confirms that finding. The demonstration of greater impairment of voluntary than of pursuit movements and of preservation of reflex ocular movements supports the diagnosis. Similar abnormalities, however, are occasionally seen in corticobasal ganglionic degeneration, cerebral multiinfarct disease, and diffuse Lewy body disease.

TREATMENT

The etiology of PSP is unknown, and there is no specific treatment. Levodopa/carbidopa and other antiparkinson medications are usually ineffective, although they are rarely helpful in alleviating the parkinsonian features of rigidity and bradykinesia. When they are helpful, benefit is short-lived or limited by toxic psychic effects, which tend to become prominent when dementia develops. Tricyclic antidepressants may suppress inappropriate crying or laughing. Anticholinergic drugs administered in modest doses may be useful in controlling drooling. Apraxia of eyelid opening and painful neck or limb dystonia may improve with botulinum toxin injections. Some patients and families choose to use an enteric feeding tube when dysphagia becomes severe.

SUGGESTED READINGS

Brooks DJ. PET studies in progressive supranuclear palsy. In: Tolosa E, Duvoisin R, Cruz-Sánchez, eds. *Progressive supranuclear palsy: diagnosis, pathology, and therapy.* New York: Springer-Verlag/Wien, 1994:119–134.

Chin SS, Goldman JE. Glial inclusions in CNS degenerative diseases. *J Neuropathol Exp Neurol* 1996;55:499–508.

Golbe LI, Davis PH, Schoenberg BS, Duvoisin RC. Prevalence and natural history of progressive supranuclear palsy. *Neurology* 1988;38:1031–1034.

Litvan I. Progressive supranuclear palsy revised. *Acta Neurol Scand* 1998;98:73–84.

Litvan I, Agid Y, eds. *Progressive supranuclear palsy: clinical and research approaches.* New York: Oxford University Press, 1992.

Litvan I, Agid Y, Calne D, et al. Clinical research criteria for the diagnosis of progressive supranuclear palsy (Steele-Richardson-Olszewski syndrome). *Neurology* 1996;47:1–9.

Litvan I, Campbell G, Mangone CA, et al. Which clinical features differentiate progressive supranuclear palsy (Steele-Richardson-Olszewski syndrome) from related disorders? *Brain* 1997;120:65–74.

Pierrot-Deseilligny C, Gaymard B, et al. Cerebral ocular motor signs. *J Neurol* 1997;244:65–70.

Pillon B, Dubois B, Ploska A, et al. Severity and specificity of cognitive impairment in Alzheimer's, Huntington's, Parkinson's diseases and progressive supranuclear palsy. *Neurology* 1991;41:634–643.

Riley DE, Fogt N, Leigh RJ. The syndrome of "pure akinesia" and its relationship to progressive supranuclear palsy. *Neurology* 1994;44:1025–1029.

Steele JC, Richardson JC, Olszewski J. Progressive supranuclear palsy: a heterogenous degeneration involving the brain stem, basal ganglia and cerebellum with vertical gaze and pseudobulbar palsy, nuchal dystonia and dementia. *Arch Neurol* 1964;10:333–359.

Tanner CM, Goetz CG, Klawans HL. Multiinfarct PSP. *Neurology* 1987;37:1819–1820.

Tetrud JW, Golbe LI, Forno LS, et al. Autopsy-proven progressive supranuclear palsy in two siblings. *Neurology* 1996;46:931–934.

Troost BT, Daroff RB. The ocular motor defects in progressive supranuclear palsy. *Ann Neurol* 1977;2:397–403.

Merritt's Neurology, 10th ed., edited by L.P. Rowland. Lippincott Williams & Wilkins, Philadelphia © 2000.

C H A P T E R
116

TARDIVE DYSKINESIA AND OTHER NEUROLEPTIC-INDUCED SYNDROMES

STANLEY FAHN
ROBERT E. BURKE

The most widely used drugs that block dopamine D2 receptors are the antipsychotic agents, such as the phenothiazines and the butyrophenones; others include metoclopramide, flunarizine hydrochloride (Sibelium), and cinnarizine. These D2 receptor–blocking agents can cause the following various adverse neurologic effects:

Acute dystonic reaction
Oculogyric crisis
Acute akathisia
Drug-induced parkinsonism
Neuroleptic malignant syndrome
Withdrawal emergent syndrome
Persistent dyskinesias (tardive dyskinesia syndromes)
    Classic orobuccolingual dyskinesia
    Tardive dystonia
    Tardive akathisia
    Tardive tics
    Tardive myoclonus
    Tardive tremor

The "atypical" neuroleptic clozapine (Clozaril), a drug that predominantly blocks the D4 receptor, is free of these complications, except for acute akathisia. The related drug quetiapine appears to be similar in being relatively free from the above list of adverse effects. Other drugs, also commonly called "atypical" neuroleptics, such as olanzapine (Zyprexa) and risperidone (Risperdal) are more readily able to induce the above adverse effects. The dopamine-depleting drugs reserpine and tetrabenazine can induce acute akathisia and drug-induced parkinsonism but have never been convincingly implicated in causing the other complications listed, other than acute dystonic reactions from tetrabenazine.

Acute dystonic reactions tend to occur within the first few days of exposure to the dopamine-receptor blocker and predominantly affect children and young adults, and males more than females. Severe twisting and uncomfortable postures of limbs, trunk, neck, tongue, and face are dramatic. *Oculogyric crisis* is a form of dystonia in which the eyes are deviated conjugately in a fixed posture for minutes or hours. Dystonic reactions are easily reversible with parenteral administration of antihistamines (e.g., diphenhydramine, 50 mg intravenously), anticholinergic drugs (e.g., benztropine mesylate [Cogentin], 2 mg intramuscularly), or diazepam (5 to 7.5 mg intramuscularly).

Acute akathisia occurs within the first few months of drug use; it may appear as the dosage is being increased. Akathisia consists of a *subjective* sense of restlessness or aversion to being still. The *motor* features of restlessness include frequent and repetitive stereotyped movements, such as pacing, repeatedly caressing the scalp, or crossing and uncrossing the legs. It can occur in subjects of any age. The beta-adrenergic blocker propranolol may be helpful in doses of 20 to 80 mg per day. Anticholinergic agents occasionally help. Acute akathisia disappears on discontinuance of the offending drug.

Drug-induced parkinsonism resembles idiopathic parkinsonism in manifesting all the cardinal signs of the syndrome. Levodopa is not effective in reversing this complication, probably because the dopamine receptors are blocked and occupied by the antipsychotic agent. Oral anticholinergic drugs and amantadine are effective. Upon withdrawal of the offending antipsychotic drug, the symptoms slowly disappear in weeks or months.

The *neuroleptic malignant syndrome* is characterized by a triad of fever, signs of autonomic dysfunction (e.g., pallor, diaphoresis, blood pressure instability, tachycardia, pulmonary congestion, tachypnea), and a movement disorder (e.g., akinesia, rigidity, or dystonia). The level of consciousness may be depressed, eventually leading to stupor or coma; death may occur. Withdrawal of antipsychotic medication and supportive therapy, including intravenous hydration and cooling, are recommended. Although controlled trials have not been conducted, numerous reports suggest that dantrolene sodium (Dantrium), a muscle relaxant, or bromocriptine mesylate (Parlodel), a direct-acting dopamine agonist, may be beneficial. Carbamazepine (Tegretol) has also been found effective. In most patients, the antipsychotic medication can be restarted later without recurrence of the syndrome.

The *withdrawal emergent syndrome* may be a variant of tardive dyskinesia. "Emergent" implies that the symptoms emerge after abrupt cessation of the chronic use of an antipsychotic drug. The syndrome is primarily one of children. The choreic movements resemble those of Sydenham chorea because the movements are flowing rather than repetitive, as occurs in classic tardive dyskinesia. The withdrawal emergent syndrome is self-limiting but may take weeks to resolve. Reintroducing the antipsychotic drug and then slowly tapering the dosage can eliminate the choreic movements.

The *persistent dyskinesia syndromes* are the most feared complications of antipsychotic medications because the symptoms are long-lasting and often permanent. *Classic tardive dyskinesia* consists of repetitive (stereotypic) rapid movements. The lower part of the face is most often involved; this orobuccolingual dyskinesia resembles continual chewing movements, with the tongue intermittently darting out of the mouth ("fly-catcher" tongue). Movements of the trunk may cause a repetitive pattern of flexion and extension (body-rocking). The distal parts of the limbs may show incessant flexion-extension movements ("piano-playing" fingers and toes). The proximal muscles are usually spared, but respiratory dyskinesias are not uncommon. When the patient stands, there may be repetitive movements of the legs ("marching-in-place"). Occasionally, the gait is short-stepped, possibly because of an associated drug-induced parkinsonism. More often, the arms tend to swing more than normal, and the stride may be lengthened. The patient may not be aware of the dyskinesia.

The prevalence of classic tardive dyskinesia increases with age; it is more severe among elderly women and more likely to occur with longer duration of exposure to antipsychotic drugs. The time of onset is difficult to discern because these drugs mask the movements. Reducing the dosage or discontinuing the offending drug can unmask the disorder, and reinstituting the drug can suppress the movements.

Not all cases of *oral dyskinesia* are classic tardive dyskinesia. There are many other choreic and nonchoreic causes. Essential to the diagnosis of tardive dyskinesia is a history of exposure to dopamine D2 receptor–blocking drugs. For this diagnosis, the symptoms should have started while the patient was still taking the drug or less than 3 months after discontinuing the drug. If oral dyskinesia is induced by other types of drugs, it is not, by definition, tardive dyskinesia. The following list outlines the classification of movement disorders affecting the face:

Chorea and stereotypes
 Encephalitis lethargica; postencephalitic
 Drug-induced
  Tardive dyskinesia (antipsychotics)
  Levodopa
  Anticholinergic drugs
  Phenytoin intoxication
  Antihistamines
  Tricyclic antidepressants
 Huntington disease
 Hepatocerebral degeneration
 Cerebellar and brainstem infarction
 Edentulous malocclusion
 Idiopathic
Dystonia
 Meige syndrome
  Complete: oromandibular dystonia plus blepharospasm
  Incomplete syndromes
   Mandibular dystonia
   Orofacial dystonia
   Lingual dystonia
   Pharyngeal dystonia
   Essential blepharospasm
 Bruxism
 As part of a segmental or generalized dystonic syndrome
Myoclonus and tics
 Facial tics
 Facial myoclonus of central origin
 Facial nerve irritability
  Hemifacial spasm
  Myokymia
  Faulty regeneration; synkinesis
Tremor
 Essential tremor of neck and jaw
 Parkinsonian tremor of jaw, tongue, and lips
 Idiopathic tremor of neck, jaw, tongue, or lips
 Cerebellar tremor of neck

Huntington disease and oromandibular dystonia are the major differential diagnoses of the oral dyskinesias. Oromandibular dystonia is probably the most common form of spontaneous oral dyskinesia. Clinical features differentiating these disorders from classic tardive dyskinesia are presented in Table 116.1. Patients with Huntington disease are frequently treated with antipsychotic drugs; a resulting tardive dyskinesia may be superimposed on the chorea. The presence of akathisia or repetitive (stereotyped) involuntary movements suggests the additional diagnosis of tardive dyskinesia. Often, oromandibular dystonia takes the appearance of a repetitive opening and closing of the jaw as the patient attempts to overcome the muscle pulling. By asking the patient not to fight the involuntary movement but to let it "do what it wants to do," one can usually discern whether the oral dystonia is of the jaw-closing or jaw-opening form.

Several important forms of tardive dyskinesia syndrome are now recognized. Unlike classic oral dyskinesia, these forms are

TABLE 116.1. CLINICAL FEATURES OF CLASSIC TARDIVE DYSKINESIA (TD), OROMANDIBULAR DYSTONIA (OMD), AND HUNTINGTON DISEASE (HD)

Clinical signs	TD	OMD	HD
Type of involuntary movements	Stereotypic	Dystonic	Choreic
Flowing movements	0	0	+++
Repetitive movements	+++	+	±
Sustained contractions	+	+++	±
Movements of mouth	+++	+++	+
Blepharospasm	+	+++	+
Forehead chorea	±	±	++
Platysma	±	+++	±
Masticatory muscles	+++	+++	±
Nuchal muscles	+	++	±
Trunk, legs	++	0	+++
Akathisia	++	0	0
Marching in place	++	0	0
Truncal rocking	++	0	+
Motor impersistence (tongue, grip)	0	0	+++
Stuttering, ataxic gait	±	0	+++
Postural instability	0	0	+++
Effect of			
Antidopaminergics	Decrease	Decrease	Decrease
Anticholinergics	Increase	Decrease	±
Effect on			
Talking, chewing	±	+++	+
Swallowing	0	++	+++

0, not seen; ±; may be seen; +, occasionally seen; ++, usually seen; +++, almost always seen.

frequently quite disabling. *Tardive dystonia* is a chronic dystonia resulting from exposure to dopamine D2 receptor blockers. Individuals of all ages are susceptible to tardive dystonia, and younger individuals are more likely to have a more severe generalized form. Tardive dystonia usually begins in the face or neck, and may remain confined to these regions or may spread to the arms and trunk. The legs are infrequently affected. Often, neck involvement consists of retrocollis, and the trunk arches backward. The arms are typically rotated internally, the elbows extended, and the wrists flexed. The differential diagnosis includes all the many causes of dystonia. Wilson disease, in particular, must be excluded specifically in any patient with psychiatric symptoms and dystonia.

Tardive akathisia is another important disabling variant of tardive dyskinesia. It is a chronic akathisia consisting of a subjective aversion to being still. Motor signs of restlessness include frequent, repeated, stereotyped movements, such as marching in place, crossing and uncrossing the legs, and repetitively rubbing the face or hair with the hand. Patients may not use the word "restless" to describe their symptoms; instead they may use expressions such as "going to jump out of my skin" or "jittery" or "exploding inside." Akathisia can appear as focal discomfort, such as pain, or as moaning sounds. It can be a distressing symptom. In contrast to acute akathisia, the delayed type tends to become worse when antipsychotic medication is withdrawn, similar to the worsening of classic tardive dyskinesia on discontinuance of these drugs. As with other types of tardive dyskinesia syndrome, tardive akathisia tends to persist. Usually, tardive akathisia is associated with classic oral dyskinesia. Classic tardive dyskinesia, tardive dystonia, and tardive akathisia may occur together. Less common variants of tardive dyskinesia include *tardive tics, tardive myoclonus,* and *tardive tremor.*

Efforts should be made to avoid the tardive dyskinesia syndromes. Antipsychotic drugs should be given only when indicated, namely, to control psychosis or a few other conditions where no other effective agent has been helpful, as in some choreic disorders or tics. These drugs should not be used indiscriminately, and when they are used, the dosage and duration should be as low and as brief as possible. If the psychosis has been controlled, the physician should attempt to reduce the dosage and even try to eliminate the drug, if possible. Once a tardive dyskinesia syndrome has appeared, treatment depends on eliminating the causative agents, the dopamine D2 receptor–blocking drugs. Unfortunately, psychosis may no longer be under control if these drugs are withdrawn; if the medication is required, increasing the dosage or adding reserpine may suppress the dyskinesia and akathisia. If the antipsychotic drug can be tapered and discontinued safely, the dyskinesia and akathisia may slowly subside in months or years. If the dyskinetic or akathitic symptoms are too distressful, treatment with dopamine-depleting drugs, such as reserpine, may suppress them. The dosage of reserpine should be increased gradually to avoid the side effects of postural hypotension and depression. A dosage of 6 mg per day or more may be required. Addition of alpha-methyltyrosine may be necessary to relieve symptoms, but this combination is more likely to cause postural hypotension and parkinsonism. With time, these dopamine-depleting drugs may eventually be tapered and discontinued. Tardive dystonia may be treated by dopamine depletion, but unlike oral tardive dyskinesia and akathisia, it may be treated with anticholinergic drugs. Clozapine may be helpful in some patients with tardive dystonia.

The pathogenesis of the tardive dyskinesia syndromes is unknown. No one hypothesis is able to explain the disorder, and more than one factor may be necessary. These factors include the development of dopamine-receptor supersensitivity, activation of dopamine D1 receptors, and loss of τ-aminobutyric acid activity in the subthalamic nucleus.

SUGGESTED READINGS

Andersson U, Haggstrom JE, Levin ED, et al. Reduced glutamate decarboxylase activity in the subthalamic nucleus in patients with tardive dyskinesia. *Mov Disord* 1989;4:37–46.

Burke RE, Kang UK, Jankovic J, et al. Tardive akathisia: an analysis of clinical features and response to open therapeutic trials. *Mov Disord* 1989;4:157–175.

Fahn S. A therapeutic approach to tardive dyskinesia. *J Clin Psychiatry* 1985;46:19–24.

Ford B, Greene P, Fahn S. Oral and genital tardive pain syndromes. *Neurology* 1994;44:2115–2119.

Friedman J, Feinberg SS, Feldman RG. A neuroleptic malignant-like syndrome due to l-dopa withdrawal. *Ann Neurol* 1984;16:126–127.

Henderson VW, Wooten GF. Neuroleptic malignant syndrome: a pathogenetic role for dopamine receptor blockade? *Neurology* 1981;31:132–137.

Kane JM, Woerner M, Borenstein M, et al. Integrating incidence and prevalence of tardive dyskinesia. *Psychopharmacol Bull* 1986;22:254–258.

Kang UJ, Burke RE, Fahn S. Natural history and treatment of tardive dystonia. *Mov Disord* 1986;1:193–208.

Kiriakakis V, Bhatia KP, Quinn NP, Marsden CD. The natural history of tardive dystonia: a long-term follow-up study of 107 cases. *Brain* 1998;121:2053–2066.

Paulsen JS, Caligiuri MP, Palmer B, McAdams LA, Jeste DV. Risk factors for orofacial and limb-truncal tardive dyskinesia in older patients: a prospective longitudinal study. *Psychopharmacology* 1996;123:307–314.

Seeman P, Tallerico T. Antipsychotic drugs which elicit little or no parkinsonism bind more loosely than dopamine to brain D2 receptors, yet occupy high levels of these receptors. *Mol Psychiatry* 1998;3:123–134.

Smith JM, Baldessarini RJ. Changes in prevalence, severity and recovery in tardive dyskinesia with age. *Arch Gen Psychiatry* 1980;37:1368–1373.

Thomas P, Maron M, Rascle C, Cottencin O, Vaiva G, Goudemand M. Carbamazepine in the treatment of neuroleptic malignant syndrome. *Biol Psychiatry* 1998;43:303–305.

Van Harten PN, Kamphuis DJ, Matroos GE. Use of clozapine in tardive dystonia. *Prog Neuropsychopharmacol Biol Psychiatry* 1996;20:263–274.

Merritt's Neurology, 10th ed., edited by L.P. Rowland. Lippincott Williams & Wilkins, Philadelphia © 2000.

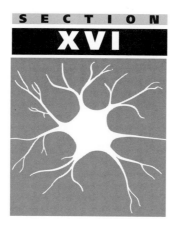

SPINAL CORD DISEASES

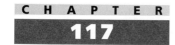

HEREDITARY AND ACQUIRED SPASTIC PARAPLEGIA

LEWIS P. ROWLAND

Several different diseases are evident solely or primarily by spastic gait disorder (spastic paraparesis), which may progress to spastic paralysis of the legs (paraplegia). Autopsy usually reveals degeneration of the corticospinal tracts with or without involvement of other motor, sensory, or cerebellar systems. Among both heritable and acquired diseases, there is heterogeneity of pathogenesis.

HEREDITARY SPASTIC PARAPLEGIA

Harding (1993) divided hereditary spastic paraplegia (HSP) syndromes into pure and complicated types, depending on the clinical manifestations. The complications include epilepsy, dementia, parkinsonism, ataxia, amyotrophy, peripheral neuropathy, and blindness or deafness. One multisystem syndrome gained the acronym CRASH (corpus callosum hypoplasia, retardation, adducted thumbs, spasticity, hydrocephalus). Even in pure HSP, sensory evoked responses may be abnormal, and the spinocerebellar tracts were affected at autopsy in Strumpell's original description in 1890.

Genetics

The syndrome is genetically heterogeneous; most families show autosomal-dominant inheritance, but some are autosomal-recessive and others are X-linked (Table 117.1). Locus heterogeneity is evident because some X-linked forms map to chromosome Xq28, others to Xq22. Some autosomal-dominant families map to 14q, 15q, or 2p, and others are unlinked (Table 117.2). Families mapped to 16q24.3 have homozygous mutations in the gene for *paraplegin*, a mitochondrial ATPase. Mutations have been found in the genes for prion protein, presenilin, or a triplet nucleotide expansion; anticipation has been found in some families. In one X-linked family, the mutation affected the gene for proteolipid protein, which is also involved in Pelizaeus-Merzbacher disease. Both pure and complicated HSP have been mapped to chromosome 2p, but the two syndromes seem mostly genetically separate. Not all familial forms are inherited because infection with human T-cell lymphotropic virus type I (HTLV-I) can affect more than one person in a family.

Clinical Manifestations

The syndrome is also clinically heterogeneous. Some cases start early, others after age 35 years. Some are mild and some are severe. The complicated forms differ in the nature of the clinical associations. All are usually slowly progressive. The spastic gait dis-

TABLE 117.1. CLASSIFICATION OF THE HEREDITARY SPASTIC PARAPLEGIAS

Pure spastic paraplegia

MIM no.	
182600	Autosomal dominant (AD), type 1, onset before age 35 yr
	Autosomal dominant, type 2, onset after age 35 yr
270800	Autosomal recessive (AR)
312900	X-linked (SPG1) Xq28
312920	X-linked (SPG2) Xp21

Complicated spastic paraplegia with

—	Peroneal muscular atrophy
275900	Amyotrophy of hands, AR, Troyer syndrome
182700	Amyotrophy of hands, AD, Silver syndrome
270200	Ichthyosis, mental retardation, retinopathy (Sjögren-Larsson syndrome)
270550	Cerebellar ataxia, Charlevoix-Sageunay syndrome
270950	Pigmentary macular degeneration, mental retardation
182830	Optic atrophy
—	Myoclonic epilepsy
312890	Choreoathetosis, dystonia
248900	Athetosis, dementia (Mast syndrome)
—	Sensory neuropathy
270750	Hypopigmentation
182690	Deafness, nephropathy
176640	Dementia (prion protein)
300100	Adrenomyeloneuropathy

Modified from Harding, 1993.

order is one of coordination; there may be no weakness in manual muscle tests. Tendon reflexes are overactive, and Babinski signs and clonus are often evident. Sensation is usually normal on routine examination, but quantitative studies may show an abnormality. Sphincter symptoms may appear in late-onset forms. Variability of manifestations often occurs within the same family.

Laboratory Data

Laboratory studies, including magnetic resonance imaging (MRI) of the brain or spinal cord, are usually unrevealing; however, one family showed white matter lesions in the brain, and some show prominent thinning of the corpus callosum. Sensory evoked potentials may be abnormal even without clinically evident sensory loss. Magnetic stimulation usually shows an abnormality of central motor conduction; responses are either absent or delayed. The cerebrospinal fluid (CSF) is not diagnostic.

TABLE 117.2. FAMILIAL SPASTIC PARAPLEGIA

Gene	Location	Families (n)	%
Autosomal dominant			
FSP2	2p	15	45
FSP1	14q	2	6
FSP3	15q	1	3
FSP4	Other	15	45
Autosomal recessive			
—	8q12–13	4	80
—	Other	1	20
X-linked			
SPG2	Xq22	2	100
SPG1	Xq28	—	—

Data from Fink et al., 1996.

Diagnosis and Treatment

Diagnosis is usually evident from the clinical and family data. Sporadic cases could be the result of new mutations, but most prove to be multiple sclerosis, as reviewed later in the differential diagnosis of primary lateral sclerosis.

Management is primarily symptomatic. Intrathecal administration of baclofen (Lioresal) seems to be gaining favor because gait may improve. Tizanidine (Zanaflex) is also reported to be beneficial but seems no better than oral administration of baclofen.

TROPICAL MYELONEUROPATHIES

The term *tropical myeloneuropathies* refers to several syndromes encountered in equatorial countries around the world. The syndromes are manifestations of lesions in the spinal cord and peripheral nerves, separately or together. These disorders have been long-standing public health problems. Some have been traced to specific etiologies, including infection with HTLV-I, or the chronic ingestion of cassava beans or lathyrogenic agents. Other exogenous toxins may play a role. In the past and perhaps still today, similar syndromes have been ascribed to nutritional deprivation.

Among the numerous names for these disorders are *Strachan syndrome, Jamaican neuropathy, tropical spastic paraparesis* (TSP), *tropical ataxic neuropathy* (TAN), *konzo*, and *lathyrism*. TSP has generated other acronyms: RAM (for retrovirus-associated myelopathy) and HAM (for HTLV-I-associated myelopathy).

History, Clinical Manifestations, and Pathology

Because the symptoms and signs of these disorders are similar and the modes of pathogenesis are only now being identified with precision, it seems reasonable to describe the several conditions together.

Strachan Syndrome (Nutritional Neuropathy)

Strachan (1897) is credited with the first description of these syndromes when he reported his observations of a disorder found on the Caribbean island of Jamaica. The symptoms included numbness and burning in the limbs, girdling pains, impairment of vision and hearing, muscle weakness and wasting, hyporeflexia, and sensory ataxia. Mucocutaneous lesions included angular stomatitis, glossitis, and scrotal dermatitis. Scott later described similar manifestations in Jamaican sugar-cane workers; identical cases were reported in World War II prisoner-of-war camps in the Middle East and Asia, in the malnourished populations of Africa, India, and Malaya, and among those besieged in Madrid in the Spanish Civil War. Most patients so afflicted with *Strachan syndrome* have a predominantly sensory neuropathy, presumably a consequence of nutritional depletion. Neuropathologic studies have demonstrated symmetric ascending (secondary) degeneration in the posterior columns, spinocerebellar tracts, optic nerves, and peripheral nerves.

Jamaican Neuropathies: Tropical Ataxic Neuropathy and Tropical Spastic Paraparesis

Montgomery and colleagues (1964) described another group of patients in Jamaica. The dominant signs were spasticity and

TABLE 117.3. NEUROLOGIC SIGNS IN TROPICAL SPASTIC PARAPARESIS

Abnormal signs	Affected (%)
Corticospinal	
Legs	100
Arms	60–90
Jaw jerk	30–70
Bladder dysfunction	70–90
Impaired position, vibration sense	10–60
Root or cord sensation	20–65
Optic atrophy	2–20
Cerebellar	3–10

Modified from Rodgers-Johnson et al., 1990.

other evidence of corticospinal tract disease, sometimes with the peripheral manifestations of Strachan syndrome.

Two seemingly distinct varieties have been identified. Both are primarily diseases of adults. The *ataxic* form seems less common in Jamaica (but is more common in Nigeria). It evolves slowly and is generally less severe than the *spastic* type. Manifestations include sensory ataxia, numbness and burning sensations in the feet, deafness, visual impairment with optic atrophy and a central or paracentral scotoma, mild spasticity with Babinski signs, and wasting and weakness of the legs, sometimes with footdrop. Patients appear undernourished but without stigmata of nutritional disorder.

TSP is the more common variety of Jamaican neuropathy. It is a subacute condition in which pyramidal tract signs predominate and are accompanied by impairment of posterior column sensibility, bladder dysfunction, and girdling lumbar pain (Table 117.3). In both varieties, histamine-fast gastric achlorhydria and positive serologic tests for syphilis are frequent; in the more common subacute form, protein elevation and lymphocytic pleocytosis are found in the CSF. Myopathy, peripheral neuropathy, and leukoencephalopathy have been seen in some patients with HTLV-I infection. Antibodies to HTLV-I have been found in more than 80% of patients with TSP, and the virus has been isolated from CSF. The serologic abnormalities are similar in tropical countries throughout the world—Colombia, the Seychelles, Martinique, and the southernmost part of Japan around the city of Kagoshima.

The pathologic basis of TAN is not clear; it is presumed to be a myelopathy, and the ataxia is attributed to sensory loss. The pathology of TSP also needs more study, but the early descriptions included symmetric and severe degeneration of the pyramidal tracts and posterior columns. The spinocerebellar and spinothalamic pathways are affected in some patients. Nerve cell loss is evident in the Clarke column and in the anterior horns. Demyelination appears in the posterior spinal roots and in the optic and auditory nerves. In more acute cases, inflammatory exudates are seen in cord and spinal roots.

Lathyrism

The clinical manifestations of lathyrism are similar to those of TSP. It is mainly a disease of adults, and the manifestations are primarily those of pyramidal tract dysfunction. It is slowly progressive but may ultimately cause paraplegia. Descriptions of the disease extend back to ancient Hindu writings and to Hippocrates. Lathyrism was once probably prevalent in Europe, as well as tropical countries, but now seems restricted to India, Bangladesh, and Ethiopia.

Etiology

Malnutrition

Nutritional deprivation has long been recognized as a cause of peripheral neuropathy, optic neuropathy, and myelopathy. Avitaminosis and lack of other dietary necessities may account for some of the original cases of TSP and TAN, but other causes are now likely.

Persistent Viral Infection

The evidence of widespread HTLV-I infection in patients with TSP has had a major impact. Theoretically, it again shows that chronic viral infection can cause chronic human disease. The pathogenesis has not been elucidated, but transmission has been linked to blood transfusion, venereal contacts, contaminated needles of intravenous drug users, and the milk of nursing mothers. People with serologic evidence of syphilis, yaws, or human immunodeficiency virus (HIV) infection have a higher frequency of antibodies to HTLV-I. The disease may occur in more than one person in a family and could be confused with hereditary spastic paraparesis.

Dietary Toxins

The cause of lathyrism has long been ascribed to chronic ingestion of the chickling pea or vetch. *Lathyrus sativus* is a nourishing and inexpensive food that has been popular in impoverished countries. The active agent, isolated by Spencer and Schaumberg (1983), has been found to be a simple amino acid: beta-(*N*)-oxalyl-amino-l-alanine.

Another dietary constituent has been implicated in the African ataxic disorder TAN. Among patients in Nigeria, ingestion of the cassava plant seems to be important. Although the essential ingredient has not been identified, some investigators suspect compounds that can generate cyanide.

Other Toxins and Nutritional Deprivation

No other toxins have been shown to be important in TSP or TAN. However, another myelopathy closely resembling *TSP clinically* was encountered in Japan until corrective measures were taken. That condition, called *subacute myelopathy-neuropathy,* was attributed to use of iodochlorhydroxyquinoline to treat traveler's diarrhea. The drug was withdrawn, and the syndrome seems to have disappeared.

Vernant disease is seen in the French West Indies and is characterized by the triad of optic neuritis, cervical myelopathy, and hypothalamic-hypophyseal abnormalities. The cause is not known. In Cuba, an epidemic of optic neuritis has been ascribed to nutritional deficiency.

Prevention and Treatment

These tropical diseases are widespread and have been called the "hidden endemias." Prevention seems more likely to have an impact than treatment. Malnutrition ought to be preventable. Venereal transmission is amenable to control (though not easily). Exogenous toxins can be excluded from the environment. Blood intended for transfusion must be monitored for HTLV-I.

Once neurologic damage exists, however, the task is more difficult. Prednisone therapy seems to be effective in TSP; however, it seems more likely to benefit motor function in Japan and Colombia and to help bladder symptoms in Jamaica. Antiviral drug therapy remains a goal. Even replacement therapy with vitamins may not restore function to normal. Rehabilitation and adaptation remain important.

PRIMARY LATERAL SCLEROSIS (PLS)

In theory, primary lateral sclerosis (PLS) should be the pure upper motor neuron component of amyotrophic lateral sclerosis (ALS), just as progressive spinal muscular atrophy is the purely lower motor neuron version of that disease. That assumption has not been proved, however, and the condition is still a diagnosis of exclusion. Before the introduction of MRI, many clinicians eschewed the clinical diagnosis of PLS because some other condition often turned up at autopsy. Now, however, MRI plays a key role in the clinical diagnosis, which concerns the differential diagnosis of spastic paraparesis of middle life.

Information about the prevalence of this condition is not available, but the syndrome accounts for less than 5% of all cases of motor neuron disease.

Clinical Manifestations

PLS commences after age 40 with a spastic gait disorder that is slowly progressive and becomes stable. In our experience, patients rarely lose the ability to walk with a cane or other assistance. No paresthesias or findings of sensory loss are evident on examination. Most patients with PLS have no sphincter symptoms.

Laboratory Data

MRI with or without gadolinium shows no consistent abnormality, but after age 40 years many asymptomatic people show white matter lesions in the brain; PLS patients are not more likely to show these changes. The CSF is usually normal, but the protein content may be increased, without a rise in gamma globulin content or oligoclonal bands. Although electromyography should not show signs of denervation, it sometimes does so without uniformly predicting the later appearance of lower motor neuron disease. Magnetic stimulation of the brain may show delayed conduction of the corticospinal tracts. Sensory evoked potentials should be normal.

Diagnosis

The clinical diagnosis is made only after other possible causes of adult-onset progressive spastic paraparesis have been excluded.

TABLE 117.4. DIFFERENTIAL DIAGNOSIS OF PRIMARY LATERAL SCLEROSIS

Disease	Tests
Multiple sclerosis	MRI of brain and cervical spinal cord with gadolinium; CSF examination with oligoclonal bands and gamma globulin synthesis; visual, somatosensory, brainstem auditory-evoked responses

Cervical cord compression
  Cervical spondylosis
  Chiari malformation
  Foramen magnum tumors
  Arteriovenous malformations
	MRI with gadolinium

Amyotrophic lateral sclerosis	EMG
Adrenoleukodystrophy	Very-long-chain fatty acids in plasma
Tropical spastic paraparesis	HTLV-I antibody titer
HIV-associated myelopathy	HIV antibody titer
Paraneoplastic myelopathy	Evidence of primary neoplasm
Combined system disease	Serum vitamin B_{12} level

Modified from Younger et al., 1988.

This process can be done with a reasonable dependence on modern imaging and a few blood tests (Table 117.4).

No reliable figures exist for the relative frequency of the different diseases that cause spastic paraparesis. Most observers agree, however, that the main cause is the chronic and progressive form of spinal multiple sclerosis (MS). That diagnosis can be excluded with more than 90% certainty if none of the characteristic abnormalities of MS show on all three modern tests: MRI with gadolinium to examine the brain and upper cervical cord, CSF examination including oligoclonal bands and gamma globulin, and evoked responses. Prominent bladder symptoms are more likely to be found in MS.

In the process of evaluating for MS, MRI also excludes other possible causes, such as cervical spondylotic myelopathy, Chiari malformation or other hindbrain anomaly, arteriovenous malformation, or tumor at the foramen magnum. Exclusion of cervical spondylosis may be difficult because the MRI findings of that condition are so prevalent in asymptomatic people. MRI also evaluates the possibility of multiinfarct brain disease. Some authorities have placed reliance of MRI evidence of atrophy of the motor cortex or high signal in the corticospinal tract. However, we and others have found MR spectroscopy more reliable in identifying pathology of the upper motor neuron in both PLS and ALS. Since PLS is likely to be heterogeneous in pathology, some cases may involve subcortical structures primarily, and MR spectroscopy may therefore be normal.

In theory, ALS sometimes should start first as a purely upper motor neuron disorder, but that seems truly exceptional. Clinical evidence of fasciculation implicates the lower motor neurons and, by definition, excludes PLS. However, PLS is truly a diagnosis of exclusion, and conversion to ALS has been reported after 20 years of PLS. Clinical signs of parkinsonism, cerebellar disorder, or orthostatic hypotension imply a multisystem central nervous system disease, such as the Machado-Joseph syndrome or multiple system atrophy (Shy-Drager syndrome). One patient with PLS proved to have Lewy body disease.

Rare causes of paraparesis are HTLV-I infection, HIV myelopathy, or adrenoleukodystrophy, which can be detected by appropriate tests. In time, some of these adult-onset cases are likely to be sporadic examples of one of the hereditary spastic paraparesis syndromes, but that possibility awaits better delineation of the specific mutations so that they can be tested. The condition is age-related, with almost all cases starting after age 40 years, so similar findings in children are likely to be due to some other disease.

SUGGESTED READINGS

Hereditary Spastic Paraplegia

Benson KF, Horwitz M, Wolff J, et al. CAG expansion in autosomal dominant familial spastic paraplegia: novel expansion in a subset of patients. *Hum Mol Genet* 1998;7:1179–1186.

Bonneau D, Rozet JM, Bulteau C, et al. X-linked spastic paraplegia (SPG2): clinical heterogeneity at a single locus. *J Med Genet* 1993;30:381–384.

Casari G, De Fusco M, Ciarmatori S, et al. Spastic parplegia and OXPHOS impairment caused by mutations in paraplegin, a nuclear-encoded mitochondrial metalloprotease. *Cell* 1998;93:973–983.

Claus D, Waddy HM, Harding AE, et al. Hereditary motor and sensory neuropathies and hereditary spastic paraplegia: a magnetic stimulation study. *Ann Neurol* 1990;28:43–49.

Fink JK. Advances in hereditary spastic paraplegia. *Curr Opin Neurol* 1997;10:313–318.

Fink JK, Heiman-Patterson T, Bird T, et al. Hereditary spastic paraplegia: advances in genetic research. Hereditary Spastic Paraplegia Working Group. *Neurology* 1996;46:1507–1514.

Gutmann DH, Fischbeck KH, Kamholz J. Complicated spastic paraparesis with cerebral white matter lesions. *Am J Med Genet* 1990;36:251–257.

Harding AE. Hereditary spastic paraplegia. *Semin Neurol* 1993; 13:333–336.

Hazan J, Lamy C, Melki J, et al. Autosomal dominant familial spastic paraplegia is genetically heterogeneous and one locus maps to 14q. *Nat Genet* 1993;5:163–167.

Kitamoto T, Amano N, Terao Y, et al. A new inherited prion disease (PrP-P105L mutation) showing spastic paraparesis. *Ann Neurol* 1993; 34:808–813.

Krabbe K, Nielsen JE, Fallentin E, Feneger K, Nerning M. MRI of autosomal dominant pure spastic paraplegia. *Neuroradiology* 1997;39:724–727.

Meyer T, Munch C, Volkel H, Booms P, Ludolph AC. The EAAT2 (GLT-1) gene in motor neuron disease: absence of point mutations in ALS and a point mutation in hereditary spastic paraplegia. *J Neurol Neurosurg Psychiatry* 1998;65:594–596.

Polo JM, Calleja J, Combaros O, Berciano J. Hereditary "pure" spastic paraplegia: study of nine families. *J Neurol Neurosurg Psychiatry* 1993;56:175–181.

Schady W, Dick JPR, Sheard A, Cramptom S. Central motor conduction studies in hereditary spastic paraplegia. *J Neurol Neurosurg Psychiatry* 1991;54:775–779.

Schady W, Sheard A. Quantitative study of sensory function in hereditary spastic paraplegia. *Brain* 1990;113:709–720.

Ueda M, Katayama Y, Kamiya T, et al. Hereditary spastic paraplegia with a thin corpus callosum and thalamic involvement in Japan. *Neurology* 1998;6:1751–1754.

Tropical Myeloneuropathies

Achiron A, Pinlas-Hamiel OP, Doll L, et al. Spastic paraparesis associated with human T-lymphotropic virus type 1: clinical, serological, and genomic study in Iranian-born Mashhadi Jews. *Ann Neurol* 1993;34:670–675.

CDC and USPHS working group guidelines for counselling persons affected with HTLV-1 and HTLV-II. *Ann Intern Med* 1993;118:448–454.

Cliff J, Lundqvist P, Martensson J, et al. Association of high cyanide and low sulphur intake in cassava-induced spastic paraparesis. *Lancet* 1985;2:1211–1212.

Cruickshank EK. Neuromuscular disease in relation to nutrition. *Fed Proc* 1961;20[Suppl 7]:345–360.

Cuetter AC. Strachan's syndrome: a nutritional disorder of the nervous system. Proceedings of the weekly seminar in neurology. Edward Hines Jr. Veterans Administration Hospital, Hines, IL. 1968;18.

Denny-Brown D. Neurological conditions resulting from prolonged and severe dietary restriction. *Medicine* 1947;26:41–113.

Domingues RB, Muniz MR, Jorge ML, et al. Human T-cell lymphotropic virus type-1-associated myelopathy/tropical spastic paraparesis in Sao Paulo, Brazil: association with blood transfusion. *Am J Trop Med Hyg* 1997;57:56–59.

Douen AG, Pringle CE, Guberman A. Human T-cell lymphotropic virus type 1 myositis, peripheral neuropathy, and cerebral white matter lesions in the absence of spastic paraparesis. *Arch Neurol* 1997;54:896–900.

Fisher CM. Residual neuropathological changes in Canadians held prisoners of war by the Japanese. *Can Service Med J* 1955;11:157–199.

Gessain A, Gout O. Chronic myelopathy associated with human T-lymphotropic virus type 1 (HTLV-1). *Ann Intern Med* 1992;117:933–946.

Hollsberg P, Hafler DA. Pathogenesis of diseases induced by human lymphotropic virus type 1 infection. *N Engl J Med* 1993;328:123–138.

Izumo S, Umehara F, Kashio N, Kubota R, Sato E, Osame M. Neuropathology of HTLV-1-associated myelopathy (HAM/TSP). *Leukemia* 1997;11[Suppl 3]:82–84.

Janssen RS, Kaplan JE, Khabbaz RF, et al. HTLV-1-associated myelopathy/tropical spastic paraparesis in the United States. *Neurology* 1991;41:1355–1357.

Kira J, Fujihara K, Itoyama Y, et al. Leucoencephalopathy in HTLV-1-associated myelopathy/tropical spastic paraparesis: MRI analysis and two-year follow-up study after corticosteroid therapy. *J Neurol Sci* 1991;106:41–49.

Montgomery RD, Cruickshank EK, Robertson WB, McMenemey WH. Clinical and pathological observations on Jamaican neuropathy. *Brain* 1964;87:425–462.

Osame M, Matsumoto M, Usuku K, et al. Chronic progressive myelopathy associated with elevated antibodies to human T-lymphotropic virus type I and adult T-cell leukemia-like cells. *Ann Neurol* 1987;21:117–123.

Osuntokun BO. An ataxic neuropathy in Nigeria: a clinical, biochemical and electrophysiological study. *Brain* 1965;91:215–248.

Rodgers-Johnson PEB, Ono SG, Asher DM, Gibbs CJ. Tropical spastic paraparesis and HTLV-1 myelopathy: clinical features and pathogenesis. In: Waksman BH, ed. *Immunologic mechanisms in neurologic and psychiatric disease.* New York: Raven Press, 1990.

Roman GC. Tropical myeloneuropathies revisited. *Curr Opin Neurol* 1998;11:539–544.

Roman GC, Spencer PS, Schoenberg BS. Tropical myeloneuropathies: the hidden endemias. *Neurology* 1985;35:1158–1170.

Roman GC, Vernant JC, Osame M, eds. *HTLV-1 and the nervous system.* New York: Alan R Liss, 1989.

Rudge P, Ali A, Cruickshank JK. Multiple sclerosis, tropical spastic paraparesis, and HTLV-1 infection in Afro-Caribbean patients in the United Kingdom. *J Neurol Neurosurg Psychiatry* 1991;54:689–694.

Salazar-Grueso EF, Holzer TJ, Gutierrez RA, et al. Familial spastic paraparesis syndrome associated with HTLV-1 infection. *N Engl J Med* 1990;108:732–737.

Smith CR, Dickson D, Samkoff L. Recurrent encephalopathy and seizures in a U.S. native with HTLV-1 associated myelopathy/tropical spastic paraparesis: clinicopathologic study. *Neurology* 1992;42:658–661.

Spencer PS, Schaumberg HH. Lathyrism: a neurotoxic disease. *Neurobehav Toxicol Teratol* 1983;5:625–629.

Strachan H. On a form of multiple neuritis prevalent in the West Indies. *Practitioner* 1897;59:477.

Tylleskar T, Howlett WP, Rwiza HT, et al. Konzo: a distinct disease entity with selective upper motor neuron damage. *J Neurol Neurosurg Psychiatry* 1993;56:638–643.

Vernant JC, Cabre P, Smadjia D, et al. Recurrent optic neuromyelitis with endocrinopathies: a new syndrome. *Neurology* 1997;48:58–64.

Vernant JC, Maurs L, Gesain A, et al. Endemic tropical spastic paraparesis associated with human T-lymphotropic virus type I: a clinical and seroepidemiological study of 25 cases. *Ann Neurol* 1987;21:123–131.

Yoshioka A, Hirose G, Ueda Y, et al. Neuropathological studies of the spinal cord in early stage HTLV-1-associated myelopathy (HAM). *J Neurol Neurosurg Psychiatry* 1993;56:1004–1007.

Primary Lateral Sclerosis

Brown WF, Ebers GC, Hudson AJ, et al. Motor-evoked responses in primary lateral sclerosis. *Muscle Nerve* 1992;15:626–629.

Forsyth PA, Dalmau J, Graus F, Cwik V, Rosenblum MK, Posner JB. Motor neuron syndromes in cancer patients. *Ann Neurol* 1997;41:722–730.

Grignani G, Gobbi PG, Piccolo G, et al. Progressive necrotic myelopathy as a paraneoplastic syndrome: report of a case and some pathogenetic considerations. *J Intern Med* 1992;231:81–85.

Hainfellner JA, Pliz P, Lassmann H, et al. Diffuse Lewy body disease as substrate of primary lateral sclerosis. *J Neurol* 1995;242:59–63.

Pringle CE, Hudson AJ, Ebers GC. Primary lateral sclerosis: the clinical and laboratory definition of a discrete syndrome. *Can J Neurol Sci* 1990;17:235–236.

Pringle CE, Hudson AJ, Munoz DG, et al. Primary lateral sclerosis: clinical features, neuropathology, and diagnostic criteria. *Brain* 1992;115:495–520.

Rowland LP. Paraneoplastic primary lateral sclerosis and amyotrophic lateral sclerosis. *Ann Neurol* 1997;41:703–705.

Rowland LP. Diagnosis of amyotrophic lateral sclerosis. *J Neurol Sci* 1998;160[Suppl 1];S6–S24.

Rowland LP. Primary lateral sclerosis: disease, syndrome, both, or neither? *J Neurol Sci* 1999;170:1–4.

Swash M, Desai J, Misra VP. What is primary lateral sclerosis? *J Neurol Sci* 1999;170:5–10.

Younger DS, Chou S, Hays AP, et al. Primary lateral sclerosis: a clinical diagnosis reemerges. *Neurology* 1988;45:1304–1307.

Baclofen Therapy

Coffey RJ, Cahill D, Steers W, et al. Intrathecal baclofen for intractable spasticity of spinal origin: results of a long-term multicenter study. *J Neurosurg* 1993;78:226–232.

McLean BN. Intrathecal baclofen in severe spasticity. *Br J Hosp Med* 1993;49:262–267.

HEREDITARY AND ACQUIRED MOTOR NEURON DISEASES

LEWIS P. ROWLAND

DEFINITIONS AND CLASSIFICATIONS

Several different diseases are characterized by progressive degeneration and loss of motor neurons in the spinal cord with or without similar lesions in the motor nuclei of the brainstem or the motor cortex, and by replacement of the lost cells by gliosis. All these can be considered *motor neuron diseases* (plural). The term *motor neuron disease* (singular), however, is used to describe an adult disease, *amyotrophic lateral sclerosis* (ALS), in which upper motor neurons are affected, as well as lower motor neurons. (The terms *motor neuron disease* and *ALS* have become equivalent in the United States.)

The term *spinal muscular atrophy* (SMA) refers to syndromes characterized solely by lower motor neuron signs. The official classification of the World Federation of Neurology lists numerous different forms of SMA in children. Some are differentiated by associated conditions, such as optic atrophy, deafness, or mental retardation. Childhood SMA is inherited and is not accompanied by upper motor neuron signs.

In adults, some patients also show only lower motor neuron signs in life (*progressive spinal muscular atrophy* [PSMA]). In two autopsy series, however, 17 of 25 patients with adult-onset PSMA showed degeneration of the corticospinal tracts (Table 118.1). For that reason, adult-onset PSMA is considered a form of ALS. Almost all adult-onset cases are sporadic, not familial.

A *motor neuropathy* is also evident by lower motor neuron signs alone, with no sensory loss, and therefore resembles PSMA. The condition is considered a neuropathy rather than a disease of the perikaryon because nerve conduction measurements show evidence of diffuse demyelination, focal demyelination (conduction block), or axonal neuropathy (see Chapter 15). Rarely, the diagnosis of motor neuropathy might depend on histologic changes in nerve rather than on physiologic criteria.

PROGRESSIVE SPINAL MUSCULAR ATROPHIES OF CHILDHOOD

Three major syndromes of SMA occur in children. They differ in age at onset and severity of symptoms. All are autosomal-recessive and map to the same locus, chromosome 5q11-q13. They are therefore regarded as examples of allelic heterogeneity;\ that is, mutations of the same gene. In theory, there ought to be some locus heterogeneity, with some families showing the same or similar phenotype but mapping to different chromosomes; in fact, however, families throughout the world map to the same locus. The gene is called survival motor neuron gene (SMN); a

TABLE 118.1. AUTOPSY FINDINGS IN CLINICAL SYNDROMES OF MOTOR NEURON DISEASE: DEGENERATION OF PYRAMIDAL TRACTS

	Brownell, Trevor-Hughes (1970)	Lawyer, Netsky (1953)	Total
Patients (n)	21	22	43
Lower motor neuron alone	11/17	6/8	17/25
Lower plus upper motor neurons	16/18	45/45	61/63
Lower motor neuron, uncertain upper	1/1	—	1/1
Total	28/36	51/53	79/89

neighboring gene is the neuronal apoptosis inhibitory protein gene (NAIP). Both have two almost identical copies, one telomeric (SMNt) and one centromeric (SMNc). If there were a conversion from the telomeric to the centromeric, SMNt would seem to have been deleted, but there would be extra copies of SMNc, as is actually found in the less severe forms of the disease.

In 98% of children with the severe infantile SMA type 1, there is a deletion of SMNt, and point mutations are found in the few who lack a deletion. The frequency of deletions of NAIP is lower, but it is also included in large deletions. Adjacent to NAIP is another gene, p44, which is sometimes deleted as well, but less often than SMN or NAIP. In general, the size of the deletion parallels clinical severity; the largest deletions may encompass all three genes. Direct deletion analysis has high sensitivity and specificity and can be used for diagnosis without muscle biopsy in suspected cases; it is also effective in antenatal diagnosis in an at-risk fetus.

The SMN protein is depleted in the spinal cord of patients, but its normal role is not known, except that it is found in the cytoplasm and in nuclear structures called "gems," where it is linked to ribonucleic acid–binding proteins and seems to be involved in the biogenesis of ribonucleoproteins. Another possibly important association of both SMN and NAIP is with Bcl-2, an antiapoptotic protein. How absence of SMN leads to the disease, however, still has to be elucidated.

Infantile SMA type 1 (Werdnig-Hoffmann syndrome) (MIM 253300) is evident at birth or soon thereafter, always before age 6 months. Mothers may notice that intrauterine movements are decreased. In the neonatal period, nursing problems may occur, and limb movements are feeble and decreased; this is one of the most common forms of the *floppy infant syndrome.* Proximal muscles are affected before distal muscles, but ultimately complete flaccid quadriplegia results. The tongue is often seen to fasciculate, but twitching is only seen rarely in limb muscles, presumably because of the ample subcutaneous fat. Sooner or later, respiration is compromised, and paradoxical movements of the chest wall are seen; the sternum may be depressed with inspiration. Tendon reflexes are absent. The condition is devastating, and 85% of the children die before age 2 years. The others may survive but never walk; their condition may remain stable for many years. Some authorities believe the survivors form a special intermediate class, *SMA type 2* (MIM 253550); this category also includes cases of onset from 6 months to 1 year.

With the introduction of electromyography (EMG) after World War II, Kugelberg and Welander noted physiologic evidence of denervation in adolescents with proximal limb weakness. The essentials of that disorder were delineated in the title of their paper, "Juvenile spinal muscular atrophy simulating muscular dystrophy;" the condition described is now called the *Kugelberg-Welander syndrome,* or *SMA type 3* (MIM 253400). Symptoms begin with a slowly progressive gait disorder in late childhood or adolescence. The onset is followed by symptoms of proximal arm weakness and wasting; tendon reflexes are lost. Unlike the Werdnig-Hoffmann syndrome, fasciculation of limb muscles, as well as of the tongue, may be visible. This condition is relatively benign; many patients continue to function socially with a normal life span. Others may be handicapped, but serious dysphagia or respiratory compromise is rare. Sensation is spared, and no other organ systems are affected.

Laboratory Data

Electrodiagnostic studies show evidence of denervation with normal nerve conductions. Muscle biopsy similarly shows evidence of denervation. The cerebrospinal fluid (CSF) shows no characteristic changes. Serum levels of sarcoplasmic enzymes, such as creatine kinase, may be increased; in the Kugelberg-Welander type, the increase may be 20 times normal, in the range of many myopathies. The electrocardiogram is normal.

Diagnosis now depends on deoxyribonucleic acid (DNA) analysis. Muscle biopsy and even EMG are not necessary if a deletion or mutation of SMN is found.

Treatment

There is no specific therapy. Treatment of survivors is analogous to that described for children with muscular dystrophy: rehabilitation measures, bracing, attention to scoliosis, and assistance in education and social adaptation. Some authorities believe that children with SMA are characteristically of high intelligence; education programs are important.

FOCAL MUSCULAR ATROPHIES OF CHILDHOOD AND ADOLESCENCE

These syndromes do not map to 5q11 and differ in the focal distribution of symptoms and signs. Most are autosomal-recessive, but some families show dominant inheritance.

Fazio-Londe Syndrome

In contrast to the sparing of cranial nerve functions in most juvenile SMA, selective dysarthria and dysphagia in Fazio-Londe syndrome (MIM 211500) begin in late childhood or adolescence. Wasting of the tongue with visible fasciculation occurs. Symptoms may be restricted for years, but weakness of the arms and legs may occur later, and respiration may be affected. There have been few documented cases and fewer autopsy-proven cases.

Scapuloperoneal and Facioscapulohumeral Forms

Scapuloperoneal (MIM 271220, 181400) and facioscapulohumeral (FSH) (MIM 182970) forms of SMA have been reported. Some may actually have had FSH muscular dystrophy with ambiguous results on EMG and biopsy that led to incorrect classification as a neurogenic disorder. The distinction now depends on DNA analysis.

Childhood Spinal Muscular Atrophy with Known Biochemical Abnormality

Hexosaminidase deficiency (MIM 272800) may cause a syndrome of SMA starting in childhood or adolescence. The pattern of inheritance is autosomal recessive. Some patients also have upper motor neuron signs, as in ALS. Associated psychosis, dementia, or cerebellar signs may appear. Other rare biochemical abnormalities seen with SMA are lysosomal diseases, phenylketonuria, hydroxyisovaleric aciduria, mutations of mitochondrial DNA, perioxosomal disease, and ceroid lipofuscinosis.

Diagnosis

Most of the childhood SMAs can be identified by the history and clinical examination. They must be differentiated from muscular dystrophies by EMG, muscle biopsy, or DNA analysis; the family history aids in classification. Hexosaminidase deficiency is suspected in families of Ashkenazi-Jewish background, especially if there are known cases of Tay-Sachs disease in the family or if some family members are known to be carriers of the gene. Kennedy syndrome is recognized by onset after age 40 years, distribution of weakness, and gynecomastia.

MOTOR NEURON DISEASES OF ADULT ONSET

X-linked Recessive Spinobulbar Muscular Atrophy (Kennedy Disease)

Symptoms of X-linked recessive spinobulbar muscular atrophy (Kennedy disease) (MIM 313200) usually begin after age 40 years with dysarthria and dysphagia; limb weakness is delayed for years. The tongue fasciculates, and twitching of limb muscles is often visible. Limb weakness is usually more severe proximally. Tendon reflexes are lost, and upper motor neuron signs are never evident. Although the condition is purely motor in life, nerve conduction studies suggest a large-fiber sensory peripheral axonopathy; sensory evoked potentials may be abnormal and sensory tracts in the spinal cord may be affected at autopsy. Exceptional cases have shown upper motor neuron signs or dementia. Gynecomastia is present in most but not all patients; reproductive fitness is only slightly decreased.

Diagnosis is aided by the characteristic distribution of signs, lack of upper motor neuron signs, slow progression, and a family history suggesting X-linkage. Nevertheless, 2% of patients diagnosed with ALS show the Kennedy mutation, so diagnosis is not always straightforward.

The gene maps to Xq11-12, the site of the androgen receptor. The mutation is an expansion of a CAG repeat. At autopsy immunochemical studies show the presence of both normal and mutant gene products, including nuclear inclusions that contain androgen receptor. It is not known how these abnormalities cause the disease. There have been no reports of a neurologic disorder in people with the testicular feminizing syndrome, the major clinical manifestation of a mutation in the gene for the androgen receptor. This and other evidence suggest that, with the expanded polyglutamine repeat, the disease results from a toxic gain of function. Kennedy syndrome was one of the first to be associated with an expansion of a trinucleotide repeat and, as in others of this class, there is an inverse relationship between the number of repeats and the severity of the disorder.

Amyotrophic Lateral Sclerosis

Definition

ALS is of unknown cause and pathogenesis, and is defined pathologically as one in which there is degeneration of both upper and lower motor neurons. Charcot made the early clinical and pathologic description, and the disease is named for him in Europe. In the United States, the disease is colloquially called "Lou Gehrig's disease" after a famous baseball player who had the disease. The SMA form is deduced from clinical observations, but few patients show only lower motor neuron changes at autopsy. In life, the disease is defined by finding evidence of both lower motor neuron disease (weakness, wasting, fasciculation) and upper motor neuron disease (hyperactive tendon reflexes, Hoffmann signs, Babinski signs, or clonus) in the same limbs. The accuracy of clinical diagnosis is assumed to be more than 95%, but that figure has not been formally tested. Nevertheless, the reliability of clinical diagnosis suffices to make the findings in the history and examination part of the definition. Problems in diagnosis are reviewed below.

Epidemiology

The disease is found worldwide in roughly the same prevalence (about 50×10^{-6}). In 1945, however, about 50 times that number were found on the island of Guam, where the findings of ALS were frequently associated with parkinsonism and dementia. With modernization of the island, the disease seems to have declined in frequency to levels found elsewhere. (Some authorities believe dementia has replaced ALS as the people now live longer, creating a different form of the same basic disease.) A few other areas of unexplained high incidence have surfaced. Apparent clusters in a building or a small community have not yet led to identification of an etiologic agent. Similarly, case–control studies have not identified consistent risk factors related to occupation, trauma, diet, or socioeconomic status.

The disease is one of middle and late life. Only 10% of cases begin before age 40 years; 5% begin before age 30. An increase in age-adjusted incidence is seen in succeeding decades, except for a decrease after age 80. In most series, men are affected one to two times more often than women. There is no known ethnic predilection.

About 5% of cases are familial in an autosomal dominant pattern (MIM 105400). About 20% of familial cases map to chromosome 21, where there are mutations in the gene for superoxide dismutase (SOD). The evidence suggests no deficiency in normal SOD; rather the mutant protein exerts a toxic effect on motor neurons. The essential elements of the disease have been reproduced in transgenic mice bearing the mutant protein, providing the first clue to the pathogenesis of motor neuron disease. The familial cases that do not map to this locus are taken as evidence of locus heterogeneity. The occurrence of dementia and parkinsonism seems to increase in first-degree relatives of patients with ALS, thus implying a possible common susceptibility to the neurodegenerative diseases of aging.

Pathogenesis

The cause of sporadic ALS is not known. Because of the high incidence in Guam, environmental factors have been suspected, but none has emerged there or anywhere else. Lead and mercury intoxication may cause similar syndromes but are no longer seen in modern societies. Excitotoxic amino acids, especially glutamate, are now held suspect, but there is no indication how the condition might arise or why the same theory should be considered for Alzheimer disease or Parkinson disease. Some authorities believe that an autoimmune disorder is present in all patients; others think there is a higher than expected frequency of monoclonal gammopathy or lymphoproliferative disease, but, together, these abnormalities are found in less than 10%. Among the sporadic cases, fewer than 5% are new SOD mutations.

Information from the transgenic mice has reinforced the theory that both sporadic and familial ALS result from excitotoxic effects. In sporadic ALS, evidence of glutamate toxicity is accumulating, and drugs with antiglutamate effects have been tested in humans and transgenic mice. The evidence is marginal but supports the excitotoxic theory.

Whether there is a paraneoplastic form of ALS has long been debated. An increased frequency of malignancy has been difficult to prove in a case–control study of patients with ALS. Several reports, however, have described ALS syndromes that improved or disappeared when a lung or renal cancer was cured. In addition, the frequency of association of ALS and lymphoma seems to be disproportionate.

The pathology of ALS implies selective vulnerability of motor neurons, which show several neuronal inclusions that include ubiquitinated skeins or Lewy-like formations and Bunina bodies. These structures are found in most patients with sporadic ALS. In familial forms, a different form is the "hyaline conglomerate", which includes neurofilaments and does not contain ubiquitin. Determination of the nature of these structures could elucidate, which pathogenesis. Some authorities believe the cellular abnormalities identify a common basic mechanism for the syndromes of ALS, adult-onset SMA, primary lateral sclerosis (PLS), and ALS-dementia.

The clinical syndrome of ALS can be induced by several known agents, including radiotherapy, lead poisoning, and lightning stroke. Less dramatic environmental effects could bring on more typical sporadic ALS in a person who is genetically susceptible. The search is on for susceptibility factors and environmental agents.

Clinical Manifestations

Weakness may commence in the legs, hands, proximal arms, or oropharynx (with slurred speech or dysarthria, or difficulty swallowing). Often, the hands are affected first, usually asymmetrically. Painless difficulty with buttons or turning a key is an ominous symptom in midlife. Gait is impaired because the muscles are weak, and footdrop is characteristic, although proximal muscles are sometimes affected first. Alternatively, a spastic gait disorder may ensue. Slowly, the weakness becomes more severe, and more areas of the body are affected, leading to an increasing state of dependency. Muscle cramps (attributed to the hypersensitivity of denervated muscle) and weight loss (resulting from the combination of muscle wasting and dysphagia) are characteristic symptoms. Respiration is usually affected late but, occasionally, may be an early or even the first manifestation; breathing is compromised by paresis of intercostal muscles and diaphragm, or the dysphagia may lead to aspiration and pneumonitis, which can be the terminal event. Sensation is not clinically affected; pain and paresthesia are impermissible with this diagnosis, unless there is a complicating disease (e.g., diabetic neuropathy) and bladder function is spared. The eye muscles are affected only exceptionally. Pain is not an early symptom but may occur later when limbs are immobile.

Lower motor neuron signs must be evident if the diagnosis is to be considered valid. Fasciculation may be seen in the tongue, even without dysarthria. If there is weakness and wasting of limb muscle, fasciculation is almost always seen. Tendon reflexes may be increased or decreased; the combination of overactive reflexes with Hoffmann signs in arms with weak, wasted, and fasciculating muscles is virtually pathognomonic of ALS (except for the syndrome of motor neuropathy, which is discussed later). Unequivocal signs of upper motor neuron disorder are Babinski signs and clonus. If a spastic gait disorder is seen without lower motor neuron signs in the legs, weakness in the legs may not be found, but incoordination is evident by clumsiness and slowness in the performance of alternating movements.

The cranial nerve motor nuclei are implicated by dysarthria, lingual wasting and fasciculation, and impaired movement of the uvula. Facial weakness and wasting can be discerned, especially in the mentalis muscle, but is usually not prominent. Dysarthria and dysphagia caused by upper motor neuron disease (*pseudobulbar palsy*) is made evident by movements of the uvula that are more vigorous on reflex innervation than on volition; that is, the uvula does not move well (or at all) on phonation, but a vigorous response is seen in the pharyngeal or gag reflex. A common manifestation of pseudobulbar palsy is *emotional lability* with inappropriate laughing or, more often, crying that can be regarded erroneously as a reactive depression because of the diagnosis; it is better regarded as a release phenomenon of the complex reflexes involved in emotional expression.

The course is relentless and progressive without remissions, relapses, or even stable plateaus. Death results from respiratory failure, aspiration pneumonitis, or pulmonary embolism after prolonged immobility. The mean duration of symptoms is about 4 years; 20% of patients live longer than 5 years. Once a tracheostomy has been placed, the patient may be kept alive for years, although totally paralyzed and unable to move anything other than the eyes; this condition can be a locked-in state. Exceptional patients die in the first year or live longer than 25 years.

About 10% of patients have associated dementia. The most common pathology is that of frontotemporal dementia; some show changes of Alzheimer disease and some show nonspecific pathology. The chromosome 17–related dementia, a tauopathy, has included amyotrophy in a few cases.

Clinical Classification

In addition to the terms *SMA* and *ALS,* two other labels have been used. *Progressive bulbar palsy* implies prominent dysarthria and dysphagia. This term, however, is falling into disfavor because almost all patients with bulbar symptoms already have fasciculations in arms and legs or display upper motor neuron signs; that is, the signs are not restricted to the cranial nerves and the syndrome is clearly ALS. *PLS* refers to a syndrome of upper motor neuron disorder only in life. At autopsy, cases of this nature are found in 5% or fewer of patients, and it is difficult to prove that the condition is really a form of ALS rather than a separate disease. PLS is described in Chapter 117 in the differential diagnosis of spastic paraparesis. Pure SMA (lower motor neuron signs alone) also accounts for fewer than 5% of cases at autopsy.

Laboratory Data

There is no pathognomonic laboratory abnormality, but the clinical diagnosis should be confirmed by EMG evidence of active denervation in at least three limbs. Nerve conduction velocities should be normal or nearly so; conduction block is rare in patients with frank upper motor neuron signs. CSF protein content is increased above 50 mg/dL in about 30% of patients and above 75 mg/dL in about 10%; the higher values seem more likely to occur in the presence of monoclonal gammopathy or lymphoma. Gammopathy is found by sensitive methods, such as immunofixation electrophoresis, in 5% to 10% of patients. Bone marrow examination is reserved for patients with monoclonal gammopathy. Magnetic resonance spectroscopy (MRS) and transcranial magnetic stimulation are emerging as effective measures of upper motor neuron dysfunction in patients who have few or no clinical corticospinal signs. Antibodies to the neuronal ganglioside GM_1 are demonstrable in 10% or less. No evidence supports the notion that ALS may be a manifestation of Lyme disease. A few cases have been found in patients with serologic evidence of human immunodeficiency virus or human T-cell lymphotropic virus type I infection.

Diagnosis

In adults, the finding of widespread lower motor neuron signs is virtually diagnostic of motor neuron disease, especially if Babinski signs or clonus appear. Even if these definite upper motor neuron signs are lacking the diagnosis is similarly secure if inappropriately active tendon reflexes or Hoffmann signs are found in arms with weak, wasted, and twitching muscles. The accuracy of clinical diagnosis has not been formally determined but, from clinical experience, is probably better than 95%. Rarely, some other condition, such as polyglucosan body disease, turns up at autopsy in a patient with clinical signs of ALS. The combination of ALS and dementia has been associated with several different pathologic changes (including Pick disease, Lewy body disease, or nonspecific subcortical gliosis).

Although clinical diagnosis can be considered reliable, several common diagnostic problems occur:

1. The most important disorder, because it is treatable, is *multifocal motor neuropathy with conduction block* (MMNCB), which is defined by finding conduction block in more than one nerve and not at sites of entrapment neuropathy. Strict criteria include more than 50% decline in amplitude between proximal and distal sites of stimulation with less than 50% increase in duration of the response. As described, MMNCB primarily affects the hands, is asymmetric, affects men much more often than women, and is "predominantly lower motor neuron." None of these features, however, clearly distinguishes the disorder from ALS. MMNCB progresses more slowly than ALS, so that relatively little disability after 5 years of symptoms would favor the diagnosis; however, that criterion is not applicable if a patient is seen soon after onset. More of a problem is the fact that about 50% of patients with MMNCB have had active tendon jerks in limbs with clear lower motor neuron signs. Regardless of the clinical similarities to ALS, the finding of conduction block is an indication for immunosuppressive drug therapy or intravenous immunoglobulin therapy because many patients with MMNCB show a good response. In the few autopsies of patients with MMNCB, there has been loss of motor neurons, suggesting that both motor neuron and peripheral nerve are affected in some cases.

2. *Myasthenia gravis* (MG) is a common cause of dysarthria and dysphagia in people who are in the age range of those afflicted with ALS. If there is concomitant ptosis or ophthalmoparesis, if diurnal fluctuation in severity is marked, or if remissions have occurred, MG is more likely. If the syndrome is compatible and if there is an unequivocal response to edrophonium chloride, high titer of antibodies to acetylcholine receptor, or evidence of thymoma on computed tomography, the diagnosis is MG. If fasciculations are evident and the patient is not taking pyridostigmine bromide, or if upper motor neuron signs appear, the syndrome cannot be caused by MG.

3. The differential diagnosis of spastic paraplegia in middle life includes multiple sclerosis (MS), ALS, cervical spondylosis, tropical spastic paraplegia, vitamin B_{12} deficiency, and adrenoleukodystrophy. The appropriate tests are described in Chapter 117. Because magnetic resonance imaging (MRI) evidence of spondylosis is so common in asymptomatic people, the findings can be seen coincidentally in patients with ALS. The differentiation of ALS from spondylotic myelopathy can therefore be vexing; the diagnosis of spondylotic myelopathy should be made cautiously if unequivocal lower motor neuron signs are found in the hands without sensory symptoms or signs. The presence of fasciculations in legs or tongue is incompatible with cervical spondylosis. In contrast, neck pain and persistent paresthesia with unequivocal sensory loss are incompatible with ALS, unless there is an additional condition. MRS and transcranial magnetic stimulation of the motor cortex may be helpful in identifying PLS.

4. *Pseudobulbar palsy* is seen in ALS and MS and after bilateral strokes. MRI is especially useful in identifying the causes other than motor neuron disease. Clinically, lower motor neuron signs are found in all patients with ALS, and they are incompatible with MS or stroke. In a patient with ALS, the liability to weeping should not be construed as a reactive depression.

5. In our center, we carry out tests for monoclonal gammopathy, conduction block, antibodies to GM_1 ganglioside and myelin-associated glycoprotein (MAG), and lymphoproliferative disease in all patients with ALS.

6. ALS is differentiated from myopathies by finding fasciculations or upper motor neuron signs on examination. If these are lacking, the differential diagnosis depends on EMG evidence of denervation.

7. The *postpolio syndrome* is important for theoretic reasons (because persistent infection by the virus might cause ALS) and for practical reasons (because survivors of acute poliomyelitis have feared that the virus might be revived and attack again). No evidence suggests that survivors of acute childhood polio are at increased risk of ALS. The postpolio syndrome takes three forms: loss of ability to compensate for residual paresis with increasing age; addition of arthritis or some other physical condition that impedes adaption and compensation; or, decades after the original paralysis, new weakness of muscles thought not to have been affected in the childhood attack. These developments are accompanied by evidence of chronic denervation on EMG, but conduction velocities are normal; the consensus is that this syndrome is a residual effect in previously paralyzed muscles and that it is not a new motor neuron disease. Progression is slow and is limited to previously paralyzed muscles. No upper motor neuron signs appear, and clinically evident fasciculations are exceptional.

8. *Monomelic muscular atrophy* (Hirayama syndrome) affects young men, not women, at about age 20 years and is restricted to one limb, usually an arm and hand rather than a leg. Although the condition was first reported in Japan, it has been seen in other countries. Many of those affected seem to be athletes, but the syndrome is not overtly related to cervical trauma. The condition progresses slowly for 1 or 2 years and then seems to become arrested. The origin of this disorder is not known. The patient must be observed for some months to be certain that other signs of motor neuron disease do not appear.

9. *Reversible motor neuron* disease is the hope of diagnosis, but cases of spontaneous recovery are so rare that it is difficult to mention the possibility to a patient with ALS. The reversible syndrome may be one of lower motor neurons alone or may include the full picture of ALS. Many patients are younger than 30, but some are older.

10. The syndrome of *benign fasciculation and cramps* is virtually restricted to medical students, physicians, and other medical workers because they are the only people in society who know the malignant implications of fasciculating muscles. The syndrome can be called the *Denny-Brown, Foley syndrome* after the discoverers. The condition has been rediscovered several times and given other names. The origin is not known, but because neither weakness nor wasting occurs, it is not ALS. In theory, ALS should sometimes start with this syndrome. For reasons unknown, however, it almost never does; only one case has been reasonably documented.

Treatment

Sadly, there is no effective drug therapy for ALS. Therapeutic trials have shown no benefit from immunosuppression, immunoenhancement, plasmapheresis, lymph node irradiation, glutamate antagonists, nerve growth factors, antiviral agents, and numerous other categories of drugs. Riluzole (Rilutek), a glutamate inhibitor, is the only drug approved by the U.S. Food and Drug Administration for the treatment of ALS. It is said to prolong life by 3 to 6 months but has no visible effect on function or quality of life. Treatment is therefore symptomatic, and emotional support is vitally important; management may be carried out most efficiently in an ALS center. Early in the course, patients should try to continue to perform routine activities as long as they can. There is difference of opinion about exercising weak muscles, but physical therapy can help maintain function as long as possible. Drooling of saliva (sialorrhea) may be helped by atropine sulfate, glycopyrrolate (Robinul), or amitriptyline. Dysphagia leads to percutaneous gastrostomy to maintain nutrition and to protect against aspiration. Antispastic agents have not been helpful in the spastic gait disorder, but intrathecal administration of baclofen (Lioresal) might be considered in a few patients.

The major decision concerns the use of tracheostomy and chronic mechanical ventilation, which can be done at home. In making the decision, patients should be informed fully about the long-term consequences of life without movement; they must decide whether they want to be kept alive or made as comfortable as possible—two choices that are not identical. Palliative care is emerging as a major option (see Chapter 165).

Immunosuppressive therapy, starting with intravenous immunoglobulin, is used for the few patients with lymphoproliferative disease, monoclonal gammopathy, conduction block, or high titers of antibodies to GM_1 or MAG. Chronic therapy with cyclophosphamide or fludarabine (Fludara) may follow.

In familial ALS, the question of presymptomatic diagnosis raises other ethical questions.

SUGGESTED READINGS

Spinal Muscular Atrophy

Biros I, Forrest S. Spinal muscular atrophy: untangling the knot? *J Med Genet* 1999;36:1–8.

Brzustowicz LM, Lehner T, Castilla LH, et al. Genetic mapping of chronic childhood-onset spinal muscular atrophy to chromosome 5q11.2-13.3. *Nature* 1990;344:540–541.

Crawford TO, Sladky JT, Hurko O, Besner-Johnson A, Kelley RJ. Abnormal fatty acid metabolism in childhood spinal muscular atrophy. *Ann Neurol* 1999;45:337–343.

Dubowitz V. Chaos in classification of the spinal muscular atrophies of childhood. *Neuromuscul Disord* 1991;1:77–80.

Gilliam TC, Brzustowicz LM, Castilla LH, et al. Genetic homogeneity between acute and chronic forms of spinal muscular atrophy. *Nature* 1990;345:823–825.

Lefebvre S, Burglen L, Frezal J, Munnich A, Melki J. The role of the SMN gene in proximal spinal muscular atrophy. *Hum Mol Genet* 1998;7:1531–1536.

McShane MA, Boyd S, Harding B, et al. Progressive bulbar paralysis of childhood: a reappraisal of Fazio-Londe disease. *Brain* 1992;115:1889–1900.

Melki J, LeFebvre S, Burglen L, et al. *De novo* and inherited deletions of the 5q13 region in spinal muscular atrophies. *Science* 1994;264:1474–1476.

Moulard B, Salachas F, Chassande B, et al. Association between centromeric deletions of the SMN gene and sporadic adult-onset lower motor neuron disease. *Ann Neurol* 1998;43:640–644.

Rowland LP. Molecular basis of genetic heterogeneity: role of the clinical neurologist. *J Child Neurol* 1998;13:122–132.

Rubi-Gozalbo ME, Smeitink JAM, Ruitenbeck W, et al. Spinal muscular atrophy-like picture, cardiomyopathy, and cytochrome-*c*-oxidase deficiency. *Neurology* 1999;52:383–386.

Stewart H, Wallace A, McGaughran J, Mountford R, Kingston H. Molecular diagnosis of spinal muscular atrophy. *Arch Dis Child* 1998;78:531–535.

Kennedy Disease

Fischbeck KH. Kennedy disease. *J Inherit Metab Dis* 1997;20:152–158.

Harding AE, Thomas PK, Baraister M, et al. X-linked bulbospinal neuronopathy: report of 10 cases. *J Neurol Neurosurg Psychiatry* 1982;45:1012–1019.

La Spada AR, Wilson EM, Lubahn DB, et al. Androgen receptor gene mutation in X-linked spinal and bulbar muscular atrophy. *Nature* 1991;352:77–79.

Li M, Miwa S, Kobayashi Y, et al. Nuclear inclusions of the androgen receptor protein in spinal and bulbar muscular atrophy. *Ann Neurol* 1998;44:249–254.

Merry DE, Kobayashi Y, Bailey CK, Taye AA, Fischbeck KH. Cleavage, aggregation and toxicity of the expanded androgen receptor in spinal and bulbar muscular atrophy. *Hum Mol Genet* 1998;7:693–701.

Paraboosingh JS, Figlwicz DA, Krizus A, et al. Spinobulbar muscular atrophy can mimic ALS: the importance of genetic testing in male patients with atypical ALS. *Neurology* 1997;49:568–572.

Shaw PJ, Thagesen H, Tomkins J, et al. Kennedy's disease: unusual molecular pathologic and clinical features. *Neurology* 1998;51:252–255.

Trojaborg W, Wulff CH. X-linked bulbospinal neuronopathy (Kennedy's syndrome): a neurophysiological study. *Acta Neurol Scand* 1994;89:214–219.

Amyotrophic Lateral Sclerosis

Armon C, Daube JR, Windebank AJ, Kurland LT. How frequently does classic amyotrophic lateral sclerosis develop in survivors of poliomyelitis? *Neurology* 1990;40:172–174.

Belsh JM, Schiffman MG, eds. *Amyotrophic lateral sclerosis.* Armonk NY: Futura Publishing, 1996.

Ben Hamida M, Hentati F, Hamida CB. Hereditary motor system disease (chronic juvenile amyotrophic lateral sclerosis). *Brain* 1990;113:347–363.

Blexrud MD, Windebank AJ, Daube JR. Long-term follow-up of 121 patients with benign fasciculations. *Ann Neurol* 1993;34:622–625.

Bonduelle M. Amyotrophic lateral sclerosis. In: Vinken PJ, Bruyn GW, de Jong JMBV, eds. *System disorders and atrophies. Handbook of clinical neurology, vol 22.* Amsterdam: North-Holland Publishing Co, 1975:281–338.

Boothby J, DeJesus PV, Rowland LP. Reversible forms of motor neuron disease: lead "neuritis." *Arch Neurol* 1974;31:18–23.

Borchelt DR, Wong PC, Sisodia SS, Price DL. Transgenic mouse models of Alzheimer's disease and amyotrophic lateral sclerosis. *Brain Pathol* 1998;8:735–757.

Bradley WG, Tobison SH, Tandan R, Besser D. Post-radiation motor neuron syndromes. *Adv Neurol* 1991;56:341–356.

Brown RH Jr. Amyotrophic lateral sclerosis and the inherited motor neuron diseases. In Martin JB, ed. *Scientific American molecular neurology.* New York: Scientific American, 1998:223–238.

Brownell B, Trevor-Hughes J. Central nervous system in motor neuron disease. *J Neurol Neurosurg Psychiatry* 1970;33:338–357.

Bruyn GW. Progressive bulbar palsy in adults. In: Vinken PJ, Bruyn GW, Klawans HL, de Jong JMBV, eds *Diseases of the motor system. Handbook of clinical neurology, vol 59.* New York: Elsevier Science 1991:217–229.

Chaudry V, Corse AM, Cornblath DR, et al. Multifocal motor neuropathy: response to human immune globulin. *Ann Neurol* 1993;33:237–242.

Cornblath DR, Kuncl RW, Mellits D, et al. Nerve conduction studies in amyotrophic lateral sclerosis. *Muscle Nerve* 1992;15:1111–1115.

Dalakas MC, Elder G, Hallet M, et al. A long-term follow-up study of patients with post-poliomyelitis neuromuscular symptoms. *N Engl J Med* 1986;314:959–963.

DeCarolis P, Montagna P, Cipiuli M, et al. Isolated lower motor neuron involvement following radiotherapy. *J Neurol Neurosurg Psychiatry* 1986;48:718–719.

Eisen A, Krieger S, eds. *Amyotrophic lateral sclerosis: a synthesis of research and clinical practice.* New York: Cambridge University Press, 1998.

Ellis CM, Simmons A, Andrews C, Dawson JM, Williams SC, Leigh PN. A proton magnetic resonance spectroscopic study in ALS: correlation with clinical findings. *Neurology* 1998;51:1104–1109.

Evans BK, Fagan C, Arnold T, et al. Paraneoplastic motor neuron disease and renal cell carcinoma. *Neurology* 1990;40:960–963.

Forsyth PA, Dalmau J, Graus F, Cwik V, Rosenblum MK, Posner JB. Motor neuron syndromes in cancer patients. *Ann Neurol* 1997;41:722–730.

Gordon PH, Rowland LP, Younger DS, et al. Lymphoproliferative disorders and motor neuron disease. *Neurology* 1997;48:1671–1678.

Ince PG, Lowe J, Shaw PJ. Amyotrophic lateral sclerosis: current issues in the classification, pathogenesis, and molecular pathology. *Neuropathol Appl Neurobiol* 1998;24:104–117.

Jubelt B. Motor neuron diseases and viruses: poliovirus, retroviruses, and lymphomas. *Curr Opin Neurol Neurosurg* 1992;5:655–658.

Kaji R, Oka N, Tsuji T, et al. Pathological findings at the site of conduction block in multifocal motor neuropathy. *Ann Neurol* 1993;33:152–158.

Kaji R, Shibasaki H, Kimura J. Multifocal demyelinating motor neuropathy: cranial nerve involvement and immunoglobulin therapy. *Neurology* 1992;42:506–509.

Kuroda Y, Sugihara H. Autopsy report of HTLV-1-associated myelopathy presenting with ALS-like manifestations. *J Neurol Sci* 1991;106:199–205.

Kurtzke JF. Risk factors in amyotrophic lateral sclerosis. *Adv Neurol* 1991;56:245–270.

Lange DJ, McDonald TD, Trojaborg W, Blake DM. Persistent and transient "conduction block" in motor neuron diseases. *Muscle Nerve* 1993;16:896–903.

Lange DJ, Trojaborg W, Latov N, et al. Multifocal motor neuropathy with conduction block: is it a distinct clinical entity? *Neurology* 1992;42:497–505.

Latov N. Antibodies to glycoconjugates in neurologic disease. *Clin Aspect Autoimmun* 1990;4:18–29.

Lawyer T, Netsky MG. Amyotrophic lateral sclerosis: clinico-anatomic study of 53 cases. *Arch Neurol Psychiatry* 1953;69:171–192.

Lin CL, Bristol LA, Jin L, et al. Aberrant RNA processing in a neurodegenerative disease: the cause for absent EAAT2, a glutamate transporter, in ALS. *Neuron* 1998;20:589–602.

Malapert D, Brugieres P, Degos JD. Motor neuron syndrome in the arms after radiation treatment. *J Neurol Neurosurg Psychiatry* 1991;54:1123–1124.

Martyn CN. Poliovirus and motor neuron disease. *J Neurol* 1990;237:336–358.

Matherson L, Barrau K, Blin O. Disease management: the example of amyotrophic lateral sclerosis. *J Neurol* 1998;245[Suppl 2]:S20–S28.

Mitsumoto H, Chad DA, Piro EP, eds. *Amyotrophic lateral sclerosis.* Philadephia: FA Davis Co, 1998.

Moss AH, Case P, Stocking CB, et al. Home ventilation for amyotrophic lateral sclerosis patients: outcomes, costs, and patient, family, and physician attitudes. *Neurology* 1993;43:438–443.

Munsat TL. *Post-polio syndrome.* Boston: Butterworth-Heinemann, 1991.

Norris F, Shepher R, Denys E, et al. Onset, natural history, and outcome in idiopathic adult motor neuron disease. *J Neurol Sci* 1993;118:48–55.

Pestronk A, Cornblath DR, Ilyas AA, et al. A treatable multifocal motor neuropathy with antibodies to GM1 ganglioside. *Ann Neurol* 1988;24:73–78.

Rosen DR, Siddique T, Patterson D, et al. Mutations in Cu/Zn superoxide dismutase gene are associated with familial amyotrophic lateral sclerosis. *Nature* 1993;362:59–62.

Rosenfeld MR, Posner JB. Paraneoplastic motor neuron disease. *Adv Neurol* 1991;56:445–463.

Rothstein JD, Martin LJ, Kuncl RW. Decreased glutamate transport by the brain and spinal cord in amyotrophic lateral sclerosis. *N Engl J Med* 1992;326:1464–1468.

Rowland LP, ed. *Amyotrophic lateral sclerosis and other motor neuron diseases.* New York: Raven Press, 1991.

Rowland LP. Ten central themes in a decade of ALS research. *Adv Neurol* 1991;56:3–23.

Rowland LP. Surgical treatment of cervical spondylotic myelopathy: time for a controlled trial. *Neurology* 1992;42:5–13.

Rowland LP. Diagnosis of amyotrophic lateral sclerosis. *J Neurol Sci* 1998;160[Suppl 1]:S6–S24.

Santoro M, Thomas FP, Fink ME, et al. IgM deposits at nodes of Ranvier in a patient with amyotrophic lateral sclerosis, anti-GM1 antibodies, and multifocal conduction block. *Ann Neurol* 1990;28:373–377.

Serratrice G. Spinal monomelic amyotrophy. *Adv Neurol* 1991;56:169–173.

Smith RG, Hamilton S, Hofmann F, et al. Serum antibodies to L-type calcium channels in patients with ALS. *N Engl J Med* 1992;327:1721–1728.

Smith RG, Henry YK, Mattson MP, Appel SH. Presence of 4-hydroxynonenal in cerebrospinal fluid of patients with sporadic amyotrophic lateral sclerosis. *Ann Neurol* 1998;44:696–699.

Smith RG, Siklos L, Alexianu ME, et al. Autoimmunity and ALS. *Neurology* 1996[Suppl 2]:S40–S46.

Tucker T, Layzer RB, Miller RG, Chad D. Subacute reversible motor neuron disease. *Neurology* 1991;41:1541–1544.

Vinken PJ, Bruyn GW, Klawans HL, DeJong JMBV, eds. *Diseases of the motor system. Handbook of clinical neurology, vol 59.* New York: Elsevier Science, 1991.

Merritt's Neurology, 10th ed., edited by L.P. Rowland. Lippincott Williams & Wilkins, Philadelphia © 2000.

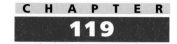

SYRINGOMYELIA

ELLIOTT L. MANCALL
PAUL C. MCCORMICK

Cavitation within the spinal cord was first described by Esteinne in 1546 in *La dissection du corps humain*. Ollivier D'Angers applied the term *syringomyelia* in 1827. This term connotes a chronic, progressive disorder that most often involves the spinal cord. The exact incidence of syringomyelia is not known, but it is rare. It occurs more frequently in men than in women. Familial cases have been described. The disease usually appears in the third or fourth decade of life, with a mean age at onset of about 30 years. It is rare in childhood or late-adult years. Syringomyelia usually progresses slowly; the course extends over many years. An acute course may be evident when the brainstem is affected (*syringobulbia*).

Syringomyelia rarely occurs *de novo* or in isolation, but usually arises as a result of an associated anomaly. Over two-thirds of cases of syringomyelia are associated with the Arnold-Chiari malformation. Less commonly, a variably sized syringomyelic cavity, or syrinx, may be found within or in proximity to an intramedullary tumor, generally a glioma. Syringomyelia may also be a late consequence of spinal cord trauma, arising *ex vacuo* after absorption of an intramedullary hematoma (*hematomyelia*). In about 5% of patients with spinal cord injury, the delayed onset of an ascending spinal cord syndrome is caused by an expanding syrinx. Cerebrospinal fluid (CSF) circulation may be impaired by dense arachnoiditis at the site of the trauma, thereby causing the delayed formation of a syrinx on an ischemic basis.

CLINICAL MANIFESTATIONS

Symptoms depend primarily on the location of the lesion, Milhorat and his colleagues have isolated several individual cavitary patterns, each producing a more or less distinctive clinical appearance. The syrinx is most commonly encountered in the lower cervical region, particularly at the base of the posterior horn, extending into the central gray matter and anterior commissure. The cyst interrupts the decussating spinothalamic fibers that mediate pain and temperature sensibility, resulting in loss of these sensations; light touch, vibratory sense, and position sense are relatively preserved, at least early in the disease, by virtue of sparing of the posterior columns. This pattern of loss of cutaneous sensibility with preservation of posterior column sensory modalities is commonly referred to as *dissociated sensory loss*. Pain and temperature sensations are typically impaired in the arm on the involved side, sometimes in both arms or in a shawl-like distribution (*en cuirasse*) across the shoulders and upper torso, front and back. When the cavity enlarges to involve the posterior columns, there is loss of position and vibratory sense in the feet,

and astereognosis may be noted in the hands. Extension of the lesion into the anterior horns with loss of motor neurons causes amyotrophy that begins in the small muscles of the hands (*brachial amyotrophy*), ascends to the forearms, and ultimately affects the shoulder girdle. The hand may be strikingly atrophied, with the development of a claw-hand deformity (*main en griffe*). Weakness appears in the hands, forearms, and shoulder girdle, and fasciculations may be seen. Because the syrinx is asymmetrically placed early in its development, manifestations in the arms and hands tend to be similarly asymmetric. Muscle stretch reflexes in the arms are characteristically lost early. As the syrinx extends into the lateral columns, spasticity appears in the legs, with paraparesis, hyperreflexia, and extensor plantar responses. Impairment of bowel and bladder functions may be a late manifestation. A Horner syndrome may appear, reflecting damage to the sympathetic neurons in the intermediolateral cell column.

Pain, generally deep and aching in quality, is sometimes experienced and may be severe. It involves the neck and shoulders or follows a radicular distribution in the arms or trunk.

The syrinx sometimes ascends into the medulla. Syringobulbia is evidenced by dysphagia, pharyngeal and palatal weakness, asymmetric weakness and atrophy of the tongue, sensory loss involving primarily pain and temperature sense in the distribution of the trigeminal nerve, and nystagmus. Signs of cerebellar dysfunction may appear. Rarely, the syrinx extends even higher in the brainstem or into the centrum semiovale as a *syringocephalus*.

Many other clinical abnormalities are evident. Scoliosis is characteristically seen, and neurogenic arthropathies (*Charcot joints*) may affect the shoulder, elbow, or wrist. Acute painful enlargement of the shoulder may appear and is associated with destruction of the head of the humerus. Painless ulcers of the hands are frequent. The hands are occasionally the site of remarkable subcutaneous edema and hyperhidrosis (*main succulente*), presumably caused by interruption of central autonomic pathways.

A cyst sometimes develops in the lumbar cord either in association with or independent of a cervical syrinx. Lumbar syringomyelia is characterized by atrophy of proximal and distal leg muscles with dissociated sensory loss in lumbar and sacral dermatomes. Stretch reflexes are lost in the legs; impairment of sphincter function is common. The plantar responses are ordinarily flexor.

PATHOLOGY AND PATHOGENESIS

As emphasized by Greenfield, syringomyelia may be defined as a tubular cavitation of the spinal cord, usually beginning within the cervical cord and generally extending over many segments. Syringomyelia should be regarded as distinct from simple cystic expansion of the central canal of the cord; the term *hydromyelia* is more appropriately applied to that condition. The syrinx may communicate with the central canal, and ependymal cells occasionally line the wall of the syrinx. The fluid within the cyst is similar to, if not identical with, CSF. The syrinx may be limited to the cervical cord or may extend the length of the cord; it tends to vary in transverse diameter from segment to segment, usually achieving maximal extent in the cervical and lumbosacral enlargements. Originally confined to the base of a posterior horn or to the anterior commissure, the cyst slowly enlarges to involve much of both gray and white matter; at times, only a narrow rim of cord parenchyma can be identified histologically. The cyst itself is surrounded by a dense glial fibril wall. Extension of the cavity into the medulla or, rarely, higher within the neuraxis may be noted. Developmental abnormalities in the cervical spine and at the base of the skull, such as platybasia, are common. Features of the Arnold-Chiari malformation, such as displacement of the cerebellar tonsils into the cervical canal, are often identified. Hydrocephalus is frequent, and cerebellar hypoplasia may be found. In a few patients, ependymoma or astrocytoma of the spinal cord is encountered, usually in juxtaposition with the syrinx itself.

The pathogenesis of syringomyelia is uncertain. Following Gardner, it is widely held that most cases of syringomyelia are of a "communicating" variety. Dilatation of the central canal is attributed to CSF pulsations directed downward from the fourth ventricle because the foramina of exit are occluded by a developmental defect in the rhombic roof or other anomalies of the medullocervical junction. According to this hydrodynamic theory, obstruction or atresia of the normal outlets of the fourth ventricle is essential; in most cases, the ventricular obstruction is associated with features of the Arnold-Chiari malformation and, often, with hydrocephalus. As a modification of Gardner's theory, Boulay and associates emphasized systolic excursions of CSF in the basal cisterns in the formation of the cystic cavity.

Alternatively, Williams proposed that the Arnold-Chiari malformation is an acquired anomaly that results from excessive molding of the head during difficult, usually high forceps, delivery. A ball-valve effect of the cerebellar tonsils in the foramen magnum could create a dissociation between cranial and spinal CSF pressures, particularly during Valsalva maneuvers, which in turn could lead to syrinx formation. Both the Gardner and Williams hypotheses are challenged by the evidence cited by Milhorat and associates to the effect that most syrinx cavities do not in fact communicate with the fourth ventricle; caudal flow of CSF from the fourth ventricle into the central canal cannot therefore be considered the explanation for the appearance of a syrinx with a lesion of the hindbrain.

In the traditional nomenclature of Greenfield, distention of the central canal is therefore designated *hydromyelia,* with the term *syringomyelia* reserved for a noncommunicating cyst. From this perspective, and in keeping with the observations of Milhorat, the syringomyelic cavity cannot be considered part of the ventricular system in what is essentially a persistent embryonic configuration; rather it is an independent development. As already stressed, noncommunicating syrinx has been attributed to several factors, including extension of CSF under pressure along the Virchow-Robin spaces, cystic degeneration of an intramedullary glioma, and ischemia with cyst formation secondary to arachnoiditis caused by meningitis or subarachnoid hemorrhage with resultant insufficiency of blood flow in the anterior spinal artery. A syrinx may also develop after spinal cord trauma either soon after resorption of an intramedullary hematoma (*hematomyelia*) or as a delayed phenomenon after cord contusion or compression with microcystic cavitation. Birth trauma may be important in the development of syringomyelia.

In the last analysis, the distinction between communicating and noncommunicating forms of syringomyelia may be artificial; the term *syringohydromyelia* has been suggested as a more inclusive term. Most instances of syringomyelia do seem to fall into the Gardner communicating variety, although the precise pathogenetic mechanisms remain incompletely understood. In some individuals, the original communication with the fourth ventricle may have been obliterated with time, resulting in the spurious appearance of a noncommunicating configuration.

LABORATORY DATA

CSF ordinarily demonstrates few abnormalities. CSF pressure is sometimes elevated, and complete subarachnoid block may be noted. The cell count is only rarely more than $10/mm^3$. A mild elevation of CSF protein content occurs in 50% of patients; in presence of subarachnoid block, CSF protein may exceed 100 mg/dL.

Magnetic resonance imaging (MRI) is the diagnostic procedure of choice for the diagnosis and evaluation of syringomyelia. Cystic enlargement of the spinal cord extends over several segments (Fig. 119.1). The signal intensity of the cyst is generally similar to that of CSF. The cyst margins are often irregular and may demonstrate periodic folds or septations that may result from turbulent flow within the cavity. If syringomyelia is identified on MRI, further evaluation should include MRI of the brain and craniovertebral junction to identify associated anomalies, such as hydrocephalus or an Arnold-Chiari malformation. If syringomyelia occurs without an Arnold-Chiari malformation or prior spinal cord injury, a complete spinal MRI with gadolinium is performed to rule out an intramedullary spinal cord tumor. Myelography and computed tomography (CT) are rarely used for the diagnosis or evaluation of syringomyelia. Plain films and CT may be useful in consideration of bony anomalies that commonly occur at the craniovertebral junction in patients with hindbrain abnormalities.

DIFFERENTIAL DIAGNOSIS

Amyotrophic lateral sclerosis (ALS) commonly causes weakness, atrophy, and reflex loss in the arms that is often asymmetric, with heightened reflexes and extensor-plantar responses in the legs. Sensory loss, however, does not occur in ALS. Multiple sclerosis (MS) may mimic syringomyelia. Early atrophy of hand muscles, however, does not occur in MS, and the lack of evidence of dissemination of lesions elsewhere argues against this diagnosis. MRI of brain and spinal cord separates MS and syringomyelia. Intrinsic tumors of the spinal cord may produce clinical signs similar to those of syringomyelia. Again, MRI generally distinguishes the two. MRI also differentiates syringomyelia from cervical spondylosis. Anomalies of the craniovertebral junction and cervical ribs may also cause symptoms reminiscent of syringomyelia; because both may be associated with true syringomyelia, identification of these abnormalities is not sufficient to exclude cavitation within the spinal cord.

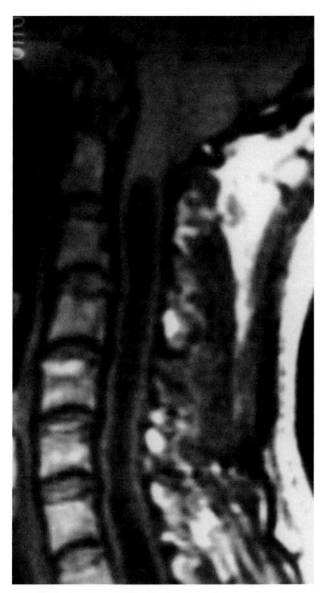

FIG. 119.1. Sagittal T1-weighted MRI shows a large syrinx. Note the associated Arnold-Chiari malformation with cerebellar tonsillar herniation below the foramen magnum. Decompression of the foramen magnum usually results in resolution of the syrinx.

TREATMENT

The treatment of syringomyelia consists of either drainage of the syrinx cavity or correction of the abnormal dynamics that allowed the syrinx to develop. In tumor-associated syringomyelia, for example, removal of the mass nearly always results in resolution of the syrinx. Syringomyelia arising as a late consequence of spinal cord trauma usually requires direct drainage because the dense arachnoiditis at the level of the trauma generally cannot be corrected. Simple drainage can consist of either percutaneous needle aspiration or open syringotomy. These maneuvers provide temporary relief at best, and the cavity usually reexpands because of spontaneous closure of the syringotomy and persistence of the filling mechanism. Prolonged successful drainage usually requires the insertion through laminectomy of a small Silastic tube directly

into the syrinx cavity. The other end of the catheter is placed in either the pleural or the peritoneal space, thereby allowing continuous drainage of the syrinx into a cavity of lower pressure.

Management of syringomyelia that occurs in association with an Arnold-Chiari malformation is more complicated. Ventriculoperitoneal shunting is generally performed initially if significant hydrocephalus is present. In the absence of hydrocephalus or if the ventriculoperitoneal shunt fails to relieve symptoms, a posterior fossa decompression with or without simultaneous shunting of the syrinx can be performed. The posterior fossa decompression consists of a wide suboccipital craniectomy and cervical laminectomy with duraplasty to enlarge the foramen magnum effectively. Plugging of the obex with muscle or the placement of a Silastic stent into the fourth ventricle to improve the CSF outflow into the basal cisterns and subarachnoid space may also be performed, but each is controversial. In most patients, adequate posterior fossa decompression results in shrinkage or even resolution of the syrinx. In refractory cases, a direct syrinx shunt may be placed.

SUGGESTED READINGS

Barnett HJM, Foster JB, Hudgson P. *Syringomyelia*. Philadelphia: WB Saunders, 1973.

Batzdorf U, Klekamp J, Johnson JP. A critical appraisal of syrinx cavity shunting procedures. *J Neurosurg* 1998;89:382–388.

Berry RG, Chambers RA, Lublin FD. Syringoencephalomyelia (syringocephalus). *J Neuropathol Exp Neurol* 1981;40:633–644.

Caplan LR, Norohna AB, Amico LL. Syringomyelia and arachnoiditis. *J Neurol Neurosurg Psychiatry* 1990;53:106–113.

Del Bigio MR, Deck JHN, MacDonald JK. Syrinx extending from conus medullaris to basal ganglia: a clinical, radiological, and pathological correlation. *Can J Neurol Sci* 1993;20:240–246.

Donauer E, Rascher K. Syringomyelia: a brief review of ontogenetic, experimental and clinical aspects. *Neurosurg Rev* 1993;16:7–13.

Dyste GN, Menezes AH, VanGilder JC. Symptomatic Chiari malformations: an analysis of presentation, management, and long-term outcome. *J Neurosurg* 1989;71:159–168.

Fischbein NJ, Dillon WP, Cobbs C, Weinstein PR. The "presyrinx state": a reversible myelopathic condition that may precede syringomyelia. *AJNR* 1999;20:7–20.

Gardner WH, McMurry FG. "Non-communicating" syringomyelia: a nonexistent entity. *Surg Neurol* 1976;6:251–256.

Gardner WJ. Hydrodynamic mechanism of syringomyelia: its relationship to myelocele. *J Neurol Neurosurg Psychiatry* 1965;28:247–259.

Goldstein JH, Kaptain GJ, Do HM, Cloft HJ, Jane JA Sr, Phillips CD. CT-guided percutaneous drainage of syringomyelia. *J Comput Assist Tomogr* 1998;22:984–988.

Graham DI, Lantos PL, eds. *Greenfields neuropathology*, vol. 1, 6th ed. Edward Arnold, 1997:486–490.

Haponik EF, Givens D, Angelo J. Syringobulbia-myelia with obstructive sleep apnea. *Neurology* 1983;33:1046–1049.

Hodge C, Jones M. Syringomyelia and spinal cord tumors. *Curr Opin Neurol Neurosurg* 1991;4:597–600.

Igbal JB, Bradey N, Macfaul R, Cameron MM. Syringomyelia in children: six case reports and review of the literature. *Br J Neurosurg* 1992;6:13–20.

Isu T, Susaki H, Takamura H, Kobayashi N. Foramen magnum decompression with removal of the outer layer of the dura as treatment for syringomyelia occurring with Chiari I malformation. *Neurosurgery* 1993;33:844–849.

Jones J, Wolf S. Neuropathic shoulder arthropathy (Charcot joint) associated with syringomyelia. *Neurology* 1998;50:825–827.

Keung YK, Cobos E, Whitehead RP, et al. Secondary syringomyelia due to intramedullary spinal cord metastasis: case report and review of literature. *Am J Clin Oncol* 1997;20:577–579.

Mariani C, Cislaghi MG, Barbieri S, et al. The natural history and results of surgery in 50 cases of syringomyelia. *J Neurol* 1991;238:433–438.

Milhorat, TH, Capocelli, AL, Anzil, AP, et al. Pathological basis of spinal cord cavitation in syringomyelia: analysis of 105 autopsy cases. *J Neurosurg* 1995;82;802–812.

Milhorat TH, Johnson WD, Miller JI, et al. Surgical treatment of syringomyelia based on magnetic resonance imaging criteria. *Neurosurgery* 1992;31:231–244.

Milhorat TH, Miller JI, Johnson WD, et al. Anatomical basis of syringomyelia occurring with hindbrain lesions. *Neurosurgery* 1993;32;748–754.

Oldfield EH, Muraszko K, Shawker TH, Patronas NJ. Pathophysiology of syringomyelia associated with Chiari I malformation of the cerebellar tonsils: implications for diagnosis and treatment. *J Neurosurg* 1994;80:3–15.

Pillay PK, Awad IA, Hahn JF. Gardner's hydrodynamic theory of syringomyelia revisited. *Cleve Clin J Med* 1992;59:373–380.

Poser CM. *The relationship between syringomyelia and neoplasm.* Springfield, IL: Charles C Thomas, 1956.

Sackellares JC, Swift TR. Shoulder enlargement as the presenting sign in syringomyelia. *JAMA* 1976;236:2878–2879.

Schurch B, Wichmann W, Rossier AB. Post-traumatic syringomyelia (cystic myelopathy): a prospective study of 449 patients with spinal cord injury. *J Neurol Neurosurg Psychiatry* 1996;60:61–67.

Vassilouthis J, Papandreou A, Anagnostaras S, Pappas J. Thecoperitoneal shunt for syringomyelia: report of three cases. *Neurosurgery* 1993;33:324–327.

Williams B. On the pathogenesis of syringomyelia: a review. *J R Soc Med* 1980;73:798–806.

Williams B. Post-traumatic syringomyelia, an update. *Paraplegia* 1990;28:296–313.

Williams B. Syringomyelia. *Neurosurg Clin N Am* 1990;1:653–685.

Merritt's Neurology, 10th ed., edited by L.P. Rowland. Lippincott Williams & Wilkins, Philadelphia © 2000.

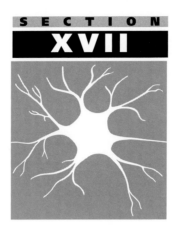

DISORDERS OF THE NEUROMUSCULAR JUNCTION

MYASTHENIA GRAVIS

AUDREY S. PENN
LEWIS P. ROWLAND

Myasthenia gravis (MG) is caused by a defect of neuromuscular transmission due to an antibody-mediated attack on nicotinic acetylcholine receptors (AchR) at neuromuscular junctions. It is characterized by fluctuating weakness that is improved by inhibitors of cholinesterase.

ETIOLOGY AND PATHOGENESIS

The pathogenesis of MG is related to the destructive effects of autoantibodies to AChR, as indicated by several lines of evidence:

1. In several species of animals, experimental immunization with AChR purified from the electric organ of the torpedo, an electric fish, induced high titers of antibody to the receptor. Overt evidence of weakness varies but may be uncovered by small doses of curare. Many animals also showed the essential electrophysiologic and pathologic features of human MG. This was first found in rabbits by Patrick and Lindstrom (1973).
2. Serum antibodies that react with human AChR are found in humans with MG.
3. Toyka and colleagues (1975) found that the electrophysiologic features of MG were reproduced by passive transfer of human immunoglobulin (Ig) G to mice. By analogy, human transient neonatal MG could then be explained by transplacental transfer of maternal antibody.
4. Pinching found that plasmapheresis reduced plasma levels of anti-AChR and ameliorated MG symptoms and signs.

The polyclonal IgG antibodies to AChR are produced by plasma cells in peripheral lymphoid organs, bone marrow, and thymus. These cells are derived from B cells that have been activated by antigen-specific T-helper (CD4+) cells. The T-cells have also been activated, in this case by binding to AChR antigenic peptide sequences (epitopes) that rest within the histocompatibility antigens on the surface of antigen-presenting cells.

The AChR antibodies react with multiple determinants, and enough antibody circulates to saturate up to 80% of all AChR sites on muscle. A small percentage of the anti-AChR molecules interfere directly with the binding of ACh, but the major damage to endplates seems to result from actual loss of receptors due to complement-mediated lysis of the membrane and to acceleration of normal degradative processes (internalization, endocytosis, lysosomal hydrolysis) with inadequate replacement by new synthesis. As a consequence of the loss of AChR and the erosion and simplification of the endplates, the amplitude of miniature endplate potentials is about 20% of normal, and patients are abnormally sensitive to the competitive antagonist curare. The characteristic decremental response to repetitive stimulation of the motor nerve reflects failure of endplate potentials to reach threshold so that progressively fewer fibers respond to arrival of a nerve impulse.

How the autoimmune disorder starts is not known. In human disease, in contrast to experimental MG in animals, the thymus gland is almost always abnormal; there are often multiple lymphoid follicles with germinal centers ("hyperplasia of the thymus"), and in about 15% of patients, there is an encapsulated benign tumor, a thymoma. These abnormalities are impressive because the normal thymus is responsible for the maturation of T-cells that mediate immune protection without promoting autoimmune responses. AChR antibodies are synthesized by B cells in cultures of hyperplastic thymus gland. The hyperplastic glands contain all the elements needed for antibody production: class II HLA-positive antigen-presenting cells, T-helper cells, B cells, and AChR antigen; that is, messenger ribonucleic acid for subunits of AChR has been detected in thymus, and "myoid cells" are found in both normal and hyperplastic thymus. The myoid cells bear surface AChR and contain other muscle proteins. When human myasthenic thymus was transplanted into severely congenitally immunodeficient mice, the animals produced antibodies to AChR that bound to their own motor endplates, even though weakness was not evident.

Excessive and inappropriately prolonged synthesis of thymic hormones that normally promote differentiation of T-helper cells may contribute to the autoimmune response. Still another possible initiating factor is immunogenic alteration of the antigen, AChR, at endplates, because penicillamine therapy in patients with rheumatoid arthritis may initiate a syndrome that is indistinguishable from MG except that it subsides when administration of the drug is stopped.

There are few familial cases of the disease, but disproportionate frequency of some HLA haplotypes (B8, DR3, DQB1) in MG patients suggests that genetic predisposition may be important. Other autoimmune diseases also seem to occur with disproportionate frequency in patients with MG, especially hyperthyroidism and other thyroid disorders, systemic lupus erythematosus, rheumatoid arthritis, pernicious anemia, and pemphigus.

Most AChR antibodies are directed against antigenic determinants other than the ACh binding site. Nevertheless, the summed effects of the polyclonal anti-AChR antibodies with differing modes of action result in destruction of the receptors. Physiologic studies indicate impaired postsynaptic responsiveness to ACh, which accounts for the physiologic abnormalities, clinical symptoms, and beneficial effects of drugs that inhibit acetylcholinesterase.

SPECIAL FORMS OF MYASTHENIA GRAVIS
Juvenile and Adult Forms

Typical MG may begin at any age, but it is most common in the second to fourth decades. It is less frequent before age 10 or after age 65 years. Circulating AChR antibodies are demonstrated in 85% to 90% of patients with generalized MG and 50% to 60% of those with restricted ocular myasthenia. Patients without antibodies do not differ clinically or in response to immunotherapy; this seronegative MG may be more common in patients who are symptomatic before puberty. These are the typical forms of MG; other forms are rare.

Neonatal Myasthenia

About 12% of infants born to myasthenic mothers have a syndrome characterized by impaired sucking, weak cry, limp limbs, and, exceptionally, respiratory insufficiency. Symptoms begin in the first 48 hours and may last several days or weeks, after which the children are normal. The mothers are usually symptomatic but may be in complete remission; in either case, AChR antibodies are demonstrable in both mother and child. Symptoms disappear as the antibody titer in the infant declines. Severe respiratory insufficiency may be treated by exchange transfusion, but the natural history of the disorder is progressive improvement and total disappearance of all symptoms within days or weeks. Respiratory support and nutrition are the key elements of treatment. Rare instances of arthrogryposis multiplex congenita have been attributed to transplacental transfer of antibodies that inhibit fetal AChR.

Congenital Myasthenia

Children with congenital MG, although rarely encountered, show several characteristics. The mothers are asymptomatic and do not have circulating anti-AChR in the blood. Usually, no problem occurs in the neonatal period; instead, ophthalmoplegia is the dominant sign in infancy. Limb weakness may be evident. The condition is often familial. Antibodies to AChR are not found, but there are decremental responses to repetitive stimulation. Ultrastructural and biochemical examination of motor endplates, microelectrode analysis, and identification of mutations have delineated a series of disorders that include both presynaptic and postsynaptic proteins. Disorders of the ion channel formed by the AChR molecule include the *slow-channel syndrome,* in which the response to ACh is enhanced because the opening episodes of the channel are abnormally prolonged. Forearm extensors tend to be selectively weak. More than 11 different mutations have been identified in different AChR subunits. Quinidine shortens the prolonged openings and gives therapeutic benefit. A *fast-channel syndrome,* with impaired response to ACh has been reported in rare patients with mutations of the epsilon subunit. Another mutation in the same subunit leads to *abnormal kinetics of AChR activation* so that the channel opens more slowly and closes more rapidly than normal. The 24 known mutations in the epsilon subunit are inherited recessively and result in severe *lack of AChR in the endplates.* One syndrome results from mutations in the collagen tail subunit of the enzyme, creating *deficiency of acetylcholinesterase.* These landmark observations were made at the Mayo Clinic by Andrew G. Engel and his colleagues. Anticholinesterase drugs may help in some of these disorders, but parents should be warned that sudden apneic spells may be induced by mild infections.

Drug-induced Myasthenia

The best example of this condition occurs in patients treated with penicillamine for rheumatoid arthritis, scleroderma, or hepatolenticular degeneration (Wilson disease). The clinical manifestations and AChR antibody titers are similar to those of typical adult MG, but both disappear when drug administration is discontinued. Cases attributed to trimethadione (Tridione) have been less thoroughly studied.

PATHOLOGY

The overt pathology of MG is found primarily in the thymus gland. About 70% of thymus glands from adult patients with MG are not involuted and weigh more than normal. The glands show lymphoid hyperplasia: In normal individuals, germinal centers are numerous in lymph nodes and spleen but are sparse in the thymus. Immunocytochemical methods indicate that these thymic germinal centers contain B cells, plasma cells, HLA class II DR-positive T cells, and interdigitating cells.

Another 10% of myasthenic thymus glands contain thymomas of the lymphoepithelial type. The lymphoid cells in these tumors are T cells; the neoplastic elements are epithelial cells. Benign thymomas may nearly replace the gland, with only residual glandular material at the edges, or they may rest within a large hyperplastic gland. Thymomas tend to occur in older patients, but in Castleman's series, 15% were found in patients between ages 20 and 29 years. They may invade contiguous pleura, pericardium, or blood vessels, or seed onto more distant thoracic structures, including the diaphragm; however, they almost never spread to other organs. In older patients without thymoma, thymus gland appears involuted, often showing hyperplastic foci within fatty tissue on microscopic examination of multiple samples.

In about 50% of cases, muscles contain *lymphorrhages,* which are focal clusters of lymphocytes near small necrotic foci without perivascular predilection. In a few cases, especially in patients with thymoma, there is diffuse muscle fiber necrosis with infiltration of inflammatory cells; similar lesions are rarely encountered in the myocardium. Lymphorrhages are not seen near damaged neuromuscular junctions (although inflammatory cells may be seen in necrotic endplates in rat experimental autoimmune MG), but morphometric studies have shown loss of synaptic folds and widened clefts. Some nerve terminals are smaller than normal, and multiple small terminals are applied to the elongated, simplified postsynaptic membrane; others are absent. Other endplates appear normal. On residual synaptic folds, immunocytochemical methods show Y-shaped antibody-like structures, IgG, complement components 2 and 9, and complement membrane attack complex.

INCIDENCE

MG is a common disease. An apparent increase in the incidence of the disease in recent years is probably due to improved diagnosis. According to Phillips and Torner (1996), the prevalence rate is 14 per 100,000 (or about 17,000 cases) in the United States. Before age 40 years, the disease is three times more common in women, but at older ages both sexes are equally affected.

Familial cases are rare; single members of pairs of fraternal twins and several sets of identical twins have been affected. Young women with MG tend to have HLA-B8, -DR3, and -DQB1* 0102 haplotypes; in young Japanese women HLA-A12 is prominent. These observations imply the presence of a linked immune response gene that encodes a protein involved in the autoimmune response. First-degree relatives show an unusual incidence of other autoimmune diseases (systemic lupus erythematosus, rheumatoid arthritis, thyroid disease) and HLA-B8 haplotype.

SYMPTOMS

The symptoms of MG have three general characteristics that, together, provide a diagnostic combination. Formal diagnosis depends on demonstration of the response to cholinergic drugs, electrophysiologic evidence of abnormal neuromuscular transmission, and demonstration of circulating antibodies to AChR.

The fluctuating nature of myasthenic weakness is unlike any other disease. The weakness varies in the course of a single day, sometimes within minutes, and it varies from day to day or over longer periods. Major prolonged variations are termed *remissions* or *exacerbations;* when an exacerbation involves respiratory muscles to the point of inadequate ventilation, it is called a *crisis.* Variations sometimes seem related to exercise; this and the nature of the physiologic abnormality have long been termed "excessive fatigability," but there are practical reasons to deemphasize fatigability as a central characteristic of MG. Patients with the disease almost never complain of fatigue or symptoms that might be construed as fatigue except when there is incipient respiratory muscle weakness. Myasthenic symptoms are *always* due to weakness and not to rapid tiring. In contrast, patients who complain of fatigue, if they are not anemic or harboring a malignant tumor, almost always have emotional problems, usually depression.

The second characteristic of MG is the distribution of weakness. Ocular muscles are affected first in about 40% of patients and are ultimately involved in about 85%. Ptosis and diplopia are the symptoms that result. Other common symptoms affect facial or oropharyngeal muscles, resulting in dysarthria, dysphagia, and limitation of facial movements. Together, oropharyngeal and ocular weakness causes symptoms in virtually all patients with acquired MG. Limb and neck weakness is also common, but in conjunction with cranial weakness. Almost never are limbs affected alone.

Crisis seems most likely to occur in patients with oropharyngeal or respiratory muscle weakness. It seems to be provoked by respiratory infection in many patients or by surgical procedures, including thymectomy, although it may occur with no apparent provocation. Both emotional stress and systemic illness may aggravate myasthenic weakness for reasons that are not clear; in patients with oropharyngeal weakness, aspiration of secretions may occlude lung passages to cause rather abrupt onset of respiratory

difficulty. Major surgery may be followed by respiratory weakness without aspiration, however, so this cannot be the entire explanation. "Spontaneous" crisis seems to be less common now than it once was.

The third characteristic of myasthenic weakness is the clinical response to cholinergic drugs. This occurs so uniformly that it has become part of the definition, but it may be difficult to demonstrate in some patients, especially those with purely ocular myasthenia.

Aside from the fluctuating nature of the weakness, MG is not a steadily progressive disease. The general nature of the disease, however, is usually established within weeks or months after the first symptoms. If myasthenia is restricted to ocular muscles for 2 years, certainly if it is restricted after 3 years, it is likely to remain restricted, and only in rare cases does it then become generalized. (Solely ocular myasthenia differs serologically from generalized MG because AChR antibodies are found in lower frequency [50%] and in low titer.) Spontaneous remissions are also more likely to occur in the first 2 years.

Before the advent of intensive care units and the introduction of positive pressure respirators in the 1960s, crisis was a life-threatening event, and the mortality of the disease was about 25%. With improved respiratory care, however, patients rarely die of MG, except when cardiac, renal, or other disease complicates the picture.

SIGNS

The vital signs and general physical examination are usually within normal limits, unless the patient is in crisis. The findings on neurologic examination depend on the distribution of weakness. Weakness of the facial and levator palpebrae muscles produces a characteristic expressionless facies with drooping eyelids. Weakness of the ocular muscles may cause paralysis or weakness of isolated muscles, paralysis of conjugate gaze, complete ophthalmoplegia in one or both eyes, or a pattern resembling internuclear ophthalmoplegia. Weakness of oropharyngeal or limb muscles, when present, can be shown by appropriate tests. Respiratory muscle weakness can be detected by pulmonary function tests, which should not be limited to measurement of vital capacity but should also include inspiratory and expiratory pressures, the measurements of which may be abnormal even before overt symptoms exist. Muscular wasting of variable degree is found in about 10% of patients, but is not focal and is usually encountered only in patients with malnutrition due to severe dysphagia. Fasciculations do not occur, unless the patient has received excessive amounts of cholinergic drugs. Sensation is normal and the reflexes are preserved, even in muscles that are weak.

LABORATORY DATA

Routine examinations of blood, urine, and cerebrospinal fluid are normal. The characteristic electrodiagnostic abnormality is progressive decrement in the amplitude of muscle action potentials evoked by repetitive nerve stimulation at 3 or 5 Hz. In generalized MG, the decremental response can be demonstrated in about 90% of patients, if at least 3 nerve–muscle systems are used (median-thenar, ulnar-hypothenar, accessory-trapezius). In microelectrode study of intercostal muscle, the amplitude of miniature endplate potentials is reduced to about 20% of normal. This is caused by a decrease in the number of AChR available to agonists applied by microiontophoresis. In single-fiber electromyography (EMG), a small electrode measures the interval between evoked potentials of the muscle fibers in the same motor unit. This interval normally varies, a phenomenon called *jitter,* and the normal temporal limits of jitter have been defined. In MG, the jitter is increased, and an impulse may not appear at the expected time; this is called *blocking,* and the number of blockings is increased in myasthenic muscle. All these electrophysiologic abnormalities are characteristic of MG, but blocking and jitter are also seen in disorders of ACh release. The standard EMG is usually normal, occasionally shows a myopathic pattern, and almost never shows signs of denervation unless some other condition supervenes. Similarly, nerve conduction velocities are normal.

Antibodies to AChR are found in 85% to 90% of patients of all ages with generalized MG if human muscle is used as the test antigen. There have been no false-positive results except for rare patients with Lambert-Eaton syndrome or thymoma without clinical or provocable MG, or in remission; these may be considered unusual forms of MG. Antibodies may not be detected in patients with strictly ocular disease, in some patients in remission (or after thymectomy), or even in some patients with severe symptoms. The titer does not match the severity of symptoms; patients in complete clinical remission may have high titers. Antibodies to myofibrillar proteins (titin, myosin, actin, actomyosin) are found in 85% of patients with thymoma and may be the first evidence of thymoma in some cases.

The different forms of congenital MG can be identified only in a few special centers that are prepared to perform microelectrode and ultrastructural analyses of intercostal muscle biopsies for miniature endplate potentials, AChR numbers, and determination of bound antibodies. It seems likely that deoxyribonucleic acid analysis may soon suffice for diagnosis.

Other serologic abnormalities are encountered with varying frequency, but in several studies, antinuclear factor, rheumatoid factor, and thyroid antibodies were encountered more often than in control populations. Laboratory (and clinical) evidence of hyperthyroidism occurs at some time in about 5% of patients with MG. Radiographs of the chest (including 10-degree oblique films) provide evidence of thymoma in about 15% of patients, especially in those older than 40 years. Computed tomography (CT) of the mediastinum demonstrates all but microscopic thymomas. Magnetic resonance imaging does not appear to be any more useful than CT.

DIAGNOSIS

The diagnosis of MG can be made without difficulty in most patients from the characteristic history and physical examination. The dramatic improvement that follows the injection of neostigmine bromide (Prostigmin) or edrophonium chloride makes the

administration of these drugs essential. Return of strength in weak muscles occurs uniformly after the injection of neostigmine or edrophonium (Fig. 120.1); if no such response occurs, the diagnosis of MG can be doubted. Demonstration of the pharmacologic response is sometimes difficult; however, if the clinical features are suggestive, the test should be repeated, perhaps with a different dosage or rate of administration. Withholding anticholinesterase medication overnight may be helpful. False-positive responses to edrophonium are exceptional but have been recorded with structural lesions, such as a brainstem tumor. (MG can also coexist with other diseases, such as Graves ophthalmopathy or the Lambert-Eaton syndrome.)

The diagnosis of MG is buttressed by the finding of high titers of antibodies to AChR, but a normal titer does not exclude the diagnosis. Somnier found that the test had a specificity of more than 99.9%; sensitivity was 88% because of the negative tests.

Responses to repetitive stimulation and single-fiber EMG also help. If a thymoma is present, the diagnosis of MG (rather than some other neuromuscular disease) is likely. In the past, clinicians used the increased sensitivity to curare as a test to prove that a syndrome simulating MG was actually psychasthenia or something else; however, the test was inconvenient and, if done without proper precautions, was even hazardous. Since the advent of the antibody test, the curare test has virtually disappeared.

In the neostigmine test, 1.5 to 2 mg of the drug and atropine sulfate, 0.4 mg, are given intramuscularly. Objective improvement in muscular power is recorded at 20-minute intervals up to 2 hours. Edrophonium is given intravenously in a dose of 1 to 10 mg. The initial dose is up to 2 mg followed in 15 seconds by an additional 3 mg and in another 15 seconds by 5 mg to a maxi-

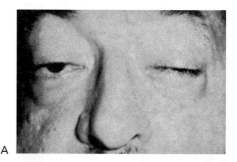

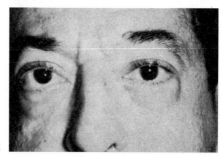

FIG. 120.1. Myasthenia gravis. **A:** Severe ptosis of the lids. **B:** Same patient 1 minute after intravenous injection of edrophonium (10 mg). (From Rowland et al., 1961; with permission.)

mum of 10 mg. Improvement is observed within 30 seconds and lasts a few minutes. Because of the immediate and dramatic nature of the response, edrophonium is preferred for evaluation of ocular and other cranial muscle weakness, and neostigmine is generally reserved for evaluation of limb or respiratory weakness, which may require more time. Placebo injections are sometimes useful in evaluating limb weakness, but placebos are not necessary in evaluating cranial muscle weakness because that abnormality cannot be simulated. For all practical purposes, a positive response is diagnostic of MG.

DIFFERENTIAL DIAGNOSIS

The differential diagnosis includes all diseases that are accompanied by weakness of oropharyngeal or limb muscles, such as the muscular dystrophies, amyotrophic lateral sclerosis, progressive bulbar palsy, ophthalmoplegias of other causes, and the asthenia of psychoneurosis or hyperthyroidism. There is usually no difficulty in differentiating these conditions from MG by the findings on physical and neurologic examination and by the failure of symptoms in these conditions to improve after parenteral injection of neostigmine or edrophonium. Occasionally, blepharospasm is thought to mimic ocular myasthenia, but the forceful eye closure in that condition involves both the upper and lower lids; the narrowed palpebral fissure and signs of active muscle activity are distinctive.

The only other conditions in which clinical improvement has been documented after use of edrophonium are other disorders of neuromuscular transmission: botulinum intoxication, snake bite, organophosphate intoxication, or unusual disorders that include features of both MG and the Lambert-Eaton syndrome. Denervating disorders, such as motor neuron disease or peripheral neuropathy, do not show a reproducible or unequivocal clinical response to edrophonium or neostigmine. The response should be unequivocal and reproducible. If a structural lesion of the third cranial nerve seems to respond, the result should be photographed (and even published).

TREATMENT

Clinicians must choose the sequence and combination of five different kinds of therapy: Anticholinesterase drug therapy and plasmapheresis are symptomatic treatments, whereas thymectomy, steroids, and other immunosuppressive drugs may alter the course of the disease.

It is generally agreed that anticholinesterase drug therapy should be given as soon as the diagnosis is made. Of the three available drugs—neostigmine, pyridostigmine bromide, and ambenonium (Mytelase)—pyridostigmine is the most popular but has not been formally assessed in controlled comparison with the other drugs. The muscarinic side effects of abdominal cramps and diarrhea are the same for all three drugs but are least severe with pyridostigmine; none has more side effects than another. The usual starting dose of pyridostigmine is 60 mg given orally every 4 hours while the patient is awake. Depending on clinical response, the dosage may be increased, but incremental benefit is

not to be expected in amounts greater than 120 mg every 2 hours. If patients have difficulty eating, doses can be taken about 30 minutes before a meal. If patients have special difficulty on waking in the morning, a prolonged-release 180-mg tablet of pyridostigmine (Mestinon Timespans) can be taken at bedtime. Muscarinic symptoms can be ameliorated by preparations containing atropine (0.4 mg) with each dose of pyridostigmine. Excessive doses of atropine can cause psychosis, but the amounts taken in this regimen have not had this effect. Other drugs may be taken if diarrhea is prominent. There is no evidence that any one of the three drugs is more effective than the others in individual patients, and there is no evidence that combinations of two drugs are better than any one drug alone.

Although cholinergic drug therapy sometimes gives impressive results, there are serious limitations. In ocular myasthenia, ptosis may be helped, but some diplopia almost always persists. In generalized MG, patients may improve remarkably, but some symptoms usually remain. Cholinergic drugs do not return function to normal, and the risk of crisis persists because the disease is not cured. Therefore, usually, one of the other treatments is used promptly to treat generalized MG.

Thymectomy was originally reserved for patients with serious disability because the operation had a high mortality. With advances in surgery and anesthesia, however, the operative mortality is now negligible in major centers. About 80% of patients without thymoma become asymptomatic or go into complete remission after thymectomy; although there has been no controlled trial of thymectomy, these results seem to diverge from the natural history of the untreated disease. Thus, thymectomy is now recommended for most patients with generalized MG. Decisions made for children or patients older than 65 must be individualized. Although it is safe, thymectomy is a major operation and is not usually recommended for patients with ocular myasthenia unless there is a thymoma. The beneficial effects of thymectomy are usually delayed for months or years. It is never an emergency measure, and other forms of therapy are usually needed in the interim.

Prednisone therapy is used by some authorities to prepare patients for thymectomy, but that function is also served by plasmapheresis or by intravenous immunoglobulin (IVIG) therapy. Exchanges of about 5% of calculated blood volume may be given several times before the day of surgery to be certain that the patient is functioning as well as possible, and to ameliorate or avoid a postoperative respiratory crisis. Plasmapheresis is also used for other exacerbations; the resulting improvement, seen in most patients, may be slight or dramatic and may last only a few days or several months. Plasmapheresis is safe but expensive and is not convenient for many patients.

IVIG therapy is usually given in five daily doses to a total of 2 g/kg body weight. Side effects include headache, aseptic meningitis, and a flulike syndrome that can be alarming but subsides in 1 or 2 days. Thromboembolic events, including stroke, have occurred but are not clearly related to the treatment, which is generally regarded as safe, less cumbersome than plasmapheresis, and less dependent on technical staff who may not be available on weekends. Both treatments are also available for management of exacerbations.

If a patient is still seriously disabled after thymectomy, most clinicians use prednisone, 60 to 100 mg every other day, to achieve a response within a few days or weeks. An equally satisfactory response can be seen with a lower dosage, but it takes longer; for instance, if the dose is 25 to 40 mg, benefit may be seen in 2 to 3 months. Once improvement is achieved, the dosage should be reduced gradually to 20 to 35 mg every other day. This has become a popular form of treatment for disabled patients, but there has been no controlled trial. If the patient does not improve in about 6 months, treatment with azathioprine (Imuran) or cyclophosphamide would be considered, in doses up to 2.5 mg/kg daily for an adult. The dosage should be increased gradually and may have to be taken with food to avert nausea. Whether steroids and immunosuppressive drugs have additive effects is uncertain, and the relative risks are difficult to assess. The numerous side effects of prednisone must be weighed against the possibilities of marrow suppression, susceptibility to infection, or delayed malignancy in patients who are taking immunosuppressive drugs.

Prednisone, 20 to 35 mg on alternate days, is also recommended by some clinicians for ocular myasthenia, weighing risks against potential benefit. For some patients in sensitive occupations, the risks of prednisone therapy may be necessary (e.g., actors, police officers, roofers or others who work on heights, or those who require stereoscopic vision). Ocular myasthenia is not a threat to life; however, pyridostigmine may alleviate ptosis. An eye patch can end diplopia, and prisms help some patients with stable horizontal diplopia. Thymectomy has become so safe that it might be considered for ocular myasthenia that is truly disabling.

Patients with thymoma are likely to have more severe MG and are less likely to improve after thymectomy; nevertheless, many of these patients also improve if the surrounding thymus gland is excised in addition to the tumor.

Myasthenic crisis is defined as the need for assisted ventilation, a condition that arises in about 10% of myasthenic patients. It is more likely to occur in patients with dysarthria, dysphagia, and documented respiratory muscle weakness, presumably because they are liable to aspirate oral secretions, but crisis may also occur in other patients after respiratory infection or major surgery (including thymectomy). The principles of treatment are those of respiratory failure in general. Cholinergic drug therapy is usually discontinued once an endotracheal tube has been placed and positive pressure respiration started; this practice avoids questions about the proper dosage or cholinergic stimulation of pulmonary secretions. Crisis is viewed as a temporary exacerbation that subsides in a few days or weeks. The therapeutic goal is to maintain vital functions and to avoid or treat infection until the patient spontaneously recovers from the crisis. Cholinergic drug therapy need not be restarted unless fever and other signs of infection have subsided, there are no pulmonary complications, and the patient is breathing without assistance.

To determine whether plasma exchange or IVIG therapy actually shortens the duration of crisis would require a controlled trial, but that has not been done. Even so, pulmonary intensive care is now so effective that crisis is almost never fatal and many patients go into a remission after recovery from crisis. Because of advances in therapy, MG is still serious, but not so grave.

SUGGESTED READINGS

Battocchi AP, Majolini L, Evoli A, Lino MM, Minisci C, Tonali P. Course and treatment of myasthenia gravis during preganancy. *Neurology* 1999;52:447–452.

Bever CT Jr, Chang HW, Penn AS, et al. Penicillamine-induced myasthenia gravis: effects of penicillamine on acetylcholine receptor. *Neurology* 1982;32:1077–1082.

Borodic G. Myasthenic crisis after botulinum toxin [Letter]. *Lancet* 1998;352:1832.

Bufler J, Pitz R, Czep M, Wick M, Franke C. Purified IgG from seropositive and seronegative patients with myasthenia gravis reversibly blocks currents through nicotinic acetylcholine receptor channels. *Ann Neurol* 1998;43:458–464.

Castleman B. The pathology of the thymus gland in myasthenia gravis. *Ann NY Acad Sci* 1966;135:496–505.

Christensen PB, Jensen TS, Tsiropoulos I, et al. Mortality and survival in myasthenia gravis: a Danish population based study. *J Neurol Neurosurg Psychiatry* 1998;64:78–83.

Donaldson JO, Penn AS, Lisak RP, et al. Antiacetylcholine receptor antibody in neonatal myasthenia gravis. *Am J Dis Child* 1981;135:222–226.

Eaton LM, Lambert EH. Electromyography and electric stimulation of nerves in diseases of motor unit: observations in myasthenic syndrome associated with malignant tumors. *JAMA* 1957;163:1117–1120.

Engel AG, ed. *Myasthenia gravis and myasthenic disorders.* New York: Oxford University Press, 1999.

Engel AG, Ohno K, Sine SM. Congenital myasthenic syndromes: recent advances. *Arch Neurol* 1999;56:163–171.

Engel AG, Ohno K, Wang HL, Milone M, Sine SM. Molecular basis of congenital myasthenic syndrome: mutations in the acetylcholine receptor. *Neuroscientist* 1998;4:185–194.

Erb W. Zur Causistik der bulbären Lähmungen: über einem neuen, wahrscheinlich bulbären Symptomencomplex. *Arch Psychiatr Nervenkr* 1879;336–350.

Gajdos P, Chervet S, Clair B, Tranchant C, Chastang C. Clinical trial of plasma exchange and high-dose intravenous immunoglobulin in myasthenia gravis. Myasthenia Gravis Clinical Study Group. *Ann Neurol* 1997;41:789–796.

Goldflam S. Über einen scheinbar heilbaren bulbärparalytischen Symptomencomplex mit Beteiligungen der Extremitäten. *Dtsch Z Nervenheilk* 1893;4:312–352.

Harper CM, Engel AG. Quinidine sulfate therapy for the slow-channel congenital myasthenic syndrome. *Ann Neurol* 1998;43:480–484.

Jaretzki A III, Penn AS, Younger DS, et al. "Maximal" thymectomy for myasthenia gravis: results. *J Thorac Cardiovasc Surg* 1988;95:747–757.

Jolly F. Über Myasthenia Gravis pseudoparalytica. *Berl Klin Wochenschr* 1895;1:1–7.

Katz JS, Wolfe GI, Bryan WW, Tintner R, Barohn RJ. Acetylcholine receptor antibodies in the Lambert-Eaton myasthenic syndrome. *Neurology* 1998;50:470–475.

Lindberg C, Andersen O, Lefvert AK. Treatment of myasthenia gravis with methylprednisolone pulse: a double-blind study. *Acta Neruol Scand* 1998;97:370–373.

Lindner A, Schalke B, Toyka KV. Outcome in juvenile onset myasthenia gravis: a retrospective study with long-term follow-up of 79 patients. *J Neurol* 1997;244:515–520.

Lindstrom J, Seybold M, Lennon VA, et al. Antibody to acetylcholine receptor in myasthenia gravis: prevalence, clinical correlates, and diagnostic value. *Neurology* 1976;26:1054–1059.

Lisak RP, ed. *Handbook of myasthenia gravis.* New York: Marcel Dekker, 1994.

Lisak RP, Barchi RL. *Myasthenia gravis.* Philadelphia: WB Saunders, 1982.

Miller RG, Filler-Katz A, Kiprov D, Roan R. Repeat thymectomy in chronic refractory myasthenia gravis. *Neurology* 1991;41:923–924.

Morel E, Eynard B, Vernet B, et al. Neonatal myasthenia gravis: clinical and immunologic appraisal in 30 cases. *Neurology* 1988;38:138–142.

Randomised clinical trial comparing prednisone and azathioprine in myasthenia gravis: results of the second interim analysis. Myasthenia Gravis Clinical Study Group. *J Neurol Neurosurg Psychiatry* 1993;56:1157–1163.

Odel JG, Winterkorn JMS, Behrens MM. The sleep test for myasthenia gravis. *J Clin Neuroophthal* 1991;11:288–292.

Oosterhuis HGJH. The natural course of myasthenia gravis: a long-term follow-up study. *J Neurol Neurosurg Psychiatry* 1989;52:1121–1127.

Palace J, Newsom-Davis J, Lecky B, and the Myasthenia Gravis Study Group. A randomized double-blind trial of pednisolone alone or with azathioprine in myasthenia gravis. *Neurology* 1998;50:1778–1783.

Pascuzzi RM. Iatrogenic disorders of the neuromuscular junction. In Biller J, ed. *Iatrogenic neurology.* Boston: Butterworth-Heinemann, 1998:283–304.

Patrick J, Lindstrom J. Autoimmune response to acetylcholine receptor. *Science* 1973;180:871–872.

Penn AS, Richman DP, Ruff RL, Lennon VA, eds. Myasthenia gravis and related disorders: experimental and clinical aspects. Conference proceedings, Washington, DC, April 12–15, 1992. *Ann N Y Acad Sci* 1993;681:1–622.

Phillips LH 2nd, Torner JC. Epidemiologic evidence for a changing natural history of myasthenia gravis. *Neurology* 1996;47:1233–1238.

Pinching AJ, Peters DK. Remission of myasthenia gravis following plasma exchange. *Lancet* 1976;2:1373–1376.

Qureshi AJ, Choudry MA, Akbar MS, et al. Plasma exchange versus intravenous immunoglobulin treatment in myasthenic crisis. *Neurology* 1999;52:629–632.

Robertson NP, Deans J, Compston DAS. Myasthenia gravis: a population-based epidemiological study in Cambridgeshire, England. *J Neurol Neurosurg Psychiatry* 1998;65:492–496.

Rowland LP. Controversies about the treatment of myasthenia gravis. *J Neurol Neurosurg Psychiatry* 1980;43:644–659.

Rowland LP, Hoefer PFR, Aranow H Jr. Myasthenic syndromes. *Res Publ Assoc Res Nerv Ment Dis* 1961;38:548–600.

Rowland LP, Hoefer PFA, Aranow H Jr, Merritt HH. Fatalities in myasthenia gravis: a review of 39 cases with 26 autopsies. *Neurology* 1956;6:307–326.

Soliven B, Lange DJ, Penn AS, et al. Seronegative myasthenia gravis. *Neurology* 1988;38:514–517.

Somnier FE. Clinical implementation of anti-acetylcholine receptor antibodies. *J Neurol Neurosurg Psychiatry* 1993;56:496–504.

Steinman L, Mantegazza R. Prospects for specific immunotherapy in myasthenia gravis. *FASEB J* 1990;4:2726–2731.

Thomas CE, Mayer SA, Gungor Y, et al. Myasthenic crisis: clinical features, mortality, complications, and risk factors for intubation. *Neurology* 1997;48:1253–1260.

Toyka KV, Drachman DB, Pestronk A, Kao I. Myasthenia gravis: passive transfer from man to mouse. *Science* 1975;190:397–399.

Vincent A, Jacobson L, Plested P, et al. Antibodies affecting ion channel function in acquired neuromyotonia, in seropositive and seronegative myasthenia gravis, and in antibody-mediated arthrogryposis multiplex congenita. *Ann N Y Acad Sci* 1998;841:482–496.

Wang ZU, Karachunski PI, Howard JF, Conti-Fine B. Myasthenia in SCID mice grafted with myasthenic patient lymphocytes: role of CD4 and CD8 cells. *Neurology* 1999;52:484–497.

Wittbrodt ET. Drugs and myasthenia gravis: an update. *Arch Intern Med* 1997;157:399–408.

Merritt's Neurology, 10th ed., edited by L.P. Rowland. Published by Lippincott Williams & Wilkins, Philadelphia, 2000.

C H A P T E R
121

LAMBERT-EATON SYNDROME

AUDREY S. PENN

The Lambert-Eaton myasthenic syndrome (LEMS) is an autoimmune disease of peripheral cholinergic synapses. Antibodies are directed against voltage-gated calcium channels in peripheral nerve terminals. A disease of adults, LEMS is found in 60% of patients with small-cell carcinoma of the lung. The neurologic symptoms almost always precede those of the tumor; the interval may be as long as 5 years. Other tumors have also been implicated, but about 33% of cases are not associated with tumor. Cell lines derived from the lung cancer show reactive antigens in the calcium channel proteins; the antibodies presumably arise in reaction to the tumor. If tumor cells are grown in the presence of immunoglobulin (Ig) G from a patient with LEMS, the number of functional channels declines. Similar antigens are found in calcium channel proteins from neuroendocrine tumors. The cultured carcinoma cells also bear receptors for dihydropyridines.

The abnormality of neurotransmission is attributed to inadequate release of acetylcholine (ACh) from nerve terminals at both nicotinic and muscarinic sites and is related to abnormal voltage-dependent calcium channels. When IgG from affected patients is injected into mice, the number ACh quanta released by nerve stimulation is reduced, and there is disarray of the active zone particles that is detected by freeze-fracture ultrastructural analysis.

Purified calcium channel proteins can be directly radiola-

beled. An alternative label can be generated by the use of a specific ligand, *omega-conotoxin,* which is prepared from a marine snail and has been used to identify P/Q-type calcium channels in extracts of small-cell carcinoma, neuroblastoma, and other neuroendocrine cell lines. A diagnostic test for the autoantibodies is based on radiolabeled preparations, but it is not fully specific. In the series of Motomura and associates (1997), 92% of 72 patients had a positive reaction. There have been a few positive tests in paraneoplastic cerebellar disorders. Some patients have both LEMS and a cerebellar syndrome.

LEMS may be suspected in patients with symptoms of proximal limb weakness who have lost knee and ankle jerks and complain of dry mouth or myalgia. Other, less common autonomic symptoms include impotence, constipation, and hypohidrosis. LEMS differs clinically from myasthenia gravis (MG) because diplopia, dysarthria, dysphagia, and dyspnea are lacking. Autonomic symptoms are more common in LEMS than in MG.

The disease is defined, and the diagnosis made, by the characteristic incremental response to repetitive nerve stimulation, a pattern that is the opposite of MG. The first evoked potential has an abnormally low amplitude, which decreases even further at low rates of stimulation. At rates greater than 10 Hz, however, there is a marked increase in the amplitude of evoked response (2 to 20 times the original value). This incremental response results from facilitation of release of transmitter at high rates of stimulation; at low rates the number of quanta released per impulse (quantal content) is inadequate to produce endplate potentials that achieve threshold. Similar abnormalities are found in preparations exposed to botulinum toxin or to a milieu low in calcium or high in magnesium.

Some patients with LEMS have ptosis with antibodies to ACh receptor. This "combined" syndrome may be an example of multiple autoimmune diseases in the same individual.

Treatment is directed to the concomitant tumor. The neuromuscular disorder is treated with drugs that facilitate release of ACh. A combination of pyridostigmine bromide and 3,4-diaminopyridine improves strength, but other aminopyridines may be hazardous. Other drugs that facilitate release of ACh have had adverse effects. Guanidine hydrochloride (20 to 30 mg/kg per day) may depress bone marrow or cause severe tremor and cerebellar syndrome. 4-Aminopyridine causes convulsions. Plasmapheresis is often helpful, but the effects are transient. Cytotoxic drugs should be used cautiously because a risk of malignancy is already present, even in patients who do not seem to have one already. Intravenous immunoglobulin therapy is another alternative.

SUGGESTED READINGS

Fetell MR, Shin HS, Penn AS, Lovelace RE, Rowland LP. Combined Eaton-Lambert syndrome and myasthenia gravis. *Neurology* 1978;28:398.

Johnson I, Lang B, Leys K, Newsom-Davis J. Heterogeneity of calcium channel autoantibodies detected using a small cell lung cancer line derived from a Lambert-Eaton myasthenic syndrome patient. *Neurology* 1994;44:334–338.

Katz JS, Wolfe GI, Bryan WW, Tintner R, Barohn RJ. Acetylcholine receptor antibodies in the Lambert-Eaton myasthenic syndrome. *Neurology* 1998;50:470–475.

Lambert EH, Rooke ED, Eaton LM, Hodgson CH. Myasthenic syndrome occasionally associated with bronchial neoplasm: neurophysiologic studies. In: Viets HR, ed. *Myasthenia gravis.* Springfield, IL: Charles C Thomas, 1961:362–410.

Lang B, Newsom-Davis J, Wray D, et al. Autoimmune etiology for myasthenic (Eaton-Lambert) syndrome. *Lancet* 1981;2:224–226.

Lennon VA, Kryzer TJ, Griesmann GE, et al. Calcium-channel antibodies in the Lambert-Eaton syndrome and other paraneoplastic syndromes. *N Engl J Med* 1995;332:1467–1474.

Leys K, Lang B, Johnston I, Newsom-Davis J. Calcium channel autoantibodies in the Lambert-Eaton myasthenic syndrome. *Ann Neurol* 1991;29:307–314.

Lund H, Nilsson O, Rosen I. Treatment of Lambert-Eaton syndrome: 3,4-diaminopyridine and pyridostigmine. *Neurology* 1984;34:1324–1330.

Mason WP, Graus F, Lang B, et al. Small-cell lung cancer, paraneoplastic cerebellar degeneration, and the Lambert-Eaton myasthenic syndrome. *Brain* 1997;120:1279–1300.

McEvoy K, Windebank AJ, Daube JR, Low PA. 3,4-Diaminopyridine in the treatment of Lambert-Eaton myasthenic syndrome. *N Engl J Med* 1989;321:1567–1571.

Motomura M, Lang B, Johnston I, Palace J, Vincent A, Newsom-Davis J. Incidence of serum anti-P/O-type and anti-N-type calcium channel autoantibodies in the Lambert-Eaton myasthenic syndrome. *J Neurol Sci* 1997;147:35–42.

Newsom-Davis J. Antibody-mediated channelopathies at the neuromuscular junction. *Neuroscientist* 1997;3:337–346.

Newsom-Davis J. A treatment algorithm for Lambert-Eaton myasthenic syndrome. *Ann N Y Acad Sci* 1998;841:817–822.

Newsom-Davis J, Leys K, Vincent A, et al. Immunological evidence for the co-existence of the Lambert-Eaton myasthenic syndrome and myasthenia gravis in two patients. *J Neurol Neurosurg Psychiatry* 1991;54:452–453.

Oh SJ, Kim DS, Head TC, Claussen GC. Low-dose guanidine and pyridostigmine: relatively safe and effective long-term symptomatic therapy in Lambert-Eaton myasthenic syndrome. *Muscle Nerve* 1997;20:1146–1152.

O'Neill JH, Murray NMF, Newsom-Davis J. The Lambert-Eaton myasthenic syndrome: a review of 50 cases. *Brain* 1988;111:577–596.

Penn AS, Richman DP, Ruff RL, Lennon VA, eds. Myasthenia gravis and related disorders: experimental and clinical aspects. Conference proceedings, Washington, DC, April 12–15, 1992. *Ann N Y Acad Sci* 1993;681:1–622.

Raymond C, Walker D, Bichet D, et al. Antibodies against the beta subunit of voltage-dependent calcium channels in Lambert-Eaton myasthenic syndrome. *Neuroscience* 1999;90:269–277.

Roberts A, Perera S, Lang B, et al. Paraneoplastic myasthenic syndrome IgG inhibits $^{45}Ca^{2+}$ flux in a small cell carcinoma line. *Nature* 1985;2:737–739.

Verschuuren JJ, Dalmau J, Tunkel R, et al. Antibodies against the calcium channel beta subunit in Lambert-Eaton myasthenic syndrome. *Neurology* 1998;50:475–479.

Vincent A. Antibodies to ion channels in paraneoplastic disorders. *Brain Pathol* 1999;9:285–291.

Waterman SA, Lang B, Newsom-Davis J. Effect of Lambert-Eaton myasthenic syndrome antibodies on autonomic neurons in the mouse. *Ann Neurol* 1997;42:147–156.

Merritt's Neurology, 10th ed., edited by L.P. Rowland. Published by Lippincott Williams & Wilkins, Philadelphia, 2000.

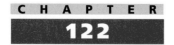

CHAPTER 122

BOTULISM AND ANTIBIOTIC-INDUCED NEUROMUSCULAR DISORDERS

AUDREY S. PENN

BOTULISM

Botulism is a disease in which nearly total paralysis of nicotinic and muscarinic cholinergic transmission is caused by botulinum toxin acting on presynaptic mechanisms for release of acetylcholine (ACh) in response to nerve stimulation. The toxin is produced by spores of *Clostridium botulinum*, which may contaminate foods grown in soil (types A, B, F, and G) or fish (type E). Intoxication results if contaminated food is inadequately cooked and the spores are not destroyed, or if fish are not eviscerated before drying or salt curing. Toxin can be produced in anaerobic wounds that have been contaminated by organisms and spores. Ingestion or inhalation of spores by infants may cause botulism when toxin type A is then produced in the gastrointestinal tract during periods of constipation. An analogous syndrome may occur in adults with persistent growth of *C. botulinum* in the intestine after surgery, from gastric achlorhydria, or from antibiotic therapy. The toxin causes destruction of the terminal twigs of cholinergic nerve endings, which require several months to regenerate and remodel after a single exposure.

Electrophysiologic evidence of severely disturbed neuromuscular transmission includes an abnormally small single-muscle action potential evoked in response to a supramaximal nerve stimulus. When the synapse is driven by repetitive stimulation at high rates (20 to 50 Hz), the evoked response is potentiated up to 400%. In affected infants, muscle action potentials are unusually brief, of low amplitude, and overly abundant. This is presumably related to involvement of terminal nerve twigs in endings of many motor units. In patients who have been treated for blepharospasm or other movement disorders by intramuscular injections of botulinum toxin, single-fiber electromyography shows increased jitter in muscles remote from those injected, and the jitter is maximally increased at low firing rates. These abnormalities are not symptomatic but imply an effect of circulating toxin.

C. botulinum toxin may be the "most poisonous poison" (the lethal dose for a mouse is 10^{-12} g/kg body weight). If the patient survives and reaches a hospital, symptoms include dry, sore mouth and throat, blurred vision, diplopia, nausea, and vomiting. Signs include hypohidrosis, total external ophthalmoplegia, and symmetric descending facial, oropharyngeal, limb, and respiratory paralysis. Pupillary paralysis, however, is not invariable. Not all patients are equally affected, suggesting variable toxin intake or variable individual responses. When cases occur in clusters, the diagnosis is usually suspected immediately.

Isolated cases in children and adolescents may be thought to be Guillain-Barré syndrome, myasthenia gravis, or even diphtheria. Ptosis has responded to intravenous edrophonium chloride in a few patients, but response to anticholinesterase drugs is neither sufficiently extensive nor sufficiently prolonged to be therapeutic. Infants with botulism are usually younger than 6 months. They show generalized weakness, decreased or absent sucking and gag reflex, facial diplegia, lethargy, ptosis, and ophthalmoparesis. Diagnosis is made by the following characteristics: clustering of cases, symmetry of signs, dry mouth or absence of secretion, pupillary paralysis, and the characteristic incremental response to repetitive nerve stimulation. The Centers for Disease Control and Prevention (CDC) (with a dedicated emergency 24-hour telephone number) or appropriate state laboratories should be notified so that the toxin can be identified in refrigerated samples of serum, stool, or residual food samples. In suspected infantile botulism, feces should be evaluated for the presence of *C. botulinum*, as well as toxin.

Patients should be treated in intensive care facilities for respiratory care. Specific therapy includes antitoxin (a horse serum product that may cause serum sickness or anaphylaxis) available from the CDC, and guanidine hydrochloride, which promotes release of transmitter from residual spared nerve endings but may depress bone marrow.

ANTIBIOTIC-INDUCED NEUROMUSCULAR BLOCKADE

Aminoglycoside antibiotics (neomycin sulfate, streptomycin sulfate, and kanamycin sulfate [Kantrex]) and polypeptide antibiotics (colistin sulfate [Coly-Mycin S] and polymyxin B sulfate) may cause symptomatic block in neuromuscular transmission in patients without any known neuromuscular disease. Antibiotics

occasionally aggravate myasthenia gravis. The problem surfaces when blood levels are excessively high, which usually occurs in patients with renal insufficiency, but levels may be within the therapeutic range. Studies of bath-applied streptomycin in nerve–muscle preparations disclosed inadequate release of ACh; the effect was antagonized by an excess of calcium ion. In addition, the sensitivity of the postjunctional membrane to ACh was reduced. Different compounds differed in relative effects on pre- and postsynaptic events. Neomycin and colistin produced the most severe derangements. The effects of kanamycin, gentamicin sulfate, streptomycin, tobramycin sulfate (Nebcin), and amikacin sulfate (Amikin) were moderate; tetracycline, erythromycin, vancomycin hydrochloride, penicillin G, and clindamycin (Cleocin) had negligible effects. Patients who fail to regain normal ventilatory effort after anesthesia or who show delayed depression of respiration after extubation and are receiving one of the more potent agents should receive ventilatory support until the agent can be discontinued or another antibiotic substituted.

SUGGESTED READINGS

Arnon SS, Midura TF, Clay SH, et al. Infant botulism: epidemiological, clinical and laboratory aspects. *JAMA* 1977;237:1946–1951.

Barrett DH. Endemic blood-borne botulism: clinical experience, 1973–1986 at Alaska Native Medical Center. *Alaska Med* 1991;33:101–108.

Cherington M. Clinical spectrum of botulism. *Muscle Nerve* 1998;21:701–710.

Davis LE, Johnson JK, Bicknell JM, Levy H, McEvoy KM. Human type A botulism and treatment with 3,4-diaminopyridine. *Electromyogr Clin Neurophysiol* 1992;32:379–383.

DeJesus PV, Slater R, Spitz LK, Penn AS. Neuromuscular physiology of wound botulism. *Arch Neurol* 1973;29:425–431.

Griffin PM, Hathaway CL, Rosenbaum RB, Sokolow R. Endogenous antibody production to botulinum toxin in an adult with intestinal colonization botulism and underlying Crohn's disease. *J Infect Dis* 1997;175:633–637.

MacDonald KL, Rutherford GW, Friedman SM, et al. Botulism and botulism-like illness in chronic drug abusers. *Ann Intern Med* 1985;102:616–618.

Maselli RA, Ellis W, Mandler RN, et al. Cluster of wound botulism in California: clinical, electrophysiological, and pathologic study. *Muscle Nerve* 1997;20:1284–1295.

Montecucco C, Schiavo G, Tugnoli V, de Grandis D. Botulism neurotoxins: mechanism of action and therapeutic applications. *Mol Med Today* 1996;2:418–424.

Pickett J, Berg B, Chaplin E, Brunstelter-Shafer M. Syndrome of botulism in infancy: clinical and electrophysiologic study. *N Engl J Med* 1976;295:770–772.

Sanders DB. Clinical neurophysiology of disorders of the neuromuscular junction. *J Clin Neurophysiol* 1993;10:167–180.

Terranova W, Palumbo JN, Breman JG. Ocular findings in botulism type B. *JAMA* 1979;241:475–477.

Woodrull BA, Griffin PM, McCroskey LM, et al. Clinical and laboratory comparison of botulism from toxin types A, B, and E in the United States, 1975–1988. *J Infect Dis* 1992;166:1281–1286.

Merritt's Neurology, 10th ed., edited by L.P. Rowland. Published by Lippincott Williams & Wilkins, Philadelphia, 2000.

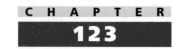

ACUTE QUADRIPLEGIC MYOPATHY

MICHIO HIRANO

In 1977, MacFarlane and Rosenthal described an acute myopathy after high-dose steroid therapy. Since then, more than 200 cases of this acute quadriparesis in critically ill patients have been reported (Table 123.1). The majority of these patients were

TABLE 123.1. CLINICAL AND LABORATORY FEATURES OF 33 REPORTED CASES OF ACUTE QUADRIPLEGIC MYOPATHY

Features	Cases (no/total)	%
Corticosteroids	33/33	100
Hydrocortisone (1–4 g/d)		
Prednisone (50–75 mg/d)		
Methylprednisolone (500–1,440 mg/d)		
Dexamethasone (40–80 mg/d)		
Nondepolarizing neuromuscular blocking agent	30/33	91
Presenting illness		
Asthma	21/33	64
Trauma	8/33	24
Peritonitis	2/33	6
Allergic vasculitis	1/33	3
Multiple medical problems	1/33	3
Weakness (onset, 4 d to 2 wk)	33/33	100
Distal	2/33	6
Proximal	5/33	15
Diffuse	26/33	79
Areflexia	11/33	33
Fasciculations	0/1	0
Creatine kinase		
Normal	6/16	38
Elevated (from 4 to 410 × control)	10/16	63
EMG/NCS		
Myopathic	9/19	47
Neuropathic	6/19	32
Normal	3/19	16
Muscle biopsy		
Myopathy	14/17	82
Neuropathy	2/17	12
Normal	1/17	6
Outcome		
Died (two of the primary illness, two unknown)	4/33	12
Improved	29/33	88
Normal	15/33	45

From Hirano et al., 1992; with permission.

given corticosteroids, nondepolarizing neuromuscular blocking agents, or both; however, the acute myopathy developed in at least two individuals who received neither agent. Most commonly, patients were being treated for status asthmaticus, after organ transplantation, and after trauma. The others had diverse disorders but rarely neuromuscular diseases.

Severe quadriplegia and muscle atrophy commence 4 days to 2 weeks after initiation of intensive care therapy. The weakness may be primarily distal or proximal but is usually diffuse; tendon reflexes are lost in many patients. Ophthalmoparesis and facial muscle weakness are sometimes present. Persistent respiratory muscle weakness makes weaning patients from ventilators difficult. Improvement is evident in 1 month to 5 years in most individuals who survive their critical illness.

Laboratory studies have shown normal or elevated serum creatine kinase levels. Nerve conduction and electromyographic studies have given normal, myogenic, or neurogenic results; however, muscle biopsies demonstrated predominantly myopathy. In some patients, direct muscle stimulation has shown a loss of excitability, which, in a rodent model, has been attributed to reductions of voltage-gated sodium channel. Enhanced expression of calcium-activated proteases (calpains) have been observed and postulated to play a pathogenic role.

Three distinct histologic features have been described in skeletal muscle biopsies; the abnormalities may be present in isolation or in variable combinations. Muscle fiber atrophy, often more prominent in type 2 fibers, is routinely seen. In patients with markedly elevated creatine kinase levels, necrosis of muscle fibers has been observed. The most striking feature revealed by electron microscopy is loss of thick (myosin) filaments. The loss of myosin has been corroborated by antimyosin-antibody stains.

Thus, acute myopathy must be distinguished from the persistent weakness that may follow administration of nondepolarizing blocking agents to a person with impaired hepatic metabolism, reduced renal excretion, or both. *Critical-illness polyneuropathy,* an axonal neuropathy in the setting of sepsis, multiorgan failure, or both, is an alternative cause of weakness in intensive care unit patients and may coexist with acute quadriplegic myopathy. In addition, an idiopathic poliomyelitis-like neurogenic disease, *Hopkins syndrome,* has been reported in children after exacerbation of bronchial asthma. Nerve or muscle histology reports in Hopkins syndrome do not appear to have determined whether that syndrome and acute quadriplegic myopathy are the same or different.

SUGGESTED READINGS

Danon MJ, Carpenter S. Myopathy with thick filament (myosin) loss following prolonged paralysis with vecuronium during steroid treatment. *Muscle Nerve* 1991;14:1131–1139.

Hirano M, Ott BR, Raps EC, et al. Acute quadriplegic myopathy: a complication of treatment with steroids, nondepolarizing blocking agents, or both. *Neurology* 1992;42:2082–2087.

Lacomis D, Petrella JT, Giuliani MJ. Causes of neuromuscular weakness in the intensive care unit: a study of ninety-two patients. *Muscle Nerve* 1997;1998:610–617.

MacFarlane IA, Rosenthal FD. Severe myopathy after status asthamaticus [Letter]. *Lancet* 1977;2:615.

Rich MM, Pinter MJ, Kraner SD, Barchi RL. Loss of electrical excitability in an animal model of acute quadriplegic myopathy. *Ann Neurol* 1998;43:171–179.

Rich MM, Teener JW, Raps EC, et al. Muscle is electrically inexcitable in acute quadriplegic myopathy. *Neurology* 1996;46:731–736.

Segredo V, Caldwell JE, Matthay MA, et al. Persistent paralysis in critically ill patients after long-term administration of vecuronium. *N Engl J Med* 1992;327:524–527.

Shahar EM, Hwang PA, Niesen CE, Murphy EG. Poliomyelitis-like paralysis during recovery from acute bronchial asthma: possible etiology and risk factors. *Pediatrics* 1991;88:276–279.

Sher JH, Shafiq SA, Schutta HS. Acute myopathy with selective lysis of myosin filaments. *Neurology* 1991;41:921–923.

Showalter CJ, Engel AG. Acute quadriplegic myopathy: analysis of myosin isoforms and evidence for calpain-mediated proteolysis. *Muscle Nerve* 1997;20:316–322.

Merritt's Neurology, 10th ed., edited by L.P. Rowland. Lippincott Williams & Wilkins, Philadelphia © 2000.

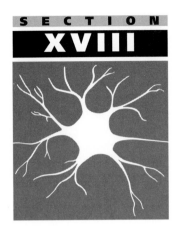

MYOPATHIES

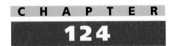

IDENTIFYING DISORDERS OF THE MOTOR UNIT

LEWIS P. ROWLAND

Muscle weakness may result from lesions of the corticospinal tract or the motor unit. Central disorders are accompanied by the distinctive and recognizable signs of upper motor neuron dysfunction. However, lesions of the motor unit (which includes the anterior horn cell, peripheral motor nerve, and muscle) are all manifested by flaccid weakness, wasting, and depression of tendon reflexes. Because the abnormalities are so similar, there may be problems identifying disorders that affect one or another of the structures of the motor unit. As a result, there has been controversy about the classification of individual cases, as well as about some of the criteria used to distinguish the disorders.

Nevertheless, for many reasons, it is still convenient to separate diseases of the motor unit according to the signs, symptoms, and laboratory data, as indicated in Table 124.1. It is necessary to oversimplify to prepare such a table; there are probably excep-

tions to each of the statements made in the table, and individual cases may be impossible to define because of ambiguities or incongruities in clinical or laboratory data. However, there is usually a satisfactory consistency between the different sets of findings. Some syndromes can be recognized clinically without recourse to laboratory tests, including typical cases of Duchenne dystrophy, Werdnig-Hoffmann disease, peripheral neuropathies, myotonic dystrophy, myotonia congenita, periodic paralysis, dermatomyositis, myasthenia gravis, and the myoglobinurias, to name a few. Controversies are mostly limited to syndromes of proximal limb weakness without clear signs of motor neuron disease (fasciculation) or peripheral neuropathy (sensory loss and high cerebrospinal fluid protein content).

LABORATORY DATA

The essential laboratory tests have been described in detail in other chapters: electrodiagnosis in Chapter 14, electromyography (EMG) and nerve conduction velocity in Chapter 15, and biopsy of muscle and nerve in Chapter 18. EMG is essential in identifying neurogenic or myopathic disorders. Measurement of nerve conduction velocities helps distinguish axonal and demyelinating sensorimotor peripheral neuropathy; slow conduction implies demyelination. In motor neuron diseases, conduction is typically normal or only slightly delayed. However,

TABLE 124.1. IDENTIFICATION OF DISORDERS OF THE MOTOR UNIT

	Anterior horn cell	Peripheral nerve	Neuromuscular junction	Muscle
Clinical				
Symptoms				
Persistent weakness	Yes	Yes	Yes	Yes
Variable weakness	No	No	Yes	Yes
Painful cramps	Often	Rare	No	Rare
Myoglobinuria	No	No	No	No
Paresthesia	No	Yes	No	No
Bladder disorder	Rare	Occasional	No	No
Signs				
Weakness	Yes	Yes	Yes	Yes
Wasting	Yes	Yes	No	Yes
Reflexes lost	Yes	Yes	No (MG)	Yes
Reflexes increased	Yes (ALS)	No	No	No
Babinski	Yes (ALS)	No	No	No
Acral sensory loss	No	Yes	No	No
Fasciculation	Common	Rare	No	No
Laboratory				
Serum enzymes ↑	No or mild	No	No	Yes
CSF protein ↑	Yes or mild	Yes	No	No
Motor nerve conduction				
Velocity slow	No or mild	Often	No	No
↑ or ↓ amplitude (repetitive stimulation)	No	No	Yes	No
EMG				
Denervation	Yes	Yes	No	No
Myopathic	No	No	No	Yes
Biopsy				
Neurogenic features	Yes	Yes	No	No
Myopathic features	No	No	No	Yes

ALS, amyotrophic lateral sclerosis; MG, myasthenia gravis.

conduction velocity is also normal in axonal forms of peripheral neuropathy. Therefore, slow conduction indicates the presence of a peripheral neuropathy, but normal values can be seen in either an axonal peripheral neuropathy or a motor neuron disease (spinal muscular atrophy).

Muscle Biopsy

Muscle biopsy helps distinguish neurogenic and myopathic disorders. Evidence of degeneration and regeneration involves fibers in a random pattern in a myopathy. Some fibers are unusually large, and fiber splitting may be evident. In chronic diseases, there is usually little or no inflammatory cellular response; however, infiltration by white blood cells may be prominent in dermatomyositis and polymyositis. In the dystrophies, there may be infiltration by fat and connective tissue, especially as the disease advances. In denervated muscle, the major fiber change is simple atrophy, and groups of small fibers are typically seen adjacent to groups of fibers of normal size. In histochemical stains, fibers of different types are normally intermixed in a random checkerboard pattern, but in denervated muscle, fibers of the same staining type are grouped, presumably because of reinnervation of adjacent fibers by one motor neuron. In denervated muscle, angular fibers may be the earliest sign. In other conditions, histochemical stains may give evidence of storage products, such as glycogen or fat, or may indicate structurally specific abnormalities, such as nemaline rods, central cores, or other unusual structures.

Serum Enzymes

Serum enzyme determination is another important diagnostic aid. Creatine kinase (CK) is the most commonly used enzyme for diagnostic purposes; it is present in high concentration in muscle and is not significantly present in liver, lung, or erythrocytes. To this extent, it is specific, and high serum content of CK usually indicates disease of the heart or skeletal muscle. The highest values are seen in Duchenne dystrophy, dermatomyositis, polymyositis, and attacks of myoglobinuria. In these conditions, other sarcoplasmic enzymes are also found in the serum, including aspartate transaminase (SGOT), alanine transaminase (SGPT), and lactate dehydrogenase. CK may also be increased in neurogenic diseases, especially Werdnig-Hoffmann disease, Kugelberg-Welander syndrome, and amyotrophic lateral sclerosis, although not to the same extent as in the myopathies named. For instance, with the normal maximum value for CK at 50 U/L, values of about 3,000 U/L are common in Duchenne dystrophy or dermatomyositis, and may reach 50,000 U/L in myoglobinuria. In the denervating diseases, CK values greater than 500 U/L would be unusual but do occur. In some individuals, CK may be inexplicably increased with no other evidence of any muscle disease. Cardiologists have used isoenzyme analysis of CK to help differentiate between skeletal muscle and heart as the source of the increased serum activity. However, in the differential diagnosis of muscle disease, isoenzyme study has not been helpful, and the appearance of the "cardiac" isoenzyme of CK does not necessarily implicate the heart when there is limb weakness.

DEFINITIONS

It is useful to define some terms. *Atrophy* is used in three ways: to denote wasting of muscle in any condition, to denote small muscle fibers under the light microscope, and to name some diseases. By historical accident, all the diseases in which the word atrophy has been used in the name proved to be neurogenic (e.g., peroneal muscular atrophy or spinal muscular atrophy). Therefore, it seems prudent to use the word *wasting* in clinical description of limb muscles, unless it is known that the disorder is neurogenic. *Myopathies* are conditions in which the symptoms are due to dysfunction of muscle and in which there is no evidence of causal emotional disorder or of denervation on clinical grounds or in laboratory tests. The symptoms of myopathies are almost always due to weakness, but other symptoms include impaired relaxation (myotonia), cramps or contracture (McArdle disease), or myoglobinuria. *Dystrophies* are myopathies with five special characteristics: (1) they are inherited; (2) all symptoms are due to weakness; (3) the weakness is progressive; (4) symptoms result from dysfunction in voluntary muscles; and (5) there are no histologic abnormalities in muscle other than degeneration and regeneration, or the reaction to those changes in muscle fibers (infiltration by fat and connective tissue). There is no storage of abnormal metabolic products. Some heritable myopathies are not called dystrophies because weakness is not the dominant symptom (e.g., familial myoglobinurias) or the syndrome is not usually progressive (e.g., periodic paralysis or static, presumably congenital myopathies), and other names are assigned.

SUGGESTED READINGS

Brooke MM. *A clinician's view of neuromuscular disease,* 2nd ed. Baltimore: Williams & Wilkins, 1986.
Engel AG, Franzini-Armstrong C, eds. *Myology,* 2nd ed. New York: McGraw-Hill, 1994.
Walton JN, ed. *Disorders of voluntary muscle,* 6th ed. Edinburgh: Churchill Livingstone, 1994.

Merritt's Neurology, 10th ed., edited by L.P. Rowland. Lippincott Williams & Wilkins, Philadelphia © 2000.

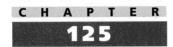

PROGRESSIVE MUSCULAR DYSTROPHIES

LEWIS P. ROWLAND

A muscular dystrophy has five essential characteristics:

1. It is a myopathy, as defined by clinical, histologic, and electromyographic (EMG) criteria. No signs of denervation or sensory loss are apparent unless there is a concomitant and separate disease.
2. All symptoms are effects of limb or cranial muscle weakness. (The heart and visceral muscles may also be involved.)
3. Symptoms become progressively worse.
4. Histologic changes imply degeneration and regeneration of muscle, but no abnormal storage of a metabolic product is evident.
5. The condition is recognized as heritable, even if there are no other cases in a particular family.

Although not part of the definition, there are two further characteristics that we hope will be reversed in the future:

1. It is not understood why muscles are weak in any of these conditions, even when the affected gene product is known.
2. As a result, there is no effective therapy for any of the dystrophies, and gene therapy has not yet been successful.

Therefore, prevention is often the best help that can be offered. The acceleration of research progress may change this state of affairs.

The definition requires some qualifications. For instance, some familial myopathies are manifest by symptoms other than limb weakness, but those conditions are not called dystrophies. Familial recurrent myoglobinuria, for example, is considered a metabolic myopathy. The several forms of familial periodic paralysis do not qualify as dystrophies, even if there is progressive limb weakness, because the attacks are the dominant manifestation in most patients. Syndromes with myotonia include that word in the name of the disease (e.g., myotonia congenita), but the condition is called *muscular dystrophy* only when there is limb weakness.

In addition, a static condition is not called a dystrophy; instead, for instance, a disease of that type is a *congenital myopathy*. This distinction has some exceptions: A slowly progressive dystrophy may seem static, and some congenital myopathies slowly become more severe. Another exception is the term *congenital muscular dystrophy*, which may be severe and static from birth.

CLASSIFICATION

The modern classification of muscular dystrophies commenced three decades ago and has not required much revision. It has served both biochemical and molecular genetics and has not been replaced, except for the gradual erosion of the category called limb-girdle muscular dystrophy (LGMD). This classification of muscular dystrophies, developed by John Walton and his associates, is based on clinical and genetic patterns, starting with three main types: Duchenne muscular dystrophy, facioscapulohumeral muscular dystrophy, and myotonic muscular dystrophy. Each type differs from the others in age at onset, distribution of weakness, rate of progression, presence or absence of calf hypertrophy or high serum levels of sarcoplasmic enzymes, such as creatine kinase (CK), and pattern of inheritance (Table 125.1).

Early investigators recognized that these three types did not include all muscular dystrophies, so they included a fourth type, LGMD. That class has been depleted, however, with the recognition of metabolic myopathies, mitochondrial myopathies, structurally specific congenital myopathies, and manifesting carriers of X-linked dystrophies. Progress has also been made in identifying polymyositis and distal myopathies. LGMD is still a diagnosis of exclusion, but classification may soon depend on deoxyribonucleic acid (DNA) analysis to demonstrate how many forms there actually are.

TABLE 125.1. FEATURES OF THE MOST COMMON MUSCULAR DYSTROPHIES

	Duchenne	Facioscapulohumeral	Myotonic
Age at onset	Childhood	Adolescence; rarely childhood	Adolescence or later; rarely congenital
Sex	Male	Either	Either
Pseudohypertrophy	Common	Never	Never
Onset	Pelvic girdle	Shoulder girdle	Distal limbs
Weakness of face	Rare and mild	Always	Common
Rate of progression	Relatively rapid	Slow	Slow (variable)
Contractures and deformity	Common	Rare	Rare
Cardiac disorder	Usually late	None	Common (conduction)
Inheritance	X-linked recessive	Dominant	Dominant
Expressivity	Full	Variable	Variable
Genetic heterogeneity	Duchenne and Becker allelic	None	Proximal myotonic myopathy

LABORATORY DIAGNOSIS

It has become conventional to perform EMG and muscle biopsy for each new patient in a family. The availability of DNA analysis in white blood cells, however, often obviates biopsy. DNA studies are needed for the diagnosis of Duchenne, Becker, facioscapulohumeral, scapuloperoneal, myotonic, and LGMDs. If no defining mutation is found in a limb-girdle syndrome, it may be useful to carry out histochemical and electrophoretic studies of dystrophin. If unusual features are encountered in the biopsy, a regional research center can be consulted. Muscle biopsy is needed to characterize most congenital and metabolic myopathies. Serum CK determination and electrocardiogram (ECG) should be included for all patients with any kind of myopathy.

X-LINKED MUSCULAR DYSTROPHIES

Definitions

Duchenne and Becker dystrophies (MIM 310200) are defined by the features listed in Table 125.1. The conditions, however, can also be defined in molecular terms. The two diseases are the result of mutations in the gene for dystrophin at Xp21. Although other diseases that map to Xp21 may differ from Duchenne or Becker dystrophies, neither disease can be diagnosed if no abnormality of the gene or gene product is found. In that sense, they are *dystrophinopathies*. Nondystrophin diseases that map to the same position can be called *Xp21 myopathies*.

Prevalence and Incidence

The incidence of Duchenne dystrophy is about 1 in 3,500 male births. There is no geographic or ethnic variation in this figure. Approximately one-third of the cases are caused by new mutations; the others are more clearly familial. Because the life span of patients with Duchenne dystrophy is shortened, the prevalence is less—about 1 in 18,000 males. Becker dystrophy is much less common, with a frequency of about 1 in 20,000.

Duchenne and Becker Muscular Dystrophies

Duchenne Muscular Dystrophy

Duchenne dystrophy is inherited as an X-linked recessive trait. Girls and women who carry the gene are *carriers;* some are *manifesting carriers* with limb weakness, calf hypertrophy, or high serum CK levels.

The condition may become evident at birth if serum enzymes are measured, for example, for an incidental respiratory infection. Authorities often state that symptoms do not begin until age 3 to 5 years, but that view may be a measure of the crudeness of muscle evaluation in infants. Walking may be delayed, and the boys probably never run normally; there is much commotion, but little forward progression because they cannot raise their knees properly. Soon, toe-walking and waddling gait are evident. Then, the condition progresses to overt difficulty in walking, climbing stairs, and rising from chairs. An exaggerated lordosis is

assumed to maintain balance (Fig. 125.1). The boys tend to fall easily if jostled, and then they have difficulty rising from the ground. In doing so, they use a characteristic maneuver called the *Gowers sign* (Fig. 125.2): They roll over to kneel, push down on the ground with extended forearms to raise the rump and straighten the legs, then move the hands to the knees and push up from there. The process has been called "climbing up himself." It is also seen in other conditions that include proximal limb and trunk weakness, such as spinal muscular atrophy. At this stage, the knee jerks may be lost, whereas ankle jerks are still present; this discrepancy is a measure of the proximal accentuation of weakness.

As the disease progresses, the arms and hands are affected. Slight facial weakness may be seen, but speech, swallowing, and ocular movements are spared. Iliotibial contractures limit hip flexion; heel cord contractures are partly responsible for toe-walking. At ages 9 to 12 years, the boys no longer walk; they use a wheelchair. Now, scoliosis may become serious; contractures at elbows and knees contribute to disability. By about age 20, respiration is compromised, and mechanical ventilation is needed.

The heart is usually spared clinically, but congestive heart failure (CHF) may result from cardiomyopathy. The ECG is abnormal in most patients, with increased RS amplitude in lead V_1 and deep, narrow Q waves in left precordial leads. Signs of CHF may supervene in a few cases.

The gastrointestinal system is usually spared, but acute gastric dilatation is an uncommon complication. Mental retardation seems to affect about one-third of boys with Duchenne dystro-

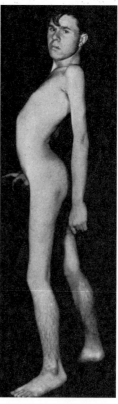

FIG. 125.1. Progressive muscular dystrophy. Lumbar lordosis. (Courtesy Dr. P.I. Yakovlev.)

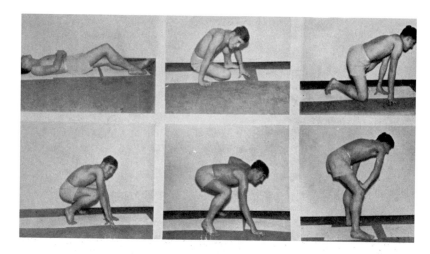

FIG. 125.2. Gowers sign in a patient with Duchenne or Becker MD. Postures assumed in attempting to rise from the supine position.

phy. However, there is no adequate control group to account for the impact on test results of the progressive social and educational isolation of the disease; in no other childhood disease does a child start out almost normal and then gradually face total disability and death. There is neither a characteristic brain pathology nor any correlation of intelligence with changes in dystrophin or the affected gene.

Becker Muscular Dystrophy

This condition resembles Duchenne dystrophy in essential characteristics: It is X-linked, calf hypertrophy is present, weakness is greatest proximally, and serum CK levels are high. EMG and muscle histology are the same. The two differences are age at onset (usually after age 12) and rate of progression (still walking after age 20, often later).

Diagnosis

The clinical diagnosis of Duchenne dystrophy is usually evident from clinical features. In sporadic and atypical cases, spinal muscular atrophy might be mistaken for Duchenne dystrophy. Clinical fasciculation and EMG evidence of denervation, however, identify the neurogenic disorder; in a few cases, dystrophin analysis has made the correct diagnosis.

High values for CK are sometimes encountered in automated chemistry analysis and have mistakenly led to the diagnosis of Duchenne dystrophy. However, values typical of Duchenne or Becker dystrophy are usually at least 20 times normal, and few other conditions attain these levels, not even interictal phosphorylase deficiency or acid maltase deficiency, which typically show high levels. Increased serum levels of CK are seen in Xp21 gene carriers, in some patients with spinal muscular atrophy, and, for unknown reasons, in some otherwise normal people (*idiopathic hyperCKemia*). High values are seen in men with the nonvacuolar form of distal myopathy. When a child with an incidental infection has routine blood tests, increased serum enzyme values may lead to a diagnosis of hepatitis; serum CK should then be assayed, and if it is elevated, a myopathy should be suspected, not a liver disease.

Molecular Genetics

The same gene is involved in both Duchenne and Becker dystrophies; they are allelic diseases. The gene was mapped, before the gene product was known, by a process called positional cloning. The gene product was inferred from DNA sequencing, and then it was identified as *dystrophin,* a cytoskeletal protein located at the plasma membrane. The brain and other organs contain slightly different isoforms. In muscle, dystrophin is associated with membrane glycoproteins that link it to laminin on the external surface of the muscle fiber (Fig. 125.3). The protein may therefore play an essential role in maintaining the integrity

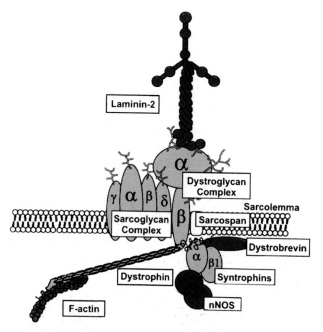

FIG. 125.3. Components of the dystrophin-glycoprotein complex are indicated by *open ellipsis* (light red shading); proteins known to be associated with the complex are in darker red shading. The complex is thought to play a role in stabilizing the sarcolemma and in protecting against stress on the surface membranes from muscle contraction. (From Lim and Campbell, 1998; with permission.)

of muscle fiber. If dystrophin is absent, as in Duchenne dystrophy, or abnormal, as in Becker dystrophy, the sarcolemma becomes unstable in contraction and relaxation, and the damage results in excessive influx of calcium, thereby leading to muscle cell necrosis. If the glycoproteins are abnormal or missing, the same problems arise, as in some LGMDs (described later).

These findings have been put to practical use in the diagnosis of Duchenne and Becker dystrophies and in providing genetic counseling. DNA analysis demonstrates a deletion or a duplication at Xp21 in 60% to 70% of patients with Duchenne or Becker dystrophy. Point mutations account for the remainder but have been difficult to identify. The presence of a deletion in a patient with compatible clinical findings is diagnostic. Carriers can be similarly identified, and the test can be used for antenatal diagnosis (Fig. 125.4).

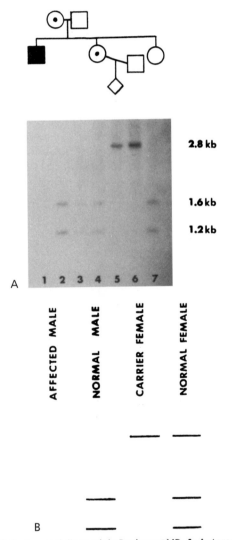

FIG. 125.4. Prenatal diagnosis in Duchenne MD. **A:** Autoradiograph of Southern blot of 1% agarose gel with DNA samples from each individual digested with the restriction enzyme XmnI and probed with pERT87-15. The affected male is deleted (no signal). His sister who was pregnant has a deleted X and an X chromosome with the 1.6/1.2 allele. Her husband's X chromosome contains the 2.8 allele. The fetus contains the husband's X and the deleted X. **B:** Diagram of the four possible outcomes of the prenatal diagnosis. The fetus is a carrier female. (Courtesy A.D. Roses.)

If there is no deletion, the diagnosis can be made by dystrophin studies, which require a muscle biopsy and are therefore not suitable for prenatal diagnosis. There are two types of studies: immunocytochemical and electrophoresis with immunochemical identification of the protein (Western blot). In Duchenne dystrophy, dystrophin is not evident by either method. In Becker dystrophy, the cytochemical method shows an interrupted pattern of staining in the surface membrane, and the Western blot shows two abnormalities: decreased abundance of dystrophin and an abnormal protein size, usually smaller than normal but sometimes larger than normal (if there is an insertion or duplication in the gene). In carriers, there is a mosaic pattern in the biopsy; some fibers contain dystrophin and others show none at all.

A relationship between the site of the deletion and the clinical syndrome is seen in analysis of Becker dystrophy. The gene contains 79 exons. More severe types tend to be related to deletions in either the C-terminal or the N-terminal regions. Milder Becker syndromes are associated with deletions in the central part of the rod domain. In most typical Becker cases, the deletion involves exon 45. A hot spot for Duchenne mutations is located in the first 20 exons.

However, it is not known why the lack of dystrophin results in the clinical syndrome or in high serum CK values, or why an abnormal amount or structure of dystrophin leads to the Becker type. In an animal model, an X-linked disease of the mdx mouse, dystrophin is also totally absent and serum CK levels are high, but weakness is not evident and histologic changes are mild.

Treatment

There is no specific drug therapy for these diseases. Prednisone therapy was better than placebo in controlled trials, but the side effects of chronic administration limit the practical usage of steroids. Oral administration of creatine is said to increase strength in several neuromuscular disorders, without mention of effects on daily function. Attempts to replace the missing gene by implantation of healthy myoblasts have been limited by inefficiency of the process; the transplanted myoblasts produce normal dystrophin, but only about 1% of the fibers are replaced. Management is therefore directed to bracing and surgical correction of spine and limb deformities to maintain ambulation as long as possible. Bracing may prevent scoliosis in wheelchair-bound patients. The children and their families need social support to aid financially, educationally, and emotionally. Genetic counseling is crucial. Heart transplantation has been used for the cardiomyopathy seen occasionally in Becker patients.

Children with Duchenne dystrophy, unlike other dystrophies, are at risk of myoglobinuria after general anesthesia. The syndrome resembles malignant hyperthermia and should be treated accordingly when it occurs.

Other Xp21 Myopathies

Dystrophinopathies

A myopathy may appear when a deletion in a neighboring gene extends into the dystrophin gene. The resulting syndrome may be dominated by *congenital adrenal insufficiency* or *glycerol kinase deficiency,* but there is also a myopathy that may be mild or severe. In addition, syndromes are customarily called *Becker variants* if the dystrophin abnormalities are compatible with that disease. This nomenclature may be confusing, however, because the original definition of Becker dystrophy was based on clinical criteria, and these syndromes are clinically different. Among them are myopathies that affect girls or women (not only manifesting carriers but girls with Turner syndrome or balanced translocations that involve Xp21), syndromes of atypical distribution of weakness (e.g., distal myopathy or quadriceps myopathy), and syndromes that lack weakness but are manifested by some other symptoms (e.g., recurrent myoglobinuria or X-linked cramps). The appearance of any of these disorders warrants appropriate study of dystrophin.

Nondystrophin-related Xp21 Myopathies

One of the mysteries of molecular genetics is *Mcleod syndrome,* a disorder first discovered in blood banks because the donors lacked a red cell antigen, the Kell antigen. These people were soon found to have abnormally shaped red blood cells (acanthocytes), and serum CK values were often 29 times normal or even higher. In addition, there was sometimes limb weakness, and the condition was linked to Xp21. Therefore, this condition, too, was expected to be a dystrophinopathy. In fact, however, dystrophin is normal. How the myopathy arises is not known.

EMERY-DREIFUSS MUSCULAR DYSTROPHY

Emery-Dreifuss muscular dystrophy (EDMD) (MIM 310300) meets the criteria previously listed for a muscular dystrophy. It is characterized clinically by several unusual manifestations:

1. The distribution of weakness is unusual, with a *humeroperoneal* emphasis; that is, the biceps and triceps are affected rather than shoulder girdle muscles, and distal muscles are affected in the legs
2. *Contractures* are disproportionately severe and are experienced before much weakness is noted; the contractures affect the elbows, knees, ankles, fingers, and spine. A rigid spine develops, and neck flexion is limited.
3. *Heart block* is common and often leads to placement of a pacemaker. The myopathy may be mild or severe.

The gene for EDMD maps to the long arm of the X chromosome, at Xq28, and more than 60 mutations have been found. The affected gene product, *emerin,* is localized to the nuclear membrane in muscle and other tissues. In patients, immunochemical methods show that emerin is absent not only in muscle nuclei but also in circulating white blood cells and skin. As a result, skin biopsy or leukocyte studies could be used diagnostically instead of muscle biopsy. The simplest alternative is to take a swab of the inner cheek and study exfoliated mucosal cells. DNA or gene product analysis is now needed for precise diagnosis because of clinical diagnostic problems and because cardiac surveillance is crucial.

EDMD must be distinguished from other conditions. First,

some patients meet the clinical criteria for EDMD, but the pattern of inheritance is autosomal dominant or recessive, not X-linked. These variants have not yet been mapped but do not involve the expression of emerin. Second, the *rigid spine syndrome* includes vertebral and limb contractures, but not cardiopathy, muscle wasting, or X-linked inheritance. Because the cardiac abnormality may not be evident in childhood, some patients with a rigid spine might be expected to have EDMD. In one study, DNA analysis showed this in one of seven rigid-spine patients. Third, Bethlem myopathy (MIM 158810) includes contractures and myopathy, but not cardiopathy. Fourth, other myopathies include cardiomyopathy with CHF rather than solely anomalies of rhythm.

Management is symptomatic.

FACIOSCAPULOHUMERAL MUSCULAR DYSTROPHY

Definition

Facioscapulohumeral muscular dystrophy (FSHMD) (MIM 158900) is defined by clinical and genetic features that differ from those of the Duchenne form in all particulars. It is inherited in autosomal-dominant fashion. The name reflects the characteristic distribution of the weakness; the face is probably always affected. Progression is slow; it may even be asymptomatic. Onset is usually in adolescence, but the disease is occasionally detected in children. Serum enzyme levels are normal or near-normal.

Molecular Genetics

The autosomal-dominant disease shows almost complete penetrance. It maps to chromosome 4q35-qter; the gene product has not been identified. Most apparently sporadic cases prove to have the same mutation; many are new mutations. Diagnosis by deletion analysis is defining, but about 10% of clinically diagnosed cases are not linked, which implies locus heterogeneity. The deletions at 4q35 do not seem to interrupt any identifiable gene. Instead, they move the telomere closer to the centromere, and this *position-effect variegation* presumably and indirectly affects some neighboring gene.

Clinical Manifestations

In full-blown FSHMD, the following features are characteristic:

1. Facial weakness is evident not only in limited movements of the lips but also in the appearance of the slightly everted lips and wide eyes. Patients state that they have never been able to whistle or blow up a balloon. Some are said to sleep with eyes open.
2. Scapular winging is prominent. This feature can be seen with the arms dependent. The traditional test is to ask the patient to push against a wall at shoulder level, exaggerating the winging. The winging also becomes more evident when the patient tries to elevate the arms laterally; in addition to exaggeration of winging, there is limitation, and the patient often cannot

raise the arms to shoulder level, even though no deltoid weakness is noted on manual testing. The limitation is the inadequate fixation of the scapula. Considerable disability may result from this problem, even though limb weakness may not be detectable.

3. The shoulder girdle has a characteristic appearance. Viewed from the front, the clavicles seem to sag and the tips of the scapulae project above the supraclavicular fossa; this abnormality becomes more marked when the subject tries to raise the arms laterally to shoulder level. Smallness of the pectorals affects the anterior axillary fold, which is ordinarily diagonal but assumes a vertical position in FSHMD.

4. Weakness of the legs may affect proximal muscles or, more often, the anterior tibials and peroneals.

In family studies, asymptomatic individuals can be identified by mild versions of these signs. We once concluded that mild facial weakness was the most reliable sign, but that impression was not put to a test by DNA diagnosis. Within a single family, the condition may vary from this mild state to disability. Progression is slow, however, and the condition may not shorten longevity. Few patients are so severely affected that they must use a wheelchair.

Associated Disorders

The childhood form seems to include an unusual frequency of deafness, oropharyngeal symptoms, and, possibly, mental retardation, as well as facial diplegia. Tortuous retinal vessels and Coats disease (exudative telangiectasia of the retina) have also been reported in children with FSHMD but do not seem to be consistent findings. How these disorders relate to the genetic abnormality remains to be elucidated.

Laboratory Studies

EMG and muscle biopsy, by definition, should show a myopathic pattern. The histologic changes are mild. Occasional diagnostic problems are reviewed later. Serum enzyme values are usually normal or trivially elevated. The ECG is normal or shows the common changes with age and atherosclerosis.

Presymptomatic diagnosis is possible in families with more than one affected member, but this procedure should be done only with appropriate counseling. Apparently sporadic cases often prove to be new mutations by DNA analysis. FSHMD is now defined by identification of deletions at 4q35.

Diagnosis

Three persistent diagnostic problems have been discussed in the literature (Table 125.2). One comprises reports of a spinal muscular atrophy of FSH distribution; this diagnosis depends entirely on the interpretation of muscle biopsy and EMG. In our experience, however, FSH manifestations, without exception, have been associated with myopathic changes in these studies (i.e., the clinical diagnosis is FSHMD).

The second problem is the tendency to see inflammatory cells in the muscle biopsy, which has led to the belief that there may be an FSH form of polymyositis. Immunosuppressive therapy has always failed in these patients, however. The significance of the inflammatory cells is not known.

TABLE 125.2. SYNDROMES RESEMBLING FACIOSCAPULOHUMERAL MUSCULAR DYSTROPHY

Autosomal dominant, different distribution of weakness
Scapuloperoneal muscular dystrophy
Rigid spine syndrome
Autosomal-dominant limb-girdle muscular dystrophy
Autosomal-dominant Emery-Dreifuss syndrome
Bethlem myopathy
Benign autosomal-dominant limb-girdle myopathy with contractures
Autosomal dominant, EMG or biopsy evidence of neurogenic
Scapuloperoneal spinal muscular atrophy
Scapuloperoneal sensorimotor peripheral neuropathy
Autosomal dominant, unusual histologic abnormality
Polymyositis
Mitochondrial myopathy
Centronuclear myopathy
Multicore myopathy
Similar distribution weakness, autosomal recessive
Saskatchewan Hutterite muscular dystrophy (Shokeir)

The third problem is evident in reports of an autosomal dominant *scapuloperoneal myopathy* or *atrophy,* thereby implying that this condition differs from FSHMD. The difference depends on the difficult determination of whether the face is affected. Both scapuloperoneal syndromes have been linked, providing new criteria for diagnosis and seemingly confirming the existence of both myopathic and neurogenic syndromes that map to different chromosomes. Additionally, EDMD has sometimes been confused with FSHMD, but the characteristic clinical features of that syndrome differ in essentials from FSH.

Another diagnostic problem is created by a *mitochondrial myopathy with FSH distribution and cardiomyopathy.* This disorder may be the most important reason to perform a muscle biopsy in the propositus of newly identified families or sporadic cases.

Infantile onset of FSHMD is rare, but facial weakness may be severe enough to simulate the *Möbius syndrome of congenital facial diplegia.*

Management

Treatment is symptomatic. Some authorities have suggested that wiring the scapulae to the chest wall makes the arms more useful, but there has been too little experience to recommend such extensive surgery. In an open trial, albuterol, a beta-2-adrenergic agonist, improved muscle strength; a blinded trial was planned.

MYOTONIC MUSCULAR DYSTROPHY

Definition

Myotonic dystrophy (MIM 160900) is an autosomal-dominant, multisystem disease that includes a dystrophy of unique distribution, myotonia, cardiopathy, ocular cataracts, and endocrinopathy. The diverse manifestations are called *pleiotropic.*

Epidemiology

Myotonic dystrophy is compatible with long life, and the penetrance of the gene is almost 100%. Because of these characteristics, myotonic dystrophy is a disease of high prevalence, about 5 per 100,000 throughout the world, with no specific geographic or ethnic variation. It is probably the most common form of muscular dystrophy. The incidence is about 13.5 per 100,000 live births.

Clinical Manifestations

Like many other autosomal-dominant diseases, there is great variation in the age at onset and severity of the different manifestations of myotonic dystrophy. Some affected people are asymptomatic but show signs of the disease on examination.

The *myopathy* is distinctive in distribution (Fig. 125.5). Unlike any of the other major forms of muscular dystrophy, it affects cranial muscles in addition to those of the face. There is ptosis; in some patients, eye movements are impaired. Dysarthria and dysphagia may be problems. The temporalis muscles are small. The overall appearance is distinctive, with a long lean face and ptosis. In men, frontal baldness contributes to the impression. (To this day, insensitive clinicians perpetuate unkind words to describe this facial appearance.) The sternomastoid muscles are characteristically small and weak in manual tests. The limb myopathy is most pronounced distally and affects the hands and feet equally. This dystrophy is one of the few neuromuscular disorders in which weakness of the finger flexors is prominent. Distal leg weakness may cause a footdrop or steppage gait. Most patients are generally thin, and focal wasting is not prominent. The tendon jerks are lost in proportion to the weakness. Muscles of respiration may be affected even before there is much limb weakness; this symptom may be manifested as hypersomnia. Sensitivity to general anesthesia may be increased, with prolonged hy-

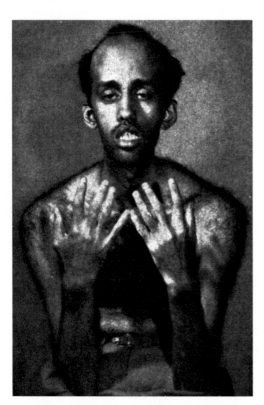

FIG. 125.5. Myotonic dystrophy. Atrophy of facial, temporal, neck, and hand muscles.

poventilation in the postoperative period. Myotonic dystrophy, however, is not a muscle disease likely to cause alveolar hypoventilation. The rate of progression is slow and longevity may not be affected, but variation is evident; some people are almost asymptomatic, and some become disabled.

Myotonia has a dual definition. First, clinically, it is a phenomenon of impaired relaxation. Second, the EMG shows a pattern of waxing and waning of high-frequency discharge that continues after relaxation begins, thus prolonging and impeding the effort. EMG activity is essential to the definition because there are other forms of impaired relaxation (see Chapter 129). Myotonia is most evident in the hands. Symptomatically, it may impair skilled movements or may embarrass the patient by complicating the attempt to shake hands or turn a doorknob because it is difficult to let go. As a sign on examination, the slow relaxation can be elicited by tapping the thenar eminence or, in the forearm, the bellies of the extensors of the fingers. Eliciting percussion myotonia in other limb muscles may be difficult for reasons unknown, but lingual myotonia may be present. The activity can also be evoked by asking the patient to grasp forcefully and then relax, which a normal person can do rapidly. In a patient with myotonia, however, the grasp is followed by slow relaxation. The abnormal activity arises in the muscle because the response to percussion persists in curarized muscle of these patients; that is, the activity persists after neuromuscular transmission has been blocked.

Cataracts are almost universal but take years to appear. Early findings include characteristic iridescent opacities and posterior opacities. Before DNA analysis became available, the finding of cataracts on slit-lamp examination was the most sensitive way to determine which members of a family were affected; cataracts were sometimes the only manifestation of the disease.

Endocrinopathy is most readily seen in men. Frontal baldness is almost universal, and testicular atrophy is common; fertility is little diminished, however, so that the disease continues to be propagated in the family. Menstrual irregularities and ovarian failure are not nearly so frequent, and fertility is little decreased in women. Diabetes mellitus is more common than in the general population, but otherwise no specific endocrine abnormalities are encountered.

The *cardiac disorder* is manifested mostly by abnormalities in the ECG. Conduction abnormalities (with first-degree heart block or bundle branch block) and sometimes abnormal rhythms are seen, but they are rarely symptomatic and pacemakers are rarely needed. CHF and syncope or sudden death may be no more common in affected individuals than in age-matched cohorts of normal people, but this risk has not been assessed by a case–control study.

Gastrointestinal disorders are not common, but pseudoobstruction or megacolon can be dramatic. There may be a tendency to constipation, but in general the autonomic nervous system is not affected. *Cerebral* symptoms are not common, but many clinicians are impressed by the personalities of some patients with myotonic dystrophy, who may seem cantankerous and ornery. Many patients, however, have normal social adjustment.

Laboratory Studies

EMG shows evidence of myopathy and the characteristic waxing and waning after-discharge of myotonia. The muscle biopsy shows mild and nonspecific changes. Serum CK level may be normal or slightly increased, but never to the extent seen in Duchenne dystrophy or polymyositis. The ECG and ocular findings were previously described. No consistent changes appear on brain imaging. DNA analysis is now obligatory for precise diagnosis but may raise sensitive questions in a family, and some individuals at risk may not wish to be tested.

Molecular Genetics and Pathophysiology

The gene for myotonic dystrophy maps to 19q13.2. The mutation is an expansion of a CTG triplet repeat within the dystrophia myotonica protein kinase (DMPK) gene. Unaffected people have 5 to 40 CTG repeats; affected individuals have more than 100. It is uncertain how the mutation exerts its effects, partly because the mutation is outside the open reading frame of the gene. Several proposals of pathogenesis have not been proved. The expansion may alter the DNA in chromatin. It may affect ribonucleic acid metabolism of DMPK or neighboring genes. It may affect the DMPK protein itself, but there seems to be no consistent deficiency of this protein. Whatever the fundamental fault, it is uncertain how this change could cause the *pleiotropic* disorder, with manifestations in so many different organs. The characteristic myotonia is an abnormality of the muscle surface membrane, but the molecular basis is not clear.

The gene was one of the first to demonstrate *expansion,* a phenomenon that allows direct DNA diagnosis. There is a correlation between the number of repeats and the severity of symptoms, with instability between generations as the explanation for anticipation (earlier age at onset in succeeding generations) and potentiation (more severe disease in the next generation). This increase is attributed to an increase in the number of trinucleotide repeats in germ cells. The most extreme example is *congenital myotonic dystrophy,* which affects children of either sex who are born to a woman with the usual adult form of the disease, which is often so mild that the woman may be asymptomatic but shows signs of the condition; the mother is almost always the affected parent. Children with the congenital disease have difficulty in the newborn period, develop slowly, are often mentally retarded, and show developmental anomalies of the face and jaws, as well as severe limb weakness and clubfeet (Table 125.3).

Diagnosis

Typical myotonic dystrophy is so characteristic that diagnosis is often evident at a glance and is confirmed by finding small sternomastoids, distal myopathy, and myotonia of grasp and percussion. Diagnostic problems may arise if a man is not bald or if the facial appearance is not typical. Footdrop may be the first symptom of myotonic dystrophy and might be confused with Charcot-Marie-Tooth neuropathy, but the EMG shows a myopathic pattern, as well as myotonia. Noting an autosomal-dominant pattern in other members of the family helps make the diagnosis. Congenital myotonic dystrophy can be mistaken for other causes of mental retardation of chromosome abnormalities. As DNA analysis is perfected, it will be used increasingly to resolve diagnostic problems, including the identification of presymptomatic individuals in a family.

TABLE 125.3. MANIFESTATIONS OF CONGENITAL MYOTONIC DYSTROPHY (54 CASES REPORTED AFTER 1977)

	Abnormal (n)/ mentioned[a] (n)	Abnormal (%)
Reduced fetal movement	28/41	68
Polyhydramnios	43/54	80
Gestation < 36 wk	28/54	52
Hypotonia	54/54	100
Facial weakness	54/54	100
Respiratory distress	46/54	85
Feeding difficulty	22/24	92
Elevated right hemidiaphragm	17/35	49
Hydrocephalus	32/41	78
Talipes	26/40	65
Tented upper lip	24/26	92
Cutaneous hematoma	13/26	50
Edema	14/26	54
Newborn death	22/54	41
Neonatal death in siblings	5/18	28
Psychomotor retardation	16/16	100

[a]Manifestation not mentioned in all reports. Modified from Hageman et al., 1993.

A syndrome called *proximal myotonic myopathy* (PROMM) is similar to myotonic dystrophy in many respects, including autosomal-dominant myopathy, myotonia, cataracts, and weakness of the sternomastoids. It differs in the distribution of limb weakness, because myotonic dystrophy is primarily a distal myopathy, and in other, less conspicuous ways. For instance, myotonia is more difficult to elicit, symptoms are less severe, and there may be calf hypertrophy. Most important, the syndrome does not map to chromosome 19. A similar syndrome was called "myotonic muscular dystrophy type 2" and mapped to chromosome 3q; soon afterward PROMM mapped to the same position.

Myotonia is found in several other conditions that are described in other chapters: hyperkalemic periodic paralysis and paramyotonia congenita (see Chapter 126), and myotonia congenita and the Schwartz-Jampel syndrome (see Chapter 127). "Pseudomyotonia," or impaired relaxation without the typical EMG pattern, is seen in Isaacs syndrome or neuromyotonia (see Chapter 129). Myotonic-like patterns are seen in the EMG of patients with acid maltase deficiency, but clinical myotonia is not seen in that syndrome. None of these other myotonic syndromes is accompanied by the characteristic myopathy of myotonic dystrophy; none of them causes diagnostic confusion.

Management and Genetic Counseling

Myotonia can be ameliorated with quinine, phenytoin sodium (Dilantin), or other anticonvulsant drugs. However, myotonia is only rarely a bothersome symptom; it is the weakness that is disabling, and little can be done about that. Rehabilitation measures are helpful in keeping the muscles functioning as best they can and in assisting the patient in the activities of daily living. Orthoses help the footdrop. The ocular and cardiac symptoms are treated as they would be in any patient. An ECG should be recorded annually for adults, and slit-lamp examination is also carried out periodically. The families are educated about the nature of the disease, inheritance, and the availability of DNA diagnosis for adults and for prenatal testing.

LIMB-GIRDLE MUSCULAR DYSTROPHY

History and Definition

LGMD (MIM 253600; 159000; 253700) is a category of muscular dystrophy that was conceived as a diagnosis of exclusion to include syndromes not meeting the diagnostic criteria for Duchenne, FSH, or myotonic dystrophy. As a result, autosomal-dominant and recessive forms were described, as well as familial disorders of proximal or distal limb weakness. These disorders were long assumed to be heterogeneous, awaiting separation on the basis of pathogenesis, and that has been forthcoming. Metabolic myopathies have been separated, especially acid maltase and debrancher enzyme deficiencies; other limb-girdle syndromes proved to be Becker dystrophy, mitochondrial myopathies, polymyositis, inclusion body myositis, or other diseases (Table 125.4). With the advance of molecular genetics, dystrophin-normal myopathies were mapped, and gene products were identified as a new class of mostly cytoskeletal proteins. Immunochemical identification of these proteins and DNA analysis now play a major role in both diagnosis and definition.

LGMD can be defined as follows: It comprises a heterogeneous group of muscular dystrophies that are predomiantly proximal in limb distribution. They are distinguished by patterns of inheritance, site of mutation, and nature of the affected protein. In all of them, dystrophin is present, and there is no mutation at Xp21. Childhood forms are related to mutations in genes for cytoskeletal proteins. In cases of adolescent or adult on-set, LGMD is still a diagnosis of exclusion and is likely to be heterogeneous in etiology.

Clinical Manifestations

Onset may be in childhood, adolescence, or adulthood, and inheritance may be autosomal dominant or recessive. The disorder may be more severe in some families than in others.

The legs are usually affected first, with difficulty climbing stairs and rising from chairs. A waddling gait then develops. Later, raising the arms becomes difficult, and winging of the scapula may be seen. Knee jerks tend to be lost before ankle jerks. Cranial muscles are usually spared. Progression is slow. EMG and muscle biopsy, by definition, show myopathic changes. Serum CK is elevated, usually less so than in Duchenne dystrophy but in the same range. Diagnosis now depends on DNA analysis.

In one late-onset disorder, *quadriceps myopathy*, symptoms are focal, as the name implies; it may be inherited as an autosomal-dominant trait. Polymyositis may be similarly restricted, and some quadriceps syndromes seem to be neurogenic. In rare cases, dystrophin is lacking. There are still some limb-girdle disorders that have not been mapped. Distal and congenital myopathies are described in later sections.

Molecular Genetics

The discovery of the affected gene product in Duchenne MD was rapidly followed by remarkable advances in the cell biology of muscle and, simultaneously, in the analysis of LGMDs. These diseases resemble the Duchenne form clinically but differ because dystrophin is normal and inheritance is autosomal dominant or recessive rather than X-linked. Starting with these diseases, Kevin Campbell and colleagues discovered new proteins by mapping the genes responsible for dystrophin-normal dystrophies and then identifying the affected gene products.

The dystrophin-associated glycoproteins include some that are extracellular (merosin, formerly called laminin, and dystroglycans), some that are located on the cytoplasmic side of the muscle plasma membrane (dystrophin, syntrophin, and utrophin), and some that span the surface membrane (sarcoglycans). They function as a group to anchor intracellular cytoskeletal components (including actin and dystrophin) to extracellular proteins supporting the surface membrane as the muscle contracts and relaxes (see Fig. 125.3).

The importance of sarcoglycans and dystroglycans is emphasized by the limb-girdle diseases that result when these glycoproteins are genetically absent. In these conditions, one of the sarcoglycans is missing (Table 125.5). All but one of these newly recognized disease-associated proteins is part of the muscle cytoskeleton; the exception is calpain, a muscle-specific calcium-activated protease. However, some families show no linkage to these loci, and identified mutations account for only about 10% of all myopathies with normal dystrophin. As a group, these LGMDs exemplify locus heterogeneity, whereby different mutant gene products are encoded on different chromosomes but give rise to clinically similar syndromes. The *sarcoglycanopathies* teach us that dystrophin is needed to anchor the sarcoglycans, but the glycoproteins are important themselves and seem to function as a com-

TABLE 125.4. CONDITIONS SIMULATING LIMB-GIRDLE MUSCULAR DYSTROPHY

Acquired disease
Inflammatory
    Polymyositis, dermatomyositis, inclusion body myositis, sarcoidosis
Toxic myopathies
    Chloroquine, steroid myopathy, vincristine, lovastatin, ethanol abuse, phenytoin
Endocrinopathies
    Hyperthyroidism, hypothyroidism, hyperadrenocorticism (Cushing syndrome), hyperparathyroidism, hyperaldosteronism
Vitamin deficiency
    Vitamin D and vitamin E malabsorption
Paraneoplastic
    Lambert-Eaton syndrome, carcinomatous myopathy
Heritable diseases
Becker muscular dystrophy
Manifesting carrier of Duchenne or Becker gene
Emery-Dreifuss muscular dystrophy
Facioscapulohumeral or scapulohumeral dystrophy
Myotonic muscular dystrophy
Congenital myopathies (centronuclear, central core, emaline, tubular aggregates, cytoplasmic body)
Metabolic myopathies: glycogen storage diseases (phosphorylase deficiency, acid maltase deficiency, debrancher deficiency), lipid storage diseases (carnitine deficiences), mitochondrial myopathies
Myopathy of periodic paralysis

Modified from Jerusalem and Sieb, 1992.

TABLE 125.5. **LIMB-GIRDLE MUSCULAR DYSTROPHIES**

	Map position	Gene product	Name	MIM no.
Autosomal dominant				
LGMD1A	5q22–34	Unknown		159000
LGMD1B	1q11–21	Unknown		159000
LGMD1C	3p25	Caveolin-3		159000
	Other	Unmapped		
Autosomal recessive				
LGMD2A	15q15	Calpain-3		253600
LGMD2B	2p	Unknown		253600
LGMD2C	13q12	γ-Sarcoglycan	SCARMD	253700
LGMD2D	17q12	α-Sarcoglycan (adhalin)	DMD-like	600119
LGMD2E	4q12	β-Sarcoglycan	DMD-like	253700
LGMD2F	5q33	δ-Sarcoglycan	DMD-like	253700
LGMD2G	17q11	Unknown	DMD-like	253700

DMD, Duchenne muscular dystrophy; LGMD, limb-girdle muscular dystrophy; MIM, Mendelian Inheritance in Man (McKusick); SCARMD, severe childhood autosomal-recessive muscular dystrophy.
Modified from Neuromuscular disorders: gene location. *Neuromuscul Disord* 1998;8:I–VII.

plex. If a key sarcoglycan is missing, dystrophin does not function properly. Further, mutation of one sarcoglycan leads to secondary loss of the other components of the complex. The nonmapped conditions indicate that still other mechanisms need to be identified. For instance, merosin deficiency is the cause of 50% of all cases of congenital muscular dystrophy but is also found in some limb-girdle syndromes starting after age 20 years.

CONGENITAL MUSCULAR DYSTROPHIES

These are the only conditions called "dystrophy" that are not clearly progressive. Instead, the appellation was taken from histologic changes in muscle. Limb weakness and floppiness are evident at bith. One type has been mapped to 6q2; the affected protein is laminin α2 (merosin); it is called *merosin-deficient congenital dystrophy.* The histology is that of a dystrophy, but inflammatory cells may be prominent. This form accounts for almost 50% of all congenital dystrophy cases. Disability may be mild or severe. Contractures and respiratory problems are common; CK values may be high in early stages. Mental development is normal. Merosin-positive cases are unmapped, and the disease is milder on all scores. In *Fukuyama congenital muscular dystrophy* (MIM 253800), severe neuromuscular symptoms are apparent at birth, with difficulty swallowing and feeble limb movements, but little change later. Additionally, congenital abnormalities of the brain, especially microcephaly and hydrocephalus, are manifested by seizures and mental retardation. The children never walk, and severe disability leads to inanition and death by age 10. Fukuyama congenital dystrophy is autosomal-recessive and maps to 9q31; the gene product is not yet known.

In the *Walker-Warburg syndrome* (MIM 236670), the myopathy and cerebral abnormalities are similar, but ocular malformations characteristically include cataracts and retinal dysplasia. Lissencephaly (agyria) is a prominent cerebral anomaly. Another congenital disorder is the *muscle-eye-brain syndrome* or *Santavuori disease.* In addition to severe limb weakness, mental retardation, malformations of the brain, retinal dysplasia and optic atrophy are all seen.

Except for merosin, the gene products are not known in congenital dystrophies, but consanguinity in many families suggests recessive inheritance. The Fukuyama syndrome seems especially prevalent in Japan but has been seen in Europe and the United States. In sporadic cases, dystrophin analysis is needed to be certain that an unusual congenital myopathy is not a variant of Duchenne dystrophy.

DISTAL MYOPATHIES (DISTAL MUSCULAR DYSTROPHIES)

Distal myopathies (distal muscular dystrophies) (MIM 160500) are defined by clinical manifestations in the feet and hands before proximal limb muscles are affected. As heritable diseases with features of myopathy and slow progression, they are properly considered muscular dystrophies The distinction from heritable neuropathies depends on the sparing of sensation, as well as histologic and electrodiagnostic features of myopathy. Most distal myopathies have been assigned to different map positions, confirming the clinical differences in patterns of inheritance, onset in leg or hands, predominant leg weakness in anterior or posterior compartments, presence or absence of vacuoles, and rise in serum CK (Table 125.6).

The most common form is *Welander distal myopathy,* which was first described in Sweden; inheritance is autosomal-dominant. Symptoms begin in adolescence or adult years and progress slowly. The legs are affected before the hands. Histologic changes are mild, but filamentous inclusions may resemble those seen in oculopharyngeal dystrophy or inclusion body myositis. Serum CK is only slightly elevated.

In the autosomal-recessive *Nonaka* variant, a vacuolar myopathy is seen, the gastrocnemius muscles are spared, and serum enzyme values are only slightly increased. Nonaka distal myopathy and hereditary inclusion body myopathy share clinical and morphologic similarities; both conditions map to 9p1-q1. *Miyoshi* distal myopathy is also autosomal recessive but differs from Nonaka in that the histologic changes are nonspecific (without vacuoles), the gastrocnemius muscles are affected

TABLE 125.6. DISTAL MYOPATHIES

Type	Heritance	Map	Site	CK	Vacuoles	MIM no.
Onset after age 40 yr						
Welander	AD	??	Hands	Normal	Sometimes	—
Markesbery-						
Griggs-Udd	AD	2q31–33	AC	Normal	Yes	600344
Onset before age 40 yr						
Nonaka	AR	9p1–q1	AC	<5×	Yes	—
Miyoshi	AR	2p12–13	PC	10–150×	No	254130
Laing	AD	14q11[a]	AC	<3×	No	160500
Feit	AD	5q31	AC	<3×	Yes	—
			VC			
Schotland-						
Satoyoshi[b]	AD	??	Eyes, hands, AC	—	Few (5% of fibers)	—

AC, anterior compartment of legs; AD, autosomal dominant; AR, autosomal recessive; CK, creatine kinase; MIM, Mendelian Inheritance in Man (McKusick); PC, posterior compartment; VC, vocal cords, pharynx; ×, times normal for CK value.
[a]Laing type at 14q11 is same position as oculopharyngeal muscular dystrophy.
[b]Schotland-Satoyoshi dystrophy is oculopharyngodistal myopathy.

first, and serum CK values are as high as those in Duchenne dystrophy; hyperCKemia may be noted before there is any symptomatic weakness. The Miyoshi variety and LGMD type 2B (proximal limb weakness) both map to 2p17. The gene product has been named *dysferlin*. Some Miyoshi families do not link to this position, which implies locus heterogeneity. Another form of distal myopathy is accompanied by vocal cord and pharyngeal weakness. Still more variants are likely to be identified.

SUGGESTED READINGS

General

Emery AEH, ed. *Neuromuscular disorders: clinical and molecular genetics.* New York: John Wiley and Sons, 1998.

Griggs RC, Mendell JR, Miller RG. *Evaluation and treatment of myopathies.* Philadelphia: FA Davis Co, 1995.

Karpati G, Carpenter S. Skeletal muscle pathology in neuromuscular diseases. In: Vinken PJ, Bruyn GW, Klawans HL, Rowland LP, DiMauro S, eds. *Myopathies. Handbook of clinical neurology, rev ser, vol 62(18).* New York: Elsevier Science, 1992:1–48.

Kissel T, Hendell J, eds. Muscular dystrophies. *Semin Neurol* 1999;19:1–100.

Tarnopolsky M, Martin J. Creatine monohydrate increases strength in patients with neuromuscular disease. *Neurology* 1999;52:854–857.

Vinken PJ, Bruyn GW, Klawans HL Rowland LP, DiMauro S, eds. *Myopathies. Handbook of clinical neurology, rev ser, vol 62(18).* New York: Elsevier Science, 1992.

Walton JN, ed. *Diseases of voluntary muscle,* 5th ed. London: Churchill Livingstone, 1994.

Walton JN, Nattrass FJ. On the classification, natural history and treatment of the myopathies. *Brain* 1954;77:170–231.

Duchenne and Becker Dystrophies and Other X-linked Diseases

Ades LC, Gedeon AK, Wilson MJ, et al. Barth syndrome: clinical features and confirmation of gene localization to distal Xq28. *Am J Med Genet* 1993;45:327–334.

Anderson MS, Kunkel LM. The molecular and biochemical basis of Duchenne muscular dystrophy. *Trends Biochem Sci* 1993;17:289–292.

Barth PG, Van Wijngaarden GK, Bethlem J. X-linked myotubular myopathy with fatal neonatal asphyxia. *Neurology* 1975;25:531–536.

Becker PE, Kiener F. Eine neue X-chromosomale Muskeldystrophie. *Arch Psychiatr Z Neurol* 1955;193:427–448.

Bush A, Dubowitz V. Fatal rhabdomyolysis complicating general anesthesia in a child with Becker dystrophy. *Neuromuscul Disord* 1991;1:201–204.

Bushby KMD. Genetic and clinical correlations of Xp21 muscular dystrophy. *J Inherit Metab Dis* 1992;15:551–564.

Bushby KMD, Gardner-Medwin S. The clinical, genetic and dystrophin characteristics of Becker muscular dystrophy. I. Natural history. *J Neurol* 1993;240:98–104.

Bushby KMD, Gardner-Medwin S, Nicholson LVB, et al. The clinical, genetic and dystrophin characteristics of Becker muscular dystrophy. II. Correlation of phenotype with genetic and protein abnormalities. *J Neurol* 1993;240:105–112.

Bushby KM, Hill A, Steele JG. Failure of early diagnosis in symptomatic Duchenne muscular dystrophy. *Lancet* 1999;353:557–558.

Case records of the Massachusetts General Hospital. Case 22-1998. Becker's muscular dystrophy involving skeletal muscle and myocardium. *N Engl J Med* 1998;339:182–190.

Dubrovsky AL, Angelini C, Bonifati DM, Pegoraro E, Mesa L. Steroids in muscular dystrophy: where do we stand? *Neuromuscul Disord* 1998;8:380–384.

Hoffman EP. Genotype/phenotype correlations in Duchenne/Becker dystrophy. In: Partridge T, ed. *Molecular and cell biology of muscular dystrophy.* London: Chapman & Hall, 1993.

Hoffman EP, Arahata K, Minetti C, et al. Dystrophinopathy in isolated cases of myopathy in females. *Neurology* 1992;42:957–975.

Hoffman EP, Brown RH, Kunkel LM. Dystrophin: the protein product of the Duchenne muscular dystrophy locus. *Cell* 1987;51:919–928.

Karpati G, Ajdukovic D, Arnold D, et al. Myoblast transfer in Duchenne muscular dystrophy. *Ann Neurol* 1993;34:8–17.

Matsumara K, Campbell KP. Dystrophin-glycoprotein complex: its role in the molecular pathogenesis of muscular dystrophies. *Muscle Nerve* 1994;17:2–15.

Nicholson LVB, Johnson MA, Bushby KMD, et al. Integrated study of 100 patients with Xp21-linked muscular dystrophy using clinical, genetic, immunochemical, and histopathological data. Part 1. Trends across the clinical groups. *J Med Genet* 1993;30:728–736.

Palmucci L, Doriguzzi C, Mongini T, et al. Dilating cardiomyopathy as the expression of Xp21 Becker type muscular dystrophy. *J Neurol Sci* 1992;111:218–221.

Quinlivan RM, Dubowitz V. Cardiac transplantation in Becker muscular dystrophy. *Neuromuscul Disord* 1992;2:165–167.

Van Ommen GJB, Scheuerbrandt G. Workshop report: neonatal screening for muscular dystrophy. *Neuromuscul Disord* 1993;3:231–239.

Emery-Dreifuss Muscular Dystrophy and Rigid Spine Syndrome

Emery AEH, Dreifuss FE. Unusual type of benign X-linked muscular dystrophy. *J Neurol Neurosurg Psychiatry* 1966;29:338–342.

Fidzianska A, Toniolo D, Hausmanowa-Petrusewicz I. Ultrastructural abnormality of sarcolemma nuclei in Emery-Dreifuss muscular dystrophy. *J Neurol Sci* 1998;159:88–93.

Kubo S, Tsukahara T, Takemitsu M, et al. Presence of emerinopathy in cases of rigid spine syndrome. *Neuromuscul Disord* 1998;8:502–507.

Miller RG, Layzer RB, Mellenthin MA, et al. Emery-Dreifuss muscular dystrophy with autosomal dominant inheritance. *Neurology* 1985;35:1230–1233.

Rowland LP, Fetell MR, Olarte MR, et al. Emery-Dreifuss muscular dystrophy. *Ann Neurol* 1979;5:111–117.

Sabatelli P, Squarzoni S, Pertini S, et al. Oral exfoliative cytology for the noninvasive diagnosis in X-linked Emery-Dreifuss muscular dystrophy patients and carriers. *Neuromuscul Disord* 1998;8:67–71.

Taylor J, Sewry CA, Dubowitz V, Muntoni F. Early-onset, autosomal-recessive muscular dystrophy with Emery-Dreifuss phenotype and normal emerin expression. *Neurology* 1998;51:1116–1120.

Toniolo D, Bione S, Arahata K. Emery-Dreifuss muscular dystrophy. In: Emery AEH, ed. *Neuromuscular disorders: clinical and molecular genetics.* New York: John Wiley and Sons, 1998:87–104.

Facioscapulohumeral Muscular Dystrophy

Brouwer OF, Padberg GW, Ruys CJM, et al. Hearing loss in facioscapulohumeral muscular dystrophy. *Neurology* 1991;41:1878–1881.

Brouwer OF, Wijmenga C, Frants RR, Padberg GW. Facioscapulohumeral muscular dystrophy: impact of genetic research. *J Neurol Sci* 1993;95:9–21.

Fisher J, Upadhyaya M. Molecular genetics of facioscapulohumeral muscular dystrophy. *Neuromuscul Disord* 1997;7:55–62.

Griggs RC, Tawil R, Storwick D, et al. Genetics of facioscapulohumeral muscular dystrophy: new mutations in sporadic cases. *Neurology* 1993;43:2369–2377.

Kissel JT, McDermott MP, Nitarajan R, et al. Pilot trial of albuterol in facioscapulohumeral muscular dystrophy. FSH-DY Group. *Neurology* 1998;50:1402–1406.

Laforet P, de Toma C, Eymard B, et al. Cardiac involvement in genetically confirmed facioscapulohumeral muscular dystrophy. *Neurology* 1998;51:1454–1456.

Letournel E, Fardeau M, Lytle JO, Serrault M, Gosselin RA. Scapulothoracic arthrodesis for patients who have facioscapulohumeral muscular dystrophy. *J Bone Joint Surg [Am]* 1990;72:78–84.

Munsat TL, Serratrice G. Facioscapulohumeral and scapuloperoneal syndromes. In: Vinken PJ, Bruyn GW, Klawans HL, Rowland LP, DiMauro S, eds. *Myopathies. Handbook of clinical neurology, rev ser, vol 62(18).* New York: Elsevier Science, 1992:161–177.

Tawil R, Figlewicz DA, Griggs RC, Weiffenbach B. Facioscapulohumeral dystrophy: a distinct regional myopathy with a novel molecular pathogenesis. FSH consortium. *Ann Neurol* 1998;43:279–282.

Tawil R, Storvick D, Weiffenbach B, et al. Extreme variability of expression in monozygotic twins with facioscapulohumeral muscular dystrophy. *Neurology* 1993;43:345–348.

Typler R, Babierato L, Menni M, et al. Identical *de novo* mutations at the D4F104S1 locus in monozygotic male twins with facioscapulohumeral muscular dystrophy with different clinical expression. *J Med Genet* 1998;35:778–786.

Wijmenga C, Padberg GW, Moerer P, et al. Mapping of facioscapulohumeral muscular dystrophy gene to chromosome 4q35-qter by multipoint linkage analysis. *Nat Genet* 1992;2:26–30.

Myotonic Muscular Dystrophy

AFM/MDA 1st international myotonic dystrophy consortium conference, 30 June–1 July, 1997, Paris. *Neuromuscul Disord* 1998;8:432–437.

Ashizawa T. Myotonic dystrophy as a brain disorder. *Arch Neurol* 1998;55:291–293.

Brook JD, McCurrach ME, Harley HG, et al. Molecular basis of myotonic muscular dystrophy: expansion of a trinucleotide (CTG) repeat at the 3′ end of a transcript encoding a protein kinase family member. *Cell* 1992;68:799–808.

Hageman ATM, Gabreels FJM, Liem KD, et al. Congenital myotonic dystrophy: report on 13 cases and review of the literature. *J Neurol Sci* 1993;115:95–101.

Harper PS. *Myotonic dystrophy.* London: WB Saunders, 1989.

Moxley RT III. Myotonic muscular dystrophy. In: Vinken PJ, Bruyn GW, Klawans HL, Rowland LP, DiMauro S, eds. *Myopathies. Handbook of clinical neurology, rev ser, vol 62(18).* New York: Elsevier Science, 1992:209–261.

Ranum LPW, Rasmussen PF, Benzow KA, Koob MD, Day JW. Genetic mapping of a second myotonic dystrophy locus. *Nat Genet* 1998;19:196–198.

Ricker K, Grimm T, Koch MC, et al. Linkage of proximal myotonic dystrophy to chromosome 3q. *Neurology* 1999;52:170–171.

Shelbourne P, Davies J, Buxton J, et al. Direct diagnosis of myotonic dystrophy with a disease-specific DNA marker. *N Engl J Med* 1993;328:471–475.

Tapscott SJ, Kiesert TR, Widrow RJ, Stöger R, Laird CD. Fragile-X syndrome and myotonic dystrophy: parallels and paradoxes. *Curr Opin Genet Dev* 1998;8:245–253.

Thornton CA, Ashizawa T. Getting a grip on the myotonic dystrophies. *Neurology* 1999;52:12–13.

Thornton CA, Griggs RC, Moxley RT III. Myotonic dystrophy with no trinucleotide expansion. *Ann Neurol* 1994;35:269–272.

Timchenko LT. Myotonic dystrophy: the role of RNA CUG triplet repeats. *Am J Hum Genet* 1999;64:360–364.

Tsilfidis C, MacKenzie AE, Mettler G, et al. Trinucleotide repeat length and frequency of severe congenital myotonic dystrophy. *Nat Genet* 1992;1:192–195.

Limb-Girdle Muscular Dystrophy

Angelini C, Fanin M, Freda MP, Duggan DJ, Siciliano G, Hoffman EP. The clinical spectrum of sarcoglycanopathies. *Neurology* 1999;52:175–179.

Brown RH Jr. Dystrophin-associated proteins and the muscular dystrophies. *Annu Rev Med* 1997;48:457–466.

Bushby K, Anderson VB, Pollitt C, Naom I, Muttoni F, Bindoff L. Abnormal merosin in adults: a new form of late-onset muscular dystrophy not linked to chromosome 6q2. *Brain* 1998;121:581–588.

Haq RU, Speer MC, Chu ML, Tandan R. Respiratory involvement in Bethlem myopathy. *Neurology* 1999;52:174–176.

Jerusalem F, Sieb JP. The limb-girdle syndromes. In: Vinken PJ, Bruyn GW, Klawans HL, Rowland LP, DiMauro S, eds. *Myopathies. Handbook of clinical neurology, rev ser, vol 62(18).* New York: Elsevier Science, 1992:179–195.

Lim LE, Campbell KP. The sarcoglycan complex in limb-girdle muscular dystrophy. *Curr Opin Neurol* 1998;11:443–452.

Matsumara K, Campbell KP. Deficiency of dystrophin-associated proteins: a common mechanism leading to muscle cell necrosis in severe childhood muscular dystrophies. *Neuromuscul Disord* 1993;3:109–118.

Smith FJD, Eady RAJ, Leigh IM, et al. Plectin deficiency results in muscular dystrophy with epidermolysis bullosa. *Nat Genet* 1996;13:450–457.

Speer MC, Tandan R, Rao PN, et al. Evidence for locus heterogeneity in the Bethlem myopathy and linkage to 2q37. *Hum Mol Genet* 1996;5:1043–1046.

Distal Muscular Dystrophies

Barohn RJ, Amato AA, Griggs RC. Overview of distal myopathies: from the clinical to the molecular. *Neuromuscul Disord* 1998;8:309–316.

Feit H, Silergleit A, Schneider LB, et al. Vocal cord and pharyngeal weakness with autosomal dominant distal myopathy: clinical description and gene localization to 5p31. *Am J Hum Genet* 1998;63:1732–1742.

Galassi G, Rowland LP, Hays AP, et al. High serum levels of creatine kinase: asymptomatic prelude to distal myopathy. *Muscle Nerve* 1987; 10:346–350.

Ikeuchi T, Asaka T, Saito M, et al. Gene locus for autosomal recessive distal myopathy with rimmed vacuoles maps to chromosome 9. *Ann Neurol* 1997;41:432–437.

Linssen WHJP, de Visser M, Notermans NC, et al. Genetic heterogeneity in Miyoshi-type distal muscular dystrophy. *Neuromuscul Disord* 1998;8:317–329.

Liu J, Aoki M, Illa I, et al. Dysferlin, a novel skeletal muscle gene, is mutated in Miyoshi myopathy and limb-girdle muscular dystrophy. *Nat Genet* 1998;20:31–36.

Miyoshi K, Iwasa M, Kawai H, et al. Autosomal recessive distal muscular dystrophy: a new variety of distal muscular dystrophy predominantly seen in Japan. *Brain* 1986;109:31–54.

Somer H, Paetau A, Udd B. Distal myopathies. In: Emery AEH, ed. *Neuromuscular disorders: clinical and molecular genetics.* New York: John Wiley and Sons, 1998:181–202.

Sunohara N, Nonaka I, Kamei N, Satoyaoshi E. Distal myopathy with rimmed vacuole formation. *Brain* 1989;112:65–83.

Udd B. Limb-girdle type muscular dystrophy in a large family with distal myopathy: homozygous manifestation or a dominant gene? *J Med Genet* 1992;29:383–389.

Udd B, Rapola J, Nkelainen P, et al. Nonvacuolar myopathy in a large family with both late adult-onset distal myopathy and severe proximal dystrophy. *J Neurol Sci* 1992;112:214–231.

Weiler T, Greenberg CR, Nylen E, et al. Limb-girdle muscular dystrophy and Miyoshi myopathy in an aboriginal Canadian kindred map to LGMD2B and segregate with the same haplotype. *Am J Hum Genet* 1996;59:872–878.

Congenital Muscular Dystrophies

Beggs AH, Neumann PE, Arahata K, et al. Possible influences on the expression of X-chromosome-linked dystrophin abnormalities by heterozygosity for autosomal recessive Fukuyama congenital muscular dystrophy. *Proc Natl Acad Sci U S A* 1992;89:623–627.

Cohn RD, Herrmann R, Sorokin L, Wewer UM, Voit T. Laminin $\alpha2$ chain-deficient congenital muscular dystrophy: variable epitope expression in severe and mild cases. *Neurology* 1998;51:94–101.

Fukuyama U, Osawa M, Suzuki H. Congenital progressive muscular dystrophy of the Fukuyama type: clinical, genetic and pathologic considerations. *Brain Dev* 1981;3:1–10.

Matsumara K, Nonaka I, Campbell KP. Abnormal expression of dystrophin-associated protein in Fukuyama-type congenital muscular dystrophy. *Lancet* 1993;341:521–522.

Pegotato E, Mancias P, Swerdlow SH, et al. Congenital muscular dystrophy wtih primary lamnin $\alpha2$ (merosin) deficiency presenting as inflammatory myopathy. *Ann Neurol* 1996;40:782–791.

Pegotato E, Marks H, Garcia CA, et al. Laminin $\alpha2$ muscular dystrophy: genotype/phenotype studies of 22 patients. *Neurology* 1998;51:101–110.

Shewell MI, Rosenblatt B, Silver K. Inflammatory myopathy and Walker-Warburg syndrome: etiologic implications. *Can J Neurol Sci* 1993;20:227–229.

Tomé FMS, Guicheney P, Fardeau M. Congenital muscular dystrophies. In: Emery AEH, ed. *Neuromuscular disorders: clinical and molecular genetics.* New York: John Wiley and Sons, 1998:21–58.

Merritt's Neurology, 10th ed., edited by L.P. Rowland. Lippincott Williams & Wilkins, Philadelphia © 2000.

CHAPTER 126

FAMILIAL PERIODIC PARALYSIS

LEWIS P. ROWLAND

Familial periodic paralysis comprises diseases characterized by episodic bouts of limb weakness. On clinical grounds, there are three main types: hypokalemic periodic paralysis (HoPP) (MIM 170400), hyperkalemic (HyPP) (MIM 170500), and periodic paralysis with cardiac arrhythmia (MIM 170390). HyPP maps to 17q13, the locus of the gene for the alpha subunit of the sodium channel. HoPP maps to the gene for the dihydropyridine-sensitive L-type calcium channel of muscle, which is localized at 1q31. A third type, with cardiac arrhythmia, maps to neither site. Locus heterogeneity validates the clinical classification, although many investigators now lump the conditions as "channelopathies," including paramyotonia congenita and other "nondystrophic myotonias."

Attacks are similar in all three conditions but differ somewhat in severity and duration (Table 126.1). The two main types were first separated by the level of serum potassium during a spontaneous or induced attack. Provocative tests can be performed by intravenous administration of glucose and insulin to drive the potassium level down or by administration of potassium salts to increase the serum level.

The greatest uncertainty concerns *paramyotonia congenita*, which most investigators consider a separate syndrome that is manifested only by myotonia, with no attacks of paralysis. Some authorities believe that there are disease-specific mutations within the sodium channel gene. The word *paramyotonia* is used because the condition is thought to differ from ordinary myotonia in two ways: Paramyotonia is brought on by cold (but so are other forms of myotonia), and it is "paradoxic" in that it becomes more severe with exercise, whereas the myotonia of other diseases is ameliorated by exercise. In families with HyPP, however, many individuals have myotonia, and in presumed families of paramyotonia congenita, some individuals have attacks of paralysis (including the original families described by Eulenberg in Germany and Rich in the United States). Some people with paramyotonia congenita are susceptible to attacks induced by administration of potassium. The diseases are allelic, mapping to the same gene. Similarly, the same gene accounts for paramyotonic variants, such as myotonia fluctuans, acetazolamide-responsive myotonia, and painful myotonia.

The third type of familial periodic paralysis, now called *Andersen syndrome*, was first thought to be normokalemic, then hyperkalemic. In fact, spontaneous attacks have been associated with high, low, or normal potassium levels. Nevertheless, patients are sensitive to administered potassium, which always provoked an attack before the provocative test was deemed dangerous. The

TABLE 126.1. CLINICAL FEATURES OF LOW- AND HIGH-SERUM POTASSIUM PERIODIC PARALYSIS AND PARAMYOTONIA

	Low-serum potassium periodic paralysis	High-serum potassium periodic paralysis	Paramyotonia congenita
Age of onset	Usually second or latter part of first decade	First decade	First decade
Sex	Male preponderance	Equal	Equal
Incidence of paralysis	Interval of weeks or months	Interval of hours or days	May not be present; otherwise, interval of weeks or months
Degrees of paralysis	Tends to be severe	Tends to be mild but can be severe	Tends to be mild but can be severe
Effect of cold	May induce an attack	May induce an attack	Tends to induce an attack
Effect of food (especially glucose)	May induce an attack	Relieves an attack	Relieves an attack
Serum potassium	Low	High	Tends to be high
Oral potassium	Prevents an attack	Precipitates an attack	Precipitates an attack

Modified from Hudson AJ. *Brain* 1963; 86:811.

hazard is feared because affected children are likely to have cardiac arrhythmias that lead to the need for a pacemaker. The syndrome was named after Andersen because she described a dysmorphic boy; since then dysmorphism has become one of five criteria for diagnosis; the others are periodic paralysis, potassium sensitivity, myotonia (usually mild), and cardiac arrhythmia. The dysrhythmia may be preceded by an asymptomatic prolonged QT interval on the ECG. The disease does not link to sodium or calcium channel genes or to the gene for the cardiac potassium channel that is responsible for most long QT syndromes.

Vacuoles are found in the muscles in the early stages of both HoPP and HyPP. These vacuoles seem to arise both from the terminal cisterns of the sarcoplasmic reticulum and from proliferation of the T tubules. In the later stage, there may be degeneration of the muscle fibers, possibly related to persistent weakness in the intervals between attacks.

HYPOKALEMIC PERIODIC PARALYSIS

In HoPP, the potassium content decreases in a spontaneous attack to values of 3.0 mEq/L or lower. Attacks may be induced by the injection of insulin, epinephrine, fluorohydrocortisone, or glucose, or they may follow ingestion of a meal high in carbohydrates. The potassium content of the urine is also decreased in an attack. It is not clear why potassium shifts into muscle to cause the attack.

Incidence

The disease is rare. There are no large series reported in the literature, and only one or two new patients are seen each year in any of the large neurologic centers in the United States. Males are affected two to three times as frequently as females. The first attack usually occurs at about the time of puberty, but it may occur as early as age 4 years or be delayed until the sixth decade.

Symptoms and Signs

An attack usually begins after a period of rest. It commonly develops during the night or is present on waking in the morning.

The extent of the paralysis varies from slight weakness of the legs to complete paralysis of all the muscles of the trunk and limbs. The oropharyngeal and respiratory muscles are usually spared, even in severe attacks. There may be retention of urine and feces during a severe attack. The duration of an individual attack varies from a few hours to 24 or 48 hours. According to some patients, strength improves if they move around and keep active ("walk it off"). The interval between attacks may be as long as 1 year, or one or more attacks of weakness may occur daily. Weakness is especially likely to be present in the morning after ingestion of a high-carbohydrate meal before retiring on the previous night. Rarely, the disease may occur in association with peroneal muscular atrophies.

In the interval between attacks, patients are usually strong, and the potassium content of the serum is normal. In some patients, mild proximal limb weakness persists. In a mild attack, tendon reflexes and electrical reactions of the muscles are diminished in proportion to the degree of weakness. In severe attacks, tendon and cutaneous reflexes are absent and the muscles do not respond to electrical stimulation. Cutaneous sensation is not disturbed.

Course

Familial HoPP is not accompanied by any impairment of general health. As a rule, the frequency of the paralytic attacks decreases with the passage of years, and they may cease altogether after age 40 or 50. Fatalities are rare, but death may occur from respiratory paralysis. The fixed myopathy, usually mild, may be severe and disabling.

Diagnosis

The diagnosis can usually be made without difficulty on the basis of the familial occurrence of transient attacks of weakness. The diagnosis is usually confirmed by finding low potassium and high sodium content in the serum during an attack, or by inducing an attack with an intravenous infusion of glucose (100 g) and regular insulin (20 U). Now, the provocative test can be avoided by DNA testing. However, if a patient is in the hospital during a spontaneous attack, it is important to determine which type of periodic paralysis is to be treated.

In sporadic cases, the first attack must be differentiated from other causes of hypokalemia (Table 126.2). Persistent hypokalemia from any cause may manifest as an acute attack of paralysis or persistent limb weakness with high levels of serum creatine kinase. Sometimes, there are attacks of myoglobinuria.

Repeated attacks of HoPP, identical clinically to the familial form, occur in patients with hyperthyroidism. Japanese and Chinese people seem to be especially susceptible to this disorder. The paralytic attacks cease when the thyroid disorder has been successfully treated.

Treatment

Acute attacks, spontaneous or induced, may be safely and rapidly terminated by ingestion of 20 to 100 mEq of potassium salts. Intravenous administration of potassium is usually avoided because of the hazard of inducing hyperkalemia.

The basis of prophylactic therapy is oral administration of the carbonic anhydrase inhibitor acetazolamide (Diamox), 250 to 1,000 mg daily. This regimen prevents attacks in about 90% of patients with HoPP and also improves the interictal weakness attributed to the vacuolar myopathy. The mechanism of action of acetazolamide is uncertain; the beneficial effect may be related to the mild metabolic acidosis it induces. For those not helped by acetazolamide, other effective agents include triamterene (Dyrenium) or spironolactone (Aldactone), which promote retention of potassium. Another carbonic anhydrase inhibitor of value is dichlorphenamide (Daranide). Dietary controls are usually not accepted by patients and are not effective.

Treatment of other forms of HoPP depends on the nature of the underlying renal disease, diarrhea, drug ingestion, or thyrotoxicosis. Patients with thyrotoxic periodic paralysis are susceptible to spontaneous or induced attacks during the period of hyperthyroidism. When the patients become euthyroid, spontaneous attacks cease and they are no longer sensitive to infusion of glucose and insulin. Glucose and insulin are useful in the interim between treatment of hyperthyroidism by drugs or radioiodine, before the euthyroid state returns. Repeated attacks can be prevented by either acetazolamide or propranolol.

HYPERKALEMIC PERIODIC PARALYSIS

In 1951, Frank Tyler recognized a form of familial periodic paralysis in which attacks were not accompanied by a decrease in the serum potassium content. In 1957, Gamstorp and colleagues drew attention to several other features of these cases that separated them from the usual cases of periodic paralysis. The disease is transmitted by an autosomal-dominant gene with almost complete penetrance. In addition to the absence of hypokalemia in the attacks, the syndrome is characterized by an early age of onset (usually before age 10). The attacks tend to occur in the daytime and are likely to be shorter and less severe than those in HoPP. Myotonia is usually demonstrable by EMG, but abnormalities of muscular relaxation are rarely symptomatic. Myotonic lid lag (Fig. 126.1) and lingual myotonia may be the sole clinical evidence of the trait. Serum potassium content and urinary excretion of potassium may be increased during an attack, possibly the result of leakage of potassium from muscle. The attacks tend to be precipitated by hunger, rest, or cold or by administration of potassium chloride.

Attacks may be terminated by administration of calcium gluconate, glucose, and insulin. Acetazolamide, 250 mg to 1 g orally daily, has been effective in reducing the number of attacks or in

TABLE 126.2. POTASSIUM AND PARALYSIS: NONINHERITED FORMS

Hypokalemic
  Excessive urinary loss
    Hyperaldosteronism
    Drugs: glycyrrhizate (licorice), thiazides, furosemide, chlorthalidone, ethacrynic acid, amphotericin, duogastrone
    Pyelonephritis, renal tubular acidosis
    Recovery from diabetic acidosis
    Ureterocolostomy
  Excessive gastrointestinal loss
    Malabsorption syndrome
    Laxative abuse
    Diarrhea
    Fistulas, vomiting, villous adenoma
    Pancreatic tumor, diarrhea
  Thyrotoxicosis
Hyperkalemia
  Uremia
  Addison disease
  Spironolactone excess
  Excessive intake
    Iatrogenic
    Geophagia

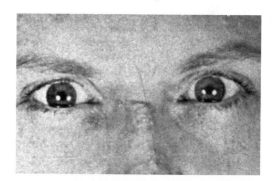

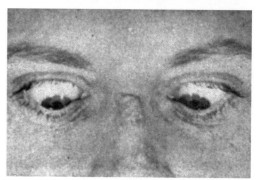

FIG. 126.1. Paramyotonia congenita. Myotonia of muscles of the upper eyelids on looking downward. (Courtesy of Dr. Robert Layzer.)

abolishing them altogether. Other diuretics that promote urinary excretion of potassium are also effective. If acetazolamide therapy fails, thiazides or fludrocortisone acetate (Florinef Acetate) may be beneficial. In addition, beta-adrenergic drugs may be effective prophylactic agents. Epinephrine, Salbutamal, and metaproterenol have been used. They presumably act by increasing the activity of Na+,K+-ATPase.

Pathophysiology

The pathophysiology of the HyPP has been analyzed by the team of Rudel, Ricker, and Lehmann-Horn (1993); their findings led to the suspicion that a sodium channel protein would be a good candidate gene. First, using microelectrode studies of intercostal muscle, they confirmed that muscle isolated from patients with HyPP is partially depolarized at rest. The abnormal depolarization was blocked by tetrodotoxin, which specifically affects the alpha subunit of the sodium channel. Patch clamp experiments showed faulty inactivation, leading to the conclusion that excessive sodium influx was accompanied by excessive efflux of potassium, thereby raising levels in extracellular fluids. They found that muscle from patients with more paramyotonia than sensitivity to potassium was more sensitive to cold.

In contrast, the calcium channel gene for HoPP was found not by physiology but by a genome-wide search. The pathophysiology of HoPP is not clear but may include an indirect effect on a sarcolemmal ATP-sensitive potassium channel.

The challenge now is to determine just how the single amino acid substitutions result in the altered function. Because periodic paralysis and potassium sensitivity are seen in families with paramyotonia, it is important to determine whether disease-specific mutations exist. Alternatively, as in myotonic muscular dystrophy and other autosomal-dominant diseases, there could be pleiotropic expression of the mutation, which is expressed by four abnormalities: paralytic attacks, myotonia, potassium sensitivity, and cold sensitivity. In the same family, one or more of these manifestations may be dominant in different individuals.

SUGGESTED READINGS

Hypokalemic Periodic Paralysis

Comi G, Testa D, Cornelio F, et al. Potassium depletion myopathy: a clinical and morphological study of six cases. *Muscle Nerve* 1985;8:17–21.

Conway MJ, Seibel JA, Eaton RP. Thyrotoxicosis and periodic paralysis: improvement with beta blockade. *Ann Intern Med* 1974;81:332–336.

Engel AG, Lambert EH, Rosevear JW, Tauxe WN. Clinical and electromyographic studies in a patient with primary hypokalemic periodic paralysis. *Am J Med* 1965;38:626–640.

Fontain B, Trofatter J, Rouleau GA, et al. Different gene loci for hyperkalemic and hypokalemic periodic paralysis. *Neuromuscul Disord* 1991;1:235–238.

Griggs RC, Engel WK, Resnik JS. Acetazolamide treatment of hypokalemic periodic paralysis: prevention of attacks and improvement of persistent weakness. *Ann Intern Med* 1970;73:39–48.

Holtzapple GE. Periodic paralysis. *JAMA* 1905;45:1224–1231.

Johnsen T. Familial periodic paralysis with hypokalemia. *Dan Med Bull* 1981;28:1–27.

Knochel JP. Neuromuscular manifestations of electrolyte disorders. *Am J Med* 1982;72:525–535.

Layzer RB, Goldfield E. Periodic paralysis caused by abuse of thyroid hormone. *Neurology* 1974;24:949–952.

Links TP, Zwarts MJ, Oosterhuis HJGH. Improvement of muscle strength in familial hypokalemic periodic paralysis with acetazolamide. *J Neurol Neurosurg Psychiatry* 1988;51:1142–1145.

Martin AR, Levinson SR. Contribution of the Na,K pump to membrane potential in familial periodic paralysis. *Muscle Nerve* 1985;8:359–362.

Marx A, Ruppersberg JP, Pietrzyk C, Rudel R. Thyrotoxic periodic paralysis and the sodium-potassium pump. *Muscle Nerve* 1989;12:810–815.

Minaker KL, Menelly GS, Flier JS, Rowe JW. Insulin-mediated hypokalemia and paralysis in familial hypokalemic periodic paralysis. *Am J Med* 1988;84:1001–1006.

Morrill JA, Brown RH Jr, Cannon SC. Gating of the L-type Ca channel in human skeletal myotubes: an activation defect caused by hypokalemic periodic paralysis mutation R528H. *J Neurosci* 1998;18:10320–10334.

Roadma JS, Reidenberg MM. Symptomatic hypokalemia resulting from surreptitious diuretic ingestion. *JAMA* 1981;246:1687–1689.

Vern BA, Danon MJ, Hanlon K. Hypokalemic periodic paralysis with unusual responses to acetazolamide and sympathomimetics. *J Neurol Sci* 1987;81:159–172.

Vroom FQ, Jarrell MA, Maren TH. Acetazolamide treatment of hypokalemic periodic paralysis: probable mechanisms of action. *Arch Neurol* 1975;32:385–392.

Yazaki K, Kuribayashi T, Yamamura Y, et al. Hypokalemic myopathy associated with 17α-hydroxylase deficiency: a case report. *Neurology* 1982;32:94–97.

Hyperkalemic Periodic Paralysis

Barchi RL. Phenotype and genotype in the myotonic disorders. *Muscle Nerve* 1998;21:1119–1120.

Bendheim PE, Reale EO, Berg BO. Beta-adrenergic treatment of hyperkalemic periodic paralysis. *Neurology* 1985;35:746–749.

Benstead TJ, Camfield PR, Ding DB. Treatment of paramyotonia congenita with acetazolamide. *Can J Neurol Sci* 1987;14:156–158.

Borg K, Hovmoller M, Larsson L, Edstrom L. Paramyotonia congenita (Eulenberg): clinical, neurophysiological and muscle biopsy observations in a Swedish family. *Acta Neurol Scand* 1993;87:37–42.

Bradley WG. Adynamia episodica hereditaria: clinical, pathological, and electrophysiological studies in an affected family. *Brain* 1969;92:345–378.

Christopher GA, Johnson JP, Palevsky PM, Greenberg A. Hyperkalemia in hospitalized patients. *Arch Intern Med* 1998;158:917–924.

De Silva S, Kuncl RW, Griffin JW, et al. Paramyotonia congenita or hyperkalemic periodic paralysis? Clinical and electrophysiological features of each entity in one family. *Muscle Nerve* 1990;13:21–26.

Eulenberg A. Über einer familiäre, durch 6 Generationen verfolgbare Form congenitaler Paramyotonie. *Neurol Centralbl* 1886;5:265–272.

Evers S, Engelien A, Karsch V, Hund M. Secondary hyperkalemic paralysis. *J Neurol Neurosurg Psychiatry* 1998;64:249–252.

Gamstorp I. Adynamia episodica hereditaria. *Acta Pediatr (Uppsala)* 1956;45(Suppl 108):1–126.

Hanna MF, Stewart J, Schapira AH, Wood NW, Morgan-Hughes JA, Murray NM. Salbutamol treatment in a patient with hyperkalaemic periodic paralysis due to a mutation in the skeletal muscle sodium channel gene (SCN4A). *J Neurol Neurosurg Psychiatry* 1998;65:248–250.

Heine R, Pika U, Lehmann-Horn F. A novel SCN4A mutation causing myotonia aggravated by cold and potassium. *Hum Mol Genet* 1991;2:1349–1353.

Hoffman EH, Wang J. Duchenne-Becker muscular dystrophy and the nondystrophic myotonias. *Arch Neurol* 1993;50:1227–1237.

Layzer RB, Lovelace RE, Rowland LP. Hyperkalemic periodic paralysis. *Arch Neurol* 1967;16:455–472.

Lisak RP, Lebeau J, Tucker SH, Rowland LP. Hyperkalemic periodic paralysis and cardiac arrhythmia. *Neurology* 1972;22:810–815.

Magee KR. A study of paramyotonia congenita. *Arch Neurol* 1963;8:461–470.

McArdle B. Adynamia episodica hereditaria and its treatment. *Brain* 1962;85:121–148.

McClatchey AI, Trofatter J, McKenna-Yasek D, et al. Dinucleotide repeat polymorphisms at the SCN4A locus suggest allelic heterogeneity of hyperkalemic periodic paralysis and paramyotonia congenita. *Am J Hum Genet* 1992;50:896–901.

Moxley RT, Ricker KM, Kingston WJ, Bohlen R. Potassium uptake in muscle during paramyotonic weakness. *Neurology* 1989;39:952–955.

Ponce SP, Jennings AE, Madias NE, Harrington JT. Drug-induced hyperkalemia. *Medicine* 1985;64:357–370.

Ptacek LJ, Griggs RC. Genetics and physiology of the myotonic muscle disorders. *N Engl J Med* 1993;328:482–489.

Ptacek LJ, Timmer JS, Agnew WS, et al. Paramyotonia congenita and hyperkalemic periodic paralysis map to the same sodium channel locus. *Am J Hum Genet* 1991;49:851–854.

Rich EC. A unique form of motor paralysis due to cold. *Med News* 1894;65:210–213.

Ricker K, Bohlen R, Rohkamm R. Different effectiveness of tocainide and hydrochlorothiazide in paramyotonia congenita with hyperkalemic episodic paralysis. *Neurology* 1983;33:1615–1618.

Riggs JE, Griggs RC, Moxley RT. Acetazolamide-induced weakness in paramyotonia congenita. *Ann Intern Med* 1977;86:169–173.

Rudel R, Ricker K, Lehmann-Horn F. Genotype-phenotype correlations in human skeletal muscle sodium channel diseases. *Arch Neurol* 1993;50:1241–1248.

Sansone V, Griggs RC, Meola G, et al. Andersen's syndrome: a distinct periodic paralysis. *Ann Neurol* 1997;42:305–312.

Streib EW. Hypokalemic paralysis in two patients with paramyotonia congenita and known hyperkalemic/exercise-induced weakness. *Muscle Nerve* 1989;12:936–937.

Tricarico D, Servidei S, Tonali P, Jurkat-Rott K, Camerino DC. Impairment of skeletal muscle adenosine triphosphate-sensitive K+ channels in patients with hypokalemic periodic paralysis. *J Clin Invest* 1999;103:675–682.

Merritt's Neurology, 10th ed., edited by L.P. Rowland. Lippincott Williams & Wilkins, Philadelphia © 2000.

CHAPTER 127

CONGENITAL DISORDERS OF MUSCLE

LEWIS P. ROWLAND

Several different categories of muscle disease are evident from birth; most of them are familial in mendelian patterns of inheritance, but some are characteristically sporadic. The cause of such cases is uncertain. Terminology is currently unsatisfactory because there is no clear distinction between congenital muscular dystrophies (see Chapter 125) and the congenital myopathies. The diseases in either group may be evident at birth or become evident because motor milestones are delayed, and then remain static or be steadily progressive. The conditions called *congenital myopathies* here are mostly static or only slowly progressive. One group is characterized by a disorder of contractility with little or no weakness (myotonia congenita); another combines myotonia with severe dysmorphic features (Schwartz-Jampel syndrome). Others are defined by structurally specific histologic characteristics (congenital myopathies).

MYOTONIA CONGENITA

Myotonia congenita (MIM 160800), often called Thomsen disease, was described by a Danish physician in 1876. He had a close view of the condition, which affected his own family in an autosomal-dominant pattern. Symptoms are caused only by myotonia or the consequences thereof. The disease differs from myotonic muscular dystrophy in that there is no muscle weakness or wasting and no systemic disorder is present (i.e., no cataracts, electrocardiogram abnormalities, or endocrinopathy). The myotonia tends to be more severe than that in myotonic MD, where myotonia is rarely sufficiently bothersome to warrant symptomatic treatment. In myotonia congenita, however, the myotonia may be a functional handicap and more often leads to treatment. Presumably as a consequence of involuntary isometric contraction, the muscles tend to hypertrophy and give the person an athletic appearance. The myotonia is also more widespread, and in addition to the characteristic difficulty in relaxing the grip, the myotonia may affect the orbicularis oculi (difficulty opening the eyes after a forceful closure), leg muscles (difficulty in starting to walk or run), or even muscles of the pharynx (difficulty in swallowing). Respiration is spared. The myotonia is painless. Patients usually adapt well to the condition and live a normal life span.

The myotonia shows the usual physiologic characteristics of other forms of myotonia, including myotonic dystrophy and hyperkalemic periodic paralysis (HyPP). A repetitive discharge of muscle fiber potentials occurs after a forceful contraction, and the myotonia originates in the muscle surface membrane, as demonstrated by experiments in which percussion myotonia could still be evoked after the muscle had been isolated from the central and peripheral nervous systems by curarization. Characteristically, the myotonia is worse on the initiation of exercise and is ameliorated by gradually increasing the vigor of movements by "warming up."

Physiologic studies in a herd of myotonic goats implied an abnormality of the chloride channel (in contrast to the dysfunctional sodium channel in HyPP). As a result, chloride conductance is decreased. The chloride channel was then found to be affected in symptomatic humans, and the gene for both channel and disease was mapped to chromosome 7q35. In almost all cases, inheritance is autosomal-dominant, but a recessive pattern (MIM 255700) has been identified in a few families in which mild weakness improves with exercise. Remarkably, both autosomal dominant and recessive forms seem to be linked to the same chloride channel gene, CLCN1; the gene product is ClC-1. Other variants, such as painful myotonia or fluctuating myotonia, have been described clinically, but the relationship of these conditions to myotonia congenita awaits clarification by genetic studies.

In contrast to the chloride channel myotonias, the sodium channel diseases are often associated with periodic paralysis and are grouped as *nondystrophic myotonias* (see Chapter 126).

Myotonia congenita can be relieved by phenytoin sodium (Dilantin), 300 to 400 mg daily for serum level of 10 to 20 μg/mL, or quinine sulfate, 200 to 1,200 mg daily. Acetazolamide (Diamox) is sometimes effective. Hexiletine, an antiarrhythmic agent, is also helpful. Procainamide hydrochloride ameliorates myotonia but may induce systemic lupus erythematosus and is therefore avoided. The mode of action of these drugs is not clear, except that they seem to stabilize muscle membranes.

CHONDRODYSTROPHIC MYOTONIA (SCHWARTZ-JAMPEL SYNDROME)

Chondrodystrophic myotonia (Schwartz-Jampel syndrome) is an autosomal-recessive syndrome that is recognizable at birth because of the facial abnormalities: narrow palpebral fissures (blepharophimosis), pinched nose, and micrognathia. Other skeletal anomalies include short neck, flexion contractures of the limbs, and kyphosis. Limb muscles are clinically stiff and often hypertrophied. On EMG, the myotonia is often continuous, with little waxing and waning. Like other forms of myotonia, the chondrodystrophic form persists after curarization. The myotonia can be treated, but the skeletal abnormalities are more disabling. The condition must be differentiated from Isaacs syndrome (see Chapter 129).

Three forms of Schwartz-Jampel syndrome are recognized. The most common is autosomal-recessive and has been mapped to chromosome 1p34-p36.1; symptoms begin in late infancy or childhood. A second, more severe type is the neonatal variety, which may be fatal and does not map to chromosome 1. The third type is autosomal-dominant and unmapped.

CONGENITAL MYOPATHIES

In the 1960s, the application of histochemical stains to muscle biopsy specimens led to the recognition of unusual structures in children with mild myopathies. The myopathies are determined by changes in the EMG and muscle biopsy, with only slight increase in serum creatine kinase. The syndromes are not usually evident in the first 2 years of life, except for delayed walking. The persistent and relatively static weakness, however, suggests that the myopathy is congenital. Sometimes, however, symptoms do appear in the neonatal period, especially difficulty in sucking. They may cause the floppy infant syndrome (see Chapter 75). Conversely, there are later-onset forms, including some that appear first in adults. Whatever the clinical course, the disorders are named after the dominant structural abnormality (Table 127.1).

In *central core disease* (MIM 117000), an amorphous area in the center of the fiber stains blue with the Gomori trichrome stain and contrasts with the red-staining peripheral fibrils. The cores are devoid of enzymatic activity histochemically, and under the electron microscope, the area lacks mitochondria. In *nemaline disease* (from the Greek word for thread) (MIM 161800),

TABLE 127.1. CONGENITAL MUSCULAR DYSTROPHIES AND CONGENITAL MYOPATHIES

Congenital muscular dystrophies
  Merosin-deficient congenital muscular dystrophy
  Merosin-positive congenital muscular dystrophy
  Fukuyama congenital muscular dystrophy
  Muscle-eye-brain disease (Santavuori disease)
  Walker-Warburg syndrome and congenital muscular dystrophy
Congenital myopathies
  Common types
    Central core disease
    Centronuclear myopathies (myotubular myopathy)
      X-linked, autosomal dominant or recessive forms
      Neonatal, childhood, juvenile, adult forms
    Nemaline (rod) myopathy
  Uncommon types
    Cylindrical spirals myopathy
    Desminopathies
    Finger print body myopathy
    Hyaline body myopathy (also called lysis of myofibrils)
    Multicore or minicore disease
    Sarcotubular myopathy
    Tubular aggregate myopathy (familial)
  Dubious types
    Cap disease
    Congenital fiber-type disproportion
    Cytoplasmic body myopathy
    Myopathy with tubular aggregates (sporadic)
    Reducing-body myopathy
    Trilaminar myopathy
    Zebra-body myopathy

Modified from Griggs et al., 1995; Tome et al. 1998; and Goebel and Anderson, 1999.

small rods near the sarcolemma stain bright red with the trichrome stain and seem to originate from Z-band material. In *myotubular* or *centronuclear myopathy* (MIM 310400), the nuclei are situated centrally instead of in the normal sarcolemmal position, and are surrounded by a pale halo. *Cytoplasmic body myopathy* is characterized by accumulations of desmin, and some authorities suggest a category of *desmin-related myopathies*. Fiber-type disproportion, fingerprint bodies, tubular aggregates, and numerous other anomalies have been seen in different families, and variants of the original anomalies include minicores and multicores. For most of these myopathies, the origin of the structure is not known. In some *nonspecific congenital myopathies*, myopathic changes are found with no specific structure.

A few clinical clues might predict findings on muscle biopsy. In some patients, the usual static or slow progression of the disease with normal life expectancy gives way to more serious weakness or even premature death. Skeletal abnormalities are seen in centronuclear or nemaline myopathies or with fiber-type disproportion; a long, lean face, prognathism, kyphoscoliosis, pedal deformities, and congenital dislocation of the hip are characteristic. Centronuclear myopathy seems to be associated more often than the other congenital disorders with progressive ophthalmoplegia. Nemaline myopathy may be the most common of the group to cause respiratory problems in infancy and throughout life. *Arthrogryposis congenita multiplex* is the name given to a condition characterized by flexion contracture of the limbs; as determined by EMG and muscle biopsy, the syndrome is sometimes neurogenic and sometimes a congenital myopathy of the non-specific type. In the *Prader-Willi syndrome* (MIM 176270), the findings include hypotonia, neonatal dysphagia, tented upper lip, depressed myotatic reflexes, and cryptorchidism; these manifestations are prominent in infancy, but there is no permanent weakness. The syndrome is later recognized by mental retardation, obesity, short stature, skeletal anomalies, and childhood diabetes.

Progress is being made in the molecular genetics of these disorders. The following have been mapped: myotubular myopathy, Xq28; central core disease, 19q13.1; and nemaline myopathy, 1q21-q23 and 2q22. The Prader-Willi syndrome has been linked to deletions at 15q11-q13 and is a disease in which imprinting is involved; the autosomal-dominant condition results if the paternal chromosome is affected. If the maternal chromosome is affected, a different clinical disorder called the *Angelman syndrome* (MIM 234400) results; it is also manifested by mental retardation, but the other Prader-Willi manifestations are lacking. Instead, characteristics are microcephaly, lack of speech, and inappropriate laughter, leading to the appellation of the "happy puppet syndrome."

Although chromosome map positions have been established, only four gene products have been identified. In X-linked myotubular myopathy, the MTM1 gene encodes *myotubularin*, which is a protein tyrosine phosphatase. The gene product for autosomal recessive, chromosome-1q21-linked nemaline disease is *slow tropomyosin*. The affected protein in autosomal dominant nemaline disease is *alpha-tropomyosin* in some families, but others lack this mutation. The fourth known gene product is that of central core disease, which maps to the *ryanodine receptor* at 19q13.1. This is also the map position noted for malignant hyperthermia (MIM 145600). Patients with central core disease are at increased risk for malignant hyperthermia, and the two conditions may be found in different people in the same family.

The diagnosis of these conditions rests on the muscle pathology. Other congenital syndromes include myasthenia gravis, congenital myotonic dystrophy, and spinal muscular atrophy. In addition, the typical morphologic structures are sometimes found in adult-onset myopathies or other conditions. For instance, a late-onset nemaline disease can cause a severe myopathy after age 50 years.

Treatment of the congenital myopathies is symptomatic.

SUGGESTED READINGS

Myotonia Congenita

Becker PE. *Myotonia congenita and syndromes associated with myotonia: clinical-genetic studies of the nondystrophic myotonias.* Stuttgart: Thieme, 1977.

Deymeer F, Cakirkaya S, Serdaroglu P, et al. Transient weakness and compound muscle action potential decrement in recessive myotonia congenita. *Muscle Nerve* 1998;21:1334–1337.

Koch MC, Steinmeyer K, Lorenz C, et al. Skeletal muscle chloride channel in dominant and recessive human myotonia. *Science* 1992;257:797–800.

Kubisch C, Schmidt-Rose T, Fontaine B, Bretag AH, Jentsch TJ. ClC-1 chloride channel mutations in myotonia congenita: variable penetrance of mutations shifting the voltage dependence. *Hum Mol Genet* 1998;7:1753–1760.

Plassart-Schliess E, Garvais A, Eymard B, et al. Novel muscle chloride channel (CLCN1) mutations in myotonia congenita with various modes of in-

heritance including incomplete dominance and penetrance. *Neurology* 1998;50:1176–1179.

Trudell RG, Kaiser KK, Griggs RC. Acetazolamide-responsive myotonia congenita. *Neurology* 1987;37:488–491.

Wagner S, Deymeer F, Kurz LL, et al. The dominant chloride channel mutant G200R causing fluctuating myotonia: clinical findings, electrophysiology, and channel pathology. *Muscle Nerve* 1998;21:1122–1128.

Chondrodystrophic Myotonia (Schwartz-Jampel Syndrome)

Brown KA, Al-Gazali LI, Moynihan M, Lench NJ, Markham AF, Mueller RF. Genetic heterogeneity in Schwartz-Jampel syndrome: two families with neonatal Schwartz-Jampel syndrome do not map to chromosome 1p34-p36.1. *J Med Genet* 1997;34:685–687.

Farrell SA, Davidson RG, Thorp P. Neonatal manifestations of Schwartz-Jampel syndrome. *Am J Med Genet* 1987;27:799–805.

Nicole S, Ben Hamida C, Beighton P, et al. Localization of the Schwartz-Jampel syndrome locus to chromosome 1p34-36.1 by homozygosity mapping. *Hum Mol Genet* 1995;4:1633–1636.

Schwartz O, Jampel RS. Congenital blepharophimosis associated with a unique generalized myopathy. *Arch Ophthalmol* 1962;68:52–57.

Spaans F, Theunissn P, Reekerss AD, et al. Schwartz-Jampel syndrome. I. Clinical, electromyographic, and histologic studies. *Muscle Nerve* 1990;13:516–527.

Taylor RG, Layzer RB, Davis HS, Fowler WM. Continuous muscle fiber activity in the Schwartz-Jampel syndrome. *Electroencepahlogr Clin Neurophysiol* 1972;33:497–502.

Congenital Myopathies

Baeta AM, Figarella-Branger D, Bille-Ture F, Lepidi H, Pellissier JF. Familial desmin myopathies and cytoplasmic body myopathies. *Acta Neuropathol* 1996;92:499–510.

De Angelis MS, Palmucci L, Leone M, Doriguzzi C. Centronucleolar myopathy: clinical, morphological, and genetics characters: a review of 288 cases. *J Neurol Sci* 1991;103:2–9.

Glenn CC, Nicholls RD, Robinson WP, et al. Modification of 15q11-q13 DNA methylation imprints in unique Angelman and Prader-Willi patients. *Hum Mol Genet* 1993;2:1377–1382.

Goebel HH, Anderson JR. Structural congenital myopathies (excluding nemaline myopathy, myotubular myopathy and desminopathies). 56th European Neuromuscular Centre (ENMC) sponsored international workshop, December 12–14, 1997, Naarden, The Netherlands. *Neuromuscul Disord* 1999;9:50–57.

Goebel HH, Lenard HG. Congenital myopathies. In: Vinken PJ, Bruyn GW, Klawans HL, Rowland LP, DiMauro S, eds. *Myopathies. Handbook of clinical neurology, rev ser, vol 62(18).* New York: Elsevier Science, 1992:331–368.

Gordon N. Arthrogryposis multplex congenita. *Brain Dev* 1998;20:507–511.

Griggs RC, Mendell JR, Miller RG. *Evaluation and treatment of myopathies.* Philadelphia: FA Davis Co, 1995.

Gyure KA, Prayson RA, Estes ML. Adult-onset nemaline myopathy: case report and review of the literature. *Arch Pathol Lab Med* 1997;121:1210–1213.

Howard RS, Wiles CM, Hirsch NP, Spencer GT. Respiratory involvement in primary muscle disorders: assessment and management. *Q J Med* 1993;86:175–189.

Laing NG, Wilton SD, Akkari PA, et al. A mutation of the alpha tropomyosin gene TPM3 associated with autosomal dominant nemaline myopathy. *Nat Genet* 1995;9:75–79. Erratum: *Nat Genet* 1995;10:249.

Romero NB, Nivoche Y, Lunardi J, et al. Malignant hyperthermia and central core disease: analysis of two families with heterogeneous clinical expression. *Neuromuscul Disord* 1993;3:547–551.

Shuaib A, Martin JME, Mitchell LB, Brownell AKW. Multicore myopathy: not always a benign entity. *Can J Neurol Sci* 1988;15:10–14.

Shuaib A, Paasuke RT, Brownell AKW. Central core disease: clinical features in 13 patients. *Medicine* 1987;66:389–396.

Shy GM, Engel WK, Somers JE, Wanko T. Nemaline myopathy: a new congenital myopathy. *Brain* 1963;86:793–810.

Spargo E, Doshi B, Whitwell HL. Fatal myopathy with cytoplasmic inclusions. *Neuropathol Appl Neurobiol* 1988;14:516.

Spiro AJ, Shy GM, Gonatas NK. Myotubular myopathy. *Arch Neurol* 1966;14:1–14.

Tanner SM, Schneider V, Thomas NST. Characterization of 34 novel and six known MTM1 gene mutations in 47 unrelated X-linked myotubular myopathy patients. *Neuromuscul Disord* 1999;9:41–49.

Tein I, Haslam RHA, Rhead WJ, Bennett MJ, Becker LE, Vockley J. Short-chain acyl-coA dehydrogenase deficiency: a cause of ophthalmoplegia and multicore myopathy. *Neurology* 1999;52:366–372.

Tome FMS, Guicheney P, Fardeau M. Congenital muscular dystrophies. In Emery AEH, ed. *Neuromuscular disorders: clinical and molecular genetics*. New York: John Wiley and Sons, 1998:21–58.

Vajsar J, Becker LE, Freedom RM, Murphy EG. Familial desminopathy: myopathy with accumulation of desmin-type intermediate filaments. *J Neurol Neurosurg Psychiatry* 1993;56:644–648.

Wallgren-Petterson C. Genetics of the nemaline myopathies and the myotubular myopathies. *Neuromuscul Disord* 1998;8:401–404.

Merritt's Neurology, 10th ed., edited by L.P. Rowland. Lippincott Williams & Wilkins, Philadelphia © 2000.

CHAPTER 128

MYOGLOBINURIA

LEWIS P. ROWLAND

When necrosis of muscle is acute, myoglobin escapes into the blood and then into the urine. In the past, the term *myoglobinuria* was reserved for grossly pigmented urine, but modern techniques can detect amounts of this protein so minute that discoloration may not be evident. (Determination of serum myoglobin content by radioimmunoassay has the same diagnostic significance as measurement of serum creatine kinase [CK] activity.) The clinically important syndromes, however, are associated with gross pigmenturia. Sometimes, the disorder can be recognized without direct demonstration of myoglobin in the urine, for instance, in cases of acute renal failure with very high levels of serum CK activity. Inexplicably, *rhabdomyolysis* has become the official (*Index Medicus*) term for these syndromes, although it is really a synonym for myoglobinuria.

No classification of the myoglobinurias is completely satisfactory, but Table 128.1 lists the most important causes. Many cases of inherited recurrent myoglobinuria are due to unidentified abnormalities. In six forms, however, the genetic defect has been recognized: lack of phosphorylase (McArdle), phosphofructokinase (Tarui), carnitine palmityltransferase (CPT) (DiMauro-Bank), phosphoglyceraldehyde kinase (DiMauro), phosphoglycerate mutase (DiMauro), and lactate dehydrogenase (Kanno). CPT is important in lipid metabolism; the others are involved in glycogenolysis or glycolysis, and are reviewed in Chapter 84. In all these conditions, there is a disorder in the metabolism of a fuel necessary for muscular work; in all six, exercise is limited by painful cramps after exertion, and myoglobinuria occurs after especially strenuous activity. There may be a subtle difference in the kinds of activity that provoke attacks, which are more prolonged in CPT deficiency than in the glycogen disorders. The glycogen disorders can be identified by a simple clinical test: A cramp is induced by ischemic exercise of forearm muscles for less than 1 minute, and venous lactate fails to rise as it does in normal individuals or those with CPT defi-

ciency. Specific diagnosis requires histochemical or biochemical analysis of muscle homogenates. Five of the conditions are inherited in autosomal-recessive pattern; phosphoglycerate kinase deficiency is X-linked.

The relative frequency of the causes of recurrent myoglobinuria differed in two studies. In the United States, samples were sent to an active referral laboratory, and almost 50% had an identifiable cause; phosphorylase, phosphorylase kinase, phosphofructokinase, CPT, and myoadenylate deaminase deficiencies accounted for almost all in the report of Tonin and colleagues (1990). In Finland, however, only 23% of 22 patients with recurrent myoglobinuria had an identifiable cause, and none had CPT deficiency or myoadenylate deaminase deficiency. Lofberg and associates (1998) gave two explanations of recurrent myoglobinuria without an enzyme defect: disappearance of some genes from the genetically isolated population in Finland and an increase in recreational distance running or body building.

Another important form of inherited myoglobinuria occurs in *malignant hyperthermia* (MIM 180901, 145600), which is attributed to succinylcholine, halothane, or both together. The characteristic syndrome includes widespread muscular rigidity, a rapid rise in body temperature, myoglobinuria, arrhythmia, and metabolic acidosis. In some cases, muscular rigidity is lacking. The pathogenesis is uncertain, but the offending drugs may interact with a defective protein in the muscle sarcoplasmic reticulum that fails to bind calcium. The muscle, flooded with calcium, shortens to create the stiff muscles and attendant muscle necrosis. The syndrome is often familial in an autosomal dominant pattern, but many cases are sporadic. In some families, the gene mapped to chromosome 19q12-13.2, the site of the gene for the *ryanodine receptor*, which is the calcium release channel and also the locus for central core disease, a congenital myopathy that seems to increase the risk of malignant hyperthermia. A similar syndrome in pigs maps to the same gene product. However, there is evidence of locus heterogeneity because only 50% of all families map to that locus. Another calcium-binding protein of the sarcoplasmic reticulum is the dihydropyridine receptor, but the disease does not map to the locus for that candidate gene product. Yet another sign of heterogeneity is the occurrence of the syndrome in children with Duchenne muscular dystrophy or myotonia congenita. A closely related disorder is the *neuroleptic malignant syndrome*, which is similar in clinical manifestations, although the offending drugs are different and the disorder has not yet appeared in a family with malignant hyperthermia.

TABLE 128.1. CLASSIFICATION OF HUMAN MYOGLOBINURIA

Hereditary myoglobinuria
  Myophosphorylase deficiency (McArdle) (MIM 232600)
  Phosphofructokinase deficiency (Tarui) (MIM 171840)
  Carnitine palmityltransferase deficiency (DiMauro) (MIM 255110, 255120)
  Phosphoglycerate kinase (DiMauro) (MIM 311800)
  Phosphoglycerate mutase (DiMauro) (MIM 261670)
  Lactate dehydrogenase (Kanno) (MIM 150000)
  Incompletely characterized syndromes
    Excess lactate production (Larsson)
  Uncharacterized
    Familial; biochemical defect unknown
      Provoked by diarrhea or infection
      Provoked by exercise
    Malignant hyperthermia (MIM 180901, 145600)
    Repeated attacks in an individual; biochemical defect unknown
Sporadic myoglobinuria
  Exertion in untrained individuals
    "Squat-jump" and related syndromes
    Anterior tibial syndrome
    Convulsions
    High-voltage electric shock, lightning stroke
    Agitated delerium, restraints
    Status asthmaticus
    Prolonged myoclonus or acute dystonia
  Crush syndrome
    Compression by fallen weights
    Compression by body in prolonged coma
  Ischemia
    Arterial occlusion
    Ischemia in compression and anterior tibial syndromes
    Coagulopathy in sickle-cell disease or disseminated intravascular coagulation
    Ligation of vena cava
  Metabolic abnormalities
    Metabolic depression
      Barbiturate, carbon monoxide, narcotic coma
      Diabetic acidosis
      General anesthesia
      Hypothermia
    Exogenous toxins and drugs
      Haff disease
      Alcoholism
      Malayan sea-snake bite poison
      Plasmocid
      Succinylcholine
      Glycyrrhizate, carbenoxolone, amphotericin B
      Heroin
      Phenylpropanolamine
      Lovastatin
      Malignant neuroleptic syndrome
    Chronic hypokalemia of any cause
    Heat stroke
    Toxic shock syndrome
  Progressive muscle disease ("polymyositis," "alcoholic myopathy")
  Cause unknown

Most attacks of *acquired myoglobinuria* occur in nonathletic individuals who are subjected to extremely vigorous exercise, a hazard faced primarily by military recruits. These individuals are otherwise normal. Even trained runners may experience myoglobinuria in marathon races. If muscle is compressed, as occurs in the crush syndrome of individuals pinned by fallen timber af-

ter bombing raids, or after prolonged coma in one position, myoglobinuria may ensue. Ischemia after occlusion of large arteries may also lead to necrosis of large amounts of muscle. Depression of muscle metabolism, especially after drug ingestion, may also be responsible in some cases. Hypokalemia from any cause may predispose to myoglobinuria, but especially after chronic licorice ingestion or abuse of thiazide diuretics. Alcoholics seem especially prone to acute attacks of myoglobinuria, which may punctuate or initiate a syndrome of chronic limb weakness (alcoholic myopathy). In children, as in adults, the attacks may be precipitated by exercise (often with an identifiable enzymatic defect); in contrast to adults, however, myoglobinuria in children seems more often associated with a nonspecific viral infection and fever.

Whatever the cause, the clinical syndrome is similar: widespread myalgia, weakness, malaise, renal pain, and fever. Pigmenturia usually ceases within a few days, but the weakness may persist for weeks, and high concentrations of serum enzymes may not return to normal for even longer. The main hazard of the syndrome is heme-induced nephropathy with anuria, azotemia, and hyperkalemia. Hypercalcemia occurs in a few patients after anuria. Occasionally, respiratory muscles are symptomatically weakened.

Treatment of an acute episode of myoglobinuria is directed primarily toward the kidneys. Promotion of diuresis with mannitol seems desirable whenever there is oliguria. Dialysis and measures to combat hyperkalemia may be necessary. In recurrent cases due to defects of glycolytic enzymes or to unknown cause, various therapeutic regimens have been tried, but patients usually learn the limits of exercise tolerance.

The treatment of malignant hyperthermia is unsatisfactory because the rigidity is not abolished by curare. Intravenous infusions of dantrolene sodium (Dantrium) are given because this drug inhibits the release of calcium from the sarcoplasmic reticulum, relaxing the hypercontracted muscle. The average dose in successfully treated patients is 2.5 mg/kg body weight.

Once a person has been identified with malignant hyperthermia, the clinician must determine whether other family members are at risk. With the mapping of the gene to chromosome 19, it was hoped that a DNA test would be available. Locus heterogeneity, however, means that other, still unidentified genes are sometimes responsible. An alternative test to identify susceptibility is the caffeine contracture test, during which bundles of fibers from a muscle biopsy are exposed to the drug and tension is measured. Individuals are deemed susceptible if the response is significantly greater than normal. Unfortunately, the test is not completely reliable. Nevertheless, the condition is now so well known to anesthesiologists that offending volatile and neuromuscular blocking agents are avoided in people who may be at risk, and the frequency of attacks has fallen.

For the malignant neuropletptic syndrome, bromocriptine mesylate (Parlodel) and carbamazepine (Tegretol) have reportedly been beneficial (see Chapter 116).

SUGGESTED READINGS

Ball SP, Johnson KJ. The genetics of malignant hyperthermia. *J Med Genet* 1993;30:89–93.

Bank WJ, DiMauro S, Bonilla E, et al. A disorder of lipid metabolism and myoglobinuria: absence of carnitine palmityl transferase. *N Engl J Med* 1975;292:443–449.

Bristow MF, Kohen D. How "malignant" is the neuroleptic malignant syndrome? *BMJ* 1993;307:1223–1224.

Britt BA, Kalow W. Malignant hyperthermia: a statistical review. *Can Anaesth Soc J* 1970;17:293–315.

Corpier CL, Jones PH, Suki WN, et al. Rhabdomyolysis and renal injury with lovastatin use: report of two cases in cardiac transplant patients. *JAMA* 1988;260:239–241.

Denborough M. Malignant hypethermia. *Lancet* 1998;352:1131–1136.

DiMauro S, Dalakas M, Miranda AF. Phosphoglycerate kinase deficiency: another cause of recurrent myoglobinuria. *Ann Neurol* 1983;13:11–19.

DiMauro S, DiMauro PMM. Muscle carnitine palmityl transferase deficiency and myoglobinuria. *Science* 1973;182:929–931.

Duthie DJR. Heat-related illness. *Lancet* 1998;352:1329–1330.

Ebadi M, Pfeiffer RF, Murrin LC. Pathogenesis and treatment of neuroleptic malignant syndrome. *Gen Pharmacol* 1990;21:367–386.

Gabow PA, Kaehny WD, Kelleher SP. The spectrum of rhabdomyolysis. *Medicine* 1982;61:141–152.

Hogan K. The anesthetic myopathies and malignant hyperthermias. *Curr Opin Neurol* 1998;11:469–476.

Knochel JP. Rhabdomyolysis and myoglobinuria. *Annu Rev Med* 1982;33:435–443.

Kolb ME, Horne ML, Matz R. Dantrolene in human malignant hyperthermia: a multicenter study. *Anaesthesiology* 1982;56:254–262.

Lofberg M, Jankala H, Paetau A, Harkonen M, Somer H. Metabolic causes of recurrent rhabdomyolysis. *Acta Neurol Scand* 1998;98:268–275.

Manning BM, Quane KA, Ording H, et al. Identification of novel mutations in the ryanodine-receptor gene (RYR1) in malignant hyperthermia: genotype-phenotype correlation. *Am J Hum Genet* 1998;62:599–609.

Melamed I, Romen Y, Keren G, et al. March myoglobinuria: a hazard to renal function. *Arch Intern Med* 1982;142:1277–1279.

Nelson TE, Butler IJ. Malignant hyperthermia: skeletal muscle defects predisposing to labile Ca^{2+} regulation? *J Child Neurol* 1992;7:329–331.

Penn AS, Rowland LP, Fraser DW. Drugs, coma, and myoglobinuria. *Arch Neurol* 1972;26:336–343.

Perkoff GT. Alcoholic myopathy. *Annu Rev Med* 1971;22:125–132.

Quane KA, Healy JMS, Keating KE, et al. Mutations in the ryanodine receptor gene in central core disease and malignant hyperthermia. *Nat Genet* 1993;5:51–55.

Romero NB, Nivoche Y, Lunardi J, et al. Malignant hyperthermia and central core disease: analysis of two families with heterogeneous clinical expression. *Neuromuscul Disord* 1993;3:547–551.

Rowland LP. Myoglobinuria. *Can J Neurol Sci* 1984;11:1–13.

Tein I, DiMauro S, Rowland LP. Myoglobinuria. In: Vinken PJ, Bruyn GW, Klawans HL, Rowland LP, DiMauro S, eds. *Myopathies. Handbook of clinical neurology, rev ser, vol 62(18).* New York: Elsevier Science, 1992:479–526.

Tonin P, Lewis P, Servidei S, DiMauro S. Metabolic causes of myoglobinuria. *Ann Neurol* 1990;27:181–185.

Ueda M, Hamamoto M, Nagayama H, et al. Susceptibility to neuroleptic malignant syndrome in Parkinson's disease. *Neurology* 1999;52:777–781.

Wedel DJ. Malignant hyperthermia and neuromuscular disease. *Neuromuscul Disord* 1993;3:157–164.

Yaqub B, Al Deeb S. Heat strokes: aetiopathogenesis, neurological characteristics, treatment and outcome. *J Neurol Sci* 1998;156:144–151.

Merritt's Neurology, 10th ed., edited by L.P. Rowland. Lippincott Williams & Wilkins, Philadelphia © 2000.

CHAPTER 129

MUSCLE CRAMPS AND STIFFNESS

ROBERT B. LAYZER
LEWIS P. ROWLAND

The term *muscle stiffness* implies a state of continuous muscle contraction at rest; *cramps* or *spasms* are transient, involuntary contractions of a muscle or group of muscles. Table 129.1 lists some of the many disorders that cause muscle stiffness or cramps.

ORDINARY MUSCLE CRAMPS

The common *muscle cramp* is a sudden, forceful, often painful muscle contraction that lasts from a few seconds to several minutes. Cramps are provoked by a trivial movement or by contracting a shortened muscle. They may occur during vigorous exercise but are more likely to occur after exercise ceases. Unusually frequent cramps tend to accompany pregnancy, hypothyroidism, uremia, profuse sweating or diarrhea, hemodialysis, and lower motor neuron disorders, especially anterior horn cell diseases. Benign fasciculations or myokymia may be associated with frequent muscle cramps in apparently healthy people.

Nocturnal cramps typically cause forceful flexion of the ankle and toes, but cramps can affect almost any voluntary muscle. A cramp often starts with fasciculations, after which the muscle becomes intermittently hard and knotlike as the involuntary contraction waxes and wanes, passing from one part of the muscle to another. Electromyography (EMG) shows brief, periodic bursts of motor unit potentials discharging at a frequency of 200 to 300 Hz, appearing irregularly and intermingling with similar discharges from adjacent motor units. Several foci within the same muscle may discharge independently. This electrical activity clearly arises within the lower motor neuron; whether it occurs in the soma, in the peripheral nerve, or in the intramuscular nerve terminals is still debated. The chemical mechanisms are not understood.

Stretching the affected muscle usually terminates a cramp. Information about prophylactic therapy is largely anecdotal, and no single agent appears to be uniformly effective. For nocturnal leg cramps, a bedtime dose of quinine, phenytoin sodium (Dilantin), carbamazepine (Tegretol), or diazepam may be used. The beneficial effects of quinine have been demonstrated by controlled trials. Serious adverse effects are uncommon; tinnitus is relieved by interrupting treatment. The conventional dosage is 300 or 600 mg at bedtime. Frequent daytime cramps sometimes respond to maintenance therapy with carbamazepine or phenytoin.

Most people have cramps at some time, but a few people have inordinately frequent cramps, often accompanied by fasciculations. The syndrome of *benign fasciculation with cramps* is disproportionately more frequent among physicians and other medical workers because they are more likely to know the ominous implications of fasciculations for the diagnosis of motor neuron dis-

TABLE 129.1. MOTOR UNIT DISORDERS CAUSING CRAMPS AND STIFFNESS

Location of abnormality	Name of disorder	Principal manifestations	Treatment
Spinal cord and brainstem	Stiff-man syndrome	Rigidity and reflex spasms	Diazepam
	Tetanus	Rigidity and reflex spasms	Diazepam
	Progressive encephalomyelitis with rigidity and spasms	Rigidity and reflex spasms, focal neurologic deficits	None
	Myelopathy with alpha rigidity	Extensor rigidity	None
	Spinal myoclonus	Segmental repetitive myoclonic jerks	Clonazepam
Peripheral nerves	Tetany	Carpopedal spasm	Correction of calcium, magnesium, or acid–base derangement
	Neuromyotonia	Stiffness, myokymia, delayed relaxation	Phenytoin, carbamazepine
Muscle	Myotonic disorders	Delayed relaxation, percussion myotonia	Phenytoin, carbamazepine, procainamide
	Schwartz-Jampel syndrome	Stiffness and myotonia	Phenytoin, carbamazepine
	Phosphorylase deficiency, phosphofructokinase deficiency	Cramps during intense or ischemic exercise	None
	Malignant hyperthermia	Rigidity during anesthesia	Dantrolene
Unknown	Ordinary muscle cramps	Cramps during sleep or ordinary activity	Quinine, phenytoin carbamazepine

ease. In fact, however, motor neuron disease almost never starts with fasciculations alone. If neither weakness nor wasting exists, motor neuron disease is essentially excluded. The syndrome of benign fasciculation has been reported many times with variations on the name. Because the syndrome and the physiologic analysis were completely described by Denny-Brown and Foley, a reasonable eponym is the *Denny-Brown, Foley syndrome.*

True cramps must be distinguished from cramplike muscle pain unaccompanied by spasm. The cramps of McArdle disease occur only during intense or ischemic exercise. Because no electrical activity is evident in the EMG during the painful shortening of muscle affected by McArdle disease, the term *contracture* is used. The origin of the contracture is not known; depletion of adenosine triphosphate has long been suspected (because of the block of glycogen metabolism) but has not been proved, even by magnetic resonance spectroscopy.

Mild dystrophinopathies, with little or no clinical weakness, may be manifested by exertional muscle pain and even myoglobinuria. These symptoms have been referred to as muscle cramps, but actual muscle spasm has not been described in such cases; the pain may simply be a measure of muscle injury.

Myalgia and cramps are believed to be especially common in *myoadenylate deaminase deficiency* (MIM 102770), but that state is common in asymptomatic people (found in 1% to 3% of all muscle biopsies). Therefore, the association is difficult to confirm. Moreover, in affected families, a poor correlation exists between the muscle enzyme deficiency and clinical symptoms. An autosomal-dominant cramp syndrome is seen without known biochemical abnormality (MIM 158400).

NEUROMYOTONIA (ISAACS SYNDROME)

Isaacs first described this disorder as a state of "continuous muscle fiber activity." The invariable clinical manifestation is

myokymia (clinically visible and continuous muscle twitching that may be difficult to distinguish from vigorous fasciculation). The word has two meanings, one clinical and the other electromyographic. Physiologically, spontaneous activity is seen at rest in the form of fasciculations, doublets, and multiplets that may lead to prolonged trains of discharges at a rate up to 60 Hz. In Isaacs syndrome, both the clinical and the EMG features are present, but myokymia may be found in the EMG of some individuals without any clinically visible twitching. Neuromyotonic discharges start and stop abruptly, and the discharge rate of 150 to 300 Hz is higher than that in myokymia.

As a result of the continuous activity, a second characteristic of the syndrome is the finding of *abnormal postures* of the limbs, which may be persistent or intermittent and are identical to carpal or pedal spasm. A third characteristic is *pseudomyotonia,* which resembles the difficulty in relaxing in true myotonia; here, however, the characteristic EMG pattern—waxing and waning of myotonic bursts—is not seen. Instead, continuous motor unit activity interferes with relaxation. In addition, there is no percussion myotonia. The fourth characteristic is *liability to cramps. Hyperhidrosis,* or increased sweating, is variable.

The syndrome affects children, adolescents, or young adults and begins insidiously, progressing slowly for months or a few years. Slow movement, clawing of the fingers, and toe-walking are later joined by stiffness of proximal and axial muscles; occasionally, oropharyngeal or respiratory muscles are affected. The stiffness and myokymia are seen at rest and persist in sleep. Voluntary contraction may induce a spasm that persists during attempted relaxation.

The EMG recorded from stiff muscles reveals prolonged, irregular discharges of action potentials that vary in amplitude and configuration; some of them resemble fibrillations. Voluntary effort triggers more intense discharges that persist during relaxation, accounting for the myotonia-like after-contraction. The condition is often attributed to a peripheral neuropathy because acral sensory loss is noted in some patients, nerve conduction may be slow, or abnormality may appear on sural nerve biopsy. Perhaps, most important, the EMG activity may persist after nerve block by injection of local anesthetic but is abolished by botulinum toxin, implying that the activity arises distal to the nerve block and proximal to the neuromuscular junction; the generator must be in the nerve terminals. In an analysis of 28 reported cases, however, only four patients had definite evidence of peripheral neuropathy (Table 129.2), and some of the features suggested a disorder of the nerve cell itself.

Sometimes, neuromyotonia is seen in association with a tumor; that is, it may be a paraneoplastic syndrome. Several patients have had thymoma with or without myasthenia gravis. Newsom-Davis, Vincent, and their associates have demonstrated antibodies to neural potassium channels in most patients.

Treatment with carbamazepine or phenytoin usually controls the symptoms and signs. Plasmapheresis and intravenous immunoglobulin therapy have been effective in some patients.

TETANY

Tetany is a clinical syndrome characterized by convulsions, paresthesia, prolonged spasms of limb muscles, or laryngospasm; it is accompanied by signs of hyperexcitability of peripheral nerves. It occurs in patients with hypocalcemia, hypomagnesemia, or alkalosis; it occasionally represents a primary neural abnormality. Hyperventilation may unmask latent hypocalcemic tetany, but respiratory alkalosis itself only rarely causes outright tetany.

Intense circumoral and digital paresthesia generally precedes the typical carpopedal spasms, which consist of adduction and extension of the fingers, flexion of the metacarpophalangeal joints, and equinovarus postures of the feet. In severe cases, the spasms spread to the proximal and axial muscles, eventually causing opisthotonus. In all forms of tetany, the nerves are hyperexcitable, as manifested by the reactions to ischemia (Trousseau sign) and percussion (Chvostek sign). The spasms are due to spontaneous firing of peripheral nerves, starting in

TABLE 129.2. MANIFESTATIONS OF ISAACS SYNDROME IN 28 PATIENTS

	Patients (n)		
	Present	Absent	Not mentioned
Clinical			
Myokymia	28	0	0
Cramps	15	2	11
Pseudomyotonia	15	3	10
Carpopedal spasm	12	2	14
Sweating	15	3	10
Chvostek sign	1	2	25
Trousseau sign	1	2	25
Response to hyperventilation	0	0	28
Electromyography			
Multiplets	18	0	10
After discharge	6	1	21
Ischemia augments	3	0	16
Ischemia decreases	9	0	16
Hyperventilation increases	0	1	27
Activity decreased by			
Sleep	0	18	10
General anesthesia	0	6	22
Spinal anesthesia	1	4	23
Nerve block	9	7	12
Curare	7	0	21
Diazepam	1	12	15
Carabamazepine	14	2	12
Phenytoin	16	5	7
Evidence of peripheral neuropathy			
Paresthesia	3	7	18
Cutaneous sensory loss	4	14	10
Limb weakness	7	16	5
Knee jerks	16	12	0
Ankle jerks	13	15	0
CSF protein 50–100 mg/dL	1	13	12
> 100 mg/dL	2	13	12
MNCV slow	9	11	8
SNCV slow	4	8	16
Denervation, muscle biopsy	5	13	10
Abnormal nerve biopsy	2	1	25
Neuropathy clear	4	22	—
Neuropathy possible	2	22	—

MNCV, motor nerve conduction velocity; SNCV, sensory nerve conduction velocity.
Modified from Rowland, 1985.

the proximal portions of the longest nerves. EMG shows individual motor units discharging independently at a rate of 5 to 25 Hz; each discharge consists of a group of two or more identical potentials.

The treatment of tetany consists of correcting the underlying metabolic disorder. In hypomagnesemia, tetany does not respond to correction of the accompanying hypocalcemia unless the magnesium deficit is also corrected.

STIFF-MAN SYNDROME (MOERSCH-WOLTMAN SYNDROME)

The catchy name for this syndrome was coined by two senior clinicians at the Mayo Clinic in 1956. The name has been perpetuated since, but the titles have sometimes been awkward (e.g., stiff-man syndrome in a woman, stiff-man syndrome in a boy, stiff-baby syndrome, or stiff-person syndrome). We now strive for gender-neutral language; the masculine version is especially inappropriate for a syndrome that occurs equally often in women and men. The eponym seems apropos.

Clinical Manifestations

The Moersch-Woltman syndrome is defined clinically, with progressive muscular rigidity and painful spasms that resemble a chronic form of tetanus. The symptoms develop over several months or years and may either increase slowly or become stable. Aching discomfort and stiffness tend to predominate in the axial and proximal limb muscles, causing awkwardness of gait and slowness of movement. Trismus does not occur, but facial and oropharyngeal muscles may be affected. The stiffness diminishes during sleep and under general anesthesia. Later, painful reflex spasms occur in response to movement, sensory stimulation, or emotion. The spasms may lead to joint deformities and are powerful enough to rupture muscles, rip surgical sutures, or fracture bones. Passive muscle stretch provokes an exaggerated reflex contraction that lasts several seconds. Whether any of the findings in Table 129.3 must be present to make the diagnosis is not clear. For instance, the response to diazepam may not be complete, or the spinal deformity may not be present. And some investigators have noted that findings on examination and EMG activity are compatible with those of voluntary behavior. A psychogenic cause has been mentioned, however, only to be derided because

TABLE 129.3. DEFINING CHARACTERISTICS OF THE MOERSCH-WOLTMAN SYNDROME

Prodromal stiffness of axial muscles
Slow progress to proximal limbs; walking awkward
Fixed deformity of the spine; lordosis; "permanent shrug" (neck drawn down to shoulder girdle)
Spasms precipitated by startle, jarring, noise, emotional upset
Otherwise normal findings on motor and sensory examination
Normal intellect and affect
Continuous motor activity in affected muscles relieved by intravenous or oral diazepam

Modified from Lorish et al., 1989.

the tin-soldier appearance of the patient is so dramatic and because the spasms may cause physical injury.

Laboratory Data

EMG recordings from stiff muscles show a continuous discharge of motor unit potentials resembling normal voluntary contraction. As in tetanus, the activity is not inhibited by voluntary contraction of the antagonist muscles; however, a normal silent period is present during the stretch reflex, indicating that there is no impairment of recurrent spinal inhibition. The rigidity is abolished by spinal anesthesia, by peripheral nerve block, or by selective block of gamma motor nerve fibers. Some authors have postulated that both alpha and gamma motor neurons are rendered hyperactive by excitatory influences descending from the brainstem. The electroencephalogram is normal. Routine cerebrospinal fluid (CSF) analysis is also normal, but immunoglobulin (Ig) G concentration may be increased and oligoclonal IgG bands may be present.

Administration of diazepam is the most effective symptomatic treatment; high doses may be required. Additional benefit can be obtained in some cases from administration of baclofen, phenytoin, clonidine hydrochloride (Catapres), or tizanidine (Zanaflex). Intrathecal baclofen (Lioresal) has been used. The long-term prognosis is still uncertain.

The pathogenesis may involve autoimmunity. Antibodies to glutamate decarboxylase have been found in both serum and CSF in this syndrome and in diabetes mellitus; the frequency of the association of the two diseases seems to be inordinately high. Plasmapheresis may be beneficial. Other autoimmune diseases may be present, and the Moersch-Woltman syndrome is sometimes paraneoplastic.

Differential Diagnosis

Evidence of corticospinal tract disease or abnormality of the CSF implies an anatomic disorder of the central nervous system (CNS), but in postmortem examination of typical cases, no CNS histopathology is revealed. Patients with similar physical findings may show CSF pleocytosis or Babinski signs. In autopsies of those patients, however, inflammation has been sufficient to warrant the term *encephalomyelitis*. Stiffness of the arms in some patients with cervical lesions is attributed to spontaneous activity of alpha motor neurons isolated from synaptic influences. That combination is best regarded as *stiff encephalomyelitis*, because the pathogenesis ought to differ in the two categories with or without clear evidence of CNS disease. However, antibodies to glutamate decarboxylase have also been found in patients with myelitis. A related disorder has been called the *stiff limb syndrome*.

The main distinction between Moersch-Woltman and Isaacs syndromes is the distribution of the symptoms, which affect the distal arms and legs in Isaacs and the trunk in Moersch-Woltman. Myokymia is seen only in Isaacs. Many of the features of Isaacs syndrome are similar to those of tetany, as are the *painful tonic spasms of multiple sclerosis* (MS). MS, however, is identified by other signs of disseminated CNS lesions. These tonic spasms, like other paroxysmal symptoms in MS, are thought to originate as ectopic activity in demyelinated CNS nerve tracts. They usually last less than 1 minute but occur many times a day. The attacks usually respond promptly to treatment with carbamazepine or phenytoin. The startle reactions of Moersch-Woltman syndrome are similar to those in the autosomal-dominant condition *hyperekplexia* or *startle disease* (MIM 149400). Hyperekplexia, however, lacks axial rigidity and has been mapped to a subunit of an inhibitory glycine receptor on chromosome 5. It is relieved by the τ-aminobutyric acid agonist clonidine. The Moersch-Woltman syndrome itself is rarely autosomal-dominant (MIM 184850). The fixed postures of the limbs in Isaacs syndrome can be simulated by the Schwartz-Jampel syndrome (SJS) (see Chapter 127). However, SJS is characterized by a unique facial appearance (blepharophimosis), short stature, and bony abnormalities. In SJS, the more frequent EMG pattern is that of myotonia, but there may be continuous motor activity with both myokymic and neuromyotonic discharges.

SUGGESTED READINGS

Cramps and Related Disorders

Blexrud MD, Windebank AJ, Daube JR. Long-term follow-up of 121 patients with benign fasciculations. *Ann Neurol* 1993;34:622–625.

Connolly PS, Shirley EA, Wasson JH, Nierenberg DW. Treatment of nocturnal leg cramps: crossover trial of quinine versus vitamin E. *Arch Intern Med* 1992;152:1877–1880.

Dressler D, Thompson PD, Gledhill RF, Marsden CD. The syndrome of painful legs and moving toes. *Mov Disord* 1994;9:13–21.

Man-Son Hing M, Wells G, Lau A. Quinine for nocturnal leg cramps: a meta-analysis including unpublished data. *J Gen Intern Med* 1998;13:600–606.

Pagni CA, Canavero D. Pain, muscle spasms, and twitching fingers following brachial plexus avulsion: three cases relieved by dorsal root entry zone coagulation. *J Neurol* 1993;240:468–470.

Rose MR, Ball JA, Thompson PD. Magnetic resonance imaging in tonic spasms of multiple sclerosis. *J Neurol* 1993;241:115–117.

Rowland LP. Cramps, spasms, and muscle stiffness. *Rev Neurol (Paris)* 1985;4:261–273.

Rowland LP, Trojaborg W, Haller RG. Muscle contracture: physiology and clinical classification. In: Serratrice G, ed. *Muscle contracture.* In press.

Neuromyotonia

Deymeer F, Oge AE, Serdaroglu P, Yaaziei J, Ozdemir C, Basio A. The use of botulinum toxin in localizing neuromyotonia to the terminal branches of the peripheral nerve. *Muscle Nerve* 1998;21:643–646.

Hart HC, Waters C, Vincent A, et al. Autoantibodies detected to K+ channels are implicated in neuromyotonia. *Ann Neurol* 1997;41:238–246.

Heidereich F, Vincent A. Antibodies to ion-channel proteins in thymoma with myasthenia, neuromyotonia, and peripheral neuropathy. *Neurology* 1998;50:1483–1485.

Jamieson PW, Katirj MB. Idiopathic generalized myokymia. *Muscle Nerve* 1994;17:42–51.

Layzer RB. Neuromyotonia: a new autoimmune disease. *Ann Neurol* 1995;38:701–702.

Newsom-Davis J, Mills KR. Immunological associations of acquired neuromyotonia (Isaacs' syndrome). *Brain* 1993;116:453–469.

Taylor RG, Layzer RB, Davis HS, Fowler WM. Continuous muscle fiber activity in the Schwartz-Jampel syndrome. *Electroencephalogr Clin Neurophysiol* 1972;33:497–509.

Torbensen T, Stalberg E, Brautaset NJ. Generator sites for spontaneous activity in neuromyotonia: an EMG study. *Electroencephalogr Clin Neurophysiol* 1996;101:69–78.

Van Dijk JG, Lammers GJ, Wintzen AR, Molenaar PC. Repetitive CMAPs: mechanisms of neural and synaptic genesis. *Muscle Nerve* 1996;19:1127–1133.

Wakayama Y, Ohbu S, Machida H. Myasthenia gravis, muscle twitch, hyperhidrosis and limb pain associated with thymoma: proposal of possible new myasthenic syndrome. *Tohoku J Exp Med* 1991;164:285–291.

Stiff-man Syndrome (Moersch-Woltman Syndrome)

Barker RA, Revesz T, Thom M, Marsden CD, Brown P. Review of 23 patients affected by the stiff man syndrome: clinical subdivision into stiff trunk (man) syndrome, stiff limb syndrome, and progressive encephalomyelitis with rigidity. *J Neurol Neurosurg Psychiatry* 1998;65:633–640.

Floeter MK, Valla-Sole J, Toro C, Jacobowitz D, Hallett M. Physiologic studies of spinal inhibitory circuits in patients with stiff-person syndrome. *Neurology* 1998;51:85–93.

Grimaldi LME, Martino G, Braghi S, et al. Heterogeneity of autoantibodies in stiff-man syndrome. *Ann Neurol* 1993;34:57–64.

Kissel JT, Elble RJ. Stiff-person syndrome: stiff opposition to a simple explanation. *Neurology* 1998;51:11–14.

Layzer RB. Stiff-man syndrome—an autoimmune disease? *N Engl J Med* 1988;53:695–696.

Layzer RB. Motor unit hyperactivity states. In: Engel AG, Franzini-Armstrong C, eds. *Myology,* 2nd ed. London: Churchill Livingstone, 1994.

Lorish TR, Thorsteinsson G, Howard FH Jr. Stiff-man syndrome updated. *Mayo Clin Proc* 1989;64:629–636.

McEvoy KM. Stiff-man syndrome. *Mayo Clin Proc* 1991;66:303–304.

Meinck HM, Ricker K, Hulser PJ, et al. Stiff man syndrome: clinical and laboratory findings in 8 patients. *J Neurol* 1993;241:157–166.

Moersch FP, Woltman HW. Progressive fluctuating muscular rigidity and spasm (stiff-man syndrome): report of a case and some observations in 13 other cases. *Proc Staff Meet Mayo Clin* 1956;31:421–427.

Penn RD, Mangieri EA. Stiff-man syndrome treated with intrathecal baclofen. *Neurology* 1993;43:2412.

Piccolo G, Martino G, Moglia A, et al. Autoimmune myasthenia gravis with thymoma following spontaneous remission of stiff-man syndrome. *Ital J Neurol Sci* 1990;11:177–180.

Rosin L, De Camilli P, Butler M, et al. Stiff-man syndrome in a woman with breast cancer: an uncommon central nervous system paraneoplastic syndrome. *Neurology* 1998;50:94–98.

Schmierer K, Valueza JM, Bender A, et al. Stiff-man syndrome with spinal MRI findings, amphiphysin autoantibodies, and immunosuppressive treatment. *Neurology* 1998;51:250–252.

Solimena M, De Camilli P. Autoimmunity to glutamic acid decarboxylase (GAD) in stiff-man syndrome and insulin-dependent diabetes mellitus. *Trends Neurosci* 1991;14:452–457.

Solimena M, Folli F, Aparisi R, et al. Autoantibodies to GABA-ergic neurons and pancreatic beta cells in stiff man syndrome. *N Engl J Med* 1990;322:1555–1560.

Thompson PD. Stiff muscles. *J Neurol Neurosurg Psychiatry* 1993;56:121–124.

Merritt's Neurology, 10th ed., edited by L.P. Rowland. Lippincott Williams & Wilkins, Philadelphia © 2000.

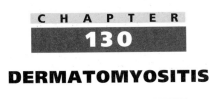

DERMATOMYOSITIS

LEWIS P. ROWLAND

Dermatomyositis, a disease of unknown etiology, is characterized by inflammatory changes in skin and muscle.

PATHOLOGY AND PATHOGENESIS

Dermatomyositis is thought to be an autoimmune disease, but there has been no consistent evidence of either antibodies or lymphocytes directed against specific muscle antigens. However, there has been growing agreement among muscle histologists that dermatomyositis is humorally mediated, characterized by more B cells than T cells in the muscle infiltrates, as well as a vasculopathy with deposits of immunoglobulins in intramuscular blood vessels. This contrasts with the predominance of T cells in polymyositis, which is attributed to a disorder of lymphocyte regulation. Some authorities believe that the pathogenesis of the disease differs in adults and children.

The acute changes of both skin and muscle are marked by signs of degeneration, regeneration, edema, and infiltration by lymphocytes. The inflammatory cells are found around small vessels or in the perimysium rather than within the muscle fiber itself. In muscle biopsies, however, lymphocytic infiltration may be lacking in 25% of patients; this probably depends on the time of sampling, as well as on the distribution and severity of the process. The lymphocytes are predominantly B cells, with some CD4 (T-helper) cells. Capillaries often show endothelial hyperplasia; deposits of immunoglobulin (Ig) G, IgM, and complement (the membrane attack complex) may be found within and occluding these vessels. Evidence of muscle degeneration and regeneration is multifocal and may be most marked at the periphery of muscle bundles (*perifascicular atrophy*), where the capillaries are occluded. Increasingly, investigators have come to believe that the primary attack is on blood vessels. A similar myopathy without skin lesions can be induced in animals by immunization with muscle extracts. Viruslike particles have been seen in some cases, but no virus has been cultured from muscle.

INCIDENCE

Dermatomyositis is rare. Together with polymyositis, the incidence has been estimated to be about seven cases each year for a population of 1 million. That figure may be too low; in our 1,200-bed hospital, we see five new cases of dermatomyositis and 15 to 20 cases of polymyositis each year.

Dermatomyositis occurs in all decades of life, with peaks of incidence before puberty and at about age 40 years. In young adults, women are more likely to be affected. Familial cases are

rare. It is generally believed that about 10% of cases starting after age 40 are associated with malignant neoplasms, most often carcinoma of lung or breast. Typical findings, including the rash, have also been seen in patients with agammaglobulinemia, graft-versus-host disease, toxoplasmosis, hypothyroidism, sarcoidosis, ipecac abuse, hepatitis B virus infection, penicillamine reactions, or vaccine reactions. Cases have even been ascribed to azathioprine (Imuran).

SYMPTOMS AND SIGNS

The first manifestations usually involve both skin and muscle at about the same time. The rash may precede weakness by several weeks, but weakness alone is almost never the first symptom. Sometimes, the rash is so typical that the diagnosis can be made even without evidence of myopathy ("amyopathic dermatomyositis"), and sometimes weakness is not evident but there is electromyographic (EMG), biopsy, or serum creatine kinase (CK) evidence of myopathy.

The rash may be confined to the face in a butterfly distribution around the nose and cheeks, but the edema and erythema are especially likely to affect the eyelids, periungual skin, and extensor surfaces of the knuckles, elbows, and knees. The upper chest is another common site. The initial redness may be replaced later by brownish pigmentation. The Gottron sign is denoted by red-purple scaly macules on the extensor surfaces of finger joints. Fibrosis of subcutaneous tissue and thickening of the skin may lead to the appearance of scleroderma. Later, especially in children, calcinosis may involve subcutaneous tissues and fascial planes within muscle. The calcium deposits may extrude through the skin.

Affected muscles may ache and are often tender. Weakness of proximal limb muscles causes difficulty in lifting, raising the arms overhead, rising from low seats, climbing stairs, or even walking on level ground. The interval from onset of weakness to most severe disability is measured in weeks. Cranial muscles are spared, except that difficulty in swallowing is noted by about one-third of patients. Some patients have difficulty in holding the head up because neck muscles are weak. Sensation is preserved, tendon reflexes may or may not be lost, and there is no fasciculation.

Systemic symptoms are uncommon. Fever and malaise may characterize the acute stage in a minority of patients. Pulmonary fibrosis has been encountered, and rarely there are cardiac symptoms. Arthralgia may be prominent, but deforming arthritis and renal failure have never been documented.

In about 10% of patients, the cutaneous manifestations have features of both scleroderma and dermatomyositis, warranting the name *sclerodermatomyositis.* These cases have sometimes been designated as *mixed connective tissue disease,* with a high incidence of antibody to extractable nuclear antigen; however, it now seems unlikely that the mixed syndrome is unique in any way.

DIAGNOSIS

The characteristic rash and myopathy usually make the diagnosis clear at a glance. Problems may arise if the rash is inconspicuous; in those cases the differential diagnosis is that of polymyositis (see Chapter 131). Other collagen-vascular diseases may cause both rash and myopathy at the same time, but systemic lupus erythematosus is likely to affect kidneys, synovia, and the CNS in patterns that are never seen in dermatomyositis. Similarly, there has never been a documented case of typical rheumatoid arthritis with typical dermatomyositis. The diagnosis of dermatomyositis is therefore clinical, based on the rash and myopathy. There is no pathognomonic laboratory test.

Except for the presence of lymphocytes and perifascicular atrophy in the muscle biopsy and increased serum CK (and other sarcoplasmic enzymes), there are no characteristic laboratory abnormalities. The EMG shows myopathic abnormalities and, often, evidence of increased irritability of muscle. Computed tomography (CT) and magnetic resonance imaging (MRI) of muscle have not been widely adopted but are useful in evaluating pulmonary fibrosis. Nonspecific serologic abnormalities include rheumatoid factor and several different kinds of antinuclear antibodies, none consistently present in patients with dermatomyositis. For instance, anti-Jo antibodies (against histidyl transfer RNA synthetase) are present in about 50% of patients with pulmonary fibrosis, but only 20% of all patients with inflammatory myopathy.

Once the diagnosis is made, many clinicians set off on a search for occult neoplasm. In preimaging days, Callen (1982) showed that in most cases a tumor was already evident or that there was an abnormality in some simple routine test (blood count, erythrocyte sedimentation rate, test for heme pigment in stool, chest film) or in findings on physical examination including pelvis and rectum. However, investigations have not yet evaluated the impact of CT or MRI of the chest, abdomen, and pelvis on the discovery of tumors in patients with dermatomyositis. Sometimes, no matter how exhaustive the search, the tumor is not discovered until an autopsy is performed.

PROGNOSIS

The natural history of dermatomyositis is now unknown because patients are automatically treated with steroids. The disease may become inactive after 5 to 10 years. Although the mortality rate 50 years ago was given as 33% to 50%, it is not appropriate to use those ancient figures for current comparison; antibiotics and respirators affect outcome as much as any presumably specific immunotherapy. Even so, in reviews published after 1982, mortality rates were 23% to 44%. Because few fatalities have occurred in children, many of the deaths are caused by the associated malignancy. Other causes of death are myocarditis, pulmonary fibrosis, or steroid-induced complications. The myopathy may also be severe. In an analysis of survivors of childhood dermatomyositis, 83% were capable of self-care, almost all were working, and 50% were married; 33% had persistent rash or weakness, and a similar number had calcinosis.

TREATMENT

The standard therapy for dermatomyositis is administration of prednisone. The recommended dose for adults is at least 60 mg daily; higher dosages are often given for severe cases. For children, the recommended dose is higher: 2 mg/kg body weight. The basic dosage is continued for at least 1 month, perhaps longer. If the patient has improved by then, the dosage can be reduced slowly. If there has been no improvement, choices include prolonging the trial of prednisone in the same or a higher dosage with or without the addition of an immunosuppressive drug chosen according to local usage.

In the past decade, improvement was reported in 80% of all steroid-treated patients in one series, but only 50% or fewer patients benefited in other studies. Apparent response to treatment of individual patients with apparent relapses on withdrawal of medication has been reported anecdotally many times. In one retrospective analysis, favorable outcome of childhood dermatomyositis seemed to be linked to early treatment (less than 4 months after onset) and use of high doses of prednisone. Dubowitz (1984), however, reported just the reverse: better outcome and fewer steroid complications with low doses of prednisone (1 mg/kg body weight).

The value of steroid treatment is still unproved, however, because there has never been a prospectively controlled study. In one retrospective analysis, untreated patients were seen many years before treated patients. In another study, there was no difference in outcome of patients treated with prednisone alone or with both prednisone and azathioprine. Moreover, it is not clear whether immunosuppressive drugs are more or less dangerous than steroids, and there is no evidence that any single immunosuppressive drug is superior to others. Azathioprine, methotrexate, cyclophosphamide, and cyclosporine have all been championed.

Plasmapheresis was of no value in a controlled trial, but intravenous immunoglobulin (IVIG) therapy was uniformly beneficial in eight patients with steroid-resistant dermatomyositis, in contrast to no improvement in seven blinded, control patients who were given placebo. IVIG therapy may therefore be the procedure of choice for acute therapy of seriously ill patients. Some long-term immunosuppressive therapy, however, would have to be added. IVIG therapy is also useful in adults or children who do not respond to other agents.

Some clinicians worry that exercising a weak muscle may be harmful, but formal tests in dermatomyositis and polymyositis have shown benefit.

SUGGESTED READINGS

Akira M, Hara H, Sakatani M. Interstitial lung disease in association with polymyositis-dermatomyositis: long-term follow-up CT evaluation in seven patients. *Radiology* 1999;210:333–338.

Amato AA, Barohn RJ. Idiopathic inflammatory myopathies. *Neurol Clin* 1997;15:615–648.

Andrews A, Hickling P, Hutton C. Familial dermatomyositis. *Br J Rheumatol* 1998;37:231–232.

Banker BQ, Victor M. Dermatomyositis (systemic angiopathy) in childhood. *Medicine* 1966;45:261–289.

Bohan A, Peter JB, Bowman RL, Pearson CM. A computer-assisted analysis of 153 patients with polymyositis and dermatomyositis. *Medicine* 1977;56:255–286.

Bowyer SL, Blane CE, Sullivan DB, Cassidy JT. Childhood dermatomyositis: factors predicting functional outcome and development of dystrophic calcification. *J Pediatr* 1983;103:882–888.

Callen JP. The value of malignancy evaluation in patients with dermatomyositis. *J Am Acad Dermatol* 1982;6:253–259.

Chalmers A, Sayson R, Walters K. Juvenile dermatomyositis: medical, social and economic status in adulthood. *Can Med Assoc J* 1982;126:31–33.

Chou SM, Mike T. Ultrastructural abnormalities and perifascicular atrophy in childhood dermatomyositis. *Arch Pathol Lab Med* 1981;105:76–85.

Dalakas MC. Molecular immunology and genetics of inflammatory muscle diseases. *Arch Neurol* 1998;55:1509–1512.

Dalakas MC, Illa I, Dambrosia JM, et al. A controlled trial of high-dose intravenous immune globulin infusions as treatment for dermatomyositis. *N Engl J Med* 1993;329:1993–2000.

Dubowitz V. Prognostic factors in dermatomyositis [Letter]. *J Pediatr* 1984;105:336–337.

Esmie-Smith AM, Engel AG. Microvascular changes in early and advanced dermatomyositis: a quantitative study. *Ann Neurol* 1990;27:343–356.

Euwer RL, Sontheimer RD. Amyopathic dermatomyositis (dermatomyositis sine myositis): six new cases. *J Am Acad Dermatol* 1991;24:959–966.

Fujino H, Kobayashi T, Goto I, Onitsuka H. MRI of muscle in patients with polymyositis and dermatomyositis. *Muscle Nerve* 1991;14:716–720.

Heffner RR. Inflammatory myopathies: a review. *J Neuropathol Exp Neurol* 1993;52:339–350.

Hochberg MC. Mortality from polymyositis and dermatomyositis in the United States, 1968–1978. *Arthritis Rheum* 1983;26:1465–1472.

Hochberg MC, Feldman D, Stevens MB. Adult-onset polymyositis/dermatomyositis: an analysis of clinical and laboratory features and survival of 76 patients. *Semin Arthritis Rheum* 1986;15:168–178.

Kissel JT, Halterman RK, Rammohan KW, Mendell JR. The relationship of complement-mediated microvasculopathy to the histologic features and clinical duration of disease in dermatomyositis. *Arch Neurol* 1991;48:26–30.

Mantegazza R, Bernasconi P, Confalonieri P, Cornelio F. Inflammatory myopathies and systemic disorders: a review of immunopathogenetic mechanisms and clinical features. *J Neurol* 1997;244:277–287.

Mastaglia FL, Phillips BA, Zilko PJ. Immunoglobulin therapy in inflammatory myopathies. *J Neurol Neuosurg Psychiatry* 1998;65:107–110.

Maugars YM, Berthelot JMM, Aabbas AA, et al. Long-term prognosis of 69 patients with dermatomyositis or polymyositis. *Clin Exp Rheumatol* 1996;14:263–274.

Medsger TA Jr, Oddis CV. Classification and diagnostic criteria for polymyositis and dermatomyositis [Editorial]. *J Rheumatol* 1995; 22:581–585.

Mease PJ, Ochs HD, Wedgwood RJ. Successful treatment of echovirus meningoencephalitis and myositis-fasciitis with intravenous immune globulin therapy in a patient with X-linked agammaglobulinemia. *N Engl J Med* 1981;304:1278–1281.

Nimmelstein SH, Brody S, McShane D, Holman HR. Mixed connective tissue disease: a subsequent evaluation of the original 25 patients. *Medicine* 1980;59:239–248.

Ollivier I, Wolkenstein P, Gheradi R, et al. Dermatomyositis-like graft-versus-host disease. *Br J Dermatol* 1998;138:358–359.

Pachman LM, Hayford JR, Chung A, et al. Juvenile dermatomyositis at diagnosis: clinical characteristics of 79 children. *J Rheumatol* 1998;25:1198–1204.

Rowland LP, Clark C, Olarte MR. Therapy for dermatomyositis and polymyositis. *Adv Neurol* 1977;17:63–97.

Sansome A, Dubowitz V. Intravenous immunoglobulin in juvenile dermatomyositis: four-year review of nine cases. *Arch Dis Child* 1995;72:25–28.

Sigurgeirsson B, Lindelof B, Edhag O, Allander E. Risk of cancer in patients with dermatomyositis or polymyositis: a population-based study. *N Engl J Med* 1992;326:363–367.

Tanimoto K, Nakano K, Kano, S et al. Classification criteria for polymyositis and dermatomyositis. *J Rheumatol* 1995;22:668–674.

Wiesinger GF, Quittan M, Graninger M, et al. Benefit of 6 months' long-term physical training in polymyositis/dermatomyositis patients. *Br J Rheumatol* 1998;37:1338–1342.

Merritt's Neurology, 10th ed., edited by L.P. Rowland. Lippincott Williams & Wilkins, Philadelphia © 2000.

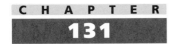

CHAPTER 131

POLYMYOSITIS, INCLUSION BODY MYOSITIS, AND RELATED MYOPATHIES

LEWIS P. ROWLAND

DEFINITION OF POLYMYOSITIS

Polymyositis is a disorder of skeletal muscle of diverse causes characterized by acute or subacute onset, possible intervals of improvement of symptoms, and typically infiltration of muscle by lymphocytes. It is one of the three major categories of inflammatory myopathy; each differs from the others clinically and in muscle pathology. The other two conditions are dermatomyositis and inclusion body myositis (IBM).

This definition is insufficiently precise, however, because there is no pathognomonic clinical syndrome, laboratory test, or combination of the two. The problem arises because lymphocytic infiltration of muscle may be lacking in an individual case or the typical pattern may not be seen; also, lymphocytic infiltration may be seen in other conditions. Additionally, polymyositis may occur alone or as part of a systemic disease, especially a collagen-vascular disease.

CLINICAL MANIFESTATIONS

The symptoms are those of a myopathy that primarily affects proximal limb muscles: difficulty climbing stairs or rising from low seats, lifting packages or dishes, or working with the arms overhead. Weakness of neck muscles may result in difficulty holding the head erect. Distal muscles are usually affected later, so difficulty using the hands is not encountered at first. Eyelids and ocular movements are spared; the only cranial symptom is dysphagia, usually without dysarthria. Respiration is only rarely affected.

Symptoms of systemic disease, malaise, or even weight loss are not evident. In many cases, arthralgia is symptomatic without objective change in the joints. Raynaud symptoms may be prominent, but by definition, there is no rash of dermatomyositis. No visceral lesions appear, other than interstitial lung disease and pulmonary fibrosis in some patients. Myocarditis may also occur. The syndrome is usually subacute in onset, reaching a nadir in months rather than weeks or years, but both acute and chronic forms are seen. Symptoms may persist for years and then the condition seems to become quiescent.

LABORATORY DATA

The findings are those of a myopathy, with characteristic electromyographic (EMG) findings of small-amplitude short-duration potentials and full recruitment. Signs of muscle "irritability" may be noted, with fibrillations and positive waves but no fasciculations. Nerve conduction studies give normal values. Serum levels of creatine kinase (CK) and other sarcoplasmic enzymes are usually increased to values 10 times normal or even more. Serum enzyme levels may be normal, however, probably depending on the stage of the disease.

A definite diagnosis requires characteristic changes in the muscle biopsy, especially infiltration around healthy muscle fibers by cells that have the immunocytochemical characteristics of CD8+ T lymphocytes. Signs of muscle necrosis and regeneration are apparent, but the pattern differs from that of dermatomyositis because neither vascular lesions nor perifascicular atrophy are seen. The pattern differs from IBM because vacuoles or the defining inclusions are not evident.

PATHOGENESIS

Polymyositis is considered an autoimmune disease of disordered cellular immunity (in contrast to the presumed humoral abnormalities of dermatomyositis). The nature of the antigen is not known, however, and the nature of the immunologic aberration is not known. The association with collagen-vascular disease increases the likelihood of autoimmune disorder, as does the association of polymyositis with other autoimmune diseases, including Crohn disease, biliary cirrhosis, sarcoidosis, myasthenia gravis with thymoma and candidiasis, or graft versus host disease. Human immunodeficiency virus and human T-cell lymphotropic virus type I are viral diseases associated with polymyositis; it is not known whether polymyositis is a viral infection of muscle or an autoimmune reaction. In contrast to dermatomyositis, myopathy without rash is uncommon in patients with concomitant malignant neoplasms.

Fibers adjacent to the T cells express the class 1 major histocompatibility complex, an antigen that is lacking in normal fibers and is a recognition factor for the activation of T cells. Circulating T cells may be cytotoxic to cultures of the patient's cultured myotubes.

In the past decade, interest has been directed to antibodies to cytoplasmic ribonucleoproteins. Because they are not disease specific, however, they neither help to explain pathogenesis nor provide a major diagnostic tool. Anti-Jo antibodies are found in about half of all patients with both polymyositis and pulmonary fibrosis.

DIAGNOSIS

In the past, polymyositis was regarded as dermatomyositis without a rash. The histologic differences are now recognized, but the clinical problem remains: How can we identify the qualities of polymyositis that are similar to those of dermatomyositis while distinguishing polymyositis from other myopathies with which it might be confused, such as muscular dystrophies, metabolic myopathies, or disorders of the neuromuscular junction? The following criteria are suggested:

1. There is no family history of similar disease and onset is usually after age 35. No familial limb-girdle dystrophy starts so late. Cases of younger onset are few, unless there is some associated collagen-vascular or other systemic disease. If there is no family history, it may be necessary to test for sarcoglycanopathies.
2. Progression from onset to peak weakness is measured in weeks or months, not years as in the muscular dystrophies.
3. Symptoms may improve spontaneously or concomitantly with the administration of drugs, unlike any muscular dystrophy.
4. In addition to proximal limb weakness, there may be dysphagia or weakness of neck flexors, but other cranial muscles are not affected. (If eyelids or ocular muscles were involved, it would be difficult or impossible to distinguish the disorder from myasthenia gravis.)
5. Arthralgia, myalgia, and Raynaud symptoms help to make the diagnosis, but lack of these symptoms does not exclude the diagnosis.
6. Muscle biopsy usually shows the abnormalities described above, especially early in the course. As in patients with dermatomyositis, however, lymphocytic infiltration may be lacking in muscle biopsies in polymyositis. Typical histologic changes help to make the diagnosis; lack of these changes does not exclude the diagnosis because the changes may be focal in the muscle or transient and not present in the muscle at the site and time of the biopsy. In histochemical stains, there must be no evidence of excess lipid or glycogen storage and there should be no signs of denervation.
7. In addition to conventional EMG signs of myopathy, increased irritability of muscle may be evident.

The problem of diagnosis is exemplified by a patient with limb weakness at age 40 when EMG and muscle biopsy indicate that the disorder is a myopathy. Search must then be made for known causes of myopathy (Table 131.1). If none is found, the diagnosis of exclusion is idiopathic polymyositis.

It seems unlikely that this residual group is all due to one disease because there is clinical heterogeneity, such as differences in rapidity of progression, distribution of weakness, or severity of disorder. In addition, if there are so many known causes of similar syndromes, it is likely that still more remain to be identified. A restricted concept of idiopathic polymyositis will emerge only when more is known about the disordered immunology of dermatomyositis itself.

If there is no family history of similar disease and, especially if there are no inflammatory cells in the muscle biopsy, a form of limb-girdle muscular dystrophy must be considered. Sometimes polymyositis is the suspected diagnosis, but muscle biopsy shows glycogen or lipid accumulation or mitochondrial disease.

RELATION OF POLYMYOSITIS TO DERMATOMYOSITIS

These conditions are usually considered together because of the similarities in course and muscle disease. There are, however, important differences, as follows:

TABLE 131.1. DIFFERENTIAL DIAGNOSIS OF POLYMYOSITIS

Etiology unknown: Idiopathic polymyositis
Collagen-vascular diseases
 SLE, rheumatoid arthritis, periarteritis nodosa, systemic sclerosis, giant cell arteritis, Sjögren syndrome
Infections
 Toxoplasmosis, trichinosis, schistosomiasis, cysticercosis, Chagas disease, legionnaires disease, candidiasis, acne fulminans, microspiradosis, AIDS, influenza virus, rubella, hepatitis B, Behçet, Kawasaki, mycoplasma, coxsackie, Echovirus
 Immunization
Drugs
 Systemic: ethanol penicillamine, clofibrate, steroids, emetine, chloroquine, kaluretics, aminocaproic acid, rifampicin, ipecac, zidovudine
 Intramuscular: meperidine, pentazocine
Systemic diseases
 Carcinoma, thymoma, sarcoid, amyloid, psoriasis, hyperglobulinemia (plasma cell dyscrasia), celiac disease, papular mucinosis, graft-vs.-host disease after transplantation, alcoholism
Endocrine diseases
 Hyperthyroidism, hypothyroidism, hyperadrenocorticism, hyperparathyroidism, Hashimoto, thyroiditis
Metabolic diseases
 Therapeutic starvation, total parenteral nutrition, anorexia nervosa
 Hypocalcemia, osteomalacia, chronic renal disease
 Chronic K^+ depletion
 Carnitine deficiency in muscle
 Lack of acid maltase, phosphorylase, phosphofructokinase
 Iron overload on maintenance hemodialysis
Toxins
 Contaminated tryptophan (eosinophilia-myalgia syndrome), contaminated rapeseed oil (toxic oil syndrome)

1. Dermatomyositis is a homogeneous condition, only rarely associated with a known cause other than carcinoma. Polymyositis is associated with some other systemic disease in about half the cases.

2. Polymyositis is often a manifestation of a specific collagen-vascular disease, such as systemic lupus erythematosus, systemic sclerosis, or different forms of vasculitis. Dermatomyositis, however, is rarely if ever associated with evidence of collagen-vascular disease other than scleroderma. When polymyositis occurs in a patient with lupus erythematosus, for instance, it can be regarded as a manifestation of lupus, not a combination of two different disorders (or an "overlap syndrome").

3. Dermatomyositis occurs at all ages, including childhood. Polymyositis is rare before puberty.

4. As assessed by inability to walk, the myopathy of dermatomyositis is severe more often than the myopathy of polymyositis.

5. Dermatomyositis is far more likely to be associated with malignant neoplasm than is myopathy without rash.

RELATION OF POLYMYOSITIS TO INCLUSION BODY MYOSITIS

The attempt to link polymyositis to a viral infection led Chou (1986) to find tubular filaments in nuclear and cytoplasmic vac-uoles in some patients with other pathologic features of polymyositis. Yunis and Samaha coined the name in 1971. These histologic findings were then related to a characteristic clinical syndrome (Table 131.2).

Polymyositis and IBM are similar in that they are inflammatory myopathies, lack a rash, and rarely affect children. IBM is slower in progression. Dysphagia is common in both. Neither IBM nor polymyositis, in contrast to dermatomyositis, is often a paraneoplastic disorder. The two conditions differ clinically and histologically.

Clinically, IBM affects proximal limb muscles but, in contrast to polymyositis, is much more likely to affect distal muscles of the legs, and IBM is one of the few myopathies that causes weakness of the long finger flexors, an early symptom and sign in most IBM patients. IBM characteristically affects men after age 50; polymyositis affects younger adults as well and women more often than men. IBM more often shows mixed neurogenic and myopathic features in conventional EMG. In contrast to polymyositis, IBM is less often seen with collagen-vascular or other autoimmune disorders. Serum CK values are normal or only slightly increased in IBM. A major distinction is the failure of IBM to respond to steroid therapy.

TABLE 131.2. DEFINITION OF INCLUSION BODY MYOSITIS IN ANALYSIS OF 48 PATIENTS

	Patients (%)
Histology	
Fibers with rimmed vacuoles	100.00
Nonnecrotic cells invaded	89.6
Necrotic fibers	79.2
Groups of atrophic fibers	91.7
Eosinophilic inclusions	58.3
Inflammation	
Endomysial	95.8
Perivascular	87.5
Perimysial	37.5
EM filaments (40/43 cases)	93.3
Symptoms	
Limb weakness	100.0
Age >50 year	83.7
Family history of same disease	0.0
Dysphagia	33.3
Myalgia	16.7
Signs	
Distal limb weakness	50.0
Distal weakness ≥ proxima	35.0
KJs and AJs absent	27.1
Brisk tendon jerks	4.2
EMG	
Insertion activity increased	100.0
Fibrillation potentials	100.0
Fasciculation potentials	10.0
Short-duration potentials	100.0
Long-duration potentials	77.5
Both short and long in same muscle	75.0
Laboratory test	
Increased sedimentation rate	17.5
Creatine kinase level increased	80.0
Blood glucose increased	35.0
Antinuclear antibody	18.8

KJs, knee jerks; AJs, ankle jerks.
Modified from Lotz, 1989.

IBM and polymyositis differ pathologically because IBM is characterized by rimmed vacuoles, with the defining cellular inclusions and vacuoles. The pathogenesis of IBM is not known. Originally, IBM was thought to be a variant of polymyositis because, in addition to the inclusions, muscle is often infiltrated by lymphocytes in distribution, number, and T-cell characteristics similar to those of polymyositis. However, the vacuoles give immunochemical stains for proteins seen in the brain of patients with Alzheimer disease (beta-amyloid precursor protein and others), which leads some investigators to regard IBM as a "degenerative disease" rather than an autoimmune disorder.

Yet another peculiar facet of IBM is the presence of ragged fibers and cytochrome *c* oxidase negative fibers, findings that imply abnormalities of mitochondria, which prove to be multiple deletions of mitochondrial DNA. How this arises or what it means in the pathogenesis of the disorder is still uncertain.

IBM may be familial with little inflammation and vacuolar histologic characteristics similar to those of autosomal dominant Welander distal muscular dystrophy or oculopharyngeal muscular dystrophy; these syndromes differ clinically, but the similarities may cause problems in classification.

RELATION OF POLYMYOSITIS TO EOSINOPHILIC MYOSITIS

Rarely, a myopathy is associated with infiltration of muscle by eosinophils in addition to or instead of lymphocytes. One is the eosinophilic myositis of trichinosis or other parasitic infestation. Another form was seen in an epidemic in Spain of the toxic oil syndrome that was attributed to ingestion of denatured rapeseed oil. In addition to rash, fever, adenopathy, and other symptoms, some patients had prominent myalgia, but serum CK values were normal. In 1989, an epidemic in the United States of similar symptoms was finally attributed to ingestion of a contaminated preparation of L-tryptophan as a sedative. As many as 10,000 cases of that eosinophilia-myalgia syndrome may have occurred. Arthralgia, limb swelling, and evidence of myopathy or sensorimotor peripheral neuropathy were prominent. Muscle biopsy showed fascitis, perimyositis, and inflammatory microangiopathy. Eosinophilic myositis was found in some cases. The neuropathy had physiologic features of axonal damage in most patients, but some had conduction block.

MYOPATHY IN ACQUIRED IMMUNODEFICIENCY SYNDROME

Myopathy may appear in patients with AIDS. Intense debate has ensued about the pathogenesis of the disorder. Some believe it is an autoimmune polymyositis or the result of viral invasion of muscle. Others believe it is virtually restricted to those taking zidovudine; in those cases most show ragged-red fibers, and depletion of mitochondrial DNA has been documented. DNA levels return to normal when the drug therapy is interrupted.

RELATION OF POLYMYOSITIS TO POLYMYALGIA RHEUMATICA

In polymyalgia rheumatica, no symptomatic weakness or elevation of serum CK levels occurs. If overt weakness or high CK levels were evident, the syndrome would be impossible to distinguish from polymyositis. Polymyalgia can be defined as a syndrome in which a person older than age 65 has joint pains, myalgia, malaise, and a high erythrocyte sedimentation rate as described in Chapter 155.

THERAPY

Polymyositis itself is treated with steroids and immunosuppressive drugs, as described for dermatomyositis in Chapter 130. The advantages and risks must be balanced against the patient's disability. In controlled trials, plasmapheresis and leukapheresis had no effect, but intravenous immunoglobulin therapy has been beneficial, at least temporarily.

IBM characteristically does not respond to steroid therapy; this feature has led to the diagnosis of IBM in patients originally thought to have polymyositis. IBM does not respond to plasmapheresis but benefit was found in a few patients participating in a trial of intravenous immunoglobulin. Favorable results have been few.

The eosinophilia-myalgia syndrome has not responded to conventional immunosuppression, steroids, or plasmapheresis.

SUGGESTED READINGS

Polymyositis (also refer to Suggested Readings in Chapter 130)

Amato AA, Barohn RJ. Idiopathic inflammatory myopathies. *Neurol Clin* 1997;15:615–648.

Arahata K, Engel AG. Monoclonal antibody analysis of mononuclear cells in myopathies. V. T8+ cytotoxic and suppressor cells. *Ann Neurol* 1988;23:493–499.

Bautista J, Gil-Necija E, Castilla J, et al. Dialysis myopathy: 13 cases. *Acta Neuropathol (Berl)* 1983;61:71–75.

Benbassat J, Gefel D, Larholt K, et al. Prognostic factors in polymyositis. A computer-assisted analysis of 92 cases. *Arthritis Rheum* 1985;28:249–255.

Cohen O, Steiner I, Argov Z, et al. Mitochondrial myopathy with atypical subacute presentation. *J Neurol Neurosurg Psychiatry* 1998;410–411.

Crennan JM, Van Scoy RE, McKenna CH, Smith TF. Echovirus polymyositis in patients with hypogammaglobulinemia: failure of high-dose intravenous gamma globulin therapy. *Am J Med* 1986;81:35–42.

Cumming WJK, Weiser R, Teoh R, et al. Localized nodular myositis: a clinical and pathological variant of polymyositis. *Q J Med* 1977;184:531–546.

Dalakas MC. Inflammatory myopathies. *Handb Clin Neurol* 1992;18:369–390.

Dewberry RG, Schneider BF, Cale WF, Phillips LH II. Sarcoid myopathy presenting with diaphragm weakness. *Muscle Nerve* 1993;16:832–835.

Gheradi RK, Coquet M, Cherin P, et al. Macrophagic myofasciitis: an emerging entity. *Lancet* 1998;352:347–352.

Hart FD. Polymyalgia rheumatica. Correct diagnosis and treatment. *Drugs* 1987;33:280–287.

Hopkinson ND, Shawe DJ, Gumpel JM. Polymyositis, not polymyalgia rheumatica. *Ann Rheum Dis* 1991;50:321–322.

Kaufman LD, Kephart GM, Seidman RJ, et al. The spectrum of eosinophilic myositis. *Arthritis Rheum* 1993;36:1014–1024.

Lampe J, Kitzler H, Walter MC, Lochmuller H, Reichmann H. Methionine homozygosity at prion gene codon 129 may predispose to sporadic inclusion-body myositis. *Lancet* 1999;353:465–466.

Lange DJ. Neuromuscular diseases associated with HIV infection. *Muscle Nerve* 1994;7:16–30.

Layzer RB. The hypereosinophilic syndromes. In: Serratrice G, Pellissier J, Desnuelle C, Pouget J, eds. *Myelopathies, neuropathies et myopathies: acquisitions recentes (advances in neuromuscular diseases).* Paris: Expansion Scientifique Francaise, 1989.

Layzer RB, Shearn MA, Satya-Murti S. Eosinophilic polymyositis. *Ann Neurol* 1977;1:65–71.

Miller FW. Myositis-specific autoantibodies. Touchstones for understanding inflammatory myopathies. *JAMA* 1993;270:1846–1849.

Moskovic E, Fisher C, Wetbury G, Parsons C. Focal myositis: a benign inflammatory pseudotumor: CT appearance. *Br J Radiol* 1991; 64:489–493.

Navarro C, Bragado FG, Lima J, Fernandez JM. Muscle biopsy findings in systemic capillary leak syndrome. *Hum Pathol* 1990;21:297–301.

Persellin ST. Polymyositis associated with jejunoileal bypass. *J Rheumatol* 1983;10:637–639.

Phillips BA, Zilko P, Garlepp MJ, Mastaglia FL. Frequency of relapses in patients with polymyositis and dermatomyositis. *Muscle Nerve* 1998;21:1668–1672.

Pickering MC, Walport MJ. Eosinophilic myopathic syndromes. *Curr Opin Rheumatol* 1998;10:504–510.

Ringel SP, Thorne EG, Phanuphak P, et al. Immune complex vasculitis, polymyositis, and hyperglobulinemic purpura. *Neurology* 1979;29:682–689.

Rowland LP, Clark C, Olarte M. Therapy for dermatomyositis and polymyositis. In: Griggs RC, Moxley RT, eds. *Treatment of neuromuscular disease.* New York: Raven Press, 1977.

Spuler S, Emslie-Smith A, Emgel AG. Amyloid myopathy: an underdiagnosed entity. *Ann Neurol* 1998;43:719–728.

Symmans WA, Beresford CH, Bruton D, et al. Cyclic eosinophilic myositis and hyperimmunoglobulin-E. *Ann Intern Med* 1986;104:26–32.

Tsokos GC, Moutsopoulos M, Steinberg AD. Muscle involvement in systemic lupus erythematosus. *JAMA* 1981;246:766–768.

Vaish AK, Mehrotra S, Kushwaha MRS. Proximal muscle weakness due to amyloid deposition. *J Neurol Neurosurg Psychiatry* 1998;409–410.

Drug-induced Myopathies

Arnaudo E, Dalakas M, Shanske S, et al. Depletion of muscle mitochondrial DNA in AIDS patients with zidovudine-induced myopathy. *Lancet* 1991;337:508–510.

Batchelor TT, Taylor LP, Thaler HT et al. Steroid myopathy in cancer patients. *Neurology* 1997;48:1234–1238.

Choucair AK, Ziter FA. Pentazocine abuse masquerading as familial myopathy. *Neurology* 1984;34:524–527.

Doyle DR, McCurley TL, Sergent JS. Fatal polymyositis in D-penicillamine-induced nephropathy and polymyositis. *N Engl J Med* 1983;308:142–145.

Giordano N, Senesesi M, Mattii G, et al. Polymyositis associated with simvastatin. *Lancet* 1997;349:1600–1601.

Haller RG, Knochel JP. Skeletal muscle disease in alcoholism. *Med Clin North Am* 1984;68:91–103.

Kalkner KM, Ronnblom L, Karlsson Parra AK, et al. Antibodies against double-stranded DNA and development of polymyositis during treatment with interferon. *Q J Med* 1998;91:393–399.

Mastaglia FL. Adverse effects of drugs on muscle. *Drugs* 1982;24:304–321.

Ojeda VJ. Necrotizing myopathy associated with steroid therapy. Report of two cases. *Pathology* 1982;14:435–438.

Schultz CE, Kincaid JC. Drug-induced myopathies. In: Biller J, ed. *Iatrogenic neurology.* Boston: Butterworth-Heinemann, 1998:305–318.

Simpson DM, Citak KA, Godfrey E, et al. Myopathies associated with HIV and zidovudine. Can their effects be distinguished? *Neurology* 1993;43:971–976.

Simpson DM, Slasor P, Dafni U, et al. Analysis of myopathy in a placebo-controlled zidovudine trial. *Muscle Nerve* 1997;20:382–385.

Takahasi K, Ogita T, Okudaira H, et al. Penicillamine-induced polymyositis in patients with rheumatoid arthritis. *Arthritis Rheum* 1986;29:560–564.

Inclusion Body Myositis

Amato AA, Gronseth GS, Jackson CE, et al. Inclusion body myositis: clinical and pathological boundaries. *Ann Neurol* 1996;40:581–586.

Askanas V. New developments in hereditary inclusion body myositis. *Ann Neurol* 1997;41:421–422.

Askanas V, Serratrice G, Engel WK, eds. *Inclusion-body myositis.* Cambridge: Cambridge University Press, 1998.

Barohn RJ. The therapeutic dilemma of inclusion body myositis. *Neurology* 1997;48:567–568.

Brannagan TH, Hays AP, Lange DJ, Trojaborg W. The role of quantitative electromyography in inclusion body myositis. *J Neurol Neurosurg Psychiatry* 1997;63:776–779.

Chou SM. Inclusion body myositis: a chronic persistent mumps myositis? *Hum Pathol* 1986;17:765–777.

Garlepp MJ, Mastaglia F. Inclusion body myositis. *J Neurol Neurosurg Psychiatry* 1996;60:251–255.

Griggs RC, Askansas V, DiMauro S, et al. Inclusion body myositis and myopathies. *Ann Neurol* 1995;38:705–713.

Lindberg C, Borg K, Edstrom L, et al. Inclusion body myositis and Welander distal myopathy: a clinical, neurophysiological, and morphological comparison. *J Neurol Sci* 1991;103:76–81.

Lotz BP, Engel AG, Nishino H, et al. Inclusion body myositis. Observations in 40 patients. *Brain* 1989;112:727–747.

Moslemi A-R, Lindberg C, Oldfors A. Analysis of multiple mitochondrial DNA deletions in inclusion body myositis. *Hum Mutat* 1997;10: 381–386.

Sadeh M, Gadoth N, Hadar H, Ben-David E. Vacuolar myopathy sparing the quadriceps. *Brain* 1993;116:217–232.

Sivakumar K, Dalakas MC. Inclusion body myositis and myopathies. *Curr Opin Neurol* 1997;10:413–420.

Merritt's Neurology, 10th ed., edited by L.P. Rowland. Lippincott Williams & Wilkins, Philadelphia © 2000.

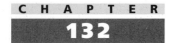

CHAPTER 132

MYOSITIS OSSIFICANS

LEWIS P. ROWLAND

The identifying characteristic of myositis ossificans (MIM 135100), a rare disorder, is the deposition of true bone in subcutaneous tissue and along fascial planes in muscle. McKusick (1974) believed that the primary disorder is in connective tissue and preferred the term *fibrodysplasia ossificans* rather than its traditional name, which implies a disease of muscle. Nevertheless, in some cases myopathic changes occur in muscle biopsy or electromyogram, and occasionally serum creatine kinase levels are increased.

Symptoms usually start in the first or second year of life.

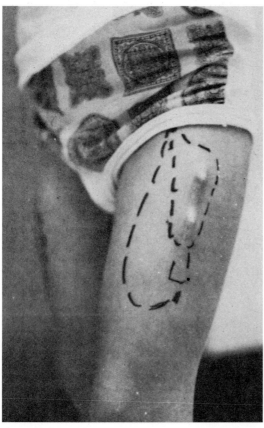

FIG. 132.1. Ossification of muscle biopsy scar in boy with myositis ossificans. The outer border of marks indicates extent of spontaneous ossification.

Transient and localized swellings of the neck and trunk are the first abnormality. Later, minor bruises are followed by deposition of solid material beneath the skin and within muscles. Plates and bars of material may be seen and felt in the limbs (Fig. 132.1), paraspinal tissues, and abdominal wall. These concretions are readily visible on radiographic examination, magnetic resonance imaging, or computed tomography; when they cross joints, a deforming ankylosis results. The cranial muscles are spared, but the remainder of the body may be encased in bone. The extent of disability depends on the extent of ossification, which varies considerably. No abnormality of calcium metabolism has been detected.

Almost all cases are sporadic, but it is suspected that the disease is inherited because minor skeletal abnormalities occur in almost all patients, and these abnormalities seem to be transmitted in the family in an autosomal dominant pattern. The most common deformity is a short great toe (*microdactyly*) and curved fingers (*clinodactyly*), and other digital variations are also seen. Most cases are attributed to new mutations because reproductive fitness is much reduced. The gene locus has not been mapped yet. Restricted ossification at the site of single severe injury may also occur in otherwise normal adults with no apparent genetic risk.

Treatment is symptomatic. Excision of ectopic bone is fruitless because local recurrence is invariable and disability may become worse. Surgery sometimes helps to refix a joint in a functionally better position. Treatment with diphosphonates inhibits calcification of new ectopic matrix but does not block production of the fibrous material and may have adverse effects on normal skeleton.

SUGGESTED READINGS

Amendola MA. Myositis ossificans circumscripta: computed tomography diagnosis. *Radiology* 1983;149:775–779.

Cohen RB, Hahn CV, Tabas JA, et al. The natural history of heterotopic ossification in patients with fibrodysplasia ossificans progressiva: 44 patients. *J Bone Joint Surg [Am]* 1993;75:215–219.

Connor JM. Fibrodysplasia ossificans progressiva. In: Royce PM, ed. *Connective tissue and its heritable disorders*. New York: Wiley Press, 1993.

Connor JM, Skirton H, Lunt PW. A three-generation family with fibrodysplasia ossificans progressiva. *J Med Genet* 1993;30:687–689.

Debene-Bruyerre C, Chikhami L, Lockhart R, et al. Myositis ossificans progressiva: five generations where the disease was exclusively limited to the maxillofacial region. *Int J Oral Maxillofac Surg* 1998;27:299–302.

DeSmet AA, Norris AA, Fisher DR. MRI of myositis ossificans: 7 cases. *Skel Radiol* 1992;21:503–507.

Kaplan FS, Tabas JA, Gauman FH, et al. The histopathology of fibrodysplasia ossificans progressiva. *J Bone Joint Surg [Am]* 1993;75:220–230.

McKusick VA. *Heritable diseases of connective tissue*, 4th ed. St Louis: CV Mosby, 1972.

Smith R. ENMC-sponsored international workshop: fibrodysplasia (myositis) ossificans progressiva (FOP). *Neuromusc Disord* 1997;7:407–410.

Merritt's Neurology, 10th ed., edited by L.P. Rowland. Lippincott Williams & Wilkins, Philadelphia © 2000.

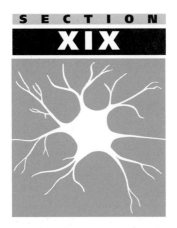

DEMYELINATING DISEASES

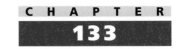

MULTIPLE SCLEROSIS

JAMES R. MILLER

DEFINITION

Multiple sclerosis (MS) is a chronic disease that begins most commonly in young adults and is characterized pathologically by multiple areas of central nervous system (CNS) white matter inflammation, demyelination, and glial scarring (sclerosis). The lesions are therefore multiple in space.

The clinical course varies from a benign, largely symptom-free disease to one that is rapidly progressive and disabling. Most patients begin with relapsing and remitting symptoms. At first, recovery from relapses is almost complete, but then neurologic disabilities accrue gradually. The lesions are therefore multiple in time and space.

The cause is elusive, although autoimmune mechanisms, possibly triggered by environmental factors in genetically susceptible individuals, are thought to be important.

INCIDENCE AND EPIDEMIOLOGY

Age at onset follows a unimodal distribution with a peak between ages 20 and 30 years; symptoms rarely begin before age 10 or after age 60. In a series of 660 patients, Bauer and Hanefeld (1993) found that almost 70% of patients had symptoms at ages 21 to 40, 12.4% at ages 16 to 20, and 12.8% at 41 to 50. The youngest patient had symptoms at age 3 and the oldest at 67 years. Younger and older cases have been reported.

In women, the incidence of MS is 1.4 to 3.1 times higher than in men. Among patients with later onset, the sex ratio tends to be equal.

The geographic distribution is uneven. In general, the disease increases in frequency with latitude in both the northern and southern hemispheres, although the rates tend to decrease above 65 degrees north or south.

Because of differences in methods of case finding and the need to rely on subjective clinical criteria in identifying cases of MS in large populations, the absolute numbers in any given area are uncertain. The distribution of MS is best considered in terms of zones. High prevalence areas are those with cases equal to or more than 30 per 100,000 population, medium prevalence areas have rates between 5 and 30 per 100,000, and low prevalence areas have rates less than 5 per 100,000. Most of northern Europe, northern United States, southern Canada, and southern Australia and New Zealand are areas of high prevalence. Southern Europe, southern United States, Asia Minor, the Middle East, India, parts of northern Africa, and South Africa have medium prevalence rates. Low prevalence areas are Japan, China, and Latin and South America. MS is virtually unknown among na-

tive Inuit in Alaska and among the indigenous people of equatorial Africa.

Although latitude may be an independent variable affecting MS prevalence rates, racial differences may explain some of the geographic distribution. This is illustrated by comparing the prevalence rate for MS in Britain (85 per 100,000) and Japan (1.4 per 100,000), although both countries lie at the same latitude. When racial differences are correlated with prevalence rates for MS worldwide, white populations are at greatest risk and both Asian and black populations have a low risk.

Studies of migrant populations provide evidence of environmental changes on the risk of MS while keeping genetic factors constant. Children born in Israel of immigrants from Asian and North African countries showed relatively higher incidence rates, like those of European immigrants, rather than the low rates characteristic of their parents. This finding implies that an environmental factor is critically important in pathogenesis. Similar differences were noted among the native-born South African whites, who had a relatively low incidence, as opposed to the high incidence among immigrants from Great Britain. Refinement of these studies suggested that age at time of immigration played an important role; an immigrant leaving the country of origin before age 15 years had nearly the same risk of acquiring MS as that of the native-born Israeli or South African. Individuals migrating after age 15 have the risk of the country of origin. These studies were confirmed by studies of people migrating from the Indian subcontinent or the West Indies to Great Britain. The data suggest that an infectious agent of long latency is acquired at the time of puberty.

Reports of epidemics of MS provide further evidence of an environmental factor. The most impressive epidemic occurred in the Faroe Islands where cases appeared shortly after the islands were occupied by British troops in World War II. Similar epidemics of cases have been seen in Iceland, in the Orkney and Shetland Islands, and in Sardinia. Rigorous epidemiologic scrutiny failed to prove, however, that these cases were true point-source epidemics. Therefore, other plausible explanations cannot be excluded.

MS is reported to occur more frequently in higher socioeconomic classes and in urban areas, but these assertions are unproved.

ETIOLOGY AND PATHOGENESIS

The cause of MS is unknown. Genetic susceptibility, autoimmune mechanisms, and viral infections may play a pathogenic role in the demyelination.

Genetic Susceptibility

Compelling data indicate that susceptibility to MS is inherited. The epidemiologic studies just summarized reveal a racial susceptibility to the development of MS. Whites appear most susceptible. Within this group are regional trends; the highest rates are associated with areas in which Nordic invasions took place. Alternatively, genetic resistance to MS in Asians and descendants of black Africans helps to explain racial variations in prevalence rates of MS. Because racial prevalence of MS changes with migration, however, definite conclusions of genetic predisposition cannot be drawn.

Studies of families and twins provide more support for genetic susceptibility. In high-prevalence regions, the lifetime risk of developing MS is about 0.00125% in the general population. Siblings of MS patients have a risk of about 2.6%, parents a risk of about 1.8%, and children a risk of about 1.5%. First-, second-, and third-degree relatives also have a higher risk. Overall, about 15% of patients with MS have an affected relative. Data from twin studies indicate a concordance rate of about 25% in monozygotic twins and of only 2.4% for same-sex dizygotic twins. These studies suggest a substantial genetic component. Rather than a single dominant gene, however, multiple genes probably confer susceptibility.

Pedigree data from families with more than one affected member are consistent with the hypothesis that multiple unlinked genes predispose to MS. The major histocompatibility complex (MHC) on chromosome 6 has been identified as one genetic determinant for MS. The MHC encodes the genes for the histocompatibility antigens (the human leukocyte antigen [HLA] system) involved in antigen presentation to T cells. Of the three classes of HLA genes, the strongest association is with the class II alleles, particularly the DR and DQ regions. In whites, the class II haplotype DR15, DQ6, Dw2 is associated with increased risk of MS. Delineation of this haplotype in patients with MS and in normal people, however, revealed no significant differences; genetic susceptibility to MS may therefore reside in functional aspects of these genes. The roles of other genes in MS, including the T-cell receptor (TCR) and immunoglobulin heavy chain genes, are reviewed later in the chapter.

Immunology

Substantial evidence from peripheral blood abnormalities, cerebrospinal fluid (CSF) findings, and CNS pathology in MS and animal models of demyelination suggests that autoimmune mechanisms are involved.

In the peripheral blood, several nonspecific changes are seen, particularly in secondary progressive MS. These changes are similar to those encountered in other autoimmune diseases, such as systemic lupus erythematosus (SLE). The activity of suppressor CD8+ T cells is reduced, as is the autologous mixed lymphocyte reaction, which seems to be an indicator of autoreactive cell suppression. In MS, as in SLE, there are fewer CD4+CD45RA+ suppressor-inducer T cells in the peripheral blood. An increase in activated T cells in MS is unlikely because cell surface molecules associated with T-cell activation are not abundant and lymphokine levels are normal.

CSF pleocytosis is common, particularly in the acute phases of MS. T cells that are helper-inducers (CD4+CDw29+ cells) constitute most of these cells and are found in higher ratios in CSF than in the peripheral circulation. By contrast, the number of CD4+CD45RA T cells, which induce suppressor cells, is decreased. Although some T lymphocytes in the CSF of patients with MS are activated, the antigenic stimulus is unclear. T-cell reactivity is found against several epitopes of myelin basic pro-

tein (MBP) and proteolipid protein. Analysis of the TCR gene, which is unique for each T-cell clone, suggests that the immune response is polyclonal and likely to have multiple antigenic specificities. Sequencing the variable regions of these cells reveals a high degree of somatic hypermutation, as is seen in chronic stimulation *in vivo*.

Antibody-secreting B cells are also activated in MS. The amount of IgG in the CSF and the rate of IgG synthesis are increased. Because only a few clones of CSF cells are activated, the response is *oligoclonal*. This seems to be a restricted response to stimulation within the neuraxis because similar oligoclonal IgGs are not found at all or are found in lower concentration in the serum than in CSF. Oligoclonal IgG is found in other inflammatory or infectious conditions, such as viral encephalitis or CNS syphilis. In these situations, however, the oligoclonal IgGs are antibodies directed against the agents of the infecting agent. In MS, an antigen for most of the oligoclonal IgG has not been identified. Therefore, the CSF IgG may be a secondary effect, possibly a result of the decrease in CD4+CD45RA+ suppressor-inducer cells, which allows a few clones of antibody-producing cells to escape suppression.

Perivascular lymphocyte and macrophage infiltration is characteristic of the CNS immunopathology. The predominant lymphocytes in MS lesions are helper-inducer cells (CD4+CDw29+). Interleukin-2 receptors are demonstrable on many of the T cells, thereby indicating that these cells are secreting cytokines and are immunologically activated. Also, astrocytes, which normally do not express MHC molecules, express class II molecules in active lesions. This pattern suggests that astrocytes are involved in antigen presentation to T cells. In more chronic lesions, γ/δ T cells are present around the edges of the plaque. Oligoclonal IgG is also present in MS plaques. Overall, the types of immunologically active cells and IgGs in the CNS lesions are similar to those found in CSF.

The cytokines produced by activated T cells and macrophages may play a role in some of the tissue damage. The cytokine called tissue necrosis factor is toxic to oligodendroglial cells and myelin and can be found in MS plaques. Further, CSF levels of tissue necrosis factor may correlate with MS disease activity.

Further evidence that MS may have an immunologic basis comes from the animal model *experimental allergic encephalomyelitis* (EAE), which is induced in genetically susceptible animals by immunization with normal CNS tissue and an adjuvant. The chronic relapsing-remitting form of EAE is pathologically similar to that of MS. EAE can also be induced by immunization with MBP or immunodominant peptide regions of MBP, thus suggesting that MBP is the putative antigen in EAE. T cells reactive against MBP and proteolipid protein mediate the CNS inflammation, as shown by "adoptive transfer": Sensitized T cells from an animal with EAE can transfer disease to a healthy syngeneic recipient. The T-cell response in EAE seems to be genetically restricted to a few families on the TCR gene, however, and removal or suppression of these T-cell lines leads to immunity from EAE. This response contrasts with the findings in human MS where the TCR gene response is more heterogeneous.

Although current understanding of MS pathogenesis derives mainly from consideration of the EAE and chronic EAE models, many features of the human disease are not understood or explained by this animal model. We do not know the precipitant antigens or even if the immune process is the primary force. There are differences in the pathology of the experimental and clinical disorders, the relative roles of cytokine activation, and antibody-mediated immunity; macrophage activity may differ. Healthy skepticism is warranted in considering theories of pathogenesis.

Viruses

Epidemiologic data imply a role for environmental exposure. Viral encephalitis in children may be followed by demyelination. In animals, the most widely studied model of viral-induced demyelinating disease is created by the Theiler virus, a murine picornavirus. Infection with some Theiler strains results in an infection of oligodendrocytes with multifocal perivascular lymphocytic infiltration and demyelination. Genetic factors influence susceptibility to development of demyelination and clinical disease; this susceptibility is linked to the immune response generated in the animals against viral determinants. Therefore, in MS, demyelination could be precipitated by a viral infection. Measles, rubella, mumps, coronavirus, parainfluenza, herpes simplex, Epstein-Barr, vaccinia, and human T-cell lymphotropic virus type I viruses all have been reported to be present in patients with MS. None of these agents, however, has been detected reproducibly. Human herpesvirus-6 has been implicated in MS disease activity; it is a ubiquitous agent that causes roseola subitum in children. Over 90% of adults have antibodies to the agent, and infection, mostly asymptomatic, probably occurs in early childhood. Human herpesvirus-6 then persists in a latent state in neural tissue. Results have not been uniform, but some investigators found an increased incidence of viral activity in areas around acute MS plaques. Activity of the virus may precipitate a flareup of symptoms. Studies are in progresss to determine if prophylactic treatment with an antiviral agent could reduce the frequency of episodes in MS. Perhaps no single virus is the trigger for demyelination in all patients with MS. Instead, several different viruses may be involved.

Other Factors

Other mechanisms have been suggested as precipitating the onset of MS or relapses. Physical trauma has been invoked as precipitating or aggravating the disease. In a population-based cohort study, however, Siva et al. (1993) found no association between MS and head injuries in 819 patients. Other studies also failed to show any causal correlation between trauma and MS. The effect of pregnancy is difficult to evaluate because MS is most common in women of childbearing age. If the pregnancy year is considered, however, exacerbations seem to cluster in the postpartum period rather than during pregnancy. Whether this clustering is related to hormonal changes or other factors is unclear. In any event, no convincing evidence has revealed that MS is worsened by pregnancy. Therefore, interruption of pregnancy in women with MS is not indicated on this basis alone.

Vaccination is also cited frequently as a precipitating event, although the evidence is anecdotal. One study with influenza vaccine found no relationship. In the absence of definitive stud-

ies, patients with MS should be advised against routine casual vaccination, especially if previous exacerbations have been preceded by vaccination. However, medically indicated inoculations should not be withheld. Surgery, anesthesia, and lumbar punctures also have been invoked in MS, but controlled studies failed to show any relationship.

PATHOLOGY

The gross appearance of the external surface of the brain is usually normal. Frequently in long-standing cases there is evidence of atrophy and widening of cerebral sulci with enlargement of the lateral and third ventricles. Brain sections reveal numerous small irregular grayish areas in older lesions and pink areas in acute lesions in the cerebral hemispheres, particularly in the white matter and in periventricular regions (Fig. 133.1). The white matter that forms the superior lateral angle of the body of the lateral ventricles is frequently and characteristically affected. Similar areas of discoloration are also found in the brainstem and cerebellum. These are the plaques of MS.

The external appearance of the spinal cord is usually normal. In a few cases, the cord is slightly shrunken and the pia arachnoid may be thickened. The cord occasionally may be swollen over several segments if death follows soon after the onset of an acute lesion of the cord. Plaques similar to those seen in the cerebrum are seen occasionally on the external surface of the cord, but they are recognized most easily on cross-section. The optic nerves may be shrunken, but the external appearance of the other cranial nerves is usually normal.

Myelin sheath stains of CNS sections show areas of demyelination in the regions that were visibly discolored in the unstained specimen. In addition, many more plaques are apparent. These plaques are sharply circumscribed and are diffusely scattered throughout all parts of the brain and spinal cord (Fig. 133.2). The lesions in the brain tend to be grouped around the lateral and third ventricles. Lesions in the cerebral hemispheres vary from the size of a pinhead to large areas that encompass the major portion of one lobe of the hemisphere. Small lesions may be found in the gray matter and in the zone between the gray and white matter. Plaques of varying size may be found in the optic nerves, chiasm, or tracts (Fig. 133.3). Lesions in the corpus callosum are not uncommon (Fig. 133.4). The lesions in the brainstem are usually numerous (Fig. 133.5), and sections from this area when stained by the Weigert method have a characteristic "Holstein cow" appearance (Fig. 133.6).

In sections of the spinal cord, the areas of demyelination vary from small lesions involving a portion of the posterior or lateral funiculi to almost complete loss of myelin in an entire cross-section of the cord (Figs. 133.7 and 133.8).

Lesions are usually characterized by sharp delimitation from the surrounding normal tissue. Within the lesion is variable destruction of the myelin and to a lesser degree damage to the neurons, proliferation of the glial cells, changes in the blood vessels, and relatively good preservation of the ground structure. Only rarely is the damage severe enough to affect the ground substance and produce a cyst (Fig. 133.6).

Most myelin sheaths within a lesion are destroyed, and many

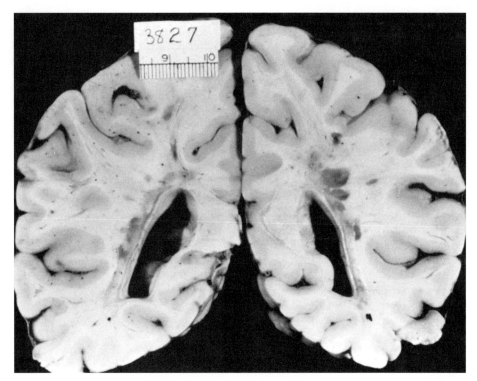

FIG. 133.1. Gross appearance, coronal section, occipital lobe. Note extensive periventricular lesions. Several small lesions are scattered elsewhere in the white matter. (Courtesy of Dr. Daniel Perl.)

of those that remain show swelling and fragmentation. The degree of damage to the neurons varies. In the more severe lesions, axons may be entirely destroyed, but more commonly only a few are severely injured and the remainder appear normal or show only minor changes. However, loss of axons is found in even the

earliest MS plaques. Secondary degeneration of long tracts occurs when the axons have been significantly destroyed. Recently, it has been appreciated that axonal loss and resulting brain atrophy are probably more closely correlated with irreversible clinical dysfunction than the number or size of plaques. When the le-

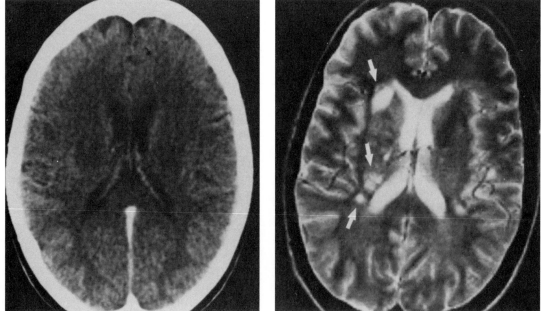

FIG. 133.2. A: Normal contrast-enhanced computed tomography. **B:** The axial T2-weighted magnetic resonance image in the same patient during the same period shows multiple white matter lesions, the largest designated by arrows.

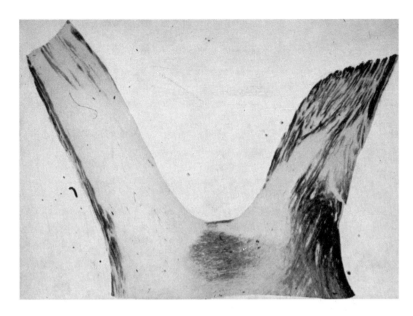

FIG. 133.3. Multiple sclerosis. Demyelinization of optic nerves and chiasm. (Courtesy of Dr. Abner Wolf.)

sion involves gray matter, nerve cells are less affected than is myelin, but some cells may be destroyed and show degenerative changes.

In the early or acute lesion there is marked hypercellularity, with macrophage infiltration and astrocytosis accompanied by perivenous inflammation with lymphocytes and plasma cells. Myelin sheaths disintegrate, and chemical breakdown of myelin occurs. It is not yet established whether the cellular response leads to, or occurs as a result of, the myelin breakdown. These acute lesions may remain active for several months with contin-

ued macrophage and astrocytic hyperactivity and breakdown of myelin. Phagocytic cells are laden with lipid degradation products of myelin. In these active but nonacute plaques, the inflammatory cell response is minimal centrally. At the edges, however, myelin disintegration is still active, and numbers of macrophages, lymphocytes, and plasma cells are increased. With time, the plaques become inactive. Demyelination is prominent, almost total oligodendrocyte cell loss occurs, and gliosis is extensive. Inactive lesions are hypocellular and devoid of myelin breakdown products.

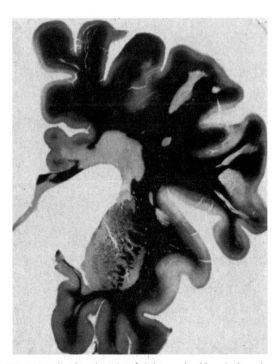

FIG. 133.4. Myelin sheath stain of right cerebral hemisphere in multiple sclerosis (celloidin). Note lesions in corpus callosum and superior lateral angle of the ventricle and several plaques in the subcortical white matter. (Courtesy of Dr. Charles Poser.)

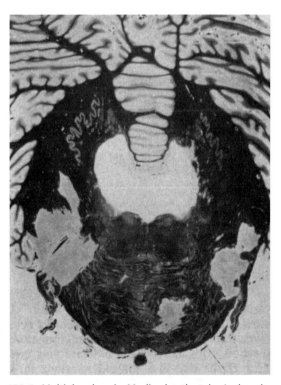

FIG. 133.5. Multiple sclerosis. Myelin sheath stain. Lesions in pons, middle cerebellum peduncle, and cerebellar white matter, typically near the dentate nuclei. (Courtesy of Dr. Charles Poser.)

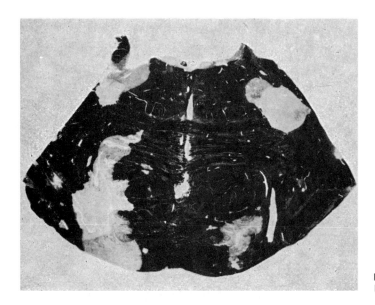

FIG. 133.6. Myelin sheath stain of brainstem in multiple sclerosis. Note sharp demarcation of lesions.

Remyelination in MS plaques, particularly after the early acute phase, is thought to result from the differentiation of a precursor cell that is common to type II astrocytes and oligodendrocytes. This remyelination, however, is usually aberrant and incomplete. Uniform areas of incomplete myelination ("shadow plaques") are evident in some chronic lesions; it is not known whether these regions result from partial demyelination or incomplete remyelination.

Electron microscopy reveals different aspects of myelin disorder in MS, including widening of the outer myelin lamellae, splitting and vacuolation of myelin sheaths, vesicular dissolution of myelin, myelin sheath fragmentation, ball and ovoid formation, filamentous accumulations in sheath, thin myelin sheaths, and macrophage-associated pinocytosis and actual peeling of layers of myelin by the processes of these microglial cells.

The peripheral nerves are usually normal. Subtle changes, however, in sural nerve biopsies include endothelial pinocytosis, expansion of the endoneurial space, mononuclear cell infiltra-

tion, or demyelination. In addition, hypertrophic neuropathy and chronic inflammatory demyelinating polyneuropathy have been reported in patients with MS.

Biochemical analysis of MS lesions reveals a decrease in both the protein and the lipid components of normal myelin. Thus, by immunocytochemistry, a decrease in staining for the MBP and myelin-associated glycoprotein and a decrease in cholesterol, glycolipids, phosphoglycerides, and sphingomyelins result. Because of phagocytosis and lysosomal activation, myelin breakdown products, including polypeptides, glycerol, fatty acids, and triglycerides, are abundant, particularly in active lesions.

Based largely on immunohistologic analysis of cell types in lesions, some investigators believe that there are variants in the pathology of MS and that individual patients tend to have one type of pathology. For example, lesions may vary in the prominence of T cells or macrophages and may vary in the extent of demyelination. This has led to the suggestion that MS may not be a single disease but rather a group of disorders all characterized by the final common pathway of inflammatory mediated demyelination. Others have found too much pathologic overlap in a single patient to warrant the view that these variants imply different forms of MS.

SYMPTOMS AND SIGNS

MS is characterized by dissemination of lesions in time and space. Exacerbations and remissions occur frequently. In addition, signs and symptoms usually indicate more than one lesion. Clinical manifestations may be transient and some may seem bizarre. The patient may experience unusual sensations that are difficult to describe and impossible to verify objectively.

The symptoms and signs (Tables 133.1 and 133.2) are diverse and seem to include all the symptoms that can result from injury to any part of the neuraxis from the spinal cord to the cerebral cortex. The chief characteristics are multiplicity and tendency to vary in nature and severity with time. Complete remis-

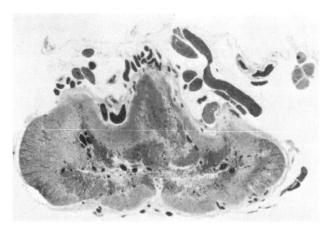

FIG. 133.7. Myelin sheath stain: tenth thoracic segment of spinal cord. Almost complete demyelination of the entire section. The gray matter is severely involved, and cystic degeneration causes obliteration of normal architecture.

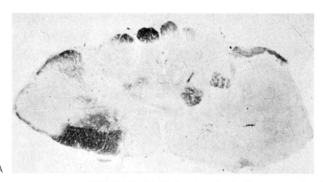
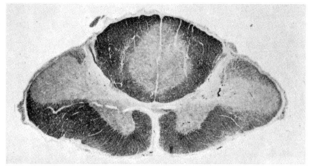

A
B

FIG. 133.8. Multiple sclerosis. **A:** Almost complete loss of myelin in transverse section of cord. **B:** Symmetric lesions in the posterior and lateral funiculi simulating distribution of lesions in combined system disease. (From Merritt HH, Mettler FA, Putnam TJ. *Fundamentals of clinical neurology.* Philadelphia: Blakiston, 1947.)

sion of the first symptoms frequently occurs, but with subsequent attacks, remissions tend not to occur or are incomplete. The clinical course extends for one or many decades in most cases, but a rare few are fatal within a few months of onset.

The clinical manifestations depend on the particular areas of

TABLE 133.1. COMMON SYMPTOMS AND SIGNS IN CHRONIC MULTIPLE SCLEROSIS

Functional system	% Frequency[a]
Motor	
Muscle weakness	65–100
Spasticity	73–100
Reflexes (hyperreflexia,Babinski, absent abdominals)	62–98
Sensory	
Impairment of vibratory/position sense	48–82
Impairment of pain, temperature, or touch	16–72
Pain (moderate to severe)	11–37
Lhermitte sign	1–42
Cerebellar	
Ataxia (limb/gait/truncal)	37–78
Tremor	36–81
Nystagmus (brainstem or cerebellar)	54–73
Dysarthria (brainstem or cerebellar)	29–62
Cranial nerve/brainstem	
Vision affected	27–55[b]
Ocular disturbances (excluding nystagmus)	18–39
Cranial nerves V, VII, VIII	5–52
Bulbar signs	9–49
Vertigo	7–27
Autonomic	
Bladder dysfunction	49–93
Bowel dysfunction	39–64
Sexual dysfunction	33–59
Others (sweating and vascular abnormalities)	38–43
Psychiatric	
Depression	8–55
Euphoria	4–18[c]
Cognitive abnormalities	11–59
Miscellaneous	
Fatigue	59–85

[a]Frequency values derived from the lowest and highest published rates. The higher frequency values are obtained mostly from studies with older patients with long-standing disease.
[b]Visual-evoked response abnormalities not included in these figures.
[c]Earlier studies suggested a much higher frequency, but these rates are not reproducible using current psychometric tests and therefore are excluded.

the CNS involved. Although no "classic" form of MS exists, for unknown reasons the disease frequently involves some areas and systems more than others. The optic chiasm, brainstem, cerebellum, and spinal cord, especially the lateral and posterior columns, are commonly involved (Table 133.1). Because of these predilections, some clinicians have classified MS into spinal, brainstem, cerebellar, and cerebral forms. These "forms" are often combined, and such classification is of no clinical value. In fact, the combination of anatomically unrelated symptoms and signs forms the basis for the clinical diagnosis of MS.

Visual symptoms include diplopia, blurred vision, diminution or loss of visual acuity on one or both sides, and visual field defects ranging from a unilateral scotoma or field contraction (Fig. 133.9) to homonymous hemianopsia. These symptoms characteristically begin over hours or days. Patients may also complain of a curious and quite distinctive problem in recognizing objects or faces, often stated as "blurry vision." This symptom is caused by optic nerve lesions that result in loss of contrasts of shade and colors. In early or mild optic or retrobulbar neuritis, color vision may be decreased, whereas black and white vision remains normal. Rarely, when color vision is affected in both eyes, either transient or permanent color blindness, almost always of the red-green type, may result. Examination of the visual fields with a red or green test object may uncover a central sco-

TABLE 133.2. SYMPTOMS AND SIGNS SEEN INFREQUENTLY IN MULTIPLE SCLEROSIS

Well-recognized associations	Rare associations
Generalized seizures	Aphasia
Tonic seizure	Anosmia
Headache	Hiccoughs
Trigeminal neuralgia	Deafness
Paroxysmal dysarthria/ataxia	Horner syndrome
Paroxysmal itching	
Chorea/athetosis	Cardiac arrhythmias
Myoclonus	Acute pulmonary edema
Facial hemispasm	Hypothalamic dysfunction
Myokymia	Narcolepsy
Spasmodic torticollis/focal dystonia	
Lower motor neuron signs—wasting, decreased tone, areflexia	
Restless legs	
Hysteria	

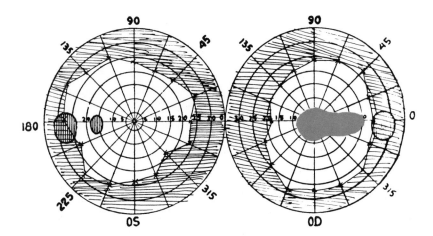

FIG. 133.9. Cecocentral scotoma in patient with acute right optic neuropathy: multiple sclerosis of 3 years' duration.

toma or field contraction that is not apparent with the usual white test object. Optic neuritis must be differentiated from papilledema because the fundoscopic appearance of both may be similar if the plaque is near the nerve head. Optic neuritis, however, is characterized by early impairment of visual acuity, which is a late manifestation of papilledema. A central or cecocentral scotoma is the most characteristic field loss. Retrobulbar neuritis, a common manifestation of MS, may not be associated with any fundoscopic abnormality but is revealed only by loss of visual acuity.

Diplopia may be caused by lesions in the medial longitudinal fasciculus that produce *internuclear ophthalmoplegia*. In young adults, internuclear ophthalmoplegia is uncommon in any other condition and is therefore an important sign in the diagnosis of MS. It is characterized by paresis of one medial rectus with failure of the eye to adduct on the side of the lesion and by nystagmus and weakness of the lateral rectus on the other side. This impairment of gaze may be present on attempts to look to one or both sides. In uncomplicated lesions of the medial longitudinal fasciculus, action of the medial rectus is preserved in reflex convergence, thus implying a supranuclear lesion. Mild diplopia may be reported as blurred vision. The true nature of the complaint is discovered only if the patient shuts one eye and vision improves.

The sudden onset of optic neuritis, without any other CNS signs or symptoms, is often interpreted as the first symptom of MS. Optic neuritis may also result, however, from a postinfectious or postvaccinal reaction or other conditions. The frequency by which MS follows a single isolated episode of optic neuritis is difficult to determine; published figures range from 15% to 85%. This spread is probably the result of differences of follow-up periods or of diagnostic and assessment measures. A critical review of published figures suggests that 35% to 40% of patients with optic neuritis ultimately develop MS.

The most common pupillary abnormalities are irregularities in the outline of the pupil, partial constriction, and partial loss of the light reflex.

Involvement of the descending root of the fifth cranial nerve occurs in some patients. Pain sensation in the face may be impaired and the corneal reflex may be diminished or lost. Paroxysmal pain indistinguishable from cryptogenic *trigeminal neuralgia* may occur. This symptom often responds to carbamazepine.

MS should be considered whenever a young adult develops trigeminal neuralgia.

Weakness of the facial muscles of the lower half of one side of the face is common, but complete peripheral facial palsy is rare. On the other hand, *hemifacial spasm* (consisting of spasmodic contractions of facial muscles) is a rare but characteristic paroxysmal disorder of MS. True vertigo, which often lasts several days and may be severe, is seen with new lesions of the floor of the fourth ventricle but is seldom a chronic symptom. Dysarthria and, rarely, dysphagia are seen in advanced MS because of cerebellar lesions or bilateral demyelination of corticobulbar tracts that cause pseudobulbar palsy, which is also characterized by emotional lability and forced laughing or crying without the accompanying affect.

Limb weakness is the most common sign, almost always present in advanced cases. Monoparesis, hemiparesis, or tetraparesis may be present; an asymmetric paraparesis is most common. Fatigability out of proportion to demonstrable muscular weakness is common. Direct testing of muscle strength alone often does not correlate with the degree of difficulty in walking. Concomitant spasticity and ataxia augment the gait disturbance. Gait ataxia is caused by a combination of lesions in the cerebellar pathways and loss of proprioception resulting from lesions in the posterior columns of the spinal cord.

In some patients, particularly those with late onset, the disease may appear as a slowly progressive spastic paraparesis, with no abnormality except corticospinal signs (spasticity, hyperreflexia, bilateral Babinski signs) and slight impairment of proprioceptive sensation.

The cerebellum and its connections with the brainstem are usually involved, thereby causing dysarthria, gait ataxia, tremor, and incoordination of the trunk or limbs. Tremor of the head and body is occasionally almost continuous when the patient is awake. The characteristic scanning speech of MS is a result of cerebellar incoordination of the palatal and labial muscles combined with dysarthria of corticobulbar origin. (The so-called *Charcot triad* of dysarthria, tremor, and ataxic gait is a combination of cerebellar symptoms.)

Urinary symptoms are also common, including incontinence and frequency or urgency of urination, and must be differentiated from manifestations of urinary tract infections or local conditions. Fecal incontinence or urgency is less common than urinary disturbances, but constipation is not unusual, especially in established cases. Loss of libido and erectile impotence are common problems in men. Almost invariably these are associated sphincter disturbances or corticospinal tract dysfunction, but psychologic problems may compound the problem. Sexual dysfunction in women is also frequent. Lack of lubrication and failure to reach orgasm are the major problems, but sensory dysesthesias are also significant.

Paresthesias and sensory impairment are common. When they are symptoms of an acute relapse, they tend to resolve completely in 6 to 8 weeks. In advanced disease, vibratory perception is commonly affected. Frequently, patients feel tingling or numbness in the limbs, trunk, or face. The *Lhermitte symptom* is a sensation of "electricity" down the back after passive or active flexion of the neck. It indicates a lesion of the posterior columns in the cervical spinal cord and may be seen in other diseases. The Lhermitte symptom is rarely elicited by flexion of the trunk. Pain is increasingly recognized as a frequent and disabling symptom. Pain may be associated with the Lhermitte phenomenon, trigeminal neuralgia, or retrobulbar neuritis. Other types of pain include painful flexor-extensor spasms; *painful tonic spasms* of the limbs (which can be evoked by hyperventilation); local pain such as constricting pain around a limb, burning pain, or pseudoradicular pain; foreign body sensation; headache; pain with pressure sores; pain caused by joint contractures and osteoporosis; pseudorheumatic pain with myalgia and arthralgia; or neuralgic pain shooting down the legs or around the abdomen, as in tabetic pain.

Psychiatric mood disorder symptoms are frequent. Depression is common. Whether it is directly related to MS lesions or a psychologic response to the disease is unclear. Both mechanisms are likely. Euphoria was once considered characteristic of MS patients. Even when this symptom exists, it appears more likely to be a frontal lobe dysinhibition syndrome, and underlying depression is often found. Some have found hypomanic behavior or bipolar disorders to be more common than expected by chance. This does not appear to be part of the disease, because the lifestyle is apparent long before neurologic symptoms occur. A genetic linkage has been suggested, but significant epidemiologic data have not been obtained.

Some have commented upon a tendency of patients to exaggerate and extend symptoms that have an obvious anatomic basis. Thus, diplopia may be transformed into triplopia, quadriplopia, or monocular double vision. However, because even the most obvious sensory symptoms often lack distinct correlates in the neurologic examination, it is dangerous to assume that unexplained sensory phenomenon are "psychogenic."

Cognitive, judgment, and memory disorders are important features in MS and may be more important than physical disorders in causing disability. These changes may range from the very obvious to subtle; even sophisticated psychometric studies may not detect early changes. Remedial training for memory problems may be helpful. Awareness of these potential difficulties may help relatives, friends, and patients cope with otherwise difficult behavior. Aphasic disorders are occasionally the major feature of an exacerbation.

Fatigue is another common symptom. It may appear as persistent fatigue, easy fatigability related to physical activity, or fatigue related to minor degrees of mental exertion. It is often the prodromal symptom of an exacerbation. Fatigue is not related to age because it is noted with the same frequency by patients under 30 or over 50. Also, fatigue is not related to the amount of physical disability because it is noted in more than 50% of patients with early MS. It is important to analyze the symptom; depression or lack of sleep due to nocturia may play a role. The fatigue of MS may respond to brief naps.

As may be seen from Table 133.1, most symptoms described occur in more than 50% of patients with MS at some time. The clinical features of MS, however, are protean; almost any part of the CNS may be affected (Table 133.2).

One of the characteristics of MS symptoms is evanescence. Diplopia may last only a few seconds. Paresthesias may last for seconds or hours; diminution of visual acuity may be equally short-lived. Transient loss of color vision may presage the onset of optic neuritis. Because of the transient and bizarre nature of these symptoms, they are frequently deemed hysterical before clearer manifestations arise. There may also be paroxysmal limb spasms, incoordination syndromes, or neuralgias. Trigeminal neuralgia in young people is most clearly associated with MS, but similar pains in other distributions may occur. Both the paroxysmal movements and neuralgias often respond to carbamazepine.

Other transient disorders may be precipitated by exercise, exposure to heat, or other stimuli. Transient dysesthesias, visual blurring or diplopia, or weakness after hot showers or exercise may occur. These episodes appear to represent derangements of the neurologic signal through previous damaged pathways and not an increase in the inflammatory process. They invariably disappear soon after the provoking activity is stopped.

Remissions are also characteristic, but clinicians have difficulty agreeing on the nature or duration of some remissions. If a remission is defined only by the complete or almost complete disappearance of a major symptom, such as loss of vision, marked weakness of a limb, or diplopia, clinical remissions occur in about 70% of all patients early in the course of the disease.

MODE OF ONSET

The onset is usually acute or subacute within days and is only rarely apoplectic. There is no characteristic mode of onset, but some symptoms and signs are more common (Table 133.3). Monosymptomatic onset is most common, but when onset is polysymptomatic, the clinical features often help to establish the diagnosis. Frequently, however, the past history reveals remote or recent episodes of other manifestations that had been ignored or not considered significant by the patient or physician. Dismissal is particularly true of transient paresthesias, mild urinary disturbances, or mild ocular manifestations, such as blurred vision or transient diminution of monocular visual acuity.

LABORATORY DATA

There is no pathognomonic test for MS, but magnetic resonance imaging (MRI), CSF examination, and evoked potential studies are of greatest diagnostic value (Table 133.4).

TABLE 133.3. COMMON SYMPTOMS AND SIGNS AT THE ONSET OF DISEASE IN PATIENTS WITH CLINICALLY DEFINITE MULTIPLE SCLEROSIS

Clinical feature	% Frequency
Monosymptomatic	45–79
Polysymptomatic	21–55
Weakness	10–40
Parasthesias	21–40
Sensory loss	13–39
Optic neuritis[a]	14–29
Diplopia	8–18
Ataxia	2–18
Bladder dysfunction	0–13
Vertigo	2–9

[a]Optic neuritis is more common in Japanese series (approximately 40%).

The most valuable laboratory aid is MRI, which shows multiple white matter lesions in 90% of patients (Fig. 133.10) and is the imaging procedure of choice in the diagnosis of MS. T2-weighted imaging has been the standard for demonstrating areas of involvement. Subsequently, proton density images and the fluid-attenuated inversion recovery technique have enhanced the ability to detect lesions, particularly in periventricular distribution. The distribution and morphology of plaques on T2-weighted MRI may be strongly suggestive of MS (Fig. 133.11) but occasionally it is difficult to distinguish from other lesions, particularly vascular disease. The MS plaques are found in the white matter in a periventricular distribution; the posterior poles of the lateral ventricles and the area of the centrum semiovale are most frequently involved. Corpus callosum lesions are characteristic and are brought out best with saggital proton density or fluid-attenuated inversion recovery. The most common appearance is of homogeneously hyperintense lesions; less commonly, ring or cystic lesions may occur. T1-imaging is not sensitive, but hypodense areas ("black holes") may be observed; these may be superimposed on active lesions or with frank tissue necrosis and glial scarring. Gadolinium enhancement is useful in defining areas of active inflammation. Triple-dose gadolinium is more sensitive than the standard dose, and delay in scanning after injection also enhances detection of inflammation. Because nonspecific white matter abnormalities are commonly seen, particularly in patients older than 50 years, a careful approach is still advisable when interpreting MRI studies despite the improvement in techniques (Table 133.4). Correlation of the MRI and the clinical history is of paramount importance.

Although MRI has been most useful diagnostically, correlation with clinical findings and disability has been disappointing. First, MRI abnormality is only an indirect measure of the actual lesions, and histologic damage may be far less than the size on the scan. This amplification factor is useful diagnostically but reduces the correlation with function. Also, much of observed mo-

TABLE 133.4. LABORATORY FINDINGS IN MULTIPLE SCLEROSIS (MS)

Magnetic resonance imaging (MRI)

  Appropriate T2-weighted scans abnormal in approximately 90% of patients.

  MRI interpretation should be conservative and correlate with the clinical findings.

  Typically, at least four white matter areas of increased signal of >3 mm diameter or three areas if at least one is periventricular should be seen.

  False-positive scans are common in patients with one or two white matter lesions, particularly in patients older than age 50 yrs

Cerebrospinal fluid findings

Protein	Normal or mildly increased in 50%.
Glucose	Normal.
Lymphocytes	Normal in 66%. In remainder, range from 5 to 20 cells/mm³.
	T/B lymphocyte ratio is 80:20.
	$CD4^+/CD8^+$ is 2:1.
IgG	Increased in about 70%.
Increased IgG synthesis	3.3 mg/day in 90% of patients.
High IgG index	0.7 in 90% of patients.
Oligoclonal IgG bands	90% of cases immunoelectrophoresis and silver staining.
Light chains	Increased ratio of kappa/lambda and free kappa light chains.
Myelin basic protein	Normally <1 ng/mL. Increased in acute relapses to 4 ng/mL in 80% of cases.

Evoked potentials

Visual-evoked responses	Very sensitive for detecting plaques in optic nerves, chiasm, or tracts.
	Abnormal responses in 85% of those with definite and 58% of those with probable MS.
	Interocular P_{100} latency difference is common feature.
Brainstem auditory	Most useful in detecting suspected pontine lesions.
	Abnormal responses in 67% of patients with definite and 41% of those with probable MS.
Somatosensory	Useful to document sensor abnormalities in patients with MS who have normal clinical sensory examinations.
	Abnormal in 77% of patients with definite and 67% of patients with probable MS.

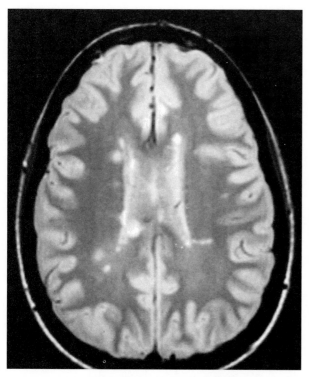
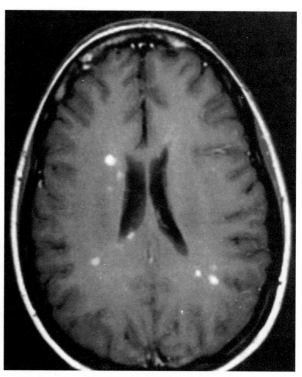

FIG. 133.10. A: Proton-density axial magnetic resonance image shows multiple hyperintense lesions within the periventricular white matter and corona radiata that are suggestive of demyelinating plaques. **B:** T1-weighted axial magnetic resonance image after gadolinium enhancement shows that some of these lesions exhibit contrast enhancement. (Precontrast T1-weighted images showed no hyperintense lesions.) Contrast enhancement of demyelinating plaques suggests active demyelination, and acute exacerbation of multiple sclerosis was evident clinically in this patient. (Courtesy of Dr. S. Chan.)

tor dysfunction is based on spinal cord lesions, which are difficult to image and are unobserved if only the brain is imaged. Volumetric MRI studies demonstrate cerebral atrophy even early in MS when obvious lesions are relatively sparse. This atrophy reflects axonal and neuronal loss and correlates better with disability than other scanning techniques, particularly with cognitive and memory dysfunction. Unfortunately, these techniques are largely clinically unavailable.

MR spectroscopy is useful for analyzing the parenchyma involved in MS lesions. Changes in tissue components may antedate by 1 week even the earliest observable MRI finding of gadolinium enhancement. Some have speculated that this may indicate the inflammatory process is only secondary to some other neuropil involvement. Further studies are required to resolve the issue.

Examination of the CSF frequently provides supportive information for the diagnosis (Table 133.4). The characteristic changes in CSF gamma globulins (IgG) are the most useful findings. The presence of oligoclonal IgG bands by electrophoretic analysis of CSF is the most frequent abnormality. A few antibody-producing plasma cell clones are thought to proliferate within the neuraxis in MS. The IgG production of these clones stands out in the electrophoretic analysis of the CSF as distinct *oligoclonal bands (OCBs)*. This pattern is not seen in normal people, in whom the CSF IgGs are passively derived from the serum and appear as diffuse broad bands in electrophoretic gels. For OCBs to be diagnostically useful, two or more bands must be seen, and these bands should be either absent from the serum or

present in lower concentrations than in CSF, implying primary intrathecal synthesis of the IgG. More than 90% of patients with clinically definite MS have CSF OCBs, but they are also detected in patients with other CNS inflammatory or infectious diseases. The other conditions, however, often reveal serum bands of at least equal intensity, thus indicating the systemic nature of the illness. For reasons unknown, OCBs are found in about 5% of patients with other (noninflammatory) neurologic problems.

The first abnormality of CSF IgG reported in MS was a relative increase in concentration of IgG compared with CSF total protein. This increase is found in only 70% of patients with clinically definite MS. Refinements of technique now compare the concentration of CSF IgG to serum IgG and take into account the relative concentrations of serum and CSF albumin, thereby increasing the sensitivity. By accounting for the relative albumin concentrations, the method can be used when the CSF total protein content is elevated, indicating breakdown of the blood–brain barrier and passive diffusion of antibody into the CSF from the serum. Formulas have been derived to estimate *intrathecal IgG synthetic rate,* which is elevated in MS. The sensitivity of these measurements now approaches the frequency of detection of CSF OCBs by electrophoresis.

The recording of *cortical-evoked responses* from visual, auditory, and somatosensory stimulation is also of great value in demonstrating clinically unsuspected lesions (Table 133.4). *Visual-evoked* responses to both flash and pattern reversal stimuli demonstrate abnormalities in many patients without symptoms

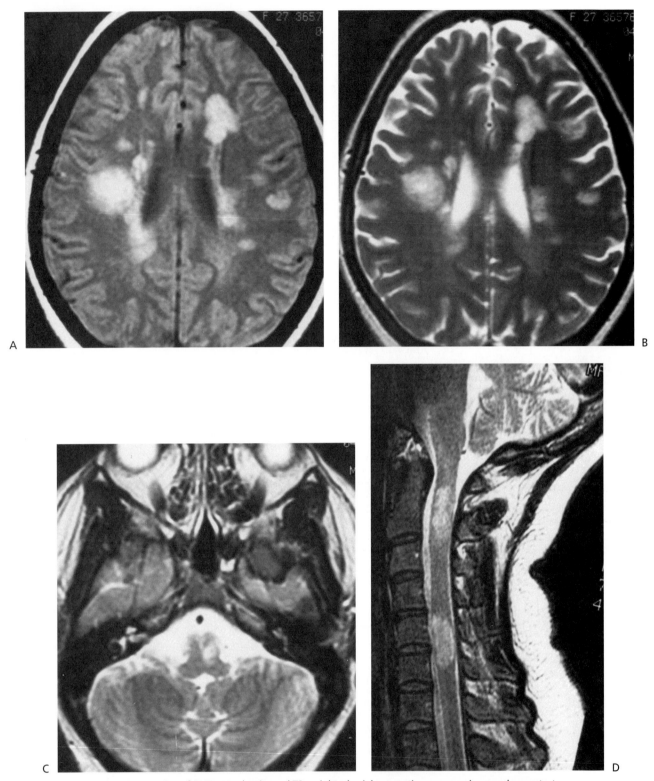

FIG. 133.11. A and B: Proton-density and T2-weighted axial magnetic resonance images demonstrate multiple periventricular hyperintense lesions, many of which abut the ependymal lining of the lateral ventricles. **C:** T2-weighted axial magnetic resonance image shows single hyperintense lesion within inferior left pons. **D:** T2-weighted sagittal magnetic resonance image shows two hyperintense lesions within cervical cord. This distribution of lesions is highly suggestive of multiple sclerosis. (Courtesy of Dr. S. Chan and Dr. A. G. Khandji.)

TABLE 133.5. CRITERIA FOR CLINICAL DIAGNOSIS OF MULTIPLE SCLEROSIS (MS)

Clinically definite	Consistent course
	Relapsing, remitting course; at least two bouts separated by at least 1 mo
	Slow or stepwise progressive course for at least 6 mo
	Documented neurologic signs of lesions in more than one site, of brain or spinal cord white matter
	Onset of symptoms between ages 10 and 50 yr
	No better neurologic explanations
Probable	History of relapsing, remitting symptoms but signs not documented and only one current sign commonly associated with MS
	Documented single bout of symptoms with signs of more than one white matter lesion; good recovery, then variable symptoms and signs
	No better neurologic explanation
Possible	History of relapsing, remitting symptoms without documentation of signs
	Objective signs insufficient to establish more than one lesion of central white matter
	No better explanation

From Rose AS, Ellison GW, Meyers LW, Tourtellotte WW. *Neurology* 1976;26:20–22.

or signs of visual impairment. *Somatosensory-evoked potentials* may help but are usually normal unless there are distinct clinical symptoms or findings. *Brainstem auditory-evoked responses* are even less sensitive in detecting abnormalities in asymptomatic patients but may be useful in confirming abnormalities in patients with brainstem symptoms or signs. These procedures are simple, noninvasive, harmless, and may be useful in providing evidence of anatomic abnormalities when clinical data are not clear. *Magnetically evoked motor potentials* detect lesions of the motor pathways from the cortex to spinal cord. This technique is not yet widely available.

DIAGNOSIS

Because no specific test for MS is available, the diagnosis rests on the multiple signs and symptoms with characteristic remissions and exacerbations (Table 133.5). The diagnosis can rarely be made with assurance at the time of the first attack. The diagnosis of MS is based on the ability to demonstrate, on the basis of the history, neurologic examination, and laboratory tests, the existence of lesions involving different parts of the CNS. The history should bring out mild and transient past events, and the examination should be detailed (e.g., testing for monocular color vision).

The advent of technologically based laboratory tests (Table 133.4) has added a new dimension to the documentation of multiple lesions. Even in patients who have had a single attack of optic neuritis or transverse myelitis, these tests may indicate more than one lesion, thereby changing the diagnosis from "probable" to laboratory-supported "definite" MS. At present, the following guidelines combine the clinical criteria of 1976 (Table 133.5) and those of 1983 (Table 133.6) with a few modifications:

TABLE 133.6. CRITERIA FOR THE DIAGNOSIS OF MULTIPLE SCLEROSIS

	Number of attacks	Evidence of more than one lesion		CSF, OCB, or IgG
		Clinical	Laboratory	
A. Clinically definite				
A1	2	2		
A2	2	1 and	1	
B. Laboratory-supported definite				
B1	2	1 or	1	+
B2	1	2		+
B3	1	1 and	1	+
C. Clinically probable				
C1	2	1		
C2	1	2		
C3	1	1 and	1	
D. Laboratory-supported probable				
D1	2	0	0	+

CSF; cerebrospinal fluid.
From Poser C, Paty DW, Scheinberg L, McDonald WI, Ebers GC. *The diagnosis of multiple sclerosis.* New York: Thieme-Stratton, 1984.

1. *Clinically definite MS* requires either evidence from both history and neurologic examination of more than one lesion or evidence from history of two episodes, signs of one lesion on examination, and evidence from evoked responses or MRI of other lesions.
2. *Laboratory-supported definite MS* requires evidence of two lesions in either history or examination. If only one lesion is evident in either of those categories, at least one more lesion must be evident in evoked response or MRI. In addition, CSF IgG content and pattern should be abnormal.
3. In *clinically probable MS*, either history or examination, but not both, provides evidence of more than one lesion. If only one lesion is evident by history and only one by neurologic examination, evoked potentials or MRI may provide evidence of one or more lesions in addition. In this category, CSF IgG studies are normal.

In practice, these criteria are overly conservative because the diagnosis can certainly be made in patients even if symptoms begin after age 50. Finally, when the diagnosis of MS cannot be made with certainty, the clinician should reevaluate the patient rather than make a hasty diagnostic decision. In some cases, however, MS may remain asymptomatic, and a firm diagnosis may be made only at autopsy.

DIFFERENTIAL DIAGNOSIS

In young adults with characteristic manifestations (Table 133.3) and laboratory abnormalities (Table 133.4), the diagnosis is easily made. Although the complete list of diagnostic possibilities may seem endless, only a few disorders have similar clinical or laboratory features that lead to diagnostic difficulties (Table 133.7).

It is difficult, if not impossible, to differentiate between the first attack of MS and acute disseminated encephalomyelitis (ADEM). ADEM follows infection or vaccination and occurs most commonly in children. A clear distinction between the two conditions may not be possible because about 25% of patients diagnosed as having ADEM later develop MS. Furthermore, the pathologic lesions of MS and ADEM are difficult to distinguish.

In endemic areas, Lyme disease is an important consideration because chronic CNS infection with *Borrelia burgdorferi* can

TABLE 133.7. DIFFERENTIAL DIAGNOSIS OF MULTIPLE SCLEROSIS

Disorder	Distinguishing clinical/laboratory features
Acute disseminated encephalomyelitis	Follows infections or vaccination in children; fever, headaches, and meningism common
Lyme disease	Antibodies to Borrelia antigens in serum and CSF by ELISA and Western blotting
HIV-associated myelopathy	HIV serology
HTLV-I myelopathy	HTLV-I serology in serum/CSF
Neurosyphilis	Serum/CSF serology
Progressive multifocal leukoencephalopathy	Immunosuppressed patients; biopsy of lesions demonstrates virus by electron microscopy
Systemic lupus erythematosus	Non-CNS manifestations of lupus; antinuclear antibodies, anti-dsDNA and anti-Sm antibodies
Polyarteritis nodosa	Systemic signs; angiography shows microaneuryms; biopsy of involved areas shows vasculitis
Sjögren syndrome	Dry eyes and mouth; anti-Ro and anti-La antibodies; lower lip biopsy helpful
Behçet disease	Oral/genital ulcers, antibodies to oral mucosa
Sarcoidosis	Non-CNS signs; increased protein in CSF; biopsy shows granuloma
Paraneoplastic syndromes	Older age group; anti-Yo antibodies; identify neoplasm
Subacute combined degeneration of cord	Peripheral neuropathy; vitamin B_{12} levels
Subacute meylooptic neuritis	Mainly in Japanese; adverse reaction to chlorhyroxyquinoline
Adrenomyeloneuropathy	Adrenal dysfunction; neuropathy; plasma very-long-chain fatty acids increased
Spinocerebellar syndromes	Familial; pes cavus; scoliosis; absent reflexes; normal CSF IgG and no bands
Hereditary spastic paraparesis/ primary lateral sclerosis	Normal CSF studies
Miscellaneous	Strokes, tumors, arteriovenous malformations, arachnoid cysts, Arnold-Chiari malformations, and cervical spondylosis all may lead to diagnostic dilemmas on occasion. These conditions may coexist; differentiation based on history, clinical follow-up and MRI features.

HIV, human immunodeficiency virus; CSF,z cerebrospinal fluid; CNS, central nervous system; MRI, magnetic resonance imaging.

cause spastic paraparesis, cerebellar signs, and cranial nerve palsies. The MRI and CSF abnormalities of MS can also be seen in Lyme disease, so the diagnosis of Lyme disease must rest on a history of characteristic acute symptoms and rash of Lyme disease, with demonstration of antibodies to *Borrelia* antigens in high titer and in both CSF and serum.

Because other infections may mimic MS, serologic tests for human immunodeficiency virus, human T-cell lymphotropic virus type I, and syphilis are required. Progressive multifocal leukoencephalopathy should be considered in immunosuppressed individuals.

Several autoimmune diseases have CNS manifestations and particularly MRI changes that can resemble MS. SLE, polyarteritis nodosa, Sjögren syndrome, Behçet disease, and sarcoidosis are the most notable. The non-CNS features of these diseases usually distinguish them from MS, but if diagnostic difficulties are encountered, specific serum antibody tests, such as anti-DNA antibodies in SLE, or a biopsy of an appropriate site, such as in sarcoidosis, are sufficient to clinch the diagnosis.

Paraneoplastic syndromes with cerebellar signs may cause diagnostic problems, particularly in older patients. Serum antibodies to Purkinje cells are useful in making the diagnosis.

Subacute combined degeneration should be excluded in all cases of spinal MS by measuring serum vitamin B_{12} levels. Similarly, women with progressive spastic paraparesis should have a test for the plasma content of very-long-chain fatty acids to exclude the heterozygous carrier state of adrenomyeloneuropathy. Subacute myelooptic neuritis is an adverse reaction to chlorhydroxyquinoline; relapses of sensory symptoms, limb weakness, and optic neuritis may occur. Subacute myelooptic neuritis is restricted almost exclusively to Japanese people, and no further cases should be seen because the drug has been withdrawn.

Hereditary spinocerebellar ataxia syndromes can cause diagnostic dilemmas. If the syndrome is Friedreich ataxia, differentiation is easily made on clinical grounds, but if only cerebellar and pyramidal signs develop, diagnosis may be difficult. The most vexing problem is to separate slowly progressive spastic paraparesis of MS from hereditary spastic paraplegia or primary lateral sclerosis, especially if CSF studies and MRI are normal.

Vascular disease, arteriovenous malformations, tumors of brain or spinal cord, and arachnoid cysts can have relapsing-remitting signs. MRI is usually defining. The effects of an Arnold-Chiari malformation can simulate MS clinically, but MRI findings are usually diagnostic. Cervical spondylotic myelopathy may simulate spinal MS; MRI of the brain and CSF changes may indicate MS.

Common neurologic conditions, including cerebrovascular disease or cervical spondylosis, may be found in a patient who also has MS. Determination of whether new symptoms are caused by relapse of MS or by the coexisting condition may be challenging. History, examination, and MRI are of greatest use in determining the cause.

COURSE AND PROGNOSIS

The clinical course of MS varies. Exceptional cases are clinically silent for a lifetime; the typical pathologic findings are discovered only at autopsy. At the other extreme, some cases are so rapidly progressive or malignant that only a few months elapse between onset and death.

Clinical observation of the course of MS led to the description of "types." *Relapsing-remitting MS* is one type. This pattern is usually present at the outset and is characterized by exacerbations followed by a variable extent of improvement, ranging from complete resolution of neurologic deficit to symptomatic residual dysfunction. About 10% of patients have relatively few attacks throughout their life and accrue minimal disability. This is referred to as *benign MS*. Relapsing-remitting MS frequently (approximately 85% of the time) evolves into a situation in which the course progresses slowly in between or in lieu of discrete attacks. This is referred to as *secondary-progressive MS*.

Subsets have also been described. These descriptions have limitations because a relapsing-remitting course may occur for several years followed by a chronic-progressive illness. Also, no universal agreement has been reached about the definition of relapse or remission. Determining if a patient is having a relapse may be difficult, especially in mild cases, and the assessment is often made in retrospect.

There is no discernible difference in MRI activity between relapsing-remitting and secondary-progressive MS, and the change of course does not indicate a change in the inflammatory process. This is supported by newer information that the β-interferons appear to be beneficial in the treatment of both these phases of MS. Primary-progressive MS has some different characteristics from the other types of MS and is discussed more fully below as a variant.

The diagnostic use of evoked potentials, CSF OCBs, and MRI has changed concepts about the course of MS. People once thought to have a mild neurologic disorder of undetermined cause are now included as having probable or definite MS, altering the incidence and prevalence data of clinical subtypes.

The question most frequently asked by patients is that of prognosis. Unfortunately, no reliable prognostic indicators are available, and the generalizations that follow may not be applicable in individual cases. The characteristics of a good prognosis in order of usefulness are minimal disability 5 years after onset, complete and rapid remission of initial symptoms, age 35 years or less at onset, only one symptom in the first year, acute onset of first symptoms, and brief duration of the most recent exacerbation. In general, onset with sensory symptoms or mild optic neuritis is also associated with a good prognosis. Poor prognostic indicators include polysymptomatic onset, cerebellar signs of ataxia or tremor, vertigo, or corticospinal tract signs.

Disability and work capacity are important concerns in any chronic disease with onset from 15 to 55 years (Table 133.8). Overall, MS has only a modest effect on life expectancy, but disability is a major issue. After 10 years, 70% of MS patients are not working full-time because of cognitive and memory disorders, spastic paraparesis, poor coordination, and sphincter dysfunction.

Death from MS itself is rare. Bronchopneumonia after aspiration or respiratory insufficiency is the most common cause of death. Other causes include cardiac failure, malignancies (as would be expected in older patients regardless of MS), septicemia (decubitus ulcers, urinary infections), and suicide.

In the last few decades, average survival has increased from 25

TABLE 133.8. WORKING CAPACITY AND SURVIVAL IN 800 PATIENTS WITH MULTIPLE SCLEROSIS

Duration	1–5 yr (%)	6–10 yr (%)	11–15 yr (%)	16–20 yr (%)	21 yr (%)
Working	71	50	31	30	28
Disabled	29	49	63	57	52
Dead	—	1	6	13	20

From Bauer HJ. *Neurology* 1978;28:8–20.

years to 35 years after onset, probably as a result of better management of infection and decubitus ulcers.

VARIANTS OF MULTIPLE SCLEROSIS

Several variants of MS are recognized. The typical form of relapsing-remitting disease, which often evolves into more progressive disease, is called the *Charcot variant. Primary-progressive MS* differs from the more common form because it is progressive from the outset and distinct exacerbations do not occur. It accounts for about 10% of MS cases and is more common in older men. Brain MRI lesions tend to be sparse or absent, and this seems to be mainly a spinal cord syndrome. Not infrequently, optic neuropathy is present as demonstrated by visual evoked responses (VERs). The pathology tends to show a less exuberant immune inflammatory component than in more typical disease. OCBs are, however, found in the CSF in over 50% of patients. The course is more relentless than that of typical MS.

A more rapidly progressive disease with severe disability and frequently death in the first year is the *Marburg variant.* The pathology usually shows more exuberant inflammation and axonal loss than in the Charcot variant. Some patients have a fulminant myelitis with optic neuritis, which is frequently bilateral; this combination is called the *Devic syndrome.* Some consider it a separate disease because of the severely necrotic lesions and a relative paucity of immune active cells. However, many cases with typical pathology of Devic syndrome have had a previous course consistent with the Charcot variant and many cases have lesions that elsewhere are indistinguishable from classic MS.

Schilder disease appears to be fulminant MS in children. The pathology is similar to that of MS, but confluent lesions involving both hemispheres are typical. The *concentric sclerosis of Balo* also occurs primarily in children. The course is similar to typical MS but the pathology is strikingly different and characterized by concentric rings of inflammation and demyelination. It is not known how this pattern comes about.

Although these variants are unusual, without clear knowledge of etiology and pathogenesis it is impossible to state authoritatively whether they are separate diseases or forms of MS.

Finally, some paroxysmal inflammatory CNS disorders in adults are equivocally related to MS. Cases of recurrent optic neuritis without any evidence of other neuraxis involvement are well known. Similarly, recurrent episodes of myelitis may occur without other CNS lesions. The CSF may be inflammatory, but OCBs are often absent. ADEM may be clinically indistinguishable from an attack of MS. Lesions tend to be more inflammatory and less demyelinating than MS plaques. ADEM is charac-

teristically a monophasic illness and may be more of a cognate for EAE than MS. Recurrences have been reported, but unless there is a distinct immune stimulant, it is hard to understand why these cases should not be classified as MS.

MANAGEMENT

MS presents a major challenge for the physician. The fact that no known cure exists is often interpreted as meaning that no treatment is effective. This error leads to neglect of symptoms and complications that are amenable to prevention and treatment. The skepticism and pessimism pervasive among physicians are based in large part on the long list of ineffective therapeutic regimens that have been tried. Although no cure is in sight, the results of controlled therapeutic trials with β-interferons suggest that the natural history of MS can be favorably altered.

Before making specific recommendations about treatment, some general guidelines are appropriate:

1. The patient and family should be informed of the diagnosis by specific name when it is firmly established, so they can begin to accept the diagnosis and can avail themselves of all accessible services.
2. The disease should be explained in understandable terms, with a realistic but best possible prognosis.
3. At first, the patient should be reevaluated at short intervals for counseling and support and then at regular intervals to monitor possible complications and to evaluate progress.
4. The patient should be given realistic information about the goals of therapy and should participate in decisions (e.g., adjustment of antispastic medication).
5. Patients with MS have complex problems, and many benefit from care at MS centers, where a team approach provides comprehensive service.
6. The patient should be informed about local and national MS societies that provide educational material, support groups, and other services.

Therapeutic regimens are either disease specific (immunosuppressive or immunomodulatory) or symptomatic. If the symptoms of an acute attack are severe enough to warrant treatment, methylprednisolone is given in a dose of 1 g by intravenous infusion daily for 7 to 10 days. This is followed by oral prednisone in a tapering schedule. A typical tapering regimen follows: prednisone 80 mg daily for 4 days; followed by 60, 40, 20, 10, and 5 mg each for 4 days; and then four doses of 5 mg on alternate days. Tapering schedules are arbitrary and are often empiric or based on speculative theoretic considerations.

They may be considerably longer or shorter than the one described.

Alternatively, corticotropin may be given, but it has lost favor because it seems to give less rapid improvement. In controlled trials, steroid therapy hastens recovery from acute attacks, but it is not clear whether it affects the eventual outcome. Both CSF pleocytosis and MRI findings are reduced in patients who receive intravenous high-dose steroid therapy. A shorter (3-day) high-dose intravenous methylprednisolone treatment was compared with oral steroids and placebo over a 2-year period in patients with a first episode of optic neuritis alone. The effect on speeding up recovery without influencing eventual outcome was confirmed. Retrospective data analysis suggested that the development of MS was delayed in the intravenous methylprednisolone group. The 3-day course of intravenous high-dose corticosteroids is a matter of convenience and has never been demonstrated to be as effective as longer courses.

In the short term, adverse effects of corticosteroids are usually minimal or transitory. Psychologic agitation is perhaps most common and should be treated if it occurs. Avascular necrosis of joints is rare but can occur regardless of the steroid dose. Patients who have frequent relapses and are treated repeatedly with steroids, however, are at risk of serious adverse effects. To minimize these effects, the steroid dosage is tapered and calcium carbonate supplements (650 mg two times per day) are given to forestall osteoporosis. Chronic oral steroid use has no merit, either daily or on alternate days, because this treatment does not alter the course of the disease.

In 1993, the first practical treatments for use in early MS that affected the course of the disease became available in the United States and subsequently in other countries. Two classes of medications are now in use. β-Interferon is available in two preparations with a third expected soon. The first released was β-interferon-1b (Betaseron), a form chemically modified from naturally occurring human β-interferon. This medication is given on alternate days subcutaneously in a dose of 0.250 mg. β-Interferon-1a (Avonex) is chemically unaltered and is given intramuscularly once week in a dose of 30 μg. Rebif is also classified as a β-interferon-1a but is not yet commercially available. In initial trials it was given three times weekly in doses of 22 or 44 μg subcutaneously. In placebo-controlled studies, all three forms of β-interferon have given remarkably similar results. They all seem to reduce the frequency of attacks in the relapsing-remitting phase by about 30%. The severity of attacks also seems to be reduced. Favorable effects on MRI changes have also been noted. Most important, a favorable effect on the development of disability is now being established for these medications. Studies in progressive disease are also being concluded; one published study of Betaseron confirms its usefulness in retarding progression. Similar results can be anticipated for the other β-interferons.

The β-interferons are well tolerated. Early in treatment a "flu-like" syndrome may follow each injection but rarely lasts longer than 24 hours. It may include myalgia, arthralgia, headache, and fever, which dissipate in about a month. Taking the medication in the evening and with acetaminophen or a nonsteroidal antiinflammatory drug often ameliorates the syndrome. Low doses of corticosteroids at the outset of treatment have also been advocated. Rarely, these symptoms persist and force discontinuation

of treatment. Some patients find that their function decreases the day after an injection, and this may also necessitate discontinuation. Hepatic abnormalities and bone marrow depression may occur but rarely necessitate discontinuation. Periodic blood studies are advisable in the first 2 years of administration. Although there is no known danger to the fetus, manufacturers have indicated pregnancy (including the period of conception and breastfeeding) as a contraindication to the use of the β-interferons. Depression is commonly thought to be caused by the β-interferons, but there is no scientific support for this contention, based solely on anecdote.

All these medications can be self-administered, if neurologic function permits. Neutralizing antibodies against β-interferon may appear and render treatment ineffective. Development of antibodies seems to be more frequent with Betaseron (approximately 25%), intermediate with Rebif, and least frequent with Avonex (5% to 10%). The subcutaneous route for injection may be a factor in antibody development. If antibodies interfere, medication should probably be stopped and alternative treatment considered.

There is now debate about the optimum route of administration and dosage, the intensity of which is matched only by the lack of directly comparable information. Unfortunately, the information is unlikely to be forthcoming, because it would require a direct comparison of the medications, and the expense of such a study would be staggering.

The other disease-specific therapy currently available is *glatiramer acetate* (Copaxone or copolymer I), a mixture of polymers of four amino acids. One of the sequences is a nonencephalitogenic peptide fragment of MBP. It has been demonstrated to have effects similar to the β-interferons on exacerbation frequency and attack severity. However, effects on MRI lesions or development of disability are less well established. Some consider this to be the drug of choice in early mild cases, as suggested by controlled studies. Its effect on progressive problems is currently being studied. Glatiramer acetate is given subcutaneously on a daily basis. It is not associated with systemic symptoms or abnormalities; some patients report chest pressure similar to angina, but there is no evidence of cardiac ischemia. The injections can be associated with intense but brief pain. When disease-specific treatment first became available, fewer patients accepted treatment then was anticipated. The reasons were diverse but included reluctance to take injections and disappointment because of the partial effect. As evidence accrued of a favorable effect on progression, the importance of early treatment became more apparent. The current recommendation of the National Multiple Sclerosis Society is that all patients with clinically definite exacerbating disease should be taking medication. In view of the information supporting the use of β-interferon in progressive illness, many experts are treating MS patients as well. A study of Avonex is designed to determine the benefit of taking β-interferon before a second attack occurs.

Severe and frequent relapses or rapidly progressive MS pose a difficult therapeutic problem. This may occur at the outset of the disease or later even with treatment with one of the prophylactic agents. Typically, these patients have no response to high-dose intravenous steroids or, more frequently, have a modest initial response and minimal responses with subsequent cycles of therapy. If a β-interferon is being administered, it is appropriate to determine the neutralizing antibody level. Alternative treatments that may be used are mainly the immunosupressants. Cyclophosphamide is used in monthly pulse doses of 800 to 1,000 mg/m^2 surface area (s.a.) in 500 mL of 0.9% sodium chloride solution infused over 2 to 4 hours. Patients are given 3 L of fluid over 24 hours to maintain adequate urinary output. Mesna, in an equal milligram quantity, may be added to the cyclophosphamide to reduce bladder irritation. Ondansetron 10 mg and dexamethasone 10 mg are given to reduce nausea and vomiting. However, clinical trials of cyclophosphamide have given conflicting results. Many use it based on anecdotal experience and believe it stabilizes the disease even though improvement is not anticipated. Another agent that has been used with some enthusiasm despite conflicting results in the literature is cladribine (Leucostatin), which is relatively specific for T$_4$ helper cells, and some consider this a theoretic advantage.

Azathioprine taken orally in a dose of 1 to 2 mg/kg body weight merits mention. As with all other such agents, its use is limited by toxicity, and reliable controlled studies are wanting. Mitoxantrone has been widely used in Europe. Methotrexate taken in doses similar to those used in rheumatoid arthritis (7.5 to 15 mg orally once a week) is modestly effective in progressive disease. It should be considered in situations when prophylactic agents or more intensive chemotherapy is not indicated.

In a disease that cannot be prevented or cured, symptomatic therapy is important to minimize functional impairment and discomfort. Spasticity with stiffness, painful flexor or extensor spasms, and clonus are major causes of disability. If untreated, contractures may develop and increase disability. Baclofen is the most commonly used drug at a dose of 40 to 80 mg/day in divided doses. If tolerated, higher doses may be used in severe cases. Diazepam or dantrolene may be added or substituted if necessary. Tizanidine in doses up to 24 mg daily may also be considered. It supposedly does not cause as much weakness as the other antispasticity agents but sedation is a major problem with tizanidine, and very slow titration is required. For localized adductor spasms, injections of botulinum toxin may be useful. However, the large muscle groups involved required large doses of medication and antibody production rapidly develops. In resistant cases, baclofen may be administered intrathecally with an indwelling catheter and implantation of a reservoir pump. Only patients who have a beneficial effect with an intrathecal test bolus dose of 50 to 100 μg baclofen should have the pump implanted. Adverse effects are not common but include meningitis and seizures. Cracks in the tubing may develop and should be considered if effect is rapidly lost. In addition to relief of spasticity, bladder symptoms frequently improve. The dosage of all antispastic agents must be monitored and titrated with the clinical response; flaccidity and unmasked weakness changes in mentation may result in functional deterioration.

Bladder management is important to prevent debilitating and life-threatening infections or stone formation and to allow maximum functional independence. The basic problem may be failure to retain urine, excessive urinary retention, or a combination of the two. In all these problems, the symptoms of urgency, frequency, and incontinence are similar. The most important measures are postvoiding residuals, urine cultures, and, occasionally, urodynamic studies or renal ultrasound studies. The atonic bladder with a residual volume over 100 mL is best managed by a program of clean intermittent self-catheterization. Cholinergic drugs, such as bethanechol, carbachol, and pyridostigmine, are marginally and transiently effective in aiding bladder emptying. For acute urinary retention during a relapse of MS, phenoxybenzamine is the drug of choice because it induces relaxation of the bladder neck. Patients with bladder atony are susceptible to urinary infections. Some authorities routinely use urine acidifiers, such as vitamin C, and urinary antiseptics, such as methenamine mandelate, for all such patients.

Detrusor muscle hyperexcitability that causes the spastic bladder is the most common cause of urinary urgency and incontinence in patients with MS. Oxybutinin is the most effective agent in relieving symptoms, but other anticholinergic medications include propantheline, hycosamine, and imipramine. Tolterodine (Detrol), a long-acting anticholinergic, has been released and decreases the frequency of dosing. A sustained-release form of oxybutinin is currently under study. The synthetic antidiuretic hormone (vasopressin), desmopressin acetate, has been used with success as an intranasal spray, particularly for patients with nocturia. The usual dose is 10 to 40 μg at night. Serum osmolality and electrolytes should be measured weekly for the first month and then monthly as a precaution in these patients. Some patients find a morning-after rebound effect that is unacceptable.

In patients with long-standing bladder disease, indwelling catheters may have to be used even though the risk of infection increases. Disposable catheters, periodic irrigation, weekly catheter renewal, and urine acidifiers minimize infections. Bladder augmentation with a section of bowel has been helpful when bladder size has diminished because of spasticity. A continent port may be placed on the abdominal wall to facilitate catheterization in appropriate situations. In late stages, suprapubic cystostomy or urinary diversion procedures may be appropriate. In all patients with urinary symptoms, a urine culture should be obtained because treatment of infection alone may suffice to relieve new symptoms.

Cerebellar symptoms are generally resistant to therapy. An occasional patient with disabling intention tremor may respond to propranolol or clonazepam. Cryothalamotomy may be effective but is reserved for severe cases.

Painful radiculopathy or neuralgia and painful parasthesias may respond to carbamazepine or, if not tolerated, to phenytoin or amitriptyline. Less specific pain syndromes may respond to nonsteroidal anti-inflammatory agents.

Fatigue may respond to amantadine or pemoline and to a change in work schedule. Methylphenidate is also used to control fatigue. Depression may contribute to fatigue and usually responds to selective serotonin reuptake inhibitor antidepressants. Whether these drugs affect fatigue independent of depression is conjectural.

Constipation responds best to changes in diet, bulk-providing substances, and stool softeners. Laxatives are reserved for resistant cases. Bowel incontinence is less common and is generally unresponsive to medication. Regularization of bowel habits seems the most useful approach. Anticholinergic drugs may be useful adjuncts.

Sexual dysfunction should be treated with counseling for both partners, but treatments exist to alleviate the problems. In the past, erectile dysfunction had been treated with papaverine injections, alprostadil intracavernosal injections, or intraurethral suppositories or less effectively with vacuum devices designed to increase penile blood flow. Although often successful, few patients continue to use these treatments. However, sildenafil citrate (Viagra) is successful in treating erectile dysfunction in MS patients. Ease of use makes it likely to be of continuing benefit. In women, lubricating agents may help. The usefulness of sildenafil in restoring orgasmic capability and lubrication is currently being studied in women with MS.

When paraparesis is severe, skin care is essential to prevent decubitus ulcers. Physical therapy and nursing care with adequate nutrition and hydration are valuable in preventing painful disabling complications, such as decubitus ulcers, renal and bladder calculi, contractures, and intercurrent infections. When these complications occur, aggressive attempts to relieve them often give gratifying results.

Diet therapy and vitamin supplements are frequently advocated, but no special supplementation or elimination diet has proved to be more beneficial than a well-balanced diet that maintains correct body weight and provides sufficient roughage for bowel management. Other therapies, such as hyperbaric oxygen, plasmapheresis, intravenous immunoglobulin, neurostimulation, cobra or bee sting venom, and acupuncture, are unproven, and any response to these treatments is usually a result of coincidental spontaneous remission so often seen early in the disease.

Physical therapy should be applied judiciously with the goals of maintaining mobility in ambulatory patients or avoiding contractures in bedridden patients. Excessive active exercise may exhaust the patient, and the increase in body temperature may cause transient symptoms. Swimming in cool water is the best active physical therapy. Occupational therapy is important to assist patients in activities of daily living.

MS is one of the few diseases for which a cure is unavailable, yet a comprehensive therapeutic regimen supervised by an experienced and sympathetic physician can give rewarding results.

SUGGESTED READINGS

Ablashi D, Lapps W, Kaplan M, Whitman J, Richert J, Pearson G. Human herpesvirus-6 (HHV-6) infection in multiple sclerosis: a preliminary report. *Multiple Sclerosis* 1998;4:490–496.

Afifi AK, Bell WE, Menezes AH, Moore SA. Myelinoclastic diffuse sclerosis (Schilder's disease): report of a case and review of the literature. *J Child Neurol* 1994;9:398–403.

Barnes MP, Bateman DE, Cleland PG, et al. Intravenous methylprednisone for multiple sclerosis in relapse. *J Neurol Neurosurg Psychiatry* 1985;48:157–159.

Bauer HJ, Hanefeld FA, eds. *Multiple sclerosis; its impact from childhood to old age*. London: Saunders, 1993.

Beck RW, Cleary PA, Anderson MM, et al. A randomized, controlled trial of corticosteroids in the treatment of acute optic neuritis. *N Engl J Med* 1992;326:581–588.

Beck RW, Cleary PA, Trobe JD, et al. The effects of corticosteroids for acute optic neuritis on the subsequent development of multiple sclerosis. *N Engl J Med* 1993;329:1764–1769.

Betts CD, D'Mello MT, Fowler, CJ. Urinary symptoms and the neurological features of bladder dysfunction in multiple sclerosis. *J Neurol Neurosurg Psychiatry* 1993;56:245–250.

Borras C, Rio J, Porcel J, Barrios M, Tintore M, Montalban X. Emotional state of patients with relapsing-remitting MS treated with interferon beta-1b. *Neurology* 1999;52:1636–1639.

Challoner P, Smith K, Parker J, et al. Plaque-associated expression of human herpesvirus 6 in multiple sclerosis. *Proc Natl Acad Sci USA* 1995;92:7440–7444.

Confavreux C, Hutchinson M, Hours MM, Cortinovis-Tourniaire P, Moreau T. Rate of pregnancy-related relapse in multiple sclerosis. Pregnancy in Multiple Sclerosis Group [see comments]. *N Engl J Med* 1998;339:285–291.

Deisenhammer F, Reindl M, Harvey J, Gasse T, Dilitz E, Berger T. Bioavailability of interferon beta 1b in MS patients with and without neutralizing antibodies. *Neurology* 1999;52:1239–1243.

Ebers G, Bulman D, Sadovnick A, et al. A population-based study of multiple sclerosis in twins. *N Engl J Med* 1986;315:1638–1642.

Ebers GC, Dyment DA. Genetics of multiple sclerosis. *Semin Neurol* 1998;18:295–299.

European Study Group on Interferon Beta-1b in Secondary Progressive MS. Placebo-controlled multicentre randomised trial of interferon beta-1b in treatment of secondary progressive multiple sclerosis. *Lancet* 1998;352:1491–1497.

Fazekas F, Deisenhammer F, Strasser-Fuchs S, et al. Randomized placebo-controlled trial of monthly intravenous immunoglobulin therapy in relapsing-remitting multiple sclerosis. *Lancet* 1997;349:589–593.

Filippi M, Iannucci G, Tortorella C, et al. Comparison of MS clinical phenotypes using conventional and magnetization transfer MRI. *Neurology* 1999;52:588–594.

Filippi M, Rocca MA, Martino G, Horsfield MA, Comi G. Magnetization transfer changes in the normal appearing white matter precede the appearance of enhancing lesions in patients with multiple sclerosis. *Ann Neurol* 1998;43:809–814.

Filippi M, Silver N, Yousry T, Miller D. Newer magnetic resonance techniques and disease activity in multiple sclerosis: new concepts and new concerns. *Multiple Sclerosis* 1998;4:469–470.

Garell PC, Menezes AH, Baumbach G, et al. Presentation, management and follow-up of Schilder's disease. *Pediatr Neurosurg* 1998;29:86–91.

Haegert DG, Francis GS. HLA-DQ polymorphisms do not explain HLA class II associations with multiple sclerosis in two Canadian patient groups. *Neurology* 1993;43:1207–1210.

The IFNB Multiple Sclerosis Study Group. Interferon beta-1b is effective in relapsing-remitting multiple sclerosis. I. Clinical results of a multicenter, randomized, double-blind, placebo-controlled trial. *Neurology* 1993;43:655–661.

The IFNB Multiple Sclerosis Study Group and The University of British Columbia MS/MRI Analysis Group. Interferon beta-1b in the treatment of multiple sclerosis: final outcome of the randomized controlled trial [see comments]. *Neurology* 1995;45:1277–1285.

Jacobs LD, Cookfair DL, Rudick RA, et al. Intramuscular interferon beta-1a for disease progression in relapsing multiple sclerosis. *Ann Neurol* 1996;39:285–294.

Johnson KP, Brooks BR, Cohen JA, et al. Copolymer 1 reduces relapse rate and improves disability in relapsing-remitting multiple sclerosis: results of a phase III multicenter, double-blind placebo-controlled trial. The Copolymer 1 Multiple Sclerosis Study Group [see comments]. *Neurology* 1995;45:1268–1276.

Johnson KP, Brooks BR, Cohen JA, et al. Extended use of glatiramer acetate (Copaxone) is well tolerated and maintains its clinical effect on multiple sclerosis relapse rate and degree of disability. Copolymer 1 Multiple Sclerosis Study Group. *Neurology* 1998;50:701–708.

Kermode AG, Thompson AJ, Tofts P, et al. Breakdown of the blood-brain barrier precedes symptoms and other MRI signs of new lesions in multiple sclerosis. Pathogenetic and clinical implications. *Brain* 1990;113[Pt 5]:1477–1489.

Kim MO, Lee SA, Choi CG, Huh JR, Lee MC. Balo's concentric sclerosis: a clinical case study of brain MRI, biopsy, and proton magnetic resonance spectroscopic findings. *J Neurol Neurosurg Psychiatry* 1997;62:655–658.

Kupersmith MJ, Kaufmann D, Paty DW, et al. Megadose corticosteroids in multiple sclerosis. *Neurology* 1994;44:1–4.

Leuzzi V, Lyon G, Cilio MR, et al. Childhood demyelinating diseases with a prolonged remitting course and their relation to Schilder's disease: report of two cases. *J Neurol Neurosurg Psychiatry* 1999;66:407–408.

Lucchinetti CF, Bruck W, Rodriguez M, Lassmann H. Distinct patterns of multiple sclerosis pathology indicates heterogeneity on pathogenesis. *Brain Pathol* 1996;6:259–274.

Lucchinetti CF, Brueck W, Rodriguez M, Lassmann H. Multiple sclerosis: lessons from neuropathology. *Semin Neurol* 1998;18:337–349.

Mandler RN, Davis LE, Jeffery DR, Kornfeld M. Devic's neuromyelitis optica: a clinicopathological study of 8 patients. *Ann Neurol* 1993;34:162–168.

Mathews WB, Compston A, Allen IV, Martyn CN, eds. *McAlpine's multiple sclerosis.* Edinburgh: Churchill-Livingstone, 1991.

Metz L. Multiple sclerosis: symptomatic therapies. *Semin Neurol* 1998;18:389–395.

Miller DH. Multiple sclerosis: use of MRI in evaluating new therapies. *Semin Neurol* 1998;18:317–325.

Miller JR, Burke AM, Bever CT. Occurrence of oligoclonal bands in multiple sclerosis and other CNS diseases. *Ann Neurol* 1983;13:53–56.

Molyneux PD, Filippi M, Barkhof F, et al. Correlations between monthly enhanced MRI lesion rate and changes in T2 lesion volume in multiple sclerosis. *Ann Neurol* 1998;43:332–339.

Murray T. Amantadine therapy of fatigue in multiple sclerosis. *Can J Neurol Sci* 1985;12:251–254.

Myhr KM, Riise T, Green Lilleas FE, et al. Interferon-alpha2a reduces MRI disease activity in relapsing-remitting multiple sclerosis. Norwegian Study Group on Interferon-alpha in Multiple Sclerosis. *Neurology* 1999;52:1049–1056.

Nelson RF. Ethical issues in multiple sclerosis. *Semin Neurol* 1997;17:227–234.

Noseworthy JH. Multiple sclerosis clinical trials: old and new challenges. *Semin Neurol* 1998;18:377–388.

Paty D, Ebers G, eds. *Multiple sclerosis.* Philadelphia: FA Davis, 1998.

Paty DW, Li DK. Interferon beta-1b is effective in relapsing-remitting multiple sclerosis. II. MRI analysis results of a multicenter, randomized, double-blind, placebo-controlled trial. UBC MS/MRI Study Group and the IFNB Multiple Sclerosis Study Group [see comments]. *Neurology* 1993;43:662–667.

Phadke J, Best P. Atypical and clinically silent multiple sclerosis: a report of 12 cases discovered unexpectedly at necropsy. *J Neurol Neurosurg Psychiatry* 1983;46:414–420.

Poser CM. Serial magnetization transfer imaging to characterize the early evolution of new MS lesions [letter]. *Neurology* 1999;52:1717.

Poser CM, Paty DW, Scheinberg L, et al. New diagnostic criteria for multiple sclerosis: guidelines for research protocols. *Ann Neurol* 1983;13:227–231.

PRISMS (Prevention of Relapses and Diability by Interferon β-1a Subcutaneouly in Multiple Sclerosis) Study Group. Randomized double-blind placebo-controlled study of interferon β-1a in relapsing/remitting multiple sclerosis. *Lancet* 1998;352:1498–1504.

Ravborg M, Liguori R, Christiansen P, et al. The diagnostic reliability of magnetically evoked motor potentials in multiple sclerosis. *Neurology* 1992;42:1296–1301.

Rice GP, Paszner B, Oger J, Lesaux J, Paty D, Ebers G. The evolution of neutralizing antibodies in multiple sclerosis patients treated with interferon beta-1b. *Neurology* 1999;52:1277–1279.

Rudick RA, Goodkin DE, Jacobs LD, et al. Impact of interferon beta-1a on neurologic disability in relapsing multiple sclerosis. The Multiple Sclerosis Collaborative Research Group (MSCRG). *Neurology* 1997;49:358–363.

Rudick RA, Simonian NA, Alam JA, et al. Incidence and significance of neutralizing antibodies to interferon beta-1a in multiple sclerosis. Multiple Sclerosis Collaborative Research Group (MSCRG) [see comments]. *Neurology* 1998;50:1266–1272.

Sadovnick AD, Ebers GC, Wilson RW, Paty DW. Life expectancy in patients attending multiple sclerosis. *Neurology* 1992;42:991–994.

Sibley WA. *Therapeutic claims in multiple sclerosis.* New York: Demos, 1992.

Siva A, Radhaskrishnan K, Kurland LT, et al. Trauma and multiple sclerosis: a population based cohort study from Olstead County, Minnesota. *Neurology* 1993;43:1878–1881.

Sorensen TL, Ransohoff RM. Etiology and pathogenesis of multiple sclerosis. *Semin Neurol* 1998;18:287–294.

Staugaitis S, Roberts JK, Sacco RL, Miller JR, Dwork AJ. Devic type multiple sclerosis in an 81 year old woman. *J Neurol Neurosurg Psychiatry* 1998;64:417–418.

Trapp BD, Peterson J, Ransohoff RM, Rudick R, Mork S, Bo L. Axonal transection in the lesions of multiple sclerosis. *N Engl J Med* 1998;338:278–285.

Weiner HL, Mackin GA, Orav EJ, et al. Intermittent cyclophosphamide pulse therapy in progressive multiple sclerosis: final report of the Northeast Cooperative Multiple Sclerosis Treatment Group. *Neurology* 1993;43:910–918.

Weinshenker BG. The natural history of multiple sclerosis. *Neurol Clin* 1995;13:119–146.

Weinshenker BG. The natural history of multiple sclerosis: update 1998. *Semin Neurol* 1998;18:301–307.

Weinshenker BG, Issa M, Baskerville J. Long-term and short-term outcome of multiple sclerosis: a 3-year follow- up study. *Arch Neurol* 1996;53:353–358.

Merritt's Neurology, 10th ed., edited by L.P. Rowland. Lippincott Williams & Wilkins, Philadelphia © 2000.

C H A P T E R
134

MARCHIAFAVA-BIGNAMI DISEASE

JAMES R. MILLER

Primary degeneration of the corpus callosum is clinically characterized by altered mental status, seizures, and multifocal neurologic signs. Demyelination of the corpus callosum without inflammation is the primary pathologic feature, but other areas of the central nervous system may be involved. The disease was first described by Marchiafava and Bignami in 1903.

ETIOLOGY

The cause is not known. The disease was first noted in middle-aged and elderly Italian men who consumed red wine. It has been described worldwide, however, and is not confined only to drinkers of red wine. In some cases, alcohol consumption was not a factor. Nutritional deficiencies also have been implicated. The syndrome is rare, however, even in severe malnutrition. Toxic factors have been suggested, but no agent has been implicated.

PATHOLOGY

The *sine qua non* is necrosis of the medial zone of the corpus callosum. The dorsal and ventral rims are spared. The necrosis varies from softening and discoloration (Fig. 134.1) to cavitation and cyst formation. Usually, all stages of degeneration are found.

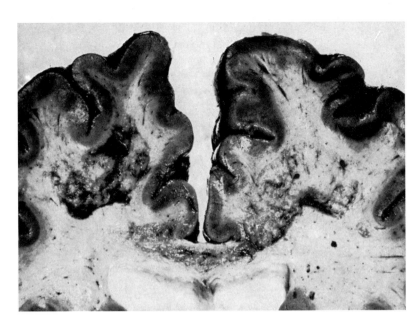

FIG. 134.1. Marchiafava-Bignami disease. Acute necrosis of corpus callosum and neighboring white matter of the frontal lobes. (From Merritt HH, Weisman AD. *J Neuropathol Exp Neurol* 1945;4:155–163.)

In most cases, the rostral position of the corpus callosum is affected first. The lesions arise as small symmetric foci that extend and become confluent. Although medial necrosis of the corpus callosum is the principal finding, there also may be degeneration of the anterior commissure (Fig. 134.2), the posterior commissure, centrum semiovale, subcortical white matter, long association bundles, and middle cerebellar peduncles. All these lesions have a constant bilateral symmetry. Usually spared are the internal capsule, corona radiata, and subgyral arcuate fibers. The gray matter is not grossly affected.

Few diseases have such a well-defined pathologic picture. The corpus callosum may be infarcted as a result of occlusion of the anterior cerebral artery, but the symmetry of the lesions, sparing of the gray matter, and occurrence of similar lesions in the anterior commissure, long association bundles, and cerebellar peduncles are found only in Marchiafava-Bignami disease.

The microscopic alterations are the result of a sharply defined necrotic process with loss of myelin but relative preservation of axis cylinders in the periphery of the lesions. There is usually no evidence of inflammation aside from a few perivascular lymphocytes. In most cases, fat-filled phagocytes are common. Gliosis is usually not well advanced. Capillary endothelial proliferation may be present in the affected area, but no thrombi are seen.

The disease has been reported with central pontine myelinolysis or Wernicke encephalopathy in alcoholics and in nonalcoholic persons, thus suggesting a possible common pathogenesis.

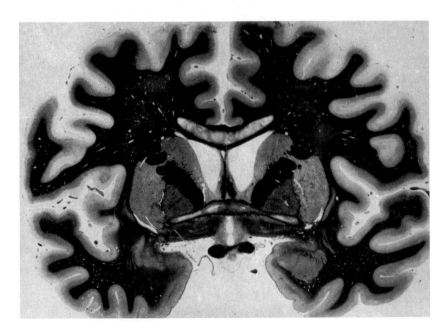

FIG. 134.2. Marchiafava-Bignami disease. Medial necrosis of the corpus callosum and anterior commissure with sparing of the margins. (Courtesy of Dr. P.I. Yakovlev.)

INCIDENCE

More than 100 cases have been reported, but the disease is probably more common. Before the advent of modern imaging, however, the diagnosis was rarely made before death because the symptoms and findings are nonspecific. Genetic predisposition has been suspected because of the frequent reports in Italian men. The onset is usually in middle age or late life.

SYMPTOMS AND SIGNS

The onset is usually insidious, and the first symptoms are so nonspecific that an accurate estimate of the exact time of onset is difficult. There is a mixture of focal and diffuse signs of cerebral disease, especially dementia. In addition to memory loss and confusion, manic, paranoid, or delusional states may occur. Depression and extreme apathy are typical.

DIAGNOSIS

Marchiafava-Bignami disease may be suspected when insidiously developing dementia, multifocal neurologic signs, and seizures occur in elderly, particularly alcoholic, men. Computed tomography and especially magnetic resonance imaging have enhanced the ability to diagnose the disease before death. Either form of imaging can show the typical callosal lesions and symmetric demyelinating lesions in other areas. Brain single-photon emission computed tomographies may also prove useful in analysis of cases.

COURSE

The disease is usually slowly progressive and results in death within 3 to 6 years. There is a rare acute fever lasting days or weeks. In an occasional patient there is a temporary remission.

Some reports of reversibility exist, but the diagnosis has only been by imaging studies.

TREATMENT

There is no known therapy.

SUGGESTED READINGS

Baron R, Heuser K, Marioth G. Marchiafava-Bignami disease with recovery diagnosed by CT and MRI: demyelination affects several CNS structures. *J Neurol* 1989;236:364–366.

Berek K, Wagner M, Chemelli AP, Aichner F, Benke T. Hemispheric disconnection in Marchiafava-Bignami disease: clinical, neuropsychological and MRI findings. *J Neurol Sci* 1994;123:2–5.

Chang KH, Cha SH, Han MH, et al. Marchiafava-Bignami disease: serial changes in corpus callosum on MRI. *Neuroradiology* 1992;34:480–482.

Gass A, Birtsch G, Olster M, Schwartz A, Hennerici MG. Marchiafava-Bignami disease: reversibility of neuroimaging abnormality. *J Comput Assist Tomogr* 1998;22:503–504.

Georgy BA, Hesselink JR, Jernigan TL. MR imaging of the corpus callosum. *AJR* 1993;160:949–955.

Ghatak N, Hadfield N, Rosenblum W. Association of central pontine myelinolysis and Marchiafava-Bignami disease. *Neurology* 1978;28:1295–1298.

Humbert T, De Guilhermier P, Maktouf C, Grasset G, Lopez FM, Chabrand P. Marchiafava-Bignami disease. A case studied by structural and functional brain imaging. *Eur Arch Psychiatry Clin Neurosci* 1992;242:69–71.

Ironside R, Bosanquet FD, McMenemey WH. Central demyelination of the corpus callosum (Marchiafava-Bignami disease). *Brain* 1961;84:212–230.

Marchiafava E, Bignami A. Sopra un'alterazione del corpo calloso osservata in soggetti alcoolisti. *Riv Patol Nerve* 1903;8:544–549.

Yamashita K, Kobayashi S, Yamaguchi S, Koide H, Nishi K. Reversible corpus callosum lesions in a patient with Marchiafava-Bignami disease: serial changes on MRI. *Eur Neurol* 1997;37:192–193.

Merritt's Neurology, 10th ed., edited by L.P. Rowland. Lippincott Williams & Wilkins, Philadelphia © 2000.

C H A P T E R
135

CENTRAL PONTINE MYELINOLYSIS

**GARY L. BERNARDINI
ELLIOTT L. MANCALL**

In 1959, Adams, Victor, and Mancall described a distinctive, previously unrecognized disease characterized primarily by the symmetric destruction of myelin sheaths in the basis pontis. They called it central pontine myelinolysis and numerous reports followed. The general term *myelinolysis* may be more appropriate because the condition affects extrapontine brain areas as well.

Most patients who develop pontine myelinolysis have had documented hyponatremia, and serum sodium levels were corrected rapidly to normal or supranormal levels. Chronic alcoholism and undernutrition are frequently associated with this condition. Pontine myelinolysis has been seen, however, in hyponatremic nonalcoholic patients, including some with dehydration resulting from vomiting, diarrhea, or diuretic therapy; with postoperative overhydration; or with compulsive water drinking. Severe malnutrition, including that resulting from extensive burn injuries, may be a predisposing condition. The main underlying factor to the development of pontine myelinolysis in these cases seems to be too rapid the correction of serum sodium levels. Correction after hypernatremia rather than hyponatremia has also been encountered. The condition has been described with increasing frequency in patients undergoing orthotopic liver transplantation. Pontine myelinolysis is found in 0.28% to 9.8% of these cases.

The clinical manifestations vary from asymptomatic to comatose, although there may be signs of a generalized encephalopathy associated with low levels of serum sodium. Neurologic signs and symptoms of myelinolysis usually appear within 2 to 3 days after rapid correction of sodium levels. Findings include dysarthria or mutism, behavioral abnormalities, ophthalmoparesis, bulbar and pseudobulbar palsy, hyperreflexia, quadriplegia, seizures, and coma. Typically, a rapidly progressive corticobulbar and corticospinal syndrome may be noted in a debilitated patient, often during an acute illness with associated electrolyte imbalance. Although the patients are mute, coma is unusual. The patients may be "locked-in"; communication by eye blinking can sometimes be established. The course is rapid, and death generally ensues within days or weeks of the onset of symptoms.

Extrapontine myelinolysis is seen in about 10% of all cases of pontine myelinolysis. Clinically, extrapontine myelinolysis can present with ataxia, irregular behavior, visual field deficits, or movement disorders such as Parkinson disease or parkinsonism, choreoathetosis, or dystonia. The movement disorders can appear with or without radiographic evidence of extrapontine myelinolysis. Bilateral symmetric involvement outside the pons may affect the cerebellum, putamen, thalamus, corpus callosum, subcortical white matter, claustrum, caudate, hypothalamus, lateral geniculate bodies, amygdala, subthalamic nuclei, substantia nigra, or medial lemnisci.

Although most cases have been diagnosed only at autopsy, the syndrome can be diagnosed in life. The clinical diagnosis is supported by radiologic studies. Computed tomography may be normal, especially early in the course, but computed tomography abnormalities include symmetric areas of hypodensity in the basis pontis and extrapontine regions without associated mass effect. Magnetic resonance imaging is more sensitive in diagnosing the condition; lesions appear hyperintense on T2-weighted images and hypointense on T1-weighted images but typically do not enhance (Fig. 135.1). The lesions may take 2 weeks to appear on magnetic resonance imaging. Brainstem auditory-evoked responses may demonstrate prolonged III-V and I-V latencies consistent with bilateral pontine lesions. An electroencephalogram may show slowing and low voltage. Cerebrospinal fluid levels of protein and myelin basic protein may be elevated.

The principal pathologic change is demyelination; within affected areas, nerve cells and axon sheaths are spared, blood vessels are unaffected, and there is no inflammation. In animal studies, the initial event after administration of hypertonic saline in hypotonic rats seems to be opening of the blood–brain barrier, followed sequentially by swelling of the inner loop of the myelin sheath, oligodendrocyte degeneration, and release of macrophage-derived factors leading to the eventual breakdown

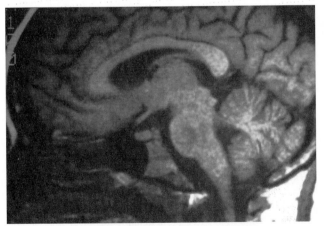

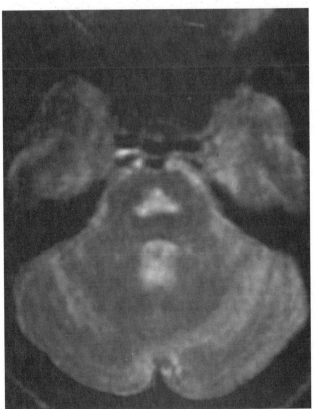

FIG. 135.1. A: T1-weighted sagittal magnetic resonance (MR) image in a 21-year-old alcoholic woman after rapid correction of severe hyponatremia, showing a hypointense area in the basis pons consistent with the lesion of pontine myelinolysis. **B:** T2-weighted axial MR image in the same patient demonstrating the characteristic centrally located hyperintense areas consistent with demyelination within the pons. (Courtesy of Dr. L. A. Heier.)

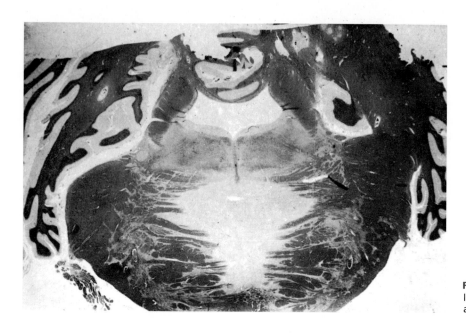

FIG. 135.2. Central pontine myelinolysis. Histologic section through rostral pons showing characteristic lesion. (Courtesy of Dr. J. Kepes.)

of myelin. Histologically, the lesion begins in the median raphe and may involve all or part of the base of the pons (Fig. 135.2). The lesion may spread into the pontine tegmentum or superiorly into the mesencephalon or involve bilateral extrapontine areas with or without concurrent basis pontis lesions. Microscopically, the lesions resemble those of Marchiafava-Bignami disease.

The cause of pontine myelinolysis is uncertain. In those with hyponatremia that has been rapidly corrected to normal or supranormal levels, it is not clear whether the low sodium, the rate of correction, or the absolute change in the serum sodium content is the causative factor. Symptoms are, however, more likely to develop with rapid correction of chronic (more than 48 hours) rather than acute hyponatremia. In experimental animals, pontine myelinolysis develops in hyponatremic rats, rabbits, or dogs treated rapidly with hypernatremic saline. Animals left with untreated hyponatremia did not develop neuropathologic changes. Therefore, attention has focused on the rate of correction of the hyponatremia rather than on the hyponatremia itself as the mechanism of injury.

Prevention of myelinolysis includes judicious correction of hyponatremia with normal saline and free water restriction, discontinuation of diuretic therapy, and correction of associated metabolic abnormalities and medical complications. Hyponatremic patients who are asymptomatic may not require saline infusion; those with agitated confusion, seizures, or coma should be treated with normal saline until the symptoms improve. Based on clinical data and animal studies, there is a low incidence of myelinolysis if the increase in serum sodium is less than or equal to 12 mmol/L in 24 hours. Late appearance of tremor and dystonia or cognitive and behavioral changes have been reported in survivors. Full recovery has also been seen.

SUGGESTED READINGS

Adams RD, Victor M, Mancall EL. Central pontine myelinolysis: a hitherto undescribed disease occurring in alcoholic and malnourished patients. *Arch Neurol Psychiatry* 1959;81:154–172.

Ayus JC, Krothpalli RK, Arieff AI. Treatment of symptomatic hyponatremia and its relation to brain damage. *N Engl J Med* 1987;317:1190–1195.

Brunner JE, Redmond JM, Haggar AM, et al. Central pontine myelinolysis and pontine lesions after rapid correction of hyponatremia: a prospective magnetic resonance imaging study. *Ann Neurol* 1990;27:61–66.

Donahue SP, Kardon RH, Thompson HS. Hourglass-shaped visual fields as a sign of bilateral lateral geniculate myelinolysis. *Am J Ophthalmol* 1995;119:378–380.

Hadfield MG, Kubal WS. Extrapontine myelinolysis of the basal ganglia without central pontine myelinolysis. *Clin Neuropathol* 1996;15:96–100.

Harris CP, Townsend JJ, Baringer JR. Symptomatic hyponatremia: can myelinolysis be prevented by treatment? *J Neurol Neurosurg Psychiatry* 1993;56:626–632.

Kandt RS, Heldrich FJ, Moser HW. Recovery from probable central pontine myelinolysis associated with Addison's disease. *Arch Neurol* 1983;40:118–119.

Kleinschmidt-Demasters BK, Norenberg MD. Rapid correction of hyponatremia causes demyelination: relation to central pontine myelinolysis. *Science* 1981;211:1068–1071.

Laureno R, Karp BI. Myelinolysis after correction of hyponatremia. *Ann Intern Med* 1997;126:57–62.

Morlan L, Rodriguez E, Gonzales J, et al. Central pontine myelinolysis following correction of hyponatremia: MRI diagnosis. *Eur Neurol* 1990;30:149–152.

Norenberg MD, Leslie KO, Robertson AS. Association between rise in serum sodium and central pontine myelinolysis. *Ann Neurol* 1982;11:128–135.

Rojiani AM, Cho ES, Sharer L, et al. Electrolyte-induced demyelination in rats. 2. Ultrastructural evolution. *Acta Neuropathol* 1994;88:293–299.

Salerno SM, Kurlan R, Joy SE, et al. Dystonia in central pontine myelinolysis without evidence of extrapontine myelinolysis. *J Neurol Neurosurg Psychiatry* 1993;56:1221–1223.

Schrier RW. Treatment of hyponatremia. *N Engl J Med* 1985;312:1121–1122.

Thompson DS, Hutton JT, Stears JC, et al. Computerized tomography in the diagnosis of central and extrapontine myelinolysis. *Arch Neurol* 1981;38:243–246.

Wright DG, Laureno R, Victor M. Pontine and extrapontine myelinolysis. *Brain* 1979;102:361–385.

Merritt's Neurology, 10th ed., edited by L.P. Rowland. Lippincott Williams & Wilkins, Philadelphia © 2000.

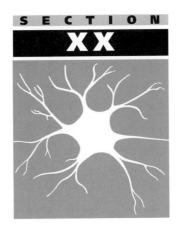

AUTONOMIC DISORDERS

CHAPTER 136

NEUROGENIC ORTHOSTATIC HYPOTENSION AND AUTONOMIC FAILURE

LOUIS H. WEIMER

MULTIPLE SYSTEM ATROPHY

In 1960, Shy and Drager described two patients with generalized autonomic failure and additional findings in other central and peripheral systems. This combination differed from the pure autonomic failure (PAF) described in 1925 by Bradbury and Eggleston. Currently, the Shy-Drager syndrome with initial or predominate autonomic failure is considered a manifestation of multiple system atrophy (MSA). Distinguishing this form of MSA from PAF or idiopathic Parkinson disease (PD) is still clinically challenging.

Clinical Manifestations

Autonomic failure is the hallmark of Shy-Drager syndrome, but demonstrable evidence of autonomic dysfunction is eventually found in 97% of patients clinically diagnosed with any form of MSA (see Chapter 114). Orthostatic hypotension (OH) or syncope is often the first recognized and most disabling symptom. However, other autonomic symptoms often predate OH, including impotence or ejaculatory dysfunction, decreased sweating, and urinary and less commonly fecal incontinence. Postprandial hypotension starting 10 to 15 minutes after a meal can be disabling. Parkinsonism is common with rigidity and bradykinesia more prominent than rest tremor but may be mild or not evident for several years after the onset of autonomic failure. Parkinsonian symptoms usually respond poorly to levodopa therapy, yet some have initial symptomatic relief. Levodopa therapy may also exacerbate or unmask underlying OH. Cerebellar and corticospinal tract signs provide evidence of multisystem involvement. Less commonly, fasciculations and amyotrophy are evident, as in one of the two original cases. Rarely, peripheral neuropathy or signs of a mild frontal lobe dementia are seen. Inspiratory stridor is a frequent feature with laryngeal muscle denervation. A variety of sleep disturbances and altered respiratory patterns are common and include apnea producing hypoxemia and paroxysmal sleep movements.

Laboratory Data

An autonomic screening battery (Table 136.1) in addition to bedside tests can aid in establishing the diagnosis, especially before the development of OH. Formal testing is also beneficial in MSA and in other cases of dysautonomia to characterize the individual autonomic problems, monitor progression, and assess

TABLE 136.1. TESTS OF AUTONOMIC FUNCTION

Well established
  Cardiovagal
    HR variability to cyclic deep breathing
    HR response to the Valsalva maneuver (Valsalva ratio)
    HR response to standing (30:15 ratio)
  Adrenergic
    BP response to the Valsalva maneuver (phases IV and late II)
    BP response to orthostatic stress
      Head-up tilt
      Standing
  Sudomotor
    Quantitative sudomotor axon reflex test (QSART)
    Thermoregulatory sweat test
    Silastic sweat imprint testing
    Sympathetic skin response
Additional or investigational methods
  Serum norepinephrine levels, supine and upright
  BP or HR response to alternate stressors
    Lower body negative pressure
    Sustained handgrip
    Mental arithmetic
    Diving reflex
    Cold pressor test
    Cough
  Spectral analysis of HR and BP signals
  Pharmacologic challenges
  Pupillary testing (pharmacologic, pupillometry, pupil cycle time)
  Urodynamics/sphincter EMG
  GI motility and manometry studies
  Salivary testing/Schirmer test
  Microneurography
  Vasomotor testing

HR, heart rate; BP, blood pressure; EMG, electromyogram; GI, gastrointestinal.

treatment effects. To enhance reliability, before testing patients should be free of autonomically active medications such as caffeine or nicotine, recovered from any acute illness, and in a relaxed euvolemic state.

The degenerative process in MSA has a special predilection for Onuf nucleus, spinal somatic motor neurons that serve voluntary urinary and anal sphincter function. Concentric needle electromyography of striated sphincters may show chronic partial denervation, an important diagnostic sign in all forms of MSA, not simply Shy-Drager syndrome. Paradoxically, these sphincter muscles are spared in amyotrophic lateral sclerosis. Formal sleep studies may document dangerous nocturnal apneic episodes or other alterations of sleep or respiratory patterns. MSA patients have normal or mildly reduced supine resting levels of norepinephrine that fail to show a normal increase on head-up tilt. PAF patients have low resting norepinephrine levels, which also fail to elevate with tilt.

Pathology

Demonstration of argyrophilic glial cytoplasmic inclusions in oligodendroglia (GCIs) has enhanced and refined the pathologic diagnosis of MSA over earlier assessments based on patterns of neuronal loss and gliosis. However, the inclusions are occasionally seen in other disorders. GCIs are prominent in vital sites of autonomic control such as the intermediolateral column of the spinal cord, dorsal vagal nucleus, solitary tract and nucleus, ponto-bulbar reticular formation, and medullary tegmentum. GCIs correlate better with clinical findings than do areas of neuronal loss.

Diagnosis

Classification of MSA cases remains inexact before autopsy. The main difficulty is separating cases with initial autonomic failure from the rare PAF cases and, more problematically, from idiopathic PD with autonomic features. Severe autonomic failure is rare in typical PD. However, autonomic symptoms and lesser degrees of autonomic dysfunction are relatively common. When more marked autonomic failure occurs in PD, it tends to be later in the disease and in elderly patients. Magalhães et al. (1995) retrospectively reviewed autonomic symptoms in 135 autopsy-proven cases of PD and MSA. One-third of the 33 MSA cases were misdiagnosed as PD before autopsy. Autonomic symptoms at onset, stridor, and cerebellar signs were rare in PD patients in this series. The degree of clonidine-induced growth hormone release has been proposed as an alternate test to separate MSA from PD.

Course and Prognosis

Prognosis studies have divided MSA into parkinsonian (striatonigral degeneration) and cerebellar (sporadic OPCA) forms, without separate data on patients with autonomic onset. In general, however, the prognosis is worse than for either PAF or PD with autonomic features or MSA without autonomic onset.

PURE AUTONOMIC FAILURE

Isolated PAF without involving other systems is rare but well described (idiopathic OH, Bradbury-Eggleston syndrome). Widespread autonomic failure is present with prominent and often disabling OH. However, approximately 10% develop into MSA within 3 to 5 years. In contrast to MSA and idiopathic chronic pandysautonomia, severe cholinergic impairment and gastrointestinal symptoms other than constipation are less apparent. Supine norepinephrine levels are reduced, and the response to norepinephrine infusion is excessive because of denervation supersensitivity. Histopathology is predominantly that of degeneration of postganglionic sympathetic neurons. Some loss of sympathetic neurons in the intermediolateral spinal cell column has been noted. Lewy bodies staining for ubiquitin may be seen in sympathetic ganglia.

Other Causes of Autonomic Failure

A multitude of peripheral neuropathies show some degree of impairment in autonomic function on formal testing, especially in distal vasomotor and sudomotor function. However, only some lead to frank clinically important autonomic failure with prominent OH. Particularly noteworthy causes include diabetes, amyloidosis, paraneoplastic, selected hereditary neuropathies, and dopamine β-hydoxylase deficiency (Table 136.2). Other disor-

ders that disrupt central or peripheral autonomic pathways may also lead to OH (Table 136.2) or less marked dysautonomia, especially lesions in the region of the third ventricle, posterior fossa, spinal cord, autonomic ganglia, and small diameter nerve fibers. In addition, processes may be pathway specific such as predominantly cholinergic, regional, or organ specific.

Treatment

Therapy of autonomic failure is aimed at symptomatic relief and improved quality of life. Treatment of OH, generally the most disabling symptom, depends on the underlying mechanism. Asymptomatic hypotension on standing usually does not require treatment. Cerebral perfusion typically does not drop signifi-

---

TABLE 136.2. SELECTED DISORDERS OF AUTONOMIC FUNCTION

Pure autonomic failure (PAF)
Multisystem disorders
  Multiple system atrophy (MSA)
    Shy-Drager syndrome
    Striatonigral degeneration (Chap. 114)
    Sporadic OPCA
  Parkinson's disease with autonomic failure
  Machado-Joseph disease
Central
  Brain tumors (posterior fossa, third ventricle, hypothalamus), syringobulbia, multiple sclerosis, tetanus, Wernicke-Korsakoff syndrome, fatal familial insomnia
Spinal cord
  Multiple scleroris, syringomyelia, transverse myelitis, transection/trauma, tumor
Peripheral
  Immune mediated
    Guillain-Barré syndrome (Chap. 105), acute and subacute pandysautonomia, acute cholinergic neuropathy, Sjögren disease, SLE, rheumatoid arthritis, Holmes-Adie syndrome
  Metabolic
    Diabetes, vitamin B_{12} and thiamine deficiency, uremia
  Paraneoplastic
    Paraneoplastic autonomic neuropathy, sensory neuronopathy with autonomic failure (ANNA antibodies), enteric neuropathy, Lambert-Eaton myasthenic syndrome (cholinergic)
  Infectious
    Chagas disease (cholinergic), tabes, leprosy, HIV, Lyme disease, diptheria
  Hereditary
    Familial amyloidosis, hereditary sensory and autonomic neuropathies (Chapter 104), dopamine β-hydroxylase deficiency, porphyria, Fabry disease
  Toxins
    Botulism, vincristine, cisplatin, taxol, amiodarone, vacor, hexacarbon, carbon disulfide, heavy metals, podophyllin, alcohol
  Drug and medication effects
Reduced orthostatic tolerance
  Neurocardiogenic syncope, POTS syndrome, mitral valve prolapse syndrome, prolonged bedrest or weightlessness
Other
  Acquired amyloidosis, chronic idiopathic autonomic neuropathies, small fiber neuropathy, idiopathic hyperhidrosis, idiopathic anhidrosis, Ross syndrome

---

OPCA, olivopontocerebellar atrophy; SLE, systemic lupus erythematosus; HN, human immunodeficiency virus; POTS, postural orthostatic tachycardia syndrome.

cantly until the systolic pressure is reduced below 80 mm Hg due to compensatory effects of cerebrovascular autoregulation. Simple maneuvers are tried initially and may be sufficient. Measures include maintaining the head and trunk at about 15 to 20 degrees higher than the legs in bed, which promotes the release of renin and stimulates baroreceptors. This can be achieved with a hospital bed with head elevation or by placing blocks under the head of an ordinary bed. Counterpressure support garments that provide abdominal and lower limb compression (such as Jobst half-body leotard) can reduce venous pooling, but patients often find these garments too uncomfortable and cumbersome to put on, especially if they are hampered by other neurologic impairment. Physical countermaneuvers such as squatting and leg crossing may provide some benefit. Particular care after situations that predictably lower blood pressure is prudent, including meals, vigorous exercise, hot temperature, and motionless standing.

No single drug is ideal for the treatment of neurogenic OH. Common useful therapies include supplemental sodium chloride (2 to 4 g/day) to increase plasma volume and, if necessary, fludrocortisone, starting at 0.1 mg/day to increase salt and water retention. The patient must be watched carefully to avoid excessive water retention, rising blood pressure, or heart failure. Oral sympathomimetics, such as ephedrine, phenylephrine, and tyramine, are usually of limited benefit; however, midodrine (a selective alpha-1 agonist now approved in the United States) is of proven benefit in OH. Anemia is a common exacerbating condition with autonomic failure. Epoetin alpha (Epogen) increases hematocrit, reduces symptoms, and elevates systolic pressure an average of 10 to 15 mm Hg. Other drugs of potential but less consistent benefit include indomethacin, somatostatin analogues, caffeine, ergot alkaloids, nocturnal desmopressin, and 3,4-dihydroxyphenylserine, which is specifically indicated in the rare but distinctive hereditary dopamine β-hydoxylase deficiency. Concomitant treatment of urinary dysfunction, gastric and intestinal dysmotility, impotence, and secretomotor dysfunction is often necessary. In MSA, inspiratory stridor may necessitate tracheostomy, and nocturnal positive pressure ventilation may be needed for sleep apnea.

SUGGESTED READINGS

Appenzeller O, Goss JE. Autonomic deficits in Parkinson's syndrome. *Arch Neurol* 1971;24:50–57.

Assessment: clinical autonomic testing report of the therapeutics and technology assessment subcommittee of the American Association of Neurology. *Neurology* 1996;46:873–880.

Biaggioni I, Robertson D, Frantz S, Krantz S, Jones M, Haile V. The anemia of primary autonomic failure and its reversal with recombinant erythropoietin. *Ann Intern Med* 1994;121:181–186.

Bradbury S, Eggleston C. Postural hypotension: a report of three cases. *Am Heart J* 1925;1:73–86.

Cohen J, Low P, Fealey R, Sheps S, Jiang N-S. Somatic and autonomic function in progressive autonomic failure and multiple system atrophy. *Ann Neurol* 1987;22:692–699.

Consensus statement on the definition of orthostatic hypotension, pure autonomic failure, and multiple system atrophy. *Neurology* 1996;46:1470.

Hague K, Lento P, Morgello S, Caro S, Kaufmann H. The distribution of Lewy bodies in pure autonomic failure: autopsy findings and review of the literature. *Acta Neuropathol (Berl)* 1997;94:192–196.

Jankovic J, Gilden JL, Hiner BC, et al. Neurogenic orthostatic hypotension: A double-blind, placebo-controlled study with Midodrine. *JAMA* 1993;95:38–48.

Kanda T, Tomimitsu H, Yokota T, Ohkoshi N, Hayashi M, Mizusawa H. Unmyelinated nerve fibers in sural nerve in pure autonomic failure. *Ann Neurol* 1998;43:267–271.

Kimber JR, Watson L, Mathias CJ. Distinction of idiopathic Parkinson's disease form multiple-system atrophy by stimulation of growth-hormone release with clonidine. *Lancet* 1997;349:1877–1881.

Kontos HA, Richardson DW, Norvell JE. Mechanisms of circulatory dysfunction in orthostatic hypotension. *Trans Am Clin Climatol Assoc* 1976;87:26–33.

Low PA, Bannister R. Multiple system atrophy and pure autonomic failure. In: Low PA, ed. *Clinical autonomic disorders*, 2nd ed. Philadelphia: Lippincott-Raven, 1997:555–575.

Magalhães M, Wenning GK, Daniel SE, Quinn NP. Autonomic dysfunction in pathologically confirmed multiple system atrophy and idiopathic Parkinson's disease—a retrospective comparison. *Acta Neurol Scand* 1995;91:98–102.

Mannen T, Iwata M, Toyokura Y, Nagashima K. The Onuf's nucleus and the external anal sphincter muscles in amyotrophic lateral sclerosis and Shy-Drager syndrome. *Acta Neuropathol* 1982;58:255–260.

Martignoni E, Pacchetti C, Godi L, Micieli G, Nappi G. Autonomic disorders in Parkinson's disease. *J Neurol Transm* 1995;45[Suppl]:11–19.

Mathias CJ. Desmopressin reduces nocturnal polyuria, reverses overnight weight loss and improves morning postural hypotension in autonomic failure. *Br Med J* 1986;293:353–354.

Mathias CJ. Orthostatic hypotension: causes, mechanisms, and influencing factors. *Neurology* 1995;45[Suppl 5]:S6–S11.

McLeod JD, Tuck RR. Disorders of the autonomic nervous system. Part I. Pathophysiology and clinical features. *Ann Neurol* 1987;21:419–430.

Papp MI, Kahn JE, Lantos PL. Glial cytoplasmic inclusion in the CNS of patients with multiple system atrophy (striatonigral degeneration, olivopontocerebellar atrophy and Shy-Drager syndrome). *J Neurol Sci* 1989;94:79–100.

Papp MI, Lantos PL. The distribution of oligodendroglial inclusions in multiple system atrophy and its relevance to clinical symptomatology. *Brain* 1994;117:235–243.

Ravits J, Hallett M, Nilsson J, Polinsky R, Dambrosia J. Electrophysiological tests of autonomic function in patients with idiopathic autonomic failure syndromes. *Muscle Nerve* 1996;19:758–763.

Robertson D, Davis RL. Recent advances in the treatment of orthostatic hypotension. *Neurology* 1995;45[Suppl 5]:S26–S32.

Sandroni P, Ahlskog JE, Fealey RD, Low PA. Autonomic involvement in extrapyramidal and cerebellar disorders. *Clin Auton Res* 1991;1:147–155.

Schatz IJ. Farewell to the "Shy-Drager" syndrome. *Ann Intern Med* 1996;125:74–75.

Shy GM, Drager GA. A neurological syndrome associated with orthostatic hypotension: a clinical-pathologic study. *Arch Neurol* 1960;2:511–527.

Sung JH, Mastri AR, Segal E. Pathology of Shy-Drager syndrome. *J Neuropathol Exp Neurol* 1979;38:353–368.

Thomas JE, Schirger A. Idiopathic orthostatic hypotension: a study of its natural history in 57 neurologically affected patients. *Arch Neurol* 1970;22:289–293.

Merritt's Neurology, 10th ed., edited by L.P. Rowland. Lippincott Williams & Wilkins, Philadelphia © 2000.

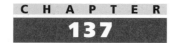

ACUTE AUTONOMIC NEUROPATHY

LOUIS H. WEIMER

Acute autonomic neuropathy (AAN) is rare, but there have been numerous reports since the initial description by Young et al. in 1975. Autonomic manifestations include orthostatic hypotension, nausea and vomiting, constipation or diarrhea, bladder atony, impotence, anhidrosis, impaired lacrimation and salivation, and pupillary abnormalities. Gastroparesis may be prominent. In pure dysautonomia, there is no somatic disturbance, but minor sensory findings are not uncommon, and in severe cases cutaneous sensation may be markedly impaired. Motor involvement is less common. Roughly one-fourth of cases have a purely cholinergic form, without orthostatic hypotension (OH), and rarely findings are restricted to gastrointestinal dysmotility. Although OH is the hallmark of the dysautonomia, exaggerated orthostatic tachycardia may be evident without change in blood pressure. This has led to the proposal that a syndrome of orthostatic intolerance without OH (postural orthostatic tachycardia syndrome) may be an attenuated form of AAN. This assertion is supported by abnormalities of sudomotor and other autonomic systems in roughly one-half of cases and an antecedent viral infection at the same percentage, as seen in AAN. Symptoms include postural dizziness, palpitations, and presyncope despite minimal changes in blood pressure. Possible etiologies are multiple, including distal loss of vasomotor control with excessive venous pooling, volume depletion, and altered cerebrovascular autoregulation.

In pure dysautonomia, electromyography, nerve conduction velocities, sural nerve biopsy, and cerebrospinal fluid are normal. In complicated cases, these studies may yield abnormalities blurring the distinction from Guillain-Barré syndrome. Additionally, autonomic involvement is common in typical Guillain-Barré syndrome and may be a prominent cause of morbidity and mortality. Functional tests in AAN usually reveal widespread abnormalities of autonomic function (Table 136.1).

The etiology of AAN is unknown, but many cases are presumed to be immune mediated and follow diverse viral infections. Sural nerve biopsies show epineural mononuclear cell infiltrates. Symptoms may evolve for several weeks, plateau for many weeks, and then slowly improve. The differential diagnosis includes other subacute neuropathies, such as paraneoplastic panautonomic neuropathy, Guillain-Barré syndrome, botulism, porphyria, and some drug or other toxic neuropathies. Treatment is symptomatic based on the involved systems. Control of OH is typically most important. Anecdotal reports suggest that intravenous immune globulin therapy may be effective. Recovery is slow and often incomplete.

SUGGESTED READINGS

Bennett JL, Mahalingam R, Wellish MC, et al. Epstein-Barr virus associated with acute autonomic neuropathy. *Ann Neurol* 1996;40:453–455.

Fagius J, Westerburg CE, Olsson Y. Acute pandysautonomia and severe sensory deficit with poor recovery. A clinical, neurophysiological and pathological case study. *J Neurol Neurosurg Psychiatry* 1983;46:725–733.

Hart RG, Kanter MC. Acute autonomic neuropathy: two cases and clinical review. *Arch Intern Med* 1990;150:2373–2376.

Heafield MTE, Gammage MD, Nightingale S, Williams AC. Idiopathic dysautonomia treated with intravenous gammaglobulin. *Lancet* 1996;347:28–29.

Laiwah ACY, MacPhee GJA, Boyle MR, Goldberg A. Autonomic neuropathy in acute intermittent porphyria. *J Neurol Neurosurg Psychiatry* 1985;48:1025–1030.

Low PA, Dyck PJ, Lambert EH, et al. Acute panautonomic neuropathy. *Ann Neurol* 1983;13:412–417.

McLeod JG, Tuck RR. Disorders of the autonomic nervous system. *Ann Neurol* 1987;21:419–430, 519–529.

Neville BG, Sladen OF. Acute autonomic neuropathy following primary herpes simplex infection. *J Neurol Neurosurg Psychiatry* 1984;47:648–650.

Schondorf R, Low PA. Idiopathic postural orthostatic tachycardia syndrome. An attenuated form of acute pandysautonomia? *Neurology* 1993;43:132–137.

Suarez GA, Fealey RD, Camilleri M, Low PA. Idiopathic autonomic neuropathy: clinical, neurophysiologic and follow-up studies on 27 patients. *Neurology* 1994;44:1675–1682.

Young RR, Asbury AK, Corbett JL, Adams RD. Pure pandysautonomia with recovery. *Brain* 1975;98:613–636.

Merritt's Neurology, 10th ed., edited by L.P. Rowland. Lippincott Williams & Wilkins, Philadelphia © 2000.

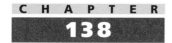

FAMILIAL DYSAUTONOMIA

ALAN M. ARON

OVERVIEW

Familial dysautonomia was described by Riley et al. in 1949. The autonomic symptoms are prominent, but the condition also affects other parts of the nervous system and general somatic growth. It is a rare autosomal recessive disease; more than 500 cases have been reported. Virtually all patients are of Eastern European (Ashkenazi) Jewish descent where the carrier rate is 1 in 30. The causative gene has been mapped to chromosome 9q31-q33. There results a sensory and autonomic neuropathy whose biochemical and genetic defects are yet to be defined. Linkage analyses using closely related markers have permitted reliable prenatal diagnosis in families with a previously affected child.

The condition can be diagnosed in the perinatal period. Clinical manifestations tend to increase with age. Biochemical alterations point to decreased synthesis of noradrenaline. Hypersensitivity to sympathomimetic drugs suggests a denervation type of supersensitivity. The exact pathophysiology has yet to be elucidated.

CLINICAL PRESENTATION

The dysautonomic infant frequently shows low birth weight and breech presentation. Neurologic abnormalities detected in the neonatal period include decreased muscle tone, diminished or absent deep tendon reflexes, absent corneal responses, poor Moro response, and weak cry and suck. The tongue tip lacks fungiform papillae and appears smooth. Uncoordinated swallowing with resultant regurgitation may cause aspiration and pneumonia. Some infants require tube feeding, gastrostomy, and fundoplication because of gastroesophageal reflux. Absence of overflow tears, which may be normal for the first 3 months, persists thereafter and becomes a consistent feature. Corneal ulceration can occur.

During the first 3 years of life, affected children show delayed physical and developmental milestones, episodic vomiting, excessive sweating, excessive drooling, blotchy erythema, and breath-holding spells. Dysautonomic crises occur after age 3, with irritability, self-mutilation, negativistic behavior, diaphoresis, tachycardia, hypertension, and thermal instability. The most outstanding symptom is episodic vomiting, which may be cyclic and require hospitalization for stabilization with parenteral hydration.

The school-aged dysautonomic child tends to have short stature, awkward gait, and nasal speech. School performance may be poor. As a group, patients score in the average range on intelligence tests but they are frequently 20 or more points below unaffected siblings. Scoliosis is frequent and can begin in childhood and progress rapidly during preadolescence. Some poorly developed patients show delayed puberty. Vomiting and vasomotor crises tend to decrease during adolescence when more frequent symptoms center on decreased exercise tolerance, poor general coordination, emotional difficulties, and postural hypotension. Vasovagal responses may occur after micturition or during laryngeal intubation for anesthesia. Up to one-third of patients have seizures during early life. These are usually associated with fever, breathholding spells, or hypoxia. Less than 10% of patients have subsequent long-standing seizure disorders.

Patients show abnormal responses to altered atmospheric air. Hypercapnia and hypoxia do not produce expected increases in ventilatory effort. Drownings have occurred, presumably because air hunger did not develop when submerged. Coma has occurred in patients at high altitudes.

DIAGNOSIS

The diagnosis should be made on the constellation of clinical symptoms and genetic background. The most distinctive sign is the absence or paucity of overflow tearing. Low doses of methacholine may restore transient tearing. Other cardinal clinical features include hyporeflexia, absent corneal responses, and the absence of the fungiform tongue papillae. This is associated with impaired taste sensation. There is relative indifference to pain, poor temperature control, and postural hypotension.

Intradermal histamine phosphate in a dosage of 1:1,000 (0.03 to 0.05 mL) normally produces pain and erythema. Within minutes, a central wheal forms and is surrounded by an axon flare that is a zone of erythema measuring 2 to 6 cm in diameter. The flare lasts for several minutes. In dysautonomic patients, pain is greatly reduced and there is no axon flare. In infants, a saline solution of 1:10,000 histamine should be used. The methacholine test involves installation of one drop of 2.5% methacholine into the eye. (One drop of dilute pilocarpine [0.0625%] is equivalent to 2.5% methacholine.) The other eye serves as control. The pupils are compared at 5-minute intervals for 20 minutes. The normal pupil remains unchanged; the dysautonomic pupil develops miosis. The pupillary responses to light and accommodation in familial dysautonomia appear normal.

The combination of axon flare response to intradermal histamine, miosis with methacholine or pilocarpine, and absent glossal fungiform pupillae are diagnostic. Frequently, there is an elevated urinary homovanillic acid–vanilylmandelic acid ratio. This assay is not required for diagnosis.

BIOCHEMICAL AND PATHOLOGIC DATA

The neuronal abnormality is probably present at birth, but subsequent degenerative changes seem to occur. The primary metabolic defect is unknown. Fibroblast study has shown normal mitochondrial DNA and respiratory chain activity. Mitochondrial dysfunctions due to glycosphingolipid accumulation, changes in mitochondrial DNA, or mutation of chromosome 9 genetic material in mitochrondial factions have not been demonstrated.

Serum levels of both norepinephrine and dopamine are markedly elevated during dysautonomic crises. Vomiting coincides with high dopamine levels; hypertension correlates with increased norepinephrine levels. Pathologic data reveal hypoplastic cervical sympathetic ganglia with diminished volume and neuronal counts. Sympathetic preganglionic spinal cord neurons seem to be reduced in number. Patients are deficient in type C fibers. The parasympathetic sphenopalatine ganglia have shown the most depleted neuronal populations with only minimal reductions in the ciliary ganglia. The lingual submucosal neurons and sensory axons are reduced. Tastebuds are scant; circumvallate papillae are hypoplastic.

PATHOPHYSIOLOGY

Gastroesophageal dysfunction, manifest by prolonged esophageal transit time, gastroesophageal reflux, and delayed gastric emptying, has been demonstrated by scintigraphic analysis, cine radiography, PH monitoring, and endoscopy. There is severe oropharyngeal incoordination.

Cardiovascular instability is a prominent manifestation. Prolonged QT intervals greater than 440 mse without shortening during exercise demonstrate a defect in autonomic regulation of cardiac conduction. Renal insufficiency, common in adult patients, can be assessed by noninvasive Doppler techniques to detect changes in renal blood flow.

Sympathetic denervation may increase the responsiveness to

regulators of cardiovascular integrity such as atrial natriuretic peptide. Medication can also influence circulating atrial natriuretic peptide and cathecol amines.

Excessive drooling and swallowing difficulties are common and can be attributable to salivary gland denervation hypersensitivity. Hypersalivation may account for the low caries rate and increased plaque formation.

Postural hypotension can be explained by peripheral sympathetic denervation. Skin blotching and hypertension are attributed to denervation supersensitivity at the sympathetic effector sites. Lack of overflow tears correlates with the diminution of neurons in the sphenopalatine ganglia. Other symptoms can be explained as manifestations of a diffuse sensory deficit and autonomic insufficiency with hypersensitivity to acetylcholine and possibly to catecholamines. In addition, there may be decreased or dysfunctional adrenoceptors and decreased denervation.

PROGNOSIS

Long-term survival has been documented. Surviving patients include women whose pregnancies terminated in the birth of normal infants. Infant and childhood fatalities may be due to aspiration pneumonia, gastric hemorrhage, or dehydration. A second cluster of fatalities between the ages of 14 and 24 showed pulmonary complications, sleep deaths, and cardiopulmonary arrests. The oldest patients are now in their fifth decade.

TREATMENT

Laparoscopic surgery for performing a modified Nissen fundoplication and gastrostomy has modified gastroesophageal reflux and the resultant pulmonary complications associated with aspiration. The use of epidural anesthesia has been advocated for surgical procedures such as Nissen fundoplication and cesarean section. This is to avoid intubation and the sometimes fatal complications of general anesthesia. Midodrine, a peripheral α-adrenergic agonist, may be useful in the management of orthostatic hypotension in a dose of 0.25 mg/kg/day. Symptomatic treatment is indicated for dysautonomic crises with parenteral fluids, diazepam, sedation, and antiemetic therapy.

SUGGESTED READINGS

Alvarez E, Ferrer T, Perez-Conde C, et al. Evaluation of congenital dysautonomia other than Riley-Day syndrome. *Neuropediatrics* 1996;27:26–31.

Axelrod FB. Familial dysautonomia: a 47-year perspective. How technology confirms clinical acumen. *J Pediatr* 1998;132[3 Pt 2]:S2–S5.

Axelrod FB, Goldstein DS, Holmes C, et al. Genotype and phenotype in familial dysautonomia. *Adv Pharmacol* 1998;42:925–928.

Axelrod FB, Krey L, Glickstein JS, et al. Atrial natriuretic peptide response to postural change and medication in familial dysautonomia. *Clin Auton Res* 1994;4:311–318.

Axelrod FB, Porges RF, Seir ME. Neonatal recognition of familial dysautonomia. *J Pediatr* 1987;110:969–948.

Blumenfeld A, Slaugenhaupt SA, Axelrod FB. Localization of the gene for familial dysautonomia on chromosome 9 and definition of DNA markers for genetic diagnosis. *Nat Genet* 1993;4:160–164.

Eng-CM, Slaugenhaupt SA, Blumenfeld A, et al. Prenatal diagnosis of familial dysautonomia by analysis of linked CA-repeat polymorphisms on chromosome 9q31-q33. *Am J Med Genet* 1995;59:349–355.

Glickstein JS, Schwartzman D, Friedman D, et al. Abnormalities of the corrected QT interval in familial dysautonomia: an indicator of autonomic dysfunction. *J Pediatr* 1993;122:925–928.

Korczyn AD, Rubenstein AE, Yahr MD, Axelrod FB. The pupil in familial dysautonomia. *Neurology* 1981;31:628–629.

Pearson J, Pytel B. Quantitative studies of sympathetic ganglia and spinal cord intermediolateral gray columns in familial dysautonomia. *J Neurol Sci* 1978;39:47–59.

Pearson J, Pytel B. Quantitative studies of ciliary and sphenopalatine ganglia in familial dysautonomia. *J Neurol Sci* 1978;39:123–130.

Riley CM, Day RL, Greely DM, Langford NS. Central autonomic dysfunction with defective lacrimation. I. Report of five cases. *Pediatrics* 1949;3:468–478.

Smith AA, Dancis J. Responses to intradermal histamine in familial dysautonomia—a diagnostic test. *J Pediatr* 1963;63:889–894.

Strasberg P, Bridge P, Merante F, Yeger H, Pereira J. Normal mitochondrial DNA and respiratory chain activity in familial dysautonomia fibroblasts. *Biochem Mol Med* 1996;59:20–27.

Szald A, Udassin R, Maayan C, et al. Laparoscopic modified Nissen fundoplication in children with familial dysautonomia. *J Pediatr Surg* 1996;31:1560–1562.

Udassin R, Seror D, Vinograd I, et al. Nissen fundoplication in the treatment of children with familial dysautonomia. *Am J Surg* 1992;164:332–336.

Weiser M, Helz MJ, Bronfin L, Axelrod FB. Assessing microcirculation in familial dysautonomia by laser Doppler flowmeter. *Clin Auton Res* 1998;8:13–23.

Merritt's Neurology, 10th ed., edited by L.P. Rowland. Lippincott Williams & Wilkins, Philadelphia © 2000.

SECTION

XXI

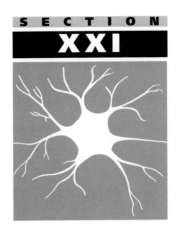

PAROXYSMAL DISORDERS

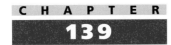

MIGRAINE AND OTHER HEADACHES

NEIL H. RASKIN

When headache is chronic, recurrent, and unattended by signs of disease, the physician confronts a challenging but ultimately gratifying problem. Previously, head pain was thought to originate from either contracted scalp and neck muscles or vascular dilatation. Neither of these mechanisms achieved scientific support; central mechanisms of head pain are of current interest. In migraine, the neurologic symptoms are attributed to neuronal dysfunction similar to that of spreading depression; a phase of vasoconstriction and vasodilatation also undoubtedly occurs, as does a final phase that results in the secretion of vasoactive peptides. Most recurring headaches are probably caused by impaired central inhibitory mechanisms at varying loci within the brain.

MIGRAINE

The term *migraine* derives from Galen's usage of *hemicrania* to describe a periodic disorder that comprises paroxysmal and blinding hemicranial pain, vomiting, photophobia, recurrence at regular intervals, and relief by darkness and sleep. Hemicrania was later corrupted into low Latin as *hemigranea* and *migranea*; eventually the French translation, migraine, gained acceptance in the 18th century and has prevailed ever since. This designation is misleading, however, because head pain is lateralized in less than 60% of those affected. Furthermore, undue emphasis on the dramatic features of migraine has often led to the illogical conclusion that a periodic headache lacking such characteristics is not migrainous in mechanism. Severe headache attacks, regardless of causation, are more likely to be throbbing and associated with vomiting and scalp tenderness. Milder headaches tend to be nondescript—tight bandlike discomfort often involving the entire head, the profile of "tension headache." These differing clinical patterns of headaches that are not caused by an intracranial structural anomaly or systemic disease are probably different points on a continuum rather than disparate clinical entities. Whether a common mechanism underlies the different headaches remains to be determined.

A working descriptive definition follows. Migraine is a benign recurring headache, recurring neurologic dysfunction, or both; it is usually attended by pain-free interludes and is almost always provoked by stereotyped stimuli. It is far more common in women; those affected have a hereditary predisposition toward attacks; and the cranial circulatory phenomena that attend attacks seem to be due to a primary brainstem disorder.

Clinical Subtypes

The designation *classic migraine* (migraine with aura) denotes the syndrome of headache associated with characteristic premonitory sensory, motor, or visual symptoms; *common migraine* (migraine without aura) denotes the syndrome in which no focal neurologic symptoms precede the headache. Focal symptoms, however, occur in only a small proportion of attacks and are more common during headache attacks than as prodromal symptoms. Focal neurologic symptoms without headache or vomiting are called *migraine equivalents or accompaniments* and seem to be more common in patients between the ages of 40 and 70 years. The term *complicated migraine* is generally used to describe migraine with dramatic focal neurologic features, thus overlapping with classic migraine; it has also been used to connote a persisting neurologic disorder after a migraine attack.

Common Migraine

Benign periodic headache lasting several hours and often attributed to tension by its sufferers is the most liberal way of describing common migraine. The fallacy intrinsic to most of the traditionally acceptable definitions is that they define severe attacks but do not include patients with more modest degrees of head pain; thus, unilateral pain, attendant nausea or vomiting, positive family history, responsiveness to ergotamine, and scalp tenderness in varying combinations have been alleged to establish a diagnosis of migraine. Each of these occurs in 60% to 80% of patients as dependent variables, however, and the validity of using these clinical features to diagnose migraine has never been established. Common migraine is the most frequent type of headache and includes the now anachronistic concept of periodic "tension headache."

Classic Migraine

The most common premonitory symptoms are visual, arising from dysfunction of occipital lobe neurons. Scotomas or hallucinations occur in about one-third of migraineurs and usually appear in the central portion of the visual fields. A highly characteristic syndrome occurs in about 10% of patients; it usually begins as a small paracentral scotoma that slowly expands into a C shape. Luminous angles appear at the enlarging outer edge and become colored as the scintillating scotoma expands and moves toward the periphery of the involved half of the visual field. It eventually disappears over the horizon of peripheral vision; the entire process consumes 20 to 25 minutes. This phenomenon never occurs during the headache phase of an attack and is pathognomonic of migraine; it has never been described with a cerebral structural anomaly. It is commonly called a "fortification spectrum" because the serrated edges of the hallucinated C seemed to Dr. Hubert Airy to resemble a "fortified town with bastions all round it"; "spectrum" is used in the sense of an apparition or specter.

Basilar Migraine

Symptoms implying altered brainstem function include vertigo, dysarthria, and diplopia; they occur as the only neurologic symptoms of migraine in about 25% of patients. Bickerstaff called attention to a stereotyped sequence of dramatic neurologic events, often comprising total blindness and sensorial clouding; this is most commonly seen in adolescent women but also occurs in others. The episodes begin with total blindness accompanied or followed by admixtures of vertigo, ataxia, dysarthria, tinnitus, and distal and perioral paresthesia. In about 25% of patients, a confusional state supervenes. The symptoms usually persist for about 30 minutes and are usually followed by a throbbing occipital headache. The basilar migraine syndrome also occurs in children or adults over age 50. Sensorial alterations, including confusional states that may be mistaken for psychotic reactions, may last as long as 5 days.

Carotidynia

The carotidynia syndrome, sometimes called "lower-half headache" or "facial migraine," is more prominent among older patients, with peak incidence at ages 30 to 69. Pain is usually located at the jaw or neck and is sometimes periorbital or maxillary. It is often continuous, deep, dull, and aching and becomes pounding or throbbing episodically. Sharp ice pick–like jabs are commonly superimposed. Attacks occur one to several times a week, each lasting minutes to hours. Tenderness and prominent pulsations of the cervical carotid artery and swelling of soft tissues over the carotid are usually present homolateral to the pain; many patients report throbbing ipsilateral headache concurrent with carotidynia and interictally. Dental trauma is a common precipitant of this syndrome. Carotid artery involvement in the more traditional forms of migraine is also common; more than 50% of patients with frequent migraine attacks show carotid tenderness at several points homolateral to the cranial side involved in most of their attacks.

Hemiplegic Migraine

Hemiparesis occasionally occurs during the prodromal phase of migraine; like the fortification spectrum, it often resolves in 20 to 30 minutes, and contralateral head pain then commences. The affected side may vary from attack to attack. A more profound form appears as hemiplegia, often affecting the same side, that persists for days to weeks after headache subsides. A clear autosomal dominant pattern of attacks may appear within a family. The gene for familial hemiplegic migraine maps to chromosome 19 in half the families; a mutation in a P/Q-type calcium channel (1-subunit gene has been identified. Dysarthria and aphasia occur in more than 50% of patients; hemihypesthesia attends hemiparesis in nearly every case. There may be cerebrospinal fluid (CSF) pleocytosis as high as 350 cells/mm^3 or transient CSF protein elevations to 200 mg/dL.

Ophthalmoplegic Migraine

Rarely, patients report infrequent attacks of periorbital pain accompanied by vomiting for 1 to 4 days. As the pain subsides, ipsilateral ptosis appears, and within hours, a complete third nerve palsy occurs, often including pupillary dilatation. The ophthalmoplegia may persist for several days to as long as 2 months. Af-

ter many attacks, some ophthalmoparesis may remain. This syndrome usually begins in childhood, whereas the Tolosa Hunt syndrome, another painful ophthalmoplegia, is a condition of adults.

Pathogenesis

Modern orientations toward migraine began with Liveing's 1873 publication, *A Contribution to the Pathology of Nerve Storms*, the first major treatise devoted to the subject of migraine. He believed that the analogy of migraine to epilepsy was obvious and that the clinically apparent circulatory phenomena of migrainous attacks were caused by cerebral discharges or nerve storms. In the 1930s, attention was focused on the vascular features of migraine by Graham and Wolff, who found that the administration of ergotamine reduced the amplitude of temporal artery pulsations in patients and that this effect was often, but not consistently, associated with a decrease in head pain. Therefore, many authorities believed for many years that the headache phase of migrainous attacks was caused by extracranial vasodilatation and that neurologic symptoms were produced by intracranial vasoconstriction, the "vascular" hypothesis of migraine. A barrage of publications by Wolff and coworkers supported the hypothesis, and observations made during the 1940s nonresonant with their hypothesis were ignored.

In 1941, K. S. Lashley, a neuropsychologist, was among the first to chart his own migrainous fortification spectrum. He estimated that the evolution of his own scotoma proceeded across the occipital cortex at a rate of 3 mm/min. He speculated that a wave front of intense excitation was followed by a wave of complete inhibition of activity across the visual cortex. Uncannily, in 1944, the phenomenon of "spreading depression" was described in the cerebral cortex of laboratory animals by the Brazilian physiologist Leão. A slowly moving (2 to 3 mm/min) potassium-liberating depression of cortical activity is preceded by a wave front of increased metabolic activity. Spreading depression can be produced by a variety of experimental stimuli, including hypoxia, mechanical trauma, and the topical application of potassium.

These observations, striking in retrospect, could not be incorporated into the vascular model of migraine. Cerebral blood flow studies, however, have rendered untenable a primary vascular mechanism and support the possibility that spreading depression, or more likely a neuronal phenomenon with similar characteristics, is important in the pathogenesis of migraine.

The mechanism of migraine can be partitioned into three phases. The first is brainstem generation; the second may be considered "vasomotor activation" in which arteries within and outside the brain may contract or dilate. In the third phase, cells of the trigeminal nucleus caudalis become active and release vasoactive neuropeptides at terminations of the trigeminal nerve on blood vessels, possibly explaining the soft tissue swelling and tenderness of blood vessels during migraine attacks. Activation of any of the three phases is *sufficient* for headache production; one phase may dominate in an individual's migrainous syndrome. For example, the fortification spectrum is probably entirely neurogenic, requiring only the first phase.

During attacks of classic migraine, studies of regional cerebral blood flow have shown a modest cortical hypoperfusion that begins in visual cortex and spreads forward at a rate of 2 to 3 mm/min. The decrease in blood flow averages 25% to 30% (too little to explain symptoms) and progresses anteriorly in a wave-like fashion that is independent of the topography of cerebral arteries. The wave of hypoperfusion persists for 4 to 6 hours, follows the convolutions of the cortex, and does not cross the central or lateral sulcus but progresses to the frontal lobe via the insula. Subcortical perfusion is normal. Contralateral neurologic symptoms appear during the period of temporoparietal hypoperfusion; at times, hypoperfusion persists in these regions after symptoms cease. More often, frontal spread continues as the headache phase begins. A few patients with classic migraine show no abnormalities of blood flow; rarely, focal ischemia is sufficient to cause symptoms. Focal ischemia, however, does not appear necessary for focal symptoms to occur. In attacks of common migraine, no abnormalities of blood flow have been seen. The changes in cerebral blood flow are attributed to alterations of cerebral neuronal function. The cortical events require a "generator," which has been identified within the brainstem.

Pharmacologic data converge on serotonin receptors. About 35 years ago, methysergide was found to antagonize peripheral actions of serotonin (5-hydroxytryptamine) and was introduced as the first drug capable of preventing migraine attacks by stabilizing the basic fault. Platelet levels of serotonin fall at the onset of headache, and migrainous episodes can be triggered by drugs that release serotonin. These changes in circulating levels proved to be pharmacologically trivial, however, and interest in the role of serotonin declined, only to be revived by the introduction of sumatriptan, which is remarkably effective for migraine attacks. Sumatriptan is a designer drug synthesized to activate selectively a particular subpopulation of serotonin receptors.

The main families of serotonin receptors are types 1, 2, 3, and 4; within each family are receptor subtypes. Sumatriptan interacts as an agonist with 1A receptors and especially with 1D and 1B receptors. By contrast, dihydroergotamine, another drug effective in aborting migraine attacks, is most potent as an agonist of 1A receptors but is an order of magnitude less potent at 1D and 1B receptors. After systemic administration, dihydroergotamine in the brain is found in highest concentrations in the midbrain dorsal raphe. The dorsal raphe contains the highest concentration of serotonin receptors in the brain and could be the generator of migraine and the main site of drug action. Raphe receptors are mainly of 1A, but 1D receptors are also present.

Electrical stimulation near dorsal raphe neurons can result in migrainelike headaches. Projections from the dorsal raphe terminate on cerebral arteries and alter cerebral blood flow. The dorsal raphe also projects to visual processing neurons in the lateral geniculate body, superior colliculus, retina, and visual cortex. These projections could provide the anatomic and physiologic bases for the circulatory and visual characteristics of migraine. The dorsal raphe cells stop firing during deep sleep, and sleep ameliorates migraine; antimigraine drugs also stop the firing of the dorsal raphe cells through a direct or indirect agonist effect (Fig. 139.1). The shutdown of an inhibitory system may enhance or stabilize neurotransmission.

Migraine may therefore be considered a hereditary perturbation of central inhibitory mechanisms. Similar perturbations

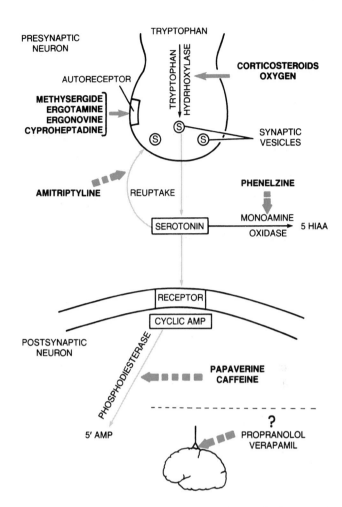

FIG. 139.1. The actions of the antimigraine drugs at brainstem and forebrain synapses. The *solid arrows* indicate agonist properties; the *segmented arrows* indicate inhibitory properties. (From Raskin NH. *Headache*, 2nd ed. New York: Churchill Livingstone, 1988.)

may underlie many types of head pain; "ordinary" periodic headaches may be the "noise" of the normally functioning system.

Treatment

Nonpharmacologic treatments have been advocated, but rigorously controlled trials have shown no benefit without concomitant drug treatment. The mainstay of therapy is the judicious use of one or more of the many drugs that are relatively specific for migraine.

Acute Treatment

In general, an adequate dose of whichever agent is chosen should be used at the onset of an attack. If additional medication is requested in 30 to 60 minutes because symptoms have returned or have not abated, the initial dosage should be increased for subsequent attacks. Drug absorption is impaired during attacks because of reduced gastrointestinal motility. Absorption may be delayed in the absence of nausea, and the delay is related to the severity of the attack but not to the duration. Therefore, when oral agents fail, the major considerations revolve about rectal administration of ergotamine, subcutaneous sumatriptan, parenteral dihydroergotamine, and intravenous chlorpromazine or prochlorperazine.

For patients with a prolonged buildup of headache, oral agents may suffice. When aspirin and acetaminophen fail, the addition of butalbital and caffeine to these analgesics is highly effective; ibuprofen (600 to 800 mg) and naproxen (375 to 750 mg) are often useful. One or two capsules of isometheptene compound are effective for mild to moderate "stress headaches." When these measures fail, more aggressive therapy is considered.

A subnauseating dose of ergotamine, if possible, should be determined for the individual patient; a dose that provokes nausea—probably a centrally mediated effect—is too high for therapy and may intensify head pain. The average oral dose of ergotamine is 3 mg (three 1-mg ergotamine-caffeine tablets); the average dose of the 2-mg suppository is one-half (1 mg). Many patients use one-fourth of a suppository (0.5 mg) with an optimal result. Sumatriptan may be given as an oral 50-mg dose, a 20-mg intranasal dose, or a 6-mg subcutaneous dose; the recurrence rate is high because of the short half-life of this drug (2 hours), and a second dose may be necessary. Rizatriptan and zolmitriptan have similar success rates, and peak blood levels are achieved more quickly. Naratriptan has the best side-effect profile of this group of drugs and the lowest recurrence rate; it is less effective than the other "triptans."

Dihydroergotamine is available as a parenteral preparation and as a nasal spray. Peak plasma levels of dihydroergotamine are achieved 45 to 60 minutes after nasal administration, 45 minutes after subcutaneous administration, 30 minutes after intramuscular administration, and 3 minutes after intravenous administration. If an attack has not already peaked, subcutaneous or intramuscular administration of 1 mg suffices for about 90% of patients. A common intravenous protocol is the mixture of prochlorperazine 5 mg and dihydroergotamine 0.5 mg given over 2 minutes (they are miscible).

When a patient's headache profile transforms into a chronic daily headache syndrome, opiate-type analgesics should be restricted to 2 days out of 7. The mainstay of therapy for these patients is daily amitriptyline (30 to 100 mg) or nortriptyline (40 to 120 mg). For recalcitrant individuals, valproate (500 to 2,000 mg) or phenelzine (45 to 90 mg) may be necessary. Drugs that

have antidepressant effects act independent of such effects in migraine.

Prophylaxis

Several drugs can stabilize migraine and prevent attacks; for this purpose, the drugs must be taken daily (Table 139.1). When to implement this approach depends on the frequency of attacks and how effective the acute treatment is. At least two or three attacks a month could signal this approach. Usually a lag of about 2 weeks must pass before an effect is seen; this may be the time needed to downregulate serotonin receptors. The major drugs and their daily dose are propranolol (60 to 240 mg), amitriptyline (30 to 100 mg), valproate (500 to 2,000 mg), verapamil (120 to 480 mg), phenelzine (45 to 90 mg), and methysergide (4 to 12 mg).

Phenelzine and methysergide are usually reserved for more recalcitrant headaches because of serious adverse effects. Because phenelzine is a monoamine oxidase inhibitor, concomitant use of tyramine-containing foods, decongestants, or meperidine is contraindicated. Methysergide may cause retroperitoneal or cardiac valvular fibrosis when it is used for more than 8 months; thus, monitoring is requisite for patients using this drug. Imaging of the pelvis and abdomen and cardiac auscultation should be carried out at least yearly. The risk of the fibrotic complications is about 1 in 1,500 and is likely to reverse after the drug is stopped.

The probability of success with any one of the antimigraine drugs is about 60% to 75%. If one drug is assessed each month, the likelihood is high that stabilization will be achieved within a few months. Most patients are managed successfully with propranolol or amitriptyline; for more urgent resolution, valproate, methysergide, or phenelzine can be implemented. Once effective, the drug is continued for about 6 months, and the dose is then tapered slowly to assess continued need. Many patients can discontinue medication and experience fewer and less severe attacks for a long time, thus suggesting that the drugs may alter the natural history of migraine.

CLUSTER HEADACHE

Recognition of this disorder has been retarded by confusing names, including *Raeder syndrome, histamine cephalalgia,* and *sphenopalatine neuralgia.* Cluster headache is firmly established

TABLE 139.1. DRUG STABILIZATION OF MIGRAINE

Drug	Tablet size (mg)	Daily dose range (mg)	Most common side effects
Propranolol	10, 20, 40, 60, 80, 90; sustained release: 60, 80, 120, 160	40–320	Fatigue, insomia, light-headedness, impotence
Amitriptyline	10, 25, 50, 75, 100	10–175	Sedation, dry mouth, appetite stimulation
Ergonovine	0.2	0.4–2.0	Nausea, abdominal pain, leg tiredness, diarrhea
Verapamil	40, 80, 120; sustained release: 120, 180, 240	160–480 320–960	Constipation, nausea, fluid retention, light-headedness, hypotension
Valproate	125, 250, 500	375–2,500	Nausea, tremor, alopecia, appetite stimulation
Phenelzine	15	30–90	Sedation, orthostatic hypotension, constipation, urinary retention
Methysergide	2	2–12	Nausea, abdominal pain, insomnia, appetite stimulation, fluid retention, limb claudication

as a distinct syndrome that is likely to respond to treatment. The episodic type, the most common, is characterized by one to three short-lived attacks of periorbital pain each day for 4 to 8 weeks, followed by a pain-free interval for a mean of 1 year. The chronic form may begin *de novo* or may appear several years after an episodic pattern has been established. The attacks are similar, but there are no sustained periods of remission. Either type may transform into the other.

Men are affected more often than women in a proportion of about 8:1. Hereditary factors are usually absent. The prevalence is 69 cases per 100,000 people. Although most patients begin experiencing headache between the ages of 20 and 50 years, the syndrome may begin as early as the first decade and as late as the eighth decade. The cluster syndrome differs from migraine genetically, biochemically, and clinically. Propranolol and amitriptyline are largely ineffective in cluster headache. However, lithium is beneficial for the cluster syndrome and ineffective in migraine. Nevertheless, the two disorders may blend into one in occasional patients, suggesting that the mechanisms include some features in common.

Clinical Features

Periorbital or, less commonly, temporal pain begins without warning and reaches a crescendo within 5 minutes. It is often excruciating in intensity and is deep, nonfluctuating, and explosive in quality; only rarely is it pulsatile. Pain is strictly unilateral and usually affects the same side in subsequent months. Attacks last from 30 minutes to 2 hours; the associated symptoms of homolateral lacrimation, reddening of the eye, nasal stuffiness, lid ptosis, and nausea often appear. Alcohol provokes attacks in about 70% of patients but has no effect when the bout remits; this on–off vulnerability to alcohol is pathognomonic of cluster headache. Only rarely do foods or emotional factors activate the mechanism, in contradistinction to migraine.

Periodicity of attacks is evident in at least 85% of patients. At least one of the daily attacks of pain recurs at about the same hour each day for the duration of a bout. This clock mechanism is set for nocturnal hours in about 50% of patients; in these circumstances, the pain usually wakens patients within 2 hours of falling asleep.

Pathogenesis

No consistent changes in cerebral blood flow attend attacks of pain. Perhaps the strongest evidence pointing to a central mechanism is the "periodicity"; reinforcing this conclusion are the bilateral autonomic symptoms that accompany the pain and are more severe on the painful side. The hypothalamus may be the site of activation. The posterior hypothalamus contains cells that regulate autonomic functions, and the anterior hypothalamus contains cells (the suprachiasmatic nuclei) that serve as the principal circadian pacemaker in mammals. Activation of both is necessary to explain the symptoms of cluster headache. The pacemaker is modulated serotonergically through projections of the dorsal raphe. Therefore, both migraine and cluster headache may result from abnormal serotonergic neurotransmission, albeit at different loci.

Treatment

The most satisfactory treatment is the administration of drugs to prevent cluster attacks until the bout is over. The major prophylactic drugs are prednisone, lithium, methysergide, ergotamine, and verapamil. Lithium (600 to 900 mg daily) appears to be particularly effective for the chronic form. A 10-day course of prednisone, beginning at 60 mg daily for 7 days and rapidly tapering, seems to curtail the bout for many patients. Ergotamine is most effective when given 1 or 2 hours before an expected attack; for patients with a single nocturnal episode, 1 mg ergotamine in suppository formulation taken at bedtime may be all that is necessary. Patients must be educated regarding the early symptoms of ergotism (limb claudication) when ergotamine is used daily; a weekly limit of 14 mg should be followed.

For the attacks themselves, oxygen inhalation (9 L/min given with a loose mask) is effective; 15 minutes of inhalation of 100% oxygen is often necessary. The self-administration of intranasal lidocaine, either 4% topical or 2% viscous, to the most caudal aspect of the inferior nasal turbinate can deliver a sphenopalatine ganglion block that is often remarkably effective for the termination of an attack. Sumatriptan, 6 mg subcutaneously, usually shortens an attack to 10 to 15 minutes.

COUGH HEADACHE

A male-dominated (4:1) syndrome, cough headache is characterized by transient severe head pain upon coughing, bending, lifting, sneezing, or stooping. Head pain persists for seconds to a few minutes. Many patients date the origin of the syndrome to a lower respiratory infection accompanied by severe coughing or to strenuous weight-lifting programs. Headache is usually diffuse but is lateralized in about one-third of patients. The incidence of serious intracranial structural anomalies causing this condition is about 25%; the Arnold-Chiari malformation is a common cause. Magnetic resonance imaging is indicated for these patients. The benign disorder may persist for a few years; it is inexplicably and remarkably ameliorated by indomethacin at doses of 50 to 200 mg daily. A large-volume (40 mL) lumbar puncture dramatically terminates the syndrome for 50% of patients so treated.

Many patients with migraine note that attacks of headache may be provoked by *sustained* physical exertion, such as during the third mile of a 5-mile run. Such headaches build up over hours and thus are distinctly different from the cough headache syndrome. The term "effort migraine" has been used for this syndrome to avoid the ambiguous term "exertional headache."

COITAL HEADACHE

In another male-dominated (4:1) syndrome, headaches occur during coitus, usually close to orgasm. They are abrupt in onset and subside in a few minutes if coitus is interrupted. These headaches are nearly always benign and usually occur sporadically; if coital headaches persist for hours or are accompanied by vomiting, subarachnoid hemorrhage must be evaluated by computed tomography or CSF examination. An unruptured aneurysm may result in a headache during coitus and can be indistinguishable from benign coital headache; therefore, angiography should be considered for the first attack of coital headache. If attacks occur frequently and are brief, however, the disorder is benign.

POSTCONCUSSION HEADACHES

After a seemingly trivial head injury and particularly after a rear-end motor vehicle collision, many people report admixtures of headache, vertigo, and impaired memory and concentration for months or years after the injury. This syndrome is usually not associated with an anatomic lesion of the brain and may occur whether or not the person was rendered unconscious by head trauma. In general, this headache is "neurobiologic" rather than "psychologic." The syndrome usually persists long after the settlement of a lawsuit. Some evidence suggests that concussion perturbs neurotransmission within the brain and that restoration of this condition is typically delayed. Understanding this common problem is contingent upon clarification of the biology of cerebral concussion. Treatment is symptomatic, including repeated encouragement that the syndrome eventually remits.

GIANT CELL ARTERITIS

This is a common disorder in elderly patients; the average annual incidence is 77 per 100,000 people aged 50 and older. Women account for 65% of cases, and the average age at onset is 70 years, with a range of 50 to 85 years. The inflammatory process may result in blindness in 50% of patients if corticosteroid treatment is not instituted; indeed, the ischemic optic neuropathy of giant cell arteritis is the major cause of rapidly developing bilateral blindness after age 60 years.

The most common initial symptoms are headache, polymyalgia rheumatica, jaw claudication, fever, and weight loss (see Chapter 155). Headache is the dominant symptom and usually appears with malaise and muscle aches. Head pain may be unilateral or bilateral and is located temporally in 50% of patients but may involve any and all aspects of the cranium. Pain usually appears gradually over a few hours before peak intensity is reached; occasionally, it is explosive in onset. The quality of pain is only seldom throbbing; it is almost invariably described as dull and boring with superimposed episodic ice pick–like lancinating pains similar to the sharp pains that appear in migraine. Most patients can recognize that the origin of their head pain is superficial, and external to the skull, rather than deep within the cranium (the site of pain in migraine). Scalp tenderness is present, often to a marked degree; brushing the hair or resting the head on a pillow may be impossible because of pain. Headache is usually worse at night and is often aggravated by exposure to cold. Reddened tender nodules or red streaking of the skin overlying the temporal arteries is found in highest frequency in patients with headache, as is tenderness of the temporal or, less commonly, the occipital arteries. Temporal artery biopsy may be followed by cessation of headache.

The erythrocyte sedimentation rate is often but not always elevated; a normal erythrocyte sedimentation rate does not exclude giant cell arteritis. After the temporal artery biopsy, prednisone is given at 80 mg daily for the first 4 to 6 weeks, when clinical suspicion is high. Because patients with migraine also report amelioration of headaches with prednisone therapy, therapeutic responses are not diagnostic. Contrary to widespread notions, the prevalence of migraine among the elderly population is substantial, considerably higher than that of giant cell arteritis.

LUMBAR PUNCTURE HEADACHE

Headache after lumbar puncture usually begins within 48 hours but may be delayed for up to 12 days. The mean incidence is about 30%. Head pain is dramatically positional; it begins when the patient sits or stands upright and subsides on reclining or with abdominal compression. The longer the patient is upright, the longer the latency before head pain subsides. It is worsened by head shaking or jugular vein compression. The pain is usually a dull ache but may be throbbing; the location is occipitofrontal. Nausea and stiff neck often accompany headache, and some patients report blurred vision, photophobia, tinnitus, and vertigo. The symptoms resolve over a few days but may persist for weeks or months.

Loss of CSF volume decreases the supportive cushion of the brain; when the patient is erect, vascular dilatation probably results and tension is placed on anchoring intracranial structures, including the pain-sensitive dural sinuses. There is often intracranial hypotension, but the full-blown syndrome may occur with normal CSF pressure.

Treatment is remarkably effective. Intravenous caffeine sodium benzoate given over a few minutes as a 500-mg dose promptly terminates headache in 75% of patients; a second dose 1 hour later brings the total success rate to 85%. An epidural blood patch accomplished by injection of 15 mL of the patient's blood rarely fails for those who do not respond to caffeine. The mechanism for these treatment effects is not clear because the blood patch has an immediate effect; thus, the sealing of a dural hole with blood clot is an unlikely mechanism of action.

BRAIN TUMOR HEADACHE

About 30% of patients with brain tumors consider headache their chief complaint. The head pain syndrome is nondescript; a deep dull aching quality of moderate intensity occurs intermittently, is worsened by exertion or change in position, and is associated with nausea and vomiting. This pattern of symptoms results from migraine far more often than from brain tumor. Headache disturbs sleep in about 10% of patients. Vomiting that precedes the appearance of headache by weeks is highly characteristic of posterior fossa brain tumors.

SUGGESTED READINGS

Cutrer FM, Sorensen AG, Weisskoff RM, et al. Perfusion-weighted imaging defects during spontaneous migrainous aura. *Ann Neurol* 1998;43:25–37.

Ferrari MD. Migraine. *Lancet* 1998;351:1043–1051.

Goadsby PJ. A triptan too far? *J Neurol Neurosurg Psychiatry* 1998;64:143–147.

Goadsby PJ, Gundlach AL. Localization of ³H-dihydroergotamine binding sites in the cat central nervous system: relevance to migraine. *Ann Neurol* 1991;29:91–94.

Grimson BS, Thompson HS. Raeder's syndrome. A clinical review. *Surg Ophthalmol* 1980;24:199–210.

Hoskin KL, Kaube H, Goadsby PJ. Sumatriptan can inhibit trigeminal afferents by an exclusively neural mechanism. *Brain* 1996;119:1419–1428.

Lance JW, Goadsby PJ. *Mechanism and management of headache*, 6th ed. London: Butterworth Scientific, 1998.

Nyholt DR, Lea RA, Goadsby PJ, et al. Familial typical migraine. *Neurology* 1998;50:1428–1432.

Olesen J. Cerebral and extracranial circulatory disturbances in migraine: pathophysiological implications. *Cerebrovasc Brain Metab Rev* 1991;3:1–28.

Raps EC, Rogers JD, Galetta SL, et al. The clinical spectrum of unruptured intracranial aneurysms. *Arch Neurol* 1993;30:265–268.

Raskin NH. Lumbar puncture headache: a review. *Headache* 1990;30:197–200.

Raskin NH. Short-lived head pains. *Neurol Clin* 1997;15:143–152.

Schraeder PL, Burns RA. Hemiplegic migraine associated with an aseptic meningeal reaction. *Arch Neurol* 1980;37:377–379.

Silberstein SD. The pharmacology of ergotamine and dihydroergotamine. *Headache* 1997;37[Suppl]:S15–S25.

Symonds C. Cough headache. *Brain* 1956;79:557–568.

Weiller C, May A, Limmroth V, et al. Brain stem activation in spontaneous human migraine attacks. *Nat Med* 1995;1:658–660.

Merritt's Neurology, 10th ed., edited by L.P. Rowland. Lippincott Williams & Wilkins, Philadelphia © 2000.

CHAPTER 140

EPILEPSY

TIMOTHY A. PEDLEY
CARL W. BAZIL
MARTHA J. MORRELL

An epileptic seizure is the result of a temporary physiologic dysfunction of the brain caused by a self-limited, abnormal, hypersynchronous electrical discharge of cortical neurons. There are many different kinds of seizures, each with characteristic behavioral changes and electrophysiologic disturbances that can usually be detected in scalp electroencephalographic (EEG) recordings. The particular manifestations of any single seizure depend on several factors: whether most or only a part of the cerebral cortex is involved at the beginning, the functions of the cortical areas where the seizure originates, the subsequent pattern of spread of the electrical ictal discharge within the brain, and the extent to which subcortical and brainstem structures are engaged.

A seizure is a transient epileptic event, a symptom of disturbed brain function. Although seizures are the cardinal manifestation of epilepsy, not all seizures imply epilepsy. For example, seizures may be self-limited in that they occur only during the course of an acute medical or neurologic illness; they do not persist after the underlying disorder has resolved. Some people, for no discoverable reason, have a single unprovoked seizure. These kinds of seizures are not epilepsy.

Epilepsy is a chronic disorder, or group of chronic disorders, in which the indispensable feature is recurrence of seizures that are typically unprovoked and usually unpredictable. About 40 million people are affected worldwide. Each distinct form of epilepsy has its own natural history and response to treatment. This diversity presumably reflects the fact that epilepsy can arise from a variety of underlying conditions and pathophysiologic mechanisms, although most cases are classified as "idiopathic" or "cryptogenic."

CLASSIFICATION OF SEIZURES AND EPILEPSY

Accurate classification of seizures and epilepsy is essential for understanding epileptic phenomena, developing a rational plan of investigation, making decisions about when and for how long to treat, choosing the appropriate antiepileptic drug, and conducting scientific investigations that require delineation of clinical and EEG phenotypes.

Classification of Seizures

The classification used today is the 1981 Classification of Epileptic Seizures developed by the International League Against Epilepsy (ILAE) (Table 140.1). This system classifies seizures by clinical symptoms supplemented by EEG data.

Inherent in the classification are two important physiologic principles. First, seizures are fundamentally of two types: those with onset limited to a part of one cerebral hemisphere (*partial or focal* seizures) and those that seem to involve the brain diffusely from the beginning (*generalized* seizures). Second, seizures are dynamic and evolving; clinical expression is determined as much by the sequence of spread of electrical discharge within the brain as by the area where the ictal discharge originates. Variations in the seizure pattern exhibited by an individual imply variability in the extent and pattern of spread of the electrical discharge.

Both generalized and partial seizures are further divided into subtypes. For partial seizures, the most important subdivision is based on consciousness, which is preserved in *simple* partial seizures or lost in *complex* partial seizures. Simple partial seizures may evolve into complex partial seizures, and either simple or complex partial seizures may evolve into secondarily generalized seizures. In adults, most generalized seizures have a focal onset whether or not this is apparent clinically. For generalized seizures, subdivisions are based mainly on the presence or absence and character of ictal motor manifestations.

The initial events of a seizure, described by either the patient or an observer, are usually the most reliable clinical indication to determine whether a seizure begins focally or is generalized from the moment of onset. Sometimes, however, a focal signature is lacking for several possible reasons:

TABLE 140.1. ILAE CLASSIFICATION OF EPILEPTIC SEIZURES

I. Partial (focal) seizures
  A. Simple partial seizures (consciousness not impaired)
    1. With motor signs (including jacksonian, versive, and postural)
    2. With sensory symptoms (including visual, somatosensory, auditory, olfactory, gustatory, and vertiginous)
    3. With psychic symptoms (including dysphasia, dysmensic, hallucinatory, and affective changes)
    4. With autonomic symptoms (including epigastric sensation, pallor, flushing, pupillary changes)
  B. Complex partial seizures (consciousness is impaired)
    1. Simple partial onset followed by impaired consciousness
    2. With impairment of consciousness at onset
    3. With automatisms
  C. Partial seizures evolving to secondarily generalized seizures
II. Generalized seizures of nonfocal origin (convulsive or nonconvulsive)
  A. Absence seizures
    1. With impaired consciousness only
    2. With one or more of the following: atonic components, tonic components, automatisms, autonomic components
  B. Myoclonic seizures
    Myoclonic jerks (single or multiple)
  C. Tonic-clonic seizures (may include clonic-tonic-clonic seizures)
  D. Tonic seizures
  E. Atonic seizures
III. Unclassified epileptic seizures

ILAE, International League Against Epilepsy.
From Commission on Classification and Terminology of the International League Against Epilepsy. Proposal for revised clinical and electroencephalographic classification of epileptic seizures. *Epilepsia* 1981;22:489–501.

1. The patient may be amnesic after the seizure, with no memory of early events.
2. Consciousness may be impaired so quickly or the seizure generalized so rapidly that early distinguishing features are blurred or lost.
3. The seizure may originate in a brain region that is not associated with an obvious behavioral function; thus, the seizure becomes clinically evident only when the discharge spreads beyond the ictal onset zone or becomes generalized.

Partial Seizures

Simple partial seizures result when the ictal discharge occurs in a limited and often circumscribed area of cortex, the *epileptogenic focus*. Almost any symptom or phenomenon can be the subjective ("aura") or observable manifestation of a simple partial seizure, varying from elementary motor ("jacksonian seizures," adversive seizures) and unilateral sensory disturbance to complex emotional, psychoillusory, hallucinatory, or dysmnesic phenomena. Especially common auras include an epigastric rising sensation, fear, a feeling of unreality or detachment, deja vu and jamais vu experiences, and olfactory hallucinations. Patients can interact normally with the environment during simple partial seizures except for limitations imposed by the seizure on specific localized brain functions.

Complex partial seizures, on the other hand, are defined by impaired consciousness and imply bilateral spread of the seizure discharge, at least to basal forebrain and limbic areas. In addition to loss of consciousness, patients with complex partial seizures usually exhibit automatisms, such as lip-smacking, repeated swallowing, clumsy perseveration of an ongoing motor task, or some other complex motor activity that is undirected and inappropriate. Postictally, patients are confused and disoriented for several minutes, and determining the transition from ictal to postictal state may be difficult without simultaneous EEG recording. Of complex partial seizures, 70% to 80% arise from the temporal lobe; foci in the frontal and occipital lobes account for most of the remainder.

Generalized Seizures

Generalized tonic-clonic (grand mal) seizures are characterized by abrupt loss of consciousness with bilateral tonic extension of the trunk and limbs (*tonic phase*), often accompanied by a loud vocalization as air is forcedly expelled across contracted vocal cords (*epileptic cry*), followed by synchronous muscle jerking (*clonic phase*). In some patients, a few clonic jerks precede the tonic-clonic sequence; in others, only a tonic or clonic phase is apparent. Postictally, patients are briefly unarousable and then lethargic and confused, often preferring to sleep. Many patients report inconsistent nonspecific premonitory symptoms (*epileptic prodrome*) for minutes to a few hours before a generalized tonic-clonic seizure. Common symptoms include ill-defined anxiety, irritability, decreased concentration, and headache or other uncomfortable feelings.

Absence (petit mal) seizures are momentary lapses in awareness that are accompanied by motionless staring and arrest of any ongoing activity. Absence seizures begin and end abruptly; they occur without warning or postictal period. Mild myoclonic jerks of the eyelid or facial muscles, variable loss of muscle tone, and automatisms may accompany longer attacks. When the beginning and end of the seizure are less distinct, or if tonic and autonomic components are included, the term *atypical absence* seizure is used. Atypical absences are seen most often in retarded children with epilepsy or in epileptic encephalopathies, such as the Lennox-Gastaut syndrome (defined later).

Myoclonic seizures are characterized by rapid brief muscle jerks that can occur bilaterally, synchronously or asynchronously, or unilaterally. Myoclonic jerks range from isolated small movements of face, arm, or leg muscles to massive bilateral spasms simultaneously affecting the head, limbs, and trunk.

Atonic (astatic) seizures, also called *drop attacks*, are characterized by sudden loss of muscle tone, which may be fragmentary (e.g., head drop) or generalized, resulting in a fall. When atonic seizures are preceded by a brief myoclonic seizure or tonic spasm, an acceleratory force is added to the fall, thereby contributing to the high rate of self-injury with this type of seizure.

Classification of Epilepsy (Epileptic Syndromes)

Attempting to classify the kind of epilepsy a patient has is often more important than describing seizures, because the formulation includes other relevant clinical data of which the seizures are only a part. The other data include historical information (e.g., a personal history of brain injury or family history of first-degree relatives with seizures); findings on neurologic examination; and results of EEG, brain imaging, and biochemical studies.

The ILAE classification separates major groups of epilepsy first on the basis of whether seizures are partial (*localization-related epilepsies*) or generalized (*generalized epilepsies*) and second by cause (*idiopathic, symptomatic,* or *cryptogenic* epilepsy). Subtypes of epilepsy are grouped according to the patient's age and, in the case of localization-related epilepsies, by the anatomic location of the presumed ictal onset zone.

Classification of the epilepsies has been less successful and more controversial than the classification of seizure types. A basic problem is that the classification scheme is empiric, with clinical and EEG data emphasized over anatomic, pathologic, or specific etiologic information. This classification is useful for some reasonably well-defined syndromes, such as *infantile spasms or benign partial childhood epilepsy with central-midtemporal spikes*, especially because of the prognostic and treatment implications of these disorders. On the other hand, few epilepsies imply a specific disease or defect. A further drawback to the ILAE classification is that the same epileptic syndrome (e.g., infantile spasms or Lennox-Gastaut syndrome) may be produced by a specific disease (e.g., tuberous sclerosis), considered "cryptogenic" on the basis of nonspecific imaging abnormalities, or categorized as "idiopathic." Another biologic incongruity is the excessive detail in which some syndromes are identified, with specific entities culled from what are more likely simply different biologic expressions of the same abnormality (e.g., childhood and juvenile forms of absence epilepsy).

With these reservations, there is little question that defining common epilepsy syndromes has practical value. Table 140.2 gives a modified version of the ILAE classification, which continues to evolve.

SELECTED GENERALIZED EPILEPSY SYNDROMES

Infantile Spasms (West Syndrome)

The term infantile spasms denotes a unique age-specific form of generalized epilepsy that may be either idiopathic or symptomatic. When all clinical data are considered, including results of imaging studies, only about 15% of patients are now classified as idiopathic. Symptomatic cases result from diverse conditions, including cerebral dysgenesis, tuberous sclerosis, phenylketonuria, intrauterine infections, or hypoxic-ischemic injury.

Seizures are characterized by sudden flexor or extensor spasms that involve the head, trunk, and limbs simultaneously. The attacks usually begin before 6 months of age. The EEG is grossly abnormal, showing chaotic high-voltage slow activity with multifocal spikes, a pattern termed *hypsarrhythmia*. The treatment of choice is corticotropin or prednisone; spasms are notoriously refractory to conventional antiepileptic drugs. Vigabatrin, an antiepileptic drug that is not approved for use in the United States but is widely available elsewhere, is an exception. Several small series indicate that vigabatrin is an effective alternative to corticotropin in selected cases. Although corticotropin therapy usually controls spasms and reverses the EEG abnormalities, it has little effect on long-term prognosis. Only about 5% to 10%

TABLE 140.2. MODIFIED CLASSIFICATION OF EPILEPTIC SYNDROMES

I. Idiopathic epilepsy syndromes (focal or generalized)
  A. Benign neonatal convulsions
    1. Familial
    2. Nonfamilial
  B. Benign childhood epilepsy
    1. With central midtemporal spikes
    2. With occipital spikes
  C. Childhood/juvenile absence epilepsy
  D. Juvenile myoclonic epilepsy (including generalized tonic-clonic seizures on awakening)
  E. Idiopathic epilepsy, otherwise unspecified
II. Symptomatic epilepsy syndromes (focal or generalized)
  A. West syndrome (infantile spasms)
  B. Lennox-Gastaut syndrome
  C. Early myoclonic encephalopathy
  D. Epilepsia partialis continua
    1. Rasmussen syndrome (encephalitic form)
    2. Restricted form
  E. Acquired epileptic aphasia (Landau-Kleffner syndrome)
  F. Temporal lobe epilepsy
  G. Frontal lobe epilepsy
  H. Posttraumatic epilepsy
  I. Other symptomatic epilepsy, focal or generalized, not specified
III. Other epilepsy syndromes of uncertain or mixed classification
  A. Neonatal seizures
  B. Febril seizures
  C. Reflex epilepsy
  D. Other unspecified

of children with infantile spasms have normal or near-normal intelligence, and more than 66% have severe disabilities.

Childhood Absence (Petit Mal) Epilepsy

This disorder begins most often between the ages of 4 and 12 years and is characterized predominantly by recurrent absence seizures, which, if untreated, can occur literally hundreds of times each day. EEG activity during an absence attack is characterized by stereotyped, bilateral, 3-Hz spike-wave discharges. Generalized tonic-clonic seizures also occur in 30% to 50% of cases. Most children are normal, both neurologically and intellectually. Ethosuximide and valproate are equally effective in treating absence seizures, but valproate or lamotrigine are preferable if generalized tonic-clonic seizures coexist. Topiramate may also be effective in generalized-onset seizures.

Lennox-Gastaut Syndrome

This term is applied to a heterogeneous group of childhood epileptic encephalopathies that are characterized by mental retardation, uncontrolled seizures, and a distinctive EEG pattern. The syndrome is not a pathologic entity, because clinical and EEG manifestations result from brain malformations, perinatal asphyxia, severe head injury, central nervous system infection, or, rarely, a progressive degenerative or metabolic syndrome. A presumptive cause can be identified in 65% to 70% of affected children. Seizures usually begin before age 4 years, and about 25% of children have a history of infantile spasms. No treatment is consistently effective, and 80% of children continue to have seizures as adults. Best results are generally obtained with broad-spectrum antiepileptic drugs, such as valproate, lamotrigine, or topiramate. Despite the higher incidence of severe side effects, felbamate is often effective when these other agents do not result in optimal seizure control. Refractory cases may be considered for corpus callosotomy.

Juvenile Myoclonic Epilepsy

This subtype of idiopathic generalized epilepsy most often begins in otherwise healthy individuals between the ages of 8 and 20 years. The fully developed syndrome comprises morning myoclonic jerks, generalized tonic-clonic seizures that occur just after waking, normal intelligence, a family history of similar seizures, and an EEG that shows generalized spikes, 4- to 6-Hz spike waves, and multiple spike ("polyspike") discharges. The myoclonic jerks vary in intensity from bilateral massive spasms and falls to minor isolated muscle jerks that many patients consider nothing more than "morning clumsiness." Valproate is the treatment of choice and controls seizures and myoclonus in more than 80% of cases. Lamotrigine or acetazolamide are alternatives, although lamotrigine can exacerbate myoclonus in some patients. Some linkage studies have identified a marker for juvenile myoclonic epilepsy on the short arm of chromosome 6; the gene product is not known.

SELECTED LOCALIZATION-RELATED EPILEPSY SYNDROMES

Benign Focal Epilepsy of Childhood

Several "benign" focal epilepsies occur in children, of which the most common is the syndrome associated with central-midtemporal spikes on EEG. This form of idiopathic focal epilepsy, also known as *benign rolandic epilepsy*, accounts for about 15% of all pediatric seizure disorders.

Onset is between 4 and 13 years; children are otherwise normal. Most children have attacks mainly or exclusively at night. Sleep promotes secondary generalization, so that parents report only generalized tonic-clonic seizures; any focal manifestations go unobserved. In contrast, seizures that occur during the day are clearly focal with twitching of one side of the face; speech arrest; drooling from a corner of the mouth; and paresthesias of the tongue, lips, inner cheeks, and face. Seizures may progress to include clonic jerking or tonic posturing of the arm and leg on one side. Consciousness is usually preserved.

The interictal EEG abnormality is distinctive and shows stereotyped di- or triphasic sharp waves over the central-midtemporal (rolandic) regions. Discharges may be unilateral or bilateral. They increase in abundance during sleep and, when unilateral, switch from side to side on successive EEGs. In about 30% of cases, generalized spike-wave activity also occurs. The EEG pattern is inherited as an autosomal dominant trait with age-dependent penetrance. The inheritance pattern of the seizures, although clearly familial, is probably multifactorial and less well understood. More than half the children who show the characteristic EEG abnormality never have clinical attacks. Linkage has recently been reported in some families to chromosome 15q14.

The prognosis is uniformly good. Seizures disappear by mid to late adolescence in all cases. Seizures in many children appear to be self-limited, and more physicians now defer treatment until after the second or third attack, a policy with which we agree. Because seizures are easily controlled and self-limited, drugs with the fewest adverse effects, such as carbamazepine or gabapentin, should be used. Low doses, often producing subtherapeutic blood concentrations, are generally effective.

Temporal Lobe Epilepsy

This is the most common epilepsy syndrome of adults. In most cases, the epileptogenic region involves mesial temporal lobe structures, especially the hippocampus, amygdala, and parahippocampal gyrus. Seizures usually begin in late childhood or adolescence, and a history of febrile seizures is common. Virtually all patients have complex partial seizures, some of which secondarily generalize. Auras are frequent; visceral sensations are particularly common. Other typical behavioral features include a motionless stare, loss of awareness that may be gradual, and oral-alimentary automatisms, such as lip-smacking. A variable but often prolonged period of postictal confusion is the rule. Interictal EEGs show focal temporal slowing and epileptiform sharp waves or spikes over the anterior temporal region. Antiepileptic drugs are usually successful in suppressing secondarily generalized seizures, but 50% or more of patients continue to have partial attacks. When seizures persist, anterior temporal lobe resection is the treatment of choice. In appropriately selected patients, complete seizure control is achieved in more than 80% of cases.

Frontal Lobe Epilepsy

The particular pattern of the many types of frontal lobe seizures depends on the specific location where the seizure discharge originates and on the pathways subsequently involved in propagation. Despite this variability, the following features, when taken together, suggest frontal lobe epilepsy:

1. Brief seizures that begin and end abruptly with little, if any, postictal period;
2. A tendency for seizures to cluster and to occur at night;
3. Prominent, but often bizarre, motor manifestations, such as asynchronous thrashing or flailing of arms and legs, pedaling leg movements, pelvic thrusting, and loud, sometimes obscene, vocalizations, all of which may suggest psychogenic seizures;
4. Minimal abnormality on scalp EEG recordings;
5. A history of status epilepticus.

Posttraumatic Seizures

Seizures occur within 1 year in about 7% of civilian and in about 34% of military head injuries. The differences relate mainly to the much higher proportion of penetrating wounds in military cases. The risk of developing posttraumatic epilepsy is directly related to the severity of the injury and also correlates with the total volume of brain lost as measured by computed tomography (CT). Depressed skull fractures may or may not be a risk; the rate of posttraumatic epilepsy was 17% in one series but not increased above control levels in another. Head injuries are classified as *severe* if they result in brain contusion, intracerebral or intracranial hematoma, unconsciousness, or amnesia for more than 24 hours or in persistent neurologic abnormalities, such as aphasia, hemiparesis, or dementia. *Mild* head injury (brief loss of consciousness, no skull fracture, no focal neurologic signs, no contusion or hematoma) do not increase the risk of seizures significantly above general population rates.

Nearly 60% of those who have seizures have the first attack in the first year after the injury. In the Vietnam Head Injury Study, however, more than 15% of patients did not have epilepsy until 5 or more years later. Posttraumatic seizures are classified as *early* (within the first 1 to 2 weeks after injury) or *late*. Only recurrent late seizures (those that occur after the patient has recovered from the acute effects of the injury) should be considered *posttraumatic epilepsy*. Early seizures, however, even if isolated, increase the chance of developing posttraumatic epilepsy. About 70% of patients have partial or secondarily generalized seizures. *Impact seizures* occur at the time of or immediately after the injury. These attacks are attributed to an acute reaction of the brain to trauma and do not increase the risk of later epilepsy.

Overt seizures should be treated according to principles reviewed later in this chapter. The most controversial issue concerns the prophylactic use of antiepileptic drugs to retard or abort the development of subsequent seizures. Based on the data of Temkin et al. (1990), we recommend treating patients with severe head trauma, as just defined, with phenytoin for the first week after injury to minimize complications from seizures occurring during acute management. Phenytoin, or fosphenytoin, should be given intravenously in a loading dose of about 20 mg/kg; subsequent doses should be adjusted to maintain blood levels of 15 to 20 μg/mL. If seizures have not occurred, we do not continue phenytoin beyond the initial 1 to 2 weeks, because evidence does not show that longer treatment prevents the development of later seizures or of posttraumatic epilepsy. Recent data have also shown that valproate is less effective than phenytoin in suppressing acute seizures and also ineffective in preventing the development of posttraumatic seizures.

Epilepsia Partialis Continua

Epilepsia partialis continua (EPC) refers to unremitting motor seizures involving part or all of one side of the body. They typically consist of repeated clonic or myoclonic jerks that may remain focal or regional or may march from one muscle group to another, with the extent of motor involvement waxing and waning in endless variation. In adults, EPC occurs in diverse settings, such as with subacute or chronic inflammatory diseases of the brain (Kozhevnikov Russian spring-summer encephalitis; Behçet disease) or with acute strokes, metastases, and metabolic encephalopathies, especially hyperosmolar nonketotic hyperglycemia.

The most distinctive form of EPC, known as the *Rasmussen syndrome*, occurs in children; it usually begins before the age of 10 years. The underlying disorder is chronic focal encephalitis, although an infectious agent has not been identified consistently. About two-thirds of patients report an infectious or inflammatory

illness 1 to 6 months before onset of EPC. Generalized tonic-clonic seizures are often the first sign and appear before the EPC establishes itself. About 20% of cases begin with an episode of convulsive status epilepticus. Slow neurologic deterioration inevitably follows, with development of hemiparesis, mental impairment, and, usually, hemianopia. If the dominant hemisphere is affected, aphasia occurs. EEGs are always abnormal, but findings are not specific, and they frequently do not correlate with clinical manifestations. Magnetic resonance imaging (MRI) may be normal early but later show unilateral cortical atrophy and signal changes consistent with gliosis. Antiepileptic drugs are usually ineffective, as are corticosteroids and antiviral agents. When seizures have not spontaneously remitted by the time hemipleiga and aphasia are complete, functional hemispherectomy can control seizures and leads to substantial improvement in many patients. Whether hemispherectomy should be performed before the maximal motor or language deficit has developed is controversial.

EPIDEMIOLOGY

In the United States, about 6.5 persons per 1,000 population are affected with recurrent unprovoked seizures, so-called *active epilepsy*. Based on 1990 census figures, age-adjusted annual incidence rates for epilepsy range from 31 to 57 per 100,000 in the United States (Fig. 140.1). Incidence rates are highest among young children and the elderly; epilepsy affects males 1.1 to 1.5 times more often than females.

Complex partial seizures are the most common seizure type among newly diagnosed cases, but age-related variability occurs in the proportions of different seizure types (Fig. 140.2). The cause of epilepsy also varies somewhat with age. Despite advances in diagnostic capabilities, however, the "unknown" etiologic category remains larger than any other for all age groups (Fig. 140.3). Cerebrovascular disease, associated developmental neurologic disorders (e.g., cerebral palsy and mental retardation), and head trauma are the other most commonly identified causes.

Although defined genetic disorders account for only about 1% of epilepsy cases, heritable factors are important. Monozygotic twins have a much higher concordance rate for epilepsy than do dizygotic twins. By age 25, nearly 9% of children of

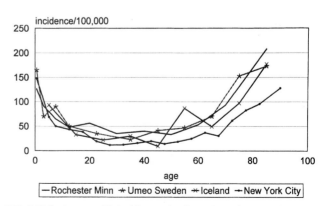

FIG. 140.1. Age-specific incidence of epilepsy in Rochester, Minnesota, 1935–1984. (From Hauser et al. [1993].)

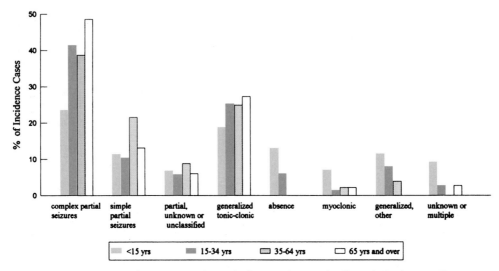

FIG. 140.2. Proportion of seizure types in newly diagnosed cases of epilepsy in Rochester, Minnesota, 1935–1984. (From Hauser et al. [1993].)

mothers with epilepsy and 2.4% of children of affected fathers develop epilepsy. The reason for an increased risk of seizures in children of women with epilepsy is not known.

Some forms of epilepsy are more heritable than others. For example, children of parents with absence seizures have a higher risk of developing epilepsy (9%) than do offspring of parents with other types of generalized seizures or partial seizures (5%). As a general rule, though, even offspring born to a "high-risk" parent have a 90% or greater chance of being unaffected by epilepsy.

Many persons who experience a first unprovoked seizure never have a second. By definition, these people do not have epilepsy and generally do not require long-term drug treatment. Unfortunately, our ability to identify such individuals with accuracy is incomplete. Treatment decisions must be based on epi-

demiologic and individual considerations. Some seizure types, such as absence and myoclonic, are virtually always recurrent by the time the patient is seen by a physician. On the other hand, patients with convulsive seizures may seek medical attention after a first occurrence because of the dramatic nature of the attack. Prospective studies of recurrence after a first seizure indicate a 2-year recurrence risk of about 40%, which is similar in children and adults. The risk is lowest in people with an idiopathic generalized first seizure and normal EEG (about 24%), higher with idiopathic generalized seizures and an abnormal EEG (about 48%), and highest with symptomatic (i.e., known preceding brain injury or neurologic syndrome) seizures and an abnormal EEG (about 65%). Epileptiform, but not nonepileptiform, EEG abnormalities impart a greater risk for recurrence. If the first seizure is a partial seizure, the relative risk of recurrence is also increased. The risk for further recurrence after a second unprovoked seizure is greater than 80%; a second unprovoked seizure is, therefore, a reliable marker of epilepsy.

About 4% of persons living to age 74 have at least one unprovoked seizure. When provoked seizures (i.e., febrile seizures or those related to an acute illness) are included, the likelihood of experiencing a seizure by age 74 increases to at least 9%. The risk of developing epilepsy is about 3% by age 74.

Of persons with epilepsy, 60% to 70% achieve remission of seizures with antiepileptic drug therapy. Factors that favor remission include an idiopathic (or cryptogenic) form of epilepsy, normal findings on neurologic examination, and onset in early to middle childhood (except neonatal seizures). Unfavorable prognostic factors include partial seizures, an abnormal EEG, and associated mental retardation or cerebral palsy (Table 140.3).

Mortality is increased in persons with epilepsy, but the risk is incurred mainly by symptomatic cases in which higher death rates are related primarily to the underlying disease rather than to epilepsy. Accidental deaths, especially drowning, are more common, however, in all patients with epilepsy. Sudden unexplained death is nearly 25 times more common in patients with epilepsy than in the general population; estimates of incidence

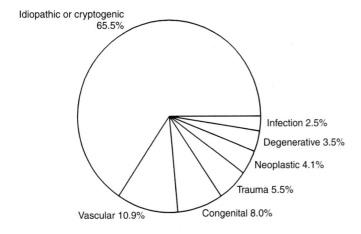

FIG. 140.3. Etiology of epilepsy in all cases of newly diagnosed seizures in Rochester, Minnesota, 1935–1984 (From Hauser et al. [1993].)

TABLE 140.3. PREDICTORS OF INTRACTABILITY

Very young age at onset (<2 yr)
Frequent generalized seizures
Failure to achieve control readily
Evidence of brain damage
A specific cause of the seizures
Severe electroencephalogram abnormality
Low IQ
Atonic atypical absence seizures

rates range from 1 in 500 to 1 in 2,000 per year. Severe epilepsy and uncontrolled generalized convulsions are risk factors.

INITIAL DIAGNOSTIC EVALUATION

The diagnostic evaluation has three objectives: to determine if the patient has epilepsy; to classify the type of epilepsy and identify an epilepsy syndrome, if possible; and to define the specific underlying cause. Accurate diagnosis leads directly to proper treatment and formulation of a rational plan of management. The differential diagnosis is considered in Chapter 3.

Because epilepsy comprises a group of conditions and is not a single homogeneous disorder, and because seizures may be symptoms of both diverse brain disorders and an otherwise normal brain, it is neither possible nor desirable to develop inflexible guidelines for what constitutes a "standard" or "minimal" diagnostic evaluation. The clinical data from the history and physical examination should allow a reasonable determination of probable diagnosis, seizure and epilepsy classification, and likelihood of underlying brain disorder. Based on these considerations, diagnostic testing should be undertaken selectively.

History and Examination

A complete history is the cornerstone for establishing a diagnosis of epilepsy. An adequate history should provide a clear picture of the clinical features of the seizures and the sequence in which manifestations evolve; the course of the epileptic disorder; seizure precipitants, such as alcohol or sleep deprivation; risk factors for seizures, such as abnormal gestation, febrile seizures, family history of epilepsy, head injury, encephalitis or meningitis, and stroke; and response to previous treatment. In children, developmental history is important.

In describing the epileptic seizure, care should be taken to elicit a detailed description of any aura. The aura was once considered to be the "warning" of an impending attack, but it is actually a simple partial seizure made apparent by subjective feelings or experiential phenomena observable only by the patient. Auras precede many complex partial or generalized seizures and are experienced by 50% to 60% of adults with epilepsy. Auras confirm the suspicion that the seizure begins locally within the brain; they may also provide direct clues about the location or laterality of the focus. Information about later events in the seizure usually are obtained from an observer because of the patient's impaired awareness or frank loss of consciousness or because of postictal amnesia even though responses to questions during the seizure indicate preserved responsiveness.

The nature of repetitive automatic or purposeless movements (automatisms), sustained postures, presence of myoclonus, and the duration of the seizure help to delineate specific seizure types or epileptic syndromes. Nonspecific postictal findings of lethargy and confusion must be distinguished from focal neurologic abnormalities, such as hemiparesis or aphasia, that point to the hemisphere of seizure onset.

Information about risk factors (Table 140.4) may suggest a particular cause and assist in prognosis. Discussion with parents may be necessary, because children or adults may be uninformed about, or may not recall, early childhood events, such as perinatal encephalopathy, febrile seizures, brain infections, head injuries, or intermittent absence seizures. Age at seizure onset and course of the seizure disorder should be clarified, because these features differ in the various epilepsy syndromes.

Findings on neurologic examination are usually normal in patients with epilepsy but occasionally may provide etiologic clues. Focal signs indicate an underlying cerebral lesion. Asymmetry of the hand or face may indicate localized or hemispheric cerebral atrophy contralateral to the smaller side. Phakomatoses are commonly associated with seizures and may be suggested by cafe-au-lait spots, facial angioma, conjunctival telangiectasia, hypopigmented macules, fibroangiomatous nevi, or lumbosacral shagreen patches.

TABLE 140.4. RISK FACTORS FOR EPILEPSY

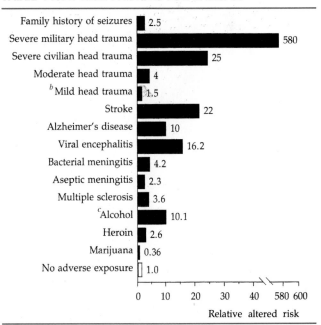

[a]Relative to people without these adverse exposures.
[b]Not statistically significant.
[c]One pint of 80 proof, 2.5 bottles of wine.
From Hauser WA, Hesdorffer DC. *Epilepsy: frequency, causes and consequences.* New York: Demos, 1990.

Electroencephalography

Because epilepsy is fundamentally a physiologic disturbance of brain function, the EEG is the most important laboratory test in evaluating patients with seizures. The EEG helps both to establish the diagnosis of epilepsy and to characterize specific epileptic syndromes. EEG findings may also help in management and in prognosis.

Epileptiform discharges (spikes and sharp waves) are highly correlated with seizure susceptibility and can be recorded on the first EEG in about 50% of patients. Similar findings are recorded in only 1% to 2% of normal adults and in a somewhat higher percentage of normal children. When multiple EEGs are obtained, epileptiform abnormalities eventually appear in 60% to 90% of adults with epilepsy, but the yield of positive studies does not increase substantially after three or four tests. It is important to remember, therefore, that 10% to 40% of patients with epilepsy do not show epileptiform abnormalities on routine EEG; a normal or nonspecifically abnormal EEG never excludes the diagnosis. Sleep, hyperventilation, photic stimulation, and special electrode placements are routinely used to increase the probability of recording epileptiform abnormalities.

Different and distinctive patterns of epileptiform discharge occur in specific epilepsy syndromes as summarized in Chapter 14.

Brain Imaging

MRI should be performed in all patients over age 18 years and in children with abnormal development, abnormal findings on physical examination, or seizure types that are likely to be manifestations of symptomatic epilepsy. CT will often miss common epileptogenic lesions such as hippocampal sclerosis, cortical dysplasia, and cavernous malformations. Because CT is very sensitive for detecting brain calcifications, a noncontrast CT (in addition to MRI) may be helpful in patients at risk for neurocysticercosis.

Routine imaging is not necessary for children with idiopathic epilepsy, including the benign focal epilepsy syndromes (see later section). Brain MRI, although more costly, is more sensitive than CT in detecting potentially epileptogenic lesions, such as cortical dysplasia, hamartomas, differentiated glial tumors, and cavernous malformations. Both axial and coronal planes should be imaged with both T1 and T2 sequences. Gadolinium injection does not increase the sensitivity for detecting cerebral lesions but may assist in differentiating possible causes.

Imaging in the coronal plane perpendicular to the long axis of the hippocampus and other variations in technique have improved the detection of hippocampal atrophy and gliosis, findings that are highly correlated with mesial temporal sclerosis (Fig. 140.4) and an epileptogenic temporal lobe. An even more sensitive measure of hippocampal atrophy is MRI measurement of the volume of the hippocampus. Hippocampal volume measurements in an individual patient then can be compared with those of normal control subjects.

Other Laboratory Tests

Routine blood tests are rarely diagnostically useful in healthy children or adults. They are necessary in newborns and in older patients with acute or chronic systemic disease to detect abnor-

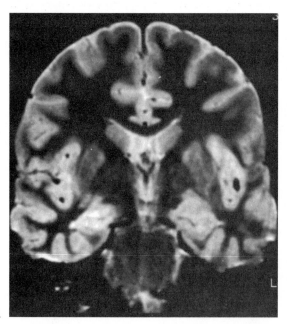
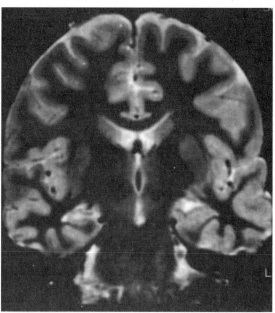

FIG. 140.4. Mesial temporal sclerosis. **A and B:** Short-tau inversion recovery (STIR) coronal magnetic resonance images through the temporal lobes show increased signal and decreased size of right hippocampus as compared with left. These findings are characteristic of mesial temporal sclerosis. Note incidental focal dilatation of left choroid fissure, which represents a choroid fissure cyst, and is a normal variant. (Courtesy of Dr. S. Chan, Columbia University College of Physicians and Surgeons, New York, NY.)

mal electrolyte, glucose, calcium, or magnesium values or impaired liver or kidney function that may contribute to seizure occurrence. In most patients, serum electrolytes, liver function tests, and a complete blood count are useful mainly as baseline studies before initiating antiepileptic drug treatment.

Any suspicion of meningitis or encephalitis mandates lumbar puncture. Urine or blood toxicologic screens should be considered when otherwise unexplained new-onset generalized seizures occur.

LONG-TERM MONITORING

The most direct and convincing evidence of an epileptic basis for a patient's episodic symptoms is the recording of an electrographic seizure discharge during a typical behavioral attack. This recording is especially necessary if the history is ambiguous, EEGs are repeatedly normal or nonspecifically abnormal, and reasonable treatment has failed. Because most patients have seizures infrequently, routine EEG rarely records an attack. Long-term monitoring permits EEG recording for a longer time, thus increasing the likelihood of recording seizures or interictal epileptiform discharges. Two methods of long-term monitoring are now widely available: simultaneous closed-circuit television and EEG (CCTV/EEG) monitoring and ambulatory EEG. Both have greatly improved diagnostic accuracy and the reliability of seizure classification and both provide continuous recordings through one or more complete waking-sleep cycles and capture ictal episodes. Each has additional specific advantages and disadvantages. The method used depends on the question posed by a particular patient.

Long-term monitoring using CCTV/EEG, usually in a specially designed hospital unit, is the procedure of choice to document psychogenic seizures and other nonepileptic paroxysmal events. It can also establish electrical-clinical correlations and localize epileptogenic foci for resective surgery. The emphasis in monitoring units is usually on behavioral events, not interictal EEG activity. The availability of full-time technical or nursing staff ensures high-quality recordings and permits examination of patients during clinical events. Antiepileptic drugs can be discontinued safely to facilitate seizure occurrence. Computerized detection programs are used to screen EEG continuously for epileptiform abnormalities and subclinical seizures.

The other method of long-term monitoring is designed for outpatient use in the patient's home, school, or work environment. Ambulatory EEG is often especially helpful in pediatrics, because children are often more comfortable in their familiar and unrestricted home environment. The major limitations of ambulatory monitoring are the limited coverage of cortical areas, variable technical quality resulting from lack of expert supervision, frequent distortion of EEG data by environmental contaminants, and the absence of video documentation of behavioral changes. Ambulatory monitoring is most useful in documenting interictal epileptiform activity when routine EEGs have been repeatedly negative or in recording ictal discharges during typical behavioral events. At present, however, ambulatory EEG is not a substitute for CCTV/EEG monitoring, especially when psychogenic seizures are an issue or when patients are being evaluated for epilepsy surgery.

MEDICAL TREATMENT

Therapy of epilepsy has three goals: to eliminate seizures or reduce their frequency to the maximum extent possible, to avoid the side effects associated with long-term treatment, and to assist the patient in maintaining or restoring normal psychosocial and vocational adjustment. No medical treatment now available can induce a permanent remission ("cure") or prevent development of epilepsy by altering the process of epileptogenesis.

The decision to institute antiepileptic drug therapy should be based on a thoughtful and informed analysis of the issues involved. Isolated infrequent seizures, whether convulsive or not, probably pose little medical risk to otherwise healthy persons. However, even relatively minor seizures, especially those associated with loss or alteration of alertness, have many psychosocial, vocational, and safety ramifications. Finally, the probability of seizure recurrence varies substantially among patients, depending on the type of epilepsy and any associated neurologic or medical problems. Drug treatment, on the other hand, carries a risk of adverse effects, which approaches 30% after initial treatment. Treatment of children raises additional issues, especially the unknown effects of long-term antiepileptic drug use on brain development, learning, and behavior.

These considerations mean that although drug treatment is indicated and beneficial for most patients with epilepsy, certain circumstances call for antiepileptic drugs to be deferred or used for only a limited time. As a rule of thumb, antiepileptic drugs should be prescribed when the potential benefits of treatment clearly outweigh possible adverse effects of therapy.

Acute Symptomatic Seizures

These seizures are caused by, or associated with, an acute medical or neurologic illness. A childhood febrile seizure is the most common example of an acute symptomatic seizure, but other frequently encountered causes include metabolic or toxic encephalopathies and acute brain infections. To the extent that these conditions resolve without permanent brain damage, seizures are usually self-limited. The primary therapeutic concern in such patients should be identification and treatment of the underlying disorder. If antiepileptic drugs are needed to suppress seizures acutely, they generally do not need to be continued after the patient recovers.

The Single Seizure

About 25% of patients with unprovoked seizures come to a physician after a single attack, nearly always a generalized tonic-clonic seizure. Most of these people have no risk factors for epilepsy, have normal findings on neurologic examination, and show a normal first EEG. Only about 25% of these patients later develop epilepsy. For this group, the need for treatment is questionable. For many years, no convincing data indicated any beneficial effect of treatment on preventing recurrence. In 1993, a large multicenter randomized study from Italy convincingly demonstrated that antiepileptic drugs reduce the risk of relapse after the first unprovoked convulsive seizure. Among nearly 400 children and adults, treatment within 7 days of a first seizure was followed by a recurrence rate of 25% at 2 years. In contrast, untreated patients had a recurrence rate of 51%. When patients with previous "uncertain spells" were excluded from the analysis, treatment benefit was still evident, but the magnitude of the effect was reduced to a recurrence rate of 30% in the treated group and 42% in untreated patients.

Although treatment of first seizures reduces the relapse rate even in low-risk patients, there is no evidence that such treatment alters the prognosis of epilepsy. Thus, treatment should not be automatic, and the decision to treat should be made only in consultation with the patient or parents after weighing the unique circumstances posed by that individual. In most patients with idiopathic epilepsy, deferring treatment until a second seizure occurs is a reasonable and often preferable decision.

Benign Epilepsy Syndromes

Several electroclinical syndromes begin in childhood and are associated with normal development, normal findings on neurologic examination, and normal brain imaging studies. They have a uniformly good prognosis for complete remission in mid to late adolescence without long-term behavioral or cognitive problems. The most common and best characterized of these syndromes is benign partial epilepsy of childhood with central-midtemporal sharp waves (rolandic epilepsy). Most seizures occur at night as secondarily generalized convulsions. Focal seizures occur during the day and are characterized by twitching of one side of the face, anarthria, salivation, and paresthesias of the face and inner mouth followed variably by hemiclonic movements or hemitonic posturing. Other benign syndromes include benign partial epilepsy with occipital spike waves and benign epilepsy with affective symptoms.

Because of the good prognosis, the sole goal of treatment in such cases is to prevent recurrence. Because many children, especially those who are older, tend to have only a few seizures, treatment is not always necessary. Antiepileptic drugs are usually reserved for children whose seizures are frequent or relatively severe or whose parents, or the children themselves, are distressed at the prospect of future episodes. With these considerations in mind, only about half the children with benign partial epilepsy require treatment.

Antiepileptic Drugs

Selection of Antiepileptic Drugs

Two nationwide collaborative Veterans Administration Cooperative Studies (1985 and 1992) compared the effectiveness of antiepileptic drugs. In the 1985 study, carbamazepine, phenytoin, primidone, and phenobarbital were equally effective in controlling complex partial and secondarily generalized seizures. In the 1992 study, carbamazepine was slightly more effective than valproate in treating complex partial seizures, but both drugs were of equal efficacy in controlling secondarily generalized seizures. These studies also demonstrated that despite their

relatively uniform ability to suppress seizures, the drugs had different risks of adverse effects. Considering both efficacy and tolerability, carbamazepine and phenytoin are drugs of first choice for patients with partial and secondarily generalized seizures. For patients who have predominantly secondarily generalized seizures, valproate is also effective.

No clinical trials have addressed the relative efficacy of antiepileptic drugs against different symptomatic localization-related epilepsies. There are also few data about the effectiveness of newer antiepileptic drugs (those approved since 1993) compared with older agents or each other. Preliminary studies from Europe indicate that lamotrigine is comparable in effectiveness with phenytoin and carbamazepine and that gabapentin shows similar efficacy to carbamazepine for treatment of new-onset partial seizures. Drugs are therefore chosen based on the patient's predominant seizure type.

In general, valproate is the drug of choice for generalized-onset seizures and can be used advantageously as monotherapy when several generalized seizure types coexist (Table 140.5). Lamotrigine and probably topiramate are alternatives if valproate is ineffective or not tolerated. Phenytoin and carbamazepine are also effective against generalized tonic-clonic seizures, but the response is less predictable than that with valproate. Carbamazepine, phenytoin, gabapentin, and sometimes lamotrigine can aggravate myoclonic seizures; all of these except lamotrigine also sometimes exacerbate absence seizures. Tiagabine can aggravate or induce absence seizures. Ethosuximide is as effective as valproate in controlling absence seizures and has fewer side effects. Ethosuximide is ineffective against tonic-clonic seizures, however, so its main use is as an alternative to valproate in patients who only have absence seizures.

Adverse Effects of Antiepileptic Drugs

All antiepileptic drugs have undesirable effects in some patients. Although interindividual variation occurs, most adverse drug effects are mild and dose related. Many are common to virtually all antiepileptic drugs, especially when treatment is started. These include sedation, mental dulling, impaired memory and concen-

TABLE 140.5. DRUGS USED IN TREATING DIFFERENT TYPES OF SEIZURES

Type of seizure	Drugs[a]
Simple and complex partial	Carbamazepine, phenytoin; valproate; gabapentin and lamotrigine as add-on; primidone, phenobarbital
Secondarily generalized	Carbamazepine, phenytoin, valproate; and gabapentin lamotrigine as add-on; phenobarbital, primidone
Primary generalized seizures	
Tonic-clonic	Valproate; lamotrigine,
Absence	carbamazepine, phenytoin;
Myoclonic	lamotrigine ethosuximide,
Tonic	valproate; clonazepam valproate, felbamate; clonazepam

tration, mood changes, gastrointestinal upset, and dizziness. Other adverse effects are relatively specific for individual agents.

Dose-related Side Effects

These typically appear when a drug is first given or when the dosage is increased. They usually, but not always, correlate with blood concentrations of the parent drug or major metabolites (Table 140.6). Dose-related side effects are always reversible on lowering the dosage or discontinuing the drug. Adverse effects frequently determine the limits of treatment with a particular drug and have a major influence on compliance with the prescribed regimen. Because dose-related side effects are broadly predictable, they are often the major differentiating feature in choosing among otherwise equally effective therapies.

Idiosyncratic Side Effects

Idiosyncratic reactions account for most serious and virtually all life-threatening adverse reactions to antiepileptic drugs. All antiepileptic drugs can cause similar serious side effects (Table 140.6), but with the exception of rash, these are fortunately rare. For example, the risk of carbamazepine-induced agranulocytosis or aplastic anemia is about 2 per 575,000; with felbamate, the risk of aplastic anemia may be as high as 1 per 5,000. Idiosyncratic reactions are not dose related; rather they arise either from an immune-mediated reaction to the drug or from poorly defined individual factors, largely genetic, that convey an unusual sensitivity to the drug. An example of the genetic mechanism is valproate-induced fatal hepatotoxicity. Valproate, like most antiepileptic drugs, is metabolized in the liver, but several biochemical pathways are available to the drug. Clinical and experimental data indicate that one of these pathways results in a hepatotoxic compound that may accumulate and lead to microvesicular steatosis with necrosis. The extent to which this pathway is involved in biotransformation is age dependent and promoted by concurrent use of other drugs that are eliminated in the liver. Thus, most patients who have had fatal hepatotoxicity were younger than 2 years of age and treated with polytherapy (Table 140.7). In addition, most had severe epilepsy associated with mental retardation, developmental delay, or congenital brain anomalies. No hepatic deaths have occurred in persons older than 10 years of age treated with valproate alone.

No laboratory test, certainly not untargeted routine blood monitoring, identifies individuals specifically at risk for valproate hepatotoxicity or any other drug-related idiosyncratic reaction. Clinical data, however, permit identification of groups of patients at increased risk for serious adverse drug reactions, including patients with known or suspected metabolic or biochemical disorders, a history of previous drug reactions, and medical illnesses affecting hematopoesis or liver and kidney function.

Antiepileptic Drug Pharmacology

Table 140.8 provides summary information about dose requirements, pharmacokinetic properties, and therapeutic concentration ranges for the major antiepileptic drugs available in the United States. Of patients with epilepsy, 60% to 70% achieve satisfactory control of seizures with currently available antiepileptic drugs, but fewer than 50% of adults achieve complete control without drug side effects. Many patients continue to have frequent seizures despite optimal medical therapy.

Therapy should start with a single antiepileptic drug chosen according to the type of seizure or epilepsy syndrome and then be modified, as necessary, by considerations of side effects, required dosing schedule, and cost. Phenytoin, phenobarbital, and

TABLE 140.6. TOXICITY OF ANTIEPILEPTIC DRUGS

Dose-Related adverse effects
  Systemic toxicity
    Gastrointestinal (dyspepsia, nausea, diarrhea)
    Benign elevation in liver enzymes
    Benign leukopenia
    Gingival hypertrophy
    Weight gain
    Anorexia
    Hair loss, change in hair texture
    Hirsutism
    Hyponatremia
    Coarsening of facial features
    Dupuytren contracture, frozen shoulder
    Osteoporosis
    Impotence.
  Neurologic toxicity
    Drowsiness, sedation
    Impaired cognition (memory, concentration)
    Depression and mood changes
    Irritability, hyperactivity
    Insomnia
    Dizziness/vertigo
    Nystagmus, diplopia
    Ataxia
    Tremor, asterixis
    Dyskinesias, dystonia, myoclonus
    Dysarthria
    Headache
    Sensory neuropathy
Idiosyncratic reactions
  Rash
  Exfoliative dermatitis
  Erythema multiforme
  Stevens-Johnson syndrome
  Agranulocytosis
  Aplastic anemia
  Hepatic failure
  Pancreatitis
  Connective tissue disorders
  Thrombocytopenia
  Pseudolymphoma syndrome

TABLE 140.7. EFFECT OF AGE AND TREATMENT ON RISK OF DEVELOPING FATAL VALPROATE HEPATOTOXICITY

Age	Monotherapy	Polytherapy
<2 yr	1/7,000	1/500
>2 yr	1/80,000	1/25,000

Modified from Dreifuss FE, Santilli N, Langer DH, et al. *Neurology* 1987;37:379–385.

TABLE 140.8. ANTIEPILEPTIC DRUGS: DOSAGE AND PHARMACOKINETIC DATA

Drug	Usual adult dose 24 hr (mg)	Half-life (hr)	Usually effective plasma concentration (μg/mL)	Time to peak concentration (hr)	Bound fraction (%)
Phenytoin	300–400	22	10–20	3–8	90–95
Carbamazepine	800–1,600	8–22	8–12	4–8	75
Phenobarbital	90–180	100	15–40	2–8	45
Valproate	1,000–3,000	15–20	50–120	3–8	80–90
Ethosuximide	750–1,500	60	40–100	3–7	<5
Felbamate	2,400–3,600	14–23	20–140	2–6	25
Gabapentin	1,800–3,600	5–7	>2[a]	2–3	<5
Lamotrigine	100–500	12–60[b]	1–4[a]	2–5	55
Topiramate	200–400	19–25[b]	2–25[a]	2–4	9–17
Vigabatrin	1,000–3,000	5–7	NE	1–4	5
Tiagabine	32–56	5–13	NE	1	95

[a]Not established; corresponds to usual range in patients treated with recommended dose.
[b]Highly dependent on concurrently administered drugs.
NE, not established.

gabapentin can be loaded acutely. In most cases, however, antiepileptic drugs should be started in low dosages to minimize acute toxicity and then increased according to the patient's tolerance and the drug's pharmacokinetics. The initial target dose should produce a serum concentration in the low-to-mid therapeutic range. Further increases can then be titrated according to the patient's clinical progress, which is measured mainly by seizure frequency and the occurrence of drug side effects. A drug should not be judged a failure unless seizures remain uncontrolled at the maximal tolerated dosage, regardless of the blood level.

Dosage changes generally should not be made until the effects of the drug have been observed at steady-state concentrations (a time about equal to five drug half-lives). If the first drug is ineffective, an appropriate alternative should be gradually substituted (Table 140.5). Combination treatment using two drugs should be attempted only when monotherapy with primary antiepileptic drugs fails. Combination therapy is sometimes effective, but the price of improved seizure control is often additional drug toxicity. Sometimes combination therapy with relatively nonsedating drugs (e.g., carbamazepine, lamotrigine, gabapentin, or valproate) is preferable to high-dose monotherapy with a sedating drug (e.g., phenobarbital or primidone). When used together, carbamazepine and lamotrigine result in a pharmacodynamic interaction that often produces neurotoxicity at dosages that are usually well tolerated when either drug is used alone.

Dosing intervals should usually be less than one-third to one-half the drug's half-life to minimize fluctuations between peak and trough blood concentrations. Large fluctuations can result in drug-induced side effects at peak levels and in breakthrough seizures at trough concentrations. Sometimes, however, a drug has a relatively long pharmacodynamic half-life, so that twice a day dosing is reasonable even if the pharmacokinetic half-life is short. This is typically the case with valproate, tiagabine, and, possibly, gabapentin.

Therapeutic drug monitoring has improved the care of patients with epilepsy, but published "therapeutic ranges" are only guidelines. Most patients who achieve drug concentrations within a standard therapeutic range usually achieve adequate seizure control with minimal side effects, but notable exceptions occur. Some patients develop unacceptable side effects at "subtherapeutic" concentrations; others benefit from "toxic" concentrations without adverse effects.

Determining serum drug concentrations when seizure control has been achieved or when side effects appear can assist in future management decisions. Drug levels are also useful in documenting compliance and in assessing the magnitude and significance of known or suspected drug interactions. Therapeutic drug monitoring is an essential guide to treating neonates, infants, young children, elderly persons, and patients with diseases (e.g., liver or kidney failure) or physiologic conditions (e.g., pregnancy) that alter drug pharmacokinetics. Although the total blood concentrations that are routinely reported are satisfactory for most indications, unbound ("free") concentrations are useful when protein binding is altered, as in renal failure, pregnancy, extensive third-degree burns, and combination therapy using two or more drugs that are highly bound to serum proteins (e.g., phenytoin, valproate, tiagabine).

Specific Drugs

Phenytoin is unique among antiepileptic drugs because it exhibits nonlinear elimination at therapeutically useful serum concentrations. That is, hepatic enzyme systems metabolizing phenytoin become increasingly saturated at plasma concentrations greater than 10 to 12 μg/mL and metabolic rate approaches a constant value at high concentrations. With increasing doses, phenytoin plasma concentrations rise exponentially (Fig. 140.5), so that steady-state concentration at one dose cannot be used to predict directly the steady-state concentration at a higher dose. Clinically, this requires cautious titration within the therapeutic range, using dose increments of 30 mg to avoid toxic effects.

Carbamazepine induces activation of the enzymes that metabolize it. The process, termed *autoinduction*, is time dependent. When carbamazepine is first introduced, the half-life ap-

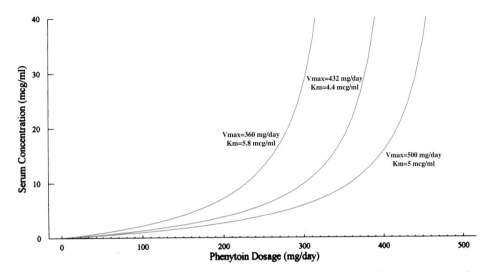

FIG. 140.5. Phenytoin dose-concentration curves from three representative adult patients. Note the markedly nonlinear relationship in the 200- to 400-mg dose range. Careful dose titration is necessary in this portion of the curve to avoid neurotoxicity. *Km*, Michaelis-Menten constant; *Vmax*, maximum elimination rate.

proximates 30 hours. With increasing hepatic clearance in the first 3 to 4 weeks of therapy, however, the half-life shortens to 11 to 20 hours. As a result, the starting dose should be low, the dosage should be increased gradually, and dosing should be frequent (three or four times daily). Recently introduced extended-release formulations now permit twice a day administration. The principal metabolite is carbamazepine-10,11-epoxide, which is pharmacologically active. Under certain circumstances (e.g., when coadministered with valproate or felbamate), the epoxide metabolite accumulates selectively, thereby producing neurotoxic effects even though the plasma concentration of the parent drug is in the therapeutic range or low.

Valproate is highly bound to plasma proteins, but the binding is concentration dependent and nonlinear. The unbound fraction increases at plasma concentrations greater than 75 μg/mL because protein binding sites become saturated. For example, doubling the plasma concentration from 75 to 150 μg/mL can result in a more than sixfold rise in concentration of free drug (from 6.5 to 45 μg/mL). Therefore, as the dose of valproate is increased, side effects may worsen rapidly because of the increasing proportion of unbound drug. Furthermore, adverse effects may vary in the course of a single day or from day to day, because concentrations of unbound drug fluctuate despite seemingly small changes in total blood levels. Additionally, circulating fatty acids displace valproate from protein binding sites. If fatty acid levels are high, the amount of unbound valproate increases. Lamotrigine and felbamate prolong valproates half-life; reduced dosage is typically necessary when these drugs are added.

Gabapentin requires an intestinal amino acid transport system for absorption. Because the transporter is saturable, the percentage of drug that is absorbed after an oral dose decreases with increasing dosage. More frequent dosing schedules using smaller amounts may therefore be necessary to increase blood levels. When dosages above 3,600 mg/day are used, blood levels can be helpful in demonstrating that an increase in dosage is reflected in an increased serum concentration. Gabapentin does not interact

to any clinically significant degree with any other drugs, which makes it especially useful when antiepileptic drug polytherapy is necessary and in patients with medical illnesses that also require drug treatment. It is not metabolized in the liver, but as it is excreted unchanged by the kidneys, dose adjustment is required in patients with renal failure.

Lamotrigine is very sensitive to coadministration of other antiepileptic drugs. Enzyme-inducing agents, such as phenytoin and carbamazepine, decrease lamotrigine's half-life from 24 to 16 hours (or less). In contrast, enzyme inhibition by valproate increases lamotrigine's half-life to 60 hours. Therefore, lamotrigine dosing depends very much on whether it is used as monotherapy or in combination with other antiepileptic drugs. Lamotrigine has little or no effect on other classes of drugs. Rash occurs in about 10% of patients; it is more common in children and rarely leads to Stevens-Johnson syndrome. The incidence of rash can be minimized by slow titration schedules.

Topiramate is also affected by coadministered antiepileptic drugs. Carbamazepine, phenytoin, and phenobarbital shorten topiramates half-life, but valproate has little effect. Topiramate does not affect most other drugs, although phenytoin blood levels may increase by 25%. Adverse cognitive effects frequently limit dosage, especially word-finding difficulties and memory impairment. These are usually dose dependent and can be minimized with slow titration schedules. Doses above 400 mg/day do not usually lead to better seizure control but are associated with an increasing incidence of side effects.

Tiagabine is highly bound to serum proteins and will therefore displace other drugs (e.g., phenytoin, valproate) that are also protein bound. Other drugs do not affect tiagabine's metabolism significantly. Gastrointestinal side effects usually limit the rate at which the dosage may be increased.

Felbamate has a much higher risk of serious adverse reactions, including aplastic anemia and hepatic failure, than other antiepileptic drugs. For this reason, its use is currently restricted to patients who are refractory to other agents and in whom the risk of continued seizures outweighs the risk of side effects. Use of felbamate is also limited by other common but less serious adverse effects, including anorexia, weight loss, insomnia, and nausea, and by numerous complex drug interactions. Nonetheless, felbamate remains useful in cases of severe epilepsy such as Lennox-Gastaut syndrome.

Gender-based differences in antiepileptic drug pharmacokinetics, sex steroid hormones, and reproductive life events raise special issues for women with epilepsy. The management of pregnancy in the woman with epilepsy is discussed in detail in Chapter 156. This section focuses on the effects of reproductive hormones on seizures and on the effects of seizures and antiepileptic drugs on reproductive health.

Although the prevalence of epilepsy is not higher in women, epilepsy in women may be specially affected by changes in reproductive steroids. Estrogen is a proconvulsant drug in animal models of epilepsy, whereas progesterone and its metabolites have anticonvulsant effects. Ovarian steroid hormones act at the neuronal membrane and on the genome to produce immediate and long-lasting effects on excitability. Estrogen reduces GABA-mediated inhibition, whereas progesterone enhances GABA effects. Estrogen also potentiates the action of excitatory neurotransmitters in some brain regions and increases the number of excitatory synapses. These dynamic and significant changes in neuronal excitability are observed with changes in estrogen and progesterone concentrations similar to those observed in the human menstrual cycle.

Approximately one-third of women with epilepsy report patterns of seizure occurrence that relate to phases of the menstrual cycle (*catamenial seizures*). Women with catamenial seizures indicate that seizures are more frequent, or more severe, just before menstruation and during the time of menstrual flow. In some women, seizures also increase at ovulation. These are times in the menstrual cycle when estrogen levels are relatively high and progesterone concentration is relatively low. Several small clinical trials have described benefit from chronic progesterone therapy in women with catamenial seizure patterns. Changes in seizures related to puberty and menopause are not well understood.

The pharmacokinetics of some antiepileptic drugs can complicate epilepsy management in women. Antiepileptic drugs that induce activity of the cytochrome P450 enzyme system (carbamazepine, phenytoin, phenobarbital, primidone, and, to a lesser extent, topiramate) interfere with the effectiveness of estrogen-based hormonal contraception. In women taking these drugs, the metabolism and binding of contraceptive steroids is enhanced, thus reducing the biologically active fraction of steroid hormone. The failure rate of oral contraceptive pills exceeds 6% per year in women taking enzyme-inducing antiepileptic drugs, in contrast to a failure rate of less that 1% per year in medication-compliant women without epilepsy. Women motivated to avoid pregnancy should consider using a contraceptive preparation containing 50 μg or more of an estrogenic compound or using an additional barrier method of contraception. Alternatively, they should discuss with their physician the possibility of selecting an antiepileptic drug that does not alter steroid metabolism or binding.

Reproductive health may be compromised in both women and men with epilepsy. Fertility rates for men and women with epilepsy are one-third to two-thirds those of men and women without epilepsy. Lower birth rates cannot be explained on the basis of lower marriage rates, because marriage rates for women with epilepsy are now similar to those of nonepileptic women. Reduced fertility appears to be the direct result of a disturbance in reproductive physiology.

Men and women with epilepsy show a higher than expected frequency of reproductive endocrine disturbances. These include abnormalities both in the cyclic release and concentration of pituitary luteinizing hormone and prolactin and in the concentration of gonadal steroid hormones. Some of these abnormalities are likely to be a consequence of seizure activity. Seizures involving mesial temporal lobe structures are associated with an immediate and significant (three- to fivefold) increase in pituitary prolactin levels. Similar disturbances have been reported with pituitary luteinizing hormone. Changes in these pituitary hormones may be one mechanism for the increased likelihood of anovulatory menstrual cycles and abnormalities in length of the menstrual cycle that are seen in about one-third of women with epilepsy. Antiepileptic drugs can also alter concentrations of gonadal steroids by affecting steroid hormone metabolism and binding. Antiepileptic drugs that increase steroid metabolism and binding reduce steroid hormone feedback at the hypothalamus and pituitary. Antiepileptic drugs that inhibit steroid metabolism (e.g., valproate) increase concentrations of steroid hormones, particularly androgens.

Polycystic ovaries are more common in women with epilepsy: Multiple ovarian cysts are detected in 25% to 40% of women with epilepsy. The basis of this association is not known but may be related to antiepileptic drugs (especially valproate) or to seizures. In nonepileptic women, polycystic ovaries are associated with infertility, carbohydrate intolerance (insulin resistance), dyslipidemia, and elevated lifetime risk for endometrial carcinoma and other gynecologic malignancies. The long-term consequences of polycystic ovaries in women with epilepsy are unknown.

Sexual dysfunction affects about one-third of men and women with epilepsy. Men report low sexual desire, difficulty achieving or maintaining an erection, or delayed ejaculation. Women with epilepsy can experience painful intercourse because of vaginismus and lack of lubrication. Although there are certainly psychosocial reasons for sexual dysfunction in some people with epilepsy, physiologic causes are demonstrable in others. Physiologic causes of sexual dysfunction include disruption of brain regions controlling sexual behavior by epileptogenic discharges, abnormalities of pituitary and gonadal hormones, and side effects of antiepileptic drugs.

Women with epilepsy who have difficulty conceiving, irregular or abnormal menstrual cycles, midcycle menstrual bleeding, sexual dysfunction, obesity, or hirsutism should undergo a reproductive endocrine evaluation. This includes pituitary luteinizing hormone and prolactin levels, estrogen, testosterone and progesterone levels, and ovarian ultrasound examination. Men with sexual dysfunction or difficulty conceiving should also have an endocrine evaluation and semen analysis. All the reproductive disorders seen in people with epilepsy are potentially treatable.

Discontinuing Antiepileptic Drugs

Epidemiologic studies indicate that 60% to 70% of patients with epilepsy become free of seizures for at least 5 years within 10 years of diagnosis. Similarly, prospective clinical trials of treated patients whose seizures were in remission for 2 years or more showed that a nearly identical percentage of patients remained seizure free after drug withdrawal. These studies also identified predictors that permit patients to be classified as being at low or high risk for seizure relapse after drug therapy ends. The risk of relapse was high if patients required more than one antiepileptic drug to control seizures, if seizure control was difficult to establish, if the patient had a history of generalized tonic-clonic seizures, and if the EEG was significantly abnormal when drug withdrawal was considered. Continued freedom from seizures is favored by longer seizure-free intervals (up to 4 years) before drug withdrawal is attempted, few seizures before remission, monotherapy, normal EEG and examination, and no difficulty establishing seizure control.

All benign epilepsy syndromes of childhood carry an excellent prognosis for permanent drug-free remission. In contrast, juvenile myoclonic epilepsy has a high rate of relapse when drugs are discontinued, even in patients who have been seizure free for years. The prognosis for most other epilepsy syndromes is largely unknown.

Discontinuing antiepileptic drug therapy in appropriate patients is reasonable when they have been seizure free for at least 2 years. The most powerful argument for stopping antiepileptic drugs is concern about long-term systemic and neurologic toxicity, which may be insidious and not apparent for many years after a drug has been introduced. On the other hand, however, is the concern of the patient or family about seizure recurrence. Even a single seizure can have disastrous psychosocial and vocational consequences, particularly in adults. Therefore, the decision to withdraw drugs must be weighed carefully in the light of individual circumstances. If a decision is made to discontinue antiepileptic drugs, we favor slow withdrawal, over 3 to 6 months, but this recommendation is controversial because few studies have been conducted of different withdrawal rates.

SURGICAL TREATMENT

Surgery should be considered when seizures are uncontrolled by optimal medical management and when they disrupt the quality of life. Quantifying these issues, however, has defied strict definition, perhaps deservedly, because intractability is clearly more than continued seizures. Only patients know how their lives differ from what they would like them to be; the concept of *disability* includes both physical and psychologic components. Some patients with refractory seizures suffer little disability; others, for whatever reason, find their lives severely compromised by infrequent attacks. Still others have had their seizures completely cured by surgery but are still disabled and incapable of functioning productively. The determination of which patients are "medically refractory" and which are "satisfactorily controlled" can always be argued in the abstract. Fortunately, there is usually general agreement in practice about which patients should be referred for surgical evaluation.

Few patients benefit from further attempts at medical treatment if seizures have not been controlled after two trials of high-dose monotherapy using two appropriate drugs and one trial of combination therapy. These therapeutic efforts can be accomplished within 1 to 2 years; the detrimental effects of continued seizures or drug toxicity warrant referral to a specialized center after that time.

There are few blanket contraindications to epilepsy surgery today, although patients with severe concurrent medical illness and progressive neurologic syndromes are usually excluded. Some centers prefer not to operate on patients with psychosis or other serious psychiatric disorder, those older than 50, and those with an IQ of less than 70. Patients in these categories, however, must be considered individually. Many patients who undergo corpus callosum section for atonic seizures associated with Lennox-Gastaut syndrome have an IQ under 70. Although surgery for epilepsy is increasingly performed in children, functional resections in infancy remain controversial for several reasons: the uncertain natural history of seizures in many of these patients; the unknown effects of surgery on the immature brain; and the lack of data about long-term neurologic, behavioral, and psychologic outcomes.

Because of technical advances in imaging and electrophysiologic monitoring, epilepsy surgery is no longer automatically contraindicated in patients with multifocal interictal epileptiform abnormalities or even foci near language or other eloquent cortical areas.

Resective Procedures

Focal brain resection is the most common type of epilepsy surgery. Resection is appropriate if seizures begin in an identifiable and restricted cortical area, if the surgical excision will encompass all or most of the epileptogenic tissue, and if the resection will not impair neurologic function. These criteria are met most often by patients with temporal lobe epilepsy, but extratemporal resections are increasingly common.

Anterior Temporal Lobe Resection

This resective procedure is the most common, but the operation varies in what is considered "standard," especially with regard to how much lateral neocortical and mesial limbic structures are removed. At our institution, most patients with unilateral temporal foci undergo Spencer's (1991) anteromedial temporal lobe resection, which includes removal of the anterior middle and inferior temporal gyri, parahippocampal gyrus, 3.5 to 4 cm of hippocampus, and a variable amount of amygdala. For nondominant foci, this approach is slightly modified to include the anterior superior temporal gyrus as well. Patients with medial temporal lobe epilepsy associated with hippocampal sclerosis are ideal candidates for anterior temporal lobe resection, because over 80% will become seizure free with the remainder having substantial improvement.

Lesionectomy

Well-circumscribed epileptogenic structural lesions (cavernous malformations, hamartomas, gangliogliomas, and other encapsulated tumors) can be removed by stereotactic microsurgery. The extent to which tissue margins surrounding the lesion are included in the resection depends on how the margins are defined (radiologic, visual, electrophysiologic, or histologic inspection) and the surgeon's preference. Seizures are controlled by this method in 50% to 60% of patients. A lesion involving the cerebral cortex should always be considered the source of a patient's seizures unless compelling EEG evidence suggests otherwise.

Nonlesional Cortical Resections

When a lesion cannot be visualized by MRI, it is difficult to demonstrate a restricted ictal onset zone outside the anterior temporal lobe. This situation almost always requires placement of intracranial electrodes to map the extent of epileptogenic tissue and to determine its relation to functional brain areas. Outcome after nonlesional cortical resections is not as good as with anterior temporal lobectomy or lesionectomy, mainly because the boundaries of epileptogenic cortical areas often cannot be delineated precisely, and removal of all the epileptogenic tissue often is not possible.

Corpus Callosotomy

Section of the corpus callosum disconnects the two hemispheres and is indicated for treatment of patients with uncontrolled atonic or tonic seizures in the absence of an identifiable focus suitable for resection. Most patients referred for corpus callosotomy have severe and frequent seizures of multiple types, usually with mental retardation and a severely abnormal EEG (the Lennox-Gastaut syndrome).

Unlike resective surgery, corpus callosotomy is palliative, not curative. Nonetheless, it can be strikingly effective for generalized seizures, with 80% of patients experiencing complete or nearly complete cessation of atonic, tonic, and tonic-clonic attacks. This outcome is often remarkably beneficial because it eliminates falls and the associated self-injury. The effect on partial seizures, however, is inconsistent and unpredictable. Complex partial seizures are reduced or eliminated in about half the patients, but simple or complex partial seizures are exacerbated in about 25%. Therefore, refractory partial seizures alone are not an indication for corpus callosotomy. Similarly, absence, atypical absence, and myoclonic seizures either do not benefit or show an inconsistent response.

Hemispherectomy

Removal or disconnection of large cortical areas from one side of the brain is indicated when the epileptogenic lesion involves most or all of one hemisphere. Because hemispherectomy guarantees permanent hemiplegia, hemisensory loss, and usually hemianopia, it can be considered only in children with a unilateral structural lesion that has already resulted in those abnormalities and who have refractory unilateral seizures. Examples of conditions suitable for hemispherectomy include infantile hemiplegia syndromes, Sturge-Weber disease, Rasmussen syndrome, and severe unilateral developmental anomalies, such as hemimegalencephaly. In appropriate patients, the results are dramatic. Seizures cease, behavior improves, and development accelerates (Table 140.9).

Preoperative Evaluation

The objective in evaluating patients for focal resection is to demonstrate that all seizures originate in a limited cortical area that can be removed safely. This determination requires more extensive evaluation than is necessary in the routine management of patients with epilepsy. The different tests used provide complementary information about normal and epileptic brain functions.

CCTV/EEG monitoring is necessary to record a representative sample of the patient's typical seizures to confirm the diagnosis and classification and also to localize the cortical area involved in ictal onset. Volumetric or other special MRI techniques may demonstrate unilateral hippocampal atrophy or other anatomic abnormalities that may be epileptogenic. Positron emission tomography and ictal single-photon emission CT are useful to demonstrate focal abnormalities in glucose metabolism or cerebral blood flow that correspond to the epileptogenic brain region. Neuropsychologic testing is useful in demonstrating focal cognitive dysfunction, especially language and memory. Intracarotid injection of amobarbital (the *Wada test*) to determine hemispheric dominance for language and memory competence is generally considered necessary before temporal lobectomy, but the implications of a failed test are uncertain.

Intracranial electrodes are necessary if noninvasive methods do not unequivocally localize the epileptogenic area or if different noninvasive tests give conflicting results. Intracranial electrode placement is also necessary when vital brain functions (language, motor cortex) must be mapped in relation to the planned resection.

Vagal Nerve Stimulation

Vagal nerve stimulation is a novel nonpharmacologic treatment for medically refractory partial seizures. Like corpus callosotomy, vagal nerve stimulation is a palliative procedure, because very few patients become seizure free. Vagal nerve stimulation is delivered via a stimulating lead attached to the left vagus nerve. The stimulus generator is implanted in the upper left chest. The device is

TABLE 140.9. OUTCOME AFTER EPILEPSY SURGICAL PROCEDURES

Procedure	Seizure free (%)	Improved (%)	Not improved (%)
Anterior temporal lobectomy (n = 3,579)	68.8	22.2	9.0
Lesionectomy (n = 293)	66.6	21.5	11.9
Nonlesional extratemporal neocortical resection (n = 805)	45.1	35.2	19.8
Hemispherectomy (n = 190)	67.4	21.1	11.6
Corpus callosum section (n = 563)	7.6	60.9	31.4

Modified from Engel J Jr. *Surgical treatment of the epilepsies,* 2nd ed. New York: Raven Press, 1993.

usually programmed to give a 3-second electrical pulse every 5 minutes, although stimulus parameters can be adjusted to the requirements of an individual patient. In patients with aura, a magnetic wand can be used to deliver vagal nerve stimulation on demand, which may abort seizure progression. About 30% to 35% of patients have at least a 50% reduction in seizure frequency, which compares favorably with the efficacy of new antiepileptic drugs. Chronic adverse effects include hoarseness and difficulty swallowing, both of which increase at the time of stimulation.

REPRODUCTIVE HEALTH ISSUES

Status Epilepticus

Convulsive status epilepticus is a medical emergency, and failure to treat the condition in a timely and appropriate manner can result in serious systemic and neurologic morbidity. At least 65,000 cases of status epilepticus occur each year in the United States. It is diagnosed if seizures last longer than 10 minutes or if two or more seizures occur in close succession without recovery of consciousness.

Status epilepticus may be either *convulsive* or *nonconvulsive*. The most life-threatening pattern, and that requiring the most urgent treatment, is convulsive status epilepticus, which, like seizures and epileptic syndromes, may be a manifestation either of idiopathic (i.e., nonfocal) epilepsy or secondary to spread from a localized epileptogenic brain region. Nonconvulsive status epilepticus occurs as a kind of twilight confusional state and is caused by either continuing generalized absence seizures or complex partial seizures.

Status epilepticus is most frequent in infants and young children and in elderly persons, but it occurs at all ages. More than 50% of those affected do not have a history of epilepsy. In about 10% of patients with epilepsy, status epilepticus is the first manifestation, and about 15% of patients with epilepsy have had one or more episodes of status at some time.

In two-thirds of cases of status epilepticus, an acute cause or precipitating factor, such as systemic metabolic derangement, alcohol or other drug abuse, hypoxia, head trauma, infection, or a cerebral lesion, such as a stroke or tumor, can be identified. Therefore, part of the emergency evaluation of patients in status is determining the probable cause (Table 140.10).

Convulsive Status Epilepticus

Convulsive status epilepticus generates metabolic and physiologic stresses that contribute to permanent brain damage, including hyperthermia, hypoxia, lactic acidosis, hypoglycemia, and hypotension. Plasma catecholamine levels are acutely elevated during the attack and may trigger fatal cardiac arrhythmias. Death usually results from the underlying condition rather than from the status epilepticus itself. Nonetheless, death from status epilepticus per se occurs in 2% to 3% of children and in 7% to 10% of adults.

The goals of treatment are to eliminate all seizure activity and to identify and treat any underlying medical or neurologic disorder. Initial management is that of any comatose patient: to ensure airway and oxygenation, to access circulation and maintain

TABLE 140.10. CAUSES OF STATUS EPILEPTICUS

Diagnosis	Children (%)	Adults (%)
Stroke	3	25
Drug change/noncompliance	20	20
Alcohol/other drugs	2	15
Central nervous system infection	5	10
Hypoxia	5	10
Metabolic	10	10
Tumor	<1	5
Trauma	3.5	5
Fever/infection	35	2
Congenital	10	<1

Modified from Hauser WA. *Neurology* 1990;40[Suppl 2]:9–13; and DeLorenzo RJ, Towne AR, Pellock JM, et al. *Epilepsia* 1992;33[Suppl 4]:S15–S25.

blood pressure, and to monitor cardiac function (Table 140.11). Blood should be obtained for antiepileptic drug levels, blood count, and routine chemistries. Brain imaging should be done in all adult patients with status epilepticus and in all children with nonfebrile status epilepticus. Patients should be in stable condition, and CT is usually sufficient to exclude an acute brain lesion. MRI should be obtained later if the CT was normal. Lumbar puncture should be performed in any febrile patient, even if

TABLE 140.11. PROTOCOL AND TIMETABLE FOR TREATING STATUS EPILEPTICUS IN ADULTS AT THE NEUROLOGICAL INSTITUTE OF NEW YORK, COLUMBIA-PRESBYTERIAN MEDICAL CENTER

Time (min)	Action
0–5	Diagnose; give O_2; ABCs; obtain i.v. access; begin ECG monitoring; draw blood for chem-7, Mg, Ca, CBC, AED levels, ABG; toxicology screen
6–10	Thiamine 100 mg i.v.; 50 mL of D50 i.v. unless adequate glucose level known
	Lorazepam (Ativan) 4 mg i.v. over 2 min; repeat once in 8–10 min p.r.n.
	Or
	Diazepam (Valium) 10 mg i.v. over 2 min; repeat once in 3–5 min p.r.n.
10–20	If status persists or if it was stopped with diazepam, immediately begin fosphenytoin (Cerebyx) 20 mg/kg i.v. at 150 mg/min, with blood pressure and ECG monitoring
20–30	If status persists, give additional 5 mg/kg fosphenytoin two times (total 30 mg/kg)
30+	If status persists, intubate and give one of the following (in order of our preference), preferably with EEG monitoring:
	1. Phenobarbital 20 mg/kg i.v. at 50–100 mg/min. Additional 5-mg/kg boluses can be given as needed; *or*
	2. Midazolam continuous infusion, 0.2 mg/kg slow bolus, then 0.1–2.0 mg/kg/hr; *or*
	3. Propofol continuous infusion, 1–5 mg/kg bolus over 5 min, then 2–4 mg/kg/hr

ABCs, airway, blood pressure, cardiac function; ECG; electrocardiogram; CBC; complete blood count; AED, antiepileptic drug; ABG, arterial blood gas; D50, 50% dextrose in water; EEG, electroencephalogram.
From Dodson et al. (1993), Lowenstein and Alldredge (1998), and Treiman et al. (1998).

signs of meningitis are not present. If brain infection is strongly suspected, the need for lumbar puncture is urgent, and the procedure should be carried out immediately. If signs of increased intracranial pressure are apparent or if a mass lesion is suspected, antibiotics should be given immediately and a CT obtained first.

If the history is at all uncertain, glucose should be given, preceded by thiamine in adults. Although several antiepileptic drug regimens are effective for treating status epilepticus, we begin with lorazepam, 0.1 mg/kg, or diazepam, 0.2 mg/kg, followed immediately by phenytoin (or fosphenytoin), 20 mg/kg. If there is no response, additional phenytoin (or fosphenytoin), 5 mg/kg, should be administered. If status persists, the patient should be intubated and anesthetized with pentobarbital or midazolam with EEG monitoring to ensure complete suppression of all electrical ictal activity.

Fosphenytoin is a phosphate ester prodrug of phenytoin. Unlike intravenous phenytoin, fosphenytoin is compatible with all intravenous solutions in common use. Because it is much less alkaline, it causes only minimal local irritation and can be infused at much faster rates than phenytoin. After entering the blood, fosphenytoin is converted rapidly to phenytoin by phosphatases in the liver and red blood cells. Fosphenytoins pharmacologic properties are identical to those of phenytoin and is dosed in phenytoin equivalents. Unique side effects are paresthesias in the low back and groin, probably due to the phosphate load.

After the patient has been stabilized and seizures controlled, a rigorous search for an underlying condition should be instituted.

Nonconvulsive Status Epilepticus

This condition is difficult to diagnose clinically and is frequently unrecognized. Patients are most often middle-aged or elderly and usually have no past history of seizures. Onset is generally abrupt, and all patients show altered mentation and behavioral changes that typically last for days to weeks. Patients in nonconvulsive status are characteristically alert (although dull), and the absence of stupor or coma contributes to misdiagnosis. A psychiatric diagnosis is often the first consideration if the condition presents as bizarre behavior and change in affect, often with hallucinations, paranoia, or catatonia. When memory loss, disorientation, and mood changes predominate, diagnostic possibilities include dementia, stroke, or metabolic/toxic encephalopathy.

Once the suspicion of nonconvulsive status epilepticus has been raised, diagnosis depends on demonstrating ictal patterns in the EEG while the patient is symptomatic. Most patients show continuous or nearly continuous 1- to 2.5-Hz generalized spike-wave ("atypical spike-wave") activity. In these cases, status epilepticus is presumed to be a manifestation of generalized-onset epilepsy akin to absence status epilepticus in children. Occasionally, the EEG ictal activity is localized, usually to the frontal or temporal lobes, thus indicating that in these patients the nonconvulsive status is a form of continuous partial seizure activity.

Diagnosis of nonconvulsive status epilepticus is confirmed by the response to intravenous diazepam (5 to 10 mg) or lorazepam (1 to 2 mg): Epileptiform EEG abnormalities disappear, and the patient's mental state reverts to normal. Long-term seizure control is achieved using valproate, phenytoin, or carbamazepine.

Laboratory studies are usually normal, but occasionally they identify a cause for the nonconvulsive status epilepticus, such as

nonketotic hyperglycemia, electrolyte imbalance, drug toxicity (e.g., lithium), or a focal cerebral lesion (e.g., frontal lobe infarction).

GENE DEFECTS IN EPILEPSY

Genetic factors have been implicated strongly in several epilepsy syndromes, and twin studies have confirmed important genetic determinants in both localization-related and generalized types of seizure disorders. Hereditary aspects are easiest to discern in childhood absence epilepsy, juvenile myoclonic epilepsy, benign rolandic epilepsy, and idiopathic grand mal seizures. However, genetic epidemiologic studies have demonstrated clearly that complex polygenic susceptibilities exist in both the idiopathic and symptomatic epilepsies. Thus, a major challenge facing investigators today is to clarify how different genes alter an individual's susceptibility to seizures and epilepsy in the presence of acquired brain pathology or as a reaction to acute or subacute cerebral dysfunction. This is no easy task, however, because the number of genes that encode molecules that regulate cortical excitability directly through membrane and synaptic functions and the second messenger cascades that indirectly regulate membrane proteins involved in signal transduction is very large.

These considerations imply a continuum between idiopathic and symptomatic epilepsies, with the development of epilepsy deriving from the complex interrelation of genetic factors and brain pathology. In any given patient, therefore, the relative contribution of genetic or acquired pathologic factors determines whether the epilepsy presents clinically as an idiopathic disorder or a symptomatic one.

Linkage studies have identified specific gene loci for several human epilepsies (Table 140.12). Genes have been identified for three autosomal recessive progressive myoclonic epilepsies (Unverricht-Lundborg disease, Lafora disease, and the form of neuronal ceroid lipofuchsinosis known as Batten's disease), an autosomal dominant idiopathic generalized epilepsy (benign familial neonatal seizures), an autosomal dominant form of febrile seizures, and one type of idiopathic partial epilepsy (autosomal dominant nocturnal frontal lobe epilepsy). The defective gene in Unverricht-Lundborg disease encodes cystatin B, a ubiquitous inhibitor of cysteine protease, a lysosomal enzyme that cannot, at the present time, be related easily to any known epileptogenic mechanism, although programmed neuronal cell death may be involved. An abnormal potassium-channel gene results in the syndrome of benign familial neonatal seizures, and an abnormal sodium channel gene leads to an autosomal dominant form of febrile seizures. Some, but not all, families with autosomal dominant frontal lobe epilepsy have an abnormality in the gene for the α 4-subunit of the neuronal nicotinic acetylcholine receptor. A point mutation in mitochondrial DNA results in myoclonic epilepsy with ragged red fibers (MERRF).

PSYCHOSOCIAL AND PSYCHIATRIC ISSUES

The impact of epilepsy on the quality of life is usually greater than the limitations imposed by the seizures alone. The diagnosis of epilepsy frequently carries other consequences that can

TABLE 140.12. HUMAN EPILEPSY GENES AND GENE DEFECTS

Syndrome	Chromosome/gene location	Gene product
Unverricht-Lundborg disease	21q22	Cystatin B
Nocturnal frontal lobe epilepsy	20q13	α-4-nicotinic Ach receptor
Benign familial infantile convulsions	20q13 and 8q24	Voltage-gated K$^+$ channel
Batten's disease	16	CLN3 gene: 1.02 kb deletion (loss of function?)
Autosomal dominant febrile seizures	19q	Voltage-gated Na$^+$ channel
Tuberous sclerosis (TSC2)	16	rasGAP-like signaling molecule
Lafora's disease	6q24	Laforin (protein tyrosine phosphate)

greatly alter the lives of many patients. For adults, the most important problems are discrimination at work and driving restrictions, which lead to loss of mobility and independence. Children and adults alike may be shunned by uninformed friends. Patients must learn to avoid situations that precipitate seizures, and a change in lifestyle may be necessary. Common factors that increase the likelihood of seizure occurrence include sleep deprivation, alcohol (and other drugs), and emotional stress (Table 140.13). Compliance with antiepileptic drug treatment is often an issue, especially with adolescents. Psychiatric symptoms, especially depression, may complicate management.

Some restrictions are medically appropriate, at least for limited times. For example, when seizures impair consciousness or judgment, driving and certain kinds of employment (working at exposed heights or with power equipment) and a few other activities (swimming alone) should be interdicted. On the other hand, legal prohibitions on driving vary in different states in the United States and in different countries and are often not medically justified. Employers frequently have unrealistic fears about the physical effects of a seizure, the potential for liability, and the impact on insurance costs. In fact, the Americans with Disabilities Act prohibits denying employment to persons with disability if the disability does not prevent them from meeting job requirements.

Children have special problems because their seizures affect the entire family. Parents may, with the best of intentions, handicap the child by being overly restrictive. The necessary and special attention received by the "sick" child may encourage passive manipulative behavior and overdependence while unintentionally exacerbating normal sibling rivalries.

TABLE 140.13. FACTORS THAT LOWER THE SEIZURE THRESHOLD

Common	Occasional
Sleep deprivation	Barbiturate withdrawal
Alcohol withdrawal	Hyperventilation
Stress	Flashing lights
Dehydration	Diet and missed meals
Drugs and drug interactions	Specific "reflex" triggers
Systemic infection	
Trauma	
Malnutrition	

The physician must be sensitive to these important quality of life concerns, even when they are not raised spontaneously by the patient or family. In fact, psychosocial issues often become the major focus of follow-up visits after the diagnosis has been made, the initial evaluation completed, and treatment started. We cannot emphasize too much the physician's responsibility to educate society to counter misperceptions and prejudices and to separate myth from medical fact. The Epilepsy Foundation (Landover, Maryland; 1-800-EFA-1000; www.efa.org) and its nationwide system of affiliates have a wealth of materials about epilepsy suitable for patient, family, and public education.

Compliance

The most common cause of breakthrough seizures is noncompliance with the prescribed therapeutic regimen. Only about 70% of patients take antiepileptic medications as prescribed. For phenytoin or carbamazepine, noncompliance can be inferred when sequential blood levels vary by more than 20%, assuming similarly timed samples and unchanged dosage. Persistently low antiepileptic drug levels in the face of increasing dosage also generally imply poor compliance. Caution is warranted with phenytoin, however, because as many as 20% of patients have low levels as a result of poor absorption or rapid metabolism.

Noncompliance is especially common in adolescents and elderly persons, when seizures are infrequent or not perceived as disabling, when antiepileptic drugs must be taken several times each day, and when toxic effects persist. Compliance can be improved by patient education, by simplifying drug regimens, and by tailoring dosing schedules to the patient's daily routines. Pill box devices that alert the patient to scheduled doses can be useful.

Depression and Psychosis

In referral centers, depression and suicide are more common in patients with epilepsy than in patients with other neurologic disorders or in disease-free control subjects. Whether this predilection is true for the epilepsy population at large is not known because few community-based population studies have been conducted. Depression in epilepsy may be influenced by several factors: the type or severity of the seizures, the location of the epileptogenic focus, associated neurologic or medical conditions, the antiepileptic drugs used, and by the personal stigma and limitations that accompany the diagnosis. Curiously, depression sometimes follows successful epilepsy surgery.

Treatment of depression begins with optimal treatment of the seizure disorder. Barbiturate and succinimide drugs may adversely affect mood, inducing symptoms that mimic endogenous depression. Although tricyclic antidepressants reduce the seizure threshold in experimental models of epilepsy, this is not a practical concern because they only rarely trigger seizures or increase seizure frequency in humans. Monoamine oxidase inhibitors neither induce seizures nor increase seizure frequency. Modern electroconvulsive therapy does not worsen epilepsy. We have used both sertraline and fluoxetine without exacerbating seizures.

The relation between psychosis and epilepsy is controversial. No convincing evidence shows that interictal psychosis is a manifestation of epilepsy, but some demographic features are overrepresented in patients with epilepsy.

Phenothiazines, butyrophenones, and clozapine lower seizure threshold in experimental animals and occasionally seem to induce seizures in nonepileptic patients. Most occurrences have been associated with high drug doses or a rapid increase in dose. With the possible exception of clozapine, however, little evidence supports the notion that reasonable and conservative use of antipsychotic medications increases seizure frequency in patients with epilepsy.

Interictal aggressive behavior is not more common in people with epilepsy. Directed aggression during seizures occurs in less than 0.02% of patients with severe epilepsy; it is almost certainly less common in the general epilepsy population. Undirected pushing or resistance occasionally occurs postictally when attempts are made to restrain confused patients.

Postictal psychosis is a limited period of psychosis that follows a flurry of seizures, usually after an interval of appropriate behavior. This uncommon condition does not lead to chronic psychosis.

SUGGESTED READINGS

American EEG Society. Guidelines for long-term neurodiagnostic monitoring in epilepsy. *J Clin Neurophysiol* 1994;11:88–110.

Annegers JF, Hauser WA, Coan SP, Rocca WA. A population-based study of seizures after traumatic brain injuries. *N Engl J Med* 1998;338:20–24.

Bazil CW, Pedley TA. Advances in the medical treatment of epilepsy. *Annu Rev Med* 1998;49:135–162.

Berg AT, Shinnar S. The risk of seizure recurrence following a first unprovoked seizure: a quantitative review. *Neurology* 1991;41:965–972.

Berkovic SF, Scheffer IE. Epilepsies with single gene inheritance. *Brain Dev* 1997;19:13–18.

Brodie MJ, Dichter MA. Antiepileptic drugs. *N Engl J Med* 1996;334:168–175.

Cascino GD, Jack CR, Parisi JE, et al. Magnetic resonance imaging-based volume studies in temporal lobe epilepsy: pathological correlations. *Ann Neurol* 1991;30:31–36.

Cendes F, Cramanos Z, Andermann F, Dubeau F, Arnold DL. Proton magnetic resonance spectroscopic imaging and magnetic resonance imaging volumetry in the lateralization of temporal lobe epilepsy: a series of 100 patients. *Ann Neurol* 1997;42:737–746.

Delgado-Escueta AV, Mattson RH, King L, et al. The nature of aggression during epileptic seizures. *N Engl J Med* 1981;305:711–716.

DeLorenzo RJ, Pellock JM, Towne AR, Boggs JG. Epidemiology of status epilepticus. *J Clin Neurophysiol* 1995;12:316–325.

Devinsky O. *A guide to understanding and living with epilepsy*. Philadelphia: FA Davis, 1994.

Dodson WE, DeLorenzo RJ, Pedley TA, et al. Treatment of convulsive status epilepticus: recommendations of the Epilepsy Foundation of America's working group on status epilepticus. *JAMA* 1993;270:854–859.

Dreifuss FE, Rosman NP, Clloyd JC, et al. A comparison of rectal diazepam gel and placebo for acute repetitive seizures. *N Engl J Med* 1998;338:1869–1875.

Dreifuss FE, Santilli N, Langer DH, et al. Valproic acid hepatic fatalities: a retrospective review. *Neurology* 1987;37:379–385.

Engel J Jr, ed. *Surgical treatment of the epilepsies*, 2nd ed. New York: Raven Press, 1993.

Engel J Jr, Pedley TA, eds. *Epilepsy: a comprehensive textbook*. Philadelphia: Lippincott-Raven, 1998.

First Seizure Trial Group. Randomized clinical trial on the efficacy of antiepileptic drugs in reducing the risk of relapse after a first unprovoked tonic-clonic seizure. *Neurology* 1993;43:478–483.

Hauser WA. Status epilepticus: epidemiologic considerations. *Neurology* 1990;40[Suppl 2]:9–13.

Hauser WA, Annegers JF, Kurland LT. Incidence of epilepsy and unprovoked seizures in Rochester, Minnesota: 1935–1984. *Epilepsia* 1993;34:453–468.

Hauser WA, Hesdorffer DC. *Epilepsy: frequency, causes and consequences*. New York: Demos, 1990.

Hauser WA, Rich SS, Annegers, JF, Anderson VE. Seizure recurrence after a 1st unprovoked seizure: an extended follow-up. *Neurology* 1990;40:1163–1170.

Hauser WA, Rich SS, Lee JR-J, Annegers JF, Anderson VE. Risk of recurrent seizures after two unprovoked seizures. *N Engl J Med* 1998;338:429–434.

Herman ST, Pedley TA. New options for the treatment of epilepsy. *JAMA* 1998;280:693–694.

Jackson GD, Berkovic SF, Tress BM, et al. Hippocampal sclerosis can be reliably detected by magnetic resonance imaging. *Neurology* 1990;40:1869–1875.

Krauss GL, Johnson MA, Miller NR. Vigabatrin-associated retinal cone system dysfunction. Electroretinogram and ophthalmologic findings. *Neurology* 1998;50:614–618.

Kuzniecky R, Hugg JW, Hetherington H, et al. Relative utility of ^{1}H spectroscopic imaging and hippocampal volumetry in the lateralization of mesial temporal lobe epilepsy. *Neurology* 1998;51:66–71.

Langendorf F, Pedley TA. Post-traumatic seizures. In: Engel J Jr, Pedley TA, eds. *Epilepsy: a comprehensive textbook*. Philadelphia: Lippincott-Raven, 1998:2469–2474.

Lee SI. Non-convulsive status epilepticus. Ictal confusion in later life. *Arch Neurol* 1985;42:778–781.

Lowenstein DH, Alldredge BK. Status epilepticus. *N Engl J Med* 1998;338:970–976.

Mattson RH, Cramer JA, Collins JF. Comparison of valproate with carbamazepine for the treatment of complex partial seizures and secondarily generalized tonic-clonic seizures in adults. *N Engl J Med* 1992;327:765–771.

Mattson RH, Cramer JA, Collins JF, et al. A comparison of carbamazepine, phenobarbital, phenytoin, and primidone in partial and secondarily generalized tonic-clonic seizures. *N Engl J Med* 1985;313:145–151.

McNamara JO. Emerging insights into the genesis of epilepsy. *Nature* 1999;399 (Suppl):A15–A22.

Medical Research Council Antiepileptic Drug Withdrawal Study Group. Randomised study of antiepileptic drug withdrawal in patients in remission. *Lancet* 1991;337:1175–1180.

Morrell MJ. Hormones, reproductive health, and epilepsy. In: Wyllie E, ed. *The treatment of epilepsy: principles and practice*, 2nd ed. Baltimore: Williams & Wilkins, 1996:179–187.

Morrell MJ. Sexuality in epilepsy. In: Engel J Jr, Pedley TA, eds. *Epilepsy: a comprehensive textbook*. New York: Lippincott-Raven, 1998:2021–2026.

Musicco M, Beghi E, Solari A, et al. Treatment of first tonic-clonic seizure does not improve the prognosis of epilepsy. *Neurology* 1997;49:991–998.

Pellock JM, Willmore LJ. A rational guide to routine blood monitoring in patients receiving antiepileptic drugs. *Neurology* 1991;41:961–964.

Prasad AN, Prasad C, Stafstrom CE, Recent advances in the genetics of epilepsy: Insights from human and animal studies. *Epilepsia* 1999;40:1329–1352.

Salazar AM, Jabbari B, Vance SC, et al. Epilepsy after penetrating head injury. I. Clinical correlates: a report of the Vietnam Head Injury Study. *Neurology* 1985;35:1406–1414.

Sillanpaa M, Jalava M, Kaleva O, Shinnar S. Long-term prognosis of seizures with onset in childhood. *N Engl J Med* 1998;338:1715– 1722.

Spencer DD. Anteromedial temporal lobectomy: directing the surgical approach to the pathologic substrate. In: Spencer SS, Spencer DD, eds. *Surgery for epilepsy.* Boston: Blackwell Scientific, 1991.

Sperling MR, Feldman H, Kirman J, et al. Seizure control and mortality in epilepsy. *Ann Neurol* 1999;46:45–50.

Temkin NR, Dikmen SS, Wilensky AJ, et al. A randomized, double blind study of phenytoin for the prevention of post-traumatic seizures. *N Engl J Med* 1990;323:497–502.

Treiman DM, Meyers PD, Walton NY, et al. A comparison of four treatments for generalized convulsive status epilepticus. *N Engl J Med* 1998;339:792–798.

Walczak TS, Radtke RA, McNamara JO, et al. Anterior temporal lobectomy for complex partial seizures: evaluation, results, and long-term follow-up of 100 cases. *Neurology* 1990;40:413–418.

Zahn CA, Morrell MJ, Collins SD, et al. Management issues for women with epilepsy: a review of the literature. American Academy of Neurology Practice Guidelines. *Neurology* 1998;51:949–956.

Merritt's Neurology, 10th ed., edited by L.P. Rowland. Lippincott Williams & Wilkins, Philadelphia © 2000.

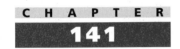

FEBRILE SEIZURES

DOUGLAS R. NORDLI, JR.
TIMOTHY A. PEDLEY

Febrile seizures are generalized convulsions that occur during a febrile illness that does not involve the brain. They represent acute symptomatic or reactive seizures, and even when recurrent they do not warrant the designation of epilepsy. Most febrile seizures occur in children between the ages of 6 months and 4 years; they are occasionally seen in children as old as 6 or 7 years.

Febrile seizures are the most frequent cause of a convulsion in a child: Between 3% and 5% of all children in the United States and Europe and 6% to 9% of children in Japan have at least one febrile seizure before age 5 years. Hauser (1994) estimated 100,000 cases of febrile seizures in the United States in 1990. Genetic factors are important; overall, siblings and offspring of affected probands have a two- to threefold increased risk of seizures with fever. Recent linkage studies in a few large families indicate that febrile seizure susceptibility genes are located on portions of chromosomes 8 and 19 (see Chapter 140). The role of such genes in sporadic febrile seizures remains to be determined.

CLINICAL MANIFESTATIONS

Febrile seizures appear typically early in the febrile illness, while the temperature is rapidly rising. In many children, the seizure is the first indication of illness. Although generalized convulsions are the rule, focal features or a Todd's paresis are seen in about 10% of patients. Febrile seizures are subdivided operationally into *simple* and *complex* types. Simple (also called benign) febrile seizures are brief isolated occurrences that lack focal manifestations. Complex febrile seizures are frequently focal, last longer than 15 minutes, and tend to occur repeatedly within 24 hours.

DIAGNOSIS

Diagnosis is made by excluding other possible causes of the convulsion, such as meningitis, metabolic abnormalities, or structural brain lesions. Depending on the manifestations and the clinician's experience, laboratory tests are not always necessary. Usually, a clinically identifiable infection, such as otitis media, roseola infantum, pharyngitis, or gastroenteritis, is present. Fever after immunization may also trigger a febrile seizure. Any suspicion of meningitis, however, mandates lumbar puncture. The typical indicators of meningeal irritation, such as nuchal rigidity and the Brudzinki sign, are not reliable in young infants. If the seizure has focal features or if the examination elicits focal neurologic abnormalities, brain imaging is necessary. Electroencephalography is not a useful test because it does not provide information regarding either risk of recurrence of febrile seizures or later development of epilepsy.

PROGNOSIS AND TREATMENT

About one-third of children with febrile seizures have more than one attack. Recurrence is highest in infants whose first febrile seizure occurred before the age of 1 year and in children with a family history of febrile seizures. When the first seizure is a typical simple febrile seizure, only 1% of patients have prolonged convulsions later.

The risk of developing epilepsy is increased in children with febrile seizures, but the magnitude of the risk depends on several factors. In children with simple febrile seizures, the risk of later epilepsy is 2% to 3%. The incidence of epilepsy increases to about 10% to 13% in children who have had complex febrile seizures, who have a family history of afebrile seizures, or who were neurologically abnormal before the first febrile seizure. Young children who have unprovoked seizures after a febrile convulsion are at much greater risk of further seizures with subsequent febrile illnesses.

Neither simple nor complex febrile seizures are associated with, nor do they lead to, mental retardation, low global IQ, poor school achievement, or behavioral problems. Some differences have been reported, however. Children with febrile seizures in the first year of life are more likely to require special schooling than those who have them later. In children with prolonged febrile convulsions, nonverbal intelligence measures may be slightly lower compared with children with simple febrile seizures. Mortality is not increased in children with febrile seizures who are neurologically normal.

Because most children with febrile seizures have no long-term consequences, most clinicians now avoid chronic prophylactic treatment with antiepileptic drugs, even after two or three isolated convulsions. Although both phenobarbital and valproate are effective in reducing recurrence, evidence does not show that treatment alters the risk of later epilepsy. In addition, adverse drug effects occur in as many as 40% of infants and children treated with phenobarbital, and valproate carries a risk of idiosyncratic fatal hepatotoxicity and pancreatitis. Phenytoin is ineffective.

If treatment is considered at all, it should be reserved for children with complex febrile seizures who are neurologically abnormal or who have a strong family history of afebrile seizures. A reasonable alternative to chronic drug therapy is intermittent treatment using rectal diazepam. Several studies have shown that rectal administration of diazepam during febrile illnesses is safe and as effective as phenobarbital in reducing seizure recurrence. A rectal formulation of diazepam (Diastat) is now available in the United States, although the U.S. Food and Drug Administration has not yet approved it for use in prolonged febrile seizures.

Watching their child have a convulsion is one of the most frightening experiences that parents can have. The physician therefore must provide reassurance to dispel any myths the family may have, emphasizing in particular that febrile seizures are neither life-threatening nor damaging to the brain.

SUGGESTED READINGS

American Academy of Pediatrics. Provisional Committee on Quality Improvement, Subcommittee on Febrile Seizures. Practice parameter: the neurodiagnostic evaluation of the child with a first simple febrile seizure. *Pediatrics* 1996;97:769–772.

Berg AT, Darefsky AS, Holford TR, Shinnar S. Seizures with fever after unprovoked seizures: an analysis in children followed from the time of a first febrile seizure. *Epilepsia* 1998;39:77–80.

Berg AT, Shinnar S, Darefsky AS, et al. Predictors of recurrent febrile seizures. A prospective cohort study. *Arch Pediatr Adolesc Med* 1997;151:371–378.

Berg AT, Shinnar S, Shapiro ED, et al. Risk factors for a first febrile seizure: a matched case-control study. *Epilepsia* 1995;36:334–341.

Johnson EW, Dubovsky J, Rich SS, et al. Evidence for a novel gene for familial febrile convulsions, FEB2, linked to chromosome 19p in an extended family from the Midwest. *Hum Mol Genet* 1998;7:63–67.

Kolfen W, Pehle K, Konig S. Is the long-term outcome of children following febrile convulsions favorable? *Dev Med Child Neurol* 1998;40:667–671.

Kugler SL, Johnson WG. Genetics of the febrile seizure susceptibility trait. *Brain Dev* 1998;20:265–274.

Nelson KB, Ellenberg JH. Prognosis in children with febrile seizures. *Pediatrics* 1978;61:720–727.

Pfeiffer A, Thompson J, Charlier C, et al. A locus for febrile seizures (FEB$_3$) maps to chromosome 2q23-24. *Ann Neurol* 1999;46:671–678.

Rosman NP, Colton T, Labazzo RNC, et al. A controlled trial of diazepam administered during febrile illnesses to prevent recurrence of febrile seizures. *N Engl J Med* 1993;329:79–84.

Tarkka R, Rantala H, Huhari M, Pokka T. Risk of recurrence and outcome after the first febrile seizure. *Pediatr Neurol* 1998;18:218–220.

Verity CM, Greenwood R, Golding J. Long-term intellectual and behavioral outcomes of children with febrile convulsions. *N Engl J Med* 1998;338:1723–1728.

Wallace RH, Wang DW, Singh R, et al. Febrile seizures and generalized epilepsy associated with a mutation in the Na$^+$-channel beta 1 subunit gene SCN1B. *Nature Genetics* 1998;19:366–370.

Merritt's Neurology, 10th ed., edited by L.P. Rowland. Lippincott Williams & Wilkins, Philadelphia © 2000.

CHAPTER 142

NEONATAL SEIZURES

DOUGLAS R. NORDLI, JR.
TIMOTHY A. PEDLEY

Seizures are the most common sign of neurologic dysfunction in the neonate. They occur in 0.5% of all newborns, more often in preterm babies, and frequently signify injury to the developing brain. They are thus an urgent clinical problem that requires prompt diagnosis and treatment.

CLASSIFICATION

The clinical semiology and electroencephalographic (EEG) features of neonatal seizures have been recognized for years to differ substantially from those of older children and adults. Therefore, the classification schemes used for seizures in older patients are inappropriate for newborns.

Neonatal seizures are almost always identified by clinical observation, and traditionally, clinical features have been used for classification. Analysis of simultaneous closed-circuit television

and EEG recordings has revealed that not all clinical seizure behaviors are accompanied by an EEG seizure discharge. Also, not all EEG ictal patterns produce clinical behavioral changes.

The current classification proposed by Volpe (1989) recognizes four general patterns of clinical behavior and describes each by the presence or absence of a consistent EEG discharge (Table 142.1). Focal clonic, focal tonic, and some myoclonic seizures are accompanied by characteristic EEG discharges. In contrast, generalized tonic seizures, most motor automatisms (mouthing, pedaling, stepping, rotary arm movements), and some myoclonic seizures have inconsistent or no reliable EEG changes. Autonomic phenomena are common, especially in term newborns, but they almost always accompany other behavioral manifestations. In preterm infants, however, isolated autonomic phenomena may be the only evidence of seizure activity. Apnea is rarely the sole manifestation of an ictal event. A complete generalized tonic-clonic sequence does not occur in newborns.

ETIOLOGY

Although the incidence of neonatal seizures has not changed much in several decades, the frequency of different causes has been modified considerably. Former frequent causes of seizures in the newborn, such as hypocalcemia and obstetric injury, are rare today. Now, hypoxic-ischemic encephalopathy is the major cause (Table 142.2). Infants at highest risk for developing seizures second to asphyxia have low 5-minute Apgar scores, re-

TABLE 142.1. CLASSIFICATION OF NEONATAL SEIZURES

Clinical seizure	Electrographic seizure	
	Common	Uncommon
Subtle (autonomic phenomena, oral-buccal lingual movements, automatisms)		+
Clonic		
Focal	+	
Multifocal	+	
Tonic		
Focal	+	
Generalized		+
Myoclonic		
Focal, multifocal		+
Generalized	+	

Modified from Volpe JJ. *Pediatrics* 1989;84:422–428.

quire intubation in the delivery room, and have severe acidemia. Other important causes of neonatal seizures include intraventricular and intracerebral hemorrhage, intrauterine or postnatal infection, cerebral malformations, and metabolic disorders, including hypoglycemia, hypocalcemia, hypomagnesemia, and inborn errors of metabolism (nonketotic hyperglycinemia, urea cycle defects). In many babies, multiple factors coexist (e.g., hypoxia and intraventricular hemorrhage), and concurrent metabolic abnormalities, especially hypoglycemia and hypocalcemia, occur frequently. A potassium channel gene defect has been identified as the cause of benign familial neonatal convulsions.

EVALUATION

As in older patients with seizures, the history is the most important component of the neurologic assessment, including the family history and details of the infant's gestation and delivery. With patience, seizures often can be observed directly. If not, the nursery attendant is a reliable source of information. Examination should assess the overall well-being of the child, the infant's resting posture and quality of spontaneous movements, and whether any abnormal postures or movements can be elicited by stimulation or positioning. The infant's head circumference should be determined, and note should be made of any congenital anomalies, signs of a neurocutaneous disorder, or organomegaly.

Laboratory tests, including lumbar puncture and blood cultures, must be obtained rapidly to identify treatable metabolic abnormalities, sepsis, and meningitis. Ultrasound, head computed tomography, or brain magnetic resonance imaging assess

TABLE 142.2. CAUSES OF NEONATAL SEIZURES

Identified causes	Frequency (%)
Hypoxia-ischemia	60
Intracranial hemorrhage	10
Infection	10
Metabolic abnormalities	10
Developmental defects	<5
Other	5

possible hydrocephalus, intracranial hemorrhage, or major anomalies. Magnetic resonance imaging is usually necessary to detect more subtle developmental abnormalities, such as partial lissencephaly, polymicrogyria, or cortical dysplasia. Properly performed, magnetic resonance imaging demonstrates brain abnormalities in two-thirds of newborns with seizures, and diffuse brain lesions, irrespective of etiology, are associated with a high mortality rate. EEG provides important information about the physiologic state of the brain and may be diagnostic if a seizure is recorded.

The timing of the first seizure helps to distinguish diagnostic possibilities. Seizures resulting from severe brain malformations, intracerebral hemorrhage, and hypoxic-ischemic injury occur within 24 to 48 hours. Seizures caused by infection and inborn errors of metabolism typically begin toward the end of the first week of life or later. Seizures related to passive drug withdrawal usually occur within the first 3 days (e.g., alcohol, short-acting barbiturates) but may not appear for 2 to 3 weeks (e.g., methadone). Seizures resulting from sepsis occur at any time.

Seizures must be distinguished from other paroxysmal phenomena in the newborn, including jitteriness, benign sleep myoclonus, dyskinesias (common with severe bronchopulmonary dysplasia), and the movements of rapid eye movement sleep. Brief generalized tonic postures occur with poor cerebral perfusion or with resolving encephalopathies; they do not signify convulsions. Epileptic (associated with an EEG ictal discharge) must be separated from nonepileptic seizures because of the therapeutic implications. Seizures without EEG changes are probably caused by subcortical or brainstem release phenomena rather than by cortical events and therefore result from different pathophysiologic mechanisms.

TREATMENT

Treatment should be based on assumed physiologic mechanism. Epileptic seizures should be treated with antiepileptic drugs. Antiepileptic drugs are probably ineffective, however, in seizures that are not associated with an EEG discharge, and drugs may worsen already depressed forebrain function. It must be recognized, however, that some clinical and experimental evidence suggests that deep subcortical or brainstem structures may give rise to seizures in newborns without an EEG correlate. More controversial is the end point of therapy. Antiepileptic drug treatment often suppresses clinical manifestations whereas electrical seizure activity persists. Although experimental evidence indicates that prolonged electrical seizures can injure the brain, there is uncertainty and debate about the extent to which EEG ictal discharges contribute, by themselves, and in the absence of hypoxia and ischemia, to permanent neurologic sequelae. We recommend using antiepileptic drugs to the point that clinical seizure activity is eliminated or a high therapeutic blood level is achieved without compromising respiratory or circulatory function. We do not attempt to suppress EEG seizure activity that continues after clinical seizures end, mainly because the drug dosages necessary to achieve this end usually lead to obtundation, ventilatory failure, or cardiac depression. More data are needed about the possible long-term deleterious effects of subclinical electrical seizure discharges.

Phenobarbital is the most frequently used antiepileptic drug in newborns. The infant should be given 20 mg/kg intravenously over 15 to 20 minutes. If seizures persist, then additional 5-mg/kg increments of phenobarbital can be given every 20 minutes up to a total loading dose of 40 mg/kg. The maintenance dose for phenobarbital is between 3 to 6 mg/kg/day. Therapeutic levels are 15 to 35 μg/mL; levels higher than 40 μg/mL produce lethargy.

Phenytoin is an alternative drug when phenobarbital fails. It is given intravenously over about 20 minutes in a loading dose of 20 mg/kg. Some clinicians advise dividing the loading dose into two 10-mg/kg increments to minimize cardiac toxicity. Maintenance doses are 3 to 4 mg/kg/day. Fosphenytoin, the water-soluble phosphorylated version of phenytoin, has been administered safely to small groups of neonates as young as 26 weeks conceptional age. Midazolam, 0.1 to 0.4 mg/kg/hr administered by continuous intravenous infusion, may be useful in suppressing seizures refractory to phenobarbital and phenytoin.

Hypoglycemia should be treated using a 10% glucose solution infused in a dosage of 2 ml/kg.

When to stop antiepileptic drugs is a matter of judgment. If the infant is normal and the EEG is normal or near normal, we generally discontinue antiepileptic drug therapy before the child is discharged from the hospital. In other cases, we wait 1 to 3 months after the last seizure.

PROGNOSIS

The long-term prognosis relates not to the seizures but to the underlying cause. Perinatal asphyxia, severe intracranial hemorrhage, and cerebral malformations all have a high correlation with permanent brain damage. Therefore, prognosis is guarded for most newborns with seizures; 33% to 50% have neurologic sequelae. Recurrent seizures from the first day of life that interfere with respiration and feeding schedules also carry a poor prognosis. Serial EEG studies assist in identifying term infants at high risk for abnormal neurologic outcome. Several EEG patterns (suppression-burst background activity, unreactive low-voltage recording, continuous multifocal ictal events) reliably predict a fatal outcome or disabling brain damage more than 90% of the time. EEG is less useful in predicting which infants will continue to have seizures beyond the neonatal period.

About 15% to 30% of infants with neonatal seizures develop epilepsy.

SUGGESTED READINGS

Bye AM, Cunningham CA, Chee KY, Flanagan D. Outcome of neonates with electrographically identified seizures, or at risk of seizures. *Pediatr Neurol* 1997;16:225–231.

Clancy RR, Legido A, Lewis D. Occult neonatal seizures. *Epilepsia* 1988;29:256–261.

Hall RT, Hall FK Daily DK. High-dose phenobarbital therapy in term newborn infants with severe perinatal asphyxia: a randomized, prospective study with three-year follow-up. *J Pediatr* 1998;132:345–348.

Holmes GL, Gairsa JL, Chevassus-Au-Louis N, Ben-Ari Y. Consequences of neonatal seizures in the rat: morphological and behavioral effects. *Ann Neurol* 1998;44:845–857.

Lanska MJ, Lanska DJ. Neonatal seizures in the United States: results of the National Hospital Discharge Survey, 1980–1991. *Neuroepidemiology* 1996;15:117–125.

Leth H, Toft PB, Herning M, et al. Neonatal seizures associated with cerebral lesions shown by magnetic resonance imaging. *Arch Dis Child Fetal Neonat Med* 1997;77:F105–F110.

Mizrahi EM, Kellaway P. Characterization and classification of neonatal seizures. *Neurology* 1987;37:1837–1844.

Ortibus EL, Sum JM, Hahn JS. Predictive value of EEG for outcome and epilepsy following neonatal seizures. *Electroencephalogr Clin Neurophysiol* 1996;98:175–185.

Perlman JM, Risser R. Can asphyxiated infants at risk for neonatal seizures be rapidly identified by current high-risk markers? *Pediatrics* 1996;97:456–462.

Ronen GM, Penney S, Andrews W. The epidemiology of clinical neonatal seizures in Newfoundland: a population-based study. *J Pediatr* 1999;134:71–75.

Sher MS. Seizures in the newborn infant. Diagnosis, treatment, and outcome. *Clin Perinatol* 1997;24:735–772.

Sher MS, Aso K, Beggarly ME, et al. Electrographic seizures in preterm and full-term neonates: Clinical correlates, associated brain lesions, and risk of neurologic sequelae. *Pediatrics* 1993;91:128–134.

Sheth RD, Buckley DJ, Gutierrez AR, et al. Midazolam in the treatment of refractory neonatal seizures. *Clin Neuropharmacol* 1996;19:156–170.

Strober JB, Bienkowski RS, Maytal J. The incidence of acute and remote seizures in children with intraventricular hemorrhage. *Clin Pediatr* 1997;36:643–647.

Volpe JJ. Neonatal seizures: current concepts and revised classification. *Pediatrics* 1989;84:422–428.

Merritt's Neurology, 10th ed., edited by L.P. Rowland. Lippincott Williams & Wilkins, Philadelphia © 2000.

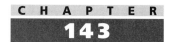

CHAPTER 143

TRANSIENT GLOBAL AMNESIA

JOHN C.M. BRUST

Transient global amnesia (TGA) is characterized by sudden inability to form new memory traces (*anterograde amnesia*) in addition to retrograde memory loss for events of the preceding days, weeks, or even years. During attacks, which affect both verbal and nonverbal memory, there is often bewilderment or anxiety and a tendency to repeat one or several questions (e.g., "Where am I?"). Physical and neurologic examinations, including mental status, are otherwise normal. Immediate registration of events (e.g., serial digits) is intact, and self-identification is preserved. Attacks last minutes or hours, rarely longer than a day, with gradual recovery. Retrograde amnesia clears in a forward fashion, often with permanent loss for events occurring within minutes or a few hours of the attack; there is also permanent amnesia for events during the attack itself. TGA sometimes seems to be precipitated by physical or emotional stress, such as sexual intercourse, driving an automobile, or swimming in cold water. Because amnesia can accompany a variety of neurologic disturbances, such as head trauma, intoxication, partial complex seizures, or dissociative states, criteria for diagnosing TGA should include observation of the attack by others.

Patients are usually middle-aged or elderly and otherwise healthy. Recurrent attacks occur in less than 25% of cases, and fewer than 3% have more than three attacks. Intervals between attacks range from 1 month to 19 years. Permanent memory loss is rare, although subtle defects have been reported after only one attack. The cause of TGA is uncertain. Case–control series and anecdotal reports variably implicate stroke, seizures, or migraine.

In a large series of patients with TGA, the cause was epileptic in 7%. Attacks in this group were nearly always less than 1 hour in duration and tended to occur on awakening; two-thirds had additional seizure types, usually simple or complex partial seizures. Sleep, but not interictal, electroencephalograms revealed temporal lobe epileptiform discharges.

Major risk factors for stroke (hypertension, diabetes mellitus, tobacco, ischemic heart disease, atrial fibrillation, and past stroke or transient ischemic attack) are no more common among patients with TGA than in age-matched controls, and TGA is not a risk factor for stroke. On the other hand, attacks have been associated with cerebral angiography (especially vertebral), polycythemia, cardiac valvular disease, and patent foramen ovale. Patients with amnestic stroke due to documented posterior cerebral artery occlusion do not report previous TGA; their neurologic signs include more than simple amnesia (e.g., visual impairment), and they do not exhibit repetitive queries. Reduced blood flow to the thalamus or temporal lobes has been documented during attacks of TGA but could be secondary to neuronal dysfunction rather than its cause.

Epidemiologic studies confirm an association of TGA with migraine, even though in the great majority of patients migraine attacks are recurrent, whereas attacks of TGA are not. Sometimes, both amnestic and migrainous attacks (including visual symptoms and vomiting) have occurred simultaneously or followed one another. Spreading depression of Leao (possibly the pathophysiologic basis of cerebral symptoms in migraine) could, by affecting the hippocampus, explain some cases of TGA, as well. Diffusion-weighted magnetic resonance imaging during or soon after an attack of TGA in several patients revealed signal abnormalities in one or both temporal lobes that were more suggestive of spreading depression than primary ischemia.

Thus, even when strict diagnostic criteria are applied, TGA probably has diverse origins. In patients in whom epilepsy and migraine can be excluded and who have risk factors for cerebrovascular disease, antiplatelet drugs may be considered, but the benign natural history makes it difficult to evaluate any preventive treatment.

SUGGESTED READINGS

Caplan LB. Transient global amnesia. In: Vinken PJ, Bruyn GW, Klawans HL, Frederiks JAM, eds. *Clinical neuropsychology. Handbook of clinical neurology, rev ser, vol 45(1).* Amsterdam: Elsevier Science, 1985:205–218.

Fisher CM, Adams RD. Transient global amnesia syndrome. *Acta Neurol Scand* 1964;40[Suppl 9]:7–82.

Hodges JR, Warlow CP. The aetiology of transient global amnesia: a case-control study of 114 cases with prospective follow-up. *Brain* 1990;113:639–658.

Inzitari D, Pantoni L, Lamassa M, et al. Emotional arousal and phobia in transient global amnesia. *Arch Neurol* 1997;54:866–873.

Melo TP, Ferro JM, Ferro H. Transient global amnesia: a case-control study. *Brain* 1992;115:261–270.

Olesen J, Jorgensen MB. Leao's spreading depression in the hippocampus explains transient global amnesia: A hypothesis. *Acta Neurol Scand* 1986;73:219–220.

Strupp M, Brüning R, Wu RH, et al. Diffusion-weighted MRI in transient global amnesia: elevated signal intensity in the left mesial temporal lobe in 7 of 10 patients. *Ann Neurol* 1998;43:164–170.

Zeman AZJ, Boniface SJ, Hodges JR. Transient epileptic amnesia: a description of the clinical and neuropsychological features in 10 cases and a review of the literature. *J Neurol Neurosurg Psychiatry*, 1998;64:435–443.

Zorzon M, Antonutti L, Masè G, et al. Transient global amnesia and transient ischemic attack: natural history, vascular risk factors, and associated conditions. *Stroke* 1995;26:1536–1542.

Merritt's Neurology, 10th ed., edited by L.P. Rowland. Lippincott Williams & Wilkins, Philadelphia © 2000.

MENIERE SYNDROME

JACK J. WAZEN

First described in 1861 by the French physician Prosper Meniere, this syndrome affects people of all ages, especially those in middle age or older. It is characterized by a recurrent and episodic triad of spinning vertigo, hearing loss, and tinnitus.

SIGNS AND SYMPTOMS

Patients with Meniere syndrome are usually asymptomatic between attacks. The acute episode may be preceded by warning symptoms of pressure sensation or fullness in one ear, which feels "blocked." Hearing then drops, accompanied by a loud roaring tinnitus. Vertigo soon follows and lasts from a few minutes to many hours, rarely lasting as long as 24 hours. The interval between the onset of symptoms and the peak of vertigo varies from a few minutes to a full day or so. Depending on the severity of the vertigo, patients may experience nausea, vomiting, or diarrhea. Pallor and cold sweat are common. Early in the disease, once the spell is over, the ear clears, hearing returns to normal, and the tinnitus may subside. The patient may feel weak and unsteady for 1 or 2 days following a severe attack. A dull unilateral headache may accompany the sensation of blockage and fullness in the ear.

Recurrence of the attacks is a cardinal feature. The attacks are of unpredictable frequency. At first, patients may have one attack per year. Then attacks may occur more frequently, once a week or even daily. The more frequent the spells, the more disabled the patient becomes; anxiety and panic reactions are generated by the fear that vertigo may occur at any moment.

The hearing loss is usually most severe in the low frequencies. At first, it fluctuates. With progression of the disease, hearing loss becomes permanent, and the high frequencies are affected, resulting in a flat sensorineural hearing loss. Despite the progressive hearing loss, patients often complain of noise intolerance, which is attributed to recruitment in the cochlea. *Recruitment* is an abnormally rapid increase in the sense of loudness as sound intensity increases. The comfortable range of hearing becomes narrow, and patients become intolerant of sounds barely above their hearing threshold. Recruitment makes it difficult but still feasible to fit a patient with a hearing aid.

Examination of a patient during a vertigo attack invariably reveals a rotatory-horizontal nystagmus beating toward the affected ear. This nystagmus of peripheral labyrinthine origin is reduced or abolished by visual fixation. A patient with Meniere syndrome does not necessarily experience all features of the syndrome with each attack, especially in the initial stages of the disease. Recurrent, fluctuating hearing loss may occur without vertigo, or recurrent vertigo may occur without hearing loss. Depending on the major symptom, the disorder may be considered primarily cochlear or vestibular. Eventually, however, the full complement of symptoms ensues.

A few patients with Meniere syndrome experience drop attacks or tumarcin crisis. The vertigo is so sudden in onset and so intense that patients find themselves on the floor as if pushed by an invisible force, even from a sitting position, with no loss of consciousness or other neurologic symptoms.

Symptoms in the contralateral ear occur in 20% to 30% of patients. The risk of bilateral disease depends on the cause of the syndrome (see below).

DIAGNOSIS

The diagnosis is usually evident from the history. Audiologic tests confirm the low-frequency sensorineural hearing loss. Repeated audiograms reveal the fluctuating nature of the loss. Electronystagmography reveals a vestibular disorder in the affected ear. Other vestibular tests, such as rotational chair testing or dynamic platform posturography, are also diagnostic of a peripheral vestibular disorder, but they do not lateralize the lesion. The auditory brainstem response is consistent with a cochlear lesion. Computed tomography and magnetic resonance imaging are usually normal.

ETIOLOGY AND PATHOGENESIS

Extensive research into the cause of this symptom complex has led to the present understanding that Meniere syndrome is not the result of any particular cause but is the reaction of the inner ear to different offending agents that cause disruption of endolymphatic homeostasis. Recognized causes include congenital inner ear deformities, labyrinthitis, physical trauma to the head and ear, acoustic trauma, congenital or acquired syphilis, allergic disorders, autoimmune disorders, and vascular disorders, including diabetes and hypertension. Most cases, however, are idiopathic. These idiopathic cases are labeled as *Meniere disease.*

Postmortem histopathologic studies of temporal bones from patients with the syndrome revealed endolymphatic hydrops, which describes dilatation and ballooning of the endolymphatic compartment in the scala media of the cochlea, as well as of the saccule, utricle, and the semicircular canals. These findings suggest that the condition is caused by oversecretion or malabsorption of the endolymph. Disorders of endolymph malabsorption through the endolymphatic duct and sac are now believed to cause the dilatation. Some investigators noted that ruptures in the Reisner membrane, with sudden decompression and mixing of perilymph with endolymph, could result in loss of endocochlear potentials or hair cell injury. The membrane ruptures, however, may be caused by fixing artifacts. Current research centers on the functions of the endolymphatic sac, including its fluid absorption and immunologic properties.

TREATMENT

Medical Management

Treatment is directed to reducing the impact of the acute attack and the frequency of spells. Controlled trials of the efficacy of any treatment of an acute attack have been difficult to complete because of the unpredictable and variable nature of the syndrome. As a result, many drugs, such as meclizine hydrochloride (Antivert), diazepam, promethazine hydrochloride, and prochlorperazine, are used as labyrinthine sedatives. Similarly, no regimen has proved effective in reducing the frequency of attacks. Some authorities advocate a strict low-salt diet and diuretics to reduce the endolymphatic hydrops. Patients are advised to discontinue the use of caffeine, tobacco, and alcohol. Vasodilator therapy with histamine and nicotinic acid offers inconsistent results. Patients whose syndrome is allergic or has immunologic factors may respond well to a course of steroids. Patients are also encouraged to address anxiety, depression, and other psychologic symptoms that result from fear of attacks.

Surgical Treatment

About 20% of patients fail to respond to medical management and become candidates for surgery to relieve disabling vertigo. Patients who have lost hearing respond well to a labyrinthectomy, which is the complete removal of the vestibular end-organ. For patients who still have serviceable hearing, vestibular neurectomy is the procedure of choice, offering a 90% to 95% success rate in vertigo control while preserving hearing. Endolymphatic sac surgery with decompression and shunting of the endolymph into the mastoid cavity is still performed despite controversies about long-term effectiveness.

Chemical Labyrinthectomy

Nonsurgical candidates and patients who refuse surgery but yet fail to respond to medical treatments may benefit from the intratympanic injection of gentamicin sulfate, an aminoglycoside known for its ototoxicity. Gentamicin has a greater affinity for vestibular hair cells and thus causes a significant loss of vestibular function before attacking the cochlear hair cells. Given in the appropriate dose and with close supervision, intratympanic gentamicin is absorbed through the round window membrane, creating a chemical labyrinthectomy with hearing preservation.

Bilateral Meniere Disease

Patients with active bilateral Meniere disease are treated with systemic injections of streptomycin sulfate. As an ototoxic agent, streptomycin has a stronger affinity for vestibular hair cells than for cochlear hair cells. Given in daily 1-g injections with close monitoring of vestibular function, treatment is interrupted after the first signs of vestibular ototoxicity and before the onset of hearing loss. Reduction in the vestibular hair cell population decreases the severity of the vertigo. Total bilateral ablation of vestibular hair cells leads to oscillopsia and permanent ataxia and therefore should be avoided.

SUGGESTED READINGS

Arenberg IK. Endolymphatic hypertension and hydrops in Meniere's disease: current perspectives. *Am J Otol* 1982;4:52–65.

Baloh RW. *Dizziness, hearing loss, and tinnitus: essentials of neurology.* Philadelphia: FA Davis Co, 1984.

Blakeley BW. Clinical forum: a review of intratympanic therapy. *Am J Otol* 1997;18:520–526.

Brackman DE. *Neurological surgery of the ear and skull base.* New York: Raven Press, 1982.

Brookes GB. The pharmacological treatment of Meniere's disease. *Clin Otolaryngol* 1996;21:3–11.

Brookes GB, Hodge RA, Booth JB, Morrison AW. The immediate effects of acetazolamide in Meniere's disease. *J Laryngol Otol* 1982;96:57–72.

Dandy WE. Treatment of Meniere's disease by section of only the vestibular portion of the acoustic nerve. *Bull Johns Hopkins Hosp* 1933;53:52–55.

Hallpike CS, Cairns H. Observations on the pathology of Meniere's syndrome. *J Laryngol* 1938;53:625–654.

Meniere P. Sur une forme particulière de surdité grave dependant d'une lesion de l'oreille interne. *Gaz Med Paris* 1861;16:29.

Pulec JL. Meniere's disease: etiology, natural history, and results of treatment. *Otolaryngol Clin North Am* 1973;6:25–39.

Stahle J, Wilbrand HF, Rask-Andersen H. Temporal bone characteristics in Meniere's disease. *Ann N Y Acad Sci* 1981;374:794–807.

Tomiyama S, Harris JP. The endolymphatic sac: its importance in inner ear immune responses. *Laryngoscope* 1986;96:685–691.

Wazen JJ, Foyt D, Huang CC. Quantitative immunochemical studies of the endolymphatic sac in Meniere's disease. In: Barbara M, Filipo R, eds. *Meniere's disease: pathogenesis, pathophysiology, diagnosis and treatment. proceedings of the third international symposium.* Amsterdam: Kugler, 1994.

Wazen JJ, Spitzer J, Kasper C, Anderson B. Long-term hearing results following vestibular surgery in Meniere's disease. *Laryngoscope* 1998;108:1470–1473.

Merritt's Neurology, 10th ed., edited by L.P. Rowland. Lippincott Williams & Wilkins, Philadelphia © 2000.

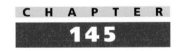

CHAPTER 145

SLEEP DISORDERS

JUNE M. FRY

The clinical application of scientific knowledge of sleep physiology and biologic rhythms led to the development of standards for normal sleep and arousal, diagnostic tests, and a classification of sleep disorders (Table 145.1). This classification is based on clinical signs, symptoms, age at onset, and natural history. Clinical polysomnography is an important diagnostic tool that provides objective confirmation of the clinical syndromes.

SLEEP PHYSIOLOGY

Sleep is an active and complex state comprising four stages of non–rapid eye movement (NREM) sleep and rapid eye movement (REM) sleep. Wakefulness and sleep stages are characterized by physiologic measures that are assessed by polysomnography. Standardized sleep scoring is based on the electroencephalogram (EEG), the electrooculogram (EOG; a

measurement of eye movements), and the electromyogram (EMG) of the mentalis muscle (chin EMG). *Stage 1* sleep is characterized by a low-voltage, mixed-frequency EEG and slow, rolling eye movements. Reactivity to outside stimuli is decreased, and mentation may occur but is no longer reality-oriented. *Stage 2* consists of a moderate low-voltage background EEG with sleep spindles (bursts of 12- to 14-Hz activity lasting 0.5 to 2 seconds) and K-complexes (brief high-voltage discharges with an initial negative deflection followed by a positive component). Heart and respiratory rates are regular and slightly slower. *Stage 3* sleep consists of high-amplitude theta (5 to 7 Hz) and delta (1 to 3 Hz) frequencies, as well as interspersed K-complexes and sleep spindles. *Stage 4* sleep is similar to stage 3, except that high-voltage delta waves make up at least 50% of the EEG and sleep spindles are few or absent. Stages 3 and 4 are often combined and referred to as *delta sleep, slow-wave sleep,* or *deep sleep.* During this deeper sleep, heart and respiratory rates are slowed and regular. During NREM sleep, the tonic chin EMG is of moderately high amplitude but less than that of quiet wakefulness.

The EEG pattern during REM sleep consists of low-voltage, mixed-frequency activity and is similar to that of stage 1 sleep. Moderately high-amplitude, 3- to 5-Hz triangular waveforms called saw-tooth waves are intermittently present and are unique to REM sleep. Intermittent bursts of rapid conjugate eye movements occur. Tonic chin EMG activity is absent or markedly reduced, and phasic muscle discharges occur in irregular bursts. The decreased EMG activity is a reflection of muscle paralysis re-

TABLE 145.1. INTERNATIONAL CLASSIFICATION OF SLEEP DISORDERS

I. Dyssomnia
  A. Intrinsic sleep disorders
    1. Psychophysiologic insomnia
    2. Sleep-state misperception
    3. Idiopathic insomnia
    4. Narcolepsy
    5. Recurrent hypersomnia
    6. Idiopathic hypersomnia
    7. Posttraumatic hypersomnia
    8. Obstructive sleep apnea syndrome
    9. Central sleep apnea syndrome
    10. Central alveolar hypoventilation syndrome
    11. Periodic limb movement disorder
    12. Restless legs syndrome
    13. Intrinsic sleep disorder NOS
  B. Extrinsic sleep disorders
    1. Inadequate sleep hygiene
    2. Environmental sleep disorder
    3. Altitude insomnia
    4. Adjustment sleep disorder
    5. Insufficient sleep syndrome
    6. Limit-setting sleep disorder
    7. Sleep-onset association disorder
    8. Food allergy insomnia
    9. Nocturnal eating (drinking) syndrome
    10. Hypnotic-dependent sleep disorder
    11. Stimulant-dependent sleep disorder
    12. Alcohol-dependent sleep disorder
    13. Toxin-induced sleep disorder
    14. Extrinsic sleep disorder NOS
  C. Circadian rhythm sleep disorders
    1. Time-zone-change (jet lag) syndrome
    2. Shift-work sleep disorder
    3. Irregular sleep–wake pattern
    4. Delayed sleep phase syndrome
    5. Advanced sleep phase syndrome
    6. Non-24-hour sleep–wake disorder
    7. Circadian rhythm sleep disorder NOS
II. Parasomnias
  A. Arousal disorders
    1. Confusional arousals
    2. Sleepwalking
    3. Sleep terrors
  B. Sleep–wake transition disorders
    1. Rhythmic movement disorder
    2. Sleep starts
    3. Sleep talking
    4. Nocturnal leg cramps
  C. Parasomnias usually associated with REM sleep
    1. Nightmares
    2. Sleep paralysis
    3. Impaired sleep-related penile erections
    4. Sleep-related painful erections

    5. REM sleep-related sinus arrest
    6. REM sleep behavior disorder
  D. Other parasomnias
    1. Sleep bruxism
    2. Sleep enuresis
    3. Sleep-related abnormal swallowing
    4. Nocturnal paroxysmal dystonia
    5. Sudden unexplained nocturnal death syndrome
    6. Primary snoring
    7. Infant sleep apnea
    8. Congenital central hypoventilation syndrome
    9. Sudden infant death syndrome
    10. Benign neonatal sleep myoclonus
    11. Other parasomnia NOS
III. Sleep disorders associated with medical/psychiatric disorders
  A. Associated with mental disorders
    1. Psychoses
    2. Mood disorders
    3. Anxiety disorders
    4. Panic disorder
    5. Alcoholism
  B. Associated with neurologic disorders
    1. Cerebral degenerative disorders
    2. Dementia
    3. Parkinsonism
    4. Fatal familial insomnia
    5. Sleep-related epilepsy
    6. Electrical status epilepticus of sleep
    7. Sleep-related headaches
  C. Associated with other medical disorders
    1. Sleeping sickness
    2. Nocturnal cardiac ischemia
    3. Chronic obstructive pulmonary disease
    4. Sleep-related asthma
    5. Sleep-related gastroesophageal reflux
    6. Peptic ulcer disease
    7. Fibrositis syndrome
IV. Proposed sleep disorders
  A. Short sleeper
  B. Long sleeper
  C. Subwakefulness syndrome
  D. Fragmentary myoclonus
  E. Sleep hyperhidrosis
  F. Menstrual-associated sleep disorder
  G. Pregnancy-associated sleep disorder
  H. Terrifying hypnagogic hallucinations
  I. Sleep-related neurogenic tachypnea
  J. Sleep-related laryngospasm
  K. Sleep choking syndrome

sulting from active inhibition of muscle activity during REM sleep. During REM sleep, heart and respiratory rates are increased and irregular, and vivid dreaming occurs.

NREM sleep alternates with REM sleep at intervals of 85 to 100 minutes. The normal healthy adult typically falls asleep within 10 minutes and goes through the sequence of stages 1 through 4 followed by the reverse (stages 4, 3, and 2). Afterward, the first REM sleep period occurs. This normal sleep pattern consists of three to five such cycles. Typically, stages 3 and 4 are more prominent during the first half of the sleep period, and the REM sleep episodes increase in duration and intensity of REM activity during the second half of the sleep period.

DIAGNOSTIC PROCEDURES

Clinical polysomnography, the simultaneous recording of sleep and multiple physiologic variables, provides objective documentation of sleep disorders. An all-night polysomnogram consists of continuous EEG, EOG, mentalis EMG, surface EMG of the anterior tibialis muscles for detection of leg movements in sleep, electrocardiogram, and measurement of nasal and oral airflow, respiratory effort, and oxygen saturation. Polysomnographic tracings are analyzed in detail to determine a patient's sleep pattern and the presence and severity of a sleep disorder.

Patients with excessive daytime sleepiness are also evaluated by the multiple sleep latency test (MSLT), a series of four or five nap opportunities with sleep recordings at 2-hour intervals throughout the day. The nap is terminated 15 minutes after sleep onset. If no sleep occurs, each recording session is terminated after 20 minutes. The sleep latency (time it takes to fall asleep) is determined for each nap and provides an objective measure of daytime sleepiness. Patients with pathologic daytime sleepiness generally fall asleep in less than 5 minutes on all naps. Normally alert individuals take more than 10 minutes to fall asleep or often remain awake. The MSLT is also used to determine the presence of sleep-onset REM periods found in narcolepsy, and REM sleep rebound.

SPECIFIC DISORDERS OF SLEEP

Only selected disorders are described, primarily the most common and those of particular interest to neurologists.

Disorders with a Complaint of Insomnia

Transient insomnia lasts less than 3 weeks, is usually situational, and is caused by emotions such as excitement, sorrow, or anxiety resulting from a specific situation, or by a schedule change, such as jet lag or a work-shift change. A short course (2 weeks or less) of a hypnotic may be indicated for treatment of transient *situational insomnia*. Benzodiazepines became the drugs of choice soon after becoming available in the 1960s. New hypnotics, the imidazopyridines, have favorable properties and are useful for sleep-onset difficulties, but because of very short half-lives, they are less useful for middle-of-the-night or early-morning awakenings.

Persistent or chronic insomnia has many underlying causes. When the cause is a psychiatric disorder, pain, gastroesophageal reflux, or drug or alcohol abuse, the underlying cause should be treated. Long-term use of hypnotic drugs is one cause of persistent insomnia.

A common dyssomnia is *psychophysiologic insomnia*. This disorder usually follows a situational insomnia and results from somatized anxiety that is manifested as restlessness, apprehension, ruminative thoughts, and hypervigilance, all of which interfere with sleep. These factors, combined with negative conditioning, lead to a vicious cycle: The more the patient tries to sleep, the less successful the attempts become. The most effective treatment for this disorder is behavioral therapy consisting of relaxation therapy, stimulus control, good sleep hygiene (Table 145.2), and sleep restriction.

Alveolar hypoventilation syndrome, a cause of sleep disruption, is associated with major changes in respiratory function during sleep, including central sleep apnea and hypopnea associated with recurrent hypoxemia, hypercapnia, and a decreased tidal and minute volume. REM sleep is the time of greatest abnor-

TABLE 145.2. PRINCIPLES OF SLEEP HYGIENE

Regulate the sleep–wake cycle
Wake regularly at a fixed time
Regulate the amount of sleep obtained each night
Exercise daily and regularly but not in the late evening
Sleep in a quiet environment
Avoid caffeinated beverages
Avoid alcohol within 3 hours of bedtime
Avoid hypnotic drugs
Do something relaxing before bedtime

mality with the longest apneic episodes and the greatest fall in oxygen saturation. This syndrome may be idiopathic or associated with other disorders; these include chronic residual poliomyelitis, muscle diseases (e.g., myotonic dystrophy, anterior horn cell disease), involvement of thoracic cage bellows action or diaphragmatic muscle weakness, cervical spinal cordotomy, brainstem lesions of structures that control ventilation, dysautonomia syndromes, and massive obesity.

Restless Legs Syndrome and Periodic Limb Movement Disorder

In the *restless legs syndrome* (RLS), the patient feels an irresistible urge to move the legs, especially when sitting or lying down. There is a discomfort deep inside the leg, most commonly between the knee and ankle, that makes the patient move the legs or walk about vigorously. The symptoms interfere with and delay sleep onset, may recur during the night, and cause an insomnia complaint. *Periodic limb movements in sleep* (PLMS) are found in most patients with RLS who are studied with polysomnography.

PLMS are stereotyped periodic movements of one or both legs and feet during sleep. The movements, which occur primarily in NREM sleep, consist of dorsiflexion of the foot, extension of the big toe, and often flexion of the leg at the knee and hip. This triple flexion movement has a mean duration of 1.5 to 2.5 seconds. Similar movements can occur in the upper extremities but are much less common. Limb movements may be accompanied by an arousal or awakening. These movements are remarkably periodic, with 20- to 40-second intervals, and may continue for minutes to hours. In contrast to most movement disorders, which are inhibited by sleep (e.g., cerebellar and extrapyramidal tremors, chorea, dystonia, hemiballism), PLMS are initiated by sleep or drowsiness. They are different from *hypnic jerks* (sleep starts), which are nonperiodic, isolated myoclonic movements that occur at sleep onset and simultaneously involve the muscles of the trunk and extremities. Hypnic jerks are considered normal.

Patients with *periodic limb movement disorder* (PLMD) complain of chronically disturbed sleep or daytime sleepiness. The severity of symptoms appears to be related to the frequency of limb movements and associated arousals and awakenings. RLS, PLMD, or both occur in association with other sleep disorders, including sleep apnea, narcolepsy-cataplexy, and drug dependency. They may develop in patients being treated with antidepressants and during withdrawal from drugs (e.g., barbiturates, benzodiazepines), and in patients with chronic uremia, anemia, and iron deficiency.

For many years, the treatment of choice for PLMD and RLS has been clonazepam (Klonopin), 0.5 to 3.0 mg in the evening, at bedtime, or both. Other benzodiazepines have also proved beneficial. Temazepam (Restoril) is often preferred for its intermediate half-life. Levodopa plus benzerazide or carbidopa is effective, but patients often experience increased or rebound daytime symptoms, when treated only at night. Dopaminergic agonists now appear to be the drugs of choice. Pergolide mesylate (Permax) and bromocriptine mesylate (Parlodel) have been used most commonly, and the doses required are very much smaller than those used for Parkinson disease. Pergolide is generally effective with doses of 0.15 to 0.50 mg daily. Opiates are also useful, especially in severe cases.

Disorders of Excessive Somnolence

The clinical neurologist is asked to evaluate symptoms of *excessive daytime sleepiness* more than any other major category of sleep complaint. Therefore, a patient's complaint and symptoms must be well-defined to provide the physician with a rational basis for a diagnostic and treatment decision. The major symptoms include sleepiness and napping during a time of day when the patient wishes to be awake. The complaint has often been present for months or years and includes an increased amount of unavoidable napping, apparent increase in total sleep during the 24-hour day, or difficulty in achieving full alertness after awakening in the morning. These symptoms should not be confused with complaints of tiredness or lack of energy, motivation, or drive, which may reflect dysphoric symptoms such as those that might accompany depression.

Excessive sleepiness is caused by an insufficient quantity of sleep or poor sleep quality resulting from a sleep disorder, other disturbance, or both. Excessive sleepiness leads to impaired performance and diminished intellectual capacity, and is often a major factor or direct cause of accidents and catastrophes.

Several common disorders must be considered in patients with a complaint of excessive daytime sleepiness (Table 145.3). Obstructive sleep apnea (OSA) syndrome and narcolepsy account for most patients with a complaint of daytime sleepiness evaluated in sleep disorders centers.

Obstructive Sleep Apnea Syndrome

A patient with OSA syndrome often falls asleep at inappropriate or dangerous times (e.g., while eating, driving a car, waiting for a red light) and has pervasive sleepiness throughout the day that seriously interferes with work, as well as leisure time. Almost all patients have loud snoring. The snoring pattern is recurrent, with pauses between snores of 20 to 50 seconds. Each cycle comprises a series of three to six loud snores and gasps followed by a relatively silent period. During the nonsnoring period, the patient makes ineffective respiratory efforts because of an obstructed upper airway. In addition to loud cyclic snoring, sleep is restless, with frequent brief arousals and unusual sleeping postures. The patient may talk during sleep, have nocturnal enuresis, fall out of bed, and wake in the morning with a generalized severe headache and a feeling of having had an unrefreshing night.

In adults, OSA syndrome occurs predominantly between the fourth and sixth decades and is about 2.5 times more common in men. The prevalence of OSA syndrome increases with age and is higher in individuals with habitual snoring and obesity. Numerous congenital and acquired abnormalities of the upper airway are associated with OSA. These include micrognathia, deviated nasal septum, narrow nasal passages from a previous fracture, enlarged adenoids or tonsils, palatopharyngeal abnormalities (e.g., Pierre-Robin syndrome, post-cleft-palate repair, Treacher Collins syndrome), enlarged tongue in acromegaly, hypothyroidism with myxedema of the upper-airway soft tissues, and temporomandibular joint abnormalities.

In addition to daytime hypersomnia and nighttime sleep disturbances, many patients with OSA syndrome have systemic hypertension, primarily diastolic, and a wide variety of cardiac arrhythmias during sleep. Recognized systemic complications of OSA syndrome are pulmonary hypertension, cardiac enlargement, myocardial infarction, stroke, elevated hematocrit, and an increased risk of sudden death during sleep.

Sleep apnea also occurs in infants and children. In infants, it has been associated with the "acute life-threatening event," as well as familial, congenital, and acquired dysautonomia syndromes and craniofacial disorders. The peak incidence in children is around age 4 years and is often associated with adenotonsillar hypertrophy.

Central sleep apnea syndrome is characterized by intermittent cessation or decreases in respiratory effort with associated decreases in oxygen saturation during sleep. It causes complaints of frequent awakenings and restless unrefreshing sleep and is much less common than OSA syndrome.

An all-night polysomnographic recording is used to diagnose OSA and to quantify the frequency, severity, and type of respiratory disturbance. An *apnea* is defined as the cessation of airflow for 10 seconds or longer. A *central apnea* is the absence of respiratory effort. An *obstructive apnea* is the absence of airflow despite the presence of respiratory effort. A *mixed apnea* consists of an initial central component followed by obstruction. A *hypopnea* is a reduction in airflow for at least 10 seconds and may be central or obstructive. These respiratory events are accompanied by oxygen desaturation and usually by arousals. During recurrent apnea episodes in severe cases, oxygen saturation often falls to less than 50% and bradycardia (less than 60 beats per minute [beats/min]) alternates with tachycardia (greater than 110 beats/min) for each snoring cycle. Stages 3 and 4 sleep are diminished or absent, and there are many stage changes and arousals. The duration of apneic episodes and the degree of oxygen desaturation usually increase in REM sleep.

TABLE 145.3. DIFFERENTIAL DIAGNOSIS FOR EXCESSIVE DAYTIME SLEEPINESS

Insufficient sleep syndrome
Sleep apnea syndromes
Narcolepsy and other hypersomnias
Drugs, e.g., antidepressants, hypnotics, and antihistamines
Periodic limb movement disorder
Circadian rhythm disorders
Depression

Nasal continuous positive airway pressure (CPAP) is the most common and effective treatment for moderate and severe OSA syndrome. Air pressure is generated by a small blower, delivered via tubing to a nasal mask, and controlled by a pressure valve. Each patient must have a treatment trial during polysomnography to determine the pressure required to alleviate airway obstruction during sleep. If successful and well tolerated, a commercially available nasal CPAP unit is prescribed for home use. Prior to nasal CPAP, tracheostomy was the only reliably effective treatment and is still indicated for severe OSA if CPAP is not tolerated.

In some patients, especially children and young adults, the removal of enlarged tonsils and adenoids relieves the obstruction. The surgical procedure, uvulopalatopharyngoplasty, has been an inconsistently beneficial treatment, and selection criteria are not well established. Hyoidplasty and mandibular advancement have successfully treated patients with structural abnormalities causing hypopharyngeal obstruction. Other treatments for less severe cases have been sustained weight loss in obese patients and use during sleep of a dental appliance that advances the lower jaw.

Narcolepsy

Narcolepsy (MIM 161400) is an incurable lifelong neurologic disorder. The classic narcolepsy tetrad consists of (1) excessive daytime sleepiness, (2) cataplexy, (3) sleep paralysis, and (4) hypnagogic hallucinations. Narcolepsy is not rare. Estimates of prevalence range between 2 and 10 per 10,000 individuals in North America and Europe. It is about five times more prevalent in Japan, and the incidence is only 1 per 500,000 in Israel.

The onset of narcolepsy typically occurs between ages 15 and 30 years, although cases have been reported with onset as early as age 5 years and as late as 63 years. Men and women are equally affected. Daytime sleepiness is usually the first symptom to appear. Recognition that the patient has a medical disorder often takes years.

Excessive daytime sleepiness is always present and is usually the most prominent symptom. Patients often complain of fatigue and impaired performance. Irresistible sleep occurs more frequently throughout the day if the patient is inactive, but also occurs at inappropriate times, such as during a conversation, eating, driving, or a monotonous or repetitious activity. These spontaneous naps are usually brief and somewhat refreshing. Patients with narcolepsy generally do not sleep more, but need to sleep more frequently. They have difficulty in sustaining wakefulness. More than 50% of narcoleptic patients have automatic behavior that they describe as memory lapses or blackouts. These episodes are caused by microsleeps that intrude into wakefulness. Patients are capable of carrying out semipurposeful activity associated with amnesia; thus, they can neither monitor the activity nor remember it later. Common examples include getting lost while driving, typing or writing gibberish, misplacing things, or walking into objects. Automatic behavior also occurs in other disorders of excessive sleepiness. Other complaints, such as poor memory and visual disturbances, appear to be related to excessive daytime sleepiness. The symptom of excessive daytime sleepiness

is disabling and often leads to personal, social, and economic problems.

In a patient with excessive daytime sleepiness, the presence of cataplexy is pathognomonic of narcolepsy. Cataplexy consists of a brief episode of paralysis or weakness of voluntary muscles without change in consciousness, and is precipitated by strong but normal emotions. The onset of cataplexy usually follows excessive daytime sleepiness by months or years. It only rarely appears before the sleepiness. The severity of cataplexy is variable. Some patients may have as few as two or three episodes in a lifetime, whereas others may have several episodes every day. A full range of severity exists between these extremes. The most common precipitant is laughter. Other strong emotions include anger, surprise, fear, and anticipation. Cataplexy may be partial and affect only certain muscles; common examples include dysarthria, drooping of the head, and slight buckling of the knees. Severe global attacks affect all skeletal muscles, except muscles of respiration, and cause collapse. Most episodes last only seconds, but severe attacks can last minutes.

REM sleep mechanisms are involved in the pathophysiology of narcolepsy. Manifestations or fragments of REM sleep appear during waking hours and at sleep onset. Cataplexy is the appearance of the paralysis of REM sleep during wakefulness. REM sleep in a narcoleptic patient often begins within 10 minutes of sleep onset instead of after 85 to 100 minutes, as in the normal individual. This abnormal timing of REM sleep is called a sleeponset REM period, which may include sleep paralysis, hypnagogic hallucinations, or both.

Sleep paralysis is a global paralysis of voluntary muscles that occurs at the entry into or emergence from sleep. This muscle weakness is thought to result from the same motor inhibition that occurs during cataplexy in the narcoleptic individual and in REM sleep in everyone. Sleep paralysis without narcolepsy can occur in an isolated form in otherwise healthy individuals or in a familial form genetically transmitted. *Isolated sleep paralysis* most frequently occurs upon awakening. *Familial sleep paralysis* and *sleep paralysis associated with narcolepsy* occur more often at sleep onset. In isolated cases, sleep paralysis may occur only when precipitated by predisposing factors, such as irregular sleep habits, sleep deprivation, work shift, jet lag, and psychologic stress. Although the familial form and that associated with narcolepsy are more chronic, the frequency of episodes can be increased by the same factors. *Hypnagogic hallucinations* are vivid dreamlike images that the narcoleptic person experiences during sleep onset and offset. They are simple or bizarre visual hallucinations that can have auditory and tactile components. The patient is usually aware of the surroundings and has difficulty in discerning the hallucinations from reality; these hallucinations are often frightening. Hypnagogic hallucinations are most likely the result of dissociated central nervous system (CNS) processes involved in dreaming during REM sleep. They can be precipitated by sleep deprivation in normal individuals.

Narcolepsy symptoms produce major social, familial, educational, and economic consequences for both patients and their family. Patients often do not achieve their intellectual potential and suffer frequent failures of occupation, education, and marriage. Family members, friends, and even patients often interpret the symptoms as indicating laziness, lack of ambition, delayed maturation, or psychologic defects. Because these symptoms begin during the crucial period of maturation from puberty to adulthood, misinterpretation and lack of a diagnosis can greatly affect a patient's personality and feelings of self-esteem.

Genetic research shows the existence of a susceptibility gene in the region of the major histocompatibility complex located on the short arm of chromosome 6. Genetic family studies suggest that this gene is not sufficient and that an additional gene or genes may be needed for disease expression. The identification of several pairs of monozygotic twins discordant for narcolepsy indicates a role for environmental factors in the development of narcolepsy.

Several clinical reports have described structural disease in the upper brainstem–hypothalamus area with narcoleptic symptoms and cataplectic-like behavior. This has been produced in cats after microinjection of cholinergic drugs in the pontine reticular formation; however, no pathology has been reported thus far in humans or animal models of narcolepsy-cataplexy.

The current treatment for the sleepiness of narcolepsy is the use of adrenergic stimulant drugs: pemoline (Cylert), methylphenidate hydrochloride (Ritalin HCl), and amphetamines. Modafinil, a new wakefuless-promoting agent that is chemically and pharmacologically distinct from the above stimulants, has been shown to be effective in reducing daytime sleepiness in patients with narcolepsy. Use of stimulant drugs should be carefully monitored; patients and physicians should cooperate in adjusting the amount and timing of doses to meet functional daytime needs and scheduling of patients' activities. Cataplexy, when present to a significant degree, is usually well controlled with the tricyclic compounds imipramine hydrochloride (e.g., imipramine, 10 to 25 mg, two or three times daily), protriptyline hydrochloride (Vivactil), or clomipramine; however, impotence can be an undesirable side effect in men. Selective serotonin reuptake inhibitors such as paroxetine hydrochloride (Paxil) and fluoxetine hydrochloride (Prozac) are also effective. These medications are thought to effectively treat cataplexy because they suppress REM sleep. An important adjunctive treatment for narcolepsy is the rational scheduling of daytime naps and the maintenance of proper sleep hygiene. The physician's role in providing the patient with a clear understanding of the nature of the symptoms and with emotional support in coping with the many adaptive difficulties cannot be overemphasized.

Recurrent hypersomnia (Kleine-Levin syndrome) consists of recurrent episodes of hypersomnia and binge eating lasting up to several weeks, with an interval of 2 to 12 months between episodes. Neurobehavioral and psychologic changes, such as disorientation, forgetfulness, depression, depersonalization, hallucinations, irritability, aggression, and sexual hyperactivity, often accompany the episodes of hypersomnia. Onset is typically in early adolescent boys, but rarely in girls and adults. Episodes decrease in frequency and severity with age and are rarely present after the fourth decade.

A definitive treatment for Kleine-Levin syndrome is not known, but there are reports of limited success with amphetamines and methylphenidate. Because of similarities between Kleine-Levin syndrome and bipolar depression, lithium has been used.

Other Conditions Associated with Excessive Daytime Somnolence

Various neurologic and medical conditions are associated with excessive daytime sleepiness; these include endocrine and metabolic disorders, liver failure, uremia, chronic pulmonary disease (with hypercapnia), hypothyroidism (severe with myxedema), incipient coma with diabetes mellitus, and severe hypoglycemia. Neurologic disorders, such as tumors in the area of the third ventricle (e.g., glioma, craniopharyngioma, dysgerminoma, pinealoma, pituitary adenoma), obstructive hydrocephalus, increased intracranial pressure, viral encephalitis, and other infections of the brain and surrounding membranes, can cause increased daytime somnolence. The postconcussion syndrome may also be associated with increased sleepiness. However, complaints of tiredness, fatigue, difficulty in concentrating, and memory impairment are usually more prominent symptoms.

Disorders of the Sleep–Wake Schedule

The study of human chronobiology has been important for the understanding of clinical disorders of the daily sleep–wake cycle. Many functions, including body temperature, plasma and urine hormones, renal functions, psychologic performance measures, and internal sleep-stage organization, all participate in this circadian rhythm. Evidence for the importance of these cyclic physiologic systems in sleep disturbances comes from studies of acute phase shifts, such as those that occur after transmeridian air flights or in shift work. The daily sleep period is disturbed after acute shifts in such a way that intrusive awakenings take place, sleep length is shortened, and REM phase advances relative to sleep onset. Adaptation is slower after an eastward flight or a phase advance in the laboratory than after a phase delay (westward flight).

Disorders of the circadian sleep–wake cycle are divided into two major categories, transient and persistent. The *transient disorders* include the temporary sleep disturbance following an acute work-shift change and a rapid time-zone change (jet lag). Both sleep deprivation and the circadian phase shift produce symptoms including frequent arousals, especially at the end of sleep episodes, and excessive sleepiness. Affected individuals are fatigued, sleepy, and intermittently inattentive when they should be awake, and have partial insomnia during the daily time for sleep. A wide range of important occupations is involved in these acute phase-shift syndromes (e.g., doctors, nurses, police, firemen, airline pilots, air-traffic controllers, diplomats, international business executives, radar operators, postal workers, long-distance truck drivers, and others).

Persistent sleep–wake cycle disorders are divided into several major clinical categories. Persons who frequently change their sleep–wake schedule (e.g., shift workers) have a mixed pattern of excessive sleepiness alternating with arousal at inappropriate times of the day. Sleep is typically shortened and disrupted. Waking is associated with a decrease in performance and vigilance. The physician caring for such patients should be aware that the syndrome often disrupts social and family life and becomes intolerable.

The *delayed-sleep-phase syndrome* is a specific chronobiologic sleep disorder characterized by a chronic inability to sleep at the desired time to meet required work or study schedules. Patients are typically unable to fall asleep until some time between 2 and 6 a.m. On weekends and vacation days, they sleep until late morning or early afternoon and feel refreshed, but have great difficulty awakening at the required 7 or 8 a.m. for work or school. These patients have a normal sleep length and internal organization of sleep when clock time of sleep onset and sleep offset coincides with the circadian timing that controls daily sleep. When sleep onset is attempted at earlier times, there is usually a long latency to sleep onset.

Successful treatment has been a phase shift of the time of the daily sleep episode by progressive phase delay of the sleep time. By delaying the time of going to sleep and awakening by 2 or 3 hours each day (i.e., a 26- or 27-hour sleep–wake cycle), the patient's sleep timing can be successfully reset to the preferred clock time. Alternatively, treatment with bright light, which phase-shifts the circadian rhythm of core body temperature, has proved helpful in achieving and maintaining a desired schedule.

The *advanced-sleep-phase syndrome* is rare and is more likely to occur in elderly persons. Typical sleep onset is between 6 and 8 p.m., with wake times between 1 and 3 a.m. despite efforts to delay sleep time. The patient with the non-24-hour sleep–wake disorder is completely out of touch with the 24-hour cycle of the rest of society. These rare individuals maintain a 25- to 27-hour biologic day despite all attempts to entrain themselves to a 24-hour cycle. A personality disorder or blindness may predispose to this condition.

An *irregular sleep–wake pattern* consists of considerable irregularity without an identifiable persistent sleep–wake rhythm. There are frequent daytime naps at irregular times and a disturbed nocturnal sleep pattern. Most patients with this syndrome have congenital, developmental, or degenerative brain dysfunction, although it does occur rarely in cognitively intact outpatients. Treatment is difficult but should include regularly scheduled activities and time in bed based on sleep hygiene principles.

Parasomnias

Parasomnias are disorders of arousal, partial arousal, and sleep-stage transition characterized by undesirable behaviors during sleep that are manifestations of CNS activation. Autonomic nervous system changes and skeletal muscle activity are prominent features.

The arousal disorders include the classic disorders of *sleep-walking* and *sleep terrors*, as well as the more recently designated disorder *confusional arousals*. These behaviors typically emerge from slow-wave sleep during the first third of the night. Confusion during and following arousal and amnesia for the episodes are features common to the three disorders. Sleepwalking consists of complex behaviors, including automatic and semipurposeful motor acts, such as sitting up in bed, walking, opening and closing doors, opening a window, climbing stairs, dressing, and even preparing food. A subgroup of patients, usually young adult men, perform acts that are destructive or harmful to themselves, such as breaking furniture, throwing objects, and climbing out or walking through a window. A small nightly dose of a benzodiazepine, such as diazepam or temazepam, is useful, especially when violent behavior is present.

A sleep terror is typically initiated with a sudden, loud, high-pitched scream and sitting up in bed. The patient appears agitated and frightened. Major autonomic changes occur, including rapid pulse and respiration, sweating, and pupillary dilation. Arousal disorders are common in children and generally benign, and decrease in frequency and severity or resolve with increasing age. These disorders, however, must be distinguished from recurrent nocturnal seizure disorders, such as partial complex seizures. Polysomnography with additional EEG channels and videotape of the behaviors is extremely useful for differentiating arousal disorders from sleep-related epilepsy.

REM sleep behavior disorder (RBD), a parasomnia occurring during REM sleep, is characterized by intermittent loss of REM sleep atonia accompanied by motor activity consistent with dream enactment. RBD appears to be uncommon, but the true incidence is unknown. It is more common in older men and often associated with degenerative neurologic disorders, especially Parkinson disease or cerebrovascular disease. Injury to self or bed partner is a significant complication. The diagnosis is usually suggested by history and confirmed by polysomnography. Recordings show persistent muscle tone and complex behaviors during REM sleep. Most patients respond to treatment with a small dose (0.5 to 2 mg) of clonazepam at bedtime. However, daytime carry-over effects causing drowsiness and cognitive dysfunction must be carefully monitored in elderly patients.

Sleep Disorders Associated with Neurologic Disorders

Degenerative neurologic disorders, including dementia and Parkinson disease, have associated sleep disturbances. Sleep may be abnormal because of involvement of brain structures that control and regulate sleep and wakefulness or because of abnormal movements or behaviors that occur during sleep.

Fatal familial insomnia is a rare prion disease (see elsewhere in this volume).

SUGGESTED READINGS

Aharon-Peretz J, Masiah A, Pillar T, et al. Sleep-wake cycles in multi-infarct dementia and dementia of the Alzheimer type. *Neurology* 1991;41:1616–1619.

American Sleep Disorders Association. *The international classification of sleep disorders: diagnostic and coding manual*, rev ed. Rochester, MN: American Sleep Disorders Association, 1997.

Billiard M. Idiopathic hypersomnia. *Neurol Clin* 1996;14:573–582.

Bresnitz EA, Goldberg R, Kosinski RM. Epidemiology of obstructive sleep apnea. *Epidemiol Rev* 1994;16:210–227.

Chesson AL, Ferber RA, Fry JM, et al. The indications for polysomnography and related procedures. *Sleep* 1997;20:423–487.

Coleman R, Pollak CP, Weitzman ED. Periodic movements in sleep (nocturnal myoclonus): relation to sleep disorders. *Ann Neurol* 1980;8:416–421.

Consensus conference. Drugs and insomnia: the use of medications to promote sleep. *JAMA* 1984;251:2410–2414.

Critchley M. Periodic hypersomnia and megaphagia in adolescent males. *Brain* 1962;85:627–656.

Dement WC, Mitler MM, Rogh T, et al. Guidelines for the multiple sleep latency test (MSLT): a standard measure of sleepiness. *Sleep* 1986;9:519–524.

Earley CJ, Allen RP. Pergolide and carbidopa/levodopa treatment of the restless legs syndrome and periodic limb movements in sleep in a consecutive series of patients. *Sleep* 1996;19:801–810.

Feber R. Childhood sleep disorders. *Neurol Clin* 1996;14:493–511.

Fry JM. Restless legs syndrome and periodic leg movements in sleep exacerbated or caused by minimal iron deficiency. *Neurology* 1986;36[Suppl 1]:276.

Fry JM, ed. Current issues in the diagnosis of and management of narcolepsy. *Neurology* 1998;50:[Suppl 1].

Guilleminault C, ed. *Sleeping and waking disorders: indications and techniques.* Menlo Park, CA: Addison-Wesley, 1981.

Hla KM, Young TB, Bidwell T, Palta M, Skatrud JB, Dempsey J. Sleep apnea and hypertension: a population study. *Ann Intern Med* 1994;120:382–388.

Kryger MH, Roth T, Dement WC, eds. *Principles and practice of sleep medicine.* Philadelphia: WB Saunders, 1994.

Lugaresi E, Medori R, Montagna P, et al. Fatal familial insomnia and dysautonomia with selective degeneration of thalamic nuclei. *N Engl J Med* 1986;315:997–1003.

Mahowald MW, Schenck CH. NREM sleep parasomnias. *Neurol Clin* 1996;14:675–696.

Martin TJ, Sanders MH. Chronic alveolar hypoventilation: a review for the clinician. *Sleep* 1995;18:617–634.

Obermeyer WH, Benca RM. Effects of drugs on sleep. *Neurol Clin* 1996;14:827–840.

Orlosky MJ. The Kleine-Levine syndrome: a review. *Psychosomatics* 1982;23:609–621.

Parish JM, Shepard JW. Cardiovascular effects of sleep disorders. *Chest* 1990;97:1220–1226.

Prinz PN. Sleep and sleep disorders in older adults. *J Clin Neurophysiol* 1995;12:139–145.

Prinzmetal M, Bloomberg W. The use of benzedrine for the treatment of narcolepsy. *JAMA* 1935;105:2051.

Randomized trial of modafinil for the treatment of pathological somnolence in narcolepsy. US Modafinil in Narcolepsy Multicenter Study Group. *Ann Neurol* 1998;43:88–97.

Richardson GS, Malin HV. Circadian rhythm sleep disorders: pathophysiology and treatment. *J Clin Neurophysiol* 1996;13:17–31.

Rosenthal NE, Joseph-Vanderpool JR, Levendosky AA, et al. Phase-shifting effect of bright morning light as treatment for delayed sleep-phase syndrome. *Sleep* 1990;13:354–361.

Schenck CH, Mahowald MW. REM sleep parasomnias. *Neurol Clin* 1996;14:697–720.

Schenck CH, Bundlie SR, Patterson AL, Mahowald MW. Rapid eye movement sleep behavior disorders: a treatable parasomnia affecting older males. *JAMA* 1987;257:1786–1789.

Schmidt-Nowara W, Lowe A, Wiegand L, et al. Oral applications for the treatment of snoring and obstructive sleep apnea: a review. *Sleep* 1995;18:501–510.

Silber MH, Shepard JW, Wisbey JA. Pergolide in the management of restless legs syndrome: an extended study. *Sleep* 1997;20:878–882.

Spielman AJ, Nunes J, Glovinsky PB. Insomnia. *Neurol Clin* 1996;14:513–543.

Spielman AJ, Saskin P, Thorpy MJ. Treatment of chronic insomnia by restriction of time in bed. *Sleep* 1987;10:45–56.

Srollo PJ, Rogers RM. Obstructive sleep apnea. *N Engl J Med* 1996;334:99–104.

Sullivan CE, Berthon-Jones M, Issa FG, et al. Reversal of obstructive sleep apnea by continuous positive airway pressure applied through the nares. *Lancet* 1981;1:862–865.

Trenkwalder C, Walters AS, Hening W. Periodic limb movements and restless legs syndrome. *Neurol Clin* 1996;14:629–650.

Weitzman ED, Czeisler CA, Coleman RM, et al. Delayed sleep phase syndrome: a chronobiological disorder with sleep-onset insomnia. *Arch Gen Psychiatry* 1981;38:737–746.

Weitzman ED, Czeisler CA, Zimmerman JC, Moore-Ede M. Biological rhythms in man: relationship of a sleep-wake, cortisol, growth hormone and temperature during temporal isolation. In: Martin JB, Reichlin S, Bick K, eds. *Neurosecretion and brain peptides.* New York: Raven Press, 1981:475–499.

Merritt's Neurology, 10th ed., edited by L.P. Rowland. Lippincott Williams & Wilkins, Philadelphia © 2000.

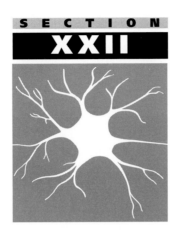

SYSTEMIC DISEASES AND GENERAL MEDICINE

CHAPTER 146

ENDOCRINE DISEASES

GARY M. ABRAMS
EARL A. ZIMMERMAN

Endocrine secretions have a profound influence on the metabolism of the nervous system. Disturbances of consciousness and cognition, along with other neurologic symptoms, may occur with endocrine diseases. This chapter considers the common structural and secretory endocrine disorders that may cause important neurologic symptoms.

PITUITARY

Hypopituitarism

Hypofunction of the pituitary may follow damage to the gland by tumors, inflammatory processes, vascular lesions, or trauma. The location of the lesion may be the pituitary itself, the stalk that connects it with the hypothalamus, or the hypothalamus. Destruction of the hypophyseal portal system in the stalk or the median eminence above by a tumor, such as a craniopharyngioma, or sarcoidosis deprives the anterior pituitary of hypothalamic regulatory hormones. In hypothalamic disease, as in pituitary disease, peripheral blood levels of all the anterior pituitary hormones may be reduced except for prolactin (PRL), which is normally under inhibitory control by hypothalamic dopamine. Diabetes insipidus (DI; see later), which may result from disruption of neurosecretory pathways terminating in the posterior pituitary, is also a feature of some structural diseases causing hypopituitarism. Additionally, neurologic manifestations of hypopituitarism are due to "neighborhood effects" resulting from the contiguous location of the pituitary to the visual pathways and cranial nerves controlling ocular motility.

Secretory and nonsecretory pituitary tumors are the most common causes of neurologic symptoms of hypopituitarism. The size of the lesion usually determines the extent of neurologic symptoms and the degree of hypopituitarism. Headache and visual loss are common when tumors are large and extend into the suprasellar region in the vicinity of the optic chiasm. Lateral extension of masses may produce syndromes involving structures in the cavernous sinus. Growth of tumors superiorly may compress the hypothalamus and obstruct the cerebrospinal fluid (CSF) pathways to cause hydrocephalus.

Vascular lesions of the pituitary may cause dramatic and life-threatening onset of hypopituitarism. In *pituitary apoplexy,* sudden hemorrhage into a pituitary tumor may cause headache, meningismus, visual loss, oculomotor abnormalities, and alteration in the level of consciousness. Hypopituitarism, including acute adrenal insufficiency, may result from a combination of vascular necrosis and compression by the enlarging pituitary

mass. Neurosurgical decompression can improve neurologic and endocrine function.

Sheehan syndrome or postpartum necrosis of the pituitary may also cause actue hypopituitarism and local neurologic symptoms. Hypotension or shock from obstetric hemorrhage or infection causes occlusive spasm of pituitary arteries with anoxic-ischemic necrosis of a pituitary gland that has hypertrophied under estrogen stimulation from pregnancy. Acutely, there may be a shock-like syndrome with obtundation, hypotension, tachycardia, and hypoglycemia. Acute and chronic Sheehan syndromes are both characterized by syndromes of anterior pituitary insufficiency, particularly amenorrhea and failure to lactate. Rarely, DI occurs. A neurologic disorder might be suspected if patients complain of lightheadedness or diminished libido.

In adults, hypopituitarism is often recognized first by impaired secretion of gonadotropins with irregular menstrual periods or amenorrhea in women or loss of libido, potency, or fertility in men. The skin is often thin, smooth, and dry; the peculiar pallor (alabaster skin) and inability to tan have been related to loss of melanotropic (melanocyte-stimulating hormone) or adrenocorticotropic (ACTH) hormones. Axillary and pubic hair may be sparse, with relatively infrequent facial shaving. Depending on the severity of the decrease of production of ACTH and thyroid-stimulating hormone (TSH), patients may note lethargy, weakness, fatigability, cold intolerance, and constipation. There may be an acute adrenal crisis with nausea, vomiting, hypoglycemia, hypotension, and circulatory collapse, particularly in response to stress. Hypothalamic hypopituitarism may additionally be accompanied by hyperprolactinemia with galactorrhea.

Evaluation of patients with pituitary insufficiency caused by an intrasellar or hypothalamic lesion depends on measurement of pituitary hormone levels in the peripheral blood, coupled with functional assessment of the target organs. The basic endocrine evaluation includes thyroid functions (triiodothyronine [T_3], thyroxine [T_4], and TSH), PRL determination, and assessment of adrenal reserve, such as ACTH stimulation for cortisol responsiveness. Pituitary hormone levels must be interpreted in the context of clinical findings. For example, normal gonadotropin levels (follicle-stimulating hormone, luteinizing hormone) may indicate pituitary insufficiency after menopause, when elevated levels would be expected. Elevated levels of gonadotropin or TSH suggest primary gonadal or thyroid failure but, rarely, may be secreted by pituitary tumors. Dynamic tests of pituitary reserve or stimulation tests with synthetic hypothalamic releasing factors are sometimes needed to detect mild hypopituitarism or to distinguish between pituitary and hypothalamic causes of hypopituitarism.

Pituitary Tumors

Most pituitary tumors are associated with oversecretion of one or more anterior pituitary hormones or their subunits. These tumors produce symptoms related to the metabolic or trophic effect of the secreted hormone. Symptoms may be associated with variable degrees of hypopituitarism, depending on the extent of destruction caused by the tumor. Microadenomas (less than 10

TABLE 146.1. CAUSES OF ELEVATED PROLACTIN LEVELS

Normal	Drugs	Diseases
Sleep	Phenothiazines	Pituitary adenoma
Stress	Butyrophenones	Pituitary stalk section
Exercise	Benzamides	Hypothalamic diseases
Coitus	Reserpine	Sarcoidosis
Nipple stimulation	Methyldopa	Tumors (e.g., craniopharyngioma)
Pregnancy	Morphine	Histiocytosis X
Nursing	Thyrotropin-releasing hormone	Primary hypothyroidism
	Estrogens	Renal failure
		Partial seizures

mm) typically cause only symptoms referable to the secreted hormone; macroadenomas (greater than 10 mm) more often cause neural or pituitary dysfunction. Fewer than 10% of microadenomas that secrete PRL show progressive enlargement.

The PRL-secreting adenoma, or *prolactinoma,* is the most common secretory adenoma of the pituitary. It is the most common cause of clinically manifest hyperprolactinemia. In women, there is often a microadenoma with amenorrhea and galactorrhea. In men, the endocrine effects of hyperprolactinemia include impotence, infertility, or, rarely, galactorrhea. In men, prolactinoma is more commonly associated with mass effects of the macroadenoma: headaches, visual-field deficits, and ocular motility problems.

The causes of hyperprolactinemia are listed in Table 146.1. In prolactinoma, serum PRL levels may be less than 200 ng/mL and must be distinguished from other causes of hyperprolactinemia. Values above 200 ng/mL, however, are nearly always associated with a prolactinoma. There is a rough positive correlation between the PRL level and the size of the tumor. Several random

PRL levels of more than 200 ng/mL establish the diagnosis of prolactinoma; more modest elevations may be caused by drugs, hypothalamic disorders, or hypothyroidism (see Table 146.1). In primary hypothyroidism, thyrotropin-releasing hormone (TRH) secretion is presumably enhanced in response to the low circulating levels of thyroid hormone; TRH is a potent stimulus for PRL release. The pituitary may be enlarged (Fig. 146.1).

Computed tomography (CT) or magnetic resonance imaging (MRI) establishes the diagnosis of sellar or parasellar mass lesions. Prolactinoma does not have specific imaging characteristics; the diagnosis is established by correlation with clinical and laboratory findings. Important diagnostic considerations include carotid aneurysm, inflammatory (e.g., lymphocytic hypophysitis) and hormonal causes of pituitary enlargement (e.g., primary hypothyroidism), and craniopharyngioma.

Treatment of hyperprolactinemia is accomplished with dopaminergic agonists, such as bromocriptine mesylate (Parlodel), which usually reduce serum PRL levels to normal, but treatment of the primary pathology (e.g., thyroid failure) may be

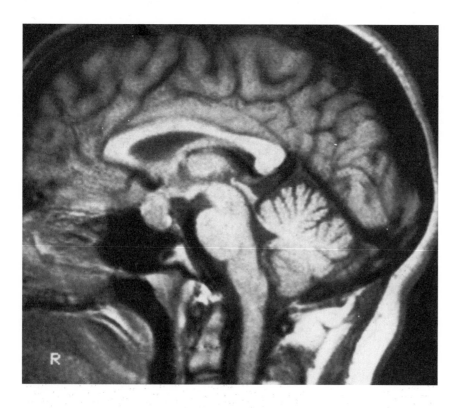

FIG. 146.1. Pituitary enlargement in association with primary hypothyroidism is shown on MRI.

more appropriate. Return of PRL levels to normal is usually associated with restoration of gonadal function and cessation of galactorrhea. In patients with a prolactinoma, bromocriptine therapy is often accompanied by reduction of tumor size, resolution of neurologic symptoms, and reversal of pituitary insufficiency. Long-term therapy is required because the tumor recurs if bromocriptine is withdrawn. Both microadenomas and macroadenomas can be removed by transsphenoidal adenomectomy. "Cure" rates are correlated with tumor size and PRL level, but surgery is most effective for rapid decompression of the optic nerves or chiasm. Surgical cures have been associated with tumor recurrence rates of 20% to 50% after 5 years. Radiotherapy alone or in combination with surgery or pharmacotherapy is also a therapeutic option.

Infertility in women as a result of hyperprolactinemia from a pituitary tumor can be successfully treated with bromocriptine. If pregnancy results, bromocriptine therapy is discontinued, although there has been no evidence of teratogenesis. Estrogen stimulation of prolactinoma during pregnancy causes tumor enlargement, but clinically significant enlargement occurs in only 10% to 15% of macroadenomas. Bromocriptine therapy may be reintroduced with successful control of symptoms; in unusual cases, transsphenoidal surgery can be used.

Excessive Growth Hormone and Acromegaly

Growth hormone (GH)-secreting pituitary tumors are the most common cause of *acromegaly* (Figs. 146.2 to 146.4). When fully developed, acromegaly is easily recognized by excessive skeletal and soft tissue growth. Facial features are coarse, with a large bulbous nose, prominent supraorbital ridges, a protruding mandible, separated teeth, and thick lips. Hands and feet are en-

larged, and sweating is frequently increased. These changes are usually slowly progressive. Patients complain of headaches, fatigue, muscular pain, visual disturbances, and impairment of gonadal function. Paresthesia, sometimes with a typical carpal tunnel syndrome, may be present. Generalized arthritis and diabetes mellitus (DM) are frequent components; mortality is increased with acromegaly. In young patients before epiphyseal closure, excessive secretion of GH results in gigantism.

The neuroendocrine regulation of GH secretion is complex. The major releasing factor is *GH-releasing hormone;* the major inhibitory agent is *somatostatin.* GH has a predominantly nocturnal pattern of secretion and is influenced by age and sleep. The diagnosis of acromegaly is most easily established by demonstrating sustained elevation of GH that cannot be suppressed by physiologic stimuli, such as glucose. Paradoxic elevation of GH may occur with glucose or TRH, suggesting hypothalamic dysfunction. Many actions of GH are mediated by insulin-like growth factor I (formerly somatomedin C), and these levels may be elevated with acromegaly.

MRI is sensitive in localizing even small GH-secreting adenomas, and surgical removal is the treatment of choice. Cure rate is highest for microadenomas. Surgical decompression and radiation therapy may be the best alternative for larger tumors. Bromocriptine therapy has been useful in some patients. The long-acting somatostatin analog octreotide acetate (Sandostatin) offers specific adjunctive therapy for control of GH secretion.

Excessive Adrenocorticotropic Hormone

Cushing disease results from hypersecretion of ACTH by a pituitary tumor. Such tumors are usually small and often difficult to detect. Cushing disease may be difficult to distinguish from

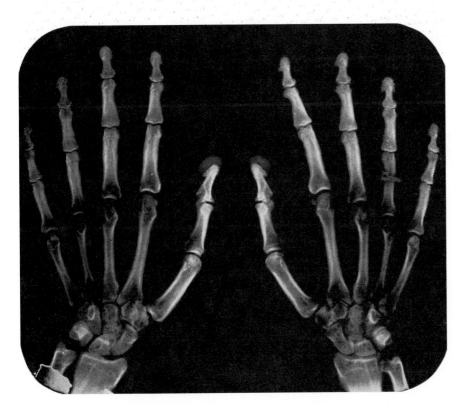

FIG. 146.2. Tufting of the terminal phalanges in acromegaly. (Courtesy of Dr. Juan Taveras.)

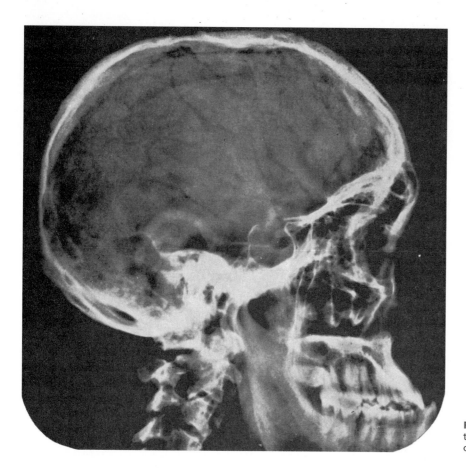

FIG. 146.3. Pituitary tumor with ballooning of the sella turcica, prognathism, and enlargement of the skull bones. (Courtesy of Dr. Juan Taveras.)

other causes of hyperadrenalism, such as adrenal adenoma or ectopic ACTH production by neoplasms. The symptoms of Cushing disease include plethoric facies, centripetal obesity, hypertension, DM, amenorrhea, hirsutism, acne, and osteoporosis. Mental status changes or myopathy may be prominent.

The differential diagnosis of Cushing syndrome can be challenging. Elevated urinary free cortisol levels and suppressibility of cortisol secretion by dexamethasone are the key tests for establishing the diagnosis of pituitary-dependent Cushing syn-

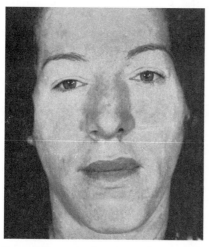

FIG. 146.4. Prognathism and enlargement of nose in acromegaly secondary to pituitary adenoma. (Courtesy of Dr. E. Herz.)

drome. Direct assay of plasma ACTH may be helpful; high levels are seen with ectopic ACTH production. The ACTH response to corticotropin-releasing factor may distinguish Cushing disease from other causes of hypercortisolism. Selective sampling of ACTH levels from the petrosal sinuses may help localize an adenoma within the pituitary.

MRI with gadolinium is the most sensitive procedure for detecting these tumors. Transsphenoidal adenomectomy is the treatment of choice. In patients treated by bilateral adrenalectomy, an aggressive ACTH-secreting pituitary tumor may develop to cause the hyperpigmentation of Nelson syndrome. The hypothalamus may play a role in the pathogenesis of both Cushing disease and Nelson syndrome. Ketoconazole (Nizoral), an inhibitor of adrenal steroidogenesis, may inhibit the adverse effects of hypercortisolism.

The *empty sella syndrome* rarely poses difficulty in the diagnosis of pituitary tumors. The syndrome develops with herniation of the subarachnoid space through the diaphragma sellae either idiopathically or following destruction or surgical removal of the pituitary gland. Remodeling and enlargement of the bony sella turcica may occur, and the sella may appear enlarged on skull x-ray film. CT or MRI usually clarifies the diagnosis. Pituitary dysfunction is uncommon and, if present, suggests that the apparently empty sella is accompanied by a pituitary tumor. The clinical accompaniments of the empty sella syndrome—obese women with headache—are similar to those of pseudotumor cerebri; chronically increased CSF pressure may precipitate the development of an empty sella.

Diabetes Insipidus

DI is characterized by excessive excretion of urine and an abnormally large fluid intake caused by impaired production of antidiuretic hormone (arginine vasopressin) in the posterior pituitary. There are two general groups of patients. In primary DI, there is no known lesion in the pituitary or hypothalamus; secondary DI is associated with lesions in the hypothalamus either in the supraoptic and paraventricular nuclei or in their tracts in the medial eminence or upper pituitary stalk. Among the lesions are tumors (e.g., pituitary adenoma, craniopharyngioma, meningioma), aneurysms, xanthomatosis (Schüller-Christian disease), sarcoidosis, trauma, infections, and vascular disease. Primary DI is rare. Heredity is a factor in some patients. Many different mutations have been found in familial autosomal-dominant DI. Autopsy studies of a few cases revealed loss of neurons in the supraoptic and paraventricular nuclei. Secondary or symptomatic DI is more frequent but still uncommon. It may follow head injury and is present in many patients with xanthomatosis and in some patients with tumors or other lesions in the hypothalamic region. The syndrome is evidence of hypothalamic disease.

Unless complicated by other symptoms associated with the lesion, the symptoms of DI are limited to polyuria and polydipsia. Eight to 20 L or even more of urine are passed in 24 hours, and there is a comparably high level of water intake. The frequent voiding and excessive water intake may interfere with normal activities and disturb sleep. Usually, however, general health is maintained if this is an isolated deficiency of the hypothalamus. The symptoms and signs in patients with tumors or other lesions in the hypothalamic region are those usually associated with these conditions (see Chapter 58). The laboratory findings are normal, except for a low specific gravity of the urine (1.001 to 1.005) and increased serum osmolality in many patients.

The diagnosis is made, based on polyuria and polydipsia. It is distinguished from DM by the glycosuria and high specific gravity of the urine in DM. A large amount of urine may be passed by patients with chronic nephritis but not the large volumes (more than 3 L per day) found in DI; the presence of albumin and casts in the urine and other findings should prevent any confusion in recognizing nephritis. Psychogenic polydipsia must be considered (see below).

A rare cause of DI is failure of the kidneys to respond to vasopressin, a hereditary defect in infant boys.

Absence of vasopressin is difficult to determine in blood by radioimmunoassay. Therefore, the diagnosis is made by clinical tests that include antidiuretic responses to exogenous vasopressin and dehydration. Administration of five pressor units of aqueous vasopressin rapidly results in a marked decrease in urinary output and an increase in osmolality (specific gravity greater than 1.011) in a patient with DI; there is no response in nephrogenic disease. Psychogenic polydipsia, however, may also show a limited response. In contrast to DI, however, there is a normal response to dehydration in psychogenic polydipsia, although the time required for an increase in urinary concentration may be 12 to 18 hours. Normal subjects dehydrated for 6 to 8 hours reduce urinary volume and concentrate urinary osmolality to roughly twice that of plasma (specific gravity greater than 1.015). Patients with severe DI do not respond and should be observed closely, with care taken to prevent loss of more than 3% of body weight during the test; otherwise, patients may become severely dehydrated. A useful clinical test, devised by Moses and Miller, that combines dehydration with the response to exogenous vasopressin distinguishes these disorders and also partial DI.

The diagnosis of DI carries with it the necessity of determining the cause. This means a thorough neurologic examination with particular attention to visual acuity and visual fields. MRI is essential. In DI, the normally bright spot outlining the posterior pituitary gland on MRI may be absent or displaced more proximally in the hypothalamic infundibular stalk (ectopic) (Fig 146.5). MRI may also show craniopharyngioma, hamartoma, dysgerminoma, or histiocytosis X.

Primary DI may persist for years. DI caused by known lesions in the hypothalamus may also be permanent, but complete remission with reversal of symptoms is not infrequent.

Treatment of DI associated with tumors or other remediable hypothalamic lesions is that appropriate to the lesion (surgical removal or radiation therapy). Symptomatic therapy of the DI, if it persists in these cases and in syndromes of unknown cause, is directed toward suppression of diuresis. No effort is made to limit fluid intake. Aqueous vasopressin (Pitressin) can be administered subcutaneously in five pressor-unit doses one to four times daily; it may also be sprayed transnasally in the form of lysine vasopressin or placed high in the nasopharynx on cotton pledgets. Vasopressin tannate in oil injected intramuscularly is slowly absorbed and may be effective for several days.

The drug of choice is now the synthetic analog of vasopressin, 1-deamino-8-D-arginine vasopressin (DDAVP). DDAVP has no smooth muscle effects and has no pressor or cardiac complications. It also avoids the nasal irritation associated with adminis-

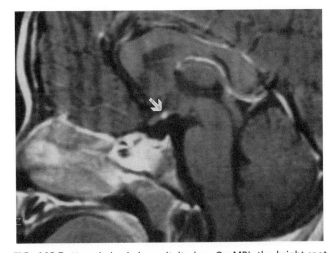

FIG. 146.5. Hypothalamic hypopituitarism. On MRI, the bright-spot *(arrow)* appearance of the posterior pituitary gland is missing from its normal location in the sella turcica. Instead, it is located in the lower hypothalamus and upper pituitary stalk in this child with congenital GH and TSH deficiency. Damage to the stalk interrupts the hypophyseal portal system and vasopressin fibers. These fibers regenerate, forming a new, usually smaller, posterior pituitary in this location (ectopic). Such patients may recover from or have partial DI. More proximal lesions in the hypothalamic nuclei and tracts to the vasopressin system do not regenerate. Interruption of the releasing-factor pathways and the portal system results in anterior pituitary deficiencies. (From Zimmerman, 1998; with permission.)

tration of lysine vasopressin nasal spray. It is given by nasal instillation or spray and provides good control for about 8 hours. An oral form is also now available; the usual dose is 300 to 600 μg per day in divided doses. Partial DI may require no therapy or may be ameliorated by oral administration of clofibrate or chlorpropamide. Chlorpropamide occasionally causes hypoglycemia and, rarely, water intoxication.

Excessive Secretion of Antidiuretic Hormone

Inappropriate secretion of antidiuretic hormone may occur with injury to the hypothalamohypophyseal system by head injury, infections, tumors, and other causes. It has been reported in association with lung carcinoma and, occasionally, with other tumors that elaborate vasopressin. It may also be associated with lung diseases that may overstimulate afferent pathways to the hypothalamus or with drugs that cause excess secretion of vasopressin, such as carbamazepine (Tegretol). Other drugs associated with the syndrome include vasopressin and its oxytocin analog, nonsteroidal antiinflammatory medications, antipsychotics, thiazides, and selective serotonin-reuptake inhibitors.

Hyponatremia and natriuresis in patients with intracranial disease may also be due to "cerebral salt wasting," which is now recognized as different from inappropriate secretion of antidiuretic hormones, as it is associated with the loss of salt and hypovolemia and responds to their replacement.

The salient features of the syndrome are hyponatremia and hypotonicity of body fluids, excessive urinary excretion of sodium despite hyponatremia, normal renal and adrenal function, absence of edema, hypotension, azotemia or dehydration, and improvement of the electrolyte disturbance and clinical symptoms on restriction of fluid intake. Evidence of cerebral dysfunction includes headache, confusion, somnolence, coma, seizures, transient focal neurologic signs, and an abnormal electroencephalogram (EEG). Mild forms clear with simple fluid restriction. Severe cases with seizures or coma are treated with furosemide (Lasix) diuresis and electrolyte replacement (3% sodium chloride). Caution should be used in rapid correction of hyponatremia to avoid central pontine demyelination. Intravenous urea and normal saline have also been used for rapid correction. In the near future, vasopressin antagonists may be useful in diagnosing and treating this condition.

THYROID

Hypothyroidism

Thyroid hormone is important in early growth and development, and the neurologic consequences of hypothyroidism depend on the age of the patient when the deficiency begins. Severe thyroid deficiency *in utero* or early life results in delayed physical and mental development or *cretinism*. Soon after birth, subcutaneous tissue thickens, the infant's cry becomes hoarse, the tongue enlarges, and the infant has widely spaced eyes, a potbelly, and an umbilical hernia. Anomalies of the cardiac and gastrointestinal system commonly accompany congenital hypothyroidism. If treatment is not prompt, dwarfism and mental

deficiency result. Despite early treatment, mild hearing and vestibular dysfunction may persist.

Juvenile myxedema is similar to cretinism, with variations that depend on age at onset of thyroid deficiency. The severity of physical and mental retardation is usually less than in infantile myxedema. Precocious puberty also occurs in juvenile hypothyroidism. Enlargement of the sella turcica has been seen in juvenile myxedema and other forms of long-standing hypothyroidism, which can be associated with hyperprolactinemia. Adult myxedema is characterized by lethargy; weakness; slowness of speech; nonpitting edema of the subcutaneous tissues; coarse, pale skin; dry, brittle hair; thick lips; macroglossia; and increased sensitivity to cold environmental temperatures.

The neurologic complications of hypothyroidism include headache, disorders of the cranial and peripheral nerves, sensorimotor abnormalities, and changes in cognition and level of consciousness. Cranial nerve abnormalities, other than visual and acoustic nerve problems, are unusual. Decreased vision and hearing loss may occur, and vertigo and tinnitus may be present. Visual and auditory evoked potentials have been reported to be abnormal and respond to treatment. The cause of headache is uncertain. Pseudotumor cerebri has been reported in hypothyroidism in children receiving thyroid replacement therapy.

Encephalopathy has recently been associated with euthyroid patients with Hashimoto thyroiditis. Two types of presentations have been noted: a strokelike pattern with mild cognitive impairment and a diffuse progressive type with seizures, psychotic episodes, and dementia. Some patients responded to steroids.

A mild polyneuritis is a rare complication characterized mainly by paresthesia in the hands and feet. Entrapment neuropathy of the median nerve (carpal tunnel syndrome) is attributed to the accumulation of acid mucopolysaccharides in the nerve and surrounding tissues. Neuromuscular findings include slowing of voluntary movements and slow relaxation of tendon reflexes, particularly the ankle jerks. Electrically silent mounding of muscles on direct percussion is called *myoidema*. There may be myopathic weakness. Enlargement of muscles is the *Hoffmann syndrome*. Neuromuscular symptoms improve with thyroid replacement.

In hypothyroid infants, a remarkable generalized enlargement or hypertrophy of muscles constitutes the Kocher-Debré-Sémélaigne syndrome, creating an "infant Hercules" (Fig. 146.6); the muscles decrease in size with replacement therapy.

Cerebellar syndromes may occur in adults, manifestly ataxic gait. In children, cell loss has been detected in the vermis.

Mental status changes may be prominent, with decreased attentiveness, poor concentration, lethargy, and dementia. Psychiatric symptoms—delirium, depression, or frank psychosis (*myxedema madness*)—may appear, depending on the severity and duration of thyroid deficiency. *Myxedema coma* may be accompanied by hypothermia, hypotension, and respiratory and metabolic disturbances, and, if untreated, has a high mortality rate.

Severe hypothyroidism or myxedema is primarily associated with thyroid failure as opposed to hypothalamic–pituitary disease. The characteristic findings are low circulating T_4 and T_3, elevated TSH, and low radioiodine uptake by the thyroid. The

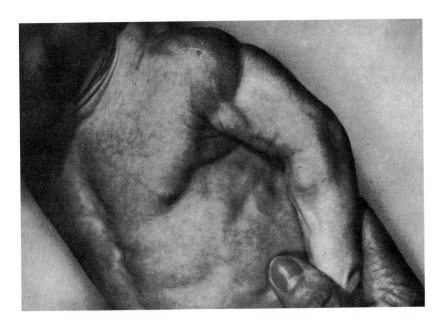

FIG. 146.6. Enlargement of muscles in Kocher-Debré-Sémélaigne syndrome. (Courtesy of Dr. Arnold Gold.)

CSF protein content increases; values greater than 100 mg/mL are not exceptional. EEG abnormalities include slowing and generalized decrease in amplitude.

The treatment of hypothyroidism depends on the severity of the deficiency. Myxedema coma should be treated rapidly with intravenous administration of levothyroxine. In other patients, gradually increasing doses of oral levothyroxine are recommended. Angina pectoris or heart failure can be precipitated by too rapid replacement in adults. In secondary hypothyroidism, thyroid replacement should not be started without concomitant corticosteroid replacement. Prophylactic treatment of cretinism is important in goiter districts, where iodine should be given to all pregnant women.

Hyperthyroidism

Hyperthyroidism or thyrotoxicosis is associated with an increased metabolic rate, abnormal cardiovascular and autonomic functions, tremor, and myopathy. It may present as atrial fibrillation in older adults. Mental disturbances range from mild irritability to psychosis. When hyperthyroidism is associated with diffuse goiter, ophthalmopathy, and dermopathy, it is termed *Graves disease,* which is an autoimmune disorder. Immunologic mechanisms probably play an important role in the thyroid, eye, and skin manifestations. Hyperthyroidism may be subtle in older patients, with apathy, myopathy, and cardiovascular disease as the most prominent symptoms.

Ocular symptoms are common in thyrotoxicosis. These may be present as infrequent blinking, lid lag, or weakness of convergence and are distinct from the infiltrative ophthalmopathy associated with thyroid disease known as *Graves ophthalmopathy.* The relationship of the eye disorder to thyroid status is unclear; it may appear in hyperthyroid patients, in euthyroid patients after thyroidectomy, or in euthyroid patients with no history of hyperthyroidism.

The pathologic changes are confined to the orbit. There is an increase in the orbital contents with edema, hypertrophy, infil-

tration, and fibrosis of the extraocular muscles (Fig. 146.7). Onset of symptoms is gradual; exophthalmos is often accompanied by diplopia secondary to paresis of one or more ocular muscles. Both eyes may be simultaneously involved, or the exophthalmos in one eye may precede the other by several months. With advance of the exophthalmos, paresis of the extrinsic muscles of the eye increases until, finally, the eyeball is almost totally fixed. Papilledema sometimes occurs, and ulcerations of the cornea may develop secondary to failure of the lid to protect the eye. The paralysis may involve all of the eye muscles concerned with the movement of the eyes in a particular plane. The symptoms progress rapidly for a few months and may lead to complete ophthalmoplegia. Occasionally, spontaneous improvement occurs; as a rule, the symptoms persist unchanged throughout a patient's life, unless relieved by therapy.

Treatment of thyroid ophthalmopathy is controversial. Radiation therapy of the pituitary or thyroid has no effect; neither does surgical removal of the thyroid. Surgical decompression of the orbit is of disputed benefit. Methylcellulose drops, shields, or partial suturing of the lids is recommended to protect the eye. Prednisone is favored by some clinicians.

Limb myopathy is common with hyperthyroidism. *Thyrotoxic myopathy* is characterized by weakness and wasting of the muscles of the pelvic girdle, particularly the iliopsoas, and, to a lesser extent, the muscles of the shoulder girdle. Tendon reflexes are normal or hyperactive, and sensation is normal. Fasciculations or myokymia may be noted. Thyrotoxic myopathy needs to be distinguished from myasthenia gravis (MG), which may accompany hyperthyroidism. Improvement of the myopathy follows effective treatment of the hyperthyroidism.

The occurrence of hyperthyroidism and periodic paralysis seems more common in people of Asian ancestry. *Thyrotoxic periodic paralysis* is similar to hypokalemic periodic paralysis in terms of precipitants and treatment. Propranolol may temporarily reduce the number of attacks. Symptoms disappear when the treated patient becomes euthyroid.

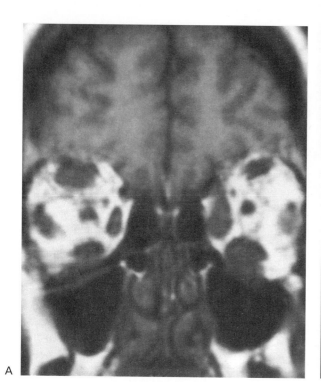
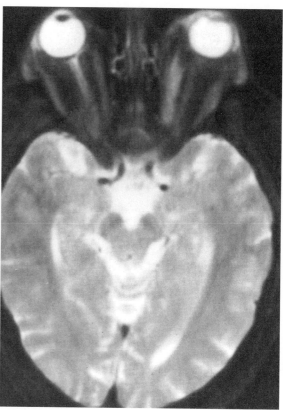

FIG. 146.7. Graves disease. Coronal T1-weighted **(A)** and axial T2-weighted fat-suppressed **(B)** MR images of the orbits show bilateral proptosis with enlargement of the medial rectus muscles (left greater than right), the left lateral and inferior rectus muscles, and the right superior rectus muscle. Although the most common pattern of extraocular muscle enlargement is symmetric, asymmetric involvement is not uncommon in Graves disease. This patient had known hyperthyroidism secondary to Graves disease. (Courtesy of Dr. S. Chan.)

There is an association between hyperthyroidism and MG. About 5% of patients with MG have hyperthyroidism. In most patients, MG precedes or occurs simultaneously with the hyperthyroidism. Differential diagnosis between thyrotoxic myopathy and MG is primarily made on the clinical features, response to edrophonium chloride, and electrophysiologic abnormalities of MG. If there are cranial symptoms (dysarthria, dysphagia, ptosis) in a hyperthyroid patient, MG should be suspected. Interpretation of ocular signs may be complicated by thyrotoxic ophthalmopathy, but even with exophthalmos, the presence of ptosis suggests concomitant MG, which may respond to edrophonium.

PARATHYROID

Hypoparathyroidism

Hypoparathyroidism results in a disturbance of calcium and phosphorus metabolism that is manifested especially by tetany. Hypoparathyroidism may be due to primary deficiency of parathyroid hormone or from lack of peripheral responses as a result of defective action at cellular hormone receptors. Hypoparathyroidism may follow thyroidectomy or may be part of an idiopathic autoimmune syndrome, which sometimes includes primary adrenal failure.

In *pseudohypoparathyroidism,* symptoms of hypocalcemia result from the ineffective action of parathyroid hormone at cellular receptors. Patients have a characteristic habitus, with short stature, stocky physique, rounded face, and shortening of the metacarpal and metatarsal bones. Common clinical features of hypoparathyroidism and pseudohypoparathyroidism include mental deficiency, cataracts, tetany, and seizures (Table 146.2). Lesions of ectodermally derived tissue include scaly skin, alopecia, or atrophic changes in the nails. Other neurologic manifestations are directly related to the effects of hypocalcemia on the nervous system.

Tetany is the most distinctive sign that may be manifested by carpopedal spasm. *Latent tetany* can be demonstrated by contracture of the facial muscles on tapping the facial nerve in front of the ear (*Chvostek sign*), evoking carpal spasm by inducing ischemia in the arm with an inflated blood pressure cuff (*Trousseau sign*), or demonstrating the lowered threshold of electrical excitability of the nerve (*Erb sign*).

Convulsions are a symptom of hypocalcemia regardless of cause. Seizures are usually generalized, tend to be frequent, and respond poorly to anticonvulsant drugs. EEG changes are nonspecific and typically revert to normal with correction of the serum calcium levels. Although hypoparathyroidism is a rare cause of seizures, the diagnosis should be considered when seizures are frequent or bizarre and difficult to control with medication.

TABLE 146.2. INCIDENCE OF SIGNS AND SYMPTOMS IN PSEUDOHYPOPARATHYROIDISM

Characteristics	Patients (%)
Biochemical	
Hypocalcemia	96
Increased alkaline phosphatase	20
Body habitus	
Short stature	80
Round face	92
Stocky or obese	50
Ocular	
Lenticular opacities	49
Dental	
Hypoplasia, enamel defects	51
Calcification	
Subcutaneous	55
Basal ganglia	50
Skeletal	
Short metacarpals	68
Thickened calvarium	62
Neurologic	
Mental retardation	75
Seizures	59
Muscle cramps, twitches	38

In: Stanbury JB, Wyngaarden JB, Fredrickson DS, eds. Pseudohypoparathyroidism. *The metabolic basis of inherited disease,* 3rd ed. New York: McGraw-Hill, 1983: 1508–1527; with permission.

Intracranial calcifications are common in hypoparathyroidism (Fig. 146.8). The basal ganglia are the predominant site for calcium deposition, but other regions may be affected. The calcifications are usually not associated with symptoms, but a variety of hypokinetic and hyperkinetic movement disorders have been seen in hypoparathyroidism. Symptoms may be reversible with appropriate treatment.

Increased intracranial pressure with papilledema has been reported with hypoparathyroidism. The mechanism is unexplained. CSF pressure returns to normal with correction of serum calcium values. Hypoparathyroid myopathy may be accompanied by high values of serum creatine kinase. The diagnosis of hypoparathyroidism is made based on clinical symptoms, hypocalcemia, and low or undetectable plasma parathyroid hormone levels. In pseudohypoparathyroidism, parathyroid hormone levels are elevated. Hypocalcemia may be associated with electrocardiogram changes, including prolongation of the QT interval and T-wave changes.

Vitamin D and calcium supplements are the primary therapy for most forms of hypoparathyroidism. They are effective in relieving tetany and in restoring the serum calcium and phosphorus values to normal. Dosage needs to be adjusted to the needs of the patient.

Hyperparathyroidism

Primary hyperparathyroidism is most commonly due to the oversecretion of parathyroid hormone by a solitary adenoma of the parathyroid glands. The classic syndrome of hyperparathyroidism is hypercalcemia with a combination of renal lithiasis, osteitis, and peptic ulcer disease (Table 146.3). Modern-day hyperparathyroidism, however, is frequently seen with minimal symptoms.

Neuromuscular symptoms include symmetric proximal limb weakness and muscle wasting. Tendon reflexes may be normal or hyperactive. Abnormal movements of the tongue may be seen. Electromyography and muscle biopsy may show evidence of neuropathic disease. Mental status changes include memory loss, irritability, and depression, which improve with return to normal of serum calcium levels.

The diagnosis of hyperparathyroidism is now often made by automated blood chemistry tests in routine examinations, before

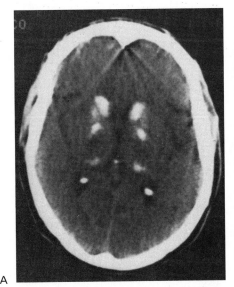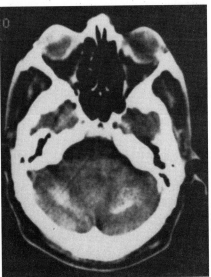

FIG. 146.8. Pseudohypoparathyroidism. **A:** Dense areas of calcification are evident in the head of the caudate nucleus (anterior putamen and globus pallidus (middle pair) and pulvinar (posterior). The fine densities in the occipital horns are calcifications in the choroid plexus. **B:** Calcification is also seen in subcortical areas of the cerebellar hemispheres. (Courtesy of Dr. S.K. Hilal and Dr. M. Mawad.)

TABLE 146.3. CLUES TO THE DIAGNOSIS OF HYPERPARATHYROIDISM IN THE FIRST 343 CASES AT THE MASSACHUSETTS GENERAL HOSPITAL

Clue	Cases (n)
Bone disease	80
Renal stones	195
Peptic ulcer	27
Pancreatitis	9
Fatigue	10
Hypertension	6
Mental disturbance	3
CNS signs	7
Multiple endocrine abnormalities	3
Lumps in neck	1
No symptoms	2

From Cope, 1966; with permission.

there are clinical signs. Calcium levels are not as elevated as in the past, and the classic neuromuscular symptoms and signs are less frequently observed. Limb weakness, paresthesia, and muscle cramps may be seen. Neurologic abnormalities are now uncommon.

Differential diagnosis includes the conditions that cause hypercalcemia, including secondary hyperparathyroidism.

PANCREAS

Hypoglycemia

The central nervous system (CNS) depends almost entirely on glucose for its metabolism; dysfunction develops rapidly when the amount of glucose in the blood falls below critical levels. Hypoglycemia may be associated with an overdose of insulin in the treatment of DM. Spontaneous hypoglycemia is usually the result of *pancreatic hyperinsulinism.* Hypersecretion of insulin by the pancreas may be due to a tumor of the islet cells or functional overactivity of these cells. Hypoglycemia may also occur when liver function is impaired or when there is severe damage to the pituitary or adrenal glands.

The symptoms of hyperinsulinism are paroxysmal, tending to occur when the blood glucose could be expected to be low (in the morning before breakfast, after a fast, or after heavy exercise). Occasionally, symptoms follow a meal. The duration of symptoms varies from minutes to hours. The severity also varies. There may be only nervousness, anxiety, or tremulousness, which is relieved by the ingestion of food. Severe attacks last for hours, during which the patient may perform automatic activity with complete amnesia for the entire period or seizures may be followed by coma. The frequency of attacks varies from several per day to infrequent episodes.

Spontaneous hypoglycemia is occasionally seen in infants. Risk factors include immaturity, low birthweight, or severe illness. Infants of diabetic mothers may exhibit hyperinsulinism. A host of genetic or metabolic defects may cause hypoglycemia, including galactosemia, fructose intolerance, or leucine sensitivity. The symptoms of infantile hypoglycemia are muscular twitching, myoclonic jerks, and seizures. Mental retardation results if

the condition is not recognized and adequately treated. Hypoglycemic symptoms can be divided into two groups: autonomic and cerebral. Sympathetic symptoms are present in most patients at the onset of hypoglycemia, usually preceding the more serious cerebral manifestations. Autonomic symptoms include lightheadedness, sweating, nausea, vomiting, pallor, palpitations, precordial oppression, headache, abdominal pain, and hunger.

Cerebral symptoms usually occur with the sympathetic phenomena but may be the only manifestations. The most common manifestations are paresthesia, diplopia, and blurred vision, which may be followed by tremor, focal neurologic abnormalities, abnormal behavior, or convulsions. After prolonged, severe hypoglycemia, coma may ensue. Episodic confusion and abnormal behavior may simulate complex partial epilepsy. Although generalized or partial seizures may be a common manifestation of hypoglycemia, hyperinsulinism only rarely causes epilepsy.

The neurologic examination is usually normal, except during attacks of hypoglycemia when there may be findings as described. The diagnosis is established by documentation of hypoglycemia during a symptomatic episode, but the timing of the specimen is important because homeostatic mechanisms may return the blood glucose level to normal. The level of blood glucose at which symptoms appear varies from person to person. The EEG shows focal or widespread dysrhythmia during an attack of hypoglycemia and, in some patients, even in the interval between attacks.

The diagnosis of hyperinsulinism is made by the paroxysmal appearance of signs of autonomic and cerebral dysfunction in association with a low blood glucose level and an inappropriately high circulating insulin level. Factitious hypoglycemia may be caused by self-administration of insulin or inappropriate use of oral hypoglycemic agents. If it is not possible to obtain a blood specimen during an attack, a diagnostic fast should be considered. After 12 to 14 hours, 80% of patients with islet cell tumors have low glucose and high insulin levels. Longer fasts may be needed. The diagnosis of *islet cell adenoma* can be difficult; additional endocrine tests and imaging studies may be needed. Hypoglycemia associated with diseases of the liver, adrenal, or pituitary can usually be distinguished by other signs and symptoms of disease in these organs.

Early, intensive treatment of acute hypoglycemia is important to prevent CNS damage. Sugar can be given orally in conscious patients. Comatose patients should be given glucose intravenously. Functional hyperinsulinism is treated by diet modifications to avoid excessive insulin secretion by the pancreas. Long-term management of hyperinsulinism is directed at identification and correction of the underlying cause.

Diabetes Mellitus

DM is a systemic metabolic disorder characterized by hypoinsulinism or peripheral resistance to the action of insulin. Current classification systems broadly divide DM into two types defined by clinical characteristics and pattern of insulin deficiency. *Insulin-dependent DM* usually occurs in young, nonobese people with insulin deficiency. *Noninsulin-dependent DM* is generally encountered in older, obese individuals with peripheral resistance to the action of insulin. The neurologic complications in both types of DM are similar; the presence of neurologic disease is roughly correlated with the duration and severity of the disease and is commonly associated with other tissue complications of DM, such as retinopathy and nephropathy.

The primary neurologic complication of DM is peripheral neuropathy. This includes mononeuropathies (peripheral and cranial nerves), polyneuropathy, autonomic neuropathy, radiculopathies, and entrapment neuropathy (median, ulnar, and peroneal) (see Chapter 105). The cause of these neuropathies is uncertain; metabolic, vascular, and hypoxic mechanisms have been advanced.

Mononeuropathies are attributed to vascular lesions of peripheral nerves. Onset of symptoms is rapid, and pain is common in both mononeuropathies and radiculopathies caused by DM. Common cranial neuropathies involve the oculomotor and abducens nerves and are also due to vascular lesions. Pupillary sparing is common but not invariable because of the pattern of vascular damage to the oculomotor nerve. The prognosis for recovery from mononeuropathy or radiculopathy is good.

Symmetric polyneuropathy of DM is the one most commonly encountered. There is typically a gradual onset of symptoms, the character of the symptoms depending on the type of peripheral nerve fiber affected. Numbness and burning are common complaints. Rarely, a patient may present with a Charcot joint or skin ulcer if nociceptive fibers have sustained the predominant damage. Distal sensory loss may be accompanied by weakness; tendon reflexes are usually lost. Diagnosis of diabetic polyneuropathy is aided by nerve conduction studies that show an axonal neuropathy. CSF protein content is usually elevated but may be normal.

Autonomic neuropathy may be prominent in DM. Cardiovascular symptoms include arrhythmias or orthostatic hypotension. These may complicate diagnosis and treatment of concurrent myocardial disease. Gastrointestinal motility problems can produce nausea, vomiting, or diarrhea, depending on the severity and distribution of the autonomic neuropathy. Diabetic neuropathy may lead to bladder dysfunction or erectile and ejaculatory failure in men.

CNS complications of DM are primarily due to the metabolic derangements of hypoinsulinism and hypoglycemia that may follow administration of insulin. Cerebrovascular disease is an important problem in diabetics because of accelerated atherosclerosis of cerebral blood vessels and related cardiovascular disorders of heart failure, hypertension, and coagulation abnormalities. Hypoinsulinism or insulin resistance may also be a secondary feature of other neurologic disorders (e.g., Friedreich ataxia) and may share common etiologic features with some genetic or familial diseases.

ADRENAL

The adrenal gland is composed of two distinct parts: the mesodermally derived cortex and the neuroectodermally derived medulla. The cortex synthesizes and secretes steroid hormones, including mineralocorticoids, glucocorticoids, progestins, estrogens, and androgens. Aldosterone is the principal mineralocorticoid and is involved in sodium and potassium homeostasis by the kidney. Glucocorticoids play an important role in metabolic and immunologic processes. Under normal circumstances, sex steroid production by the adrenal plays a relatively minor role compared with the contribution by the gonads. The adrenal medulla contains chromaffin cells, the most important source of circulating catecholamines. These catecholamines, epinephrine and norepinephrine, have important cardiovascular, metabolic, and neural effects.

Hypoadrenalism

Hypofunction of the adrenal cortex is usually due to atrophy of the gland of unknown cause. The gland may be destroyed by tuberculosis, neoplasms, amyloidosis, hemochromatosis, or fungal or human immunodeficiency virus infection. Addison disease, or chronic insufficiency of the adrenal cortex, is characterized by weakness, weight loss, increased pigmentation of the skin, hypotension, behavioral changes, and hypoglycemia. Chronic adrenal insufficiency may be an autoimmune disorder, occasionally in association with other autoimmune disorders, such as MG. It may also be a feature of the abnormal metabolism of long-chain fatty acids in X-linked adrenoleukodystrophy. It may be the only clinical expression in about 10% of cases, including both the cerebral and adrenomyelopathic forms of the disease. In one study, one-third of young males diagnosed with primary adrenal failure (Addison disease) were found to have adrenoleukodystrophy after measurement of long-chain fatty acids. Secondary adrenal insufficiency follows pituitary failure, in which symptoms are less severe because of the relative preservation of mineralocorticoid function, which is not regulated by ACTH.

CNS manifestations of Addison disease are common, primarily in cognition and behavior. Psychotic symptoms are rare. Elevated CSF pressure is sometimes accompanied by cerebral edema. Autopsy studies of the brain in Addison disease indicate that glucocorticoids play an important trophic function in the CNS, sustaining the granule cells of the hippocampus. (The loss of hippocampal neurons with adrenocortical hormone receptors in aging is accelerated in Alzheimer disease and appears to be associated with hypercortisolism.)

Diagnosis is suggested by the clinical features and is confirmed by low plasma levels of cortisol with elevated ACTH levels (in primary adrenal failure), decreased excretion of 17-hydroxycorticosteroids, and failure of the adrenal cortex to respond to ACTH. Treatment is based on administration of a glucocorticoid preparation and replacement of mineralocorticoids with sodium. The latter may not be needed if the pituitary is the source of adrenal insufficiency.

Hyperadrenalism

Hyperfunction of the adrenal cortex produces *Cushing syndrome,* which was attributed by Cushing to a basophilic adenoma of the pituitary. The clinical symptoms of Cushing disease can be reproduced by the administration of corticosteroids. Mental status changes, including difficulties with memory, and myopathy are two of the more common neurologic symptoms. The syndrome of idiopathic intracranial hypertension with headache, nausea, vomiting, and papilledema may occur with reduction or withdrawal of corticosteroids being used as therapy. Symptoms resolve with reinstatement of steroid dosage, and withdrawal is accomplished more gradually.

The differential diagnosis of Cushing syndrome may be difficult because there are several potential sources of hyperadrenalism (pituitary, adrenal, or ectopic source of ACTH production) and also because of the effects of common clinical conditions, such as obesity and depression, on the production and suppressibility of corticosteroids. These conditions may make interpretation of diagnostic tests challenging (Table 146.4). Treatment is directed at control of corticosteroid secretion and the underlying pathology.

Primary Hyperaldosteronism

In 1955, Conn described a syndrome caused by production of aldosterone from a tumor of the adrenal cortex. The clinical manifestations include recurrent attacks of muscular weakness simulating periodic paralysis, tetany, polyuria, hypertension, and a striking imbalance of electrolytes with hypokalemia, hypernatremia, and alkalosis. Paresthesia may occur as a result of the alkalosis. Diagnosis is made by finding increased aldosterone secretion and excretion, with reduced activity of plasma renin. Treatment involves removal of the adrenal tumor coupled with use of an aldosterone inhibitor. Familial glucocorticoid-remediable aldosteronism may be associated with intracranial aneurysms at about the same frequency as in inherited polycystic kidney disease.

Bartter syndrome is a related disorder characterized by hyperreninemia, hyperaldosteronism, and hypokalemic alkalosis without hypertension or peripheral edema. Hypomagnesemia is often present, and treatment with potassium chloride and magnesium may restore potassium levels. Recent genetic studies have begun to define the nature of the ion channel defects in these renal tubular disorders of the Bartter-like syndromes, including the Gitelman variant, which also has hypocalciuria.

Pheochromocytoma

Hyperfunction of the adrenal medulla as a result of a tumor of the chromaffin cells is accompanied by increased secretion of catecholamines. The tumor may be familial, alone or in conjunction with other endocrine tumors. Pheochromocytoma may be seen with neurofibromatosis, von Hippel-Lindau disease, ataxia-telangiectasia, or Sturge-Weber syndrome, consistent with the neuroectodermal origin of the adrenal medulla. Familial pheochromocytoma is associated with bilateral adrenal tumors, while sporadic cases are nearly always unilateral.

Hypertension of a moderate or severe degree is characteristic. The hypertension may be paroxysmal or sustained and is associated with palpitations, episodic hyperhidrosis, headaches, and other nonspecific systemic symptoms, such as nausea, emesis, or diarrhea. Anxiety attacks are common. Death may result from cerebral hemorrhage, pulmonary edema, or cardiac failure in one of the acute attacks or as a result of one of these complications from sustained hypertension.

Diagnosis and treatment are directed at establishing the increased excretion of catecholamine metabolites in the urine and localization and removal of the tumor. The tumor may occur in sites other than the adrenal; imaging techniques are helpful in localization.

GONADS

Neurologic disorders associated with diseases of the ovary or testes are not well-defined. However, the primary secretions of the gonads—estrogens, progestins, and androgens—have been reported to influence a variety of neurologic symptoms. Cyclic or phasic fluctuations in gonadal secretion (during the menstrual cycle or pregnancy) have been linked to common problems such as migraine headache and epilepsy and to less common disorders such as porphyria. Therapeutic use of estrogen–progestin preparations in oral contraceptives poses potential risks for neurologic complications, notably cerebrovascular disease.

Although migraine has been frequently reported in association with menstrual periods, the true incidence of *catamenial migraine* is difficult to determine. Somerville (1975) demonstrated that some women have headaches precipitated by the rapid decline in circulating estradiol during the late-luteal phase and that these headaches can be prevented by administration of estrogen, but not progesterone. The mechanism of action is not clear, but the role of estrogens in catamenial migraine may explain the onset and variation of headaches during pregnancy or with the use of oral contraceptives. Although long-term estrogen treatment is said to be useful in catamenial migraine, this is not practical for most women. Premenstrual administration of prostaglandin inhibitors may be helpful. Discontinuation of estrogen-containing oral contraceptives usually relieves the symptoms.

TABLE 146.4. EVALUATION OF HYPERCORTISOLISM (CUSHING SYNDROME)

Clinical presentation	Morning cortisol level after overnight dexamethasone	Urinary corticosteroids after high-dose dexamethasone (8 mg/24h)	Plasma ACTH
Obesity	Suppress to normal	Suppress	—
Adrenal hyperplasia (Cushing disease)	Does not suppress	Suppress	Often elevated
Adrenal tumor (adenoma or carcinoma)	Does not suppress	Does not suppress	Low
Ectopic ACTH secretion	Does not suppress	Does not supress	High

The relation of oral contraceptive use and the occurrence of stroke has been a controversial topic. Numerous epidemiologic studies indicate that age greater than 35 years and cigarette smoking increase the risk of ischemic and hemorrhagic stroke in women using oral contraceptives. Contraceptive preparations with lower doses of synthetic estrogens are thought to be safest. Hypercoagulability associated with estrogens is thought to be an important etiologic factor in arterial strokes, as well as in the syndromes of cerebral venous thrombosis that may complicate pregnancy or contraceptive use.

Direct effects of sex steroids on the CNS may explain the effects of estrogens (epileptogenic) and progestins (anticonvulsant) on seizure frequency in epilepsy. Oral contraceptives or pregnancy may unmask latent chorea (*chorea gravidarum*), and menstrual cyclicity or exogenous administration of estrogen has been reported to be associated with functional changes in parkinsonism, myoclonus, and other movement disorders. Sex steroid receptors on CNS neoplasms may influence growth characteristics of the tumor. Clinically evident enlargement of meningioma may be seen with pregnancy.

The developmental effects of estrogens and androgens on the brain are extensive. Many behavioral characteristics, sexual and otherwise, may be directed by the influence of these hormones on the morphology of neurons and the creation of neural networks. Studies of cognitive function in hypothalamic hypogonadism emphasize the linkages between endocrine and neural function. Clinical interventions may be forthcoming.

SUGGESTED READINGS

Pituitary

Abrams GM, Schipper HM. Neuroendocrine syndromes of the hypothalamus. *Neurol Clin* 1986;4:769–782.

Barzilay J, Heatley GJ, Cushing GW. Benign and malignant tumors in patients with acromegaly. *Arch Intern Med* 1991;151:1629–1632.

Bauer HG. Endocrine and other clinical manifestations of hypothalamic disease: a survey of 60 cases with autopsies. *J Clin Endocrinol Metab* 1954;14:13–31.

Brada M, Ford D, Ashley S, et al. Risk of second brain tumour after conservative surgery and radiotherapy for pituitary adenoma. *BMJ* 1992;304:1343–1346.

Brunner HO, Ollen BJ. Precocious puberty in boys. *N Eng J Med* 1999;341.

Chan TY. Drug-induced syndrome of inappropriate antidiuretic hormone secretion: causes, diagnosis and management. *Drugs Aging* 1998;11:27–44.

Chanson P, Weinbraub BD, Harris AG. Octreotide therapy for thyroid-stimulating hormone-secreting pituitary adenomas: a follow-up of 52 patients. *Ann Intern Med* 1993;119:236–240.

Damaraju SC, Rajshekhar V, Chandy MJ. Validation study of a central venous pressure-based protocol for the management of neurosurgical patients with hypontremia and natriuresis. *Neurosurgery* 1997;40:312–317.

Dash RJ, Gupta V, Suri S. Sheehan's syndrome: clinical profile, pituitary hormone responses and computed sellar tomography. *Aust N Z J Med* 1993;23:26–31.

DeSouza B, Brunetti A, Fulham MJ, et al. Pituitary microadenomas: a PET Study. *Radiology* 1990;177:39–44.

Doppmen JL, Frank JA, Dwyer AJ, et al. Gadolinium DTPA-enhanced MR imaging of ACTH-secreting microadenomas of the pituitary gland. *J Comput Assist Tomogr* 1988;12:728–735.

Harrigan MR. Cerebral salt wasting syndrome: a review. *Neurosurgery* 1996;38:152–160.

Hartog M, Hull MG. Hyperprolactinaemia. *BMJ* 1988;297:701–702.

Hirshberg B, Ben-Yehuda A. The syndrome of inappropriate antidiuretic hormone secretion in the elderly. *Am J Med* 1997;103:270–273.

Hua F, Asati R, Miki Y, et al. Differentiation of suprasellar non-neoplastic cysts from cystic neoplasms by Gd-DTPA MRI. *J Comput Asst Tomogr* 1992;16:744–749.

Khaleeli A, Lerg RD, Edwards RHT, et al. The neuromuscular features of acromegaly: a clinical and pathological study. *J Neurol Neurosurg Psychiatry* 1984;47:1009–1015.

Kivela T, Pelkonen R, Heiskanen O. Diabetes indipidus and blindness caused by a suprasellar tumor: Pieter Pauw's observations from the 16th century. *JAMA* 1998;279:48–50.

Kleinberg DL, Noel GL, Frantz AG. Galactorrhea: a study of 235 cases including 48 with pituitary tumors. *N Engl J Med* 1977;296:589–600.

Klibanski A, Zervas NT. Diagnosis and management of hormone-secreting pituitary adenomas. *N Engl J Med* 1991;342:822–830.

Kovacs K. Necrosis of anterior pituitary in humans. I *Neuroendocrinology* 1969;4:170–199.

Kovacs K. Necrosis of anterior pituitary in humans. II. *Neuroendocrinology* 1969;4:201–241.

Lam KS, Wat MS, Choi KL, Ip TP, Pang RW, Kumana CR. Pharmacokinetics, pharmacodynamics, long-term efficacy and safety of oral 1-deamino-8-D-arginine vasopressin in adult patients with central diabetes insipidus. *Br J Clin Pharmacol* 1996;42:379–385.

Lee BCP, Deck MDF. Sellar and juxtasellar lesion detection with MR. *Radiology* 1985;157:143–147.

Loli P, Berselli ME, Tagliaferri M. Use of ketoconazole in the treatment of Cushing's syndrome. *J Clin Endocrinol Metab* 1986;63:1365–1371.

Mantello MT, Schwartz RB, Jones KM, et al. Imaging of neurologic complications associated with pregnancy. *AJR* 1993;160:843–847.

Martin JB, Reichlin S. *Clinical neuroendocrinology*, 2nd ed. Philadelphia: FA Davis Co, 1987.

Melmed S. Acromegaly. *N Engl J Med* 1990;322:966–977.

Molitch ME. Pituitary incidentalomas. *Endocrinol Metab Clin North Am* 1997;26;724–740.

Molitch ME, Thorner MO, Wilson C. Management of prolactinomas. *J Clin Endocrinol Metab* 1997;26:996–1000.

Moses AM, Notman DD. Diabetes insipidus and syndrome of inappropriate antidiuretic hormone secretion (SIADH). *Adv Intern Med* 1982;27:73–100.

Newman CB, Melmed S, Snyder PJ, et al. Safety and efficacy of long-term octreotide therapy of acromegaly: results of a multicenter trial of 105 patients—a clinical research center study. *J Clin Endocrinol Metab* 1995;80:2668–2675. Erratum: *J Clin Endocrinol Metab* 1995;80:3238.

Oldfield EH, Chrousas GP, Schulte HM. Preoperative lateralization of ACTH-secreting pituitary microadenomas by bilateral and simultaneous inferior petrosal sinus sampling. *N Engl J Med* 1985;312:100–103.

Onesti ST, Wisniewski T, Post KD. Clinical versus subclinical pituitary apoplexy: presentation, surgical management, and outcome in 21 patients. *Neurosurgery* 1990;26:980–986.

Ozbev N, Inanc S, Aral F, et al. Clinical and laboratory evaluation of 40 patients with Sheehan's syndrome. *Isr J Med Sci* 1994;11:826–829.

Papastolou C, Mantzoros CS, Evagelopoulou C, et al. Imaging of the sella in the syndrome of inappropriate secretion of antidiuretic hormone. *J Intern Med* 1995;237:181–185.

Plum F, Van Uitert R. Nonendocrine diseases and disorders of the hypothalamus. In: Reichlin S, Baldessarini RJ, Martin JB, eds. *The hypothalamus.* New York: Raven Press, 1978.

Repaske DR, Phillips JA 3d. The molecular biology of human hereditary central diabetes insipidus. *Prog Brain Res* 1992;93:295–306.

Rittig S, Robertson GL, Siggaard C, et al. Identification of 13 new mutations in the vasopressin-neurophysin II gene in 17 kindreds with familial autosomal dominant neurohypophyseal diabetes insipidus. *Am J Hum Genet* 1996;58:107–117.

Robinson DB, Michaels RD. Empty sella resulting from the spontaneous resolution of a pituitary macroadenoma. *Arch Intern Med* 1992;152:1920–1923.

Ruitshauser J, Boni-Schnetzler M, Boni J, et al. A novel point mutation in the translation initiation codon of the pre-pro-vasopressin-neurophysin II gene: cosegregation with morphological abnormalities and clinical aymptoms in autosomal dominant neurohypophyseal diabetes insipidus. *J Clin Endocrinol Metab* 1996;81:192–198.

Saito T, Ishikawa S, Abe K, et al. Acute aquaresis by the nonpeptide arginine vasopressin (AVP) antagonist OPC-31260 improves hyponatremia in patients with the syndrome of inappropriate secretion of antidiuretic hormone (SIADH). *J Clin Endocrinol Metab* 1997;82:1054–1057.

Singer I, Oster JR, Fishman LM. The management of diabetes insipidus in adults. *Arch Intern Med* 1997;157:1293–1301.

Styne D, Grumbach MM, Kaplan SL, et al. Treatment of Cushing's disease in childhood and adolescence by transsphenoidal microadenomectomy. *N Engl J Med* 1984;310:889–893.

Tanigawa K, Yamashita S, Nagataki S. Acute quadriplegia in acromegaly. *Ann Intern Med* 1992;117:94–95.

Vidal E, Cevallos R, Vidal J, et al. Twelve cases of pituitary apoplexy. *Arch Intern Med* 1992;152:1893–1899.

Woo MH, Smythe MA. Association of SIADH with selective serotonin reuptake inhibitors. *Ann Pharmacother* 1997;31:108–110.

Young WF, Scheithauer BW, Kovacs KT, et al. Gonadotropin adenoma of the pituitary gland: a clinicopathologic analysis of 100 cases *Mayo Clin Proc* 1996;71:649–656.

Zimmerman EA. Neuroendocrine disorders. In: Rosenberg R, ed. *Atlas of clinical neurology.* Philadelphia: Current Medicine, 1998:3.1–3.15.

Thyroid

Anasti JN, Flack MR, Nelson LM, et al. A potential novel mechanism for precocious puberty in juvenile hypothyroidism. *J Clin Endocrinol Metab* 1995;80:276–279.

Atchison JA, Lee PA, Albright AL. Reversible suprasellar pituitary mass secondary to hypothyroidism. *JAMA* 1989;262:3175–3177.

Barnard RD, Campbell MJ, McDonald MI. Pathologic findings in a case of hypothyroidism with ataxia. *J Neurol Neurosurg Psychiatry* 1971;34:755–760.

Beghi E, Delodovici ML, Bogliun G, et al. Hypothyroidism and polyneuropathy. *J Neurol Neurosurg Psychiatry* 1989;52:1420–1423.

Bellman SC, Davies A, Fuggle PW, et al. Mild impairment of neuro-oto-logical function in early treated congenital hypothyroidism. *Arch Dis Child* 1996;74:215–218.

Brody IE, Dudley AW Jr. Thyrotoxic hypokalemic periodic paralysis. *Arch Neurol* 1969;21:1–6.

Bulens C. Neurologic complications of hyperthyroidism. *Arch Neurol* 1981;38;669–670.

Burstein B. Psychoses associated with thyrotoxicosis. *Arch Gen Psychiatry* 1961;4:267–273.

Chao T, Wang JR, Hwang B. Congenital hypothyroidism and concomitant anomalies. *J Pediatr Endocrinol Metab* 1997;10:217–221.

Dresner S, Kennerdell JS. Dysthyroid orbitopathy. *Neurology* 1985;35:1628–1634.

Dyck PJ, Lambert EH. Polyneuropathy associated hypothyroidism. *J Neuropathol Exp Neurol* 1970;29:631–658.

Fells P. Thyroid-associated eye disease: clinical management. *Lancet* 1991;338:29–31.

Fidler SM, O'Rourke RA, Buchsbaum W. Choreoathetosis as a manifestation of thyrotoxicosis. *Neurology* 1971;21:55–57.

Fort P, Lipschitz, F, Pugliese M, et al. Neonatal thyroid disease: differential expression in three successive offspring. *J Clin Endocrinol Metab* 1988;66:645–647.

Gamblin GT, Harper DG, Galentine P, et al. Prevalence of increased intraocular pressure in Graves' disease: evidence of frequent subclinical ophthalmopathy. *N Engl J Med* 1983;308:420–424.

Garcia CA, Fleming H. Reversible corticospinal tract disease due to hyperthyroidism. *Arch Neurol* 1977;34:647–648.

Glorieux J, Dussault JH, Letarte J, et al. Preliminary results on the mental development of hypothyroid infants detected by the Quebec Screening Program. *J Pediatr* 1983;102:19–22.

Hagberg B, Westphal O. Ataxic syndrome in congenital hypothyroidism. *Acta Paediatr Scand* 1970;59:323–327.

Haggerty JJ Jr, Prange AJ Jr. Borderline hypothyroidism and depression. *Annu Rev Med* 1995;46:37–46.

Kaminski HJ, Ruff RL. Neurologic complications of endocrine diseases. *Neurol Clin* 1989;7:489–508.

Kelley DE, Gharib H, Kennedy FP, et al. Thyrotoxic periodic paralysis: report of 10 cases and review of electromyographic findings. *Arch Intern Med* 1989;149:2597–2600.

Kennerdell JS, Rosenbaum AE, El-Hoshy MH. Apical optic nerve compression of dysthyroid optic neuropathy on computed tomography. *Arch Ophthalmol* 1982;100:324–328.

Klein I, Parker M, Shebert R, et al. Hypothyroidism presenting as muscle stiffness and pseudohypertrophy: Hoffmann's syndrome. *Am J Med* 1981;70:891–894.

Kodama K, Bandy-Dafoe P, Sokorska H, et al. Circulating autoantibody against a soluble eye-muscle antigen in Graves' ophthalmopathy. *Lancet* 1982;2:1353–1356.

Kothbauer-Margreiter I, Sturzenegger M, Komor J, et al. Encephalopathy associated with Hashimoto thyroiditis: diagnosis and treatment. *J Neurol* 1996;243:585–593.

Lindberger K. Myxoedema coma. *Acta Med Scand* 1975;198:87–90.

Nordgren L, von Scheele C. Myxedematous madness without myxedema: selective defect of TSH release on TRF loading in a young woman with a history of severe depressive illness cured with thyroid hormone replacement therapy. *Acta Med Scand* 1976;199:233–236.

Ober KP. Thyrotoxic periodic paralysis in the United States: report of 7 cases and review of the literature. *Medicine* 1992;71:109–120.

Rao SN, Katiyar BC, Nair KRP, et al. Neuromuscular status in hypothyroidism. *Acta Neurol Scand* 1980;61:167–177.

Reidl S, Frisch H. Pituitary hyperplasia in a girl with gonadal dysgenesis and primary hypothyroidism. *Horm Res* 1997;47:126–130.

Rosman NP. Neurological and muscular aspects of thyroid dysfunction in childhood. *Pediatr Clin North Am* 1976;23:575–594.

Sanders V. Neurologic manifestations of myxedema. *N Engl J Med* 1962;266:547–552.

Satoyoshi E, Murakami K, Kowa H, et al. Periodic paralysis in hyperthyroidism. *Neurology* 1963;13:746–752.

Savoic JC, Fardeau M, Leger F, et al. Hyperthyroidism without hypermetabolism in two cases of diffuse muscular atrophy. *Ann Endocrinol* 1975;36:175–176.

Shaw PJ, Bates D, Kendall-Taylor P. Hyperthyroidism presenting as pyramidal tract disease. *BMJ* 1988;297:1395–1396.

Solomon DJ, Chopra IJ, Smith FJ. Identification of subgroups of euthyroid Graves' ophthalmopathy. *N Engl J Med* 1977;296:340–349.

Spiro AJ, Hirano A, Beilin RL, et al. Cretinism with muscular hypertrophy (Kocher-Debre-Semelaigne syndrome). *Arch Neurol* 1970;23:340–349.

Strakosch CR, Wenzel BE, Row VV, et al. Immunology of autoimmune thyroid diseases. *N Engl J Med* 1982;307:1499–1507.

Swanson JW, Kelly JJ Jr, McConahey WM. Neurologic aspects of thyroid dysfunction. *Mayo Clin Proc* 1981;56:504–512.

Tallstedt L, Lundell G, Torring O, et al. Occurrence of ophthalmopathy after treatment for Graves' hyperthyroidism. *N Engl J Med* 1992;326:1733–1738.

Trobe JD, Glaser JS, Laflamme P. Dysthyroid optic neuropathy. *Arch Ophthalmol* 1978;96:1199–1209.

Trokel SL, Hilal SK. Recognition and differential diagnosis of enlarged extraocular muscles in computed tomography. *Am J Ophthalmol* 1979;87:503–512.

Van Dop C, Conte FA, Koch TK. Pseudotumor cerebri with initiation of levothyroxine therapy for juvenile hypothyroidism. *N Engl J Med* 1983;308:1076–1080.

Wise MP, Blunt S, Lane RJ. Neurological presentations of hypothyroidism: the importance of slow-relaxing reflexes. *J R Soc Med* 1995;88:272–274.

Wong PS, Hee FL, Lip GY. Atrial fibrillation and the thyroid. *Heart* 1997;78:623–624.

Parathyroid

Abe S, Tojo K, Ichida K, et al. A rare case of idiopathic hypoparathyroidism with varied neurological manifestations. *Intern Med* 1996;35:129–134.

Burch WM, Posillico JT. Hypoparathyroidism after I-131 therapy with subsequent return of parathyroid function. *J Clin Endocrinol Metab* 1983;57:398–401.

Cogan MG, Covey CM, Arieff AI, et al. Central nervous system manifestations of hyperparathyroidism. *Am J Med* 1978;65:563–630.

Cope O. The story of hyperparathyroidism at the Massachusetts General Hospital. *N Engl J Med* 1966;274:1174–1182.

Mallette LE, Bilezikian JP, Heath DA, Aurback GD. Primary hyperparathyroidism: clinical and biochemical features. *Medicine (Baltimore)* 1974;53:127–146.

Mallette LE, Patten BM, Engel WK. Neuromuscular disease in secondary hyperparathyroidism. *Ann Intern Med* 1975;82:474–483.

McKinney AS. Idiopathic hypoparathyroidism presenting as chorea. *Neurology* 1962;12:485–491.

Muenter MD, Whisnant JP. Basal ganglia calcification, hypoparathyroidism and extrapyramidal motor manifestations. *Neurology* 1968;18:1075–1083.

Nusynowitz ML, Frame B, Kolb PO. The spectrum of hypoparathyroid states. *Medicine* 1976;55:105–119.

Patten BM, Bilezikian JP, Mallette LE, et al. Neuromuscular disease in primary hyperparathyroidism. *Ann Intern Med* 1974;80:182–194.

Roisin AJ. Ectopic calcification around joints of paralyzed limbs in hemiplegia, diffuse brain damage and other neurological diseases. *Ann Rheum Dis* 1975;34:499–505.

Spiegel AM, Weinstein LS. Pseudohypoparathyroidism. In: Scriver CR, Beaudet AL, Sly WS, Valle, D, eds. *The metabolic and molecular basis of inherited disease,* 5th ed. New York: McGraw-Hill 1995;3073–3089.

Tabaee-Zadeh MJ, Frame B, Kappahn K. Kinesiogenic choreoathetosis and idiopathic hypoparathyroidism. *N Engl J Med* 1972;286:762–763.

Turken SA, Cafferty M, Silverberg S, et al. Neuromuscular involvement in mild asymptomatic primary hyperparathyroidism. *Am J Med* 1989;87:553–557.

Pancreas

Cryer PE, Polonsky KS. Glucose homeostasis and hypoglycemia. In: Wilson JD, Foster DW, Kronenberg HM, Larsen PR, eds. *Williams' textbook of endocrinology,* 9th ed. Philadelphia: WB Saunders, 1998:939–971.

Dyck PJ, Thomas PK, Asbury AK, et al., eds. *Diabetic neuropathy.* Philadelphia: WB Saunders, 1987.

Gale E. Hypoglycaemia. *Clin Endocrinol Metab* 1980;9:461–475.

Harati Y. Diabetes and the nervous system. *Endocrinol Metab Clin North Am* 1996;25:325–359.

Harrison MJ. Muscle wasting after prolonged hypoglycaemic coma: case report with electrophysiological data. *J Neurol Neurosurg Psychiatry* 1976;39:465–470.

Kalimo H, Olsson Y. Effects of severe hypoglycemia on the human brain: neuropathologic case reports. *Acta Neurol Scand* 1980;62:345–356.

Mabry CC, DiGeorge AM, Auerbach VH. Leucine-induced hypoglycemia. *J Pediatr* 1970;57:526–538.

Malouf R, Brust JCM. Hypoglycemia: causes, neurological manifestations and outcome. *Ann Neurol* 1985;17:421–430.

Merimee TJ. Spontaneous hypoglycemia in man. *Adv Intern Med* 1977;22:301–307.

Mooradian A. Pathophysiology of central nervous system complications of diabetes mellitus. *Clin Neurosci* 1997;4:322–326.

Pagliara AS, Karl IE, Haymond M, et al. Hypoglycemia in childhood. *J Pediatr* 1973;82:365–379.

Richardson ML, Kinard RE, Gray MB. CT of generalized gray matter infarction due to hypoglycemia. *AJNR* 1981;2:366–367.

Silas JH, Grant DS, Maddocks JL. Transient hemiparetic attacks due to unrecognized nocturnal hypoglycemia. *BMJ* 1981;282:132–133.

Adrenal

Abbas DH, Schlagenhauff RE, Strong HE. Polyradiculoneuropathy in Addison's disease: case report and review of literature. *Neurology* 1977;27:494–495.

Atsumi T, Ishikawa S, Miyatake T, et al. Myopathy and primary aldosteronism: electron microscopic study. *Neurology* 1979;29:1348–1358.

Bravo EL, Gifford RW. Pheochromocytoma: diagnosis, localization and management. *N Engl J Med* 1984;311:1298–1303.

Brennemann W, Kohler W, Zierz S, Klingmuller D. Occurrence of adrenocortical insufficiency in adrenomyeloneuropathy. *Neurology* 1996;47:605.

Brennemann W, Kohler W, Zierz S, et al. Testicular dysfunction in adrenomyeloneuropathy. *Eur J Endocrinol* 1997;137:34–39.

Bridgewater GR, Starling JR. Pheochromocytoma: paroxysmal hypertensive headaches. *Headache* 1982;22:84–85.

Britton C, Boxhill C, Brust JC, et al. Pseudotumor cerebri, empty sella syndrome, and adrenal adenoma. *Neurology* 1980;30:292–296.

Carpenter PC. Cushing's syndrome: update of diagnosis and management. *Mayo Clin Proc* 1986;61:49–58.

Condulis N, Germain G, Charest N, et al. Pseudotumor cerebri: a presenting manifestation of Addison's disease. *Clin Pediatr* 1997;36:711–713.

Cook DM, Loriaux DL. Cushing's syndrome: medical approach. In: Bardin CW, ed. *Current therapy in endocrinology and metabolism,* 6th ed. St. Louis: Mosby, 1997:59–62.

De Kloet ER, Vreugdenhil E, Oitzl MS, et al. Brain corticosteroid receptor balance in health and disease. *Endocr Rev* 1998;19:269–301.

Doppman JL. CT findings in Addison's disease. *J Comput Assist Tomogr* 1982;6:757–761.

Drake FR. Neuropsychiatric-like symptomatology of Addison's disease: a review of the literature. *Am J Med Sci* 1957;234:106–113.

Ganguly A, Grim CE, Weinberger MH. Primary aldosteronism: the etiologic spectrum of disorders and their clinical differentiation. *Arch Intern Med* 1982;142:813–815.

Greenwald RA. Complications of steroid therapy. *Del Med J* 1981;53:451–460.

Huang YY, Hsu BR, Tsai JS. Paralytic myopathy: a leading clinical presenetation for primary aldosteronism in Taiwan. *J Clin Endocrinol Metab* 1997;82:2377–2378.

Hoffman RW, Gardner DW, Mitchell FL. Intrathoracic and multiple abdominal pheochromocytomas in von Hippel-Lindau disease. *Arch Intern Med* 1982;142:1962–1964.

Jefferson A. A clinical correlation between encephalopathy and papilloedema in Addison's disease. *J Neurol Neurosurg Psychiatry* 1956;19:21–26.

Kandt RS, Heldrich FJ, Moser HW. Recovery from probable central pontine myelinolysis associated with Addison's disease. *Arch Neurol* 1983;40:118–119.

Krieger DT. Pathophysiology and treatment of Cushing disease. *Prog Clin Biol Res* 1982;87:19–32.

Laureti S, Casucci G, Santeusania F, et al. X-linked adrenoleukodystrophy is a frequent cause of idiopathic Addison's disease in young adult male patients. *J Clin Endocrinol Metab* 1996;81:470–474.

Litchfield WR, Anderson BF, Weiss RJ, et al. Intracranial aneurysm and hemorrhagic stroke in glucocorticoid-remediable aldosteronism. *Hypertension* 1998;31:445–450.

Machlen J, Torvik A. Necrosis of granule cells of hippocampus in adrenocortical failure. *Acta Neuropathol* 1990;80:85–87.

Malik GH, al-Wakeel J, al-Mohaya S, et al. Bartter's syndrome in two successive generations of a Saudi family. *Am J Nephrol* 1997;17:495–498.

Manger WM. Psychiatric manifestations in patients with pheochromocytoma. *Arch Intern Med* 1985;145:229–230.

Mutations in the gene encoding the inwardly-rectifying renal potassium channel, ROMK, cause the antenatal variant of Bartter syndrome: evidence for genetic heterogeneity. International Collaborative Study Group for Bartter-like Syndromes. *Hum Mol Genet* 1997;6:17–26.

Neufeld M, Maclaren NK, Blizzard RM. Two types of autoimmune Addison's disease associated with different polyglandular autoimmune (PGA) syndromes. *Medicine* 1981;60:355–362.

Newman PK, Snow M, Hudgson P. Benign intracranial hypertension and Cushing's disease. *BMJ* 1980;281:113.

Pomares FJ, Canas R, Rodriguez JM, et al. Differences between sporadic and multiple endocrine neoplasia type 2A phaeochromocytoma. *Clin Endocrinol (Oxf)* 1998;48:195–200.

Simon DB, Bindra RS, Mansfield TA, et al. Mutations in the chloride channel gene, CLCNKB, cause Bartter's syndrome type III. *Nat Genet* 1997;17:171–178.

Thomas JE, Rooke ED, Kvale WF. The neurologists's experience with pheochromocytoma: a review of 100 cases. *JAMA* 1966;197:754–758.

Vaughan NJA, Slater JD, Lightman SL, et al. The diagnosis of primary aldosteronism. *Lancet* 1981;1:120–125.

Gonads

Estanol B, Ridriquez A, Conte G, et al. Intracranial venous thrombosis in young women. *Stroke* 1979;10:680–684.

Mattson RH, Cramer JA, Darney PD, et al. Use of oral contraceptives by women with epilepsy. *JAMA* 1986;256:238–240.

Oral contraception and increased risk of cerebral ischemia or thrombosis. Collaborative Group for the Study of Stroke in Young Women. *N Engl J Med* 1973;288:871–878.

Oral contraceptives and stroke in young women: associated risk factors. Collaborative Group for the Study of Stroke in Young Women. *JAMA* 1975;231:718–722.

Schipper H. Neurology of sex steroids and oral contraceptives. *Neurol Clin* 1986;4:721–752.

Schwartzhaus JD, Currie J, Jaffe MJ, et al. Neurologic findings in men with isolated hypogonadotropic hypogonadism. *Neurology* 1989;39:223–226.

Somerville BW. Estrogen withdrawal migraine. I. Duration of exposure required and attempted prophylaxis by premenstrual estrogen administration. *Neurology* 1975;25:239–244.

Somerville BW. Estrogen withdrawal migraine. II. Attempted prophylaxis by continuous estradiol administration. *Neurology* 1975;25:245–250.

Stadel BV. Oral contraceptives and cardiovascular disease (first of two parts). *N Engl J Med* 1981;305:612–618.

Stadel BV. Oral contraceptives and cardiovascular disease (second of two parts). *N Engl J Med* 1981;305:672–677.

Tang MX, Jacobs D, Stern Y, et al. Effect of oestrogen during menopause on risk and age at onset of Alzheimer's disease. *Lancet* 1996;348:429–432.

Merritt's Neurology, 10th ed., edited by L.P. Rowland. Lippincott Williams & Wilkins, Philadelphia © 2000.

C H A P T E R

147

HEMATOLOGIC AND RELATED DISEASES

KYRIAKOS P. PAPADOPOULOS
CASILDA M. BALMACEDA

ERYTHROCYTE DISORDERS

Sickle Cell Disease

Sickle hemoglobin (HbS) is characterized by an abnormal β-globin chain in which the sixth amino acid valine is substituted by glutamic acid. The disorder is prevalent in blacks of African descent. Individuals with *sickle cell anemia* are homozygous for HbS (SS); their hemoglobin contains two normal alpha chains and two abnormal beta chains. In the deoxygenated condition, the hemoglobin tetramer polarizes and the cell shape becomes distorted, resulting in rigid red blood cells. Cell damage leads to hemolytic anemia and to occlusion of vessels in the kidney, bone, lung, liver, heart, spleen, peripheral nerves, and brain. Other common sickle genotypes having neurologic sequelae include *sickle cell-hemoglobin C* (SC) disease and the *sickle-β-thalassemia* syndromes.

Stroke is the second leading cause of death after infection, occurring in 7% to 15% of homozygous children. According to the Cooperative Study of Sickle Cell Disease, the incidence of first cerebrovascular accident is 0.6 per 100 patient years for SS, 0.15 per 100 patient years for SC, and 0.08 per 100 patient years for sickle-β-thalassemia. Isolated case reports describe patients with *sickle cell trait* as having otherwise unexplained strokes, particularly with subcortical infarction. In large series, however, the incidence of cerebrovascular disease in these patients was the same as for the general African-American population.

The risk of stroke in children with sickle cell disease is 250 to

400 times more than in the general population. The cumulative risk of stroke by age 45 is about 24% for SS patients and 10% for SC patients. About 60% of strokes are ischemic; the others are hemorrhagic. Mean age at development of cerebral infarcts is 8 years, but they also occur in older patients, whereas hemorrhage is most frequent in patients between ages 20 and 29 years.

Most strokes do not occur at the time of painful crisis, dehydration, fever, or infection. Preceding transient ischemic attacks (TIAs) are uncommon. Low hemoglobin concentration and high leukocyte count are risk factors for hemorrhagic stroke.

In ischemic stroke, the primary vascular lesion is occlusive disease of the intracranial portion of the distal internal carotid, proximal middle cerebral, or anterior cerebral artery. Vascular damage includes segmental thickening caused by intimal proliferation of fibroblasts and smooth muscle. Both large and small vessels are affected.

Many infarcts occur in watershed distributions, attributed to large vessel disease compounded by anemia and hemodynamic insufficiency or hypoperfusion in the border zone. Cerebral blood flow studies show hyperemia, but the vessels fail to dilate further with hypercapneic stimulation. The vessels may be maximally dilated, and a drop in perfusion cannot be compensated by further vasodilatation. Therefore, damage is attributed to a combination of both perfusion failure and intraarterial embolization. Strokes occur when the hypoperfusion exceeds adaptive mechanisms and further vasodilatation is not possible. The second mechanism of stroke is the resistance to the passage of sickle cells in the small distal penetrating arterioles, with rigid red cell sludge and stasis. Small vessels in the distal fields are the most vulnerable because the cells adhere and are trapped in the areas of already decreased perfusion. In large vessels, damage from the abnormal red cells leads to large vessel hyperplasia and thrombus formation at the bifurcation.

Subarachnoid hemorrhage is more common in children, whereas intraparenchymal hemorrhage is seen in adults. The causes of hemorrhage include aneurysmal dilatation of large vessels, *moyamoya*-like disease with fragile collateral circulation, and hemorrhage into infarcted tissue. Aneurysms are found at the bifurcation points of large vessels, which are also the sites of endothelial hyperplasia. The chronically abnormal rheology is thought to weaken the mural integrity of the blood vessel walls, leading to aneurysmal dilatation and rupture.

Magnetic resonance imaging (MRI) shows infarcts, often asymptomatic, in small vessel territory in 28% and large vessel territory in 72%. Angiography shows a high incidence of large vessel pathology, but intraarterial injections increase the risk of stroke or sickle cell crisis. Preparation for angiography includes transfusions to reduce the HbS concentration to less than 30%. An 11% incidence of stenosis has been shown by MR angiography in children younger than 4 years. Carotid and transcranial Doppler studies are sensitive in detecting arterial vasculopathy. Positron emission tomography shows higher regional blood flow in sickle cell patients than in age-matched control subjects.

The incidence of stroke recurrence is lower in patients who receive transfusions regularly. In those who receive chronic transfusion therapy, 10% have recurrent stroke; without transfusions, stroke recurrence is 46% to 90% usually within 3 years of the first event. The goal of transfusion with HbA cells is an HbS concentration less than 30% of the total hemoglobin. The transfusion regimen is maintained for 2 to 4 years; some advocate long-term transfusion indefinitely.

Younger patients with strokes tend to have residual symptoms, and survivors may be neuropsychologically impaired. Cognitive abnormalities occur even in the absence of MRI abnormalities or clinical stroke, and the IQ may be lower than in asymptomatic carriers.

Transcranial Doppler ultrasonography identifies SS children at risk of stroke. Elevated time-averaged mean blood flow velocity in the intracranial internal carotid or middle cerebral artery is associated with a 46% risk of cerebral infarction in 39 months. The randomized Stroke Prevention Trial in Sickle Cell Anemia of prophylactic transfusion for prevention of first stroke in patients with abnormal transcranial Doppler ultrasonography showed a 92% decrease in stroke occurrence. Ultimately, the benefits of long-term transfusion in preventing a first or recurrent stroke must be weighed against the complications of transfusions, including alloimmunization, infection, and iron overload. Other therapies include efforts to increase the concentration of fetal hemoglobin with butyric acid and hydroxyurea and bone marrow transplantation.

The incidence of seizures varies from 6% to 12%. Seizures may accompany strokes or meningitis and may be precipitated by dehydration or by commonly used medications such as meperidine. Computed tomography (CT) or MRI only rarely shows a lesion responsible for the seizures. Infections are common for several reasons: splenic infarction, local tissue hypoxia, or abnormalities in complement activation. Bacterial meningitis, most commonly caused by streptococcus pneumonia, cerebral abscesses, and tuberculomas, have all been seen.

Headache is reported in 28% of children. It is often not associated with sickle cell crisis, intracerebral hemorrhage, skull infarction, or osteomyelitis. An acute or chronic progressive encephalopathy may be seen. In individuals with SC disease, visual disturbances due to retinopathy is seen in 58% and hearing loss is more common than with SS disease.

Myelopathy is rare but may follow spinal cord infarction or spinal cord compression by extramedullary hematopoiesis. Pe-

ripheral neuropathy is also unusual but may manifest as an acute mononeuropathy affecting the mental, peroneal, or multiple cranial nerves.

Thalassemia

β-Thalassemia is an inherited hemolytic anemia resulting from defective β-globin chain synthesis. It usually occurs in individuals of Mediterranean or Asian extraction and is characterized by hepatosplenomegaly, skin changes, and growth retardation. Transient dizziness and visual blurring are seen in up to 20%. The transient symptoms characteristically occur between transfusions and improve when the anemia is ameliorated. Other manifestations are headaches (13%) and seizures (13%). Twenty percent develop a mild peripheral, mainly motor, neuropathy in the second decade of life. A syndrome consisting of myalgia, paroxysmal muscle weakness, and myopathic electromyography changes has also been reported. Stroke is rare, seen in those receiving multiple transfusions and attributed to thrombocytosis after splenectomy or to intravascular hemolysis. Spinal cord and cauda equina compression resulting from extramedullary hematopoiesis responds to transfusion and radiation therapy. Skull x-ray films show characteristic abnormalities (Fig. 147.1).

Polycythemia

Polycythemia, an abnormal increase in the number of circulating erythrocytes, occurs with the myeloproliferative disorder *polycythemia vera* or may be secondary to pulmonary hypoventilation or high altitude. Rarely, cerebellar hemangioblastoma or hepatoma causes polycythemia by elaborating erythropoietin. Blood viscosity increases and may cause headache. Other symptoms, occurring in 50% to 80% of patients, include dizziness, tinnitus, visual disturbances, and cognitive impairment. These symptoms respond to reduction in the red blood cell count by phlebotomy or chemotherapy. Circulation returns to normal as the hematocrit is reduced to 40% to 45% and blood viscosity is lowered.

Hyperviscosity also predisposes to large and small vessel cerebral infarction and may accelerate atherosclerosis. In polycythemia vera, transient ischemic attacks and ischemic stroke account for 70% of arterial thromboses. Aseptic cavernous sinus thrombosis is rare. Both thrombocytosis and a platelet disorder that leads to a hemorrhagic diathesis may be seen. Cerebral thrombosis is fatal in 15% and cerebral hemorrhage in 3% of patients with this condition. Patients may complain of limb pain or paresthesias that are attributed to ischemia and often recede promptly with phlebotomy. Peripheral neuropathy, predominantly sensory axonal, occurs in up to 46% of patients.

PLATELET DISORDERS

Essential Thrombocytosis (Thrombocythemia)

Essential thrombocytosis is an acquired myeloproliferative disorder characterized by splenomegaly, elevated platelet count, platelet dysfunction, and a predisposition to both hemorrhage and thrombosis involving the arterial and venous circulation.

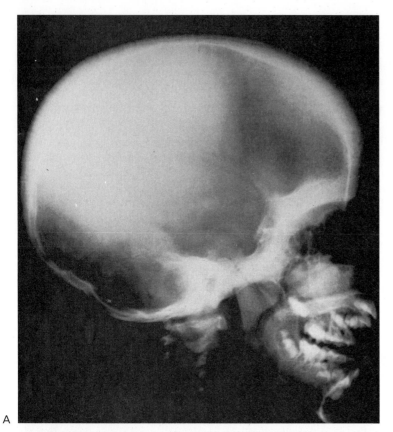

A

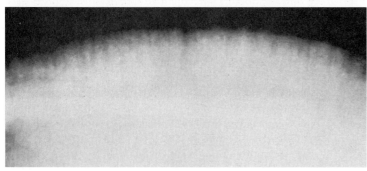

B

FIG. 147.1. Skull in chronic hemolytic anemia (thalassemia). **A:** Thickening of vault. **B:** Magnified view of "hair-on-end" appearance as a result of extramedullary hematopoiesis in the widened diploic space. (Courtesy of Dr. William H. McAlister.)

The Polycythemia Vera Study Group established specific criteria for diagnosis: persistent thrombocytosis (platelet count greater than 600,000/mm³), megakaryocytic hyperplasia in the bone marrow, absence of the Philadelphia chromosome, marrow fibrosis or myeloid metaplasia, and absence of increased erythrocyte mass in the presence of normal iron stores. Other causes of secondary thrombocytosis, such as underlying systemic illness, iron deficiency, and neoplasia, must be excluded. Onset is in the sixth or seventh decade of life, and the mean platelet count at diagnosis is $1 \times 10^6/mm^3$. Neurologic episodes occur in about 30% of patients. The most common neurologic manifestation is headache, followed by paresthesias, TIAs, cerebral infarction, and seizures. Bleeding complications are mild, primarily gastrointestinal, and rarely of neurologic consequence.

It is not known whether the qualitative platelet abnormalities or the thrombocytosis is responsible for symptoms. Most neurologic episodes occur at onset or with hematologic relapse. Microvasculature occlusion may be responsible. Some authorities recommend treatment with aspirin or dipyridamole in asymptomatic patients. After serious thromboembolic events, urgent platelet pheresis is recommended. Hydroxyurea and anagralide are effective in reducing the platelet count. The clinician should check the platelet count in all patients with ischemic episodes and in those with headaches, visual symptoms, or paresthesias.

Thrombotic Thrombocytopenic Purpura

Thrombotic thrombocytopenic purpura (TTP) is characterized by microangiopathic hemolytic anemia, thrombocytopenia, fever, nephropathy, and neurologic manifestations. The mean age at onset is 40 years as an acute process that causes damage by microvasculature occlusion, with anoxic injury, in kidney and brain.

Seventy percent of the patients have neurologic symptoms, most commonly as hemiparesis in 25% or an organic mental syndrome in 50%. Aphasia, hemisensory loss, seizures, ataxia, and field defects are less common. The symptoms are transient, usually lasting less than 48 hours. Permanent neurologic symptoms occur in a few patients. Hemiparesis tends to improve more readily than mental status changes.

Neuropathologic changes may or may not be symptomatic. Hyaline thrombotic occlusion of arterioles and capillaries without inflammation results in small infarcts and petechial hemorrhages, usually in the gray matter (Fig. 147.2). Rarely, there is large vessel occlusion or subarachnoid or subdural hemorrhage. Symptoms are attributed to episodes of focal ischemia. The majority of cases of TTP are associated with an acquired IgG inhibitor of von Willebrand factor cleaving protease. Ticlopidine therapy has been associated with TTP.

Normal findings on CT suggest the possibility of full clinical recovery in 70% of the patients. If CT findings are abnormal, death or permanent neurologic disorder follows in 80% of the patients. Cerebrospinal fluid (CSF) is usually normal except for elevated protein content.

Treatment includes chemotherapy, steroids, or plasma exchange, leading to remission in 75%. Dialysis is used to treat the renal dysfunction, and heparin may be used but may cause cerebral hemorrhage. Death from neurologic complications in TTP is not as common as from other organ failure. Malaria may be mimicked by TTP.

Heparin-induced Thrombocytopenia

Heparin-induced thrombocytopenia is an immune-mediated disorder typically occurring 5 or more days after initiation of therapy in a patient not previously exposed to heparin. The pathogenic IgG immunoglobulin binds a heparin/platelet factor 4 complex, causing platelet activation. This prothrombotic state is characterized by a 50% or greater decrease in platelet count, and up to 50% of patients develop thrombotic complications, including cerebral infarction in 3% to 4% of all patients. Heparin therapy should be discontinued immediately, and warfarin withheld until platelets recover to avoid venous limb gangrene. Danaparoid, a heparinoid mixture of anticoagulant glycosaminoglycans, is an effective therapy.

BLOOD CELL DYSCRASIAS

Leukemia

All forms of leukemia may lead indirectly to neurologic symptoms because of complications of therapy, especially hemorrhage due to thrombocytopenia or infection due to low white blood cell counts. With markedly elevated white blood counts (greater than 150,000/mm^3), *leukostasis* may occlude cerebral blood vessels. Furthermore, leukemic blasts can infiltrate the arteriole endothelial walls to cause hemorrhage. Patients at risk for central nervous system (CNS) leukostasis are treated with emergency leukapheresis to lower the blast count. Leukemic nodules may also predispose to intracerebral hemorrhage, which may be fatal.

Direct CNS manifestations of leukemia depend on the specific cell type involved. In *acute myelogenous leukemias*, CNS involvement is uncommonly the first manifestation. Patients at risk for CNS symptoms include those with high circulating blast counts and the monocytic M4 subtype. The M4 Eo variant in particular, with eosinophilia and the inv(16)(p13q22) inversion of chromosome 16, is commonly associated with leptomeningeal and intracerebral lesions. Cranial nerve palsies due to infiltration are rare

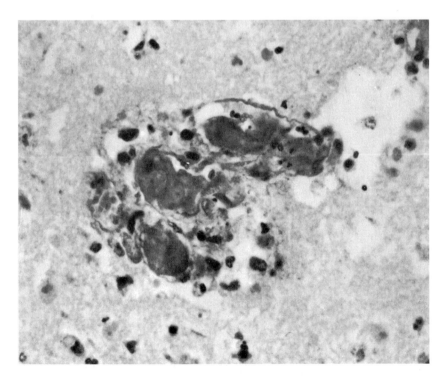

FIG. 147.2. Thrombotic thrombocytopenic purpura. Occlusion of small cerebral vessels by amorphous hyaline material. (Courtesy of Dr. Abner Wolf.)

in acute myelogenous leukemias, mostly involving the fifth and seventh nerves. Unless CNS symptoms require therapy, lumbar puncture is deferred until the peripheral blood is cleared of blast cells to avoid possible CNS seeding. Acute myelogenous leukemias may affect the CNS in the form of a *chloroma* (or *granulocytic sarcoma*), a local collection of blast cells that appears green because of a high myeloperoxidase content. Chloromas may be seen 1 year before the overt onset of acute leukemia, originating in subperiosteal sites in bone and characteristically causing unilateral or bilateral exophthalmos simulating orbital lymphoma. Other sites include the cranial and facial bones, commonly causing facial palsy, and the spinal epidural space, causing paraplegia.

Acute lymphocytic leukemia involves the CNS in 5% to 10% of patients at time of diagnosis, often without symptoms. Risk factors for CNS leukemia include a high lymphocyte count, T-ALL phenotype, and L3 (Burkitt) morphology. Without prophylactic chemotherapy directed at the CNS, the CNS relapse rate is up to 50%. Leukemic cells invade the meninges; tumor spreads from the bone marrow centripetally along arachnoid veins, giving rise to leptomeningeal metastases. The infiltrate spreads along the arachnoid into the Virchow-Robin spaces, secondarily affecting the adventitia of arterioles. With leptomeningeal seeding, the CSF cytology is invariably abnormal. As with meningeal involvement by carcinoma, all levels of the CNS are affected, with cranial nerve signs (IIIrd, IVth, VIth, and VIIth), seizures, cognitive deficit, or hydrocephalus. Uncommon syndromes with leukemic infiltration include hypothalamic infiltration with *hyperphagia and obesity* or diabetes insipidus.

The prognosis for acute leukemia was poor before therapy directed at eradication of leptomeningeal metastasis was introduced in the early 1960s. The CNS is a sanctuary because most systemic antileukemic chemotherapy does not achieve adequate therapeutic CSF levels to eradicate tumor cells. Surviving leukemia cells in the CSF may reenter the marrow and reestablish the disease. With combined craniospinal radiation and intrathecal chemotherapy (methotrexate or cytosine arabinoside), the incidence of CNS relapse has declined dramatically, with improved quality of life and survival. Although cranial irradiation is neurotoxic (see Chapter 71), intrathecal chemotherapy is less satisfactory. Current protocols attempt to eliminate spinal radiation, reduce the cranial dose, and treat more intensively with intrathecal medications. Bone marrow transplantation in patients with leukemia may be complicated by posttransplant leukoencephalopathy.

In contrast, chronic leukemia rarely affects the CNS. When *chronic myelogenous leukemia* enters into blast crisis, leptomeningeal metastases may occur. *Chronic lymphocytic leukemia* is common but only exceptionally invades the meninges or brain, most often with late-stage disease.

Plasma Cell Dyscrasias

Several conditions, both neoplastic and nonneoplastic, are characterized by the appearance of monoclonal gamma globulins (M protein) in the serum. The monoclonal proteins are produced by cells of B-cell lineage, and the associated *plasma cell dyscrasias* include multiple myeloma, Waldenström macroglobulinemia (with IgM paraprotein), and amyloidosis.

If monoclonal gammopathy is the only manifestation, this is termed *monoclonal gammopathy of unknown significance* (MGUS). MGUS may persist in asymptomatic people for years or decades. In 20% of patients, a plasma cell dyscrasia or one of the lymphoproliferative diseases (chronic lymphocytic leukemia [CLL], lymphoma) later appears. Differentiation of MGUS from more serious disease depends on bone marrow examination, urinary excretion of light chains (Bence-Jones protein), and survey for bone lesions.

Peripheral neuropathy is a common neurologic manifestation of MGUS. In most cases the paraprotein is IgM and less commonly IgG or IgA. In about half of the patients with IgM neuropathy, the monoclonal protein has antibody activity against *myelin-associated glycoprotein* and results in a demyelinating peripheral neuropathy. These patients show large-fiber sensory loss and late-onset distal limb weakness. Some patients with a sensory axonal neuropathy have IgM antibodies that recognize axonal sulfatides or chondroitin sulfate. The role of the M protein in the pathogenesis of these syndromes is debated, but experimentally antibodies to myelin-associated glycoprotein can induce peripheral nerve demyelination.

In myeloma, the most frequent neurologic complication is thoracic or lumbosacral radiculopathy, resulting from nerve compression by a vertebral lesion or collapsed bone. A syndrome of spinal cord compression may appear when there are *epidural myeloma masses* within the spinal canal. The intraspinal lesions are treated with combinations of radiotherapy or chemotherapy. Intracranial *plasmacytomas* are usually extensions of myeloma skull lesions. Characteristic multiple osteolytic lesions are seen on radiographs of the skull and other bones (Fig. 147.3). Leptomeningeal invasion is also seen with myeloma. Peripheral neuropathy is uncommon and usually associated with axonal degeneration and amyloidosis. One unusual multisystem disease is POEMS (*p*olyneuropathy, *o*rganomegaly, *e*ndocrinopathy, *M* protein, and *s*kin changes), which is associated with osteosclerotic myeloma or plasmacytoma. The M protein is usually IgG or IgA, invariably associated with a lambda light chain. Surgical removal of the plasmacytoma may reverse the neuropathy.

The peripheral neuropathy in *Waldenström macroglobulinemia* is similar to the demyelinating neuropathy of MGUS. Leukoencephalopathy with macroglobulinemia is called the *Bing-Neel syndrome*; there may be plasma cell invasion of perivascular spaces, but there is no cerebral mass lesion. A *hyperviscosity syndrome* with IgM paraproteinemia is associated with headache, blurred vision, tinnitus, vertigo, and ataxia. Serum viscosity can be reduced by chemotherapy or by plasmapheresis to lower the paraprotein concentration.

The neuropathies are treated with immunosuppressive drugs, intravenous immunoglobulin therapy, or plasmapheresis.

Myelofibrosis

Extramedullary hematopoiesis often accompanies myelofibrosis or polycythemia vera and may cause extradural spinal cord compression, cerebral compression by calvarial-based intracranial masses, or orbital lesions with exophthalmos. The neurologic signs are usually painless and develop insidiously. The syndrome occurs more frequently after splenectomy and responds to radiotherapy.

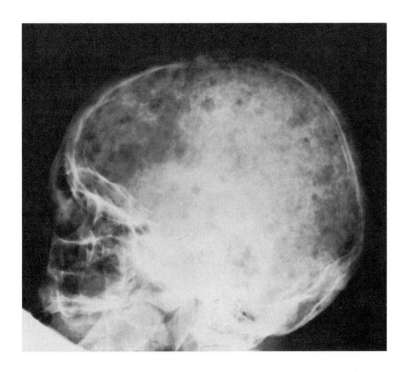

FIG. 147.3. Multiple myeloma. Myriads of osteolytic lesions. (Courtesy of Dr. Lowell G. Lubic.)

COAGULATION DISORDERS

Hematologic disorders or coagulopathies may be responsible for stroke in 4% to 17% of young patients and 1% of all patients with ischemic stroke. The role of prothrombotic disorders in older stroke patients is not known. Most prothrombotic disorders are associated with venous thrombosis in unusual sites (mesentery, sagittal sinus), but arterial thrombosis, mainly in the carotid artery, has been described. Women with hereditary prothrombotic conditions using oral contraception are at a three- to fourfold risk of cerebral sinus thrombosis. Cerebral thrombosis can occur without systemic manifestations. A hematologic abnormality is attributed a causal role in stroke if the abnormality persists months after the event or is seen in other family members.

Antithrombin III Deficiency

Antithrombin III (ATIII) is a plasma glycoprotein synthesized by the liver and endothelial cells. It binds to endogenous heparan on the surface of endothelial cells or to exogenous heparin. ATIII is required for the anticoagulant action of heparin, increasing its ability to inhibit thrombin and other activated clotting factors. The activity of ATIII can be measured by its ability to inactivate factor Xa or thrombin. Heparin accelerates this interaction.

Deficiency of ATIII is inherited or acquired, with a prevalence of 1:2,000 to 1:5,000 in the general population. There are two types of familial ATIII deficiency. Type I accounts for about 90% of inherited cases; both antigen level and functional activity of ATIII are decreased. In type II, levels are normal, but there is dysfunction of ATIII. The disease is inherited in an autosomal dominant fashion, affecting both sexes equally. Penetrance is variable. The most common manifestation is leg thrombosis and pulmonary embolus. In heterozygote individuals, symptomatic

thrombosis increases after the age of 15, and by age 55 it is estimated to occur in 85% of gene carriers. More than half of the thrombotic episodes occur with triggering events: pregnancy, surgery, or infection. It is an isolated event in 42%. Cerebral venous thrombosis is more common, but arterial thrombosis may occur. For homozygotes, venous thrombosis is usually seen during the first year of life. Clues to diagnosis are family history of thromboembolism, thrombosis during pregnancy, resistance to heparin therapy, or unusual sites of thrombosis (brain, mesentery).

There are several causes of acquired ATIII deficiency. Decreased synthesis is seen with liver cirrhosis. Drug-induced ATIII deficiency occurs with L-asparaginase, heparin, or oral contraceptives containing estrogen. Increased excretion in protein-losing enteropathy, inflammatory bowel disease, or nephrotic syndrome results in low ATIII levels. Accelerated consumption in disseminated intravascular coagulopathy (DIC) or after major surgery can lead to ATIII deficiency.

ATIII deficiency is resistant to anticoagulation with heparin. ATIII concentrate is given to deficient patients with a thrombotic event or at times of maximal risk, such as surgery or delivery. After a thrombotic event, lifelong warfarin therapy is indicated. The value of prophylactic anticoagulation for all carriers during high-risk events is debated.

Protein S Deficiency

Protein S is a vitamin K–dependent plasma protein synthesized in the liver. It facilitates the binding of protein C to the platelet membrane, acting as a nonenzymatic cofactor for the anticoagulant activity of activated protein C. Only 40% of protein S is in a free form; the rest is in an inactive form, bound to C4-binding protein. C4-binding protein levels are elevated during acute inflammation or stress, increasing the inactivation of protein S and thus the risk of thrombosis. The complex of proteins C and S inhibits the clotting cascade. Protein S deficiency can be acquired or congenital, inherited as autosomal dominant with partial expressivity. Acquired deficiency is caused by liver dysfunction, vitamin K deficiency, warfarin therapy, nephrotic syndrome, oral contraceptives, or chemotherapy.

Up to 20% of patients with stroke have protein S deficiency, but the significance of this figure has been challenged by case-control studies. Thrombosis, both cerebral venous and arterial system, has been described. In evaluating protein S deficiency, it is necessary to determine both the free and the total protein S levels. Most patients with protein S deficiency and stroke are given anticoagulation therapy for a predetermined period. Prophylactic anticoagulation is not advocated for asymptomatic protein S deficiency.

Protein C Deficiency

Protein C is a serine protease and an important inhibitor of plasma coagulation. Similar to protein S, its synthesis by the liver depends on vitamin K. Protein C in the plasma is inactive; it is activated by a thrombin–thrombomodulin complex when clotting is initiated at the endothelial surface. Protein S enhances the activity of protein C. Once activated, protein C inactivates factors Va and VIIIa, inhibiting coagulation and enhancing fibrinolytic activity. Deficiency can be inherited or acquired. The trait is autosomal dominant with incomplete penetrance. Homozygous individuals develop *purpura fulminans* and severe thrombotic complications in the neonatal period. Heterozygotes have recurrent thrombosis in early adult years. Members of the family may have subnormal protein C levels but may be asymptomatic. Additional risk factors for thromboembolism, such as smoking or oral contraceptives, may be contributory. Acquired protein C deficiency may occur with vitamin K malabsorption or warfarin therapy or with malignancy or chemotherapy. Either quantitative or qualitative protein C deficiency can lead to cerebral thrombosis.

Protein C deficiency is found in 6% to 8% of patients who have a stroke before age 40. Strokes are usually attributed to venous thrombosis. Occlusion of the cerebral arteries is rare, as is cerebral sinus thrombosis.

Anticoagulation with heparin or warfarin is recommended only for clinical thrombosis and not for those with subnormal levels. *Warfarin necrosis* of skin and subcutaneous tissues, particularly breast and adipose tissue, may be seen in patients 2 to 5 days into treatment and has been attributed to loading doses. Protein C deficiency may be associated with homocysteinemia, which itself can lead to thrombosis.

Factor V Leiden and Prothrombin G20210A Mutations

Factor V Leiden is the most common known genetic risk factor for thrombosis. A mutation of the factor V gene causing replacement of arginine 506 by glycine results in factor Va resistance to degradation by activated protein C. The resultant imbalance between pro- and anticoagulant factors predisposes to venous thrombosis. The incidence of heterozygous factor V Leiden is

2% to 8.5%, depending on the ethnicity and geographic location of the population studied. Heterozygosity for the factor V mutation alone does not appear to increase the risk for ischemic stroke.

There is conflicting data as to whether the prothrombin G20210A mutation, which is associated with thrombosis, confers an increased risk of ischemic stroke in young patients heterozygous for this mutation. Spinal cord infarction in young women smokers on oral contraception having the prothrombin G20210A mutation has been described.

Recent data suggest that the frequent coexistence of factor V Leiden; the prothrombin 20210A allele; and hereditary deficiencies of ATIII, protein C, and protein S may significantly contribute to the risk of thrombotic events.

Hereditary Abnormalities of Fibrinolysis

There are four inherited abnormalities of fibrinolysis. *Plasminogen* deficiency is autosomal dominant, with patients predisposed to venous thrombosis, including cortical vein thrombosis. *Tissue plasminogen activator* deficiency has been associated with venous thrombosis but not stroke. Patients with *dysfibrinogenemia* can have strokes rarely. Those with *factor XII deficiency* have elevated activated partial thromboplastin time, and some have had strokes.

Autoantibodies

Antiphospholipid antibodies, encompassing the *lupus anticoagulant* and *anticardiolipin antibodies*, are the most common acquired defects associated with thrombosis. IgG anticardiolipin antibodies have been associated with ischemic stroke, often recurrent, particularly in young adults. Other neurologic presentations in patients with antiphospholipid antibodies include cerebral venous sinus thrombosis, dementia, and chorea. The presence of a lupus anticoagulant should be suspected if the activated partial thromboplastin time (and prothrombin time in some cases) is prolonged and fails to correct with mixing studies.

Paroxysmal Nocturnal Hemoglobinuria

This clonal myelodysplastic syndrome is characterized by the absence of glycosylphosphatidylinositol, which anchors proteins to the cell surface. Patients are prone to hepatic vein and sagittal sinus thrombosis and may have hemolytic anemia, cytopenia, and headache.

Hemophilia

Twenty-five percent of hemorrhagic deaths in hemophiliacs are due to intracranial bleeding, often without precedent trauma. Bleeding can be subdural, epidural, intracerebral, or infrequently intraspinal. In a study of 2,500 patients followed for 10 years, the incidence of intracranial bleeding was 3%, with a 34% mortality rate and 47% of survivors having residual mental retardation, motor impairment, or seizures. Treatment with factor concentrate should not be delayed for diagnostic procedures if there is a clinical suspicion of intracranial bleeding. Peripheral neuropathies may follow intaneural bleeding or nerve compression by hematomas.

CEREBROVASCULAR COMPLICATIONS OF CANCER

At autopsy, as many as 15% of patients with systemic malignancy have evidence of cerebrovascular disease. Cancers cause vascular complications by several indirect or direct mechanisms.

Nonbacterial thrombotic endocarditis with sterile platelet-fibrin heart valve vegetations is the most common cause of cerebral infarction in patients with systemic malignancy. Most patients have disseminated malignancy and have multiple strokes, with ischemic or hemorrhagic infarctions in different vascular territories, often preceded by TIAs. The lesions are differentiated from brain metastases by CT or MRI. The most common tumors are lymphomas and adenocarcinomas, particularly mucin-producing adenocarcinomas. Emboli to other organs (pulmonary embolism, limb arterial emboli, or myocardial infarction) may call attention to the diagnosis, especially in patients with neurologic symptoms. There is thought to be a coagulopathy, but this has not been clarified. Therapy is directed toward eradication of the primary tumor; the role of anticoagulation is unsettled.

Tumor emboli uncommonly cause cerebral infarction, usually with atrial myxoma or lung carcinoma. *Neoplastic angioendotheliomatosis* was formerly attributed to tumor emboli or diffuse spread of endothelial cells with strokelike symptoms, but neoplastic angioendotheliomatosis is a systemic lymphoma with intravascular dissemination (see Chapter 56).

Coagulation disorders may be due to the underlying tumor, chemotherapy, or radiotherapy. Coagulopathy is often seen with hepatic metastases and depletion of coagulation factors. Many chemotherapeutic agents depress stem cell function to cause thrombocytopenia. *Colony-stimulating factors* stimulate leukocyte production and permit more intensive chemotherapy, but thrombocytopenia may require platelet transfusions. Spontaneous intraparenchymal or subarachnoid hemorrhage may occur when the platelet count is less than 20,000/mm^3, a common problem in the cancer patient with sepsis. The combination of coagulopathy and thrombocytopenia, often seen with leukemia, predisposes to *cerebral hemorrhage*. In contrast, *subdural hemorrhage* is less common than parenchymal or subarachnoid hemorrhage in patients with coagulopathy or thrombocytopenia and occurs more frequently in the presence of dural metastases from carcinoma of breast, lung, or prostate.

Even with normal coagulation and platelet function, some metastatic tumors (melanomas, lung carcinomas, choriocarcinomas, and hypernephromas) are likely to cause hemorrhage into a tumor. With gliomas, the likelihood of *intratumor hemorrhage* increases with increasing grade of malignancy. To avert intratumor hemorrhage, patients with known primary or metastatic brain tumors should receive platelet transfusions if the count falls below 20,000/mm^3, and coagulation functions should be maintained with transfusions of fresh frozen plasma. Intracranial or subarachnoid hemorrhage may result from rupture of a *neoplastic (oncotic) aneurysm* caused by atrial myxomas or direct de-

struction of arterial walls as a result of invasion by a metastatic lung carcinoma or choriocarcinoma or glioblastoma.

DIC is readily detected in its acute fulminant form when patients bleed profusely after venipuncture and have intracranial hemorrhage. *Acute promyelocytic leukemia* is associated with fulminant DIC, probably secondary to release of granules from leukemic cells. A more indolent form of DIC may also cause neurologic manifestations. Autopsy examinations reveal evidence of thrombosis *in situ*, intravascular coagulation. In contrast to nonbacterial thrombotic endocarditis, in which multifocal neurologic signs predominate, the main neurologic manifestation of DIC is diffuse encephalopathy. The diagnosis of chronic DIC is difficult but should be considered if the level of *fibrin split products* is elevated. Heparin anticoagulation is a logical but unproven therapy.

Occlusion of the superior sagittal sinus may follow direct spread of tumor to the dura. The cardinal symptoms of *venous sinus thrombosis* include headache secondary to increased intracranial pressure and seizures. It may also be a *nonmetastatic complication*, presumably caused by coagulopathy. The diagnosis is made by MRI, which shows loss of the typical signal flow void in the superior sagittal sinus at the site of the thrombosis. Heparin therapy is frequently beneficial but must be monitored, particularly if there is hemorrhagic cortical infarction. *Leptomeningeal metastasis* infrequently produces TIA or infarction by compromising vessels near the meningeal infiltrate.

Radiation-induced vasculopathy of the carotid artery may be delayed for years after radiation therapy for tumors of the head or neck. Symptoms of TIAs or infarction point to the involved vessel, and angiography reveals intimal irregularity. Radiotherapy may accelerate atherosclerosis, and appropriate patients benefit from endarterectomy.

OTHER DISORDERS

Hypereosinophilic Syndrome

Hypereosinophilia has been associated with a number of disorders, including allergies, parasitic infections, Hodgkin and T-cell lymphomas, and some forms of vasculitis. When eosinophilia (greater than 1,500/mm^3) persists for more than 6 months without an apparent underlying cause, with evidence of tissue damage by eosinophils, the disorder is termed the *hypereosinophilic syndrome*. The pathogenesis may be related to T-cell overexpression of cytokines, particularly interleukin-5. Eosinophils contain a number of granule proteins that damage tissue, including the eosinophil-derived neurotoxin that can cause Purkinje cell degeneration, ataxia, and paralysis in experimental animals. Multiple organs are affected, including the heart (endomyocardial fibrosis), lungs, liver, spleen, and skin. The CNS is affected in 15% of cases as encephalopathy, TIA, embolic infarction, or peripheral neuropathy. Behavioral changes, confusion, memory loss, ataxia, and upper motor neuron signs may be the first manifestation. Cerebral embolism is attributed to the cardiac disorder and responds poorly to anticoagulation. Patients with hypereosinophilia and peripheral neuropathy raise the possibility of the *Churg-Strauss syndrome*. Steroids and hydroxyurea are the mainstay of therapy for the eosinophilic syndrome.

Langerhans Cell Histiocytosis

Histiocytes include the antigen-presenting dendritic cells and antigen-processing phagocytic cells. Disorders of dendritic cells, previously called histiocytosis X, are now termed *Langerhans cell histiocytosis*. They may arise from clonal proliferation of cells but malignant histiocytosis, a true neoplasm, is rare. A localized form is the *eosinophilic granuloma* (Fig. 147.4); a multifocal form is the *Hand-Schüller-Christian disease*, and a disseminated disease in children under age 2 is the *Letterer-Siwe disease*. The diagnosis of Langerhans cell histiocytosis is made by biopsy of affected tissues and immunohistochemical analysis with surface markers that are expressed by Langerhans cells.

Eosinophilic granuloma is a painless destructive bone lesion that frequently involves the calvarium but is detected on CT performed for other reasons. Excision and local radiation therapy are often curative.

Hand-Schüller-Christian disease is characterized by the triad of calvarial lesions, exophthalmos, and diabetes insipidus. Otitis media and constitutional symptoms of fever or weight loss may occur. The hypothalamus is likely to be affected, most often with diabetes insipidus, especially in children and young adults. CT or MRI reveals both gray and white matter contrast and non-contrast-enhancing intraparenchymal lesions that are not specific; biopsy is needed unless tissue diagnosis can be obtained from a calvarial lesion. Therapy consists of localized irradiation and corticosteroids. Chemotherapy is given for those with resistant disease.

Letterer-Siwe disease causes a granulomatous rash, lymphadenopathy, hepatosplenomegaly, fever, and weight loss, usually without neurologic involvement. The prognosis for this form is quite poor; cytotoxic chemotherapy has been recommended.

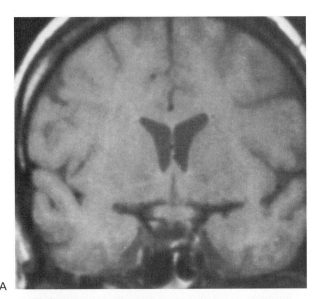

A

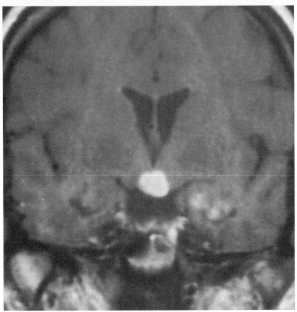

B

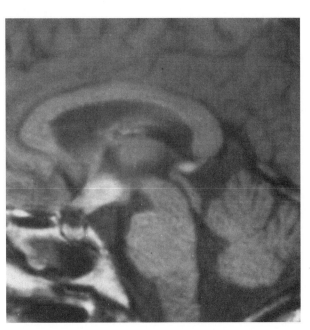

C

FIG. 147.4. Eosinophilic granuloma of optic chiasm. **A:** T1-weighted coronal magnetic resonance (MR) image shows enlargement of optic chiasm. **B and C:** T1-weighted coronal and sagittal MR images after gadolinium enhancement demonstrate focal enhancing nodule involving optic chiasm and hypothalamus, consistent with known eosinophilic granuloma. Incidentally noted are several small enhancing lesions in left temporal lobe (an unusual site for eosinophilic granuloma). (Courtesy of Drs. S. Chan and S.K. Hilal.)

Neurolymphomatosis

In 1934, Lhermitte and Trelles described lymphomatous infiltration of peripheral nerves or neurolymphomatosis. Of more than 40 histologically proven cases reported subsequently, most have had non-Hodgkin lymphoma with progressive sensorimotor peripheral neuropathy. Some also had cranial neuropathy (45%), bowel or bladder incontinence (25%), gait ataxia (18%), or mental change (13%). The CSF protein content was above 100 mg/dL in 57% of patients, and 70% had lymphocytic CSF pleocytosis. CSF cytology was abnormal in 33%. Electrodiagnostic studies show axonal neuropathy, mixed, or pure demyelinating neuropathy. Sural nerve biopsy shows equal numbers of patients with purely axonal degeneration or demyelinating lesions. MRI may be useful in identifying appropriate biopsy sites. At postmortem examination, there is often B-lymphocytic infiltration of leptomeninges, dorsal root ganglia, and spinal roots. The histopathologic pattern is indistinguishable from that of primary leptomeningeal lymphoma. Neurolymphomatosis is readily discernible from the polyclonal T-cell infiltration in human immunodeficiency virus-associated diffuse infiltrative lymphocytosis syndrome. The neurologic disorder sometimes improves with corticosteroids, chemotherapy, or radiation therapy.

Angiocentric Immunoproliferative Lesions

These disorders are discussed in Chapter 56.

Chediak-Higashi Syndrome

This rare autosomal recessive disorder is characterized by partial oculocutaneous albinism, immunologic defects, a bleeding diathesis, and progressive neurologic dysfunction. Mutation of the CHS1 gene on chromosome 1q42-q44 appears to result in defective transport of intracellular proteins, producing giant lysosomal granules in granule-containing cells, including neutrophils, monocytes, hepatocytes, and renal tubular cells. The granules are easily recognized on a peripheral blood smear. Impaired neutrophil function and defective T-cell and natural killer cell cytotoxicity predisposes to infections that lead to death, usually within the first decade of life. Neurologic syndromes include a spinocerebellar disorder and peripheral neuropathy. The neurologic symptoms may be associated with neuronal or Schwann cell inclusions or by lymphohistiocytic infiltration of peripheral nerves. CT brain findings include diffuse atrophy and decreased periventricular density. Bone marrow transplant is a potentially curative avenue for therapy.

SUGGESTED READINGS

Sickle Cell

Adams RJ, McKie VC, Hsu L, et al. Prevention of a first stroke by transfusions in children with sickle cell anemia and abnormal results on transcranial Doppler ultrasonography. *N Engl J Med* 1998;339:5–11.

Earley CJ, Kittner SJ, Feeser BR, et al. Stroke in children and sickle-cell disease: Baltimore-Washington Cooperative Young Stroke Study. *Neurology* 1998;51:169–176.

Fabian R, Peters B. Neurological complications of hemoglobin SC disease. *Arch Neurol* 1984;41:289–292.

Greenberg J, Massey E. Cerebral infarction in sickle cell trait. *Ann Neurol* 1985;18:354–355.

Hart RG, Kanter MC. Hematologic disorders and ischemic stroke. A selective review. *Stroke* 1990;21:1111–1121.

Liu JE, Gzesh DJ, Ballas SK. The spectrum of epilepsy in sickle cell anemia. *J Neurol Sci* 1994;123:6–10.

Moser FG, Miller ST, Bello JA, et al. The spectrum of brain MR abnormalities in sickle-cell disease: a report from the Cooperative Study of Sickle Cell Disease. *AJNR* 1996;17:965–972.

Ohene-Frempong K, Weiner SJ, Sleeper LA, et al. Cerebrovascular accidents in sickle cell disease: rates and risk factors. *Blood* 1998;91:288–294.

Preul MC, Cendes F, Just N, Mohr G. Intracranial aneurysms and sickle cell anemia: multiplicity and propensity for the vertebrobasilar territory. *Neurosurgery* 1998;42:971–977.

Reyes M. Subcortical cerebral infarctions in sickle cell trait. *J Neurol Neurosurg Psychiatry* 1989;52:516–518.

Wang WC, Langston JW, Steen RG, et al. Abnormalities of the central nervous system in very young children with sickle cell anemia. *J Pediatr* 1998;132:994–998.

Thalassemia

Kaufmann T, Coleman M, Giardina P, Nisce LZ. The role of radiation therapy in the management of hematopoietic neurologic complications in thalassemia. *Acta Haematol* 1991;85:156–159.

Logothetis J, Constantoulakis M, Economidou J, et al. Thalassemia major (homozygous beta-thalassemia). A survey of 138 cases with emphasis on neurologic and muscular aspects. *Neurology* 1972;22:294–304.

Papanastasiou DA, Papanicolaou D, Magiakou AM, et al. Peripheral neuropathy in patients with beta-thalassaemia. *J Neurol Neurosurg Psychiatry* 1991;54:997–1000.

Wong V, Yu Y, Liang R, et al. Cerebral thrombosis in β-thalassemia/hemoglobin E disease. *Stroke* 1990;21:812–816.

Polycythemia

Gruppo Italiano Studio Policitemia. Polycythemia vera: the natural history of 1213 patients followed for 20 years. *Ann Intern Med* 1995;123:656–664.

Newton LK. Neurologic complications of polycythemia and their impact on therapy. *Oncology* 1990;4:59–64.

Poza JJ, Cobo AM, Marti-Masso JF. Peripheral neuropathy associated with polycythemia vera. *Neurologia* 1996;11:276–279.

Yiannikas C, McLeod JG, Walsh JC. Peripheral neuropathy associated with polycythemia vera. *Neurology* 1983;33:139–143.

Essential Thrombocytosis (Thrombocythemia)

Koudstaal PJ, Koudstaal A. Neurologic and visual symptoms in essential thrombocythemia: efficacy of low-dose aspirin. *Semin Thromb Hemost* 1997;23:365–370.

Martin EA, Lavin PJ, Thompson AJ. Painful extremities and neurological disorder in essential thrombocythaemia. *J R Soc Med* 1984;77:372–374.

Mitus AJ, Tiziano B, Shulman LN, et al. Hemostatic complications in young patients with essential thrombocythemia. *Am J Med* 1990;88:371–375.

Thrombotic Thrombocytopenic Purpura

Bennett CL, Weinberg PD, Rozenberg-Ben-Dror K, et al. Thrombotic thrombocytopenic purpura associated with ticlopidine. A review of 60 cases. *Ann Intern Med* 1998;128:541–544.

Kay AC, Solberg LA Jr, Nichols DA, Petitt RM. Prognostic significance of computed tomography of the brain in thrombotic thrombocytopenic purpura. *Mayo Clin Proc* 1991;66:602–607.

Tardy B, Page Y, Convers P, et al. Thrombotic thrombocytopenic purpura: MR findings. *AJNR* 1993;14:489–490.

Tsai HM, Lian EC. Antibodies to von Willebrand factor-cleaving protease in acute thrombotic thrombocytopenic purpura. *N Engl J Med* 1998;339:1585–1594.

Heparin-induced Thrombocytopenia

Becker PS, Miller VT. Heparin-induced thrombocytopenia. *Stroke* 1989;20:1449–1459.

Magnani HN. Heparin-induced thrombocytopenia (HIT): an overview of 230 patients treated with Organan (Org 10172). *Thromb Haemost* 1993;70:554–561.

Warkentin TE, Kelton JG. A 14-year study of heparin-induced thrombocytopenia. *Am J Med* 1996;101:502–507.

Myelofibrosis

Landolfi R, Colosimo CJ, De Candia E, et al. Meningeal hematopoiesis causing exophthalmos and hemiparesis in myelofibrosis: effect of radiotherapy. *Cancer* 1988;62:2346–2349.

Rice GPA, Assis LJP, Barr RM, et al. Extramedullary hematopoiesis and spinal cord compression complicating polycythemia rubra vera. *Ann Neurol* 1980;7:81–84.

Leukemia

Azzarelli B, Roessmann U. Pathogenesis of central nervous system infiltration in acute leukemia. *Arch Pathol Lab Med* 1977;101:203–205.

Balis FM, Savitch JL, Bleyer WA, et al. Remission induction of meningeal leukemia with high-dose intravenous methotrexate. *J Clin Oncol* 1985;3:485–489.

Cramer SC, Glaspy JA, Efird JT, Louis DN. Chronic lymphocytic leukemia and the central nervous system: a clinical and pathological study. *Neurology* 1996;46:19–25.

Dekker AW, Elderson A, Punt K, Sixma JJ. Meningeal involvement in patients with acute nonlymphocytic leukemia. Incidence, management, and predictive factors. *Cancer* 1985;56:2078–2082.

Freeman AI, Weinberg V, Breecher ML, et al. Comparison of intermediate-dose methotrexate with cranial irradiation for the post-induction treatment of acute lymphocytic leukemia in children. *N Engl J Med* 1983;308:477–484.

Holmes R, Keating MJ, Cork A, et al. A unique pattern of central nervous system leukemia in acute myelomonocytic leukemia associated with inv(16)(p13q22). *Blood* 1985;65:1071–1078.

McCarthy LJ. Leukostasis thrombi. *JAMA* 1985;254:613.

McKee LC, Collins RD. Intravascular leukocyte thrombi and aggregates as a cause of morbidity and mortality in leukemia. *Medicine (Baltimore)* 1974;53:463–478.

Pinkel D, Woo S. Prevention and treatment of meningeal leukemia in children. *Blood* 1994;84:355–366.

Pui CH, Dahl GV, Kalwinsky DK, et al. Central nervous system leukemia in children with acute nonlymphoblastic leukemia. *Blood* 1985;66:1062–1067.

Steinherz PG, Miller LP, Ghavimi F, et al. Dural sinus thrombosis in children with acute lymphoblastic leukemia. *JAMA* 1981;246:2837–2839.

Plasma Cell Dyscrasias

Delauche-Cavallier MC, Laredo JD, Wybier M, et al. Solitary plasmacytoma of the spine. *Cancer* 1988;61:1707–1714.

Gordon PH, Rowland LP, Younger DS, et al. Lymphoproliferative disorders and motor neuron disease: an update. *Neurology* 1997;48:1671–1678.

Kelly JJ Jr, Kyle RA, Miles JM, et al. Osteosclerotic myeloma and peripheral neuropathy. *Neurology* 1983;33:202–210.

Latov N. Pathogenesis and therapy of neuropathies associated with monoclonal gammopathies. *Ann Neurol* 1995;37[Suppl 1]:S32–S42.

Neau JP, Guilhot F, Dumas P, et al. Formes nerologiques centrales de la maladie de Waldenstrom. Syndrome de Bing-Neel. Trois cas. *Rev Neurol (Paris)* 1991;147:56–60.

Nobile-Orazio E, Barbieri S, Baldini L, et al. Peripheral neuropathy in monoclonal gammopathy of undetermined significance: prevalence and immunopathogenetic studies. *Acta Neurol Scand* 1992;85:383–390.

Ropper AH, Gorson KC. Neuropathies associated with paraproteinemia. *N Engl J Med* 1998;338:1601–1607.

Schey S. Osteosclerotic myeloma and "POEMS" syndrome. *Blood Rev* 1996;10:75–80.

Schulman P, Sun T, Shareer L, et al. Meningeal involvement in IgD myeloma with cerebrospinal fluid paraprotein analysis. *Cancer* 1980;46:152–155.

Sherman WH, Olarte MR, McKiernan G, et al. Plasma exchange treatment of peripheral neuropathy associated with plasma cell dyscrasia. *J Neurol Neurosurg Psychiatry* 1984;47:813–819.

Spiers ASD, Halpern R, Ross SC, et al. Meningeal myelomatosis. *Arch Intern Med* 1980;140:256–259.

West SG, Pittman DL, Coggin JT. Intracranial plasma cell granuloma. *Cancer* 1980;46:330–335.

Disorders of Coagulation

Antiphospholipid Antibodies in Stroke Study (APASS) Group. Anticardiolipin antibodies are an independent risk factor for first ischemic stroke. *Neurology* 1993;43:2069–2073.

de Bruijn SF, Stam J, Koopman MM, Vandenbroucke JP. Case-control study of risk of cerebral sinus thrombosis in oral contraceptive users and in [correction of who are] carriers of hereditary prothrombotic conditions. The Cerebral Venous Sinus Thrombosis Study Group. *BMJ* 1998;316:589–592.

De Stefano V, Chiusolo P, Paciaroni K, et al. Prothrombin G20210A mutant genotype is a risk factor for cerebrovascular ischemic disease in young patients. *Blood* 1998;91:3562–3565.

Grewal RP, Goldberg MA. Stroke in protein C deficiency. *Am J Med* 1990;89:538–539.

Harris M, Exner T, Rickard K, et al. Multiple cerebral thrombosis in Fletcher factor (prekallikrein) deficiency: a case report. *Am J Hematol* 1985;19:387–393.

Hathaway WE. Clinical aspects of antithrombin III deficiency. *Semin Hematol* 1991;28:19–23.

Israel S, Seshia S. Childhood stroke associated with protein C or S deficiency. *J Pediatr* 1987;111:562–564.

Jorens PG, Hermans CR, Haber I, et al. Acquired protein C and S deficiency, inflammatory bowel disease and cerebral arterial thrombosis. *Blut* 1990;61:307–310.

Kohler J, Kasper J, Witt I, et al. Ischemic stroke due to protein C deficiency. *Stroke* 1990;21:1077–1080.

Kwaan HC. Protein C and protein S. *Semin Thromb Hemost* 1989;15:353–355.

Lee MK, Ng SC. Cerebral venous thrombosis associated with antithrombin III deficiency. *Aust N Z J Med* 1991;21:772–773.

Leone G, Graham JA, Daly HM, Carson PJ. Antithrombin III deficiency and cerebrovascular accidents in young adults. *J Clin Pathol* 1992;45:921–922.

Levine SR, Brey RL, Sawaya KL, et al. Recurrent stroke and thrombo-occlusive events in the phospholipid syndrome. *Ann Neurol* 1995;38:119–124.

Martinez HR, Rangel-Guerra R, Marfil LJ. Ischemic stroke due to deficiency of coagulation inhibitors. Report of 10 young adults. *Stroke* 1993;24:19–45.

Matsushita K, Kuriyama Y, Sawada T, et al. Cerebral infarction associated with protein C deficiency. *Stroke* 1992;23:108–111.

Mayer S, Sacco R, Hurlet-Jensen A, et al. Free protein S deficiency in acute ischemic stroke. A case-control study. *Stroke* 1993;24:224–227.

Munts AG, van Genderen PJ, Dippel DW, et al. Coagulation disorders in young adults with acute cerebral ischaemia. *J Neurol* 1998;245:21–25.

Prats JM, Garaizar C, Zuazo E, et al. Superior sagittal sinus thrombosis in a child with protein S deficiency. *Neurology* 1992;42:2303–2305.

Pratt CW, Church FC. Antithrombin: structure and function. *Semin Hematol* 1991;28:3–9.

Rich C, Gill JC, Wernick S, et al. An unusual cause of cerebral venous thrombosis in a four-year-old child. *Stroke* 1993;24:603–605.

Ridker PM, Hennekens CH, Lindpaintner K, et al. Mutation in the gene coding for coagulation factor V and the risk of myocardial infarction, stroke, and venous thrombosis in apparently healthy men. *N Engl J Med* 1995;332:912–917.

Shinmyozu K, Ohkatsu Y, Maruyama Y, et al. A case of congenital antithrombin III deficiency complicated by an internal carotid artery occlusion. *Clin Neurol* 1986;26:162–165.

Vomberg P, Breederveld C. Cerebral thromboembolism due to antithrombin III deficiency in two children. *Neuropediatrics* 1987;18:42–44.

Cerebrovascular Complications of Cancer

Amico L, Caplan LR, Thomas C. Cerebrovascular complications of mucinous cancers. *Neurology* 1989;39:522–526.

Atkinson JL, Sundt TM, Dale AJD, et al. Radiation associated atheromatous disease of the cervical carotid artery: report of seven cases and review of the literature. *Neurosurgery* 1989;24:171.

Biller J, Challa VR, Toole JF, et al. Nonbacterial thrombotic endocarditis: a neurologic perspective of clinicopathologic correlations in 99 patients. *Arch Neurol* 1982;39:95–98.

Edoute Y, Haim N, Rinkevich D, et al. Cardiac valvular vegetations in cancer patients: a prospective echocardiographic study of 200 patients. *Am J Med* 1997;102:252–258.

Feehs RS, McGuirt WF, Bond MG, et al. Irradiation. A significant risk factor for carotid atherosclerosis. *Arch Otolaryngol Head Neck Surg* 1991;117:1135–1137.

Graus F, Rogers LR, Posner JB. Cerebrovascular complications in patients with cancer. *Medicine (Baltimore)* 1985;64:16–35.

Green KB, Silverstein RL. Hypercoagulability in cancer. *Hematol Oncol Clin North Am* 1996;10:499–530.

Helmer FA. Oncotic aneurysm. *J Neurosurg* 1976;45:98–100.

Hickey WF, Garnick MB, Henderson IC, et al. Primary cerebral venous thrombosis in patients with cancer—a rarely diagnosed paraneoplastic syndrome. *Am J Med* 1982;73:740–750.

Ho K-L. Neoplastic aneurysm and intracranial hemorrhage. *Cancer* 1982;50:2935–2940.

Klein P, Haley EC, Wooten GF, et al. Focal cerebral infarctions associated with perivascular tumor infiltrates in carcinomatous leptomeningeal metastases. *Arch Neurol* 1989;46:1149.

Murros KE, Toole JF. The effect of radiation on carotid arteries. *Arch Neurol* 1989;46:449.

O'Neill BP, Dinapoli RP, Okazaki H. Cerebral infarction as a result of tumor emboli. *Cancer* 1987;60:90–95.

Rogers LR, Cho E, Kempin S, et al. Cerebral infarction from non-bacterial thrombotic endocarditis. *Am J Med* 1987;83:746.

Hypereosinophilic Syndrome

Bell D, Mackay IG, Pentland B. Hypereosinophilic syndrome presenting as peripheral neuropathy. *Postgrad Med J* 1985;61:429–432.

Brito-Babapulle F. Clonal eosinophilic disorders and the hypereosinophilic syndrome. *Blood Rev* 1997;11:129–145.

Durack DT, Sumi SM, Klebanoff SJ. Neurotoxicity of human eosinophils. *Proc Natl Acad Sci USA* 1979;76:1443–1447.

Monaco S, Lucci B, Laperchia N, et al. Polyneuropathy in hypereosinophilic syndrome. *Neurology* 1988;38:494–496.

Rosenberg HF, Tenen DG, Ackerman SJ. Molecular cloning of the human eosinophil-derived neurotoxin: a member of the ribonuclease gene family. *Proc Natl Acad Sci USA* 1989;86:4460–4464.

Langerhans Cell Histiocytosis

Adornato BT, Eil C, Head GL, Loriaus L. Cerebellar involvement in multifocal eosinophilic granuloma: demonstration by computerized tomographic scanning. *Ann Neurol* 1980;7:125–129.

George JC, Edwards MK, Smith RR, et al. MR of intracranial Langerhans cell histiocytosis. *J Comput Assist Tomogr* 1994;18:295–297.

Grois NG, Favara BE, Mostbeck GH, Prayer D. Central nervous system disease in Langerhans cell histiocytosis. *Hematol Oncol Clin North Am* 1998;12:287–305.

Ladisch S. Langerhans cell histiocytosis. *Curr Opin Hematol* 1998;5:54–58.

Neurolymphomatosis

Diaz-Arrastia R, Younger DS, Hair L, et al. Neurolymphomatosis: a clinicopathologic syndrome re-emerges. *Neurology* 1992;42:1136–1141.

Gherardi RK, Chretien F, Delfau-Larue MH, et al. Neuropathy in diffuse infiltrative lymphocytosis syndrome: an HIV neuropathy, not a lymphoma. *Neurology* 1998;50:1041–1044.

Gordon PH, Younger DS. Neurolymphomatosis. *Neurology* 1996;46:1191–1192.

Van den Bent MJ, de Bruin HG, Beun GD, Vecht CJ. Neurolymphomatosis of the median nerve. *Neurology* 1995;45:1403–1405.

Chediak-Higashi Syndrome

Ballard R, Tien RD, Nohria V, Juel V. The Chediak-Higashi syndrome: CT and MR findings. *Pediatr Radiol* 1994;24:266–267.

Misra VP, King RHM, Harding AE, et al. Peripheral neuropathy in the Chediak-Higashi syndrome. *Acta Neuropathol* 1991;81:354–358.

Pettit RE, Berdal KG. Chediak-Higashi syndrome. *Arch Neurol* 1984;41:1001–1002.

Spitz RA. Genetic defects in Chediak-Higashi syndrome and the beige mouse. *J Clin Immunol* 1998;18:97–105.

Merritt's Neurology, 10th ed., edited by L.P. Rowland. Lippincott Williams & Wilkins, Philadelphia © 2000.

HEPATIC DISEASE

**NEIL H. RASKIN
LEWIS P. ROWLAND**

The terms *hepatic coma* and *encephalopathy* have led to imprecision of both clinical and pathophysiologic concepts. The often fatal comatose state associated with acute hepatic necrosis is usually attended by striking elevation of serum ammonia content; coma is usually a single event of rapid onset and fulminant course that is characterized by delirium, convulsions, and, occasionally, decerebrate rigidity. The mechanism of this encephalopathy is not clear.

Hepatic encephalopathy usually develops in patients with chronic liver disease when portal hypertension induces an extensive portal collateral circulation; portal venous blood bypasses the detoxification site, which is the liver, and drains directly into the systemic circulation to produce the cerebral intoxication that is properly termed *portal-systemic encephalopathy*. Several examples of portal-systemic encephalopathy have been reported in which the hepatic parenchyma was normal, underlining the anatomic importance of bypassing the liver as the mechanism. The offending nitrogenous substance arising in the intestine has not been identified with precision, but ammonia is the prime suspect.

The clinical syndrome resulting from shunting is an episodic encephalopathy comprising admixtures of ataxia, action tremor, dysarthria, sensorial clouding, and asterixis. The episodes are usually reversible, although they may recur. Cerebral morphologic changes are few except for an increase in large Alzheimer type II astrocytes. In a few patients with this disorder, a relentlessly progressing neurologic disorder occurs in addition to the fluctuating intoxication syndrome, including dementia, ataxia, dysarthria, intention tremor, and a choreoathetotic movement. The brains of these patients show zones of pseudolaminar necrosis in cerebral and cerebellar cortex, cavitation and neuronal loss in the basal ganglia and cerebellum, and glycogen-staining inclusions in enlarged astrocytes. This irreversible disorder has been termed *acquired chronic hepatocerebral degeneration*, but it is probably the ultimate morphologic destruction that may result from the chronic metabolic defect that attends portal-systemic shunting.

CLINICAL FEATURES

Thought processes are usually compromised insidiously, although an acute agitated delirium may occasionally usher in the syndrome. Mental dullness and drowsiness are usually the first symptoms; patients yawn frequently and drift off to sleep easily yet remain arousable. Cognitive defects eventually appear. Asterixis almost always accompanies these modest changes of con-

sciousness. As encephalopathy progresses, bilateral paratonia appears, and the stretch reflexes become brisk; bilateral Babinski signs are usually found when obtundation becomes profound. Convulsions are decidedly uncommon in this disorder, in contrast to uremic encephalopathy. Spastic paraparesis may be seen. Decerebrate and decorticate postures and diffuse spasticity of the limbs frequently accompany deeper stages of coma.

In the patient with overt hepatocellular failure with jaundice or ascites, the diagnosis of this disorder is not difficult. When parenchymal liver disease is mild or nonexistent, however, an elevated serum ammonia level or an elevation of cerebrospinal fluid glutamine content has high diagnostic sensitivity. The cerebrospinal fluid is otherwise bland. The ultimate diagnostic test is clinical responsiveness to ammonium loading; the risks of this procedure in patients with intact hepatocellular function are minimal. Ten grams of ammonium chloride is given in daily divided doses for 3 days; the appearance or worsening of asterixis, dysarthria, or ataxia or a further slowing of the electroencephalogram is diagnostic. Early in the course of encephalopathy, when the only evidence is seen on neuropsychologic tests, computed tomography may show cortical atrophy, cerebral edema, or normal patterns. Magnetic resonance imaging usually shows increased signal in the globus pallidus in T1-weighted studies. Manganese deposition may account for this. Sometimes there is calcification, and there may be abnormalities in the mesencephalon and pons. Cerebral edema is more common in chronic encephalopathy than once believed.

PATHOPHYSIOLOGY

Several substances have been considered the putative neurotoxin in portal-systemic encephalopathy. These include methionine, other amino acids, short-chain fatty acids, biogenic amines, indoles and skatoles, and ammonia. None of these has succeeded in explaining the condition better than ammonia.

Ammonia, a highly neurotoxic substance, is ordinarily converted to urea by the liver; when this detoxification mechanism is bypassed, levels of ammonia in the brain and blood increase. Occasionally, blood ammonia levels are normal or only slightly elevated in the face of full-blown coma. This has been used as a powerful argument against the implication of ammonia in this disorder; however, at physiologic pH, almost all serum ammonia in the $NH_4^+ \leftrightarrow NH_3 + H^+$ system is in the form of NH_4^+, with only traces of NH_3 present. NH_3 crosses membranes with facility and is far more toxic than NH_4^+; thus, it is possible that when methods become available to measure circulating free ammonia levels in portal-systemic encephalopathy, they will be strikingly consistently elevated. Ammonia is detoxified in brain astrocytes by conversion to the nontoxic glutamine.

Following up on the observation that levodopa benefited patients in hepatic coma, Fischer and Baldessarini (1971) proposed the false neurotransmitter hypothesis to explain the mechanism of this effect and other features of the disorder. They suggested that amines such as octopamine (or their aromatic amino acid precursors tyrosine and phenylalanine), which are derived from protein by gut bacterial action, might escape oxidation by the liver and flood the systemic and cerebral circulations. Octopamine could then replace norepinephrine and dopamine in nerve endings and act as a false neurotransmitter; the accumulation of false neurotransmitters might then account for the encephalopathy, and the amelioration could be achieved by restoring "true" neurotransmitters through an elevation of tissue dopamine levels. L-Dopa administration, however, has a powerful peripheral effect, inducing the renal excretion of ammonia and urea; this probably accounts for the beneficial effects of L-dopa in some encephalopathic patients. Further, octopamine concentration in rat brain has been elevated more than 20,000-fold, along with depletion of both norepinephrine and dopamine, without any detectable alteration of consciousness. Although false neurotransmitters do accumulate in portal-systemic encephalopathy, there is little reason to hold them responsible for the encephalopathy. It has also been suggested that increased sensitivity to inhibitory neurotransmitters such as GABA and glycine may underlie the encephalopathy.

DIFFERENTIAL DIAGNOSIS

Among the numerous causes of encephalopathy, several affect abusers of alcohol, including acute ethanolic intoxication and delerium tremens, Wernicke encephalopathy, Korsakoff syndrome, drug intoxication, other metabolic disorders (uremia, hyponatremia), and consequences of head injury, such as subdural hematoma. Another consideration is Wilson disease.

TREATMENT

Administration of antibiotics (especially neomycin or metronidazole) decreases the population of intestinal organisms to decrease production of ammonia and other cerebrotoxins. Lactulose is also beneficial for reasons that are not clear, but it lowers colonic pH, increases incorporation of ammonia into bacterial protein, and is a cathartic. The effects of neomycin and lactulose, given together, seem better than the effects either gives alone.

Although recovery is expected in patients with mild acute encephalopathy, cerebral edema occurs in about 75% of patients in acute coma and may be the cause of death. Intracranial pressure monitoring is often carried out in transplantation centers despite the risk of bleeding. If cerebral perfusion pressure is less than 40 mm Hg and does not respond to mannitol therapy, transplantation is deemed futile. In some cases of fulminant hepatic failure, emergency hepatectomy has been performed, followed by support with an extracorporeal bioartificial liver and then orthoptic liver transplantation.

NEUROLOGIC COMPLICATIONS OF LIVER TRANSPLANTATION

Neurologic problems arise in 8% to 47% of liver transplant recipients. The complications range from mild encephalopathy to akinetic mutism or coma. Psychiatric syndromes range from mild anxiety or depression to hallucinatory psychosis. Other syndromes include seizures, myoclonus, tremor, cortical blindness,

TABLE 148.1. NEUROLOGIC COMPLICATIONS OF LIVER TRANSPLANTATION

Total number	Number of patients	
	Adults[a] (n = 40)	Children[b] (n = 24)
Central nervous system		
Seizures	8	9
Cerebrocerebellar syndrome	4	8
Coma	2	0
Cortical blindness	2	0
Delusions, visual hallucinations	2	0
Psychosis without hallucinations	3	0
Headache	3	0
Intracerebral hemorrhage	1	1
Tremor, myoclonus	2	2
Meningitis	0	1
Peripheral nerves		
Brachial plexopathy	2	0
Polyneuropathy	1	0
Partial third nerve palsy	1	0

[a]Thirteen of 40 adults (33%) had one or more neurologic complications
[b]Eleven of 24 children (46%) had one or more neurologic complications.
Modified from Stein et al. 1992, and Garg et al. 1993.

brachial plexopathy, and peripheral neuropathy (Table 148.1). Cerebral hemorrhage is sometimes responsible. Recovery from these disorders is often excellent and has no effect on survival, which is the same for those with or without neurologic syndromes. The acute leukoencephalopathy caused by tacrolimus (FK506) is reversed promptly on withdrawal of drug.

The necessary immunosuppression may lead to the opportunistic infections, and cyclosporine itself is held responsible for some cerebral disorders, possibly including central pontine myelinosis and leukoencephalopathy. Instead of the intravenous administration of cyclosporine, use of an oral formulation has reduced the severity of neurotoxicity. Both cyclosporine and OKT3 may cause seizures, and OKT3 may cause aseptic meningitis.

Epileptiform activity in the electroencephalogram is seen much more often in patients who die than in those who survive. In an autopsy study of 21 patients who had seizures, Estol et al. (1989) found combinations of ischemic or hemorrhagic strokes in 18, central pontine myelinosis in 5, and central nervous system infections in 5. Metabolic abnormalities were also responsible for the seizures in these patients. Graft-versus-host reactions may include polyneuropathy, myasthenia gravis, and polymyositis. Infected donor tissue may transmit cytomegalovirus or Creutzfeldt-Jakob disease.

SUGGESTED READINGS

Hepatic Encephalopathy

Asconape JJ. Use of antiepileptic drugs in the presence of liver and kidney diseases: a review. *Epilepsia* 1982;23[Suppl 1]:S65–S79.
Butterworth RF, Spahr L, Fontaine S, Layrargues GP. Manganese toxicity, dopaminergic dysfunction and hepatic encephalopathy. *Metab Brain Dis* 1995;10:259–267.

Crippen JS, Gross JB Jr, Lindor KD. Increased intracranial pressure and hepatic encephalopathy in chronic liver disease. *Am J Gastroenterol* 1992;87:879–882.

Donovan JP, Schafer DF, Shaw BW, Sorrell MF. Cerebral oedema and increased intracranial pressure in chronic liver disease. *Lancet* 1998;351:719–721.

Ferenci P, Pappas SC, Munson PJ, et al. Changes in the status of neurotransmitter receptors in a rabbit model of hepatic encephalopathy. *Hepatology* 1984;4:186–191.

Fischer JE, Baldessarini RJ. False neurotransmitters and hepatic failure. *Lancet* 1971;2:75–80.

Haseler LJ, Sibbitt WL Jr, Mojtahedzadeh HN, Reddy S, Agarwal VF, McCarthy DM. Proton MR spectroscopic measurement of neurometabolites in hepatic encephalopathy during oral lactulose therapy. *AJNR* 1998;19:1681–1686.

Jones EA, Weissenborn K. Neurology and the liver. *J Neurol Neurosurg Psychiatry* 1997;63:279–293.

Lockwood AH, Yap EW, Wong WH. Cerebral ammonia metabolism in patients with severe liver disease and minimal hepatic encephalopathy. *J Cereb Blood Flow Metab* 1991;11:337–341.

Lunzer M, James IM, Weinman J, et al. Treatment of chronic hepatic encephalopathy with levodopa. *Gut* 1974;15:555–561.

Raskin NH, Bredesen D, Ehrenfeld WK, et al. Periodic confusion caused by congenital extrahepatic portacaval shunt. *Neurology* 1984;34:666–669.

Riordan SM, Williams R. Treatment of hepatic encephalopathy. *N Engl J Med* 1997;337:473–479.

Rozga J, Podesta L, LePage E, et al. Control of cerebral oedema by total hepatectomy and extracorporeal liver support in fulminant hepatic failure. *Lancet* 1993;342:898–899.

Shady H, Lieber CS. Blood ammonia levels in relationship to hepatic encephalopathy after propranolol. *Am J Gastroenterol* 1988;83:249–255.

Sherlock S. Chronic portal systemic encephalopathy: update 1987. *Gut* 1987;28:1043–1048.

Summerskill WHJ, Davidson EA, Sherlock S, et al. The neuropsychiatric syndrome associated with hepatic cirrhosis and an extensive portal collateral circulation. *Q J Med* 1956;25:245–266.

Victor M, Adams RD, Cole M. The acquired (non-Wilsonian) type of chronic hepatocerebral degeneration. *Medicine (Baltimore)* 1965;44:345–396.

Zieve L, Doizai M, Derr RF. Reversal of ammonia coma in rats by L-dopa: a peripheral effect. *Gut* 1979;20:28–32.

Liver Transplantation

Bird GLA, Meadows J, Goka J, et al. Cyclosporin-associated akinetic mutism and extrapyramidal syndrome after liver transplantation. *J Neurol Neurosurg Psychiatry* 1990;53:1068–1071.

Campellone JV, Lacomis D, Kramer DJ, Van Cott AC, Giuliani MJ. Acute myopathy after liver transplantation. *Neurology* 1998;50:45–53.

De Groen PC, Aksamit AJ, Rakela J, et al. Central nervous system toxicity after liver transplantation: role of cyclosporin and cholesterol. *N Engl J Med* 1987;317:861–866.

Estol CJ, Faris AA, Martinez AJ, et al. Central pontine myelinosis after liver transplantation. *Neurology* 1989;39:493–498.

Estol CJ, Lopez O, Brenner RP, et al. Seizures after liver transplantation: a clinicopathologic study. *Neurology* 1989;39:1297–1301.

Fisher NC, Ruban E, Carey M et al. Late-onset fatal acure leukoencephalopathy in liver transplant recipient. *Lancet* 1997;349:1884–1885.

Garg BP, Walsh LE, Pescovitz MD, et al. Neurologic complications of pediatric liver transplantation. *Pediatr Neurol* 1993;9:44–48.

Martin MA, Massanari RM, Ngheim DD, et al. Nosocomial aseptic meningitis associated with administration of OKT3. *JAMA* 1988;259:2002–2005.

Small SL, Fukui MB, Bramblett GT, et al. Immunosuppression-induced leukoencephalopathy from Tacrolimus (FK506). *Ann Neurol* 1996;40:575–580.

Stein DP, Lederman RJ, Vogt DP, et al. Neurological complications following liver transplantation. *Ann Neurol* 1992;31:644–649.

Torocsik HV, Curless RG, Post J, et al. FK506-induced leukoencephalopathy in children with organ transplants. *Neurology* 1999;52:1497–1500.

Truwit CL, Denaro CP, Lake JR, et al. MRI of reversible cyclosporin A-induced neurotoxicity. *AJNR* 1991;12:651–659.

Wijdicks EFM, Dahlke LJ, Wiesner RH. Oral cyclosporine decreases severity of neurotoxicity in liver transplant recipients. *Neurology* 1999;52:1708–1710.

Wijdicks EFM, Wiesner RH, Krom RAF. Neurotoxicity in liver transplant recipients with cyclosporine immunosuppression. *Neurology* 1995;45:1962–1964.

Wszolek ZK, Aksamit AJ, Ellingson RJ, et al. Epileptiform EEG abnormalities in liver transplant recipients. *Ann Neurol* 1991;130:37–41.

Merritt's Neurology, 10th ed., edited by L.P. Rowland. Lippincott Williams & Wilkins, Philadelphia © 2000.

CEREBRAL COMPLICATIONS OF CARDIAC SURGERY

ERIC J. HEYER
LEWIS P. ROWLAND

MAGNITUDE OF THE PROBLEM

In one series of 1,487 cardiac operations performed between 1984 and 1989, the mortality rate was 8.54%. Additionally, 16 patients (1.1%) had major neurologic syndromes of four types: unresponsive after surgery, awoke with signs of cerebral infarction, initially intact but had a stroke later, or dementia without focal signs. Among those who were unresponsive in the postop-

erative period, half died or remained comatose. The problems were attributed to atheromatous embolism, perioperative hypotension, or air embolism. In another series, up to 4% had cerebral symptoms if reactions included chronic anxiety and depression. Clinically detectable encephalopathy results in 3% to 12% of operations, but permanent cognitive disability is less common.

DISORDERS OF COGNITION

In the early days of heart surgery, intellectual decline seemed inordinately common after operations performed with cardiopulmonary bypass support, even when the procedure seemed to be uncomplicated. In prospective studies, cognitive problems were seen in up to 70% of survivors, depending on the criteria used; neuropsychologic testing is most sensitive. Six months after surgery, Shaw et al. (1987) found that 3 of 259 (2%) patients seemed seriously disabled and were dependent on family members.

The pathogenesis of this disorder is probably influenced by more than one of the following during cardiopulmonary bypass: type of oxygenator, type of cardiopulmonary bypass circuit, body temperature, arterial blood gas management, and use of arterial line filters.

Before 1985, cardiopulmonary bypass was achieved with bubble oxygenators that produced particulate or gaseous bubbles, which could have occluded small cerebral vessels. Capillary membrane oxygenators were substituted to avoid this complication, and the frequency of serious intellectual loss occurs less often. Also, hypothermia is maintained as a protective measure, but there is uncertainty about the exact temperature ("mild," 32 to 34°C, versus "moderate," 28 to 32°C) to be used, although normothermia (37°C) is potentially harmful. Solid emboli are held responsible for the cerebral injury. Arterial line filters, however, reduce the number of emboli from the cardiopulmonary bypass system. The fraction of cardiac output going to the brain also determines the fraction of the embolic load reaching the brain.

Maintaining cerebral blood flow by supporting autoregulation would provide sufficient but not excessive flow to support cerebral metabolism. To maintain autoregulation during cardiopulmonary bypass, blood gas values must be kept near normal when measured at 37°C even though the patient may actually be colder. In contrast, correcting the blood gases for the lower temperature would lead to the addition of carbon dioxide to the cardiopulmonary bypass system to normalize the blood gas values at the patient's hypothermic temperature; under those conditions, autoregulation would be lost. If heparin is bonded to the cardiopulmonary bypass circuit there is considerably less activation of platelets, white cells, and endothelial cells, resulting in attenuation of coagulation and the inflammatory response. Consequently, less anticoagulation may be required and blood loss decreases. The incidence of cerebral dysfunction may also decrease.

Despite these precautions, however, some patients note forgetfulness, mental slowing, or difficulty concentrating. Performance on neuropsychologic tests is worst in the first week or so after surgery; months later, most patients have returned to preoperative levels.

Moody et al. (1990) found many focal dilatations or small aneurysms in 90% of patients who died after cardiac surgery on bypass. The dilated areas were empty and were therefore assumed to have been sites of gas bubbles or fat emboli. In living patients, continuous transcranial or carotid Doppler measurements have detected emboli in operations performed with either membrane or bubble oxygenators. With either membrane or bubble oxygenators, emboli also arise when the aortic cannula is inserted and when the aorta is unclamped. Emboli also arise during bypass when the bubble oxygenator is used.

In coronary artery bypass graft (CABG) operations, carotid Doppler studies demonstrated a mean of 62 emboli for each operation. In open-chamber cardiac operations, carotid and transcranial Doppler studies demonstrated even more cerebrally directed emboli. Times of danger included removal of the aortic side clamp, aortic cannulation, onset of cardiopulmonary bypass, and resumption of ventricular contraction. Emboli and cerebral injuries are even more numerous with aortic disease.

Other monitoring systems have not been successful. Quantitative electroencephalogram does not detect impending brain damage, partly because cerebral hypothermia reduces the electroencephalogram amplitude. Infrared detection of cerebral oxygenation is beset by technical problems, including contamination of the signal with extracranial blood.

OTHER COMPLICATIONS OF OPEN-HEART SURGERY

Patients with active infective endocarditis and those having a second cardiac operation are at high risk for stroke or other cerebral complications. Risk factors include impaired left ventricular function, low cardiac output, sepsis, toxemia, and impaired hemostasis. Use of aprotinin for hemostasis may decrease morbidity. Heparin-bonded cardiopulmonary bypass circuits may circumvent this issue. Controversy exists about the advantages of pulsatile or nonpulsatile perfusion during bypass.

INTERVENTIONAL CARDIAC PROCEDURES

Cardiac Catheterization

Strokes or transient ischemic attacks after cardiac catheterization are rare, encountered in 0.1% to 1.0% of procedures. The posterior circulation is affected more than the carotid territory. Cerebral blindness and visual field defects result. About half of those with occipital symptoms have a confusional state or memory problems that are attributed to temporal lobe ischemia. Carotid syndromes of hemiparesis, with or without language disorders, occur in 30% to 40%. About half of the syndromes abate within 48 hours. The episodes are attributed to emboli released by the guidewire or in flushing the catheter in the ascending aorta. Systemic hypotension may be responsible for some.

Showers of cholesterol emboli after catheterization or cardiac surgery can cause peripheral occlusive vascular disease, with gangrene and peripheral neuropathy (*cholesterol emboli syndrome*).

Coronary Angioplasty

Transient ischemic attacks occur in about 0.2% of these procedures, presumably embolic in origin.

Valvuloplasty

Percutaneous balloon valvuloplasty is used to treat stenosis of pulmonary, mitral, and aortic valves. In one series, embolic stroke occurred in 3 of 26 aortic valve procedures and none of 6 mitral procedures.

Coronary Artery Bypass Graft

Stroke is the major complication of CABG, and although the rate has declined, it is still reported in 1% to 5% of operations, affecting 1,000 to 3,000 people annually in the United States. Many of these patients are elderly. More than half of the episodes are transient or mild, but that leaves many with serious disability. The major recognized factors are cardiac arrhythmia during surgery, carotid artery disease, and air embolism from the left ventricle.

Attention has focused on the carotid arteries, assuming that hypotension during surgery in the presence of arterial narrowing induces focal cerebral ischemia. Many strokes, however, occur in people with normal carotids or after, not during, surgery. There seems to be no advantage to defer CABG for prophylactic endarterectomy. In one series, stroke occurred in 1 of 90 patients with 50% to 90% asymptomatic carotid stenosis and 1 of 16 with 90% stenosis. Even symptomatic carotid stenosis does not seem to increase the risk prohibitively, but conclusive data are not available.

A history of stroke increases the likelihood of a second stroke as a complication of CABG. Among 127 CABG patients with a history of stroke, 17 (13.4%) had a new one with surgery; 3.2% were deemed serious. Many were thought to be embolic because of atrial fibrillation. Postoperative cardiac arrhythmia is a common problem even in patients who have not had prior stroke.

Persistent postoperative coma is encountered in 1% of patients. In half the cases, the cause is not apparent. The others are attributed to global ischemia or hypoxia, major hemisphere infarction with herniation, or multiple infarcts.

Cardiac Transplantation

In the early days of heart transplantation, neurologic complications were seen in 54% of the cases, and 20% were fatal. With time, both figures have been much reduced. Because the patients have advanced atherosclerosis, stroke is still a major risk, occurring in up to 9%. Other problems include reversible encephalopathy and seizures. Cerebral hemorrhage is rare, linked to anticoagulation or uncontrolled hypertension. Vascular headache is common.

Encephalopathy occurs in about 10% of cases and is attributed to renal or hepatic failure or sepsis. Later, because of the necessary immunosuppression, opportunistic infection is the most common cause of neurologic disorder; with new antibiotics, the rate has dropped from 15% to 5%. Aspergillus, toxoplasma, and other uncommon organisms are encountered. Cytomegalovirus and herpes zoster may cause problems. Aseptic meningitis may have no detectable cause. The incidence of primary central nervous system lymphoma is increased. Osteoporosis and other complications of steroid therapy are common, and cyclosporine may cause tremor, seizures, and confusional states.

SUGGESTED READINGS

Aldea GS, O'Gara P, Shapira OM, et al. Effect of anticoagulation protocol on outcome in patients undergoing CABG with heparin-bonded cardiopulmonary bypass circuits. *Ann Thorac Surg* 1998;65:425–433.

Barbut D, Lo YW, Hartman GS, et al. Aortic atheroma is related to outcome but not numbers of emboli during coronary bypass. *Ann Thorac Surg* 1997;64:454–459.

Bendixen BH, Younger DS, Hair LS, et al. Cholesterol emboli neuropathy. *Neurology* 1992;42:428–430.

Fessatidis I, Prapas S, Havas A, et al. Prevention of perioperative neurological dysfunction: six year prospective study of cardiac surgery. *J Cardiovasc Surg* 1991;32:570–574.

Furlan AJ, Sila CA, Chimowitz MI, et al. Neurologic complications related to cardiac surgery. *Neurol Clin* 1992;10:145–166.

Grote CL, Shanahan PT, Salmon P, et al. Cognitive outcome after cardiac operations. *J Thorac Cardiovasc Surg* 1992;104:1405–1409.

Heyer EJ. Neurologic assessment and cardiac surgery. *J Cardiothorac Vasc Anesth* 1996;10:99–103.

Hotson JR, Enzman DR. Neurological complications of cardiac transplantation. *Neurol Clin* 1988;6:349–365.

Kirkham FJ. Recognition and prevention of neurological complications in pediatric cardiac surgery. *Pediatr Cardiol* 1998;19:331–345.

Kosmororsky G, Hanson MR, Tomsak RL. Neuro-ophthalmic complications of cardiac catheterization. *Neurology* 1988;38:483–485.

Lane RJM, Roche SW, Leung AAW, et al. Cyclosporine neurotoxicity in cardiac transplant recipients. *J Neurol Neurosurg Psychiatry* 1988;51:1434–1437.

Montero C, Martinez AJ. Neuropathology of heart transplantation. *Neurology* 1986;36:1149–1156.

Moody DM, Bell MA, Challa VA, et al. Brain microemboli during cardiac surgery or aortography. *Ann Neurol* 1990;28:477–486.

Prevost S, Deshotels A. Quality of life after cardiac surgery. *AACN Clin Issues Crit Care Nurs* 1993;4:320–328.

Riggle KP, Oddi MA. Spinal cord necrosis and paraplegia as complications of the intra-aortic balloon. *Crit Care Med* 1989;17:75–76.

Roach GW, Kanchuger M, Mangano CM, et al. Adverse cerebral outcomes after coronary bypass surgery. *N Engl J Med* 1996;335:1857–1863.

Robinson M, Blumenthal JA, Burker EJ, et al. Coronary artery bypass grafting and cognitive function; a review. *J Cardiopulm Rehab* 1990;10:180–189.

Rorick M, Furlan AJ. Risk of cardiac surgery in patients with prior stroke. *Neurology* 1990;40:835–837.

Shapira OM, Aldea GS, Zelingher J, et al. Enhanced blood conservation and improved clinical outcome after valve surgery using heparin-bonded cardiopulmonary bypass circuits. *J Cardiol Surg* 1996;11:307–317.

Shaw PJ, Bates D, Cartilidge NEF, et al. Long-term intellectual dysfunction following coronary artery bypass graft surgery: a six-month follow-up study. *Q J Med* 1987;62:259–268.

Shaw PJ, Bates D, Cartilidge NEF, et al. An analysis of factors predisposing to neurological injury in patients undergoing coronary bypass operations. *Q J Med* 1989;267:633–646.

Sila CA. Spectrum of neurologic events following cardiac transplantation. *Stroke* 1989;20:1586–1589.

Sotaniemi KA, Mononen H, Hokkanen TE. Long-term cerebral outcome after open-heart surgery. Five-year neuropsychological follow-up study. *Stroke* 1986;17:410–416.

Taylor KM. Improved outcome of seriously ill open-heart surgery patients: focus on reoperation and endocarditis. *J Heart Lung Transplant* 1993;12:S14–S18.

Van der Linden J, Casimir-Ahn H. When do cerebral emboli appear during open-heart operations? Transcranial Doppler study. *Ann Thorac Surg* 1991;51:237–241.

Merritt's Neurology, 10th ed., edited by L.P. Rowland. Lippincott Williams & Wilkins, Philadelphia © 2000.

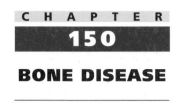

CHAPTER 150

BONE DISEASE

ROGER N. ROSENBERG

OSTEITIS DEFORMANS (PAGET DISEASE)

This chronic disease of the adult skeleton is characterized by bowing and irregular flattening of the bones. Any or all skeletal bones may be affected, but the tibia, skull, and pelvis are the most frequent sites. Except for the skeletal deformities and pain, the disease causes disability only when the skull or spine is involved.

Pathology

In affected bones, there is an imbalance between formation and resorption of bone. In most cases, there is a mixture of excessive bone formation and bone destruction. The areas of bone destruction are filled with hyperplastic vascular connective tissue. New bone formation may occur in the destroyed areas in an irregular disorganized manner. The metabolic disturbance is unknown.

Incidence

There is a postmortem incidence of 3% in patients over 40 years of age. Men and women are equally affected. The common age at onset is in the fourth to sixth decades; it is rare before age 30.

Symptoms and Signs

Two types of neurologic symptoms appear: those due to the abnormalities in bone and those due to arteriosclerosis, a common accompaniment. The cerebral manifestations that occur with arteriosclerosis are identical to those seen in patients with arteriosclerosis in the absence of Paget disease.

The neurologic defects of osteitis deformans are usually related to pressure on the central nervous system or the nerve roots by the overgrowth of bone. Convulsive seizures, generalized or neuralgic head pain, cranial nerve palsies, and paraplegia occur in a few cases. Deafness caused by pressure on the auditory nerves is the most common symptom; unilateral facial palsy is the next most common symptom. Loss of vision in one eye, visual field defects, or exophthalmos may occur when the sphenoid bone is affected. Compression of the spinal cord is more common than compression of the cerebral substance, which is extremely rare except when there is sarcomatous degeneration of the lesions. Platybasia may occur in advanced cases. Paget disease has been described in a patient with basilar impression and Arnold-Chiari type 1 malformation.

Laboratory Data

The serum calcium content is normal, and the serum phosphorus is normal or only slightly increased. Serum alkaline phosphatase activity is increased; the level varies with the extent and activity of the process. It may be only slightly elevated when the disease is localized to one or two bones.

Diagnosis

The diagnosis of Paget disease is made from the patient's appearance and the characteristic radiographic changes. Involvement of the skull in advanced cases is manifested by a generalized enlargement of the calvarium, anteroflexion of the head, and depression of the chin on the chest. When the spine is involved, the patient's stature is shortened; the spine is flexed forward and its mobility is greatly reduced.

Radiographically, the skull shows areas of increased bone density with loss of normal architecture, mingled with areas in which the density of the bone is decreased (Fig. 150.1). The margins of the bones are fuzzy and indistinct. The general appearance is that of an enormous skull with the bones of the vault covered with "cotton wool." In advanced cases, there may be a flattening of the base of the skull on the cervical vertebrae (*platybasia*) with signs of damage to the lower cranial nerves, medulla, or cerebellum. Both computed tomography (CT) and magnetic resonance imaging (MRI) aid diagnosis (Fig. 150.2).

Diagnosis may be difficult if the clinical symptoms are mainly neurologic. In these instances, radiographs of the pelvis and legs or a general survey of the entire skeleton may establish the diagnosis. Rarely, it may be impossible to distinguish monophasic Paget disease of the skull from osteoblastic metastases. Search for a primary neoplasm, particularly in the prostate or biopsy of one of the lesions in the skull may be necessary in those cases.

Course

The course is variable but usually extends over decades. The neurologic lesions seldom lead to serious disability other than deafness, convulsive seizures, or compression of the spinal cord.

Treatment

There is no specific therapy. Calcitonin is given to inhibit the osteolytic process. Salmon calcitonin is given in subcutaneous injections of 50 to 100 units daily. Improvement of osteolytic lesions and reversal of neurologic manifestations have been noted with long-term therapy. About 25% of the patients develop serum antibodies to salmon calcitonin, sometimes in titers high enough to make the person resistant to the hormonal action of calcitonin; under these circumstances, human calcitonin may be effective.

An alternate therapy is disodium editronate in a dosage of 5.0 mg/kg body weight daily for 6 months. The value of either medical therapy can be evaluated by reduction of serum levels of alkaline phosphatase measured at 4-month intervals and annual radiographs of specific lesions.

Decompression of the spinal cord may be indicated for

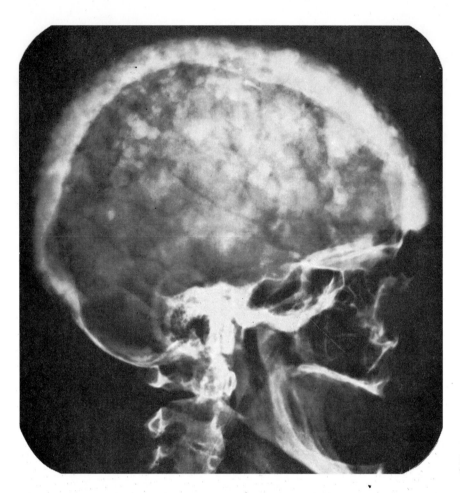

FIG. 150.1. Osteitis deformans (Paget disease) of the skull. (Courtesy of Dr. Juan Taveras.)

myelopathy secondary to stenosis created by the enlarged vertebrae. Similarly, platybasia may lead to decompression of the posterior fossa.

FIBROUS DYSPLASIA

The skull and the bones in other parts of the body are occasionally involved by a process characterized by small areas of bone destruction or massive sclerotic overgrowth. The clinical picture of fibrous dysplasia is related to the site and extent of the bone overgrowth. Sassin and Rosenberg (1968) described involvement of bones of the skull in 50 cases as follows: frontal, 28; sphenoid, 24; frontal and sphenoid, 18; temporal, 8; facial, 15; parietal, 6; and occipital, 8. Diffuse involvement of the entire skull produces leontiasis ossea, with exophthalmos, optic atrophy, and cranial nerve palsies (Fig. 150.3).

In addition to the disfiguration of the skull in the polyostotic form, symptoms of the monostotic form of the disease include headache, convulsions, exophthalmos, optic atrophy, and deafness. Symptoms may begin at any age, but onset usually occurs in early adult life. The family history is negative, and there is no racial or sexual predominance.

A polyostotic form of the disease is characterized by cafe-au-lait spots, endocrine dysfunction with precocious puberty in girls, and involvement of the femur (shepherd's crook deformity). Mutations in the Arg201 codon of the Ys G protein subunit have been described in patients with fibrous dysplasia. These Ys G as mutations may be seen in monostotic or polyostotic patients and in the McCune-Albright syndrome that includes multiple endocrinopathies and cafe-au-lait lesions with fibrous dysplasia.

ACHONDROPLASIA

Achondroplasia (*chondrodystrophy*) is the most frequent form of skeletal dysplasia causing dwarfism. It is characterized by short arms and legs, lumbar lordosis, and enlargement of the head caused by mutations in the fibroblast growth factor receptor 3 gene (FGFR3). The disease is rare and is estimated to occur in 15 of 1 million births in the United States. It is usually inherited as an autosomal dominant trait.

Symptoms of involvement of the nervous system sometimes develop as a result of hydrocephalus, compression of the medulla and cervical cord at the level of the foramen magnum, compression of the spinal cord by ruptured intervertebral disk, and bone compression of the lower thoracic or lumbar cord. Convulsive seizures, ataxia, and paraplegia are the most common symptoms. Mental development is usually normal.

The diagnosis is made from the characteristic body configuration of short arms and legs, normal-size trunk, enlargement of

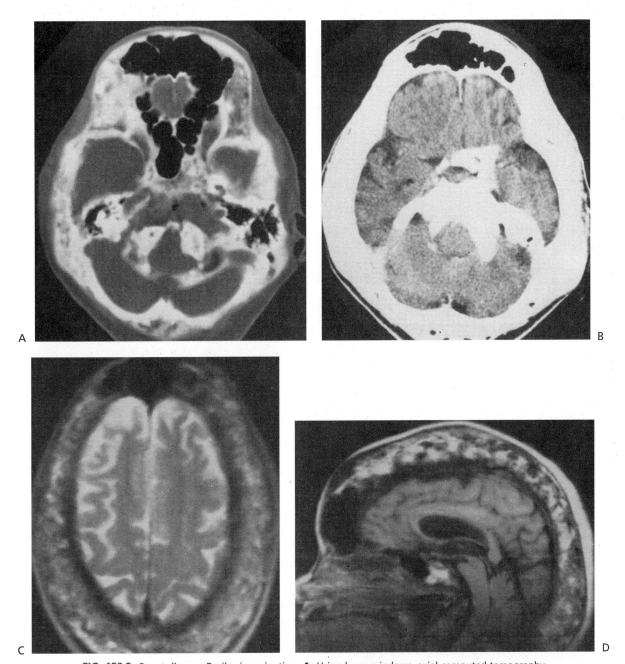

FIG. 150.2. Paget disease. Basilar invagination. **A:** Using bone windows, axial computed tomography shows the foramen magnum projected within the posterior fossa. Intradiploic calcific density with "cotton wool" appearance is typical of Paget disease. **B:** Higher section, using soft tissue windows, demonstrates obliteration of basal cisterns and brainstem compression caused by basilar invagination. **C:** Axial T2-weighted magnetic resonance image shows prominent mottled signal in the diploic space. **D:** Sagittal T1-weighted magnetic resonance image confirms impingement of brainstem by dens. (Courtesy of Drs. J.A. Bello and S.K. Hilal.)

the head, and changes in the radiographs of the skeleton (Fig. 150.4). Many affected infants die in the perinatal period, although a normal lifespan is possible for patients with less severe involvement of the bones.

Shunting procedures may be needed for hydrocephalus caused by involvement of the bones at the base of the skull. Laminectomy is indicated for signs of cord compression.

The mutations described in 1994 in the FGFR3 gene at 4p are usually new mutations and result in autosomal dominant inheritance. The gene product is expressed in cartilage. A frequent FGFR3 mutation is a G1138A codon mutation with GGG to AGG or CGG substitutions, resulting in an exchange of glycine at position 380 in the FGFR3 protein to arginine. As a result of this mutation, a gain of negative function results, producing an inactive fibroblast growth factor receptor and resultant dwarfism.

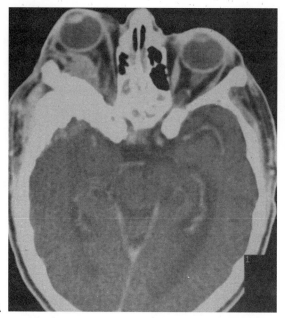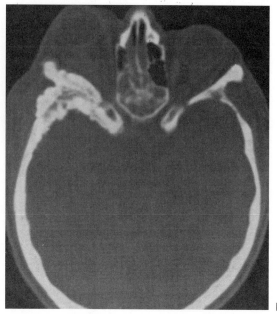

FIG. 150.3. Fibrous dysplasia. Computed tomographies. **A:** Axial contrast-enhanced scan shows proptosis on right with abnormal soft tissue enhancement within orbit and middle cranial fossa. **B:** Bone window depicts pronounced thickening of sphenoid bone. (Courtesy of Dr. T.L. Chi.)

ANKYLOSING SPONDYLITIS

This inflammatory disorder affects ligamentous insertions into bones; at first, it usually affects the sacroiliac joints and lumbar spine. In some patients, the entire spine is involved, with ossification of the ligaments and fusion of the vertebra. The spine becomes rigid and susceptible to a variety of disorders that may affect the spinal cord, including fractures and dislocations, atlantooccipital dislocation, and spinal stenosis. The condition is common, affecting an estimated 1.4% of the general population. It only rarely, however, causes symptoms and signs of myelopathy.

A cauda equina syndrome may appear in patients with long-standing spondylitis. Signs and symptoms are symmetric, with weakness, wasting, and sensory loss in lumbosacral myotomes. Bladder and bowel are commonly affected, and pain may be severe. The mechanism is not clear.

Although concomitant arachnoiditis has been suspected as the cause, the syndrome appears late, when there is little evidence that the underlying spondylitis is active. Moreover, there is little inflammation at postmortem examination, which is likely to show chronic fibrosis. There is erosion of posterior bone elements, and, in earlier days, myelography showed enlargement of the caudal sac and prominent diverticulae of the arachnoid. CT shows similar pathology, but MRI is more illuminating, showing nerve root thickening and sometimes enhancement of dura and nerve roots; that pattern suggests inflammation of the arachnoid structures, supporting the earlier theory. Surgery is generally ineffective and has sometimes been deleterious, although there have been rare reports of some relief. Steroid therapy has been similarly without benefit.

ATLANTOAXIAL DISLOCATION

Subluxation of C-1 on C-2 occurs in many conditions that render the odontoid process of C-2 ineffective as a stabilizing post. This occurs most often as a complication of cervical trauma but also occurs as a congenital malformation (alone or in combination with other anomalies of the cervical spine or cranium) and is seen with disproportionate frequency with Down syndrome, ankylosing spondylitis, and rheumatoid arthritis. It can be demonstrated with plain spine films, CT, or MRI. There is risk of cervical myelopathy or medullary compression, and sudden death has been reported. For symptomatic cases, surgical stabilization is indicated. For asymptomatic cases, there has to be consideration of the risks of surgery against uncertain risks of no

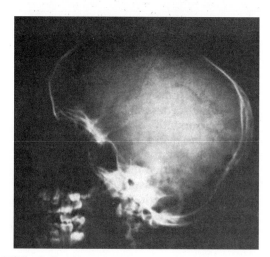

FIG. 150.4. Skull radiograph showing typical malformation of achondroplasia. The clivus is shortened.

surgery. A general recommendation is to consider stabilization or decompression if imaging shows deformation of the neuroaxis, symptomatic or not. A closed reduction and brace immobilization was successfully applied to a patient with traumatic bilateral rotatory dislocation of the atlantoaxial joints.

SUGGESTED READINGS

Osteitis Deformans (Paget Disease)

Boutin RD, et al. Complications in Paget disease at MR imaging. *Radiology* 1998;209:641–651.

Chen J-R, Rhee RSC, Wallach S, et al. Neurologic disturbances in Paget disease of bone: response to calcitonin. *Neurology* 1979;29:448–457.

Davis DP, et al. Coccygeal fracture and Paget's disease presenting as acute cauda equina syndrome. *J Emerg Med* 1999;17:251–254.

Douglas DL, Duckworth T, Kanis JA, et al. Spinal cord dysfunction in Paget's disease of bone. Has medical treatment a vascular basis? *J Bone Joint Surg Br* 1981;63B:495–503.

Douglas DL, Kanis JA, Duckworth T, et al. Paget's disease: improvement of spinal cord dysfunction with diphosphate and calcitonin. *Metab Bone Dis Relat Res* 1981;3:327–335.

Gandolfi A, Brizzi R, Tedesghi F, et al. Fibrosarcoma arising in Paget's disease of the vertebra: review of the literature. *Surg Neurol* 1983;13:72–76.

Ginsberg LE, Elster AD, Moody DM. MRI of Paget disease with temporal bone involvement presenting with sensorineural hearing loss. *J Comput Assist Tomogr* 1992;16:314–316.

Goldhammer V, Braham J, Kosary IZ. Hydrocephalic dementia in Paget's disease of the skull: treatment by ventriculoatrial shunt. *Neurology* 1979;29:513–516.

Hadjipavlou A, Lander P. Paget disease of the spine. *J Bone Joint Surg Am* 1991;73:1376–1381.

Iglesias-Osma C. Paget's disease of bone and basilar impression with an Arnold-Chiari type-1 malformation. *Ann Med Intern* 1997;14:519–522.

Roberts MC, Kressel HY, Fallon MD, et al. Paget disease: MR imaging findings. *Radiology* 1989;173:341–345.

Singer F, Krane S. Paget's disease of bone. In: Avioli L, Krane S, eds. *Metabolic bone disease and clinically related disorders*, 2nd ed. Philadelphia: WB Saunders, 1990.

Wallach S. Treatment of Paget's disease. *Adv Neurol* 1982;27:1–43.

Weisz GM. Lumbar spinal canal stenosis in Paget's disease. *Spine* 1983;8:192–198.

Fibrous Dysplasia

Albright F. Polyostotic fibrous dysplasia: a defense of the entity. *J Clin Endocrinol Metab* 1947;7:307–324.

Candeliere GA, Roughley PJ, Glorieux FH. Polymerase chain reaction-based technique for the selective enrichment and analysis of mosaic Arg201 mutations in G alpha S from patients with fibrous dysplasia of bone. *Bone* 1997;21:201–206.

Casselman JW, DeJong I, Neyt L, et al. MRI in craniofacial fibrous dysplasia. *Neuroradiology* 1993;35:234–237.

Cole DE, Fraser FC, Glorieux FH, et al. Panostotic fibrous dysplasia: a congenital disorder of bone with unusual facial appearance, bone fragility, hyperphosphatasemia, and hypophosphatemia. *Am J Med Genet* 1983;14:725–735.

Finney HL, Roberts JS. Fibrous dysplasia of the skull with progressive cranial nerve involvement. *Surg Neurol* 1976;6:341–343.

Katz BJ, Nerad JA. Ophthalmic manifestations of fibrous dysplasia: a disease of children and adults. *Ophthalmology* 1998;105:2207–2215.

Mohammadi-Araghi H, Haery C. Fibro-osseous lesions of craniofacial bones. The role of imaging. *Radiol Clin North Am* 1993;31:121–134.

Saper JR. Disorders of bone and the nervous system: the dysplasias and premature closure syndromes. In: Vinken PJ, Bruyn GW, eds. *Handbook of clinical neurology.* New York: Elsevier-North Holland, 1979.

Sassin JF, Rosenberg RN. Neurologic complications of fibrous dysplasia of the skull. *Arch Neurol* 1968;18:363–376.

Tehranzadeh J, et al. Computed tomography of Paget disease of the skull versus fibrous dysplasia. *Skeletal Radiol* 1998;27:664–672.

Achondroplasia

Aryanpur J, Hurko O, Francomano C, et al. Craniocervical decompression for cervicomedullary compression in pediatric patients with achondroplasia. *J Neurosurg* 1990;73:375–382.

Dandy WF. Hydrocephalus in chondrodystrophy. *Bull Johns Hopkins Hosp* 1921;32:5–10.

Denis JP, Rosenberg HS, Ellsworth CA Jr. Megalocephaly, hydrocephalus and other neurological aspects of achondroplasia. *Brain* 1961;84:427–445.

Duvoisin RC, Yahr MD. Compressive spinal cord and root systems in achondroplastic dwarfs. *Neurology* 1962;12:202–207.

Hamamci N, Hawran S, Biering-Sorensen F. Achondroplasia and spinal cord lesion. Three case reports. *Paraplegia* 1993;31:375–379.

Hecht JT, Butler IJ. Neurologic morbidity associated with achondroplasia. *J Child Neurol* 1990;5:84–97.

Horton WA. Fibroblast growth factor receptor 3 and the human chondrodysplasias. *Curr Opin Pediatr* 1997;9:437–442.

Kahandovitz N, Rimoin DL, Sillence DO. The clinical spectrum of lumbar spine disease in achondroplasia. *Spine* 1982;7:137–140.

McKusick VA. 1997 Albert Lasker Award for Special Achievement in Medical Science. Observations over 50 years concerning intestinal polyposis, Marfan syndrome, and achondroplasia. *Nat Med* 1997;3:1065–1068.

Shiang R, Thompson LH, Zhu Y-Z, et al. Mutations in the transmembrane domain of FGFR3 cause the most common genetic form of dwarfism, achondroplasia. *Cell* 1994;78:335–342.

Thomas IT, Frias JL. The prospective management of cervicomedullary compression in achondroplasia. *Birth Defects* 1989;25:83–90.

Thompson NM, et al. Neuroanatomic and neuropsychological outcome in school-age children with achondroplasia. *Am J Med Genet* 1999;88:145–153.

Wynne-Davies R, Walsh WK, Gormley J. Achondroplasia and hypochondroplasia. Clinical variation and spinal stenosis. *J Bone Joint Surg Br* 1981;63B:508–515.

Ankylosing Spondylitis

Bruining K, Weiss K, Zelfer B, et al. Arachnoiditis in the cauda equina syndrome of longstanding ankylosing spondylitis. *J Neuroimag* 1993;3:55–57.

Fox MW, Onofrio BM, Kilgore JE. Neurological complications of ankylosing spondylitis. *J Neurosurg* 1993;78:871–878.

Mitchell MJ, Sartoris DJ, Moody D, et al. Cauda equina syndrome complicating ankylosing spondylitis. *Radiology* 1990;175:521–525.

Rowed DW. Management of cervical spinal cord injury in ankylosing spondylitis: intervertebral disc as a cause of cord compression. *J Neurosurg* 1992;77:241–246.

Rubenstein DJ, Alvarez O, Ghelman B, et al. Cauda equina syndrome complicating ankylosing spondylitis. *J Comput Assist Tomogr* 1989;13:511–513.

Shaw PJ, Allcutt DA, Bates D, et al. Cauda equina syndrome with multiple lumbar arachnoid cysts in ankylosing spondylitis: improvement following surgical therapy. *J Neurol Neurosurg Psychiatry* 1990;53:1076–1079.

Sparling M, Bartelson JD, McLeod RA, et al. MRI of arachnoid diverticula associated with cauda equina syndrome in ankylosing spondylitis. *J Rheumatol* 1989;16:1335–1337.

Tullous MW, Skerhut HEI, Story JL, et al. Cauda equina syndrome of long-lasting ankylosing spondylitis. *J Neurosurg* 1990;73:441–447.

Atlantoaxial Dislocation

Crockard HA, Heiman AE, Stevens JM. Progressive myelopathy secondary to odontoid fractures: clinical, radiological, and surgical features. *J Neurosurg* 1993;78:579–586.

Elliott S, Morton RE, Whitelaw RA. Atlantoaxial instability and abnormalities of the odontoid in Down's syndrome. *Arch Dis Child* 1988; 63:1484–1489.

Floyd AS, Learmouth ID, Mody G, et al. Atlantoaxial instability and neurologic indicators in rheumatoid arthritis. *Clin Orthop* 1989;241:177–182.

Martich V, Ben Ami T, Yousefzadeh DK, et al. Hypoplastic posterior arch of C1 in children with Down syndrome: a double jeopardy. *Radiology* 1992;183:125–128.

Rowland LP, Shapiro JH, Jacobson HG. Neurological syndromes associated with congenital absence of the odontoid process. *Arch Neurol Psychiatry* 1958;80:286–291.

Sorin S, Askari I, Moskowitz RW. Atlantoaxial subluxation as a complication of early ankylosing spondylitis. *Arthritis Rheum* 1979;22:273–276.

Stevens JM, Chong WK, Barber C, et al. A new appraisal of abnormalities of the odontoid process associated with atlantoaxial subluxation and neurological disability. *Brain* 1994;117:133–148.

Wise JJ, Cheney R, Fischgrund J. Traumatic bilateral rotatory dislocation of the atlanto-axial joints: a case report and review of the literature. *J Spinal Disord* 1997;10:451–453.

Yamashita Y, Takahashi M, Sakamoto Y, et al. Atlantoaxial subluxation. Radiography and MRI correlated to myelopathy. *Acta Radiol* 1989;10:135–140.

Merritt's Neurology, 10th ed., edited by L.P. Rowland. Lippincott Williams & Wilkins, Philadelphia © 2000.

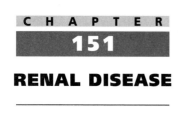

CHAPTER 151

RENAL DISEASE

NEIL H. RASKIN

Uremia is a term used to describe a constellation of signs and symptoms in patients with severe azotemia caused by acute or chronic renal failure; symptomatic renal failure is an acceptable definition. The clinical features of the neurologic consequences of renal failure do not correlate well with any single biochemical abnormality but seem to be related to the rate of development of renal failure. This chapter summarizes the features of uremic encephalopathy and neuropathy and the distinctive neurologic complications of dialysis and renal transplantation.

UREMIC ENCEPHALOPATHY

In uremia, as in other metabolic encephalopathies, there is a continuum of signs of neurologic dysfunction, including dysarthria, instability of gait, asterixis, action tremor, multifocal myoclonus, and sensorial clouding. One or more of these signs may predominate, but fluctuation of clinical signs from day to day is characteristic. The earliest most reliable indication of uremic encephalopathy is sensorial clouding. Patients appear fatigued, preoccupied, and apathetic; they have difficulty concentrating. Obtundation becomes more apparent as perceptual errors, defective memory, and mild confusion become evident. Illusions and perceptions sometimes progress to frank visual hallucinations.

Asterixis is almost always present once sensorial clouding appears: It is most effectively elicited by having the patient hold the arms outstretched in fixed hyperextension at the elbow and wrist, with the fingers spread apart. After a latency of up to 30 seconds, flexion-extension ("flapping") of the fingers at the metacarpophalangeal joints and at the wrist appears arrhythmically and at irregular intervals.

Multifocal myoclonus refers to visible twitching of muscles that is sudden, arrhythmic, and asymmetric, involving muscles first in one locus and then in another and affecting chiefly the face and proximal limbs. It is a strong indication of a severe metabolic disturbance and usually does not appear until stupor or coma has supervened. In uremia, asterixis and myoclonus may be so intense that muscles appear to fasciculate, giving rise to the term *uremic twitching.* This form of myoclonus probably signifies cortical irritability; it is, at times, difficult to distinguish from a multifocal seizure. *Tetany* is commonly associated with myoclonus and other signs of encephalopathy. It may be overt, with spontaneous carpopedal spasms, or latent, manifested by a Trousseau sign. The spasms originate in abnormal peripheral nerve discharges. In uremic patients, tetany does not usually respond to injections of calcium and occurs despite metabolic acidosis (which inhibits hypocalcemic tetany).

The *restless-legs syndrome* occurs in 40% of uremic patients and probably is an encephalopathic symptom. This syndrome comprises creeping, crawling, prickling, and pruritic sensations deep within the legs. These sensations are almost always worse in the evening; they are relieved by movement of the limbs. Clonazepam, levodopa, dopamine agonists, opioids, and some anticonvulsants are effective in terminating this syndrome.

Alterations in limb tone appear as encephalopathy progresses and brainstem function is compromised. Muscle tone is usually heightened and is sometimes asymmetric. Eventually, decorticate posturing may appear in preference to decerebrate attitudes. Focal motor signs are present in about 20% of patients; these signs often clear after hemodialysis.

Convulsions are usually a late manifestation of uremic encephalopathy. In the older literature, convulsions were thought to occur far more often than is now reported; this may have been the result of failing to distinguish hypertensive encephalopathy from uremia, which may coexist. Hypertensive retinopathy and papilledema are major signs that distinguish the two conditions; further, focal signs such as aphasia or cortical blindness are much more common in hypertensive brain disease than in uremia. The treatment of recurring uremic convulsions is not straightforward because the pharmacokinetics of phenytoin are altered in uremic patients. In uremia, plasma protein binding of phenytoin is decreased so much that the unbound fraction of the drug is two to three times more than that found in normal plasma. In uremic patients, however, the volume of distribution of the drug is larger, and there is an increased rate of conversion of phenytoin to hydroxylated derivatives, resulting in lower total serum concentrations of the drug for any given dose. This combination of factors allows the physician to administer the usual dosage of phenytoin (300 to 400 mg daily) to a uremic patient and attain therapeutic unbound levels of the drug despite lower total serum levels (i.e., 5 to 10 mg/L rather than 10 to 20 mg/L).

Meningeal signs occur in about 35% of uremic patients; half of those affected have cerebrospinal fluid (CSF) pleocytosis. CSF protein elevations greater than 60 mg/dL occur in 60% of uremic patients; in 20%, the CSF protein exceeds 100 mg/dL. CSF protein content may return to normal in the immediate posthemodialysis period. The increase in CSF protein is caused by an alteration in the permeability properties of the brain's capillary endothelial cells adjacent to the CSF, which have tight intercellular junctions.

There are no specific pathologic alterations of brain in uremic encephalopathy; cerebral use of oxygen is depressed, as it is in other metabolic encephalopathies, because of a primary interference with synaptic transmission. Depressed cerebral metabolic rate and clinical state usually change together but are probably independent reflections of generally impaired neuronal functions. The profundity of uremic encephalopathy correlates only in a general way, and sometimes poorly, with biochemical abnormalities in the blood. Cerebral acidosis has been suggested as a possible mechanism, but CSF pH is usually normal. Brain calcium is increased by 50% and seems to be due to excess circulating parathyroid hormone, which is nondialyzable. It is not clear whether calcium changes are related to the cerebral dysfunction.

The rapid clearing of uremic encephalopathy after dialysis suggests that small to moderately sized water-soluble molecules are responsible for the encephalopathy. Excessive accumulation of toxic organic acids overwhelms the normal mechanisms for excluding such compounds from the brain and may be important. These organic acids may block transport systems of the choroid plexus and of glia that normally remove metabolites of some neurotransmitters in brain. Furthermore, there is a nonspecific increase in cerebral membrane permeability in uremia, and this may permit greater entry into brain of uremic toxins such as the organic acids, which further derange cerebral function.

Erythropoietin is often given to patients on long-term dialysis to correct the anemia. In the process, cognitive functions may improve.

UREMIC NEUROPATHY

Peripheral neuropathy is the most common neurologic consequence of chronic renal failure. It is a distal, symmetric, mixed sensorimotor neuropathy affecting the legs more than the arms. It is clinically indistinguishable from the neuropathies of chronic alcohol abuse or diabetes mellitus. The rate of progression, severity, prominence of motor or sensory signs, and prevalence of dysesthesia vary. It is several times more common in men than in women. The symptom of burning feet was considered a common feature of uremic neuropathy but probably resulted from removal of water-soluble thiamine by hemodialysis, and with near universal B vitamin replacement, this syndrome is now rare.

The rate of progression of uremic neuropathy varies widely; in general, it evolves over several months but may be fulminant. Among most patients who enter chronic hemodialysis programs, the neuropathy stabilizes or improves slowly. Patients with mild

neuropathy often recover completely, but those who begin dialysis with severe neuropathy rarely recover even after several years. Lack of improvement or progression of symptoms while on hemodialysis may suggest an alternative diagnosis, such as chronic inflammatory demyelinating polyneuropathy. Patients in chronic renal failure are also more susceptible to drugs that are normally excreted in the urine; for this reason, there may be prolonged paralysis after administration of neuromuscular blocking agents as an aid to endotracheal intubation, and the prolonged paralysis may be mistaken for peripheral neuropathy. An *accelerated neuropathy of renal failure* may progress so rapidly that it is mistaken for the Guillain-Barré syndrome.

Successful renal transplantation has a clear, predictable, and beneficial effect on uremic neuropathy. Motor nerve conduction velocities increase within days of transplantation. There is progressive improvement for 6 to 12 months, often with complete recovery, even in patients with severe neuropathy before transplantation.

Pathologically, this neuropathy is usually a primary axonal degeneration with secondary segmental demyelination, probably as a result of a metabolic failure of the perikaryon; there is also a predominantly demyelinative type. Because uremic neuropathy improves with hemodialysis, it seems evident that the neuropathy results from the accumulation of dialyzable metabolite. These substances may be in the "middle molecule" (300 to 2,000 Da) range; compounds of this size cross dialysis membranes more slowly than smaller molecules such as creatinine and urea, which are the usual measures of chemical control of uremia. Supporting this contention are observations that control of neuropathy in some patients depends on increased hours of dialysis each week (beyond that necessary for chemical control of uremia) and that peritoneal dialysis seems to be associated with a lower incidence of neuropathy. The peritoneal membrane seems to permit passage of some molecules more readily and selectively than the cellophane membrane used in hemodialysis. The transplanted kidney deals effectively with substances of different molecular size; the resulting elimination of middle molecules could explain the invariable improvement of the neuropathy after transplantation.

There is a parathormone-induced increase in calcium in peripheral nerves in experimental uremia, which causes slowed nerve conduction velocity; these changes can be prevented by prior parathyroidectomy. In human uremic patients, circulating parathormone levels correlate inversely with nerve conduction velocities. It seems unlikely, however, that parathormone is involved in uremic neuropathy because the hormone is nondialyzable, and hyperparathyroidism itself is not usually associated with neuropathy.

DIALYSIS DYSEQUILIBRIUM SYNDROME

Headache, nausea, and muscle cramps attend hemodialysis in more than 50% of patients; in somewhat over 5%, obtundation, convulsions, or delirium may occur. The cerebral sequelae are usually seen with rapid dialysis at the outset of a dialysis program; symptoms usually appear toward the third or fourth hour of a dialysis run but occasionally appear 8 to 24 hours later. The syndrome is usually self-limited, subsiding in hours, but delirium may persist for several days. Some patients become exophthalmic because of increased intraocular pressure at the height of the syndrome. Other clinical correlates include increased intracranial pressure, papilledema, and generalized electroencephalographic slowing.

Shift of water into brain is probably the proximate cause of dysequilibrium. Rapid reduction of blood solute content cannot be paralleled by brain solutes because of the blood–brain barrier. An osmotic gradient is produced between blood and brain causing movement of water into brain, which results in encephalopathy, cerebral edema, and increased intracranial pressure. The osmotically active substances retained in brain have not yet been identified.

DIALYSIS DEMENTIA

A distinctive, progressive, usually fatal encephalopathy may occur in patients who are chronically dialyzed for periods that exceed 3 years. The first symptom is usually a stammering, hesitancy of speech, and, at times, speech arrest. The speech disorder is intensified during and immediately after dialysis and at first may be seen only during these periods. A thought disturbance is usually evident, and there is a consistent electroencephalogram abnormality, with bursts of high-voltage slowing in the frontal leads. As the disorder progresses, speech becomes more dysarthric and aphasic; dementia and myoclonic jerks usually become apparent (Table 151.1) at this time. The other elements of the encephalopathy include delusional thinking, convulsions, asterixis, and occasionally focal neurologic abnormalities. Early in the course, diazepam is effective in lessening myoclonus and seizures and in improving speech; it becomes less effective later. The CSF is unremarkable. Increased dialysis time and renal transplantation do not seem to alter the course of the disease. No distinctive abnormalities have been found in brain at autopsy.

The geographic variation in the incidence of dialysis dementia suggests a neurotoxin. Aluminum content is consistently elevated in the cerebral gray matter of patients who die from this condition. Municipal water supplies heavily contaminated with aluminum have been linked to the syndrome in epidemiologic studies. Another possible source is absorption of aluminum from orally administered phosphate-binding agents that are given to uremic patients. Plasma protein binding of aluminum retards the removal of aluminum during dialysis even when an aluminum-free dialysate is used. Nevertheless, there have been several reports of remission of dialysis dementia when deferoxamine was used to remove aluminum from the diet, from the dialysate, or from the patient. Cerebral aluminum intoxication, still an unconfirmed hypothesis, seems to be the most likely possibility at this time. Brain GABA levels are reduced in numerous regions, but the meaning of this finding is not clear.

PSEUDOTUMOR CEREBRI

Patients in chronic renal failure may be at increased risk for benign intracranial hypertension. There has been no formal epidemiologic study, but several cases have been reported. In the experience of Guy et al. (1990), patients in renal failure seem more likely to lose vision, but fenestration of the optic nerve sheath was effective in improving vision in several of them.

NEUROLOGIC COMPLICATIONS OF RENAL TRANSPLANTATION

A curious vulnerability to certain brain tumors and unusual infections of the nervous system occur in patients who have undergone transplantation; however, cerebral infarction is the most common neurologic complication.

The risk that a lymphoma will develop after a transplant is about 35 times greater than normal; this increased risk depends almost entirely on the increased incidence of primary central nervous system lymphoma. Brain tumors appear between 5 and 46 months after transplantation. The resulting clinical syndromes include increased intracranial pressure, rapidly evolving focal neurologic signs, or combinations of these. Convulsions are rare. A remarkable characteristic of primary lymphomas is the response to radiotherapy; survivals of 3 to 5 years are not unusual.

Systemic fungal infections are found at autopsy in about 45% of patients who have been treated with renal transplantation and immunosuppression; brain abscess formation occurs in about 35% of these patients. In almost all cases, the primary source of infection is in the lung. Chest radiographs and the presence of fever aid in differentiating fungal brain abscess from brain tumor in recipients of transplants. *Aspergillus* has a unique predilection for dissemination to brain and accounts for most fungal brain abscesses; candida, nocardia, and histoplasma are found in the others. The clinical syndrome resulting from these infections is usually delirium accompanied by seizures. Headache, stiff neck, and focal signs also occur but not commonly. The CSF is often remarkably bland, and brain biopsy may be the only reliable way to establish a diagnosis. The distinction of fungal brain abscess from possibly radiosensitive brain tumor makes it important to consider this procedure.

TABLE 151.1. CLINICAL FEATURES OF DIALYSIS DEMENTIA

Feature	Totals in 42 patients
Age at onset, yr	21–68 (average, 45)
Months on hemodialysis at onset	9–84 (average, 37)
Duration of illness until death, mo	1–15 (average, 6)
Sex	21 M, 21 F
Dementia, %	98
Speech impairment, %	95
Myoclonus, %	81
Seizures, %	57
Behavioral abnormalities, %	52
Gait disorder, %	17
Tremor, %	7

Modified from Lederman RJ and Henry CF (1978).

SUGGESTED READINGS

Adams HP, Dawson G, Coffman TJ, Corry RI. Stroke in renal transplant recipients. *Arch Neurol* 1986;43:113–115.

Altmann P, Al-Salihi F, Butter K, et al. Serum aluminum levels and erythrocyte dihydropteridine reductase activity in patients on hemodialysis. *N Engl J Med* 1987;317:80–84.

Babb AL, Ahmad S, Bergstrom J, Scribner BH. The middle molecule hypothesis in perspective. *Am J Kidney Dis* 1981;1:46–50.

Bolton CF, Young GB. *Neurological complications of renal disease.* London: Butterworths, 1990.

Bucher SF, Seelos KC, Oertel WH, et al. Cerebral generators involved in the pathogenesis of the restless legs syndrome. *Ann Neurol* 1997;41:639–645.

Guy J, Johnston PK, Corbett JJ, et al. Treatment of visual loss in pseudotumor cerebri with uremia. *Neurology* 1990;40:28–32.

Hamed LM, Winward KE, Glaser JS, et al. Optic neuropathy in uremia. *Am J Ophthalmol* 1989;108:30–35.

Healton EB, Brust JCM, Feinfeld DA, Thomson GE. Hypertensive encephalopathy and the neurologic manifestations of malignant hypertension. *Neurology* 1982;32:127–132.

Lederman RJ, Henry CF. Progressive dialysis encephalopathy. *Ann Neurol* 1978;4:199–204.

Mattana J, Effiong C, Gooneratne R, Singhal PC. Outcome of stroke in patients undergoing hemodialysis. *Arch Intern Med* 1998;158:537–541.

McCarthy JT, Milliner DS, Johnson WJ. Clinical experience with desferrioxamine in dialysis patients with aluminum toxicity. *Q J Med* 1990;74:257–276.

Nissenson AR, Nimer SD, Wolcott DL. Recombinant human erythropoietin and renal anemia: molecular biology, clinical efficacy, and nervous system effects. *Ann Intern Med* 1991;114:402–416.

Pastan S, Bailey J. Dialysis therapy. *N Engl J Med* 1998;338:1428–1437.

Patchell RA. Neurological complications of organ transplantation. *Ann Neurol* 1994;36:688–703.

Raskin NH, Fishman RA. Neurologic disorders in renal failure. *N Engl J Med* 1976;294:143–148, 204–210.

Ropper AH. Accelerated neuropathy of renal failure. *Arch Neurol* 1993;50:536–539.

Russo LS, Beale G, Sandroni S, et al. Aluminum intoxication in undialyzed adults with chronic renal failure. *J Neurol Neurosurg Psychiatry* 1992;55:697–700.

Said G, Boudier L, Selva J, et al. Patterns of uremic polyneuropathy. *Neurology* 1983;33:567–574.

Sidhom OA, Odeh YK, Krumlovsky FA, et al. Low-dose prazosin in patients with muscle cramps during hemodialysis. *Clin Pharm Ther* 1994;56:445–451.

Wills MR, Savory J. Aluminum and chronic renal failure; sources, absorption, transport, and toxicity. *Crit Rev Clin Lab Sci* 1989;27:59–107.

Merritt's Neurology, 10th ed., edited by L.P. Rowland. Lippincott Williams & Wilkins, Philadelphia © 2000.

C H A P T E R
152

RESPIRATORY CARE: DIAGNOSIS AND MANAGEMENT

STEPHAN A. MAYER
MATTHEW E. FINK

Many different problems are encountered in a neurologic intensive care unit (ICU); all patients share a common need for meticulous nursing care and cardiorespiratory monitoring to prevent a life-threatening complication. Diagnosis is rarely a problem; the major concern in the ICU is treatment of neurologic disease and the medical complications that determine survival and recovery. Neurologic patients who require ICU treatment frequently have a depressed level of consciousness, impaired airway protection due to depressed cough and gag reflexes, immobilization and paralysis, or oropharyngeal and respiratory muscle weakness, all of which predispose to pulmonary complications and respiratory failure. In fact, respiratory monitoring and support is the most common reason for admission of neurologic patients to the ICU.

RESPIRATORY PHYSIOLOGY

Respiratory failure occurs when gas exchange is impaired. The diagnosis of respiratory failure depends on arterial blood gas analysis. PaO_2 less than 60 mm Hg or $PaCO_2$ greater than 50 mm Hg unequivocally defines respiratory failure. There are warning signs, however, of deteriorating ventilatory function before respiratory failure is overt. Patients with neurologic disease often do not complain of dyspnea. The premonitory signs of mild respiratory failure include restlessness, insomnia, confusion, tachycardia, tachypnea, diaphoresis, asterixis, and headache. When muscle weakness is the problem, use of accessory muscles, dysynchronous breathing, and paradoxical respirations (inward movement of the abdomen with inspiration) may be observed. Advanced respiratory failure leads to cyanosis, hypotension, and coma. It is impossible to predict PaO_2 and $PaCO_2$ from clinical signs; measurement of arterial blood gases is essential. Normal PaO_2 is a function of age. A healthy 20 year old has a PaO_2 of 90 to 95 mm Hg. With each decade, PaO_2 decreases by 3 mm Hg. Normal $PaCO_2$ is 37 to 43 mm Hg and is not affected by age.

Hypoxemia is caused by five conditions: a low inspired oxygen concentration, alveolar hypoventilation, ventilation-perfusion mismatch, intracardiac right-to-left shunting, and impaired diffusion. Accurate interpretation of PaO_2 requires calculation of the alveolar-arterial (A-a) oxygen tension difference, or "A-a gradient." Alveolar oxygen tension (PAO_2) can be calculated from the equation $PAO_2 = (FiO_2 - 713) - (PaCO_2/0.8)$, where FiO_2 is the inspired fraction of oxygen (0.21 in room air) and $PaCO_2$ is the arterial carbon dioxide tension.

An A-a gradient exceeding 20 mm Hg usually results from *ventilation-perfusion mismatching*, which in turn comes in two forms. "Dead space ventilation" occurs when ventilated lung segments do not come in contact with pulmonary capillary blood flow; this occurs when the alveolar-capillary interface is destroyed (e.g., emphysema) or when blood flow is reduced (e.g., pulmonary embolism). "Intrapulmonary shunting" occurs when perfused lung segments do not come in contact with ventilated alveoli; this occurs when small airways are occluded (e.g., asthma, chronic bronchitis), when alveoli are filled with fluid (e.g., pulmonary edema, pneumonia), or when alveoli collapse (atelectasis). In most conditions, these two processes occur in combination. Hypoxemia with an A-a gradient less than 20 mm

TABLE 152.1. PULMONARY FUNCTION TESTS IN NEUROMUSCULAR RESPIRATORY FAILURE

	Normal	Criteria for intubation and weaning	Criteria for extubation
Vital capacity	40–70 mL/kg	15 mL/kg	25 mL/kg
Negative inspiratory pressure	>80 cm H_2O	20 cm H_2O	40 cm H_2O
Positive expiratory pressure	>140 cm H_2O	40 cm H_2O	50 cm H_2O

Adapted from Mayer (1997).

Hg strongly suggests an extrapulmonary cause of hypoxemia (hypoventilation or a low inspired oxygen concentration).

Hypercapnia is caused by three conditions: increased CO_2 production or inhalation, alveolar hypoventilation, and ventilation-perfusion mismatching with dead space ventilation. Hypoventilation is identified by high $PaCO_2$ with a normal A-a gradient. Acute hypercapnia leads to acidosis and cerebral vasodilation, which in turn can cause depressed level of consciousness ("CO_2 narcosis"), aggravation of elevated intracranial pressure, and blunted respiratory drive leading to further hypoventilation.

Pulmonary function testing is the simplest and most reliable way to evaluate respiratory function in patients with neuromuscular respiratory failure (Table 152.1). Arterial blood gases are also important to monitor, but abnormalities (hypoxia and hypercarbia) usually develop late in the cycle of respiratory decompensation and thus are not sensitive for detecting early ventilatory failure. Vital capacity, the volume of exhaled air after maximal inspiration, normally ranges from 40 to 70 mL/kg. Reduction of vital capacity to 30 mL/kg is associated with a weak cough, accumulation of oropharyngeal secretions, atelectasis, and hypoxemia. A vital capacity of 15 mL/kg (1 L in a 70-kg person) is generally considered the level at which intubation is required (Table 152.2). Negative inspiratory pressure, normally more than 80 cm H_2O, measures the strength of the diaphragm and other muscles of inspiration and generally reflects the ability to maintain normal lung expansion and avoid atelectasis. Positive expiratory force, normally more than 140 cm H_2O, measures the strength of the muscles of expiration and correlates with strength of cough and the ability to clear secretions from the airway.

The pathophysiology of neuromuscular respiratory failure resembles a vicious cycle. Mild hypoxemia usually precedes hypercapnia because atelectasis (and mild intrapulmonary shunting) is an early development. As weakness progresses, inability to maintain normal lung expansion results in reduced lung compliance and an increase in the work of breathing, which is often further aggravated by a weak cough and inability to clear secretions from the airway. As vital capacity approaches 15 mL/kg, rapid shallow breathing and hypercapnia develop. At this stage, the situation can rapidly and unexpectedly deteriorate once muscle fatigue develops and the patient can no longer compensate with increased respiratory effort.

NEUROLOGIC DISEASES WITH PRIMARY RESPIRATORY DYSFUNCTION

Brainstem Disease

Reticular formation neurons, sensitive to hypoxemia and hypercarbia, are located in the brainstem and may be affected by ischemia, hemorrhage, inflammation, or neoplasms. The medullary center is responsible for initiation and maintenance of spontaneous respirations, whereas the pontine pneumotaxic center helps to coordinate cyclic respirations. Forebrain damage, often from metabolic causes, can lead to Cheyne-Stokes respirations (regular, cyclic crescendo-decrescendo respiratory pattern with intervening apnea), as respiratory drive becomes dependent on changes in PCO_2. Hypothalamic or midbrain damage, particularly in the setting of brainstem herniation, may cause central neurogenic hyperventilation (low PCO_2 with normal A-a gradient). Lower pontine tegmental damage may lead to apneustic (inspiratory breath holding) or cluster breathing (irregular bursts of rapid breathing alternating with apneic periods). Medullary damage may cause ataxic breathing (irregular pattern with hypoxemia and hypercarbia), gasping, or apnea.

Documentation of total apnea in the face of a hypercarbic stimulus is an essential component in the diagnosis of brain death. Formal apnea testing requires preoxygenating the patient with 100% oxygen and normalizing the PCO_2 to 40 mm Hg, turning off the ventilator, and allowing the PCO_2 to rise above 55 mm Hg (the PCO_2 will rise 3 to 6 mm Hg/min). Arterial blood gases are checked at both the beginning and end of the test to confirm the eventual extent of hypercarbia. The physician must stand at the bedside during the apnea test to observe the chest wall and diaphragm to confirm the absence of respiratory muscle movement.

In addition to abnormalities in respiratory rate and pattern and synchronization of diaphragm and intercostal muscles, brainstem damage often alters consciousness and causes paralysis of pharyngeal and laryngeal musculature, predisposing to aspiration pneumonitis. Patients with severe brainstem dysfunction should have nasotracheal or orotracheal intubation, electively, to prevent respiratory complications.

TABLE 152.2. CRITERIA FOR INTUBATION AND MECHANICAL VENTILATION

Respiratory rate > 35/min
Vital capacity < 15 mL/kg
Peak inspiratory pressure < 25 cm H_2O
PaO_2 < 70 mm Hg with maximum oxygen by face mask
$PaCO_2$ > 50 mm Hg associated with acidosis (pH < 7.35)
Severe oropharyngeal paresis with inability to protect the airway

These physiologic criteria are intended to serve only as guidelines; treatment decisions must be individualized. As a general rule, intubation in neurologic patients with impending respiratory failure should be performed *before* significant blood gas abnormalities develop.

Brainstem respiratory centers may be depressed (lose responsiveness to CO_2 or O_2) by narcotics or barbiturates, metabolic abnormalities such as hypothyroidism, and by starvation or metabolic alkalosis. Idiopathic primary alveolar hypoventilation and "central sleep apnea syndrome" are due to brainstem malfunction. These disorders are easily distinguished from structural brainstem pathology by the lack of associated neurologic signs.

Spinal Cord Disease

The respiratory system is affected depending on the segmental level and severity of the spinal injury. In spinal cord trauma, the most common cause of death is acute respiratory failure due to apnea, aspiration pneumonia, or pulmonary embolism. The long-term care of a quadraplegic patient heavily depends on the degree of respiratory impairment.

A lesion at C-3 abolishes both diaphragmatic and intercostal muscle activity, leaving only accessory muscle function. The result is severe hypercapnic respiratory failure. Acute spinal cord lesions at the C-5 to C-6 level produce an immediate fall in vital capacity to 30% of normal. Several months after injury, however, the vital capacity will increase to 50% to 60% of normal. High thoracic lesions will compromise intercostal and abdominal muscles, causing a limitation of inspiratory capacity and active expiration. Midthoracic lesions have little impact on respiratory muscle function because only the abdominal muscles are affected.

Most spinal cord diseases cause respiratory impairment by interrupting the suprasegmental impulses that drive the diaphragm and intercostal muscles. There are two notable exceptions, however, strychnine poisoning and tetanus. Both of these toxins block the inhibitory interneurons within the spinal cord, causing simultaneous increases in the activity of muscles that are normally antagonists. Apnea and respiratory failure can result from intense muscle spasms of the upper airway muscles, diaphragm, and intercostal muscles. In rare cases, severe generalized dystonia can lead to a similar picture.

Motor Neuron Diseases

Amyotrophic lateral sclerosis is the main form of motor neuron disease that causes respiratory failure (see Chapter 117). Respiratory failure usually develops late in course of amyotrophic lateral sclerosis, as the respiratory muscles and strength of cough progressively weaken. If symptoms begin with limb weakness, the disorder may progress to respiratory failure in 2 to 5 years. If oropharyngeal symptoms appear first, respiratory complications may be caused by recurrent aspiration pneumonitis. Frequent pulmonary function testing can identify patients at risk for respiratory complications. The earliest changes are decreases in maximum inspiratory and expiratory muscle pressures, followed by reduced vital capacity. When vital capacity falls below 30 mL/kg, the ability to cough and maintain lung expansion is impaired, increasing the risk of aspiration pneumonia. Blood gases remain normal until the patient is near respiratory arrest.

Peripheral Neuropathies

The Guillain-Barré syndrome, or acute inflammatory demyelinating polyneuropathy, is the prototype neuropathy with respiratory complications (see Chapter 105). Of patients with this syndrome, 20% require tracheal intubation and mechanical ventilation. There is a 5% mortality rate with the best possible treatment. Most deaths are due to pulmonary embolism, severe pneumonia, or other medical complications. Some degree of respiratory insufficiency must be expected in all patients with severe disease; therefore, during the 2- to 4-week period of progression, there should be frequent measurements of inspiratory and expiratory pressures and vital capacity. Intubation is usually required when the vital capacity falls below 15 mL/kg. Plasmapheresis or intravenous immunoglobulin therapy should be initiated as soon as possible in all Guillain-Barré patients with respiratory muscle weakness.

Critical illness neuropathy is an acquired axonal neuropathy that usually presents as failure to wean from mechanical ventilation. Sepsis and multisystem organ failure are risk factors. Neurologic examination reveals flaccid, areflexic quadraparesis, or quadraplegia. Recovery occurs gradually over months, if the patient's underlying medical problems are stabilized.

Disorders of Neuromuscular Transmission

Myasthenia gravis, botulism, and neuromuscular blocking drugs may affect respiratory muscles. Myasthenia gravis almost always affects cranial muscles, causing ptosis, weakness in the ocular and oropharyngeal muscles, and symmetric facial weakness (see Chapter 120). As in Guillain-Barré syndrome and other neuromuscular diseases, blood gas abnormalities are a late manifestation of respiratory failure. Frequent measurement of inspiratory and expiratory pressures and vital capacity is essential; tracheal intubation is carried out if the vital capacity is less than 15 mL/kg. Myasthenia gravis is a treacherous disease because fluctuations may be sudden and unpredictable. Patients with severe dysarthria and dysphagia are at greatest risk.

Myasthenic crisis is defined an exacerbation of weakness that requires mechanical ventilation. It occurs in 15% to 20% of patients overall, and one-third of these will experience two or more episodes of crisis. As with Guillain-Barré syndrome, mortality is approximately 5%. Infection (usually pneumonia or viral upper respiratory infection) is the most common precipitant (40%), followed by no obvious cause (30%) and aspiration (10%). As a general rule, 25% of patients in crisis can be extubated after 1 week, 50% after 2 weeks, and 75% after 1 month. Plasmapheresis leads to short-term improvement of weakness in 75% of patients and should be performed in all patients unless otherwise contraindicated, although its efficacy for reducing the duration of crisis has not been tested in a randomized controlled trial.

Muscle Disease

Muscular dystrophies, myotonic disorders, inflammatory myopathies, periodic paralyses, metabolic myopathies (especially acid maltase deficiency), endocrine disorders, infectious myopathies, mitochondrial myopathies, toxic myopathies, myoglobinuria, critical illness myopathy, and electrolyte disorders may cause widespread skeletal muscle weakness. Respiratory failure may appear in acute fulminant attacks or after a period of progression. Rarely, respiratory failure may be the first manifestation of a generalized myopathy.

MANAGEMENT OF RESPIRATORY FAILURE IN NEUROLOGIC DISEASES

Examination

The initial management of the patient with impending neuromuscular respiratory failure is directed toward assessing the adequacy of ventilation and possible need for immediate intubation. The patient's overall comfort level and the rapidity with which the dyspnea has developed are both important. Rapid shallow breathing, with inability to generate adequate tidal volumes, is a danger sign of significant respiratory muscle fatigue. Diaphragmatic strength can be estimated by palpating for normal outward movement of the abdomen with inspiration; with severe weakness, inspiration is associated with spontaneous inward movement of the diaphragm (paradoxical respirations). Ventilatory reserve can be assessed by checking the patient's ability to count from 1 to 25 in a single breath. The strength of the patient's cough should be observed. A wet gurgled voice and pooled oropharyngeal secretions are the best clinical signs of significant dysphagia. When severe, weakness of the glottic and oropharyngeal muscles can lead to stridor, which is indicative of potentially life-threatening upper airway obstruction. Dysphagia is best screened for by asking the patient to sip 3 ounces of water; coughing is diagnostic of aspiration, and if present, oral feedings should be held until swallowing can be formally assessed.

Mechanical Ventilation

Mechanical ventilation may be positive pressure or negative pressure. Until the mid-1950s, all mechanical ventilation was negative pressure. The most common device was the Drinker tank respirator ("iron lung"), which created a cyclical subatmospheric pressure around the patient's chest, causing chest expansion. Today, there are several types of negative-pressure devices, cuirass ventilators, that can be used on a long-term basis to assist the patient's own respiratory efforts without tracheal intubation. Patients with motor neuron disease and chronic myopathies are sometimes able to live at home with these devices.

Small suitcase-sized portable and battery-powered volume-cycled ventilators are also available for ambulatory use. Ventilator-dependent patients may go home and remain mobile.

Mechanical ventilation is the primary treatment for respiratory failure. The trachea may be intubated orally or nasally; a soft air-filled cuff is then inflated in the trachea to prevent leakage of air around the tube. Indications for endotracheal intubation include physiologic parameters (Table 152.2) and the rate of respiratory deterioration and the patient's overall comfort level. In some cases, positive-pressure ventilation can be delivered for short periods (e.g., overnight) with the use of a tight-fitting face mask.

Positive pressure ventilation may be pressure cycled or volume cycled; the latter mode is usually preferred because it delivers a precise tidal volume over a wide range of pressures. Synchronous intermittent mandatory ventilation is the initial mode of ventilation in most patients. With this mode, a predetermined number of volume-cycled positive pressure breaths are delivered per minute. The patient can initiate a spontaneous breath at any time and receive either a volume-assisted breath or an unsupported breath, depending on the phase of the ventilator cycle. Initially, the tidal volume is set at 10 mL/kg with a respiratory rate of 8 to 12 breaths/min, and 3 to 5 cm H_2O of positive end-expiratory pressure is maintained to prevent atelectasis. The fraction of inspired air is gradually adjusted downward from 100% until the PaO_2 is 70 to 90 mm Hg.

Weaning from the ventilator can be considered when pulmonary function tests show improvement and there are no significant medical complications (Table 152.3). Weaning can be accomplished in three ways: a gradual reduction of the rate of intermittent mandatory ventilation, enabling the patient to take over the spontaneous respirations; "pressure support" weaning with continuous positive airway pressure; and complete removal of the patient from the respirator, allowing free breathing for short periods with oxygen supplementation alone (weaning with a T-tube). Breathing through a ventilator circuit can sometimes increase the work of breathing because of the internal resistance of the machine. Thus, some patients with respiratory muscle weakness wean more easily on a T-tube. Pressure support is a preset level of airway pressure delivered with each inspiratory effort, which reduces the overall work of breathing; the level (usually 5 to 15 cm H_2O) should be adjusted to attain spontaneous tidal volumes of 300 to 500 mL and a comfortable breathing pattern. Whatever the mode of weaning, an increasing respiratory rate with decreasing tidal volumes indicates tiring, at which point the weaning trial should be stopped and the patient returned to synchronous intermittent mandatory ventilation for rest overnight. The ability of the patient to tolerate a T-tube or continuous positive airway pressure with minimal pressure support (5 cm H_2O) for extended periods of time, while maintaining a ratio of respiratory rate (breaths/min) to tidal volume (L) below 100, is probably the single best predictor of successful extubation.

Most clinicians perform a tracheostomy if mechanical ventilation is required for more that 2 weeks. Tracheostomy has several advantages over long-term endotracheal intubation, including increased comfort, reduced risk of permanent tracheolaryngeal injury, increased ease of weaning from the ventilator (reduced dead space and less resistance to flow from the endotracheal tube), and improved ability to manage and suction secretions. The latter two considerations are of particular importance when weaning patients with neuromuscular respiratory failure from mechanical ventilation. If some patients with severe persistent oropharyngeal muscle weakness, a tracheostomy is necessary to manage secretions and prevent aspiration, even though respiratory muscle function is adequate.

TABLE 152.3. CRITERIA FOR WEANING FROM MECHANICAL VENTILATION

Neurologic condition is stable or improving
Vital capacity > 15 mL/kg
Negative inspiratory pressure > 20 mm Hg
PaO_2 > 80 mm Hg with 40% oxygen
Patient is free of fever, infection, fluid overload, anemia, gastric distention, or other medical complications

SUGGESTED READINGS

American Thoracic Society Symposium Summary. Respiratory muscles: structure and function. *Am Rev Respir Dis* 1986;134:1078–1093.

Bach JR, O'Brien J, Krotenberg R, Alba A, et al. Management of end stage respiratory failure in Duchenne muscular dystrophy. *Muscle Nerve* 1987;10:177–182.

Bolton CF. Assessment of respiratory function in the intensive care unit. *Can J Neurol Sci* 1994;21:S28–S34.

Borel CO, Tilford C, Nichols DG, et al. Diaphragmatic performance during recovery from acute ventilatory failure in patients with Guillain-Barre syndrome and myasthenia gravis. *Chest* 1991;99:444–451.

Chevrolet JC, Deleamont P. Repeated vital capacity measurements as predictive parameters for mechanical ventilation and weaning success in the Guillain-Barré syndrome. *Am Rev Respir Dis* 1991;144:814–818.

Cohen CA, Zagelbaum G, Gross D, et al. Clinical manifestations of inspiratory muscle fatigue. *Am J Med* 1982;73:308–316.

Hall JB, Wood LDH. Liberation of the patient from mechanical ventilation. *JAMA* 1987;257:1621–1628.

Hirano M, Ott BR, Raps EC, et al. Acute quadriplegic myopathy: complication of treatment with steroids, nondepolarizing blocking agents, or both. *Neurology* 1992;42:2082–2087.

Howard RS, Wiles CM, Hirsch NP, et al. Respiratory involvement in primary muscle disorders: assessment and management. *Q J Med* 1993;86:175–189.

Hughes RAC, Bihari D. Acute neuromuscular respiratory paralysis. *J Neurol Neurosurg Psychiatry* 1993;56:334–343.

Hund EF, Borel CO, Cornblath DR, et al. Intensive management and treatment of severe Guillain-Barre syndrome. *Crit Care Med* 1993;21:433–446.

Karpel JP, Aldrich TK. Respiratory failure and mechanical ventilation: pathophysiology and methods of promoting weaning. *Lung* 1986;164:309–324.

Kelley BJ, Luce JM. The diagnosis and management of neuromuscular diseases causing ventilatory failure. *Chest* 1991;99:1485–1494.

Make BJ, Gilmartin ME. Rehabilitation and home care for ventilator-assisted individuals. *Clin Chest Med* 1986;7:679–691.

Mayer SA. Intensive care of the myasthenic patient. *Neurology* 1997;48[Suppl 5]:S70–S75.

Ropper AH, Kehne SM. Guillain-Barré syndrome: management of respiratory failure. *Neurology* 1985;35:1662–1665.

Strumpf DA, Millman RP, Hill NS. The management of chronic hypoventilation. *Chest* 1990;98:474–480.

Thomas CE, Mayer SA, Gungor Y, et al. Myasthenic crisis: clinical features, mortality, complications, and risk factors for prolonged intubation. *Neurology* 1997;48:1253–1260.

Tobin MJ. Mechanical ventilation. *N Engl J Med* 1994;330:1056–1061.

Wijdicks EFM, Borel CO. Respiratory management in acute neurologic illness. *Neurology* 1998;50:11–20.

Yang KL, Tobin MJ. A prospective study of indexes predicting the outcome of trials of weaning from mechanical ventilation. *N Engl J Med* 1991;324:1445–1450.

Merritt's Neurology, 10th ed., edited by L.P. Rowland. Lippincott Williams & Wilkins, Philadelphia © 2000.

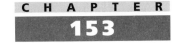

CHAPTER 153

PARANEOPLASTIC SYNDROMES

LEWIS P. ROWLAND

DEFINITION

A paraneoplastic syndrome is one that occurs more frequently than expected by chance in association with neoplasm, most often a malignant tumor. It is called "paraneoplastic" because the neurologic disorder is not the result of tumor invasion or metastasis, chemotherapy, radiotherapy, malnutrition, or coincidental infection.

EPIDEMIOLOGY

If only clinically symptomatic syndromes are considered (and not, say, subclinical peripheral neuropathy determined by nerve conduction studies), all syndromes are rare. For instance, all syndromes together occur in less than 1% of all patients with small cell lung cancer. Conversely, among patients diagnosed with a recognized paraneoplastic syndrome, 10% to 60% prove to have a tumor (Table 153.1). The possible presence of a tumor cannot be totally eliminated without postmortem examination.

PATHOGENESIS

The dominant theory holds that most paraneoplastic disorders are autoimmune in origin. This is based primarily on the frequent presence of characteristic antibodies against neuronal antigens. Presumably, the host mounts an antibody attack against antigens in the tumor and, by a process of molecular mimicry, the immune response is directed against central or peripheral neural antigens. However, the antibodies have limited specificity and sensitivity. Also, there is no evidence of complement-mediated autoimmunity. Attention has therefore been directed to the possibility of T-cell–mediated neurotoxicity. Because the syndromes are so rare, genetic susceptibility is thought to play a role.

TABLE 153.1. FREQUENCY OF ASSOCIATED TUMOR WITH CLINICAL SYNDROMES THAT ARE OFTEN PARANEOPLASTIC

Syndrome[a]	Paraneoplastic (%)
Lambert-Eaton myasthenic syndrome	60
Subacute cerebellar degeneration	50
Opsoclonus/myoclonus (children)	50
Opsoclonus/myoclonus (adults)	20
Subacute sensory neuropathy	20
Myasthenia gravis after age 40 (thymoma)	20
Dermatomyositis after age 40	20
Sensorimotor peripheral neuropathy after age 50	10
Encephalomyelitis	10

[a]Figures are for adults unless age specifically mentioned; particular tumors described in text.
Modified from Posner JB. *Neurologic complications of cancer.* Philadelphia: FA Davis, 1995:353–385.

In contrast to the central nervous system syndromes, antibodies are thought to be pathogenic in the peripheral neuromuscular disorders of the Lambert-Eaton syndrome with neoplasm and myasthenia gravis with thymoma and the anti–myelin-associated glycoprotein (MAG) peripheral neuropathies with lymphoproliferative disease. These syndromes are discussed in Chapters 103, 120, and 121.

Other recognized paraneoplastic mechanisms include hormones secreted by a tumor, such as corticotropin, resulting in Cushing syndrome, or parathyroid hormone-related protein, causing hypercalcemic encephalopathy. Carcinoid tumors may compete with tryptophan to cause a pellagra-like encephalopathy. Immunodeficiency may lead to opportunistic infection, especially by the JC virus in progressive multifocal leukoencephalopathy.

CLINICAL SYNDROMES

Paraneoplastic Cerebellar Degeneration

Symptoms and signs are dominated by cerebellar pathways: ataxia of gait and limbs, dysarthria, nystagmus, and oscillopsia. Other manifestations are encountered in half the cases, with hearing loss, bulbar syndromes, corticospinal tract signs, dementia, and peripheral neuropathy. Computed tomography (CT) and magnetic resonance imaging (MRI) show no specific lesions. Cerebrospinal fluid (CSF) abnormalities may include modest pleocytosis and high protein content, sometimes with high IgG and oligoclonal bands. Associated antibodies may be anti-Yo (with cancer of the ovary), anti-Hu (with small cell lung cancer), Hodgkin antibody with Hodgkin disease, or anti-Ri with cancer of the breast. The differential diagnosis includes viral encephalitis, multiple sclerosis, Creutzfeldt-Jakob disease, alcoholic cerebellar degeneration, and hereditary spinocerebellar atrophy. Treatment is not satisfactory.

Subacute Sensory Neuropathy/Encephalitis

Among patients with idiopathic sensory neuropathy, at least one-third prove to have an associated malignant tumor. Neurologic symptoms usually precede those of the tumor, which is likely to be small. Painful paresthesias are the dominant symptoms and progress for days or weeks on all four limbs, the trunk, and sometimes the face. Unlike cisplatinum neuropathy, which spares pain and temperature, paraneoplastic neuropathy affects all forms of sensation, resulting in a severe sensory ataxia. Tendon reflexes are lost and CSF pleocytosis is characteristic. Nerve conduction studies show loss of sensory evoked potentials, with normal motor functions. Inflammation is seen in the dorsal root ganglia.

Limbic Encephalitis

Personality and mood changes progress rapidly, and within weeks the syndrome is dominated by delirium and dementia with severe memory loss. The disorder may occur alone or with other signs of encephalitis or sensory neuropathy. Computed tomography and magnetic resonance imaging are usually normal at first, but enhancing lesions may be seen in the temporal lobes. CSF pleocytosis is characteristic. Pathologic signs of inflammation are limited at first to the limbic and insular cortex, but other gray matter may be affected. The changes include loss of neurons, perivascular infiltration by leukocytes, and microglial proliferation.

Brainstem Encephalitis

Symptoms of brainstem encephalitis are usually part of a more widespread encephalitis but may be the first manifestations. The manifestations are those of the cranial nerves or basal ganglia. Common findings are oculomotor disorders, including nystagmus and supranuclear vertical gaze palsy as well as hearing loss, dysarthria, dysphagia, and abnormal respiration. Movement disorders may be prominent.

Opsoclonus-Myoclonus

This syndrome is seen most often in children with neuroblastoma, which has a favorable prognosis. The term implies constant motion of the eyes—arrhytmic, irregular in direction, or tempo. There may be evidence of encephalomyelitis or cerebellar disorder. The disorder of eye movements is attributed to dysfunction of the paramedian pontine reticular formation. In adults, opsoclonus may be part of a complex syndrome with cerebellar signs and encephalomyelitis, tumors of several types, and anti-Ri antibodies.

Myelitis

Spinal cord symptoms evolve in days or weeks with clinical evidence of a level lesion. The CSF may show pleocytosis with high protein content and normal sugar; oligoclonal bands may be present. Myelitis may occur with or without encephalomyelitis. Acute necrotizing myelopathy may be an extreme form of the inflammatory demyelinating myelitis.

Motor Neuron Diseases

It is uncertain whether there is a higher frequency of malignant tumor in patients with forms of motor neuron disease. Most epidemiologic studies have shown no such relation. Yet there have been reports of patients whose neurologic symptoms disappeared with treatment of the tumor. Also, there have been more than 60 reports of patients with motor neuron diseases and lymphoproliferative disease. Lower motor neuron signs ("amyotrophy"), including fasciculation, are seen in combination with paraneoplastic encephalomyelitis. A pure upper motor neuron syndrome ("primary lateral sclerosis") has been reported in women with breast cancer, but several patients also developed lower motor neuron signs (i.e., they developed amyotrophic lateral sclerosis).

Sensorimotor Peripheral Neuropathy

Sensorimotor peripheral neuropathy with or without slow conduction velocity is common after age 50. Among the diverse causes are anti-MAG paraproteinemic peripheral neuropathy and paraneoplastic neuropathy. Prominent features may include glove-stocking paresthesias and sensory loss, distal limb weakness, or both. Autonomic failure may be prominent, with disorders of gastrointestinal motility, especially diarrhea or pseudo-obstruction. Cranial symptoms are lacking and the syndrome is slow in evolution; it may responde to immunotherapy, as described in Chapter 105. Vasculitis is found in some acute neuropathies.

Neuromuscular Disorders

The association of myasthenia gravis with thymoma is described in Chapter 120. There is no known paraneoplastic form of myasthenia with cancers; the neuromuscular disorder may occur by chance with a malignant tumor. Lambert-Eaton myasthenic syndrome (LEMS) is discussed in Chapter 121. Paraneoplastic neuromyotonia, as described in Chapter 129, is associated most often with thymoma but also with small cell lung cancer or other tumors. The Moersch-Woltman or stiff-man syndrome is sometimes associated with cancer of lung or other organs.

Myopathies

About 20% patients with dermatomyositis starting after age 40 have an associated tumor, which can be almost any type. Whether there is a higher than expected association of tumor with polymyositis has not been proven. These syndromes are described in Chapters 130 and 131.

LABORATORY DATA

Few laboratory tests point to the diagnosis of a paraneoplastic syndrome. MRI may or may not show abnormalities of white or gray matter; scans are often normal. Similarly, the CSF may or may not show high CSF protein or pleocytosis, but the CSF sugar content should be normal or some other diagnosis suspected. The diagnosis of peripheral neuropathy depends in part on the demonstration of conduction abnormalities, and LEMS is virtually defined by the demonstration of an incrementing response to repetitive nerve stimulation, as described in Chapter 121. Demonstration of a characteristic antibody can accelerate diagnosis of the several paraneoplastic syndromes.

Antibodies

Anti-amphiphysin is found in nerve terminals. Antibodies are found in diverse syndromes, including LEMS, sensory neuropathy, and limbic encephalitis. The associated tumors are also diverse, including lung, breast, and ovary.

Anti-Hu was the first antibody to be identified with small cell lung carcinoma. Like several of the others that followed, it was named after the patient who provided the first serum. It is also called "type 1 antineuronal nuclear autoantibody" or ANNA-1. In a few patients, the tumor was one other than small cell lung cancer. Specificity for sensory neuropathy is given as 99%, with a sensitivity of 82%. The clinical syndrome is most often encephalomyelitis or sensory neuropathy, and the neurologic symptoms usually precede discovery of the tumor.

Anti-Ri is an RNA-binding protein. The clinical syndrome is opsoclonus-myoclonus and the tumors are mostly breast and small cell lung cancer.

In anti-ta, the antigen, Ma2, is a member of a family of proteins in brain, testis, and some tumors. The antibody has been found primarily in patients with testicular cancer associated with limbic and brainstem encephalitis.

Anti-Tr reacts with Purkinje cells of the cerebellum. The clinical syndrome is primarily a subacute cerebellar disorder, often with dysarthria and nystagmus. The neoplasm is almost always Hodgkin disease.

Anti-VGCC reacts with voltage-gated calcium channel of muscle and is found in patients with LEMS. The antibody is not found in other types of paraneoplastic syndromes.

Anti-Yo is a DNA-binding protein, and the antibody is found most often with a cerebellar disorder or brainstem encephalitis in association with a tumor of the ovary, uterus, or breast.

TREATMENT

The peripheral disorders of sensorimotor polyneuropathy and LEMS often respond to intravenous immunoglobulin therapy or immunosuppressive drug therapy. The central nervous system syndromes are refractory to treatment. Corticosteroid therapy is often effective for the opsoclonus-myoclonus syndrome in children, and treatment of the associated tumor may ameliorate the syndrome in adults.

SUGGESTED READINGS

Albert M, Darnell JC, Bender A, Francisco LM, Bhardwaj N, Darnell RB. Tumor-specific killer cells in paraneoplastic cerebellar degeneration. *Nat Med* 1998;4:1321–1324.

Antoine JC, Absi L, Honnorat J, et al. Antiamphiphysin antibodies ae associated with various paraneoplastic neurological syndromes and tumors. *Arch Neurol* 1999;56:172–177.

Bennett JL, Galetta SL, Friedman LP, et al. Neuro-ophthalmologic manifestations of a paraneoplastic syndrome and testicular carcinoma. *Neurology* 1999;52:864–867.

Burns TM, Juel VC, Sanders DB, Phillips LH II. Neuroendocrine lung tumors and disorders of the neuromuscular junction. *Neurology* 1999;52:1480–1491.

Camerlingo M, Nemni R, Ferraro B, et al. Malignancy and sensory: neuropathy of unexplained cause. *Arch Neurol* 1998;55:981–984.

Dalmau J, Gultekin SH, Posner JB. Paraneoplastic neurologic syndromes: pathogenesis and pathophysiology. *Brain Pathol* 1999;9:275–284.

Dalmau J, Gultekin SH, Voltz R, et al. Ma1, a novel neuron- and testis-specific protein, is recognized by the serum of patients with paraneoplastic neurological disorders. *Brain* 1999;122:27–39.

Dropcho EJ. Neurologic paraneoplastic syndromes. *J Neurol Sci* 1998;153:264–278.

Forsyth PA, Dalmau J, Graus F, Cwik V, Rosenblum MK, Posner JB. Motor neuron syndromes in cancer patients. *Ann Neurol* 1997;41:722–730.

Giometto B, Taraloto B, Graus F. Autoimmunity in paraneoplastic neurological syndromes. *Brain Pathol* 1999;9:261–273.

Gordon PH, Rowland LP, Younger DS, et al. Lymphoproliferative disorders and motor neuron disease. *Ann Neurol* 1997;48:1671–1678.

Ichimura M, Yamamoto M, Kobayashi Y, et al. Tissue distribution of pathological lesions and Hu antigen expression in paraneoplastic sensory neuropathy. *Acta Neuropathol* 1998;95:641–648.

Klawaja S, Sripathi N, Ahmad BK, Lemmon VA. Paraneoplastic motor neuron disease with type 1 Purkinje cell antibodies. *Muscle Nerve* 1998;2:943–945.

Lieberman FS, Odel J, Hirsch J, Heinemann M, Michaaeli J, Posner J. Bilateral optic neuropathy with IgGk multiple myeloma improved after myeloablative chemotherapy. *Neurology* 1999;52:414–416.

Lucchinetti CF, Kimmel DW, Lennon VA. Paraneoplastic and oncologic profiles of patients seropositive for type 1 antineuronal nuclear autoantibodies. *Neurology* 1998;50:652–657.

Molinuevo JL, Graus F, Serrano C, Rene R, Guerrero A, Illa I. Utility of anti-Hu antibodies in the diagnosis of paraneoplastic sensory neuropathy. *Ann Neurol* 1998;44:976–980.

Posner JB. *Neurologic complications of cancer.* Philadelphia: FA Davis, 1995:353–385.

Posner JB, Dalmau JO. Paraneoplastic syndromes affecting the central nervous system. *Annu Rev Med* 1997;48:157–166.

Rees J. Paraneoplastic syndromes. *Curr Opin Neurol* 1998;11:623–637.

Ropper AH, Gorson KC. Neuropathies associated with paraproteinemia. *N Engl J Med* 1998;338:1601–1607.

Russo C, Cohn SL, Petruzzi MJ, de Alarcon PA. Long-term neurologic outcome in children with opsoclonus-myoclonus associated with neuroblas-

toma: a report from the Pediatric Oncology Group. *Med Pediatr Oncol* 1997;28:284–288.

Scaravilli F, An SF, Groves M, Thom M. The neuropathology of paraneoplastic syndromes. *Brain Pathol* 1999;9:251–260.

Sodeyama N, Ishida K, Jaeckle KA, et al. Pattern of epitopic reactivity of the anti-Hu antibody on HuD with and without paraneoplastic syndrome. *J Neurol Neurosurg Psychiatry* 1999;66:97–99.

Tabarki B, Palmer P, Lebon P, Sebire G. Spontaneous recovery of opsoclonus-myoclonus syndrome caused by enterovirus infection. *J Neurol Neurosurg Psychiatry* 1998;64:406–407.

Voltz R, Carpentier AF, Rosenfeld MR, Posner JB, Dalmau J. P/Q type voltage-gated calcium channel antibodies in paraneoplastic disorders of the central nervous system. *Muscle Nerve* 1999;22:119–122.

Wakabyashi K, Horikawa Y, Oyake M, Suzuki S, Morita T, Takahashi H. Sporadic motor neuron disease with severe sensory neuronopathy. *Acta Neuropathol* 1998;95:426–430.

Merritt's Neurology, 10th ed., edited by L.P. Rowland. Lippincott Williams & Wilkins, Philadelphia © 2000.

CHAPTER 154

NUTRITIONAL DISORDERS: VITAMIN B₁₂ DEFICIENCY, MALABSORPTION, AND MALNUTRITION

LEWIS P. ROWLAND
BRADFORD P. WORRALL

Many neurologic syndromes are ascribed to lack of vitamins or other essential nutrients. The most common are pernicious anemia (lack of vitamin B_{12}), malnutrition, and malabsorption syndromes.

VITAMIN B₁₂ (COBALAMIN) DEFICIENCY

History

Although not the first to describe the disorder, in 1849 Thomas Addison made pernicious anemia well known. By the turn of the century, the diagnostic triad was recognized: anemia, neurologic symptoms, and atrophy of the epithelial covering of the tongue. In 1900, Russell, Batten, and Collier introduced the term *combined degeneration of the spinal cord.* The disease was lethal until 1926, when Minot and Murphy used replacement therapy without knowing what had to be replaced; they found that supplementing the diet with liver was therapeutic. Castle administered liver extract parenterally, and in 1948 vitamin B_{12} completely reversed the symptoms. Additionally, the automation of blood counts and measurement of blood vitamin B_{12} levels has made early diagnosis the rule. As a result, the neurologic disorder is now rarely seen in major medical centers of industrialized coun-

tries. Although the condition was once thought to affect Nordic people primarily, it is seen in all racial groups. The prevalence of undiagnosed pernicious anemia after age 60 is about 2%.

Physiology

Cobalamin is synthesized only in specific microorganisms, and animal products are the sole dietary sources for humans. Gastric acid is needed for peptic digestion to release the vitamin from proteins. Achlorhydria of the elderly may suffice to cause B_{12} deficiency, but an intrinsic factor is usually missing as well.

The freed B_{12} is bound by R proteins (R for "rapid" movement on electrophoresis) and then by gastric intrinsic factor, a glycoprotein produced by gastric parietal cells, which is needed for absorption of B_{12} and which is absent in people with pernicious anemia. The combined intrinsic factor–cobalamin complex is transported across the terminal ileum and binds to transcobalamin, with a half-life of 6 to 9 minutes. The complex enters cells by endocytosis, and the vitamin enters red blood cells in an energy-dependent process.

Cobalamin is converted to adenosyl or methyl coenzymes, which are necessary for normal neural metabolism. If they are missing, abnormal fatty acids may accumulate in myelin or methylating reactions may be defective. A congenital form of methylcobalamin deficiency leads to developmental delay, microcephaly, and seizures, with delayed myelination. However, the details of B_{12} dependency in the mature nervous system are not well known, and it is not clear why the spinal cord and peripheral nerves are so vulnerable when B_{12} levels are low.

Pathogenesis

About 80% of adult-onset pernicious anemia is attributed to lack of gastric intrinsic factor secondary to atrophic gastritis (Table 154.1). The disorder is thought to be autoimmune in origin because antibodies to gastric parietal cells are found in 90% and antibodies to intrinsic factor occur in up to 76%. The parietal cell

TABLE 154.1. CAUSES OF COBALAMIN DEFICIENCY IN 143 PATIENTS

Etiology	No. patients	Percent
Pernicious anemia		
Proven	95	66.4
Probable	17	11.9
Tropical sprue	8	5.6
Gastric resection	6	4.2
Ileal resection	4	2.5
Jejunal diverticula	3	2.1
Dietary B$_{12}$ malabsorption	3	2.1
Multiple etiologies	4	2.8
Etiology unknown	3	2.1
Total	143	100

Modified from Healton et al. (1991).

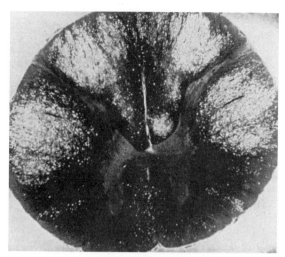

FIG. 154.2. Subacute combined degeneration. Destruction of myelin predominating in the posterior and lateral columns. Swelling of affected myelin sheaths causes spongy appearance.

antigen is gastric H$^+$/K$^+$-ATPase. Supporting the view that autoimmunity is important is the frequent association of pernicious anemia with some other autoimmune disease, such as myasthenia gravis, Hashimoto thyroiditis, vitiligo, or polyglandular deficiency. A murine model of the immune disorder has been developed. In those with normal intrinsic factor, the vitamin is not absorbed because of jejunal diverticulosis, tropical sprue, or loss of the stomach or ileum by surgical resection. Rarely, the vitamin cannot be liberated from dietary animal proteins because peptic digestion is inadequate.

Pathology

In the spinal cord, white matter is affected more than gray. Symmetric loss of myelin sheaths occurs more often than axonal loss; changes are most prominent in the posterior and lateral columns (*combined system disease*) (Figs. 154.1 and 154.2). The thoracic cord is affected first and then the process extends in either direction. Patchy demyelination may be seen in the frontal white matter (Fig. 154.3).

Clinical Features

Today most patients are probably asymptomatic. If the deficiency persists, symptoms may be those of anemia, neurologic

disorder, or other problems such as vitiligo, sore tongue, or prematurely gray hair. Anorexia and weight loss may be prominent.

About 40% of all patients with B$_{12}$ deficiency are said to have some neurologic symptoms or signs, and these are often the first or most prominent manifestations of the disease. Only 20% of patients are younger than age 50; most are over 60. Usually, there are features of both myelopathy and peripheral neuropathy. The most common symptom, attributed to the neuropathy, is acroparesthesia, burning and painful sensations that affect the hands and feet. There may be sensory ataxia. Memory loss, visual loss (due to optic neuropathy), orthostatic hypotension, anosmia, impaired taste (dysgeusia), sphincter symptoms, and impotence are other symptoms.

On examination, there is glove-stocking sensory loss, and almost all patients show loss of vibratory sensation and of position sense. The *Romberg sign* is often present; the patient can stand with feet together if the eyes are open but sways and falls on closing the eyes because of the loss of position sense. There may or may not be weakness of limb muscles; the neuropathy is predominantly sensory, but there are upper motor neuron signs: increased tone, impaired alternating movements, and hyperactive

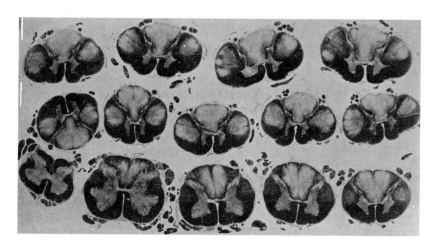

FIG. 154.1. Subacute combined degeneration. Sections of spinal cord at various levels showing segmental loss of myelin, which is most intense in the dorsal and lateral columns.

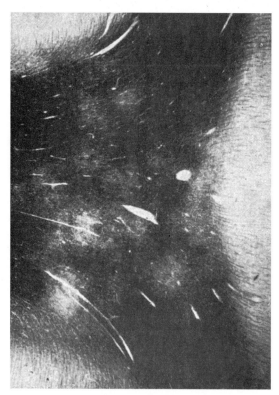

FIG. 154.3. Subacute combined degeneration. Partial loss of myelin of white matter of frontal lobe. (Courtesy of Dr. L. Roizin.)

tendon jerks, with Babinski and Hoffmann signs. Cognitive loss may be evident as florid dementia or may be manifest only on neuropsychologic tests. Optic atrophy is found in fewer than 1% of patients.

As a measure of the efficacy of modern diagnosis and treatment, even symptomatic patients are usually independent in activities of daily living. Fewer than 10% are restricted to chair or bed.

Diagnosis

The diagnosis rests on demonstration of blood levels of vitamin B_{12} less than 200 pg/mL, but low normal values (200 to 350 pg/mL) may be found in people who respond to therapy. Some people with low values are not deficient, and additional tests may be useful. Both methylmalonic acid and homocysteine accumulate when there is impairment of cobalamin-dependent reactions; both metabolites are abnormally increased in serum in more than 99% of patients with true cobalamin deficiency. The *Schilling test*, a measure of the absorption of orally ingested labeled B_{12}, is technically difficult and unreliable because it may be normal in vegetarians and nitrous oxide abusers. Sometimes a therapeutic trial is the only way to determine whether a neurologic syndrome is in fact due to B_{12} deficiency. Magnetic resonance imaging (MRI) may show increased T2-weighted signal and contrast enhancement of the posterior and lateral columns of the spinal cord, with return to normal on treatment.

Nerve conduction tests show a sensorimotor neuropathy that may be either axonal or demyelinating. Visual, brainstem, and somatosensory evoked responses may be normal or abnormal. Computed tomography and MRI may show no abnormality, or there may be cerebral atrophy in patients with dementia.

In patients with neurologic signs, only about 20% show severe anemia. Both the hematocrit and mean corpuscular volume may be normal, although they are the traditional abnormalities. Bone marrow biopsy, however, reliably shows megaloblastic abnormalities. B_{12} deficiency must be considered in any sensorimotor neuropathy, myelopathy, autonomic neuropathy, dementia, or optic neuropathy. Several of these disorders arise in acquired immunodeficiency syndrome, but a possible role of B_{12} is doubted.

Dentists may be at special risk because recreational abuse of nitrous oxide can interfere with cobalamin metabolism and cause neuropathy or combined system disease.

Treatment

B_{12} is given intramuscularly in a dosage of 1,000 μg daily for the first week, followed by weekly injections for the first month, and then monthly injections for life. Oral therapy is less reliable largely because absorption without intrinsic factor is inefficient. After parenteral injection of B_{12}, hematologic improvement may be evident within 48 hours, and there is a subjective sense of general improvement. Paresthesias are often the first neurologic symptoms to improve and do so within 2 weeks; corticospinal abnormalities are slower to respond. If there is no response in 3 months, the condition is probably not due to B_{12} deficiency. About half of the patients are left with some abnormality on examination; the residual disability depends on the duration of symptoms.

MALNUTRITION

Malnutrition is still a serious problem throughout the world. In poor countries, dietary deficiency is common. In industrial countries, nutritional syndromes are more likely to be seen in alcoholics, in patients with chronic bowel disease, or in patients after some medical treatment that interferes with essential elements of diet (Table 154.2). Even if the acute disorders are corrected, there may be long-term effects. Maternal malnutrition may affect the fetus and cause mental retardation; on another level, chronic neurologic syndromes persisted in World War II prisoners long after they had resumed a normal diet.

Dietary therapy may be important in the management of some inborn errors of metabolism to prevent accumulation of some toxic substances (as in phenylketonuria) or to amplify the activity of a mutant enzyme (as in vitamin B_6-responsive homocystinuria).

Diseases of malnutrition may arise if essential nutrients are not provided because the diet is inadequate. The result may be the same if nutrients are lost by vomiting or diarrhea, if there is malabsorption, if use of a nutrient is impaired, or if the target organ is unresponsive to a mediating hormone.

Examples of different syndromes are found in other chapters of this book; a simple listing or table is a gross oversimplification for two reasons. First, vitamin deficiency is likely to be multiple

TABLE 154.2. NEUROLOGIC SYNDROMES ATTRIBUTED TO NUTRITIONAL DEFICIENCY

Site of major syndrome	Name
Encephalon	Hypocalcemia (lack of vitamin D), tetany, seizures
	Mental retardation (protein-calorie deprivation)
	Cretinism (lack of iodine)
	Wernicke-Korsakoff syndrome (thiamine)
Corpus callosum	Marchiafava-Bignami disease
Optic nerve	Nutritional deficiency optic neuropathy ("tobacco-alcohol amblyopia")
Brainstem	Central pontine myelinolysis
Cerebellum	Alcoholic cerebellar degeneration
	Vitamin E deficiency in bowel disease
Spinal cord	Combined system disease (B_{12} deficiency)
	Tropical spastic paraparesis (some forms?)
Peripheral nerves	Beriberi (thiamine), pellagra (nicotinic acid)
	Hypophosphatemia (?)
	Tetany (vitamin D deficiency)
Muscle	Myopathy of osteomalacia

and often accompanied by protein-calorie malnutrition and thus the resulting syndromes are complex. Second, it is possible to tabulate the major target system of a particular syndrome, although most involve more than one system; spinal cord syndromes and encephalopathy, for example, may be more prominent than the peripheral neuropathy of pellagra. In contrast, peripheral neuropathy, optic neuropathy, or dementia may be seen in patients with combined system disease of the spinal cord secondary to vitamin B_{12} deficiency. Some neurologic syndromes are attributable to dietary excess (Table 154.3). For this reason, too, the syndromes are likely to be complex.

A common cause of malnutrition in industrialized countries is *anorexia nervosa*. In addition to the conventional neuropathy and other syndromes of multiple vitamin deficiency, there may be a myopathy. Here, however, the nutritional disorder is often complicated by the ingestion of *emetine* to induce vomiting.

An epidemic of *peripheral and optic neuropathy* in Cuba was seen in 1991 after the collapse of support from the Soviet Union

and enforcement of an embargo by the United States. As many as 50,000 may have been affected. This combination of disorders had earlier been seen in prisoners of war and other malnourished populations. In Cuba, some patients had mutations of mitochondrial DNA of the kind seen in Leber hereditary optic neuropathy, which may have made them more susceptible to dietary deprivation. Many patients improved with supplemental vitamin therapy. Viral infection may have been responsible for some cases.

Only a brief overview is offered of disorders of the stomach and intestine. The major neurologic syndrome of stomach disease results from lack of intrinsic factor and B_{12} deficiency. There are no major neurologic consequences of peptic ulcer (other than those that might result from shock after massive hemorrhage), but treatment of the ulcer may lead to a neurologic disorder. Antacids may cause a partial malabsorption syndrome. Cimetidine therapy avoids these problems but may cause an acute confusional state. Antacids that contain aluminum or phosphate-binders can cause encephalopathy, especially in the presence of renal disease. Surgical therapy may cure the ulcer but may also create a neurologic disorder as a result of malabsorption.

MALABSORPTION

Malabsorption syndromes may arise for any of several reasons (Table 154.4). In patients with these disorders, neurologic abnormalities seem to be disproportionately frequent. Alone or in combination, there may be evidence of myopathy, sensorimotor peripheral neuropathy, degeneration of corticospinal tracts and posterior columns, and cerebellar abnormality. Optic neuritis, atypical pigmentary degeneration of the retina, and dementia are less common signs of malabsorption syndromes.

There have been three waves of explanation. First, the syndromes were attributed to vitamin B_{12} deficiency, which probably accounted for some but not all cases; many patients had normal serum B_{12} levels and did not respond to vitamin B_{12} therapy. Second, there was considerable interest in the relation of the neurologic abnormality to osteomalacia, which often appeared in the same patients. Osteomalacia also accompanied similar neurologic syndromes in patients who had dietary problems other than malabsorption (e.g., lack of sunlight or dietary vitamin D, resis-

TABLE 154.3. NEUROLOGIC SYNDROMES ATTRIBUTED TO DIETARY EXCESS

Syndrome	Condition	Agent
Increased intracranial pressure	Self-medication	Vitamin A
Encephalopathy	Phenylketonuria	Phenylalanine
	Water intoxication	Water
	Hepatic encephalopathy	Protein (and NH_3)
	Ketotic or nonketotic coma in diabetes	Glucose
Strokes	Hyperlipidemia	Lipid
Peripheral neuropathy	Hypochondriasis	Pyridoxine
	Insomnia, anxiety	Tryptophan, contaminated
Myopathy	Anorexia nervosa, bulimia	Emetine, ipecac
Myoglobinuria	Constipation	Licorice

TABLE 154.4. SOME CAUSES OF NEUROLOGIC DISORDER DUE TO MALABSORPTION

Defective intraluminal hydrolysis	Gastric resection
	Pancreatic insufficiency
	Exclusion or deficiency of bile salts
Primary mucosal cell abnormality	Celiac disease
	Abetalipoproteinemia
Inadequate absorption surface	Massive small gut resection
	Ileal resection or bypass
	Jejunal bypass
	Jejunocolic fistula
	Gastroileostomy
Abnormalities of intestinal wall	Ileojejunitis
	Amyloidosis
	Radiation injury
Lymphatic obstruction and stasis	Lymphoma
	Tuberculosis
Bacterial overgrowth and parasitic infections	Blind loops
	Jejunal diverticula
	Scleroderma
	Whipple disease
	Tropical sprue
	D-Lactic acidosis
Miscellaneous	Diabetic neuropathy
	Hypoparathyroidism
	Hypothyroidism

From Glickman R. In: Wyngaarden JB, Smith LH Jr, eds. *Cecil's textbook of medicine,* 16th ed. Philadelphia: WB Saunders, 1982:678–690.

TABLE 154.5. NEUROLOGIC SYNDROMES IN 19 PATIENTS WITH INFLAMMATORY BOWEL DISEASE

Syndrome	Number of patients
Myelopathy	5
Acute inflammatory demyelinating polyneuropathy	3
Dermatomyositis	2
Recurrent stroke or TIA	2
Sinus thrombosis	2
Mononeuritis multiplex	1
Brachial plexopathy	1
Mlkersson-Rosenthal syndrome	1
Myasthenia gravis	1
Vacuolar myopathy	1

TIA, transient ischemic attack.
Modified from Lossos et al. (1995).

tance to vitamin D, renal disease, ingestion of anticonvulsant drugs). Osteomalacia or vitamin D deficiency, however, was hard to prove in some cases, and there was often no response to vitamin D therapy. Third, now the main culprit is lack of vitamin E, which can arise in several different ways: fat malabsorption, colestatic liver disease, abetalipoproteinemia, and autosomal recessive absence of the tocopherol transfer protein. In these disorders, ataxia and sensorimotor polyneuropathy are prominent clinical signs and may improve with vitamin E replacement, giving up to 4 g daily of alpha tocopherol.

The main bowel diseases associated with neurologic symptoms are celiac disease and inflammatory bowel disease (Crohn disease or ulcerative colitis). *Celiac disease* is characterized by the triad of malabsorption, abnormal small bowel mucosa, and intolerance to gluten, a complex of wheat proteins. Gluten sensitivity can be documented by finding antibodies to gliadin. Neurologic complications arise from osteomalacic myopathy, B_{12} deficiency with neuropathy or myelopathy, hypokalemia, or hypocalcemia. In some patients, severe ataxia of gait has been related to the gluten sensitivity, with changes in peripheral nerves, posterior columns, and cerebellum.

Both *Crohn disease* and *ulcerative colitis* are associated with increased risk of thromboembolism that may affect other parts of the body but includes arteries and veins of the brain or spinal cord. Neuromuscular disorders are diverse (Table 154.5). Peripheral neuropathy is found with Crohn disease for reasons that are uncertain; acute or chronic demyelinating neuropathy is found more often with ulcerative colitis. Myopathy may occur with either disorder, but symptomatic central nervous system disease is exceptional even though white matter lesions are found by MRI.

Another unusual syndrome of malabsorption is episodic ab-

normality of sleep, thirst, hunger, and mood, a combination that suggests a hypothalamic disorder. Other manifestations are episodes of weakness, ataxia, slurred speech, confusion, and nausea. This is attributed to bacterial overgrowth with production of D-lactic acid. *D*-Lactic acidosis is seen in patients with a short small intestine and an intact colon. Excessive production of D-lactate by abnormal bowel flora overwhelms normal metabolism of D-lactate and leads to an accumulation of this enantiomer in the blood. The condition may be fatal, but oral antibiotic treatment has abolished the syndrome in some patients.

Chronic diarrhea from any cause, including malabsorption or abuse of laxatives, may cause hypokalemia with resulting chronic myopathy, acute paralysis, or acute myoglobinuria. Acute hypophosphatemia may arise in alcohol abusers treated for loss of fluids and electrolytes, after treatment of diabetic ketoacidosis, or after hyperalimentation. In these circumstances, limb weakness may simulate Guillain-Barré syndrome, or the acute electrolyte disorder may actually precipitate the neuropathy; seizures and coma may be part of the picture.

In some conditions, diarrhea accompanies but is not thought to cause the neurologic disorder. The combination of diarrhea, orthostatic hypotension, and peripheral neuropathy suggests the possibility of amyloid disease or diabetes mellitus. The combination of chronic diarrhea, arthritis, and dementia or other cerebral disorder suggests *Whipple disease* (see Chapter 34). The disease is often diagnosed only at autopsy because there is no characteristic clinical picture and steatorrhea may be lacking. An unusual sign is *oculomasticatory myorhythmia,* a term that describes rhythmic convergence of the eyes and synchronous contractions of the masticatory muscles. Diagnosis can be made reliably by a polymerase chain reaction test. Recognition is important because Whipple disease can be cured by treatment with trimethoprim-sulfamethoxazole.

SUGGESTED READINGS

General

Glickman R. Malabsorption syndromes. In: Wyngaarden JB, Smith LH Jr, eds. *Cecil's textbook of medicine,* 16th ed. Philadelphia: WB Saunders, 1982.

Keane JR. Neurologic symptoms mistaken for gastrointestinal disease. *Neurology* 1998;50:1189–1190.

Malouf R, Brust JCM. Hypoglycemia: causes, neurological manifestations, and outcome. *Ann Neurol* 1985;17:321–430.

Pallis CA, Lewis PD. *The neurology of gastrointestinal disease.* Philadelphia: WB Saunders, 1974.

Perkin GD, Murray-Lyon I. Neurology and the gastrointestinal system. *J Neurol Neurosurg Psychiatry* 1998;65:291–300.

Winick M. *Malnutrition and the brain.* New York: Oxford University Press, 1976.

Vitamin B$_{12}$ Deficiency

Al-Shubali AF, Farah SA, Hussein JM, Trontelj JV, Khuraibet AJ. Axonal and demyelinating neuropathy with reversible proximal conduction block, an unusual feature of vitamin B$_{12}$ deficiency. *Muscle Nerve* 1998;21:1341–1343.

Anonymous Editorial. Still time for rational debate about vitamin B$_{12}$. *Lancet* 1998;351:1523.

Brantigan CO. Folate supplementation and the risk of making vitamin B$_{12}$ deficiency. *JAMA* 1997;277:884–885.

Chanarin I, Metz J. Diagnosis of cobalamin deficiency: the old and the new. *Br J Haematol* 1997;97:695–700.

Elia M. Oral or parenteral therapy for B$_{12}$ deficiency. *Lancet* 1998;352:1721–1722.

Green R, Kinsella LJ. Current concepts in the diagnosis of cobalamin therapy. *Neurology* 1995;45:1435–1440.

Hall CA. Function of vitamin B$_{12}$ in the central nervous system as revealed by congenital defects. *Am J Hematol* 1990;34:121–127.

Healton EH, Savage DG, Brust JCM, et al. Neurologic aspects of cobalamin deficiency. *Medicine (Baltimore)* 1991;70:228–245.

Holloway KL, Alberico AM. Postoperative myelopathy: a preventable complication in patients with B$_{12}$ deficiency. *Neurosurgery* 1990;72:732–736.

Kinsella LJ, Green R. "Anesthesia paresthetica": nitrous oxide-induced cobalamin deficiency. *Neurology* 1995;45:1608–1610.

Layzer RB. Myeloneuropathy after prolonged exposure to nitrous oxide. *Lancet* 1978;2:1227–1230.

Layzer RB, Fishman RA, Schafer JA. Neuropathy following abuse of nitrous oxide. *Neurology* 1978;28:504–506.

Lindenbaum J, Healton EB, Savage DG, et al. Neuropsychiatric disorders caused by cobalamin deficiency in the absence of anemia or macrocytosis. *N Engl J Med* 1988;318:1720–1728.

Lindenbaum J, Savage DG, Stabler SP, et al. Diagnosis of cobalamin deficiency. II. Relative sensitivities of serum cobalamin, methylmalonic acid, and total homocysteine concentrations. *Am J Hematol* 1990;34:99–107.

Locatelli ER, Laureno R, Ballard P, Mark AS. MRI in vitamin B$_{12}$ deficiency myelopathy. *Can J Neurol Sci* 1999;26:60–62.

Robertson KR, Stern RA, Hall CD, et al. Vitamin B$_{12}$ deficiency and nervous system disease in HIV infection. *Arch Neurol* 1993;50:807–811.

Russell JSR, Batten FE, Collier J. Subacute combined degeneration of the spinal cord. *Brain* 1900;23:39–110.

Sigal SH, Hall CA, Antel JP. Plasma R binder deficiency and neurologic disease. *N Engl J Med* 1987;317:1330–1332.

Stabler SP. Vitamin B$_{12}$ deficiency in older people: improving diagnosis and preventing disability. *J Am Geriatr Soc* 1998;46:1199–1206.

Stojsavljevic N, Levic Z, Drulovic J. 44-month clinical-brain MRI follow-up in a patient with B$_{12}$ deficiency. *Neurology* 1997;49:878–881.

Toh B-H, van Driel IR, Gleeson PA. Pernicious anemia. *N Engl J Med* 1997;337:1441–1448.

Victor M, Lear AA. Subacute combined degeneration of the spinal cord. *Am J Med* 1956;20:896–911.

Malnutrition and Malabsorption

Albers JW, Nostrant TT, Riggs JE. Neurologic manifestations of gastrointestinal disease. *Neurol Clin* 1989;7:525–548.

Alloway R, Reynolds EH, Spargo E, et al. Neuropathy and myopathy in two patients with anorexia and bulimia nervosa. *J Neurol Neurosurg Psychiatry* 1985;48:1015–1020.

Dastur DK, Manghani DK, Osuntokun BO, et al. Neuromuscular and related changes in malnutrition. A review. *J Neurol Sci* 1982;55:207–230.

Flannelly G, Turner MJ, Connolly R, et al. Persistent hyperemesis gravidarum complicated by Wernicke's encephalopathy. *Irish J Med Sci* 1990;159:89.

Gill GV, Bell DR. Persisting nutritional neuropathy amongst former war prisoners. *J Neurol Neurosurg Psychiatry* 1982;45:861–865.

Hadjivassiliou M, Grunewald RA, Chattopadhyay AK, et al. Clinical, radiological, neurophysiological, and neuropathological characteristics of gluten ataxia. *Lancet* 1998;352:1582–1585.

Hart PE, Gould SR, MacSweeney JE, Clifton A, Schon F. Brain white matter lesions in inflammatory bowel disease. *Lancet* 1998;351:1558.

Hedges TR 3rd, Hirano M, Tucker K, Caballero B. Epidemic optic and peripheral neuropathy in Cuba: a unique geopolitical public health problem. *Surv Ophthalmol* 1997;41:341–353.

Hirano M, Cleary JM, Stewart AM, et al. Mitochondrial DNA mutations in an outbreak of optic neuropathy in Cuba. *Neurology* 1994; 44:843–845.

Johns DR. Cerebrovascular complications of inflammatory bowel disease. *Am J Gastroenterol* 1991;86:367–370.

Lloyd-Still JD, Tomasi L. Neurovascular and thromboembolic complications of inflammatory bowel disease in childhood. *J Paediatr Gastroenterol Nutr* 1989;9:461–466.

Lossos A, River Y, Eliakim A, Steiner I. Neurologic aspects of inflammatory bowel disease. *Neurology* 1995;45:416–421.

Mitchell JE, Seim HC, Colon E, et al. Medical complications and medical management of bulimia. *Ann Intern Med* 1987;107:71–77.

Palmer EP, Guary AT. Reversible myopathy secondary to abuse of ipecac in patients with major eating disorders. *N Engl J Med* 1985;313:1457–1459.

Patchell RA, Fellows HA, Humphries LL. Neurologic complications of anorexia nervosa. *Acta Neurol Scand* 1994;89:111–116.

Pellecchia MT, Scala R, Filla A, De Michele G, Ciacci C, Barone P. Idiopathic cerebellar ataxia associated with celiac disease: lack of distinctive neurological features. *J Neurol Neurosurg Psychiatry* 1999;66:32–35.

Roman GC. Epidemic neuropathy in Cuba: a public health problem related to the Cuban Democracy Act of the United States. *Neuroepidemiology* 1998;17:111–115.

Schwartz MA, Selhorst JB, Ochs AL, et al. Oculomasticatory myorhythmia: a unique movement disorder occurring in Whipple's disease. *Ann Neurol* 1986;20:677–681.

Smiddy WE, Green WR. Nutritional amblyopia. A histopathologic study with retrospective clinical correlation. *Graefe's Arch Clin Exp Ophthalmol* 1987;225:321–324.

Vitamin E Deficiency

Cavalier L, Ouahchi K, Kayden HJ, et al. Ataxia wih isolated vitamin E deficiency: heterogeneity of mutations and phenotypic variability in a large number of families. *Am J Hum Genet* 1998;62:301–310.

Harding AE, Muller DPR, Thomas PK, et al. Spinocerebellar degeneration secondary to chronic intestinal malabsorption: a vitamin E deficiency syndrome. *Ann Neurol* 1982;12:419–424.

Mauro A, Orsi L, Mortara P, et al. Cerebellar syndrome in adult celiac disease with vitamin E deficiency. *Acta Neurol Scand* 1991;84:167–170.

Sitrin MD, Lieberman F, Jensen WE, et al. Vitamin E deficiency and neurologic disease in adults with cystic fibrosis. *Ann Intern Med* 1987;107:51–54.

Sokol RJ. Vitamin E and neurologic deficits. *Adv Pediatr* 1990;37:119–148.

D-Lactic Acidosis

Carr DB, Shih VE, Richter JM, et al. D-lactic acidosis simulating a hypothalamic syndrome after bowel bypass. *Ann Neurol* 1982;11:195–197.

Vella A, Farrugia G. D-Lactic acidosis: pathologic consequence of saprophytism. *Mayo Clin Proc* 1998;73:451–456.

Vitamins and Minerals

Insogna KL, Bordley DR, Caro JF, et al. Osteomalacia and weakness from excessive antacid ingestion. *JAMA* 1980;244:2544–2546.

Parry GJ, Bredsen DE. Sensory neuropathy with low-dose pyridoxine. *Neurology* 1985;35:1466–1468.

Rosenberg M, McCarten JR, Snyder BD, et al. Hypophosphatemia with reversible ataxia and quadriparesis. *Am J Med Sci* 1987;293:261–264.

Schott GD, Wills MR. Muscle weakness in osteomalacia. *Lancet* 1976;1:626–629.

Weintraub MI. Hypophosphatemia mimicking acute Guillain-Barré-Strohl syndrome. A complication of parenteral alimentation. *JAMA* 1980;235:1040–1041.

Merritt's Neurology, 10th ed., edited by L.P. Rowland. Lippincott Williams & Wilkins, Philadelphia © 2000.

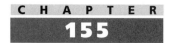

CHAPTER 155

VASCULITIS SYNDROMES

LEWIS P. ROWLAND

Several syndromes are commonly linked because they are characterized by a combination of arthritis, rash, and visceral disease. Because arthritis is common to all and fibrinoid degeneration of blood vessels is common, they are called *collagen-vascular diseases*. Inflammatory lesions of the blood vessels, however, are the dominant pathologic changes in some syndromes. Periarteritis nodosa was the model vasculitis, but the classification of related syndromes depended on autopsy evaluation of histologic changes in the arteries, whether large or small vessels were involved, and which organs were most affected. Similar classifications were applied to clinical diagnosis, but overlap between syndromes and lack of knowledge of pathogenesis obscured the area. Some of these diseases were attributed to the deposition of circulating immune complexes within vessel walls, and some

seemed related to viral infection. With the discovery of antineuronal cytoplasmic autoantibodies (ANCA) and other antibodies, a new classification was adopted by an international consensus conference in 1994 (Table 155.1). An older classification describes syndromes that have characteristic clinical and neurologic manifestations and warrant individual discussion (Table 155.2). Clinical disorders of brain, spinal cord, peripheral nerve, and muscle are prominent in these diseases. All these conditions are said to be rare except for temporal arteritis and polymyalgia rheumatica after age 60 and Kawasaki disease in children.

ANCA tests have had a major impact in clinical practice and in theory, bolstering the view that these diseases are autoimmune in origin. In the United Kingdom, the annual incidence of systemic vasculitis other than temporal arteritis was 42 per million population, and 50% of patients tested positive for ANCA. They are especially prevalent in Wegener granulomatosis, microscopic polyangiitis, and the Churg-Strauss syndrome. The test depends on immunofluorescence that gives either of two patterns, cytoplasmic ANCA or perinuclear ANCA. The cytoplasmic antigen is a proteinase (PR3-ANCA) and the perinuclear antigen is myeloperoxidase (MPO-ANCA); 90% of patients with Wegener disease have the cytoplasmic PR3-ANCA, and 90% of patients with Churg-Strauss have the perinuclear MPO-ANCA. However, the missing 10% is important because a negative test does not exclude either diagnosis.

TABLE 155.1. VASCULITIS SYNDROMES: CHAPEL HILL CONSENSUS CRITERIA

Syndromes	Pathologies
Large-vessel vasculitis	
Giant cell (temporal) arteritis	Granulomatous arteritis of aorta and its major branches; predilection for extracarnial branches of carotid artery. Often involves temporal artery; patients older than 50 yr; with polymyalgia rheumatica.
Takeyusu arteritis	Granulomatous arteritis of aorta and major branches; patients younger than age 50.
Medium-sized vessel vasculitis	
Polyarteritis nodosa	Necrotizing inflammation of medium- or small-sized arteries; no glomerulonephritis or vasculitis of arterioles, capillaries, venules.
Kawasaki disease	Arteritis of large, medium-sized, small arteries plus mucocutaneous-lymph node syndrome. Coronary arteries often involved; aorta and veins may be involved; usually in children
Small-vessel vasculitis	
Wegener granulomatosis[a]	Granulomatous inflammation including respiratory tract and necrotizing vasculitis of small-to-medium vessels (capillaries, venules, arterioles, arteries). Necrotizing glomerulonephritis common.
Churg-Strauss syndrome[a]	Eosinophil-rich granulomatous inflammation of respiratory tract and necrotizing vasculitis of small-to-medium-sized vessels; with asthma and eosinophilia.
Microscopic polyangiitis[a]	Necrotizing vasculitis with few or no immune deposits; affects small vessels (capillaries, venules, arterioles). May involve small- and medium-sized arteries. Common features: necrotizing glomerulonephritis and involvement of pulmonary capillaries.
Henoch-Schönlein purpura	Vasculitis with IgA-dominant immune deposits on small vessels (capillaries, venules, arterioles). Affects skin, gut, glomeruli plus arthritis or arthralgia.
Essential cryoglobulinemic vasculitis	Vasculitis with immune deposits on small vessels (capillaries, venules, arterioles); cryoglobulins in serum; skin and glomeruli often involved.
Cutaneous leukocytoclastic angiitis	Isolated cutaneous leukocytoclastic angiitis without systemic vasculitis or glomerulonephritis.

[a]Antineuronal cytoplasmic autoantibodies present in most patients with Wegener granulomatosis, Churg-Strauss syndrome, and microscopic polyangiitis.
Modified from Jennette et al. (1994) and Jennette and Falk (1997).

TABLE 155.2. SYNDROMES ASSOCIATED WITH SYSTEMIC VASCULITIS

Syndrome	Systemic manifestations	Laboratory abnormalities	Neurologic syndromes
Systemic vasculitis (periarteritis nodosa)	Skin, kidneys, joints, lungs, hypertension; abdominal pain; heart	Serum complement decreased; immune complexes; hepatitis B antigen and antibody rheumatoid factor	Peripheral neuropathy; mononeuritis multiplex; stroke; polymyositis
Wegener granulomatosis	Nose, paranasal sinuses, lungs, other viscera	As above; also increased serum IgE	Peripheral or cranial neuropathy encephalopathy
Churg-Strauss vasculitis	Lungs, other viscera	As above; also eosinophilia	
Temporal arteritis (giant cell arteritis)	Fever, malaise, myalgia, weight loss, claudication of chewing	Increased ESR	Visual loss due to lesions of optic nerve or retina; papilledema; stroke rare
Polymyalgia rheumatica	Fever, malaise; myalgia weight loss	Increased ESR	None
Cogan syndrome	Interstitial keratitis, aortic insufficiency; occasionally other viscera	Increased ESR; CSF pleocytosis	Vestibular or auditory loss; peripheral neuropathy; stroke; encephalomyelopathy
Takayasu syndrome (aortic arch disease; pulseless disease)	Cataracts, retinal atrophy; cranial muscular wasting; claudication loss of peripheral pulses; heart	Increased ESR	Stroke; amaurosis fugax; visual loss
Granulomatous angiitis of the brain	None	CSF pleocytosis, increased protein content, normal sugar	Somnolence, confusion; encephalomyelopathy; myeloradiculoneuropathy
Systemic lupus erythematosus	Skin, lungs, kidneys, joints, liver, heart, Raynaud, fever	Leukopenia, multiple autoantibodies, increased ESR; evidence of renal or hepatic disease	Organic psychosis; seizures; chorea; myelopathy; peripheral neuropathy; polymyositis; aseptic meningitis
Systemic sclerosis	Skin, lungs, gastrointestinal tract, kidneys, heart, joints, Raynaud	None characteristic except disordered mobility of esophagus and bowel	Polymyositis
Rheumatoid arthritis	Joints; viscera occasionally	Rheumatoid factor	Polymyositis; mononeuritis multiplex peripheral neuropathy
Dermatomyositis	Skin, by definition; lungs; gastrointestinal tract, rare	Inflammatory cells in muscle	Polymyositis
Mixed connective tissue disease (sclerodermatomyositis?)	Skin lesions of dermatomyositis or scleroderma; joints; Raynaud; lungs; esophagus	Antibody to extractable nuclear ribonucleoprotein	Polymyositis

ESR, erythracyte sedimentation rate; CSF, cerebrospinal fluid.
From Cupps and Fauci (1982).

POLYARTERITIS NODOSA

Polyarteritis nodosa is an inflammatory arteritis that affects primarily the medium-sized arteritis. It is characterized by nonspecific symptoms commonly associated with an infection or signs and symptoms involving abdominal organs, joints, peripheral nerves, muscles, or central nervous system (CNS).

Etiology

The cause of periarteritis is unknown; reactions to bacterial or viral infection have been postulated. Association of the disorder with asthma, serum sickness, or drug reactions suggests autoimmunity. Rich reproduced the lesions in rabbits by repeated injections of horse serum. Immune complexes may play a role; in some cases, immune complexes have been found in vessel walls without vasculitis but with chronic aggressive hepatitis attributed to hepatitis B virus.

Pathology

There is widespread panarteritis. The pathology in the nervous system includes infiltrates in the adventitia and vasa vasorum, polymorphonuclear leukocytes, and eosinophils. Necrosis of the media and elastic membrane occurs and may lead to formation of multiple small aneurysms. As these become fibrotic, they may rupture; proliferation of intima may lead to thrombosis of vessels. Repair and fibrosis of the aneurysms lead to a characteristic beading appearance caused by the nodules.

Incidence

Polyarteritis nodosa is rare, but when it occurs, the CNS is involved in about 25% of cases. Both sexes are affected. The disease may occur at any age, but more than 50% of the reported cases are in the third or fourth decades of life.

Signs and Symptoms

Onset may be acute or insidious. Fever; malaise; tachycardia; sweating; fleeting edema; weakness; and pains in the joints, muscles, or abdomen are common early symptoms (Tables 155.3 and 155.4). Blood pressure may be elevated, and there may be a moderate or severe anemia with leukocytosis.

Visceral lesions occur in most cases. Kidney involvement produces symptoms and signs of acute glomerular nephritis. Cutaneous hemorrhages, erythematous eruptions, and tender red subcutaneous nodules may appear in the skin of the trunk or limbs. Gastrointestinal, hepatic, renal, or cardiac symptoms may develop.

Peripheral neuropathy is the most common neurologic disorder. Periarteritis is probably one of the most common causes of

TABLE 155.3. CLINICAL FEATURES IN PATIENTS^a WITH POLYARTERITIS NODOSA

Clinical manifestation	Percent	No. patients
Fever	71	460
Weight loss	54	405
Organ system involvement		
Kidney	70	375
Musculoskeletal system	64	301
Arthritis/arthralgia	53	301
Myalgias	31	238
Hypertension	54	356
Peripheral neuropathy	51	495
Gastrointestinal tract	44	507
Abdominal pain	43	122
Nausea/vomiting	40	30
Cholecystitis	17	64
Bleeding	6	205
Bowel perforation	5	64
Bowel infarction	1.4	140
Skin	43	476
Rash/purpura	30	259
Nodules	15	369
Livedo reticularis	4	194
Heart	36	413
Congestive heart failure	12	204
Myocardial infarct	6	64
Pericarditis	4	204
Brain	23	184
Stroke	11	90
Altered mental status	10	90
Seizure	4	90

^aMean age of patients was 45; the male-to-female ratio was 2.5:1.
From Cupps TR and Fauci AS (1982).

TABLE 155.4. SYMPTOMS AT ONSET IN PATIENTS WITH POLYARTERITIS NODOSA

Symptoms	Percent of patients
Malaise/weakness	13
Abdominal pain	12
Leg pain	12
Neurologic signs/symptoms	10
Fever	8
Cough	8
Myalgias	5
Peripheral neuropathy	5
Headache	5
Arthritis/arthralgia	4
Skin involvement	4
Painful arms	4
Painful feet	4

From Cupps TR and Fauci AS (1982).

mononeuritis multiplex, but there may also be a diffuse sensorimotor peripheral neuropathy. Both forms of neuropathy are attributed to ischemia effected by the arteritis of nutrient vessels.

Damage to cerebral arteries may lead to thrombosis or hemorrhage; spinal syndromes are exceptional. The most common manifestations of cerebral involvement are headache, convulsions, blurred vision, vertigo, sudden loss of vision in one eye, and confusional states or organic psychosis.

A disorder characterized by keratitis and deafness in nonsyphilitic individuals is called the *Cogan syndrome*. It occurs predominantly in young adults with negative blood and cerebrospinal fluid (CSF) tests for syphilis and no stigmata of congenital syphilis. The cause of the keratitis and deafness is not known, but in some cases, the syndrome was one feature of polyarteritis nodosa. Symptoms begin suddenly, involving the cornea and both divisions of the eighth nerve. The eye and the eighth nerve are usually involved simultaneously, but there may be weeks or months between the onset of symptoms in the eye and the ear. Involvement of the eighth nerve is usually signaled by nausea, vomiting, tinnitus, and loss of hearing. With progression of the hearing loss to complete deafness, the vestibular symptoms subside.

Laboratory Data

There is a leukocytosis with an inconstant eosinophilia. Nontreponemal serologic tests for syphilis may be positive, and there may be positive skin and serologic tests for trichinosis. CSF is normal unless there has been a meningeal hemorrhage.

Diagnosis

Diagnosis of polyarteritis nodosa should be considered in all patients with an obscure febrile illness with systemic symptoms and chronic peripheral neuropathy. The diagnosis can often be established by biopsy of sural nerve, muscle, or testicle.

Course and Prognosis

Prognosis is poor. Death usually occurs because of lesions of the kidneys, other abdominal viscera, or the heart; occasionally, lesions in the brain or peripheral nerves may cause death. Duration of life after onset of symptoms varies from a few months to several years. Spontaneous healing of the arteritis may occur and is followed by remission of all symptoms and signs, including those due to involvement of the peripheral nerves.

Treatment

There is no specific therapy. Treatment is chiefly supportive, including blood transfusions and symptomatic therapy for associated conditions. Corticosteroids may be of temporary benefit in some cases.

TEMPORAL ARTERITIS AND POLYMYALGIA RHEUMATICA (GIANT CELL ARTERITIS)

Temporal arteritis and polymyalgia rheumatica are inextricably linked because they overlap in clinical features, high erythrocyte sedimentation rate (ESR), pathology in the temporal artery (giant cell arteritis), course, and response to steroid therapy. Both affect people older than age 50, and dominant features include malaise and myalgia. The major difference is the prominent headache in temporal arteritis and the threat of visual loss. However, temporal artery biopsy may be positive in patients who lack the cranial symptoms. It is not clear whether the two syndromes are slightly different manifestations of the same etiology and pathogenesis or there are two separate conditions with overlapping manifestations. Doppler studies may provide a noninvasive mode of diagnosis, but sensitivity and specificity must be assessed.

The lesions are characterized by the presence of activated CD4+ T cells, macrophages that produce transforming growth factor-β, and absence of B cells. If temporal artery biopsy samples are implanted in severe combined immunodeficiency mice, patterns suggest that persistence of the transforming growth factor-β macrophages accounts for the chronicity of disease and that steroid therapy suppresses the function of these cells as assessed by histology and also by interleukin production.

TEMPORAL ARTERITIS

This syndrome was first described by Horton in 1934. The pathology is similar to that of periarteritis nodosa except that the inflammatory reaction is more severe and there are more multinucleated giant cells in the media (*giant cell arteritis*). It is usually restricted to the temporal artery, but other vessels are sometimes affected. The syndrome occurs after age 50 equally in men and women.

It is said to occur exclusively in whites and primarily those of Nordic descent. In Sweden, the incidence rate was 18.3 cases per 100,000 inhabitants over age 50. In Italy, the comparable figure was 6.9 per 100,000. The low frequency in blacks parallels the distribution of HLA-DR4.

The pathogenesis is uncertain. Immune complexes are not found consistently, and it is thought that local T cells are activated, many bearing receptors for interleukin-2. There is also evidence, however, of depletion of circulating T-suppressor CD8

cells, implying a general abnormality of immune function. Also, the antigen is unknown.

Symptoms include headache, which is typically centered on the affected temporal artery but may be more generalized. Systemic symptoms include malaise, fever, anorexia, weight loss, and myalgia. The ESR is almost always above 50 mm/hr. The affected temporal artery may be prominent, nodular, tender, and noncompressible. Unilateral visual loss, found in 14% to 33% of patients in different series, is attributed to occlusion of the central retinal artery. The disk may appear pale, normal, or swollen with retinal hemorrhages. Ophthalmoparesis may be prominent, but other cranial nerve palsies are uncommon. Coronary and limb arteries are sometimes affected. Cerebral symptoms are mostly those of cerebral infarction, which is seen in few cases. However, it is also one of the rare forms of *reversible dementia*.

Diagnosis is simple when all typical findings are present. The ESR, however, may not be elevated, and the temporal artery biopsy specimen may be normal in otherwise typical cases. The diagnosis should be considered whenever a person older than 50 begins to have new headaches, unilateral visual loss, or ophthalmoparesis. Diagnosis is then made by the high ESR or typical findings on biopsy. Typical abnormalities on temporal artery biopsy are diagnostic because inflammatory cells are not seen at autopsy of control subjects. If the clinical picture includes headache, jaw claudication, and myalgia with high ESR, it is more likely that the biopsy will support the diagnosis, but not always. It is difficult to substantiate the diagnosis if clinical manifestations are not typical and the ESR or biopsy is normal.

It is now difficult to determine the natural history because the threat of visual loss leads to steroid treatment as soon as the diagnosis is made; it is truly emergency treatment. It is difficult to justify a placebo-controlled trial under these circumstances. However, it is believed that the disease is self-limited, lasting months or a year or two. In the past, when daily prednisone doses were about 60 mg, few patients could stop steroid therapy. In the 1980s, the dose gradually dropped without losing efficacy. The adverse effects of steroid therapy are dose and duration dependent; with "standard" doses, at least a third of the patients had serious adverse effects of steroids. With maintenance doses of 5 to 10 mg prednisone, the frequency of side effects is much less, and therapy can often be discontinued in 6 to 12 months. In the past decade, the recommended starting dose has dropped from 60 mg daily to 20 to 40 mg daily.

Taylor and Samanta recommend a starting dose of 40 mg daily if there has been no visual loss. They reduce the dose by 10 mg/day each month for 3 months, then from 20 to 10 mg daily over another 3 months, and slower tapering thereafter. If vision is already affected, the dose is 60 to 80 mg daily, and some add 250 mg hydrocortisone intravenously if vision has already been affected; there is no evidence that these higher doses are more effective. In the only controlled trial of steroids and cyclophosphamide, neither was superior.

Early steroid therapy seems to prevent the most feared consequence of temporal arteritis, loss of vision. If therapy is started when one eye is affected, vision in the other eye is protected. If vision has already been lost, chances of recovery are low. Aiello et al. (1993) found that 34 of 245 patients (14%) lost vision; in 32 of them, the visual loss occurred before steroid therapy commenced.

The mortality rate is low, and most deaths that do occur are encountered in the first 4 months of the disease.

POLYMYALGIA RHEUMATICA

This condition is defined by the combination of myalgia, malaise, weight loss, and increased ESR in a person older than 50. In many patients, temporal artery biopsy shows the changes of temporal arteritis, even if there is no headache or other symptomatic indication that cranial vessels are affected. The threat of visual loss is lower if there are no cranial symptoms, but the similarities require the same steroid therapy.

The symptoms of polymyalgia rheumatica are nonspecific and could be reproduced by someone with an occult malignant tumor. It becomes a matter of clinical judgment to decide whether there is time for a diagnostic therapeutic trial of steroid therapy (as described for temporal arteritis) with or without search for the possible tumor. The other major consideration in differential diagnosis is *polymyositis*. In polymyalgia, however, there is no limb weakness, serum levels of creatine kinase are normal, and there are no myopathic changes in muscle biopsy or electromyography; if any of these tests gave abnormal results, the syndrome would be indistinguishable from polymyositis.

Treatment is the same as for temporal arteritis, but there may be more consistent symptomatic relief with even smaller doses of prednisolone, 15 to 20 mg daily, dropping to 10 mg daily by 3 months. The long-term outlook is excellent, but there are recurrences in some patients.

ANTINEURONAL CYTOPLASMIC AUTOANTIBODY-POSITIVE GRANULOMATOUS GIANT CELL ARTERITIS: CHURG-STRAUSS SYNDROME AND WEGENER GRANULOMATOSIS

The arterial lesions in these rare syndromes differ from those of periarteritis in that granuloma formation is more prominent, and they may be more necrotizing. There are other differences. For instance, eosinophilia and asthma define the *Churg-Strauss syndrome*. Sensorimotor neuropathy is seen in about 70% of patients and, sometimes, visual loss. *Microscopic polyangiitis* resembles periarteritis nodosa clinically and neurologically but affects smaller vessels, especially in the kidneys and lungs (Table 155.5).

Wegener granulomatosis has a predilection for the respiratory system and kidneys. According to criteria of the American Academy of Rheumatology, the diagnosis can be made if there are two of the following four criteria: oral ulcers or purulent bloody nasal discharge; abnormal chest film showing nodules, fixed infiltrates, or cavities; microhematuria; and biopsy evidence of granulomatous inflammation in the wall of an artery or perivascular tissue. "Limited" Wegemer disease shows the typical pathology but spares lungs and kidney. Ninety percent of typical Wegener patients are ANCA positive; 50% to 80% have the C-ANCA pattern with anti-proteinase 3, and 10% to 18% show the P-ANCA pattern with anti-myeloperoxidase. Neurologic manifestations, as in other vasculitis syndromes, more often indicate a sensorimotor peripheral neuropathy than a CNS syndrome. The disease was once thought to be uniformly fatal, but survival is reported with modern immunosuppressive therapy, including cyclophosphamide.

GRANULOMATOUS ANGIITIS OF THE BRAIN

In one form of granulomatous angiitis, clinical manifestations are restricted to the brain. Thus, this is appropriately called *granulomatous angiitis of the brain* (GAB). In a few cases, the spinal cord is similarly affected, alone or with cerebral lesions. Therefore, the more comprehensive term is *granulomatous angiitis of the nervous system* (GANS). This disorder is essentially defined by the characteristic histologic lesion, a granulomatous change that includes multinucleated giant cells; it is seen in small or larger named cerebral blood vessels.

Lesions of this nature are found in some patients with clinical evidence of a cerebral infarct ipsilateral to herpes zoster ophthalmicus. Otherwise, there is no clinical clue to the nature of the disease. A few patients have had evidence of immunosuppression with sarcoidosis, Hodgkin disease, or acquired immunodeficiency syndrome.

After herpes zoster, the clinical manifestations may be those of an uncomplicated stroke, with severe or mild manifestations in different cases. When there is no evidence of zosterian infection, the symptoms include two invariable but nonspecific sets, focal cerebral signs and mental obtundation, which may be preceded by dementia. The course is subacute, so this can be regarded as a progressive encephalopathy.

Characteristically, there is CSF pleocytosis, up to 500 mononuclear cells per high-power field. CSF protein content is

TABLE 155.5. FREQUENCY OF MANIFESTATIONS IN SMALL-VESSEL VASCULITIS (PERCENT OF PATIENTS)

Organ	Cryoglobulin vasculitis	Microscopic polyarteritis	Wegener granumoatosus	Churg-Strauss syndrome
Cutaneous	90	40	40	60
Renal	55	90	80	45
Pulmonary	<5	50	90	70
Ear, Nose, Throat	<5	35	90	60
Musculoskeletal	70	60	60	50
Neurologic	40	30	50	70
Gastrointestinal	30	50	50	50

Modified from Jennette and Falk (1997).

usually increased, exceeding 100 mg/dL in 75% of cases, but CSF glucose content is normal.

There has been doubt about the necessity or desirability of brain biopsy for diagnosis. Advocates believe that pathologic proof is needed and that the risks of meningeal biopsy are about 1%. On the other hand, the risks of immunotherapy are much higher and may be given for an erroneous diagnosis. Analyzing 30 biopsies for presumed GANS, Goldstein and associates found that 50% had some other disease. Moreover, angiographic evidence of arteritis is unreliable when "positive" and is absent in most cases of histologically proven granulomatous angiitis of the brain.

Others contend that a negative biopsy does not exclude the diagnosis and believe that sufficient evidence is given by angiographic "beading" of arteries. Cases so diagnosed have been treated with cyclophosphamide, and, if the outcome was favorable, the authors concluded that the likely catastrophic outcome had been averted. In autopsy-proven cases, however, the arteriogram is usually normal or shows evidence of an infarct or local tissue swelling but not beading. Moreover, the clinical, arteriographic, and CSF manifestations can be caused by infiltration of meninges by tumor cells or viral infection; beading of cerebral arteries is a nonspecific finding.

These different perspectives can be seen in a comparison of series defined by pathologic diagnosis (the "neurologist's view") or by cerebral angiography and pathology (the "rheumatologist's view") (Table 155.5). Neurologists do not consider diagnosis by arteriography reliable because beading is found in only 10% of pathologically proven cases. Strokes are found in only 15%. In contrast to arteriographic diagnosis, pathologic diagnosis leads to a reasonably consistent picture: encephalopathy (obtundation, cognitive loss); headache; onset over days or weeks, not apoplectic; and CSF protein content greater than 100 mg/dL.

Other problems of diagnosis include subacute bacterial, yeast, or neoplastic meningitis; these conditions are more likely if CSF glucose content is less than 40 mg/dL, and if the glucose content is normal, CSF cytology is needed. GAB may simulate prion disease by causing severe dementia within a few weeks. If GAB produces a mass lesion, brain biopsy makes the distinction from tumor. The diagnosis of GANS implies myelopathy, which is difficult to diagnose in life unless there is concomitant evidence of herpes zoster or sarcoid.

The neurologists' consensus is that diagnosis in living patients can be verified only by a brain biopsy that includes meningeal vessels. In histologically proven cases (without zoster), the outcome has been fatal in most cases within a few years. About half the patients die within 6 weeks, but a third live longer than 1 year after onset. Treatment with immunosuppressive drugs has not been effective in most proven cases, but control of GAB has been documented in patients with biopsy-proven GAB who were treated with immunosuppression, died later, and had no autopsy evidence of lingering inflammation; two of those patients also had amyloid angiopathy.

SYSTEMIC LUPUS ERYTHEMATOSUS

Systemic lupus erythematosus (SLE) is characterized by widespread inflammatory change in the connective tissue (collagen) of the skin and systemic organs. The primary damage is to the subendothelial connective tissue of capillaries, small arteries, and veins; the endocardium; and the synovial and serous membranes.

Etiology and Incidence

The cause is not known, but immune complexes are deposited in small vessels. The initiating event could be a persistent viral infection, but sometimes serologic and clinical manifestations follow administration of drugs, such as procainamide. Although rare, the incidence may be increasing. Most cases begin between ages 20 and 40, but the disease may be seen in children. Some 95% of adult patients are women.

Symptoms and Signs

The chief clinical manifestations are prolonged irregular fever, with remissions of variable duration (weeks, months, or even years); erythematous rash; recurrent attacks with evidence of involvement of synovial and serous membranes (polyarthritis, pleuritis, pericarditis); depression of bone marrow function (leukopenia, hypochromic anemia, moderate thrombocytopenia); and, in advanced stages, clinical evidence of vascular alteration in the skin, kidneys, and other viscera.

Neurologic manifestations can be divided into several major categories. The most common form, affecting up to 25% of all patients with SLE, is *cerebral lupus*, an encephalopathy manifest by seizures, psychosis, dementia, chorea, or cranial nerve disorder. SLE is one of the few remaining causes of chorea in young women. Other neurologic syndromes are transverse myelopathy, sensorimotor peripheral neuropathy, and polymyositis (Table 155.6). These symptoms are often attributed to thrombosis of small vessels or petechial hemorrhages. Microinfarcts may be related to fibrinoid degeneration of small vessels with deposition of antibodies to a platelet membrane glycoprotein. The same neurologic symptoms are encountered in pediatric lupus.

Evidence of cerebral vasculitis is meager. The cause of cerebral symptoms is not known but they are attributed to mixed pathogenesis: antineuronal antibodies of unknown type, microvascular occlusions from vasculitis, antiphospholipid antibodies, and noninflammatory vasculopathy. Although strokes are a feature of the "antiphospholipid syndrome," there is little evidence they are responsible for cerebral lupus. Antibodies to ribosomal protein P are said to be highly specific for cerebral lupus but of poor sensitivity, found in only 20% of patients.

Stroke caused by occlusion of large cerebral vessels is distinctly uncommon. In 1994, Mitsias and Levine found only 30 reported cases, and they were due to diverse mechanisms, including thrombus, dissection, fibromuscular dysplasia, vasculitis, and premature atherosclerosis. The short-term death rate was 40%, and recurrences occurred in 13% of the survivors. Venous sinus thrombosis is also recognized. In general, little information has been provided by brain imaging of any kind, including positron emission tomography and single-photon emission computed tomography.

The cause of cerebral lupus is therefore uncertain. In some cases, cerebral emboli arise from endocarditis or thrombotic thrombocytopenia.

TABLE 155.6. COMPARISON OF TWO CONCEPTS OF GRANULOMATOSIS ANGIITIS OF THE BRAIN: DIAGNOSIS BY HISTOPATHOLOGY OR ARTERIOGRAPHY

	Mode of diagnosis	
	Pathology[a]	Pathology or arteriography[b]
Reference	58	54
Number of patients	78	48
Clinical features		
Onset	"Days or weeks"	"Typically sudden"
Mental changes	61 (78%)	13 (27)
Headache	42 (53%)	28 (58)
Coma	42 (53%)	3 (6)
Focal weakness (hemiparesis)	33 (42%)	17 (35)
Clinical stroke	12 (15%)	
Seizures	18 (23%)	6 (13)
Fever	16 (20%)	5 (10)
Aphasia	10 (12%)	7 (15)
Altered vision	9 (11%)	6 (13)
Quadriparesis or paraparesis (spinal)	8 (10%)	5 (10)
Fatal	68 (87%)	27/38 (71)
Laboratory findings		
CSF examination		
WBC < 3	17/55 (30)	12/40 (30)
3–250	38/55 (69)	28/40 (70)
50–250	24/55 (43)	—
Protein normal	9/55 (16)	12/40 (30)
50–600	39/55 (70)	28/40 (70)
> 100	25/55 (45)	—
CT		
Normal	4/11 (36)	—
Enhancing mass	3/11 (27)	—
Infarct	3/11 (27)	—
Hematoma	1/11 (9)	—
Angiography		
Normal	13/33 (39)	4/31 (13)
Avascular mass	6/33 (18)	—
Diffuse narrowing	5/33 (15)	—
Other abnormality	—	6/31 (19)
Beading	3/33 (9)	20/31 (65)
Brain biopsy		
Normal	4/20 (20)	—
Diagnostic	10/20 (50)	4/14 (29)
Not diagnostic	6/20 (30)	4/14 (29)
Autopsy diagnostic	64/74 (86)	26/48 (54)

[a]Data from Younger et al. (1988).
[b]Data from Calabrese and Mallek (1988).
CSI, Cerebrospinal fluid; WBC, white blood cell count.
From Rowland LP. *Merritt's textbook of neurology, update 12.* Philadelphia: Lea & Febiger, 1992.

Laboratory Data

In addition to anemia and leukopenia, there is often hematuria or proteinuria, signs of renal damage. Biologic false-positive tests for syphilis may be encountered. The most important diagnostic test is the search for *antinuclear antibodies* (ANA), especially antibodies to double-stranded DNA, which are also used as a measure of activity of the disease. Antibodies to a particular antigen ("Sm" for Smith) may be found more often in patients with cerebral disease. Although not used often these days, phagocytic polymorphonuclear leukocytes (*LE cells*) are found in 80% of all cases and

are considered pathognomonic by some authorities. Serum complement levels may be decreased in patients with renal disease; deposits of globulin and complement may be found in renal biopsy specimens. CSF is usually normal, but there may be a modest increase in protein content. For reasons not known, the CSF glucose content is often decreased in SLE patients with myelitis.

Computed tomography and magnetic resonance imaging show nonspecific changes in cerebral lupus. Positron emission tomography may show lesions in brain in SLE patients with normal magnetic resonance imaging; functional abnormality may precede structural abnormality.

Diagnosis

Diagnosis may be difficult. Fever; weight loss; arthritis; anemia; leukopenia; pleuritis; and cardiac, renal, or neurologic symptoms in a young woman should lead to a consideration of this diagnosis. An erythematous rash on the bridge of the nose and the malar eminences in a butterfly-like distribution facilitates the diagnosis. Finding LE cells or ANA in the blood is of value in establishing the diagnosis. Neurologic manifestations are only rarely the first manifestation of SLE, but the diagnosis should be kept in mind when there is an acute encephalopathy in a young woman. Acute psychosis in a woman with known SLE may be due to the disease or the effects of steroid therapy, which may be difficult to unravel.

Mixed connective tissue disease is an overlap syndrome with features of SLE, systemic sclerosis, and polymyositis. At first, there seemed to be an association with antibodies to ribonucleoprotein, but the specificity disappeared. Also, polymyositis can be a manifestation of any collagen-vascular or vasculitis syndrome, with little specificity. It is primarily systemic sclerosis that overlaps with both SLE and dermatomyositis. For instance, the multisystem disease described in Case Record 24-1995 may show polymyositis, with evidence of SLE (rash more like that of SLE than that of dermatomyositis) and high titer of ANA, and features of systemic sclerosis (esophageal dysmotility, Raynaud phenomenon, and severe lung disease), but no skin lesions of scleroderma. SLE patients may also show features of rheumatoid arthritis or Sjögren syndrome. It seems unlikely that mixed connective tissue disease is a unique condition, but the multisystem diseases are a diagnostic and therapeutic challenge.

Course, Prognosis, and Therapy

Cerebral lupus is a medical catastrophe with poor prognosis. Recommendations include intravenous doses of methylprednisolone (1 g daily for 3 days), followed by low-dose oral prednisolone. Some authorities add intravenous cyclophosphamide in the initial treatment. Plasmapheresis has not been established as beneficial, and intravenous immunoglobulin therapy is still experimental. Cases are so few and the disease is so devastating that it has been difficult to carry out a therapeutic trial.

Treatment is equally uncertain for the less-threatening syndromes of peripheral neuropathy, myelitis, or polymyositis. Steroid therapy is the accepted treatment but not established by therapeutic trial. In the long run, death may result from renal failure or infection.

OTHER COLLAGEN-VASCULAR DISEASES

Neurologic syndromes may complicate other collagen-vascular diseases, usually when the systemic disorder is evident. Sometimes, there are characteristic syndromes. For instance, an aggressive polyneuropathy may be seen in patients with rheumatoid arthritis. Some clinicians believe the neuropathy may be precipitated by steroid therapy. Another neurologic syndrome of rheumatoid arthritis is atlantoaxial dislocation with resulting cord compression; the syndrome is attributed to resorption of the odontoid process.

Sjögren syndrome is defined clinically by internationally accepted criteria. There must be at least two of the following: xerostomia (dry mouth), which can be documented by scintigraphy; xerophthalmia (dry eyes; pathologic documentation of abnormality in salivary gland biopsy); or keratoconjunctivitis sicca, as demonstrated by the *Shirmer test* for tear production. Lip biopsy may show sialoadenitis. If the neurologic manifestations dominate, the term "sicca complex" has been used. Sensorimotor peripheral neuropathy (primarily sensory or sensorimotor) and polymyositis are the most common neurologic manifestations. Sjögren disease is one of the causes of trigeminal sensory neuropathy. CNS complications are rare, but venous sinus thrombosis, myelopathy, a form of motor neuron disease, or aseptic meningitis is seen. The origin of the neuropathy is not known. Antineuronal antibodies have been found in some cases. Treatment, as usual in these diseases, focuses on steroids in uncontrolled trials.

In Sjögren syndrome, peripheral neuropathy and polymyositis may be prominent. Peripheral neuropathy is also seen in more than half the patients with the idiopathic hypereosinophilic syndrome, and there may be evidence of vasculitis in the nerve biopsy.

SUGGESTED READINGS

General

Cupps TR, Fauci AS. The vasculitic syndromes. *Adv Intern Med* 1982;27:315–344.

Jennette JC, Falk RJ. Small-vessel vasculitis. *N Engl J Med* 1997; 337:1512–1523.

Jennette JC, Falk RJ, Andrassy K, et al. Nomenclature of systemic vasculitides:proposal of an international consensus conference. *Arthritis Rheum* 1994;37:187–192.

Olney RK. Neuropathies associated with connective tissue disease. *Semin Neurol* 1998;18:63–72.

Savage COS, Harper L, Adu D. Primary systemic vasculitis. *Lancet* 1997;349:553–558.

Polyarteritis Nodosa

Bicknell JM, Holland JV. Neurologic manifestations of Cogan syndrome. *Neurology* 1978;28:278–281.

Ford RG, Siekert RG. Central nervous system manifestations of periarteritis nodosa. *Neurology* 1965;15:114–122.

Gayraud M, Guillevin L, Cohen P, et al. Treatment of good-prognosis polyarteritis nodosa and Churg-Strauss syndrome: comparison of steroids and oral or pulse cyclophosphamide in 25 patients. French Cooperative Study Group for Vasculitides. *Br J Rheumatol* 1997;36:1290–1297.

Lande A, Rossi P. The value of total aortography in diagnosis of Takayasu arteritis. *Radiology* 1975;114:287–297.

Lovelace RE. Mononeuritis multiplex in polyarteritis nodosa. *Neurology* 1964;14:434–442.

Moore PM, Cupps TR. Neurological complications of vasculitis. *Ann Neurol* 1983;14:155–167.

Oren S, Besbas N, Saatci U, et al. Diagnostic criteria for polyarteritis nodosa in childhood. *J Pediatr* 1992;120:206–209.

Rose AG, Sinclair-Smith CC. Takayasu's arteritis? A study of 16 autopsy cases. *Arch Pathol Lab Med* 1980;104:231–234.

Wicki J, Olivieri J, Pizzolato G, et al. Successful treatment of polyarteritis nodosa related to hepatitis B virus with a combination of lamivudine and interferon alpha. *Rheumatology (Oxford)* 1999;38:183–185.

Temporal Arteritis and Polymyalgia Rheumatica

Aiello PD, Traumann JC, McPhee TJ, et al. Visual prognosis in giant cell arteritis. *Ophthalmology* 1993;100:550–555.

Andersson R, Malmvall BE, Bengtsson BA. Long-term survival in giant cell arteritis including temporal arteritis and polymyalgia rheumatica. *Acta Med Scand* 1986;220:361–364.

Barricks ME, Traviesa DB, Glaser JS, Levy IS. Ophthalmoplegia in cranial arteritis. *Brain* 1977;100:209–221.

Black A, Rittner HL, Younge BR, Kaltschmidt C, Weyand C, Goronzy JJ. Glucocorticoid-mediated repression of cytokine gene transcription in human arteritis-SCID chimeras. *J Clin Invest* 1997;99:2842–2850.

Brack A, Martinez-Taboada V, Stanson A, Goronzy JJ, Weyand CM Disease pattern in cranial and large-vessel giant cell arteritis. *Arthritis Rheum* 1999;42:311–317.

Brooks RC, McGee SR. Diagnostic dilemmas in polymyalgia rheumatica. *Arch Intern Med* 1997;157:162–168.

Caselli RJ, Hunder GG, Whisnant JP. Neurologic disease in biopsy-proven giant cell (temporal) arteritis. *Neurology* 1988;38:352–357.

Cullen JF, Coleiro JA. Ophthalmic complications of giant cell arteritis. *Surv Ophthalmol* 1976;20:247–260.

Duhaut P, Pinede L, Bornet H, et al. Biopsy proven and biopsy negative temporal arteritis: differences in clinical spectrum at the onset of the disease. *Ann Rheum Dis* 1999;58:335–341.

Grodum E, Petersen HA. Temporal arteritis with normal erythrocyte sedimentation rate. *J Intern Med* 1990;227:279–280.

Hall S, Hunder CC. Is temporal artery biopsy prudent? *Mayo Clin Proc* 1984;59:309–314.

Hamilton CR Jr, Shelley WM, Tumulty PA. Giant cell arteritis: including temporal arteritis and polymyalgia rheumatica. *Medicine (Baltimore)* 1971;50:1–27.

Hauser WA, Ferguson RH, Holley KE, et al. Temporal arteritis in Rochester, Minnesota. *Mayo Clin Proc* 1981;46:597–602.

Healy LA. On the epidemiology of polymyalgia rheumatica and temporal arteritis. *J Rheumatol* 1993;20:1639–1640.

Heathcote JG. Update in pathology: temporal arteritis and its ocular manifestations. *Can J Ophthalmol* 1999;34:63–68.

Horton BT, Magath TB, Brown GE. Arteritis of the temporal vessels. *Arch Intern Med* 1934;53:400–409.

Hunder GG, Weyand CM. Sonography in giant-cell arteritis. *N Engl J Med* 1997;337:1385–1386.

Kyle V, Hazleman BL. Treatment of polymyalgia rheumatica and giant cell arteritis. II. Relation between steroid dose and steroid-associated side effects. *Ann Rheum Dis* 1989;48:662–666.

Kyle V, Hazleman BL. Stopping steroids in polymyalgia rheumatica and giant cell arteritis. Treatment usually lasts for two to five years. *BMJ* 1990;300:344–345.

Lundberg J, Hedfors E. Restricted dose and duration of corticosteroid treatment in patients with polymyalgia rheumatica and temporal arteritis. *J Rheumatol* 1990;17:1340–1345.

Matheson EL, Gold KN, Bock DA, Hunder GG. Long-term survival of patients with giant cell arteritis in the American College of Rheumatology giant cell arteritis classification criteria cohort. *Am J Med* 1996; 100:193–196.

Redlich FC. A new medical diagnosis of Adolf Hitler. Giant cell arteritis-temporal arteritis. *Arch Intern Med* 1993;153:693–697.

Samantray SK. Takayasu arteritis: 45 cases. *Aust N Z J Med* 1978;8:68–73.

Taylor HG, Samanta A. Treatment of vasculitis. *Br J Clin Pharmacol* 1993;35:93–104.

Vilaseca J, Gonzalez A, Cid MC, et al. Clinical usefulness of temporal artery biopsy. *Ann Rheum Dis* 1987;46:282–285.

ANCA-Positive Vasculitis

Case Records of the Massachusetts General Hospital. Case 28-1998. Wegener granulomatosis. *N Engl J Med* 1998;339:755–763.

Case Records of the Massachusetts General Hospital. Case 9-1999. Wegener granulomatosis with pachymeningeal granulomatous inflammation. *N Engl J Med* 1998;340:945–953.

Chumbley LC, Harrison EG, DeRemee RA. Allergic granulomatosis and angiitis (Churge-Strauss syndrome): 30 cases. *Mayo Clin Proc* 1977;52:477–484.

Green RL, Vayonis AG. Churg-Strauss syndrome after zafirklast in two patients not receiving systemic steroid treatment. *Lancet* 1999;353:725–726.

Marazzi R, Pareyson D, Boardi A, et al. Peripheral nerve involvement in Churg-Strauss syndrome. *J Neurol* 1992;239:317–321.

Nishino H, Rubino FA, DeRenee RA, et al. Neurological involvement in Wegener's granulomatosis; analysis of 324 consecutive patients at the Mayo Clinic. *Ann Neurol* 1993;33:4–9.

Tahmoush AJ, Liu JE, Amir MS, Heiman-Patterson T. Myopathy, antineutrophil cytoplasmic antibodies, and glomerulonephritis. *Muscle Nerve* 1995;18:475–477.

Granulomatous Giant Cell Arteritis

Berlitt P. Clinical and laboratory findings with giant cell arteritis. *J Neurol Sci* 1992;111:1–12.

Börnke C, Hays N, Büttner T. Rapidly progressive dementia. *Lancet* 1999:353:1150.

Cupps TR, Moore PM, Fauci AS. Isolated angiitis of the central nervous system. Prospective diagnostic and therapeutic experience. *Am J Med* 1983;74:97–105.

Gilden DH, Kleinschmidt-DeMasters BK, Wellish M, Hedley-Whyte ET, Rentier B, Mahalingam R. Varicella zoster virus, a cause of waxing and waning vasculitis: the New England Journal of Medicine case 51995 revisited. *Neurology* 1996;47:1441–1446.

Hawke SH, Davies L, Pamphlett A, et al. Vasculitis neuropathy. A clinical and pathological study. *Brain* 1991;114:2175–2190.

Sigal LH. The neurologic presentation of vasculitic and rheumatologic syndromes. A review. *Medicine (Baltimore)* 1987;66:157–180.

Granulomatous Angiitis of the Brain

Calabrese LH, Mallek JA. Primary angiitis of the central nervous system; report of 8 new cases, review of the literature, and proposal for diagnostic criteria. *Medicine (Baltimore)* 1988;67:20–39.

Chu CT, Gray LT, Goldstein LB, Hulette CM. Diagnosis of intracranial vasculitis: a multidisciplinary approach. *J Neuropathol Exp Neurol* 1998;57:30–38.

Fountain NB, Lopes MBS. Control of primary angiitis of the CNS associated with cerebral amyloid angiopathy by cyclophosphamide alone. *Neurology* 1999;52:660–662.

Greenan TJ, Grossman RI, Goldberg HI. Cerebral vasculitis: MR imaging and angiographic correlation. *Radiology* 1992;182:65–72.

Hankey GJ. Isolated angiitis/angiopathy of the central nervous system. *Cerebrovasc Dis* 1991;1:2–15.

Harris KG, Tran DD, Sickels WJ, et al. Diagnosing intracranial vasculitis: the roles of MR and angiography. *AJNR* 1994;15:317–330.

Moore PM. Central nervous system vasculitis. *Curr Opin Neurol* 1998;11:241–246.

Riemer G, Lamaszus K, Zschbar R, Freitag HJ, Eggers C, Pfeiffer G. Isolated angiitis of the central nervous system: lack of inflammation after long-term treatment. *Neurology* 1999;52:196–199.

Rowland LP. The need for reliable diagnostic laboratory tests: problems in clinical diagnosis illustrated by inclusion body myositis, granulomatous angiitis of the brain, and the stiff-man syndrome (Moersch-Woltman syndrome). In Rowland LP, ed.: *Merritt's textbook of neurology*, 8th ed. Philadelphia: Lea & Febiger, 1992.

Wolfenden AB, Teng DC, Marks MP, Ali AO, Albers GW. Angiographically defined primary angiitis of the CNS: is it really benign? *Neurology* 1998;51:183–185.

Younger DS, Hays AP, Brust JCM, et al. Granulomatous angiitis of the brain: an inflammatory reaction of diverse etiology. *Arch Neurol* 1988;45:514–518.

Systemic Lupus Erythematosus

Asherson RA, Lubbe WF. Cerebral and valve lesions in SLE: association with antiphospholipid antibodies. *J Rheumatol* 1988;15:539–543.

Boumpas DT, Scott DE, Balow JE. Neuropsychiatric lupus: a case for guarded optimism. *J Rheumatol* 1993;20:1641–1643.

Cabral AR, Alacron-Segovia D. Autoantibodies in systemic lupus erythematosus. *Curr Opin Rheumatol* 1997;8:403–407.

Case Records of the Massachusetts General Hospital. Case 24-1995. Mixed connective tissue disease. *N Engl J Med* 1995;333:369–377.

Devinsky O, Petito CK, Alonso DR. Clinical and neuropathological findings in systemic lupus erythematosus: the role of vasculitis, heart emboli, and thrombotic thrombocytopenic purpura. *Ann Neurol* 1988;23:380–384.

Ellison D, Gatter K, Heryet A, et al. Intramural platelet deposition in cerebral vasculopathy of systemic lupus erythematosus. *J Clin Pathol* 1993;46:37–40.

Eustace S, Hutchinson M, Bresnihan B. Acute cerebrovascular episodes in systemic lupus erythematosus. *Q J Med* 1991;293:739–750.

Feinglass EJ, Arnett FC, Dorsch CA. Neuropsychiatric manifestations of systemic lupus erythematosus: diagnosis, clinical spectrum, and relationship to other features of the disease. *Medicine (Baltimore)* 1976;55:323–339.

Friedman SD, Stidley CA, Brooks WM, Hart BL, Sibbitt WL Jr. Brain injury and neurometabolic abnormalities in systemic lupus erythematosus. *Radiology* 1998;209:79–84.

Haris EN, Pierangeli S. Antiphospholipid antibodies and cerebral lupus. *Ann N Y Acad Sci* 1997;823:270–278.

Johnson RT, Richardson EP. The neurological manifestations of systemic lupus erythematosus. *Medicine (Baltimore)* 1968;47:337–369.

McLean BN. Neurological involvement in systemic lupus erythematosus. *Curr Opin Neurol* 1998;11:247–251.

Mitchell I, Hughes RAC, Maidey M, et al. Cerebral lupus. *Lancet* 1994;343:579–582.

Mukerji B, Hardin JG. Undifferentiated, overlapping, and mixed connective tissue diseases. *Am J Med Sci* 1993;305:114–119.

Penn AS, Rowan AJ. Myelopathy in systemic lupus erythematosus. *Arch Neurol* 1968;18:337–349.

Prockop LD. Myotonia, procaine amide, and lupus-like syndrome. *Arch Neurol* 1966;14:326–330.

Steinlin MI, Blaser SI, Gilday DL, et al. Neurologic manifestations of pediatric systemic lupus erythematosus. *Pediatr Neurol* 1995;13:191–197.

Strand V. Approaches to the management of systemic lupus erythematosus. *Curr Opin Rheumatol* 1996;9:410–420.

Wong KL, Woo EK, Yu YL, et al. Neurological manifestations of systemic lupus erythematosus: a prospective study. *Q J Med* 1991;88:857–870.

Sjögren Syndrome and Sicca Complex

Alexander EL, Ranzenbach AJ, Kumar AJ, et al. Anti-Ro(SS-A) autoantibodies in central nervous system disease associated with Sjögren's syndrome (CNS-SS): clinical, neuroimaging, and angiographic correlates. *Neurology* 1994;44:899–908.

Fox RI, Robinson CA, Curd JG, et al. Sjögren's syndrome. Proposed criteria for classification. *Arthritis Rheum* 1986;29:577–585.

Hietaharju A, Yli-Kertutula U, Hakkinen V, et al. Nervous system manifestations in Sjögren's syndrome. *Acta Neurol Scand* 1990;81:144–152.

Katz JS, Houroupian D, Ross MA. Multisystem neuronal involvement and sicca complex: broadening the spectrum of complications. *Muscle Nerve* 1999;22:404–407.

Mausch E, Volk C, Kratzsch G, et al. Neurological and neuropsychiatric dysfunction in primary Sjögren's syndrome. *Acta Neurol Scand* 1994;89:31–35.

Mellgren SI, Conn DL, Stevens JC, Dyck PJ. Peripheral neuropathy in primary Sjögren's syndrome. *Neurology* 1989;39:390–394.

Moll JWB, Maarkusse HM, Pijnenburg JJJM, et al. Antineuronal antibodies in patients with neurologic complications of primary Sjögren's syndrome. *Neurology* 1993;43:2574–2581.

Vitali C, Bombardieri S, Moutsopoulos HM, et al. Preliminary criteria for the classification of Sjögren's syndrome. *Arthritis Rheum* 1993;36:340–347.

Wright RA, O'Duffy JD, Rodriguez M. Improvement of myelopathy in Sjögren's syndrome with chlorambucil and prednisone therapy. *Neurology* 1999;52:386–388.

Other Collagen-Vascular Diseases

Cogan DG. Syndrome of nonsyphilitic interstitial keratitis and vestibuloauditory symptoms. *Arch Ophthalmol* 1945;33:144–149.

Herrick AL. Advances in treatment of systemic sclerosis. *Lancet* 1998;352:1874–1875.

Kothare SV, Chu CC, VanLandingham K, Richards KC, Hosford DA, Radtke RA. Migratory leptomeningeal inflammation with relapsing polychondritis. *Neurology* 1998;51:614–617.

Krieg T, Meurer M. Systemic scleroderma: clinical and pathophysiologic aspects. *J Am Acad Dermatol* 1988;18:457–484.

Mikulowski P, Wolheim FA, Rotmil P, Olsen I. Sudden death in rheumatoid arthritis with atlanto-axial dislocation. *Acta Med Scand* 1975;198:445–451.

Moore PM, Harley JB, Fauci AS. Neurologic dysfunction in the idiopathic hypereosinophilic syndrome. *Ann Intern Med* 1985;102:109–114.

Sundaran MBM, Rajput AH. Nervous system complications of relapsing polychondritis. *Neurology* 1983;33:513–515.

Vollersten RS, Conn DL, Ballard DJ, et al. Rheumatoid vasculitis: survival and associated risk factors. *Medicine (Baltimore)* 1986;65:365–374.

Merritt's Neurology, 10th ed., edited by L.P. Rowland. Lippincott Williams & Wilkins, Philadelphia © 2000.

C H A P T E R

156

NEUROLOGIC DISEASE DURING PREGNANCY

ALISON M. PACK
MARTHA J. MORRELL

Pregnancy and the postpartum period are times of major biologic and social changes. Pregnancy may be associated with alterations in preexisting neurologic conditions, such as epilepsy or migraine, or herald the emergence of neurologic disorders such as peripheral nerve entrapment or a movement disorder. This chapter addresses the diagnosis, management, and treatment of neurologic disorders arising in or altered by pregnancy.

BIOLOGY OF PREGNANCY

Some physiologic changes during pregnancy may influence the expression of neurologic disease and complicate management. Alterations in neuroactive steroid hormones may influence the phenotypic appearance of the disease. Changes in pharmacokinetics, compliance, and sleep patterns may make disease management more challenging.

The concentration and type of circulating steroid hormones change during pregnancy. Estrogen production increases. In the nonpregnant state, the main circulating estrogens are estradiol, which is synthesized by ovarian thecal cells, and estrone, which is produced by the extraglandular conversion of androstenedione. Estriol is a peripheral metabolite of estrone and estradiol. In pregnancy, the concentrations of all these estrogens, particularly estriol, increase. As pregnancy progresses, maternal steroids and dihydroisoandrostene from developing fetal adrenal glands

are converted principally to estriol. Progesterone production also increases dramatically. These hormonal changes may affect neurologic conditions that are hormone-responsive, including migraine, epilepsy, and multiple sclerosis.

Drug pharmacokinetics are affected by the physiologic changes of pregnancy (Table 156.1). Renal blood flow and glomerular filtration increase as a function of increased cardiac output. Plasma volume, extravascular fluid, and adipose tissue increase to create a larger volume of distribution. Serum albumin decreases, which reduces drug-binding and increases drug clearance. These pharmacokinetic alterations may affect drug concentrations. The changes are most important for drugs that are highly protein bound, hepatically metabolized, or renally cleared.

Other events of pregnancy that may compromise management are hyperemesis gravidarum, sleep deprivation, and poor compliance. Hyperemesis gravidarum can make it difficult to maintain adequate concentrations of oral medications. Sleep deprivation aggravates many neurologic conditions and can be a particular problem in the third trimester. Compliance may deteriorate because of a woman's concern that taking medication might harm her baby. Women are often advised by friends, relatives, and even medical personnel to minimize fetal drug exposure. This may lead to skipped doses, reduced doses, or even self-discontinuation of an indicated medication.

TABLE 156.1. PHYSIOLOGIC CHANGES DURING PREGNANCY

Variable	Change
Extracellular volume	Increases 4–6 L
Plasma volume	Increases 40%
Renal blood flow	Increases 30%–50%
Glomerular filtration rate	Increases 30%–50%
Cardiac output	Increases 30%–50%
Serum albumin	Decreases 20%–30%

Adapted from Silberstein, 1998.

EPILEPSY

Each year 20,000 women with epilepsy become pregnant. This number has grown as marriage rates have increased for women with epilepsy, as parenting has become more socially supported, and as the medical management of pregnancy in women with epilepsy has improved.

Seizure frequency may change during pregnancy. In women with preexisting epilepsy, 35% experience an increase in seizure frequency, 55% have no change, and 10% have fewer seizures. Changes responsible for this include changes in sex hormones, antiepileptic drug (AED) metabolism, sleep schedules, and medication compliance. AED concentrations may change. The total AED concentration falls because of an increase in volume of distribution, decreased drug absorption, and increased drug clearance. Although the total concentration decreases, the proportion of unbound or free drug increases because albumin levels and protein binding decline. Therefore, it is necessary to follow the nonprotein-bound drug concentrations for AEDs that are highly protein-bound, including carbamazepine (Tegretol), phenytoin sodium (Dilantin), and sodium valproate (Depakene). Dose adjustments should maintain a stable nonprotein-bound fraction.

The older AEDs (benzodiazepines, phenytoin, carbamazepine, phenobarbital, and valproate) are teratogenic in humans. Major malformations related to AED exposure include cleft lip and palate and cardiac defects (atrial septal defect, tetralogy of Fallot, ventricular septal defect, coarctation of the aorta, patent ductus arteriosus, and pulmonary stenosis). The incidence of these major malformations in infants born to mothers with epilepsy is 4% to 6%, compared to 2% to 4% for the general population. These malformations can occur with exposure to any of the older AEDs. Neural tube defects (spina bifida and anencephaly) occur in 0.5% to 1% of infants exposed to carbamazepine and 1% to 2% of infants exposed to valproate during the first month of gestation. Minor congenital anomalies associated with AED exposure include facial dysmorphism and digital anomalies, which arise in 6% to 20% of infants exposed to AEDs *in utero*. This is a twofold increase over the rate in the general population. However, these anomalies are usually subtle and may often be outgrown.

Since 1993, seven new AEDs have been introduced, with little information about effects on the developing fetus. A prospective registry has been established to learn more about pregnancy and fetal outcome in women using AEDs (Table 156.2). The registry should be contacted regarding any woman who becomes pregnant while taking AEDs.

Several mechanisms have been postulated to explain the teratogenicity of AEDs. Some may be teratogenic because of free radical intermediates that may bind with ribonucleic acid and disrupt deoxyribonucleic acid synthesis and organogenesis. Higher concentrations of oxide metabolites increase the risk of fetal malformations. Some AEDs may cause folic acid deficiency, which is associated with higher occurrence and recurrence rates of neural tube defects. The American Academy of Neurology (AAN) and the American College of Obstetric and Gynecologic Physicians (1996) recommend that all women of childbearing age taking AEDs should receive folic acid supplementation of 0.4 to 5.0 mg per day.

TABLE 156.2. NORTH AMERICAN ANTIEPILEPTIC DRUG PREGNANCY REGISTRY

This is a prospective registry to gather information on pregnancy and fetal outcome from pregnancies in which the mother has used an antiepileptic drug. Women should contact the registry directly; they will receive information and be requested to provide informed consent.
Genetics and Teratology Unit
14CNY-MGH East
Room 5022A
Charlestown, MA 02129-2000
Telephone: 1-888-233-2334
Web site: neuro-www2.mgh.harvard.edu/aed/registry.nclk

Management of epilepsy in women of reproductive age should focus on maintaining effective control of seizures while minimizing fetal exposure to AEDs. This applies to dosage and to number of AEDs. Medication reduction or substitution should be achieved prior to conception. Altering medication during pregnancy increases the risk of breakthrough seizures and exposes the fetus to an additional AED. The recommended AED management in pregnancy is monotherapy at the lowest effective dose. The drug of choice is the one most likely to be effective and well tolerated. Current information is not sufficient to identify a particular AED as favored in pregnancy. If there is a family history of neural tube defects, an agent other than carbamazepine or valproate might be considered.

Once a woman is pregnant, prenatal diagnostic testing includes a maternal serum alpha-fetoprotein and a level II (anatomic) ultrasound at 14 to 18 weeks. This combination will identify more than 95% of infants with neural tube defects. In some instances, amniocentesis may be indicated.

AEDs have also been associated with an increased risk for early fetal hemorrhage. This may be due to an AED-drug related vitamin K deficiency. Therefore, the AAN recommends vitamin K supplementation (vitamin K_1 at 10 mg per day) for the last month of gestation.

For pregnant women with new-onset seizures, the diagnostic strategy is similar to that for any patient with a first-time seizure. A complete neurologic history and examination should be obtained, with attention to signs of a specific etiology, such as acute intracranial hemorrhage or central nervous system (CNS) infection. The evaluation should also screen for hypertension, proteinuria, and edema to exclude eclampsia. Follow-up studies include serologic tests for syphilis and human immunodeficiency virus, electroencephalogram (EEG), and magnetic resonance imaging (MRI). MRI is the preferred imaging technique for pregnant woman. As in nonpregnant women with a first-time seizure, treatment depends on seizure type and etiology.

PREECLAMPSIA AND ECLAMPSIA

Preeclampsia and eclampsia are most often seen in young primigravida women. Preeclampsia is a multisystem disorder that is diagnosed clinically by hypertension, proteinuria, and edema. Preeclampsia is associated with hepatic and coagulation abnormalities, hypoalbuminemia, increased urate levels, and hemoconcentration. Eclampsia is manifested by seizures, cerebral bleeding, and death. The incidence in Europe and other developed countries is 1 per 2,000. In developing countries, the incidence varies from 1 in 100 to 1 in 1,700. Worldwide, eclampsia probably accounts for 50,000 deaths annually.

Neurologic abnormalities associated with eclampsia include confusion, seizures, cortical blindness, visual-field defects, headaches, and blurred vision. Seizures are most often generalized but may be partial. Cortical blindness and visual-field defects may occur with bilateral occipital lobe involvement.

The differential diagnosis of eclampsia includes subarachnoid hemorrhage and cerebral venous thrombosis. The diagnosis is established by increased blood pressure plus proteinuria, edema, or both. A significant increase in blood pressure is defined as an increase of more than 15 mm Hg diastolic or 30 mm Hg systolic above baseline measurements obtained before or early in pregnancy. If no early reading is available, a blood pressure of 140/90 mm Hg or higher in late pregnancy is significant.

Neuroimaging, EEG, cerebrospinal fluid (CSF) analysis, and angiography may help in diagnosis. Computed tomography (CT) is usually normal in eclampsia but may show hypodense regions in areas of cerebral edema. MRI permits better detection of edema in the cortical mantle. During an eclamptic convulsion, the EEG shows spike-and-wave discharges. The CSF is usually normal in preeclampsia. In eclampsia, the CSF protein content is often moderately elevated, and the pressure may be increased. In some patients, angiography shows arterial spasm.

Pathologic examination of eclamptic brains reveals petechial hemorrhages in cortical and subcortical patches. Microscopically, these petechial hemorrhages are ring hemorrhages about capillaries and precapillaries occluded by fibrinoid material. Areas that are predisposed include the parietooccipital and occipital regions.

Treatment of eclampsia is controversial. The most accepted treatment is delivery of the fetus, if appropriate. Hypertension should be treated with antihypertensive agents. The National Blood Pressure Education Program recommends magnesium sulfate for the treatment and prevention of eclamptic seizures. In the United States, obstetricians have traditionally used magnesium sulfate. However, in the United Kingdom, they use phenytoin or diazepam. Randomized trials have compared these agents for seizure prevention in women with preeclampsia/eclampsia. The results suggest that magnesium is the agent of choice, but no study has evaluated the treatment of eclamptic seizures with both magnesium sulfate and an AED.

STROKE

Pregnancy is a risk factor for stroke, and the postpartum period is the most vulnerable time. Presumptive mechanisms include changes in the coagulation and fibrinolytic systems leading to a hypercoagulable state and an increase in viscosity and stasis, which can promote thrombosis. In the postpartum period, the large decrease in blood volume at childbirth, rapid changes in hormone status that alter hemodynamics and coagulation, and the strain of delivery may predispose to a stroke.

Arterial occlusion causes 50% to 80% of ischemic strokes in pregnant women. Cerebral venous thrombosis is the next most common etiology. Arterial occlusion occurs primarily in the second and third trimesters, whereas venous thrombosis most often occurs in the postpartum period. Arterial strokes most often occur as a consequence of identifiable risk factors, including premature atherosclerosis, moyamoya disease, Takayasu arteritis, fibromuscular dysplasia, and primary CNS vasculitis. Hematologic disorders can play an etiologic role in arterial and venous strokes. Such disorders include sickle-cell disease, antiphospholipid syndrome, thrombotic thrombocytopenic purpura, and deficiencies in antithrombin III, protein C, protein S, and factor V Leiden. Other etiologies are cardiogenic and paradoxic emboli.

Treatment of strokes in pregnancy is directed to the specific cause. Heparin does not cross the placenta and is the anticoagulant of choice in pregnancy. However, long-term use (greater than 1 month) is associated with osteoporosis. Warfarin sodium (Coumadin) crosses the placenta and is a known teratogen. It is therefore recommended only for women who cannot tolerate heparin or who have recurrent thromboembolic events. Aspirin complications in pregnancy include teratogenic effects and bleeding in the neonate. However, low-dose aspirin (less than 150 mg) is safe in the second and third trimesters, with no increase in maternal or neonatal adverse effects. Use of low-molecular-weight heparin is gaining acceptance during pregnancy. Like heparin, low-molecular-weight heparin does not cross the placenta. The risk of bleeding with these compounds is small, and the development of osteoporosis is less likely, although there is little information about appropriate doses in pregnancy.

CEREBRAL HEMORRHAGE

The risk of cerebral hemorrhage increases in pregnancy. Cerebral hemorrhage occurs in 1 to 5 pregnancies per 10,000, with an associated mortality of 30% to 40%. Factors that predispose to hemorrhage include physiologic changes of pregnancy such as hypertension, high concentrations of estrogens causing arterial dilation, and increases in cardiac output, blood volume, and venous pressure. Pregnancy-related conditions also increase the risk of hemorrhage. These include eclampsia, metastatic choriocarcinoma, cerebral emboli, and coagulopathies.

Subarachnoid hemorrhage accounts for 50% of all intracranial bleeding in pregnancy and carries a high mortality. Cerebral aneurysms and arteriovenous malformations cause most subarachnoid hemorrhages in pregnancy. Other causes include eclampsia, cocaine use, coagulopathies, ectopic endometriosis, moyamoya disease, and choriocarcinoma. Aneurysmal bleeding usually occurs in older patients in the second and third trimesters. In contrast, hemorrhages from arteriovenous malformations occur in younger women throughout gestation, with the highest risk during labor and the puerperium.

The diagnosis and treatment of subarachnoid hemorrhage and intracerebral hemorrhage in pregnant women are similar to those in nonpregnant patients. Subarachnoid hemorrhage is diagnosed by clinical manifestations and CT. If brain CT is normal and the clinical signs are consistent with intracranial hemorrhage, lumbar puncture should be performed. Once intracranial hemorrhage is detected, follow-up studies include MRI and four-vessel angiography. Noncontrast CT is also the most sensitive means of diagnosing intracerebral hemorrhage. Treatment of these conditions is directed to supporting the mother and fetus and preventing complications. Blood pressure should be carefully monitored, and fetal monitoring is indicated. The specific treatment depends on the etiology of the hemorrhage.

MULTIPLE SCLEROSIS

Multiple sclerosis (MS) affects 1 in 10,000 people in Western countries, primarily women in the childbearing years. A multicenter, prospective observational study (Pregnancy in Multiple Sclerosis Study; Confavreux, 1998) and other surveys found that the rate of relapse declines in pregnancy, especially in the third trimester, and increases in the first 3 months postpartum. Longterm disability was not affected.

The mechanisms responsible for the change in the rate of relapses include humoral and immunologic changes, as seen also in pregnant women with other autoimmune diseases such as rheumatoid arthritis or systemic lupus erythematosus. There is no correlation of relapse rate with the physical stress of childbirth and caring for the newborn, sleep deprivation, type and dose of anesthesia, breast-feeding, or socioeconomic factors.

Many women with relapsing-remitting MS are treated with interferon beta-1b (Betaseron), interferon beta-1a (Avonex), or glatiramer acetate (Copaxone). None of these has been tested formally in pregnant women and discontinuation of these agents is recommended. In addition, there have been no controlled trials addressing the safety of medication for MS relapses. If a severe relapse does occur with pregnancy, a short course of corticosteroid therapy is recommended. However, neonatal adrenal suppression may follow maternal corticosteroid use, and large prenatal doses in animals caused growth retardation and compromised development of the CNS.

MIGRAINE

Migraine is diagnosed in 18% of women of childbearing years, and 60% to 80% of migraine headaches improve during pregnancy. Women who had migraine onset at menarche or who have had menstrual migraines are more likely to experience improvement, especially in the first or second trimester. Higher levels of estrogen are probably responsible for this improvement during pregnancy. The subsequent fall in estrogen levels may cause postpartum headaches. It is not known why migraine may start or become worse in pregnancy.

If migraine arises in pregnancy, the differential diagnosis must be considered. A new-onset migraine with aura can be a symptom of vasculitis, brain tumor, or occipital arteriovenous malformation. Subarachnoid hemorrhage can cause headache any time during pregnancy or delivery. Other disorders with headache include stroke, cerebral venous thrombosis, eclampsia, pituitary tumor, and choriocarcinoma.

Medication use during pregnancy should be limited. If neces-

sary, acetaminophen, nonsteroidal antiinflammatory drugs, codeine, or other narcotics may be used; low-dose aspirin may also be given. Antiemetics such as metoclopramide or prochlorperazine may relieve the headache and associated nausea and vomiting. These agents are generally safe and effective. Ergotamine, dihydroergotamine mesylate (D.H.E. 45), and sumatriptan succinate (Imitrex) should be avoided. For someone with recurrent headaches, a beta-adrenergic blocker, such as propanolol, may be used prophylactically. However, adverse effects including intrauterine growth retardation have been reported with beta-adrenergic blockers. Therefore, the choice of medication for migraine in pregnant women should balance the the mother's comfort with the least fetal risk.

NEOPLASMS

Brain tumors rarely become symptomatic during pregnancy. The types of tumors arising in pregnancy differ from those in nonpregnant women. Glioma is the most common, followed by meningioma, acoustic neuroma, and then a variety of other tumors, including pituitary tumors. Tumor growth may be exacerbated by pregnancy, especially meningioma. Possible mechanisms include increased blood volume, fluid retention, and stimulation of tumor growth by hormones.

Systemic cancer is unusual in young women and rarely begins during pregnancy. Choriocarcinoma is the only systemic tumor specifically associated with pregnancy. Brain metastases are common in choriocarcinoma; among patients diagnosed with choriocarcinoma, 3% to 20% have brain disease at diagnosis.

Cerebral neoplasms cause headaches, seizures, focal signs, or symptoms of increased intracranial pressure. The seizures may be partial or generalized. Nausea and vomiting in the first trimester can be confused with morning sickness. All women suspected of having a brain tumor should be examined with MRI.

NEUROPATHIES

During pregnancy and the puerperium, women are at an increased risk for peripheral neuropathy. Backache or poorly localized paresthesia is common. At least 50% of pregnant women have back pain, Among the specific rare neuropathies that occur with a higher incidence during pregnancy are carpal tunnel syndrome, facial nerve palsy, meralgia paresthetica, and chronic inflammatory demyelinating polyneuropathy (CIDP) (see Chapters 63 and 105).

Carpal tunnel syndrome is the most frequent neuropathy of pregnancy. It usually begins in the third trimester and disappears after delivery; it is attributed to generalized edema. *Bell palsy* appears with a slightly higher frequency during pregnancy, mostly in the third trimester. Prognosis for recovery is excellent and is similar to that in nonpregnant women. Treatment is symptomatic, including protection of the eye. *Meralgia paresthetica,* a sensory neuropathy of the lateral femoral cutaneous nerve of the thigh, is attributed to compression of the nerve under the lateral part of the inguinal ligament. Swelling during pregnancy, increased body weight, and increased lordosis during pregnancy are possible causes. Numbness, burning, tingling, or pain in the lateral thigh suggests the diagnosis. A local anesthetic with or without steroids is usually all that is necessary. Most women improve in the postpartum period. The incidence of *CIDP* is slightly higher during pregnancy. As in nonpregnant women, treatment includes plasmapheresis, intravenous gamma globulin, or steroids.

MYASTHENIA GRAVIS

Symptoms of myasthenia gravis (MG) may increase during menstruation, pregnancy, or the puerperium. About one-third of MG patients become worse, one-third show no change, and one-third show improvement. If symptoms begin during pregnancy, the diagnosis is established, and treatment is symptomatic, with plasmapheresis and intravenous immunoglobulin. Thymectomy is deferred until long after delivery.

Neonatal MG affects 12% to 20% of infants born to mothers with MG. The symptoms clear within a few weeks.

MOVEMENT DISORDERS

Movement disorders are unusual in young women, but those that specifically occur during pregnancy include the restless leg syndrome, chorea, and drug-induced movement disorders.

The *restless leg syndrome* is probably the most common movement disorder of pregnancy. It is characterized by a crawling, burning, or aching sensation in the calves with an irresistible urge to move the legs. It occurs in 10% to 20% of pregnant women. Treatment includes massage, flexion and extension, walking, benzodiazepines, opiates, or levodopa. *Chorea gravidarum* occurs in pregnancy (see Chapter 109). Treatment is reserved for those with violent and disabling chorea and includes haloperidol or benzodiazepines.

Drugs that block dopamine receptors are often used to treat the nausea and vomiting of pregnancy. These drugs can cause new-onset chorea, tremor, dystonia, or parkinsonism. *Idiopathic Parkinson disease* is uncommon in women younger than 40 years. More common is secondary parkinsonism caused by medication or toxins. There is no definite evidence that Parkinson disease worsens during pregnancy, and there is little information about the toxicity of antiparkinson medications. Successful pregnancies have been reported in women taking levodopa.

SUGGESTED READINGS

Biology of Pregnancy

Harris RZ, Benet LZ, Schwartz JB. Gender effects in pharmacokinetics and pharmacodynamics. *Drugs* 1995;50:222–239.

Neuroendocrinology. In: Speroff L, Glass RH, Kase NG, eds. *Clinical gynecologic endocrinology and fertility.* Baltimore: Williams & Wilkins, 1994:141–182.

Silberstein SD. Drug treatment and trials in women. In: Kaplan PW, ed. *Neurologic disease in women.* New York: Demos Medical Publishing, 1998:25–44.

Epilepsy

Brown JE, Jacobs DR, Hartman TJ, et al. Predictors of red cell folate level in women attempting pregnancy. *JAMA* 1997;277:548–552.

Buehler BA, Delimont D, Van Waes M, Finnell RH. Prenatal prediction of risk of the fetal hydantoin syndrome. *N Engl J Med* 1990;322:1567–1572.

Cornelissen M, Steegers-Theunissen R, Kollee L, et al. Increased incidence of neonatal vitamin K deficiency resulting from maternal anticonvulsant therapy. *Am J Obstet Gynecol* 1993;168:923–928.

Czeizel AE, Dudas I. Prevention of the first occurrence of neural-tube defects by periconceptional vitamin supplementation. *N Engl J Med* 1992;327:1832–1835.

Daly LE, Kirke PN, Molloy A, Weir DG, Scott JM. Folate levels and neural tube defects: implications for treatment. *JAMA* 1995;274:1698–1702.

Dansky L, Andermann E, Roseblatt D, Sherwin AL, Andermann F. Anticonvulsants, folate levels, and pregnancy outcome. *Ann Neurol* 1987;21:176–182.

Delgado-Escueta AV, Janz D. Consensus guidelines: preconception counseling, management, and care of the pregnant woman with epilepsy. *Neurology* 1992;42[Suppl 5]:149–160.

Finnell RH, Buehler BA, Kerr BM, Agler PL, Levy RH. Clinical and experimental studies linking oxidative metabolism to phenytoin-induced teratogenesis. *Neurology* 1992;42:25–31.

Gaily E, Granstrom ML. Minor anomalies in children of mothers with epilepsy. *Neurology* 1992;42[Suppl 5]:128–131.

Gordon N. Folate metabolism and neural tube defects. *Brain Dev* 1995;17:307–311.

Guidelines for the care of women of childbearing age with epilepsy. Commission on Genetics, Pregnancy, and the Child, International League Against Epilepsy. *Epilepsia* 1993;34:588–589.

Kaneko S, Otani K, Fukushima Y, et al. Teratogenicity of antiepilepsy drugs: analysis of possible risk factors. *Epilepsia* 1988;29:459–467.

Koch S, Loesche G, Jager-Roman E, et al. Major birth malformations and antiepileptic drugs. *Neurology* 1992;42[Suppl 5]:83–88.

Laurence KM, James N, Miller MH, Tennant GB, Campbell H. Double-blind, randomised controlled trial of folate before conception to prevent the recurrence of neural tube defects. *BMJ* 1981;282:1509–1511.

Milunsky A, Jick H, Jick SS, et al. Multivitamin/folic acid supplementation in early pregnancy reduces the prevalence of neural tube defects. *JAMA* 1988;262:2847–2852.

Morrell MJ. Pregnancy and epilepsy. In: Porter RJ, Chadwick D, eds. *The epilepsies 2.* Boston: Butterworth-Heinemann, 1997:313–332.

Morrell MJ. Guidelines for the care of women with epilepsy. *Neurology* 1998;51[Suppl 4]:21–27.

Morrell MJ. Seizures and epilepsy in women. In: Kaplan PW, ed. *Neurologic disease in women.* New York: Demos Medical Publishing, 1998:189–206.

Mulinare J, Cordero JF, Erickson JD, Berry RJ. Periconceptional use of multivitamins and the occurrence of neural tube defects. *JAMA* 1988;260:3141–3145.

Ogawa Y, Kaneko S, Otani K, Fukushima Y. Serum folic acid levels in epileptic mothers and their relationship to congenital malformations. *Epilepsy Res* 1991;8:75–78.

Omtzigt JGC, Los FJ, Grobee DE, et al. The risk of spina bifida aperta after first-trimester exposure to valproate in a prenatal cohort. *Neurology* 1992;42[Suppl 5]:119–125.

Prevention of neural tube defects: results of the Medical Research Council Vitamin Study. MRC Vitamin Study Research Group. *Lancet* 1991;338:131–137.

Recommendations for the use of folic acid to reduce the number of cases of spina bifida and other neural tube defects. *MMWR* 1992;41:1–7.

Rosa FW. Spina bifida in infants of women treated with carbamazepine during pregnancy. *N Engl J Med* 1991;324:674–677.

Schmidt D, Beck-Mannagetta G, Janz D, Koch S. The effect of pregnancy on the course of epilepsy: a prospective study. In: Janz D, Dam M,

Richens A, eds. *Epilepsy, pregnancy, and the child.* New York: Raven Press, 1982:39–49.

Seizure disorders in pregnancy. *ACOG Physicians Educ Bull* 1996;231:1–13.

Strickler SM, Dansky LV, Miller MA, et al. Genetic predisposition to phenytoin-induced birth defects. *Lancet* 1985;2:746–749.

Thorp JA, Gaston L, Caspers DR, Pal ML. Current concepts and controversies in the use of vitamin K. *Drugs* 1995;49:376–387.

Tomson T, Lindbom U, Ekqvist B, Sundqvist A. Disposition of carbamazepine and phenytoin in pregnancy. *Epilepsia* 1994;35:131–135.

Tomson T, Lindbom U, Sundqvist A, Berg A. Red cell folate levels in pregnant epileptic women. *Eur J Clin Pharmacol* 1995;48:305–308.

Van Allen M, Fraser FC, Dallaire L, et al. Recommendations on the use of folic acid supplementation to prevent the occurrence of neural tube defects. *Can Med Assoc J* 1993;149:1239–1243.

Wegner C, Nau H. Alteration of embryonic folate metabolism by valproic acid during organogenesis: implications for the mechanism of teratogenesis. *Neurology* 1992;42[Suppl 5]:17–24.

Werler MM, Shapiro S, Mitchell AA. Periconceptional folic acid exposure and the risk of occurrent neural tube defects. *JAMA* 1993;269:1257–1261.

Yerby MS, Friel PN, McCormick K. Pharmacokinetics of anticonvulsants in pregnancy: alterations in protein binding. *Epilepsy Res* 1990;5:223–228.

Preeclampsia and Eclampsia

Burrows RF, Burrows EA. The feasibility of a control population for a randomized control trial of seizure prophylaxis in the hypertensive disorders of pregnancy. *Am J Obstet Gynecol* 1995;173:929–935.

Donaldson JO. Eclampsia. In: Devinsky O, Feldmann E, Hainline B, eds. *Neurological complications of pregnancy.* New York: Raven Press, 1994:25–33.

Duley L, Johanson R. Magnesium sulphate for pre-eclampsia and eclampsia: the evidence so far. *Br J Obstet Gynaecol* 1994;101:565–567.

Hutton JD, James DK, Stirrat GM, Douglas KA, Redman CW. Management of severe pre-eclampsia and eclampsia by UK consultants. *Br J Obstet Gynaecol* 1992;99:554–556.

Lenfant C, Gifford RW, Zuspan FP. Report of the National High Blood Pressure Education Program working group on high blood pressure in pregnancy. *Am J Obstet Gynecol* 1990;163:1691–1712.

Lucas MJ, Leveno KJ, Cunningham FG. A comparison of magnesium sulfate with phenytoin for the prevention of eclampsia. *N Engl J Med* 1995;333:201–205.

Repke JT, Friedman SA, Kaplan PW. Prophylaxis of eclamptic seizures: current controversies. *Clin Obstet Gynecol* 1992;35:365–374.

Roberts JM, Redman CWG. Pre-eclampsia: more than pregnancy-induced hypertension. *Lancet* 1993;341:1447–1451.

Sibai BM, Spinnato JA, Watson DL, Lewis JA, Anderson GD. Eclampsia. IV. Neurological findings and future outcome. *Am J Obstet Gynecol* 1985;152:184–192.

Thomas SV, Somanathan N, Radhakumari R. Interictal EEG changes in eclampsia. *Electroencephalogr Clin Neurophysiol* 1995;94:271–275.

Which anticonvulsant for women with eclampsia? Evidence from the Collaborative Eclampsia Trial. *Lancet* 1995;345:1455–1463. Erratum: *Lancet* 1995;346:258.

Stroke

Cross JN, Castro PO, Jennett WB. Cerebral strokes associated with pregnancy and the puerperium. *BMJ* 1968;3:214–218.

Gilmore J, Pennell PB, Stern BJ. Medication use during pregnancy for neurologic conditions. *Neurol Clin* 1998;16:189–206.

Kittner SJ, Stern BJ, Feeser BR, et al. Pregnancy and the risk of stroke. *N Engl J Med* 1996;335:768–774.

Lanska DJ, Kryscio RJ. Stroke and intracranial venous thrombosis during pregnancy and the puerperium. *Neurology* 1998;51:1622–1628.

Mabie WC, DiSessa TG, Crocker LG, Sibai BM, Arheart KL. A longitudinal study of cardiac output in normal human pregnancy. *Am J Obstet Gynecol* 1994;170:849–856.

Mas JL, Lamy C. Stroke in pregnancy and the puerperium. *J Neurol* 1998;245:305–313.

Sharshar T, Lamy C, Mas JL. Incidence and cause of strokes associated with pregnancy and the puerperium: a study in public hospitals of Ile de France. Stroke in Pregnancy Study Group. *Stroke* 1995;26:930–936.

Simolke GA, Cox SM, Cunningham FG. Cerebrovascular accidents complicating pregnancy and the puerperium. *Obstet Gynecol* 1991;78:37–42.

Srinivasan K. Cerebral venous thrombosis in pregnancy and the puerperium: a study of 135 patients. *Angiology* 1983;34:731–746.

Wiebers D. Ischemic cerebrovascular complications of pregnancy. *Arch Neurol* 1985;42:1106–1113.

Wiebers DO, Whisnant JP. The incidence of stroke among pregnant women in Rochester, Minn, 1955 through 1979. *JAMA* 1985;254:3055–3057.

Wilterdink JL, Feldmann E. Cerebral ischemia. In: Devinsky O, Feldmann E, Hainline B, eds. *Neurological complications of pregnancy.* New York: Raven Press, 1994:1–11.

Headache

Bousser MG, Ratinahirana H, Darbois X. Migraine and pregnancy: a prospective study in 703 women after delivery. *Neurology* 1990;40:437(abst).

Callaghan N. The migraine syndrome in pregnancy. *Neurology* 1968;18:197–201.

Chanceller MD, Wroe SJ. Migraine occurring for the first time during pregnancy. *Headache* 1990;30:224–227.

Granella F, Sances G, Zanferrari C, Costa A, Martignoni E, Manzoni GC. Migraine without aura and reproductive life events: a clinical epidemiological study in 1,300 women. *Headache* 1993;33:385–389.

Lance JW, Anthony M. Some clinical aspects of migraine: a prospective study of 500 patients. *Arch Neurol* 1966;15:356–361.

Scharff L, Marcus DA, Turk DC. Headache during pregnancy and in the postpartum: a prospective study. *Headache* 1997;37:203–210.

Silberstein S. Migraine and pregnancy. *Neurol Clin* 1997;15:209–231.

Somerville B. A study of migraine in pregnancy. *Neurology* 1972;22:824–828.

Stein GS. Headaches in the first post-partum week and their relationships to migraine. *Headache* 1981;21:201–205.

Welch KMA. Migraine and pregnancy. In: Devinsky O, Feldmann E, Hainline B, eds. *Neurological complications of pregnancy.* New York: Raven Press, 1994:77–82.

Welch KM, Darnley D, Simkins RT. The role of estrogen in migraine: a review and hypothesis. *Cephalalgia* 1984;4:227–236.

Cerebral Hemorrhage

Sharshar T, Lamy C, Mas JL. Incidence and causes of stroke associated with pregnancy and puerperium: a study in public hospitals of Ile de France. Stroke in Pregnancy Study Group. *Stroke* 1995;25:930–936.

Wiebers DO, Whisnant JP. The incidence of stroke among pregnant women in Rochester, Minn, 1955 through 1979. *JAMA* 1985; 254:3055–3057.

Wilterdink JL, Feldmann E. Cerebral hemorrhage. In: Devinsky O, Feldmann E, Hainline B, eds. *Neurological complications of pregnancy.* New York: Raven Press, 1994:13–23.

Wong C, Guiliani M, Haley E. Cerebrovascular disease and stroke in women. *Cardiology* 1990;77[Suppl 2]:80–90.

Multiple Sclerosis

Abramsky O. Pregnancy and multiple sclerosis. *Ann Neurol* 1994;36[Suppl]:S39–S41.

Bernardi S, Grasso MG, Bertollini R, Orzi F, Fieschi C. The influence of pregnancy on relapses in multiple sclerosis: a cohort study. *Acta Neurol Scand* 1991;84:403–406.

Birk K, Ford C, Smeltzer S, Ryan D, Miller R, Rudick RA. The clinical course of multiple sclerosis during pregnancy and the puerperium. *Arch Neurol* 1990;47:738–742.

Birk K, Rudick R. Pregnancy and multiple sclerosis. *Arch Neurol* 1986;43:719–726.

Confavreux C, Hutchinson M, Hours MM, Cortinovis-Tournaire P, Moreau T, and the Pregnancy in Multiple Sclerosis Group. Rate of pregnancy-related relapse in multiple sclerosis. *N Engl J Med* 1998;339:285–291.

Cook SD, Troiano R, Bansil S, Dowling PC. Multiple sclerosis and pregnancy. In: Devinsky O Feldmann E, Hainline B, eds. *Neurological complications of pregnancy.* New York: Raven Press, 1994:139–152.

Douglass LH, Jorgensen CL. Pregnancy and multiple sclerosis. *Am J Obstet Gynecol* 1948;55:332–336.

Frith JA, McLeod JG. Pregnancy and multiple sclerosis. *J Neurol Neurosurg Psychiatry* 1988;51:495–498.

Ghezzi A, Caputo D. Pregnancy: a factor influencing the course of multiple sclerosis? *Eur Neurol* 1981;20:115–117.

Hutchinson M. Pregnancy in multiple sclerosis. *J Neurol Neurosurg Psychiatry* 1993;56:1043–1045.

Korn-Lubetzki I, Kahana E, Cooper G, Abramsky O. Activity of multiple sclerosis during pregnancy and the puerperium. *Ann Neurol* 1984;16:229–231.

Millar JHD, Allison RS, Cheeseman EA, Merrett JD. Pregnancy as a factor influencing relapse in disseminated sclerosis. *Brain* 1959;82:417–426.

Nelson LM, Franklin GM, Jones MC. Risk of multiple sclerosis exacerbation during pregnancy and breast-feeding. *JAMA* 1988;259:3441–3443.

Poser CM. MS and postpartum stress [Letter]. *Neurology* 1984;34:704–705.

Poser S, Poser W. Multiple sclerosis and gestation. *Neurology* 1983;33:1422–1427.

Roullet E, Verdier-Taillerfer MH, Amarenco P, Gharbi G, Alperovitch A, Marteau R. Pregnancy and multiple sclerosis: a longitudinal study of 125 remittent patients. *J Neurol Neurosurg Psychiatry* 1993;56:1062–1065.

Sadovnick AD, Ebers GC. Epidemiology of multiple sclerosis: a critical overview. *Can J Neurol Sci* 1993;20:17–29.

Sadovnick AD, Eisen K, Hashimoto SA, et al. Pregnancy and multiple sclerosis: a prospective study. *Arch Neurol* 1994;51:1120–1124.

Schapira K, Poskanzer DC, Newell DJ, Miller H. Marriage, pregnancy and multiple sclerosis. *Brain* 1996;89:419–428.

Sweeney WJ. Pregnancy and multiple sclerosis. *Am J Obstet Gynecol* 1953;66:124–130.

Thompson DS, Nelson IM, Burns A, Burks JS, Franklin GM. The effects of pregnancy in multiple sclerosis: a retrospective study. *Neurology* 1986;36:1097–1099.

Tillman AJB. The effect of pregnancy on multiple sclerosis and its management. *Res Publ Assoc Res Nerv Ment Dis* 1950;28:548–582.

Van Walderveen MAA, Tas MW, Barkhof F, et al. Magnetic resonance evaluation of disease activity during pregnancy in multiple sclerosis. *Neurology* 1994;44:327–329.

Wegmann TG, Lin H, Guilbert L, Mosmann TR. Bidirectional cytokine interactions in the maternal-fetal relationship: is successful pregnancy a TH2 phenomenon? *Immunol Today* 1993;14:353–356.

Worthington J, Jones R, Crawford M, Forti A. Pregnancy and multiple sclerosis: a 3-year prospective study. *J Neurol* 1994;241:228–233.

Neoplasia

DeAngelis LM. Central nervous system neoplasms in pregnancy. In: Devinsky O, Feldmann E, Hainline B, eds. *Neurological complications of pregnancy.* New York: Raven Press, 1994:139–152.

Isla A, Alvarez F, Gonzalez A, et al. Brain tumor and pregnancy. *Obstet Gynecol* 1997;89:19–23.

Weinreb HJ. Demyelinating diseases and neoplastic diseases in pregnancy. *Neurol Clin* 1994;12:509–526.

Peripheral Nerve Disorders

Beric A. Peripheral nerve disorders in pregnancy. In: Devinsky O, Feldmann E, Hainline B, eds. *Neurological complications of pregnancy.* New York: Raven Press, 1994:179–192.

Conwit RA, Good JL. Peripheral nerve disease. In: Kaplan PW, ed. *Neurologic disease in women.* New York: Demos Medical Publishing, 1998:295–305.

Rosenbaum RB, Donaldson JO. Peripheral nerve and neuromuscular disorders. *Neurol Clin* 1994;12:461–478.

Myasthenia Gravis

Ahisten G, Lefvert AK, Osterman PO, et al. Follow-up study of muscle function in children of mothers with myasthenia gravis during pregnancy. *J Child Neurol* 1992;7:264–269.

Eymard B, Vernet-der Garabedian B, Berrih-Aknin S, Pannier C, Bach JF. Anti-acetylcholine receptor antibodies in neonatal myasthenia gravis: heterogeneity and pathogenic significance. *J Autoimmun* 1991;4:185–195.

Mitchell PJ, Bebbington M. Myasthenia gravis in pregnancy. *Obstet Gynecol* 1992;80:178–181.

Papazian O. Transient neonatal myasthenia gravis. *J Child Neurol* 1992;7:135–141.

Rosenbaum RB, Donaldson JO. Peripheral nerve and neuromuscular disorders. *Neurol Clin* 1994;12:461–478.

Movement Disorders

Golbe LI. Pregnancy and movement disorders. *Neurol Clin* 1994;12:497–508.

Rogers JD, Fahn S. Movement disorders and pregnancy. In: Devinsky O, Feldmann E, Hainline B, eds. *Neurological complications of pregnancy.* New York: Raven Press, 1994:163–178.

Merritt's Neurology, 10th ed., edited by L.P. Rowland. Lippincott Williams & Wilkins, Philadelphia © 2000.

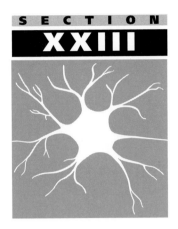

ENVIRONMENTAL NEUROLOGY

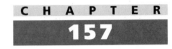

ALCOHOLISM

JOHN C.M. BRUST

In the United States, 7% of all adults and 19% of adolescents are "problem drinkers": addicted to ethanol or, even if abstinent most of the time, likely to get into trouble when they drink. Ethanol-related deaths exceed 100,000 each year, accounting for 5% of all deaths in the United States. The devastation is direct (from intoxication, addiction, and withdrawal) or indirect (from nutritional deficiency or other ethanol-related diseases).

ETHANOL INTOXICATION

Ethanol acts at many levels of the neuraxis and affects a number of neurotransmitter systems, especially τ-aminobutyric acid and glutamate. Like general anesthetics, ethanol disrupts ("fluidizes") the phospholipid bilayer of cell membranes. How much of its actions on neurotransmitter receptors and protein channels is indirectly the result of this less specific effect is uncertain.

To obtain a mildly intoxicating blood ethanol concentration (BEC) of 100 mg/dL, a 70-kg person must drink about 50 g (2 oz) of 100% ethanol. Following zero-order kinetics, ethanol is metabolized at about 70 to 150 mg/kg of body weight per hour, with a fall in BEC of 10 to 25 mg/dL per hour. Thus, most adults require 6 hours to metabolize a 50-g dose, and the ingestion of only 8 g of additional ethanol per hour would maintain the BEC at 100 mg/dL.

Symptoms and signs of acute ethanol intoxication are due to cerebral depression, possibly at first of the reticular formation with cerebral disinhibition and later of the cerebral cortex itself. Manifestations depend not only on the BEC but also on the rate of climb and the person's tolerance, which is related less to increased metabolism than to poorly understood adaptive changes in the brain. At any BEC, intoxication is more severe when the level is rising than when it is falling, when the level is reached rapidly, and when the level has only recently been achieved. A single BEC determination therefore is not a reliable indicator of drunkenness, and the correlations of Table 157.1 are broad generalizations. Death from respiratory paralysis may occur with a BEC of 400 mg/dL and survival may occur at 700 mg/dL; a level of 500 mg/dL would be fatal in 50% of individuals.

Low-to-moderate BECs cause slow saccadic eye movements and interrupted jerky pursuit movements that may impair visual acuity. Esophoria and exophoria cause diplopia. With a BEC of 150 to 250 mg/dL, there is increased electroencephalogram (EEG) beta activity ("beta buzz"); higher BECs cause EEG slowing. During sleep, suppression of the rapid eye movement (REM) stage is followed by REM rebound after a few hours.

The term *pathologic intoxication* refers to sudden extreme excitement with irrational or violent behavior after even small

TABLE 157.1. CORRELATION OF SYMPTOMS WITH BLOOD ETHANOL CONCENTRATION (BEC)

BEC	Symptoms
50–150 mg/dL	Euphoria or dysphoria, shyness or expansiveness, friendliness or argumentativeness Impaired concentration, judgment, and sexual inhibitions
150–250 mg/dL	Slurred speech and ataxic gait, diplopia, nausea, tachycardia, drowsiness, or labile mood with sudden bursts of anger or antisocial acts
300 mg/dL	Stupor alternating with combativeness or incoherent speech, heavy breathing, vomiting
400 mg/dL	Coma
500 mg/dL	Respiratory paralysis

doses of ethanol. Episodes are said to last for minutes or hours, followed by sleep and, on awakening, amnesia for the events that took place. Delusions, hallucinations, and homicide may occur during bouts of pathologic intoxication. Some cases are probably psychologic dissociative reactions; others may be due to the kind of paradoxic excitation that sometimes follows barbiturate administration.

The term *alcoholic blackout* refers to amnesia for periods of intoxication, sometimes lasting several hours, even though consciousness at the time did not seem to be disturbed. Although sometimes considered a sign of physiologic dependence, blackouts also occur in occasional drinkers. Their nature is uncertain.

Acute ethanol poisoning causes more than 1,000 deaths each year in the United States. In stuporous alcoholic patients, subdural hematoma, meningitis, and hypoglycemia are important diagnostic considerations, but it is equally important to remember that ethanol intoxication alone can be fatal.

Blood ethanol causes a rise of blood osmolality, about 22 mOsm/L for every 100 mg/dL of ethanol; however, there are no transmembrane shifts of water, and the hyperosmolarity does not cause symptoms. Ethanol overdose should be considered in any comatose patient whose serum osmolarity is higher than predicted by calculation of the sum of serum sodium, glucose, and urea.

Patients stuporous or comatose from ethanol intoxication are generally managed similarly to those poisoned by other depressant drugs (Table 157.2). Death comes from respiratory depression, and artificial ventilation in an intensive care unit is the mainstay of treatment. Hypovolemia, acid–base or electrolyte imbalance, and abnormal temperature require attention, and if there is any uncertainty about the blood glucose level, 50% glucose is given intravenously, along with parenteral thiamine. Because ethanol is rapidly absorbed, gastric lavage does not help unless other drugs have been ingested. In obstreperous or violent patients, sedatives (including phenothiazines and haloperidol) should be avoided because they may push patients into stupor and respiratory depression. When a patient is being addressed, he or she may be alert but then lapse into stupor or coma when stimuli are decreased.

In a nonhabitual drinker, a BEC of 400 mg/dL takes 20 hours

TABLE 157.2. TREATMENT OF ACUTE ETHANOL INTOXICATION

For obstreperous or violent patients
  Isolation, calming environment, reassurance—avoid sedatives
  Close observation

For stuporous or comatose patients
  If hypoventilation, artificial respiration in an intensive care unit
  If serum glucose in doubt, intravenous 50% glucose with parenteral thiamine
  Careful monitoring of blood pressure; correction of hypovolemia or acid–base imbalance
  Consider hemodialysis if patient apneic or deeply comatose
  Avoid emetics or gastric lavage
  Avoid analeptics
  Do not forget other possible causes of coma in an alcoholic

to return to zero. The only practical agent that might accelerate ethanol metabolism and elimination is fructose, but this causes gastrointestinal upset, lactic acidosis, and osmotic diuresis. (An imidazobenzodiazepine drug has been developed that reverses symptoms of mild-to-moderate ethanol intoxication; it is available for experimental use only.) Hemodialysis or peritoneal dialysis can be used for BECs greater than 600 mg/dL; for severe acidosis; for concurrent ingestion of methanol, ethylene glycol, or other dialyzable drugs; or for severely intoxicated children. Analeptic agents such as ethamivan, caffeine, or amphetamine have no useful role and can cause seizures and cardiac arrhythmia. Although patients are often depleted of magnesium, administration of magnesium sulfate may further depress the sensorium in intoxicated patients. Reports suggesting that naloxone hydrochloride (Narcan) benefits patients with ethanol intoxication require confirmation.

ETHANOL–DRUG INTERACTIONS

The combination of ethanol with other drugs, often in suicide attempts, causes 2,500 deaths annually, or 13% of all drug-related fatalities. Ethanol is often taken with marijuana, barbiturates, opiates, cocaine, hallucinogens, and inhalants—with varying interactions. Alcoholics often abuse barbiturates, and although ethanol and barbiturates are cross-tolerant, they lower the lethal dose of either alone or when taken acutely in combination. Ethanol with chloral hydrate (Mickey Finn) may be especially dangerous.

Impaired judgment and respiratory depression are also hazards when ethanol is combined with hypnotics, such as methaqualone (Quaalude), sedating antihistamines, antipsychotic agents, and tranquilizers such as meprobamate and benzodiazepines. Hypnotic drugs with long half-lives may cause potentially dangerous incoordination when ethanol is consumed the following day.

The cross-tolerance of ethanol with general anesthetics such as ether, chloroform, or fluorinated agents raises the threshold to sleep induction, but synergistic interaction then increases the depth and length of the anesthetic stage reached. Tricyclic antidepressants do not have a consistent effect; desipramine hydrochloride antagonizes the effects of ethanol, and amitriptyline

potentiates them. Ethanol and morphine, repeatedly used, can increase each other's potency, and methadone addicts not only frequently become alcoholics but also can then develop a characteristic encephalopathy. Death has followed ethanol taken with propoxyphene hydrochloride. A mild reaction resembling that caused by disulfiram (Antabuse) occurs when patients combine ethanol with sulfonylureas such as tolbutamide (Orinase) or with some antibiotics, including chloramphenicol, griseofulvin, isoniazid, metronidazole, and quinacrine hydrochloride.

ETHANOL DEPENDENCE AND WITHDRAWAL

The term *hangover* refers to the headache, nausea, vomiting, malaise, nervousness, tremulousness, and sweating that can occur in anyone after brief but excessive drinking. Hangover does not imply ethanol addiction, but *ethanol withdrawal* does imply addiction and encompasses several disorders (Table 157.3), which may occur alone or in combination after reduction or cessation of drinking. Severity depends on the length and degree of a particular binge.

Tremulousness, the most common ethanol withdrawal symptom, usually appears in the morning after several days of drinking. It is promptly relieved by ethanol, but if drinking cannot continue, tremor becomes more intense, with insomnia, easy startling, agitation, facial and conjunctival flushing, sweating, anorexia, nausea, retching, weakness, tachypnea, tachycardia, and systolic hypertension. Except for inattentiveness and inability to fully recall the events that occurred during the binge, mentation is usually intact. Symptoms subside in a few days, but it may be 2 weeks before they completely disappear.

Perceptual disturbances, with variable insight, occur in about 25% of ethanol-addicted patients and include nightmares, illusions, and hallucinations, which are most often visual but may be auditory, tactile, olfactory, or a combination of these. Imagery includes insects, animals, or people. Hallucinations are usually fragmentary, lasting minutes at a time for several days. Sometimes, however, auditory hallucinations of threatening content last much longer, and occasionally, a persistent state of auditory hallucinosis with paranoid delusions that resembles schizophrenia develops in these patients and may require care in a mental hospital. Repeated bouts of acute auditory hallucinosis may predispose to the chronic form.

Ethanol can precipitate *seizures* in any epileptic; seizures usually occur the morning after weekend or even single-day drinking rather than during inebriation. Alcohol-related seizures affecting alcoholics not otherwise epileptic have traditionally been

TABLE 157.3. ETHANOL WITHDRAWAL SYNDROMES

Early
  Tremulousness
  Hallucinosis
  Seizures

Late
  Delirium tremens

considered a withdrawal phenomenon, usually occurring within 48 hours of the last drink in persons who have abused ethanol chronically or in binges for months or years. The minimal duration of drinking sufficient to cause seizures is uncertain, but the risk is dose-related, beginning at only 50-g absolute ethanol daily. Seizures usually occur singly or in a brief cluster; status epilepticus is infrequent. Focal features are present in 25% and do not consistently correlate with evidence of previous head injury or other structural cerebral pathology. Alcohol seizures sometimes accompany tremulousness or hallucinosis, but they may occur in otherwise asymptomatic individuals. Their frequent appearance during active drinking or after more than 1 week of abstinence suggests that mechanisms other than withdrawal play a role in some individuals.

The diagnosis of alcohol-related seizures depends on an accurate history and exclusion of other cerebral lesions. Because reliable follow-up is unlikely, a seizure workup should be done, including computed tomography (CT) or magnetic resonance imaging and examination of cerebrospinal fluid (CSF). Fewer than 10% of patients with rum fits have spontaneous EEG abnormalities, compared with 50% of those with idiopathic epilepsy. A reported high frequency of electrographic photomyoclonic and photoconvulsant responses during ethanol withdrawal was not borne out by subsequent studies.

In contrast to tremor, hallucinosis, or seizures, which usually occur within 1 or 2 days of abstinence, *delirium tremens* usually begins from 48 to 72 hours after the last drink. Patients with delirium tremens are often hospitalized for other reasons. Delirium tremens may follow withdrawal seizures either before the postictal period has cleared or after 1 or 2 asymptomatic days, but when seizures occur during a bout of delirium tremens, some other diagnosis (e.g., meningitis) should be considered.

Symptoms typically begin and end abruptly, lasting from hours to a few days. There may be alternating periods of confusion and lucidity. Infrequently, relapses may prolong the disorder for a few weeks. Patients are typically agitated, inattentive, and grossly tremulous, with fever, tachycardia, and profuse sweating. They pick at the bed clothes or stare wildly about and intermittently shout at or try to fend off hallucinated people or objects. "Quiet" delirium is infrequent. Mortality is as high as 15%; death is usually due to other diseases (e.g., pneumonia or cirrhosis), but it may be attributed to unexplained shock, lack of response to therapy, or no apparent cause.

Treatment of ethanol withdrawal includes prevention or reduction of early symptoms, prevention of delirium tremens, and management of delirium tremens after it starts (Table 157.4). Sedatives have been recommended for recently abstinent alcoholics or those with mild early withdrawal symptoms, with theoretical consideration given to cross-tolerance with ethanol. Popular agents include paraldehyde, barbiturates, and benzodiazepines. With any of these agents, the aim is to give a loading dose likely to cause symptoms of mild intoxication (calming, dysarthria, ataxia, fine nystagmus), and then to adjust subsequent doses to avoid intoxication and tremulousness. After 1 or 2 days, dosage is gradually tapered, with reinstitution of intoxicating doses should withdrawal symptoms reappear. Beta-adrenergic blocking agents dampen alcohol withdrawal tremor and have been reported to decrease agitation and autonomic

TABLE 157.4. TREATMENT OF ETHANOL WITHDRAWAL

Prevention or reduction of early symptoms

Diazepam, 10–40 mg, or chlordiazepoxide, 25–100 mg, p.o. or i.v., repeated hourly until sedation or mild intoxication. Successive daily doses tapered by about one-fourth of preceding day's with resumption of higher dose if withdrawal symptoms recur

Alternatively, pentobarbital, 200 mg, p.o., i.m., or i.v., and then 100 mg hourly prn. Maintenance dose and duration determined by symptoms. Subsequent tapering at about 100 mg/day

Alternatively, paraldehyde, 5–15 mg, p.o. or p.r., repeated hourly prn. Maintenance and tapering titrated with symptoms. Thiamine, 100 mg, and multivitamins, i.m. or i.v.

Magnesium, potassium, and calcium replacement as needed

Delirium tremens

Diazepam, 10 mg i.v., then 5 mg or more (up to 40 mg) every 5 min until calming. Maintenance diazepam, 5 mg or more i.v. (or i.m.) every 1–4 h, prn

Careful attention to fluid and electrolyte balance; several liters of saline per day, or even pressors, may be needed

Cooling blanket or alcohol sponges for high fever

Prevent or correct hypoglycemia

Thiamine and multivitamin replacement

Consider coexisting illness (e.g., liver failure, pancreatitis, meningitis, subdural hematoma)

signs as well, reducing the need for benzodiazepines or other sedatives.

Ethanol, when used parenterally, has the disadvantage of a low therapeutic index. Because ethanol is directly toxic to many organs, it should be avoided during hospitalization, even though most patients resume drinking on discharge. Neither haloperidol nor phenothiazines have a specific effect on hallucinations; theoretically, they are less likely to prevent hallucinosis or delirium tremens than drugs cross-tolerant with ethanol, and they can exacerbate seizures.

Phenytoin sodium (Dilantin) appears to be of no value in preventing seizures during withdrawal. Status epilepticus during ethanol withdrawal is treated as in other situations; intravenous phenobarbital or diazepam has an advantage, compared with phenytoin, of reducing other withdrawal symptoms when the patient awakens. Long-term anticonvulsants in patients with ethanol withdrawal seizures are superfluous; abstainers do not need them, and drinkers do not take them. An epileptic whose seizures are often precipitated by ethanol abuse unfortunately does need treatment, even though compliance is unlikely.

Hypomagnesemia is common during early ethanol withdrawal, and although it may not be the primary cause of symptoms, magnesium sulfate should be given to hypomagnesemic patients. Hypokalemia and hypocalcemia may also be present, and the latter may respond to treatment only when hypomagnesemia is corrected. Parenteral thiamine and multivitamins are given even if there are no clinical signs of depletion.

Delirium tremens, once it appears, cannot be abruptly reversed by any agent, and specific cross-tolerance of a sedative with ethanol is less important in full-blown delirium tremens than in early abstinence. Parenteral diazepam is more effective than paraldehyde in rapid calming and has fewer adverse reactions (including apnea) and lower mortality. The required doses might be fatal in a normal person (see Table 157.4), but one cannot predict in any individual patient how high the tolerable dose is. Liver disease decreases the metabolism of diazepam, and patients with cirrhosis are more vulnerable to the depressant effects of sedatives; as delirium tremens clears, hepatic encephalopathy takes its place.

General medical management in delirium tremens is intensive. Although dehydration may be severe enough to cause shock, patients with liver damage may retain sodium and water. Hypokalemia can cause cardiac arrhythmias. Hypoglycemia may be masked, as may other serious coexisting illnesses, such as alcoholic hepatitis, pancreatitis, meningitis, or subdural hematoma. Occasionally encountered during abstinence is either parkinsonism or chorea, which tends to clear over days or weeks. Such movement disorders are presumably related to ethanol effects on striatal dopamine.

WERNICKE-KORSAKOFF SYNDROME

Although pathologically indistinguishable, Wernicke and Korsakoff syndromes are clinically distinct. Wernicke syndrome, when full-blown, consists of mental, eye movement, and gait abnormalities. Korsakoff syndrome is only a mental disorder that differs qualitatively from Wernicke syndrome (Table 157.5). Both are the result of thiamine deficiency.

In acute Wernicke syndrome, mental symptoms most often consist of a global confusional state that appears over days or weeks; there is inattentiveness, indifference, decreased spontaneous speech, disorientation, impaired memory, and lethargy. Stupor and coma are unusual, as is selective amnesia. Disordered perception is common; a patient might identify the hospital room as his or her apartment or a bar. In fewer than 10%, mentation is normal.

Abnormal eye movements include nystagmus (horizontal with or without vertical or rotatory components), lateral rectus palsy (bilateral but usually asymmetric), and conjugate gaze palsy (horizontal with or without vertical), progressing to complete external ophthalmoplegia. Although sluggishness of pupillary reaction is common, total loss of reactivity to light does not seem to occur, and ptosis is rare. Whether mental symptoms in acute Wernicke syndrome ever occur without abnormal eye movements is uncertain.

Truncal ataxia, present in more than 80% of patients, may prevent standing or walking. Dysarthria and limb ataxia, especially in the arms, are infrequent. Peripheral neuropathy, which occurs to some degree in most patients, may cause weakness sufficient to mask the ataxia. Abnormalities of caloric testing are common, with gradual improvement, often incomplete, over several months.

Patients with Wernicke syndrome frequently have signs of nutritional deficiency (e.g., skin changes, tongue redness, cheilosis) or liver disease. Autonomic signs are common. Although beriberi heart disease is rare, acute tachycardia, dyspnea on exertion, and postural hypotension unexplained by hypovolemia are common, and sudden circulatory collapse may follow mild exertion. Hypothermia is less frequent; fever usually indicates infection.

In acute Wernicke syndrome, the EEG may show diffuse slowing, or it may be normal. CSF is normal except for occasional mild protein elevation. Elevated blood pyruvate, falling with treatment, is not specific. Decreased blood transketolase (which requires thiamine pyrophosphate as cofactor) more reliably indicates thiamine deficiency.

In most patients, the more purely amnestic syndrome of Korsakoff emerges as the other mental symptoms of Wernicke syndrome respond to treatment. How often Korsakoff syndrome occurs without a background of Wernicke syndrome is disputed and bound up with the question of "alcoholic dementia" (see below). Pathologic changes of Wernicke-Korsakoff are sometimes encountered unexpectedly at autopsy, suggesting the presence of subclinical or atypical forms, including unexplained coma.

The amnesia of Korsakoff syndrome is both anterograde, with inability to retain new information, and retrograde, with rather randomly lost recall for events months or years old. Alertness, attentiveness, and behavior are relatively preserved, but there tends to be a lack of spontaneous speech or activity. Confabulation is not invariable and, if initially present, tends gradually to disappear. Insight is usually impaired, and there may be flagrant anosognosia for the mental disturbance.

The histopathologic lesions of Wernicke-Korsakoff syndrome consist of variable degrees of neuronal, axonal, and myelin loss; prominent blood vessels; reactive microglia, macrophages, and astrocytes; and, infrequently, small hemorrhages. Nerve cells may be relatively preserved in the presence of extensive myelin destruction and gliosis, and astrocytosis may predominate chronically.

Lesions affect the thalamus (especially the dorsomedial nucleus and the medial pulvinar), the hypothalamus (especially the mamillary bodies), the midbrain (especially the oculomotor and periaqueductal areas), and the pons and medulla (especially the abducens and medial vestibular nuclei). In the anterosuperior vermis of the cerebellum, severe Purkinje cell loss and astrocytosis accompany lesser degrees of neuronal loss and gliosis in the molecular and granular layers.

TABLE 157.5. MAJOR NUTRITIONAL DISTURBANCES IN ALCOHOLICS

Disorder	Clinical features	Deficiency
Wernicke syndrome	Dementia with lethargy, inattentiveness, apathy, and amnesia Ophthalmoparesis Gait ataxia	Thiamine
Korsakoff syndrome	Dementia, mainly amnesia, with or without confabulation	Thiamine
Cerebellar degeneration	Gait ataxia; limb coordination relatively preserved	?
Polyneuropathy	Distal limb sensory loss and weakness; less often autonomic dysfunction	?
Amblyopia	Optic atrophy, decreased visual acuity, central scotoms; total blindness rare	?

The traditional view that the memory impairment of Korsakoff syndrome is the result of lesions in the mamillary body has been challenged by others who attribute amnesia to lesions in the dorsomedial nucleus of the thalamus. The global confusion of Wernicke syndrome may occur without visible thalamic lesions and may be a biochemical disorder. Periaqueductal, oculomotor, or abducens nucleus lesions may explain ophthalmoparesis, which is also seen in patients whose eye movement disorders resolved before death. The cerebellar and vestibular lesions probably contribute to ataxia.

Experimental and clinical evidence ascribes a specific role to thiamine in the Wernicke-Korsakoff syndrome. A genetic influence is implied because only a few alcoholic or otherwise malnourished people are affected, and whites seem more susceptible than blacks.

Untreated Wernicke-Korsakoff syndrome is fatal, and the mortality rate is 10% among treated patients. Concomitant liver failure, infection, or delirium tremens often makes the cause of death unclear. Postural hypotension and tachycardia call for strict bedrest; associated medical problems may require intensive care. The cornerstone of treatment is thiamine, 50 to 100 mg daily, until a normal diet can be taken; intramuscular or intravenous administration is preferred because thiamine absorption is impaired in chronic alcoholics. Hypomagnesemia may retard improvement after thiamine treatment; magnesium is therefore replaced, along with other vitamins. Protein intake may have to be titrated against the patient's liver status.

With thiamine treatment, the ocular abnormalities (especially abducens and gaze palsies) improve within a few hours and usually resolve within 1 week; in about 35% of the patients, horizontal nystagmus persists indefinitely. Global confusion may improve in hours or days and usually resolves within 1 month, leaving Korsakoff amnesia in more than 80%. In less than 25% of these patients, there is eventual clearing of the memory deficit. Ataxia may improve in a few days, but recovery is complete in less than 50% of patients, and nearly 35% do not show improvement at all.

ALCOHOLIC CEREBELLAR DEGENERATION

Cerebellar cortical degeneration may occur in nutritionally deficient alcoholics without Wernicke-Korsakoff syndrome (see Table 157.5). Instability of the trunk is the major symptom, often with incoordination of leg movements. Arm ataxia is less prominent; nystagmus and dysarthria are rare. Symptoms evolve in weeks or months and eventually stabilize, sometimes even with continued drinking and poor nutrition. Ataxia without Wernicke disease is less likely to appear abruptly or to improve.

Pathologically, the superior vermis is invariably involved, with nerve cell loss and gliosis in the molecular, granular, and especially the Purkinje cell layers. There may be secondary degeneration of the olives and of the fastigial, emboliform, globose, and vestibular nuclei. Involvement of the cerebellar hemispheric cortex is exceptional and limited to the anterior lobes. Pathologic evidence of Wernicke disease may coexist, even though it is unsuspected clinically. CT and autopsies, moreover, have revealed cerebellar atrophy in alcoholics who were not clinically ataxic.

Alcoholic cerebellar degeneration is probably nutritional in origin. Identical lesions occur in malnourished nonalcoholics, and ataxia may begin in malnourished alcoholics after weeks of abstinence. The clinical and pathologic similarity to the cerebellar component of Wernicke syndrome suggests shared mechanisms, but most patients with alcoholic cerebellar degeneration do not have pathologic evidence of Wernicke disease.

ALCOHOLIC POLYNEUROPATHY

Alcoholic polyneuropathy is a sensorimotor disorder, probably of nutritional origin, that stabilizes or improves with abstinence and an adequate diet (see Table 157.5). Neuropathy is found in most patients with Wernicke-Korsakoff syndrome but more often occurs alone. Paresthesia is usually the first symptom; there may be burning or lancinating pain and exquisite tenderness of the calves or soles. Impaired vibratory sense is usually the earliest sign; proprioception tends to be preserved until other sensory loss is substantial. Loss of ankle jerks is another early sign; eventually, there is diffuse areflexia. Weakness appears at any time and may be severe. Distal leg muscles are affected first, although proximal weakness may be marked. Radiologically demonstrable neuropathic arthropathy of the feet is common, as are skin changes (e.g., thinning, glossiness, reddening, cyanosis, hyperhidrosis). Peripheral autonomic abnormalities are usually less prominent than in diabetic neuropathy but may cause urinary and fecal incontinence, hypotension, hypothermia, cardiac arrhythmia, dysphagia, dysphonia, impaired esophageal peristalsis, altered sweat patterns, or abnormal Valsalva ratio. Pupillary parasympathetic denervation is rare. The CSF is usually normal except for occasional mild elevation of protein content.

Pathologically, there is degeneration of both myelin and axons; it is not certain which occurs first. Clinical and experimental evidence suggests that alcoholic polyneuropathy is nutritional in origin and that more than thiamine may be lacking.

Peripheral nerve pressure palsies, especially radial and peroneal, are common in alcoholics. Nutritional polyneuropathy may increase the vulnerability of peripheral nerves to compression injury in intoxicated individuals, who tend to sleep deeply in unusual locations and positions. Recovery usually takes days or weeks; splints during this period can prevent contractures.

ALCOHOLIC AMBLYOPIA

Alcoholic amblyopia is a visual impairment that progresses over days or weeks, with development of central or centrocecal scotomas and temporal disc pallor (see Table 157.5). Demyelination affects the optic nerves, chiasm, and tracts, with predilection for the maculopapular bundle. Retinal ganglion cell loss is secondary. Ethanol (or tobacco) toxicity plays little or no role; amblyopia clears in patients who receive dietary supplements but continue to smoke and drink ethanol. Alcoholic amblyopia does not progress to total blindness; it may remain stable without change in drinking or eating habits. Improvement, which is often incomplete, nearly always follows nutritional replacement.

PELLAGRA

Nicotinic acid deficiency in alcoholics causes pellagra, with dermatologic, gastrointestinal, and neurologic symptoms. Altered mentation progresses over hours, days, or weeks to amnesia, delusions, hallucinations, or delirium. Nicotinic acid therapy (plus other vitamins, deficiency of which can be contributory) usually results in prompt improvement.

ALCOHOLIC LIVER DISEASE

Cirrhosis is the sixth leading cause of death in the United States, and nearly all deaths from cirrhosis in people older than 45 years are caused by ethanol. Altered mentation in an alcoholic therefore always raises the possibility of hepatic encephalopathy, which may accompany intoxication, withdrawal, Wernicke syndrome, meningitis, subdural hematoma, hypoglycemia, or other alcohol states. Hepatic encephalopathy is discussed in detail in Chapter 148. Other neurologic disorders encountered in alcoholic cirrhotics include a poorly understood syndrome of altered mentation, myoclonus, and progressive myelopathy following portacaval shunting, as well as acquired chronic hepatocerebral degeneration, a characteristic syndrome of dementia, dysarthria, ataxia, intention tremor, choreoathetosis, muscular rigidity, and asterixis, which usually occurs in patients who have had repeated bouts of hepatic coma.

HYPOGLYCEMIA

Metabolism of ethanol by alcohol dehydrogenase and of acetaldehyde by mitochondrial aldehyde dehydrogenase utilizes nicotinamide adenine dinucleotide (NAD). The resulting elevated NADH-to-NAD ratio impairs gluconeogenesis, and if food is not being eaten and liver glycogen is depleted, there may be severe hypoglycemia with altered behavior, seizures, coma, or focal neurologic deficit. Residual symptoms are common, including dementia. Even after appropriate treatment with intravenous 50% dextrose, these patients require close observation; blood glucose may fall again, with the return of symptoms and possibly permanent brain damage.

Ethanol stimulates intestinal release of secretin, which aggravates reactive hypoglycemia, especially in children, by enhancing glucose-stimulated insulin release.

ALCOHOLIC KETOACIDOSIS

In alcoholic ketoacidosis, β-hydroxybutyric acid and lactic acid accumulate in association with heavy drinking. The mechanism is unclear. Typical patients are chronic alcoholic young women who increase their ethanol consumption for days or weeks and then stop drinking when they are overcome by anorexia. Vomiting, dehydration, confusion, obtundation, and Kussmaul respiration ensue. Blood glucose may be normal, low, or moderately elevated, with little or no glycosuria. A large anion gap is accounted for by β-hydroxybutyrate, lactate, and lesser amounts of

pyruvate and acetoacetate. Serum insulin levels are low, and serum levels of growth hormone, epinephrine, glucagon, and cortisol are high, but glucose intolerance usually clears without insulin and is not demonstrable on recovery. It is not unusual for patients to have repeated attacks of alcoholic ketoacidosis.

Alcoholics may have other reasons for metabolic acidosis with a large anion gap (e.g., methanol or ethylene glycol poisoning). When β-hydroxybutyrate is the major ketone present, the nitroprusside test (Acetest) may be negative. Treatment includes infusion of glucose (and thiamine), correction of dehydration or hypotension, and replacement of electrolytes such as potassium, magnesium, and phosphate. Small amounts of bicarbonate may be given. Insulin is usually not needed.

INFECTION IN ALCOHOLICS

Alteration of white blood cell function contributes to the alcoholic's predisposition to infection (e.g., bacterial and tuberculous meningitis). Infectious meningitis must always be considered in alcoholics with seizures or altered mental status, even when the clinical picture seems to be that of intoxication, withdrawal, thiamine deficiency, hepatic encephalopathy, hypoglycemia, or other alcoholic disturbances. Alcoholic intoxication is a risk factor for human immunodeficiency virus infection.

TRAUMA IN ALCOHOLICS

Thrombocytopenia, a direct effect of ethanol and a consequence of cirrhosis, increases the likelihood of intracranial hematomas after head injury. Abnormalities of clotting factors also increase the possibility of intracranial hematomas. Experimentally, moreover, acute ethanol enhances blood–brain barrier leakage around areas of cerebral trauma. Close observation is essential after even mild head injury in intoxicated patients; an abnormal sensorium must not be dismissed as drunkenness.

ALCOHOL AND CANCER

Independently of tobacco, ethanol in moderate amounts increases the risk of carcinoma of the mouth, esophagus, pharynx, larynx, liver, and breast.

ALCOHOL AND STROKE

As with coronary artery disease, epidemiologic studies suggest that low-to-moderate amounts of ethanol decrease stroke risk, whereas higher amounts increase it. Reports have been inconsistent, however. Some studies indicate increased risk for hemorrhagic stroke at any dose; some find ethanol protective in whites but not Japanese; and some observe increased stroke risk temporally related to binge drinking. Ethanol could either prevent or cause stroke by several mechanisms. Acutely and chronically, ethanol causes hypertension. It reportedly lowers blood levels of low-density lipoproteins, raises levels of high-density lipoproteins, decreases fibrinolytic activity, increases or inhibits platelet reactivity, dilates or constricts cerebral vessels, and indirectly reduces cerebral blood flow through dehydration. Alcoholic cardiomyopathy predisposes to embolic stroke.

ALCOHOLIC MYOPATHY

Alcoholic myopathy is of three types. Subclinical myopathy consists of elevated serum creatine kinase levels and electromyographic changes, sometimes with intermittent cramps or weakness. With chronic myopathy, there is progressive proximal weakness. Acute rhabdomyolysis causes sudden severe weakness, muscle pain, swelling, and myoglobinuria with renal shutdown. Ethanol toxicity rather than nutritional deficiency is the likely cause of myopathy, and symptoms sometimes emerge during a binge. Alcoholic cardiomyopathy often coexists. Whether subclinical, chronic, or acute, myopathy improves with abstinence.

CENTRAL PONTINE MYELINOLYSIS AND MARCHIAFAVA-BIGNAMI DISEASE

Central pontine myelinolysis occurs in both alcoholics and nondrinkers and is a consequence of overvigorous correction of hyponatremia. Marchiafava-Bignami disease is nearly always associated with alcoholism (including wine, beer, and whiskey). It is of unknown origin and causes symptoms, including death, that are scarcely explained by the characteristic callosal lesions. Marchiafava-Bignami disease and central pontine myelinolysis are discussed in detail in Chapters 134 and 135, respectively.

ALCOHOLIC DEMENTIA

Alcoholic dementia refers to progressive mental decline in alcoholics without apparent cause, nutritional or otherwise. Symptoms are said to correlate with enlarged cerebral ventricles and widened sulci, and both cognition and radiographic changes allegedly improve with abstinence. The subject is controversial, however. True brain atrophy should not be radiographically reversible, and some workers maintain that most or all cases of alleged alcoholic dementia actually represent other conditions, such as nutritional deficiency, previous trauma, or liver failure. In animals, prolonged administration of moderate amounts of ethanol causes behavioral and neuropathologic abnormalities not found in pair-fed controls. Some studies suggest synergism between ethanol toxicity and thiamine deficiency. The clinical relevance of animal studies to humans is uncertain. If ethanol is indeed neurotoxic, it remains to be seen what constitutes a safe dose.

FETAL ALCOHOL SYNDROME

Ethanol ingestion during pregnancy causes congenital malformations and delayed psychomotor development. Major clinical features of the fetal alcohol syndrome include cerebral dysfunc-tion, growth deficiency, and distinctive facies (Table 157.6); less often, there are abnormalities of the heart, skeleton, urogenital organs, skin, and muscles. Neuropathologic abnormalities include absence of the corpus callosum, hydrocephalus, and abnormal neuronal migration, with cerebellar dysplasia, heterotopic cell clusters, and microcephaly. These changes occur independently of other potentially incriminating factors, such as maternal malnutrition, smoking, other drug use, or age. Binge drinking, which may produce high ethanol levels at a critical fetal period, may be more important than chronic ethanol exposure, and early gestation appears to be the most vulnerable period.

Children of alcoholic mothers are often intellectually borderline or retarded without other features of the fetal alcohol syndrome; fetal effects of ethanol thus cover a broad spectrum. Stillbirth and attention deficit disorder seem especially frequent among offspring of heavy drinkers, and each anomaly of the fetal alcohol syndrome may occur alone or in combination with others. The face of a typical patient with the fetal alcohol syndrome is distinctive and as easily recognized at birth as that of the infant with Down syndrome. Irritability and tremulousness with poor suck reflex and hyperacusis are usually present at birth and last weeks or months. Of these children, 85% perform more than two standard deviations below the mean on tests of mental performance; those who are not grossly retarded rarely have even average mental ability. Older children are often hyperactive and clumsy, and there may be hypotonia or hypertonia. Except for neonatal seizures, epilepsy is not a component of the syndrome.

Ethanol is directly teratogenic to many animals, but the mechanism is not known. In humans, the risk of alcohol-induced birth defects is established with more than 3 oz of absolute alcohol daily. Below that, the risk is uncertain; a threshold of safety has not been defined. The incidence of fetal alcohol syndrome may be as high as 1 to 2 per 1,000 live births, with partial expression in 3 to 5 per 1,000. It may affect 1% of infants born to women who drink 1 oz of ethanol daily early in pregnancy. More than 30% of the offspring of heavy drinkers are affected by fetal alcohol syndrome, which thus may be the leading teratogenic cause of mental retardation in the Western world.

TREATMENT OF CHRONIC ALCOHOLISM

The literature on the treatment of alcoholism is voluminous, and strong opinions outweigh scientific data. Not all problem drinkers consume physically addicting quantities of ethanol, no personality type defines an alcoholic, and the relative roles of genetics and social deprivation vary from patient to patient. (Animal and human studies indicate genetic influences in alcoholism, but the association is complex and undoubtedly involves more than one gene.) Of course, such variability of alcoholic populations means that no treatment modality (e.g., psychotherapy, group psychotherapy, family or social network therapy, drug therapy, behavioral [aversion] therapy) or no single therapeutic setting (e.g., general hospital, halfway house, vocational rehabilitation clinic, Alcoholics Anonymous) is appropriate for all. For example, the success rate of Alcoholics Anonymous has been estimated to be 34%.

TABLE 157.6. CLINICAL FEATURES OF FETAL ALCOHOL SYNDROME

Feature	Majority	Minority
CNS	Mental retardation Microcephaly Hypotonia Poor coordination Hyperactivity	
Impaired growth	Prenatal for length and weight Postnatal for length and weight Diminished adipose tissue	
Abnormal face		
Eyes	Short palpebral fissures	Ptosis Strabismus Epicanthal folds Myopia Microphthalmia Blepharophimosis Cataracts Retinal pigmentary abnormalities
Nose	Short, upturned Hypoplastic philtrum	
Mouth	Thin vermilion lip borders Retrognathia in infancy Micrognathia or prognathia in adolescence	Prominent lateral palatine ridges Cleft lip or palate Small teeth with faulty enamel
Maxilla	Hypoplastic	
Ears		Posteriorly rotated Poorly formed concha
Skeletal		Pectus excavatum or carinatum Syndactyly, clinodactyly, or campodactyly Limited joint movements Nail hypoplasia Radiolunar synostosis Bifid xiphoid Scoliosis Klippel-Feil anomaly
Cardiac		Septal defects Great vessel anomalies
Cutaneous		Abnormal palmar creases Hemangiomas Infantile hirsutism
Muscular		Diaphragmatic, inguinal, or umbilical hernias Diastasis recti
Urogenital		Labial hypoplasia Hypospadias Small rotated kidneys Hydronephrosis

Use of tranquilizing and sedating drugs is especially controversial because they may lead to switching of dependency or to drug–ethanol interactions. Some clinicians espouse short-term use of these drugs in doses high enough to reduce the psychologic tensions that lead to ethanol use but low enough not to block symptoms of ethanol withdrawal.

Disulfiram inhibits aldehyde dehydrogenase and reduces the rate of oxidation of acetaldehyde, accumulation of which accounts for the symptoms that appear soon after someone taking disulfiram drinks ethanol. Within 5 to 10 minutes, there is warmth and flushing of the face and chest, throbbing headache, dyspnea, nausea, vomiting, sweating, thirst, chest pain, palpitations, hypotension, anxiety, confusion, weakness, vertigo, and blurred vision. The severity and duration of these symptoms depend on the amount of ethanol drunk; a few milliliters can cause mild symptoms followed by drowsiness, sleep, and recovery; severe reactions can last hours or be fatal and require hospital admission, with careful management of hypotension and cardiac arrhythmia.

Taken in the morning, when the urge to drink is least, disulfiram, 0.25 to 0.5 g daily, does not alter the taste for ethanol and helps only patients who strongly desire to abstain. In the United States, 150,000 to 200,000 patients are maintained on disulfiram, although controlled studies demonstrating substantial long-term benefit are lacking. Side effects of disulfiram that are unrelated to ethanol ingestion include drowsiness, psychiatric symptoms, and cardiovascular problems. Paranoia, impaired memory, ataxia, dysarthria, and even major motor seizures may be difficult to distinguish from ethanol effects, as may peripheral neuropathy. Hypersensitivity hepatitis also occurs.

Approved by the U.S. Federal Drug Administration in 1994 as adjunctive therapy for alcoholism, the opiate antagonist naltrexone hydrochloride (ReVia) probably acts at the level of the mesolimbic "reward" circuit to blunt the pleasurable effects of ethanol. In Europe, acamprosate, a drug with an uncertain mechanism of action, is available. Other proposed treatments for alcoholism include lithium, serotonin-uptake inhibitors, dopaminergic agonists, opiates, and psychotherapy. None is scientifically accredited.

SUGGESTED READINGS

Alcohol-related mortality and years of potential life lost—United States. *MMWR* 1990;39:173–178.

Alldredge BK, Lowenstein DH, Simon RP. A placebo-controlled trial of intravenous diphenylhydantoin for short-term treatment of alcohol withdrawal seizures. *Am J Med* 1989;87:645–648.

Brust JCM. Ethanol. In: *Neurological aspects of substance abuse.* Boston: Butterworth-Heinemann, 1993:190–252.

Brust JCM. Ethanol. In: Schaumburg HH, Spencer PS, eds. *Experimental and clinical neurotoxicology,* 2nd ed. Baltimore: Williams & Wilkins, 1999.

Brust JCM. Stroke and substance abuse. In: Barnett HJM, Mohr JP, Stein BM, et al., eds. *Stroke: pathophysiology, diagnosis, and management,* 3rd ed. Philadelphia: WB Saunders, 1998:979–1000.

Camargo CA. Moderate alcohol consumption and stroke: the epidemiologic evidence. *Stroke* 1989;20:1611–1626.

Charness ME, Simon RP, Greenberg DA. Ethanol and the nervous system. *N Engl J Med* 1989;321:442–454.

Cloninger CR. D2 dopamine receptor gene is associated but not linked with alcoholism. *JAMA* 1991;266:1793–1800.

Day NL, Jasperse D, Richardson D, et al. Prenatal exposure to alcohol: effect on infant growth and morphologic characteristics. *Pediatrics* 1989;84:536–541.

Fisch BJ, Hauser WA, Brust JCM, et al. The EEG response to diffuse and patterned photic stimulation during acute untreated alcohol withdrawal. *Neurology* 1989;39:434–436.

Fuller RK, Branhey L, Brightwell DR, et al. Disulfiram treatment of alcoholism. A Veterans Administration Cooperative Study. *JAMA* 1986;256:1449–1455.

Goldstein DB. Effects of alcohol on cellular membranes. *Ann Emerg Med* 1986;15:1013–1018.

Joyce EM. Aetiology of alcoholic brain damage: alcoholic neurotoxicity or thiamine malnutrition? *Br Med Bull* 1994;50:99–114.

Lemoine P, Lemoine P. Avenir des infants de meres alcooliques (etude de 105 case retrouves a l'age adult) et quelques constatations d'interet prophylactique. *Ann Pediatr* 1992;29:226–230.

Neiman J, Lang AE, Fornazarri L, Carlen PL. Movement disorders in alcoholism: a review. *Neurology* 1990;40:741–746.

Ng SKC, Hauser WA, Brust JCM, et al. Alcohol consumption and withdrawal in new-onset seizures. *N Engl J Med* 1988;319:666–673.

O'Connor PG, Schottenfeld RS. Patients with alcohol problems. *N Engl J Med* 1998;338:592–602.

Suzdak PD, Glowa JR, Crawley JN, et al. A selective imidazobenodiazepine antagonist of ethanol in the rat. *Science* 1986;234:1243–1247.

Tabakoff B, Hoffman PL. Alcohol addiction: an enigma among us. *Neuron* 1996;16:909–912.

Thompson WL, Johnson AD, Maddrey WL, et al. Diazepam and paraldehyde for treatment of severe delirium tremens: a controlled trial. *Ann Intern Med* 1975;82:175–180.

Thun MJ, Peto R, Lopez AD, et al. Alcohol consumption and mortality among middle-aged and elderly U.S. adults. *N Engl J Med* 1997; 24:1705–1714.

Urbano-Marquez AM, Estruch R, Navarro-Lopez F, et al. The effects of alcoholism on skeletal and cardiac muscle. *N Engl J Med* 1989; 320:409–415.

Victor M. Persistent altered mentation due to ethanol. *Neurol Clin* 1993;11:639–661.

Victor M, Adams RD. The effect of alcohol on the nervous system. *Res Publ Assoc Res Nerv Ment Dis* 1953;32:526–573.

Victor M, Adams RD, Collins GH. *The Wernicke-Korsakoff syndrome,* 2nd ed. Philadelphia: FA Davis Co, 1989.

Victor M, Adams RD, Mancall EL. A restricted form of cerebellar cortical degeneration occurring in alcoholic patients. *Arch Neurol* 1959;1:579–688.

Merritt's Neurology, 10th ed., edited by L.P. Rowland. Lippincott Williams & Wilkins, Philadelphia © 2000.

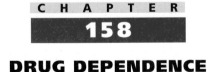

CHAPTER 158

DRUG DEPENDENCE

JOHN C.M. BRUST

There are two kinds of drug dependence. *Psychic dependence* leads to craving and drug-seeking behavior. *Physical dependence* produces somatic withdrawal symptoms and signs. Depending on the particular drug and the circumstances of its administration, psychic and physical dependence can coexist or occur alone. *Addiction* is psychic dependence.

In the United States, dependence of one or both types is encountered with a variety of agents, licit and illicit (Table 158.1).

Different classes of drugs produce diverse symptoms of intoxication and withdrawal, as well as medical and neurologic complications. Their legal status has little to do with potential harmfulness.

DRUGS OF DEPENDENCE

Opioids

Opioids include agonists (e.g., morphine, heroin, methadone, fentanyl citrate [Sublimaze], meperidine hydrochloride (Demerol HCl), hydromorphone hydrochloride (Dilaudid), codeine, propoxyphene hydrochloride [Darvon]), antagonists (e.g., naloxone hydrochloride [Narcan], naltrexone hydrochloride [ReVia]), and mixed agonist-antagonists (e.g., pentazocine [Talwin], buprenorphine hydrochloride [Buprenex], butorphanol tartrate [Stadol]). At desired levels of intoxication, agonist opioids produce drowsy euphoria, analgesia, cough suppres-

TABLE 158.1. DRUGS OF DEPENDENCE

Opioids
Psychostimulants
Sedatives/hypnotics
Marijuana
Hallucinogens
Inhalants
Phencyclidine
Anticholinergics
Ethanol
Tobacco

sion, miosis, and often nausea, vomiting, sweating, pruritus, hypothermia, postural hypotension, constipation, and decreased libido. Taken parenterally, they produce a "rush," a brief ecstatic feeling followed by euphoria and either relaxed "nodding" or garrulous hyperactivity. Overdose causes coma, respiratory depression, and pinpoint (but reactive) pupils. For adults with respiratory depression, treatment consists of respiratory support and naloxone, 2 mg intravenously, repeated as needed up to 20 mg; for those with normal respirations, smaller doses (0.4 to 0.8 mg) are given to avoid precipitation of withdrawal signs. Naloxone is short-acting, and so patients receiving it require admission and close observation.

Opioid agonist withdrawal symptoms include irritability, lacrimation, rhinorrhea, sweating, yawning, mydriasis, myalgia, muscle spasms, piloerection, nausea, vomiting, abdominal cramps, fever, hot flashes, tachycardia, hypertension, and orgasm. In adults, seizures and delirium are not features of opioid withdrawal, which is rarely life-threatening and can usually be prevented or treated with methadone, 20 mg once or twice daily. By contrast, untreated opioid withdrawal in newborns is severe, protracted, and often fatal; treatment is with titrated doses of methadone, paregoric, or, if additional drug withdrawal is suspected, a barbiturate.

Psychostimulants

Psychostimulants include amphetamines, methamphetamine, methylphenidate hydrochloride (Ritalin HCl), ephedrine, phenylpropanolamine hydrochloride, other anorectics and decongestants, and cocaine (which, in contrast to other psychostimulants, is also a local anesthetic). Desired effects include alert euphoria with increased motor activity and physical endurance. Taken parenterally or smoked as alkaloidal cocaine ("crack") or methamphetamine ("ice"), psychostimulants produce a rush clearly distinguishable from that of opioids. With repeated use, there is stereotypic activity progressing to bruxism or other dyskinesias and paranoia progressing to frank hallucinatory psychosis. Overdose causes headache, chest pain, tachycardia, hypertension, flushing, sweating, fever, and excitement. There may be delirium, cardiac arrhythmia, seizures, myoglobinuria, shock, coma, and death. Treatment includes benzodiazepine sedation, bicarbonate for acidosis, anticonvulsants, cooling, an antihypertensive (preferably a direct vasodilator such as sodium nitroprusside [Nitropress]), respiratory and blood pressure support, and cardiac monitoring.

Psychostimulant withdrawal produces fatigue, depression, and increased hunger and sleep. Objective signs are few, but depression can require treatment or even hospitalization.

Sedatives

Sedative agents include barbiturates (e.g., phenobarbital, pentobarbital sodium, amobarbital, secobarbital [Seconal]), benzodiazepines (e.g., diazepam, chlordiazepoxide hydrochloride [Librium], alprazolam [Xanax], lorazepam (Ativan), triazolam [Halcion], flunitrazepam), and miscellaneous products (e.g., glutethimide, ethchlorvynol [Placidyl], methaqualone [Quaalude]). Desired effects and overdose both resemble ethanol intoxication, although respiratory depression is much milder with benzodiazepines. Treatment is supportive; for severe benzodiazepine poisoning, there is a specific antagonist, flumazenil (Romazicon). Withdrawal causes tremor and seizures, which can be prevented or treated with titrated doses of a barbiturate or benzodiazepine. Delirium tremens is a medical emergency requiring intensive care.

Marijuana

Marijuana, from the hemp plant *Cannabis sativa,* contains many cannabinoid compounds, of which the principal psychoactive agent is Δ^9-tetrahydrocannabinol. Hashish refers to preparations made from the plant resin, which contains most of the psychoactive cannabinoids. Usually smoked, marijuana produces a relaxed dreamy euphoria, often with jocularity, disinhibition, depersonalization, subjective slowing of time, conjunctival injection, tachycardia, and postural hypotension. High doses cause auditory or visual hallucinations, confusion, and psychosis, but fatal overdose has not been documented. Withdrawal symptoms, other than craving, are minimal; there may be jitteriness, anorexia, and headache.

Hallucinogens

Hallucinogenic plants are used ritualistically or recreationally around the world. In the United States, the most popular agents are the indolealkylamines psilocybin and psilocin (from several mushroom species), the phenylalkylamine mescaline (from the peyote cactus), and the synthetic ergot compound lysergic acid diethylamide (LSD). Several synthetic phenylalkylamines are also available, including 3,4-methylenedioxymethamphetamine (MDMA; "ecstasy"), which has both hallucinogenic and amphetamine-like effects. The acute effects of hallucinogens are perceptual (distortions or hallucinations, usually visual and elaborately formed), psychologic (depersonalization or altered mood), and somatic (dizziness, tremor, and paresthesia). Some users experience paranoia or panic, and some, days to months after use, have "flashbacks," the spontaneous recurrence of drug symptoms without taking the drug. High doses of LSD cause hypertension, obtundation, and seizures, but fatalities have usually been the result of accidents or suicide. Treatment of overdose consists of a calm environment, reassurance, and, if necessary, a benzodiazepine. Withdrawal symptoms do not occur.

Inhalants

Recreational inhalant use is especially popular among children and adolescents, who sniff a wide variety of products, including aerosols, spot removers, glues, lighter fluid, fire-extinguishing agents, bottled fuel gas, marker pens, paints, and gasoline. Compounds include aliphatic hydrocarbons such as n-hexane, aromatic hydrocarbons such as toluene, and halogenated hydrocarbons such as trichloroethylene; in addition, nitrous oxide is sniffed from whipped-cream dispensers and butyl or amyl nitrite from "room odorizers." Despite such chemical diversity, desired subjective effects are similar to those of ethanol intoxication. Overdose can cause hallucinations, seizures, and coma; death has resulted from cardiac arrhythmia, accidents, and aspiration of vomitus. Symptoms tend to clear within a few hours, and treatment consists of respiratory and cardiac monitoring. There is no predictable abstinence syndrome other than craving.

Phencyclidine

Developed as an anesthetic, phencyclidine hydrochloride (PCP or "angel dust") was withdrawn because it caused psychosis. As a recreational drug, it is usually smoked. Low doses cause euphoria or dysphoria and a feeling of numbness; with increasing intoxication, there is agitation, nystagmus, tachycardia, hypertension, fever, sweating, ataxia, paranoid or catatonic psychosis, hallucinations, myoclonus, rhabdomyolysis, seizures, coma, respiratory depression, and death. Treatment includes a calm environment with benzodiazepine sedation and restraints as needed, gastric suctioning, activated charcoal, forced diuresis, cooling, antihypertensives, anticonvulsants, monitoring of cardiorespiratory and renal function, and, for frank psychosis, haloperidol. Symptoms can persist for hours or days. Withdrawal signs are not seen.

Anticholinergics

The recreational use of anticholinergics includes ingestion of the plant *Datura stramonium,* popular among American adolescents, as well as use of antiparkinson drugs and the tricyclic antidepressant amitriptyline. Intoxication produces decreased sweating, tachycardia, dry mouth, dilated unreactive pupils, and delirium with hallucinations. Severe poisoning causes myoclonus, seizures, coma, and death. Treatment includes intravenous physostigmine salicylate (Antilirium), 0.5 to 3 mg, repeated as needed every 30 minutes to 2 hours, plus gastric lavage, cooling, bladder catheterization, respiratory and cardiovascular monitoring, and, if necessary, anticonvulsants. Neuroleptics, which have anticholinergic activity, are contraindicated. There is no withdrawal syndrome.

TRAUMA

Trauma may be a consequence of a drug's acute effects, for example, automobile and other accidents during marijuana, inhalant, or anticholinergic intoxication; violence in psychostimu-

lant or PCP users; and self-mutilation during hallucinogen psychosis. Trauma among users of illicit drugs, however, is most often the result of the illegal activities necessary to distribute and procure them. Overprescribing of sedatives is a major contributor to falls in the elderly.

INFECTION

Parenteral users of any drug are subject to an array of local and systemic infections, which in turn can affect the nervous system. Hepatitis leads to encephalopathy or hemorrhagic stroke. Cellulitis and pyogenic myositis produce more distant infection, including vertebral osteomyelitis with myelopathy or radiculopathy. Endocarditis, bacterial or fungal, leads to meningitis, cerebral infarction or abscess, and septic or mycotic aneurysm. Tetanus, often severe, affects heroin users, and botulism occurs at injection sites or, among cocaine users, in the nasal sinuses. Malaria has occurred in heroin users from endemic areas.

By 1998, nonhomosexual parenteral drug users composed 26% of acquired immunodeficiency syndrome (AIDS) cases reported to the Centers for Disease Control and Prevention; male homosexual drug users accounted for another 6%. Nearly two-thirds of patients receiving methadone maintenance treatment are seropositive for human immunodeficiency virus (HIV). Parenteral drug users experience the same neurologic complications of AIDS as do other groups and are particularly susceptible to syphilis and tuberculosis, including drug-resistant forms. Because of promiscuity and associated sexually transmitted diseases, nonparenteral cocaine users are also at increased risk for AIDS. Heroin and cocaine are themselves immunosuppressants (heroin users were vulnerable to unusual fungal infections before the AIDS epidemic), yet their use in HIV-seropositive individuals does not seem to accelerate the development of AIDS.

SEIZURES

Seizures are a feature of withdrawal from sedatives, including, infrequently, benzodiazepines. Methaqualone and glutethimide have reportedly caused seizures during intoxication. Opioids lower seizure threshold, but seizures are seldom encountered during heroin overdose. Myoclonus and seizures more often occur in meperidine users, a consequence of the active metabolite normeperidine. Seizures are also frequent in parenteral users of pentazocine combined with the antihistamine tripelennamine ("T's and blues"). Seizures may occur in cocaine users without other evidence of overdose. In animals, repeated cocaine administration produces seizures in a pattern suggestive of "kindling." Amphetamine and other psychostimulants are less epileptogenic than cocaine, but seizures have occurred in users of the over-the-counter anorectic phenylpropanolamine hydrochloride. A case–control study found that marijuana was protective against the development of new-onset seizures. In animal studies, the nonpsychoactive cannabinoid compound cannabidiol is anticonvulsant.

STROKE

Illicit drug users frequently abuse ethanol and tobacco, increasing their risk for ischemic and hemorrhagic stroke. Parenteral drug users are subject to stroke through systemic complications such as hepatitis, endocarditis, and AIDS. Heroin users develop nephropathy with secondary hypertension, uremia, and bleeding. Heroin has also caused stroke in the absence of other evident risk factors, perhaps through immunologic mechanisms. Stroke in injectors of pentazocine combined with tripelennamine has resulted from embolism of foreign particulate material passing through secondary pulmonary arteriovenous shunts.

Amphetamine users are prone to intracerebral hemorrhage following acute hypertension and fever. They are also at risk for occlusive stroke secondary to cerebral vasculitis affecting either medium-sized arteries (resembling polyarteritis nodosa) or smaller arteries and veins (resembling hypersensitivity angiitis). Ischemic and hemorrhagic stroke is also a frequent consequence of cocaine use, regardless of route of administration. Whether stroke is ischemic or hemorrhagic, a common mechanism may be acute hypertension and direct cerebral vasoconstriction, with hemorrhage occurring during reperfusion. Cerebral saccular aneurysms and vascular malformations have been found in more than 50% of patients undergoing angiography for cocaine-related intracranial hemorrhage. LSD and PCP are vasoconstrictive, and occlusive and hemorrhagic strokes have followed their use.

ALTERED MENTATION

Dementia in illicit drug users may be the result of concomitant ethanol abuse, malnutrition, head trauma, or infection. Parenteral drug users are at risk for HIV encephalopathy. Whether the drugs themselves cause lasting cognitive or behavioral change is more difficult to establish, for predrug mental status is nearly always uncertain and many drug users are probably self-medicating preexisting psychiatric conditions (e.g., cocaine for depression). The weight of evidence is against chronic mental abnormalities secondary to opioids, marijuana, or hallucinogens. Controversy exists over whether psychostimulants predispose to lasting depression or PCP to schizophrenia. Cerebral atrophy and irregularly decreased cerebral blood flow have been reported in chronic cocaine users. Sedatives can cause "reversible dementia" in the elderly, and their use in small children has been associated with delayed learning. Lead encephalopathy has developed in gasoline sniffers, and toluene sniffers have had cerebral white matter lesions with dementia.

FETAL EFFECTS

The effects of illicit drugs on intrauterine development are also difficult to separate from damage secondary to ethanol, tobacco, malnutrition, and inadequate prenatal care. Infants exposed *in utero* to heroin have reportedly been small for gestational age, at risk for respiratory distress, and cognitively impaired later in life. Marijuana exposure has been associated with decreased birthweight and length. Cocaine exposure has reportedly caused abruptio placentae, decreased birthweight, congenital anomalies, microcephaly, tremor, perinatal stroke, and developmental delay. A prospective study found diffuse or axial hypertonia more often among cocaine-exposed neonates than controls; this "spastic tetraparesis" cleared by 24 months of age, and there were no differences in mental or motor development.

MISCELLANEOUS EFFECTS

Guillain-Barré-type neuropathy and *brachial* or *lumbosacral plexopathy,* probably immunologic in origin, have been associated with heroin use. (Brachial plexopathy has also resulted from septic aneurysm of the subclavian artery.) Severe sensorimotor polyneuropathy occurs in sniffers of glue containing n-hexane. *Rhabdomyolysis* and renal failure have followed use of heroin, amphetamine, cocaine, and PCP. *Myeloneuropathy* indistinguishable from cobalamin deficiency occurs in nitrous oxide sniffers. Anemia is absent, and serum vitamin B_{12} levels are usually normal. The mechanism is inactivation of the cobalamin-dependent enzyme methionine synthetase. *Severe irreversible parkinsonism* developed in Californians exposed to a meperidine analog contaminated with 1-methyl-4-phenyl-1,2,3,6-tetrahydropyridine (MPTP), a metabolite of which is toxic to neurons in the substantia nigra. Symptoms respond to levodopa. *Dementia, ataxia, quadriparesis, blindness,* and *death* have occurred in European smokers of heroin pyrolysate. Autopsies show spongiform changes in the central nervous system white matter. The responsible toxin has not been identified. *Blindness* developed in a heavy heroin user whose mixture contained quinine; however, it improved when he resumed using a quinine-free preparation. Chronic cocaine users experience *dystonia* and *chorea,* and cocaine has precipitated symptoms in patients with *Tourette syndrome.* Marijuana inhibits luteinizing and follicle-stimulating hormones, causing *reversible impotence* and *sterility* in men and *menstrual irregularity* in women. *Ataxia* and *cerebellar white matter* changes have occurred in toluene sniffers.

SUGGESTED READINGS

Breiter HC, Gollub RI, Weisskoff RM, et al. Acute effects of cocaine on human brain activity and emotion. *Neuron* 1997;19:591–611.

Brust JCM. *Neurological aspects of substance abuse.* Boston: Butterworth-Heinemann, 1993.

Brust JCM. Stroke and substance abuse. In: Barnett HJM, Mohr JP, Stein BM, et al., eds. *Stroke: pathophysiology, diagnosis, and management,* 3rd ed. Philadelphia: WB Saunders, 1998:979–1000.

Chiriboga CA. Fetal effects. *Neurol Clin* 1993;11:707–728.

Chiriboga CA, Brust JCM, Bateman D, et al. Dose-response effect of fetal cocaine exposure on newborn neurological function. *Pediatrics* 1999;103:79–85.

Khanzian EJ, McKenna GJ. Acute toxic and withdrawal reactions associated with drug use and abuse. *Ann Intern Med* 1979;90:361–372.

Levine SR, Brust JCM, Futrell N, et al. Cerebrovascular complications of the use of the "crack" form of alkaloidal cocaine. *N Engl J Med* 1990;323:699–704.

Lowenstein DH, Massa SM, Rowbotham MC, et al. Acute neurologic and psychiatric complications associated with cocaine abuse. *Am J Med* 1987;83:841–846.

Nestler EJ, Aghajanian GK. Molecular and cellular basis of addiction. *Science* 1997;278:58–63.

Ng SKC, Brust JCM, Hauser WA, et al. Illicit drug use and the risk of new onset seizures: contrasting effects of heroin, marijuana, and cocaine. *Am J Epidemiol* 1990;132:47–57.

Pascual-Leone A, Dhuna A, Anderson DC. Cerebral atrophy in habitual cocaine abusers: a planimetric CT study. *Neurology* 1991;41:34–38.

Sloan MA, Kittner SJ, Feeser BR, et al. Illicit drug-associated ischemic stroke in the Baltimore-Washington Stroke Study. *Neurology* 1998;50:1688–1698.

Stolerman I. Drugs of abuse: behavioral principles, methods and terms. *Trends Pharmacol Sci* 1992;13:170–176.

Weinrieb RM, O'Brien CP. Persistent cognitive deficits attributed to substance abuse. *Neurol Clin* 1993;11:663–691.

Merritt's Neurology, 10th ed., edited by L.P. Rowland. Lippincott Williams & Wilkins, Philadelphia © 2000.

C H A P T E R

159

IATROGENIC DISEASE

LEWIS P. ROWLAND

The growing number of drugs used to treat human disease and the growing number of invasive procedures used for diagnosis and therapy have generated a new class of illness. Twenty years ago, 3% of admissions to Boston hospitals were due to adverse drug reactions, and 30% of all patients in those hospitals had at least one adverse drug reaction. Neurologic reactions accounted for 20% of all adverse reactions in another study. In 1996, Nelson and Talbert found that 16% of admissions to an intensive care unit in Texas were drug-related. In Australia, according to Roughead and associates (1996), 12% of all admissions to medical wards were drug-related, as were 15% to 22% of all emergency admissions.

A partial list of the neurologic syndromes seems formidable at first glance (Table 159.1), and it is important to keep some perspective. The drugs listed do not cause an adverse reaction every time they are used. For example, penicillin is high on the list of drugs that cause convulsive encephalopathies, but only a few cases have been recorded. Most of the other disorders are rare.

Some reactions, however, are common. Tardive dyskinesia is a price paid by many individuals for control of mental disorders, and levodopa-induced dyskinesia is the exchange many make for control of parkinsonism. Cerebral hemorrhage or femoral neuropathy due to retroperitoneal hemorrhage is the price a few patients pay for the prevention of stroke in many other patients. Drug-induced confusion and ataxia are common effects of anticonvulsants, and mental dulling or poor school performance are matters of concern for those who treat epilepsy. The adverse effects of radiotherapy limit our treatment of brain tumors. Control or elimination of these effects by alternative agents or procedures therefore has high priority in the therapeutic needs of neurology. The same must be said for the adverse effects of drugs used to treat neurologic disease that may damage other organs (e.g., corticosteroids, immunosuppressive drugs, antineoplastic drugs). There is even concern that levodopa may accelerate the course of Parkinson disease; on balance this seems unlikely.

It is sometimes difficult to list the rare side effects of a drug without inappropriately frightening patients or physicians. When considering the list of adverse reactions, one must consider the relative risks and the benefits expected from the use of specific drugs or specific procedures; patients must understand the tradeoffs involved if they are to be able to give truly *informed consent.*

There is another aspect of these drug reactions: Some have had what might be considered beneficial effects. For instance, the neuroparalytic accidents that followed the use of rabies vaccine led to the discovery of experimental autoimmune encephalomyelitis, and this in turn has had a lasting impact on our concepts of multiple sclerosis. In the meantime, rabies vaccine has been revised and now rarely leads to neurologic disease. Similarly, penicillamine-induced myasthenia gravis (MG) is a rare syndrome, but it has led to valuable observations about the nature of MG. Penicillin has also become important in the study of experimental epileptic neurons. Other drugs have been used to analyze the nature of peripheral neuropathies; some act on Schwann cells or myelin, others on the perikaryon, and others distally on the axon. Understanding the pathogenesis of some adverse reactions may lead to improved medical care in areas beyond the direct impact of the drugs involved.

New syndromes have arisen from these reactions. For instance, *epidural lipomatosis* was first recognized as a complication of steroid therapy, then a consequence of obesity, then an idiopathic disorder and finally a complication of anabolic steroid abuse by body builders. Another example is the *serotonin syndrome,* which is most often caused by use of serotonin-reuptake inhibitors. The Sternbach (1991) criteria for diagnosis are three: (1) After a serotoninergic drug is started or its dosage increased, three of the following appear: altered mental state, agitation, myoclonus, hyperreflexia, shivering, tremor, diarrhea, or incoordination. (2) Other possible etiologies are excluded, including infection, metabolic aberration, or substance abuse. (3) No other antipsychotic drug has been started or increased in dosage. Although numerous drugs can be responsible, several are often used by neurologists, such as sumatriptan succinate (Imitrex) for migraine and selegeline hydrochloride (Eldepryl) for Parkinson disease. Recognition of the syndrome and withdrawal of the offending drug are followed by reversal of symptoms.

The problems do not stop with drugs. Many procedures generate their own problems, including bone marrow transplantation, organ transplantation, brain implants, plasmapheresis, intravenous immunoglobulin therapy, pumps for intrathecal delivery of drugs, and more. The complications of a single therapy may take diverse forms; for instance, bone marrow transplantation may cause a graft-versus-host reaction and immunosuppression may also lead to central nervous system infections by bacteria, fungi, or viruses. Intensive care units are life-saving but also fraught with hazards.

TABLE 159.1. ADVERSE NEUROLOGIC REACTIONS DUE TO DRUGS OR PROCEDURES FOR DIAGNOSIS OR THERAPY

Adverse reaction	Drug or procedure
Aseptic meningitis	Trimethoprim, sulfadiazine, ibuprofen, intravenous immunoglobulin azathio-prine, sulin-dac, tolmetin, naproxen, OKT3
Basal ganglia syndromes (parkinsonism, tardive dyskinesia, other dyskinesias)	Butyrophenones, levodopa, phenothiazines, reserpine
Brain tumor	Immunosuppression (CNS lymphoma)
	Radiotherapy (meningioma)
Central pontine myelinolysis	Rapid correction of hyponatremia
Encephalopathy	Anticonvulsant drugs, cimetidine, corticosteroids, hemodialysis, insulin (hypoglycemia), lithium, methotrexate, metrizamide, monoamine oxidase inhibitors, overhydration (water intoxication), penicillin, pentazocine, propoxyphene, radiotherapy, vincristine
Leukoencephalopathy	Methotrexate, radiation, vaccines
Malignant neuroleptic syndrome	Neuroleptic drugs
Meningoencephalitis (viral, yeast, toxoplasmosis)	Immunosuppression
Malignant hyperthermia	Succinylcholine, halothane, others
Myopathies and myoglobinuria	Anticonvulsants (with osteomalacia), bacterial toxins with tampon use (toxic shock syndrome), chloroquine, corticosteroids, emetine, epsilon caproic acid, hypophosphatemia, ipecac, kaliuretic diuretics (furosemide, thiazides), licorice (glycyrrhizate), lovastatin, penicillamine, zidovudine
Muscle fibrosis	Meperidine, pentazocine
Myotonia	Diazacholesterol
Myelopathy	Intrathecal injections, delayed arachnoiditis after myelography, radiotherapy, spinal anesthesia, spinal angiography, vaccination
Neuromuscular disorders	
Myasthenia gravis	Antiepileptic drugs, penicillamine
Other neuromuscular blockade	Aminoglycoside antibiotics, succinylcholine
Optic neuropathy	Chloroquine, ethambutol, isoniazid, penicillamine, vincristine
Peripheral neuropathy	Anticoagulants (nerve compression by hematoma), barbiturates (in acute porphyria), disopyramide, disulfiram, ethambutol, hypophosphatemia, isoniazid, metronidazole, nitrofurantoin, nitrous oxide, perihexilene, phenytoin, procarbazine, vincristine, vitamin B_6 excess
Pseudotumor cerebri	Corticosteroids, nalidixic acid, tetracycline, vitamin A
Stroke	Amphetamines, anticoagulants, cerebral angiography and intraarterial interventional therapies, chiropractic manipulation of neck, induced hypotension for surgery induced cardiac arrest, insulin-induced hypoglycemia, massage of carotid sinus, open heart surgery and cardiopulmonary bypass, oral contraceptives, overcorrection of hypertension, radiotherapy of neck or cranium

Drugs and procedures are not the only iatrogenic disorders. The attitude and behavior of a physician can also contribute to chronic disability in patients. Both physicians and patients seem to prefer a serious diagnosis of nerve or muscle rather than confront the possibility that symptoms may be psychogenic. Modern epidemics of chronic fatigue syndrome, chronic Epstein-Barr syndrome, and chronic Lyme disease are new incarnations of psychasthenia and neurasthenia; physicians have a responsibility in propagating these disorders by emphasizing immunologic and other hypothetical disorders, even though study after study has shown the importance of psychosocial factors.

SUGGESTED READINGS

Allain T. Dialysis myelopathy: quadriparesis due to extradural amyloid of beta-microglobulin origin. *BMJ* 1988;296:752–753.

Atkinson JLD, Sundt TM Jr, Kazmier FJ, et al. Heparin-induced thrombocytopenia and thrombosis in ischemic stroke. *Mayo Clin Proc* 1988;63:353–361.

Baker GL, Kahl LE, Zee BC, et al. Malignancy following treatment of rheumatoid arthritis with cyclophosphamide: long-term case-control follow-up study. *Am J Med* 1987;83:1–10.

Batchelor TT, Taylor LP, Thaler HT, Posner JB, DeAngelis LM. Steroid myopathy in cancer patients. *Neurology* 1997;48:1234–1238.

Bertorini TE. Myoglobinuria, malignant hyperthermia, neuroleptic malignant syndrome and serotonin syndrome. *Neurol Clin* 1997;15:649–671.

Biller J, ed. *Iatrogenic neurology.* Boston: Buttterworth-Heinemann, 1998.

Bowyer SL, LaMothe MP, Hollister JR. Steroid myopathy: incidence and detection in a population with asthma. *J Allergy Clin Immunol* 1985;76:234–242.

Brannagan TH 3rd, Nagle KJ, Lange DJ, Rowland LP. Complications of intravenous immunoglobulin treatment in neurologic disease. *Neurology* 1996;47:674–677.

Caranasos GJ, Stewart RB, Cluff LE. Drug-induced illness leading to hospitalization. *JAMA* 1974;228:713–717.

Chaudry HJ, Cunha BA. Drug-induced aseptic meningitis. *Postgrad Med* 1991;90:65–70.

Cryer PE. Iatrogenic hypoglycemia as a cause of hypoglycemia-associated autonomic failure in IDDM: a vicious cycle. *Diabetes* 1992;41:255–260.

Cybulski GR, D'Angelo CM. Neurological deterioration after laminectomy for spondylotic cervical myeloradiculopathy: the putative role of spinal cord ischaemia. *J Neurol Neurosurg Psychiatry* 1988;51:717–718.

Dahlquist NR, Perrault J, Callaway CW, et al. D-lactic acidosis and encephalopathy after jejunoileostomy: response to overfeeding and to fasting in humans. *Mayo Clin Proc* 1984;59:141–145.

Denicoff KD, Rubinow DR, Papa MZ, et al. The neuropsychiatric effects of treatment with interleukin-2 and lymphokine-activated killer cells. *Ann Intern Med* 1987;107:293–300.

Ericsson M, Alges G, Schliamser SE. Spinal epidural abscess in adults: review and report of iatrogenic cases. *Scand J Infect Dis* 1990;22:249–257.

Evans CDH, Lacey JH. Toxicity of vitamins: complications of a health movement. *BMJ* 1986;292:509–510.

Fadul CE, Lemann W, Thaler HT, et al. Perforations of the gastrointestinal tract in patients receiving steroids for neurologic disease. *Neurology* 1988;38:348–352.

Fahn S. Welcome news about levodopa, but uncertainty remains. *Ann Neurol* 1998;43:551–554.

Fessler RG, Johnson DL, Brown FD, et al. Epidural lipomatosis in steroid-treated patients. *Spine* 1992;17:183–188.

Gardner DM, Lynd LD. Sumatriptan contraindications and the serotonin syndrome. *Ann Pharmacother* 1998;32:33–38.

Gibbons KJ, Guterman LR, Hopkins LN. Iatrogenic intracerebral hemorrhage. *Neurosurg Clin N Am* 1992;3:667–683.

Gilman PK. Serotonin syndrome: history and risk. *Fundam Clin Pharmacol* 1998;12:482–501.

Grafman J, Schwartz V, Dale JK, et al. Analysis of neuropsychological functioning in patients with chronic fatigue syndrome. *J Neurol Neurosurg Psychiatry* 1993;56:684–689.

Graus F, Saiz A, Sierra J, et al. Neurologic complications of autologous and allogeneic bone marrow transplantation in patients with leukemia: a comparative study. *Neurology* 1996;46:1004–1009.

Hunter JM. Adverse effects of neuromuscular blocking drugs. *Br J Anaesthiol* 1987;59:46–60.

Junck L, Marshall WH. Neurotoxicity of radiological contrast agents. *Ann Neurol* 1983;13:469–484.

Kaplan JG, Barasch E, Hirschfeld A, et al. Spinal epidural lipomatosis: a serious complication of iatrogenic Cushing's syndrome. *Neurology* 1989;39:1031–1034.

Kramer J, Klawans HL. Iatrogenic neurology: neurologic complications of nonneuropsychiatric agents. *Clin Neuropharmacol* 1979;4:175–198.

Lacomis D, Petrella JT, Giuliani MJ. Causes of neuromuscular weakness in the intensive care unit: a study of 92 patients. *Muscle Nerve* 1998;21:610–617.

Lane RJM, Mastaglia F. Drug-induced myopathies in man. *Lancet* 1978;2:562–566.

Laschinger JC, Izumoto H, Kouchoukos NT. Evolving concepts in prevention of spinal cord injury during operations on the descending thoracic and thoracoabdominal aorta. *Ann Thorac Surg* 1987;44:667–674.

Lawrie SM, Pelosi AJ. Chronic fatigue syndrome: prevalence and outcome. Psychosocial factors are important for management. *BMJ* 1994;308:732–733.

Lee P, Smith I, Piesowicz A, Brenton D. Spastic paraparesis after anaesthesia. *Lancet* 1999;353:554.

Mack EE, Wilson CB. Meningiomas induced by high-dose cranial irradiation. *J Neurosurg* 1993;79:28–31.

Malouf R, Brust JCM. Hypoglycemia: causes, neurological manifestations and outcome. *Ann Neurol* 1985;17:421–430.

Mattle AH, Sieb JP, Rohner M, et al. Nontraumatic spinal epidural and subdural hematomas. *Neurology* 1987;37:1351–1356.

Miller RR. Hospital admissions due to adverse drug reactions: a report from the Boston Collaborative Drug Surveillance Program. *Arch Intern Med* 1974;134:219–223.

Nelson KM, Talbert RL. Drug-related hospital admissions. *Pharmacotherapy* 1996;16:701–707.

Padovan CS, Yousry TA, Schleuning M, Holler E, Kolb HJ, Straube A. Neurological and neuroradiological findings in long-term survivors of allogeneic bone marrow transplantation. *Ann Neurol* 1998;43:627–633.

Pohl KRE, Farley JD, Jan JE, et al. Ataxia-telangiectasia in a child with vaccine-associated paralytic poliomyelitis. *J Pediatr* 1992;121:405–407.

Rampling R, Symonds P. Radiation myelopathy. *Curr Opin Neurol* 1998;11:627–632.

Richard IH. Acute, drug-induced, life-threatening neurologic syndromes. *Neurologist* 1998;4:196–210.

Richard IH, Kurlan R, Tanner C, et al. Serotonin syndrome and the combined use of deprenyl and an antidepressant in Parkinson's disease. Parkinson Study Group. *Neurology* 1997;48:1070–1077.

Rosenberg M, McCarten JR, Snyder BD, et al. Case report: hypophosphatemia with reversible ataxia and quadriparesis. *Am J Med Sci* 1987;293:261.

Roughead EE, Gilbert AL, Primrose JG, Sansom LN. Drug-related hospital admissions: a review of Australian studies published in 1988-1996. *Med J Aust* 1998;168:405–408.

Schaumberg H, Kaplan J, Windebank A, et al. Sensory neuropathy from pyridoxine abuse: a new megavitamin syndrome. *N Engl J Med* 1983;309:445–448.

Shintani S, Tanaka H, Irifune A, et al. Iatrogenic acute spinal epidural abscess with septic meningitis: MR findings. *Clin Neurol Neurosurg* 1992;94:253–255.

Siddiqui MF, Bertorini TE. Hypophosphatemia-induced neuropathy: clinical and electrophysiological findings. *Muscle Nerve* 1998;21:650–652.

Steere AC, Taylor E, McHugh GL, et al. The overdiagnosis of Lyme disease. *JAMA* 1993;269:1812–1816.

Sternbach H. The serotonin syndrome. *Am J Psychiatry* 1991;148:705–713.

Sterns RH, Riggs JE, Schochet SS Jr. Osmotic demyelination syndrome following correction of hyponatremia. *N Engl J Med* 1986;314:1535–1542.

Watanabe T, Trusler GA, Williams WG, et al. Phrenic nerve paralysis after pediatric cardiac surgery. *J Thorac Cardiovasc Surg* 1987;94:383–388.

Yuen EC, Layzer RB, Weitz SR, Olney RK. Neurologic complications of lumbar epidural anesthesia and analgesia. *Neurology* 1995;45:1795–1801.

Merritt's Neurology, 10th ed., edited by L.P. Rowland. Lippincott Williams & Wilkins, Philadelphia © 2000.

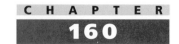

COMPLICATIONS OF CANCER CHEMOTHERAPY

MASSIMO CORBO
CASILDA M. BALMACEDA

ANTINEOPLASTIC DRUGS

Antitumor chemotherapy may be toxic to both the peripheral and central nervous system (CNS). Several antineoplastic drugs may induce more than one side effect, causing different neurologic disorders (Table 160.1). The incidence of neurotoxicity may depend on dosage, route and schedule of administration, patient age and general medical condition, and the combination with other neurotoxic drugs or with radiation therapy.

Peripheral Nervous System Toxicity

The vinca alkaloids, *vincristine sulfate* and *vinblastine sulfate* (Velban), may cause a sensorimotor neuropathy. Vincristine binds to tubulin and disrupts microtubules of the mitotic apparatus of cell division, arresting cells in metaphase. The effect on microtubules involved in axoplasmic transport may be responsible for axonal neuropathy. The severity of symptoms is related to total dose and duration of therapy. Distal paresthesia is the most common symptom, occurring in about 50% of patients. Later, there is distal sensory loss with weakness of the intrinsic hand muscles and the foot and toe dorsiflexors. Sensation is impaired more than motor function. Tendon reflexes are depressed. Although sensory loss tends to persist, paresthesia and weakness improve when dosage is reduced or therapy stopped. Cranial neuropathies tend to be bilateral; unilateral symptoms may suggest metastatic disease. Oculomotor paresis and transient vocal cord paralysis have been reported. Jaw pain results from trigeminal nerve toxicity, occurs suddenly or within 3 days after administration, and resolves spontaneously in a few days, usually without recurring with subsequent doses. An autonomic neuropathy may affect the gastrointestinal tract, causing abdominal pain and constipation in 45% to 60% of patients. Paralytic ileus

may follow. Other manifestations include urinary retention, impotence, and orthostatic hypotension. Vincristine neurotoxicity may be more severe in patients with increased age, preexisting neuropathy, and liver dysfunction and in combination with with asparaginase (Elspar) or etoposide (VePesid). Muscle cramps may be the first symptom of neurotoxicity. Patients previously treated with other spindle poisons, such as paclitaxel (Taxol), may not tolerate vincristine. *Vinorelbine* (Navelbine), a new semisynthetic vinca alkaloid, has less severe neurotoxicity, presumably because of weaker activity on axonal microtubules.

Cisplatin (Platinol) causes a dose-dependent, predominantly sensory polyneuropathy when given intravenously or after intraarterial treatment. Neuropathy follows a total cumulative dose greater than 300 to 500 mg/kg and is usually reversible by terminating therapy. Rarely, symptoms begin and progress when cisplatin is discontinued. The dorsal root ganglia are the most vulnerable structures, followed by peripheral nerves. Large myelinated fibers are most susceptible; proprioceptive sensory loss may be profound, with marked sensory ataxia. The motor system is spared. The adrenocorticotropic hormone analogs, glutathione, and nimodipine (Nimotop) may be neuroprotective when given concomitantly. Autonomic neuropathy is rare. Hearing loss is due to toxic effects on cochlear hair cells and may be irreversible. Neuropathies of cranial nerves III, V, and VI may follow intracarotid infusion. Lhermitte symptom is due to drug effects or may suggest spinal cord metastasis.

Carboplatin (Paraplatin), a cisplatin analog, has less severe neurologic toxicity but more pronounced hematologic toxicity. *Oxaliplatin* has a dose-limiting neurotoxicity, producing an acute neuropathy at a dose of 135 mg/m^2. The taxanes, *paclitaxel* and *docetaxel* (Taxotere), make microtubules excessively stable and thereby inhibit cell division. Paclitaxel produces a predominantly axonal sensory neuropathy after a single dose of 250 mg/m^2 or at lower doses with repeated treatment. Of treated patients, 50% to 90% are affected, depending on dosing regimens, and axonal sensory neuropathy may be the main dose-limiting toxicity. Early symptoms include distal numbness and tingling; examination reveals loss of tendon jerks and impaired perception of vibration. Proximal limb weakness and myalgia have been described. The neurotoxicity of the combination of docetaxel and cisplatin is more severe than when either medication is given alone. Less frequently, peripheral nerve dysfunction may also be caused by other antineoplastic agents, including *suramin, cytarabine* (Cytosar-U), *fludarabine phosphate* (Fludara), *procarbazine hydrochloride* (Matulane), and *etoposide*.

TABLE 160.1. NEUROTOXICITY OF ANTINEOPLASTIC DRUGS

Neurologic disorder	Drug
Peripheral neuropathy	Carboplatin, cisplatin, cytarabine, docetaxel, etoposide, fludarabine, oxaliplatin, paclitaxel, procarbazine, suramin, vinblastine, vincristine, vinorelbine
Cranial neuropathy	Carmustine, cisplatin, 5-fluorouracil, ifosfamide, vinblastine, vincristine
Autonomic neuropathy	Cisplatin, paclitaxel, procarbazine, vinblastine, vincristine, vinorelbine
Encephalopathy	Asparaginase, busulfan, carmustine, cisplatin, cytarabine, 5-fluorouracil, fludarabine, ifosfamide, methotrexate, procarbazine
Cerebellar syndrome	Cytarabine, 5-fluorouracil, procarbazine
Acute myelopathy	Cytarabine, methotrexate, thiotepa

Central Nervous System Toxicity

Most chemotherapeutic agents penetrate the blood–brain barrier poorly, and acute neurotoxicity is uncommon. However, symptoms and signs of CNS dysfunction may be induced by *ifosfamide* (IFEX) (10% to 30%), *fludarabine* (10% to 38%), *asparaginase* (15% to 40%), and *procarbazine* (less than 14%). *5-Fluorouracil* (5-FU) neurotoxicity is rare (5%) but includes an acute cerebellar syndrome with dysarthria, dysmetria, ataxia, vertigo, and nystagmus. The symptoms usually clear within 1 to 6 weeks after drug withdrawal. An inflammatory leukoencephalopathy with enhancing white matter lesions on magnetic resonance imaging (MRI) may follow combined administration of 5-FU and levamisole hydrochloride (Ergamisol). Vacuolar and necrotic lesions are found particularly in the brainstem and cerebellum. A cerebellar syndrome is also the most common neurologic adverse effect of high-dose *cytarabine* therapy (3 g/m^2 every 12 hours for 12 doses per course). Other manifestations are anosmia, somnolence, optic atrophy, bulbar and pseudobulbar palsies, and hemiparesis. The frequency of CNS side effects is 6% to 47%, usually within 1 week after the first dose. Patients older than 60 years may be at increased risk. Symptoms often subside within weeks. Complications after intrathecal administration of cytarabine include meningismus, seizures, or paraparesis, often with pain and loss of sensation. Although CNS toxicity is uncommon with *vincristine* treatment, intrathecal administration may cause seizures, encephalopathy, or myelopathy.

High doses of chemotherapy in conjunction with stem cell support or bone marrow transplantation may result in neurotoxicity that is not seen with conventional doses. This occurs with the alkylating agents *busulfan* (Myleran), the *nitrosoureas,* or *thiotepa* (Thioplex), as well as with *etoposide.* High-dose or intracarotid therapy with *carmustine* (BiCNU) may cause encephalopathy or retinopathy. Carotid artery injection of *cisplatin* may cause loss of vision or seizures. Drug streaming after intraarterial infusion may expose local areas of brain to extremely high concentrations of the drug, resulting in focal cerebral necrosis.

Methotrexate in conventional doses has little or no neurotoxicity when given intravenously, but high-dose therapy may cause an acute strokelike encephalopathy. This syndrome usually occurs abruptly several days after the initiation of therapy and resolves within days after treatment stops. It is characterized by seizures, confusion, hemiparesis, speech disorders, and loss of consciousness. A vascular or embolic etiology has been postulated. Intrathecal methotrexate therapy, used in the prophylaxis of meningeal leukemia and in the treatment of leptomeningeal carcinomatosis, may induce an acute arachnoiditis in 5% to 40% of patients. Starting a few hours after drug administration, the syndrome includes headache, nausea, vomiting, fever, back pain, dizziness, meningismus, and signs of increased intracranial pressure. It usually resolves within a few days. If methotrexate is given intrathecally two to three times a week, a subacute myelopathy or encephalopathy may follow. Subacute methotrexate neurotoxicity seems to be mediated by release of adenosine, and it is relieved by giving aminophylline, which displaces adenosine from its receptor.

A chronic delayed leukoencephalopathy may be caused by intravenous high-dose methotrexate, with symptoms beginning several months after the start of treatment and involving personality changes followed by dementia, focal seizures, spasticity, and alterations in consciousness. Most patients show improvement if treatment ceases. A progressive leukoencephalopathy may also be seen in patients given methotrexate intrathecally combined with prophylactic cranial radiotherapy. Computed tomography (CT) or MRI shows extensive, deep, bilateral white matter lesions. Calcification may be observed in children. The syndrome typically follows a delay of 1 to 2 years and is a major problem in patients successfully treated for leukemia. Although the combined effects of methotrexate and radiation are held responsible rather than the methotrexate alone, this combination is still considered an important strategy for the treatment of acute lymphoblastic leukemia. However, the incidence of leukoencephalopathy (18%) following treatment with intrathecal moderate-dose methotrexate (8 to 12 mg/m^2; cumulative dose, 24 to 90 mg) and prophylactic radiotherapy (18 to 24 Gy) appears to be less than that following treatment with intravenous high-dose methotrexate (50% to 68%). Rarely, a focal leukoencephalopathy is seen if the Ommaya reservoir tip is misplaced in the white matter. Leukoencephalopathy has also been described after oral methotrexate therapy for rheumatoid arthritis.

IMMUNOSUPPRESSANT DRUGS

Cyclosporine (Sandimmune) is the mainstay therapy in preventing organ transplant rejection. It acts by inhibiting interleukin-2 (IL-2) production by T cells and is successful in suppressing T-cell response to transplantation antigens and thus prolonging graft survival. In addition to nephrotoxicity and hypertension, neurotoxicity in 8% to 47% of patients includes tremor, paresthesias, seizures, lethargy, ataxia, and quadriparesis. Toxicity, more frequently observed with serum levels greater than 500 ng/mL, may also cause a cerebral blindness that is usually reversible, improving with cessation of therapy or dose reduction. Reversible cerebral white matter lesions are seen on CT or MRI; cortical lesions in both occipital lobes may be present. Hemiparesis may suggest that cyclosporine focally damages blood vessels, but the frequency of cyclosporine neurotoxicity increases in HLA-mismatched and unrelated donor transplants, suggesting that immune factors play a role. Cyclosporine induces activity of the hepatic cytochrome P-450, which also mediates drug oxidation. Consequently, hepatic dysfunction or concomitant administration of agents that induce the P-450 system can cause increased or reduced concentrations of cyclosporine in blood. In the circulation, cyclosporine is bound to lipoproteins; a reduction in serum cholesterol to less than 120 mg/dL may increase free-drug levels and neurotoxicity. Corticosteroids also increase plasma cyclosporine levels.

OKT3, a powerful immunosuppressive drug, is the first monoclonal murine antibody to become available for therapy in humans. It is used to treat acute allograft rejection. An asymptomatic cerebrospinal fluid pleocytosis occurs in most patients so treated. Neurologic complications may develop within hours of administration and include altered mental function, seizures, and lethargy. Contrast-enhancing cerebral lesions may be seen on MRI. Aseptic meningitis, visual loss, and transient sensorineural hearing loss are other adverse effects.

Tacrolimus (Prograf) has cyclosporine-like activity and is approved for immunosuppression in organ transplantation, particularly if organ rejection is not responsive to OKT3 therapy. It may cause acute tremor, headache, and paresthesias, but neurotoxicity occurs in only 5% to 10% of patients. Neurologic symptoms begin when the tacrolimus level in blood is at a peak, and eventually resolve after the dose is reduced or stopped. In a tacrolimus-related leukoencephalopathy, demyelination in the parietooccipital region and centrum semiovale may be seen on MRI, as in the syndrome caused by cyclosporine. Clinical recovery is usually accompanied by reversal of radiologic abnormalities. Transient cortical blindness and cerebellar symptoms have been described.

BIOLOGIC RESPONSE MODIFIERS

Cytokines, such as interferons and IL-2, are used as biologic response modifiers to treat cancer. Neurotoxic effects include vertigo, memory loss, confusion, emotional instability, somnolence, depression, seizures, and hemiparesis. Cytokine-related encephalopathy is self-limited and probably related to increased levels of circulating cytokines after renal allografting. Risk factors include delayed graft function, cadaveric transplantation, and diabetes. Corticosteroid treatment may be helpful.

BONE MARROW TRANSPLANTATION

Bone marrow transplantation (BMT) of cells from an HLA-matched donor is widely used to treat refractory leukemia or myelodysplastic conditions. It often results in an immunologic reaction of donor T lymphocytes against recipient tissues, called *graft-versus-host-disease* (GVHD). Acute GVHD involves the skin, gastrointestinal tract, and liver. Chronic GVHD occurs in 30% to 40% of patients who survive more than 100 days. Manifestations include altered immune function, hypergammaglobulinemia, increased susceptibility to viral infection, and symptoms of collagen-vascular disease. Neurologic disorders of chronic GVHD are polymyositis, myasthenia gravis, sensorimotor neuropathy, aseptic meningitis, or leukoencephalopathy. Remission of neurologic toxicity may follow successful treatment of GVHD with steroids and immunosuppressive drugs.

The most common neurologic complications in patients who undergo allogeneic or autologous BMT are cerebral hemorrhage (4%), metabolic encephalopathy (3%), and CNS infections (2%). Hemorrhages are most common with autologous BMT, are mostly subdural, and are attributed to thrombocytopenia. A post-BMT leukoencephalopathy occurs particularly in patients who have had prior cerebral irradiation. It is characterized by focal signs, lethargy, confusion, and progressive deterioration. An acute parkinsonian syndrome has been described. Progressive multifocal leukoencephalopathy may occur in immunocompromised patients after autologous or allogeneic BMT for chronic myelogenous leukemia. The most common neuropathologic

findings in patients undergoing BMT are cerebrovascular lesions, including areas of hemorrhagic necrosis and infarction.

SUGGESTED READINGS

Antineoplastic Drugs

Baker WJ, Royer GL Jr, Weiss RB. Cytarabine and neurologic toxicity. *J Clin Oncol* 1991;9:67–93.

Berger T, Malayeri R, Doppelbauer A, et al. Neurological monitoring of neurotoxicity induced by paclitaxel/cisplatin chemotherapy. *Eur J Cancer* 1997;33:1393–1399.

Bernini JC, Fort DW, Griener JC, et al. Aminophylline for methotrexate-induced neurotoxicity. *Lancet* 1995;345:544–547.

Blay JY, Conroy T, Chevreau C, et al. High-dose methotrexate for the treatment of primary cerebral lymphomas: analysis of survival and late neurologic toxicity in a retrospective series. *J Clin Oncol* 1998;16:864–871.

Cain JW, Bender CM. Ifosfamide-induced neurotoxicity: associated symptoms and nursing implications. *Oncol Nurs Forum* 1995;22:659–666.

Cain MS, Burton GV, Holcombe RF. Fatal leukoencephalopathy in a patient with non-Hodgkin's lymphoma treated with CHOP chemotherapy and high-dose steroids. *Am J Med Sci* 1998;315:202–207.

Cavaletti G, Bogliun G, Marzorati L, et al. Peripheral neurotoxicity of Taxol in patients previously treated with cisplatin. *Cancer* 1995;75:1141–1150.

Chaudhry V, Rowinsky EK, Sartorious SE, et al. Peripheral neuropathy from Taxol and cisplatin combination chemotherapy: clinical and electrophysiological studies. *Ann Neurol* 1994;35:304–311.

Fazeny B, Zifko U, Meryn S, et al. Vinorelbine-induced neurotoxicity in patients with advanced breast cancer pretreated with paclitaxel: a phase II study. *Cancer Chemother Pharmacol* 1996;39:150–156.

Figueredo AT, Fawcet SE, Molloy DW, et al. Disabling encephalopathy during 5-fluorouracil and levamisole adjuvant therapy for resected colorectal cancer: a report of two cases. *Cancer Invest* 1995;13:608–611.

Forman AR. Peripheral neuropathy in cancer patients: clinical types, etiology and presentation. *Oncology* 1990;4:85–89.

Gregg RW, Molepo JM, Monpetit VJ, et al. Cisplatin neurotoxicity: the relationship between dosage, time, and platinum concentration in neurologic tissues, and morphologic evidence of toxicity. *J Clin Oncol* 1992;10:795–803.

Hilkens PH, Pronk LC, Verweij J, et al. Peripheral neuropathy induced by combination chemotherapy of docetaxel and cisplatin. *Br J Cancer* 1997;75:417–422.

Kimmel DW, Wijdicks EF, Rodriguez M. Multifocal inflammatory leukoencephalopathy associated with levamisole therapy. *Neurology* 1995;45:374–376.

Lovblad K, Kelkar P, Ozdoba C, et al. Pure methotrexate encephalopathy presenting with seizures: CT and MRI features. *Pediatr Radiol* 1998;28:86–91.

Lyass O, Lossos A, Hubert A, et al. Cisplatin-induced non-convulsive encephalopathy. *Anticancer Drugs* 1998;9:100–104.

Macdonald DR. Neurologic complications of chemotherapy. *Neurol Clin* 1991;9:955–967.

Matsumoto K, Takahashi S, Sato A, et al. Leukoencephalopathy in childhood hematopoietic neoplasm caused by moderate-dose methotrexate and prophylactic cranial radiotherapy: an MR analysis. *Int J Radiat Oncol Biol Phys* 1995;32:913–918.

New PZ, Jackson CE, Rinaldi D, et al. Peripheral neuropathy secondary to docetaxel (Taxotere). *Neurology* 1996;46:108–111.

Resar LMS, Phillips PC, Kastan MB, et al. Acute neurotoxicity after intrathecal cytosine arabinoside in two adolescents with acute lymphoblastic leukemia of B-cell type. *Cancer* 1993;71:117–123.

Tuxen MK, Hansen SW. Neurotoxicity secondary to antineoplastic drugs. *Cancer Treat Rev* 1994;20:191–214.

Verschraegen C, Conrad CA, Hong WK. Subacute encephalopathic toxicity of cisplatin. *Lung Cancer* 1995;13:305–309.

Waber DP, Tarbell NJ. Toxicity of CNS prophylaxis for childhood leukemia. *Oncology* 1997;11:259–265.

Worthley SG, McNeil JD. Leukoencephalopathy in a patient taking low-dose oral methotrexate therapy for rheumatoid arthritis. *J Rheumatol* 1995;22:335–337.

Immunosuppressant Drugs: General

Martinez AJ. The neuropathology of organ transplantation: comparison and contrast in 500 patients. *Pathol Res Pract* 1998;194:473–486.

Cyclosporine and Tacrolimus

Appignani BA, Bhadelia RA, Blacklow SC, et al. Neuroimaging findings in patients on immunosuppressive therapy: experience with tacrolimus toxicity. *AJR* 1996;166:683–688.

Devine SM, Newman NJ, Siegel JL, et al. Tacrolimus (FK506)-induced cerebral blindness following bone marrow transplantation. *Bone Marrow Transplant* 1996;18:569–572.

Hughes RL. Cyclosporine-related central nervous system toxicity in cardiac transplantation. *N Engl J Med* 1990;323:420–421.

Lanzino G, Cloft H, Hemstreet MK, et al. Reversible posterior leukoencephalopathy following organ transplantation: description of two cases. *Clin Neurol Neurosurg* 1997;99:222–226.

Memon M, deMagalhaes-Silverman M, Bloom EJ, et al. Reversible cyclosporine-induced cortical blindness in allogeneic bone marrow transplant recipients. *Bone Marrow Transplant* 1995;15:283–286.

Pace MT, Slovis TL, Kelly JK, Abella SD. Cyclosporin A toxicity: MRI appearance of the brain. *Pediatr Radiol* 1995;25:180–183.

Shutter LA, Green JP, Newman NJ, et al. Cortical blindness and white matter lesions in a patient receiving FK506 after liver transplantation. *Neurology* 1993;43:2417–2418.

Small SL, Fukui MB, Bramblett GT, Eidelman BH. Immunosuppression-induced leukoencephalopathy from tacrolimus (FK506). *Ann Neurol* 1996;40:575–580.

Tezcan H, Zimmer W, Fenstermaker R, et al. Severe cerebellar swelling and thrombotic purpura associated with FK506. *Bone Marrow Transplant* 1998;21:105–109.

Zimmer WE, Hourihane JM, Wang HZ, Schriber JR. The effect of human leukocyte antigen disparity on cyclosporine neurotoxicity after allogeneic bone marrow transplantation. *AJNR* 1998;19:601–610.

OKT3

Coleman AR, Norman DJ. OKT3 encephalopathy. *Ann Neurol* 1990;28:837–838.

Parizel PM, Snoeck HW, van den Hauwe L, et al. Cerebral complications of murine monoclonal CD3 antibody (OKT3): CT and MR findings. *AJNR* 1997;18:1935–1938.

Seifeldin RA, Lawrence KR, Rahamtulla AF, Monaco AP. Generalized seizures associated with the use of muromonab-CD3 in two patients after kidney transplantation. *Ann Pharmacother* 1997;31:586–589.

Shihab F, Barry JM, Bennet WM, et al. Cytosine-related encephalopathy induced by OKT3: incidence and predisposing factors. *Transplant Proc* 1993;25:564–565.

Biologic Response Modifiers

Bender CM, Monti EJ, Kerr ME. Potential mechanisms of interferon toxicity. *Cancer Pract* 1996;4:35–39.

Licinio J, Kling MA, Hauser P. Cytokines and brain function: relevance to interferon-alpha-induced mood and cognitive changes. *Semin Oncol* 1998;25:30–38.

Michel M, Vincent F, Sigal R, et al. Cerebral vasculitis after interleukin-2 therapy for renal cell carcinoma. *J Immunother Emphasis Tumor Immunol* 1995;18:124–126.

Bone Marrow Transplantation

Amato AA, Barohn RJ, Sahenk Z, et al. Polyneuropathy complicating bone marrow and solid organ transplantation. *Neurology* 1993;43:1513–1518.

Anderson BA, Young PV, Kean WF, et al. Polymyositis in chronic graft-versus-host disease. *Arch Neurol* 1982;39:188–190.

Bolger GB, Sullivan KM, Spence AM, et al. Myasthenia gravis after allogeneic bone marrow transplantation: relationship to chronic graft-versus-host disease. *Neurology* 1986;36:1087–1091.

Ferrara JLM, Deeg HJ. Graft-versus-host disease. *N Engl J Med* 1991;324:667–674.

Graus F, Saiz A, Sierra J, et al. Neurologic complications of autologous and allogeneic bone marrow transplantation in patients with leukemia: a comparative study. *Neurology* 1996;46:1004–1009.

Lockman LA, Sung JH, Krivit W. Acute parkinsonian syndrome with demyelinating leukoencephalopathy in bone marrow transplant recipients. *Pediatr Neurol* 1991;7:457–463.

Owen RG, Patmore RD, Smith GM, Barnard DL. Cytomegalovirus-induced T-cell proliferation and the development of progressive multifocal leucoencephalopathy following bone marrow transplantation. *Br J Haematol* 1995;89:196–198.

Provenzale JM, Graham ML. Reversible leukoencephalopathy associated with graft-versus-host disease: MR findings. *AJNR* 1996;17:1290–1294.

Seong D, Bruner JM, Lee KH, et al. Progressive multifocal leukoencephalopathy after autologous bone marrow transplantation in a patient with chronic myelogenous leukemia. *Clin Infect Dis* 1996;23:402–403.

Snider S, Bashir R, Bierman P. Neurologic complications after high-dose chemotherapy and autologous bone marrow transplantation for Hodgkin's disease. *Neurology* 1994;44:681–684.

Tahsildar HI, Remler BF, Creger RJ, et al. Delayed, transient encephalopathy after marrow transplantation: case reports and MRI findings in four patients. *J Neurooncol* 1996;27:241–250.

Merritt's Neurology, 10th ed., edited by L.P. Rowland. Lippincott Williams & Wilkins, Philadelphia © 2000.

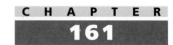

OCCUPATIONAL AND ENVIRONMENTAL NEUROTOXICOLOGY

LEWIS P. ROWLAND

Neurotoxicology commands newspaper attention these days. Is there a Gulf War syndrome? Did exposure there to anticholinesterase nerve gases cause amyotrophic lateral sclerosis (ALS)? Do silicon breast implants cause autoimmune disorders, including multiple sclerosis? Are behavioral changes due to subclinical occupational exposure? Do nearby petrochemical plants or high power electrical lines increase the incidence of brain tumors? Can mercury intoxication result from inhalation of the element from dental amalgams and can that cause multiple sclerosis, ALS, or other diseases? These and similar questions have been debated in an atmosphere of contentious uncertainty. In this chapter we focus on the particular clinical syndromes that result from exposure to heavy metals, solvents, and natural neurotoxins (Table 161.1). Clinical diagnosis, laboratory proof of diagnosis, and treatment are the practical issues. We bypass detailed discussion of behavioral effects from chronic low-level exposures as beyond the scope of this chapter. More detailed information is provided in the General section of Suggested Readings.

HEAVY METAL INTOXICATION

Pathogenesis

The heavy metals have diverse toxic effects on cell nuclei, mitochondria, other organelles, cytoplasmic enzymes, and membrane lipids. Clinical syndromes may result from combinations of these effects that do not readily explain the real-life disorders or why the assault should affect the central nervous system (CNS) in some people, peripheral nerves in others, or both.

Lead provides an example of the complexity. It interferes with the sulfhydryl enzymes of heme biosynthesis, especially δ-aminolevulinic acid dehydratase, coproporphyrin oxidase, and ferrochetalase. As a result of these partial blocks, several metabolites accumulate in blood and urine: δ-aminolevulinic acid, coprophorphyrin III, and zinc protoporphyrin. Other heme-containing enzymes are also affected, including cytochrome P450 in the liver and mitochondrial cytochrome c oxidase. Lead also interferes with calcium-activated enzymes, calcium channels, and Ca^{2+}-ATPase. Lead has similarly multiple and diverse biochemical ill effects on cell metabolism. Sorting out these interactions and their relationship to the clinical syndromes is not a simple task, and there is even less basic information about other neurointoxicants.

Nevertheless, metals and biologic toxins have been used experimentally to analyze the pathogenesis of the neuropathies according to effects on axons, myelin, or Schwann cells.

Recognizing Intoxication Clinically

The clinical manifestations of an intoxication can result from diverse causes. Other possible causes must therefore be excluded (Table 161.2) by considering systemic or metabolic disease and evaluating therapeutic drugs the patient may be taking. More reliable diagnosis depends on the recognition of exposure by occupation or recreation, recognition of a specific syndrome and elimination of other causes (as in the acute lead encephalopathy of childhood), or associated laboratory abnormalities. Outbreaks or clusters may be encountered with the relatively mild symptoms of glue sniffing or the devastating encephalomyelopathy of Minamata disease in Japan, which was caused by methyl mercury. The circumstances of attempted suicide or fire usually identify carbon monoxide exposure; a motor running in a parked automobile or a faulty gasoline-fueled heater are most often responsible. For the following discussions, the primary at-risk occupations are listed in Table 161.1 and are not repeated in the text.

Acute Encephalopathy

Syndromes of confusion, hyperactivity or somnolence, memory impairment, and behavioral change arise from many different disorders, as described under delirium in Chapter 1. The acute encephalopathy of lead poisoning is one that affects children; seizures and increased intracranial pressure without a mass lesion may be clues to diagnosis. The circumstances of intoxication may be evident as in glue sniffing or dialysis dementia. Heavy metal intoxication is not encountered frequently among the causes of delirium but may be the result of attempted murder by poisoning.

Chronic Encephalopathy

Dementia with or without tremor can be a manifestation of occupational exposure to heavy metals. Therefore, when confronted with a patient who may have been poisoned, it may be more important to know the occupational history than to order a sweeping laboratory survey of blood and urine. Mercury intoxication may be more often associated with tremor than other exposures, but this is probably not a reliable guide. Parkinsonism can arise in workers in manganese smelters; monitoring guidelines are not always heeded. Parkinsonism may also follow chronic exposure to carbon disulfide.

Peripheral Neuropathy

Neuropathy may be caused by any heavy metal, almost always the result of occupational exposure. The symptoms are those of any sensorimotor neuropathy with acroparesthesia and distal limb weakness. Optic and autonomic neuropathies seem to be rare. A hallmark of thallium neuropathy is baldness. The neuropathy of organophosphate poisoning may be accompanied by upper motor neuron signs that imply a myelopathy; sometimes the residual signs include those of the lower motor neuron but the occupational history and the sensory loss differentiate the syndrome from motor neuron disease.

TABLE 161.1. NEUROTOXIC SYNDROMES

Agent	Occupational or other exposure	Syndrome	
		Acute	Chronic
Metals			
Arsenic	Pesticides, pigments, paint, electroplating, seafood, smelter, semiconductors	Encephalopathy	Neuropathy
Lead	Solder, lead shot, illicit whiskey, insecticides, auto body shop, storge battery manufacture, smelter, paint, water pipes, gasoline sniffing	Encephalopathy	Encephalopathy, neuropathy, motor neuron disease-like syndrome
Manganese	Iron industry, welding, mining smelter, fireworks, fertilizer, dry cell batteries	Encephalopathy	Parkinsonism
Mercury	Thermometers, other gauges; dental office (amalgams); felt hat manufacture	Headache, tremor	Electroplating, photography
			Neuropathy, encephalopathy with dementia, tremor
Tin	Canning industry, solder, electronics, plastics, fungicides	Delerium	Encephalomyelopathy
Solvents			
Carbon disulfide	Rayon manufacture, preservatives, textiles, rubber cement, varnish, electroplating	Encephalopathy	Neuropathy, parkinsonism
Trichlorethylene	Paints, degreasers, spot removers, decaffeination, dry cleaning, rubber solvents	Narcosis	Encephalopathy, trigeminal neuropathy
Hexacarbons[a]	Paints, pain removers, varnish, degreasers, rapid-drying ink, glues, cleaning agents, glues for making shoes in poorly vented cottage industry, glue sniffing, MNBK in plastics	Narcosis	Neuropathy, encephalopathy, ataxia
Insecticides			
Organophosphates, carbamates	Manufacture, application	Cholinergic syndrome	Ataxia, neuropathy, myelopathy
Carbon monoxide	Accidental or deliberate exposure in motor vehicles, faulty gasoline-fueled heaters	Anoxic encephalopathy	
Methyl alcohol	Contaminated illicit whiskey	Retinal blindess	
Recreation abuse			
Nitrous oxide	Dental offices	Encephalopathy	B_{12}-deficient myelopathy
Seafood			
Ciguartera		Sensory neuropathy with temperature inversion	
Shellfish		Acute neuropathy	

[a]Hexacarbons: n-hexane, methyl-n-butyl ketone (MNBK).

Cranial Neuropathy

Trichlorethylene causes a selective sensory neuropathy of the trigeminal nerve; the syndrome is so specific that it was once seriously evaluated as a treatment for idiopathic trigeminal neuralgia. Visual loss from optic neuropathy or retinopathy is a manifestation of methanol toxicity and many therapeutic drugs.

Specific Clinical Syndromes of Intoxication

Lead

Acute lead encephalopathy in children was first recognized in 1904 and even then was attributed to lead-containing house paint. The syndrome also occurs in adults who are occupationally exposed. The childhood syndrome has been linked to pica, the in-

TABLE 161.2. CLUES TO THE DIAGNOSIS OF INTOXICATIONS

Nature of exposure	Occupation with known hazard
	Recreational use of known hazard
	Accidental exposure to hazard
	Dialysis (aluminum)
	Cluster or epidemic of syndrome (seafood, "huffing")
	Dietary exposure to known hazard (seafood)
	Diagnosis of exclusion
	Therapeutic drugs
	Alcohol abuse
	Illicit drug abuse
	Infection
	Systemic disease: renal, pulmonary, calcium, liver, endocrine, electrolytes
	Inherited metabolic diseases
Age of Patient	Children—lead encephalopathy
	Adolescents, young adults—sniffing, nitrous oxide
Associated symptoms, signs or laboratory abnormalities	
Lead	Gastrointesinal symptoms: colic, constipation
	Anemia
	Basophilic sippling
	↑ urinary δ-aminolevulinic acid
Thallium	Alopecia
Arsenic	Mees lines (horizontal stratifications of fingernails or leuconychia)
Nitrous oxide	B_{12} deficiency
Specific syndromes	
Optic neuropathy and retinopathy	Methyl alcohol
SMON	Clioquinol
Methyl mercury	Minamata disease
NMBK	Trigeminal neuropathy

NMBK, n-methyl butyl ketone; SMON, subacute myelo-optic neuropathy.

gestion of flaking lead-containing paint on the walls of old houses. Inhalation of dust from the ancient paint is another important source of household contamination and makes paint removal hazardous, especially when the paint is burned.

Because symptoms are difficult to detect in toddlers, the Centers for Disease Control and Prevention advocates periodic screening of blood lead for all children aged 9 to 36 months. That policy has been debated, but recognition and treatment can prevent the sometimes devastating cerebral consequences. Blood lead levels in U.S. children declined by 78% largely because lead was removed from automobile gasoline and also because lead has been eliminated from house paint. Acute lead encephalopathy is now rare in the United States. However, it is feared that early lead exposure can adversely affect later behavior and school performance. Evidence from several sources suggests that higher blood lead levels are associated with lower IQ. Because of increasing doubt about the efficacy of chelation therapy, prevention is now the goal, as described below.

Lead neuropathy is probably restricted to heavy occupational exposure, which is monitored by regulations established by the Occupational Safety and Health Administration; overt neuropathy is rare. Cases attributed to retained bullets in the abdomen or drinking from lead-lined glasses require confirmation by biochemical markers lacking in published reports. Traditionally, the characteristic syndrome of lead neuropathy is confined to motor fibers restricted to or especially involving the radial nerve. However, the presence of visible fasciculation and brisk reflexes or frank upper motor neuron signs suggests that this could be a myelopathy similar to that of ALS. However, there have been no convincing case reports of an ALS-like syndrome in lead workers since 1974.

Mercury

The relations between elemental, inorganic, and organic forms of mercury involve transformations from one form to another. Chronic occupational exposure to mercury may lead to the "Mad Hatter syndrome," which is dominated by a tremor resembling essential tremor but which can be severe, even affecting head and trunk. Memory loss, social withdrawal, and emotional lability may be prominent. Similar symptoms may result from exposure to inorganic mercury, which is presumably broken down to elemental mercury in the environment. Inorganic mercury is more likely to cause a sensorimotor neuropathy.

Mercury was held responsible for *Minamata disease*, which affected 2,500 people near the bay of that name in Japan. The outbreak illustrates the conversion of inorganic mercury to more toxic organic mercury by fish. A factory was using mercuric chloride in the manufacture of vinyl chloride. Waste material from the plant was discharged into the bay, ingested by fish, and converted into more toxic methylmercury. The fish were eaten by people, who were also intoxicated. The syndrome comprised cognitive change, cerebellar ataxia, and sensorimotor neuropathy. Visual loss was often severe and may be related to damage of the occipital cortex. Symptoms progressed for 3 to 10 years.

Arsenic

Acute arsenic poisoning is a multisystem disaster: vomiting, bloody diarrhea, myoglobinuria, renal failure, arrhythmias, hypotension, seizures, coma, and death. In survivors, Mees lines on the fingernails and sensorimotor neuropathy appear in 7 to 14 days. Sensory symptoms dominate, and weakness is more profound in the legs than in the arms and hands. Slow and incomplete recovery takes years. Nerve conduction velocities are typically slow. Cognition may be impaired in some survivors, depending on the severity of the acute encephalopathy.

Intoxication by inhalation may be acute or chronic. The chronic version is "blackfoot disease" with vascular changes and gangrene and a less severe peripheral neuropathy. Most arsenic exposure is occupational, but arsenic contamination of groundwater is a growing problem in poverty areas of India and elsewhere. The use of arsenic trioxide to treat leukemia may also be followed by arsenic neuropathy.

Thallium

A rare syndrome, thallium intoxication is usually the result of unwittingly ingesting a rat poison. The acute episode is dominate by gastrointestinal symptoms. Paresthesias may be noted soon afterward, but overt signs of neuropathy may take 2 weeks to appear. The encephalopathy may include cognitive impairment and choreoathetosis, myoclonus, or other involuntary movements. The unique clue to diagnosis is loss of hair, which begins 1 to 3 weeks after exposure. Neuropathy and dermatitis may be prominent in chronic exposure.

Manganese

George Cotzias, discoverer of the therapeutic value of levodopa in Parkinson disease, followed an unusual path to that achievement. He was a biochemist, interested in the role of metals in enzyme activity. Manganese was one such metal and that took him to an outbreak of parkinsonism in South American miners. At about that time, Hornykewicz identified the lack of dopamine in the substantia nigra of patients with Parkinson disease; Cotzias gave the precursor in amounts larger than others had used previously.

Manganese intoxication reproduces the essential motor features of Parkinson disease but with sufficient clinical and pathologic differences to indicate the conditions are not identical. The outlook is gloomy, including severe cognitive loss. Responses to levodopa and to chelation therapy are limited.

Aluminum

Dialysis dementia has been attributed to the presence of aluminum in the dialysis water and also in ingested phosphate binders used to control blood phosphorus levels. Treatment of the water and avoidance of the binders have decreased the incidence of the syndrome. Encephalopathy, however, has also occurred in uremic patients dialyzed with deionized water and also in some who took the binders without dialysis, implying that abnormal retention of aluminum is a characteristic of uremia.

Paresthesias and weakness were part of *potroom palsy*, a complex syndrome in workers in a smelter who were exposed to pots that had not been vented properly. Other manifestations included ataxia, tremor, and memory loss.

Biochemical Diagnosis

Measurement of blood lead levels is the time-honored diagnostic method even though technical variations render values somewhat uncertain in individual cases. The mean whole blood level in adults who are not exposed to occupational hazards is less than 5 μg/dL. Standard recommendations now consider levels safe up to 30 μg/dL; some consider a higher safe limit, 50 μg/dL. Workers are monitored closely if levels exceed 40 μg/dL. The upper limit of lead in urine is 150 μg/g creatinine. Peripheral neuropathy is usually accompanied by blood lead levels greater than 70 μg/dL.

In children, the warning mark is a blood lead level of 10 μg/dL, and estimates suggest that 1.7 million children still have higher levels. Children with levels exceeding 10 μg/dL are more likely to be African-American, poor, and living in large cities. For them, the major source of poisoning is lead paint, followed by contaminated soils and dust. Chelation therapy commences with levels of 40 μg/dL. Testing blood lead levels is recommended for children with presumed autism, attention deficit disorder, pervasive development disorder, mental retardation, or language problems. The blood lead level is considered a more reliable indicator than the biochemical tests mentioned below.

A provocative test with Ca-EDTA has been advocated but has been used less and less often. The patient is given 500 mg/m^2 Ca-EDTA in 5% glucose infused in 1 hour. If urinary lead excretion in the next 8 hours exceeds 60% of the amount of EDTA given, the test is positive, that is, the chelator is presumed to have combined with and mobilized excessive body stores of lead. The test is cumbersome, and reliability is debated.

A diagnosis of lead intoxication is supported if blood zinc protoporphyrin exceeds 100 μg/dL or if urinary aminolevulinic acid excretion is higher than 15 mg/L. With blood lead levels of 10 μg/dL, the activity of aminolevulinic acid dehydratase is low. At higher lead levels, the activities of coproporphyrinogen oxidase and ferrochetalase are also low. Anemia and basophilic stippling of erythrocytes are characteristic. No other neurotoxin generates similarly specific biochemical abnormalities that can be used diagnostically. Nerve conduction velocities are nonspecifically slow in lead and other neuropathies.

The diagnosis of arsenic intoxication is confirmed by urinary levels greater than 75 μg/dL. Hair analysis has been used but is not deemed reliable. The length-dependent neuropathy is primarily axonal with secondary demyelination.

After acute exposure, blood tests are not useful for detecting *thallium* because the metal is taken up by cells so rapidly that blood levels do not rise. Urinary thallium can be detected by atomic absorption spectrometry. Normal urinary values are 0.3 to 0.8 μg/L and levels of 200 to 300 are seen in overt poisoning. A provocative test depends on KCl, which is given orally in a dose of 45 mEq. Potassium displaces thallium from tissue stores and blood levels rise, which can be detected by serial measurement of urinary content.

Prevention and Treatment

Preventive measures have been most publicized for lead with special concern for the welfare of children. Education programs, paint removal, and deleading house paints have all played a role. Personnel involved in deleading must be protected. Workers in industries at risk have been increasingly monitored and removed from exposure when blood lead levels begin to rise. Motor nerve conduction studies have also been used.

Once symptoms of intoxication appear and the diagnosis of lead poisoning is clear, removal from exposure is mandatory. Chelation therapy can be instituted. For children with blood levels less than 45 μg/dL, oral treatment can be instituted with 2,3-dimercaptosuccinic acid and penicillamine. For acute encephalopathy and blood levels more than 70 μg/dL, Ca-EDTA and dimercaprol (2,3-dimercaptopropanol), also called British anti-Lewisite (BAL), can be used together, starting with BAL, 3 to 5 mg/kg intramuscularly; this is followed by simultaneous but separate intramuscular injections of both chelators given every 4 hours for the next 3 to 5 days. For symptomatic neuropathy, Ca-EDTA can be used alone at doses of 50 to 75 mg/kg every 12 hours in a 3- to 5-day course and a 2- to 3-week rest between courses until the blood level is normal. Treatment of the encephalopathy is also symptomatic or surgical.

Prevention of mercury intoxication requires monitoring in high-risk occupations, including dental offices, and correction of inadequate ventilation, avoiding vacuuming of spilled mercury, and removal of workers whose urinary level has increased fourfold or is more than 50 μg/L. Control of industrial pollution may require major effort. If the person is symptomatic, treatment commences with dimercaprol, which is given intramuscularly 3 to 5 mg/kg every 4 hours for day 1, every 12 hours on day 2, and then once a day for the next 3 days, followed by a 2-day interruption. Other agents are 2,3-dimercaptosuccinic acid and 2,3-dimercapto-propane-1-sulfonate, a water-soluble form of BAL. All agents are somewhat effective for organic and inorganic mercury poisoning.

BAL therapy is also used for acute arsenic poisoning and is most effective before symptoms of neuropathy appear. BAL is considered more effective than penicillamine in treating the chronic neuropathy. Hemodialysis is another treatment for the acute episode.

Aside from monitoring occupational exposure to thallium, an important preventive measure is protection of children against the ingestion of candylike pellets. Treatment of acute poisoning depends in part on enhancing urinary and fecal excretion of thallium by giving laxatives and using Prussian Blue or activated charcoal to retard absorption. Urinary excretion is enhanced by forced diuresis and administration of KCl; hemodialysis may be effective.

OTHER INTOXICATIONS

Organophosphates

Organophosphates, sometimes in combination with carbamates, are used as pesticides by more than 2.5 million agriculture workers and also by amateur gardeners. Also exposed are those engaged in the manufacture of these compounds and military personnel who use or store compounds designed for chemical warfare. It is estimated that 150,000 to 300,000 people have pesticide-induced illness each year. Popular compounds include malathion, parathion, and others. Most are lipid soluble and readily absorbed after ingestion, inhalation, or application to the skin. They are powerful inhibitors of acetylcholinesterase.

Three clinical stages follow in sequence. First, *acute cholinergic crisis* comprises nicotinic effects (limb weakness, fasciculation, tachycardia) and muscarinic manifestations (miosis, lacrimation, salivation). CNS signs include ataxia, seizures, altered consciousness, and sometimes coma. Second, the *intermediate syndrome* appears in 2 to 4 days after exposure. Weakness may be profound, affecting the proximal limbs, cranial muscles, neck flexors, and respiration; tendon reflexes are lost. The differential diagnosis includes the Guillain-Barré syndrome, periodic paralysis, and myasthenia gravis. Among survivors, recovery may be slow but is the rule. Third, *organophosphate-induced delayed neuropathy* appears 1 to 5 weeks after exposure. The syndrome was first described during the period of prohibition in the United States when illicit whiskey was made in home stills: 50,000 people consumed "Jamaica Ginger" or "Jinger Jake" that was later found to contain triorthocresyl phosphate. Paresthesias and distal leg weakness appeared weeks later. Triorthocresyl phosphate is not an anticholinesterase, but the syndrome was then seen after exposure to cholinergic organophosphates. The disorder as been attributed to inhibition of "neuropathy target esterase," disruption of axonal transport, and a dying back neuropathy. Although paresthesias may be noted, the disorder is dominantly motor. Among survivors, upper motor neuron signs implicate the CNS, which in combination with profound lower motor neuron signs may simulate ALS except that there is no progression for years.

Exposure can be documented by levels of the drug or its metabolites in blood or urine. Measurement of red cell or plasma cholinesterase is an indirect marker. In electrodiagnostic studies there may be a repetitive response to a single nerve stimulus.

The acute disorder is a medical emergency risking death from respiratory paralysis. If the patient has been splashed, clothing must be stripped and the skin washed thoroughly to prevent further absorption. Gastric lavage may be needed. Airway control and ventilation must be ensured and cardiac function monitored. Atropine is the best antidote; subcutaneous doses of 0.5 to 1.0 mg are given every 15 minutes until an effect is observed in the form of dilated pupils, flushed face, dry mouth, and dry skin with cessation of sweating. To suppress airway secretions, some give intravenous doses up to 2 mg every hour. Glycopyrrolate can be added to atropine.

Oxime therapy is also recommended in seriously ill patients. These compounds reactivate acetylcholinesterase and should be given as soon as possible after exposure by continuous intravenous infusion.

Solvents and Organic Compounds

Hexacarbon neuropathy results from mixtures that produce 2,5-hexanedione. Outbreaks arise from industrial exposure to n-hexane, recreational abuse, and industrial exposure to methyl-n-butyl ketone. Paresthesias and weakness appear distally in the legs and only later are the hands affected. Acutely, the syndrome may resemble the Guillain-Barré syndrome, including slow conduction velocity. Alternatively, progression may be slow. Optic neuropathy is rare. The characteristic pathologic change is neurofilamentous axonal swelling and distal axonal degeneration. Effective measures have been taken to reduce industrial exposure and to eliminate the toxins from glues formerly used for glue sniffing. Epidemics have largely disappeared.

Other organic compounds that induce axonal neuropathy by industrial exposure are acrylamide, carbon disulfide, methyl bromide, and triorthocresyl phosphate. A current debate is whether house painters are at risk for solvent-induced behavioral disorders.

Carbon Monoxide

Carbon monoxide intoxication is more often deliberate than accidental, about 600 a year accidentally in the United States and 5 to 10 times more often in suicide attempts. Accidents are caused predominantly by automobile exhausts and poorly ventilated gasoline-powered heaters. Methylene chloride, a paint remover, is another source. Toxicity results from issue hypoxia and direct damage to cellular structures. CO competes with oxygen for binding to hemoglobin; it binds to other proteins, including myoglobin and cytochrome *c* oxidase.

Symptoms may be mild, simulating viral infection, or it may occur with another emergency, smoke inhalation. Nonspecific symptoms may comprise headache, malaise, dizziness, nausea, difficulty concentrating, and dyspnea. A delayed neuropsychiatric syndrome may follow acute exposure by 3 to 240 days, with cognitive and personality changes, parkinsonism, and psychotic behavior. Although the syndrome seems ominous, 50% to 75% of patients recover.

Diagnosis is made by finding high levels of carboxyhemoglobin. However, serum levels may have fallen by the time the patient reaches the emergency room. Measurement of CO in expired air can therefore be useful. Blood taken at the scene by emergency technicians can be used.

Rescue from fires is of prime importance. Hospital admission is reserved for the more seriously affected or those with other medical problems. Oxygen is administered because it shortens the half-life of carboxyhemoglobin. Hyperbaric oxygen therapy has been used with increasing frequency, but it is uncertain whether it hastens recovery or reduces the rate of late sequelae. Coma is a clear indication for hyperbaric therapy. Prevention is largely a matter of monitoring equipment, monitoring workers, and education about the hazards of running a motor vehicle in a closed space.

Nitrous Oxide Myelopathy (Layzer Syndrome)

In 1978, Layzer described 15 patients; 14 were dentists. Thirteen had abused nitrous oxide for 3 months to several years; 2 patients had been exposed only professionally, working in poorly ventilated offices. Symptoms included early paresthesias, Lhermitte symptoms, ataxia, leg weakness, impotence, and sphincter disturbances. Examination showed signs of sensorimotor polyneuropathy, often combined with signs implicating the posterior and lateral columns of the spinal cord in a pattern identical to that of subacute combined system disease (SCD) due to B_{12} deficiency. Electrodiagnostic tests showed axonal polyneuropathy; cerebrospinal fluid and other laboratory results were normal. Layzer surmised that the gas interfered with the action of B_{12}.

Subsequent experience proved him correct. Additional cases were reported in abusers of nitrous oxide, and improvement was seen in weeks or months after exposure ceased. Another version of the disorder was seen in people, including a vegetarian, who had hematologic evidence of B_{12} deficiency but were asymptomatic until the neurologic disorder was precipitated by nitrous oxide anesthesia for surgery. Magnetic resonance imaging shows the characteristic distribution of lesions in the spinal cord.

Scott et al. (1981) reproduced the syndrome by maintaining monkeys in an atmosphere of nitrous oxide. If the diet was supplemented with methionine, the disorder was prevented, but in controls, symptoms progressed to a moribund state; the spinal cord and peripheral nerves of the unsupplemented monkeys showed changes of SCD. Inability to resynthesize methionine from homocysteine seemed responsible, and the primary lesion producing SCD in humans with pernicious anemia may also be impaired synthesis of methionine biosynthesis. Cyanocobalamin is involved in the conversion of L-methylmalonyl coenzyme A to succinyl coenzyme A and the formation of methionine by methylation of homocysteine, a reaction essential for DNA synthesis and for maintenance of the myelin sheath by the methylation of myelin basic protein. Active vitamin B_{12} contains cobalt and nitrous oxide produces irreversible oxidation of the Co^{2+}, rendering B_{12} inactive.

Seafood Intoxication

Ciguatera or the *marine neurotoxic syndrome* is the most common nonbacterial form of food poisoning in the United States and Canada. It is caused by eating tropical reef fish that contain several toxins in edible parts; the toxins are thought to arise in dinoflagellates. It is endemic in subtropical regions, and food shipped to other parts of the world spreads the disease. The acute symptoms are gastrointestinal followed by sensory symptoms, paresthesias, and pruritus. "Sensory inversion" describes the peculiarity that cold feels hot and vice versa. Myalgia, fasciculations, areflexia, trismus, and carpopedal spasm may be noted. Respiratory failure is exceptional. Other systems may be involved prominently, including pain on sexual activity.

None of the physical findings is diagnostic, and there are no formal criteria for diagnosis. Most associated toxins open sodium channels, but at least one affects calcium channels. Peripheral nerve conduction velocities are often slow. Bioassays for the ciguatoxins or immunochemical methods are being developed, but none has yet achieved approval by consensus. Treatment is therefore symptomatic.

Shellfish poisoning can result from contamination of mollusks by saxitoxin, which blocks sodium channels. The symptoms are similar to ciguatera but more severe, and respiratory depression is a threat. The toxin originates in a dinoflagellate. In the series of De Carvalho et al. (1998), cerebellar ataxia was the dominant finding and peripheral nerve conduction was normal. Recovery was rapid in those patients, but among those described by Gessner et al., 3 of 11 patients were treated with mechanical ventilation and 1 died. Hypertension was also prominent. Binding assays and liquid chromatography identified the toxin in serum and urine. In Japan, the agent of puffer fish poisoning is tetrodotoxin. Treatment of these conditions is symptomatic.

Methanol (Methyl Alcohol)

Methanol intoxication is seen in drinkers who take it as a substitute for ethanol. Acute poisoning was dominated by gastrointestinal symptoms, drunkenness, and coma. Severe acidosis results from the conversion of methanol to formaldehyde and formic acid. Viscera and brain show petechial hemorrhages and edema. In the series of Liu et al. (1998), the mortality rate was 36%; coma, seizures, and high methanol concentrations were predictors of poor prognosis. Visual loss is attributed to retinal metabolism of methanol (rather than an action of circulating formic acid) because the local oxidation of methanol to formic acid parallels the depletion of retinal ATP. Retinal glial cells may be the first target. It has therefore been suggested that inhibitors of aldehyde dehydrogenase could be therapeutic; here it would mean the administration of ethanol to block the first step of the toxic metabolic pathway. For similar reasons, administration of ethanol blocks the metabolism of methanol in the liver and unchanged toxin is excreted in the urine. 4-Methylpyrazole (fomepizole) has also been used for this purpose. Correction of acidosis and hemodialysis may be used. Exposure to large amounts is fatal within 72 hours. Vision is usually restored in survivors, who incur no other chronic neurologic symptoms.

Obsolete Epidemics

Many syndromes described here could be eliminated if care were taken to protect the environment. In fact, some epidemics pointed the way to correction. For instance, the outbreak of *subacute myelo-optic neuropathy* was attributed to an oral antiparasitic agent, clioquinol. The resulting peripheral neuropathy and blindness affected an estimated 10,000 people in Japan. The practice has ceased, and there have been no new cases; investigations indicate that the drug is converted to a potent mitochondrial toxin. Another transient outbreak was the *eosinophilia-myalgia syndrome*, which involved skin, muscle, lungs, and blood vessels and axonal neuropathy. The disorder was attributed to a toxic contaminant in the preparation of tryptophan, which was taken as a health supplement. That syndrome has also largely disappeared, but it seems likely that new epidemics will appear as new industries and new health fads arise.

SUGGESTED READINGS

General

Baker EL, Feldman RG, French JG. Environmentally related disorders of the nervous system. *Med Clin North Am* 1990;74:325–345.

Bleecker ML, ed. *Occupational neurology and clinical neurotoxicology*. Baltimore: Williams & Wilkins, 1994.

Feldman RG. *Occupational and environmental neurology*. Baltimore: Lippincott-Raven, 1998.

Goyer RA, Klaassen CD, Waalkes MP. *Metal toxicology*. San Diego: Academic Press, 1995.

Kuncl RW, George EB. Toxic neuropathies and myopathies. *Curr Opin Neurol* 1993;6:695–704.

Rom WN, ed. *Environmental and occupational medicine*, 3rd ed. Philadelphia: Lippincott-Raven, 1998.

Slikker W, Chang W, eds. *Handbook of developmental neurotoxicology*. New York: Academic Press, 1998.

Spencer PS, Schaumburg HH, Ludolph A. *Experimental and clinical neurotoxicology*, 2nd ed. New York: Oxford University Press, 1999.

Weiss B, O'Donaghue J. *Neurobehavioral toxicity. Analysis and intervention*. New York: Raven Press, 1994.

Aluminum

Alfrey AC, Le Gendre GR, Kaehny WD. The dialysis encephalopathy syndrome: possible aluminum intoxication. *N Engl J Med* 1976; 294:184–188.

Cannata JB, Briggs JD, Junor BJR, et al. Aluminum hydroxide intake: real risk of aluminum toxicity. *Br Med J* 1983;286:1937–1938.

Garruto RM, Strong MJ, Yanagihara R. Experimental models of aluminum-induced motor neuron degeneration. *Adv Neurol* 1991;56:327–340.

Longstreth WT Jr, Rosenstock L, Heyer NJ. Potroom palsy? Neurologic disorders in three aluminum smelter workers. *Arch Intern Med* 1985;145:1972–1975.

Murray JC, Tanner CM, Sprague SM. Aluminum neurotoxicity: a re-evaluation. *Clin Neuropharmacol* 1991;14:179–185.

Rastegar A. *Dialysis dementia. Neurobase*. La Jolla, CA: Arbor, 1999.

Van Der Voet GB, Marani E, Tio S, et al. Aluminum neurotoxicity. *Prog Histochem Cytochem* 1991;23:235–241.

White DM, Longstreth WT Jr, Rosenstock L, et al. Neurologic syndrome in 25 workers from an aluminum smelting plant. *Arch Intern Med* 1992;152:1443–1448.

Arsenic

Aposhian HV. DMSA and DMPS—water soluble antidotes for heavy metal poisoning. *Annu Rev Pharmacol Toxicol* 1983;23:193–215.

Beckett WS, Moore JL, Keogh JP, et al. Acute encephalopathy due to occupational exposure to arsenic. *Br J Ind Med* 1986;43:66–67.

Gerhardt RE, Crecelius EA, Hudson JB. Moonshine-related arsenic poisoning. *Arch Intern Med* 1980;140:211–213.

Huang SY, Chang CS, Tang JL, et al. Acute and chronic arsenic poisoning associated with treatment of acute promyelocytic leukemia. *Br J Haematol* 1998;103:1092–1095.

Nickson R, McArthur J, Burgess W, et al. Arsenic poisoning of Bangladesh groundwater [letter]. *Nature* 1998;395:338.

Quecedo E, Samartin O, Ferber MI, et al. Mees lines: a clue for the diagnosis of arsenic poisoning [Letter]. *Arch Dermatol* 1996;132:349–350.

Lead

Aub, JC, Fairhall LT, Minot A, et al. Lead poisoning. *Medicine (Baltimore)* 1925;4:1–250.

Boothby JA, deJesus PV, Rowland LP. Reversible forms of motor neuron disease—lead "neuritis." *Arch Neurol* 1974;31:18–23.

Byers RK. Lead poisoning, review of the literature and report of 45 cases. *Pediatrics* 1959;23:585–603.

Davoli CT. *Childhood lead poisoning. Neurobase*. La Jolla, CA: Arbor, 1999.

Lifshitz M, Hashkanazi R, Phillip M. The effect of 2,3-dimercaptosuccinic acid in the treatment of lead poisoning in adults. *Ann Med* 1997;29:83–85.

Needleman HL. Lead at low dose and the behavior of children. *Acta Psychiatr Scand* 1983;303[Suppl]:38–48.

Pinkle JL, Brody DJ, Gunter EW, et al. The decline in blood lead levels in the United States. *JAMA* 1994;272:284–291.

Porru S, Alessio L. The use of chelating agents in occupational lead poisoning. *Occup Med* 1996;46:41–48.

Preuss HG. A review of persistent, low-grade lead challenge: neurological and cardiovascular consequences. *J Am Coll Nutr* 1993;12:246–254.

Rutter M. Raised lead levels and impaired cognitive/behavioural functioning: a review of the evidence. *Dev Med Child Neurol* 1980; 42[Suppl]:1–36.

Ryan D, Levy B, Pollack S, Walker B Jr. Protecting children from lead poisoning and building healthy communities. *Am J Public Health* 1999;89:822–827.

Silbergeld EK. Preventing lead poisoning in children. *Annu Rev Public Health* 1997;18:187–210.

Staudinger KC, Roth VS. Occupational lead poisoning. *Am Fam Physician* 1998;57:719–726, 731–732.

Warren MJ, Cooper JB, Wood SP, Shoolingin-Jordan PM. Lead poisoning, haem synthesis, and 5-aminolevulinic acid dehydratase. *Trends Biochem Sci* 1998;23:217–221.

Manganese

Abd El Naby S, Hassanein M. Neuropsychiatric manifestations of chronic manganese poisoning. *J Neurol Neurosurg Psychiatry* 1965;28:282–288.

Aschner M, Aschner JL. Manganese neurotoxicity: cellular effects and blood-brain barrier transport. *Neurosci Behav Rev* 1991;15:333–340.

Canavan MM, Cobb S, Drinker CK. Chronic manganese poisoning. *Arch Neurol Psychiatry* 1934;32:501–512.

Chandra SV. Psychiatric illness due to manganese poisoning. *Acta Psychiatr Scand* 1983;303[Suppl]:49–54.

Huang C, Chu NS, Lu CS, et al. Long-term progression in chronic manganism;10 years of follow-up. *Neurology* 1998;50:698–700.

Rosenstock HA, Simons DG, Meyer JS. Chronic manganism. Neurologic and laboratory studies during treatment with levodopa. *JAMA* 1971;217:1354–1358.

Schuler P, Oyanguren H, Maturana V, et al. Manganese poisoning. Environmental and medical study at a Chilean mine. *Ind Med Surg* 1957;26:167–173.

Mercury

Adams CR, Ziegler DK, Lin JT. Mercury intoxication simulating amyotrophic lateral sclerosis. *JAMA* 1983;250:642–643.

Albers JW, Kallenbach LR, Fine LJ, et al. Neurologic abnormalities and remote occupational elemental mercury exposure. *Ann Neurol* 1988;24:651–659.

Eto K. Pathology of Minamata disease. *Toxicol Pathol* 1997;25:614–623.

Eyl TB. Organic-mercury food poisoning. *N Engl J Med* 1971; 284:706–709.

Haley RM, Hom J, Roland PS, et al. Evaluation of neurologic function in Gulf War veterans: a blinded case-control study. *JAMA* 1997;277:259–261.

Hay WJ, Rickards AG, McMenemey WH, et al. Organic mercurial encephalopathy. *J Neurol Neurosurg Psychiatry* 1963;26:199–202.

Korogi Y, Takahashi M, Okajima T, Eto K. MR findings of Minamata disease—organic mercury poisoning. *J Magn Reson Imaging* 1998; 8:308–316.

Kurland LT, Faro SN, Siedler H. Minamata disease. *World Neurol* 1960;1:370–390.

Thallium

Bank WJ, Pleasure DE, Suzuki K, et al. Thallium poisoning. *Arch Neurol* 1972;26:456–464.

Mahoney W. Retrobulbar neuritis due to thallium poisoning from depilatory cream. *JAMA* 1932;98:618–620.

Nordentoft T, Andersen EB, Mogensen PH. Initial sensorimotor and delayed autonomic neuropathy in acute thallium poisoning. *Neurotoxicology* 1998;19:421–426.

Passarge C, Wieck HH. Thallium polyneuritis. *Fortschr Neurol Psychiatr* 1965;33:477–557.

Rambar AC. Acute thallium poisoning. *JAMA* 1932;98:1372–1373.

Rauws AG, van Heyst AN. Check of Prussian blue for antidotal efficacy in thallium intoxication [Letter]. *Arch Toxicol* 1979;43:153–154.

Shabalina LP, Spiridonova VS. Thallium as an industrial poison (review of literature). *J Hyg Epidemiol Microbiol Immunol* 1979;23:247–255.

Smith DH, Doherty RA. Thallotoxicosis: report of three cases in Massachusetts. *Pediatrics* 1964;34:480–490.

Stein MD, Perlstein MA. Thallium poisoning. *Am J Dis Child* 1959;98:80–85.

Methyl Alcohol

Bennet IL Jr, Cary FM, Mitchell GL, et al. Acute methyl alcohol poisoning: a review based on experience in an outbreak of 323 cases. *Medicine (Baltimore)* 1953;32:431–463.

Burns MJ, Graudins A, Aaron CK, McMartin K, Brent J. Treatment of methanol poisoning with intravenous 4-methylpyrazole. *Ann Emerg Med* 1997;30:829–832.

Harrop GA Jr, Benedict EM. Acute methyl alcohol poisoning associated with acidosis. *JAMA* 1920;74:25–27.

Liu JJ, Daya MR, Carrasquillo O, Kales SN. Prognostic factors in patients with methanol intoxication. *J Toxicol Clin Toxicol* 1998;36:175–181.

Organic Solvents

Allen N, Mendell JR, Billmaier DJ, et al. Toxic polyneuropathy due to methyl n-butyl ketone. *Arch Neurol* 1975;32:209–218.

Baker EL, Fine LJ. Solvent neurotoxicity: the current evidence. *J Med* 1986;28:126–129.

Griffin JW. *Hexacarbon neuropathy. Neurobase.* La Jolla, CA: Arbor, 1999.

Juntunen J, Matikainen E, Antti-Poika M, et al. Nervous system effects of long-term occupational exposure to toluene. *Acta Neurol Scand* 1985;72:512–517.

Lees-Haley PR, Williams CW. Neurotoxicity of chronic low-dose exposure to organic solvents: a skeptical review. *J Clin Psychology* 1997; 53:699–712.

Schaumberg HH, Spencer PS. Clinical and experimental studies of distal axonopathy—a frequent form of brain and nerve damage produced by environmental chemical hazards. *Ann N Y Acad Sci* 1979;329:14–29.

Struwe G. Psychiatric and neurological symptoms in workers occupationally exposed to organic solvents—results of a differential epidemiological study. *Acta Psychiatr Scand* 1983;303[Suppl]:100–104.

Organophosphate Insecticides

Choi PT, Quinonez LG, Cook DJ, Baxter F, Whitehead L. The use of glycopyrrolate in a case of intermediate syndrome following acute organophosphate poisoning. *Can J Anesth* 1998;45:337–340.

De Bleeker J. The intermediate syndrome in organophosphate poisoning: an overview of experimental and clinical observations. *Clin Toxicol* 1995;33:683–686.

de Jager AEJ, van Weerden TW, Houthoff HJ, et al. Polyneuropathy after massive exposure to parathion. *Neurology* 1981;31:603–605.

Ecobichon DJ, Davies JE, Doull J, et al. Neurotoxic effects of pesticides. In: Baker SR, Wilkinson CF, eds. *The effects of pesticides on human health.* Princeton, NJ: Princeton Scientific, 1990:131–199.

Ecobichon DJ, Joy RM. *Pesticides and neurological diseases,* 2nd ed. Boca Raton, FL: CRC Press, 1994.

Good JL, Khurana RK, Mayer RF, et al. Pathophysiological studies of neuromuscular function in subacute organophosphate poisoning induced by phosmet. *J Neurol Neurosurg Psychiatry* 1993;56:290–294.

Landrigan P. Illness in Gulf War veterans. *JAMA* 1997;277:238–245.

Lotti M, Moretto A, Zoppelari R, et al. Inhibition of lymphocytic neuropathy target esterase predicts the development of organophosphate-induced delayed polyneuropathy. *Arch Toxicol* 1986;59:176–179.

Moretto A, Lotti M. Poisoning by organophosphorus insecticides and sensory neuropathy. *J Neurol Neurosurg Psychiatry* 1998;64:463–468.

Morgan JP, Penovich P. Jamaica ginger paralysis. 47-year follow-up. *Arch Neurol* 1978;35:530–532.

Singh G, Mahajan R, Whig J. The importance of electrodiagnostic studies in acute organophosphate poisoning. *J Neurol Sci* 1998;157:191–200.

Steenland K, Jenkins B, Ames RG, et al. Chronic neurologic sequelae to organophosphate pesticide poisoning. *Am J Public Health* 1994; 84:731–736.

Taylor JR, Selhorst JB, Houff S, et al. Chlordecone intoxication in man. *Neurology* 1978;28:626–630.

Thiermann H, Mast U, Klimmeck R, et al. Cholinesterase status, pharmacokinetics, and laboratory findings during obidoxime therapy in organophosphate poisoned patients. *Hum Exp Toxicol* 1997;16:473–480.

Tush GM, Anstead MI. Pralidoxime continuous infusion in the treatment of organophosphorus poisoning. *Ann Pharmacother* 1997;31:441–444.

Wadia RS, Chitra S, Amin RB, et al. Neurological manifestations of organophosphate insecticide poisoning. *J Neurol Neurosurg Psychiatry* 1987;50:1442–1448.

Carbon Monoxide

Ernst A, Zibrak JD. Carbon monoxide poisoning. *N Engl J Med* 1998;339:1603–1608.

Neurotoxic Seafood Poisoning

DeCarvalho M, Jacinto J, Ramos N, et al. Paralytic shellfish poisoning. Clinical and electrophysiological observations. *J Neurol* 1998; 2245:551–554.

DiNubile MJ, Hokama Y. The ciguatera poisoning syndrome from farm-raised salmon. *Ann Intern Med* 1995;122:113–114.

Gessner BD, Bell P, Doucette GJ, et al. Hypertension and identification of toxin in human urine and serum following a cluster of mussel-associated paralytic shellfish poisoning outbreaks. *Toxicon* 1997;35:711–722

Payne CA, Payne SN. *Ciguatera. Neurobase.* La Jolla, CA: Arbor, 1999.

Yasumoto T, Satake M. Chemistry, etiology and determination methods of ciguatera toxins. *Annu Rev Pharmacol Toxicol* 1988;28:141–161.

Nitrous Oxide

Beltramello A, Puppini G, Cerini R, et al. Subacute combined degeneration of the spinal cord after nitrous oxide anaesthesia: role of magnetic resonance imaging. *J Neurol Neurosurg Psychiatry* 1998;64:563–564.

Flippo TS, Holder WD Jr. Neurologic degeneration associated with nitrous oxide anesthesia in patients with vitamin B_{12} deficiency. *Arch Surg* 1993;128:1391–1395.

Gutmann L, Farrell B, Crosby TW, Johnsen D. Nitrous oxide-induced myelopathy-neuropathy: potential for chronic misuse by dentists. *J Am Dent Assoc* 1979;98:58–59.

Hadzic A, Glab K, Sanborn KV, Thys DM. Severe neurologic deficit after nitrous oxide anesthesia. *Anesthesiology* 1995;83:863–866.

Layzer RB. Myeloneuropathy after prolonged exposure to nitrous oxide. *Lancet* 1978;2:1227–1230.

Pema PJ, Horak HA, Wyatt RH. Myelopathy caused by nitrous oxide toxicity. *AJNR* 1998;19:894–896.

Rosener M, Dichgans J. Severe combined degeneration of the spinal cord after nitrous oxide anaesthesia in a vegetarian [Letter]. *J Neurol Neurosurg Psychiatry* 1996;60:354.

Scott JM, Dinn JJ, Wilson P, Weir DG. Pathogenesis of subacute combined degeneration: a result of methyl group deficiency. *Lancet* 1981; 2:334–337.

Obsolete Epidemics

Anonymous. Eosinophilia-myalgia syndrome: review and reappraisal of clinical, epidemiologic and animal studies symposium. *J Rheumatol* 1996;46[Suppl]:1–110.

Arbiser JL, Kraeft SK, van Leeuwen R, et al. Clioquinol-zinc chelate: a candidate causative agent of subacute myelo-optic neuropathy. *Mol Med* 1998;4:665–670.

Burns SM, Lange DJ, Jaffe IA, Hays AP. Axonal neuropathy in eosinophilia-myalgia syndrome. *Muscle Nerve* 1994;17:293–298.

Emslie-Smith AM, Mayeno AN, Nakano S, Gleich GJ. 1,1-Ethylidenebis-[tryptophan] induces pathologic alterations in muscle similar to those observed in the eosinophilia-myalgia syndrome. *Neurology* 1994; 44:2390–2392.

Martin RW, Duffy J, Engel AG, et al. The clinical spectrum of the eosinophilis-myalgia syndrome associated with L-tryptophan ingestion. *Ann Intern Med* 1990;113:124–134.

Merritt's Neurology, 10th ed., edited by L.P. Rowland. Lippincott Williams & Wilkins, Philadelphia © 2000.

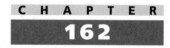

C H A P T E R

162

ABUSE OF CHILDREN

CLAUDIA A. CHIRIBOGA

PEDIATRIC ACQUIRED IMMUNODEFICIENCY SYNDROME AND HUMAN IMMUNODEFICIENCY VIRUS INFECTION

Woman and children are the fastest-growing population affected by the acquired immunodeficiency syndrome (AIDS) and the human immunodeficiency virus (HIV). Most children with AIDS in the United States are infected perinatally. In inner cities, about 2% to 4% of live births are HIV-1 antibody positive. Intravenous drug abuse and sexual contact with HIV-infected partners are the maternal risk factors in more than 85% of perinatal cases. Most infections occur during the last trimester of pregnancy and time of delivery. Risk factors for vertical transmission are recent maternal HIV seroconversion, high viral load, and maternal AIDS. Premature infants are also at increased risk of infection. Infection may result from exposure to blood and other body fluids at delivery or transmitted in breast milk. Mother-to-child HIV transmission rates range from 14% to 30%; rates decrease to 8% with prenatal and neonatal zidovudine treatment.

Determination of HIV infection in children is complicated because maternal HIV antibody transfers across the placenta and may persist up to age 18 months. HIV-seropositive children are considered HIV infected if they test positive for HIV on two separate occasions by either HIV culture or HIV polymerase chain reaction (PCR) or if they develop AIDS. HIV-seropositive children who do not meet these criteria are considered perinatally exposed, and HIV-seropositive children without AIDS and without laboratory evidence of infection who on testing after age 6 months have negative antibody are seroreverters. The 1994 revised classification system for HIV infection in children has four clinical categories: N, not symptomatic; A, mildly symptomatic;

TABLE 162.1. REVISED CENTERS FOR DISEASE CONTROL AND PREVENTION CLINICAL CATEGORIES FOR CHILDREN WITH HUMAN IMMUNODEFICIENCY VIRUS (HIV) INFECTION

Category	Characteristics
N	Not symptomatic
A	Mildly symptomatic: two or more conditions listed below, not listed in categories B and C Lymphadenopathy Hepatomegaly Splenomegaly Dermatitis Parotitis Recurrent persistent infection
B	Moderately symptomatic Anemia Bacterial meningitis Candidiasis Cardiomyopathy Cytomegalovirus infection onset before 1 mo Diarrhea, chronic recurrent Hepatitis HSV stomatitis recurrent HSV bronchitis, pneumonia, or esophagitis, onset before 1 mo Herpes zoster (shingles) at least two separate episodes or more than one dermatone Leiomyosarcoma Lymphoid interstial pneumonia Nephropathy Nocardiosis Persistent fevers (>1 mo) Toxoplasmosis, onset before age 1 mo Varicella, disseminated
C	Severely symptomatic Children who have any condition listed in the 1987 surveillance case definition for acquired immunodeficiency syndrome (e.g., *Pneumocystis carinii* pneumonia, toxoplasmosis, mycobacterium, cytomegalovirus, progressive multifocal leukoencephalopathy, HIV encephalopathy, wasting syndrome)

HSV, herpes simplex virus.
From MMWR (1995).

B, moderately symptomatic; and C, severely symptomatic, which includes all AIDS-defining conditions except lymphoid hyperplasia (Table 162.1). These clinical categories are further classified immunologically depending on the child's age and absolute CD4 count: no evidence of suppression, moderate sup-pression, and severe suppression (Table 162.2). For example, A2 indicates mild signs and symptoms of infection with moderate immunosuppression.

Diagnostic Tests

Because of early testing, most HIV-positive children are identified soon after birth. Viral load (i.e., quantified HIV DNA or RNA PCR) is more sensitive than viral cultures and p24 antigen in identifying HIV infection in asymptomatic newborns and infants. By age 4 to 6 months, over 95% of HIV-infected children are identified by a positive PCR. In newborns, a negative PCR test for HIV does not exclude infection but decreases the risk of HIV infection to 3%. Viral load runs higher in asymptomatic children than in asymptomatic adults. Sustained high viral load in adults predicts progression to AIDS. High viral loads in early infancy predict early onset of symptomatic HIV disease. HIV-1 syncytial-inducing phenotypes are linked to aggressive early symptomatic disease.

Clinical Manifestations

Mild HIV infection includes diarrhea, unexplained persistent fever, lymphadenopathy, and parotitis. Table 162.1 lists the range of signs of symptomatic HIV infection. Lymphoid interstitial pneumonitis and recurrent bacterial infections are seen in children with AIDS but not in adults. Severe manifestations in early infancy, such as progressive encephalopathy or opportunistic infections (e.g., *Pneumocystis carinii*), carry a poor prognosis for survival.

Mechanism of Action

HIV infection is maintained by viral persistence in helper T lymphocytes and macrophages. HIV strains with tropism for monocyte-derived macrophages have a predilection to infect cerebral vascular endothelium and central nervous system (CNS). Infected macrophages traverse the blood–brain barrier and infect microglial cells; neurons are spared from direct infestation. Nonproductive infection of astrocytes is reported, but infection of other glial cells has not been firmly established. Neuronal dropout is seen as the disease advances, but it is not known how HIV induces neural damage. Postulated mechanisms include release of soluble neurotoxins by HIV-infected macrophages and lymphocytes (e.g., cytokines, quinolinic acid, viral antigens, or undefined viral products), neurotoxin amplification by astrocyte–macrophage interaction, and impaired blood–brain barrier

TABLE 162.2. IMMUNOLOGICAL CATEGORIES BASED ON CHILD'S AGE-SPECIFIC CD4 + T LYMPHOCYTE COUNT AND PERCENT OF TOTAL LYMPHOCYTES

Immunologic category	<12 mo	1–5 yr	8–12 yr
No evidence of suppression	>1,500 (>25)	>1,000 (>25)	>500 (>25)
Moderate suppression	750–1,499 (15–24)	500–999 (15–24)	200–499 (15–24)
Severe suppression	<750 (<15)	<500 (<15)	<200 (<15)

Values are expressed in μL; with percents in parentheses.
From MMWR (1995).

function secondary to HIV-related endothelial damage. These neurotoxins are thought to produce a reversible metabolic encephalopathy that may disappear with effective antiretroviral treatment. Children with HIV encephalopathy who respond to antiretroviral therapy may show nonprogressive corticospinal tract sequelae.

Pathology

Glial nodules and endothelial hyperplasia with calcification, dystrophic calcification, and perivascular mononuclear inflammation are common pathologic findings of subacute encephalitis in HIV-infected brains. The glial nodule comprises a cluster of chronic inflammatory cells in the neurophil and is often associated with multinucleated giant cells that are presumed to arise from coalescent microglia.

Human Immunodeficiency Virus Encephalopathy

Two types of encephalopathy are seen in children: progressive and static. The evolution of the progressive encephalopathy may be fulminant, inexorably progressive, or stepwise. Progressive encephalopathy is characterized by loss of developmental milestones, progressive pyramidal tract dysfunction, and acquired microcephaly or impaired brain growth. The static encephalopathy is less well defined, and not all cases may be HIV induced.

The neurologic abnormalities commonly include abnormalities of muscle tone, hyperreflexia, clonus, and impaired head growth. Hypotonia with corticospinal tract dysfunction may be seen in infants early in the course of the encephalopathy and evolves into a spastic diparesis; with newer antiretroviral treatments, progression to a spastic tetraparesis, with or without pseudobulbar palsy, is seldom seen. Ataxia and rigidity are uncommon. Progressive neurologic dysfunction is the first evidence of progression to AIDS in 10% of infected children. There is always evidence of underlying HIV infection, such as immunologic compromise (low CD4 counts) or high viral load, at the time of onset of neurologic symptoms. Many infected children exhibit global developmental delay, regardless of neurologic findings. In young children, motor development is more impaired than mental development.

The incidence of neurologic abnormalities reported in HIV-infected cohorts before the advent of antiretroviral treatments was 30%. Older HIV-infected children may show problems in visual-spatial processing functions and expressive language and may develop AIDS-dementia complex indistinguishable from that described in adults.

HIV-associated myelopathy, polyneuropathy, and myopathy are rare in children. Spinal cord pathology shows demyelinating changes of the corticospinal tracts, vacuolar changes, or myelitis attributable to HIV. Acute inflammatory demyelinating polyneuropathy is a rare complication in pediatric HIV. Low-dose treatment with dideoxyinosine causes a painful sensory neuropathy in less than 10% of patients treated. The neuropathy is dose related and usually reverts with cessation of treatment. The mitochondrial myopathy induced by zidovudine has not been seen in children.

Focal Manifestations

HIV brain infection is nonfocal and subcortical. Seizures are not common. Focal signs or seizures raises the possibility of neoplasm, strokes, or, less likely, opportunistic infections.

Primary Central Nervous System Lymphoma

This is the most common cause of focal cerebral signs in HIV-infected children, found in 3% to 4% of cases. Seizures are reported in about 33% of patients. It may be difficult to differentiate this tumor from toxoplasma brain abscess; diagnosis requires brain biopsy. Magnetic resonance imaging (MRI) spectroscopy may prove helpful in distinguishing CNS toxoplasmosis from lymphoma.

Stroke

HIV infection produces inflammation of cerebral vessels, increasing the risk of stroke, which occurs at a rate of 1.3% a year in HIV-infected children. More than 50% of strokes are hemorrhagic and occur with thrombocytopenia (especially immune thrombocytopenic purpura) or CNS neoplasia. Nonhemorrhagic stroke and subarachnoid hemorrhage are attributable to an arteriopathy affecting the large vessels of the circle of Willis or meninges. HIV-related strokes may be clinically silent, so the true incidence is probably higher.

Opportunistic Central Nervous System Infection

Compared with adults, opportunistic CNS infection is infrequent in HIV-infected children, affecting primarily older children and adolescents. Only a few have had progressive multifocal leukoencephalopathy.

Imaging

In children with HIV encephalopathy, computed tomography or MRI may show diffuse cerebral atrophy or may be normal. There may be foci of demyelination. Frontal lobe or basal ganglia enhancement and calcifications are late manifestations of HIV encephalopathy and occur primarily in symptomatic infants (Fig. 162.1). HIV-related myelopathy on spinal MRI may show a high signal but is usually normal. Bilateral cerebral lesions may mimic myelopathy and must be excluded with MRI or computed tomography. Lesions of progressive multifocal leukoencephalopathy are commonly located in the parietooccipital or frontal region affecting both periventricular and subcortical white matter. These lesions may be difficult to distinguish from HIV demyelination.

Cerebrospinal Fluid

Cerebrospinal fluid (CSF) examination is commonly normal in children with HIV infection. In the absence of opportunistic infection, CSF findings in children with progressive encephalopathy are nonspecific, with a lymphocytic pleocytosis and elevated protein content. Intra-blood–brain barrier synthesis of HIV-specific antibody or antigen detection in CSF has not been useful in predicting

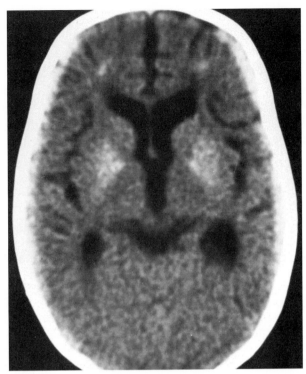

FIG. 162.1. Computed tomography of an infant with human immunodeficiency virus encephalopathy showing cortical and subcortical atrophy, basal ganglia, and frontal lobe calcifications. (Courtesy of Dr. Ram Kairam.)

encephalopathy. CSF viral load, although still experimental, may prove useful in determining HIV encephalopathy in children.

Antiretroviral Therapy

Combination antiretroviral therapy is needed to avoid emergence of resistant HIV strains. Triple combination antiretroviral therapies that include a protease inhibitor are effective in diminishing viral load and suppressing active viral replication. This in turn correlates with increases in CD4 count, weight gain, improved morbidity (including CNS symptomatology), and mortality. Whether high systemic viral load predicts the development of HIV encephalopathy has not been firmly established.

FETAL ALCOHOL SYNDROME

The fetal alcohol syndrome (FAS) affects children of chronic alcoholic women but also occurs with binge drinking, as defined by five drinks or more on one occasion. Fetal susceptibility to the effects of alcohol is greatest during the first trimester of pregnancy. FAS is characterized by abnormalities of growth, CNS, and facial features; birth defects are common (Table 162.3). FAS rates in the United States are 2 to 4 per 1,000 live births and 2% to 4% among children of *alcohol-abusing* women. FAS is confined to infants of alcohol-abusing women. Most children with FAS are mildly or moderately retarded, with mean IQ scores of 65 to 70, but intellectual ability varies widely. In families with several affected siblings, the youngest child is usually the most cognitively impaired.

Learning disabilities—in particular difficulty with arithmetic, speech delay, and hyperactivity—are commonly observed.

Less severe alcohol-related effects are associated with wide patterns of drinking. These fetal alcohol effects are probably a lower point on the continuum of alcohol effects on the fetus. Maternal alcohol abuse is associated with increased risk of spontaneous abortions, infant mortality, intrauterine growth retardation, and prematurity. Birth defects are common. Minor or major congenital anomalies occur in about a third of infants born to heavy drinkers, compared with 9% of minor anomalies in infants of women who abstain from alcohol. Depressed birth weight has been seen with ingestion of as little as 100 g of alcohol a week (about 1 drink a day); hampered brain growth may be seen with 20 mL (1.5 drinks) a day. Decrease of alcohol intake during pregnancy is beneficial to the offspring, reducing rates of growth retardation and dysmorphic features. Heavy alcohol exposure prenatally, but not mild or moderate exposure, has been linked to decrease in IQ scores, hyperactive behavior, attention problems, learning difficulties, and speech disorders.

Postnatal Alcohol Exposure

Alcohol transferred through breast milk impairs motor development but not mental development at age 1 year. Ingestion of alcohol by children may lead to hypoglycemic seizures.

Withdrawal Syndrome

Infants born to women who drink large amounts of alcohol during pregnancy may rarely exhibit signs of withdrawal. Restless-

TABLE 162.3. FETAL ALCOHOL SYNDROME

Typical features
  Prenatal and postnatal growth retardation (weight, length, and/or head size < 10th percentile)
  Cerebral involvement (neurologic or cognitive impairment, developmental delay)
  Dysmorphic features
    Microcephaly (head circumference < 3rd percentile)
    Microphthalmia and/or short palpebral fissures
    Poorly developed philtrum, thin upper lip, and/or flattening of the maxillary area

Associated malformations
  Common
    Ptosis, strabismus
    Hemangiomas
    Cardiac (septal) defects
    Minor joint and limb abnormalities
    Genital abnormalities
    Single palmar creases
  Uncommon
    Cleft lip or palate
    Renal hypoplasia or dysplasia
    Horseshoe kidney, hydronephrosis
    Polydactyly
    Blepharophimosis
    Pulmonary artery stenosis
    Atrioventricular canal, right aortic arch
    Klippel-Feil anomaly
    Neural tube defects

From Jones KL, Smith DW. *Lancet* 1973;2:999–1001.

ness, agitation, tremulousness, opisthotonus, and seizures are seen shortly after birth and disappear within a few days.

FETAL COCAINE EFFECTS

In U.S. cities, about 1 in every 10 newborns is exposed prenatally to cocaine. The long-term consequences of fetal cocaine exposure to the developing nervous system are not well known.

Cocaine use during pregnancy has been linked to spontaneous abortion, abruptio placentae, stillbirth, and premature delivery. These events may immediately follow large intakes of cocaine and are attributed to drug-induced vasoconstriction of intrauterine vessels. Women who use cocaine tend to resort to prostitution, increasing risks for syphilis and HIV. They also tend to lack prenatal care, adding to the risks of infant death, low birth weight, and prematurity.

Low birth weight and intrauterine growth retardation are common among cocaine-exposed infants. Fetal brain growth is impaired independently of birth weight or gestational age. Sudden infant death syndrome has also been linked to cocaine exposure *in utero.*

Neurobehavior

State regulation difficulties are well described among cocaine-exposed newborns, although findings are inconsistent. Some reports describe irritability, excitability, poor feeding, and sleep disturbances among cocaine and cocaine/methamphetamine infants, whereas others describe decreased organizational response and interactive behavior, even if the exposure to cocaine was limited to the first trimester of pregnancy. Modulation of attention is impaired among cocaine-exposed infants who, unlike unexposed infants, prefer higher rates of stimuli when in a high level of arousal. Exposed infants also show motor and movement abnormalities, including excessive tremor and hypertonia. Dose-response effects of cocaine on state regulation and neurologic findings are reported in newborns. Some studies show no neurobehavioral effects, however.

Strokes

Experimentally, cocaine has a vasoconstrictive effect on fetal cerebral vessels and decreases cerebral blood flow. Neonatal stroke and porencephaly have been associated with prenatal cocaine exposure. Some cases may be related to other neonatal stroke risk factors that accompany fetal cocaine exposure, such as abruptio placentae or birth asphyxia. Intracranial hemorrhage was not associated with cocaine in a prospective study of prematures.

Seizures

Focal seizures may occur in cocaine-exposed newborns with strokes. Electroencephalograms in cocaine-exposed infants show bursts of sharp waves and spikes that are often multifocal. These findings do not correlate with clinical seizures or neurologic abnormalities and may disappear in 3 to 12 months. Cocaine-ex-

posed premature infants are at increased risk of neonatal seizures. Seizures are rare if there is no stroke.

Malformations

Prenatal cocaine exposure has been linked with urogenital malformations, limb reduction deformities, and intestinal atresia and infarction. Agenesis of the corpus callosum and septooptic dysplasia have also been noted. These teratogenic effects may result from cocaine-induced vasoconstriction and fetal vascular disruption in early organogenesis.

Neurodevelopmental Impact

In experiment models, prenatal cocaine has been reported to affect serotonin, norepinephrine, and dopaminergic systems. Lower CSF levels of homovanillic acid found in human newborns exposed to cocaine suggest dopaminergic involvement. In infancy, there may be a high incidence of spastic tetraparesis and diparesis that resolves by age 24 months (Table 162.4). In toddlers and school-aged children, prenatal cocaine exposure did not decrease cognitive abilities, except as mediated through cocaine effects on brain growth. Cocaine-exposed children seem to suffer from an excess of neurobehavioral abnormalities, including irritability, impulsivity, and aggressive behavior, which may reflect coexisting maternal psychopathology rather than direct cocaine effects.

Cocaine Exposure in Childhood

Passive intoxication with cocaine may be caused by breast-feeding or passive inhalation of free-base cocaine ("crack"). Seizures

TABLE 162.4. COCAINE-RELATED EFFECTS

Pregnancy
 Spontaneous abortions
 Abruptio placentae
 Stillbirths
 Premature delivery

Growth
 Low birth weight
 Intrauterine growth retardation
 Small head size

Infections
 Perinatal human immunodeficiency virus
 Congenital syphilis

Malformations

Neurodevelopmental findings
 Neonates
  Impaired neurobehavior
  Abnormal neurologic function
  Strokes
  Seizures
  Brainstem conduction delays
 Infants and children
  Hypertonia in infancy
  Autistic-like features
  Abnormal behaviors

are the chief manifestation of symptomatic intoxication, but intoxication may be unsuspected. Urine toxicology screen to detect illicit substances is indicated in evaluating seizures in infants and children, regardless of socioeconomic status.

Withdrawal Symptoms

There is no evidence of a cocaine-induced withdrawal syndrome. Even with remote prenatal cocaine exposure, cocaine-exposed infants may show hypertonicity and tremor, which are probably cerebral manifestations of fetal cocaine effects.

THE BATTERED CHILD

Child abuse may be physical or psychological. Physical abuse includes skin burns, welts, bruises, bone fractures, head trauma, and failure to thrive. Psychological abuse frequently accompanies physical abuse and may lead to growth, behavioral, and developmental impairments. The shaken baby syndrome, an increasingly recognized form of physical abuse, is characterized by bilateral subdural hematomas or subarachnoid hemorrhage, retinal hemorrhages, and the absence of external signs of trauma. It is seen in infants mostly under age 1 year who are shaken repeatedly and violently. The aggressor, usually a parent, shakes the crying infant until he or she quiets and later denies doing so.

Depressed mental status, seizures, and signs of increased intracranial pressure are common. Neurogenic pulmonary edema may occur rarely. Bilateral retinal hemorrhages, in the absence of a coagulopathy, are the most specific signs of shaken baby syndrome. Hemorrhages may be flame shaped, round and intraretinal, preretinal, or vitreal. The speed with which blood disappears varies by type: Flame-shaped hemorrhage disappears within a few days, but round intraretinal hemorrhage may last 2 weeks. Retinal folds occasionally are seen. A dilated funduscopic examination should be performed quickly in any child with suspected child abuse to identify retinal hemorrhages before they disappear.

Shaken baby syndrome should be suspected with sudden infant death syndrome or near-miss sudden infant death syndrome, with sudden lethargy, with seizures of unknown cause, or if there is a discrepancy between the history and the clinical signs. Broken ribs and chest bruises may be seen in infants held by the chest during shaking, and spiral fractures of the long bones or epiphysial separation may be seen in those shaken by the arms or legs. A skeletal survey showing old fractures helps confirm abuse. Infants with shaken baby syndrome may suffer neurologic sequelae, including hydrocephalus, blindness, developmental delay, mental retardation, microcephaly, and spastic tetraparesis.

SUGGESTED READINGS

Caffey J. The whiplash shaken baby syndrome: manual shaking by the extremities with whiplashed-induced intracranial and intraocular bleedings, linked with residual permanent brain damage and mental retardation. *Pediatrics* 1974;54:396–403.

Chasnoff IJ, Griffith DR, Freier C, et al. Cocaine/polydrug use in pregnancy. *Pediatrics* 1992;89:284–289.

Chiriboga CA. Neurological correlates of fetal cocaine exposure in cocaine and the developing brain. *Ann N Y Acad Sci* 1998;846:109–125.

Chiriboga CA, Brust JCM, Bateman D, Hauser WA. Dose-response effect of fetal cocaine exposure on newborn neurological function. *Pediatrics* 1999;103:79–85.

Forsyth BW Primary care of children with HIV infection. *Curr Opin Pediatr* 1995;7:502–512.

Gendelman HE, Epstein LG. HIV encephalopathy in children. *Curr Opin Pediatr* 1995;7:655–662.

Park YD, Belman AL, Kim TS, et al. Stroke in pediatric acquired immunodeficiency syndrome. *Ann Neurol* 1990;28:303–311.

Pizzo PA, Wilfert CM. Markers and determinant of disease progression in children with HIV infection. The Pediatric AIDS Siena Workshop II. *J Acquir Immune Def Syndr Hum Retrovir* 1995;8:30–44.

1994 Revised classification system for human immunodeficiency virus (HIV) infection in children less than 13 years of age. *MMWR Morb Mortal Wkly Rep* 1994;43:RR12.

Streissguth AP. Fetal alcohol syndrome: early and long-term consequences. *NIDA Res Monogr* 1992;119:126–130.

Merritt's Neurology, 10th ed., edited by L.P. Rowland. Lippincott Williams & Wilkins, Philadelphia © 2000.

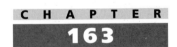

C H A P T E R
163

FALLS IN THE ELDERLY

LEWIS P. ROWLAND

Falls in the elderly are often taken for granted and considered an inevitable consequence of aging. Analysis of the factors that lead to falls, however, raises the possibility of prevention. The problem is certainly serious for individuals, families, and society (Table 163.1).

EPIDEMIOLOGY

It is estimated that 5% to 10% of falls in the elderly result in injury. Most falls occur at home, but the rate of falling is higher in long-term care facilities. Injury is the sixth leading cause of death after age 65, and most injuries result from a fall. Although people over 65 comprise about 12% of the total population, they account for 74% of all deaths caused by falls. Fatality rates increase with age in both men and women (Table 163.2).

The likelihood of admission to a nursing home increases with the number of falls an elderly person has had. Once a person is in a nursing home, the use of antidepressants increases the likelihood of falls. Falls are as likely among those who take selective serotonin reuptake inhibitors as among those taking tricyclics; use of newer drugs does not reduce the higher rates of falling.

TABLE 163.1. FALLS IN THE ELDERLY

Fall rate	33–50% of those >65
Injury due to falls	5–10% of falls
Proportion of deaths > age 65	33%
Fatalities due to falls	
Proportion total population > 65	12%
Proportion of all death due to falls; people > 65	74%
Site of fatal falls	
Home	60%
Public places	30%
Health care facilities	10%
Fatality rates	
Ages 65–74	8.5 per 100,000
> 75	56.7 per 100,000
Proportion falls resulting in hip fracture in people > 65	1%
Annual number hip fractures in United States	150,000
Cost of hip fractures (1980)	$2 billion

From Hindmarsh JJ, Estes EF Jr. *Arch Intern Med* 1989;149:2217–2222; Sorock (1988).

NEUROLOGY OF FALLS

Few falls seem to be related to syncope, drop attacks, transient ischemic attacks, or overt myopathy. Instead, a propensity to falls is generated by the cumulative handicaps of poor vision, poor balance, unsteady gait, stooped posture, and impaired proprioception. Sensitivity to drugs is another factor; falls are more frequent in people who take more than one drug. Intuitively, it seems likely that the motor impairment of Parkinson disease or previous stroke would increase the likelihood of falls and so would the physical impediments of arthritis or the intellectual failure of dementia.

Disequilibrium of unknown cause increases the likelihood of falling. The condition is identified as a triad: Impaired balance is

TABLE 163.2. DEATH RATES FROM ACCIDENTAL FALLS IN 1982

Age (yr)	Rate per 100,000 population	
	Men	Women
65–69	11.1	5.3
70–74	16.2	10.6
75–79	35.9	23.5
80–84	73.0	54.7
85+	186.3	148.9
Total 65+	35.0	32.4

From Sorock (1988).

a symptom; gait is impaired on examination; and no cause is discerned by medical, neurologic, and vestibular examination.

ENVIRONMENTAL FACTORS

Most falls in the elderly are "accidental." Examples include missing the last step on descent, slippery surfaces, poor lighting, unexpected appearance of a child or pet, and poorly fitting shoes.

PREVENTION

In one study, 46% of fallers were repeaters. The first fall led to loss of mobility and loss of confidence, making the next one more likely. Interventions included walking aids, home nursing visits to assess environmental hazards (including lighting, stairs, bathrooms, and rugs), educating patients, care in taking medications, and physical therapy for gait and balance. The list of medications should be reviewed periodically to be certain that all are needed; this is especially true of all psychoactive drugs. In the Prevention of Falls in the Elderly Trial, these measures reduced the risk of falling and of recurrent falls and the likelihood of hospital admission. Death rates from falls among people over 75 decreased by 50% between 1960 and 1980.

SUGGESTED READINGS

Avorn J. Depression in the elderly—falls and pitfalls. *N Engl J Med* 1998;339:918–20.

Close J, Ellis M, Hooper R, Glucksman E, Jackson S, Swift C. Prevention of Falls in the Elderly Trial (PROFET): a randomized controlled trial. *Lancet* 1999;353:93–97.

Fife TD, Baloh RW. Disequilibrium of unknown cause in older people. *Ann Neurol* 1993;34:694–702.

Kerber KA, Enrietto JA, Jacobson KM, Baloh RW. Disequilibrium in older people: a prospective study. *Neurology* 1998;51:574–580.

Lacomis D, Chad DA, Smith TW. Myopathy in the elderly: evaluation of the histopathologic spectrum and the accuracy of clinical diagnosis. *Neurology* 1993;43:825–828.

Nutt JG, Marsden CD, Thompson PD. Human walking and higher-level gait disorders, particularly in the elderly. *Neurology* 1993;43:268–279.

Saper CB. "All fall down": the mechanism of orthostatic hypotension in multiple systems atrophy and Parkinson's disease. *Ann Neurol* 1998;43:149–151.

Sorock GS. Falls among the elderly: epidemiology and prevention. *Am J Prevent Med* 1988;4:282–288.

Thajeb P. Gait disorders and multi-infarct dementia. *Acta Neurol Scand* 1993;87:239–242.

Thapa PB, Gideon P, Cost TW, Milam AB, Ray WA. Antidepressants and the risk of falls among nursing homs residents. *N Engl J Med* 1998;339:875–882.

Tinetti ME, Speechley M. Prevention of falls among the elderly. *N Engl J Med* 1989;320:1055–1059.

Tinetti ME, Williams CS. Falls, injuries due to falls and the risk of admission to a nursing home. *N Engl J Med* 1997;337:1279–1284.

Merritt's Neurology, 10th ed., edited by L.P. Rowland. Lippincott Williams & Wilkins, Philadelphia © 2000.

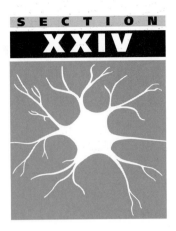

REHABILITATION

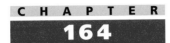

NEUROLOGIC REHABILITATION

LAURA LENNIHAN
GLENN M. SELIGER

Neurologic disorders commonly cause temporary or permanent impairments that impede simple daily functions and complex intellectual and physical activities. Neurologists play an important role in prescribing rehabilitation therapies to maximize functional recovery. The proper selection and timing of these therapies make a substantial contribution to optimum quality of life for patient and family despite persistent neurologic impairments. Although it is preferable for rehabilitation to begin soon after a neurologic injury, many people with chronic neurologic conditions have never received adequate rehabilitation therapy. Nevertheless, if they are given proper training and equipment, they may still improve in personal independence, access to the community, or ease with which a caregiver assists them. At a time when neurologists are assuming the role of principal care physicians, experience in neurorehabilitation is essential in the management continuum from acute to chronic neurologic disorders.

The World Health Organization definitions of impairment, disability, and handicap (Table 164.1) provide a structure for understanding the impact of disease on personal independence and integration into society. These criteria help to identify patients who may benefit from rehabilitation. The planning and prescription of a rehabilitation program for a neurologically impaired individual requires characterization of the neurologic disorder with regard to natural history, localization, and extent of nervous system involvement; determination of functional disabilities caused by cognitive and physical impairments; and definition of these disabilities in the context of the patient's physi-

TABLE 164.1. WORLD HEALTH ORGANIZATION DEFINITION OF IMPAIRMENT, DISABILITY, AND HANDICAP

Impairment
   In the context of health experience, an impairment is any loss or abnormality of psychologic, physiologic, or anatomic structure or function.

Disability
   In the context of health experience, a disability is any restriction or lack (resulting from an impairment) of ability to perform an activity in the manner or within the range considered normal for a human being.

Handicap
   In the context of health experience, a handicap is a disadvantage for a given individual, resulting from an impairment or a disability, that limits or prevents the fulfillment of a role that is normal (depending on age, sex, and social and cultural factors) for that individual.

World Health Organization (1980).

cal and social environment. With this information, the type and intensity of rehabilitation therapies can be planned.

Two principal approaches are used in rehabilitation therapy. The first is to bypass the neurologic impediment by teaching adaptive techniques using preserved neurologic function. For example, a person with a paralyzed arm can be trained in one-handed activities using the normal arm. The second approach is to facilitate the return of neurologic function. For example, the person with a paralyzed arm is given tasks to increase effective movement of that arm. Both methods are usually applied in rehabilitation programs. The efficacy of the first approach in improving functional independence and reducing disability is accepted. The second approach is the focus of active clinical research. In a primate model, restraint of the normal arm resulting in forced use of the paretic arm after motor cortex injury leads to better functional recovery of the affected arm than when the normal arm is unrestrained. No functional recovery occurs if the paretic arm is restrained. Case reports in humans similarly support the efficacy of this forced-use paradigm. Gait training on a treadmill while a harness provides partial body weight support is thought to recruit spinal pattern generators for walking. This technique may produce better balance, motor recovery, walking speed, and endurance compared with conventional gait training with patients bearing their full body weight.

Current research on the neurobiology of recovery from central nervous system injury and the efficacy of treatments to improve the speed and completeness of recovery is relevant to the practice of neurorehabilitation. For example, norepinephrine plays an important role in modulating central nervous system recovery. In animal models of focal brain injury and in people with strokes, amphetamine administered coincident with physical therapy has resulted in better motor recovery than in placebo-treated subjects. Drugs with central catecholamine antagonist activity, such as haloperidol, prazosin, or clonidine, interfere with motor recovery in animals. Enhancement of activity of the inhibitory neurotransmitter GABA by drugs such as diazapam, phenytoin, or phenobarbital also reduces neurologic recovery in animals. In a retrospective study, stroke patients who received either class of drug had poorer motor recovery than those who did not.

Functional outcome is improved by treatment in a comprehensive rehabilitation program. Stroke patients who receive rehabilitation therapies on a stroke rehabilitation unit have better functional outcomes and shorter hospital stays than those treated on a general neurology ward. Similarly, stroke patients admitted to hospital-based acute rehabilitation programs have better functional recovery and are more likely to return home than those treated in a subacute rehabilitation program at a skilled nursing facility.

A comprehensive inpatient neurorehabilitation program requires an interdisciplinary team: physician, physical therapist, occupational therapist, speech therapist, neuropsychologist, social worker, and rehabilitation nurse. The physician, as team leader, defines the type and prognosis of the neurologic disorder; is responsible for coordination of rehabilitation services and setting of realistic treatment goals; and provides medical care, especially for the prevention and treatment of complications of a disabling disorder, for instance, deep vein thrombosis or reflex sympathetic dystrophy.

The physical therapist's role is to maximize leg function and mobility. The occupational therapist promotes maximum independence in activities of daily living by improving arm function and cognitive skills. The speech therapist characterizes and treats specific language-based cognitive dysfunction and evaluates and treats dysphagia and dysarthria. The neuropsychologist defines cognitive problems and monitors improvement. The rehabilitation nurse, in addition to providing medical nursing care, incorporates into the patients' daily routines skills learned in therapy and institutes treatments to restore sphincter continence. The social worker implements the discharge plan. All team members participate in formulating a discharge plan and in educating and training patient and family in preparation for return home.

OCCUPATIONAL THERAPY

Neurologic injury that interferes with use of the arms and hands can be profoundly disabling. Weakness, loss of sensation, ataxia, abnormal tone, and involuntary movements, alone or in combination, can lead to inability to carry out basic activities of daily living, to drive a car, or to work. Occupational therapy promotes recovery from neurologic injury; prevents permanent disability from complications of temporary neurologic impairments, such as wrist-flexor contractures from a radial nerve palsy; teaches new techniques to perform self-care and other tasks; prescribes equipment to increase use of the impaired arm and hand; and, when the impairment is unilateral, teaches performance of one-handed techniques by the normal arm.

The approach to restoring function to the neurologically impaired arm is determined in part by central or peripheral site of injury. For example, treatment of weakness caused by an upper motor neuron lesion focuses on reestablishing movement at one joint in isolation from movement at other joints; strengthening exercises follow later. Strengthening programs are usually instituted early for peripheral injuries, but it is important not to overwork muscles recovering from a nerve injury because weakness may worsen. Wrist and ankle weights can be used to dampen arm and leg ataxia.

Improving motor skills is only one of the important components in enhancing performance of the activities of daily living, such as dressing, toileting, washing, grooming, feeding, and community skills. Training to overcome visual and perceptual difficulties, unilateral spatial neglect, memory impairment, inattentiveness, and poor safety judgment may also be important. The occupational therapist selects adaptive equipment and trains patient and family to compensate. Advanced programs may include learning special occupational skills or to drive with the left hand and foot.

PHYSICAL THERAPY

Interference with mobility by neurologic disease can be reduced or eliminated by strengthening exercises, gait and balance training, spasticity reduction through stretching or medication, surgical release of shortened tendons, bracing, assistive devices (e.g., cane, walker), and use of a wheelchair. Techniques and orthotics are chosen to maximize safe and independent mobility; to optimize energy efficiency; to prevent decubitus skin ulcers, tendon contractures, and falls; and to enhance recovery. Leg and trunk weakness, impaired postural reflexes, ataxia, proprioceptive loss, and hemineglect may all interfere with walking. Even though a person may not be able to walk immediately after neurologic injury, ambulation usually becomes possible through a combination of bracing at the ankle and sometimes the knee and use of a walker or cane. When ambulation is not possible, mobility is attained through training in the use of a wheelchair of the correct size and height, with a special seat to prevent skin breakdown and cushions for trunk support.

DYSPHAGIA THERAPY

Facial, lingual, masticatory, pharyngeal, esophageal, and respiratory muscles participate in swallowing. Neurologic disorders that disturb coordinated contraction of any of these muscles can cause dysphagia and, secondarily, airway obstruction, aspiration pneumonia, and malnutrition. Dysphagia evaluation is indicated for patients with any of these complications; who report coughing, choking, or nasal regurgitation while eating; are dysarthric; or have a disease commonly associated with dysphagia, such as motor neuron disease or myasthenia gravis. This evaluation includes characterization of the neurologic disorder and bedside and fluoroscopic observation of swallowing foods of different consistencies, from thin liquids to chewy meat. Restriction of the diet to consistencies that can be swallowed without aspiration reduces the risk of dysphagia complications. The speech therapist teaches techniques that improve coordinated swallowing and reduce the risk of aspiration, such as tucking the chin before swallowing to close the larynx and open the upper esophagus and swallowing twice after each bite of food to clear the pharynx.

LANGUAGE AND COGNITIVE THERAPIES

Brain injuries that cause behavioral, language, and other cognitive dysfunctions may be focal and discrete or generalized and diffuse. In focal injuries, the neurologic dysfunctions may be restricted, with other brain functions preserved, for instance, Broca aphasia with intact attention, memory, and concentration. In contrast, diffuse injury may affect several areas of cognitive function. The therapeutic approach needs to be tailored to the nature and complexity of the symptoms. The first step in implementing a cognitive rehabilitation program is to define the neurobehavioral impediments and how they interfere with function. For example, a short attention span may prevent participation in group activities such as business meetings, or memory impairment may lead to failure at school.

Speech therapy for aphasia is a specialized part of cognitive rehabilitation. The speech therapist defines receptive and expressive dysfunction and identifies areas of strength and weaknesses in language. Areas of strength may then be used for compensatory purposes. For instance, if an aphasic patient's written language skills are preserved better than verbal expression, writing may be useful for communication. Training in use of visual imagery as an internal cue may help to overcome the word blocking of Broca aphasia. A picture board may circumvent an expressive language deficit. The use of computer-assisted communication for aphasia is an area of active rehabilitation research. Visual imagery to create memory cues may improve performance on memory tests. Breaking a task into individual steps and then teaching one step at a time helps to overcome constructional problems.

In diffuse or multifocal brain injury that impairs attention and behavior and many aspects of cognition and language, a structured program that permits few distractions is necessary. Speech and occupational therapists collaborate on program development and implementation, and all members of the rehabilitation team contribute. Several strategies may compensate for multiple problems. For example, sensory reduction minimizes distractions by controlling the noise and activity in the environment; development of a rigidly structured daily routine helps to overcome poor planning and organizational skills. Education of patient and family about aphasia and other cognitive problems helps to reduce frustration with impaired communication, memory, and abnormal behavior.

INCONTINENCE THERAPY

Loss of control of bladder or bowel emptying is a devastating condition and should be addressed by any comprehensive neurorehabilitation program. The cause of impaired emptying or sphincter incompetence, and therefore the treatment, depends on the site of the neural injury. Evaluation includes clinical observations about incontinence and retention; search for nonneurologic factors, such as cystitis or mechanical problems, particularly urethral obstruction by prostatic enlargement; and cystometrographic measurements of bladder and sphincter functions. The neurorehabilitation nurse plays a crucial role in the treatment of bladder and bowel disorders, including implementation of voiding programs and training patient and family to use urethral catheters.

Incontinence characterized by bladder hyperreflexia, in which the bladder contracts at low urine volumes and voluntary inhibition of bladder contraction and sphincter relaxation fails, commonly complicates cerebral, particularly frontal lobe, injury. Lack of awareness or indifference may impede achievement of continence, but neurologic recovery usually reduces inconti-

nence. Scheduled voidings at 2-hour intervals contribute to regaining continence. Bladder dyssynergia, in which bladder contraction and sphincter relaxation are dissociated and the bladder contracts against a closed sphincter, is usually a consequence of lower brainstem or spinal cord disorders. Bladder emptying, if it occurs at all, is incomplete and occurs at high pressure. Treatment includes bladder antispasmodic drugs and intermittent catheterization. Hydronephrosis and renal failure are potential complications. Peripheral nerve diseases involving the nerves innervating the bladder may cause bladder flaccidity. Bladder emptying, at low pressures, is incomplete, and incontinence occurs between voluntary voidings. Cholinergic agents may improve emptying, but intermittent catheterization is often necessary.

Immobility from any neurologic disorder and loss of cortical control over bowel movements due to spinal cord injury may cause severe obstipation and even bowel obstruction. Prevention combines a high-fiber diet and stool softeners with laxatives or enemas timed to stimulate evacuation on a regular schedule.

SUGGESTED READINGS

Bennett L, Knowlton GC. Overwork weakness in partially denervated skeletal muscle. *Clin Orthop* 1958;12:22–29.

Goldstein LB, Matchar DB, Morgenlander JC, Davis JN. Influence of drugs on the recovery of sensorimotor function after stroke. *J Neurol Rehab* 1990;4:137–144.

Good DC, Couch JR, eds. *Handbook of neurorehabilitation.* New York: Marcel Dekker, 1994.

International classification of impairments, disabilities, and handicaps. Geneva: World Health Organization, 1980.

Kalra L, Dale P, Crome P. Improving stroke rehabilitation: a controlled study. *Stroke* 1993;24:1462–1467.

Kramer AM, Steiner JF, Schlenker RE, et al. Outcomes and costs after hip fracture and stroke. A comparison of rehabilitation settings. *JAMA* 1997;277:396–404.

Selzer ME. Neurological rehabilitation. *Ann Neurol* 1992;32:695–699.

Taub E, Miller NE, Novack TA, et al. Technique to improve chronic motor deficit after stroke. *Arch Phys Med Rehabil* 1993;74:347–354.

Visintin M, Barbeau H, Korner-Bitensky N, Mayo NE. A new approach to retrain gait in stroke patients through body weight support and treadmill stimulation. *Stroke* 1998;29:1122–1128.

Walker-Batson D, Smith P, Curtis S, Unwin H, Greenlee R. Amphetamine paired with physical therapy accelerates motor recovery after stroke. *Stroke* 1995;26:2254–2259.

Merritt's Neurology, 10th ed., edited by L.P. Rowland. Lippincott Williams & Wilkins, Philadelphia © 2000.

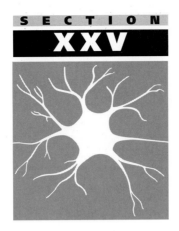

ETHICAL AND LEGAL GUIDELINES

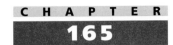

END-OF-LIFE ISSUES IN NEUROLOGY

LEWIS P. ROWLAND

Neurologic diseases have been at the center of discussions on issues at the end of life. The American Academy of Neurology has set standards for the determination of cerebral death and for the persistent vegetative state (see Chapter 4). Amyotrophic lateral sclerosis and Alzheimer disease have been the focus of debates about assisted suicide. Neurologic intensive care units face the issue of discontinuing mechanical ventilation. Presymptomatic diagnosis is available for incurable conditions like Huntington disease, creating an ethical challenge.

These ethical issues could fill a separate book. Here, we set forth some principles and definitions as an introduction for students and physicians as they learn to deal with the problems. The fundamental ethical and legal guidelines are the basis for actions taken or avoided.

INFORMED CONSENT

One basis for patient autonomy in decision making is informed consent. A patient may accept or refuse a treatment or diagnostic test after learning about the anticipated benefits and risks and alternative choices. This requires accurate information about prognosis.

ADVANCE DIRECTIVES

Individuals may prepare legal documents that specify their preferences for end-of-life treatments under specific circumstances, and they may also appoint surrogate decision makers if the individual is not competent to make decisions at some future time. Most states recognize living wills as instruments for these advance directives, which usually provide a prohibition against life-sustaining treatments that prolong the dying process if the person is in a terminal condition and can no longer make decisions. In the interim, a competent person can change the advance directive at any time.

REFUSAL OF LIFE-SUSTAINING TREATMENT

The *doctrine of informed consent* includes the patient's *right to refuse life-sustaining treatment*. Refusal is a decision not to provide consent, without which the physician usually cannot continue treatment. Respect for *patients' autonomy* does not require acceptance of all decisions; the decision must be based on adequate understanding of the nature and consequences of the choice (*informed consent*) without coercion and with capacity to make a reasoned decision.

The patient's right to consent or refuse is not abrogated when the patient loses the capacity to make decisions. It becomes transferred to a legally authorized *surrogate decision maker* and the physician must ask the surrogate for consent or refusal on behalf of the patient.

The surrogate must follow the patient's previously expressed wishes as expressed in *advance directives* or other reliable statements. If the patient's expressed wishes have not been explicitly stated, the surrogate must use the *doctrine of substituted judgment*, based on knowledge of the patient's general values and preferences. If the surrogate has no such information, the surrogate must assess the anticipated benefits and burdens, based on the *doctrine of best interest*. This may be problematic, however, because it is not based on the desires of the patient.

Despite widely held beliefs to the contrary, it is not necessary to consult legal counsel before withdrawing life-sustaining therapy.

DOUBLE EFFECT

Some actions are morally and ethically acceptable and may have foreseeable but unintended and undesirable outcomes; the morality of the action depends on the morality of the intended outcome, not the unintended one. According to the American Academy of Neurology Ethics Committee statement on assisted suicide, several conditions must be met: the action to be carried out must be morally or ethically acceptable or at least neutral, the good effect must not depend on the undesired or bad effect, and the good effect must be sufficient to justify the risk of the unintended outcome.

In practice, this principle makes it possible to administer sufficient analgesic and sedative medication to keep a patient comfortable even though the treatment will not prolong life. The principle of *double effect* is the basis of the hospice program.

PALLIATIVE CARE

According to the World Health Organization definition, palliative care is "the active total care of patients whose disease is not responsive to curative treatment, where the control of pain, of other symptoms and of psychological, social, and spiritual problems is paramount, and where the goal is the achievement of the best quality of life for patients and their families." More directly stated, palliative care is "comfort care" or treatment intended to relieve pain and suffering rather than to cure the disease, restore the patient to health, or prolong life at all costs. Oral or parenteral morphine is used in amounts sufficient to control pain and maintain comfort.

A *hospice program* is often the venue for palliative care. This is sometimes carried out in a hospital or separate physical facility but is increasingly a home care program. In the United States, a Medicare Disease-Related Group (DRG) provides reimbursement for the care of patients who are not expected to survive for more than 6 months. However, hospice care is used by only 17%

of people who are dying, and three reasons are adduced: physicians are uncomfortable about talking with patients about terminal events long enough in advance, sometimes it is difficult to determine precisely the expected time of death, and hospices emphasize home care and family members may not be able to commit the time required or there may be no family members. Most Americans die in hospitals (61%) or nursing homes (17%).

Another drawback to the use of home or hospice care is the insensitivity of U.S. physicians to the advance directives of their patients, as detected by the Study to Understand Prognoses and Preferences for Outcomes and Risks of Treatment (SUPPORT). Fifty percent of the physicians polled did not respect or did not know the advance directives; most do-not-resuscitate (DNR) orders were not written until 24 hours before death; and 40% of the patients had severe pain for several days before death. In a follow-up study, there was no improvement in communication about patients' desires for resuscitation; in the time before death in an intensive care unit; or the incidence or timing of do not resuscitate orders, which were not written in 50% of the patients surveyed. Physicians misunderstood the desires of their patients against do not resuscitate (80%) or the level of pain.

PHYSICIAN-ASSISTED SUICIDE

As specified by law in the state of Oregon, it is permissible for a physician to prescribe medication to be used by a patient for the purpose of suicide. The physician may not actually administer the drug. This law is restricted to Oregon and the practice is not legal in any other state.

Neurologic diseases generate problems for this policy. Patients may be incompetent with Alzheimer disease and would be unable to give consent. Other patients may lose the use of their hands from multiple sclerosis or amyotrophic lateral sclerosis. Under these circumstances, the patients themselves cannot fill the prescription and take the drug; someone else must assist them physically, which would be euthanasia and specifically banned by the Oregon law.

Many authorities have debated the desirability of assisted suicide. Medical and nursing organizations have uniformly opposed legalization.

TERMINAL SEDATION

The right to forgo treatment includes food and water. Pain or other discomfort can be ameliorated by standard palliative measures that may include sedation to unconsciousness. The patient then dies as a result of the underlying disease, dehydration, or both. It is believed that some form of terminal sedation is applied in up to 40% of deaths in U.S. hospitals. Discontinuing mechanical ventilation in an intensive care unit is another situation that calls for prevention or relief of suffering. Some believe that terminal dehydration has a stronger moral basis than assisted suicide, based as it is on the right to refuse treatment. A physician is morally obligated to honor a competent patient's refusal of food and water but is not obligated by a request for a lethal drug. Nev-

ertheless, detractors consider terminal sedation a form of "slow euthanasia."

EUTHANASIA

If in compliance with a patient's request a physician administers a lethal drug by injection or other means, the act is "euthanasia," which is illegal in the United States. The public, physicians, and courts have had difficulty separating refusal or discontinuation of therapy, which are legal, from assisted suicide and euthanasia, which are not. The distinction between assisted suicide and euthanasia is the most controversial of all. The Supreme Court concluded that palliative care and terminal sedation are permissible but referred the question of physician-assisted suicide back to legislation by the states.

AN OVERALL VIEW

The issues discussed here are among the most controversial in modern life. Consensus is not easy to achieve, but views are changing and current practices are likely to change as well. Already, pain control and palliative care have come to the fore and provide effective alternatives to assisted suicide. Legal changes may be anticipated but do not seem imminent.

SUGGESTED READINGS

Almqvist EW, Block M, Brinkman R, Crauford D, Hayden M. A worldwide assessment of the frequency of suicide, suicide attempts, or psychiatric hospitalization after predictive testing for Huntington disease. *Am J Hum Genet* 1999;64:1293–1304.

American Academy of Neurology Ethics and Humanities Subcommittee. Certain aspects of the care and management of profoundly and irreversibly paralyzed patients with retained consciousness and cognition. *Neurology* 1993;43:222–223.

American Academy of Neurology Ethics and Humanities Subcommittee. Palliative care in neurology. *Neurology* 1996;46:870–872.

American Academy of Neurology Ethics and Humanities Subcommittee. Ethical issues in the management of the demented patient. *Neurology* 1996;46:1180–1183.

American Academy of Neurology Ethics and Humanities Subcommittee. Assisted suicide, euthanasia, and the neurologist. *Neurology* 1998;50:596–598.

American Academy of Neurology Quality Standards Subcommittee. Practice parameter: assessment and management of patients in the persistent vegetative state. *Neurology* 1995;45:1015–1018.

Angell M. The Supreme Court and assisted suicide—the ultimate right. *N Engl J Med* 1997;336:50–53.

Bernat JL. *Ethical issues in neurology*. Boston: Butterworth-Heinemann, 1994.

Bernat JL. The problem of physician-assisted suicide. *Semin Neurol* 1997;17:271–280.

Bird TD. Outrageous fortune: the risk of suicide in genetic testing for Huntington disease. *Am J Hum Genet* 1999;64:1289–1292.

Burt RA. The Supreme Court speaks—not assisted suicide but a constitutional right to palliative care. *N Engl J Med* 1997;337:1234–1236.

Doyle D, Hanks GC, Mac Donald N, eds. *Oxford textbook of palliative care*, 2nd ed. New York: Oxford University Press, 1998.

Field MJ, Cassel CK, eds. Institute of Medicine. *Approaching death: improving care at the end of life*. Washington, DC: National Academy Press, 1997.

Foley KM. Competent care for the dying instead of physician assisted suicide. *N Engl J Med* 1997;336:54–58.

Ganzini L, Johnston WS, McFarland BH, Tolle SW, Lee MA. Attitudes of patients with amyotrophic lateral sclerosis and their care givers toward assisted suicide. *N Engl J Med* 1998;339:967–973.

Gostin LO Deciding life and death in the courtroom: from Quinlan to Cruzan, Glucksberg, and Vacco—a brief history and analysis of constitutional protection of the "right to die." *JAMA* 1997:278:1523–1528.

Mayer SA, Kossoff SB. Withdrawal of life support in the neurological intensive care unit. *Neurology* 1999;52:1602–1609.

Meier DE, Morrison RS, Cassel CK. Improving palliative care. *Ann Intern Med* 1997;127:223–230.

Miller FG, Meier DE. Voluntary death: a comparison of terminal dehydration and physician-assisted suicide. *Ann Intern Med* 1998;128:559–562.

Multisociety task force on persistent vegetative state. *N Engl J Med* 1994;330:1499–1508, 1572–1579.

Newton HB, Malkin MG. Ethical issues in neuro-oncology. *Semin Neurol* 1997;17:219–226.

Orentlicher D. The Supreme Court and physician-assisted suicide—rejecting assisted suicide but embracing euthanasia. *N Engl J Med* 1997;337:1236–1239.

Payne SK, Taylor RM. The persistent vegetative state and anencephaly: problematic paradigms for discussing futility and rationing. *Semin Neurol* 1997;17:257–264.

Quill TE, Lo B, Brock DW. Palliative options of last resort: a comparison of voluntarily stopping eating and drinking, terminal sedation, physician-assisted suicide, and voluntary active euthanasia. *JAMA* 1997; 278:2099–2104.

Quill TE, Meier DE, Block SD, Billings JA. The debate over physician-assisted suicide: empirical data and convergent views. *Ann Intern Med* 1998;128:552–558.

Rowland LP. Assisted suicide and alternatives in amyotrophic lateral sclerosis. *N Engl J Med* 1998;339:987–989.

Ruffin TA. Withdrawing life support. How is the decision made? *JAMA* 1995;273:738–739.

Youngner SJ. Beyond DNR: Fine-tuning end-of-life decision making. *Neurology* 1995;45:615–616.

Merritt's Neurology, 10th ed., edited by L.P. Rowland. Lippincott Williams & Wilkins, Philadelphia © 2000.

SUBJECT INDEX

Note: Page numbers in *italics* indicate figures; page numbers followed by t indicate tables.

A

Abacavir (Ziagen)
  for treatment of AIDS, 173
Abducens nerve
  injury to, 438–439, 439t
Abetalipoproteinemia (Bassen-Kornzweig syndrome), 552–553
  diagnosis, 553
  laboratory data, 553
  neurologic anomalies, 553t
  pathogenesis, 552
  symptoms and signs, 552–553, 553t
  treatment, 553
Abscess
  brain, 128–133
  brainstem, *131*
  intracranial epidural, 112–113, *113*
  spinal epidural, *114,* 114–115, *116*
  tuberculous, 386
Acanthamoeba infections, 200
Acanthocytes
  neurological syndromes with, 552–554
Acetaminophen
  for treatment of migraine, 810
Acetazolamide
  for treatment of hyperkalemic periodic paralysis, 751–752
  for treatment of idiopathic intracranial hypertension, 289
  for treatment of septic thrombosis, 271
Acetazolamide (Diamox)
  for treatment of hydrocephalus, 283
  for treatment of hypokalemic periodic paralysis, 751
  for treatment of myotonia congenita, 754
  for treatment of primary subarachnoid supratentorial hemorrhage, 468
Achondroglasia, 885
Achondroplasia (chondrodystrophy), 882–883, *884*
  macrocephaly and, 488t
Acidurias
  organic, 541–542
Acoustic neuroma
  cranial nerves and, 308–311, *309,* 309t, *310*
Acquired cerebellar ataxias, 654
Acquired chronic hepatocerebral degeneration, 876
Acquired immunodeficiency syndrome (AIDS), 163–175
  central nervous system pathogenesis, 166
  in children, 164
  classification of HIV disease, 163, 163t
  clinical syndromes, 166–173
    drug-induced, 172–173

HIV-related, 166–169, 167t, *168*
  opportunistic infections and neoplasms, 169–172, 170t, *171, 172*
dementia and, 4t
diagnostic evaluation, 173
drug dependence and, 931
epidemiology, 164, 164t
etiology, 164–165
fungal infections and, 175
history, 163
myopathy in, 768
neurosyphilis and, 187–188
pathogenesis, 165–166
precautions for clinical and laboratory services, 173–174
treatment, course, and prognosis, 173
Acrocephalosyndactyly (Apert syndrome), 487t, *491,* 491t
Acromegalic neuropathy, 627, 1619
Acromegaly, 851, *851, 852*
Acrylamide monomer
  neuropathies caused by, 623, 628
Actinomycosis, 178
Action dystonia, 39, 669
Acute akathisia, 696
Acute autonomic neuropathy, 802
Acute cholinergic crisis, 944
Acute disseminated encephalomyelitis (ADE), 151–153, 161, 786
  diagnosis, 153
  epidemiology, 152
  etiology, 151
  laboratory studies, 152–153, *153*
  pathogenesis, 151
  pathology, 151–152
  prognosis and course, 153
  symptoms and signs, 152
  treatment, 153
Acute dystonic reactions, 696
Acute encephalopathy
  neurotoxicology and, 940
Acute intermittent porphyria (AIP), 549–552
  clinical manifestations, 550t
  diagnosis, 550
  incidence, 549–550
  laboratory data, 550
  molecular genetics, 549
  pathogenesis, 549
  pathology, 549
  symptoms and signs, 550
  treatment, 550–551, 551t
Acute ischemic brachial neuropathy, 459
Acute lymphocytic leukemia, 868
Acute motor axonal neuropathy (AMAN), 615

Acute purulent meningitis
  causes, 103, 104t
  of unknown cause, 107
Acute quadriplegic myopathy, 730–731
Acute subdural hematoma, 403–404
Acute transverse myelitis, 152
Acute transverse myelopathy (ATM), 152
Acyclovir (Zovirax)
  for treatment of herpes simplex encephalitis, 148
  for treatment of herpes zoster, 149, 621
  for treatment of HSV, 136
  for treatment of neonatal herpes encephalitis, 470
  for treatment of varicella-zoster virus, 136
ADC. *See* Apparent diffusion coefficient maps
ADD. *See* Attention deficit disorder and ADHD
Addison disease, 288, 859
ADE. *See* Acute disseminated encephalomyelitis; Encephalomyelitis, acute disseminated
Adefovir dipivoxil
  for treatment of AIDS, 173
Adenoma
  islet cell, 858
Adenoma sebaceum, 596, *597*
Adenosine deaminase deficiency, 513
Adenovirus infections, 145–146, 160
ADHD, *See. See* Attention deficit hyperactivity disorder
Adolescents
  headache and, 38
  idiopathic intracranial hypertension in, 288
  location of central nervous system tumors in, 355t
  rubella vaccine and, 142
  seizures and
    differential diagnosis, 15t
  syncope and, 12–13
Adrenal diseases, 859–860, 863–864
Adrenal insufficiency, 741
Adrenergic stimulant drugs
  for treatment of narcolepsy, 844
Adrenocorticotrophic hormone
  deficiency, 460
  excessive, 851–852
Adrenoleukodystrophy, 538–539, 540
Adrenomyeloneuropathy, 538–539, 539t
Adriamycin
  for treatment of primary central nervous system lymphoma, 335
Adult polyglucosan body disease (APBD), 532
Adults, young
  stroke in, 245–246
Adult variant neuronal ceroid lipofuscinosis disease, 521